D0472221

Pediatric Clinical Practice Guidelines & Policies

· ·

A Compendium of Evidence-based Research for Pediatric Practice

14th Edition

American Academy of Pediatrics
141 Northwest Point Blvd
Elk Grove Village, IL 60007-1019
www.aap.org

14th Edition—2014
13th Edition—2013
12th Edition—2012
11th Edition—2011
10th Edition—2010
9th Edition—2009
8th Edition—2008
7th Edition—2007
6th Edition—2006
5th Edition—2005
4th Edition—2004
3rd Edition—2003
2nd Edition—2002
1st Edition—2001

ISBN: 978-1-58110-843-9
ISSN: 1942-2024

MA0697

9-5/0214

The recommendations in this publication do not indicate an exclusive course of treatment or serve as a standard of medical care. Variations, taking into account individual circumstances, may be appropriate.

For permission to reproduce material from this publication, visit www.copyright.com and search for "Pediatric Clinical Practice Guidelines."

INTRODUCTION TO
PEDIATRIC CLINICAL PRACTICE GUIDELINES & POLICIES: A COMPENDIUM OF EVIDENCE-BASED RESEARCH FOR PEDIATRIC PRACTICE

Clinical practice guidelines have long provided physicians with evidence-based decision-making tools for managing common pediatric conditions. Policy statements issued and endorsed by the American Academy of Pediatrics (AAP) are developed to provide physicians with a quick reference guide to the AAP position on child health care issues. We have combined these 2 authoritative resources into one comprehensive manual/CD-ROM resource to provide easy access to important clinical and policy information.

This manual contains
- Clinical practice guidelines from the AAP, plus related recommendation summaries, *ICD-9-CM/ICD-10-CM* coding information, and AAP patient education handouts
- Technical report summaries
- Clinical practice guidelines endorsed by the AAP, including abstracts where applicable
- Policy statements, clinical reports, and technical reports issued or endorsed through December 2013, including abstracts where applicable
- Full text of all 2013 AAP policy statements, clinical reports, and technical reports

The CD-ROM, which is located on the inside back cover of this manual, builds on the content of the manual and includes full text of all AAP
- Clinical practice guidelines
- Policy statements
- Clinical reports
- Technical reports
- Endorsed clinical practice guidelines and policies

For easy reference within this publication, the dates when AAP clinical practice guidelines, policy statements, clinical reports, and technical reports first appeared in the AAP journal *Pediatrics* are provided. In 2009, the online version of *Pediatrics* at http://pediatrics.aappublications.org became the official journal of record; therefore, the date of online publication is given for policies from 2010 to present.

Additional information about AAP policy can be found in a variety of professional publications such as
Care of the Young Athlete, 2nd Edition
Guidelines for Perinatal Care, 7th Edition
Pediatric Environmental Health, 3rd Edition
Pediatric Nutrition, 7th Edition
Red Book®, 29th Edition, and *Red Book® Online*
 (www.aapredbook.org)
School Health: Policy & Practice, 6th Edition

For more information on these titles and similar resources or for ordering information, please call 888/227-1770 or visit our online Bookstore at www.aap.org/bookstore.

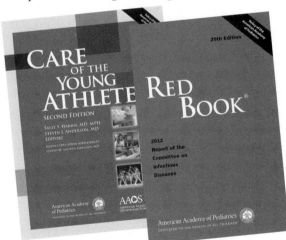

AMERICAN ACADEMY OF PEDIATRICS

The American Academy of Pediatrics (AAP) and its member pediatricians dedicate their efforts and resources to the health, safety, and well-being of infants, children, adolescents, and young adults. The AAP has approximately 62,000 members in the United States, Canada, and Latin America. Members include pediatricians, pediatric medical subspecialists, and pediatric surgical specialists.

Core Values. *We believe*
- In the inherent worth of all children; they are our most enduring and vulnerable legacy.
- Children deserve optimal health and the highest quality health care.
- Pediatricians are the best qualified to provide child health care.

The American Academy of Pediatrics is the organization to advance child health and well-being.

Vision. Children have optimal health and well-being and are valued by society. Academy members practice the highest quality health care and experience professional satisfaction and personal well-being.

Mission. The mission of the American Academy of Pediatrics is to attain optimal physical, mental, and social health and well-being for all infants, children, adolescents, and young adults. To accomplish this mission, the Academy shall support the professional needs of its members.

Table of Contents

SECTION 5

CURRENT POLICIES FROM THE AMERICAN ACADEMY OF PEDIATRICS

AAP Partnership for Policy Implementation   See Appendix 2.

APPENDIX 1

POLICIES BY COMMITTEE

APPENDIX 2

**PPI: AAP PARTNERSHIP FOR POLICY
IMPLEMENTATION** 1131

APPENDIX 3

**AMERICAN ACADEMY OF PEDIATRICS
ACRONYMS**... 1135

Clinical Practice Guidelines

From the American Academy of Pediatrics

• • • • • • • • • • • • • • • • • • •

- *Clinical Practice Guidelines*
  EVIDENCE-BASED DECISION-MAKING TOOLS FOR MANAGING COMMON PEDIATRIC CONDITIONS

- *Technical Reports and Summaries*
  BACKGROUND INFORMATION TO SUPPORT AMERICAN ACADEMY OF PEDIATRICS POLICY

- *Quick Reference Tools*
  TOOLS FOR IMPLEMENTING AMERICAN ACADEMY OF PEDIATRICS GUIDELINES IN YOUR
  PRACTICE AND AT THE POINT OF CARE

FOREWORD

In response to the growing trend toward the practice of evidence-based medicine, the American Academy of Pediatrics (AAP) created an organizational process and methodology for developing clinical practice guidelines. These guidelines provide physicians with an evidence-based decision-making tool for managing common pediatric conditions.

The evidence-based approach to developing clinical practice guidelines requires carefully defining the problem and identifying interventions and health outcomes. An extensive literature review and data analysis provide the basis for guideline recommendations. Clinical practice guidelines are also subjected to a thorough peer-review process prior to publication and subsequent dissemination, implementation, and evaluation. They are periodically reviewed to ensure that they are based on the most current data available.

American Academy of Pediatrics clinical practice guidelines are designed to provide physicians with an analytic framework for evaluating and treating common pediatric conditions and are not intended as an exclusive course of treatment or standard of care. When using AAP clinical practice guidelines, physicians should continue to consider other sources of information as well as variations in individual circumstances. The AAP recognizes the incompleteness of data and acknowledges the use of expert consensus in cases in which data do not exist; thus, AAP clinical practice guidelines allow for flexibility and adaptability at the local level and should not replace sound clinical judgment.

This manual contains clinical practice guidelines, technical reports, and technical report summaries developed and published by the AAP. Full technical reports are available on the companion CD-ROM. Each full technical report contains a summary of the data reviewed, results of data analysis, complete evidence tables, and a bibliography of articles included in the review. This manual also contains abstracts and introductions for evidence-based clinical practice guidelines from other organizations that the AAP has endorsed. Clinical practice guidelines will continually be added to this compendium as they are released or updated. We encourage you to look forward to these future guidelines. Additionally, this edition includes the full text of all policy statements, clinical reports, and technical reports published in 2013 by the AAP as well as abstracts of all active AAP and endorsed policy statements and reports. The full text of all endorsed clinical practice guidelines, as well as all active AAP and endorsed policy statements and reports published prior to 2013, is included on the companion CD-ROM.

If you have any questions about current or future clinical practice guidelines, please contact Caryn Davidson at the AAP at 800/433-9016, extension 4317. To order copies of the patient education resources that accompany each guideline, please call the AAP at 888/227-1770 or visit the online AAP Bookstore at www.aap.org/bookstore.

Xavier D. Sevilla, MD, FAAP
Chairperson, Council of Quality Improvement and Patient Safety

FOREWORD

ADHD: Clinical Practice Guideline for the Diagnosis, Evaluation, and Treatment of Attention-Deficit/Hyperactivity Disorder in Children and Adolescents

- *Clinical Practice Guideline*

    - *PPI: AAP Partnership for Policy Implementation*
      See Appendix 2 for more information.

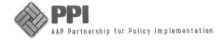

CLINICAL PRACTICE GUIDELINE

ADHD: Clinical Practice Guideline for the Diagnosis, Evaluation, and Treatment of Attention-Deficit/ Hyperactivity Disorder in Children and Adolescents

SUBCOMMITTEE ON ATTENTION-DEFICIT/HYPERACTIVITY DISORDER, STEERING COMMITTEE ON QUALITY IMPROVEMENT AND MANAGEMENT

KEY WORDS
attention-deficit/hyperactivity disorder, children, adolescents, preschool, behavioral therapy, medication

ABBREVIATIONS
AAP—American Academy of Pediatrics
ADHD—attention-deficit/hyperactivity disorder
DSM-PC—*Diagnostic and Statistical Manual for Primary Care*
CDC—Centers for Disease Control and Prevention
FDA—Food and Drug Administration
DSM-IV—*Diagnostic and Statistical Manual of Mental Disorders, Fourth Edition*
MTA—Multimodal Therapy of ADHD

www.pediatrics.org/cgi/doi/10.1542/peds.2011-2654

doi:10.1542/peds.2011-2654

All clinical practice guidelines from the American Academy of Pediatrics automatically expire 5 years after publication unless reaffirmed, revised, or retired at or before that time.

PEDIATRICS (ISSN Numbers: Print, 0031-4005; Online, 1098-4275).

abstract

Attention-deficit/hyperactivity disorder (ADHD) is the most common neurobehavioral disorder of childhood and can profoundly affect the academic achievement, well-being, and social interactions of children; the American Academy of Pediatrics first published clinical recommendations for the diagnosis and evaluation of ADHD in children in 2000; recommendations for treatment followed in 2001. *Pediatrics* 2011;128: 1007–1022

Summary of key action statements:

1. The primary care clinician should initiate an evaluation for ADHD for any child 4 through 18 years of age who presents with academic or behavioral problems and symptoms of inattention, hyperactivity, or impulsivity (quality of evidence B/strong recommendation).

2. To make a diagnosis of ADHD, the primary care clinician should determine that *Diagnostic and Statistical Manual of Mental Disorders, Fourth Edition* criteria have been met (including documentation of impairment in more than 1 major setting); information should be obtained primarily from reports from parents or guardians, teachers, and other school and mental health clinicians involved in the child's care. The primary care clinician should also rule out any alternative cause (quality of evidence B/strong recommendation).

3. In the evaluation of a child for ADHD, the primary care clinician should include assessment for other conditions that might coexist with ADHD, including emotional or behavioral (eg, anxiety, depressive, oppositional defiant, and conduct disorders), developmental (eg, learning and language disorders or other neurodevelopmental disorders), and physical (eg, tics, sleep apnea) conditions (quality of evidence B/strong recommendation).

4. The primary care clinician should recognize ADHD as a chronic condition and, therefore, consider children and adolescents with ADHD as children and youth with special health care needs. Management of children and youth with special health care needs should follow the principles of the chronic care model and the medical home (quality of evidence B/strong recommendation).

5. Recommendations for treatment of children and youth with ADHD vary depending on the patient's age:

   a. For *preschool-aged children (4–5 years of age)*, the primary care clinician should prescribe evidence-based parent- and/or teacher-administered behavior therapy as the first line of treatment (quality of evidence A/strong recommendation) and may prescribe methylphenidate if the behavior interventions do not provide significant improvement and there is moderate-to-severe continuing disturbance in the child's function. In areas where evidence-based behavioral treatments are not available, the clinician needs to weigh the risks of starting medication at an early age against the harm of delaying diagnosis and treatment (quality of evidence B/recommendation).

   b. For *elementary school–aged children (6–11 years of age)*, the primary care clinician should prescribe US Food and Drug Administration–approved medications for ADHD (quality of evidence A/strong recommendation) and/or evidence-based parent- and/or teacher-administered behavior therapy as treatment for ADHD, preferably both (quality of evidence B/strong recommendation). The evidence is particularly strong for stimulant medications and sufficient but less strong for atomoxetine, extended-release guanfacine, and extended-release clonidine (in that order) (quality of evidence A/strong recommendation). The school environment, program, or placement is a part of any treatment plan.

   c. For *adolescents (12–18 years of age)*, the primary care clinician should prescribe Food and Drug Administration–approved medications for ADHD with the assent of the adolescent (quality of evidence A/strong recommendation) and may prescribe behavior therapy as treatment for ADHD (quality of evidence C/recommendation), preferably both.

6. The primary care clinician should titrate doses of medication for ADHD to achieve maximum benefit with minimum adverse effects (quality of evidence B/strong recommendation).

INTRODUCTION

This document updates and replaces 2 previously published clinical guidelines from the American Academy of Pediatrics (AAP) on the diagnosis and treatment of attention-deficit/hyperactivity disorder (ADHD) in children: "Clinical Practice Guideline: Diagnosis and Evaluation of the Child With Attention-Deficit/Hyperactivity Disorder" (2000)[1] and "Clinical Practice Guideline: Treatment of the School-aged Child With Attention-Deficit/Hyperactivity Disorder" (2001).[2] Since these guidelines were published, new information and evidence regarding the diagnosis and treatment of ADHD has become available. Surveys conducted before and after the publication of the previous guidelines have also provided insight into pediatricians' attitudes and practices regarding ADHD. On the basis of an increased understanding regarding ADHD and the challenges it raises for children and families and as a source for clinicians seeking to diagnose and treat children, this guideline pays particular attention to a number of areas.

Expanded Age Range

The previous guidelines addressed diagnosis and treatment of ADHD in children 6 through 12 years of age. There is now emerging evidence to expand the age range of the recommendations to include preschool-aged children and adolescents. This guideline addresses the diagnosis and treatment of ADHD in children 4 through 18 years of age, and attention is brought to special circumstances or concerns in particular age groups when appropriate.

Expanded Scope

Behavioral interventions might help families of children with hyperactive/impulsive behaviors that do not meet full diagnostic criteria for ADHD. Guidance regarding the diagnosis of problem-level concerns in children based on the *Diagnostic and Statistical Manual for Primary Care* (DSM-PC), *Child and Adolescent Version*,[3] as well as suggestions for treatment and care of children and families with problem-level concerns, are provided here. The current DSM-PC was published in 1996 and, therefore, is not consistent with intervening changes to *International Classification of Diseases, Ninth Revision, Clinical Modification* (ICD-9-CM). Although this version of the DSM-PC should not be used as a definitive source for diagnostic codes related to ADHD and comorbid conditions, it certainly may continue to be used as a resource for enriching the understanding of ADHD manifestations. The DSM-PC will be revised when both the DSM-V and ICD-10 are available for use.

A Process of Care for Diagnosis and Treatment

This guideline and process-of-care algorithm (see Supplemental Fig 2 and Supplemental Appendix) recognizes evaluation, diagnosis, and treatment as a continuous process and provides recommendations for both the guideline and the algorithm in this single publication. In addition to the formal recommendations for assessment, diagnosis, and treatment, this guideline provides a single algorithm to guide the clinical process.

Integration With the Task Force on Mental Health

This guideline fits into the broader mission of the AAP Task Force on Mental Health and its efforts to provide a base from which primary care providers can develop alliances with families, work to prevent mental health conditions and identify them early, and collaborate with mental health clinicians.

The diagnosis and management of ADHD in children and youth has been particularly challenging for primary care clinicians because of the limited payment provided for what requires more time than most of the other conditions they typically address. The procedures recommended in this guideline necessitate spending more time with patients and families, developing a system of contacts with school and other personnel, and providing continuous, coordinated care, all of which is time demanding. In addition, relegating mental health conditions exclusively to mental health clinicians also is not a viable solution for many clinicians, because in many areas access to mental health clinicians to whom they can refer patients is limited. Access in many areas is also limited to psychologists when further assessment of cognitive issues is required and not available through the education system because of restrictions from third-party payers in paying for the evaluations on the basis of them being educational and not health related.

Cultural differences in the diagnosis and treatment of ADHD are an important issue, as they are for all pediatric conditions. Because the diagnosis and treatment of ADHD depends to a great extent on family and teacher perceptions, these issues might be even more prominent an issue for ADHD. Specific cultural issues

are beyond the scope of this guideline but are important to consider.

METHODOLOGY

As with the 2 previously published clinical guidelines, the AAP collaborated with several organizations to develop a working subcommittee that represented a wide range of primary care and subspecialty groups. The subcommittee included primary care pediatricians, developmental-behavioral pediatricians, and representatives from the American Academy of Child and Adolescent Psychiatry, the Child Neurology Society, the Society for Pediatric Psychology, the National Association of School Psychologists, the Society for Developmental and Behavioral Pediatrics, the American Academy of Family Physicians, and Children and Adults With Attention-Deficit/Hyperactivity Disorder (CHADD), as well as an epidemiologist from the Centers for Disease Control and Prevention (CDC).

This group met over a 2-year period, during which it reviewed the changes in practice that have occurred and issues that have been identified since the previous guidelines were published. Delay in completing the process led to further conference calls and extended the years of literature reviewed in order to remain as current as possible. The AAP funded the development of this guideline; potential financial conflicts of the participants were identified and taken into consideration in the deliberations. The guideline will be reviewed and/or revised in 5 years unless new evidence emerges that warrants revision sooner.

The subcommittee developed a series of research questions to direct an extensive evidence-based review in partnership with the CDC and the University of Oklahoma Health Sciences Center. The diagnostic review was conducted by the CDC, and the evidence was evaluated in a combined effort of

the AAP, CDC, and University of Oklahoma Health Sciences Center staff. The treatment-related evidence relied on a recent evidence review by the Agency for Healthcare Research and Quality and was supplemented by evidence identified through the CDC review.

The diagnostic issues were focused on 5 areas:

1. ADHD prevalence—specifically: (a) What percentage of the general US population aged 21 years or younger has ADHD? (b) What percentage of patients presenting at pediatricians' or family physicians' offices in the United States meet diagnostic criteria for ADHD?

2. Co-occurring mental disorders— of people with ADHD, what percentage has 1 or more of the following co-occurring conditions: sleep disorders, learning disabilities, depression, anxiety, conduct disorder, and oppositional defiant disorder?

3. What are the functional impairments of children and youth diagnosed with ADHD? Specifically, in what domains and to what degree do youth with ADHD demonstrate impairments in functional domains, including peer relations, academic performance, adaptive skills, and family functioning?

4. Do behavior rating scales remain the standard of care in assessing the diagnostic criteria for ADHD?

5. What is the prevalence of abnormal findings on selected medical screening tests commonly recommended as standard components of an evaluation of a child with suspected ADHD? How accurate are these tests in the diagnosis of ADHD compared with a reference standard (ie, what are the psychometric properties of these tests)?

The treatment issues were focused on 3 areas:

1. What new information is available

regarding the long-term efficacy and safety of medications approved by the US Food and Drug Administration (FDA) for the treatment of ADHD (stimulants and nonstimulants), and specifically, what information is available about the efficacy and safety of these medications in preschool-aged and adolescent patients?

2. What evidence is available about the long-term efficacy and safety of psychosocial interventions (behavioral modification) for the treatment of ADHD for children, and specifically, what information is available about the efficacy and safety of these interventions in preschool-aged and adolescent patients?

3. Are there any additional therapies that reach the level of consideration as evidence based?

Evidence-Review Process for Diagnosis

A multilevel, systematic approach was taken to identify the literature that built the evidence base for both diagnosis and treatment. To increase the likelihood that relevant articles were included in the final evidence base, the reviewers first conducted a scoping review of the literature by systematically searching literature using relevant key words and then summarized the primary findings of articles that met standard inclusion criteria. The reviewers then created evidence tables that were reviewed by content-area experts who were best able to identify articles that might have been missed through the scoping review. Articles that were missed were reviewed carefully to determine where the abstraction methodology failed, and adjustments to the search strategy were made as required (see technical report to be published). Finally, although published literature reviews did not contribute directly to the evidence

base, the articles included in review articles were cross-referenced with the final evidence tables to ensure that all relevant articles were included in the final evidence tables.

For the scoping review, articles were abstracted in a stratified fashion from 3 article-retrieval systems that provided access to articles in the domains of medicine, psychology, and education: PubMed (www.ncbi.nlm.nih.gov/sites/entrez), PsycINFO (www.apa.org/pubs/databases/psycinfo/index.aspx), and ERIC (www.eric.ed.gov). English-language, peer-reviewed articles published between 1998 and 2009 were queried in the 3 search engines. Key words were selected with the intent of including all possible articles that might have been relevant to 1 or more of the questions of interest (see the technical report to be published). The primary abstraction included the following terms: "attention deficit hyperactivity disorder" or "attention deficit disorder" or "hyperkinesis" and "child." A second, independent abstraction was conducted to identify articles related to medical screening tests for ADHD. For this abstraction, the same search terms were used as in the previous procedure along with the additional condition term "behavioral problems" to allow for the inclusion of studies of youth that sought to diagnose ADHD by using medical screening tests. Abstractions were conducted in parallel fashion across each of the 3 databases; the results from each abstraction (complete reference, abstract, and key words) were exported and compiled into a common reference database using EndNote 10.0.[4] References were subsequently and systematically deduplicated by using the software's deduplication procedure. References for books, chapters, and theses were also deleted from the library. Once a deduplicated library was developed, the semifinal

database of 8267 references was reviewed for inclusion on the basis of inclusion criteria listed in the technical report. Included articles were then pulled in their entirety, the inclusion criteria were reconfirmed, and then the study findings were summarized in evidence tables. The articles included in relevant review articles were revisited to ensure their inclusion in the final evidence base. The evidence tables were then presented to the committee for expert review.

Evidence-Review Process for Treatment

In addition to this systematic review, for treatment we used the review from the Agency for Healthcare Research and Quality (AHRQ) Effective Healthcare Program "Attention Deficit Hyperactivity Disorder: Effectiveness of Treatment in At-Risk Preschoolers; Long-term Effectiveness in All Ages; and Variability in Prevalence, Diagnosis, and Treatment."[5] This review addressed a number of key questions for the committee, including the efficacy of medications and behavioral interventions for preschoolers, children, and adolescents. Evidence identified through the systematic evidence review for diagnosis was also used as a secondary data source to supplement the evidence presented in the AHRQ report. The draft practice guidelines were developed by consensus of the committee regarding the evidence. It was decided to create 2 separate components. The guideline recommendations were based on clear characterization of the evidence. The second component is a practice-of-care algorithm (see Supplemental Fig 2) that provides considerably more detail about how to implement the guidelines but is, necessarily, based less on available evidence and more on consensus of the committee members. When data were lacking, particularly in the

Evidence Quality	Preponderance of Benefit or Harm	Balance of Benefit and Harm
A. Well-designed RCTs or diagnostic studies on relevant population	Strong recommendation	
B. RCTs or diagnostic studies with minor limitations; overwhelmingly consistent evidence from observational studies		Option
C. Observational studies (case-control and cohort design)	Recommendation	
D. Expert opinion, case reports, reasoning from first principles	Option	No Rec
X. Exceptional situations in which validating studies cannot be performed and there is a clear preponderance of benefit or harm	Strong recommendation / Recommendation	

FIGURE 1

Integrating evidence-quality appraisal with an assessment of the anticipated balance between benefits and harms if a policy is conducted leads to designation of a policy as a strong recommendation, recommendation, option, or no recommendation. The evidence is discussed in more detail in a technical report that will follow in a later publication. RCT indicates randomized controlled trial; Rec, recommendation.

process-of-care algorithmic portion of the guidelines, a combination of evidence and expert consensus was used. Action statements labeled "strong recommendation" or "recommendation" were based on high- to moderate-quality scientific evidence and a preponderance of benefit over harm.[6] Option-level action statements were based on lesser-quality or limited data and expert consensus or high-quality evidence with a balance between benefits and harms. These clinical options are interventions that a reasonable health care provider might or might not wish to implement in his or her practice. The quality of evidence supporting each recommendation and the strength of each recommendation were assessed by the committee member most experienced in epidemiology and graded according to AAP policy (Fig 1).[6]

The guidelines and process-of-care algorithm underwent extensive peer review by committees, sections, councils, and task forces within the AAP; numerous outside organizations; and other individuals identified by the subcommittee. Liaisons to the subcommittee also were invited to distribute the draft to entities within their organizations. The re-

sulting comments were compiled and reviewed by the chairperson, and relevant changes were incorporated into the draft, which was then reviewed by the full committee.

ABOUT THIS GUIDELINE

Key Action Statements

In light of the concerns highlighted previously and informed by the available evidence, the AAP has developed 6 action statements for the evaluation, diagnosis, and treatment of ADHD in children. These action statements provide for consistent and quality care for children and families with concerns about or symptoms that suggest attention disorders or problems.

Context

This guideline is intended to be integrated with the broader algorithms developed as part of the mission of the AAP Task Force on Mental Health.[7]

Implementation: A Process-of-Care Algorithm

The AAP recognizes the challenge of instituting practice changes and adopting new recommendations for care. To address the need, a process-of-care algorithm has been devel-

oped and has been used in the revision of the AAP ADHD toolkit.

Implementation: Preparing the Practice

Full implementation of the action statements described in this guideline and the process-of-care algorithm might require changes in office procedures and/or preparatory efforts to identify community resources. The section titled "Preparing the Practice" in the process-of-care algorithm and further information can be found in the supplement to the Task Force on Mental Health report.[7] It is important to document all aspects of the diagnostic and treatment procedures in the patients' records. Use of rating scales for the diagnosis of ADHD and assessment for comorbid conditions and as a method for monitoring treatment as described in the process algorithm (see Supplemental Fig 2), as well as information provided to parents such as management plans, can help facilitate a clinician's accurate documentation of his or her process.

Note

The AAP acknowledges that some primary care clinicians might not be confident of their ability to successfully diagnose and treat ADHD in a child because of the child's age, co-existing conditions, or other concerns. At any point at which a clinician feels that he or she is not adequately trained or is uncertain about making a diagnosis or continuing with treatment, a referral to a pediatric or mental health subspecialist should be made. If a diagnosis of ADHD or other condition is made by a subspecialist, the primary care clinician should develop a management strategy with the subspecialist that ensures that the child will continue to receive appropriate care consistent with a medical home model wherein the pediatrician partners with parents so that both health and mental health needs are integrated.

KEY ACTION STATEMENTS FOR THE EVALUATION, DIAGNOSIS, TREATMENT, AND MONITORING OF ADHD IN CHILDREN AND ADOLESCENTS

Action statement 1: The primary care clinician should initiate an evaluation for ADHD for any child 4 through 18 years of age who presents with academic or behavioral problems and symptoms of inattention, hyperactivity, or impulsivity (quality of evidence B/strong recommendation).

Evidence Profile

- **Aggregate evidence quality:** B.
- **Benefits:** In a considerable number of children, ADHD goes undiagnosed. Primary care clinicians' systematic identification of children with these problems will likely decrease the rate of undiagnosed and untreated ADHD in children.
- **Harms/risks/costs:** Children in whom ADHD is inappropriately diagnosed might be labeled inappropriately, or another condition might be missed, and they might receive treatments that will not benefit them.
- **Benefits-harms assessment:** The high prevalence of ADHD and limited mental health resources require primary care pediatricians to play a significant role in the care of their patients with ADHD so that children with this condition receive the appropriate diagnosis and treatment. Treatments available have shown good evidence of efficacy, and lack of treatment results in a risk for impaired outcomes.
- **Value judgments:** The committee considered the requirements for establishing the diagnosis, the prevalence of ADHD, and the efficacy and adverse effects of treatment as well as the long-term outcomes.

- **Role of patient preferences:** Success with treatment depends on patient and family preference, which has to be taken into account.
- **Exclusions:** None.
- **Intentional vagueness:** The limits between what can be handled by a primary care clinician and what should be referred to a subspecialist because of the varying degrees of skills among primary care clinicians.
- **Strength: strong recommendation.**

The basis for this recommendation is essentially unchanged from that in the previous guideline. ADHD is the most common neurobehavioral disorder in children and occurs in approximately 8% of children and youth[8–10]; the number of children with this condition is far greater than can be managed by the mental health system. There is now increased evidence that appropriate diagnosis can be provided for preschool-aged children[11] (4–5 years of age) and for adolescents.[12]

Action statement 2: To make a diagnosis of ADHD, the primary care clinician should determine that *Diagnostic and Statistical Manual of Mental Disorders, Fourth Edition* (DSM-IV-TR) criteria have been met (including documentation of impairment in more than 1 major setting), and information should be obtained primarily from reports from parents or guardians, teachers, and other school and mental health clinicians involved in the child's care. The primary care clinician should also rule out any alternative cause (quality of evidence B/strong recommendation).

Evidence Profile

- **Aggregate evidence quality:** B.
- **Benefits:** The use of DSM-IV criteria has lead to more uniform categorization of the condition across professional disciplines.

- **Harms/risks/costs:** The DSM-IV system does not specifically provide for developmental-level differences and might lead to some misdiagnoses.
- **Benefits-harms assessment:** The benefits far outweigh the harm.
- **Value judgments:** The committee took into consideration the importance of coordination between pediatric and mental health services.
- **Role of patient preferences:** Although there is some stigma associated with mental disorder diagnoses resulting in some families preferring other diagnoses, the need for better clarity in diagnoses was felt to outweigh this preference.
- **Exclusions:** None.
- **Intentional vagueness:** None.
- **Strength: strong recommendation.**

As with the findings in the previous guideline, the DSM-IV criteria continue to be the criteria best supported by evidence and consensus. Developed through several iterations by the American Psychiatric Association, the DSM-IV criteria were created through use of consensus and an expanding research foundation.[13] The DSM-IV system is used by professionals in psychiatry, psychology, health care systems, and primary care. Use of DSM-IV criteria, in addition to having the best evidence to date for criteria for ADHD, also affords the best method for communication across clinicians and is established with third-party payers. The criteria are under review for the development of the DSM-V, but these changes will not be available until at least 1 year after the publication of this current guideline. The diagnostic criteria have not changed since the previous guideline and are presented in Supplemental Table 2. An anticipated change in the DSM-V is increasing the age limit for when ADHD needs to have first presented from 7 to 12 years.[14]

Special Circumstances: Preschool-aged Children (4–5 Years Old)

There is evidence that the diagnostic criteria for ADHD can be applied to preschool-aged children; however, the subtypes detailed in the DSM-IV might not be valid for this population.[15–21] A review of the literature, including the multisite study of the efficacy of methylphenidate in preschool-aged children, revealed that the criteria could appropriately identify children with the condition.[11] However, there are added challenges in determining the presence of key symptoms. Preschool-aged children are not likely to have a separate observer if they do not attend a preschool or child care program, and even if they do attend, staff in those programs might be less qualified than certified teachers to provide accurate observations. Here, too, focused checklists can help physicians in the diagnostic evaluation, although only the Conners Comprehensive Behavior Rating Scales and the ADHD Rating Scale IV are DSM-IV–based scales that have been validated in preschool-aged children.[22]

When there are concerns about the availability or quality of nonparent observations of a child's behavior, physicians may recommend that parents complete a parent-training program before confirming an ADHD diagnosis for preschool-aged children and consider placement in a qualified preschool program if they have not done so already. Information can be obtained from parents and teachers through the use of validated DSM-IV–based ADHD rating scales. The parent-training program must include helping parents develop age-appropriate developmental expectations and specific management skills for problem behaviors. The clinician may obtain reports from the parenting class instructor about the parents' ability to manage their children, and if the children are

in programs in which they are directly observed, instructors can report information about the core symptoms and function of the child directly. Qualified preschool programs include programs such as Head Start or other public prekindergarten programs. Preschool-aged children who display significant emotional or behavioral concerns might also qualify for Early Childhood Special Education services through their local school districts, and the evaluators for these programs and/or Early Childhood Special Education teachers might be excellent reporters of core symptoms.

Special Circumstances: Adolescents

Obtaining teacher reports for adolescents might be more challenging, because many adolescents will have multiple teachers. Likewise, parents might have less opportunity to observe their adolescent's behaviors than they had when their children were younger. Adolescents' reports of their own behaviors often differ from those of other observers, because they tend to minimize their own problematic behaviors.[23–25] Adolescents are less likely to exhibit overt hyperactive behavior. Despite the difficulties, clinicians need to try to obtain (with agreement from the adolescent) information from at least 2 teachers as well as information from other sources such as coaches, school guidance counselors, or leaders of community activities in which the adolescent participates. In addition, it is unusual for adolescents with behavioral/attention problems not to have been previously given a diagnosis of ADHD. Therefore, it is important to establish the younger manifestations of the condition that were missed and to strongly consider substance use, depression, and anxiety as alternative or co-occurring diagnoses. Adolescents with ADHD, especially when untreated, are at greater risk of substance abuse.[26] In addition, the risks of

mood and anxiety disorders and risky sexual behaviors increase during adolescence.[12]

Special Circumstances: Inattention or Hyperactivity/Impulsivity (Problem Level)

Teachers, parents, and child health professionals typically encounter children with behaviors relating to activity level, impulsivity, and inattention who might not fully meet DSM-IV criteria. The DSM-PC[3] provides a guide to the more common behaviors seen in pediatrics. The manual describes common variations in behavior as well as more problematic behaviors at levels of less impairment than those specified in the DSM-IV.

The behavioral descriptions of the DSM-PC have not yet been tested in community studies to determine the prevalence or severity of developmental variations and problems in the areas of inattention, hyperactivity, or impulsivity. They do, however, provide guidance to clinicians regarding elements of treatment for children with problems with mild-to-moderate inattention, hyperactivity, or impulsivity. The DSM-PC also considers environmental influences on a child's behavior and provides information on differential diagnosis with a developmental perspective.

Action statement 3: In the evaluation of a child for ADHD, the primary care clinician should include assessment for other conditions that might coexist with ADHD, including emotional or behavioral (eg, anxiety, depressive, oppositional defiant, and conduct disorders), developmental (eg, learning and language disorders or other neurodevelopmental disorders), and physical (eg, tics, sleep apnea) conditions (quality of evidence B/strong recommendation).

Evidence Profile

- **Aggregate evidence quality:** B.
- **Benefits:** Identifying coexisting conditions is important for developing the most appropriate treatment plan.
- **Harms/risks/costs:** The major risk is misdiagnosing the conditions and providing inappropriate care.
- **Benefits-harms assessment:** There is a preponderance of benefit over harm.
- **Value judgments:** The committee members took into consideration the common occurrence of coexisting conditions and the importance of addressing them in making this recommendation.
- **Role of patient preferences:** None.
- **Exclusions:** None.
- **Intentional vagueness:** None.
- **Strength: strong recommendation.**

A variety of other behavioral, developmental, and physical conditions can coexist in children who are evaluated for ADHD. These conditions include, but are not limited to, learning problems, language disorder, disruptive behavior, anxiety, mood disorders, tic disorders, seizures, developmental coordination disorder, or sleep disorders.[23,24,27–38] In some cases, the presence of a coexisting condition will alter the treatment of ADHD. The primary care clinician might benefit from additional support and guidance or might need to refer a child with ADHD and coexisting conditions, such as severe mood or anxiety disorders, to subspecialists for assessment and management. The subspecialists could include child psychiatrists, developmental-behavioral pediatricians, neurodevelopmental disability physicians, child neurologists, or child or school psychologists.

Given the likelihood that another condition exists, primary care clinicians should conduct assessments that determine or at least identify the risk of coexisting conditions. Through its Task Force on Mental Health, the AAP has developed algorithms and a toolkit[39] for assessing and treating (or comanaging) the most common developmental disorders and mental health concerns in children. These resources might be useful in assessing children who are being evaluated for ADHD. Payment for evaluation and treatment must cover the fixed and variable costs of providing the services, as noted in the AAP policy statement "Scope of Health Care Benefits for Children From Birth Through Age 26.[40]

Special Circumstances: Adolescents

Clinicians should assess adolescent patients with newly diagnosed ADHD for symptoms and signs of substance abuse; when these signs and symptoms are found, evaluation and treatment for addiction should precede treatment for ADHD, if possible, or careful treatment for ADHD can begin if necessary.[25]

Action statement 4: The primary care clinician should recognize ADHD as a chronic condition and, therefore, consider children and adolescents with ADHD as children and youth with special health care needs. Management of children and youth with special health care needs should follow the principles of the chronic care model and the medical home (quality of evidence B/strong recommendation).

Evidence Profile

- **Aggregate evidence quality:** B.
- **Benefits:** The recommendation describes the coordinated services most appropriate for managing the condition.
- **Harms/risks/costs:** Providing the services might be more costly.
- **Benefits-harms assessment:** There is a preponderance of benefit over harm.
- **Value judgments:** The committee members considered the value of medical home services when deciding to make this recommendation.
- **Role of patient preferences:** Family preference in how these services are provided is an important consideration.
- **Exclusions:** None.
- **Intentional vagueness:** None.
- **Strength: strong recommendation.**

As in the previous guideline, this recommendation is based on the evidence that ADHD continues to cause symptoms and dysfunction in many children who have the condition over long periods of time, even into adulthood, and that the treatments available address symptoms and function but are usually not curative. Although the chronic illness model has not been specifically studied in children and youth with ADHD, it has been effective for other chronic conditions such as asthma,[23] and the medical home model has been accepted as the preferred standard of care.[41] The management process is also helped by encouraging strong family-school partnerships.[42]

Longitudinal studies have found that, frequently, treatments are not sustained despite the fact that long-term outcomes for children with ADHD indicate that they are at greater risk of significant problems if they discontinue treatment.[43] Because a number of parents of children with ADHD also have ADHD, extra support might be necessary to help those parents provide medication on a consistent basis and institute a consistent behavioral program. The medical home and chronic illness approach is provided in the process algorithm (Supplemental Fig 2). An important process in ongoing care is bidirectional communication with teachers and other school and mental health clinicians involved in the child's care as well as with parents and patients.

Special Circumstances: Inattention or Hyperactivity/Impulsivity (Problem Level)

Children with inattention or hyperactivity/impulsivity at the problem level (DSM-PC) and their families might also benefit from the same chronic illness and medical home principles.

Action statement 5: Recommendations for treatment of children and youth with ADHD vary depending on the patient's age.

Action statement 5a: For *preschool-aged children (4–5 years of age)*, the primary care clinician should prescribe evidence-based parent- and/or teacher-administered behavior therapy as the first line of treatment (quality of evidence A/strong recommendation) and may prescribe methylphenidate if the behavior interventions do not provide significant improvement and there is moderate-to-severe continuing disturbance in the child's function. In areas in which evidence-based behavioral treatments are not available, the clinician needs to weigh the risks of starting medication at an early age against the harm of delaying diagnosis and treatment (quality of evidence B/recommendation).

Evidence Profile

- **Aggregate evidence quality:** A for behavior; B for methylphenidate.
- **Benefits:** Both behavior therapy and methylphenidate have been demonstrated to reduce behaviors associated with ADHD and improve function.
- **Harms/risks/costs:** Both therapies increase the cost of care, and behavior therapy requires a higher level of family involvement, whereas methylphenidate has some potential adverse effects.
- **Benefits-harms assessment:** Given the risks of untreated ADHD, the benefits outweigh the risks.
- **Value judgments:** The committee mem-

bers included the effects of untreated ADHD when deciding to make this recommendation.

- **Role of patient preferences:** Family preference is essential in determining the treatment plan.
- **Exclusions:** None.
- **Intentional vagueness:** None.
- **Strength: strong recommendation.**

Action statement 5b: For *elementary school-aged children (6–11 years of age)*, the primary care clinician should prescribe FDA-approved medications for ADHD (quality of evidence A/strong recommendation) and/or evidence-based parent- and/or teacher-administered behavior therapy as treatment for ADHD, preferably both (quality of evidence B/strong recommendation). The evidence is particularly strong for stimulant medications and sufficient but less strong for atomoxetine, extended-release guanfacine, and extended-release clonidine (in that order) (quality of evidence A/strong recommendation). The school environment, program, or placement is a part of any treatment plan.

Evidence Profile

- **Aggregate evidence quality:** A for treatment with FDA-approved medications; B for behavior therapy.
- **Benefits:** Both behavior therapy and FDA-approved medications have been demonstrated to reduce behaviors associated with ADHD and improve function.
- **Harms/risks/costs:** Both therapies increase the cost of care, and behavior therapy requires a higher level of family involvement, whereas FDA-approved medications have some potential adverse effects.
- **Benefits-harms assessment:** Given the risks of untreated ADHD, the benefits outweigh the risks.
- **Value judgments:** The committee members included the effects of untreated

ADHD when deciding to make this recommendation.

- **Role of patient preferences:** Family preference, including patient preference, is essential in determining the treatment plan.
- **Exclusions:** None.
- **Intentional vagueness:** None.
- **Strength: strong recommendation.**

Action statement 5c: For *adolescents (12–18 years of age)*, the primary care clinician should prescribe FDA-approved medications for ADHD with the assent of the adolescent (quality of evidence A/strong recommendation) and may prescribe behavior therapy as treatment for ADHD (quality of evidence C/recommendation), preferably both.

Evidence Profile

- **Aggregate evidence quality:** A for medications; C for behavior therapy.
- **Benefits:** Both behavior therapy and FDA-approved medications have been demonstrated to reduce behaviors associated with ADHD and improve function.
- **Harms/risks/costs:** Both therapies increase the cost of care, and behavior therapy requires a higher level of family involvement, whereas FDA-approved medications have some potential adverse effects.
- **Benefits-harms assessment:** Given the risks of untreated ADHD, the benefits outweigh the risks.
- **Value judgments:** The committee members included the effects of untreated ADHD when deciding to make this recommendation.
- **Role of patient preferences:** Family preference, including patient preference, is essential in determining the treatment plan.
- **Exclusions:** None.
- **Intentional vagueness:** None.
- **Strength: strong recommendation/ recommendation.**

Medication

Similar to the recommendations from the previous guideline, stimulant medications are highly effective for most children in reducing core symptoms of ADHD.[44] One selective norepinephrine-reuptake inhibitor (atomoxetine[45,46]) and 2 selective α_2-adrenergic agonists (extended-release guanfacine[47,48] and extended-release clonidine[49]) have also demonstrated efficacy in reducing core symptoms. Because norepinephrine-reuptake inhibitors and α_2-adrenergic agonists are newer, the evidence base that supports them—although adequate for FDA approval—is considerably smaller than that for stimulants. None of them have been approved for use in preschool-aged children. Compared with stimulant medications that have an effect size [effect size = (treatment mean − control mean)/control SD] of approximately 1.0,[50] the effects of the nonstimulants are slightly weaker; atomoxetine has an effect size of approximately 0.7, and extended-release guanfacine and extended-release clonidine also have effect sizes of approximately 0.7.

The accompanying process-of-care algorithm provides a list of the currently available FDA-approved medications for ADHD (Supplemental Table 3). Characteristics of each medication are provided to help guide the clinician's choice in prescribing medication.

As was identified in the previous guideline, the most common stimulant adverse effects are appetite loss, abdominal pain, headaches, and sleep disturbance. The results of the Multimodal Therapy of ADHD (MTA) study revealed a more persistent effect of stimulants on decreasing growth velocity than have most previous studies, particularly when children were on higher and more consistently administered doses. The effects diminished by the third year of treatment, but no com-pensatory rebound effects were found.[51] However, diminished growth was in the range of 1 to 2 cm. An uncommon additional significant adverse effect of stimulants is the occurrence of hallucinations and other psychotic symptoms.[52] Although concerns have been raised about the rare occurrence of sudden cardiac death among children using stimulant medications,[53] sudden death in children on stimulant medication is extremely rare, and evidence is conflicting as to whether stimulant medications increase the risk of sudden death.[54–56] It is important to expand the history to include specific cardiac symptoms, Wolf-Parkinson-White syndrome, sudden death in the family, hypertrophic cardiomyopathy, and long QT syndrome. Preschool-aged children might experience increased mood lability and dysphoria.[57] For the nonstimulant atomoxetine, the adverse effects include initial somnolence and gastrointestinal tract symptoms, particularly if the dosage is increased too rapidly; decrease in appetite; increase in suicidal thoughts (less common); and hepatitis (rare). For the nonstimulant α_2-adrenergic agonists extended-release guanfacine and extended-release clonidine, adverse effects include somnolence and dry mouth.

Only 2 medications have evidence to support their use as adjunctive therapy with stimulant medications sufficient to achieve FDA approval: extended-release guanfacine[26] and extended-release clonidine. Other medications have been used in combination off-label, but there is currently only anecdotal evidence for their safety or efficacy, so their use cannot be recommended at this time.

Special Circumstances: Preschool-aged Children

A number of special circumstances support the recommendation to initiate ADHD treatment in preschool-aged children (ages 4–5 years) with behavioral therapy alone first.[57] These circumstances include:

- The multisite study of methylphenidate[57] was limited to preschool-aged children who had moderate-to-severe dysfunction.

- The study also found that many children (ages 4–5 years) experience improvements in symptoms with behavior therapy alone, and the overall evidence for behavior therapy in preschool-aged children is strong.

- Behavioral programs for children 4 to 5 years of age typically run in the form of group parent-training programs and, although not always compensated by health insurance, have a lower cost. The process algorithm (see Supplemental pages s15-16) contains criteria for the clinician to use in assessing the quality of the behavioral therapy. In addition, programs such as Head Start and Children and Adults With Attention Deficit Hyperactivity Disorder (CHADD) (www.chadd.org) might provide some behavioral supports.

Many young children with ADHD might still require medication to achieve maximum improvement, and medication is not contraindicated for children 4 through 5 years of age. However, only 1 multisite study has carefully assessed medication use in preschool-aged children. Other considerations in the recommendation about treating children 4 to 5 years of age with stimulant medications include:

- The study was limited to preschool-aged children who had moderate-to-severe dysfunction.

- Research has found that a number of young children (4–5 years of age) experience improvements in symptoms with behavior therapy alone.

- There are concerns about the possible effects on growth during this rapid growth period of preschool-aged children.

- There has been limited information about and experience with the effects of stimulant medication in children between the ages of 4 and 5 years.

Here, the criteria for enrollment (and, therefore, medication use) included measures of severity that distinguished treated children from the larger group of preschool-aged children with ADHD. Thus, before initiating medications, the physician should assess the severity of the child's ADHD. Given current data, only those preschool-aged children with ADHD who have moderate-to-severe dysfunction should be considered for medication. Criteria for this level of severity, based on the multisite-study results,[57] are (1) symptoms that have persisted for at least 9 months, (2) dysfunction that is manifested in both the home and other settings such as preschool or child care, and (3) dysfunction that has not responded adequately to behavior therapy. The decision to consider initiating medication at this age depends in part on the clinician's assessment of the estimated developmental impairment, safety risks, or consequences for school or social participation that could ensue if medications are not initiated. It is often helpful to consult with a mental health specialist who has had specific experience with preschool-aged children if possible.

Dextroamphetamine is the only medication approved by the FDA for use in children younger than 6 years of age. This approval, however, was based on less stringent criteria in force when the medication was approved rather than on empirical evidence of its safety and efficacy in this age group. Most of the evidence for the safety and efficacy of treating preschool-aged children with stimulant medications has been

from methylphenidate.[57] Methylphenidate evidence consists of 1 multisite study of 165 children and 10 other smaller single-site studies that included from 11 to 59 children (total of 269 children); 7 of the 10 single-site studies found significant efficacy. It must be noted that although there is moderate evidence that methylphenidate is safe and efficacious in preschool-aged children, its use in this age group remains off-label. Although the use of dextroamphetamine is on-label, the insufficient evidence for its safety and efficacy in this age group does not make it possible to recommend at this time.

If children do not experience adequate symptom improvement with behavior therapy, medication can be prescribed, as described previously. Evidence suggests that the rate of metabolizing stimulant medication is slower in children 4 through 5 years of age, so they should be given a lower dose to start, and the dose can be increased in smaller increments. Maximum doses have not been adequately studied.[57]

Special Circumstances: Adolescents

As noted previously, before beginning medication treatment for adolescents with newly diagnosed ADHD, clinicians should assess these patients for symptoms of substance abuse. When substance use is identified, assessment when off the abusive substances should precede treatment for ADHD (see the Task Force on Mental Health report[7]). Diversion of ADHD medication (use for other than its intended medical purposes) is also a special concern among adolescents[58]; clinicians should monitor symptoms and prescription-refill requests for signs of misuse or diversion of ADHD medication and consider prescribing medications with no abuse potential, such as atomoxetine (Strattera [Ely Lilly Co, Indianapolis, IN]) and

extended-release guanfacine (Intuniv [Shire US Inc, Wayne, PA]) or extended-release clonidine (Kapvay [Shionogi Inc, Florham Park, NJ]) (which are not stimulants) or stimulant medications with less abuse potential, such as lisdexamfetamine (Vyvanse [Shire US Inc]), dermal methylphenidate (Daytrana [Noven Therapeutics, LLC, Miami, FL]), or OROS methylphenidate (Concerta [Janssen Pharmaceuticals, Inc, Titusville, NJ]). Because lisdexamfetamine is dextroamphetamine, which contains an additional lysine molecule, it is only activated after ingestion, when it is metabolized by erythrocyte cells to dexamphetamine. The other preparations make extraction of the stimulant medication more difficult.

Given the inherent risks of driving by adolescents with ADHD, special concern should be taken to provide medication coverage for symptom control while driving. Longer-acting or late-afternoon, short-acting medications might be helpful in this regard.[59]

Special Circumstances: Inattention or Hyperactivity/Impulsivity (Problem Level)

Medication is not appropriate for children whose symptoms do not meet DSM-IV criteria for diagnosis of ADHD, although behavior therapy does not require a specific diagnosis, and many of the efficacy studies have included children without specific mental behavioral disorders.

Behavior Therapy

Behavior therapy represents a broad set of specific interventions that have a common goal of modifying the physical and social environment to alter or change behavior. Behavior therapy usually is implemented by training parents in specific techniques that improve their abilities to modify and

TABLE 1 Evidence-Based Behavioral Treatments for ADHD

Intervention Type	Description	Typical Outcome(s)	Median Effect Size[a]
Behavioral parent training (BPT)	Behavior-modification principles provided to parents for implementation in home settings	Improved compliance with parental commands; improved parental understanding of behavioral principles; high levels of parental satisfaction with treatment	0.55
Behavioral classroom management	Behavior-modification principles provided to teachers for implementation in classroom settings	Improved attention to instruction; improved compliance with classroom rules; decreased disruptive behavior; improved work productivity	0.61
Behavioral peer interventions (BPI)[b]	Interventions focused on peer interactions/relationships; these are often group-based interventions provided weekly and include clinic-based social-skills training used either alone or concurrently with behavioral parent training and/or medication	Office-based interventions have produced minimal effects; interventions have been of questionable social validity; some studies of BPI combined with clinic-based BPT found positive effects on parent ratings of ADHD symptoms; no differences on social functioning or parent ratings of social behavior have been revealed	

[a] Effect size = (treatment median − control median)/control SD.

[b] The effect size for behavioral peer interventions is not reported, because the effect sizes for these studies represent outcomes associated with combined interventions. A lower effect size means that they have less of an effect. The effect sizes found are considered moderate.

Adapted from Pelham W, Fabiano GA. *J Clin Child Adolesc Psychol.* 2008;37(1):184–214.

shape their child's behavior and to improve the child's ability to regulate his or her own behavior. The training involves techniques to more effectively provide rewards when their child demonstrates the desired behavior (eg, positive reinforcement), learn what behaviors can be reduced or eliminated by using planned ignoring as an active strategy (or using praising and ignoring in combination), or provide appropriate consequences or punishments when their child fails to meet the goals (eg, punishment). There is a need to consistently apply rewards and consequences as tasks are achieved and then to gradually increase the expectations for each task as they are mastered to shape behaviors. Although behavior therapy shares a set of principles, individual programs introduce different techniques and strategies to achieve the same ends.

Table 1 lists the major behavioral intervention approaches that have been demonstrated to be evidence based for the management of ADHD in 3 different types of settings. The table is based on 22 studies, each completed between 1997 and 2006.

Evidence for the effectiveness of behavior therapy in children with ADHD is derived from a variety of studies[60–62] and an Agency for Healthcare Research and Quality review.[5] The diversity of interventions and outcome measures makes meta-analysis of the effects of behavior therapy alone or in association with medications challenging. The long-term positive effects of behavior therapy have yet to be determined. Ongoing adherence to a behavior program might be important; therefore, implementing a chronic care model for child health might contribute to the long-term effects.[63]

Study results have indicated positive effects of behavior therapy when combined with medications. Most studies that compared behavior therapy to stimulants found a much stronger effect on ADHD core symptoms from stimulants than from behavior therapy. The MTA study found that combined treatment (behavior therapy and stimulant medication) was not significantly more efficacious than treatment with medication alone for the core symptoms of ADHD after correction for multiple tests in the primary analysis.[64] However, a secondary analysis of a combined measure of parent and teacher ratings of ADHD symptoms revealed a significant advantage for the combination with a small effect size of $d = 0.26$.[65] However, the same study also found that the combined treatment compared with medication alone did offer greater improvements on academic and conduct measures when ADHD coexisted with anxiety and when children lived in low socioeconomic environments. In addition, parents and teachers of children who were receiving combined therapy were significantly more satisfied with the treatment plan. Finally, the combination of medication management and behavior therapy allowed for the use of lower dosages of stimulants, which possibly reduced the risk of adverse effects.[66]

School Programming and Supports

Behavior therapy programs coordinating efforts at school as well as home might enhance the effects. School programs can provide classroom adaptations, such as preferred seating, modified work assignments, and test modifications (to the location at which it is administered and time allotted for taking the test), as well as behavior plans as part of a 504 Rehabilitation Act Plan or special education Individualized Education Program (IEP) under the "other health impairment" designation as part of the Individuals With

Disability Education Act (IDEA).[67] It is helpful for clinicians to be aware of the eligibility criteria in their state and school district to advise families of their options. Youths documented to have ADHD can also get permission to take college-readiness tests in an untimed manner by following appropriate documentation guidelines.[68]

The effect of coexisting conditions on ADHD treatment is variable. In some cases, treatment of the ADHD resolves the coexisting condition. For example, treatment of ADHD might resolve oppositional defiant disorder or anxiety.[68] However, sometimes the co-occurring condition might require treatment that is in addition to the treatment for ADHD. Some coexisting conditions can be treated in the primary care setting, but others will require referral and co-management with a subspecialist.

Action statement 6: Primary care clinicians should titrate doses of medication for ADHD to achieve maximum benefit with minimum adverse effects (quality of evidence B/strong recommendation).

Evidence Profile

- **Aggregate evidence quality:** B.
- **Benefits:** The optimal dose of medication is required to reduce core symptoms to or as close to the levels of children without ADHD.
- **Harms/risks/costs:** Higher levels of medication increase the chances of adverse effects.
- **Benefits-harms assessment:** The importance of adequately treating ADHD outweighs the risk of adverse effects.
- **Value judgments:** The committee members included the effects of untreated ADHD when deciding to make this recommendation.
- **Role of patient preferences:** The families' preferences and comfort need to be taken into consideration in developing a titration plan.
- **Exclusions:** None.

- **Intentional vagueness:** None.
- **Strength: strong recommendation.**

The findings from the MTA study suggested that more than 70% of children and youth with ADHD respond to one of the stimulant medications at an optimal dose when a systematic trial is used.[65] Children in the MTA who were treated in the community with care as usual from whomever they chose or to whom they had access received lower doses of stimulants with less frequent monitoring and had less optimal results.[65] Because stimulants might produce positive but suboptimal effects at a low dose in some children and youth, titration to maximum doses that control symptoms without adverse effects is recommended instead of titration strictly on a milligram-per-kilogram basis.

Education of parents is an important component in the chronic illness model to ensure their cooperation in efforts to reach appropriate titration (remembering that the parents themselves might be challenged significantly by ADHD).[69,70] The primary care clinician should alert parents and children that changing medication dose and occasionally changing a medication might be necessary for optimal medication management, that the process might require a few months to achieve optimal success, and that medication efficacy should be systematically monitored at regular intervals.

Because stimulant medication effects are seen immediately, trials of different doses of stimulants can be accomplished in a relatively short time period. Stimulant medications can be effectively titrated on a 3- to 7-day basis.[65]

It is important to note that by the 3-year follow-up of 14-month MTA interventions (optimal medications management, optimal behavioral management, the combination of the 2, or community treatment), all differences among the initial 4

groups were no longer present. After the initial 14-month intervention, the children no longer received the careful monthly monitoring provided by the study and went back to receiving care from their community providers. Their medications and doses varied, and a number of them were no longer taking medication. In children still on medication, the growth deceleration was only seen for the first 2 years and was in the range of 1 to 2 cm.

CONCLUSION

Evidence continues to be fairly clear with regard to the legitimacy of the diagnosis of ADHD and the appropriate diagnostic criteria and procedures required to establish a diagnosis, identify co-occurring conditions, and treat effectively with both behavioral and pharmacologic interventions. However, the steps required to sustain appropriate treatments and achieve successful long-term outcomes still remain a challenge. To provide more detailed information about how the recommendations of this guideline can be accomplished, a more detailed but less strongly evidence-based algorithm is provided as a companion article.

AREAS FOR FUTURE RESEARCH

Some specific research topics pertinent to the diagnosis and treatment of ADHD or developmental variations or problems in children and adolescents in primary care to be explored include:

- identification or development of reliable instruments suitable to use in primary care to assess the nature or degree of functional impairment in children/adolescents with ADHD and monitor improvement over time;
- study of medications and other therapies used clinically but not approved by the FDA for ADHD, such as

electroencephalographic biofeedback;

- determination of the optimal schedule for monitoring children/adolescents with ADHD, including factors for adjusting that schedule according to age, symptom severity, and progress reports;

- evaluation of the effectiveness of various school-based interventions;

- comparisons of medication use and effectiveness in different ages, including both harms and benefits;

- development of methods to involve parents and children/adolescents in their own care and improve adherence to both behavior and medication treatments;

- standardized and documented tools that will help primary care providers in identifying coexisting conditions;

- development and determination of effective electronic and Web-based systems to help gather information to diagnose and monitor children with ADHD;

- improved systems of communication with schools and mental health professionals, as well as other community agencies, to provide effective collaborative care;

- evidence for optimal monitoring by

some aspects of severity, disability, or impairment; and

- long-term outcomes of children first identified with ADHD as preschool-aged children.

SUBCOMMITTEE ON ATTENTION DEFICIT HYPERACTIVITY DISORDER (OVERSIGHT BY THE STEERING COMMITTEE ON QUALITY IMPROVEMENT AND MANAGEMENT, 2005–2011)

WRITING COMMITTEE

Mark Wolraich, MD, Chair – *(periodic consultant to Shire, Eli Lilly, Shinogi, and Next Wave Pharmaceuticals)*

Lawrence Brown, MD – *(neurologist; AAP Section on Neurology; Child Neurology Society) (Safety Monitoring Board for Best Pharmaceuticals for Children Act for National Institutes of Health)*

Ronald T. Brown, PhD – *(child psychologist; Society for Pediatric Psychology) (no conflicts)*

George DuPaul, PhD – *(school psychologist; National Association of School Psychologists) (participated in clinical trial on Vyvanse effects on college students with ADHD, funded by Shire; published 2 books on ADHD and receives royalties)*

Marian Earls, MD – *(general pediatrician with QI expertise, developmental and behavioral pediatrician) (no conflicts)*

Heidi M. Feldman, MD, PhD – *(developmental and behavioral pediatrician; Society for Developmental and Behavioral Pediatricians) (no conflicts)*

Theodore G. Ganiats, MD – *(family physician; American Academy of Family Physicians) (no conflicts)*

Beth Kaplanek, RN, BSN – *(parent advocate, Children and Adults With Attention Deficit Hyperactivity Disorder [CHADD]) (no conflicts)*

Bruce Meyer, MD – *(general pediatrician) (no conflicts)*

James Perrin, MD – *(general pediatrician; AAP Mental Health Task Force, AAP Council on Children With Disabilities) (consultant to Pfizer not related to ADHD)*

Karen Pierce, MD – *(child psychiatrist; American Academy of Child and Adolescent Psychiatry) (no conflicts)*

Michael Reiff, MD – *(developmental and behavioral pediatrician; AAP Section on Developmental and Behavioral Pediatrics) (no conflicts)*

Martin T. Stein, MD – *(developmental and behavioral pediatrician; AAP Section on Developmental and Behavioral Pediatrics) (no conflicts)*

Susanna Visser, MS – *(epidemiologist) (no conflicts)*

CONSULTANT

Melissa Capers, MA, MFA – *(medical writer) (no conflicts)*

STAFF

Caryn Davidson, MA

ACKNOWLEDGMENTS

This guideline was developed with support from the Partnership for Policy Implementation (PPI) initiative. Physicians trained in medical informatics were involved with formatting the algorithm and helping to keep the key action statements actionable, decidable, and executable.

REFERENCES

1. American Academy of Pediatrics, Committee on Quality Improvement and Subcommittee on Attention-Deficit/Hyperactivity Disorder. Clinical practice guideline: diagnosis and evaluation of the child with attention-deficit/hyperactivity disorder. *Pediatrics.* 2000;105(5):1158–1170

2. American Academy of Pediatrics, Subcommittee on Attention-Deficit/Hyperactivity Disorder, Committee on Quality Improvement. Clinical practice guideline: treatment of the school-aged child with attention-deficit/hyperactivity disorder. *Pediatrics.* 2001;108(4):1033–1044

3. Wolraich ML, Felice ME, Drotar DD. *The Classification of Child and Adolescent Mental Conditions in Primary Care: Diagnostic and Statistical Manual for Primary Care (DSM-PC), Child and Adolescent Version.* Elk Grove, IL: American Academy of Pediatrics; 1996

4. *EndNote* [computer program]. 10th ed. Carlsbad, CA: Thompson Reuters; 2009

5. Charach A, Dashti B, Carson P, Booker L, Lim CG, Lillie E, Yeung E, Ma J, Raina P, Schachar R. *Attention Deficit Hyperactivity Disorder: Effectiveness of Treatment in At-Risk Preschoolers; Long-term Effectiveness in All Ages; and Variability in Prevalence, Diagnosis, and Treatment.* Comparative Effectiveness Review No. 44. (Prepared by the McMaster University Evidence-based Practice Center under Contract No. MME2202 290-02-0020.)

AHRQ Publication No. 12-EHC003-EF. Rockville, MD: Agency for Healthcare Research and Quality. October 2011.

6. American Academy of Pediatrics, Steering Committee on Quality Improvement. Classifying recommendations for clinical practice guidelines. *Pediatrics.* 2004;114(3):874–877

7. Foy JM; American Academy of Pediatrics Task Force on Mental Health. Enhancing pediatric mental health care: report from the American Academy of Pediatrics Task Force on Mental Health. Introduction. *Pediatrics.* 2010;125(suppl 3)S69–S174

8. Visser SN, Lesesne CA, Perou R. National estimates and factors associated with medication treatment for childhood

attention-deficit/hyperactivity disorder. *Pediatrics.* 2007;119(suppl 1):S99–S106

9. Centers for Disease Control and Prevention. Mental health in the United States: prevalence of diagnosis and medication treatment for attention-deficit/hyperactivity disorder—United States, 2003. *MMWR Morb Mortal Wkly Rep.* 2005;54(34):842–847

10. Centers for Disease Control and Prevention. Increasing prevalence of parent-reported attention deficit/hyperactivity disorder among children: United States, 2003–2007. *MMWR Morb Mortal Wkly Rep.* 2010;59(44):1439–1443

11. Egger HL, Kondo D, Angold A. The epidemiology and diagnostic issues in preschool attention-deficit/hyperactivity disorder. *Infant Young Child.* 2006;19(2):109–122

12. Wolraich ML, Wibbelsman CJ, Brown TE, et al. Attention-deficit/hyperactivity disorder among adolescents: a review of the diagnosis, treatment, and clinical implications. *Pediatrics.* 2005;115(6):1734–1746

13. American Psychiatric Association. *Diagnostic and Statistical Manual of Mental Disorders, 4th ed, Text Revision (DSM-IV-TR).* Washington, DC: American Psychiatric Association; 2000

14. American Psychiatric Association. Diagnostic criteria for attention deficit/hyperactivity disorder. Available at: www.dsm5.org/ProposedRevision/Pages/proposedrevision.aspx?rid=383. Accessed September 30, 2011

15. Lahey BB, Pelham WE, Stein MA, et al. Validity of DSM-IV attention-deficit/hyperactivity disorder for younger children [published correction appears in *J Am Acad Child Adolesc Psychiatry.* 1999;38(2):222]. *J Am Acad Child Adolesc Psychiatry.* 1998;37(7):695–702

16. Pavuluri MN, Luk SL, McGee R. Parent reported preschool attention deficit hyperactivity: measurement and validity. *Eur Child Adolesc Psychiatry.* 1999;8(2):126–133

17. Harvey EA, Youngwirth SD, Thakar DA, Errazuriz PA. Predicting attention-deficit/hyperactivity disorder and oppositional defiant disorder from preschool diagnostic assessments. *J Consult Clin Psychol.* 2009;77(2):349–354

18. Keenan K, Wakschlag LS. More than the terrible twos: the nature and severity of behavior problems in clinic-referred preschool children. *J Abnorm Child Psychol.* 2000;28(1):33–46

19. Gadow KD, Nolan EE, Litcher L, et al. Comparison of attention-deficit/hyperactivity disorder symptoms subtypes in Ukrainian schoolchildren. *J Am Acad Child Adolesc Psychiatry.* 2000;39(12):1520–1527

20. Sprafkin J, Volpe RJ, Gadow KD, Nolan EE, Kelly K. A DSM-IV-referenced screening instrument for preschool children: the Early Childhood Inventory-4. *J Am Acad Child Adolesc Psychiatry.* 2002;41(5):604–612

21. Poblano A, Romero E. ECI-4 screening of attention deficit-hyperactivity disorder and co-morbidity in Mexican preschool children: preliminary results. *Arq Neuropsiquiatr.* 2006;64(4):932–936

22. McGoey KE, DuPaul GJ, Haley E, Shelton TL. Parent and teacher ratings of attention-deficit/hyperactivity disorder in preschool: the ADHD Rating Scale-IV Preschool Version. *J Psychopathol Behav Assess.* 2007;29(4):269–276

23. Young J. Common comorbidities seen in adolescents with attention-deficit/hyperactivity disorder. *Adolesc Med State Art Rev.* 2008;19(2):216–228, vii

24. Freeman R; Tourette Syndrome International Database Consortium. Tic disorders and ADHD: answers from a worldwide clinical dataset on Tourette syndrome [published correction appears in *Eur Child Adolesc Psychiatry.* 2007;16(8):536]. *Eur Child Adolesc Psychiatry.* 2007;16(1 suppl):15–23

25. Riggs P. Clinical approach to treatment of ADHD in adolescents with substance use disorders and conduct disorder. *J Am Acad Child Adolesc Psychiatry.* 1998;37(3):331–332

26. Kratochvil CJ, Vaughan BS, Stoner JA, et al. A double-blind, placebo-controlled study of atomoxetine in young children with ADHD. *Pediatrics.* 2011;127(4). Available at: www.pediatrics.org/cgi/content/full/127/4/e862

27. Rowland AS, Lesesne CA, Abramowitz AJ. The epidemiology of attention-deficit/hyperactivity disorder (ADHD): a public health view. *Ment Retard Dev Disabil Res Rev.* 2002;8(3):162–170

28. Cuffe SP, Moore CG, McKeown RE. Prevalence and correlates of ADHD symptoms in the national health interview survey. *J Atten Disord.* 2005;9(2):392–401

29. Pastor PN, Reuben CA. Diagnosed attention deficit hyperactivity disorder and learning disability: United States, 2004–2006. *Vital Health Stat 10.* 2008;(237):1–14

30. Biederman J, Faraone SV, Wozniak J, Mick E, Kwon A, Aleardi M. Further evidence of unique developmental phenotypic correlates of pediatric bipolar disorder: findings from a large sample of clinically referred preadolescent children assessed over the last 7 years. *J Affect Disord.* 2004;82(suppl 1):S45–S58

31. Biederman J, Kwon A, Aleardi M. Absence of gender effects on attention deficit hyperactivity disorder: findings in nonreferred subjects. *Am J Psychiatry.* 2005;162(6):1083–1089

32. Biederman J, Ball SW, Monuteaux MC, et al. New insights into the comorbidity between ADHD and major depression in adolescent and young adult females. *J Am Acad Child Adolesc Psychiatry.* 2008;47(4):426–434

33. Biederman J, Melmed RD, Patel A, McBurnett K, Donahue J, Lyne A. Long-term, open-label extension study of guanfacine extended release in children and adolescents with ADHD. *CNS Spectr.* 2008;13(12):1047–1055

34. Crabtree VM, Ivanenko A, Gozal D. Clinical and parental assessment of sleep in children with attention-deficit/hyperactivity disorder referred to a pediatric sleep medicine center. *Clin Pediatr (Phila).* 2003;42(9):807–813

35. LeBourgeois MK, Avis K, Mixon M, Olmi J, Harsh J. Snoring, sleep quality, and sleepiness across attention-deficit/hyperactivity disorder subtypes. *Sleep.* 2004;27(3):520–525

36. Chan E, Zhan C, Homer CJ. Health care use and costs for children with attention-deficit/hyperactivity disorder: national estimates from the medical expenditure panel survey. *Arch Pediatr Adolesc Med.* 2002;156(5):504–511

37. Newcorn JH, Miller SR, Ivanova I, et al. Adolescent outcome of ADHD: impact of childhood conduct and anxiety disorders. *CNS Spectr.* 2004;9(9):668–678

38. Sung V, Hiscock H, Sciberras E, Efron D. Sleep problems in children with attention-deficit/hyperactivity disorder: prevalence and the effect on the child and family. *Arch Pediatr Adolesc Med.* 2008;162(4):336–342

39. American Academy of Pediatrics, Task Force on Mental Health. *Addressing Mental Health Concerns in Primary Care: A Clinician's Toolkit* [CD-ROM]. Elk Grove Village, IL: American Academy of Pediatrics; 2010

40. American Academy of Pediatrics, Committee on Child Health Financing. Scope of health care benefits for children from birth through age 26. *Pediatrics.* 2012; In press

41. Brito A, Grant R, Overholt S, et al. The enhanced medical home: the pediatric standard of care for medically underserved children. *Adv Pediatr.* 2008;55:9–28

42. Homer C, Klatka K, Romm D, et al. A review of the evidence for the medical home for children with special health care needs. *Pediatrics.* 2008;122(4). Available at: www.pediatrics.org/cgi/content/full/122/4/e922

43. Ingram S, Hechtman L, Morgenstern G. Outcome issues in ADHD: adolescent and adult long-term outcome. *Ment Retard Dev Disabil Res Rev.* 1999;5(3):243–250

44. Barbaresi WJ, Katusic SK, Colligan RC, Weaver AL, Jacobsen SJ. Modifiers of long-term school outcomes for children with attention-deficit/hyperactivity disorder: does treatment with stimulant medication make a difference? Results from a population-based study. *J Dev Behav Pediatr.* 2007;28(4):274–287

45. Cheng JY, Cheng RY, Ko JS, Ng EM. Efficacy and safety of atomoxetine for attention-deficit/hyperactivity disorder in children and adolescents-meta-analysis and meta-regression analysis. *Psychopharmacology.* 2007;194(2):197–209

46. Michelson D, Allen AJ, Busner J, Casat C, Dunn D, Kratochvil CJ. Once daily atomoxetine treatment for children and adolescents with ADHD: a randomized, placebo-controlled study. *Am J Psychiatry.* 2002; 159(11):1896–1901

47. Biederman J, Melmed RD, Patel A, et al; SPD503 Study Group. A randomized, double-blind, placebo-controlled study of guanfacine extended release in children and adolescents with attention-deficit/hyperactivity disorder. *Pediatrics.* 2008;121(1). Available at: www.pediatrics.org/cgi/content/full/121/1/e73

48. Sallee FR, Lyne A, Wigal T, McGough JJ. Long-term safety and efficacy of guanfacine extended release in children and adolescents with attention-deficit/hyperactivity disorder. *J Child Adolesc Psychopharmacol.* 2009;19(3):215–226

49. Jain R, Segal S, Kollins SH, Khayrallah M. Clonidine extended-release tablets for pediatric patients with attention-deficit/hyperactivity disorder. *J Am Acad Child Adolesc Psychiatry.* 2011;50(2):171–179

50. Newcorn J, Kratochvil CJ, Allen AJ, et al. Atomoxetine and osmotically released methylphenidate for the treatment of attention deficit hyperactivity disorder: acute comparison and differential response. *Am J Psychiatry.* 2008;165(6):721–730

51. Swanson J, Elliott GR, Greenhill LL, et al. Effects of stimulant medication on growth rates across 3 years in the MTA follow-up. *J Am Acad Child Adolesc Psychiatry.* 2007; 46(8):1015–1027

52. Mosholder AD, Gelperin K, Hammad TA, Phelan K, Johann-Liang R. Hallucinations and other psychotic symptoms associated with the use of attention-deficit/hyperactivity disorder drugs in children. *Pediatrics.* 2009;123(2):611–616

53. Avigan M. *Review of AERS Data From Marketed Safety Experience During Stimulant Therapy: Death, Sudden Death, Cardiovascular SAEs (Including Stroke)*. Silver Spring, MD: Food and Drug Administration, Center for Drug Evaluation and Research; 2004. Report No. D030403

54. Perrin JM, Friedman RA, Knilans TK, et al; American Academy of Pediatrics, Black Box Working Group, Section on Cardiology and Cardiac Surgery. Cardiovascular monitoring and stimulant drugs for attention-deficit/hyperactivity disorder. *Pediatrics.* 2008;122(2):451–453

55. McCarthy S, Cranswick N, Potts L, Taylor E, Wong IC. Mortality associated with attention-deficit hyperactivity disorder (ADHD) drug treatment: a retrospective cohort study of children, adolescents and young adults using the general practice research database. *Drug Saf.* 2009;32(11):1089–1110

56. Gould MS, Walsh BT, Munfakh JL, et al. Sudden death and use of stimulant medications in youths. *Am J Psychiatry.* 2009;166(9):992–1001

57. Greenhill L, Kollins S, Abikoff H, McCracken J, Riddle M, Swanson J. Efficacy and safety of immediate-release methylphenidate treatment for preschoolers with ADHD. *J Am Acad Child Adolesc Psychiatry.* 2006;45(11):1284–1293

58. Low K, Gendaszek AE. Illicit use of psychostimulants among college students: a preliminary study. *Psychol Health Med.* 2002;7(3):283–287

59. Cox D, Merkel RL, Moore M, Thorndike F, Muller C, Kovatchev B. Relative benefits of stimulant therapy with OROS methylphenidate versus mixed amphetamine salts extended release in improving the driving performance of adolescent drivers with attention-deficit/hyperactivity disorder. *Pediatrics.* 2006;118(3). Available at: www.pediatrics.org/cgi/content/full/118/3/e704

60. Pelham W, Wheeler T, Chronis A. Empirically supported psychological treatments for attention deficit hyperactivity disorder. *J Clin Child Psychol.* 1998;27(2):190–205

61. Sonuga-Barke E, Daley D, Thompson M, Laver-Bradbury C, Weeks A. Parent-based therapies for preschool attention-deficit/hyperactivity disorder: a randomized, controlled trial with a community sample. *J Am Acad Child Adolesc Psychiatry.* 2001;40(4):402–408

62. Pelham W, Fabiano GA. Evidence-based psychosocial treatments for attention-deficit/hyperactivity disorder. *J Clin Child Adolesc Psychol.* 2008;37(1):184–214

63. Van Cleave J, Leslie LK. Approaching ADHD as a chronic condition: implications for long-term adherence. *J Psychosoc Nurs Ment Health Serv.* 2008;46(8):28–36

64. A 14-month randomized clinical trial of treatment strategies for attention-deficit/hyperactivity disorder. The MTA Cooperative Group. Multimodal Treatment Study of Children With ADHD. *Arch Gen Psychiatry.* 1999;56(12):1073–1086

65. Jensen P, Hinshaw SP, Swanson JM, et al. Findings from the NIMH multimodal treatment study of ADHD (MTA): implications and applications for primary care providers. *J Dev Behav Pediatr.* 2001;22(1):60–73

66. Pelham WE, Gnagy EM. Psychosocial and combined treatments for ADHD. *Ment Retard Dev Disabil Res Rev.* 1999;5(3):225–236

67. Davila RR, Williams ML, MacDonald JT. Memorandum on clarification of policy to address the needs of children with attention deficit disorders within general and/or special education. In: Parker HC *The ADD Hyperactivity Handbook for Schools*. Plantation, FL: Impact Publications Inc; 1991:261–268

68. The College Board. Services for Students With Disabilities (SSD). Available at: www.collegeboard.com/ssd/student. Accessed July 8, 2011

69. Bodenheimer T, Wagner EH, Grumbach K. Improving primary care for patients with chronic illness. *JAMA* 2002;288:1775–1779

70. Bodenheimer T, Wagner EH, Grumbach K. Improving primary care for patients with chronic illness: the chronic care model, Part 2. *JAMA* 2002;288:1909–1914

Attention-Deficit/Hyperactivity Disorder Clinical Practice Guideline Quick Reference Tools

- Action Statement Summary
  — ADHD: Clinical Practice Guideline for the Diagnosis, Evaluation, and Treatment of Attention-Deficit/Hyperactivity Disorder in Children and Adolescents
- *ICD-9-CM/ICD-10-CM* Coding Quick Reference for ADHD
- Bonus Features
  — ADHD Coding Fact Sheet for Primary Care Physicians
  — Continuum Model for ADHD
- AAP Patient Education Handouts
  — *Understanding ADHD: Information for Parents About Attention-Deficit/Hyperactivity Disorder*
  — *Medicines for ADHD: Questions From Teens Who Have ADHD*
  — *What Is ADHD? Questions From Teens*

Action Statement Summary

ADHD: Clinical Practice Guideline for the Diagnosis, Evaluation, and Treatment of Attention-Deficit/Hyperactivity Disorder in Children and Adolescents

Action statement 1

The primary care clinician should initiate an evaluation for ADHD for any child 4 through 18 years of age who presents with academic or behavioral problems and symptoms of inattention, hyperactivity, or impulsivity (quality of evidence B/strong recommendation).

Action statement 2

To make a diagnosis of ADHD, the primary care clinician should determine that *Diagnostic and Statistical Manual of Mental Disorders, Fourth Edition* (DSM-IV-TR) criteria have been met (including documentation of impairment in more than 1 major setting), and information should be obtained primarily from reports from parents or guardians, teachers, and other school and mental health clinicians involved in the child's care. The primary care clinician should also rule out any alternative cause (quality of evidence B/strong recommendation).

Action statement 3

In the evaluation of a child for ADHD, the primary care clinician should include assessment for other conditions that might coexist with ADHD, including emotional or behavioral (eg, anxiety, depressive, oppositional defiant, and conduct disorders), developmental (eg, learning and language disorders or other neurodevelopmental disorders), and physical (eg, tics, sleep apnea) conditions (quality of evidence B/strong recommendation).

Action statement 4

The primary care clinician should recognize ADHD as a chronic condition and, therefore, consider children and adolescents with ADHD as children and youth with special health care needs. Management of children and youth with special health care needs should follow the principles of the chronic care model and the medical home (quality of evidence B/strong recommendation).

Action statement 5

Recommendations for treatment of children and youth with ADHD vary depending on the patient's age.

Action statement 5a

For *preschool-aged children (4–5 years of age)*, the primary care clinician should prescribe evidence-based parent and/or teacher-administered behavior therapy as the first line of treatment (quality of evidence A/strong recommendation) and may prescribe methylphenidate if the behavior interventions do not provide significant improvement and there is moderate-to-severe continuing disturbance in the child's function. In areas in which evidence-based behavioral treatments are not available, the clinician needs to weigh the risks of starting medication at an early age against the harm of delaying diagnosis and treatment (quality of evidence B/recommendation).

Action statement 5b

For *elementary school-aged children (6–11 years of age)*, the primary care clinician should prescribe FDA-approved medications for ADHD (quality of evidence A/strong recommendation) and/or evidence based parent- and/or teacher-administered behavior therapy as treatment for ADHD, preferably both (quality of evidence B/strong recommendation). The evidence is particularly strong for stimulant medications and sufficient but less strong for atomoxetine, extended-release guanfacine, and extended-release clonidine (in that order) (quality of evidence A/strong recommendation). The school environment, program, or placement is a part of any treatment plan.

Action statement 5c

For *adolescents (12–18 years of age)*, the primary care clinician should prescribe FDA-approved medications for ADHD with the assent of the adolescent (quality of evidence A/strong recommendation) and may prescribe behavior therapy as treatment for ADHD (quality of evidence C/recommendation), preferably both.

Action statement 6

Primary care clinicians should titrate doses of medication for ADHD to achieve maximum benefit with minimum adverse effects (quality of evidence B/strong recommendation).

Coding Quick Reference for ADHD	
ICD-9-CM	*ICD-10-CM*
314.00 Attention deficit disorder without hyperactivity	**F90.0** Attention-deficit hyperactivity disorder, predominantly inattentive type
314.01 Attention deficit disorder with hyperactivity	**F90.1** Attention-deficit hyperactivity disorder, predominantly hyperactive type

ADHD Coding Fact Sheet for Primary Care Physicians

Current Procedural Terminology (CPT®) (Procedure) Codes

Initial assessment usually involves a lot of time determining the differential diagnosis, a diagnostic plan, and potential treatment options. Therefore, most pediatricians will report either an office or outpatient evaluation and management (E/M) code using time as the key factor or a consultation code for the initial assessment.

Physician Evaluation and Management Services

99201	Office or other outpatient visit, *new*[a] patient; self limited or minor problem, 10 min.
99202	low to moderate severity problem, 20 min.
99203	moderate severity problem, 30 min.
99204	moderate to high severity problem, 45 min.
99205	high severity problem, 60 min.
99211	Office or other outpatient visit, *established* patient; minimal problem, 5 min.
99212	self limited or minor problem, 10 min.
99213	low to moderate severity problem, 15 min.
99214	moderate severity problem, 25 min.
99215	moderate to high severity problem, 40 min.
99241	Office or other outpatient *consultation*,[b–d] new or established patient; self-limited or minor problem, 15 min.
99242	low severity problem, 30 min.
99243	moderate severity problem, 45 min.
99244	moderate to high severity problem, 60 min.
99245	moderate to high severity problem, 80 min.
+99354	Prolonged physician services in office or other outpatient setting, with direct patient contact; first hour (*use in conjunction with time-based codes* **99201–99215, 99241–99245, 99301–99350, 90837**)
+99355	each additional 30 min. (*use in conjunction with* **99354**)

- Used when a physician provides prolonged services beyond the usual service (ie, beyond the typical time).
- Time spent does not have to be continuous.
- Prolonged service of less than 15 minutes beyond the first hour or less than 15 minutes beyond the final 30 minutes is not reported separately.
- If reporting E/M service based on time and not key factors (history, examination, medical decision-making), the physician must reach the typical time in the highest code in the code set being reported (eg, **99205, 99215, 99245**) before face-to-face prolonged services can be reported.

---

[a] A new patient is one who has not received any professional services (face-to-face services) rendered by physicians and other qualified health care professionals who may report E/M services using one or more specific CPT codes from the physician/qualified health care professional or another physician/qualified health care professional of the exact same specialty and subspecialty who belongs to the same group practice, within the past 3 years (*CPT 2014 Professional Edition*, American Medical Association, p 4).

[b] Use of these codes (**99241–99245**) requires the following actions:
1. Written or verbal request for consultation is documented in the patient chart.
2. Consultant's opinion as well as any services ordered or performed are documented in the patient chart.
3. Consultant's opinion and any services that are performed are prepared in a written report, which is sent to the requesting physician or other appropriate source.

[c] Patients/parents may not initiate a consultation.

[d] For more information on consultation code changes for 2010, see www.aap.org/moc/loadsecure.cfm/reimburse/PositiononMedicareConsultationPolicy.doc.

+ Codes are *add-on codes*, meaning they are reported separately in addition to the appropriate code for the service provided.

Reporting E/M Services Using "Time"

- When counseling or coordination of care dominates (more than 50%) the physician/patient or family encounter (face-to-face time in the office or other outpatient setting or floor/unit time in the hospital or nursing facility), time shall be considered the key or controlling factor to qualify for a particular level of E/M services (*CPT 2014 Professional Edition*, p 10).
- This includes time spent with parties who have assumed responsibility for the care of the patient or decision-making, whether or not they are family members (eg, foster parents, person acting in loco parentis, legal guardian). The extent of counseling or coordination of care must be documented in the medical record (*CPT 2014 Professional Edition*, p 10).
- For coding purposes, face-to-face time for these services is defined as only that time that the physician spends face-to-face with the patient or family. This includes the time in which the physician performs such tasks as obtaining a history, performing an examination, and counseling the patient (*CPT 2014 Professional Edition*, p 8).
- When codes are ranked in sequential typical times (eg, office-based E/M services, consultation codes) and the actual time is between 2 typical times, the code with the typical time closest to the actual time is used (*CPT 2014 Professional Edition*, p xv).
  - **Example:** A physician sees an established patient in the office to discuss the current attention-deficit/hyperactivity disorder (ADHD) medication the patient was placed on. The total face-to-face time was 22 minutes, of which 15 minutes was spent in counseling the mom and patient. Because more than 50% of the total time was spent in counseling, the physician would report the E/M service based on time. The physician would report **99214** instead of **99213** because the total face-to-face time was closer to **99214** (25 minutes) than **99213** (15 minutes).

ADHD Follow-up During a Routine Preventive Medicine Service

- A good time to follow up with a patient regarding his or her ADHD could be during a preventive medicine service.
- If the follow-up requires little additional work on behalf of the physician, it should be reported under the preventive medicine service rather than as a separate service.
- If the follow-up work requires an additional E/M service in addition to the preventive medicine service, it should be reported as a separate service.
- Chronic conditions should only be reported if they are separately addressed.
- When reporting a preventive medicine service in addition to an office-based E/M service and the services are significant and separately identifiable, modifier **25** will be required on the office-based E/M service.
  - **Example:** A 12-year-old established patient presents for his routine preventive medicine service and while he and Mom are there, Mom asks about changing his ADHD medication because of some side effects he is experiencing. The physician completes the routine preventive medicine check and then addresses the mom's concerns in a separate service. The additional E/M service takes 15 minutes, of which the physician spends about 10 minutes in counseling and coordinating care; therefore, the E/M service is reported based on time.
    - ~ Code **99394** and **99213-25** account for both E/M services and link each to the appropriate *ICD-9-CM* code.
    - ~ Modifier **25** is required on the problem-oriented office visit code (eg, **99213**) when it is significant and separately identifiable from another service.

Physician Non–Face-to-Face Services

99339 Care Plan Oversight—Individual physician supervision of a patient (patient not present) in home, domiciliary or rest home (e.g., assisted living facility) requiring complex and multidisciplinary care modalities involving regular physician development and/or revision of care plans, review of subsequent reports of patient status, review of related laboratory and other studies, communication (including telephone calls) for purposes of assessment or care decisions with health care professional(s), family member(s), surrogate decision maker(s) (e.g., legal guardian) and/or key caregiver(s) involved in patient's care, integration of new information into the medical treatment plan and/or adjustment of medical therapy, within a calendar month; 15–29 minutes

99340 30 minutes or more

99358[a] Prolonged physician services without direct patient contact; first hour

+99359 each additional 30 min. (+ *designated add-on code, use in conjunction* with **99358**)

99367 Medical team conference by physician with interdisciplinary team of health care professionals, patient and/or family not present, 30 minutes or more

99441 Telephone evaluation and management to patient, parent or guardian not originating from a related E/M service within the previous 7 days nor leading to an E/M service or procedure within the next 24 hours or soonest available appointment; 5–10 minutes of medical discussion

99442 11–20 minutes of medical discussion

99443 21–30 minutes of medical discussion

99444 Online E/M service provided by a physician or other qualified health care professional to an established patient, guardian or health care provider not originating from a related E/M service provided within the previous 7 days, using the internet or similar electronic communications network

---

[a] This code **(99358)** is no longer an add-on service and can be reported alone.

Psychiatry

+90785 Interactive complexity (Use in conjunction with codes for diagnostic psychiatric evaluation **[90791, 90792]**, psychotherapy **[90832, 90834, 90837]**, psychotherapy when performed with an evaluation and management service **[90833, 90836, 90838, 99201–99255, 99304–99337, 99341–99350]**, and group psychotherapy **[90853]**)

Psychiatric Diagnostic or Evaluative Interview Procedures

90791 Psychiatric diagnostic interview examination evaluation

90792 Psychiatric diagnostic evaluation with medical services

Psychotherapy

90832 Psychotherapy, 30 min with patient and/or family;

+90833 with medical E/M (Use in conjunction with **99201–99255, 99304–99337, 99341–99350**)

90834 Psychotherapy, 45 min with patient and/or family;

+90836 with medical E/M services (Use in conjunction with **99201–99255, 99304–99337, 99341–99350**)

90837 Psychotherapy, 60 min with patient and/or family;

+90838 with medical E/M services (Use in conjunction with **99201–99255, 99304–99337, 99341–99350**)

+90785 Interactive complexity (Use in conjunction with codes for diagnostic psychiatric evaluation **[90791, 90792]**, psychotherapy **[90832, 90834, 90837]**, psychotherapy when performed with an evaluation and management service **[90833, 90836, 90838, 99201–99255, 99304–99337, 99341–99350]**, and group psychotherapy **[90853]**)
  - Refers to specific communication factors that complicate the delivery of a psychiatric procedure. Common factors include more difficult communication with discordant or emotional family members and engagement of young and verbally undeveloped or impaired patients. Typical encounters include
    — Patients who have other individuals legally responsible for their care
    — Patients who request others to be present or involved in their care such as translators, interpreters, or additional family members
    — Patients who require the involvement of other third parties such as child welfare agencies, schools, or probation officers

90846 Family psychotherapy (without patient present)

90847 Family psychotherapy (conjoint psychotherapy) (with patient present)

Other Psychiatric Services/Procedures

90863 Pharmacologic management, including prescription and review of medication, when performed with psychotherapy services (Use in conjunction with **90832, 90834, 90837**)
  - For pharmacologic management with psychotherapy services performed by a physician or other qualified health care professional who may report E/M codes, use the appropriate E/M codes **99201–99255, 99281–99285, 99304–99337, 99341–99350** and the appropriate psychotherapy with E/M service **90833, 90836,90838**).
  - Note code **90862** was deleted.

90887 Interpretation or explanation of results of psychiatric, other medical exams, or other accumulated data to family or other responsible persons, or advising them how to assist patient

90889 Preparation of reports on patient's psychiatric status, history, treatment, or progress (other than for legal or consultative purposes) for other physicians, agencies, or insurance carriers

Psychological Testing

96101 Psychological testing (includes psychodiagnostic assessment of emotionality, intellectual abilities, personality and psychopathology, e.g., MMPI, Rorschach, WAIS), per hour of the *psychologist's or physician's time*, both face-to-face time administering tests to the patient and time interpreting these test results and preparing the report

96102 Psychological testing (includes psychodiagnostic assessment of emotionality, intellectual abilities,

---

+ Codes are *add-on codes,* meaning they are reported separately in addition to the appropriate code for the service provided.

Current Procedural Terminology® 2013 American Medical Association. All Rights Reserved.

personality and psychopathology, e.g., MMPI, Ror-schach, WAIS), with *qualified health care professional* interpretation and report, administered by technician, per hour of technician time, face-to-face

96103 Psychological testing (includes psychodiagnostic assessment of emotionality, intellectual abilities, personality and psychopathology, e.g., MMPI, Ror-schach, WAIS), administered by a computer, with *qualified health care professional* interpretation and re-port

96110 Developmental screening, per standardized screen, with interpretation and report

96111 Developmental testing (includes assessment of motor, language, social, adaptive and/or cognitive function-ing by standardized instruments) with interpretation and report

96116 Neurobehavioral status exam (clinical assessment of thinking, reasoning and judgment, eg, acquired knowledge, attention, language, memory, planning and problem solving, and visual spatial abilities), per hour of the psychologist's or physician's time, both face-to-face time with the patient and time interpret-ing test results and preparing the report

Nonphysician Provider (NPP) Services

99366 Medical team conference with interdisciplinary team of health care professionals, face-to-face with patient and/or family, 30 minutes or more, participation by a nonphysician qualified health care professional

99368 Medical team conference with interdisciplinary team of health care professionals, patient and/or family not present, 30 minutes or more, participation by a nonphysician qualified health care professional

96120 Neuropsychological testing (eg, Wisconsin Card Sort-ing Test), administered by a computer, with qualified health care professional interpretation and report

96150 Health and behavior assessment performed by nonphysician provider (health-focused clinical inter-views, behavior observations) to identify psychologi-cal, behavioral, emotional, cognitive or social factors important to management of physical health prob-lems, 15 min., initial assessment

96151 re-assessment

96152 Health and behavior intervention performed by non-physician provider to improve patient's health and well-being using cognitive, behavioral, social, and/or psychophysiological procedures designed to amelio-rate specific disease-related problems, individual, 15 min.

96153 group (2 or more patients)

96154 family (with the patient present)

96155 family (without the patient present)

Non–Face-to-Face Services: NPP

98966 Telephone assessment and management service provided by a qualified nonphysician health care pro-fessional to an established patient, parent or guardian not originating from a related assessment and man-agement service provided within the previous seven days nor leading to an assessment and management service or procedure within the next 24 hours or soonest available appointment;

5–10 minutes of medical discussion

98967 11–20 minutes of medical discussion

98968 21–30 minutes of medical discussion

98969 Online assessment and management service provided by a qualified nonphysician health care professional to an established patient or guardian not originating from a related assessment and management service provided within the previous seven days nor using the internet or similar electronic communications net-work

Miscellaneous Services

99071 Educational supplies, such as books, tapes, or pam-phlets, provided by the physician for the patient's education at cost to the physician

International Classification of Diseases, Ninth Revision, Clinical Modification (ICD-9-CM)/ Diagnostic and Statistical Manual for Primary Care (DSM-PC) (Diagnosis) Codes

- Use as many diagnosis codes that apply to document the patient's complexity and report the patient's symptoms or adverse environmental circumstances.
- Once a definitive diagnosis is established, report the appro-priate definitive diagnosis code(s) as the primary code, plus any other symptoms that the patient is exhibiting as second-ary diagnoses.
- Counseling diagnosis codes can be used when the patient is present or when counseling the parent(s) or guardian(s) when the patient is not physically present.

285.9	Anemia, unspecified
292.84	Drug-induced mood disorder (Add E-code to identify the drug)
293.84	Anxiety disorder in conditions classified elsewhere
296.81	Atypical manic disorder
296.90	Unspecified episodic mood disorder
299.00	Autistic disorder, current or active state
299.01	Autistic disorder, residual state
300.00	Anxiety state, unspecified
300.01	Panic disorder
300.02	Generalized anxiety disorder
300.20	Phobia, unspecified
300.23	Social phobia
300.29	Other isolated or specific phobia
300.4	Dysthymic disorder
300.9	Unspecified nonpsychotic mental disorder
304.3	Cannabis dependence
304.4	Amphetamine and other psychostimulant depen-dence
304.9	Unspecified drug dependence

Substance Dependence/Abuse

For the following codes (305.0X–305.9X), fifth-digit subclassifica-tion is as follows:

0 unspecified
1 continuous
2 episodic
3 in remission

+ Codes are *add-on codes*, meaning they are reported separately in addition to the appropriate code for the service provided.

Current Procedural Terminology® 2013 American Medical Association. All Rights Reserved.

Nondependent Abuse of Drugs

305.0X	Alcohol abuse
305.1X	Tobacco use disorder
305.2X	Cannabis abuse
305.3X	Hallucinogenic abuse
305.4X	Sedative, hypnotic or anxiolytic abuse
305.5X	Opioid abuse
305.6X	Cocaine abuse
305.7X	Amphetamine or related acting sympathomimetic abuse
305.8X	Antidepressant type abuse
305.9X	Other mixed, or unspecified drug abuse (eg, caffeine intoxication, laxative habit)
307.0	Stuttering
307.20	Tic disorder, unspecified
307.21	Transient tic disorder
307.22	Chronic motor or vocal tic disorder
307.23	Tourette's disorder
307.40	Nonorganic sleep disorder, unspecified
307.41	Transient disorder of initiating or maintaining sleep
307.42	Persistent disorder of initiating or maintaining sleep
307.46	Sleep arousal disorder
307.49	Other sleep disorder
307.50	Eating disorder, unspecified
307.52	Pica
307.6	Enuresis
307.9	Other and unspecified special symptoms or syndromes, not elsewhere classified (NEC)
308.0	Predominant disturbance of emotions
309.0	Adjustment disorder with depressed mood
309.21	Separation anxiety disorder
309.24	Adjustment disorder with anxiety
309.3	Adjustment reaction; with disturbance of conduct
309.9	Unspecified adjustment reaction
310.2	Postconcussion syndrome
310.8	Other specified nonpsychotic mental disorders following organic brain damage
310.9	Unspecified nonpsychotic mental disorders following organic brain damage
312.00	Undersocialized conduct disorder, aggressive type; unspecified
312.30	Impulse control disorder, unspecified
312.81	Conduct disorder, childhood onset type
312.82	Conduct disorder, adolescent onset type
312.9	Unspecified disturbance of conduct
313.3	Relationship problems
313.81	Oppositional defiant disorder
313.83	Academic underachievement disorder
313.9	Unspecified emotional disturbance of childhood or adolescence
314.00	Attention-deficit disorder, without mention of hyperactivity
314.01	Attention-deficit disorder, with mention of hyperactivity
314.1	Hyperkinesis with developmental delay (Use additional code to identify any associated neurological disorder)
314.2	Hyperkinetic conduct disorder
314.8	Other specified manifestations of hyperkinetic syndrome
314.9	Unspecified hyperkinetic syndrome
315.00	Reading disorder, unspecified

315.01	Alexia
315.02	Developmental dyslexia
315.09	Specific reading disorder; other
315.1	Mathematics disorder
315.2	Specific learning difficulties; other
315.31	Expressive language disorder
315.32	Mixed receptive-expressive language disorder
315.34	Speech and language developmental delay due to hearing loss
315.39	Developmental speech or language disorder; other
315.4	Developmental coordination disorder
315.5	Mixed development disorder
315.8	Specified delays in development; other
315.9	Unspecified delay in development
317	Mild mental retardation
318.0	Moderate mental retardation
318.1	Severe mental retardation
318.2	Profound mental retardation
319	Unspecified mental retardation
389.03	Conductive hearing loss, middle ear
527.7	Disturbance of salivary secretion (eg, dry mouth/xerostomia)
564.00	Constipation, unspecified
780.4	Dizziness
780.50	Sleep disturbances, unspecified
781.0	Abnormal involuntary movement (eg, tremor)
781.3	Lack of coordination
782.1	Rash and other nonspecific skin eruptions
783.1	Abnormal weight gain
783.21	Loss of weight
783.3	Feeding difficulties and mismanagement
783.42	Delayed milestones
783.43	Short stature
784.0	Headache
787.01	Nausea with vomiting
787.03	Vomiting
787.91	Diarrhea
788.36	Nocturnal enuresis
789.00	Abdominal pain, unspecified
984.9	Toxic effect of lead, unspecified lead compound (Use E code in addition)

The following diagnosis codes (V11.1–V79.9) are used to deal with occasions when circumstances other than a disease or an injury are recorded as diagnoses or problems. Some carriers may request supporting documentation for the reporting of V codes. These codes may also be reported in addition to the primary ICD-9-CM code to list any contributing factors or those factors that influence the person's health status but are not in themselves a current illness or injury.

V11.1	Personal history of affective disorders
V11.8	Personal history of other mental disorders
V11.9	Personal history of unspecified mental disorders
V12.1	Personal history of a nutritional deficiency
V12.2	Personal history of endocrine, metabolic, and nutritional disorders
V12.3	Personal history of diseases of blood and blood-forming organs
V12.40	Unspecified disorder of the neurological system and sense organs
V12.49	Other disorders of the nervous system and sense organs
V12.69	Other disorders of the respiratory system

+ Codes are *add-on codes*, meaning they are reported separately in addition to the appropriate code for the service provided.

V12.79	Other diseases of the digestive system
V13.6	Congenital malformations
V14.9	Personal history of allergy to unspecified medicinal agent
V15.0	Allergy, other than to medicinal agents
V15.41	History of physical abuse
V15.42	History of emotional abuse
V15.49	Other psychological trauma
V15.52	History of traumatic brain injury
V15.81	Noncompliance with medical treatment
V15.82	History of tobacco use
V15.86	Contact with and (suspected) exposure to lead
V17.0	Family history of psychiatric disorder
V18.2	Family history of anemia
V18.4	Family history of mental retardation
V40.0	Problems with learning
V40.1	Problems with communication (including speech)
V40.2	Mental problems; other
V40.3	Behavioral problems; other
V40.9	Mental or behavioral problems; unspecified
V58.69	Long-term (current) use of other medications
V60.0	Lack of housing
V60.1	Inadequate housing
V60.2	Inadequate material resources (eg, economic problem, poverty, NOS)
V60.81	Foster care
V61.20	Counseling for parent-child problem; unspecified
V61.23	Counseling for parent-biological child problem
V61.24	Counseling for parent-adopted child problem
V61.25	Counseling for parent (guardian)-foster child problem
V61.29	Counseling for parent-child problem; other
V61.41	Health problems within family; alcoholism
V61.42	Health problems within family; substance abuse
V61.49	Health problems within family; other
V61.8	Health problems within family; other specified family circumstances
V61.9	Health problems within family; unspecified family circumstances
V62.3	Educational circumstances
V62.4	Social maladjustment
V62.5	Legal circumstances
V62.81	Interpersonal problems, NEC
V62.89	Other psychological or physical stress; NEC, other
V62.9	Other psychosocial circumstance
V65.40	Counseling NOS
V65.49	Other specified counseling
V79.0	Special screening for depression
V79.2	Special screening for mental retardation
V79.3	Special screening for developmental handicaps in early childhood
V79.8	Special screening for other specified mental disorders and developmental handicaps
V79.9	Unspecified mental disorder and developmental handicapped

International Classification of Diseases, 10th Revision, Clinical Modification (ICD-10-CM) Codes

- Use as many diagnosis codes that apply to document the patient's complexity and report the patient's symptoms and/or adverse environmental circumstances.

- Once a definitive diagnosis is established, report the appropriate definitive diagnosis code(s) as the primary code, plus any other symptoms that the patient is exhibiting as secondary diagnoses that are not part of the usual disease course or are considered incidental.

- *ICD-10-CM codes are only valid on or after October 1, 2014.*

Depressive Disorders

F34.1	Dysthymic disorder (depressive personality disorder, dysthymia neurotic depression)
F39	Mood (affective) disorder, unspecified
F30.8	Other manic episode

Anxiety Disorders

F06.4	Anxiety disorder due to known physiological conditions
F40.10	Social phobia, unspecified
F40.11	Social phobia, generalized
F40.8	Phobic anxiety disorders, other (phobic anxiety disorder of childhood)
F40.9	Phobic anxiety disorder, unspecified
F41.1	Generalized anxiety disorder
F41.9	Anxiety disorder, unspecified

Feeding and Eating Disorders/Elimination Disorders

F50.8	Eating disorders, other
F50.9	Eating disorder, unspecified
F98.0	Enuresis not due to a substance or known physiological condition
F98.1	Encopresis not due to a substance or known physiological condition
F98.3	Pica (infancy or childhood)

Impulse Disorders

F63.9	Impulse disorder, unspecified

Trauma- and Stressor-Related Disorders

F43.20	Adjustment disorder, unspecified
F43.21	Adjustment disorder with depressed mood
F43.22	Adjustment disorder with anxiety
F43.23	Adjustment disorder with mixed anxiety and depressed mood
F43.24	Adjustment disorder with disturbance of conduct

Neurodevelopmental/Other Developmental Disorders

F70	Mild intellectual disabilities
F71	Moderate intellectual disabilities
F72	Severe intellectual disabilities
F73	Profound intellectual disabilities
F79	Unspecified intellectual disabilities
F80.0	Phonological (speech) disorder
F80.1	Expressive language disorder
F80.2	Mixed receptive-expressive language disorder
F80.4	Speech and language developmental delay due to hearing loss (code also hearing loss)
F80.81	Stuttering
F80.89	Other developmental disorders of speech and language
F80.9	Developmental disorder of speech and language, unspecified
F81.0	Specific reading disorder

F81.2	Mathematics disorder
F81.89	Other developmental disorders of scholastic skills
F82	Developmental coordination disorder
F88	Specified delays in development; other
F89	Unspecified delay in development
F81.9	Developmental disorder of scholastic skills, unspecified

Behavioral/Emotional Disorders

F90.0	Attention-deficit hyperactivity disorder, predominantly inattentive type
F90.1	Attention-deficit hyperactivity disorder, predominantly hyperactive type
F90.8	Attention-deficit hyperactivity disorder, other type
F90.9	Attention-deficit hyperactivity disorder, unspecified type
F91.1	Conduct disorder, childhood-onset type
F91.2	Conduct disorder, adolescent-onset type
F91.3	Oppositional defiant disorder
F91.9	Conduct disorder, unspecified
F93.0	Separation anxiety disorder
F93.8	Other childhood emotional disorders (relationship problems)
F93.9	Childhood emotional disorder, unspecified
F94.9	Childhood disorder of social functioning, unspecified
F95.0	Transient tic disorder
F95.1	Chronic motor or vocal tic disorder
F95.2	Tourette's disorder
F95.9	Tic disorder, unspecified
F98.8	Other specified behavioral and emotional disorders with onset usually occurring in childhood and adolescence (nail-biting, nose-picking, thumb-sucking)

Other

F07.81	Postconcussional syndrome
F07.89	Personality and behavioral disorders due to known physiological condition, other
F07.9	Personality and behavioral disorder due to known physiological condition, unspecified
F48.8	Nonpsychotic mental disorders, other (neurasthenia)
F48.9	Nonpsychotic mental disorders, unspecified
F45.41	Pain disorder exclusively related to psychological factors
F51.01	Primary insomnia
F51.02	Adjustment insomnia
F51.03	Paradoxical insomnia
F51.04	Psychophysiologic insomnia
F51.05	Insomnia due to other mental disorder (Code also associated mental disorder)
F51.09	Insomnia, other (not due to a substance or known physiological condition)
F51.3	Sleepwalking [somnambulism]
F51.4	Sleep terrors [night terrors]
F51.8	Other sleep disorders
F93.8	Childhood emotional disorders, other
R46.89	Other symptoms and signs involving appearance and behavior

Substance-Related and Addictive Disorders

If a provider documents multiple patterns of use, only one should be reported. Use the following hierarchy: use–abuse–dependence (eg, if use and dependence are documented, only code for dependence).

When a minus symbol (-) is included in codes **F10–F17,** a last digit is required. Be sure to include the last digit from the following list:

0 anxiety disorder
2 sleep disorder
8 other disorder
9 unspecified disorder

Alcohol

F10.10	Alcohol abuse, uncomplicated
F10.14	Alcohol abuse with alcohol-induced mood disorder
F10.159	Alcohol abuse with alcohol-induced psychotic disorder, unspecified
F10.18-	Alcohol abuse with alcohol-induced
F10.19	Alcohol abuse with unspecified alcohol-induced disorder
F10.20	Alcohol dependence, uncomplicated
F10.21	Alcohol dependence, in remission
F10.24	Alcohol dependence with alcohol-induced mood disorder
F10.259	Alcohol dependence with alcohol-induced psychotic disorder, unspecified
F10.28-	Alcohol dependence with alcohol-induced
F10.29	Alcohol dependence with unspecified alcohol-induced disorder
F10.94	Alcohol use, unspecified with alcohol-induced mood disorder
F10.959	Alcohol use, unspecified with alcohol-induced psychotic disorder, unspecified
F10.98-	Alcohol use, unspecified with alcohol-induced
F10.99	Alcohol use, unspecified with unspecified alcohol-induced disorder

Cannabis

F12.10	Cannabis abuse, uncomplicated
F12.18-	Cannabis abuse with cannabis-induced
F12.19	Cannabis abuse with unspecified cannabis-induced disorder
F12.20	Cannabis dependence, uncomplicated
F12.21	Cannabis dependence, in remission
F12.28-	Cannabis dependence with cannabis-induced
F12.29	Cannabis dependence with unspecified cannabis-induced disorder
F12.90	Cannabis use, unspecified, uncomplicated
F12.98-	Cannabis use, unspecified with
F12.99	Cannabis use, unspecified with unspecified cannabis-induced disorder

Sedatives

F13.10	Sedative, hypnotic or anxiolytic abuse, uncomplicated
F13.129	Sedative, hypnotic or anxiolytic abuse with intoxication, unspecified
F13.14	Sedative, hypnotic or anxiolytic abuse with sedative, hypnotic or anxiolytic-induced mood disorder

---

+ Codes are *add-on codes,* meaning they are reported separately in addition to the appropriate code for the service provided.

Current Procedural Terminology® 2013 American Medical Association. All Rights Reserved.

F13.18- Sedative, hypnotic or anxiolytic abuse with sedative, hypnotic or anxiolytic-induced

F13.21 Sedative, hypnotic or anxiolytic dependence, in remission

F13.90 Sedative, hypnotic, or anxiolytic use, unspecified, uncomplicated

F13.94 Sedative, hypnotic or anxiolytic use, unspecified with sedative, hypnotic or anxiolytic-induced mood disorder

F13.98- Sedative, hypnotic or anxiolytic use, unspecified with sedative, hypnotic or anxiolytic-induced

F13.99 Sedative, hypnotic or anxiolytic use, unspecified with unspecified sedative, hypnotic or anxiolytic-induced disorder

Stimulants (eg, Caffeine, Amphetamines)

F15.10 Other stimulant (amphetamine-related disorders or caffeine) abuse, uncomplicated

F15.14 Other stimulant (amphetamine-related disorders or caffeine) abuse with stimulant-induced mood disorder

F15.18- Other stimulant (amphetamine-related disorders or caffeine) abuse with stimulant-induced

F15.19 Other stimulant (amphetamine-related disorders or caffeine) abuse with unspecified stimulant-induced disorder

F15.20 Other stimulant (amphetamine-related disorders or caffeine) dependence, uncomplicated

F15.21 Other stimulant (amphetamine-related disorders or caffeine) dependence, in remission

F15.24 Other stimulant (amphetamine-related disorders or caffeine) dependence with stimulant-induced mood disorder

F15.28- Other stimulant (amphetamine-related disorders or caffeine) dependence with stimulant-induced

F15.29 Other stimulant (amphetamine-related disorders or caffeine) dependence with unspecified stimulant-induced disorder

F15.90 Other stimulant (amphetamine-related disorders or caffeine) use, unspecified, uncomplicated

F15.94 Other stimulant (amphetamine-related disorders or caffeine) use, unspecified with stimulant-induced mood disorder

F15.98- Other stimulant (amphetamine-related disorders or caffeine) use, unspecified with stimulant-induced

F15.99 Other stimulant (amphetamine-related disorders or caffeine) use, unspecified with unspecified stimulant-induced disorder

Nicotine (eg, Cigarettes)

F17.200 Nicotine dependence, unspecified, uncomplicated
F17.201 Nicotine dependence, unspecified, in remission
F17.203 Nicotine dependence unspecified, with withdrawal
F17.20- Nicotine dependence, unspecified, with
F17.210 Nicotine dependence, cigarettes, uncomplicated
F17.211 Nicotine dependence, cigarettes, in remission
F17.213 Nicotine dependence, cigarettes, with withdrawal
F17.218- Nicotine dependence, cigarettes, with

Symptoms, Signs, and Ill-Defined Conditions

- Use these codes in absence of a definitive mental diagnosis or when the sign or symptom is not part of the disease course or considered incidental.

G47.9 Sleep disorder, unspecified
H90.0 Conductive hearing loss, bilateral
H90.11 Conductive hearing loss, unilateral, right ear, with unrestricted hearing on the contralateral side
H90.12 Conductive hearing loss, unilateral, left ear, with unrestricted hearing on the contralateral side
K11.7 Disturbance of salivary secretions
K59.00 Constipation, unspecified
N39.44 Nocturnal enuresis
R10.0 Acute abdomen pain
R11.11 Vomiting without nausea
R11.2 Nausea with vomiting, unspecified
R19.7 Diarrhea, unspecified
R21 Rash, NOS
R25.0 Abnormal head movements
R25.1 Tremor, unspecified
R25.3 Twitching, NOS
R25.8 Other abnormal involuntary movements
R25.9 Unspecified abnormal involuntary movements
R27.8 Other lack of coordination (excludes ataxia)
R27.9 Unspecified lack of coordination
R41.83 Borderline intellectual functioning
R42 Dizziness
R48.0 Alexia/dyslexia, NOS
R51 Headache
R62.0 Delayed milestone in childhood
R62.52 Short stature (child)
R63.3 Feeding difficulties
R63.4 Abnormal weight loss
R63.5 Abnormal weight gain
R68.2 Dry mouth, unspecified
T56.0X1A Toxic effect of lead and its compounds, accidental (unintentional), initial encounter

Z Codes

Z codes represent reasons for encounters. Categories **Z00–Z99** are provided for occasions when circumstances other than a disease, injury, or external cause classifiable to categories **A00–Y89** are recorded as *diagnoses* or *problems*. This can arise in 2 main ways.

1. When a person who may or may not be sick encounters the health services for some specific purpose, such as to receive limited care or service for a current condition, to donate an organ or tissue, to receive prophylactic vaccination (immunization), or to discuss a problem that is in itself not a disease or an injury.

2. When some circumstance or problem is present which influences the person's health status but is not in itself a current illness or injury.

Z13.89 Encounter for screening for other disorder
Z55.0 Illiteracy and low-level literacy
Z55.2 Failed school examinations
Z55.3 Underachievement in school
Z55.4 Educational maladjustment and discord with teachers and classmates
Z55.8 Other problems related to education and literacy
Z55.9 Problems related to education and literacy, unspecified (**Z55** codes exclude those conditions reported with **F80–F89**)
Z62.0 Inadequate parental supervision and control
Z60.4 Social exclusion and rejection

+ Codes are *add-on* codes, meaning they are reported separately in addition to the appropriate code for the service provided.

Current Procedural Terminology® 2013 American Medical Association. All Rights Reserved.

Z60.8	Other problems related to social environment
Z60.9	Problem related to social environment, unspecified
Z62.21	Foster care status (child welfare)
Z62.6	Inappropriate (excessive) parental pressure
Z62.810	Personal history of physical and sexual abuse in childhood
Z62.811	Personal history of psychological abuse in childhood
Z62.820	Parent-biological child conflict
Z62.821	Parent-adopted child conflict
Z62.822	Parent-foster child conflict
Z63.72	Alcoholism and drug addiction in family
Z63.8	Other specified problems related to primary support group
Z65.3	Problems related to legal circumstances
Z71.89	Counseling, other specified
Z71.9	Counseling, unspecified
Z72.0	Tobacco use
Z77.011	Contact with and (suspected) exposure to lead
Z79.899	Other long term (current) drug therapy
Z81.0	Family history of intellectual disabilities (conditions classifiable to **F70–F79**)
Z81.8	Family history of other mental and behavioral disorders
Z83.2	Family history of diseases of the blood and blood-forming organs (anemia) (conditions classifiable to **D50–D89**)
Z86.2	Personal history of diseases of the blood and blood-forming organs
Z86.39	Personal history of other endocrine, nutritional, and metabolic disease
Z86.59	Personal history of other mental and behavioral disorders
Z86.69	Personal history of other diseases of the nervous system and sense organs
Z87.09	Personal history of other diseases of the respiratory system
Z87.19	Personal history of other diseases of the digestive system
Z87.798	Personal history of other (corrected) congenital malformations
Z87.820	Personal history of traumatic brain injury
Z88.9	Allergy status to unspecified drugs, medicaments, and biological substances status
Z91.09	Other allergy status, other than to drugs and biological substances
Z91.128	Patient's intentional underdosing of medication regimen for other reason (report drug code)
Z91.138	Patient's unintentional underdosing of medication regimen for other reason (report drug code)
Z91.14	Patient's other noncompliance with medication regimen
Z91.19	Patient's noncompliance with other medical treatment and regimen
Z91.411	Personal history of adult psychological abuse

+ Codes are *add-on codes,* meaning they are reported separately in addition to the appropriate code for the service provided.

Current Procedural Terminology® 2013 American Medical Association. All Rights Reserved.

Continuum Model for ADHD

The following continuum model from *Coding for Pediatrics 2014* has been devised to express the various levels of service for ADHD. This model demonstrates the cumulative effect of the key criteria for each level of service using a single diagnosis as the common denominator. It also shows the importance of other variables, such as patient age, duration and severity of illness, social contexts, and comorbid conditions that often have key roles in pediatric cases.

Quick Reference for Office or Other Outpatient Codes Used in Continuum for ADHD[a]				
E/M Code Level	**History**	**Examination**	**MDM**	**Time**
99211[b]	NA	NA	NA	5 minutes
99212	Problem-focused	Problem-focused	Straightforward	10 minutes
99213	Expanded problem-focused	Expanded problem-focused	Low	15 minutes
99214	Detailed	Detailed	Moderate	25 minutes
99215	Comprehensive	Comprehensive	High	40 minutes

Abbreviations: E/M, evaluation and management; MDM, medical decision-making; NA, not applicable.
[a] Use of a code level requires that you meet or exceed 2 of the 3 key components based on medical necessity.
[b] Low level E/M service that may not require the presence of a physician.

Continuum Model for Attention-Deficit/Hyperactivity Disorder (ADHD)

CPT Code Vignette	History	Physical Examination	Medical Decision-making
99211* Nurse visit to follow up growth or blood pressure prior to renewing prescription for psychoactive drugs *There are no required key components; however, the nurse must document his or her history, physical examination, and assessment to support medical necessity.*	1. Chief complaint 2. Brief HPI, existing medications, and desired/undesired effects	1. Weight, blood pressure 2. Overall appearance	1. Refill existing prescription
99212 Follow-up visit to recheck prior weight loss in patient with established ADHD otherwise stable on stimulant medication	Problem focused 1. Chief complaint 2. Document brief HPI, existing medications, and desired/undesired effects	Problem focused 1. Weight, blood pressure 2. Overall appearance	Straightforward 1. Refill existing prescription
99213 3- to 6-month follow-up of child with ADHD who is presently doing well using medication and without other problems	Expanded problem focused 1. Reason for the visit 2. Review of medications 3. Effect of medication on appetite, mood, sleep 4. Quality of schoolwork (eg, review report cards) 5. Absence of tics 6. Problem-pertinent ROS	Expanded problem focused 1. General multisystem examination or single organ system examination with special reference to neurologic examination 2. Rating Scale Review: Teacher Vanderbilt ADHD Rating Scale results reviewed	Low complexity 1. Review rating scale results and feedback materials from teacher. 2. Discuss 6-month treatment plan with adjustment of medication. 3. Plan for further monitoring.

Continuum Model for Attention-Deficit/Hyperactivity Disorder (ADHD), continued

CPT Code Vignette	History	Physical Examination	Medical Decision-making
99214 Follow-up evaluation of an established patient with ADHD with failure to improve on medication and/or weight loss	Detailed All data implicit in **99213** expanded plus pertinent review of PFSH and extended ROS including gastrointestinal and psychiatric	Detailed 1. General multisystem examination or detailed single organ system examination of the neurologic system 2. Rating Scale Review: Parent and Teacher Vanderbilt ADHD Rating Scales results reviewed	Moderate complexity Discussion of possible interventions including, but not limited to, 1. Educational intervention 2. Alteration in medications 3. Obtaining drug levels 4. Psychiatric intervention 5. Behavioral modification program
99215 Initial evaluation of an established patient experiencing difficulty in classroom, home, or social situation and suspected of having ADHD This could be billed as a consultation if the established patient is referred by school for opinion or advice (not transfer of care) and the criteria for reporting a consultation are met.	Comprehensive 1. Chief complaint 2. History of the problem, extended 3. Complete PFSH 4. Complete ROS	Comprehensive 1. General multisystem examination with special attention to neurologic examination and mental health status 2. Rating Scale Review: Parent and Teacher Vanderbilt ADHD Rating Scales results reviewed	High complexity Review of Vanderbilt scores, school record, any other formal evaluations completed to date, discussion of differential diagnoses, possible interventions including, but not limited to, 1. Educational interventions 2. Initiation of medications 3. Obtaining drug levels or rule out substance abuse, if appropriate 4. Laboratory tests as indicated (eg, complete blood cell count and iron studies, serum lead levels) 5. Psychological and/or psychiatric interventions 6. Behavioral modification program 7. Consideration of neurology consultation 8. Coordination of care services with school, family, and other providers

Understanding ADHD:
Information for Parents About Attention-Deficit/Hyperactivity Disorder

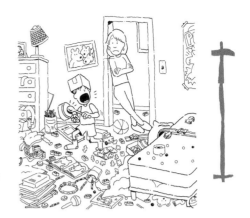

Almost all children have times when their behavior veers out of control. They may speed about in constant motion, make noise nonstop, refuse to wait their turn, and crash into everything around them. At other times they may drift as if in a daydream, failing to pay attention or finish what they start.

However, for some children, these kinds of behaviors are more than an occasional problem. Children with attention-deficit/hyperactivity disorder (ADHD) have behavior problems that are so frequent and severe that they interfere with their ability to live normal lives.

These children often have trouble getting along with siblings and other children at school, at home, and in other settings. Those who have trouble paying attention usually have trouble learning. An impulsive nature may put them in actual physical danger. Because children with ADHD have difficulty controlling this behavior, they may be labeled "bad kids" or "space cadets."

Left untreated, some of the children with ADHD will continue to have serious, lifelong problems, such as poor grades in school, run-ins with the law, failed relationships, and the inability to keep a job.

Effective treatment is available. If your child has ADHD, your pediatrician can offer a long-term treatment plan to help your child lead a happy and healthy life. As a parent, you have a very important role in this treatment.

What is ADHD?

ADHD is a condition of the brain that makes it difficult for children to control their behavior. It is one of the most common chronic conditions of childhood. It affects 4% to 12% of school-aged children. About 3 times more boys than girls are diagnosed with ADHD.

The condition affects behavior in specific ways.

What are the symptoms of ADHD?

ADHD includes 3 groups of behavior symptoms: inattention, hyperactivity, and impulsivity. Table 1 explains these symptoms.

Are there different types of ADHD?

Not all children with ADHD have all the symptoms. They may have one or more of the symptom groups listed in Table 1. The symptoms usually are classified as the following types of ADHD:

- **Inattentive only** (formerly known as attention-deficit disorder [ADD])— Children with this form of ADHD are not overly active. Because they do not disrupt the classroom or other activities, their symptoms may not be noticed. Among girls with ADHD, this form is more common.
- **Hyperactive/Impulsive**—Children with this type of ADHD show both hyperactive and impulsive behavior, but can pay attention. They are the least common group and are frequently younger.
- **Combined Inattentive/Hyperactive/Impulsive**—Children with this type of ADHD show a number of symptoms in all 3 dimensions. It is the type that most people think of when they think of ADHD.

Table 1. Symptoms of ADHD

Symptom	How a child with this symptom may behave
Inattention	Often has a hard time paying attention, daydreams
	Often does not seem to listen
	Is easily distracted from work or play
	Often does not seem to care about details, makes careless mistakes
	Frequently does not follow through on instructions or finish tasks
	Is disorganized
	Frequently loses a lot of important things
	Often forgets things
	Frequently avoids doing things that require ongoing mental effort
Hyperactivity	Is in constant motion, as if "driven by a motor"
	Cannot stay seated
	Frequently squirms and fidgets
	Talks too much
	Often runs, jumps, and climbs when this is not permitted
	Cannot play quietly
Impulsivity	Frequently acts and speaks without thinking
	May run into the street without looking for traffic first
	Frequently has trouble taking turns
	Cannot wait for things
	Often calls out answers before the question is complete
	Frequently interrupts others

How can I tell if my child has ADHD?

Remember, it is normal for all children to show some of these symptoms from time to time. Your child may be reacting to stress at school or home. She may be bored or going through a difficult stage of life. It does not mean she has ADHD.

Sometimes a teacher is the first to notice inattention, hyperactivity, and/or impulsivity and bring these symptoms to the parents' attention.

Perhaps questions from your pediatrician raised the issue. At routine visits, pediatricians often ask questions such as

- How is your child doing in school?
- Are there any problems with learning that you or your child's teachers have seen?

- Is your child happy in school?
- Is your child having problems completing class work or homework?
- Are you concerned with any behavior problems in school, at home, or when your child is playing with friends?

Your answers to these questions may lead to further evaluation for ADHD. If your child has shown symptoms of ADHD on a regular basis for more than 6 months, discuss this with your pediatrician.

Keep safety in mind

If your child shows any symptoms of ADHD, it is very important that you pay close attention to safety. A child with ADHD may not always be aware of dangers and can get hurt easily. Be especially careful around

- Traffic
- Firearms
- Swimming pools
- Tools such as lawn mowers
- Poisonous chemicals, cleaning supplies, or medicines

Diagnosis

Your pediatrician will determine whether your child has ADHD using standard guidelines developed by the American Academy of Pediatrics. These diagnosis guidelines are specifically for children 4 to 18 years of age.

It is difficult to diagnose ADHD in children younger than 4 years. This is because younger children change very rapidly. It is also more difficult to diagnose ADHD once a child becomes a teenager.

There is no single test for ADHD. The process requires several steps and involves gathering a lot of information from multiple sources. You, your child, your child's school, and other caregivers should be involved in assessing your child's behavior.

Children with ADHD show signs of inattention, hyperactivity, and/or impulsivity in specific ways. (See the behaviors listed in Table 1.) Your pediatrician will look at how your child's behavior compares to that of other children her own age, based on the information reported about your child by you, her teacher, and any other caregivers who spend time with your child, such as coaches or child care workers.

To confirm a diagnosis of ADHD, symptoms

- Occur in more than one setting, such as home, school, and social situations and cause some impairment
- Significantly impair your child's ability to function in some of the activities of daily life, such as schoolwork, relationships with you and her brothers and/or sisters, and relationships with friends or in her ability to function in groups such as sports teams
- Start before the child reaches 7 years of age (However, these may not be recognized as ADHD symptoms until a child is older.)
- Have continued for more than 6 months

In addition to looking at your child's behavior, your pediatrician will do a physical and neurologic examination. A full medical history will be needed to put your child's behavior in context and screen for other conditions that may affect her behavior. Your pediatrician also will talk with your child about how she acts and feels.

Your pediatrician may refer your child to a pediatric subspecialist or mental health clinician if there are concerns in one of the following areas:

- Intellectual disability (mental retardation)
- Developmental disorder such as speech problems, motor problems, or a learning disability
- Chronic illness being treated with a medication that may interfere with learning
- Trouble seeing and/or hearing
- History of abuse
- Major anxiety or major depression
- Severe aggression
- Possible seizure disorder
- Possible sleep disorder

How can parents help with the diagnosis?

As a parent, you will provide crucial information about your child's behavior and how it affects her life at home, in school, and in other social settings. Your pediatrician will want to know what symptoms your child is showing, how long the symptoms have occurred, and how the behavior affects your child and your family. You may need to fill in checklists or rating scales about your child's behavior.

In addition, sharing your family history can offer important clues about your child's condition.

How will my child's school be involved?

For an accurate diagnosis, your pediatrician will need to get information about your child directly from your child's classroom teacher or another school professional. Children at least 4 years of age and older spend many of their waking hours at preschool or school. Teachers provide valuable insights. Your child's teacher may write a report or discuss the following with your pediatrician:

- Your child's behavior in the classroom
- Your child's learning patterns
- How long the symptoms have been a problem
- How the symptoms are affecting your child's progress at school
- Ways the classroom program is being adapted to help your child
- Whether other conditions may be affecting the symptoms

In addition, your pediatrician may want to see report cards, standardized tests, and samples of your child's schoolwork.

How will others who care for my child be involved?

Other caregivers may also provide important information about your child's behavior. Former teachers, religious and scout leaders, or coaches may have valuable input. If your child is homeschooled, it is especially important to assess his behavior in settings outside of the home.

Your child may not behave the same way at home as he does in other settings. Direct information about the way your child acts in more than one setting is required. It is important to consider other possible causes of your child's symptoms in these settings.

In some cases, other mental health care professionals may also need to be involved in gathering information for the diagnosis.

Coexisting conditions

As part of the diagnosis, your pediatrician will look for other conditions that show the same types of symptoms as ADHD. Your child may simply have a different condition or ADHD and another condition. Most children who have been diagnosed with ADHD have at least one coexisting condition.

Common coexisting conditions include

- **Learning disabilities**—Learning disabilities are conditions that make it difficult for a child to master specific skills such as reading or math. ADHD is not a learning disability. However, ADHD can make it hard for a child to do well in school. Diagnosing learning disabilities requires evaluations, such as IQ and academic achievement tests, and requires educational interventions.
- **Oppositional defiant disorder or conduct disorder**—Up to 35% of children with ADHD also have oppositional defiant disorder or conduct disorder. Children with oppositional defiant disorder tend to lose their temper easily and annoy people on purpose and are defiant and hostile toward authority figures. Children with conduct disorder break rules, destroy property, get suspended or expelled from school, and violate the rights of other people. Children with coexisting conduct disorder are at much higher risk for getting into trouble with the law or having substance abuse problems than children who have only ADHD. Studies show that this type of coexisting condition is more common among children with the primarily hyperactive/impulsive and combination types of ADHD. Your pediatrician may recommend behavioral therapy for your child if she has this condition.
- **Mood disorders/depression**—About 18% of children with ADHD also have mood disorders such as depression or bipolar disorder (formerly called manic depression). There is frequently a family history of these types of disorders. Coexisting mood disorders may put children at higher risk for suicide, especially during the teenage years. These disorders are more common among children with inattentive and combined types of ADHD. Children with mood disorders or depression often require additional interventions or a different type of medication than those normally used to treat ADHD.
- **Anxiety disorders**—These affect about 25% of children with ADHD. Children with anxiety disorders have extreme feelings of fear, worry, or panic that make it difficult to function. These disorders can produce physical symptoms such as racing pulse, sweating, diarrhea, and nausea. Counseling and/or different medication may be needed to treat these coexisting conditions.
- **Language disorders**—Children with ADHD may have difficulty with how they use language. It is referred to as a pragmatic language disorder. It may not show up with standard tests of language. A speech and language clinician can detect it by observing how a child uses language in her day-to-day activities.

Are there other tests for ADHD?

You may have heard theories about other tests for ADHD. There are no other proven tests for ADHD at this time.

Many theories have been presented, but studies have shown that the following tests have little value in diagnosing an individual child:

- Screening for high lead levels in the blood
- Screening for thyroid problems
- Computerized continuous performance tests
- Brain imaging studies such as CAT scans, MRIs, etc
- Electroencephalogram (EEG) or brain-wave test

While these tests are not helpful in diagnosing ADHD, your pediatrician may see other signs or symptoms in your child that warrant blood tests, brain imaging studies, or an EEG.

What causes ADHD?

ADHD is one of the most studied conditions of childhood, but ADHD may be caused by a number of things.

Research to date has shown

- ADHD is a neurobiological condition whose symptoms are also dependent on the child's environment.
- A lower level of activity in the parts of the brain that control attention and activity level may be associated with ADHD.
- ADHD frequently runs in families. Sometimes a parent is diagnosed with ADHD at the same time as the child.
- In very rare cases, toxins in the environment may lead to ADHD. For instance, lead in the body can affect child development and behavior. Lead may be found in many places, including homes built before 1978 when lead was added to paint.
- Significant head injuries may cause ADHD in some cases.
- Prematurity increases the risk of developing ADHD.
- Prenatal exposures, such as alcohol or nicotine from smoking, increase the risk of developing ADHD.

There is little evidence that ADHD is caused by

- Eating too much sugar
- Food additives
- Allergies
- Immunizations

Treatment

Once the diagnosis is confirmed, the outlook for most children who receive treatment for ADHD is encouraging. There is no specific cure for ADHD, but there are many treatment options available.

Each child's treatment must be tailored to meet his individual needs. In most cases, treatment for ADHD should include

- A long-term management plan with
  - Target outcomes for behavior
  - Follow-up activities
  - Monitoring
- Education about ADHD
- Teamwork among doctors, parents, teachers, caregivers, other health care professionals, and the child
- Medication
- Behavior therapy including parent training
- Individual and family counseling

Treatment for ADHD uses the same principles that are used to treat other chronic conditions like asthma or diabetes. Long-term planning is needed because these conditions are not cured. Families must manage them on an ongoing basis. In the case of ADHD, schools and other caregivers must also be involved in managing the condition.

Educating the people involved about ADHD is a key part of treating your child. As a parent, you will need to learn about ADHD. Read about the condition and talk to people who understand it. This will help you manage the ways ADHD affects your child and your family on a day-to-day basis. It will also help your child learn to help himself.

Setting target outcomes

At the beginning of treatment, your pediatrician should help you set around 3 target outcomes (goals) for your child's behavior. These target outcomes will guide the treatment plan. Your child's target outcomes should focus on helping her function as well as possible at home, at school, and in your community. You need to identify what behaviors are most preventing your child from success.

The following are examples of target outcomes:

- Improved relationships with parents, siblings, teachers, and friends (eg, fewer arguments with brothers or sisters or being invited more frequently to friends' houses or parties)
- Better schoolwork (eg, completing class work or homework assignments)
- More independence in self-care or homework (eg, getting ready for school in the morning without supervision)
- Improved self-esteem (eg, increase in feeling that she can get her work done)
- Fewer disruptive behaviors (eg, decrease in the number of times she refuses to obey rules)
- Safer behavior in the community (eg, when crossing streets)

The target outcomes should be

- Realistic
- Something your child will be able to do
- Behaviors that you can observe and count (eg, with rating scales)

Your child's treatment plan will be set up to help her achieve these goals.

Medication

For most children, stimulant medications are a safe and effective way to relieve ADHD symptoms. As glasses help people focus their eyes to see, these medications help children with ADHD focus their thoughts better and ignore distractions. This makes them more able to pay attention and control their behavior.

Stimulants may be used alone or combined with behavior therapy. Studies show that about 80% of children with ADHD who are treated with stimulants improve a great deal once the right medication and dose are determined.

Two forms of stimulants are available: immediate-release (short-acting) and extended-release (intermediate-acting and long-acting). (See Table 2.) Immediate-release medications usually are taken every 4 hours, when needed. They are the cheapest of the medications. Extended-release medications usually are taken once in the morning.

Children who use extended-release forms of stimulants can avoid taking medication at school or after school. It is important not to chew or crush extended-release capsules or tablets. However, extended-release capsules that are made up of beads can be opened and sprinkled on food for children who have difficulties swallowing tablets or capsules.

There are 2 newer medications that have been approved by the Food and Drug Administration (FDA) that are non-stimulants. Non-stimulants can be tried when stimulant medications don't work or cause bothersome side effects.

Which medication is best for my child?

It may take some time to find the best medication, dosage, and schedule for your child.

Your child may need to try different types of stimulants or other medication. Some children respond to one type of stimulant but not another.

Table 2. Common medications

Type of medication	Brand name	Generic name	Duration
Short-acting amphetamine stimulants	Adderall	Mixed amphetamine salts	4 to 6 hours
	Dexedrine	Dextroamphetamine	4 to 6 hours
	Dextrostat	Dextroamphetamine	4 to 6 hours
Short-acting methylphenidate stimulants	Focalin	Dexmethylphenidate	4 to 6 hours
	Methylin	Methylphenidate (tablet, liquid, and chewable tablets)	3 to 5 hours
	Ritalin	Methylphenidate	3 to 5 hours
Intermediate-acting methylphenidate stimulants	Metadate CD	Extended-release methylphenidate	6 to 8 hours
	Ritalin LA	Extended-release methylphenidate	6 to 8 hours
Long-acting amphetamine stimulants	Adderall-XR	Extended-release amphetamine	10 to 12 hours
	Dexedrine Spansule	Extended-release amphetamine	6+ hours
	Vyvanse	Lisdexamfetamine	10 to 12 hours
Long-acting methylphenidate stimulants	Concerta	Extended-release methylphenidate	10 to 12 hours
	Daytrana	Extended-release methylphenidate (skin patch)	11 to 12 hours
	Focalin XR	Extended-release dexmethylphenidate	8 to 12 hours
Long-acting non-stimulants	Intuniv	Guanfacine	24 hours
	Strattera	Atomoxetine	24 hours

Products are mentioned for informational purposes only and do not imply an endorsement by the American Academy of Pediatrics. Your doctor or pharmacist can provide you with important safety information for the products listed.

The amount of medication (dosage) that your child needs also may need to be adjusted. The dosage is not based solely on his weight. Your pediatrician will vary the dosage over time to get the best results and control possible side effects.

The medication schedule also may be adjusted depending on the target outcome. For example, if the goal is to get relief from symptoms mostly at school, your child may take the medication only on school days.

It is important for your child to have regular medical checkups to monitor how well the medication is working and check for possible side effects.

What side effects can stimulants cause?

Side effects occur sometimes. These tend to happen early in treatment and are usually mild and short-lived, but in rare cases can be prolonged or more severe.

The most common side effects include

- Decreased appetite/weight loss
- Sleep problems
- Social withdrawal

Some less common side effects include

- Rebound effect (increased activity or a bad mood as the medication wears off)
- Transient muscle movements or sounds called tics
- Minor growth delay

Very rare side effects include

- Significant increase in blood pressure or heart rate
- Bizarre behaviors

The same sleep problems do not exist for atomoxetine, but initially it may make your child sleepy or upset her stomach. There have been very rare cases of atomoxetine needing to be stopped because it was causing liver damage. Rarely atomoxetine increased thoughts of suicide. Guanfacine can cause drowsiness, fatigue, or a decrease in blood pressure.

More than half of children who have tic disorders, such as Tourette syndrome, also have ADHD. Tourette syndrome is an inherited condition associated with frequent tics and unusual vocal sounds. The effect of stimulants on tics is not predictable, although most studies indicate that stimulants are safe for children with ADHD and tic disorders in most cases. It is also possible to use atomoxetine or guanfacine for children with ADHD and Tourette syndrome. Most side effects can be relieved by

- Changing the medication dosage
- Adjusting the schedule of medication
- Using a different stimulant or trying a non-stimulant (See Table 2.)

Close contact with your pediatrician is required until you find the best medication and dose for your child. After that, periodic monitoring by your doctor is important to maintain the best effects. To monitor the effects of the medication, your pediatrician will probably have you and your child's teacher(s) fill out behavior rating scales; observe changes in your child's target goals; notice any side effects; and monitor your child's height, weight, pulse, and blood pressure.

Stimulants, atomoxetine, and guanfacine may not be an option for children who are taking certain other medications or who have some medical conditions, such as congenital heart disease.

Behavior therapy

Most experts recommend using both medication and behavior therapy to treat ADHD. This is known as a multimodal treatment approach.

There are many forms of behavior therapy, but all have a common goal—to change the child's physical and social environments to help the child improve his behavior.

Under this approach, parents, teachers, and other caregivers learn better ways to work with and relate to the child with ADHD. You will learn how to set and enforce rules, help your child understand what he needs to do, use discipline effectively, and encourage good behavior. Your child will learn better ways to control his behavior as a result. You will learn how to be more consistent.

Table 3 shows specific behavior therapy techniques that can be effective with children with ADHD.

Behavior therapy recognizes the limits that having ADHD puts on a child. It focuses on how the important people and places in the child's life can adapt to encourage good behavior and discourage unwanted behavior. It is different from play therapy or other therapies that focus mainly on the child and his emotions.

Principles for behavior therapy

Behavior therapy has 3 basic principles.

1. **Set specific doable goals.** Set clear and reasonable goals for your child, such as staying focused on homework for a certain time or sharing toys with friends.
2. **Provide rewards and consequences.** Give your child a specified reward (positive reinforcement) every time she shows the desired behavior. Give your child a consequence (unwanted result or punishment) consistently when she has inappropriate behaviors.
3. **Keep using the rewards and consequences.** Using the rewards and consequences consistently for a long time will shape your child's behavior in a positive way.

How can I help my child control her behavior?

As the child's primary caregivers, parents play a major role in behavior therapy. Parent training is available to help you learn more about ADHD and specific, positive ways to respond to ADHD-type behaviors. This will help your child improve. In many cases parenting classes with other parents will be sufficient, but with more challenging children, individual work with a counselor/coach may be needed.

Taking care of yourself also will help your child. Being the parent of a child with ADHD can be tiring and trying. It can test the limits of even the best parents. Parent training and support groups made up of other families who are dealing with ADHD can be a great source of help. Learn stress-management techniques to help you respond calmly to your child. Seek counseling if you feel overwhelmed or hopeless.

Ask your pediatrician to help you find parent training, counseling, and support groups in your community. Additional resources are listed at the end of this publication.

Table 3. Behavior therapy techniques

Technique	Description	Example
Positive reinforcement	Complimenting and providing rewards or privileges in response to desired behavior.	Child completes an assignment and is permitted to play on the computer.
Time-out	Removing access to desired activity because of unwanted behavior.	Child hits sibling and, as a result, must sit for 5 minutes in the corner of the room.
Response cost	Withdrawing rewards or privileges because of unwanted behavior.	Child loses free-time privileges for not completing homework.
Token economy	Combining reward and consequence. Child earns rewards and privileges when performing desired behaviors. She loses the rewards and privileges as a result of unwanted behavior.	Child earns stars or points for completing assignments and loses stars for getting out of seat. The child cashes in the sum of her stars at the end of the week for a prize.

How can my child's school help?

Your child's school is a key partner in providing effective behavior therapy for your child. In fact, these principles work well in the classroom for most students.

Classroom management techniques may include

- Keeping a set routine and schedule for activities
- Using a system of clear rewards and consequences, such as a point system or token economy (See Table 3.)
- Sending daily or weekly report cards or behavior charts to parents to inform them about the child's progress
- Seating the child near the teacher
- Using small groups for activities
- Encouraging students to pause a moment before answering questions
- Keeping assignments short or breaking them into sections
- Close supervision with frequent, positive cues to stay on task
- Changes to where and how tests are given so students can succeed (For example, allowing students to take tests in a less distracting environment or allowing more time to complete tests.)

Tips for helping your child control his behavior

- **Keep your child on a daily schedule.** Try to keep the time that your child wakes up, eats, bathes, leaves for school, and goes to sleep the same each day.
- **Cut down on distractions.** Loud music, computer games, and TV can be overstimulating to your child. Make it a rule to keep the TV or music off during mealtime and while your child is doing homework. Don't place a TV in your child's bedroom. Whenever possible, avoid taking your child to places that may be too stimulating, like busy shopping malls.
- **Organize your house.** If your child has specific and logical places to keep his schoolwork, toys, and clothes, he is less likely to lose them. Save a spot near the front door for his school backpack so he can grab it on the way out the door.
- **Reward positive behavior.** Offer kind words, hugs, or small prizes for reaching goals in a timely manner or good behavior. Praise and reward your child's efforts to pay attention.
- **Set small, reachable goals.** Aim for slow progress rather than instant results. Be sure that your child understands that he can take small steps toward learning to control himself.
- **Help your child stay "on task."** Use charts and checklists to track progress with homework or chores. Keep instructions brief. Offer frequent, friendly reminders.
- **Limit choices.** Help your child learn to make good decisions by giving him only 2 or 3 options at a time.
- **Find activities at which your child can succeed.** All children need to experience success to feel good about themselves.
- **Use calm discipline.** Use consequences such as time-out, removing the child from the situation, or distraction. Sometimes it is best to simply ignore the behavior. Physical punishment, such as spanking or slapping, is *not* helpful. Discuss your child's behavior with him when both of you are calm.
- **Develop a good communication system with your child's teacher** so that you can coordinate your efforts and monitor your child's progress.

Your child's school should work with you and your pediatrician to develop strategies to assist your child in the classroom. When a child has ADHD that is severe enough to interfere with her ability to learn, 2 federal laws offer help. These laws require public schools to cover the costs of evaluating the educational needs of the affected child and providing the needed services.

1. The Individuals with Disabilities Education Act, Part B (IDEA) requires public schools to cover the costs of evaluating the educational needs of the affected child and providing the needed special education services if your child qualifies because her learning is impaired by his ADHD.
2. Section 504 of the Rehabilitation Act of 1973 does not have strict qualification criteria but is limited to changes in the classroom and modifications in homework assignments and taking tests in a less distracting environment or allowing more time to complete tests.

If your child has ADHD and a coexisting condition, she may need additional special services such as a classroom aide, private tutoring, special classroom settings or, in rare cases, a special school.

It is important to remember that once diagnosed and treated, children with ADHD are more likely to achieve their goals in school.

Keeping the treatment plan on track

Ongoing monitoring of your child's behavior and medications is required to find out if the treatment plan is working. Office visits, phone conversations, behavior checklists, written reports from teachers, and behavior report cards are common tools for following the child's progress.

Treatment plans for ADHD usually require long-term efforts on the part of families and schools. Medication schedules may be complex. Behavior therapies require education and patience. Sometimes it can be hard for everyone to stick with it. Your efforts play an important part in building a healthy future for your child.

Ask your pediatrician to help you find ways to keep your child's treatment plan on track.

What if my child does not reach his target outcomes?

Most school-aged children with ADHD respond well when their treatment plan includes both medication and behavior therapy. If your child is not achieving his goals, your pediatrician will assess the following factors:

- Were the target outcomes realistic?
- Is more information needed about the child's behavior?
- Is the diagnosis correct?
- Is another condition hindering treatment?
- Is the treatment plan being followed?
- Has the treatment failed?

While treatment for ADHD should improve your child's behavior, **it may not completely eliminate the symptoms** of inattention, hyperactivity, and impulsivity. Children who are being treated successfully may still have trouble with their friends or schoolwork.

However, if your child clearly is not meeting his specific target outcomes, your pediatrician will need to reassess the treatment plan.

Unproven treatments

You may have heard media reports or seen advertisements for "miracle cures" for ADHD. Carefully research any such claims. Consider whether the source of the information is valid. At this time, there is no scientifically proven cure for this condition.

The following methods **need more scientific evidence to prove that they work**:

- Megavitamins and mineral supplements
- Anti–motion-sickness medication (to treat the inner ear)
- Treatment for candida yeast infection
- EEG biofeedback (training to increase brain-wave activity)
- Applied kinesiology (realigning bones in the skull)
- Reducing sugar consumption
- Optometric vision training (asserts that faulty eye movement and sensitivities cause the behavior problems)

Always tell your pediatrician about any alternative therapies, supplements, or medications that your child is using. These may interact with prescribed medications and harm your child.

Will there be a cure for ADHD soon?

While there are no signs of a cure at this time, research is ongoing to learn more about the role of the brain in ADHD and the best ways to treat the disorder. Additional research is looking at the long-term outcomes for people with ADHD.

Frequently asked questions

Will my child outgrow ADHD?

ADHD continues into adulthood in most cases. However, by developing their strengths, structuring their environments, and using medication when needed, adults with ADHD can lead very productive lives. In some careers, having a high-energy behavior pattern can be an asset.

Why do so many children have ADHD?

The number of children who are being treated for ADHD has risen. It is not clear whether more children have ADHD or more children are being diagnosed with ADHD. Also, more children with ADHD are being treated for a longer period. ADHD is now one of the most common and most studied conditions of childhood. Because of more awareness and better ways of diagnosing and treating this disorder, more children are being helped. It may also be the case that school performance has become more important because of the higher technical demand of many jobs, and ADHD frequently interferes with school functioning.

Are schools putting children on ADHD medication?

Teachers are often the first to notice behavior signs of possible ADHD. However, only physicians can prescribe medications to treat ADHD. The diagnosis of ADHD should follow a careful process.

Are children getting high on stimulant medications?

When taken as directed by a doctor, there is no evidence that children are getting high on stimulant drugs such as methylphenidate and amphetamine. At therapeutic doses, these drugs also do not sedate or tranquilize children and do not increase the risk of addiction.

Stimulants are classified as Schedule II drugs by the US Drug Enforcement Administration because there is abuse potential of this class of medication. If your child is on medication, it is always best to supervise the use of the medication closely. Atomoxetine and guanfacine are not Schedule II drugs because they don't have abuse potential, even in adults.

Teenagers with ADHD

The teenage years can be a special challenge. Academic and social demands increase. In some cases, symptoms may be better controlled as the child grows older; however, frequently the demands for performance also increase so that in most cases, ADHD symptoms persist and continue to interfere with their ability to function adequately. According to the National Institute of Mental Health, about 80% of those who required medication for ADHD as children still need it as teenagers.

Parents play an important role in helping teenagers become independent. Encourage your teenager to help herself with strategies such as

- Using a daily planner for assignments and appointments
- Making lists
- Keeping a routine
- Setting aside a quiet time and place to do homework
- Organizing storage for school supplies, clothes, CDs, sports equipment, etc
- Being safety conscious (eg, always wearing seat belts, using protective gear for sports)
- Talking about problems with someone she trusts
- Getting enough sleep
- Understanding her increased risk of abusing substances such as tobacco and alcohol

Activities such as sports, drama, and debate teams can be good places to channel excess energy and develop friendships. Find what your teenager does well and support her efforts to "go for it."

Milestones such as learning to drive and dating offer new freedom and risks. Parents must stay involved and set limits for safety. Your child's ADHD increases her risk of incurring traffic violations and accidents.

It remains important for parents of teenagers to keep in touch with teachers and make sure that their teenager's schoolwork is going well.

Talk with your pediatrician if your teenager shows signs of severe problems such as depression, drug abuse, or gang-related activities.

Are stimulant medications "gateway" drugs leading to illegal drug or alcohol abuse?

People with ADHD are naturally impulsive and tend to take risks. But those patients with ADHD who are taking stimulants are not at greater risk and actually may be at a lower risk of using other drugs. Children and teenagers who have ADHD and also have coexisting conditions may be at higher risk for drug and alcohol abuse, regardless of the medication used.

Resources

The following is a list of support groups and additional resources for further information about ADHD. Check with your pediatrician for resources in your community.

National Resource Center on AD/HD
www.help4adhd.org/

Children and Adults with Attention-Deficit/Hyperactivity Disorder (CHADD)
800/233-4050
www.chadd.org

Attention Deficit Disorder Association

856/439-9099

www.add.org

National Dissemination Center for Children with Disabilities

800/695-0285

www.nichcy.org

National Institute of Mental Health

866/615-6464

www.nimh.nih.gov

National Tourette Syndrome Association, Inc

800/237-0717

www.tsa-usa.org

Inclusion on this list does not imply an endorsement by the American Academy of Pediatrics (AAP). The AAP is not responsible for the content of the resources mentioned above. Phone numbers and Web site addresses are as current as possible, but may change at any time.

Products are mentioned for informational purposes only and do not imply an endorsement by the American Academy of Pediatrics.

The information contained in this publication should not be used as a substitute for the medical care and advice of your pediatrician. There may be variations in treatment that your pediatrician may recommend based on individual facts and circumstances

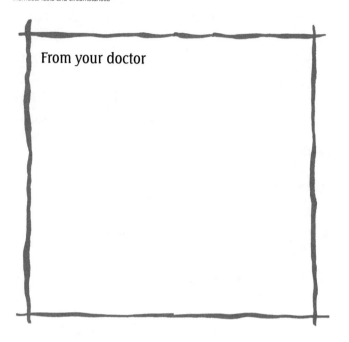

From your doctor

American Academy
of Pediatrics

DEDICATED TO THE HEALTH OF ALL CHILDREN™

The American Academy of Pediatrics is an organization of 60,000 primary care pediatricians, pediatric medical subspecialists, and pediatric surgical specialists dedicated to the health, safety, and well-being of infants, children, adolescents, and young adults.

American Academy of Pediatrics
Web site — www.HealthyChildren.org

Copyright © 2007
American Academy of Pediatrics, Updated 4/11
All rights reserved.

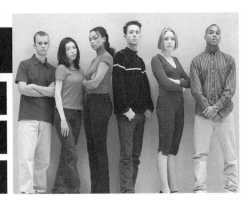

medicines for ADHD questions from teens who have ADHD

Q: What can I do besides taking medicines?

A: Medicines and behavior therapies are the only treatments that have been shown by scientific studies to work consistently for ADHD symptoms. Medicines are prescribed by a doctor, while behavior therapies usually are done with a trained counselor in behavior treatment. These 2 treatments are probably best used together, but you might be able to do well with one or the other. You can't rely on other treatments such as biofeedback, allergy treatments, special diets, vision training, or chiropractic because there isn't enough evidence that shows they work.

Counseling may help you learn how to cope with some issues you may face. And there are things you can do to help yourself. For example, things that may help you stay focused include using a daily planner for schoolwork and other activities, making to-do lists, and even getting enough sleep. Counseling can help you find an organization system or a checklist.

Q: How can medicines help me?

A: There are several different ADHD medicines. They work by causing the brain to have more *neurotransmitters* in the right places. Neurotransmitters are chemicals in the brain that help us focus our attention, control our impulses, organize and plan, and stick to routines. Medicines for ADHD can help you focus your thoughts and ignore distractions so that you can reach your full potential. They also can help you control your emotions and behavior. Check with your doctor to learn more about this.

Q: Are medicines safe?

A: For most teens with ADHD, stimulant medicines are safe and effective if taken as recommended. However, like most medicines, there could be side effects. Luckily, the side effects tend to happen early on, are usually mild, and don't last too long. If you have any side effects, tell your doctor. Changes may need to be made in your medicines or their dosages.

- **Most common side effects** include decreased appetite or weight loss, problems falling asleep, headaches, jitteriness, and stomachaches.
- **Less common side effects** include a bad mood as medicines wear off (called the rebound effect) and facial twitches or tics.

Q: Will medicines change my personality?

A: Medicines won't change who you are and should not change your personality. If you notice changes in your mood or personality, tell your doctor. Occasionally when medicines wear off, some teens become more irritable for a short time. An adjustment of the medicines by your doctor may be helpful.

Q: Will medicines affect my growth?

A: Medicines will not keep you from growing. Significant growth delay is a very rare side effect of some medicines prescribed for ADHD. Most scientific studies show that taking these medicines has little to no long-term effect on growth in most cases.

Q: Do I need to take medicines at school?

A: There are 3 types of medicines used for teens with ADHD: **short acting** (immediate release), **intermediate acting,** and **long acting.** You can avoid taking medicines at school if you take the intermediate- or long-acting kind. Long-acting medicines usually are taken once in the morning or evening. Short-acting medicines usually are taken every 4 hours.

Q: Does taking medicines make me a drug user?

A: No! Although you may need medicines to help you stay in control of your behavior, medicines used to treat ADHD do not lead to drug abuse. In fact, taking medicines as prescribed by your doctor and doing better in school may help you avoid drug use and abuse. (But never give or share your medicines with anyone else.)

Q: Will I have to take medicines forever?

A: In most cases, ADHD continues later in life. Whether you need to keep taking medicines as an adult depends on your own needs. The need for medicines may change over time. Many adults with ADHD have learned how to succeed in life without medicines by using behavior therapies or finding jobs that suit their strengths and weaknesses.

The persons whose photographs are depicted in this publication are professional models. They have no relation to the issues discussed. Any characters they are portraying are fictional.

The information contained in this publication should not be used as a substitute for the medical care and advice of your pediatrician. There may be variations in treatment that your pediatrician may recommend based on individual facts and circumstances.

American Academy of Pediatrics

DEDICATED TO THE HEALTH OF ALL CHILDREN™

The American Academy of Pediatrics is an organization of 60,000 primary care pediatricians, pediatric medical subspecialists, and pediatric surgical specialists dedicated to the health, safety, and well-being of infants, children, adolescents, and young adults.

American Academy of Pediatrics
Web site—www.HealthyChildren.org

what is ADHD?
questions from teens

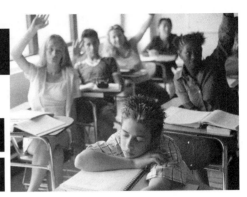

Attention-deficit/hyperactivity disorder (ADHD) is a condition of the brain that makes it difficult for people to concentrate or pay attention in certain areas where it is easy for others, like school or homework. The following are quick answers to some common questions:

Q: What causes ADHD?

A: There isn't just one cause. Research shows that
- ADHD is a medical condition caused by small changes in how the brain works. It seems to be related to 2 chemicals in your brain called *dopamine* and *norepinephrine.* These chemicals help send messages between nerve cells in the brain—especially those areas of the brain that control attention and activity level.
- ADHD most often runs in families.
- In a few people with ADHD, being born prematurely or being exposed to alcohol during the pregnancy can contribute to ADHD.
- Immunizations and eating too much sugar do NOT cause ADHD. And there isn't enough evidence that shows allergies and food additives cause ADHD.

Q: How can you tell if someone has ADHD?

A: You can't tell if someone has ADHD just by looks. People with ADHD don't look any different, but how they act may make them stand out from the crowd. Some people with ADHD are very hyperactive (they move around a lot and are not able to sit still) and have behavior problems that are obvious to everyone. Other people with ADHD are quiet and more laid back on the outside, but on the inside struggle with attention to schoolwork and other tasks. They are distracted by people and things around them when they try to study; they may have trouble organizing schoolwork or forget to turn in assignments.

Q: Can ADHD cause someone to act up or get in trouble?

A: Having ADHD can cause you to struggle in school or have problems controlling your behavior. Some people may say or think that your struggles and problems are because you are bad, lazy, or not smart. But they're wrong. It's important that you get help so your impulses don't get you into serious trouble.

Q: Don't little kids who have ADHD outgrow it by the time they are teens?

A: Often kids with the hyperactive kind of ADHD get less hyperactive as they get into their teens, but usually they still have a lot of difficulty paying attention, remembering what they have read, and getting their work done. They may or may not have other behavior problems. Some kids with ADHD have never been hyperactive at all, but usually their attention problems also continue into their teens.

Q: If I have trouble with homework or tests, do I have ADHD?

A: There could be many reasons why a student struggles with schoolwork and tests. ADHD could be one reason. It may or may not be, but your doctor is the best person to say for sure. Kids with ADHD often say it's hard to concentrate, focus on a task (for example, schoolwork, chores, or a job), manage their time, and finish tasks. This could explain why they may have trouble with schoolwork and tests. Whatever the problem, there are many people willing to help you. You need to find the approach that works best for you.

Q: Does having ADHD mean a person is not very smart?

A: Absolutely not! People who have trouble paying attention may have problems in school, but that doesn't mean they're not smart. In fact, some people with ADHD are very smart, but may not be able to reach their potential in school until they get treatment.

ADHD is a common problem. Teens with ADHD have the potential to do well in school and live a normal life with the right treatment.

Q: Is ADHD more common in boys?

A: More boys than girls are diagnosed with ADHD—about 2 or 3 boys to every 1 girl. However, these numbers do not include the number of girls with the inattentive type of ADHD who are not diagnosed. Girls with the inattentive type of ADHD tend to be overlooked entirely or do not attract attention until they are older.

Q: What do I do if I think I have ADHD?

A: Don't be afraid to talk with your parents or other adults that you trust. Together you can meet with your doctor and find out if you really have ADHD. If you do, your doctor will help you learn how to live with ADHD and find ways to deal with your condition.

The persons whose photographs are depicted in this publication are professional models. They have no relation to the issues discussed. Any characters they are portraying are fictional.

The information contained in this publication should not be used as a substitute for the medical care and advice of your pediatrician. There may be variations in treatment that your pediatrician may recommend based on individual facts and circumstances.

From your doctor

American Academy of Pediatrics

DEDICATED TO THE HEALTH OF ALL CHILDREN™

The American Academy of Pediatrics is an organization of 60,000 primary care pediatricians, pediatric medical subspecialists, and pediatric surgical specialists dedicated to the health, safety, and well-being of infants, children, adolescents, and young adults.

American Academy of Pediatrics
Web site—www.HealthyChildren.org

Diagnosis and Management of Bronchiolitis

- *Clinical Practice Guideline*

  - *PPI: AAP Partnership for Policy Implementation*
    See Appendix 2 for more information.

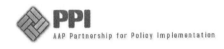

American Academy
of Pediatrics

DEDICATED TO THE HEALTH OF ALL CHILDREN™

CLINICAL PRACTICE GUIDELINE

Diagnosis and Management of Bronchiolitis

Subcommittee on Diagnosis and Management of Bronchiolitis

Organizational Principles to Guide and
Define the Child Health Care System and/or
Improve the Health of All Children

Endorsed by the American Academy of Family Physicians, the American College of Chest Physicians, and the American Thoracic Society.

ABSTRACT

Bronchiolitis is a disorder most commonly caused in infants by viral lower respiratory tract infection. It is the most common lower respiratory infection in this age group. It is characterized by acute inflammation, edema, and necrosis of epithelial cells lining small airways, increased mucus production, and bronchospasm.

The American Academy of Pediatrics convened a committee composed of primary care physicians and specialists in the fields of pulmonology, infectious disease, emergency medicine, epidemiology, and medical informatics. The committee partnered with the Agency for Healthcare Research and Quality and the RTI International-University of North Carolina Evidence-Based Practice Center to develop a comprehensive review of the evidence-based literature related to the diagnosis, management, and prevention of bronchiolitis. The resulting evidence report and other sources of data were used to formulate clinical practice guideline recommendations.

This guideline addresses the diagnosis of bronchiolitis as well as various therapeutic interventions including bronchodilators, corticosteroids, antiviral and antibacterial agents, hydration, chest physiotherapy, and oxygen. Recommendations are made for prevention of respiratory syncytial virus infection with palivizumab and the control of nosocomial spread of infection. Decisions were made on the basis of a systematic grading of the quality of evidence and strength of recommendation. The clinical practice guideline underwent comprehensive peer review before it was approved by the American Academy of Pediatrics.

This clinical practice guideline is not intended as a sole source of guidance in the management of children with bronchiolitis. Rather, it is intended to assist clinicians in decision-making. It is not intended to replace clinical judgment or establish a protocol for the care of all children with this condition. These recommendations may not provide the only appropriate approach to the management of children with bronchiolitis.

INTRODUCTION

THIS GUIDELINE EXAMINES the published evidence on diagnosis and acute management of the child with bronchiolitis in both outpatient and hospital settings, including the roles of supportive therapy, oxygen, bronchodilators, antiinflammatory agents, antibacterial agents, and antiviral agents and make recommendations to influence clinician behavior on the basis of the evidence. Methods of prevention

www.pediatrics.org/cgi/doi/10.1542/
peds.2006-2223

doi:10.1542/peds.2006-2223

All clinical practice guidelines from the American Academy of Pediatrics automatically expire 5 years after publication unless reaffirmed, revised, or retired at or before that time.

The recommendations in this guideline do not indicate an exclusive course of treatment or serve as a standard of care. Variations, taking into account individual circumstances, may be appropriate.

Key Word
bronchiolitis

Abbreviations
CAM—complementary and alternative medicine
LRTI—lower respiratory tract infection
AHRQ—Agency for Healthcare Research and Quality
RSV—respiratory syncytial virus
AAP—American Academy of Pediatrics
AAFP—American Academy of Family Physicians
RCT—randomized, controlled trial
CLD—chronic neonatal lung disease
SBI—serious bacterial infection
UTI—urinary tract infection
AOM—acute otitis media
Spo$_2$—oxyhemoglobin saturation
LRTD—lower respiratory tract disease

PEDIATRICS (ISSN Numbers: Print, 0031-4005;
Online, 1098-4275). Copyright © 2006 by the
American Academy of Pediatrics

are reviewed, as is the potential role of complementary and alternative medicine (CAM).

The goal of this guideline is to provide an evidence-based approach to the diagnosis, management, and prevention of bronchiolitis in children from 1 month to 2 years of age. The guideline is intended for pediatricians, family physicians, emergency medicine specialists, hospitalists, nurse practitioners, and physician assistants who care for these children. The guideline does not apply to children with immunodeficiencies including HIV, organ or bone marrow transplants, or congenital immunodeficiencies. Children with underlying respiratory illnesses such as chronic neonatal lung disease (CLD; also known as bronchopulmonary dysplasia) and those with significant congenital heart disease are excluded from the sections on management unless otherwise noted but are included in the discussion of prevention. This guideline will not address long-term sequelae of bronchiolitis, such as recurrent wheezing, which is a field with distinct literature of its own.

Bronchiolitis is a disorder most commonly caused in infants by viral lower respiratory tract infection (LRTI). It is the most common lower respiratory infection in this age group. It is characterized by acute inflammation, edema and necrosis of epithelial cells lining small airways, increased mucus production, and bronchospasm. Signs and symptoms are typically rhinitis, tachypnea, wheezing, cough, crackles, use of accessory muscles, and/or nasal flaring.[1] Many viruses cause the same constellation of symptoms and signs. The most common etiology is the respiratory syncytial virus (RSV), with the highest incidence of RSV infection occurring between December and March.[2] Ninety percent of children are infected with RSV in the first 2 years of life,[3] and up to 40% of them will have lower respiratory infection.[4,5] Infection with RSV does not grant permanent or long-term immunity. Reinfections are common and may be experienced throughout life.[6] Other viruses identified as causing bronchiolitis are human metapneumovirus, influenza, adenovirus, and parainfluenza. RSV infection leads to more than 90 000 hospitalizations annually. Mortality resulting from RSV has decreased from 4500 deaths annually in 1985 in the United States[2,6] to an estimated 510 RSV-associated deaths in 1997[6] and 390 in 1999.[7] The cost of hospitalization for bronchiolitis in children less than 1 year old is estimated to be more than $700 million per year.[8]

Several studies have shown a wide variation in how bronchiolitis is diagnosed and treated. Studies in the United States,[9] Canada,[10] and the Netherlands[11] showed variations that correlated more with hospital or individual preferences than with patient severity. In addition, length of hospitalization in some countries averages twice that of others.[12] This variable pattern suggests a lack of consensus among clinicians as to best practices.

In addition to morbidity and mortality during the acute illness, infants hospitalized with bronchiolitis are more likely to have respiratory problems as older children, especially recurrent wheezing, compared with those who did not have severe disease.[13–15] Severe disease is characterized by persistently increased respiratory effort, apnea, or the need for intravenous hydration, supplemental oxygen, or mechanical ventilation. It is unclear whether severe viral illness early in life predisposes children to develop recurrent wheezing or if infants who experience severe bronchiolitis have an underlying predisposition to recurrent wheezing.

METHODS

To develop the clinical practice guideline on the diagnosis and management of bronchiolitis, the American Academy of Pediatrics (AAP) convened the Subcommittee on Diagnosis and Management of Bronchiolitis with the support of the American Academy of Family Physicians (AAFP), the American Thoracic Society, the American College of Chest Physicians, and the European Respiratory Society. The subcommittee was chaired by a primary care pediatrician with expertise in clinical pulmonology and included experts in the fields of general pediatrics, pulmonology, infectious disease, emergency medicine, epidemiology, and medical informatics. All panel members reviewed the AAP Policy on Conflict of Interest and Voluntary Disclosure and were given an opportunity to declare any potential conflicts.

The AAP and AAFP partnered with the AHRQ and the RTI International-University of North Carolina Evidence-Based Practice Center (EPC) to develop an evidence report, which served as a major source of information for these practice guideline recommendations.[1] Specific clinical questions addressed in the AHRQ evidence report were the (1) effectiveness of diagnostic tools for diagnosing bronchiolitis in infants and children, (2) efficacy of pharmaceutical therapies for treatment of bronchiolitis, (3) role of prophylaxis in prevention of bronchiolitis, and (4) cost-effectiveness of prophylaxis for management of bronchiolitis. EPC project staff searched Medline, the Cochrane Collaboration, and the Health Economics Database. Additional articles were identified by review of reference lists of relevant articles and ongoing studies recommended by a technical expert advisory group. To answer the question on diagnosis, both prospective studies and randomized, controlled trials (RCTs) were used. For questions related to treatment and prophylaxis in the AHRQ report, only RCTs were considered. For the cost-effectiveness of prophylaxis, studies that used economic analysis were reviewed. For all studies, key inclusion criteria included outcomes that were both clinically relevant and able to be abstracted. Initially, 744 abstracts were identified for possible inclusion, of which 83 were retained for systematic review. Results of the literature review were presented in evidence tables and published in the final evidence report.[1]

An additional literature search of Medline and the Cochrane Database of Systematic Reviews was performed in July 2004 by using search terms submitted by the members of the Subcommittee on the Diagnosis and Management of Bronchiolitis. The methodologic quality of the research was appraised by an epidemiologist before consideration by the subcommittee.

The evidence-based approach to guideline development requires that the evidence in support of a policy be identified, appraised, and summarized and that an explicit link between evidence and recommendations be defined. Evidence-based recommendations reflect the quality of evidence and the balance of benefit and harm that is anticipated when the recommendation is followed. The AAP policy statement "Classifying Recommendations for Clinical Practice Guidelines"[16] was followed in designating levels of recommendation (Fig 1; Table 1).

A draft version of this clinical practice guideline underwent extensive peer review by committees and sections within the AAP, American Thoracic Society, European Respiratory Society, American College of Chest Physicians, and AAFP, outside organizations, and other individuals identified by the subcommittee as experts in the field. Members of the subcommittee were invited to distribute the draft to other representatives and committees within their specialty organizations. The resulting comments were reviewed by the subcommittee and, when appropriate, incorporated into the guideline.

This clinical practice guideline is not intended as a sole source of guidance in the management of children with bronchiolitis. Rather, it is intended to assist clinicians in decision-making. It is not intended to replace clinical judgment or establish a protocol for the care of all children with this condition. These recommendations may not provide the only appropriate approach to the management of children with bronchiolitis.

All AAP guidelines are reviewed every 5 years.

Definitions used in the guideline are:

- Bronchiolitis: a disorder most commonly caused in infants by viral LRTI; it is the most common lower respiratory infection in this age group and is characterized by acute inflammation, edema and necrosis of epithelial cells lining small airways, increased mucus production, and bronchospasm.

- CLD, also known as bronchopulmonary dysplasia: an infant less than 32 weeks' gestation evaluated at 36 weeks' postmenstrual age or one of more than 32 weeks' gestation evaluated at more than 28 days but less than 56 days of age who has been receiving supplemental oxygen for more than 28 days.[17]

- Routine: a set of customary and often-performed procedures such as might be found in a routine admission order set for children with bronchiolitis.

- Severe disease: signs and symptoms associated with poor feeding and respiratory distress characterized by tachypnea, nasal flaring, and hypoxemia.

- Hemodynamically significant congenital heart disease: children with congenital heart disease who are receiving medication to control congestive heart failure, have moderate to severe pulmonary hypertension, or have cyanotic heart disease.

RECOMMENDATION 1a

Clinicians should diagnose bronchiolitis and assess disease severity on the basis of history and physical examination. Clinicians should not routinely order laboratory and radiologic studies for diagnosis (recommendation: evidence level B; diagnostic studies with minor limitations and observational studies with consistent findings; preponderance of benefits over harms and cost).

RECOMMENDATION 1b

Clinicians should assess risk factors for severe disease such as age less than 12 weeks, a history of prematurity, underlying cardiopulmonary disease, or immunodeficiency when making decisions about evaluation and management of children with bronchiolitis (recommendation: evidence level B; observational studies with consistent findings; preponderance of benefits over harms).

The 2 goals in the history and physical examination of infants presenting with cough and/or wheeze, particularly in the winter season, are the differentiation of infants with probable bronchiolitis from those with other disorders and the estimation of the severity of illness. Most clinicians recognize bronchiolitis as a constellation of clinical symptoms and signs including a viral upper respiratory prodrome followed by increased respi-

Evidence quality	Preponderance of benefit or harm	Balance of benefit and harm
A. Well-designed RCTs or diagnostic studies on relevant populations	Strong recommendation	Option
B. RCTs or diagnostic studies with minor limitations; overwhelmingly consistent evidence from observational studies		
C. Observational studies (case-control and cohort design)	Recommendation	
D. Expert opinion, case reports, reasoning from first principles	Option	No recommendation

X. Exceptional situations in which validating studies cannot be performed and there is a clear preponderance of benefit or harm	Strong recommendation
	Recommendation

FIGURE 1

Integrating evidence quality appraisal with an assessment of the anticipated balance between benefits and harms if a policy is carried out leads to designation of a policy as a strong recommendation, recommendation, option, or no recommendation.

TABLE 1	Guideline Definitions for Evidence-Based Statements	
Statement	Definition	Implication
Strong recommendation	A strong recommendation in favor of a particular action is made when the anticipated benefits of the recommended intervention clearly exceed the harms (as a strong recommendation against an action is made when the anticipated harms clearly exceed the benefits) and the quality of the supporting evidence is excellent. In some clearly identified circumstances, strong recommendations may be made when high-quality evidence is impossible to obtain and the anticipated benefits strongly outweigh the harms.	Clinicians should follow a strong recommendation unless a clear and compelling rationale for an alternative approach is present.
Recommendation	A recommendation in favor of a particular action is made when the anticipated benefits exceed the harms but the quality of evidence is not as strong. Again, in some clearly identified circumstances, recommendations may be made when high-quality evidence is impossible to obtain but the anticipated benefits outweigh the harms.	Clinicians would be prudent to follow a recommendation but should remain alert to new information and sensitive to patient preferences.
Option	Options define courses that may be taken when either the quality of evidence is suspect or carefully performed studies have shown little clear advantage to one approach over another.	Clinicians should consider the option in their decision-making, and patient preference may have a substantial role.
No recommendation	No recommendation indicates that there is a lack of pertinent published evidence and that the anticipated balance of benefits and harms is presently unclear.	Clinicians should be alert to new published evidence that clarifies the balance of benefit versus harm.

ratory effort and wheezing in children less than 2 years of age. Clinical signs and symptoms of bronchiolitis consist of rhinorrhea, cough, wheezing, tachypnea, and increased respiratory effort manifested as grunting, nasal flaring, and intercostal and/or subcostal retractions.

Respiratory rate in otherwise healthy children changes considerably over the first year of life, decreasing from a mean of approximately 50 breaths per minute in term newborns to approximately 40 breaths per minute at 6 months of age and 30 breaths per minute at 12 months.[18–20] Counting respiratory rate over the course of 1 minute may be more accurate than measurements extrapolated to 1 minute but observed for shorter periods.[21] The absence of tachypnea correlates with the lack of LRTIs or pneumonia (viral or bacterial) in infants.[22,23]

The course of bronchiolitis is variable and dynamic, ranging from transient events such as apnea or mucus plugging to progressive respiratory distress from lower airway obstruction. Important issues to assess include the impact of respiratory symptoms on feeding and hydration and the response, if any, to therapy. The ability of the family to care for the child and return for further care should be assessed. History of underlying conditions such as prematurity, cardiac or pulmonary disease, immunodeficiency, or previous episodes of wheezing should be identified.

The physical examination reflects the variability in the disease state and may require serial observations over time to fully assess the child's status. Upper airway obstruction may contribute to work of breathing. Nasal suctioning and positioning of the child may affect the assessment. Physical examination findings of importance

include respiratory rate, increased work of breathing as evidenced by accessory muscle use or retractions, and auscultatory findings such as wheezes or crackles.

The evidence relating the presence of specific findings in the assessment of bronchiolitis to clinical outcomes is limited. Most studies are retrospective and lack valid and unbiased measurement of baseline and outcome variables. Most studies designed to identify the risk of severe adverse outcomes such as requirement for intensive care or mechanical ventilation have focused on inpatients.[24–26] These events are relatively rare among all children with bronchiolitis and limit the power of these studies to detect clinically important risk factors associated with disease progression.

Several studies have associated premature birth (less than 37 weeks) and young age of the child (less than 6–12 weeks) with an increased risk of severe disease.[26–28] Young infants with bronchiolitis may develop apnea, which has been associated with an increased risk for prolonged hospitalization, admission to intensive care, and mechanical ventilation.[26] Other underlying conditions that have been associated with an increased risk of progression to severe disease or mortality include hemodynamically significant congenital heart disease,[26,29] chronic lung disease (bronchopulmonary dysplasia, cystic fibrosis, congenital anomaly),[26] and the presence of an immunocompromised state.[26,30]

Findings on physical examination have been less consistently associated with outcomes of bronchiolitis. Tachypnea, defined as a respiratory rate of 70 or more breaths per minute, has been associated with increased risk for severe disease in some studies[24,27,31] but not others.[32] An AHRQ report[1] found 43 of 52 treatment trials that used clinical scores, all of which included measures of respiratory rate, respiratory effort, severity of wheezing, and oxygenation. The lack of uniformity of scoring systems made comparison between studies difficult.[1] The most widely used clinical score, the Respiratory Distress Assessment Instrument,[33] is reliable with respect to scoring but has not been validated for clinical predictive value in bronchiolitis. None of the other clinical scores used in the various studies have been assessed for reliability and validity. Studies that have assessed other physical examination findings have not found clinically useful associations with outcomes.[27,32] The substantial temporal variability in physical findings as well as potential differences in response to therapy may account for this lack of association. Repeated observation over a period of time rather than a single examination may provide a more valid overall assessment.

Pulse oximetry has been rapidly adopted into clinical assessment of children with bronchiolitis on the basis of data suggesting that it can reliably detect hypoxemia that is not suspected on physical examination.[27,34] Few studies have assessed the effectiveness of pulse oximetry to predict clinical outcomes. Among inpatients, perceived need for supplemental oxygen that is based on pulse oximetry has been associated with higher risk of prolonged hospitalization, ICU admission, and mechanical ventilation.[24,26,35] Among outpatients, available evidence differs on whether mild reductions in pulse oximetry (less than 95% on room air) predict progression of disease or need for a return visit for care.[27,32]

Radiography may be useful when the hospitalized child does not improve at the expected rate, if the severity of disease requires further evaluation, or if another diagnosis is suspected. Although many infants with bronchiolitis have abnormalities that show on chest radiographs, data are insufficient to demonstrate that chest radiograph abnormalities correlate well with disease severity.[16] Two studies suggest that the presence of consolidation and atelectasis on a chest radiograph is associated with increased risk for severe disease.[26,27] One study showed no correlation between chest radiograph findings and baseline severity of disease.[36] In prospective studies including 1 randomized trial, children with suspected LRTI who received radiographs were more likely to receive antibiotics without any difference in time to recovery.[37,38] Current evidence does not support routine radiography in children with bronchiolitis.

The clinical utility of diagnostic testing in infants with suspected bronchiolitis is not well supported by evidence.[39–41] The occurrence of serious bacterial infections (SBIs; eg, urinary tract infections [UTIs], sepsis, meningitis) is very low.[42,43] The use of complete blood counts has not been shown to be useful in either diagnosing bronchiolitis or guiding its therapy.[1]

Virologic tests for RSV, if obtained during peak RSV season, demonstrate a high predictive value. However, the knowledge gained from such testing rarely alters management decisions or outcomes for the vast majority of children with clinically diagnosed bronchiolitis.[1] Virologic testing may be useful when cohorting of patients is feasible.

Evidence Profile 1a: Diagnosis

- Aggregate evidence quality: B; diagnostic studies with minor limitations and observational studies with consistent findings
- Benefit: cost saving, limitation of radiation and blood tests
- Harm: risk of misdiagnosis
- Benefits-harms assessment: preponderance of benefit over harm
- Policy level: recommendation

Evidence Profile 1b: Risk Factors

- Aggregate evidence quality: B; observational studies with consistent findings
- Benefit: improved care of patients with risk factors for severe disease
- Harm: increased costs, increased radiation and blood testing
- Benefits-harms assessment: preponderance of benefit over harm
- Policy level: recommendation

RECOMMENDATION 2a

Bronchodilators should not be used routinely in the management of bronchiolitis (recommendation: evidence level B; RCTs with limitations; preponderance of harm of use over benefit).

RECOMMENDATION 2b

A carefully monitored trial of α-adrenergic or β-adrenergic medication is an option. Inhaled bronchodilators should be continued only if there is a documented positive clinical response to the trial using an objective means of evaluation (option: evidence level B; RCTs with limitations and expert opinion; balance of benefit and harm).

The use of bronchodilator agents continues to be controversial. RCTs have failed to demonstrate a consistent benefit from α-adrenergic or β-adrenergic agents. Several studies and reviews have evaluated the use of bronchodilator medications for viral bronchiolitis. A Cochrane systematic review[44] found 8 RCTs involving 394 children.[33,45–50] Some of the studies included infants who had a history of previous wheezing. Several used agents other than albuterol/salbutamol or epinephrine/adrenaline (eg, ipratropium and metaproterenol). Overall, results of the meta-analysis indicated that, at most, 1 in 4 children treated with bronchodilators might have a transient improvement in clinical score of unclear clinical significance. This needs to be weighed against the potential adverse effects and cost of these agents and the fact that most children treated with bronchodilators will not benefit from their use. Studies assessing the impact of bronchodilators on long-term outcomes have found no impact on the overall course of the illness.[1,44,51]

Albuterol/Salbutamol

Some outpatient studies have demonstrated modest improvement in oxygen saturation and/or clinical scores. Schweich et al[52] and Schuh et al[53] evaluated clinical scores and oxygen saturation after 2 treatments of nebulized albuterol. Each study showed improvement in the clinical score and oxygen saturation shortly after completion of the treatment. Neither measured outcomes over time. Klassen et al[47] evaluated clinical score and oxygen saturation 30 and 60 minutes after a single salbutamol treatment. Clinical score, but not oxygen saturation, was significantly improved at 30 minutes, but no difference was demonstrated 60 minutes after a treatment. Gadomski et al[54] showed no difference between those in groups on albuterol or placebo after 2 nebulized treatments given 30 minutes apart.

Studies of inpatients have not shown a clinical change that would justify recommending albuterol for routine care. Dobson et al[55] conducted a randomized clinical trial in infants who were hospitalized with moderately severe viral bronchiolitis and failed to demonstrate clinical improvement resulting in enhanced recovery or an attenuation of the severity of illness. Two meta-analyses[1,56] could not directly compare inpatient studies of albuterol because of widely differing methodology. Overall, the studies reviewed did not show the use of albuterol in infants with bronchiolitis to be beneficial in shortening duration of illness or length of hospital stay.

Epinephrine/Adrenaline

The AHRQ evidence report[1] notes that the reviewed studies show that nebulized epinephrine has "some potential for being efficacious." In contrast, a later multi-center controlled trial by Wainwright et al[51] concluded that epinephrine did not impact the overall course of the illness as measured by hospital length of stay. Analysis of outpatient studies favors nebulized epinephrine over placebo in terms of clinical score, oxygen saturation, and respiratory rate at 60 minutes[57] and heart rate at 90 minutes.[58] However, the differences were small, and it could not be established that they are clinically significant in altering the course of the illness. One study[59] found significant improvement in airway resistance (but no change in oxygen need), suggesting that a trial of this agent may be reasonable for such infants.

Several studies have compared epinephrine to albuterol (salbutamol) or epinephrine to placebo. Racemic epinephrine has demonstrated slightly better clinical effect than albuterol. It is possible that the improvement is related to the α effect of the medication.[60] Hartling et al[61] performed a meta-analysis of studies comparing epinephrine to albuterol and also participated in the Cochrane review of epinephrine.[62] The Cochrane report concluded: "There is insufficient evidence to support the use of epinephrine for the treatment of bronchiolitis among inpatients. There is some evidence to suggest that epinephrine may be favorable to salbutamol (albuterol) and placebo among outpatients."

Although there is no evidence from RCTs to justify routine use of bronchodilators, clinical experience suggests that, in selected infants, there is an improvement in the clinical condition after bronchodilator administration.[47,52,53,57,58] It may be reasonable to administer a nebulized bronchodilator and evaluate clinical response. Individuals and institutions should assess the patient and document pretherapy and posttherapy changes using an objective means of evaluation. Some of the documentation tools that have been used can be found in articles by Alario et al,[45] Bierman and Pierson,[63] Gadomski et al,[54] Lowell et al,[33] Wainwright et al,[51] Schuh et al,[64] and Gorelick et al.[65] In addition, a documentation tool has been developed by Cincinnati Children's Hospital (Cincinnati, OH).[66]

Extrapolation from the studies discussed above suggests that epinephrine may be the preferred bronchodilator for this trial in the emergency department and in hospitalized patients. In the event that there is documented clinical improvement, there is justification for continuing the nebulized bronchodilator treatments. In the absence of a clinical response, the treatment should not be continued.

Because of a lack of studies, short duration of action, and potential adverse effects, epinephrine is usually not used in the home setting. Therefore, it would be more appropriate that a bronchodilator trial in the office or clinic setting use albuterol/salbutamol rather than racemic epinephrine. Parameters to measure its effectiveness include improvements in wheezing, respiratory rate, respiratory effort, and oxygen saturation.

Anticholinergic agents such as ipratropium have not been shown to alter the course of viral bronchiolitis. Although a minority of individual patients may show a positive clinical response to anticholinergic agents, studies have shown that the groups as a whole showed no significant improvement. At this point there is no justification for using anticholinergic agents, either alone or in combination with β-adrenergic agents, for viral bronchiolitis.[67–69]

Evidence Profile 2a: Routine Use of Bronchodilators

- Aggregate evidence quality: B; RCTs with limitations
- Benefit: short-term improvement in clinical symptoms

- Harm: adverse effects, cost of medications, cost to administer
- Benefits-harms assessment: preponderance of harm over benefit
- Policy level: recommendation

Evidence Profile 2b: Trial of Bronchodilators

- Aggregate evidence quality: B; RCTs with limitations
- Benefit: some patients with significant symptomatic improvement
- Harm: adverse effects, cost of medications, cost to administer
- Benefits-harms assessment: preponderance of benefit over harm in select patients
- Policy level: option

RECOMMENDATION 3

Corticosteroid medications should not be used routinely in the management of bronchiolitis (recommendation: evidence level B; based on RCTs with limitations and a preponderance of risk over benefit).

Reports indicate that up to 60% of infants admitted to the hospital for bronchiolitis receive corticosteroid therapy.[9,12,70] Systematic review and meta-analyses of RCTs involving close to 1200 children with viral bronchiolitis have not shown sufficient evidence to support the use of steroids in this illness.[1,71,72]

A Cochrane database review on the use of glucocorticoids for acute bronchiolitis[71] included 13 studies.[37,50,64,73–82] The 1198 patients showed a pooled decrease in length of stay of 0.38 days. However, this decrease was not statistically significant. The review concluded: "No benefits were found in either LOS [length of stay] or clinical score in infants and young children treated with systemic glucocorticoids as compared with placebo. There were no differences in these outcomes between treatment groups; either in the pooled analysis or in any of the sub analyses. Among the three studies evaluating hospital admission rates following the initial hospital visit there was no difference between treatment groups. There were no differences found in respiratory rate, hemoglobin oxygen saturation, or hospital revisit or readmission rates. Subgroup analyses were significantly limited by the low number of studies in each comparison. Specific data on the harm of corticosteroid therapy in this patient population are lacking. Available evidence suggests that corticosteroid therapy is not of benefit in this patient group."[71]

The 2 available studies that evaluated inhaled corticosteroids in bronchiolitis[83,84] showed no benefit in the course of the acute disease. Because the safety of high-dose inhaled corticosteroids in infants is still not clear,

their use should be avoided unless there is a clear likelihood of benefit.

There are insufficient data to make a recommendation regarding the use of leukotriene modifiers in bronchiolitis. Until additional randomized clinical trials are completed, no conclusions can be drawn.

Evidence Profile 3: Corticosteroids

- Aggregate evidence quality: B; randomized clinical trials with limitations
- Benefit: possibility that corticosteroid may be of some benefit
- Harm: exposure to unnecessary medication
- Benefits-harms assessment: preponderance of harm over benefit
- Policy level: recommendation

RECOMMENDATION 4

Ribavirin should not be used routinely in children with bronchiolitis (recommendation: evidence level B; RCTs with limitations and observational studies; preponderance of harm over benefit).

The indications for specific antiviral therapy for bronchiolitis are controversial. A recent review of 11 randomized clinical trials of ribavirin therapy for RSV LRTIs, including bronchiolitis, summarized the reported outcomes.[85] Nine of the studies measured the effect of ribavirin in the acute phase of illness.[86–94] Two evaluated the effect on long-term wheezing and/or pulmonary function.[95,96] Three additional studies were identified with similar results. Two of these evaluated effectiveness in the acute phase[97,98] and one on subsequent respiratory status.[99]

Each of the 11 studies that addressed the acute treatment effects of ribavirin included a small sample size ranging from 26 to 53 patients and cumulatively totaling 375 subjects. Study designs and outcomes measured were varied and inconsistent. Seven of the trials demonstrated some improvement in outcome attributed to ribavirin therapy, and 4 did not. Of those showing benefit, 4 documented improved objective outcomes (eg, better oxygenation, shorter length of stay), and 3 reported improvement in subjective findings such as respiratory scores or subjective clinical assessment. The quality of the studies was highly variable.

Of the studies that focused on long-term pulmonary function, one was an RCT assessing the number of subsequent wheezing episodes and LRTIs over a 1-year period.[96] Two others were follow-up studies of previous randomized trials and measured subsequent pulmonary function as well as wheezing episodes.[95,99] The first study[96] found fewer episodes of wheezing and infections in the ribavirin-treated patients, and the latter 2 studies[95,99] found no significant differences between groups.

No randomized studies of other antiviral therapies of bronchiolitis were identified.

Specific antiviral therapy for RSV bronchiolitis remains controversial because of the marginal benefit, if any, for most patients. In addition, cumbersome delivery requirements,[100] potential health risks for caregivers,[101] and high cost[102] serve as disincentives for use in the majority of patients. Nevertheless, ribavirin may be considered for use in highly selected situations involving documented RSV bronchiolitis with severe disease or in those who are at risk for severe disease (eg, immunocompromised and/or hemodynamically significant cardiopulmonary disease).

Evidence Profile 4: Ribavirin

- Aggregate evidence quality: B; RCTs with limitations and observational studies

- Benefit: some improvement in outcome

- Harm: cost, delivery method, potential health risks to caregivers

- Benefits-harms assessment: preponderance of harm over benefit

- Policy level: recommendation

RECOMMENDATION 5

Antibacterial medications should be used only in children with bronchiolitis who have specific indications of the coexistence of a bacterial infection. When present, bacterial infection should be treated in the same manner as in the absence of bronchiolitis (recommendation: evidence level B; RCTs and observational studies; preponderance of benefit over harm).

Children with bronchiolitis frequently receive antibacterial therapy because of fever,[103] young age,[104] or the concern over secondary bacterial infection.[105] Early RCTs[106,107] showed no benefit from antibacterial treatment of bronchiolitis. However, concern remains regarding the possibility of bacterial infections in young infants with bronchiolitis; thus, antibacterial agents continue to be used.

Several retrospective studies[41,108–113] identified low rates of SBI (0%–3.7%) in patients with bronchiolitis and/or infections with RSV. When SBI was present, it was more likely to be a UTI than bacteremia or meningitis. In a study of 2396 infants with RSV bronchiolitis, 69% of the 39 patients with SBI had a UTI.[110]

Three prospective studies of SBI in patients with bronchiolitis and/or RSV infections also demonstrated low rates of SBI (1%–12%).[42,43,114] One large study of febrile infants less than 60 days of age[43] with bronchiolitis and/or RSV infections demonstrated that the overall risk of SBI in infants less than 28 days of age, although significant, was not different between RSV-positive and RSV-negative groups (10.1% and 14.2%, respectively). All SBIs in children between 29 and 60 days of age with RSV-positive bronchiolitis were UTIs. The rate of UTIs in RSV-positive patients between 28 and 60 days old was significantly lower than those who were RSV-negative (5.5% vs 11.7%).

Approximately 25% of hospitalized infants with bronchiolitis will have radiographic evidence of atelectasis or infiltrates, often misinterpreted as possible bacterial infection.[115] Bacterial pneumonia in infants with bronchiolitis without consolidation is unusual.[116]

Although acute otitis media (AOM) in bronchiolitic infants may be caused by RSV alone, there are no clinical features that permit viral AOM to be differentiated from bacterial. Two studies address the frequency of AOM in patients with bronchiolitis. Andrade et al[117] prospectively identified AOM in 62% of 42 patients who presented with bronchiolitis. AOM was present in 50% on entry to the study and developed in an additional 12% within 10 days. Bacterial pathogens were isolated from 94% of middle-ear aspirates, with *Streptococcus pneumoniae*, *Haemophilus influenzae*, and *Moraxella catarrhalis* being the most frequent isolates. A subsequent report[118] followed 150 children hospitalized for bronchiolitis for the development of AOM. Seventy-nine (53%) developed AOM, two thirds within the first 2 days of hospitalization. Tympanocentesis was performed on 64 children with AOM, and 33 middle-ear aspirates yielded pathogens. *H influenzae*, *S pneumoniae*, and *M catarrhalis* were the ones most commonly found. AOM did not influence the clinical course or laboratory findings of bronchiolitis. When found, AOM should be managed according to the AAP/AAFP guidelines for diagnosis and management of AOM.[119]

Evidence Profile 5: Antibacterial Therapy

- Aggregate evidence quality: B; RCTs and observational studies with consistent results

- Benefit: appropriate treatment of bacterial infections, decreased exposure to unnecessary medications and their adverse effects when a bacterial infection is not present, decreased risk of development of resistant bacteria

- Harm: potential to not treat patient with bacterial infection

- Benefits-harms assessment: preponderance of benefit over harm

- Policy level: recommendation

RECOMMENDATION 6a

Clinicians should assess hydration and ability to take fluids orally (strong recommendation: evidence level X; validating studies cannot be performed; clear preponderance of benefit over harm).

RECOMMENDATION 6b

Chest physiotherapy should not be used routinely in the management of bronchiolitis (recommendation: evidence level B; RCTs with limitations; preponderance of harm over benefit).

The level of respiratory distress caused by bronchiolitis guides the indications for use of other treatments.

Intravenous Fluids

Infants with mild respiratory distress may require only observation, particularly if feeding remains unaffected. When the respiratory rate exceeds 60 to 70 breaths per minute, feeding may be compromised, particularly if nasal secretions are copious. Infants with respiratory difficulty may develop nasal flaring, increased intercostal or sternal retractions, and prolonged expiratory wheezing and be at increased risk of aspiration of food into the lungs.[120] Children who have difficulty feeding safely because of respiratory distress should be given intravenous fluids. The possibility of fluid retention related to production of antidiuretic hormone has been reported in patients with bronchiolitis.[121,122] Clinicians should adjust fluid management accordingly.

Airway Clearance

Bronchiolitis is associated with airway edema and sloughing of the respiratory epithelium into airways, which results in generalized hyperinflation of the lungs. Lobar atelectasis is not characteristic of this disease, although it can be seen on occasion. A Cochrane review[123] found 3 RCTs that evaluated chest physiotherapy in hospitalized patients with bronchiolitis.[124–126] No clinical benefit was found using vibration and percussion techniques. Suctioning of the nares may provide temporary relief of nasal congestion. There is no evidence to support routine "deep" suctioning of the lower pharynx or larynx.

Evidence Profile 6a: Fluids

- Aggregate evidence quality: evidence level X; validating studies cannot be performed
- Benefit: prevention of dehydration
- Harm: overhydration, especially if syndrome of inappropriate secretion of antidiuretic hormone (SIADH) is present
- Benefits-harms assessment: clear preponderance of benefit over harm
- Policy level: strong recommendation

Evidence Profile 6b: Chest Physiotherapy

- Aggregate evidence quality: B; RCTs with limitations
- Benefit: clearance of secretions, prevention of atelectasis

- Harm: stress to infant during procedure, cost of administering chest physiotherapy
- Benefits-harms assessment: preponderance of harm over benefit
- Policy level: recommendation

RECOMMENDATION 7a

Supplemental oxygen is indicated if oxyhemoglobin saturation (Sp_{O_2}) falls persistently below 90% in previously healthy infants. If the Sp_{O_2} does persistently fall below 90%, adequate supplemental oxygen should be used to maintain Sp_{O_2} at or above 90%. Oxygen may be discontinued if Sp_{O_2} is at or above 90% and the infant is feeding well and has minimal respiratory distress (option: evidence level D; expert opinion and reasoning from first principles; some benefit over harm).

RECOMMENDATION 7b

As the child's clinical course improves, continuous measurement of Sp_{O_2} is not routinely needed (option: evidence level D; expert opinion; balance of benefit and harm).

RECOMMENDATION 7c

Infants with a known history of hemodynamically significant heart or lung disease and premature infants require close monitoring as the oxygen is being weaned (strong recommendation: evidence level B; observational studies with consistent findings; preponderance of benefit over harm).

Healthy infants have an Sp_{O_2} greater than 95% on room air, although transient decreases to an Sp_{O_2} of less than 89% occur.[127,128] In bronchiolitis, airway edema and sloughing of respiratory epithelial cells cause mismatching of ventilation and perfusion and subsequent reductions in oxygenation (Pa_{O_2} and Sp_{O_2}).

In the clinical setting, pulse oximeters are convenient, safe tools to measure oxygenation status. Clinicians ordering pulse oximetry should understand that the shape of the oxyhemoglobin dissociation curve dictates that when Sp_{O_2} is above 90%, large increases in Pa_{O_2} are associated with small increases in Sp_{O_2}. In contrast, when Sp_{O_2} is below 90%, a small decrease in Pa_{O_2} is associated with large decreases in Sp_{O_2} (Fig 2). This raises the question of whether there is a single value for Sp_{O_2} that can serve as a decision point to hospitalize or initiate supplemental oxygen in infants with bronchiolitis.

In studies that examined treatment for bronchiolitis in hospitalized infants, some investigators started supplemental oxygen when Sp_{O_2} fell below 90%, and others started oxygen before the Sp_{O_2} reached 90%.[98,129]

Although data are lacking to codify a single value of Sp_{O_2} to be used as a cutoff point for initiating or discontinuing supplemental oxygen, these studies and the relationship between Pa_{O_2} and Sp_{O_2} support the position that otherwise healthy infants with bronchiolitis who have Sp_{O_2} at or above 90% at sea level while breathing

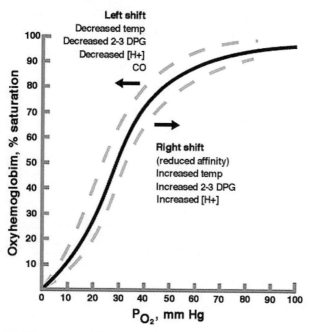

FIGURE 2
Oxyhemoglobin dissociation curve showing percent saturation of hemoglobin at various partial pressures of oxygen. Note that the position of the curve and the affinity of hemoglobin for oxygen changes with changing physiologic conditions. (Reproduced with permission from the educational website www.anaesthesiauk.com.)

room air likely gain little benefit from increasing Pao_2 with supplemental oxygen, particularly in the absence of respiratory distress and feeding difficulties. Because several factors including fever, acidosis, and some hemoglobinopathies shift the oxyhemoglobin dissociation curve so that large decreases in Pao_2 begin to occur at an Spo_2 of more than 90%, clinicians should consider maintaining a higher Spo_2 in children with these risk factors.[130,131]

Although widely used pulse oximeters have some shortcomings, under normal circumstances the accuracy of Spo_2 may vary slightly (most oximeters are accurate to ±2%). More importantly, poorly placed probes and motion artifact will lead to inaccurate measurements and false readings and alarms.[132] Before instituting O_2 therapy, the accuracy of the initial reading should be verified by repositioning the probe and repeating the measurement. The infant's nose and, if necessary, oral airway should be suctioned. If Spo_2 remains below 90%, O_2 should be administered. The infant's clinical work of breathing should also be assessed and may be considered as a factor in a decision to use oxygen supplementation.

Premature or low birth weight infants and infants with bronchopulmonary dysplasia or hemodynamically significant congenital heart disease merit special attention because they are at risk to develop severe illness that requires hospitalization, often in the ICU.[7,29,133–135] These infants often have abnormal baseline oxygenation coupled with an inability to cope with the pulmonary inflammation seen in bronchiolitis. This can result in more severe and prolonged hypoxia compared with nor-

mal infants, and clinicians should take this into account when developing strategies for using and weaning supplemental oxygen.

Evidence Profile 7a: Supplemental Oxygen

- Aggregate evidence quality: D; expert opinion and reasoning from first principles
- Benefit: use of supplemental oxygen only when beneficial, shorter hospitalization
- Harm: inadequate oxygenation
- Benefits-harms assessment: some benefit over harm
- Policy level: option

Evidence Profile 7b: Measurement of Spo_2

- Aggregate evidence quality: D; expert opinion
- Benefit: shorter hospitalization
- Harm: inadequate oxygenation between measurements
- Benefits-harms assessment: some benefit over harm
- Policy level: option

Evidence Profile 7c: High-Risk Infants

- Aggregate evidence quality: B; observational studies with consistent findings
- Benefit: improved care of high-risk infants
- Harm: longer hospitalization, use of oxygen when not beneficial
- Benefits-harms assessment: preponderance of benefit over harm
- Policy level: Strong recommendation

RECOMMENDATION 8a

Clinicians may administer palivizumab prophylaxis to selected infants and children with CLD or a history of prematurity (less than 35 weeks' gestation) or with congenital heart disease (recommendation: evidence level A; RCT; preponderance of benefit over harm).

RECOMMENDATION 8b

When given, prophylaxis with palivizumab should be given in 5 monthly doses, usually beginning in November or December, at a dose of 15 mg/kg per dose administered intramuscularly (recommendation: evidence level C; observational studies and expert opinion; preponderance of benefit over cost).

The 2006 Report of the Committee on Infectious Disease (*Red Book*) included the following recommendations for the use of palivizumab[136]:

- Palivizumab prophylaxis should be considered for infants and children younger than 24 months of age with chronic lung disease of prematurity who have required medical therapy (supplemental oxygen, bronchodilator or diuretic or corticosteroid therapy) for CLD within 6 months before the start of the RSV season. Patients with more severe CLD who continue to require medical therapy may benefit from prophylaxis during a second RSV season. Data are limited regarding the effectiveness of palivizumab during the second year of life. Individual patients may benefit from decisions made in consultation with neonatologists, pediatric intensivists, pulmonologists, or infectious disease specialists.

- Infants born at 32 weeks of gestation or earlier may benefit from RSV prophylaxis, even if they do not have CLD. For these infants, major risk factors to consider include their gestational age and chronologic age at the start of the RSV season. Infants born at 28 weeks of gestation or earlier may benefit from prophylaxis during their first RSV season, whenever that occurs during the first 12 months of life. Infants born at 29 to 32 weeks of gestation may benefit most from prophylaxis up to 6 months of age. For the purpose of this recommendation, 32 weeks' gestation refers to an infant born on or before the 32nd week of gestation (ie, 32 weeks, 0 days). Once a child qualifies for initiation of prophylaxis at the start of the RSV season, administration should continue throughout the season and not stop at the point an infant reaches either 6 months or 12 months of age.

- Although palivizumab has been shown to decrease the likelihood of hospitalization in infants born between 32 and 35 weeks of gestation (ie, between 32 weeks, 1 day and 35 weeks, 0 days), the cost of administering prophylaxis to this large group of infants must be considered carefully. Therefore, most experts recommend that prophylaxis should be reserved for infants in this group who are at greatest risk of severe infection and who are younger than 6 months of age at the start of the RSV season. Epidemiologic data suggest that RSV infection is more likely to lead to hospitalization for these infants when the following risk factor are present: child care attendance, school-aged siblings, exposure to environmental air pollutants, congenital abnormalities of the airways, or severe neuromuscular disease. However, no single risk factor causes a very large increase in the rate of hospitalization, and the risk is additive as the number of risk factors for an individual infant increases. Therefore, prophylaxis should be considered for infants between 32 and 35 weeks of gestation only if 2 or more of these risk factors are present. Passive household exposure to tobacco smoke has not been associated with an increased risk of RSV hospitalization on a consistent basis. Furthermore, exposure to tobacco smoke is a risk factor that can be controlled by the family of an infant at increased risk of severe RSV disease, and

preventive measures will be far less costly than palivizumab prophylaxis. High-risk infants never should be exposed to tobacco smoke. In contrast to the well-documented beneficial effect of breastfeeding against many viral illnesses, existing data are conflicting regarding the specific protective effect of breastfeeding against RSV infection. High-risk infants should be kept away from crowds and from situations in which exposure to infected individuals cannot be controlled. Participation in group child care should be restricted during the RSV season for high-risk infants whenever feasible. Parents should be instructed on the importance of careful hand hygiene. In addition, all high-risk infants and their contacts should be immunized against influenza beginning at 6 months of age.

- In the Northern hemisphere and particularly within the United States, RSV circulates predominantly between November and March. The inevitability of the RSV season is predictable, but the severity of the season, the time of onset, the peak of activity, and the end of the season cannot be predicted precisely. There can be substantial variation in timing of community outbreaks of RSV disease from year to year in the same community and between communities in the same year, even in the same region. These variations, however, occur within the overall pattern of RSV outbreaks, usually beginning in November or December, peaking in January or February, and ending by the end of March or sometime in April. Communities in the southern United States tend to experience the earliest onset of RSV activity, and Midwestern states tend to experience the latest. The duration of the season for western and northeast regions typically occurs between that noted in the South and the Midwest. In recent years, the national median duration of the RSV season has been 15 weeks and even in the South, with a seasonal duration of 16 weeks, the range is 13 to 20 weeks. Results from clinical trials indicate that palivizumab trough serum concentrations >30 days after the fifth dose will be well above the protective concentration for most infants. If the first dose is administered in November, 5 monthly doses of palivizumab will provide substantially more than 20 weeks of protective serum antibody concentrations for most of the RSV season, even with variation in season onset and end. Changes from this recommendation of 5 monthly doses require careful consideration of the benefits and costs.

- Children who are 24 months of age or younger with hemodynamically significant cyanotic and acyanotic congenital heart disease will benefit from palivizumab prophylaxis. Decisions regarding prophylaxis with palivizumab in children with congenital heart disease should be made on the basis of the degree of physiologic cardiovascular compromise. Children younger than 24 months of age with congenital heart disease who are most likely to benefit from immunoprophylaxis include:

- Infants who are receiving medication to control congestive heart failure
- Infants with moderate to severe pulmonary hypertension
- Infants with cyanotic heart disease

Results from 2 blinded, randomized, placebo-controlled trials with palivizumab involving 2789 infants and children with prematurity, CLD, or congenital heart disease demonstrated a reduction in RSV hospitalization rates of 39% to 78% in different groups.[137,138] Results from postlicensure observational studies suggest that monthly immunoprophylaxis may reduce hospitalization rates to an even greater extent than that described in the prelicensure clinical trials.[139] Palivizumab is not effective in the treatment of RSV disease and is not approved for this indication.

Several economic analyses of RSV immunoprophylaxis have been published.[140–147] The primary benefit of immunoprophylaxis with palivizumab is a decrease in the rate of RSV-associated hospitalization. None of the 5 clinical RCTs have demonstrated a significant decrease in rate of mortality attributable to RSV infection in infants who receive prophylaxis. Most of the economic analyses fail to demonstrate overall savings in health care dollars because of the high cost if all at-risk children were to receive prophylaxis. Estimates of cost per hospitalization prevented have been inconsistent because of considerable variation in the baseline rate of hospitalization attributable to RSV in different high-risk groups. Other considerations that will influence results include the effect of prophylaxis on outpatient costs and a resolution of the question of whether prevention of RSV infection in infancy decreases wheezing and lower respiratory tract problems later in childhood.

Evidence Profile 8a: Palivizumab Prophylaxis

- Aggregate evidence quality: A; RCTs
- Benefit: prevention of morbidity and mortality in high-risk infants
- Harm: cost
- Benefits-harms assessment: preponderance of benefit over harm
- Policy level: recommendation

Evidence Profile 8b: Five-Dose Regimen

- Aggregate evidence quality: C; observational studies and expert opinion
- Benefit: decreased cost resulting from using minimal number of needed doses

- Harm: risk of illness from RSV outside the usual season
- Benefits-harms assessment: preponderance of benefit over harm
- Policy level: recommendation

RECOMMENDATION 9a

Hand decontamination is the most important step in preventing nosocomial spread of RSV. Hands should be decontaminated before and after direct contact with patients, after contact with inanimate objects in the direct vicinity of the patient, and after removing gloves (strong recommendation: evidence level B; observational studies with consistent results; strong preponderance of benefit over harm).

RECOMMENDATION 9b

Alcohol-based rubs are preferred for hand decontamination. An alternative is hand-washing with antimicrobial soap (recommendation: evidence level B; observational studies with consistent results; preponderance of benefit over harm).

RECOMMENDATION 9c

Clinicians should educate personnel and family members on hand sanitation (recommendation: evidence level C; observational studies; preponderance of benefit over harm).

Efforts should be made to decrease the spread of RSV and other causative agents of bronchiolitis in medical settings, especially in the hospital. RSV RNA has been identified in air samples as much as 22 feet from the patient's bedside.[148] Secretions from infected patients can be found on beds, crib railings, tabletops, and toys. Organisms on fomites may remain viable and contagious for several hours.[149]

It has been shown that RSV as well as many other viruses can be carried and spread to others on the hands of caregivers.[150] Frequent hand-washing by health care workers has been shown to reduce RSV's nosocomial spread.[150] The Centers for Disease Control and Prevention published an extensive review of the hand-hygiene literature and made recommendations as to indications for hand-washing and hand antisepsis.[151] Among the recommendations are that hands should be decontaminated before and after direct contact with patients, after contact with inanimate objects in the direct vicinity of the patient, and after removing gloves. If hands are not visibly soiled, an alcohol-based rub is preferred. An alternative is to wash hands with an antimicrobial soap. The guideline also describes the appropriate technique for using these products.

Other methods that have been shown to be effective in controlling the spread of RSV are education of personnel and family members; surveillance for the onset of RSV season; use of gloves, with frequent changes to avoid the spread of organisms on the gloves; and wearing gowns for direct contact with the patient. It has not been clearly shown that wearing masks offers additional benefit to the above-listed measures.[149] Isolation and/or cohorting of RSV-positive patients, including assignment of personnel to care only for these patients, is effective[152,153] but may not be feasible. Strict hand decontamination and education of staff and families about prevention of spread of organisms is essential regardless of whether isolation is used.

Programs that implement the above-mentioned principles have been shown to decrease the nosocomial spread of RSV. Johns Hopkins Hospital (Baltimore, MD) instituted a program of pediatric droplet precaution for all children less than 2 years old with respiratory symptoms during RSV season until the child is shown to not have RSV. Nosocomial transmission of RSV decreased by approximately 50%. Before intervention, a patient was 2.6 times more likely to have nosocomially transmitted RSV than after the intervention.[154] A similar program at Children's Hospital of Philadelphia (Philadelphia, PA) resulted in a decrease of nosocomial RSV infections of 39%.[155]

Evidence Profile 9a: Hand Decontamination

- Aggregate evidence quality: B; observational studies with consistent findings
- Benefit: decreased spread of infection
- Harm: time
- Benefits-harms assessment: strong preponderance of benefit over harm
- Policy level: strong recommendation

Evidence Profile 9b: Alcohol-Based Rubs

- Aggregate evidence quality: B; observational studies with consistent findings
- Benefit: decreased spread of infection
- Harm: irritative effect of alcohol-based rubs
- Benefits-harms assessment: preponderance of benefit over harm
- Policy level: recommendation

Evidence Profile 9c: Education

- Aggregate evidence quality: C; observational studies
- Benefit: decreased spread of infection
- Harm: time, cost of gloves and gowns if used, barriers to parental contact with patient
- Benefits-harms assessment: preponderance of benefit over harm
- Policy level: recommendation

RECOMMENDATION 10a

Infants should not be exposed to passive smoking (strong recommendation: evidence level B; observational studies with consistent results; strong preponderance of benefit over harm).

RECOMMENDATION 10b

Breastfeeding is recommended to decrease a child's risk of having lower respiratory tract disease (LRTD) (recommendation: evidence level C; observational studies; preponderance of benefit over harm).

Tobacco Smoke

Passive smoking increases the risk of having an RSV infection with a reported odds ratio of 3.87.[156] There have been numerous studies on the effect of passive smoking on respiratory illness in infants and children. In a systematic review of passive smoking and lower respiratory illness in infants and children, Strachan and Cook[157] showed a pooled odds ratio of 1.57 if either parent smoked and an odds ratio of 1.72 if the mother smoked. Stocks and Dezateux[158] reviewed 20 studies of pulmonary function in infants. These studies showed a significant decrease in pulmonary function in infants of mothers who smoked during and after pregnancy. Forced expiratory flow was decreased by approximately 20%. Other measures of pulmonary function were likewise abnormal.

Paternal smoking also has an effect. The prevalence of upper respiratory tract illness increased from 81.6% to 95.2% in infants under 1 year of age in households where only the father smoked.[159]

Breastfeeding

Breast milk has been shown to have immune factors to RSV including immunoglobulin G and A antibodies[160] and interferon-α.[161] Breast milk has also been shown to have neutralizing activity against RSV.[162] In one study the relative risk of hospital admission with RSV was 2.2 in children who were not being breastfed.[163] In another study, 8 (7%) of 115 children hospitalized with RSV were breastfed, and 46 (27%) of 167 controls were breastfed.[164]

A meta-analysis of the relationship of breastfeeding and hospitalization for LRTD in early infancy[165] examined 33 studies, all of which showed a protective association between breastfeeding and the risk of hospitalization for LRTD. Nine studies met all inclusion criteria for analysis. The conclusion was that infants who were not breastfed had almost a threefold greater risk of being hospitalized for LRTD than those exclusively breastfed for 4 months (risk ratio: 0.28).

Evidence Profile 10a: Secondhand Smoke

- Aggregate evidence quality: B; observational studies with consistent findings
- Benefit: decreased risk of LRTI

- Harm: none
- Benefits-harms assessment: strong preponderance of benefit over harm
- Policy level: strong recommendation

Evidence Profile 10b: Breastfeeding

- Aggregate evidence quality: C; observational studies
- Benefit: improved immunity, decreased risk of LRTI, improved nutrition
- Harm: implied inadequacy of mothers who cannot or prefer to not breastfeed
- Benefits-harms assessment: preponderance of benefit over harm
- Policy level: recommendation

RECOMMENDATION 11

Clinicians should inquire about use of CAM (option: evidence level D; expert opinion; some benefit over harm).

No recommendations for CAM for treatment of bronchiolitis are made because of limited data. Clinicians now recognize that an increasing number of parents/caregivers are using various forms of nonconventional treatment for their children. Treatments that have been used specifically for bronchiolitis include homeopathy, herbal remedies, osteopathic manipulation, and applied kinesiology. Substantially more data are available regarding the use of homeopathic and herbal remedies for the treatment of bronchitis and the common cold. Whether these therapies would prevent the development of bronchiolitis is unknown. A single recent trial indicated that an herbal preparation containing *Echinacea*, propolis, and vitamin C prevented the development of upper respiratory infections in children between the ages of 1 and 5 years.[166] Bronchiolitis was not specifically studied.

To date, there are no studies that conclusively show a beneficial effect of alternative therapies used for the treatment of bronchiolitis. Recent interest in the use of CAM has led to research efforts to investigate its efficacy. It is difficult to design and conduct studies on certain forms of CAM because of the unique nature of the treatment. Any study conducted will need to show proof of effectiveness of a specific therapy when compared with the natural history of the disease. Conclusions regarding CAM cannot be made until research evidence is available. However, because of the widespread use of CAM, clinicians should ask parents what alternative forms of treatment they are using and be ready to discuss potential benefits or risks.

Evidence Profile 11: Asking About CAM

- Aggregate evidence quality: D; expert opinion
- Benefit: improved parent-physician communication,

awareness of other, possibly harmful treatments being used
- Harm: time required for discussion, lack of knowledge about CAM by many pediatricians
- Benefits-harms assessment: some benefit over harm
- Policy level: option

FUTURE RESEARCH

The AHRQ evidence report[1] points out that outcomes measured in future studies of bronchiolitis should be clinically relevant and of interest to parents, clinicians, and health systems. Among the recommended outcomes are rates of hospitalization, need for more intensive services in the hospital, costs of care, and parental satisfaction with treatment.[1] One of the difficulties with the bronchiolitis literature is the absence of validated clinical scoring scales that are objective, replicable, and can be easily be performed in the hospital, emergency department, and outpatient settings. Studies should also be of sufficient size to be able to draw meaningful conclusions for the above-mentioned outcomes. Because bronchiolitis is a self-limited disease, large numbers of patients would need to be enrolled to observe small changes in outcome. This would necessitate large multicenter study protocols. Currently, such multicentered studies are being conducted in the United States and Canada on the use of corticosteroids in the emergency department.

Future research should include:

- development of rapid, cost-effective tests for viruses other than RSV that may also play a role in bronchiolitis;
- studies to determine if there are selected patients who may benefit from bronchodilators or corticosteroids;
- clinical studies of the target Spo_2 for the most efficient use of oxygen and oxygen monitoring;
- development of new therapies including new antiviral medications;
- continued research into the development of an RSV vaccine; and
- continued development of immunoprophylaxis that would require fewer doses and decreased cost.

SUMMARY

This clinical practice guideline provides evidence-based recommendations on the diagnosis and management of bronchiolitis in infants less than 2 years of age. It emphasizes using only diagnostic and management modalities that have been shown to affect clinical outcomes.

Bronchiolitis is a clinical diagnosis that does not require diagnostic testing. Many of the commonly used management modalities have not been shown to be effective in improving the clinical course of the illness. This includes the routine use of bronchodilators, corticosteroids, ribavirin, antibiotics, chest radiography, chest physiotherapy, and complementary and alternative therapies. Options for the appropriate use of oxygen and oxygen monitoring have been presented. Specific prevention with palivizumab and general prevention, particularly the use of hand decontamination to prevent nosocomial spread, were also discussed.

CONCLUSIONS

1a. Clinicians should diagnose bronchiolitis and assess disease severity on the basis of history and physical examination. Clinicians should not routinely order laboratory and radiologic studies for diagnosis (recommendation).

1b. Clinicians should assess risk factors for severe disease such as age less than 12 weeks, a history of prematurity, underlying cardiopulmonary disease, or immunodeficiency when making decisions about evaluation and management of children with bronchiolitis (recommendation).

2a. Bronchodilators should not be used routinely in the management of bronchiolitis (recommendation).

2b. A carefully monitored trial of α-adrenergic or β-adrenergic medication is an option. Inhaled bronchodilators should be continued only if there is a documented positive clinical response to the trial using an objective means of evaluation (option).

3. Corticosteroid medications should not be used routinely in the management of bronchiolitis (recommendation).

4. Ribavirin should not be used routinely in children with bronchiolitis (recommendation).

5. Antibacterial medications should only be used in children with bronchiolitis who have specific indications of the coexistence of a bacterial infection. When present, bacterial infection should be treated in the same manner as in the absence of bronchiolitis (recommendation).

6a. Clinicians should assess hydration and ability to take fluids orally (strong recommendation).

6b. Chest physiotherapy should not be used routinely in the management of bronchiolitis (recommendation).

7a. Supplemental oxygen is indicated if Spo_2 falls persistently below 90% in previously healthy infants. If the Spo_2 does persistently fall below 90%, adequate supplemental oxygen should be used to maintain an Spo_2 at or above 90%. Oxygen may be discontinued if Spo_2 is at or above 90% and the infant is feeding well and has minimal respiratory distress (option).

7b. As the child's clinical course improves, continuous measurement of Spo_2 is not routinely needed (option).

7c. Infants with a known history of hemodynamically significant heart or lung disease and premature infants require close monitoring as oxygen is being weaned (strong recommendation).

8a. Clinicians may administer palivizumab prophylaxis for selected infants and children with CLD or a history of prematurity (less than 35 weeks' gestation) or with congenital heart disease (recommendation).

8b. When given, prophylaxis with palivizumab should be given in 5 monthly doses, usually beginning in November or December, at a dose of 15 mg/kg per dose administered intramuscularly (recommendation).

9a. Hand decontamination is the most important step in preventing nosocomial spread of RSV. Hands should be decontaminated before and after direct contact with patients, after contact with inanimate objects in the direct vicinity of the patient, and after removing gloves (strong recommendation).

9b. Alcohol-based rubs are preferred for hand decontamination. An alternative is hand-washing with antimicrobial soap (recommendation).

9c. Clinicians should educate personnel and family members on hand sanitation (recommendation).

10a. Infants should not be exposed to passive smoking (strong recommendation).

10b. Breastfeeding is recommended to decrease a child's risk of having LRTD (recommendation).

11. Clinicians should inquire about use of CAM (option).

SUBCOMMITTEE ON THE DIAGNOSIS AND MANAGEMENT OF BRONCHIOLITIS, 2004–2006
Allan S. Lieberthal, MD, Chairperson
Howard Bauchner, MD
Caroline B. Hall, MD
David W. Johnson, MD
Uma Kotagal, MD
Michael J. Light, MD (on the AstraZeneca and MedImmune speakers' bureaus; research grant from MedImmune)
Wilbert Mason, MD (on the MedImmune speakers' bureau)
H. Cody Meissner, MD
Kieran J. Phelan, MD
Joseph J. Zorc, MD

LIASONS

Mark A. Brown, MD (on the GlaxoSmithKline, AstraZeneca, and MedImmune speakers' bureaus)
American Thoracic Society

Richard D. Clover, MD (continuing medical education presenter for institutions that received unrestricted educational grants from Sanofi Pasteur and Merck)
American Academy of Family Physicians

Ian T. Nathanson, MD
American College of Chest Physicians

Matti Korppi, MD
European Respiratory Society

CONSULTANTS

Richard N. Shiffman, MD
Danette Stanko-Lopp, MA, MPH

STAFF

Caryn Davidson, MA

REFERENCES

1. Agency for Healthcare Research and Quality. *Management of Bronchiolitis in Infants and Children.* Evidence Report/Technology Assessment No. 69. Rockville, MD: Agency for Healthcare Research and Quality; 2003. AHRQ Publication No. 03-E014

2. Mullins JA, Lamonte AC, Bresee JS, Anderson LJ. Substantial variability in community respiratory syncytial virus season timing. *Pediatr Infect Dis J.* 2003;22:857–862

3. Greenough A, Cox S, Alexander J, et al. Health care utilisation of infants with chronic lung disease, related to hospitalisation for RSV infection. *Arch Dis Child.* 2001;85:463–468

4. Parrott RH, Kim HW, Arrobio JO, et al. Epidemiology of RSV infection in Washington DC II: infection and disease with respect to age, immunologic status, race and sex. *Am J Epidemiol.* 1973;98:289–300

5. Meissner HC. Selected populations at increased risk from respiratory syncytial virus infection. *Pediatr Infect Dis J.* 2003; 22(2 suppl):S40–S44; discussion S44–S45

6. Shay DK, Holman RC, Roosevelt GE, Clarke MJ, Anderson LJ. Bronchiolitis-associated mortality and estimates of respiratory syncytial virus-associated deaths among US children, 1979–1997. *J Infect Dis.* 2001;183:16–22

7. Leader S, Kohlhase K. Recent trends in severe respiratory syncytial virus (RSV) among US infants, 1997 to 2000. *J Pediatr.* 2003;143(5 suppl):S127–S132

8. Stang P, Brandenburg N, Carter B. The economic burden of respiratory syncytial virus-associated bronchiolitis hospitalizations. *Arch Pediatr Adolesc Med.* 2001;155:95–96

9. Willson DF, Horn SD, Hendley JO, Smout R, Gassaway J. Effect of practice variation on resource utilization in infants for viral lower respiratory illness. *Pediatrics.* 2001;108: 851–855

10. Wang EE, Law BJ, Boucher FD, et al. Pediatric Investigators Collaborative Network on Infections in Canada (PICNIC) study of admission and management variation in patients hospitalized with respiratory syncytial viral lower respiratory tract infection. *J Pediatr.* 1996;129:390–395

11. Brand PLP, Vaessen-Verberne AAPH. Differences in management of bronchiolitis between hospitals in the Netherlands. *Eur J Pediatr.* 2000;159:343–347

12. Behrendt CE, Decker MD, Burch DJ, Watson PH. International variation in the management of infants hospitalized with respiratory syncytial virus. International RSV Study Group. *Eur J Pediatr.* 1998;157:215–220

13. Martinez FD. Respiratory syncytial virus bronchiolitis and the pathogenesis of childhood asthma. *Pediatr Infect Dis J.* 2003; 22(2 suppl):S76–S82

14. Stein RT, Sherrill D, Morgan WJ, et al. Respiratory syncytial virus in early life and risk of wheeze and allergy by age 13 years. *Lancet.* 1999;354:541–545

15. Schauer U, Hoffjan S, Bittscheidt J, et al. RSV bronchiolitis and risk of wheeze and allergic sensitization in the first year of life. *Eur Respir J.* 2002;20:1277–1283

16. American Academy of Pediatrics, Steering Committee on Quality Improvement and Management. Classifying recommendations for clinical practice guidelines. *Pediatrics.* 2004; 114:874–877

17. Jobe AH, Bancalari E. Bronchopulmonary dysplasia. *Am J Respir Crit Care Med.* 2001;163:1723–1729

18. Ashton R, Connolly K. The relation of respiration rate and heart rate to sleep states in the human newborn. *Dev Med Child Neurol.* 1971;13:180–187

19. Iliff A, Lee VA. Pulse rate, respiratory rate, and body temperature of children between two months and eighteen years of age. *Child Dev.* 1952;23:237–245

20. Rogers MC. Respiratory monitoring. In: Rogers MC, Nichols DG, eds. *Textbook of Pediatric Intensive Care.* Baltimore, MD: Williams & Wilkins; 1996:332–333

21. Berman S, Simoes EA, Lanata C. Respiratory rate and pneumonia in infancy. *Arch Dis Child.* 1991;66:81–84

22. Margolis P, Gadomski A. The rational clinical examination: does this infant have pneumonia? *JAMA.* 1998;279:308–313

23. Mahabee-Gittens EM, Grupp-Phelan J, Brody AS, et al. Identifying children with pneumonia in the emergency department. *Clin Pediatr (Phila).* 2005;44:427–435

24. Brooks AM, McBride JT, McConnochie KM, Aviram M, Long C, Hall CB. Predicting deterioration in previously healthy infants hospitalized with respiratory syncytial virus infection. *Pediatrics.* 1999;104:463–467

25. Navas L, Wang E, de Carvalho V, Robinson J. Improved outcome of respiratory syncytial virus infection in a high-risk hospitalized population of Canadian children. Pediatric Investigators Collaborative Network on Infections in Canada. *J Pediatr.* 1992;121:348–354

26. Wang EE, Law BJ, Stephens D. Pediatric Investigators Collaborative Network on Infections in Canada (PICNIC) prospective study of risk factors and outcomes in patients hospitalized with respiratory syncytial viral lower respiratory tract infection. *J Pediatr.* 1995;126:212–219

27. Shaw KN, Bell LM, Sherman NH. Outpatient assessment of infants with bronchiolitis. *Am J Dis Child.* 1991;145:151–155

28. Chan, PW, Lok FY, Khatijah SB. Risk factors for hypoxemia and respiratory failure in respiratory syncytial virus bronchiolitis. *Southeast Asian J Trop Med Public Health.* 2002;33: 806–810

29. MacDonald NE, Hall CB, Suffin SC, Alexson C, Harris PJ, Manning JA. Respiratory syncytial viral infection in infants with congenital heart disease. *N Engl J Med.* 1982;307: 397–400

30. Hall CB, Powell KR, MacDonald NE, et al. Respiratory syncytial viral infection in children with compromised immune function. *N Engl J Med.* 1986;315:77–81

31. McMillan JA, Tristram DA, Weiner LB, Higgins AP, Sandstrom C, Brandon R. Prediction of the duration of hospitalization in patients with respiratory syncytial virus infection: use of clinical parameters. *Pediatrics.* 1988;81:22–26

32. Roback MG, Baskin MN. Failure of oxygen saturation and clinical assessment to predict which patients with bronchioli-

tis discharged from the emergency department will return requiring admission. *Pediatr Emerg Care.* 1997;13:9–11

33. Lowell DI, Lister G, Von Koss H, McCarthy P. Wheezing in infants: the response to epinephrine. *Pediatrics.* 1987;79: 939–945

34. Hall CB, Hall WJ, Speers DM. Clinical and physiological manifestations of bronchiolitis and pneumonia: outcome of respiratory syncytial virus. *Am J Dis Child.* 1979;133:798–802

35. Schroeder AR, Marmor AK, Pantell RH, Newman TB. Impact of pulse oximetry and oxygen therapy on length of stay in bronchiolitis hospitalizations. *Arch Pediatr Adolesc Med.* 2004; 158:527–530

36. Dawson KP, Long A, Kennedy J, Mogridge N. The chest radiograph in acute bronchiolitis. *J Paediatr Child Health.* 1990; 26:209–211

37. Roosevelt G, Sheehan K, Grupp-Phelan J, Tanz RR, Listernic R. Dexamethasone in bronchiolitis: a randomized controlled trial. *Lancet.* 1996;348:292–305

38. Swingler GH, Hussey GD, Zwarenstein M. Randomised controlled trial of clinical outcome after chest radiograph in ambulatory acute lower-respiratory infection in children. *Lancet.* 1998;351:404–408

39. Mallory MD, Shay DK, Garrett J, Bordley WC. Bronchiolitis management preferences and the influence of pulse oximetry and respiratory rate on the decision to admit. *Pediatrics.* 2003; 111(1). Available at: www.pediatrics.org/cgi/content/full/111/1/e45

40. Bordley WC, Viswanathan M, King VJ, et al. Diagnosis and testing in bronchiolitis: a systematic review. *Arch Pediatr Adolesc Med.* 2004;158:119–126

41. Liebelt E, Qi K, Harvey K. Diagnostic testing for serious bacterial infections in infants aged 90 days or younger with bronchiolitis. *Arch Pediatr Adolesc Med.* 1999;153:525–530

42. Kuppermann N, Bank DE, Walton EA, Senac MO Jr, McCaslin I. Risks for bacteremia and urinary tract infections in young febrile children with bronchiolitis. *Arch Pediatr Adolesc Med.* 1997;151:1207–1214

43. Levine DA, Platt SL, Dayan PS, et al. Risk of serious bacterial infection in young febrile infants with respiratory syncytial virus infections. *Pediatrics.* 2004;113:1728–1734

44. Kellner JD, Ohlsson A, Gadomski AM, Wang EE. Bronchodilators for bronchiolitis. *Cochrane Database Syst Rev.* 2000;(2): CD001266

45. Alario AJ, Lewander WJ, Dennehy P, Seifer R, Mansell AL. The efficacy of nebulized metaproterenol in wheezing infants and young children. *Am J Dis Child.* 1992;146:412–418

46. Henry RL, Milner AD, Stokes GM. Ineffectiveness of ipratropium bromide in acute bronchiolitis. *Arch Dis Child.* 1983;58: 925–926

47. Klassen TP, Rowe PC, Sutcliffe T, Ropp LJ, McDowell IW, Li MM. Randomized trial of salbutamol in acute bronchiolitis. *J Pediatr.* 1991;118:807–811

48. Lines DR, Kattampallil JS, Liston P. Efficacy of nebulized salbutamol in bronchiolitis. *Pediatr Rev Commun.* 1990;5: 121–129

49. Mallol J, Barrueo L, Girardi G, et al. Use of nebulized bronchodilators in infants under 1 year of age: analysis of four forms of therapy. *Pediatr Pulmonol.* 1987;3:298–303

50. Tal A, Bavilski C, Yohai D, Bearman JE, Gorodischer R, Moses SW. Dexamethasone and salbutamol in the treatment of acute wheezing in infants. *Pediatrics.* 1983;71:13–18

51. Wainwright C, Altamirano L, Cheney M, et al. A multicenter, randomized, double-blind, controlled trial of nebulized epinephrine in infants with acute bronchiolitis. *N Engl J Med.* 2003;349:27–35

52. Schweich PJ, Hurt TL, Walkley EI, Mullen N, Archibald LF.

The use of nebulized albuterol in wheezing infants. *Pediatr Emerg Care.* 1992;8:184–188

53. Schuh S, Canny G, Reisman JJ, et al. Nebulized albuterol in acute bronchiolitis. *J Pediatr.* 1990;117:633–637

54. Gadomski AM, Lichtenstein R, Horton L, King J, Keane V, Permutt T. Efficacy of albuterol in the management of bronchiolitis. *Pediatrics.* 1994;93:907–912

55. Dobson JV, Stephens-Groff SM, McMahon SR, Stemmler MM, Brallier SL, Bay C. The use of albuterol in hospitalized infants with bronchiolitis. *Pediatrics.* 1998;101:361–368

56. Flores G, Horwitz RI. Efficacy of beta2-agonists in bronchiolitis: a reappraisal and meta-analysis. *Pediatrics.* 1997;l00: 233–239

57. Kristjansson S, Lodrup Carlsen KC, Wennergren G, Strannegard IL, Carlsen KH. Nebulised racemic adrenaline in the treatment of acute bronchiolitis in infants and toddlers. *Arch Dis Child.* 1993;69:650–654

58. Menon K, Sutcliffe T, Klassen TP. A randomized trial comparing the efficacy of epinephrine with salbutamol in the treatment of acute bronchiolitis. *J Pediatr.* 1995;126:1004–1007

59. Numa AH, Williams GD, Dakin CJ. The effect of nebulized epinephrine on respiratory mechanics and gas exchange in bronchiolitis. *Am J Respir Crit Care Med.* 2001;164:86–91

60. Wohl ME, Chernick V. State of the art: bronchiolitis. *Am Rev Respir Dis.* 1978;118:759–781

61. Hartling L, Wiebe N, Russell K, Patel H, Klassen T. A meta-analysis of randomized controlled trials evaluating the efficacy of epinephrine for the treatment of acute viral bronchiolitis. *Arch Pediatr Adolesc Med.* 2003;157:957–967

62. Hartling L, Wiebe N, Russell K, Patel H, Klassen TP. Epinephrine for bronchiolitis. *Cochrane Database Syst Rev.* 2004;(1): CD003123

63. Bierman CW, Pierson WE. The pharmacological management of status asthmaticus in children. *Pediatrics.* 1974;54:245–247

64. Schuh S, Coates AL, Binnie R, et al. Efficacy of oral dexamethasone in outpatients with acute bronchiolitis. *J Pediatr.* 2002;140:27–32

65. Gorelick MH, Stevens MW, Schultz TR, Scribano PV. Performance of a novel clinical score, the Pediatric Asthma Severity Score (PASS) in the evaluation of acute asthma. *Acad Emerg Med.* 2004;11:10–18

66. Cincinnati Children's Hospital Medical Center. Evidence-based clinical practice guideline for the medical management of infants less than 1 year with a first episode of bronchiolitis. Available at: www.cincinnatichildrens.org/NR/rdonlyres/B3EC347E-65AC-490A-BC4C-55C3AF4B76D5/0/BronchRS.pdf. Accessed June 21, 2006

67. Goh A, Chay OM, Foo AL, Ong EK. Efficacy of bronchodilators in the treatment of bronchiolitis. *Singapore Med J.* 1997; 38:326–328

68. Chowdhury D, al Howasi M, Khalil M, al-Frayh AS, Chowdhury S, Ramia S. The role of bronchodilators in the management of bronchiolitis: a clinical trial. *Ann Trop Paediatr.* 1995;15:77–84

69. Wang EE, Milner R, Allen U, Maj H. Bronchodialtors for treatment of mild bronchiolitis: a factorial randomized trial. *Arch Dis Child.* 1992;67:289–293

70. Shay DK, Holman RC, Newman RD, Liu LL, Stout JW, Anderson LJ. Bronchiolitis associated hospitalizations among US children, 1980–1996. *JAMA.* 1999;282:1440–1446

71. Patel H, Platt R, Lozano JM, Wang EE. Glucocorticoids for acute viral bronchiolitis in infants and young children. *Cochrane Database Syst Rev.* 2004;(3):CD004878

72. Garrison MM, Christakis DA, Harvey E, Cummings P, Davis RL. Systemic corticosteroids in infant bronchiolitis: a meta-analysis. *Pediatrics.* 2000;105(4). Available at: www.pediatrics.org/cgi/content/full/105/4/e44

73. Berger I, Argaman Z, Schwartz SB, et al. Efficacy of corticosteroids in acute bronchiolitis: short-term and long-term follow-up. *Pediatr Pulmonol.* 1998;26:162–166

74. Bulow SM, Nir M, Levin E, et al. Prednisolone treatment of respiratory syncytial virus infection: a randomized controlled trial of 147 infants. *Pediatrics.* 1999;104(6). Available at: www.pediatrics.org/cgi/content/full/105/6/e77

75. Connolly JH, Field CMB, Glasgoe JFT, Slattery M, MacLynn DM. A double blind trial of prednisolone in epidemic bronchiolitis due to respiratory syncytial virus. *Acta Paediatr Scand.* 1969;58:116–120

76. Dabbous JA, Tkachyk JS, Stamm SJ. A double blind study on the effects of corticosteroids in the treatment of bronchiolitis. *Pediatrics.* 1966;37:477–484

77. DeBoeck K, Van der Aa N, Van Lierde S, Corbeel L, Eeckels R. Respiratory syncytial virus bronchiolitis: a double-blind dexamethasone efficacy study. *J Pediatr.* 1997;131:919–921

78. Goebel J, Estrada B, Quinonez J, Nagji N, Sanford D, Boerth RC. Prednisolone plus albuterol versus albuterol alone in mild to moderate bronchiolitis. *Clin Pediatr (Phila).* 2000;39:213–220

79. Klassen TP, Sutcliffe T, Watters LK, Wells GA, Allen UD, Li MM. Dexamethasone in salbutamol-treated inpatients with acute bronchiolitis: a randomized controlled trial. *J Pediatr.* 1997;130:191–196

80. Leer JA, Bloomfield N, Green JL, et al. Corticosteroid treatment in bronchiolitis. *Am J Dis Child.* 1969;117:495–503

81. Springer C, Bar-Yishay E, Uwayyed K, Avital A, Vilozni D, Godfrey S. Corticosteroids do not affect the clinical or physiological status of infants with bronchiolitis. *Pediatr Pulmonol.* 1990;9:181–185

82. Van Woensel JBM, Wolfs TFW, van Aaldersen WMC, Brand PLP, Kimpen JLL. Randomised double blind placebo controlled trial of prednisolone in children admitted to hospital with respiratory syncytial virus bronchiolitis. *Thorax.* 1997;52:634–637

83. de Blic J. Use of corticoids in acute bronchiolitis in infants [in French]. *Arch Pediatr.* 2001;9 (suppl 1):49S–54S

84. Chao LC, Lin YZ, Wu WF, Huang FY. Efficacy of nebulized budesonide in hospitalized infants and children younger than 24 months with bronchiolitis. *Acta Paediatr Taiwan.* 2003;44:332–335

85. King VJ, Viswanathan M, Bordley WC, et al. Pharmacologic treatment of bronchiolitis in infants and children. *Arch Pediatr Adolesc Med.* 2004;158:127–137

86. Hall CB, McBride JT, Walsh EE, et al. Aerosolized ribavirin treatment of infants with respiratory syncytial viral infection: a randomized double-blind study. *N Engl J Med.* 1983;308:1443–1447

87. Taber LH, Knight V, Gilbert BE, et al. Ribavirin aerosol treatment of bronchiolitis associated with respiratory syncytial virus infection in infants. *Pediatrics.* 1983;72:613–618

88. Barry W, Cockburn F, Cornall R, et al. Ribavirin aerosol for acute bronchiolitis. *Arch Dis Child.* 1986;61:593–597

89. Rodriguez WJ, Kim HW, Brandt CD, et al. Aerosolized ribavirin in the treatment of patients with respiratory syncytial virus disease. *Pediatr Infect Dis J.* 1987;6:159–163

90. Smith DW, Frankel LR, Mathers LH, Tang AT, Ariagno RL, Prober CG. A controlled trial of aerosolized ribavirin in infants receiving mechanical ventilation for severe respiratory syncytial virus infection. *N Engl J Med.* 1991;325:24–29

91. Janai HK, Stutman HR, Zeleska M, et al. Ribavirin effect on pulmonary function in young infants with respiratory syncytial virus bronchiolitis. *Pediatr Infect Dis J.* 1993;12:214–218

92. Meert KL, Sarnaik AP, Gelmini MJ, Lieh-Lai MW. Aerosolized ribavirin in mechanically ventilated children with respiratory syncytial virus lower respiratory tract disease: a double-blind, randomized trial. *Crit Care Med.* 1994;22:566–572

93. Guerguerian AM, Gauthier M, Lebel MH, Farrell CA, Lacroix J. Ribavirin in ventilated respiratory syncytial virus bronchiolitis. *Am J Respir Crit Care Med.* 1999;160:829–834

94. Everard ML, Swarbrick A, Rigby AS, Milner AD. The effect of ribavirin to treat previously healthy infants admitted with acute bronchiolitis on acute and chronic respiratory morbidity. *Respir Med.* 2001;95:275–280

95. Rodriguez WJ, Arrobio J, Fink R, Kim HW, Milburn C. Prospective follow-up and pulmonary functions from a placebo-controlled randomized trial of ribavirin therapy in respiratory syncytial virus bronchiolitis. *Arch Pediatr Adolesc Med.* 1999;153:469–474

96. Edell D, Khoshoo V, Ross G, Salter K. Early ribavirin treatment of bronchiolitis. *Chest.* 2002;122:935–939

97. Hall CB, McBride JT, Gala CL, Hildreth SW, Schnabel KC. Ribavirin treatment of respiratory syncytial viral infection in infants with underlying cardiopulmonary disease. *JAMA.* 1985;254:3047–3051

98. Groothuis JR, Woodin KA, Katz R, et al. Early ribavirin treatment of respiratory syncytial virus infection in high-risk children. *J Pediatr.* 1990;117:792–798

99. Long CE, Voter KZ, Barker WH, Hall CB. Long term follow-up of children hospitalized with respiratory syncytial virus lower respiratory tract infection and randomly treated with ribavirin and placebo. *Pediatr Infect Dis J.* 1997;16:1023–1028

100. Bradley JS, Conner JD, Compagiannis LS, Eiger LL. Exposure of health care workers to ribavirin during therapy for respiratory syncytial virus infections. *Antimicrob Agents Chemother.* 1990;34:668–670

101. Rodriguez WJ, Bui RHD, Conner JD, et al. Environmental exposure of primary care personnel to ribavirin aerosol when supervising treatment of infants with respiratory syncytial virus infections. *Antimicrob Agents Chemother.* 1987;31:1143–1146

102. Feldstein TJ, Swegarden JL, Atwood GF, Peterson CD. Ribavirin therapy: implementation of hospital guidelines and effect on usage and cost of therapy. *Pediatrics.* 1995;96:14–17

103. Putto A, Ruuskanen O, Meruman O. Fever in respiratory virus infections. *Am J Dis Child.* 1986;140:1159–1163

104. LaVia W, Marks MI, Stutman HR. Respiratory syncytial virus puzzle: clinical features, pathophysiology, treatment, and prevention. *J Pediatr.* 1992;121:503–510

105. Nichol KP, Cherry JD. Bacterial-viral interrelations in respiratory infections in children. *N Engl J Med.* 1967;277:667–672

106. Field CM, Connolly JH, Murtagh G, Slattery CM, Turkington EE. Antibiotic treatment of epidemic bronchiolitis. *Br Med J.* 1966;5479:83–85

107. Friis B, Andersen P, Brenoe E, et al. Antibiotic treatment of pneumonia and bronchiolitis. A prospective randomised study. *Arch Dis Child.* 1984;59:1038–1045

108. Antonow JA, Hansen K, McKinstry CA, Byington CL. Sepsis evaluations in hospitalized infants with bronchiolitis. *Pediatr Infect Dis J.* 1998;17:231–236

109. Greenes DS, Harper MB. Low risk of bacteremia in febrile children with recognizable viral syndromes. *Pediatr Infect Dis J.* 1999;18:258–261

110. Purcell K, Fergie J. Concurrent serious bacterial infections in 2396 infants and children hospitalized with respiratory syncytial virus lower respiratory tract infections. *Arch Pediatr Adolesc Med.* 2002;156:322–324

111. Purcell K, Fergie J. Concurrent serious bacterial infections in 912 infants and children hospitalized for treatment of respiratory syncytial virus lower respiratory tract infection. *Pediatr Infect Dis J.* 2004;23:267–269

112. Titus MO, Wright SW. Prevalence of serious bacterial infec-

tions in febrile infants with respiratory syncytial virus infections. *Pediatrics.* 2003;112:282–284

113. Melendez E, Harper MB. Utility of sepsis evaluation in infants 90 days of age or younger with fever and clinical bronchiolitis. *Pediatr Infect Dis J.* 2003;22:1053–1056

114. Hall CB, Powell KR, Schnabel KC, Gala CL, Pincus PH. Risk of serious bacterial infection in infants hospitalized with respiratory syncytial viral infection. *J Pediatr.* 1988;113:266–271

115. Hall CB. Respiratory syncytial virus: a continuing culprit and conundrum. *J Pediatr.* 1999;135(2 pt 2):2–7

116. Davies HD, Matlow A, Petric M, Glazier R, Wang EE. Prospective comparative study of viral, bacterial and atypical organisms identified in pneumonia and bronchiolitis in hospitalized Canadian infants. *Pediatr Infect Dis J.* 1996;15:371–375

117. Andrade MA, Hoberman A, Glustein J, Paradise JL, Wald ER. Acute otitis media in children with bronchiolitis. *Pediatrics.* 1998;101:617–619

118. Shazberg G, Revel-Vilk S, Shoseyov D, Ben-Ami A, Klar A, Hurvitz H. The clinical course of bronchiolitis associated with otitis media. *Arch Dis Child.* 2000;83:317–319

119. American Academy of Pediatrics, Subcommittee on Management of Acute Otitis Media. Diagnosis and management of acute otitis media. *Pediatrics.* 2004;113:1451–1465

120. Khoshoo V, Edell D. Previously healthy infants may have increased risk of aspiration during respiratory syncytial viral bronchiolitis. *Pediatrics.* 1999;104:1389–1390

121. Gozal D, Colin AA, Jaffe M, Hochberg Z. Water, electrolyte, and endocrine homeostasis in infants with bronchiolitis. *Pediatr Res.* 1990;27:204–209

122. van Steensel-Moll HA, Hazelzet JA, van der Voort E, Neijens HJ, Hackeng WH. Excessive secretion of antidiuretic hormone in infections with respiratory syncytial virus. *Arch Dis Child.* 1990;65:1237–1239

123. Perotta C, Ortiz Z, Roque M. Chest physiotherapy for acute bronchiolitis in paediatric patients between 0 and 24 months old. *Cochrane Database Syst Rev.* 2005;(2):CD004873

124. Nicholas KJ, Dhouieb MO, Marshal TG, Edmunds AT, Grant MB. An evaluation of chest physiotherapy in the management of acute bronchiolitis: changing clinical practice. *Physiotherapy.* 1999;85:669–674

125. Webb MS, Martin JA, Cartlidge PH, Ng YK, Wright NA. Chest physiotherapy in acute bronchiolitis. *Arch Dis Child.* 1985;60:1078–1079

126. Bohe L, Ferrero ME, Cuestas E, Polliotto L, Genoff M. Indications of conventional chest physiotherapy in acute bronchiolitis [in Spanish]. *Medicina (B Aires).* 2004;64:198–200

127. O'Brien LM, Stebbens VA, Poets CF, Heycock EG, Southall DP. Oxygen saturation during the first 24 hours of life. *Arch Dis Child Fetal Neonatal Ed.* 2000;83:F35–F38

128. Hunt CE, Corwin MJ, Lister G, et al. Longitudinal assessment of hemoglobin oxygen saturation in healthy infants during the first 6 months of age. Collaborative Home Infant Monitoring Evaluation (CHIME) Study Group. *J Pediatr.* 1999;135:580–586

129. Young S, O'Keeffe PT, Arnott J, Landau LI. Lung function, airway responsiveness, and respiratory symptoms before and after bronchiolitis. *Arch Dis Child.* 1995;72:16–24

130. Forster RE II, Dubois AB, Briscoe WA, Fisher AB. *The Lung: Physiologic Basis of Pulmonary Function Tests.* Chicago, IL: Year Book Medical Publishers, Inc; 1986

131. Chernick V, Boat TF. *Kendig's Disorders of the Respiratory Tract in Children.* Philadelphia, PA: W. B. Saunders Co; 1998

132. Salyer JW. Neonatal and pediatric pulse oximetry. *Respir Care.* 2003;48:386–396; discussion 397–398

133. Groothuis JR, Gutierrez KM, Lauer BA. Respiratory syncytial virus infection in children with bronchopulmonary dysplasia. *Pediatrics.* 1988;82:199–203

134. Grimaldi M, Gouyon B, Michaut F, Huet F, Gouyon J; Burgundy Perinatal Network. Severe respiratory syncytial virus bronchiolitis: epidemiologic variations associated with the initiation of palivizumab in severely premature infants with bronchopulmonary dysplasia. *Pediatr Infect Dis J.* 2004;23:1081–1085

135. Horn SD, Smout RJ. Effect of prematurity on respiratory syncytial virus hospital resource use and outcomes. *J Pediatr.* 2003;143(5 suppl):S133–S141

136. American Academy of Pediatrics. *Red Book: 2006 Report of the Committee on Infectious Diseases.* 27th ed. Elk Grove Village, IL: American Academy of Pediatrics; 2006

137. The IMpact-RSV study group. Palivizumab, a humanized respiratory syncytial virus monoclonal antibody, reduces hospitalization from respiratory syncytial virus infection in high-risk infants. *Pediatrics.* 1998;102:531–537

138. Feltes TF, Cabalka AK, Meissner HC, et al. Palivizumab prophylaxis reduces hospitalization due to respiratory syncytial virus in young children with hemodynamically significant congenital heart disease. *J Pediatr.* 2003;143:532–540

139. Romero JR. Palivizumab prophylaxis of respiratory syncytial virus disease from 1998 to 2002: results from four years of palivizumab usage. *Pediatr Infect Dis J.* 2003;22(2 suppl): S46–S54

140. Hay JW, Ernst RL, Meissner HC. RSV-IGIV: a cost effectiveness analysis. *Am J Manag Care.* 1996;2:851–861

141. O'Shea TM, Sevick MA, Givner LB. Costs and benefits of respiratory syncytial virus immunoglobulin to prevent hospitalization for lower respiratory tract illness in very low birth weight infants. *Pediatr Infect Dis J.* 1998;17:587–593

142. Robbins JM, Tilford JM, Jacobs RF, Wheeler JG, Gillaspy SR, Schutze GE. A number-needed-to-treat analysis of respiratory syncytial virus immune globulin intravenous to prevent hospitalization [published correction appears in *Arch Pediatr Adolesc Med.* 1998;152:577]. *Arch Pediatr Adolesc Med.* 1998; 152:358–366

143. Atkins JT, Karimi P, Morris BH, McDavid G, Shim S. Prophylaxis for RSV with RSV-IGIV among preterm infants of thirty-two weeks gestation and less: reduction in incidence, severity of illness and cost. *Pediatr Infect Dis J.* 2002;19:138–143

144. Thomas M, Bedford-Russell A, Sharland M. Hospitalization for RSV infection in ex-preterm infants: implications for use of RSV-IGIV. *Arch Dis Child.* 2000;83:122–127

145. Joffe S, Ray GT, Escobar GJ, Black SB, Lieu TA. Cost-effectiveness of RSV prophylaxis among preterm infants. *Pediatrics.* 1999;104:419–427

146. Stevens TP, Sinkin RA, Hall CB, Maniscalco WM, McConnochie KM. Respiratory syncytial virus and premature infants born at 32 weeks' gestation or earlier: hospitalization and economic implications of prophylaxis. *Arch Pediatr Adolesc Med.* 2000;154:55–61

147. Kamal-Bahl S, Doshi J, Campbell J. Economic analysis of respiratory syncytial virus immunoprophylaxis in high-risk infants. *Arch Pediatr Adolesc Med.* 2002;156:1034–1041

148. Aintablian N, Walpita P, Sawyer MH. Detection of *Bordetella pertussis* and respiratory synctial virus in air samples from hospital rooms. *Infect Control Hosp Epidemiol.* 1998;19:918–923

149. Hall CB. Nosocomial respiratory syncytial virus infections: the "Cold War" has not ended. *Clin Infect Dis.* 2000;31:590–596

150. Sattar SA, Terro J, Vashon R, Keswick B. Hygienic hand antiseptics: should they not have activity and label claims against viruses? *Am J Infect Control.* 2002;30:355–372

151. Boyce JM, Pittet D; Healthcare Infection Control Practices Advisory Committee, HICPAC/SHEA/APIC/IDSA Hand Hygiene Task Force. Guideline for hand hygiene in health-care settings. Recommendations of the Healthcare Infection Control Practices Advisory Committee and the HICPAC/SHEA/

APIC/IDSA Hand Hygiene Task Force. Society for Healthcare Epidemiology of America/Association for Professionals in Infection Control/Infectious Diseases Society of America. *MMWR Recomm Rep.* 200225;51(RR-16):1–45; quiz CE1–CE4

152. Isaacs D, Dickson H, O'Callaghan C, Sheaves R, Winter A, Moxon ER. Handwashing and cohorting in prevention of hospital acquired infections with respiratory syncytial virus. *Arch Dis Child.* 1991;66:227–231

153. Krasinski K, LaCouture R, Holzman RS, Waithe E, Bonk S, Hanna B. Screening for respiratory syncytial virus and assignment to a cohort at admission to reduce nosocomial transmission. *J Pediatr.* 1990;116:894–898

154. Karanfil LV, Conlon M, Lykens K, et al. Reducing the rate of nosocomially transmitted respiratory syncytial virus [published correction appears in *Am J Infect Control.* 1999;27:303]. *Am J Infect Control.* 1999;27:91–96

155. Macartney KK, Gorelick MH, Manning ML, Hodinka RL, Bell LM. Nosocomial respiratory syncytial virus infections: the cost-effectiveness and cost-benefit of infection control. *Pediatrics.* 2000;106:520–526

156. McConnochie KM, Roghmann KJ. Breast feeding and maternal smoking as predictors of wheezing in children age 6 to 10 years. *Pediatr Pulmonol.* 1986;2:260–268

157. Strachan DP, Cook DG. Health effects of passive smoking. 1. Parental smoking and lower respiratory illness in infancy and early childhood. *Thorax.* 1997;52:905–914

158. Stocks J, Dezateux C. The effect of parental smoking on lung function and development during infancy. *Respirology.* 2003; 8:266–285

159. Shiva F, Basiri M, Sadeghi B, Padyab M. Effects of passive smoking on common respiratory symptoms in young children. *Acta Paediatr.* 2003;92:1394–1397

160. Nandapalan N, Taylor C, Scott R, Toms GL. Mammary immunity in mothers of infants with respiratory syncytial virus infection. *J Med Virol.* 1987;22:277–287

161. Chiba Y, Minagawa T, Mito K, et al. Effect of breast feeding on responses of systemic interferon and virus-specific lymphocyte transformation in infants with respiratory syncytial virus infection. *J Med Virol.* 1987;21:7–14

162. Laegreid A, Kolsto Otnaess AB, Orstavik I, Carlsen KH. Neutralizing activity in human milk fractions against respiratory syncytial virus. *Acta Paediatr Scand.* 1986;75:696–701

163. Pullan CR, Toms GL, Martin AJ, Gardner PS, Webb JK, Appleton DR. Breastfeeding and respiratory syncytial virus infection. *Br Med J.* 1980;281:1034–1036

164. Downham MAPS, Scott R, Sims DG, Webb JKG, Gardner PS. Breast-feeding protects against respiratory syncytial virus infections. *Br Med J.* 1976;2(6030):274–276

165. Bachrach VR, Schwarz E, Bachrach LR. Breastfeeding and the risk of hospitalization for respiratory disease in infancy: a meta-analysis. *Arch Pediatr Adolesc Med.* 2003;157:237–243

166. Cohen HA, Varsano I, Kahan E, Sarrell EM, Uziel Y. Effectiveness of an herbal preparation containing echinacea, propolis, and vitamin C in preventing respiratory tract infections in children: a randomized, double-blind, placebo-controlled, multicenter study. *Arch Pediatr Adolesc Med.* 2004; 158:217–221

Bronchiolitis Clinical Practice Guideline Quick Reference Tools

- Recommendation Summary
  — Diagnosis and Management of Bronchiolitis
- *ICD-9-CM/ICD-10-CM* Coding Quick Reference for Bronchiolitis
- AAP Patient Education Handout
  — *Bronchiolitis and Your Young Child*

Recommendation Summary

Diagnosis and Management of Bronchiolitis

Recommendation 1a
Clinicians should diagnose bronchiolitis and assess disease severity on the basis of history and physical examination. Clinicians should not routinely order laboratory and radiologic studies for diagnosis (recommendation: evidence level B; diagnostic studies with minor limitations and observational studies with consistent findings; preponderance of benefits over harms and cost).

Recommendation 1b
Clinicians should assess risk factors for severe disease such as age less than 12 weeks, a history of prematurity, underlying cardiopulmonary disease, or immunodeficiency when making decisions about evaluation and management of children with bronchiolitis (recommendation: evidence level B; observational studies with consistent findings; preponderance of benefits over harms).

Recommendation 2a
Bronchodilators should not be used routinely in the management of bronchiolitis (recommendation: evidence level B; RCTs with limitations; preponderance of harm of use over benefit).

Recommendation 2b
A carefully monitored trial of α-adrenergic or ß-adrenergic medication is an option. Inhaled bronchodilators should be continued only if there is a documented positive clinical response to the trial using an objective means of evaluation (option: evidence level B; RCTs with limitations and expert opinion; balance of benefit and harm).

Recommendation 3
Corticosteroid medications should not be used routinely in the management of bronchiolitis (recommendation: evidence level B; based on RCTs with limitations and a preponderance of risk over benefit).

Recommendation 4
Ribavirin should not be used routinely in children with bronchiolitis (recommendation: evidence level B; RCTs with limitations and observational studies; preponderance of harm over benefit).

Recommendation 5
Antibacterial medications should be used only in children with bronchiolitis who have specific indications of the coexistence of a bacterial infection. When present, bacterial infection should be treated in the same manner as in the absence of bronchiolitis (recommendation: evidence level B; RCTs and observational studies; preponderance of benefit over harm).

Recommendation 6a
Clinicians should assess hydration and ability to take fluids orally (strong recommendation: evidence level X; validating studies cannot be performed; clear preponderance of benefit over harm).

Recommendation 6b
Chest physiotherapy should not be used routinely in the management of bronchiolitis (recommendation: evidence level B; RCTs with limitations; preponderance of harm over benefit).

Recommendation 7a
Supplemental oxygen is indicated if oxyhemoglobin saturation (Spo_2) falls persistently below 90% in previously healthy infants. If the Spo_2 does persistently fall below 90%, adequate supplemental oxygen should be used to maintain Spo_2 at or above 90%. Oxygen may be discontinued if Spo_2 is at or above 90% and the infant is feeding well and has minimal respiratory distress (option: evidence level D; expert opinion and reasoning from first principles; some benefit over harm).

Recommendation 7b
As the child's clinical course improves, continuous measurement of Spo_2 is not routinely needed (option: evidence level D; expert opinion; balance of benefit and harm).

Recommendation 7c
Infants with a known history of hemodynamically significant heart or lung disease and premature infants require close monitoring as the oxygen is being weaned (strong recommendation: evidence level B; observational studies with consistent findings; preponderance of benefit over harm).

Recommendation 8a

Clinicians may administer palivizumab prophylaxis to selected infants and children with CLD or a history of prematurity (less than 35 weeks' gestation) or with congenital heart disease (recommendation: evidence level A; RCT; preponderance of benefit over harm).

Recommendation 8b

When given, prophylaxis with palivizumab should be given in 5 monthly doses, usually beginning in November or December, at a dose of 15 mg/kg per dose administered intramuscularly (recommendation: evidence level C; observational studies and expert opinion; preponderance of benefit over cost).

Recommendation 9a

Hand decontamination is the most important step in preventing nosocomial spread of RSV. Hands should be decontaminated before and after direct contact with patients, after contact with inanimate objects in the direct vicinity of the patient, and after removing gloves (strong recommendation: evidence level B; observational studies with consistent results; strong preponderance of benefit over harm).

Recommendation 9b

Alcohol-based rubs are preferred for hand decontamination. An alternative is hand-washing with antimicrobial soap (recommendation: evidence level B; observational studies with consistent results; preponderance of benefit over harm).

Recommendation 9c

Clinicians should educate personnel and family members on hand sanitation (recommendation: evidence level C; observational studies; preponderance of benefit over harm).

Recommendation 10a

Infants should not be exposed to passive smoking (strong recommendation: evidence level B; observational studies with consistent results; strong preponderance of benefit over harm).

Recommendation 10b

Breastfeeding is recommended to decrease a child's risk of having lower respiratory tract disease (LRTD) (recommendation: evidence level C; observational studies; preponderance of benefit over harm).

Recommendation 11

Clinicians should inquire about use of CAM (option: evidence level D; expert opinion; some benefit over harm).

Coding Quick Reference for Bronchiolitis	
ICD-9-CM	*ICD-10-CM*
466.11 Acute bronchiolitis due to respiratory syncytial virus (RSV)	**J21.0** Acute bronchiolitis due to syncytial virus
466.19 Acute bronchiolitis due to other infectious organisms	**J21.8** Acute bronchiolitis due to other specified organisms

Bronchiolitis and Your Young Child

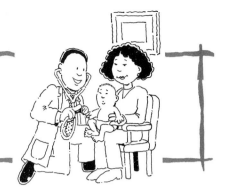

Bronchiolitis is a common respiratory illness among infants. One of its symptoms is trouble breathing, which can be scary for parents and children. Read on for more information from the American Academy of Pediatrics about bronchiolitis, its causes, signs and symptoms, how to treat it, and how to prevent it.

What is bronchiolitis?

Bronchiolitis is an infection that causes the small breathing tubes of the lungs (bronchioles) to swell. This blocks airflow through the lungs, making it hard to breathe. It occurs most often in infants because their airways are smaller and more easily blocked than in older children. Bronchiolitis is not the same as *bronchitis*, which is an infection of the larger, more central airways that typically causes problems in adults.

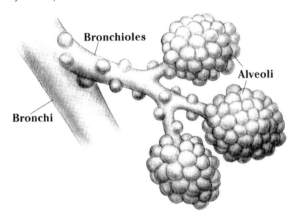

What causes bronchiolitis?

Bronchiolitis is caused by one of several viruses. *Respiratory syncytial virus* (RSV) is the most likely cause from October through March. Other viruses can also cause bronchiolitis.

Infants with RSV infection are more likely to get bronchiolitis with wheezing and difficulty breathing. Most adults and many older children with RSV infection only get a cold. RSV is spread by contact with an infected person's mucus or saliva (respiratory droplets produced during coughing or wheezing). It often spreads through families and child care centers. (See "How can you prevent your baby from getting bronchiolitis?")

What are the signs and symptoms of bronchiolitis?

Bronchiolitis often starts with signs of a cold, such as a runny nose, mild cough, and fever. After a day or two, the cough may get worse and the infant will begin to breathe faster. The following signs may mean that the infant is having trouble breathing:

- He may widen his nostrils and squeeze the muscles under his rib cage to try to get more air in and out of his lungs.
- When he breathes, he may grunt and tighten his stomach muscles.
- He will make a high-pitched whistling sound, called a wheeze, when he breathes out.
- He may have trouble drinking because he may have trouble sucking and swallowing.
- If it gets very hard for him to breathe, you may notice a bluish tint around his lips and fingertips. This tells you that his airways are so blocked that there is not enough oxygen getting into his blood.

If your baby shows any of these signs of troubled breathing, call your child's doctor.

Your child may become dehydrated if he cannot comfortably drink fluids. Call your child's doctor if your baby develops any of the following signs of dehydration:

- Drinking less than normal
- Dry mouth
- Crying without tears
- Urinating less often than normal

Bronchiolitis may cause more severe illness in children who have a chronic illness. If you think your child has bronchiolitis *and* your child has any of the following conditions, call your child's doctor:

- Cystic fibrosis
- Congenital heart disease
- Chronic lung disease (seen in some infants who were on breathing machines or respirators as newborns)
- Immune deficiency disease (like acquired immunodeficiency syndrome [AIDS])
- Organ or bone marrow transplant
- A cancer for which he is receiving chemotherapy

Can bronchiolitis be treated at home?

There is no specific treatment for RSV or the other viruses that cause bronchiolitis. Antibiotics are not helpful because they treat illnesses caused by bacteria, not viruses. However, you can try to ease your child's symptoms.

To relieve a stuffy nose

- **Thin the mucus** using saline nose drops recommended by your child's doctor. *Never use nonprescription nose drops that contain any medicine.*
- **Clear your baby's nose** with a suction bulb. Squeeze the bulb first. Gently put the rubber tip into one nostril, and slowly release the bulb. This suction will draw the clogged mucus out of the nose. This works best when your baby is younger than 6 months.

To relieve fever

- **Give your baby acetaminophen.** (Follow the recommended dosage for your child's age.) Do not give your baby aspirinbecause it has been associated with Reye syndrome, a disease that affects the liver and brain. Check with your child's doctor first before giving any other cold medicines.

To prevent dehydration

- **Make sure your baby drinks lots of fluid.** She may want clear liquids rather than milk or formula. She may feed more slowly or not feel like eating because she is having trouble breathing.

How will your pediatrician treat bronchiolitis?

If your baby is having mild to moderate trouble breathing, your child's doctor may try using a drug that opens up the breathing tubes. This may help some infants.

Some children with bronchiolitis need to be treated in a hospital for breathing problems or dehydration. Breathing problems may need to be treated with oxygen and medicine. Dehydration is treated with a special liquid diet or intravenous (IV) fluids.

In very rare cases when these treatments aren't working, an infant might have to be put on a respirator. This usually is only temporary until the infection is gone.

How can you prevent your baby from getting bronchiolitis?

The best steps you can follow to reduce the risk that your baby becomes infected with RSV or other viruses that cause bronchiolitis include

- Make sure everyone washes their hands before touching your baby.
- Keep your baby away from anyone who has a cold, fever, or runny nose.
- Avoid sharing eating utensils and drinking cups with anyone who has a cold, fever, or runny nose.

If you have questions about the treatment of bronchiolitis, call your child's doctor.

The information contained in this publication should not be used as a substitute for the medical care and advice of your pediatrician. There may be variations in treatment that your pediatrician may recommend based on individual facts and circumstances.

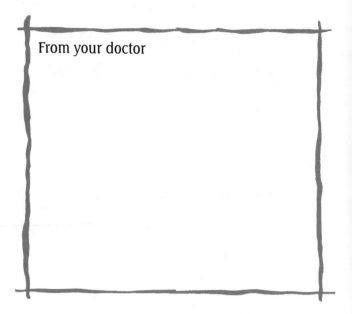

From your doctor

American Academy of Pediatrics

DEDICATED TO THE HEALTH OF ALL CHILDREN™

The American Academy of Pediatrics is an organization of 60,000 primary care pediatricians, pediatric medical subspecialists, and pediatric surgical specialists dedicated to the health, safety, and well-being of infants, children, adolescents, and young adults.

American Academy of Pediatrics
Web site — www.HealthyChildren.org

Management of Newly Diagnosed Type 2 Diabetes Mellitus (T2DM) in Children and Adolescents

- *Clinical Practice Guideline*
- *Technical Report*

  – *PPI: AAP Partnership for Policy Implementation*
  See Appendix 2 for more information.

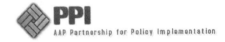

Readers of this clinical practice guideline are urged to review the technical report to enhance the evidence-based decision-making process. The full technical report is available following the clinical practice guideline and on the companion CD-ROM.

CLINICAL PRACTICE GUIDELINE

Management of Newly Diagnosed Type 2 Diabetes Mellitus (T2DM) in Children and Adolescents

abstract

Over the past 3 decades, the prevalence of childhood obesity has increased dramatically in North America, ushering in a variety of health problems, including type 2 diabetes mellitus (T2DM), which previously was not typically seen until much later in life. The rapid emergence of childhood T2DM poses challenges to many physicians who find themselves generally ill-equipped to treat adult diseases encountered in children. This clinical practice guideline was developed to provide evidence-based recommendations on managing 10- to 18-year-old patients in whom T2DM has been diagnosed. The American Academy of Pediatrics (AAP) convened a Subcommittee on Management of T2DM in Children and Adolescents with the support of the American Diabetes Association, the Pediatric Endocrine Society, the American Academy of Family Physicians, and the Academy of Nutrition and Dietetics (formerly the American Dietetic Association). These groups collaborated to develop an evidence report that served as a major source of information for these practice guideline recommendations. The guideline emphasizes the use of management modalities that have been shown to affect clinical outcomes in this pediatric population. Recommendations are made for situations in which either insulin or metformin is the preferred first-line treatment of children and adolescents with T2DM. The recommendations suggest integrating lifestyle modifications (ie, diet and exercise) in concert with medication rather than as an isolated initial treatment approach. Guidelines for frequency of monitoring hemoglobin A1c (HbA1c) and finger-stick blood glucose (BG) concentrations are presented. Decisions were made on the basis of a systematic grading of the quality of evidence and strength of recommendation. The clinical practice guideline underwent peer review before it was approved by the AAP. This clinical practice guideline is not intended to replace clinical judgment or establish a protocol for the care of all children with T2DM, and its recommendations may not provide the only appropriate approach to the management of children with T2DM. Providers should consult experts trained in the care of children and adolescents with T2DM when treatment goals are not met or when therapy with insulin is initiated. The AAP acknowledges that some primary care clinicians may not be confident of their ability to successfully treat T2DM in a child because of the child's age, coexisting conditions, and/or other concerns. At any point at which a clinician feels he or she is not adequately trained or is uncertain about treatment, a referral to a pediatric medical subspecialist should be made. If a diagnosis of T2DM is made by a pediatric medical subspecialist, the primary care clinician should develop a comanagement strategy with the subspecialist to ensure that the child continues to receive appropriate care consistent with a medical home model in which the pediatrician partners with parents to ensure that all health needs are met. *Pediatrics* 2013;131:364–382

Kenneth C. Copeland, MD, Janet Silverstein, MD, Kelly R. Moore, MD, Greg E. Prazar, MD, Terry Raymer, MD, CDE, Richard N. Shiffman, MD, Shelley C. Springer, MD, MBA, Vidhu V. Thaker, MD, Meaghan Anderson, MS, RD, LD, CDE, Stephen J. Spann, MD, MBA, and Susan K. Flinn, MA

KEY WORDS
diabetes, type 2 diabetes mellitus, childhood, youth, clinical practice guidelines, comanagement, management, treatment

ABBREVIATIONS
AAP—American Academy of Pediatrics
AAFP—American Academy of Family Physicians
BG—blood glucose
FDA—US Food and Drug Administration
HbA1c—hemoglobin A1c
PES—Pediatric Endocrine Society
T1DM—type 1 diabetes mellitus
T2DM—type 2 diabetes mellitus
TODAY—Treatment Options for type 2 Diabetes in Adolescents and Youth

www.pediatrics.org/cgi/doi/10.1542/peds.2012-3494

doi:10.1542/peds.2012-3494

PEDIATRICS (ISSN Numbers: Print, 0031-4005; Online, 1098-4275).

Key action statements are as follows:

1. Clinicians must ensure that insulin therapy is initiated for children and adolescents with T2DM who are ketotic or in diabetic ketoacidosis and in whom the distinction between types 1 and 2 diabetes mellitus is unclear and, in usual cases, should initiate insulin therapy for patients

   a. who have random venous or plasma BG concentrations ≥250 mg/dL; or

   b. whose HbA1c is >9%.

2. In all other instances, clinicians should initiate a lifestyle modification program, including nutrition and physical activity, and start metformin as first-line therapy for children and adolescents at the time of diagnosis of T2DM.

3. The committee suggests that clinicians monitor HbA1c concentrations every 3 months and intensify treatment if treatment goals for finger-stick BG and HbA1c concentrations are not being met (intensification is defined in the Definitions box).

4. The committee suggests that clinicians advise patients to monitor finger-stick BG (see Key Action Statement 4 in the guideline for further details) concentrations in patients who

   a. are taking insulin or other medications with a risk of hypoglycemia; or

   b. are initiating or changing their diabetes treatment regimen; or

   c. have not met treatment goals; or

   d. have intercurrent illnesses.

5. The committee suggests that clinicians incorporate the Academy of Nutrition and Dietetics' *Pediatric Weight Management Evidence-Based Nutrition Practice Guidelines* in their dietary or nutrition counseling of patients with T2DM at the time of diagnosis and as part of ongoing management.

6. The committee suggests that clinicians encourage children and adolescents with T2DM to engage in moderate-to-vigorous exercise for at least 60 minutes daily and to limit nonacademic "screen time" to less than 2 hours a day.

Definitions

Adolescent: an individual in various stages of maturity, generally considered to be between 12 and 18 years of age.

Childhood T2DM: disease in the child who typically

- is overweight or obese (BMI ≥85th–94th and >95th percentile for age and gender, respectively);
- has a strong family history of T2DM;
- has substantial residual insulin secretory capacity at diagnosis (reflected by normal or elevated insulin and C-peptide concentrations);
- has insidious onset of disease;
- demonstrates insulin resistance (including clinical evidence of polycystic ovarian syndrome or acanthosis nigricans);
- lacks evidence for diabetic autoimmunity (negative for autoantibodies typically associated with T1DM). These patients are more likely to have hypertension and dyslipidemia than are those with T1DM.

Clinician: any provider within his or her scope of practice; includes medical practitioners (including physicians and physician extenders), dietitians, psychologists, and nurses.

Diabetes: according to the American Diabetes Association criteria, defined as

1. HbA1c ≥6.5% (test performed in an appropriately certified laboratory); or

2. fasting (defined as no caloric intake for at least 8 hours) plasma glucose ≥126 mg/dL (7.0 mmol/L); or

3. 2-hour plasma glucose ≥200 mg/dL (11.1 mmol/L) during an oral glucose tolerance test performed as described by the World Health Organization by using a glucose load containing the equivalent of 75 g anhydrous glucose dissolved in water; or

4. a random plasma glucose ≥200 mg/dL (11.1 mmol/L) with symptoms of hyperglycemia.

(In the absence of unequivocal hyperglycemia, criteria 1–3 should be confirmed by repeat testing.)

Diabetic ketoacidosis: acidosis resulting from an absolute or relative insulin deficiency, causing fat breakdown and formation of β hydroxybutyrate. Symptoms include nausea, vomiting, dehydration, Kussmaul respirations, and altered mental status.

Fasting blood glucose: blood glucose obtained before the first meal of the day and after a fast of at least 8 hours.

Glucose toxicity: The effect of high blood glucose causing both insulin resistance and impaired β-cell production of insulin.

Intensification: Increase frequency of blood glucose monitoring and adjustment of the dose and type of medication in an attempt to normalize blood glucose concentrations.

Intercurrent illnesses: Febrile illnesses or associated symptoms severe enough to cause the patient to stay home from school and/or seek medical care.

Microalbuminuria: Albumin:creatinine ratio ≥30 mg/g creatinine but <300 mg/g creatinine.

Moderate hyperglycemia: blood glucose = 180–250 mg/dL.

Moderate-to-vigorous exercise: exercise that makes the individual breathe hard and perspire and that raises his or her heart rate. An easy way to define exercise intensity for patients is the "talk test": during moderate physical activity a person can talk, but not sing. During vigorous activity, a person cannot talk without pausing to catch a breath.

Obese: BMI ≥95th percentile for age and gender.

Overweight: BMI between the 85th and 94th percentile for age and gender.

Prediabetes: Fasting plasma glucose ≥100–125 mg/dL or 2-hour glucose concentration during an oral glucose tolerance test ≥126 but <200 mg/dL or an HbA1c of 5.7% to 6.4%.

Severe hyperglycemia: blood glucose >250 mg/dL.

Thiazolidinediones (TZDs): Oral hypoglycemic agents that exert their effect at least in part by activation of the peroxisome proliferator-activated receptor γ.

Type 1 diabetes mellitus (T1DM): Diabetes secondary to autoimmune destruction of β cells resulting in absolute (complete or near complete) insulin deficiency and requiring insulin injections for management.

Type 2 diabetes mellitus (T2DM): The investigators' designation of the diagnosis was used for the purposes of the literature review. The committee acknowledges the distinction between T1DM and T2DM in this population is not always clear cut, and clinical judgment plays an important role. Typically, this diagnosis is made when hyperglycemia is secondary to insulin resistance accompanied by impaired β-cell function resulting in inadequate insulin production to compensate for the degree of insulin resistance.

Youth: used interchangeably with "adolescent" in this document.

INTRODUCTION

Over the past 3 decades, the prevalence of childhood obesity has increased dramatically in North America,[1–5] ushering in a variety of health problems, including type 2 diabetes mellitus (T2DM), which previously was not typically seen until much later in life. Currently, in the United States, up to 1 in 3 new cases of diabetes mellitus diagnosed in youth younger than 18 years is T2DM (depending on the ethnic composition of the patient population),[6,7] with a disproportionate representation in ethnic minorities[8,9] and occurring most commonly among youth between 10 and 19 years of age.[5,10] This trend is not limited to the United States but is occurring internationally[11]; it is projected that by the year 2030, an estimated 366 million people worldwide will have diabetes mellitus.[12]

The rapid emergence of childhood T2DM poses challenges to many physicians who find themselves generally ill-equipped to treat adult diseases encountered in children. Most diabetes education materials designed for pediatric patients are directed primarily to families of children with type 1 diabetes mellitus (T1DM) and emphasize insulin treatment and glucose monitoring, which may or may not be appropriate for children with

T2DM.[13,14] The National Diabetes Education Program TIP sheets (which can be ordered or downloaded from www.yourdiabetesinfo.org or ndep.nih.gov) provide guidance on healthy eating, physical activity, and dealing with T2DM in children and adolescents, but few other resources are available that are directly targeted at youth with this disease.[15] Most medications used for T2DM have been tested for safety and efficacy only in people older than 18 years, and there is scant scientific evidence for optimal management of children with T2DM.[16,17] Recognizing the scarcity of evidence-based data, this report provides a set of guidelines for the management and treatment of children with T2DM that is based on a review of current medical literature covering a period from January 1, 1990, to July 1, 2008.

Despite these limitations, the practicing physician is likely to be faced with the need to provide care for children with T2DM. Thus, the American Academy of Pediatrics (AAP), the Pediatric Endocrine Society (PES), the American Academy of Family Physicians (AAFP), American Diabetes Association, and the Academy of Nutrition and Dietetics (formerly the American Dietetic Association) partnered to develop a set of guidelines that might benefit endocrinologists and generalists, including pediatricians and family physicians alike. This clinical practice guideline may not provide the only appropriate approach to the management of children with T2DM. It is not expected to serve as a sole source of guidance in the management of children and adolescents with T2DM, nor is it intended to replace clinical judgment or establish a protocol for the care of all children with this condition. Rather, it is intended to assist clinicians in decision-making.

Primary care providers should endeavor to obtain the requisite skills to care for children and adolescents with

T2DM, and should communicate and work closely with a diabetes team of subspecialists when such consultation is available, practical, and appropriate. The frequency of such consultations will vary, but should usually be obtained at diagnosis and then at least annually if possible. When treatment goals are not met, the committee encourages clinicians to consult with an expert trained in the care of children and adolescents with T2DM.[18,19] When first-line therapy (eg, metformin) fails, recommendations for intensifying therapy should be generally the same for pediatric and adult populations. The picture is constantly changing, however, as new drugs are introduced, and some drugs that initially appeared to be safe demonstrate adverse effects with wider use. Clinicians should, therefore, remain alert to new developments with regard to treatment of T2DM. Seeking the advice of an expert can help ensure that the treatment goals are appropriately set and that clinicians benefit from cutting-edge treatment information in this rapidly changing area.

The Importance of Family-Centered Diabetes Care

Family structure, support, and education help inform clinical decision-making and negotiations with the patient and family about medical preferences that affect medical decisions, independent of existing clinical recommendations. Because adherence is a major issue in any lifestyle intervention, engaging the family is critical not only to maintain needed changes in lifestyle but also to foster medication adherence.[20–22] The family's ideal role in lifestyle interventions varies, however, depending on the child's age. Behavioral interventions in younger children have shown a favorable effect. With adolescents, however, interventions based on target-age behaviors (eg, including phone or Internet-based

interventions as well as face-to-face or peer-enhanced activities) appear to foster better results, at least for weight management.[23]

Success in making lifestyle changes to attain therapeutic goals requires the initial and ongoing education of the patient and the entire family about healthy nutrition and exercise. Any behavior change recommendations must establish realistic goals and take into account the families' health beliefs and behaviors. Understanding the patient and family's perception of the disease (and overweight status) before establishing a management plan is important to dispel misconceptions and promote adherence.[24] Because T2DM disproportionately affects minority populations, there is a need to ensure culturally appropriate, family-centered care along with ongoing education.[25–28] Several observational studies cite the importance of addressing cultural issues within the family.[20–22]

Restrictions in Creating This Document

In developing these guidelines, the following restrictions governed the committee's work:

- Although the importance of diabetes detection and screening of at-risk populations is acknowledged and referenced, the guidelines are restricted to patients meeting the diagnostic criteria for diabetes (eg, this document focuses on treatment postdiagnosis). Specifically, this document and its recommendations do not pertain to patients with impaired fasting plasma glucose (100–125 mg/dL) or impaired glucose tolerance (2-hour oral glucose tolerance test plasma glucose: 140–200 mg/dL) or isolated insulin resistance.

- Although it is noted that the distinction between types 1 and 2 diabetes mellitus in children may be difficult,[29,30] these recommendations pertain specifically to patients 10 to less than 18 years of age with T2DM (as defined above).

- Although the importance of high-risk care and glycemic control in pregnancy, including pregravid glycemia, is affirmed, the evidence considered and recommendations contained in this document do not pertain to diabetes in pregnancy, including diabetes in pregnant adolescents.

- Recommended screening schedules and management tools for select comorbid conditions (hypertension, dyslipidemia, nephropathy, microalbuminuria, and depression) are provided as resources in the accompanying technical report.[31] These therapeutic recommendations were adapted from other recommended guideline documents with references, without an independent assessment of their supporting evidence.

METHODS

A systematic review was performed and is described in detail in the accompanying technical report.[31] To develop the clinical practice guideline on the management of T2DM in children and adolescents, the AAP convened the Subcommittee on Management of T2DM in Children and Adolescents with the support of the American Diabetes Association, the PES, the AAFP, and the Academy of Nutrition and Dietetics. The subcommittee was co-chaired by 2 pediatric endocrinologists preeminent in their field and included experts in general pediatrics, family medicine, nutrition, Native American health, epidemiology, and medical informatics/guideline methodology. All panel members reviewed the AAP policy on Conflict of Interest and Voluntary Disclosure and declared all potential conflicts (see conflicts statements in the Task Force member list).

These groups partnered to develop an evidence report that served as a major source of information for these practice guideline recommendations.[31] Specific clinical questions addressed in the evidence review were as follows: (1) the effectiveness of treatment modalities for T2DM in children and adolescents, (2) the efficacy of pharmaceutical therapies for treatment of children and adolescents with T2DM, (3) appropriate recommendations for screening for comorbidities typically associated with T2DM in children and adolescents, and (4) treatment recommendations for comorbidities of T2DM in children and adolescents. The accompanying technical report contains more information on comorbidities.[31]

Epidemiologic project staff searched Medline, the Cochrane Collaboration, and Embase. MESH terms used in various combinations in the search included diabetes, mellitus, type 2, type 1, treatment, prevention, diet, pediatric, T2DM, T1DM, NIDDM, metformin, lifestyle, RCT, meta-analysis, child, adolescent, therapeutics, control, adult, obese, gestational, polycystic ovary syndrome, metabolic syndrome, cardiovascular, dyslipidemia, men, and women. In addition, the Boolean

operators NOT, AND, OR were included in various combinations. Articles addressing treatment of diabetes mellitus were prospectively limited to those that were published in English between January 1990 and June 2008, included abstracts, and addressed children between the ages of 120 and 215 months with an established diagnosis of T2DM. Studies in adults were considered for inclusion if >10% of the study population was 45 years of age or younger. The Medline search limits included the following: clinical trial; meta-analysis; randomized controlled trial; review; child: 6–12 years; and adolescent: 13–18 years. Additional articles were identified by review of reference lists of relevant articles and ongoing studies recommended by a technical expert advisory group. All articles were reviewed for compliance with the search limitations and appropriateness for inclusion in this document.

Initially, 199 abstracts were identified for possible inclusion, of which 52 were retained for systematic review. Results of the literature review were presented in evidence tables and published in the final evidence report. An additional literature search of Medline and the Cochrane Database of

Evidence Quality	Preponderance of Benefit or Harm	Balance of Benefit and Harm
A. Well-designed RCTs or diagnostic studies on relevant population	Strong Recommendation	
B. RCTs or diagnostic studies with minor limitations; overwhelmingly consistent evidence from observational studies		Option
C. Observational studies (case-control and cohort design)	Recommendation	
D. Expert opinion, case reports, reasoning from first principles	Option	No Rec
X. Exceptional situations where validating studies cannot be performed and there is a clear preponderance of benefit or harm	Strong Recommendation / Recommendation	

FIGURE 1

Evidence quality. Integrating evidence quality appraisal with an assessment of the anticipated balance between benefits and harms if a policy is carried out leads to designation of a policy as a strong recommendation, recommendation, option, or no recommendation.[32] RCT, randomized controlled trial; Rec, recommendation.

TABLE 1 Definitions and Recommendation Implications

Statement	Definition	Implication
Strong recommendation	A *strong recommendation* in favor of a particular action is made when the anticipated benefits of the recommended intervention clearly exceed the harms (as a strong recommendation against an action is made when the anticipated harms clearly exceed the benefits) and the quality of the supporting evidence is excellent. In some clearly identified circumstances, strong recommendations may be made when high-quality evidence is impossible to obtain and the anticipated benefits strongly outweigh the harms.	Clinicians should follow a strong recommendation unless a clear and compelling rationale for an alternative approach is present.
Recommendation	A *recommendation* in favor of a particular action is made when the anticipated benefits exceed the harms but the quality of evidence is not as strong. Again, in some clearly identified circumstances, recommendations may be made when high-quality evidence is impossible to obtain but the anticipated benefits outweigh the harms.	Clinicians would be prudent to follow a recommendation but should remain alert to new information and sensitive to patient preferences.
Option	*Options* define courses that may be taken when either the quality of evidence is suspect or carefully performed studies have shown little clear advantage to 1 approach over another.	Clinicians should consider the option in their decision-making, and patient preference may have a substantial role.
No recommendation	*No recommendation* indicates that there is a lack of pertinent published evidence and that the anticipated balance of benefits and harms is presently unclear.	Clinicians should be alert to new published evidence that clarifies the balance of benefit versus harm.

It should be noted that, because childhood T2DM is a relatively recent medical phenomenon, there is a paucity of evidence for many or most of the recommendations provided. In some cases, supporting references for a specific recommendation are provided that do not deal specifically with childhood T2DM, such as T1DM, childhood obesity, or childhood "prediabetes," or that were not included in the original comprehensive search. Committee members have made every effort to identify those references that did not affect or alter the level of evidence for specific recommendations.

Systematic Reviews was performed in July 2009 for articles discussing recommendations for screening and treatment of 5 recognized comorbidities of T2DM: cardiovascular disease, dyslipidemia, retinopathy, nephropathy, and peripheral vascular disease. Search criteria were the same as for the search on treatment of T2DM, with the inclusion of the term "type 1 diabetes mellitus." Search terms included, in various combinations, the following: diabetes, mellitus, type 2, type 1, pediatric, T2DM, T1DM, NIDDM, hyperlipidemia, retinopathy, microalbuminuria, comorbidities, screening, RCT, meta-analysis, child, and adolescent. Boolean operators and search limits mirrored those of the primary search.

An additional 336 abstracts were identified for possible inclusion, of which 26 were retained for systematic review. Results of this subsequent literature review were also presented in evidence tables and published in

the final evidence report. An epidemiologist appraised the methodologic quality of the research before it was considered by the committee members.

The evidence-based approach to guideline development requires that the evidence in support of each key action statement be identified, appraised, and summarized and that an explicit link between evidence and recommendations be defined. Evidence-based recommendations reflect the quality of evidence and the balance of benefit and harm that is anticipated when the recommendation is followed. The AAP policy statement, "Classifying Recommendations for Clinical Practice Guidelines,"[32] was followed in designating levels of recommendation (see Fig 1 and Table 1).

To ensure that these recommendations can be effectively implemented, the Guidelines Review Group at Yale Center for Medical Informatics provided feedback

on a late draft of these recommendations, using the GuideLine Implementability Appraisal.[33] Several potential obstacles to successful implementation were identified and resolved in the final guideline. Evidence was incorporated systematically into 6 key action statements about appropriate management facilitated by BRIDGE-Wiz software (Building Recommendations in a Developer's Guideline Editor; Yale Center for Medical Informatics).

A draft version of this clinical practice guideline underwent extensive peer review by 8 groups within the AAP, the American Diabetes Association, PES, AAFP, and the Academy of Nutrition and Dietetics. Members of the subcommittee were invited to distribute the draft to other representatives and committees within their specialty organizations. The resulting comments were reviewed by the subcommittee and incorporated into the guideline, as appropriate. All AAP guidelines are reviewed every 5 years.

KEY ACTION STATEMENTS

Key Action Statement 1

Clinicians must ensure that insulin therapy is initiated for children and adolescents with T2DM who are ketotic or in diabetic ketoacidosis and in whom the distinction between T1DM and T2DM is unclear; and, in usual cases, should initiate insulin therapy for patients:

a. who have random venous or plasma BG concentrations ≥250 mg/dL; or

b. whose HbA1c is >9%.

(Strong Recommendation: evidence quality X, validating studies cannot be performed, and C, observational studies and expert opinion; preponderance of benefit over harm.)

process, blood glucose (BG) concentrations may be normal much of the time and the patient likely will be asymptomatic. At this stage, the disease may only be detected by abnormal BG concentrations identified during screening. As insulin secretion declines further, the patient is likely to develop symptoms of hyperglycemia, occasionally with ketosis or frank ketoacidosis. High glucose concentrations can cause a reversible toxicity to islet β cells that contributes further to insulin deficiency. Of adolescents in whom T2DM is subsequently diagnosed, 5% to 25% present with ketoacidosis.[34]

Diabetic ketoacidosis must be treated with insulin and fluid and electrolyte replacement to prevent worsening

T2DM. Patients in whom ketoacidosis is diagnosed require immediate treatment with insulin and fluid replacement in an inpatient setting under the supervision of a physician who is experienced in treating this complication.

Youth and adolescents who present with T2DM with poor glycemic control (BG concentrations ≥250 mg/dL or HbA1c >9%) but who lack evidence of ketosis or ketoacidosis may also benefit from initial treatment with insulin, at least on a short-term basis.[34] This allows for quicker restoration of glycemic control and, theoretically, may allow islet β cells to "rest and recover."[35,36] Furthermore, it has been noted that initiation of insulin may increase long-term adherence to treatment in children and adolescents with T2DM by enhancing the patient's perception of the seriousness of the disease.[7,37–40] Many patients with T2DM can be weaned gradually from insulin therapy and subsequently managed with metformin and lifestyle modification.[34]

As noted previously, in some children and adolescents with newly diagnosed diabetes mellitus, it may be difficult to distinguish between type 1 and type 2 disease (eg, an obese child presenting with ketosis).[39,41] These patients are best managed initially with insulin therapy while appropriate tests are performed to differentiate between T1DM and T2DM. The care of children and adolescents who have either newly diagnosed T2DM or undifferentiated-type diabetes and who require initial insulin treatment should be supervised by a physician experienced in treating diabetic patients with insulin.

Key Action Statement 2

In all other instances, clinicians should initiate a lifestyle modification program, including nutrition

Action Statement Profile KAS 1

Aggregate evidence quality	X (validating studies cannot be performed)
Benefits	Avoidance of progression of diabetic ketoacidosis (DKA) and worsening metabolic acidosis; resolution of acidosis and hyperglycemia; avoidance of coma and/or death. Quicker restoration of glycemic control, potentially allowing islet β cells to "rest and recover," increasing long-term adherence to treatment; avoiding progression to DKA if T1DM. Avoiding hospitalization. Avoidance of potential risks associated with the use of other agents (eg, abdominal discomfort, bloating, loose stools with metformin; possible cardiovascular risks with sulfonylureas).
Harms/risks/cost	Potential for hypoglycemia, insulin-induced weight gain, cost, patient discomfort from injection, necessity for BG testing, more time required by the health care team for patient training.
Benefits-harms assessment	Preponderance of benefit over harm.
Value judgments	Extensive clinical experience of the expert panel was relied on in making this recommendation.
Role of patient preferences	Minimal.
Exclusions	None.
Intentional vagueness	None.
Strength	Strong recommendation.

The presentation of T2DM in children and adolescents varies according to the disease stage. Early in the disease, before diabetes diagnostic criteria are met, insulin resistance predominates with compensatory high insulin secretion, resulting in normoglycemia. Over time, β cells lose their ability to secrete adequate amounts of insulin to overcome insulin resistance, and hyperglycemia results. Early in this

metabolic acidosis, coma, and death. Children and adolescents with symptoms of hyperglycemia (polyuria, polydipsia, and polyphagia) who are diagnosed with diabetes mellitus should be evaluated for ketosis (serum or urine ketones) and, if positive, for ketoacidosis (venous pH), even if their phenotype and risk factor status (obesity, acanthosis nigricans, positive family history of T2DM) suggests

and physical activity, and start metformin as first-line therapy for children and adolescents at the time of diagnosis of T2DM. (Strong recommendation: evidence quality B; 1 RCT showing improved outcomes with metformin versus lifestyle; preponderance of benefits over harms.)

Action Statement Profile KAS 2

Aggregate evidence quality	B (1 randomized controlled trial showing improved outcomes with metformin versus lifestyle combined with expert opinion).
Benefit	Lower HbA1c, target HbA1c sustained longer, less early deterioration of BG, less chance of weight gain, improved insulin sensitivity, improved lipid profile.
Harm (of using metformin)	Gastrointestinal adverse effects or potential for lactic acidosis and vitamin B_{12} deficiency, cost of medications, cost to administer, need for additional instruction about medication, self-monitoring blood glucose (SMBG), perceived difficulty of insulin use, possible metabolic deterioration if T1DM is misdiagnosed and treated as T2DM, potential risk of lactic acidosis in the setting of ketosis or significant dehydration. It should be noted that there have been no cases reported of vitamin B_{12} deficiency or lactic acidosis with the use of metformin in children.
Benefits-harms assessment	Preponderance of benefit over harm.
Value judgments	Committee members valued faster achievement of BG control over not medicating children.
Role of patient preferences	Moderate; precise implementation recommendations likely will be dictated by patient preferences regarding healthy nutrition, potential medication adverse reaction, exercise, and physical activity.
Exclusions	Although the recommendation to start metformin applies to all, certain children and adolescents with T2DM will not be able to tolerate metformin. In addition, certain older or more debilitated patients with T2DM may be restricted in the amount of moderate-to-vigorous exercise they can perform safely. Nevertheless, this recommendation applies to the vast majority of children and adolescents with T2DM.
Intentional vagueness	None.
Policy level	Strong recommendation.

Metformin as First-Line Therapy

Because of the low success rate with diet and exercise alone in pediatric patients diagnosed with T2DM, metformin should be initiated along with the promotion of lifestyle changes, unless insulin is needed to reverse glucose toxicity in the case of significant hyperglycemia or ketoacidosis (see Key Action Statement 1). Because gastrointestinal adverse effects are common with metformin therapy, the committee recommends starting the drug at a low dose of 500 mg daily, increasing by 500 mg every 1 to 2 weeks, up to an ideal and maximum dose of 2000 mg daily in divided doses.[41] It should be noted that the main gastrointestinal adverse effects (abdominal pain, bloating, loose stools) present at initiation of metformin often are transient and often disappear completely if medication is continued. Generally, doses higher than 2000 mg daily do not provide additional therapeutic benefit.[34,42,43] In addition, the use of extended-release metformin, especially with evening dosing, may be considered, although data regarding the frequency of adverse effects with this preparation are scarce. Metformin is generally better tolerated when taken with food. It is important to recognize the paucity of credible RCTs in adolescents with T2DM. The evidence to recommend initiating metformin at diagnosis along with lifestyle changes comes from 1 RCT, several observational studies, and consensus recommendations.

Lifestyle modifications (including nutrition interventions and increased physical activity) have long been the cornerstone of therapy for T2DM. Yet, medical practitioners recognize that effecting these changes is both challenging and often accompanied by regression over time to behaviors not conducive to maintaining the target range of BG concentrations. In pediatric patients, lifestyle change is most likely to be successful when a multidisciplinary approach is used and the entire family is involved. (Encouragement of healthy eating and physical exercise are discussed in Key Action Statements 5 and 6.) Unfortunately, efforts at lifestyle change often fail for a variety of reasons, including high rates of loss to follow-up; a high rate of depression in teenagers, which affects adherence; and peer pressure to participate in activities that often center on unhealthy eating.

Expert consensus is that fewer than 10% of pediatric T2DM patients will attain their BG goals through lifestyle interventions alone.[6,35,44] It is possible that the poor long-term success rates observed from lifestyle interventions stem from patients' perception that the intervention is not important because medications are not being prescribed. One might speculate that prescribing medications, particularly insulin therapy, may convey a greater degree of concern for the patient's health and the seriousness of the diagnosis, relative to that conveyed when medications are not needed, and that improved treatment adherence and follow-up may result from the use of medication. Indeed, 2 prospective observational studies revealed that treatment with lifestyle modification alone is associated with a higher rate of loss to follow-up than that found in patients who receive medication.[45]

Before initiating treatment with metformin, a number of important considerations must be taken into account. First, it is important to determine whether the child with a new diagnosis has T1DM or T2DM, and it is critical to err on the side of caution if there is any uncertainty. The 2009 *Clinical Practice Consensus Guidelines on Type 2 Diabetes in Children and Adolescents* from the International Society for Pediatric and Adolescent Diabetes provides more information on the classification of diabetes in children and adolescents with new diagnoses.[46] If the diagnosis is unclear (as may be the case when an obese child with diabetes presents also with ketosis), the adolescent must be treated with insulin until the T2DM diagnosis is confirmed.[47] Although it is recognized that some children with newly diagnosed T2DM may respond to metformin alone, the committee believes that the presence of either ketosis or ketoacidosis dictates an absolute initial requirement for insulin replacement. (This is addressed in Key Action Statement 1.)

Although there is little debate that a child presenting with significant hyperglycemia and/or ketosis requires insulin, children presenting with more modest levels of hyperglycemia (eg, random BG of 200–249 mg/dL) or asymptomatic T2DM present additional therapeutic challenges to the clinician. In such cases, metformin alone, insulin alone, or metformin with insulin all represent reasonable options. Additional agents are likely to become reasonable options for initial pharmacologic management in the near future. Although metformin and insulin are the only antidiabetic agents currently approved by the US Food and

Drug Administration (FDA) for use in children, both thiazolidinediones and incretins are occasionally used in adolescents younger than 18 years.[48]

Metformin is recommended as the initial pharmacologic agent in adolescents presenting with mild hyperglycemia and without ketonuria or severe hyperglycemia. In addition to improving hepatic insulin sensitivity, metformin has a number of practical advantages over insulin:

- Potential weight loss or weight neutrality.[37,48]
- Because of a lower risk of hypoglycemia, less frequent finger-stick BG measurements are required with metformin, compared with insulin therapy or sulfonylureas.[37,42,49–51]
- Improves insulin sensitivity and may normalize menstrual cycles in females with polycystic ovary syndrome. (Because metformin may also improve fertility in patients with polycystic ovary syndrome, contraception is indicated for sexually active patients who wish to avoid pregnancy.)
- Taking pills does not have the discomfort associated with injections.
- Less instruction time is required to start oral medication, making it easier for busy practitioners to prescribe.
- Adolescents do not always accept injections, so oral medication might enhance adherence.[52]

Potential advantages of insulin over metformin for treatment at diabetes onset include the following:

- Metabolic control may be achieved more rapidly with insulin compared with metformin therapy.[37]
- With appropriate education and targeting the regimen to the individual, adolescents are able to accept and use insulin therapy with improved metabolic outcomes.[53]

- Insulin offers theoretical benefits of improved metabolic control while preserving β-cell function or even reversing β-cell damage.[34,35]
- Initial use of insulin therapy may convey to the patient a sense of seriousness of the disease.[7,53]

Throughout the writing of these guidelines, the authors have been following the progress of the National Institute of Diabetes and Digestive and Kidney Diseases–supported Treatment Options for type 2 Diabetes in Adolescents and Youth (TODAY) trial,[54] designed to compare standard (metformin alone) therapy versus more aggressive therapy as the initial treatment of youth with recent-onset T2DM. Since the completion of these guidelines, results of the TODAY trial have become available and reveal that metformin alone is inadequate in effecting sustained glycemic control in the majority of youth with diabetes. The study also revealed that the addition of rosiglitazone to metformin is superior to metformin alone in preserving glycemic control. Direct application of these findings to clinical practice is problematic, however, because rosiglitazone is not FDA-approved for use in children, and its use, even in adults, is now severely restricted by the FDA because of serious adverse effects reported in adults. Thus, the results suggest that therapy that is more aggressive than metformin monotherapy may be required in these adolescents to prevent loss of glycemic control, but they do not provide specific guidance because it is not known whether the effect of the additional agent was specific to rosiglitazone or would be seen with the addition of other agents. Unfortunately, there are limited data for the use of other currently available oral or injected hypoglycemic agents in this age range, except for insulin. Therefore, the writing group for these guidelines continues to recommend metformin as first-line therapy in this age group but with close monitoring for glycemic deterioration and the early addition of insulin or another pharmacologic agent if needed.

Lifestyle Modification, Including Nutrition and Physical Activity

Although lifestyle changes are considered indispensable to reaching treatment goals in diabetes, no significant data from RCTs provide information on success rates with such an approach alone.

A potential downside for initiating lifestyle changes alone at T2DM onset is potential loss of patients to follow-up and worse health outcomes. The value of lifestyle modification in the management of adolescents with T2DM is likely forthcoming after a more detailed analysis of the lifestyle intervention arm of the multicenter TODAY trial becomes available.[54] As noted previously, although it was published after

plus-rosiglitazone intervention in maintaining glycemic control over time.[54]

Summary

As noted previously, metformin is a safe and effective agent for use at the time of diagnosis in conjunction with lifestyle changes. Although observational studies and expert opinion strongly support lifestyle changes as a key component of the regimen in addition to metformin, randomized trials are needed to delineate whether using lifestyle options alone is a reasonable first step in treating any select subgroups of children with T2DM.

Key Action Statement 3

The committee suggests that clinicians monitor HbA1c concentrations every 3 months and intensify treatment if treatment goals for BG and HbA1c concentrations are not being met. (Option: evidence quality D; expert opinion and studies in children with T1DM and in adults with T2DM; preponderance of benefits over harms.)

Action Statement Profile KAS 3

Aggregate evidence quality	D (expert opinion and studies in children with T1DM and in adults with T2DM; no studies have been performed in children and adolescents with T2DM).
Benefit	Diminishing the risk of progression of disease and deterioration resulting in hospitalization; prevention of microvascular complications of T2DM.
Harm	Potential for hypoglycemia from overintensifying treatment to reach HbA1c target goals; cost of frequent testing and medical consultation; possible patient discomfort.
Benefits-harms assessment	Preponderance of benefits over harms.
Value judgments	Recommendation dictated by widely accepted standards of diabetic care.
Role of patient preferences	Minimal; recommendation dictated by widely accepted standards of diabetic care.
Exclusions	None.
Intentional vagueness	Intentional vagueness in the recommendation as far as setting goals and intensifying treatment attributable to limited evidence.
Policy level	Option.

this guideline was developed, the TODAY trial indicated that results from the metformin-plus-lifestyle intervention were not significantly different from either metformin alone or the metformin-

HbA1c provides a measure of glycemic control in patients with diabetes mellitus and allows an estimation of the individual's average BG over the previous 8 to 12 weeks. No RCTs have

evaluated the relationship between glycemic control and the risk of developing microvascular and/or macrovascular complications in children and adolescents with T2DM. A number of studies of children with T1DM[55–57] and adults with T2DM have, however, shown a significant relationship between glycemic control (as measured by HbA1c concentration) and the risk of microvascular complications (eg, retinopathy, nephropathy, and neuropathy).[58,59] The relationship between HbA1c concentration and risk of microvascular complications appears to be curvilinear; the lower the HbA1c concentration, the lower the downstream risk of microvascular complications, with the greatest risk reduction seen at the highest HbA1c concentrations.[57]

It is generally recommended that HbA1c concentrations be measured every 3 months.[60] For adults with T1DM, the American Diabetes Association recommends target HbA1c concentrations of less than 7%; the American Association of Clinical Endocrinologists recommends target concentrations of less than 6.5%. Although HbA1c target concentrations for children and adolescents with T1DM are higher,[13] several review articles suggest target HbA1c concentrations of less than 7% for children and adolescents with T2DM.[40,61–63] The committee concurs that, ideally, target HbA1c concentration should be less than 7% but notes that specific goals must be achievable for the individual patient and that this concentration may not be applicable for all patients. For patients in whom a target concentration of less than 7% seems unattainable, individualized goals should be set, with the ultimate goal of reaching guideline target concentrations. In addition, in the absence of hypoglycemia, even lower HbA1c target concentrations can be considered on the basis of an absence of hypoglycemic events and other individual considerations.

When concentrations are found to be above the target, therapy should be intensified whenever possible, with the goal of bringing the concentration to target. Intensification activities may include, but are not limited to, increasing the frequency of clinic visits, engaging in more frequent BG monitoring, adding 1 or more antidiabetic agents, meeting with a registered dietitian and/or diabetes educator, and increasing attention to diet and exercise regimens. Patients whose HbA1c concentrations remain relatively stable may only need to be tested every 6 months. Ideally, real-time HbA1c concentrations should be available at the time of the patient's visit with the clinician to allow the physician and patient and/or parent to discuss intensification of therapy during the visit, if needed.

Key Action Statement 4

The committee suggests that clinicians advise patients to monitor finger-stick BG concentrations in those who

a. are taking insulin or other medications with a risk of hypoglycemia; or

b. are initiating or changing their diabetes treatment regimen; or

c. have not met treatment goals; or

d. have intercurrent illnesses.

(Option: evidence quality D; expert consensus. Preponderance of benefits over harms.)

Glycemic control correlates closely with the frequency of BG monitoring in adolescents with T1DM.[64,65] Although studies evaluating the efficacy of frequent BG monitoring have not been conducted in children and adolescents with T2DM, benefits have been described in insulin-treated adults with T2DM who tested their BG 4 times per day, compared with adults following a less frequent monitoring regimen.[66] These data support the value of BG monitoring in adults treated with insulin, and likely are relevant to youth with T2DM as well, especially those treated with insulin, at the onset of the disease, when treatment goals are not met, and when the treatment regimen is changed. The committee believes that current (2011) ADA recommendations for finger-stick BG monitoring apply to most youth with T2DM[67]:

- Finger-stick BG monitoring should be performed 3 or more times daily for patients using multiple insulin injections or insulin pump therapy.

- For patients using less-frequent insulin injections, noninsulin therapies, or medical nutrition therapy alone, finger-stick BG monitoring may be useful as a guide to the success of therapy.

- To achieve postprandial glucose targets, postprandial finger-stick BG monitoring may be appropriate.

Recognizing that current practices may not always reflect optimal care, a 2004 survey of practices among members of the PES revealed that 36% of pediatric endocrinologists asked their pediatric patients with T2DM to monitor BG concentrations twice daily; 12% asked patients to do so once daily; 13% asked patients to do so 3 times per day; and 12% asked patients to do so 4 times daily.[61] The questionnaire provided to the pediatric endocrinologists did not ask about the frequency of BG monitoring in relationship to the diabetes regimen, however.

Although normoglycemia may be difficult to achieve in adolescents with T2DM, a fasting BG concentration of 70 to 130 mg/dL is a reasonable target for most. In addition, because postprandial hyperglycemia has been associated with increased risk of cardiovascular events in adults, postprandial BG testing may be valuable in select patients. BG concentrations obtained 2 hours after meals (and paired with pre-meal concentrations) provide an index of glycemic excursion, and may be useful in improving glycemic control, particularly for the patient whose fasting plasma glucose is normal but whose HbA1c is not at target.[68] Recognizing the limited evidence for benefit of FSBG testing in this population, the committee provides suggested guidance for testing frequency, tailored to the medication regimen, as follows:

*Fasting
3.9 – 7.2*

BG Testing Frequency for Patients With Newly Diagnosed T2DM: Fasting, Premeal, and Bedtime Testing

The committee suggests that all patients with newly diagnosed T2DM, regardless of prescribed treatment plan, should perform finger-stick BG monitoring before meals (including a morning fasting concentration) and

Action Statement Profile KAS 4

Aggregate evidence quality	D (expert consensus).
Benefit	Potential for improved metabolic control, improved potential for prevention of hypoglycemia, decreased long-term complications.
Harm	Patient discomfort, cost of materials.
Benefits-harms assessment	Benefit over harm.
Value judgments	Despite lack of evidence, there were general committee perceptions that patient safety concerns related to insulin use or clinical status outweighed any risks from monitoring.
Role of patient preferences	Moderate to low; recommendation driven primarily by safety concerns.
Exclusions	None.
Intentional vagueness	Intentional vagueness in the recommendation about specific approaches attributable to lack of evidence and the need to individualize treatment.
Policy level	Option.

at bedtime until reasonable metabolic control is achieved.[69] Once BG concentrations are at target levels, the frequency of monitoring can be modified depending on the medication used, the regimen's intensity, and the patient's metabolic control. Patients who are prone to marked hyperglycemia or hypoglycemia or who are on a therapeutic regimen associated with increased risk of hypoglycemia will require continued frequent BG testing. Expectations for frequency and timing of BG monitoring should be clearly defined through shared goal-setting between the patient and clinician. The adolescent and family members should be given a written action plan stating the medication regimen, frequency and timing of expected BG monitoring, as well as follow-up instructions.

BG Testing Frequency for Patients on Single Insulin Daily Injections and Oral Agents

Single bedtime long-acting insulin: The simplest insulin regimen consists of a single injection of long-acting insulin at bedtime (basal insulin only). The appropriateness of the insulin dose for patients using this regimen is best defined by the fasting/prebreakfast BG test. For patients on this insulin regimen, the committee suggests daily fasting BG measurements. This regimen is associated with some risk of hypoglycemia (especially overnight or fasting hypoglycemia) and may not provide adequate insulin coverage for mealtime ingestions throughout the day, as reflected by fasting BG concentrations in target, but daytime readings above target. In such cases, treatment with meglitinide (Prandin [Novo Nordisk Pharmaceuticals] or Starlix [Novartis Pharmaceuticals]) or a short-acting insulin before meals (see below) may be beneficial.

Oral agents: Once treatment goals are met, the frequency of monitoring can be decreased; however, the committee recommends some continued BG testing for all youth with T2DM, at a frequency determined within the clinical context (e.g. medication regimen, HbA1c, willingness of the patient, etc.). For example, an infrequent or intermittent monitoring schedule may be adequate when the patient is using exclusively an oral agent associated with a low risk of hypoglycemia and if HbA1c concentrations are in the ideal or non-diabetic range. A more frequent monitoring schedule should be advised during times of illness or if symptoms of hyperglycemia or hypoglycemia develop.

Oral agent plus a single injection of a long-acting insulin: Some youth with T2DM can be managed successfully with a single injection of long-acting insulin in conjunction with an oral agent. Twice a day BG monitoring (fasting plus a second BG concentration – ideally 2-hour post prandial) often is recommended, as long as HbA1c and BG concentrations remain at goal and the patient remains asymptomatic.

BG Testing Frequency for Patients Receiving Multiple Daily Insulin Injections (eg, Basal Bolus Regimens): Premeal and Bedtime Testing

Basal bolus regimens are commonly used in children and youth with T1DM and may be appropriate for some youth with T2DM as well. They are the most labor intensive, providing both basal insulin plus bolus doses of short-acting insulin at meals. Basal insulin is provided through either the use of long-acting, relatively peak-free insulin (by needle) or via an insulin pump. Bolus insulin doses are given at meal-time, using one of the rapid-acting insulin analogs. The bolus dose is calculated by using a correction algorithm for the premeal BG concentration as well as a "carb ratio," in which 1 unit of

a rapid-acting insulin analog is given for "X" grams of carbohydrates ingested (see box below). When using this method, the patient must be willing and able to count the number of grams of carbohydrates in the meal and divide by the assigned "carb ratio (X)" to know how many units of insulin should be taken. In addition, the patient must always check BG concentrations before the meal to determine how much additional insulin should be given as a correction dose using an algorithm assigned by the care team if the fasting BG is not in target. Insulin pumps are based on this concept of "basal-bolus" insulin administration and have the capability of calculating a suggested bolus dosage, based on inputted grams of carbohydrates and BG concentrations. Because the BG value determines the amount of insulin to be given at each meal, the recommended testing frequency for patients on this regimen is before every meal.

Box 1 Example of Basal Bolus Insulin Regimen

If an adolescent has a BG of 250 mg/dL, is to consume a meal containing 60 g of carbohydrates, with a carbohydrate ratio of 1:10 and an assigned correction dose of 1:25>125 (with 25 being the insulin sensitivity and 125 mg/dL the target blood glucose level), the mealtime bolus dose of insulin would be as follows:

60 g/10 "carb ratio" =

6 units rapid-acting insulin for meal

plus

(250−125)/25 = 125/25 =

5 units rapid-acting insulin for correction

Thus, total bolus insulin coverage at mealtime is: **11 U** (6 + 5) of rapid-acting insulin.

Key Action Statement 5

The committee suggests that clinicians incorporate the Academy of Nutrition and Dietetics' *Pediatric Weight Management Evidence-Based Nutrition Practice Guidelines* in the nutrition counseling of patients with T2DM both at the time of diagnosis and as part of ongoing management. (Option; evidence quality D; expert opinion; preponderance of benefits over harms. Role of patient preference is dominant.)

Action Statement Profile KAS 5

Aggregate evidence quality	D (expert opinion).
Benefit	Promotes weight loss; improves insulin sensitivity; contributes to glycemic control; prevents worsening of disease; facilitates a sense of well-being; and improves cardiovascular health.
Harm	Costs of nutrition counseling; inadequate reimbursement of clinicians' time; lost opportunity costs vis-a-vis time and resources spent in other counseling activities.
Benefits-harms assessment	Benefit over harm.
Value judgments	There is a broad societal agreement on the benefits of dietary recommendations.
Role of patient preference	Dominant. Patients may have different preferences for how they wish to receive assistance in managing their weight-loss goals. Some patients may prefer a referral to a nutritionist while others might prefer accessing online sources of help. Patient preference should play a significant role in determining an appropriate weight-loss strategy.
Exclusions	None.
Intentional vagueness	Intentional vagueness in the recommendation about specific approaches attributable to lack of evidence and the need to individualize treatment.
Policy level	Option.

Consuming more calories than one uses results in weight gain and is a major contributor to the increasing incidence of T2DM in children and adolescents. Current literature is inconclusive about a single best meal plan for patients with diabetes mellitus, however, and studies specifically addressing the diet of children and adolescents with T2DM are limited. Challenges to making recommendations stem from the small sample size of these studies, limited specificity for children and adolescents, and difficulties in generalizing the data from dietary research studies to the general population.

Although evidence is lacking in children with T2DM, numerous studies have been conducted in overweight children and adolescents, because the great majority of children with T2DM are obese or overweight at diagnosis.[26] The committee suggests that clinicians encourage children and adolescents with T2DM to follow the Academy of Nutrition and Dietetics' recommendations for maintaining healthy weight to promote health and reduce obesity in this population. The committee recommends that clinicians refer patients to a registered dietitian who has expertise in the nutritional needs of youth with T2DM. Clinicians should incorporate the Academy of Nutrition and Dietetics' *Pediatric Weight Management Evidence-Based Nutrition Practice Guidelines*, which describe effective, evidence-based treatment options for weight management, summarized below (A complete list of these recommendations is accessible to health care professionals at: http://www.andevidencelibrary.com/topic.cfm?cat=4102&auth=1.)

According to the Academy of Nutrition and Dietetics' guidelines, when incorporated with lifestyle changes, balanced macronutrient diets at 900 to 1200 kcal per day are associated with both short- and long-term (eg, ≥ 1 year) improvements in weight status and body composition in children 6 to 12 years of age.[70] These calorie recommendations are to be incorporated with lifestyle changes, including increased activity and possibly medication. Restrictions of no less than 1200 kcal per day in adolescents 13 to 18 years old result in improved weight status and body composition as well.[71] The Diabetes Prevention Program demonstrated that participants assigned to the intensive lifestyle-intervention arm had a reduction in daily energy intake of 450 kcal and a 58% reduction in progression to diabetes at the 2.8-year follow-up.[71] At the study's end, 50% of the lifestyle-arm participants had achieved the goal weight loss of at least 7% after the 24-week curriculum and 38% showed weight loss of at least 7% at the time of their most recent visit.[72] The Academy of Nutrition and Dietetics recommends that protein-sparing, modified-fast (ketogenic) diets be restricted to children who are >120% of their ideal body weight and who have a serious medical complication that would benefit from rapid weight loss.[71] Specific recommendations are for the intervention to be short-term (typically 10 weeks) and to be conducted under the supervision of a multidisciplinary team specializing in pediatric obesity.

Regardless of the meal plan prescribed, some degree of nutrition education must be provided to maximize adherence and positive results. This education should encourage patients to follow healthy eating patterns, such as consuming 3 meals with planned snacks per day, not eating while watching television or using computers, using smaller plates to make portions appear larger, and leaving small amounts of food on the plate.[73] Common dietary recommendations to reduce calorie intake and to promote weight loss in children include the following: (1) eating regular meals and snacks; (2) reducing portion sizes; (3) choosing calorie-free beverages, except for milk; (4) limiting juice to 1 cup per day; (5) increasing consumption of fruits and vegetables; (6) consuming 3 or 4 servings of low-fat dairy products per day; (7) limiting intake of high-fat foods; (8) limiting frequency and size of snacks; and (9) reducing calories consumed in fast-food meals.[74]

Key Action Statement 6

The committee suggests that clinicians encourage children and adolescents with T2DM to engage in moderate-to-vigorous exercise for at least 60 minutes daily and to limit nonacademic screen time to less than 2 hours per day. (Option: evidence quality D, expert opinion and evidence from studies of metabolic syndrome and obesity; preponderance of benefits over harms. Role of patient preference is dominant.)

Action Statement Profile KAS 6

Aggregate evidence quality	D (expert opinion and evidence from studies of metabolic syndrome and obesity).
Benefit	Promotes weight loss; contributes to glycemic control; prevents worsening of disease; facilitates the ability to perform exercise; improves the person's sense of well-being; and fosters cardiovascular health.
Harm	Cost for patient of counseling, food, and time; costs for clinician in taking away time that could be spent on other activities; inadequate reimbursement for clinician's time.
Benefits-harms assessment	Preponderance of benefit over harm.
Value judgments	Broad consensus.
Role of patient preference	Dominant. Patients may seek various forms of exercise. Patient preference should play a significant role in creating an exercise plan.
Exclusions	Although certain older or more debilitated patients with T2DM may be restricted in the amount of moderate-to-vigorous exercise they can perform safely, this recommendation applies to the vast majority of children and adolescents with T2DM.
Intentional vagueness	Intentional vagueness on the sequence of follow-up contact attributable to the lack of evidence and the need to individualize care.
Policy level	Option.

Recommendations From the Academy of Nutrition and Dietetics

Pediatric Weight Management Evidence-Based Nutrition Practice Guidelines

Recommendation	Strength
Interventions to reduce pediatric obesity should be multicomponent and include diet, physical activity, nutritional counseling, and parent or caregiver participation.	Strong
A nutrition prescription should be formulated as part of the dietary intervention in a multicomponent pediatric weight management program.	Strong
Dietary factors that may be associated with an increased risk of overweight are increased total dietary fat intake and increased intake of calorically sweetened beverages.	Strong
Dietary factors that may be associated with a decreased risk of overweight are increased fruit and vegetable intake.	Strong
A balanced macronutrient diet that contains no fewer than 900 kcal per day is recommended to improve weight status in children aged 6–12 y who are medically monitored.	Strong
A balanced macronutrient diet that contains no fewer than 1200 kcal per day is recommended to improve weight status in adolescents aged 13–18 y who are medically monitored.	Strong
Family diet behaviors that are associated with an increased risk of pediatric obesity are parental restriction of highly palatable foods, consumption of food away from home, increased meal portion size, and skipping breakfast.	Fair

Engaging in Physical Activity

Physical activity is an integral part of weight management for prevention and treatment of T2DM. Although there is a paucity of available data from children and adolescents with T2DM, several well-controlled studies performed in obese children and adolescents at risk of metabolic syndrome and T2DM provide guidelines for physical activity. (See the Resources section for tools on this subject.) A summary of the references supporting the evidence for this guideline can be found in the technical report.[31]

At present, moderate-to-vigorous exercise of at least 60 minutes daily is recommended for reduction of BMI and improved glycemic control in patients with T2DM.[75] "Moderate to vigorous exercise" is defined as exercise that makes the individual breathe hard and perspire and that raises his or her heart rate. An easy way to define exercise intensity for patients is the "talk test"; during moderate physical activity a person can talk but not sing. During vigorous activity, a person cannot talk without pausing to catch a breath.[76]

Adherence may be improved if clinicians provide the patient with a written prescription to engage in physical activity, including a "dose" describing ideal duration, intensity, and frequency.[75] When prescribing physical exercise, clinicians are encouraged to be sensitive to the needs of children, adolescents, and their families. Routine, organized exercise may be beyond the family's logistical and/or financial means, and some families may not be able to provide structured exercise programs for their children. It is most helpful to recommend an individualized approach that can be incorporated into the daily routine, is tailored to the patients' physical abilities and preferences, and recognizes the families' circumstances.[77] For example, clinicians might recommend only daily walking, which has been shown to improve weight loss and insulin sensitivity in adults with T2DM[78] and may constitute "moderate to vigorous activity" for some children with T2DM. It is also important to recognize that the recommended 60 minutes of exercise do not have to be accomplished in 1 session but can be completed through several, shorter increments (eg, 10–15 minutes). Patients should be encouraged to identify a variety of forms of activity that can be performed both easily and frequently.[77] In addition, providers should be cognizant of the potential need to adjust the medication dosage, especially if the patient is receiving insulin, when initiating an aggressive physical activity program.

Reducing Screen Time

Screen time contributes to a sedentary lifestyle, especially when the child or adolescent eats while watching television or playing computer games. The US Department of Health and Human Services recommends that individuals limit "screen time" spent watching television and/or using computers and handheld devices to less than 2 hours per day unless the use is related to work or homework.[79] Physical activity may be gained either through structured games and sports or through everyday activities, such as walking, ideally with involvement of the parents as good role models.

Increased screen time and food intake and reduced physical activity are associated with obesity. There is good evidence that modifying these factors can help prevent T2DM by reducing the individual's rate of weight gain. The evidence profile in pediatric patients with T2DM is inadequate at this time, however. Pending new data, the committee suggests that clinicians follow the AAP Committee on Nutrition's guideline, *Prevention of Pediatric Overweight and Obesity*. The guideline recommends restricting nonacademic screen time to a maximum of 2 hours per day and discouraging the presence of video screens and television sets in children's bedrooms.[80–82] The American Medical Association's Expert Panel on Childhood Obesity has endorsed this guideline.

Valuable recommendations for enhancing patient health include the following:

- With patients and their families, jointly determining an individualized plan that includes specific goals to reduce sedentary behaviors and increase physical activity.

- Providing a written prescription for engaging in 60-plus minutes of moderate-to-vigorous physical activities per day that includes

dose, timing, and duration. It is important for clinicians to be sensitive to the needs of children, adolescents, and their families in encouraging daily physical exercise. Graded duration of exercise is recommended for those youth who cannot initially be active for 60 minutes daily, and the exercise may be accomplished through several, shorter increments (eg, 10–15 minutes).

- Incorporating physical activities into children's and adolescents' daily routines. Physical activity may be gained either through structured games and sports or through everyday activities, such as walking.

- Restricting nonacademic screen time to a maximum of 2 hours per day.

- Discouraging the presence of video screens and television sets in children's bedrooms.

Conversations pertaining to the Key Action Statements should be clearly documented in the patient's medical record.

AREAS FOR FUTURE RESEARCH

As noted previously, evidence for medical interventions in children in general is scant and is especially lacking for interventions directed toward children who have developed diseases not previously seen commonly in youth, such as childhood T2DM. Recent studies such as the Search for Diabetes in Youth Study (SEARCH)—an observational multicenter study in 2096 youth with T2DM funded by the Centers for Disease Control and Prevention and the National Institute of Diabetes and Digestive and Kidney Diseases—now provide a detailed description of childhood diabetes. Subsequent trials will describe the short-term and enduring effects of specific interventions on the progression of the disease with time.

Although it is likely that children and adolescents with T2DM have an aggressive form of diabetes, as reflected by the age of onset, future research should determine whether the associated comorbidities and complications of diabetes also are more aggressive in pediatric populations than in adults and if they are more or less responsive to therapeutic interventions. Additional research should explore whether early introduction of insulin or the use of particular oral agents will preserve β-cell function in these children, and whether recent technologic advances (such as continuous glucose monitoring and insulin pumps) will benefit this population. Additional issues that require further study include the following:

- To delineate whether using lifestyle options without medication is a reliable first step in treating selected children with T2DM.

- To determine whether BG monitoring should be recommended to all children and youth with T2DM, regardless of therapy used; what the optimal frequency of BG monitoring is for pediatric patients on the basis of treatment regimen; and which subgroups will be able to successfully maintain glycemic goals with less frequent monitoring.

- To explore the efficacy of school- and clinic-based diet and physical activity interventions to prevent and manage pediatric T2DM.

- To explore the association between increased "screen time" and reduced physical activity with respect to T2DM's risk factors.

RESOURCES

Several tools are available online to assist providers in improving patient adherence to lifestyle modifications, including examples of activities to be recommended for patients:

- The American Academy of Pediatrics:
  - www.healthychildren.org
  - www.letsmove.gov
  - Technical Report: Management of Type 2 Diabetes Mellitus in Children and Adolescents.[31]
    - Includes an overview and screening tools for a variety of comorbidities.
  - Gahagan S, Silverstein J; Committee on Native American Child Health and Section on Endocrinology. Clinical report: prevention and treatment of type 2 diabetes mellitus in children, with special emphasis on American Indian and Alaska Native Children. *Pediatrics*. 2003;112 (4):e328–e347. Available at: http://www.pediatrics.org/cgi/content/full/112/4/e328[63]
    - Fig 3 presents a screening tool for microalbumin.
  - Bright Futures: http://brightfutures.aap.org/
  - Daniels SR, Greer FR; Committee on Nutrition. Lipid screening and cardiovascular health in childhood. *Pediatrics*. 2008;122 (1):198–208. Available at:
- The American Diabetes Association: www.diabetes.org
  - Management of dyslipidemia in children and adolescents with diabetes. *Diabetes Care*. 2003;26(7):2194–2197. Available at: http://care.diabetesjournals.org/content/26/7/2194.full
- Academy of Nutrition and Dietetics:
  - http://www.eatright.org/childhoodobesity/
  - http://www.eatright.org/kids/
  - http://www.eatright.org/cps/rde/xchg/ada/hs.xsl/index.html

- Pediatric Weight Management Evidence-Based Nutrition Practice Guidelines: http://www.adaevidencelibrary.com/topic.cfm?cat=2721
- American Heart Association:
  - American Heart Association *Circulation*. 2006 Dec 12;114(24):2710-2738. Epub 2006 Nov 27. Review.
- Centers for Disease Control and Prevention:
  - http://www.cdc.gov/obesity/childhood/solutions.html
  - BMI and other growth charts can be downloaded and printed from the CDC Web site: http://www.cdc.gov/growth-charts.
  - Center for Epidemiologic Studies Depression Scale (CES-D): http://www.chcr.brown.edu/pcoc/cesdscale.pdf; see attachments
- *Diagnostic and Statistical Manual of Mental Disorders*. 4th ed. Washington, DC: American Psychiatric Association; 1994
- Let's Move Campaign: www.letsmove.gov
- The Reach Institute. *Guidelines for Adolescent Depression in Primary Care (GLAD-PC) Toolkit*, 2007. Contains a listing of the criteria for major depressive disorder as defined by the DSM-IV-TR. Available at: http://www.gladpc.org
- The National Heart, Lung, and Blood Institute (NHLBI) hypertension guidelines: http://www.nhlbi.nih.gov/guidelines/hypertension/child_tbl.htm
- The National Diabetes Education Program and TIP sheets (including tip sheets on youth transitioning to adulthood and adult providers, Staying Active, Eating Healthy, Ups and Downs of Diabetes, etc): www.ndep.nih.gov or www.yourdiabetesinfo.org

- National High Blood Pressure Education Program Working Group on High Blood Pressure in Children and Adolescents, The Fourth Report on the Diagnosis, Evaluation, and Treatment of High Blood Pressure in Children and Adolescents: *Pediatrics.* 2004;114:555–576. Available at: http://pediatrics.aappublications. org/content/114/Supplement_2/555. long

- National Initiative for Children's Healthcare Quality (NICHQ): childhood obesity section: http://www.nichq. org/childhood_obesity/index.html

- The National Institute of Child Health and Human Development (NICHD): www.NICHD.org

- President's Council on Physical Fitness and Sports: http://www.presidentschallenge.org/home_kids. aspx

- US Department of Agriculture's "My Pyramid" Web site:

- http://www.choosemyplate.gov/
- http://fnic.nal.usda.gov/lifecycle-nutrition/child-nutrition-and-health

SUBCOMMITTEE ON TYPE 2 DIABETES (OVERSIGHT BY THE STEERING COMMITTEE ON QUALITY IMPROVEMENT AND MANAGEMENT, 2008–2012)

Kenneth Claud Copeland, MD, FAAP: Co-chair—Endocrinology and Pediatric Endocrine Society Liaison (2009: Novo Nordisk, Genentech, Endo [National Advisory Groups]; 2010: Novo Nordisk [National Advisory Group]); published research related to type 2 diabetes

Janet Silverstein, MD, FAAP: Co-chair—Endocrinology and American Diabetes Association Liaison (small grants with Pfizer, Novo Nordisk, and Lilly; grant review committee for Genentech; was on an advisory committee for Sanofi Aventis, and Abbott Laboratories for a 1-time meeting); published research related to type 2 diabetes

Kelly Roberta Moore, MD, FAAP: General Pediatrics, Indian Health, AAP Committee on Native American Child Health Liaison (board member of the Merck Company Foundation

Alliance to Reduce Disparities in Diabetes. Their national program office is the University of Michigan's Center for Managing Chronic Disease.)

Greg Edward Prazar, MD, FAAP: General Pediatrics (no conflicts)

Terry Raymer, MD, CDE: Family Medicine, Indian Health Service (no conflicts)

Richard N. Shiffman, MD, FAAP: Partnership for Policy Implementation Informatician, General Pediatrics (no conflicts)

Shelley C. Springer, MD, MBA, FAAP: Epidemiologist (no conflicts)

Meaghan Anderson, MS, RD, LD, CDE: Academy of Nutrition and Dietetics Liaison (formerly a Certified Pump Trainer for Animas)

Stephen J. Spann, MD, MBA, FAAFP: American Academy of Family Physicians Liaison (no conflicts)

Vidhu V. Thaker, MD, FAAP: QuIIN Liaison, General Pediatrics (no conflicts)

CONSULTANT

Susan K. Flinn, MA: Medical Writer (no conflicts)

STAFF

Caryn Davidson, MA

REFERENCES

1. Centers for Disease Control and Prevention. Data and Statistics. Obesity rates among children in the United States. Available at: www.cdc.gov/obesity/childhood/prevalence. html. Accessed August 13, 2012

2. Copeland KC, Chalmers LJ, Brown RD. Type 2 diabetes in children: oxymoron or medical metamorphosis? *Pediatr Ann.* 2005;34 (9):686–697

3. Narayan KM, Boyle JP, Thompson TJ, Sorensen SW, Williamson DF. Lifetime risk for diabetes mellitus in the United States. *JAMA.* 2003;290(14):1884–1890

4. Chopra M, Galbraith S, Darnton-Hill I. A global response to a global problem: the epidemic of overnutrition. *Bull World Health Organ.* 2002;80(12):952–958

5. Liese AD, D'Agostino RB, Jr, Hamman RF, et al; SEARCH for Diabetes in Youth Study Group. The burden of diabetes mellitus among US youth: prevalence estimates from the SEARCH for Diabetes in Youth Study. *Pediatrics.* 2006;118(4):1510–1518

6. Silverstein JH, Rosenbloom AL. Type 2 diabetes in children. *Curr Diab Rep.* 2001;1 (1):19–27

7. Pinhas-Hamiel O, Zeitler P. Clinical presentation and treatment of type 2 diabetes in children. *Pediatr Diabetes.* 2007;8(suppl 9):16–27

8. Dabelea D, Bell RA, D'Agostino RB Jr, et al; Writing Group for the SEARCH for Diabetes in Youth Study Group. Incidence of diabetes in youth in the United States. *JAMA.* 2007; 297(24):2716–2724

9. Mayer-Davis EJ, Bell RA, Dabelea D, et al; SEARCH for Diabetes in Youth Study Group. The many faces of diabetes in American youth: type 1 and type 2 diabetes in five race and ethnic populations: the SEARCH for Diabetes in Youth Study. *Diabetes Care.* 2009;32(suppl 2):S99–S101

10. Copeland KC, Zeitler P, Geffner M, et al; TODAY Study Group. Characteristics of adolescents and youth with recent-onset type 2 diabetes: the TODAY cohort at baseline. *J Clin Endocrinol Metab.* 2011;96(1):159–167

11. Narayan KM, Williams R. Diabetes—a global problem needing global solutions. *Prim Care Diabetes.* 2009;3(1):3–4

12. Wild S, Roglic G, Green A, Sicree R, King H. Global prevalence of diabetes: estimates

for the year 2000 and projections for 2030. *Diabetes Care.* 2004;27(5):1047–1053

13. Silverstein J, Klingensmith G, Copeland K, et al; American Diabetes Association. Care of children and adolescents with type 1 diabetes: a statement of the American Diabetes Association. *Diabetes Care.* 2005;28 (1):186–212

14. Pinhas-Hamiel O, Zeitler P. Barriers to the treatment of adolescent type 2 diabetes—a survey of provider perceptions. *Pediatr Diabetes.* 2003;4(1):24–28

15. Moore KR, McGowan MK, Donato KA, Kollipara S, Roubideaux Y. Community resources for promoting youth nutrition and physical activity. *Am J Health Educ.* 2009;40(5):298–303

16. Zeitler P, Epstein L, Grey M, et al; The TODAY Study Group. Treatment Options for type 2 diabetes mellitus in Adolescents and Youth: a study of the comparative efficacy of metformin alone or in combination with rosiglitazone or lifestyle intervention in adolescents with type 2 diabetes mellitus. *Pediatr Diabetes.* 2007;8(2):74–87

17. Kane MP, Abu-Baker A, Busch RS. The utility of oral diabetes medications in type 2

diabetes of the young. *Curr Diabetes Rev.* 2005;1(1):83–92

18. De Berardis G, Pellegrini F, Franciosi M, et al. Quality of care and outcomes in type 2 diabetes patientes. *Diabetes Care.* 2004;27 (2):398–406

19. Ziemer DC, Miller CD, Rhee MK, et al. Clinical inertia contributes to poor diabetes control in a primary care setting. *Diabetes Educ.* 2005;31(4):564–571

20. Bradshaw B. The role of the family in managing therapy in minority children with type 2 diabetes mellitus. *J Pediatr Endocrinol Metab.* 2002;15(suppl 1):547–551

21. Pinhas-Hamiel O, Standiford D, Hamiel D, Dolan LM, Cohen R, Zeitler PS. The type 2 family: a setting for development and treatment of adolescent type 2 diabetes mellitus. *Arch Pediatr Adolesc Med.* 1999; 153(10):1063–1067

22. Mulvaney SA, Schlundt DG, Mudasiru E, et al. Parent perceptions of caring for adolescents with type 2 diabetes. *Diabetes Care.* 2006;29(5):993–997

23. Summerbell CD, Ashton V, Campbell KJ, Edmunds L, Kelly S, Waters E. Interventions for treating obesity in children. *Cochrane Database Syst Rev.* 2003;(3):CD001872

24. Skinner AC, Weinberger M, Mulvaney S, Schlundt D, Rothman RL. Accuracy of perceptions of overweight and relation to self-care behaviors among adolescents with type 2 diabetes and their parents. *Diabetes Care.* 2008;31(2):227–229

25. American Diabetes Association. Type 2 diabetes in children and adolescents. *Diabetes Care.* 2000;23(3):381–389

26. Pinhas-Hamiel O, Zeitler P. Type 2 diabetes in adolescents, no longer rare. *Pediatr Rev.* 1998;19(12):434–435

27. Fagot-Campagna A, Pettitt DJ, Engelgau MM, et al. Type 2 diabetes among North American children and adolescents: an epidemiologic review and a public health perspective. *J Pediatr.* 2000;136(5):664–672

28. Rothman RL, Mulvaney S, Elasy TA, et al. Self-management behaviors, racial disparities, and glycemic control among adolescents with type 2 diabetes. *Pediatrics.* 2008;121(4). Available at: www.pediatrics. org/cgi/content/full/121/4/e912

29. Scott CR, Smith JM, Cradock MM, Pihoker C. Characteristics of youth-onset noninsulin-dependent diabetes mellitus and insulin-dependent diabetes mellitus at diagnosis. *Pediatrics.* 1997;100(1):84–91

30. Libman IM, Pietropaolo M, Arslanian SA, LaPorte RE, Becker DJ. Changing prevalence of overweight children and adolescents at onset of insulin-treated diabetes. *Diabetes Care.* 2003;26(10):2871–2875

31. Springer SC, Copeland KC, Silverstein J, et al. Technical report: management of type 2 diabetes mellitus in children and adolescents. *Pediatrics.* 2012, In press

32. American Academy of Pediatrics Steering Committee on Quality Improvement and Management. Classifying recommendations for clinical practice guidelines. *Pediatrics.* 2004;114(3):874–877

33. Shiffman RN, Dixon J, Brandt C, et al. The GuideLine Implementability Appraisal (GLIA): development of an instrument to identify obstacles to guideline implementation. *BMC Med Inform Decis Mak.* 2005;5:23

34. Gungor N, Hannon T, Libman I, Bacha F, Arslanian S. Type 2 diabetes mellitus in youth: the complete picture to date. *Pediatr Clin North Am.* 2005;52(6):1579–1609

35. Daaboul JJ, Siverstein JH. The management of type 2 diabetes in children and adolescents. *Minerva Pediatr.* 2004;56(3):255–264

36. Kadmon PM, Grupposo PA. Glycemic control with metformin or insulin therapy in adolescents with type 2 diabetes mellitus. *J Pediatr Endocrinol.* 2004;17(9):1185–1193

37. Owada M, Nitadori Y, Kitagawa T. Treatment of NIDDM in youth. *Clin Pediatr (Phila).* 1998;37(2):117–121

38. Pinhas-Hamiel O, Zeitler P. Advances in epidemiology and treatment of type 2 diabetes in children. *Adv Pediatr.* 2005;52: 223–259

39. Jones KL, Haghi M. Type 2 diabetes mellitus in children and adolescence: a primer. *Endocrinologist.* 2000;10:389–396

40. Kawahara R, Amemiya T, Yoshino M, et al. Dropout of young non-insulin-dependent diabetics from diabetic care. *Diabetes Res Clin Pract.* 1994;24(3):181–185

41. Kaufman FR. Type 2 diabetes mellitus in children and youth: a new epidemic. *J Pediatr Endocrinol Metab.* 2002;15(suppl 2): 737–744

42. Garber AJ, Duncan TG, Goodman AM, Mills DJ, Rohlf JL. Efficacy of metformin in type II diabetes: results of a double-blind, placebo-controlled, dose-response trial. *Am J Med.* 1997;103(6):491–497

43. Dabelea D, Pettitt DJ, Jones KL, Arslanian SA. Type 2 diabetes mellitus in minority children and adolescents: an emerging problem. *Endocrinol Metabo Clin North Am.* 1999;28(4):709–729

44. Miller JL, Silverstein JH. The management of type 2 diabetes mellitus in children and adolescents. *J Pediatr Endocrinol Metab.* 2005;18(2):111–123

45. Reinehr T, Schober E, Roth CL, Wiegand S, Holl R; DPV-Wiss Study Group. Type 2 diabetes in children and adolescents in a 2-year

follow-up: insufficient adherence to diabetes centers. *Horm Res.* 2008;69(2):107–113

46. Rosenbloom AL, Silverstein JH, Amemiya S, Zeitler P, Klingensmith GJ. Type 2 diabetes in children and adolescents. *Pediatr Diabetes.* 2009;10(suppl 12):17–32

47. Zuhri-Yafi MI, Brosnan PG, Hardin DS. Treatment of type 2 diabetes mellitus in children and adolescents. *J Pediatr Endocrinol Metab.* 2002;15(suppl 1):541–546

48. Rapaport R, Silverstein JH, Garzarella L, Rosenbloom AL. Type 1 and type 2 diabetes mellitus in childhood in the United States: practice patterns by pediatric endocrinologists. *J Pediatr Endocrinol Metab.* 2004;17 (6):871–877

49. Glaser N, Jones KL. Non-insulin-dependent diabetes mellitus in children and adolescents. *Adv Pediatr.* 1996;43:359–396

50. Miller JL, Silverstein JH. The treatment of type 2 diabetes mellitus in youth: which therapies? *Treat Endocrinol.* 2006;5(4):201–210

51. Silverstein JH, Rosenbloom AL. Treatment of type 2 diabetes mellitus in children and adolescents. *J Pediatr Endocrinol Metab.* 2000;13(suppl 6):1403–1409

52. Dean H. Treatment of type 2 diabetes in youth: an argument for randomized controlled studies. *Paediatr Child Health (Oxford).* 1999;4(4):265–270

53. Sellers EAC, Dean HJ. Short-term insulin therapy in adolescents with type 2 diabetes mellitus. *J Pediatr Endocrinol Metab.* 2004; 17(11):1561–1564

54. Zeitler P, Hirst K, Pyle L, et al; TODAY Study Group. A clinical trial to maintain glycemic control in youth with type 2 diabetes. *N Engl J Med.* 2012;366(24):2247–2256

55. White NH, Cleary PA, Dahms W, Goldstein D, Malone J, Tamborlane WV; Diabetes Control and Complications Trial (DCCT)/Epidemiology of Diabetes Interventions and Complications (EDIC) Research Group. Beneficial effects of intensive therapy of diabetes during adolescence: outcomes after the conclusion of the Diabetes Control and Complications Trial (DCCT). *J Pediatr.* 2001;139(6):804–812

56. The Diabetes Control and Complications Trial Research Group. The effect of intensive treatment of diabetes on the development and progression of long-term complications in insulin-dependent diabetes mellitus. *N Engl J Med.* 1993;329(14):977–986

57. Orchard TJ, Olson JC, Erbey JR, et al. Insulin resistance-related factors, but not glycemia, predict coronary artery disease in type 1 diabetes: 10-year follow-up data from the Pittsburgh Epidemiology of Diabetes Complications Study. *Diabetes Care.* 2003;26(5):1374–1379

58. UK Prospective Diabetes Study Group. U.K. prospective diabetes study 16. Overview of 6 years' therapy of type II diabetes: a progressive disease. *Diabetes.* 1995;44(11): 1249–1258

59. Shichiri M, Kishikawa H, Ohkubo Y, Wake N. Long-term results of the Kumamoto Study on optimal diabetes control in type 2 diabetic patients. *Diabetes Care.* 2000;23 (suppl 2):B21–B29

60. Baynes JW, Bunn HF, Goldstein D, et al; National Diabetes Data Group. National Diabetes Data Group: report of the expert committee on glucosylated hemoglobin. *Diabetes Care.* 1984;7(6):602–606

61. Dabiri G, Jones K, Krebs J, et al. Benefits of rosiglitazone in children with type 2 diabetes mellitus [abstract]. *Diabetes.* 2005; A457

62. Ponder SW, Sullivan S, McBath G. Type 2 diabetes mellitus in teens. *Diabetes Spectrum.* 2000;13(2):95–119

63. Gahagan S, Silverstein J, and the American Academy of Pediatrics Committee on Native American Child Health. Prevention and treatment of type 2 diabetes mellitus in children, with special emphasis on American Indian and Alaska Native children. *Pediatrics.* 2003;112(4). Available at: www.pediatrics.org/cgi/content/full/112/ 4/e328

64. Levine BS, Anderson BJ, Butler DA, Antisdel JE, Brackett J, Laffel LM. Predictors of glycemic control and short-term adverse outcomes in youth with type 1 diabetes. *J Pediatr.* 2001;139(2):197–203

65. Haller MJ, Stalvey MS, Silverstein JH. Predictors of control of diabetes: monitoring may be the key. *J Pediatr.* 2004;144(5):660–661

66. Murata GH, Shah JH, Hoffman RM, et al; Diabetes Outcomes in Veterans Study (DOVES). Intensified blood glucose monitoring improves glycemic control in stable, insulin-treated veterans with type 2 diabetes: the Diabetes Outcomes in Veterans Study (DOVES). *Diabetes Care.* 2003;26(6): 1759–1763

67. American Diabetes Association. Standards of medical care in diabetes—2011. *Diabetes Care.* 2011;34(suppl 1):S11–S61

68. Hanefeld M, Fischer S, Julius U, et al. Risk factors for myocardial infarction and death in newly detected NIDDM: the Diabetes Intervention Study, 11-year follow-up. *Diabetologia.* 1996;39(12):1577–1583

69. Franciosi M, Pellegrini F, De Berardis G, et al; QuED Study Group. The impact of blood glucose self-monitoring on metabolic control and quality of life in type 2 diabetic patients: an urgent need for better educational strategies. *Diabetes Care.* 2001;24 (11):1870–1877

70. American Dietetic Association. Recommendations summary: pediatric weight management (PWM) using protein sparing modified fast diets for pediatric weight loss. Available at: www.adaevidencelibrary. com/template.cfm?template=guide_- summary&key=416. Accessed August 13, 2012

71. Knowler WC, Barrett-Connor E, Fowler SE, et al; Diabetes Prevention Program Research Group. Reduction in the incidence of type 2 diabetes with lifestyle intervention or metformin. *N Engl J Med.* 2002;346(6): 393–403

72. Willi SM, Martin K, Datko FM, Brant BP. Treatment of type 2 diabetes in childhood using a very-low-calorie diet. *Diabetes Care.* 2004;27(2):348–353

73. Berry D, Urban A, Grey M. Management of type 2 diabetes in youth (part 2). *J Pediatr Health Care.* 2006;20(2):88–97

74. Loghmani ES. Nutrition therapy for overweight children and adolescents with type 2 diabetes. *Curr Diab Rep.* 2005;5(5):385–390

75. McGavock J, Sellers E, Dean H. Physical activity for the prevention and management of youth-onset type 2 diabetes mellitus: focus on cardiovascular complications. *Diab Vasc Dis Res.* 2007;4(4):305–310

76. Centers for Disease Control and Prevention. Physical activity for everyone: how much physical activity do you need? Atlanta, GA: Centers for Disease Control and Prevention; 2008. Available at: www. cdc.gov/physicalactivity/everyone/guidelines/children.html. Accessed August 13, 2012

77. Pinhas-Hamiel O, Zeitler P. A weighty problem: diagnosis and treatment of type 2 diabetes in adolescents. *Diabetes Spectrum.* 1997;10(4):292–298

78. Yamanouchi K, Shinozaki T, Chikada K, et al. Daily walking combined with diet therapy is a useful means for obese NIDDM patients not only to reduce body weight but also to improve insulin sensitivity. *Diabetes Care.* 1995;18(6):775–778

79. National Heart, Lung, and Blood Institute, US Department of Health and Human Services, National Institutes of Health. Reduce screen time. Available at: www.nhlbi. nih.gov/health/public/heart/obesity/wecan/ reduce-screen-time/index.htm. Accessed August 13, 2012

80. Krebs NF, Jacobson MS; American Academy of Pediatrics Committee on Nutrition. Prevention of pediatric overweight and obesity. *Pediatrics.* 2003;112(2):424–430

81. American Academy of Pediatrics Committee on Public Education. American Academy of Pediatrics: children, adolescents, and television. *Pediatrics.* 2001;107(2):423–426

82. American Medical Association. Appendix. Expert Committee recommendations on the assessment, prevention, and treatment of child and adolescent overweight and obesity. Chicago, IL: American Medical Association; January 25, 2007. Available at: www. ama-assn.org/ama1/pub/upload/mm/433/ ped_obesity_recs.pdf. Accessed August 13, 2012

ERRATA

Several inaccuracies occurred in the American Academy of Pediatrics "Clinical Practice Guideline: Management of Newly Diagnosed Type 2 Diabetes Mellitus (T2DM) in Children and Adolescents" published in the February 2013 issue of *Pediatrics* (2013;131[2]:364–382).

On page 366 in the table of definitions, "Prediabetes" should be defined as "Fasting plasma glucose ≥100–125 mg/dL or 2-hour glucose concentration during an oral glucose tolerance test of ≥140 but <200 mg/dL or an HbA1c of 5.7% to 6.4%."

On page 378, middle column, under "Reducing Screen Time," the second sentence should read as follows: "The US Department of Health and Human Services reflects the American Academy of Pediatrics policies by recommending that individuals limit "screen time" spent watching television and/or using computers and handheld devices to <2 hours per day unless the use is related to work or homework."[79–81,83]

Also on page 378, middle column, in the second paragraph under "Reducing Screen Time," the fourth sentence should read: "Pending new data, the committee suggests that clinicians follow the policy statement 'Children, Adolescents, and Television' from the AAP Council on Communications and Media (formerly the Committee on Public Education)." The references cited in the next sentence should be 80–83.

Reference 82 should be replaced with the following reference: Barlow SE; Expert Committee. Expert committee recommendations regarding the prevention, assessment, and treatment of child and adolescent overweight and obesity: summary report. *Pediatrics*. 2007;120(suppl 4):S164–S192

Finally, a new reference 83 should be added: American Academy of Pediatrics, Council on Communications and Media. Policy statement: children, adolescents, obesity, and the media. *Pediatrics*. 2011;128(1):201–208

doi:10.1542/peds.2013-0666

TECHNICAL REPORT

Management of Type 2 Diabetes Mellitus in Children and Adolescents

abstract

OBJECTIVE: Over the last 3 decades, the prevalence of childhood obesity has increased dramatically in North America, ushering in a variety of health problems, including type 2 diabetes mellitus (T2DM), which previously was not typically seen until much later in life. This technical report describes, in detail, the procedures undertaken to develop the recommendations given in the accompanying clinical practice guideline, "Management of Type 2 Diabetes Mellitus in Children and Adolescents," and provides in-depth information about the rationale for the recommendations and the studies used to make the clinical practice guideline's recommendations.

METHODS: A primary literature search was conducted relating to the treatment of T2DM in children and adolescents, and a secondary literature search was conducted relating to the screening and treatment of T2DM's comorbidities in children and adolescents. Inclusion criteria were prospectively and unanimously agreed on by members of the committee. An article was eligible for inclusion if it addressed treatment (primary search) or 1 of 4 comorbidities (secondary search) of T2DM, was published in 1990 or later, was written in English, and included an abstract. Only primary research inquiries were considered; review articles were considered if they included primary data or opinion. The research population had to constitute children and/or adolescents with an existing diagnosis of T2DM; studies of adult patients were considered if at least 10% of the study population was younger than 35 years. All retrieved titles, abstracts, and articles were reviewed by the consulting epidemiologist.

RESULTS: Thousands of articles were retrieved and considered in both searches on the basis of the aforementioned criteria. From those, in the primary search, 199 abstracts were identified for possible inclusion, 58 of which were retained for systematic review. Five of these studies were classified as grade A studies, 1 as grade B, 20 as grade C, and 32 as grade D. Articles regarding treatment of T2DM selected for inclusion were divided into 4 major subcategories on the basis of type of treatment being discussed: (1) medical treatments (32 studies); (2) nonmedical treatments (9 studies); (3) provider behaviors (8 studies); and (4) social issues (9 studies). From the secondary search, an additional 336 abstracts relating to comorbidities were identified for possible inclusion, of which 26 were retained for systematic review. These articles included the following: 1 systematic review of literature regarding comorbidities of T2DM in adolescents; 5 expert

Shelley C. Springer, MD, MBA, MSc, JD, Janet Silverstein, MD, Kenneth Copeland, MD, Kelly R. Moore, MD, Greg E. Prazar, MD, Terry Raymer, MD, CDE, Richard N. Shiffman, MD, Vidhu V. Thaker, MD, Meaghan Anderson, MS, RD, LD, CDE, Stephen J. Spann, MD, MBA, and Susan K. Flinn, MA

KEY WORDS
childhood, clinical practice guidelines, comanagement, diabetes, management, treatment, type 2 diabetes mellitus, youth

ABBREVIATIONS
AAP—American Academy of Pediatrics
ACE—angiotensin-converting enzyme
ADA—American Diabetes Association
AHA—American Heart Association
BG—blood glucose
CAM—complementary and alternative medicine
CES-D—Center for Epidemiologic Studies Depression Scale
CVD—cardiovascular disease
HbA1c—hemoglobin A1c
LDL-C—low-density lipoprotein cholesterol
PCP—primary care provider
QDS—Quality Data Set
RCT—randomized controlled trial
T1DM—type 1 diabetes mellitus
T2DM—type 2 diabetes mellitus

www.pediatrics.org/cgi/doi/10.1542/peds.2012-3496

doi:10.1542/peds.2012-3496

PEDIATRICS (ISSN Numbers: Print, 0031-4005; Online, 1098-4275).

opinions presenting global recommendations not based on evidence; 5 cohort studies reporting natural history of disease and comorbidities; 3 with specific attention to comorbidity patterns in specific ethnic groups (case-control, cohort, and clinical report using adult literature); 3 reporting an association between microalbuminuria and retinopathy (2 case-control, 1 cohort); 3 reporting the prevalence of nephropathy (cohort); 1 reporting peripheral vascular disease (case series); 2 discussing retinopathy (1 case-control, 1 position statement); and 3 addressing hyperlipidemia (American Heart Association position statement on cardiovascular risks; American Diabetes Association consensus statement; case series). A breakdown of grade of recommendation shows no grade A studies, 10 grade B studies, 6 grade C studies, and 10 grade D studies. With regard to screening and treatment recommendations for comorbidities, data in children are scarce, and the available literature is conflicting. Therapeutic recommendations for hypertension, dyslipidemia, retinopathy, microalbuminuria, and depression were summarized from expert guideline documents and are presented in detail in the guideline. The references are provided, but the committee did not independently assess the supporting evidence. Screening tools are provided in the Supplemental Information. *Pediatrics* 2013;131:e648–e664

INTRODUCTION

This technical report details the procedures undertaken to develop the recommendations given in the accompanying clinical practice guideline, "Management of Type 2 Diabetes Mellitus in Children and Adolescents." What follows is a description of the process, including the committee's objectives; methods of evidence identification, retrieval, review, and analysis; and summaries of the committee's conclusions.

Statement of the Issue

Over the last 3 decades, type 2 diabetes mellitus (T2DM), a disease previously confined to adult patients, has markedly increased in prevalence among children and adolescents. Currently, in the United States, approximately 1 in 3 new cases of diabetes mellitus diagnosed in patients younger than 18 years is T2DM,[1,2] with a disproportionate representation in ethnic minorities,[3,4] especially among adolescents.[5] This trend is not limited to the United States but is occurring internationally as well.[6]

The rapid emergence of childhood T2DM poses challenges to the physician who is unequipped to treat adult diseases encountered in children. Most diabetes training and educational materials designed for pediatric patients address type 1 diabetes mellitus (T1DM) and emphasize insulin treatment and glucose monitoring, which may or may not be appropriate for children with T2DM.[7,8] Most medications used for T2DM have been tested for safety and efficacy only in individuals older than 18 years, and there is scant scientific evidence for optimal management of children with T2DM.[9,10] Extrapolation of data from adult studies to pediatric populations may not be valid because the hormonal milieu of the prepubescent and pubescent patient with T2DM can affect treatment goals and modalities in ways heretofore unencountered in adult patients.[11]

The United States has a severe shortage of pediatric endocrinologists, making access to these specialists difficult or, in some cases, impossible.[12] Vast geographic areas lack a pediatric endocrinologist: in 2011, 3 states had no pediatric endocrinologists, and 22 had fewer than 10, and the situation is unlikely to improve in the near future.[13] In 2004, the National Association of Children's Hospitals and Related Institutions performed a workforce survey and found that patients had to wait almost 9 weeks for an appointment to see an endocrinologist.[14] Because the number of patients with T1DM and T2DM has increased since then, this situation is presumably worse today. Regardless of their age, most patients in the United States who have T2DM are cared for by primary care providers (PCPs).[15]

Furthermore, given the expected increases in the national and global incidence of T2DM and the near impossibility that the pediatric endocrine workforce will increase proportionately, PCPs must be prepared for and capable of managing children and adolescents who have uncomplicated T2DM.

Numerous experts have argued that the ideal care of a child with T2DM is provided through a team approach, with care shared among a pediatric endocrinologist, diabetes nurse educator, nutritionist, and behavioral specialist.[16–18] In areas of limited access to pediatric endocrinologists, however, contact with the pediatric endocrinology team might involve contact at diagnosis for initial diabetes education and intermittently thereafter; annually, with interval care by a PCP and interval communication with the pediatric endocrinology team; or at every visit, for those patients who are either doing poorly or are taking insulin.

In areas where access to subspecialists is hampered by geographic distances and/or professional shortages, care provided by local generalists who are skilled in treating children and youth with T2DM is likely to improve access to medical care. Although there are no pediatric studies evaluating this issue, the committee believes that this improved access to care might result in:

- Reduced wait times and increased timeliness of care.

- Reduced economic burden to the patient, including reduced need to travel and reduced time lost from work and/or school.

- Potentially improved patient retention. Kawahara et al[19] reported that 56.9% of patients with T2DM stopped coming to their hospital diabetes clinic appointments, most commonly because they were "too busy" to keep their appointments.

Recent advances in medical technology have the potential to ameliorate limited access to specialists. Reporting on the provision of clinical specialty diabetes care to remote locations using telemedicine, Malasanos et al[20] found that weekly telemedicine clinics were able to effectively replace quarterly face-to-face clinics after an initial face-to-face clinic visit. This more frequent contact provided by the telemedicine clinics resulted in improved hemoglobin A1c (HbA1c) concentrations, better patient satisfaction, fewer days missed from work or school, more time spent with the patient during clinic visits, and fewer subsequent hospitalizations and emergency department visits. Telemedicine is costly, however, and requires equipment to be in place at both the subspecialist's office and the remote clinic; it is, therefore, not appropriate for every practice. It is possible that a similar model of service could be provided by a generalist working locally and in close communication with a specialist.

For family physicians and others who care for adult patients, managing T2DM in children poses potential challenges. The first is that what works for adults may not work for children. Experiences and results observed in adults do not necessarily apply to children. Children (and even adolescents) are not small adults; they have a changing hormonal environment, have differences in physiology, and their growth can have effects on medication doses, toxicity, and responses.[11] As a result, generalists who are confident in caring for adults with diabetes may attempt to apply adult practice experiences to children, in whom these may not necessarily be appropriate. Kaufman cited data on various drugs' effects in children and argued that harm may occur if children with T2DM are treated like adults with T2DM.[11] The author called for treatment trials for children with T2DM, to "better define the risk-benefit ratio in children and youth, since this may differ substantially from that in the adult type 2 diabetic population." In contrast, others have noted that most adolescents with T2DM are similar to adults in terms of size and reproductive maturity and argued that, in the absence of studies specifically targeted to adolescents, treatment regimens can be extrapolated from studies of adults with T2DM; they do agree, however, that more randomized controlled trials (RCTs) are needed in the pediatric population.[1]

A second challenge is presented by the conflicting evidence regarding outcomes in patients with diabetes who are managed by generalists versus subspecialists. Some studies in adult patients indicate that generalists are capable of achieving outcomes similar to those of subspecialists. Greenfield et al[21] observed that physiologic and functional status (ie, physical, psychological, social functioning) were similar at both 2 and 4 years and mortality was similar at 7 years in adult hypertensive patients with diabetes treated in multispecialty groups versus health maintenance organization general practices. Other studies indicate that generalists may achieve outcomes similar to those of diabetes specialists, as long as they have input from subspecialists.

Indeed, unlike diseases in several other specialties, care for children with diabetes that is conducted by generalists without input from specialists may be inferior to that provided by specialists. Ziemer et al[22] used an RCT design to examine the effect of providing 5 minutes of direct feedback from an endocrinologist to a PCP every 2 weeks. Performance in the feedback group was sustained after 3 years, and performance decayed in a comparison group that received computer-generated decision support reminders, including a flow-sheet section showing previous clinical data and a recommendations section. Specialist feedback contributed independently to intensification of diabetes management. In addition, "clinical inertia" (defined as failure by providers to intensify pharmacologic therapy for hyperglycemia) was more likely in a primary care versus a diabetes clinic setting (91% vs 52%) and resulted in higher HbA1c concentrations among patients.[23]

How these observations might be applied to the child who has T2DM is not entirely clear, but they suggest that regular, direct contact between the generalist and a specialist can have a positive outcome on these patients. De Berardis et al[24] reported that, compared with adult patients with diabetes mellitus who were seen in general practice offices, patients cared for in diabetes clinics were more likely to conform with process-of-care measures, including HbA1c concentrations, blood pressure, total cholesterol and low-density lipoprotein cholesterol (LDL-C) levels, microalbuminuria testing, and foot and eye examinations and were more likely to have adequate concentrations of total cholesterol. No differences were found in glycemic, blood pressure, or LDL-C control, however. In that same study, all process-of-care measures improved when the patient was seen by a single physician as opposed to being seen by several different physicians. No similar studies have been performed in children, and it is therefore unknown whether similar outcomes can be achieved in the pediatric population.

A third challenge is presented by the fact that children with T2DM are overrepresented among racial and ethnic minority populations and are more likely to be living in poverty; therefore, they may face significant challenges in accessing specialists, even under the best situations.[25] Recognizing these barriers to care and patients' real-world needs, it is the committee's consensus that it is impractical to expect every patient with T2DM to be able to access a pediatric endocrinologist on a regular basis. It is also unreasonable to assume that these visits will be frequent enough to provide the level of care needed to maintain the best possible metabolic control. For this reason alone, PCPs must have a thorough knowledge of the management of T2DM, including its unique aspects related to childhood and adolescence.

The committee also believes it is the PCP's responsibility to obtain the requisite skills for such care and to communicate and work closely with a diabetes team of subspecialists whenever possible. For this reason, when treatment goals are not met, the committee encourages clinicians to consult with an expert trained in the care of children and adolescents with T2DM. When first-line therapy fails (eg, metformin), recommendations for intensifying therapy should be generally the same for pediatric and adult populations. The picture is constantly changing, however, as new drugs are being introduced, and some drugs that initially seemed to be safe exhibit adverse effects with wider use. Clinicians should, therefore, remain alert to new developments in this area. Seeking the advice of an expert can help ensure that the treatment goals are appropriately set and that clinicians benefit from cutting-edge treatment information in this rapidly changing area.

Stated Objective of the American Academy of Pediatrics

Because the PCP caring for children will likely encounter T2DM, the American Academy of Pediatrics (AAP), the Pediatric Endocrine Society, the American Academy of Family Physicians, the American Diabetes Association (ADA), and the American Dietetic Association undertook a cooperative effort to develop clinical guidelines for the treatment of T2DM in children and adolescents, for the benefit of subspecialists and generalists alike. Representatives from these groups collaborated on developing an evidence profile that served as a major source of information for the accompanying clinical practice guideline recommendations. This report, based on a review of the current medical literature covering a period from January 1, 1990, to July 1, 2009, provides a set of evidence-based guidelines for the management and treatment of T2DM in children and adolescents.

It should be noted that, because childhood T2DM is a relatively recent medical phenomenon, there is a paucity of evidence for many or most of the recommendations provided in the accompanying guideline. Committee members have made every effort to demarcate in the guideline those references that were not identified in the original literature search and are not included in this technical report. Although provided for the reader's information, these references not identified in the literature search did not affect or alter the level of evidence for specific recommendations.

Composition of the Committee

The ad hoc multidisciplinary committee was cochaired by 2 pediatric endocrinologists pre-eminent in their field and included experts in general pediatrics, family medicine, nutrition, Native American health, epidemiology, and medical informatics. All panel members reviewed the AAP Policy on Conflict of Interest and Voluntary Disclosure and declared all potential conflicts.

Definitions

- Children and adolescents: patients ≥10 and ≥18 years of age.

- Childhood T2DM: disease in the child who typically: is obese (BMI ≥85th to 94th percentile and >95th percentile for age and gender, respectively); has a strong family history of T2DM; has substantial residual insulin secretory capacity at diagnosis (reflected by normal or elevated insulin and C-peptide concentrations); has insidious onset of disease; demonstrates insulin resistance (including clinical evidence of polycystic ovarian syndrome or acanthosis nigricans); and lacks evidence of diabetic auto-immunity. These patients are more likely to have hypertension and dyslipidemia than those with T1DM.

- Hyperglycemia: definition as accepted by the ADA. Specifically: fasting blood glucose (BG) concentration >126 mg/dL, random or 2-hour post-Glucola (Ames Co, Elkhart, IN) BG concentration >200 mg/dL.

- Clinician: any provider within his or her scope of practice; includes medical practitioners (including physicians and physician extenders), dietitians, psychologists, and nurses.

- Comorbidities: specifically limited to cardiovascular disease (CVD), hypertension, dyslipidemias and hypercholesterolemias, atherosclerosis, peripheral neuropathy, retinopathy, and nephropathy (microvascular and macrovascular). Obesity was considered a prediabetic condition and was specifically excluded.

- Diabetes: according to the ADA criteria, defined as:

  1. HbA1c concentration $\geq$6.5% (test performed in an appropriately certified laboratory); or

  2. Fasting (defined as no caloric intake for at least 8 hours) plasma glucose concentration $\geq$126 mg/dL (7.0 mmol/L); or

  3. Two-hour plasma glucose concentration $\geq$200 mg/dL (11.1 mmol/L) during an oral glucose tolerance test (test performed as described by the World Health Organization by using a glucose load containing the equivalent of 75 g of anhydrous glucose dissolved in water); or

  4. A random plasma glucose concentration $\geq$200 mg/dL (11.1 mmol/L) with symptoms of hyperglycemia.

  (In the absence of unequivocal hyperglycemia, criteria 1–3 should be confirmed by repeat testing.)

- Diabetic ketoacidosis: the absolute or relative insulin deficiency resulting in fat breakdown with resultant formation of β-hydroxybutyrate and accompanying acidosis. Symptoms include nausea, vomiting, Kussmaul respirations, dehydration, and altered mental status.

- Fasting BG: BG concentration obtained before the first meal of the day and after a fast of at least 8 hours.

- Glucose toxicity: the effect of high BG causing both insulin resistance and impaired β-cell production of insulin.

- Intensification: increasing frequency of BG monitoring and adjustment of the dose and type of medication to decrease BG concentrations.

- Intercurrent illnesses: febrile illnesses or associated symptoms severe enough to cause the patient to stay home from school and/or seek medical care.

- Microalbuminuria: albumin-to-creatinine ratio $\geq$30 mg/g creatinine but <300 mg/g creatinine.

- Moderate hyperglycemia: BG concentration of 180 to 250 mg/dL.

- Moderate to vigorous exercise: exercise that makes the individual breathe hard and perspire and which raises his or her heart rate. An easy way to define exercise intensity for patients is the "talk test": during moderate physical activity a person can talk but not sing. During vigorous activity, a person cannot talk without pausing to catch a breath.

- Obese: BMI $\geq$95th percentile for age and gender.

- Overweight: BMI between 85th and 94th percentile for age and gender.

- Prediabetes: Fasting plasma glucose concentration $\geq$100 to 125 mg/dL or 2-hour glucose concentration during an oral glucose tolerance test $\geq$126 mg/dL but <200 mg/dL or HbA1c of 5.7% to 6.4%.

- Severe hyperglycemia: BG concentration >250 mg/dL.

- Thiazolidinediones: oral hypoglycemic agents that exert their effect at least in part by activation of the peroxisome proliferator-activated receptor-γ.

- T1DM: diabetes secondary to autoimmune destruction of β-cells resulting in absolute (complete or near complete) insulin deficiency and requiring insulin injections for management.

- T2DM: The investigators' designation of the diagnosis was used for the purposes of the literature review. The committee acknowledges that the distinction between T1DM and T2DM in this population is not always clear-cut, and clinical judgment plays an important role. Typically, this diagnosis is made when hyperglycemia is secondary to insulin resistance accompanied by impaired β-cell function, resulting in inadequate insulin production to compensate for the degree of insulin resistance.

- Youth: used interchangeably with "adolescent" in this document.

FORMULATION AND ARTICULATION OF THE QUESTION ADDRESSED BY THE COMMITTEE

The committee first formulated explicit questions for which evidence would be queried by the epidemiologist. Specific clinical questions addressed by the committee included: (1) the effectiveness of treatment modalities for T2DM in children and adolescents; (2) the efficacy of pharmaceutical therapies for treatment of children and adolescents with T2DM; (3) appropriate recommendations for screening for comorbidities typically associated with T2DM in children and adolescents; and (4) treatment recommendations for comorbidities of T2DM in children and adolescents.

These recommendations pertain specifically to patients at least 10 but younger than 18 years of age with T2DM. Although the distinction between T1DM and T2DM in children may be difficult,[26,27] for purposes of this report, the definition of childhood T2DM includes the child who typically is overweight or obese (defined as having a BMI $\geq$85th to 94th percentile and >95th percentile for age and gender, respectively); has a strong family history of T2DM; has substantial residual insulin secretory capacity at diagnosis (reflected by normal or elevated insulin and C-peptide concentrations); has insidious onset of disease; demonstrates insulin resistance (including clinical evidence of polycystic ovarian syndrome or acanthosis nigricans); and lacks evidence of diabetic autoimmunity (negative for autoantibodies typically associated with T1DM). Patients with T2DM are more likely to have hypertension and dyslipidemia than are those with T1DM.

Methods

Primary Literature Search: Treatment of T2DM

The committee unanimously agreed on the objectives of the guideline and scope of the evidence search. A primary literature search was conducted by the consulting epidemiologist, using the strategy as described in the following text.

An article was eligible for inclusion if it addressed treatment of T2DM, was published in 1990 or later, was written in English, and included an abstract. Only primary research inquiries were considered; review articles were considered if they included primary data or opinion. Children and/or adolescents with an existing diagnosis of T2DM were required to constitute the research population; studies of adult patients were considered if $\geq$10% of their population was younger than 35 years.

The electronic databases PubMed, Cochrane Collaboration, and Embase were searched using the following Medical Subject Headings, alone and in various combinations: diabetes, mellitus, type 2, type 1, treatment, prevention, insipidus, diet, pediatric, T2DM, T1DM, non–insulin dependent diabetes mellitus (NIDDM), metformin, lifestyle, RCT, meta-analysis, child, adolescent, therapeutics, control, adult, obese, gestational, polycystic ovary syndrome, metabolic syndrome, cardiovascular, dyslipidemia, men, and women. In addition, the Boolean operators NOT, AND, and OR were used with the aforementioned terms, also in various combinations. Search limits included clinical trial, meta-analysis, randomized controlled trial, review, child: 6–12 years, and adolescent: 13–18 years.

Reference lists of identified articles were searched for additional studies using the same criteria for inclusion enumerated earlier. Finally, articles personally known to members of the committee that were not identified by other means were submitted for consideration and were included if they fulfilled the inclusion criteria.

A total of 196 articles were identified by using these search criteria. Of those, 58 were accepted as evidence for the guideline, and 138 were rejected as not meeting all requirements. A summary evidence table for the accepted articles can be found in Supplemental Information A.

Secondary Literature Search: Comorbidities of T2DM

After completion of the primary literature review, at the request of the committee, a second literature review was conducted to identify evidence relating to screening, diagnosis, and treatment of comorbidities of T2DM in children and adolescents. Similar to inclusion criteria for the primary review, an article relating to comorbidities was eligible for inclusion if it was published in 1990 or later, was written in English, and included an abstract. Again, only primary research inquiries were considered; review articles were considered if they included primary data or opinion. Children and/or adolescents in whom either T1DM or T2DM was diagnosed were required to constitute the research population; studies of adult patients were considered if $\geq$10% of the population was younger than 35 years. The focus of the research article must be hyperlipidemia, microalbuminuria, retinopathy, or "comorbidities of diabetes mellitus."

The electronic databases PubMed, Cochrane Collaboration, and Embase were searched using the following Medical Subject Headings, alone and in various combinations: diabetes,

mellitus, type 2, type 1, pediatric, T2DM, T1DM, NIDDM, hyperlipidemia, retinopathy, microalbuminuria, comorbidities, screening, RCT, meta-analysis, child, and adolescent. In addition, the Boolean operators NOT, AND, and OR were used with the aforementioned terms, also in various combinations. Search limitations included clinical trial, meta-analysis, randomized controlled trial, review, child: 6–12 years, and adolescent: 13–18 years. Reference lists of identified articles were searched for additional studies, with the use of the same criteria for inclusion enumerated earlier. Finally, articles personally known to members of the committee that were not identified by other means were submitted for consideration and were included if they fulfilled the inclusion criteria.

A total of 75 articles were identified by using these search criteria. Of those, 26 were accepted as evidence for the guideline, and 49 were rejected as not meeting all requirements. A summary evidence table for the accepted comorbidity articles can be found in Supplemental Information B.

Analysis of Available Evidence

A strict evidence-based approach was used to extract data used to develop the recommendations presented in the accompanying clinical practice guideline. Individual articles meeting the prospective search criteria were critically appraised for strength of methodology, and they were assigned an evidence level grade on the basis of guidelines published by the University of Oxford's Centre for Evidence-based Medicine, which are synthesized in the next discussion.[28]

Levels of Evidence (Based on Methodology)

- Level 1A: Systematic review with homogeneity of included RCTs.

- Level 1B: Individual RCT with narrow CI and >80% follow-up.
- Level 2A: Systematic review with homogeneity of cohort studies.
- Level 2B: Individual cohort study, follow-up of untreated controls in an RCT, or low-quality RCT (ie, less than 80% follow-up).
- Level 2C: "Outcomes research."
- Level 3A: Systematic review with homogeneity of case-control studies.
- Level 3B: Individual case-control studies.
- Level 4: Case series; poor-quality cohort and/or case-control studies.
- Level 5: Expert opinion without explicit critical appraisal or based on physiology, bench research, or "first principles."

Grades of Evidence Supporting the Recommendations

The AAP policy statement, "Classifying Recommendations for Clinical Practice Guidelines," was followed in designating grades of recommendation (Fig 1, Table 1), based on the levels of available evidence. AAP policy stipulates that the evidence in support of each key action statement be prospectively identified, appraised, and summarized and that an explicit link between level of evidence and grade of recommendation be defined.

Possible grades of recommendations range from A to D, with A being the highest. Some qualification of the grade is further allowed on the basis of subtle characteristics of the level of supporting evidence. The AAP policy statement is consistent with the grading recommendations advanced by the University of Oxford's Centre for Evidence-based Medicine. The AAP policy statement "Classifying Recommendations for Clinical Practice Guidelines" offers further details.[29]

- Grade A: Consistent level 1 studies. (Examples include meta-analyses

with appropriate adjustments for heterogeneity, well-designed RCTs, or high-quality diagnostic studies on relevant populations.)
- Grade B: Consistent level 2 or level 3 studies or extrapolations from level 1 studies. (Examples include RCTs or diagnostic studies with methodologic flaws or performed in less relevant populations; consistent and persuasive evidence from well-designed observational trials.)
- Grade C: Level 4 studies or extrapolations from level 2 or level 3 studies. (Examples include poor-quality observational studies, including case-control and cohort design methodologies, as well as case series.)
- Grade D: Level 5 evidence, or troublingly inconsistent or inconclusive studies of any level. (Examples include case reports, expert opinion,

reasoning from first principles, or methodologically troubling studies with questionable validity.)
- Level X: Not an explicit level of evidence as outlined by the Centre for Evidence-based Medicine. Reserved for interventions that are unethical or impossible to test in a controlled or scientific fashion, in which the preponderance of benefit or harm is overwhelming, precluding rigorous investigation.

The relationship between grades of evidence supporting recommendations and recommended key action statements is depicted in Fig 1. Note that any given recommended key action statement may only be as strong as its supporting evidence will allow.

Recommended Key Action Statements

After considering the available levels of evidence and grades of recommendations, the committee formulated

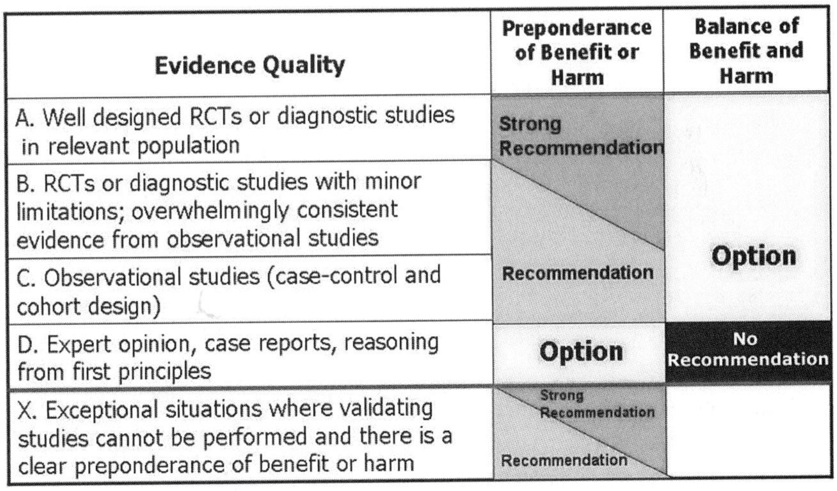

FIGURE 1
Evidence quality. Integrating evidence quality appraisal with an assessment of the anticipated balance between benefits and harms if a policy is carried out leads to designation of a policy as a strong recommendation, recommendation, option, or no recommendation.

TABLE 1 Grades of Study According to Subdivision

Evidence Quality	Medical Treatment	Nonmedical Treatment	Provider Behaviors	Social Issues
A	4	1	0	0
B	0	1	0	0
C	4	3	7	6
D	24	4	1	3

several recommended key action statements, published in the companion clinical practice guideline. As discussed previously, recommended key action statements vary in strength on the basis of the quality of the supporting evidence.

- Strong recommendation: The highest level of recommendation, this category is reserved for recommendations supported by grade A or grade B evidence demonstrating a preponderance of benefit or harm. Interventions based on level X evidence may also be categorized as strong on the basis of their risk/benefit profile. A strong recommendation in favor of a particular action is made when the anticipated benefits of the recommended intervention clearly exceed the harms (as a strong recommendation against an action is made when the anticipated harms clearly exceed the benefits) and the quality of the supporting evidence is excellent. In some clearly identified circumstances, strong recommendations may be made when high-quality evidence is impossible to obtain and the anticipated benefits strongly outweigh the harms. The implication for clinicians is that they should follow a strong recommendation unless a clear and compelling rationale for an alternative approach is present.

- Recommendation: A recommended key action statement is made when the anticipated benefit exceeds the harms but the evidence is not as methodologically sound. Recommended key action statements must be supported by grade B or grade C evidence; level X evidence may also result in a recommendation depending on risk/benefit considerations. A recommendation in favor of a particular action is made when the anticipated benefits exceed the harms, but the quality of evidence is not as strong. Again, in some clearly identified circumstances, recommendations may be made when high-quality evidence is impossible to obtain but the anticipated benefits outweigh the harms. The implication for clinicians is that they would be prudent to follow a recommendation but should remain alert to new information and sensitive to patient preferences.

- Option: Option statements are offered when the available evidence is grade D or the anticipated benefit is balanced with the potential harm. Options define courses that may be taken when either the quality of evidence is suspect or carefully performed studies have shown little clear advantage to 1 approach over another. The implication for clinicians is that they should consider the option in their decision-making, and patient preference may have a substantial role.

- No recommendation: When published evidence is lacking, and/or what little evidence is available demonstrates an equivocal risk/benefit profile, no recommended key action can be offered. No recommendation indicates that there is a lack of pertinent published evidence and that the anticipated balance of benefits and harms is presently unclear. The implication for clinicians is that they should be alert to new published evidence that clarifies the balance of benefit versus harm.

Implementation Strategy

Implementing the guideline's recommendations to improve care processes involves identifying potential barriers to the use of the knowledge, creating strategies to address those barriers, and selecting appropriate quality improvement methods (eg, education, audit and feedback, computer-based decision support).

Computer-mediated decision support offers an implementation mode that has been demonstrated to be effective[30] and that is expected to be of increasing relevance to pediatricians with the adoption of electronic health records. To facilitate translation of the recommendations into computable statements, the guideline recommendations were transformed into declarative production rule (eg, IF-THEN) statements.[31] The Key Action Statements are displayed as production rules in Supplemental Information C. The concepts required to describe antecedent and consequent clauses in these rules were translated into the following standardized coding systems: SNOMED-CT,[32] RxNorm,[33] and LOINC.[34]

In addition, the concepts described in the guideline recommendations were translated, where possible, into elements of the National Quality Forum's Quality Data Set (QDS).[35] The QDS provides a framework from which performance measurement data can be derived. The QDS is intended to serve as a standard set of reusable data elements that can be used to promote quality measurement. Each QDS element includes a name, a quality data type that describes part of the clinical care process, quality data type specific attributes, a standard code set name, and a code listing. The Methods for Developing the Guidelines section displays the relevant decision variables and actions as well as coding information. A QDS listing of decision variables and actions is provided in Supplemental Information D.

RESULTS

Primary Literature Search: Treatment of T2DM

Thousands of articles were retrieved and considered on the basis of the aforementioned criteria. From those,

199 abstracts were identified for possible inclusion, and 58 were retained for systematic review. Results of the literature review are presented in the following text and listed in the evidence tables in the Supplemental Information.

Of the 58 articles retained for systematic review, 5 studies were classified as grade A studies, 1 as grade B, 20 as grade C, and 32 as grade D. Articles regarding the treatment of T2DM selected for inclusion were divided into 4 major subcategories on the basis of type of treatment being discussed: (1) medical treatments (32 studies); (2) nonmedical treatments (9 studies); (3) provider behaviors (8 studies); and (4) social issues (9 studies). Detailed information about these articles is presented in Supplemental Information A. A graphic depiction of the grades of study according to subdivision is given in Table 1.

Rejected Articles

Of the 257 articles meeting search criteria, 199 were rejected, categorized as follows:

- Comorbidities: 69 studies. (Note: these articles were rejected within the context of the primary search string relating to treatment of T2DM. A second prospective literature search was conducted solely addressing comorbidities, the results of which are presented in the next section.)
- Medical treatment: 99 articles.
- Nonmedical treatment: 16 articles.
- Social issues: 12 articles.
- Provider behaviors: 3 articles.

To view the recommendations related to management of T2DM, please see the accompanying clinical practice guideline.[36]

Secondary Literature Search: Comorbidities of T2DM

Evidence is sparse in children and adolescents regarding the risks for developing various comorbidities of diabetes that are well recognized in adult patients. Numerous reports have documented the occurrence of comorbidities in adolescents with T2DM, but no randomized clinical trials have examined the progression and treatment of comorbidities in youth with T2DM.[29] The evidence that does exist is contradictory with regard to both screening and treatment recommendations. After applying the previously described search criteria and screening to thousands of articles, an additional 336 abstracts relating to comorbidities were identified for possible inclusion, of which 26 were retained for systematic review. Results of this subsequent literature review are presented in Supplemental Information E.

Articles discussing comorbidities ran the gamut of study focus, type, level of evidence, and grade of recommendation. The 26 articles that met the revised objective criteria had the following characteristics:

- Expert opinion global recommendations not based on evidence (5 articles).
- Cohort studies reporting natural history of disease and comorbidities (5 articles).
- Specific attention to comorbidity patterns in specific ethnic groups (case-control, cohort, and clinical report by using adult literature: 3 articles).
- Association between microalbuminuria and retinopathy (2 case-control, 1 cohort: 3 articles).
- Prevalence of nephropathy (cohort: 3 articles).
- Hyperlipidemia (American Heart Association [AHA] position statement on cardiovascular risks, ADA consensus statement, case series: 3 articles).
- Retinopathy (1 case-control, 1 position statement: 2 articles).

- Peripheral vascular disease (case series: 1 article).
- Systematic review of literature regarding comorbidities of T2DM in adolescents (1 article).

A graphic depiction of the grades of recommendation is given in Table 2.

Rejected Articles

A total of 310 articles did not meet primary inclusion criteria and were rejected; details are presented in Supplemental Information F. Profiles of the rejected articles are:

- Articles relating to T1DM (125 articles); specifically on the following topics:
  - Retinopathy (42 articles).
  - Vascular complications (34 articles).
  - Nephropathy (29 articles).
  - Natural history and epidemiology of T1DM (8 articles).
  - Hyperlipidemia (5 articles).
  - Risk factors for comorbidities (ie, ethnicity, puberty: 4 articles).
  - Neuropathy (3 articles).
- Articles involving adults, practice management issues, and other nonpertinent topics (118 articles).
- Articles about nondiabetic subjects, prediabetic subjects, or adults, including recommendations for testing for conditions such as hyperlipidemias and CVD (36 articles).
- Reviews, published trials, guidelines, and position statements not meeting criteria (19 articles).
- Studies addressing methods of testing for comorbidities (12 articles).

The initial search strategy for comorbidities included patients diagnosed with T1DM. The committee thus assumed that (with the exception of initiating screening) the pattern of comorbidities—and the need to screen for and treat them—would be similar between T1DM and T2DM. It was also assumed that comorbidities would be similar between pediatric and adult patients, with length and severity of disease the driving factors. During the search, articles addressing the following themes were identified and reviewed:

- The pattern of comorbidities in T1DM versus T2DM and the role of puberty (9 articles).

- Differences in comorbidity patterns in children with T2DM compared with adults (8 articles).

Although not included in the final list of studies, these articles are included in the Supplemental Information because they resulted in an alteration to the original inclusion criteria. The results of these articles indicate that the pattern of comorbidities in children and adolescents with T2DM may not resemble that of either T1DM patients (possibly because of the influence of puberty) or adults, as was hypothesized by the committee when identifying the primary search parameters. Accordingly, the search string was modified to include only children and adolescents with the diagnosis of T2DM.

Recommendations Regarding Comorbidities

Unlike T2DM in adult patients, data are scarce in children and adolescents regarding the diagnosis, natural history, progression, screening recommendations, and treatment recommendations. Numerous reports have documented the occurrence of comorbidities in adolescents with T2DM, but no RCTs have examined the progression and treatment of comorbidities in youth with T2DM.

TABLE 2 Grades of Recommendation

Evidence Quality	No. of Studies
A	0
B	10
C	6
D	10

The available literature is conflicting regarding whether clinical signs of pathology in adults are variants of normal for adolescents, the role of puberty in diagnosis and progression of various comorbidities, the screening tests that should be performed and how they should be interpreted, when screenings should be initiated, how often screening should be performed and by whom, and how abnormal results should be treated. Medications commonly prescribed in adult patients have not been rigorously tested in children or adolescents for safety or efficacy. The peculiarities of the developing adolescent brain, typical lifestyle, and social issues confound issues of treatment effectiveness.

Despite the limited evidence available, the committee provides information on expert recommendations for the following selected comorbidities: hypertension, dyslipidemia, retinopathy, microalbuminuria, and depression. These therapeutic recommendations were summarized from expert guideline documents and are presented in detail in the following sections. The references are provided, but the committee did not independently assess the supporting evidence. Sample screening tools are provided in the Supplemental Information (see Supplemental Information H and I).

Hypertension

Hypertension is a significant comorbidity associated with endothelial dysfunction, vessel stiffness, and increased risk of future CVD and chronic kidney disease for the child with diabetes.[37,38] It is present in 36% of youth with T2DM within 1.3 years of diagnosis[39] and was present in 65% of youth with T2DM enrolled in the SEARCH for Diabetes in Youth Study (SEARCH study).[40] Because development of CVD is associated with hypertension, recognition and treatment of this comorbidity are essential, especially in youth with T2DM.

Unfortunately, health care providers underdiagnose hypertension in children and adolescents (both with and without diabetes), resulting in a lack of appropriate treatment.[41]

Screening:

- Blood pressure should be measured with an appropriate-sized cuff and reliable equipment, monitored at every clinic visit, and plotted against norms for age, gender, and height provided in tables available at the following Web site: http://www.nhlbi. nih.gov/guidelines/hypertension/ child_tbl.htm[42] or in "The Fourth Report on the Diagnosis, Evaluation, and Treatment of High Blood Pressure in Children and Adolescents."[43] (See the Supplemental Information for the National Institutes of Health table.)

Treatment:

- Once a diagnosis of hypertension is established, the clinician can institute appropriate treatment, which might include lifestyle change and/or pharmacologic agents. Although a complete discussion of this topic is beyond the scope of these guidelines, rational treatment guidelines exist.[43,44] In adult patients with T2DM, concomitant treatment of hypertension has been shown to improve microvascular and macrovascular outcomes at least as much as control of BG concentrations.[45,46] Therefore, it is the consensus of this committee that similar benefits are likely with early recognition and treatment of hypertension in the child or adolescent with increased CVD risk secondary to T2DM.[47,48] The committee recommends appropriate surveillance and therapy as outlined in "The Fourth Report on the Diagnosis, Evaluation, and Treatment of High Blood Pressure in Children and Adolescents."[43]

- Initial treatment of blood pressure consistently at, or above, the 95th percentile on at least 3 occasions should consist of efforts at weight loss reduction, limitation of dietary salt, and increased activity.

- If, after 6 months, blood pressure is still above the 95th percentile for age, gender, and height, initiation of an angiotensin-converting enzyme (ACE) inhibitor should be considered to achieve blood pressure values that are less than the 90th percentile.

- If ACE inhibitors are not tolerated because of adverse effects (most commonly cough), an angiotensin receptor blocker should be used.

- If adequate control of hypertension is not achieved, referral to a physician specialist trained in the treatment of hypertension in youth is recommended.

Dyslipidemia

Long-term complications of T2DM in children and adolescents are not as well documented as those found in adults. It should be noted that the pediatric experience with niacin and fibrates is limited. In a review, however, Pinhas-Hamiel and Zeitler[49] noted the presence of dyslipidemia in a substantial proportion of young patients with T2DM in various populations worldwide. The SEARCH study found that 60% to 65% of 2096 youth with T2DM had hypertriglyceridemia, and 73% had a low high-density lipoprotein cholesterol level.[50] Thus, although variations exist in the criteria used for defining hyperlipidemia, there is unequivocal evidence that screening for dyslipidemia is imperative in pediatric patients with T2DM.[49,51,52] Hyperglycemia and insulin resistance may play a direct role in dyslipidemia, and cardiovascular risk is further enhanced by the presence of other risk factors, including obesity and a family history of early CVD.[49,53] The AHA classifies T2DM as a tier 2 condition (moderate risk) in which accelerated atherosclerosis has been documented in patients younger than 30 years.[51] The presence of 2 other risk factors, including obesity, smoking, family history of CVD, and poor exercise history, can accelerate this status to tier 1 (high risk), which is relevant to many young patients with T2DM.

Screening:

- On the basis of current recommendations by the ADA and the AHA, at the initial evaluation, all patients with T2DM should have baseline lipid screening (after initial glycemic control has been established) consisting of a complete fasting lipid profile, with follow-up testing based on the findings or every 2 years thereafter, if initial results are normal.[51–53] (See the Supplemental Information for screening tools.)

Treatment:

The committee suggests following the AHA position statement, "Cardiovascular Risk Reduction in High-risk Pediatric Patients," for management of dyslipidemia.[51] This position statement recommends:

- Evaluation and dietary education by a registered dietitian for all patients, with initiation of intensive therapy and follow-up for patients with a BMI >95th percentile.

- Lipid targets:
  - LDL-C: Initial concentration ≥130 mg/dL: nutritionist training with diet <30% calories from fat, <7% calories from saturated fat, cholesterol intake <200 mg/day, and avoidance of trans fats. LDL measurements should be repeated after 6 months. If concentrations are still 130 to 160 mg/dL, statin therapy should be initiated, with a goal of <130 mg/dL and an ideal target of <100 mg/dL.
  - Triglycerides: If initial concentrations are between 150 and 600 mg/dL, patients should decrease intake of simple carbohydrates and fat, with weight loss management for those who are overweight. If levels are >700 to 1000 mg/dL at initial or follow-up visit, fibrate or niacin should be considered if the patient is older than 10 years because of increased risk of pancreatitis at these concentrations.

- Control of hypertension, per guidelines referenced previously.

- Intensification of management of hyperglycemia.

- Assessment of parental smoking history and patient smoking history if the patient is older than 10 years; active antismoking counseling at every visit and referral to a smoking cessation program, if required.

- Assessment of family history of early CVD along with current family lifestyle habits; a positive family history increases the level of risk.

- Promotion of physical exercise and limitation of sedentary activities.

Retinopathy

The eye has been called a unique window into the neural and vascular health in patients with diabetes.[54] Retinopathy is well documented in adults, both alone and in association with other comorbidities,[55] but descriptions of its frequency and associations with other comorbidities in youth are limited. Some observational and case-control studies show that retinopathy in adolescents with T2DM is present earlier than in adults, whereas others indicate that it appears much later.[56–60]

The review by Pinhas-Hamiel and Zeitler[49] of complications of T2DM among adolescents cited studies in which the diagnosis of retinopathy appeared to occur strikingly early in the disease process. Two large studies in the Japanese population documented early development of retinopathy in young adults, some even before the diagnosis of diabetes mellitus. In a study of 1065 patients diagnosed with T2DM before 30 years of age, Okudaira et al[57] reported the presence of retinopathy in 99 patients (9.3%) before the first visit. One hundred thirty-five patients (12.7%) developed proliferative retinopathy before 35 years of age, and 32 (23.7%) of these patients were blind by a mean age of 32 years. Bronson-Castain et al[54] used sophisticated techniques to evaluate the neural and vascular health of the retina and reported a much higher incidence of focal retinal neuropathy, retinal thinning, and retinal venular dilation in a cohort of 15 adolescent patients with T2DM matched with 26 controls. Okudaira et al observed the development of retinopathy in 394 patients diagnosed with T2DM before 30 years of age. Of the 322 patients who were free of retinopathy at entry, 88 developed background diabetic retinopathy over 5.7 years, an incidence of 57.7 per 1000 person-years. Fifty of the 160 patients with background retinopathy developed proliferative retinopathy over 7.1 years, an incidence of 17.9 per 1000 person-years. Poor glycemic control, duration of disease, and high blood pressure seemed to be the primary risk factors.

Conversely, the study by Krakoff et al[58] of 178 youth that used the proportional hazards model showed a lower risk for retinopathy in Pima Indians (compared with the Japanese study cited previously), even after adjusting for glucose concentrations and blood pressure. Similar results were reported by Farah et al[59] in 40 African American and Hispanic youth and by Karabouta et al[60] in 7 adolescent patients. It is unclear whether these differences in results arise from variations in study design, population demographic characteristics, and/or techniques used in diagnosis. Given the variability in the results of epidemiologic studies and absence of long-term data, the committee considers it prudent for providers to follow the ADA "Standards of Medical Care in Diabetes" for identification and management of retinopathy in adolescents with T2DM, as follows[61]:

Screening:

- Patients with T2DM should have an initial dilated and comprehensive eye examination performed by an ophthalmologist or optometrist shortly after diabetes diagnosis.

- Subsequent examinations by an ophthalmologist should be repeated annually. Less frequent examinations may be considered (eg, every 2–3 years) after 1 or more normal eye examinations. More frequent examinations are required if retinopathy is progressing.

Treatment:

- Providers should promptly refer patients with any level of macular edema, severe nonproliferative diabetic retinopathy, or any proliferative diabetic retinopathy to an ophthalmologist who is knowledgeable and experienced in the management and treatment of diabetic retinopathy.

- Laser photocoagulation therapy is indicated to reduce the risk of vision loss in patients with high-risk proliferative diabetic retinopathy, clinically significant macular edema, and some cases of severe nonproliferative diabetic retinopathy.

Microalbuminuria

Microalbuminuria is a marker of vascular inflammation and a sign of early nephropathy; it has been found to be associated with CVD risk in adults. It may be present at diagnosis in youth with T2DM.[49] Higher rates of microalbuminuria have been reported among youth with T2DM than in their peers with T1DM.[39,59] Diabetic nephropathy may also be more frequent and severe among youth with T2DM.[62,63]

According to the ADA statement "Care of Children and Adolescents with Type 1 Diabetes," the definition of microalbuminuria is either:

- "Albumin-to-creatinine ratio 30–299 mg/g in a spot urine sample; slightly higher values can be used in females because of the difference in creatinine excretion,"[7,64] or

- "Timed overnight or 24-hour collections: albumin excretion rate of 20–199 mcg/min."[7]

According to the ADA, "an abnormal value should be repeated as exercise, smoking, and menstruation can affect results and albumin excretion can vary from day to day. The diagnosis of persistent abnormal microalbumin excretion requires documentation of two of three consecutive abnormal values obtained on different days."[7,65] In addition, nondiabetes-related causes of renal disease should be excluded; consultation with specialists trained in the care of children with renal diseases should be considered as required. It should be noted that orthostatic proteinuria is not uncommon in adolescents and usually is considered benign. For that reason, all patients with documented microalbuminuria should have a first morning void immediately on arising to determine if this is the case. Orthostatic proteinuria does not require treatment with medication.

The committee considers it prudent for providers to follow the ADA "Standards of Medical Care in Diabetes" for the identification and management of microalbuminuria in adolescents with T2DM, as described here. Note that monitoring should always be done on a first morning void specimen:

Screening:

- Screening for microalbuminuria should begin at the time of T2DM diagnosis and be repeated annually.

- An annual random spot urine sample for microalbumin-to-creatinine ratio is recommended.[66]

Treatment:

- Treatment with an ACE inhibitor should be initiated in nonpregnant individuals with confirmed persistent microalbuminuria from 2 additional urine specimens, even if blood pressure is not elevated.

- If possible, treatment with an ACE inhibitor should be titrated to normalization of microalbumin excretion. "Microalbumin excretion should be monitored at three- to six-month intervals to assess both the patient's response to therapy and the disease progression, and therapy should be titrated to achieve as normal an albumin-to-creatinine ratio as possible."[7]

Additional relevant issues noted in the ADA statement "Care of Children and Adolescents with Type 1 Diabetes" include[7]:

- Concomitant hypertension should be addressed. If present, hypertension should be aggressively treated to achieve normotension for age, sex, and height.

- Patients should be educated about the importance of attention to glycemic control and avoidance or cessation of smoking in preventing and/or reversing diabetic nephropathy.

- If medical treatment is unsatisfactory, referral to a nephrologist should be considered.

Depression

Depression is a significant comorbidity that can complicate the medical management of diabetes and is associated with poor adherence. Longitudinal studies of the association between T2DM and depression among youth are not available. In a longitudinal study among youth with T1DM, however, Kovacs et al[67] estimated the rate of psychiatric disorders to be 3 times higher in youth with diabetes than in those without diabetes, with the increased morbidity primarily attributable to major depression.[7,67,68] In addition, cross-sectional data from the SEARCH study have shown the prevalence of depressed mood to be higher among males with T2DM than among males with T1DM.[67] Lawrence et al[68] also found higher levels of depressed mood to be associated with poor glycemic control and number of emergency department visits among participants with both T1DM and T2DM, compared with youth with T1DM and T2DM who had "minimal" levels of depressed mood.

Because depression is associated with poor adherence to diabetic treatment recommendations, its identification and proper management are essential for maximizing therapeutic success. Given the serious nature of this comorbidity and its propensity for poor metabolic control, the committee recommends that clinicians assess youth with T2DM for depression at diagnosis; perform periodic, routine screening for depression on all youth with T2DM, especially those with frequent emergency department visits or poor glycemic control; and promptly refer youth who have positive screenings to appropriate mental health care providers for treatment. Addressing a family history of diabetes and its effect on the family unit can be a major factor in depression as well as compliance with the disease management needs.

Screening:

- According to the American Psychiatric Association, a diagnosis of major depressive disorder requires[69]:

  (a). The presence of 5 or more of the following symptoms within the same 2-week period and represents a change from previous functioning. At least 1 of the symptoms is either depressed mood or loss of interest or pleasure.

- Depressed mood most of the day, nearly every day, as indicated by either substantive report or observation made by others. (Note that in children and adolescents, this can be irritable mood.)

- Markedly diminished interest or pleasure in all, or nearly all, activities most of the day, nearly every day.

- Significant weight loss when not dieting or weight gain (eg, more than 5% of body weight in a month), or increased or decreased appetite nearly every day. (Note that in children and adolescents, this should include failure to make expected weight gains.)

- Insomnia or hypersomnia nearly every day.

- Psychomotor agitation or retardation nearly every day (observable by others, not merely the subject's feeling restless or slowed down).

- Fatigue or loss of energy nearly every day.

- Feelings of worthlessness or inappropriate guilt (which may be delusional) nearly every day.

- Diminished ability to think or to concentrate, or indecisiveness, nearly every day.

- Recurrent thoughts of death (not just fear of dying), recurrent suicidal ideation without a specific plan, or a suicide attempt, or a specific plan to commit suicide.

(b). The symptoms do not meet the criteria for a mixed episode (defined as a specific time period in which the individual experiences nearly daily fluctuations in mood that qualify for diagnoses of manic episode and major depressive episode).

(c). The symptoms cause clinically significant distress or impairment in social, occupational, or other important areas of functioning.

(d). The symptoms are not due to the direct physiologic effects of a substance (eg, a drug of abuse, medication) or a general medical condition (eg, hypothyroidism).

(e). The symptoms are not better accounted for by bereavement (ie, after the loss of a loved one), symptoms persist longer than 2 months, or symptoms are characterized by marked functional impairment, morbid preoccupation with worthlessness, suicidal ideation, psychotic symptoms, or psychomotor retardation.

- Another potentially valuable screening tool for depression is the Center for Epidemiologic Studies Depression Scale (CES-D), a 20-item scale originally developed for use in adults[70] but which has been used subsequently in studies of youth as young as 12 years.[71–74] (See Supplemental Information G for this scale.)

Treatment:

- Recognition of depression should trigger a referral to a mental health care provider skilled in addressing this condition in children and adolescents.

Other Comorbidities or Associated Medical Conditions

In addition to the comorbidities mentioned previously, T2DM is associated with other obesity-related medical conditions, many of which, when discovered, necessitate consultation with specialists who have specific expertise in the field. These associated conditions include:

- Nonalcoholic fatty liver disease: Baseline aspartate aminotransferase and alanine aminotransferase concentrations should be obtained, especially if treatment with lipid-lowering drugs is instituted. Referral to a pediatric or internal medicine gastroenterologist may be indicated.

- Obstructive sleep apnea: The diagnosis of obstructive sleep apnea can only be made reliably by using a sleep study. If the diagnosis is made, an electrocardiogram and possibly an echocardiogram should be obtained to rule out right ventricular hypertrophy. Referral to a pediatric cardiologist, internal medicine cardiologist, or sleep specialist may be indicated.

- Orthopedic problems: These comorbidities (especially slipped capital femoral epiphysis and Blount disease) require immediate referral to a specialist in orthopedics and will limit the physical activity that can be prescribed to the individual.

COMPLEMENTARY AND ALTERNATIVE MEDICINE

The clinical practice guidelines do not present any evidence-based recommendations for the use of complementary and alternative medicine (CAM) to treat T2DM in children and adolescents. Limited data are available on CAM, and none is specific to this age group. However, noting that adult patients with diabetes are 1.6 times more likely to use CAM than are individuals without diabetes, the committee believes it is important for clinicians to encourage their patients to communicate openly about the use of CAM (especially because the parents may have diabetes themselves) and, when acknowledged, to differentiate between coadministration with the prescribed therapy versus replacement of (and, thus, noncompliance with) the prescribed therapy.[75]

CAM is most likely to be used by West Indian, African, Indian, Latin American, and Asian subjects.[76] CAM is also more common in families with higher income and education levels and an increased interest in self-care. One multicenter study conducted in Germany found that, among 228 families with a T1DM diagnosis, 18.4% reported using at least 1 form of CAM.[77] Reported parental motivators for using CAM for their children included the hope of improving their well-being (92.1%); the desire to try every available treatment option (77.8%); and the assumption that CAM has fewer adverse effects than conventional therapy (55.2%). Many forms of CAM are used because of patient-perceived inadequacies of current treatments.[75]

A wide variety of CAM dietary supplements are targeted at patients with diabetes and promise to lower BG concentrations or prevent and/or treat complications associated with the disease. Common supplements used by individuals with diabetes include aloe, bitter melon, chromium, cinnamon, fenugreek, ginseng, gymnema, and nopal.[78] These products lack product standardization and are not regulated by the US Food and Drug Administration for either safety or possible complications. Although these supplements may or may not have proven beneficial effects on diabetes, many might have harmful adverse effects and/or lead to medication interactions. Adverse effects from dietary supplements can include gastrointestinal discomfort, hypoglycemia, favism, insomnia, and increased blood pressure.[78]

In addition to dietary supplements, patients may use forms of CAM that include prayer, acupuncture, massage, hot tub therapy, biofeedback, and yoga. The University of Chicago's Division of Pediatric Endocrinology interviewed 106 families with T1DM and found that 33% of children had tried CAM in the past year; the most common form used was faith-healing or prayer.[79] Parents who reported the use of CAM for their children were also more likely to report having experienced struggles with adherence to conventional medicine.

It is the committee's opinion that providers should question patients on their use of CAM and also educate patients on potential adverse effects, review evidence for efficacy, and discourage the use of potentially dangerous or ineffective products.

SUMMARY

The clinical practice guideline that this technical report accompanies provides evidence-based recommendations on the management of patients between 10 and 18 years of age who have been diagnosed with T2DM. The document does not pertain to patients with impaired glucose tolerance, isolated insulin resistance, or prediabetes, nor does it pertain to obese but nondiabetic youth. It emphasizes the use of management modalities that have been shown to affect clinical outcomes in this pediatric population. The clinical practice guideline addresses situations in which either insulin or metformin is the preferred first-line treatment of children and adolescents with T2DM. It suggests integrating lifestyle modifications (ie, diet and exercise) in concert with medication rather than as an isolated initial treatment approach. Guidelines for frequency of monitoring HbA1c and finger-stick BG concentrations are presented. The clinical practice guideline is intended to assist clinician decision-making rather than replace clinical judgment and/or establish a protocol for the care of all children with this condition. These recommendations may not provide the only appropriate approach to the management of children with T2DM. Providers should consult experts trained in the care of children and adolescents with T2DM when treatment goals are not met or when therapy with insulin is initiated.

ACKNOWLEDGMENTS

The committee acknowledges the work of Edwin Lomotan, MD, FAAP, and George Michel, MS, in creating the reports.

SUBCOMMITTEE ON TYPE 2 DIABETES (OVERSIGHT BY THE STEERING COMMITTEE ON QUALITY IMPROVEMENT AND MANAGEMENT, 2008–2012)

Kenneth Claud Copeland, MD, FAAP: Co-chair—Endocrinology and Pediatric Endocrine Society Liaison (2009: Novo Nordisk, Genentech, Endo [National Advisory Groups]; 2010: Novo Nordisk [National Advisory Group]); published research related to type 2 diabetes

Janet Silverstein, MD, FAAP: Co-chair—Endocrinology and American Diabetes Association Liaison (small grants with Pfizer, Novo Nordisk, and Lilly; grant review committee for Genentech; was on an advisory committee for Sanofi Aventis, and Abbott Laboratories for a 1-time meeting); published research related to type 2 diabetes

Kelly Roberta Moore, MD, FAAP: General Pediatrics, Indian Health, AAP Committee on Native American Child Health Liaison (board member of the Merck Company Foundation Alliance to Reduce Disparities in Diabetes. Their national program office is the University of Michigan's Center for Managing Chronic Disease.)

Greg Edward Prazar, MD, FAAP: General Pediatrics (no conflicts)

Terry Raymer, MD, CDE: Family Medicine, Indian Health Service (no conflicts)

Richard N. Shiffman, MD, FAAP: Partnership for Policy Implementation Informatician, General Pediatrics (no conflicts)

Shelley C. Springer, MD, MBA, MSc, JD, FAAP: Epidemiologist, neonatologist (no conflicts)

Meaghan Anderson, MS, RD, LD, CDE: Academy of Nutrition and Dietetics Liaison (formerly a Certified Pump Trainer for Animas)

Stephen J. Spann, MD, MBA, FAAFP: American Academy of Family Physicians Liaison (no conflicts)

Vidhu V. Thaker, MD, FAAP: QuIIN Liaison, General Pediatrics (no conflicts)

CONSULTANT

Susan K. Flinn, MA: Medical Writer (no conflicts)

STAFF

Caryn Davidson, MA

REFERENCES

1. Silverstein JH, Rosenbloom AL. Type 2 diabetes in children. *Curr Diab Rep*. 2001;1(1):19–27

2. Pinhas-Hamiel O, Zeitler P. Clinical presentation and treatment of type 2 diabetes in children. *Pediatr Diabetes*. 2007;8(9 suppl 9):16–27

3. Dabelea D, Bell RA, D'Agostino RB Jr, et al; Writing Group for the SEARCH for Diabetes in Youth Study Group. Incidence of diabetes in youth in the United States. *JAMA*. 2007;297(24):2716–2724

4. Mayer-Davis EJ, Bell RA, Dabelea D, et al; SEARCH for Diabetes in Youth Study Group. The many faces of diabetes in American youth: type 1 and type 2 diabetes in five race and ethnic populations: the SEARCH for Diabetes in Youth Study. *Diabetes Care*. 2009;32(2 suppl 2):S99–S101

5. Liese AD, D'Agostino RB, Jr, Hamman RF, et al; SEARCH for Diabetes in Youth Study Group. The burden of diabetes mellitus among US youth: prevalence estimates from the SEARCH for Diabetes in Youth Study. *Pediatrics*. 2006;118(4):1510–1518

6. Narayan KM, Williams R. Diabetes—a global problem needing global solutions. *Prim Care Diabetes*. 2009;3(1):3–4

7. Silverstein J, Klingensmith G, Copeland K, et al; American Diabetes Association. Care of children and adolescents with type 1 diabetes: a statement of the American Diabetes Association. *Diabetes Care*. 2005;28(1):186–212

8. Pinhas-Hamiel O, Zeitler P. Barriers to the treatment of adolescent type 2 diabetes—a survey of provider perceptions. *Pediatr Diabetes.* 2003;4(1):24–28

9. TODAY Study Group, Zeitler P, Epstein L, Grey M, et al Treatment options for type 2 diabetes in adolescents and youth: a study of the comparative efficacy of metformin alone or in combination with rosiglitazone or lifestyle intervention in adolescents with type 2 diabetes. *Pediatr Diabetes.* 2007;8 (2):74–87

10. Kane MP, Abu-Baker A, Busch RS. The utility of oral diabetes medications in type 2 diabetes of the young. *Curr Diabetes Rev.* 2005;1(1):83–92

11. Kaufman FR. Type 2 diabetes mellitus in children and youth: a new epidemic. *J Pediatr Endocrinol Metab.* 2002;15(suppl 2): 737–744

12. Silverstein JH. Workforce issues for pediatric endocrinology. *J Pediatr.* 2006;149(1): A3

13. American Board of Pediatrics. 2011 Endocrinology examination. Available at: https:// www.abp.org/abpwebsite/stats/wrkfrc/endo. ppt. Accessed December 20, 2012

14. National Association of Children's Hospitals and Related Institutions. *Pediatric Subspecialists Survey Results.* Alexandria, VA: National Association of Children's Hospitals and Related Institutions; 2004

15. Saudek CD. The role of primary care professionals in managing diabetes. *Clin Diabetes.* 2002;20(2):65–66

16. Libman IM, Arslanian SA. Prevention and treatment of type 2 diabetes in youth. *Horm Res.* 2007;67(1):22–34

17. Gungor N, Hannon T, Libman I, Bacha F, Arslanian S. Type 2 diabetes mellitus in youth: the complete picture to date. *Pediatr Clin North Am.* 2005;52(6):1579–1609

18. Hannon TS, Rao G, Arslanian SA. Childhood obesity and type 2 diabetes mellitus. *Pediatrics.* 2005;116(2):473–480

19. Kawahara R, Amemiya T, Yoshino M, Miyamae M, Sasamoto K, Omori Y. Dropout of young non-insulin-dependent diabetics from diabetic care. *Diabetes Res Clin Pract.* 1994;24 (3):181–185

20. Malasanos TH, Burlingame JB, Youngblade L, Patel BD, Muir AB. Improved access to subspecialist diabetes care by telemedicine: cost savings and care measures in the first two years of the FITE diabetes project. *J Telemed Telecare.* 2005;11(suppl 1):74–76

21. Greenfield S, Rogers W, Mangotich M, Carney MF, Tarlov AR. Outcomes of patients with hypertension and non-insulin dependent diabetes mellitus treated by different systems and specialties. Results from the medical outcomes study. *JAMA.* 1995;274(18):1436–1444

22. Ziemer DC, Tsui C, Caudle J, Barnes CS, Dames F, Phillips LS. An informatics-supported intervention improves diabetes control in a primary care setting. *AMIA Annu Symp Proc.* 2006:1160

23. Ziemer DC, Miller CD, Rhee MK, et al. Clinical inertia contributes to poor diabetes control in a primary care setting. *Diabetes Educ.* 2005;31(4):564–571

24. De Berardis G, Pellegrini F, Franciosi M, et al; QuED Study. Quality of care and outcomes in type 2 diabetic patients: a comparison between general practice and diabetes clinics. *Diabetes Care.* 2004;27(2): 398–406

25. Copeland KC, Zeitler P, Geffner M, et al; TODAY Study Group. Characteristics of adolescents and youth with recent-onset type 2 diabetes: the TODAY cohort at baseline. *J Clin Endocrinol Metab.* 2011;96(1):159–167

26. Scott CR, Smith JM, Cradock MM, Pihoker C. Characteristics of youth-onset noninsulin-dependent diabetes mellitus and insulin-dependent diabetes mellitus at diagnosis. *Pediatrics.* 1997;100(1):84–91

27. Libman IM, Pietropaolo M, Arslanian SA, LaPorte RE, Becker DJ. Changing prevalence of overweight children and adolescents at onset of insulin-treated diabetes. *Diabetes Care.* 2003;26(10):2871–2875

28. Centre for Evidence-based Medicine. *Levels of Evidence.* Oxford, England: Centre for Evidence-based Medicine; March 2009

29. American Academy of Pediatrics Steering Committee on Quality Improvement and Management. Classifying recommendations for clinical practice guidelines. *Pediatrics.* 2004;114(3):874–877

30. Garg AX, Adhikari NK, McDonald H, et al. Effects of computerized clinical decision support systems on practitioner performance and patient outcomes: a systematic review. *JAMA.* 2005;293(10):1223–1238

31. Shiffman RN, Michel G, Essaihi A. Bridging the guideline implementation gap: a systematic, document-centered approach to guideline implementation. *J Am Med Inform Assoc.* 2004;11(5):418–426

32. National Library of Medicine. SNOMED clinical terms. Available at: www.nlm.nih.gov/ research/umls/Snomed/snomed_main.html. Accessed August 13, 2012

33. National Library of Medicine. RxNorm. Available at: www.nlm.nih.gov/research/ umls/rxnorm/. Accessed August 13, 2012

34. Regenstrief Institute. Logical observations identifiers names and codes. Available at: http://loinc.org/. Accessed August 13, 2012

35. National Quality Forum. *Health Information Technology Automation of Quality Measurement: Quality Data Set and Data Flow.* Washington, DC: National Quality Forum; 2009

36. American Academy of Pediatrics. Subcommittee on Type 2 Diabetes. Diabetes mellitus, type 2: clinical practice guideline for the management of newly diagnosed type 2 diabetes mellitus (T2DM) in children and adolescents. *Pediatrics.* 2013, In press

37. Shear CL, Burke GL, Freedman DS, Berenson GS. Value of childhood blood pressure measurements and family history in predicting future blood pressure status: results from 8 years of follow-up in the Bogalusa Heart Study. *Pediatrics.* 1986;77(6):862–869

38. Williams CL, Hayman LL, Daniels SR, et al; American Heart Association. Cardiovascular health in childhood: a statement for health professionals from the Committee on Atherosclerosis, Hypertension, and Obesity in the Young (AHOY) of the Council on Cardiovascular Disease in the Young, American Heart Association [published correction appears in *Circulation.* 2002;106 (9):1178]. *Circulation.* 2002;106(1):143–160

39. Eppens MC, Craig ME, Cusumano J, et al. Prevalence of diabetes complications in adolescents with type 2 compared with type 1 diabetes. *Diabetes Care.* 2006;29(6): 1300–1306

40. Mayer-Davis EJ, Ma B, Lawson A, et al; SEARCH for Diabetes in Youth Study Group. Cardiovascular disease risk factors in youth with type 1 and type 2 diabetes: implications of a factor analysis of clustering. *Metab Syndr Relat Disord.* 2009;7(2): 89–95

41. Hansen ML, Gunn PW, Kaelber DC. Underdiagnosis of hypertension in children and adolescents. *JAMA.* 2007;298(8):874–879

42. National Heart, Lung and Blood Institute. Blood pressure tables for children and adolescents. Available at: www.nhlbi.nih. gov/guidelines/hypertension/child_tbl.htm. Accessed August 13, 2012

43. National High Blood Pressure Education Program Working Group on High Blood Pressure in Children and Adolescents. The fourth report on the diagnosis, evaluation, and treatment of high blood pressure in children and adolescents. *Pediatrics.* 2004; 114(2 suppl 4th report):555–576

44. Brady TM, Feld LG. Pediatric approach to hypertension. *Semin Nephrol.* 2009;29(4): 379–388

45. Hansson L, Zanchetti A, Carruthers SG, et al. Effects of intensive blood-pressure lowering and low-dose aspirin in patients

with hypertension: principal results of the Hypertension Optimal Treatment (HOT) randomised trial. *Lancet.* 1998;351(9118): 1755–1762

46. UK Prospective Diabetes Study Group. Tight blood pressure control and risk of macrovascular and microvascular complications in type 2 diabetes: UKPDS 38. *BMJ.* 1998;317(7160):703–713

47. Yoon EY, Davis MM, Rocchini A, Kershaw D, Freed GL. Medical management of children with primary hypertension by pediatric subspecialists. *Pediatr Nephrol.* 2009;24(1): 147–153

48. Zanchetti A, Hansson L, Ménard J, et al. Risk assessment and treatment benefit in intensively treated hypertensive patients of the Hypertension Optimal Treatment (HOT) study. *J Hypertens.* 2001;19(4):819–825

49. Pinhas-Hamiel O, Zeitler P. Acute and chronic complications of type 2 diabetes mellitus in children and adolescents. *Lancet.* 2007;369(9575):1823–1831

50. Rodriguez BL, Fujimoto WY, Mayer-Davis EJ, et al. Prevalence of cardiovascular disease risk factors in U.S. children and adolescents with diabetes: the SEARCH for Diabetes in Youth Study. *Diabetes Care.* 2006; 29(8):1891–1896

51. Kavey RE, Allada V, Daniels SR, et al; American Heart Association Expert Panel on Population and Prevention Science; American Heart Association Council on Cardiovascular Disease in the Young; American Heart Association Council on Epidemiology and Prevention; American Heart Association Council on Nutrition, Physical Activity and Metabolism; American Heart Association Council on High Blood Pressure Research; American Heart Association Council on Cardiovascular Nursing; American Heart Association Council on the Kidney in Heart Disease; Interdisciplinary Working Group on Quality of Care and Outcomes Research. Cardiovascular risk reduction in high-risk pediatric patients: a scientific statement from the American Heart Association Expert Panel on Population and Prevention Science; the Councils on Cardiovascular Disease in the Young, Epidemiology and Prevention, Nutrition, Physical Activity and Metabolism, High Blood Pressure Research, Cardiovascular Nursing, and the Kidney in Heart Disease; and the Interdisciplinary Working Group on Quality of Care and Outcomes Research: endorsed by the American Academy of Pediatrics. *Circulation.* 2006;114(24):2710–2738

52. American Diabetes Association. Management of dyslipidemia in children and adolescents with diabetes. *Diabetes Care.* 2003; 26(7):2194–2197

53. Taha D. Hyperlipidemia in children with type 2 diabetes mellitus. *J Pediatr Endocrinol Metab.* 2002;15(suppl 1):505–507

54. Bronson-Castain KW, Bearse MA, Jr, Neuville J, et al. Adolescents with type 2 diabetes: early indications of focal retinal neuropathy, retinal thinning, and venular dilation. *Retina.* 2009;29(5):618–626

55. Mokdad AH, Bowman BA, Ford ES, Vinicor F, Marks JS, Koplan JP. The continuing epidemics of obesity and diabetes in the United States. *JAMA.* 2001;286(10):1195–1200

56. Yokoyama H, Okudaira M, Otani T, et al. Existence of early-onset NIDDM Japanese demonstrating severe diabetic complications. *Diabetes Care.* 1997;20(5):844–847

57. Okudaira M, Yokoyama H, Otani T, Uchigata Y, Iwamoto Y. Slightly elevated blood pressure as well as poor metabolic control are risk factors for the progression of retinopathy in early-onset Japanese type 2 diabetes. *J Diabetes Complications.* 2000;14(5):281–287

58. Krakoff J, Lindsay RS, Looker HC, Nelson RG, Hanson RL, Knowler WC. Incidence of retinopathy and nephropathy in youth-onset compared with adult-onset type 2 diabetes. *Diabetes Care.* 2003;26(1):76–81

59. Farah SE, Wals KT, Friedman IB, Pisacano MA, DiMartino-Nardi J. Prevalence of retinopathy and microalbuminuria in pediatric type 2 diabetes mellitus. *J Pediatr Endocrinol Metab.* 2006;19(7):937–942

60. Karabouta Z, Barnett S, Shield JP, Ryan FJ, Crowne EC. Peripheral neuropathy is an early complication of type 2 diabetes in adolescence. *Pediatr Diabetes.* 2008;9(2):110–114

61. Executive summary: standards of medical care in diabetes—2009 [published correction appears in *Diabetes Care.* 2009;32(4): 754]. *Diabetes Care.* 2009;32(suppl 1):S6–S12

62. Svensson M, Sundkvist G, Arnqvist HJ, et al; Diabetes Incidence Study in Sweden (DISS). Signs of nephropathy may occur early in young adults with diabetes despite modern diabetes management: results from the nationwide population-based Diabetes Incidence Study in Sweden (DISS). *Diabetes Care.* 2003;26(10):2903–2909

63. Yokoyama H, Okudaira M, Otani T, et al. Higher incidence of diabetic nephropathy in type 2 than in type 1 diabetes in early-onset diabetes in Japan. *Kidney Int.* 2000;58 (1):302–311

64. Mogensen CE, Keane WF, Bennett PH, et al. Prevention of diabetic renal disease with special reference to microalbuminuria. *Lancet.* 1995;346(8982):1080–1084

65. Molitch ME, DeFronzo RA, Franz MJ, et al; American Diabetes Association. Nephropathy in diabetes. *Diabetes Care.* 2004;27 (suppl 1):S79–S83

66. American Diabetes Association. Standards of medical care in diabetes—2010. *Diabetes Care.* 2010;33(suppl 1):S11–S61

67. Kovacs M, Goldston D, Obrosky DS, Bonar LK. Psychiatric disorders in youths with IDDM: rates and risk factors. *Diabetes Care.* 1997;20(1):36–44

68. Lawrence JM, Standiford DA, Loots B, et al; SEARCH for Diabetes in Youth Study. Prevalence and correlates of depressed mood among youth with diabetes: the SEARCH for Diabetes in Youth study. *Pediatrics.* 2006; 117(4):1348–1358

69. American Psychiatric Association. *Diagnostic and Statistical Manual of Mental Disorders.* 4th ed. Washington, DC: American Psychiatric Association; 1994

70. Radloff LS. The CES-D scale: a self report depression scale for research in the general population. *Appl Psychol Meas.* 1977;1:385–401

71. Garrison CZ, Jackson KL, Marsteller F, McKeown R, Addy C. A longitudinal study of depressive symptomatology in young adolescents. *J Am Acad Child Adolesc Psychiatry.* 1990;29(4):581–585

72. Killen JD, Hayward C, Wilson DM, et al. Factors associated with eating disorder symptoms in a community sample of 6th and 7th grade girls. *Int J Eat Disord.* 1994; 15(4):357–367

73. Roberts RE, Chen YW. Depressive symptoms and suicidal ideation among Mexican-origin and Anglo adolescents. *J Am Acad Child Adolesc Psychiatry.* 1995;34(1):81–90

74. Schoenbach VJ, Kaplan BH, Wagner EH, Grimson RC, Miller FT. Prevalence of self-reported depressive symptoms in young adolescents. *Am J Public Health.* 1983;73(11):1281–1287

75. Egede LE, Ye X, Zheng D, Silverstein MD. The prevalence and pattern of complementary and alternative medicine use in individuals with diabetes. *Diabetes Care.* 2002;25(2): 324–329

76. Dham S, Shah V, Hirsch S, Banerji MA. The role of complementary and alternative medicine in diabetes. *Curr Diab Rep.* 2006;6 (3):251–258

77. Dannemann K, Hecker W, Haberland H, et al. Use of complementary and alternative medicine in children with type 1 diabetes mellitus —prevalence, patterns of use, and costs. *Pediatr Diabetes.* 2008;9(3 pt 1):228–235

78. Geil P, Shane-McWhorter L. Dietary supplements in the management of diabetes: potential risks and benefits. *J Am Diet Assoc.* 2008;108(4 suppl 1):S59–S65

79. Miller JL, Cao D, Miller JG, Lipton RB. Correlates of complementary and alternative medicine (CAM) use in Chicago area children with diabetes (DM). *Prim Care Diabetes.* 2009;3(3):149–156

ERRATUM

An error occurred in the American Academy of Pediatrics "Technical Report: Management of Type 2 Diabetes Mellitus in Children and Adolescents" published in the February 2013 issue of *Pediatrics* (2013;131[2]:e648–e664).

On page e651, third column, under "Definitions," the first sentence should read as follows: "Children and adolescents: children <10 years of age; adolescents ≥10 years but ≤18 years of age."

doi:10.1542/peds.2013-0667

Diabetes Clinical Practice Guideline Quick Reference Tools

- Action Statement Summary
  — Management of Newly Diagnosed Type 2 Diabetes Mellitus (T2DM) in Children and Adolescents
- *ICD-9-CM/ICD-10-CM* Coding Quick Reference for Type 2 Diabetes Mellitus
- AAP Patient Education Handout
  — *Type 2 Diabetes: Tips for Healthy Living*

Action Statement Summary

Management of Newly Diagnosed Type 2 Diabetes Mellitus (T2DM) in Children and Adolescents

Key Action Statement 1

Clinicians must ensure that insulin therapy is initiated for children and adolescents with T2DM who are ketotic or in diabetic ketoacidosis and in whom the distinction between T1DM and T2DM is unclear; and, in usual cases, should initiate insulin therapy for patients:
- who have random venous or plasma BG concentrations ≥250 mg/dL; or
- whose HbA1c is >9%.

(Strong Recommendation: evidence quality X, validating studies cannot be performed, and C, observational studies and expert opinion; preponderance of benefit over harm.)

Key Action Statement 2

In all other instances, clinicians should initiate a lifestyle modification program, including nutrition and physical activity, and start metformin as first-line therapy for children and adolescents at the time of diagnosis of T2DM. (Strong recommendation: evidence quality B; 1 RCT showing improved outcomes with metformin versus lifestyle; preponderance of benefits over harms.)

Key Action Statement 3

The committee suggests that clinicians monitor HbA1c concentrations every 3 months and intensify treatment if treatment goals for BG and HbA1c concentrations are not being met. (Option: evidence quality D; expert opinion and studies in children with T1DM and in adults with T2DM; preponderance of benefits over harms.)

Key Action Statement 4

The committee suggests that clinicians advise patients to monitor finger-stick BG concentrations in those who
are taking insulin or other medications with a risk of hypoglycemia; or
- are initiating or changing their diabetes treatment regimen; or
- have not met treatment goals; or
- have intercurrent illnesses.

(Option: evidence quality D; expert consensus. Preponderance of benefits over harms.)

Key Action Statement 5

The committee suggests that clinicians incorporate the Academy of Nutrition and Dietetics' *Pediatric Weight Management Evidence-Based Nutrition Practice Guidelines* in the nutrition counseling of patients with T2DM both at the time of diagnosis and as part of ongoing management. (Option; evidence quality D; expert opinion; preponderance of benefits over harms. Role of patient preference is dominant.)

Key Action Statement 6

The committee suggests that clinicians encourage children and adolescents with T2DM to engage in moderate-to-vigorous exercise for at least 60 minutes daily and to limit nonacademic screen time to less than 2 hours per day. (Option: evidence quality D, expert opinion and evidence from studies of metabolic syndrome and obesity; preponderance of benefits over harms. Role of patient preference is dominant.)

Coding Quick Reference for Type 2 Diabetes Mellitus	
ICD-9-CM	*ICD-10-CM*
250.00 Type 2 diabetes mellitus, controlled	**E11.8** Type 2 diabetes mellitus with unspecified complications **E11.9** Type 2 diabetes mellitus without complications **E11.649** Type 2 diabetes mellitus with hypoglycemia without coma **E11.65** Type 2 diabetes mellitus with hyperglycemia **E13.9** Other specified diabetes mellitus without complications
250.02 Type 2 diabetes mellitus, uncontrolled	Use codes above (**E11.8–E13.9**). *ICD-10-CM* does not discern between controlled and uncontrolled.

Type 2 Diabetes: Tips for Healthy Living

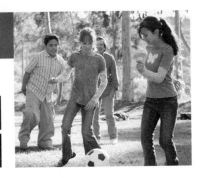

Children with type 2 diabetes can live a healthy life. If your child has been diagnosed with type 2 diabetes, your child's doctor will talk with you about the importance of lifestyle and medication in keeping your child's blood glucose (blood sugar) levels under control.

Read on for information from the American Academy of Pediatrics (AAP) about managing blood glucose and creating plans for healthy living.

What is blood glucose?

Glucose is found in the blood and is the body's main source of energy. The food your child eats is broken down by the body into glucose. Glucose is a type of sugar that gives energy to the cells in the body.

The cells need the help of insulin to take the glucose from the blood to the cells. Insulin is made by an organ called the pancreas.

In children with type 2 diabetes, the pancreas does not make enough insulin and the cells don't use the insulin very well.

Why is it important to manage blood glucose levels?

Glucose will build up in the blood if it cannot be used by the cells. High blood glucose levels can damage many parts of the body, such as the eyes, kidneys, nerves, and heart.

Your child's blood glucose levels may need to be checked on a regular schedule to make sure the levels do not get too high. Your child's doctor will tell you what your child's blood glucose level should be. You and your child will need to learn how to use a glucose meter. Blood glucose levels can be quickly and easily measured using a glucose meter. First, a lancet is used to prick the skin; then a drop of blood from your child's finger is placed on a test strip that is inserted into the meter.

Are there medicines for type 2 diabetes?

Insulin in a shot or another medicine by mouth may be prescribed by your child's doctor if needed to help control your child's blood glucose levels. If your child's doctor has prescribed a medicine, it's important that your child take it as directed. Side effects from certain medicines may include bloating or gassiness. Check with your child's doctor if you have questions.

Along with medicines, your child's doctor will suggest changes to your child's diet and encourage your child to be physically active.

Tips for healthy living

A healthy diet and staying active are especially important for children with type 2 diabetes. Your child's blood glucose levels are easier to manage when you child is at a healthy weight.

Create a plan for eating healthy

Talk with your child's doctor and registered dietitian about a meal plan that meets the needs of your child. The following tips can help you select foods that are healthy and contain a high content of nutrients (protein, vitamins, and minerals):

- Eat at least 5 servings of fruits and vegetables each day.
- Include high-fiber, whole-grain foods such as brown rice, whole-grain pasta, corns, peas, and breads and cereals at meals. Sweet potatoes are also a good choice.
- Choose lower-fat or fat-free toppings like grated low-fat parmesan cheese, salsa, herbed cottage cheese, nonfat/low-fat gravy, low-fat sour cream, low-fat salad dressing, or yogurt.
- Select lean meats such as skinless chicken and turkey, fish, lean beef cuts (round, sirloin, chuck, loin, lean ground beef—no more than 15% fat content), and lean pork cuts (tenderloin, chops, ham). Trim off all visible fat. Remove skin from cooked poultry before eating.
- Include healthy oils such as canola or olive oil in your diet. Choose margarine and vegetable oils without trans fats made from canola, corn, sunflower, soybean, or olive oils.
- Use nonstick vegetable sprays when cooking.
- Use fat-free cooking methods such as baking, broiling, grilling, poaching, or steaming when cooking meat, poultry, or fish.
- Serve vegetable- and broth-based soups, or use nonfat (skim) or low-fat (1%) milk or evaporated skim milk when making cream soups.
- Use the Nutrition Facts label on food packages to find foods with less saturated fat per serving. Pay attention to the serving size as you make choices. Remember that the percent daily values on food labels are based on portion sizes and calorie levels for adults.

Create a plan for physical activity

Physical activity, along with proper nutrition, promotes lifelong health. Following are some ideas on how to get fit:

- **Encourage your child to be active at least 1 hour a day.** Active play is the best exercise for younger children! Parents can join their children and have fun while being active too. School-aged child should participate every day in 1 hour or more of moderate to vigorous physical activity that is right for their age, is enjoyable, and involves a variety of activities.
- **Limit television watching and computer use.** The AAP discourages TV and other media use by children younger than 2 years and encourages interactive play. For older children, total entertainment screen time should be limited to less than 1 to 2 hours per day.
- **Keep an activity log.** The use of activity logs can help children and teens keep track of their exercise programs and physical activity. Online tools can be helpful.

- **Get the whole family involved.** It is a great way to spend time together. Also, children who regularly see their parents enjoying sports and physical activity are more likely to do so themselves.
- **Provide a safe environment.** Make sure your child's equipment and chosen site for the sport or activity are safe. Make sure your child's clothing is comfortable and appropriate.

For more information

National Diabetes Education Program

http://ndep.nih.gov

From your doctor

American Academy
of Pediatrics

DEDICATED TO THE HEALTH OF ALL CHILDREN™

The American Academy of Pediatrics is an organization of 60,000 primary care pediatricians, pediatric medical subspecialists, and pediatric surgical specialists dedicated to the health, safety, and well-being of infants, children, adolescents, and young adults.

American Academy of Pediatrics
Web site—www.HealthyChildren.org

Early Detection of Developmental Dysplasia of the Hip

- *Clinical Practice Guideline*
- *Technical Report Summary*

Readers of this clinical practice guideline are urged to review the technical report to enhance the evidence-based decision-making process. The full technical report is available on the companion CD-ROM.

AMERICAN ACADEMY OF PEDIATRICS

Committee on Quality Improvement, Subcommittee on Developmental Dysplasia of the Hip

Clinical Practice Guideline: Early Detection of Developmental Dysplasia of the Hip

ABSTRACT. *Developmental dysplasia of the hip* is the preferred term to describe the condition in which the femoral head has an abnormal relationship to the acetabulum. Developmental dysplasia of the hip includes frank dislocation (luxation), partial dislocation (subluxation), instability wherein the femoral head comes in and out of the socket, and an array of radiographic abnormalities that reflect inadequate formation of the acetabulum. Because many of these findings may not be present at birth, the term *developmental* more accurately reflects the biologic features than does the term *congenital*. The disorder is uncommon. The earlier a dislocated hip is detected, the simpler and more effective is the treatment. Despite newborn screening programs, dislocated hips continue to be diagnosed later in infancy and childhood,[1–11] in some instances delaying appropriate therapy and leading to a substantial number of malpractice claims. The objective of this guideline is to reduce the number of dislocated hips detected later in infancy and childhood. The target audience is the primary care provider. The target patient is the healthy newborn up to 18 months of age, excluding those with neuromuscular disorders, myelodysplasia, or arthrogryposis.

ABBREVIATIONS. DDH, developmental dysplasia of the hip; AVN, avascular necrosis of the hip.

BIOLOGIC FEATURES AND NATURAL HISTORY

Understanding the developmental nature of developmental dysplasia of the hip (DDH) and the subsequent spectrum of hip abnormalities requires a knowledge of the growth and development of the hip joint.[12] Embryologically, the femoral head and acetabulum develop from the same block of primitive mesenchymal cells. A cleft develops to separate them at 7 to 8 weeks' gestation. By 11 weeks' gestation, development of the hip joint is complete. At birth, the femoral head and the acetabulum are primarily cartilaginous. The acetabulum continues to develop postnatally. The growth of the fibrocartilaginous rim (the labrum) that surrounds

The recommendations in this statement do not indicate an exclusive course of treatment or serve as a standard of medical care. Variations, taking into account individual circumstances, may be appropriate.

The Practice Guideline, "Early Detection of Developmental Dysplasia of the Hip," was reviewed by appropriate committees and sections of the American Academy of Pediatrics (AAP) including the Chapter Review Group, a focus group of office-based pediatricians representing each AAP District: Gene R. Adams, MD; Robert M. Corwin, MD; Diane Fuquay, MD; Barbara M. Harley, MD; Thomas J. Herr, MD, Chair; Kenneth E. Matthews, MD; Robert D. Mines, MD; Lawrence C. Pakula, MD; Howard B. Weinblatt, MD; and Delosa A. Young, MD. The Practice Guideline was also reviewed by relevant outside medical organizations as part of the peer review process.

PEDIATRICS (ISSN 0031 4005). Copyright © 2000 by the American Academy of Pediatrics.

the bony acetabulum deepens the socket. Development of the femoral head and acetabulum are intimately related, and normal adult hip joints depend on further growth of these structures. Hip dysplasia may occur in utero, perinatally, or during infancy and childhood.

The acronym DDH includes hips that are unstable, subluxated, dislocated (luxated), and/or have malformed acetabula. A hip is *unstable* when the tight fit between the femoral head and the acetabulum is lost and the femoral head is able to move within (subluxated) or outside (dislocated) the confines of the acetabulum. A *dislocation* is a complete loss of contact of the femoral head with the acetabulum. Dislocations are divided into 2 types: teratologic and typical.[12] *Teratologic dislocations* occur early in utero and often are associated with neuromuscular disorders, such as arthrogryposis and myelodysplasia, or with various dysmorphic syndromes. The *typical dislocation* occurs in an otherwise healthy infant and may occur prenatally or postnatally.

During the immediate newborn period, laxity of the hip capsule predominates, and, if clinically significant enough, the femoral head may spontaneously dislocate and relocate. If the hip spontaneously relocates and stabilizes within a few days, subsequent hip development usually is normal. If subluxation or dislocation persists, then structural anatomic changes may develop. A deep concentric position of the femoral head in the acetabulum is necessary for normal development of the hip. When not deeply reduced (subluxated), the labrum may become everted and flattened. Because the femoral head is not reduced into the depth of the socket, the acetabulum does not grow and remodel and, therefore, becomes shallow. If the femoral head moves further out of the socket (dislocation), typically superiorly and laterally, the inferior capsule is pulled upward over the now empty socket. Muscles surrounding the hip, especially the adductors, become contracted, limiting abduction of the hip. The hip capsule constricts; once this capsular constriction narrows to less than the diameter of the femoral head, the hip can no longer be reduced by manual manipulative maneuvers, and operative reduction usually is necessary.

The hip is at risk for dislocation during 4 periods: 1) the 12th gestational week, 2) the 18th gestational week, 3) the final 4 weeks of gestation, and 4) the postnatal period. During the 12th gestational week, the hip is at risk as the fetal lower limb rotates medially. A dislocation at this time is termed teratologic. All elements of the hip joint develop abnormally. The hip muscles develop around the 18th gestational week. Neuromuscular problems at this time, such as myelodysplasia and arthrogryposis, also lead to teratologic dislocations. During the final 4 weeks of pregnancy, mechanical forces have a role. Conditions such as oligohydramnios or breech position predispose to DDH.[13] Breech position occurs in ~3% of births, and DDH occurs more frequently in breech presentations, reportedly in as many as 23%. The frank breech position of hip flexion and knee extension places a newborn or infant at the highest risk. Postnatally, infant positioning such as swaddling, combined with ligamentous laxity, also has a role.

The true incidence of dislocation of the hip can only be presumed. There is no "gold standard" for diagnosis during the newborn period. Physical examination, plane radiography, and ultrasonography all are fraught with false-positive and false-negative results. Arthrography (insertion of contrast medium into the hip joint) and magnetic resonance imaging, although accurate for determining the precise hip anatomy, are inappropriate methods for screening the newborn and infant.

The reported incidence of DDH is influenced by genetic and racial factors, diagnostic criteria, the experience and training of the examiner, and the age of the child at the time of the examination. Wynne-Davies[14] reported an increased risk to subsequent children in the presence of a diagnosed dislocation (6% risk with healthy parents and an affected child, 12% risk with an affected parent, and 36% risk with an affected parent and 1 affected child). DDH is not always detectable at birth, but some newborn screening surveys suggest an incidence as high as 1 in 100 newborns with evidence of instability, and 1 to 1.5 cases of dislocation per 1000 newborns. The incidence of DDH is higher in girls. Girls are especially susceptible to the maternal hormone relaxin, which may contribute to ligamentous laxity with the resultant instability of the hip. The left hip is involved 3 times as commonly as the right hip, perhaps related to the left occiput anterior positioning of most non-breech newborns. In this position, the left hip resides posteriorly against the mother's spine, potentially limiting abduction.

PHYSICAL EXAMINATION

DDH is an evolving process, and its physical findings on clinical examination change.[12,15,16] The newborn must be relaxed and preferably examined on a firm surface. Considerable patience and skill are required. The physical examination changes as the child grows older. No signs are pathognomonic for a dislocated hip. The examiner must look for asymmetry. Indeed, bilateral dislocations are more difficult to diagnose than unilateral dislocations because symmetry is retained. Asymmetrical thigh or gluteal folds, better observed when the child is prone, apparent limb length discrepancy, and restricted motion, especially abduction, are significant, albeit not pathognomonic signs. With the infant supine and the pelvis stabilized, abduction to 75° and adduction to 30° should occur readily under normal circumstances.

The 2 maneuvers for assessing hip stability in the newborn are the Ortolani and Barlow tests. The Ortolani elicits the sensation of the dislocated hip reducing, and the Barlow detects the unstable hip dislocating from the acetabulum. The Ortolani is performed with the newborn supine and the examiner's index and middle fingers placed along the greater trochanter with the thumb placed along the inner thigh. The hip is flexed to 90° but not more, and the leg is held in neutral rotation. The hip is gently abducted while lifting the leg anteriorly. With this maneuver, a "clunk" is felt as the dislocated femoral head reduces into the acetabulum. This is a positive Ortolani sign. The Barlow provocative test is performed with the newborn positioned supine and the hips flexed to 90°. The leg is then gently adducted while posteriorly directed pressure is placed on the knee. A palpable clunk or sensation of movement is felt as the femoral head exits the acetabulum posteriorly. This is a positive Barlow sign. The Ortolani and Barlow maneuvers are performed 1 hip at a time. Little force is required for the performance of either of these tests. The goal is not to prove that the hip can be dislocated. Forceful and repeated examinations can break the seal between the labrum and the femoral head. These strongly positive signs of Ortolani and Barlow are distinguished from a large array of soft or equivocal physical findings present during the newborn period. High-pitched clicks are commonly elicited with flexion and extension and are inconsequential. A dislocatable hip has a rather distinctive clunk, whereas a subluxable hip is characterized by a feeling of looseness, a sliding movement, but without the true Ortolani and Barlow clunks. Separating true dislocations (clunks) from a feeling of instability and from benign adventitial sounds (clicks) takes practice and expertise. This guideline recognizes the broad range of physical findings present in newborns and infants and the confusion of terminology generated in the literature. By 8 to 12 weeks of age, the capsule laxity decreases, muscle tightness increases, and the Barlow and Ortolani maneuvers are no longer positive regardless of the status of the femoral head. In the 3-month-old infant, limitation of abduction is the most reliable sign associated with DDH. Other features that arouse suspicion include asymmetry of thigh folds, a positive Allis or Galeazzi sign (relative shortness of the femur with the hips and knees flexed), and discrepancy of leg lengths. These physical findings alert the examiner that abnormal relationships of the femoral head to the acetabulum (dislocation and subluxation) *may* be present.

Maldevelopments of the acetabulum alone (acetabular dysplasia) can be determined only by imaging techniques. Abnormal physical findings may be absent in an infant with acetabular dysplasia but no subluxation or dislocation. Indeed, because of the confusion, inconsistencies, and misuse of language in the literature (eg, an Ortolani sign called a click by some and a clunk by others), this guideline uses the following definitions.

- A *positive examination* result for DDH is the Barlow or Ortolani sign. This is the clunk of dislocation or reduction.
- An *equivocal examination* or *warning signs* include an array of physical findings that may be found in children with DDH, in children with another orthopaedic disorder, or in children who are completely healthy. These physical findings include asymmetric thigh or buttock creases, an apparent or true short leg, and limited abduction. These signs, used singly or in combination, serve to raise the pediatrician's index of suspicion and act as a threshold for referral. Newborn soft tissue hip clicks are not predictive of DDH[17] but may be confused with the Ortolani and Barlow clunks by some screening physicians and thereby be a reason for referral.

IMAGING

Radiographs of the pelvis and hips have historically been used to assess an infant with suspected DDH. During the first few months of life when the femoral heads are composed entirely of cartilage, radiographs have limited value. Displacement and instability may be undetectable, and evaluation of acetabular development is influenced by the infant's position at the time the radiograph is performed. By 4 to 6 months of age, radiographs become more reliable, particularly when the ossification center develops in the femoral head. Radiographs are readily available and relatively low in cost.

Real-time ultrasonography has been established as an accurate method for imaging the hip during the first few months of life.[15,18–25] With ultrasonography, the cartilage can be visualized and the hip can be viewed while assessing the stability of the hip and the morphologic features of the acetabulum. In some clinical settings, ultrasonography can provide information comparable to arthrography (direct injection of contrast into the hip joint), without the need for sedation, invasion, contrast medium, or ionizing radiation. Although the availability of equipment for ultrasonography is widespread, accurate results in hip sonography require training and experience. Although expertise in pediatric hip ultrasonography is increasing, this examination may not always be available or obtained conveniently. Ultrasonographic techniques include *static evaluation* of the morphologic features of the hip, as popularized in Europe by Graf,[26] and a *dynamic evaluation*, as developed by Harcke[20] that assesses the hip for stability of the femoral head in the socket, as well as static anatomy. Dynamic ultrasonography yields more useful information. With both techniques, there is considerable interobserver variability, especially during the first 3 weeks of life.[7,27]

Experience with ultrasonography has documented its ability to detect abnormal position, instability, and dysplasia not evident on clinical examination. Ultrasonography during the first 4 weeks of life often reveals the presence of minor degrees of instability and acetabular immaturity. Studies[7,28,29] indicate that nearly all these mild early findings, which will not be apparent on physical examination, resolve spontaneously without treatment. Newborn screening with ultrasonography has required a high frequency of reexamination and results in a large number of hips being unnecessarily treated. One study[23] demonstrates that a screening process with higher false-positive results also yields increased prevention of late cases. Ultrasonographic screening of all infants at 4 to 6 weeks of age would be expensive, requiring considerable resources. This practice is yet to be validated by clinical trial. *Consequently, the use of ultrasonography is recommended as an adjunct to the clinical evaluation.* It is the technique of choice for clarifying a physical finding, assessing a high-risk infant, and monitoring DDH as it is observed or treated. Used in this selective capacity, it can guide treatment and may prevent overtreatment.

PRETERM INFANTS

DDH may be unrecognized in prematurely born infants. When the infant has cardiorespiratory problems, the diagnosis and management are focused on providing appropriate ventilatory and cardiovascular support, and careful examination of the hips may be deferred until a later date. The most complete examination the infant receives may occur at the time of discharge from the hospital, and this single examination may not detect subluxation or dislocation. Despite the medical urgencies surrounding the preterm infant, it is critical to examine the entire child.

METHODS FOR GUIDELINE DEVELOPMENT

Our goal was to develop a practice parameter by using a process that would be based whenever possible on available evidence. The methods used a combination of expert panel, decision modeling, and evidence synthesis[30] (see the Technical Report available on *Pediatrics electronic pages* at www.pediatrics.org). The predominant methods recommended for such evidence synthesis are generally of 2 types: a *data-driven* method and a *model-driven*[31,32] method. In data-driven methods, the analyst finds the best data available and induces a conclusion from these data. A model-driven method, in contrast, begins with an effort to define the context for evidence and then searches for the data as defined by that context. Data-driven methods are useful when the quality of evidence is high. A careful review of the medical literature revealed that the published evidence about DDH did not meet the criteria for high quality. There was a paucity of randomized clinical trials.[8] We decided, therefore, to use the model-driven method.

A decision model was constructed based on the perspective of practicing clinicians and determining the best strategy for screening and diagnosis. The target child was a full-term newborn with no obvious orthopaedic abnormalities. We focused on the various options available to the pediatrician* for the detection of DDH, including screening by physical examination, screening by ultrasonography, and episodic screening during health supervision. Because

---

*In this guideline, the term *pediatrician* includes the range of pediatric primary care providers, eg, family practitioners and pediatric nurse practitioners.

the detection of a dislocated hip usually results in referral by the pediatrician, and because management of DDH is not in the purview of the pediatrician's care, treatment options are not included. We also included in our model a wide range of options for detecting DDH during the first year of life if the results of the newborn screen are negative.

The outcomes on which we focused were a dislocated hip at 1 year of age as the major morbidity of the disease and avascular necrosis of the hip (AVN) as the primary complication of DDH treatment. AVN is a loss of blood supply to the femoral head resulting in abnormal hip development, distortion of shape, and, in some instances, substantial morbidity. Ideally, a gold standard would be available to define DDH at any point in time. However, as noted, no gold standard exists except, perhaps, arthrography of the hip, which is an inappropriate standard for use in a detection model. Therefore, we defined outcomes in terms of the *process of care*. We reviewed the literature extensively. The purpose of the literature review was to provide the probabilities required by the decision model since there were no randomized clinical trials. The article or chapter title and the abstracts were reviewed by 2 members of the methodology team and members of the subcommittee. Articles not rejected were reviewed, and data were abstracted that would provide evidence for the probabilities required by the decision model. As part of the literature abstraction process, the evidence quality in each article was assessed. A computer-based literature search, hand review of recent publications, or examination of the reference section for other articles ("ancestor articles") identified 623 articles; 241 underwent detailed review, 118 of which provided some data. Of the 100 ancestor articles, only 17 yielded useful articles, suggesting that our accession process was complete. By traditional epidemiologic standards,[33] the quality of the evidence in this set of articles was uniformly low. There were few controlled trials and few studies of the follow-up of infants for whom the results of newborn examinations were negative. When the evidence was poor or lacking entirely, extensive discussions among members of the committee and the expert opinion of outside consultants were used to arrive at a consensus. No votes were taken. Disagreements were discussed, and consensus was achieved.

The available evidence was distilled in 3 ways.

First, estimates were made of DDH at birth in infants without risk factors. These estimates constituted the baseline risk. Second, estimates were made of the rates of DDH in the children with risk factors. These numbers guide clinical actions: rates that are too high might indicate referral or different follow-up despite negative physical findings. Third, each screening strategy (pediatrician-based, orthopaedist-based, and ultrasonography-based) was scored for the estimated number of children given a diagnosis of DDH at birth, at mid-term (4–12 months of age), and at late-term (12 months of age and older) and for the estimated number of cases of AVN incurred, assuming that all children given a diagnosis of DDH would be treated. These numbers suggest the best strategy, balancing DDH detection with incurring adverse effects.

The baseline estimate of DDH based on orthopaedic screening was 11.5/1000 infants. Estimates from pediatric screening were 8.6/1000 and from ultrasonography were 25/1000. The 11.5/1000 rate translates into a rate for not-at-risk boys of 4.1/1000 boys and a rate for not-at-risk girls of 19/1000 girls. These numbers derive from the facts that the relative risk— the rate in girls divided by the rate in boys across several studies—is 4.6 and because infants are split evenly between boys and girls, so $.5 \times 4.1/1000 + .5 \times 19/1000 = 11.5/1000$.[34,35] We used these baseline rates for calculating the rates in other risk groups. Because the relative risk of DDH for children with a positive family history (first-degree relatives) is 1.7, the rate for boys with a positive family history is $1.7 \times 4.1 = 6.4/1000$ boys and for girls with a positive family history, $1.7 \times 19 = 32/1000$ girls. Finally, the relative risk of DDH for breech presentation (of all kinds) is 6.3, so the risk for breech boys is $7.0 \times 4.1 = 29/1000$ boys and for breech girls, $7.0 \times 19 = 133/1000$ girls. These numbers are summarized in Table 1.

These numbers suggest that boys without risk or those with a family history have the lowest risk; girls without risk and boys born in a breech presentation have an intermediate risk; and girls with a positive family history, and especially girls born in a breech presentation, have the highest risks. Guidelines, considering the risk factors, should follow these risk profiles. Reports of newborn screening for DDH have included various screening techniques. In some, the screening clinician was an orthopaedist, in

TABLE 1.   Relative and Absolute Risks for Finding a Positive Examination Result at Newborn Screening by Using the Ortolani and Barlow Signs

Newborn Characteristics	Relative Risk of a Positive Examination Result	Absolute Risk of a Positive Examination Result per 1000 Newborns With Risk Factors
All newborns	. . .	11.5
Boys	1.0	4.1
Girls	4.6	19
Positive family history	1.7	
Boys	. . .	6.4
Girls	. . .	32
Breech presentation	7.0	
Boys	. . .	29
Girls	. . .	133

TABLE 2. Newborn Strategy*

Outcome	Orthopaedist PE	Pediatrician PE	Ultrasonography
DDH in newborn	12	8.6	25
DDH at ~6 mo of age	.1	.45	.28
DDH at 12 mo of age or more	.16	.33	.1
AVN at 12 mo of age	.06	.1	.1

* PE indicates physical examination. Outcome per 1000 infants initially screened.

others, a pediatrician, and in still others, a physiotherapist. In addition, screening has been performed by ultrasonography. In assessing the expected effect of each strategy, we estimated the newborn DDH rates, the mid-term DDH rates, and the late-term DDH rates for each of the 3 strategies, as shown in Table 2. We also estimated the rate of AVN for DDH treated before 2 months of age (2.5/1000 treated) and after 2 months of age (109/1000 treated). We could not distinguish the AVN rates for children treated between 2 and 12 months of age from those treated later. Table 2 gives these data. The total cases of AVN per strategy are calculated, assuming that all infants with positive examination results are treated.

Table 2 shows that a strategy using pediatricians to screen newborns would give the lowest newborn rate but the highest mid- and late-term DDH rates. To assess how much better an ultrasonography-only screening strategy would be, we could calculate a cost-effectiveness ratio. In this case, the "cost" of ultrasonographic screening is the number of "extra" newborn cases that probably include children who do not need to be treated. (The cost from AVN is the same in the 2 strategies.) By using these cases as the cost and the number of later cases averted as the effect, a ratio is obtained of 71 children treated neonatally because of a positive ultrasonographic screen for each later case averted. Because this number is high, and because the presumption of better late-term efficacy is based on a single study, we do not recommend ultrasonographic screening at this time.

RECOMMENDATIONS AND NOTES TO ALGORITHM (Fig 1)

1. **All newborns are to be screened by physical examination**. The evidence† for this recommendation is good. The expert consensus‡ is strong. Although initial screening by orthopaedists§ would be optimal (Table 2), it is doubtful that if widely practiced, such a strategy would give the same good results as those published from pediatric orthopaedic research centers. **It is recommended that screening be done by a properly trained health care provider** (eg, physician, pediatric nurse practitioner, physician assistant, or physical therapist). (Evidence for this recommendation is strong.) A number of studies performed by properly trained nonphysicians report results

indistinguishable from those performed by physicians.[36] The examination after discharge from the neonatal intensive care unit should be performed as a newborn examination with appropriate screening. **Ultrasonography of all newborns is not recommended.** (Evidence is fair; consensus is strong.) Although there is indirect evidence to support the use of ultrasonographic screening of all newborns, it is not advocated because it is operator-dependent, availability is questionable, it increases the rate of treatment, and interobserver variability is high. There are probably some increased costs. We considered a strategy of "no newborn screening." This arm is politically indefensible because screening newborns is inherent in pediatrician's care. The technical report details this limb through decision analysis. Regardless of the screening method used for the newborn, DDH is detected in 1 in 5000 infants at 18 months of age.[3] The evidence and consensus for newborn screening remain strong.

Newborn Physical Examination and Treatment

2. **If a positive Ortolani or Barlow sign is found in the newborn examination, the infant should be referred to an orthopaedist.** Orthopaedic referral is recommended when the Ortolani sign is unequivocally positive (a clunk). Orthopaedic referral is not recommended for any softly positive finding in the examination (eg, hip click without dislocation). The precise time frame for the newborn to be evaluated by the orthopaedist cannot be determined from the literature. However, the literature suggests that the majority of "abnormal" physical findings of hip examinations at birth (clicks and clunks) will resolve by 2 weeks; therefore, consultation and possible initiation of treatment are recommended by that time. The data recommending that all those with a positive Ortolani sign be referred to an orthopaedist are limited, but expert panel consensus, nevertheless, was strong, because pediatricians do not have the training to take full responsibility and because true Ortolani clunks are rare and their management is more appropriately performed by the orthopaedist.

If the results of the physical examination at birth are "equivocally" positive (ie, soft click, mild asymmetry, but neither an Ortolani nor a Barlow sign is present), then a follow-up hip examination by the pediatrician in 2 weeks is recommended. (Evidence is good; consensus is strong.) The available data suggest that most clicks resolve by 2 weeks and that these "benign hip clicks" in the newborn period do

---

†In this guideline, evidence is listed as *good*, *fair*, or *poor* based on the methodologist's evaluation of the literature quality. (See the Technical Report.)

‡Opinion or consensus is listed as *strong* if opinion of the expert panel was unanimous or *mixed* if there were dissenting points of view.

§In this guideline, the term *orthopaedist* refers to an orthopaedic surgeon with expertise in pediatric orthopaedic conditions.

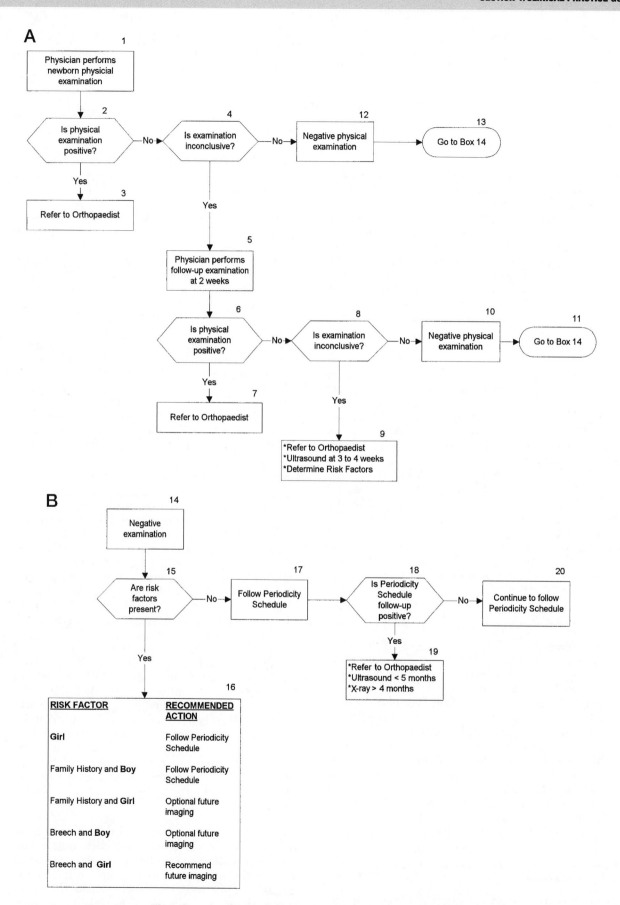

Fig 1. Screening for developmental hip dysplasia—clinical algorithm.

not lead to later hip dysplasia.[9,17,28,37] Thus, for an infant with softly positive signs, the pediatrician should reexamine the hips at 2 weeks before making referrals for orthopaedic care or ultrasonography. We recognize the concern of pediatricians about adherence to follow-up care regimens, but this concern regards all aspects of health maintenance and is not a reason to request ultrasonography or other diagnostic study of the newborn hips.

3. **If the results of the newborn physical examination are positive (ie, presence of an Ortolani or a Barlow sign), ordering an ultrasonographic examination of the newborn is not recommended.** (Evidence is poor; opinion is strong.) Treatment decisions are not influenced by the results of ultrasonography but are based on the results of the physical examination. The treating physician may use a variety of imaging studies during clinical management. **If the results of the newborn physical examination are positive, obtaining a radiograph of the newborn's pelvis and hips is not recommended** (evidence is poor; opinion is strong), because they are of limited value and do not influence treatment decisions.

The use of triple diapers when abnormal physical signs are detected during the newborn period is not recommended. (Evidence is poor; opinion is strong.) Triple diaper use is common practice despite the lack of data on the effectiveness of triple diaper use; and, in instances of frank dislocation, the use of triple diapers may delay the initiation of more appropriate treatment (such as with the Pavlik harness). Often, the primary care pediatrician may not have performed the newborn examination in the hospital. The importance of communication cannot be overemphasized, and triple diapers may aid in follow-up as a reminder that a possible abnormal physical examination finding was present in the newborn.

2-Week Examination

4. **If the results of the physical examination are positive (eg, positive Ortolani or Barlow sign) at 2 weeks, refer to an orthopaedist.** (Evidence is strong; consensus is strong.) Referral is urgent but is not an emergency. Consensus is strong that, as in the newborn, the presence of an Ortolani or Barlow sign at 2 weeks warrants referral to an orthopaedist. An Ortolani sign at 2 weeks may be a new finding or a finding that was not apparent at the time of the newborn examination.

5. **If at the 2-week examination the Ortolani and Barlow signs are absent but physical findings raise suspicions, consider referral to an orthopaedist or request ultrasonography at age 3 to 4 weeks.** Consensus is mixed about the follow-up for softly positive or equivocal findings at 2 weeks of age (eg, adventitial click, thigh asymmetry, and apparent leg length difference). Because it is necessary to confirm the status of the hip joint, the pediatrician can consider referral to an orthopaedist or for ultrasonography if the constellation of physical findings raises a high level of suspicion.

However, if the physical findings are minimal, continuing follow-up by the periodicity schedule with focused hip examinations is also an option, provided risk factors are considered. (See "Recommendations" 7 and 8.)

6. **If the results of the physical examination are negative at 2 weeks, follow-up is recommended at the scheduled well-baby periodic examinations.** (Evidence is good; consensus is strong.)

7. **Risk factors. If the results of the newborn examination are negative (or equivocally positive), risk factors may be considered.**[13,21,38–41] Risk factors are a study of thresholds to act.[42] Table 1 gives the risk of finding a positive Ortolani or Barlow sign at the time of the initial newborn screening. If this examination is negative, the absolute risk of there being a true dislocated hip is greatly reduced. Nevertheless, the data in Table 1 may influence the pediatrician to perform confirmatory evaluations. Action will vary based on the individual clinician. The following recommendations are made (evidence is strong; opinion is strong):

   • **Girl** (newborn risk of 19/1000). When the results of the newborn examination are negative or equivocally positive, hips should be reevaluated at 2 weeks of age. If negative, continue according to the periodicity schedule; if positive, refer to an orthopaedist or for ultrasonography at 3 weeks of age.

   • **Infants with a positive family history of DDH** (newborn risk for boys of 9.4/1000 and for girls, 44/1000). When the results of the newborn examination in boys are negative or equivocally positive, hips should be reevaluated at 2 weeks of age. If negative, continue according to the periodicity schedule; if positive, refer to an orthopaedist or for ultrasonography at 3 weeks of age. In girls, the absolute risk of 44/1000 may exceed the pediatrician's threshold to act, and imaging with an ultrasonographic examination at 6 weeks of age or a radiograph of the pelvis at 4 months of age is recommended.

   • **Breech presentation** (newborn risk for boys of 26/1000 and for girls, 120/1000). **For negative or equivocally positive newborn examinations, the infant should be reevaluated at regular intervals (according to the periodicity schedule) if the examination results remain negative.** Because an absolute risk of 120/1000 (12%) probably exceeds most pediatricians' threshold to act, imaging with an ultrasonographic examination at 6 weeks of age or with a radiograph of the pelvis and hips at 4 months of age is recommended. In addition, because some reports show a high incidence of hip abnormalities detected at an older age in children born breech, this imaging strategy remains an option for all children born breech, not just girls. These hip abnormalities are, for the most part, inadequate development of the acetabulum. Acetabular dysplasia is best found by a radiographic examination at 6 months of age or older. A suggestion of poorly formed acetabula may be observed at 6 weeks of age by ultrasonography, but the best study remains a radiograph performed closer to 6 months of age. Ultrasonographic newborn screening of all breech infants will not eliminate the possibility of later acetabular dysplasia.

8. **Periodicity. The hips must be examined at every well-baby visit according to the recommended periodicity schedule for well-baby examinations (2–4 days for newborns discharged in less than 48 hours after delivery, by 1 month, 2 months, 4 months, 6 months, 9 months, and 12 months of age).** If at any time during the follow-up period DDH is suspected because of an abnormal physical examination or by a parental complaint of difficulty diapering or abnormal appearing legs, the pediatrician must confirm that the hips are stable, in the sockets, and developing normally. Confirmation can be made by a focused physical examination when the infant is calm and relaxed, by consultation with another primary care pediatrician, by consultation with an orthopaedist, by ultrasonography if the infant is younger than 5 months of age, or by radiography if the infant is older than 4 months of age. (Between 4 and 6 months of age, ultrasonography and radiography seem to be equally effective diagnostic imaging studies.)

DISCUSSION

DDH is an important term because it accurately reflects the biologic features of the disorder and the susceptibility of the hip to become dislocated at various times. Dislocated hips always will be diagnosed later in infancy and childhood because not every dislocated hip is detectable at birth, and hips continue to dislocate throughout the first year of life. Thus, this guideline requires that the pediatrician follow *a process of care for the detection of DDH*. The process recommended for early detection of DDH includes the following:

- Screen all newborns' hips by physical examination.
- Examine all infants' hips according to a periodicity schedule and follow-up until the child is an established walker.
- Record and document physical findings.
- Be aware of the changing physical examination for DDH.
- If physical findings raise suspicion of DDH, or if parental concerns suggest hip disease, confirmation is required by expert physical examination, referral to an orthopaedist, or by an age-appropriate imaging study.

When this process of care is followed, the number of dislocated hips diagnosed at 1 year of age should be minimized. However, the problem of late detection of dislocated hips will not be eliminated. The results of screening programs have indicated that 1 in 5000 children have a dislocated hip detected at 18 months of age or older.[3]

TECHNICAL REPORT

The Technical Report is available from the American Academy of Pediatrics from several sources. The Technical Report is published in full-text on *Pediatrics electronic pages.* It is also available in a compendium of practice guidelines that contains guidelines and evidence reports together. The objective was to create a recommendation to pediatricians and other primary care providers about their role as screeners for detecting DDH. The patients are a theoretical cohort of newborns. A model-based method using decision analysis was the foundation. Components of the approach include:

- Perspective: primary care provider
- Outcomes: DDH and AVN
- Preferences: expected rates of outcomes
- Model: influence diagram assessed from the subcommittee and from the methodology team with critical feedback from the subcommittee
- Evidence sources: Medline and EMBase (detailed in "Methods" section)
- Evidence quality: assessed on a custom, subjective scale, based primarily on the fit of the evidence in the decision model

The results are detailed in the "Methods" section. Based on the raw evidence and Bayesian hierarchical meta-analysis,[34,35] estimates for the incidence of DDH based on the type of screener (orthopaedist vs pediatrician); the odds ratio for DDH given risk factors of sex, family history, and breech presentation; and estimates for late detection and AVN were determined and are detailed in the "Methods" section and in Tables 1 and 2.

The decision model (reduced based on available evidence) suggests that orthopaedic screening is optimal, but because orthopaedists in the published studies and in practice would differ in pediatric expertise, the supply of pediatric orthopaedists is relatively limited, and the difference between orthopaedists and pediatricians is statistically insignificant, we conclude that pediatric screening is to be recommended. The place for ultrasonography in the screening process remains to be defined because of the limited data available regarding late diagnosis in ultrasonography screening to permit definitive recommendations.

These data could be used by others to refine the conclusion based on costs, parental preferences, or physician style. Areas for research are well defined by our model-based method. All references are in the Technical Report.

RESEARCH QUESTIONS

The quality of the literature suggests many areas for research, because there is a paucity of randomized clinical trials and case-controlled studies. The following is a list of possibilities:

1. Minimum diagnostic abilities of a screener. Although there are data for pediatricians in general, few, if any, studies evaluated the abilities of an individual examiner. What should the minimum

sensitivity and specificity be, and how should they be assessed?

2. Intercurrent screening. There were few studies on systemic processes for screening after the newborn period.[2,43,44] Although several studies assessed postneonatal DDH, the data did not specify how many examinations were performed on each child before the abnormal result was found.

3. Trade-offs. Screening always results in false-positive results, and these patients suffer the adverse effects of therapy. How many unnecessary AVNs are we—families, physicians, and society—willing to tolerate from a screening program for every appropriately treated infant in whom late DDH was averted? This assessment depends on people's values and preferences and is not strictly an epidemiologic issue.

4. Postneonatal DDH after ultrasonographic screening. Although we concluded that ultrasonographic screening did not result in fewer diagnoses of postneonatal DDH, that conclusion was based on only 1 study.[36] Further study is needed.

5. Cost-effectiveness. If ultrasonographic screening reduces the number of postneonatal DDH diagnoses, then there will be a cost trade-off between the resources spent up front to screen everyone with an expensive technology, as in the case of ultrasonography, and the resources spent later to treat an expensive adverse event, as in the case of physical examination-based screening. The level at which the cost per case of postneonatal DDH averted is no longer acceptable is a matter of social preference, not of epidemiology.

ACKNOWLEDGMENTS

We acknowledge and appreciate the help of our methodology team, Richard Hinton, MD, Paola Morello, MD, and Jeanne Santoli, MD, who diligently participated in the literature review and abstracting the articles into evidence tables, and the subcommittee on evidence analysis.

We would also like to thank Robert Sebring, PhD, for assisting in the management of this process; Bonnie Cosner for managing the workflow; and Chris Kwiat, MLS, from the American Academy of Pediatrics Bakwin Library, who performed the literature searches.

REFERENCES

1. Bjerkreim I, Hagen O, Ikonomou N, Kase T, Kristiansen T, Arseth P. Late diagnosis of developmental dislocation of the hip in Norway during the years 1980–1989. *J Pediatr Orthop B*. 1993;2:112–114
2. Clarke N, Clegg J, Al-Chalabi A. Ultrasound screening of hips at risk for CDH: failure to reduce the incidence of late cases. *J Bone Joint Surg Br*. 1989;71:9–12
3. Dezateux C, Godward C. Evaluating the national screening programme for congenital dislocation of the hip. *J Med Screen*. 1995;2:200–206
4. Hadlow V. Neonatal screening for congenital dislocation of the hip: a prospective 21-year survey. *J Bone Joint Surg Br*. 1988;70:740–743
5. Krikler S, Dwyer N. Comparison of results of two approaches to hip screening in infants. *J Bone Joint Surg Br*. 1992;74:701–703
6. Macnicol M. Results of a 25-year screening programme for neonatal hip instability. *J Bone Joint Surg Br*. 1990;72:1057–1060
7. Marks DS, Clegg J, Al-Chalabi AN. Routine ultrasound screening for neonatal hip instability: can it abolish late-presenting congenital dislocation of the hip? *J Bone Joint Surg Br*. 1994;76:534–538
8. Rosendahl K, Markestad T, Lie R. Congenital dislocation of the hip: a prospective study comparing ultrasound and clinical examination. *Acta Paediatr*. 1992;81:177–181
9. Sanfridson J, Redlund-Johnell I, Uden A. Why is congenital dislocation of the hip still missed? Analysis of 96,891 infants screened in Malmo 1956–1987. *Acta Orthop Scand*. 1991;62:87–91
10. Tredwell S, Bell H. Efficacy of neonatal hip examination. *J Pediatr Orthop*. 1981;1:61–65
11. Yngve D, Gross R. Late diagnosis of hip dislocation in infants. *J Pediatr Orthop*. 1990;10:777–779
12. Aronsson DD, Goldberg MJ, Kling TF, Roy DR. Developmental dysplasia of the hip. *Pediatrics*. 1994;94:201–212
13. Hinderaker T, Daltveit AK, Irgens LM, Uden A, Reikeras O. The impact of intra-uterine factors on neonatal hip instability: an analysis of 1,059,479 children in Norway. *Acta Orthop Scand*. 1994;65:239–242
14. Wynne-Davies R. Acetabular dysplasia and familial joint laxity: two etiological factors in congenital dislocation of the hip: a review of 589 patients and their families. *J Bone Joint Surg Br*. 1970;52:704–716
15. De Pellegrin M. Ultrasound screening for congenital dislocation of the hip: results and correlations between clinical and ultrasound findings. *Ital J Orthop Traumatol*. 1991;17:547–553
16. Stoffelen D, Urlus M, Molenaers G, Fabry G. Ultrasound, radiographs, and clinical symptoms in developmental dislocation of the hip: a study of 170 patients. *J Pediatr Orthop B*. 1995;4:194–199
17. Bond CD, Hennrikus WL, Della Maggiore E. Prospective evaluation of newborn soft tissue hip clicks with ultrasound. *J Pediatr Orthop*. 1997;17:199–201
18. Bialik V, Wiener F, Benderly A. Ultrasonography and screening in developmental displacement of the hip. *J Pediatr Orthop B*. 1992;1:51–54
19. Castelein R, Sauter A. Ultrasound screening for congenital dysplasia of the hip in newborns: its value. *J Pediatr Orthop*. 1988;8:666–670
20. Clarke NMP, Harcke HT, McHugh P, Lee MS, Borns PF, MacEwen GP. Real-time ultrasound in the diagnosis of congenital dislocation and dysplasia of the hip. *J Bone Joint Surg Br*. 1985;67:406–412
21. Garvey M, Donoghue V, Gorman W, O'Brien N, Murphy J. Radiographic screening at four months of infants at risk for congenital hip dislocation. *J Bone Joint Surg Br*. 1992;74:704–707
22. Langer R. Ultrasonic investigation of the hip in newborns in the diagnosis of congenital hip dislocation: classification and results of a screening program. *Skeletal Radiol*. 1987;16:275–279

23. Rosendahl K, Markestad T, Lie RT. Ultrasound screening for developmental dysplasia of the hip in the neonate: the effect on treatment rate and prevalence of late cases. *Pediatrics*. 1994;94:47–52

24. Terjesen T. Ultrasound as the primary imaging method in the diagnosis of hip dysplasia in children aged <2 years. *J Pediatr Orthop B*. 1996;5: 123–128

25. Vedantam R, Bell M. Dynamic ultrasound assessment for monitoring of treatment of congenital dislocation of the hip. *J Pediatr Orthop*. 1995;15: 725–728

26. Graf R. Classification of hip joint dysplasia by means of sonography. *Arch Orthop Trauma Surg*. 1984;102:248–255

27. Berman L, Klenerman L. Ultrasound screening for hip abnormalities: preliminary findings in 1001 neonates. *Br Med J (Clin Res Ed)*. 1986;293: 719–722

28. Castelein R, Sauter A, de Vlieger M, van Linge B. Natural history of ultrasound hip abnormalities in clinically normal newborns. *J Pediatr Orthop*. 1992;12:423–427

29. Clarke N. Sonographic clarification of the problems of neonatal hip stability. *J Pediatr Orthop*. 1986;6:527–532

30. Eddy DM. The confidence profile method: a Bayesian method for assessing health technologies. *Operations Res*. 1989;37:210–228

31. Howard RA, Matheson JE. Influence diagrams. In: Matheson JE, ed. *Readings on the Principles and Applications of Decision Analysis*. Menlo Park, CA: Strategic Decisions Group; 1981:720–762

32. Nease RF, Owen DK. Use of influence diagrams to structure medical decisions. *Med Decis Making*. 1997;17:265–275

33. Guyatt GH, Sackett DL, Sinclair JC, Hayward R, Cook DJ, Cook RJ. Users' guide to the medical literature, IX: a method for grading health care recommendations. *JAMA*. 1995;274:1800–1804

34. Gelman A, Carlin JB, Stern HS, Rubin DB. *Bayesian Data Analysis*. London, UK: Chapman and Hall; 1997

35. Spiegelhalter D, Thomas A, Best N, Gilks W. *BUGS 0.5: Bayesian Inference Using Gibbs Sampling Manual, II*. Cambridge, MA: MRC Biostatistics Unit, Institute of Public Health; 1996. Available at: http://www.mrc-bsu.cam.ac.uk/bugs/software/software.html

36. Fiddian NJ, Gardiner JC. Screening for congenital dislocation of the hip by physiotherapists: results of a ten-year study. *J Bone Joint Surg Br*. 1994;76:458–459

37. Dunn P, Evans R, Thearle M, Griffiths H, Witherow P. Congenital dislocation of the hip: early and late diagnosis and management compared. *Arch Dis Child*. 1992;60:407–414

38. Holen KJ, Tegnander A, Terjesen T, Johansen OJ, Eik-Nes SH. Ultrasonographic evaluation of breech presentation as a risk factor for hip dysplasia. *Acta Paediatr*. 1996;85:225–229

39. Jones D, Powell N. Ultrasound and neonatal hip screening: a prospective study of "high risk" babies. *J Bone Joint Surg Br*. 1990;72:457–459

40. Teanby DN, Paton RW. Ultrasound screening for congenital dislocation of the hip: a limited targeted programme. *J Pediatr Orthop*. 1997;17: 202–204

41. Tonnis D, Storch K, Ulbrich H. Results of newborn screening for CDH with and without sonography and correlation of risk factors. *J Pediatr Orthop*. 1990;10:145–152

42. Pauker SG, Kassirer JP. The threshold approach to clinical decision making. *N Engl J Med*. 1980;302:1109–1117

43. Bower C, Stanley F, Morgan B, Slattery H, Stanton C. Screening for congenital dislocation of the hip by child-health nurses in western Australia. *Med J Aust*. 1989;150:61–65

44. Franchin F, Lacalendola G, Molfetta L, Mascolo V, Quagliarella L. Ultrasound for early diagnosis of hip dysplasia. *Ital J Orthop Traumatol*. 1992;18:261–269

ADDENDUM TO REFERENCES FOR THE DDH GUIDELINE

New information is generated constantly. Specific details of this report must be changed over time.

New articles (additional articles 1–7) have been published since the completion of our literature search and construction of this Guideline. These articles taken alone might seem to contradict some of the Guideline's estimates as detailed in the article and in the Technical Report. However, taken in context with the literature synthesis carried out for the construction of this Guideline, our estimates remain intact and no conclusions are obviated.

ADDITIONAL ARTICLES

1. Bialik V, Bialik GM, Blazer S, Sujov P, Wiener F, Berant M. Developmental dysplasia of the hip: a new approach to incidence. *Pediatrics*. 1999;103:93–99

2. Clegg J, Bache CE, Raut VV. Financial justification for routine ultrasound screening of the neonatal hip. *J Bone Joint Surg*. 1999;81-B:852–857

3. Holen KJ, Tegnander A, Eik-Nes SH, Terjesen T. The use of ultrasound in determining the initiation in treatment in instability of the hips in neonates. *J Bone Joint Surg*. 1999;81-B:846–851

4. Lewis K, Jones DA, Powell N. Ultrasound and neonatal hip screening: the five-year results of a prospective study in high risk babies. *J Pediatr Orthop*. 1999;19:760–762

5. Paton RW, Srinivasan MS, Shah B, Hollis S. Ultrasound screening for hips at risk in developmental dysplasia: is it worth it? *J Bone Joint Surg*. 1999;81-B:255–258

6. Sucato DJ, Johnston CE, Birch JG, Herring JA, Mack P. Outcomes of ultrasonographic hip abnormalities in clinically stable hips. *J Pediatr Orthop*. 1999;19:754–759

7. Williams PR, Jones DA, Bishay M. Avascular necrosis and the aberdeen splint in developmental dysplasia of the hip. *J Bone Joint Surg*. 1999;81-B:1023–1028

Technical Report Summary:
Developmental Dysplasia of the Hip Practice Guideline

Authors:

Harold P. Lehmann, MD, PhD; Richard Hinton, MD, MPH;
Paola Morello, MD; and Jeanne Santoli, MD
in conjunction with the
American Academy of Pediatrics
Subcommittee on Developmental
Dysplasia of the Hip

American Academy of Pediatrics
PO Box 927, 141 Northwest Point Blvd
Elk Grove Village, IL 60009-0927

For the complete technical report, including tables, figures, and references, please see the companion CD-ROM.

ABSTRACT

Objective. To create a recommendation for pediatricians and other primary care providers about their role as screeners for detecting developmental dysplasia of the hip (DDH) in children.

Patients. Theoretical cohorts of newborns.

Method. Model-based approach using decision analysis as the foundation. Components of the approach include the following:

Perspective: Primary care provider.

Outcomes: DDH, avascular necrosis of the hip (AVN).

Options: Newborn screening by pediatric examination; orthopaedic examination; ultrasonographic examination; orthopaedic or ultrasonographic examination by risk factors. Intercurrent health supervision-based screening.

Preferences: 0 for bad outcomes, 1 for best outcomes.

Model: Influence diagram assessed by the Subcommittee and by the methodology team, with critical feedback from the Subcommittee.

Evidence Sources: Medline and EMBASE search of the research literature through June 1996. Hand search of sentinel journals from June 1996 through March 1997. Ancestor search of accepted articles.

Evidence Quality: Assessed on a custom subjective scale, based primarily on the fit of the evidence to the decision model.

Results. After discussion, explicit modeling, and critique, an influence diagram of 31 nodes was created. The computer-based and the hand literature searches found 534 articles, 101 of which were reviewed by 2 or more readers. Ancestor searches of these yielded a further 17 articles for evidence abstraction. Articles came from around the globe, although primarily Europe, British Isles, Scandinavia, and their descendants. There were 5 controlled trials, each with a sample size less than 40. The remainder were case series. Evidence was available for 17 of the desired 30 probabilities. Evidence quality ranged primarily between one third and two thirds of the maximum attainable score (median: 10–21; interquartile range: 8–14).

Based on the raw evidence and Bayesian hierarchical meta-analyses, our estimate for the incidence of DDH revealed by physical examination performed by pediatricians is 8.6 per 1000; for orthopaedic screening, 11.5; for ultrasonography, 25. The odds ratio for DDH, given breech delivery, is 5.5; for female sex, 4.1; for positive family history, 1.7, although this last factor is not statistically significant. Postneonatal cases of DDH were divided into mid-term (younger than 6 months of age) and late-term (older than 6 months of age). Our estimates for the mid-term rate for screening by pediatricians is 0.34/1000 children screened; for orthopaedists, 0.1; and for ultrasonography, 0.28. Our estimates for late-term DDH rates are 0.21/1000 newborns screened by pediatricians; 0.08, by orthopaedists; and 0.2 for ultrasonography. The rates of AVN for children referred before 6 months of age is estimated at 2.5/1000 infants referred. For those referred after 6 months of age, our estimate is 109/1000 referred infants.

The decision model (reduced, based on available evidence) suggests that orthopaedic screening is optimal, but because orthopaedists in the published studies and in practice would differ, the supply of orthopaedists is relatively limited, and the difference between orthopaedists and pediatricians is statistically insignificant, we conclude that pediatric screening is to be recommended. The place of ultrasonography in the screening process remains to be defined because there are too few data about postneonatal diagnosis by ultrasonographic screening to permit definitive recommendations. These data could be used by others to refine the conclusions based on costs, parental preferences, or physician style. Areas for research are well defined by our model-based approach. *Pediatrics* 2000;105(4). URL: http://www.pediatrics.org/cgi/content/full/105/4/e57; keywords: *developmental dysplasia of the hip, avascular necrosis of the hip, newborn.*

I. GUIDELINE METHODS

A. Decision Model

The steps required to build the model were taken with the Subcommittee as a whole, with individuals in the group, and with members of the methodology team. Agreement on the model was sought from the Subcommittee as a whole during face-to-face meetings.

1. Perspective

Although there are a number of perspectives to take in this problem (parental, child's, societal, and payer's), we opted for the view of the practicing clinician: What are the clinician's obligations, and what is the best strategy for the clinician? This choice of perspective meant that the focus would be on screening for developmental dysplasia of the hip (DDH) and obviated the need to review the evidence for efficacy or effectiveness of specific strategies.

2. Context

The target child is a full-term newborn with no obvious orthopaedic abnormalities. Children with such findings would be referred to an orthopaedist, obviating the need for a practice parameter.

3. Options

We focused on the following options: screening by physical examination (PE) at birth by a pediatrician, orthopaedist, or other care provider; ultrasonographic screening at birth; and episodic screening during health supervision. Treatment options are not included.

We also included in our model a wide range of options for managing the screening process during the first year of life when the newborn screening was negative.

4. Outcomes

Our focus is on dislocated hips at 1 year of age as the major morbidity of the disease and on avascular necrosis of the hip (AVN), as the primary sentinel complication of DDH therapy.

Ideally, we would have a "gold standard" that would define DDH at any point in time, much as cardiac output can be obtained from a pulmonary-artery catheter. However, no gold standard exists. Therefore, we defined our outcomes in terms of the process of care: a pediatrician and an ultrasonographer perform initial or confirmatory examinations and refer the patient, whereas the orthopaedist treats the patient. It is the treatment that has the greatest effect on postneonatal DDH or on complications, so we focus on that intermediate outcome, rather than the orthopaedist's stated diagnosis. We operationalized the definitions of these outcomes for use in abstracting the data from articles. A statement that a "click" was found on PE was considered to refer to an intermediate result, unless the authors defined their "click" in terms of our definition of a positive examination. Dynamic ultrasonographic examinations include those of Harcke et al, and static refers primarily to that of Graf. The radiologic focus switches from ultrasonography to plain radiographs after 4 months of age, in keeping with the development of the femoral head.

5. Decision Structure

We used an influence diagram to represent the decision model. In this representation, nodes refer to actions to be taken or to states of the world (the patient) about which we are uncertain. We devoted substantial effort to the construction of a model that balanced the need to represent the rich array of possible screening pathways with the need to be parsimonious. We constructed the master influence diagram and determined its construct validity through consensus by the Subcommittee before data abstraction. However, the available evidence could specify only a portion of the diagram. The missing components suggest research questions that need to be posed.

6. Probabilities

The purpose of the literature review was to provide the probabilities required by the decision model. The initial number of individual probabilities was 55. (Sensitivity and specificity for a single truth-indicator pair are counted as a single probability because they are garnered from the same table.) Although this is a large number of parameters, the structure of the model helped the team of readers. As 1 reader said, referring to the influence diagram, "Because we did the picture together, it was easy to find the parameters." What follows are some operational rules for matching the data to our parameters. The list is not complete. If an orthopaedic clinic worked at case finding, we used our judgment to determine whether to accept such reports as representing a population incidence.

Risk factors were included generally only if a true control group was used for comparison. For postneonatal diagnoses, no study we reviewed included the examination of all children without DDH, say, 1 year of age, so there is always the possibility of missed cases (false-negative diagnoses) in the screen,

which leads to a falsely elevated estimate of the denominator. For studies originating in referral clinics, the data on the reasons for referrals were not usable for our purposes.

7. Preferences

Ideally, we would have cost data for the options, as well as patient data on the human burden of therapy and of DDH itself. We have deferred these assessments to later research. Therefore, we assigned a preference score of 0 to DDH at 1 year of age and 1 to its absence; for AVN, we assigned 0 for presence at 1 year of age and 1 for absence at 1 year of age.

B. Literature Review

For the literature through May 1995, the following sources were searched: Books in Print, CAT-LINE, Current Contents, EMBASE, Federal Research in Progress, Health Care Standards, Health Devices Alerts, Health Planning and Administration, Health Services/Technology Assessment, International Health Technology Assessment, and Medline. Medline and EMBASE were searched through June 1996. The search terms used in all databases included the following: hip dislocation, congenital; hip dysplasia; congenital hip dislocation; developmental dysplasia; ultrasonography/adverse effects; and osteonecrosis. Hand searches of leading orthopaedic journals were performed for the issues from June 1996 to March 1997. The bibliographies of journals accepted for use in formulating the practice parameter also were perused.

The titles and the abstracts were then reviewed by 2 members of the methodology team to determine whether to accept or reject the articles for use. Decisions were reviewed by the Subcommittee, and conflicts were adjudicated. Similarly, articles were read by pairs of reviewers; conflicts were resolved in discussion.

The focus of the data abstraction process was on data that would provide evidence for the probabilities required by the decision model.

As part of the literature abstraction process, the evidence quality in each article was assessed. The scoring process was based on our decision model and involved traditional epidemiologic concerns, like outcome definition and bias of ascertainment, as well as influence–diagram-based concerns, such as how well the data fit into the model.

Cohort definition: Does the cohort represented by the denominator in the study match a node in our influence diagram? Does the cohort represented by the numerator match a node in our influence diagram? The closer the match, the more confident we are that the reported data provide good evidence of the conditional probability implied by the arrow between the corresponding nodes in the influence diagram.

Path: Does the implied path from denominator to numerator lead through 1 or more nodes of the influence diagram? The longer the path, the more likely that uncontrolled biases entered into the study, making us less confident about accepting the raw data as a conditional probability in our model. Assignment and comparison: Was there a control group? How was assignment made to experimental or control arms? A randomized, controlled study provides the best quality evidence.

Follow-up: Were patients with positive and negative initial findings followed up? The best studies should have data on both.

Outcome definition: Did the language of the outcome definitions (PE, orthopaedic examination, ultrasonography, and radiography) match ours, and, in particular, were PE findings divided into 3 categories or 2? The closer the definition to ours, the more we could pool the data. Studies with only 2 categories do not help to distinguish clicks from "clunks."

Ascertainment: When the denominator represented more than 1 node, to what degree was the denominator a mix of nodes? The smaller the contamination, the more confident we were that the raw data represented a desired conditional probability.

Results: Did the results fill an entire table or were data missing? This is related to the follow-up category but is more general.

C. Synthesis of Evidence

There are 3 levels of evidence synthesis.

1. Listing evidence for individual probabilities
2. Summarizing evidence across probabilities
3. Integrating the pooled evidence for individual probabilities into the decision model

A list of evidence for an individual probability (or arc) is called an *evidence table* and provides the reader a look at the individual pieces of data. The probabilities are summarized in 3 ways: by averaging, by averaging weighted by sample size (pooled), and by meta-analysis. We chose Bayesian meta-analytic techniques, which allow the representation of *prior belief* in the evidence and provide an explicit portrayal of the uncertainty of our conclusions. The framework we used was that of a hierarchical Bayesian model, similar to the random effects model in traditional meta-analysis. In this hierarchical model, each study has its own parameter, which, in turn, is sampled from a wider population parameter. Because there are 2 stages (ie, population to sample and sample to observation), and, therefore, the population parameter of interest is more distant from the data, the computed estimates in the population parameters are, in general, less certain (wider confidence interval) than simply pooling the data across studies. This lower certainty is appropriate in the DDH content area because the studies vary so widely in their raw estimates because of the range in time and geography over which they were performed. In the Bayesian model, the observations were assumed to be Poisson distributed, given the study DDH rates. Those rates, in turn, were assumed to be Gamma distributed, given the population rate. The prior belief on that rate was set as Gamma (α, β), with mean α/β, and variance α/β^2 (as defined in the BUGS software). In this parameterization, α has the semantics closest to that of location, and β has the semantics of certainty: the higher its value, the narrower the distribution and the more certain we are of the estimate. The parameter, α, was modeled as Exponential (1), and β, as Gamma (0.01, 1), with a mean of 0.01. Together, these correspond to a prior belief in the rate of a mean of 100 per

1000, and a standard deviation (SD) of 100, representing ignorance of the true rate.

As an example of interpretation, for pediatric newborn screening, the posterior α was 1.46, and the posterior β was 0.17, to give a posterior rate of 8.6/1000, with a variance of 50, or an SD of 7.1. The value of β rose from 0.01 to 0.17, indicating a higher level of certainty.

The Bayesian confidence interval is the narrowest interval that contains 95% of the area under the posterior-belief curve. The confidence interval for the prior curve is 2.53 to 370. The confidence interval for the posterior curve is 0.25 to 27.5, a significant shrinking and increase in certainty but still broad.

The model for the odds ratios is more complicated and is based on the Oxford data set and analysis in the BUGS manual.

D. Thresholds

In the course of discussions about results, the Subcommittee was surveyed about the acceptable risks of DDH for different levels of interventions.

E. Recommendations

Once the evidence and thresholds were obtained, a decision tree was created from the evidence available and was reviewed by the Subcommittee. In parallel, a consensus guideline (flowchart) was created. The Subcommittee evaluated whether evidence was available for links within the guidelines, as well as their strength of consensus. The decision tree was evaluated to check consistency of the evidence with the conclusions.

F. "Cost"-Effectiveness Ratios

To integrate the results, we defined cost-effectiveness ratios, in which cost was excess neonatal referrals or excess cases of AVNs, and *effectiveness* was a decrease in the number of later cases. The decision tree from section E ("Recommendations") was used to calculate the expected outcomes for each of pediatric, orthopaedic, and ultrasonographic strategies. Pediatric strategy was used as the baseline, because its neonatal screening rate was the lowest. The cost-effectiveness ratios then were calculated as the quotient of the difference in cost and the difference in effect.

RESULTS

A. Articles

The peak number of articles is for 1992, with 10 articles. The articles are from sites all over the world, although the Nordic, Anglo-Saxon, and European communities and their descendants are the most represented.

B. Evidence

By traditional epidemiologic standards, the quality of evidence in this set of articles is uniformly low. There are few controlled trials and few studies in which infants with negative results on their newborn examinations are followed up. (A number of studies attempted to cover all possible places where an affected child might have been ascertained.)

We found data on all chance nodes, for a total of 298 distinct tables. *Decision* nodes were poorly represented: beyond the neonatal strategy, there were almost no data clarifying the paths for the diagnosis children after the newborn period. Thus, although communities like those in southeast Norway have a postnewborn screening program, it is unclear what the program was, and it was unclear how many examination results were normal before a child was referred to an orthopaedist.

The mode is a score of 10, achieved in 16 articles. The median is 9.9, with an interquartile range of 8 to 14, suggesting that articles with scores below 8 are poor sources of evidence. Note that the maximum achievable quality score is 21, so half the articles do not achieve half the maximum quality score.

Graphing evidence quality against publication year suggests an improvement in quality over time, as shown in Fig 9, but the linear fit through the data is statistically indistinguishable from a flat line. (A nonparametric procedure yields the same conclusion).

The studies include 5 in which a comparative arm was designed into the study. The remainder are divided between prospective and retrospective studies. Surprisingly, the evidence quality is not higher in the former than in the latter (data not shown).

Of the 298 data tables, half the data tables relate to the following:
- probabilities of DDH in different screening strategies
- relative risk of DDH, given risk factors
- the incidence of postneonatal DDH, and
- the incidence of AVN.

The remainder of our discussion will focus on these probabilities.

C. Evidence Tables

The evidence table details are found in the appendix of the full technical report.

1. Newborn Screening

a. Pediatric Screening

There were 51 studies, providing 57 arms, for pediatric screening. However, of these, 17 were unclear on how the intermediate examinations were handled, and, unsurprisingly, their observed rates of positivity (clicks) were much higher than the studies that distinguished 3 categories, as we had specified. Therefore, we included only the 34 studies that used 3 categories.

For pediatric screening, the rate is about 8 positive cases per 1000 examinations. The rates are distributed almost uniformly between 0 and 20 per 1000. All studies represent a large experience: a total of 2 149 972 subjects. Although their methods may not have been the best, the studies demand attention simply because of their size.

In looking for covariates or confounding variables, we studied the relationship between positivity rate and the independent variables, year of publication, evidence quality, and sample size. Year and evidence quality show a positive effect: the higher the year (slope: 0.2; P 5 .018) or evidence quality (slope: 0.6; P 5 .046), the higher the observed rate. A model with both factors has evidence that suggests that most of the effect is in the factor, year

(slope for year: 0.08; P 5 .038; slope for quality of evidence: 0.49; P 5 .09). Note that a regression using evidence quality is improper, because our evidence scale is not properly ratio (eg, the distance between 6 and 7 is not necessarily equivalent to the distance between 14 and 15), but the regression is a useful exploratory device.

b. Orthopaedic Screening

Evidence was found in 25 studies. Three studies provided 2 arms each.

The positivity rate for orthopaedic screening is between 7 and 11/1000. One outlier study, with an observed rate of more than 300/1000, skews the unweighted and meta-analytic averages. The estimate (between 7.1 and 11) is just below that of pediatric screening and is statistically indistinguishable. Note, however, that a fair number of studies have rates near 22/1000 or higher.

Unlike with pediatric screening, there are no correlations with other factors.

c. Ultrasonographic Screening

Evidence was found in 17 studies, each providing a single arm.

The rate for ultrasonographic screening is 20/1000 or more. Although the estimates are sensitive to pooling and to the outlier, the positivity rate is clearly higher than in either PE strategy. There are no correlating factors. In particular, studies that use the Graf method 2 or those that use the method of Harcke et al show comparable rates.

2. Postneonatal Cases

We initially were interested in all postneonatal diagnoses of DDH. However, the literature did not provide data within the narrow time frames initially specified for our model. Based on the data that were available, we considered 3 classes of postneonatal DDH: DDH diagnosed after 12 months of age ("late-term"), DDH diagnosed between 6 and 12 months of age ("mid-term"), and DDH diagnosed before 6 months of age. There were few data for the latter group, which often was combined with the newborn screening programs. Therefore, we collected data on only the first 2 groups.

a. After Pediatric Screening

Evidence was found in 24 studies. The study by Dunn and O'Riordan provided 2 arms. It is difficult to discern an estimate rate for mid-term DDH, because the study by Czeizel et al is such an outlier, with a rate of 3.73/1000, and because the weighted and unweighted averages also differ greatly. The meta-analytic estimate of 0.55/1000 seems to be an upper limit.

The late-term rate is easier to estimate at ~0.3/1000. Although it is intuitive that the late-term rate should be lower than the mid-term rate, our data do not allow us to draw that conclusion.

b. After Orthopaedic Screening

There were only 4 studies. The rates were comparable for mid- and late-term: 0.1/1000 newborns. A meta-analytic estimate was not calculated.

c. After Ultrasonographic Screening

Only 1 study, by Rosendahl et al is available; it reported rates for infants with and without initial risk factors (eg, family history and breech presentation). The mid-term rate was 0.28/1000 newborns in the non-risk group, and the late-term rate was 0/1000 in the same group.

3. AVN After Treatment

For these estimates, we grouped together all treatments, because from the viewpoint of the referring primary care provider, orthopaedic treatment is a "black box:" A literature synthesis that teased apart the success and complications of particular *therapeutic* strategies is beyond the scope of the present study.

The complication rate should depend only on the age of the patient at time of orthopaedic referral and on the type of treatment received. We report on the complication rates for children treated before and after 12 months of age.

a. After Early Referral

There were 17 studies providing evidence. Infants were referred to orthopaedists during the newborn period in each study except 2. In the study by Pool et al, infants were referred during the newborn period and before 2 months of age; in the study by Sochart and Paton, infants were referred between 2 weeks and 2 months of age.

The range of AVN rates per 1000 infants referred was huge, from 0 to 123. The largest rate occurred in the study by Pool et al, a sample-based study that included later referrals. Its evidence quality was 8, within the 7 to 13 interquartile range of the other studies in this group. As in earlier tables, the meta-analytic estimate lies between the average and weighted (pooled) average of the studies.

b. After Later Referral

Evidence was obtained from 6 studies. Some of the studies included children referred during the newborn period or during the 2-week to 2-month period, but even in these, the majority of infants were referred later during the first year of life.

There were no outlier rates, although the highest rate (216/1000 referred children) occurred in the study with the oldest referred children in the sample with children referred who were older than 12 months of age. One study contributed 5700 patients to the analysis, more than half of the 9270 total, so its AVN rate of 27/1000 brought the unweighted rate of 116/1000 to 54. A meta-analytic estimate was not computed.

4. Risk Factors

A number of factors are known to predispose infants to DDH. We sought evidence for 3 of these: sex, obstetrical position at birth, and family history. Studies were included in these analyses only if a control group could be ascertained from the available study data.

The key measure is the odds ratio, an estimate of the relative risk. The meaning of the odds ratio is that if the DDH rate for the control group is known, then the DDH rate for the at-risk group is the product of the control-group DDH rate and the odds ratio for the risk factor. An odds ratio statistically significantly greater than 1 indicates that the factor is a risk factor. The Bayesian meta-analysis produces estimates between the average of the odds ratios and the pooled odds ratio and is, therefore, the estimate we used in our later analyses.

a. Female

The studies were uniform in discerning a risk to girls ~4 times that of boys for being diagnosed with DDH. This risk was seen in all 3 screening environments.

b. Breech

The studies for breech also were confident in finding a risk for breech presentation, on the order of fivefold. One study found breech presentation to be protective, but the study was relatively small and used ultrasonography rather than PE as its outcome measure.

c. Family History

Although some studies found family history to be a risk factor, the range was wide. The confidence intervals for the pooled odds ratio and for the Bayesian analysis contained 1.0, suggesting that family history is *not* an independent risk factor for DDH. However, because of traditional concern with this risk factor, we kept it in our further considerations.

D. Evidence Summary and Risk Implications

To bring all evidence tables together, we constructed a summary table, which contains the estimates we chose for our recommendations. The intervals are asymmetric, in keeping with the intuition that rates near zero cannot be negative, but certainly can be very positive.

Risk factors are based on the pediatrician population rate of 8.6 labeled cases of DDH per 1000 infants screened. In the Subcommittee's discussion, 50/1000 was a cutoff for automatic referral during the newborn period. Hence, girls born in the breech position are classified in a separate category for newborn strategies than infants with other risk factors.

If we use the orthopaedists' rate as our baseline, numbers suggest that boys without risks or those with a family history have the lowest risk; girls without risks and boys born in the breech presentation have an intermediate risk; and girls with a positive family history, and especially girls born in the breech presentation, have the highest risks. Guidelines that consider risk factors should follow these risk profiles.

E. Decision Recommendations

With the evidence synthesized, we can estimate the expected results of the target newborn strategies for postneonatal DDH and AVN.

If a case of DDH is observed in an infant with an initially negative result of screening by an orthopaedist in a newborn screening program, that case is "counted" against the orthopaedist strategy.

The numbers are combined using a simple decision tree, which is not the final tree represented by our influence diagram but is a tree that is supported by our evidence. The results show that pediatricians diagnose fewer newborns with DDH and perhaps have a higher postneonatal DDH rate than orthopaedists but one that is comparable to ultrasonography (acknowledging that our knowledge of postneonatal DDH revealed by ultrasonographic screening is limited). The AVN rates are comparable with pediatrician and ultrasonographic screening and less than with orthopaedist screening.

F. Cost-Effectiveness Ratios

In terms of excess neonatal referrals, the ratios suggest that there is a trade-off: for every case that these strategies detect beyond the pediatric strategy, they require more than 7000 or 16 000 extra referrals, respectively.

DISCUSSION

A. Summary

We derived 298 evidence tables from 118 studies culled from a larger set of 624 articles. Our literature review captured most in our model-based approach, if not all, of the past literature on DDH that was usable. The decision model (reduced based on available evidence) suggests that orthopaedic screening is optimal, but because orthopaedists in the published studies and in practice would differ, the supply of orthopaedists is relatively limited, and the difference between orthopaedists and pediatricians is relatively small, we conclude that pediatric screening is to be recommended. The place of ultrasonography in the screening process remains to be defined because there are too few data about postneonatal diagnosis by ultrasonographic screening to permit definitive recommendations.

Our conclusions are tempered by the uncertainties resulting from the wide range of the evidence. The confidence intervals are wide for the primary parameters. The uncertainties mean that, even with all the evidence collected from the literature, we are left with large doubts about the values of the different parameters.

Our data do not bear directly on the issue about the earliest point that any patient destined to have DDH will show signs of the disease. Our use of the terms *mid-term* and *late-term* DDH addresses that ignorance.

Our conclusions about other areas of the full decision model are more tentative because of the paucity of data about the effectiveness of periodicity examinations. Even the studies that gave data on mid-term and late-term case findings by pediatricians were sparse in their details about how the screening was instituted, maintained, or followed up.

Our literature search was weakest in addressing the European literature, where results about ultrasonography are more prevalent. We found, however, that many of the seminal articles were republished in English or in a form that we could assess.

B. Specific Issues

1. Evidence Quality

Our measure of evidence quality is unique, although it is based on solid principles of study design and decision modeling. In particular, our measure was based on the notion that if the data conform poorly to how we need to use it, we downgrade its value.

However, throughout the analyses, there was never a correlation with the results of a study (in terms of the values of outcomes) and with evidence quality, so we never needed to use the measure for weighting the values of the outcome or for culling articles from our review. Had this been so, the measures would have needed further scrutiny and validation.

2. Outliers

Perhaps the true surrogates for study quality were the outlying values of outcomes. In general, however, there were few cases in which the outliers were clearly the result of poor-quality studies. One example is that of the outcomes of pediatric screening (1⊠3), in which the DDH rates in studies using only 2 categories were generally higher than those that explicitly specified 3 levels of outcomes.

Our general justification for using estimates that excluded outliers is that the outliers so much drove the results that they dominated the conclusion out of proportion to their sample sizes. As it is, our estimates have wide ranges.

3. Newborn Screening

The set of studies labeled "pediatrician screening" includes studies with a variety of examiners. We could not estimate the sensitivity and specificity of pediatricians' examinations versus those of other primary care providers versus orthopaedists. There are techniques for extracting these measures from agreement studies, but they are beyond the scope of the present study. It is intuitive that the more cases that one examines, the better an examiner one will be, regardless of professional title.

We were surprised that the results did not show a clear difference in results between the Graf and Harcke et al ultrasonographic examinations. Our data make no statement about the relative advantages of these methods for following up children or in addressing treatment.

4. Postneonatal Cases

As mentioned, our data cannot say when a postneonatal case is established or, therefore, the best time to screen children. We established our initial age categories for postneonatal cases based on biology, treatment changes, and optimal imaging and examination strategies. It is frustrating that the data in the literature are not organized to match this pathophysiological way of thinking about DDH. Similarly, as mentioned, the lack of details by authors on the methods of intercurrent screening means that we cannot recommend a preferred method for mid-term or late-term screening.

5. AVN

We used AVN as our primary marker for treatment morbidity. We acknowledge that the studies we grouped together may reflect different philosophies and results of orthopaedic practice. The hierarchical meta-analysis treats every study as an individual case, and the wide range in our confidence intervals reflects the uncertainty that results in grouping disparate studies together.

C. Comments on Methods

This study is unique in its strong use of decision modeling at each step in the process. In the end, our results are couched in traditional terms (estimated rates of disease or morbidity outcomes), although the context is relatively nontraditional: attaching the estimates to strategies rather than to treatments. In this, our study is typical of an *effectiveness* study, which studied results in the real world, rather than of an *efficacy* study, which examines the biological effects of a treatment.

We made strong and recurrent use of the Bayesian hierarchical meta-analysis. A review of the tables will confirm that the Bayesian results were in the same "ballpark" as the average and pooled average estimates and had a more solid grounding.

The usual criticism of using Bayesian methods is that they depend on prior belief. The usual response is to show that the final estimates are relatively insensitive to the prior belief. In fact, for the screening strategies, a wide range of prior beliefs had no effect on the estimate. However, the prior belief used for the screening strategies—with a mean of 100 cases/1000 with a variance of 100—was too broad for the postneonatal case and AVN analyses; when data were sparse, the prior belief overwhelmed the data. For instance, in late-term DDH revealed by orthopaedic screening (53 30), in an analysis not shown, the posterior estimate from the 4 studies was a rate of 0.345 cases per 1000, despite an average and a pooled average on the order of 0.08. Four studies were insufficient to overpower a prior belief of 100.

D. Research Issues

The place of ultrasonography in DDH screening needs more attention, as does the issue of intercurrent pediatrician screening. In the latter case, society and health care systems must assess the effectiveness of education and the "return on investment" for educational programs. The place of preferences—of the parents, of the clinician—must be established.

We hope that the framework we have delineated—of a decision model and of data—can be useful in these future research endeavors.

Dysplasia of the Hip Clinical Practice Guideline
Quick Reference Tools

- Recommendation Summary
  — Early Detection of Developmental Dysplasia of the Hip
- *ICD-9-CM/ICD-10-CM* Coding Quick Reference for Dysplasia of the Hip
- AAP Patient Education Handout
  — *Hip Dysplasia (Developmental Dysplasia of the Hip)*

Recommendation Summary
Early Detection of Developmental Dysplasia of the Hip

Recommendation 1

A. All newborns are to be screened by physical examination. (The evidence for this recommendation is good. The expert consensus is strong.)
B. It is recommended that screening be done by a properly trained health care provider (eg, physician, pediatric nurse practitioner, physician assistant, or physical therapist). (Evidence for this recommendation is strong.)
C. Ultrasonography of all newborns is not recommended. (Evidence is fair; consensus is strong.)

Recommendation 2

A. If a positive Ortolani or Barlow sign is found in the newborn examination, the infant should be referred to an orthopaedist. (The data recommending that all those with a positive Ortolani sign be referred to an orthopaedist are limited, but expert panel consensus, nevertheless, was strong….)
B. If the results of the physical examination at birth are "equivocally" positive (ie, soft click, mild asymmetry, but neither an Ortolani nor a Barlow sign is present), then a follow-up hip examination by the pediatrician in 2 weeks is recommended. (Evidence is good; consensus is strong.)

Recommendation 3

A. If the results of the newborn physical examination are positive (ie, presence of an Ortolani or a Barlow sign), ordering an ultrasonographic examination of the newborn is not recommended. (Evidence is poor; opinion is strong.)
B. If the results of the newborn physical examination are positive, obtaining a radiograph of the newborn's pelvis and hips is not recommended. (Evidence is poor; opinion is strong.)
C. The use of triple diapers when abnormal physical signs are detected during the newborn period is not recommended. (Evidence is poor; opinion is strong.)

Recommendation 4

If the results of the physical examination are positive (eg, positive Ortolani or Barlow sign) at 2 weeks, refer to an orthopaedist. (Evidence is strong; consensus is strong.)

Recommendation 5

If at the 2-week examination the Ortolani and Barlow signs are absent but physical findings raise suspicions, consider referral to an orthopaedist or request ultrasonography at age 3 to 4 weeks.

Recommendation 6

If the results of the physical examination are negative at 2 weeks, follow-up is recommended at the scheduled well-baby periodic examinations. (Evidence is good; consensus is strong.)

Recommendation 7

Risk factors. If the results of the newborn examination are negative (or equivocally positive), risk factors may be considered. The following recommendations are made (evidence is strong; opinion is strong):

A. Girl (newborn risk of 19/1000). When the results of the newborn examination are negative or equivocally positive, hips should be reevaluated at 2 weeks of age. If negative, continue according to the periodicity schedule; if positive, refer to an orthopaedist or for ultrasonography at 3 weeks of age.
B. Infants with a positive family history of DDH (newborn risk for boys of 9.4/1000 and for girls, 44/1000). When the results of the newborn examination in boys are negative or equivocally positive, hips should be reevaluated at 2 weeks of age. If negative, continue according to the periodicity schedule; if positive, refer to an orthopaedist or for ultrasonography at 3 weeks of age. In girls, the absolute risk of 44/1000 may exceed the pediatrician's threshold to act, and imaging with an ultrasonographic examination at 6 weeks of age or a radiograph of the pelvis at 4 months of age is recommended.
C. Breech presentation (newborn risk for boys of 26/1000 and for girls, 120/1000). For negative or equivocally positive newborn examinations, the infant should be reevaluated at regular intervals (according to the periodicity schedule) if the examination results remain negative.

Recommendation 8

Periodicity. The hips must be examined at every well-baby visit according to the recommended periodicity schedule for well-baby examinations (2–4 days for newborns discharged in less than 48 hours after delivery, by 1 month, 2 months, 4 months, 6 months, 9 months, and 12 months of age).

Coding Quick Reference for Dysplasia of the Hip	
ICD-9-CM	*ICD-10-CM*
755.63 Dysplasia, hip, congenital	**Q65.89** Other specified congenital deformities of hip **Q65.0-** Congenital dislocation of hip, unilateral **Q65.1** Congenital dislocation of hip, bilateral **Q65.2** Congenital dislocation of hip, unspecified **Q65.3-** Congenital partial dislocation of hip, unilateral **Q65.4** Congenital partial dislocation of hip, bilateral **Q65.5** Congenital partial dislocation of hip, unspecified **Q65.6** Congenital unstable hip (Congenital dislocatable hip)

ICD-10-CM Symbol: "-" Requires a fifth digit: 0 = unspecified; 1 = right; 2 = left

Hip Dysplasia

(Developmental Dysplasia of the Hip)

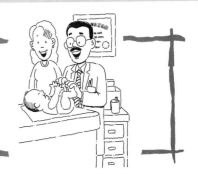

Hip dysplasia (developmental dysplasia of the hip) is a condition in which a child's upper thighbone is dislocated from the hip socket. It can be present at birth or develop during a child's first year of life.

Hip dysplasia is not always detectable at birth or even during early infancy. In spite of careful screening of children for hip dysplasia during regular well-child exams, a number of children with hip dysplasia are not diagnosed until after they are 1 year old.

Hip dysplasia is rare. However, if your baby is diagnosed with the condition, quick treatment is important.

What causes hip dysplasia?

No one is sure why hip dysplasia occurs (or why the left hip dislocates more often than the right hip). One reason may have to do with the hormones a baby is exposed to before birth. While these hormones serve to relax muscles in the pregnant mother's body, in some cases they also may cause a baby's joints to become too relaxed and prone to dislocation. This condition often corrects itself in several days, and the hip develops normally. In some cases, these dislocations cause changes in the hip anatomy that need treatment.

Who is at risk?

Factors that may increase the risk of hip dysplasia include
- Sex—more frequent in girls
- Family history—more likely when other family members have had hip dysplasia
- Birth position—more common in infants born in the breech position
- Birth order—firstborn children most at risk for hip dysplasia

Detecting hip dysplasia

Your pediatrician will check your newborn for hip dysplasia right after birth and at every well-child exam until your child is walking normally.

During the exam, your child's pediatrician will carefully flex and rotate your child's legs to see if the thighbones are properly positioned in the hip sockets. This does not require a great deal of force and will not hurt your baby.

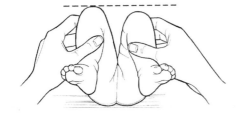

© Molly Borman

Your child's pediatrician also will look for other signs that may suggest a problem, including
- Limited range of motion in either leg
- One leg is shorter than the other
- Thigh or buttock creases appear uneven or lopsided

If your child's pediatrician suspects a problem with your child's hip, you may be referred to an orthopedic specialist who has experience treating hip dysplasia.

Treating hip dysplasia

Early treatment is important. The sooner treatment begins, the simpler it will be. In the past parents were told to double or triple diaper their babies to keep the legs in a position where dislocation was unlikely. *This practice is not recommended.* The diapering will not prevent hip dysplasia and will only delay effective treatment. Failure to treat this condition can result in permanent disability.

If your child is diagnosed with hip dysplasia before she is 6 months old, she will most likely be treated with a soft brace (such as the Pavlik harness) that holds the legs flexed and apart to allow the thighbones to be secure in the hip sockets.

The orthopedic consultant will tell you how long and when your baby will need to wear the brace. Your child also will be examined frequently during this time to make sure that the hips remain normal and stable.

In resistant cases or in older children, hip dysplasia may need to be treated with a combination of braces, casts, traction, or surgery. Your child will be admitted to the hospital if surgery is necessary. After surgery, your child will be placed in a hip spica cast for about 3 months. A hip spica cast is a hard cast that immobilizes the hips and keeps them in the correct position. When the cast is removed, your child will need to wear a removable hip brace for several more months.

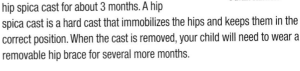

Pavlik Harness

Remember

If you have any concerns about your child's walking, talk with his pediatrician. If the cause is hip dysplasia, prompt treatment is important.

American Academy of Pediatrics

DEDICATED TO THE HEALTH OF ALL CHILDREN™

The American Academy of Pediatrics is an organization of 60,000 primary care pediatricians, pediatric medical subspecialists, and pediatric surgical specialists dedicated to the health, safety, and well-being of infants, children, adolescents, and young adults.

American Academy of Pediatrics
Web site—www.aap.org

Copyright © 2003
American Academy of Pediatrics

Febrile Seizures: Clinical Practice Guideline for the Long-term Management of the Child With Simple Febrile Seizures

• •

- *Clinical Practice Guideline*

Febrile Seizures: Clinical Practice Guideline for the Long-term Management of the Child With Simple Febrile Seizures

Steering Committee on Quality Improvement and Management, Subcommittee on Febrile Seizures

ABSTRACT

Febrile seizures are the most common seizure disorder in childhood, affecting 2% to 5% of children between the ages of 6 and 60 months. Simple febrile seizures are defined as brief (<15-minute) generalized seizures that occur once during a 24-hour period in a febrile child who does not have an intracranial infection, metabolic disturbance, or history of afebrile seizures. This guideline (a revision of the 1999 American Academy of Pediatrics practice parameter [now termed clinical practice guideline] "The Long-term Treatment of the Child With Simple Febrile Seizures") addresses the risks and benefits of both continuous and intermittent anticonvulsant therapy as well as the use of antipyretics in children with simple febrile seizures. It is designed to assist pediatricians by providing an analytic framework for decisions regarding possible therapeutic interventions in this patient population. It is not intended to replace clinical judgment or to establish a protocol for all patients with this disorder. Rarely will these guidelines be the only approach to this problem. *Pediatrics* 2008;121:1281–1286

www.pediatrics.org/cgi/doi/10.1542/peds.2008-0939

doi:10.1542/peds.2008-0939

All clinical reports from the American Academy of Pediatrics automatically expire 5 years after publication unless reaffirmed, revised, or retired at or before that time.

The guidance in this report does not indicate an exclusive course of treatment or serve as a standard of medical care. Variations, taking into account individual circumstances, may be appropriate.

Key Word
fever

Abbreviation
AAP—American Academy of Pediatrics

PEDIATRICS (ISSN Numbers: Print, 0031-4005; Online, 1098-4275). Copyright © 2008 by the American Academy of Pediatrics

The expected outcomes of this practice guideline include:

1. optimizing practitioner understanding of the scientific basis for using or avoiding various proposed treatments for children with simple febrile seizures;

2. improving the health of children with simple febrile seizures by avoiding therapies with high potential for adverse effects and no demonstrated ability to improve children's long-term outcomes;

3. reducing costs by avoiding therapies that will not demonstrably improve children's long-term outcomes; and

4. helping the practitioner educate caregivers about the low risks associated with simple febrile seizures.

The committee determined that with the exception of a high rate of recurrence, no long-term effects of simple febrile seizures have been identified. The risk of developing epilepsy in these patients is extremely low, although slightly higher than that in the general population. No data, however, suggest that prophylactic treatment of children with simple febrile seizures would reduce the risk, because epilepsy likely is the result of genetic predisposition rather than structural damage to the brain caused by recurrent simple febrile seizures. Although antipyretics have been shown to be ineffective in preventing recurrent febrile seizures, there is evidence that continuous anticonvulsant therapy with phenobarbital, primidone, or valproic acid and intermittent therapy with diazepam are effective in reducing febrile-seizure recurrence. The potential toxicities associated with these agents, however, outweigh the relatively minor risks associated with simple febrile seizures. As such, the committee concluded that, on the basis of the risks and benefits of the effective therapies, neither continuous nor intermittent anticonvulsant therapy is recommended for children with 1 or more simple febrile seizures.

INTRODUCTION

Febrile seizures are seizures that occur in febrile children between the ages of 6 and 60 months who do not have an intracranial infection, metabolic disturbance, or history of afebrile seizures. Febrile seizures are subdivided into 2 categories: simple and complex. Simple febrile seizures last for less than 15 minutes, are generalized (without a focal component), and occur once in a 24-hour period, whereas complex febrile seizures are prolonged (>15 minutes), are focal, or occur more than once in 24 hours.[1] Despite the frequency of febrile seizures (2%–5%), there is no unanimity of opinion about management options. This clinical practice guideline addresses potential therapeutic interventions in neurologically normal children with simple febrile seizures. It is not intended for patients with complex febrile seizures and does not pertain to children with previous neurologic insults, known central nervous system abnormalities, or a history of afebrile seizures. This clinical practice guideline is a revision of a 1999 American Academy of Pediatrics (AAP) clinical practice parameter, "The Long-term Treatment of the Child With Simple Febrile Seizures."[2]

For a child who has experienced a simple febrile seizure, there are potentially 4 adverse outcomes that theoretically may be altered by an effective therapeutic agent: (1) decline in IQ; (2) increased risk of epilepsy; (3) risk of recurrent febrile seizures; and (4) death. Neither a decline in IQ, academic performance or neurocognitive inattention nor behavioral abnormalities have been shown to be a consequence of recurrent simple febrile seizures.[3] Ellenberg and Nelson[4] studied 431 children who experienced febrile seizures and observed no significant difference in their learning compared with sibling controls. In a similar study by Verity et al,[5] 303 children with febrile seizures were compared with control children. No difference in learning was identified, except in those children who had neurologic abnormalities before their first seizure.

The second concern, increased risk of epilepsy, is more complex. Children with simple febrile seizures have approximately the same risk of developing epilepsy by the age of 7 years as does the general population (ie, 1%).[6] However, children who have had multiple simple febrile seizures, are younger than 12 months at the time of their first febrile seizure, and have a family history of epilepsy are at higher risk, with generalized afebrile seizures developing by 25 years of age in 2.4%.[7] Despite this fact, no study has demonstrated that successful treatment of simple febrile seizures can prevent this later development of epilepsy, and there currently is no evidence that simple febrile seizures cause structural damage to the brain. Indeed, it is most likely that the increased risk of epilepsy in this population is the result of genetic predisposition.

In contrast to the slightly increased risk of developing epilepsy, children with simple febrile seizures have a high rate of recurrence. The risk varies with age. Children younger than 12 months at the time of their first simple febrile seizure have an approximately 50% probability of having recurrent febrile seizures. Children older than 12 months at the time of their first event have an approximately 30% probability of a second febrile seizure; of those who do have a second febrile seizure, 50% have a chance of having at least 1 additional recurrence.[8]

Finally, there is a theoretical risk of a child dying during a simple febrile seizure as a result of documented injury, aspiration, or cardiac arrhythmia, but to the committee's knowledge, it has never been reported.

In summary, with the exception of a high rate of recurrence, no long-term adverse effects of simple febrile seizures have been identified. Because the risks associated with simple febrile seizures, other than recurrence, are so low and because the number of children who have febrile seizures in the first few years of life is so high, to be commensurate, a proposed therapy would need to be exceedingly low in risks and adverse effects, inexpensive, and highly effective.

METHODS

To update the clinical practice guideline on the treatment of children with simple febrile seizures, the AAP reconvened the Subcommittee on Febrile Seizures. The committee was chaired by a child neurologist and consisted of a neuroepidemiologist, 2 additional child neurologists, and a practicing pediatrician. All panel members reviewed and signed the AAP voluntary disclosure and conflict-of-interest form. The guideline was reviewed by members of the AAP Steering Committee on Quality Improvement and Management; members of the AAP Sections on Neurology, Pediatric Emergency Medicine, Developmental and Behavioral Pediatrics, and Epidemiology; members of the AAP Committees on Pediatric Emergency Medicine and Medical Liability and Risk Management; members of the AAP Councils on Children With Disabilities and Community Pediatrics; and members of outside organizations including the Child Neurology Society and the American Academy of Neurology.

A comprehensive review of the evidence-based literature published since 1998 was conducted with the aim of addressing possible therapeutic interventions in the management of children with simple febrile seizures. The review focused on both the efficacy and potential adverse effects of the proposed treatments. Decisions were made on the basis of a systematic grading of the quality of evidence and strength of recommendations.

The AAP established a partnership with the University of Kentucky (Lexington, KY) to develop an evidence report, which served as a major source of information for these practice-guideline recommendations. The specific issues addressed were (1) effectiveness of continuous anticonvulsant therapy in preventing recurrent febrile seizures, (2) effectiveness of intermittent anticonvulsant therapy in preventing recurrent febrile seizures, (3) effectiveness of antipyretics in preventing recurrent febrile seizures, and (4) adverse effects of either continuous or intermittent anticonvulsant therapy.

In the original practice parameter, more than 300 medical journal articles reporting studies of the natural history of simple febrile seizures or the therapy of these seizures were reviewed and abstracted.[2] An additional 65 articles were reviewed and abstracted for the update. Emphasis was placed on articles that differentiated simple febrile seizures from other types of seizures, that carefully matched treatment and control groups, and that described adherence to the drug regimen. Tables were constructed from the 65 articles that best fit these criteria. A more comprehensive review of the literature on which this report is based can be found in a forthcoming technical report (the initial technical report can be accessed at http://aappolicy.aappublications.org/cgi/content/full/pediatrics;103/6/e86). The technical report also will contain dosing information.

The evidence-based approach to guideline development requires that the evidence in support of a recommendation be identified, appraised, and summarized and that an explicit link between evidence and recommendations be defined. Evidence-based recommendations reflect the quality of evidence and the balance of benefit and harm that is

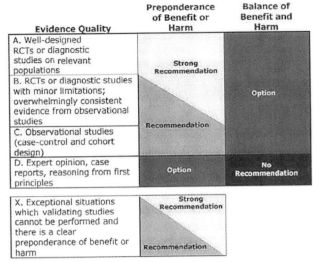

FIGURE 1
Integrating evidence-quality appraisal with an assessment of the anticipated balance between benefits and harms if a policy is conducted leads to designation of a policy as a strong recommendation, recommendation, option, or no recommendation. RCT indicates randomized, controlled trial.

anticipated when the recommendation is followed. The AAP policy statement "Classifying Recommendations for Clinical Practice Guidelines"[9] was followed in designating levels of recommendations (see Fig 1 and Table 1).

RECOMMENDATION

On the basis of the risks and benefits of the effective therapies, neither continuous nor intermittent anticonvulsant therapy is recommended for children with 1 or more simple febrile seizures.

- Aggregate evidence quality: B (randomized, controlled trials and diagnostic studies with minor limitations).

- Benefit: prevention of recurrent febrile seizures, which are not harmful and do not significantly increase the risk for development of future epilepsy.

- Harm: adverse effects including rare fatal hepatotoxicity (especially in children younger than 2 years who are also at greatest risk of febrile seizures), thrombocytopenia, weight loss and gain, gastrointestinal disturbances, and pancreatitis with valproic acid and hyperactivity, irritability, lethargy, sleep disturbances, and hypersensitivity reactions with phenobarbital; lethargy, drowsiness, and ataxia for intermittent diazepam as well as the risk of masking an evolving central nervous system infection.

- Benefits/harms assessment: preponderance of harm over benefit.

- Policy level: recommendation.

BENEFITS AND RISKS OF CONTINUOUS ANTICONVULSANT THERAPY

Phenobarbital

Phenobarbital is effective in preventing the recurrence of simple febrile seizures.[10] In a controlled double-blind study, daily therapy with phenobarbital reduced the rate of subsequent febrile seizures from 25 per 100 subjects per year to 5 per 100 subjects per year.[11] For the agent to be effective, however, it must be given daily and maintained in the therapeutic range. In a study by Farwell et al,[12] for example, children whose phenobarbital levels were in the therapeutic range had a reduction in recurrent seizures, but because noncompliance was so high, an overall benefit with phenobarbital therapy was not identified.

The adverse effects of phenobarbital include hyperactivity, irritability, lethargy, sleep disturbances, and hypersensitivity reactions. The behavioral adverse effects

TABLE 1	**Guideline Definitions for Evidence-Based Statements**	
Statement	Definition	Implication
Strong recommendation	A strong recommendation in favor of a particular action is made when the anticipated benefits of the recommended intervention clearly exceed the harms (as a strong recommendation against an action is made when the anticipated harms clearly exceed the benefits) and the quality of the supporting evidence is excellent. In some clearly identified circumstances, strong recommendations may be made when high-quality evidence is impossible to obtain and the anticipated benefits strongly outweigh the harms.	Clinicians should follow a strong recommendation unless a clear and compelling rationale for an alternative approach is present.
Recommendation	A recommendation in favor of a particular action is made when the anticipated benefits exceed the harms but the quality of evidence is not as strong. Again, in some clearly identified circumstances, recommendations may be made when high-quality evidence is impossible to obtain but the anticipated benefits outweigh the harms.	Clinicians would be prudent to follow a recommendation but should remain alert to new information and sensitive to patient preferences.
Option	Options define courses that may be taken when either the quality of evidence is suspect or carefully performed studies have shown little clear advantage to 1 approach over another.	Clinicians should consider the option in their decision-making, and patient preference may have a substantial role.
No recommendation	No recommendation indicates that there is a lack of pertinent published evidence and that the anticipated balance of benefits and harms is presently unclear.	Clinicians should be alert to new published evidence that clarifies the balance of benefit versus harm.

may occur in up to 20% to 40% of patients and may be severe enough to necessitate discontinuation of the drug.[13–16]

Primidone

Primidone, in doses of 15 to 20 mg/kg per day, has also been shown to reduce the recurrence rate of febrile seizures.[17,18] It is of interest that the derived phenobarbital level in a Minigawa and Miura study[17] was below therapeutic (16 μg/mL) in 29 of the 32 children, suggesting that primidone itself may be active in preventing seizure recurrence. As with phenobarbital, adverse effects include behavioral disturbances, irritability, and sleep disturbances.[18]

Valproic Acid

In randomized, controlled studies, only 4% of children taking valproic acid, as opposed to 35% of control subjects, had a subsequent febrile seizure. Therefore, valproic acid seems to be at least as effective in preventing recurrent simple febrile seizures as phenobarbital and significantly more effective than placebo.[19–21]

Drawbacks to therapy with valproic acid include its rare association with fatal hepatotoxicity (especially in children younger than 2 years, who are also at greatest risk of febrile seizures), thrombocytopenia, weight loss and gain, gastrointestinal disturbances, and pancreatitis. In studies in which children received valproic acid to prevent recurrence of febrile seizures, no cases of fatal hepatotoxicity were reported.[15]

Carbamazepine

Carbamazepine has not been shown to be effective in preventing the recurrence of simple febrile seizures. Antony and Hawke[13] compared children who had been treated with therapeutic levels of either phenobarbital or carbamazepine, and 47% of the children in the carbamazepine-treated group had recurrent seizures compared with only 10% of those in the phenobarbital group. In another study, Camfield et al[22] treated children (whose conditions failed to improve with phenobarbital therapy) with carbamazepine. Despite good compliance, 13 of the 16 children treated with carbamazepine had a recurrent febrile seizure within 18 months. It is theoretically possible that these excessively high rates of recurrences might have been attributable to adverse effects of carbamazepine.

Phenytoin

Phenytoin has not been shown to be effective in preventing the recurrence of simple febrile seizures, even when the agent is in the therapeutic range.[23,24] Other anticonvulsants have not been studied for the continuous treatment of simple febrile seizures.

BENEFITS AND RISKS OF INTERMITTENT ANTICONVULSANT THERAPY

Diazepam

A double-blind controlled study of patients with a history of febrile seizures demonstrated that administration of oral diazepam (given at the time of fever) could reduce the recurrence of febrile seizures. Children with a history of febrile seizures were given either oral diazepam (0.33 mg/kg, every 8 hours for 48 hours) or a placebo at the time of fever. The risk of febrile seizures per person-year was decreased 44% with diazepam.[25] In a more recent study, children with a history of febrile seizures were given oral diazepam at the time of fever and then compared with children in an untreated control group. In the oral diazepam group, there was an 11% recurrence rate compared with a 30% recurrence rate in the control group.[26] It should be noted that all children for whom diazepam was considered a failure had been noncompliant with drug administration, in part because of adverse effects of the medication.

There is also literature that demonstrates the feasibility and safety of interrupting a simple febrile seizure lasting less than 5 minutes with rectal diazepam and with both intranasal and buccal midazolam.[27,28] Although these agents are effective in terminating the seizure, it is questionable whether they have any long-term influence on outcome. In a study by Knudsen et al,[29] children were given either rectal diazepam at the time of fever or only at the onset of seizure. Twelve-year follow-up found that the long-term prognosis of the children in the 2 groups did not differ regardless of whether treatment was aimed at preventing seizures or treating them.

A potential drawback to intermittent medication is that a seizure could occur before a fever is noticed. Indeed, in several of these studies, recurrent seizures were likely attributable to failure of method rather than failure of the agent.

Adverse effects of oral and rectal diazepam[26] and both intranasal and buccal midazolam include lethargy, drowsiness, and ataxia. Respiratory depression is extremely rare, even when given by the rectal route.[28,30] Sedation caused by any of the benzodiazepines, whether administered by the oral, rectal, nasal, or buccal route, have the potential of masking an evolving central nervous system infection. If used, the child's health care professional should be contacted.

BENEFITS AND RISKS OF INTERMITTENT ANTIPYRETICS

No studies have demonstrated that antipyretics, in the absence of anticonvulsants, reduce the recurrence risk of simple febrile seizures. Camfield et al[11] treated 79 children who had had a first febrile seizure with either a placebo plus antipyretic instruction (either aspirin or acetaminophen) versus daily phenobarbital plus antipyretic instruction (either aspirin or acetaminophen). Recurrence risk was significantly lower in the phenobarbital-treated group, suggesting that antipyretic instruction, including the use of antipyretics, is ineffective in preventing febrile-seizure recurrence.

Whether antipyretics are given regularly (every 4 hours) or sporadically (contingent on a specific body-temperature elevation) does not influence outcome. Acetaminophen was either given every 4 hours or only for temperature elevations of more than 37.9°C in 104 children. The incidence of febrile episodes did not differ significantly between the 2 groups, nor did the early recurrence of febrile seizures. The authors determined that administering prophylactic acetaminophen during febrile episodes was ineffective in preventing or reducing fever and in preventing febrile-seizure recurrence.[31]

In a randomized double-blind placebo-controlled trial, acetaminophen was administered along with low-dose oral diazepam.[32] Febrile-seizure recurrence was not reduced, compared with control groups. As with acetaminophen, ibuprofen also has been shown to be ineffective in preventing recurrence of febrile seizures.[33–35]

In general, acetaminophen and ibuprofen are considered to be safe and effective antipyretics for children. However, hepatotoxicity (with acetaminophen) and respiratory failure, metabolic acidosis, renal failure, and coma (with ibuprofen) have been reported in children after overdose or in the presence of risk factors.[36,37]

CONCLUSIONS

The subcommittee has determined that a simple febrile seizure is a benign and common event in children between the ages of 6 and 60 months. Nearly all children have an excellent prognosis. The committee concluded that although there is evidence that both continuous antiepileptic therapy with phenobarbital, primidone, or valproic acid and intermittent therapy with oral diazepam are effective in reducing the risk of recurrence, the potential toxicities associated with antiepileptic drugs outweigh the relatively minor risks associated with simple febrile seizures. As such, long-term therapy is not recommended. In situations in which parental anxiety associated with febrile seizures is severe, intermittent oral diazepam at the onset of febrile illness may be effective in preventing recurrence. Although antipyretics may improve the comfort of the child, they will not prevent febrile seizures.

SUBCOMMITTEE ON FEBRILE SEIZURES, 2002–2008

Patricia K. Duffner, MD, Chairperson
Robert J. Baumann, MD, Methodologist
Peter Berman, MD
John L. Green, MD
Sanford Schneider, MD

STEERING COMMITTEE ON QUALITY IMPROVEMENT AND MANAGEMENT, 2007–2008

Elizabeth S. Hodgson, MD, Chairperson
Gordon B. Glade, MD
Norman "Chip" Harbaugh, Jr, MD
Thomas K. McInerny, MD
Marlene R. Miller, MD, MSc
Virginia A. Moyer, MD, MPH
Xavier D. Sevilla, MD
Lisa Simpson, MB, BCh, MPH
Glenn S. Takata, MD

LIAISONS

Denise Dougherty, PhD
    Agency for Healthcare Research and Quality
Daniel R. Neuspiel, MD
    Section on Epidemiology

Ellen Schwalenstocker, MBA
    National Association of Children's Hospitals and
    Related Institutions

STAFF

Caryn Davidson, MA

REFERENCES

1. Nelson KB, Ellenberg JH. Prognosis in children with febrile seizures. *Pediatrics.* 1978;61(5):720–727
2. American Academy of Pediatrics, Committee on Quality Improvement, Subcommittee on Febrile Seizures. The long-term treatment of the child with simple febrile seizures. *Pediatrics.* 1999;103(6 pt 1):1307–1309
3. Chang YC, Guo NW, Huang CC, Wang ST, Tsai JJ. Neurocognitive attention and behavior outcome of school age children with a history of febrile convulsions: a population study. *Epilepsia.* 2000;41(4):412–420
4. Ellenberg JH, Nelson KB. Febrile seizures and later intellectual performance. *Arch Neurol.* 1978;35(1):17–21
5. Verity CM, Butler NR, Golding J. Febrile convulsions in a national cohort followed up from birth. II: medical history and intellectual ability at 5 years of age. *BMJ.* 1985;290(6478):1311–1315
6. Nelson KB, Ellenberg JH. Predictors of epilepsy in children who have experienced febrile seizures. *N Engl J Med.* 1976;295(19):1029–1033
7. Annegers JF, Hauser WA, Shirts SB, Kurland LT. Factors prognostic of unprovoked seizures after febrile convulsions. *N Engl J Med.* 1987;316(9):493–498
8. Berg AT, Shinnar S, Darefsky AS, et al. Predictors of recurrent febrile seizures: a prospective cohort study. *Arch Pediatr Adolesc Med.* 1997;151(4):371–378
9. American Academy of Pediatrics, Steering Committee on Quality Improvement and Management. Classifying recommendations for clinical practice guidelines. *Pediatrics.* 2004;114(3):874–877
10. Wolf SM, Carr A, Davis DC, Davidson S, et al. The value of phenobarbital in the child who has had a single febrile seizure: a controlled prospective study. *Pediatrics.* 1977;59(3):378–385
11. Camfield PR, Camfield CS, Shapiro SH, Cummings C. The first febrile seizure: antipyretic instruction plus either phenobarbital or placebo to prevent recurrence. *J Pediatr.* 1980;97(1):16–21
12. Farwell JR, Lee JY, Hirtz DG, Sulzbacher SI, Ellenberg JH, Nelson KB. Phenobarbital for febrile seizures: effects on intelligence and on seizure recurrence [published correction appears in *N Engl J Med.* 1992;326(2):144]. *N Engl J Med.* 1990;322(6):364–369
13. Antony JH, Hawke SHB. Phenobarbital compared with carbamazepine in prevention of recurrent febrile convulsions. *Am J Dis Child.* 1983;137(9):892–895
14. Knudsen Fu, Vestermark S. Prophylactic diazepam or phenobarbitone in febrile convulsions: a prospective, controlled study. *Arch Dis Child.* 1978;53(8):660–663
15. Lee K, Melchior JC. Sodium valproate versus phenobarbital in the prophylactic treatment of febrile convulsions in childhood. *Eur J Pediatr.* 1981;137(2):151–153
16. Camfield CS, Chaplin S, Doyle AB, Shapiro SH, Cummings C, Camfield PR. Side effects of phenobarbital in toddlers: behavioral and cognitive aspects. *J Pediatr.* 1979;95(3):361–365
17. Minagawa K, Miura H. Phenobarbital, primidone and sodium valproate in the prophylaxis of febrile convulsions. *Brain Dev.* 1981;3(4):385–393
18. Herranz JL, Armijo JA, Arteaga R. Effectiveness and toxicity of phenobarbital, primidone, and sodium valproate in the pre-

vention of febrile convulsions, controlled by plasma levels. *Epilepsia*. 1984;25(1):89–95

19. Wallace SJ, Smith JA. Successful prophylaxis against febrile convulsions with valproic acid or phenobarbitone. *BMJ*. 1980; 280(6211):353–354

20. Mamelle N, Mamelle JC, Plasse JC, Revol M, Gilly R. Prevention of recurrent febrile convulsions: a randomized therapeutic assay—sodium valproate, phenobarbitone and placebo. *Neuropediatrics*. 1984;15(1):37–42

21. Ngwane E, Bower B. Continuous sodium valproate or phenobarbitone in the prevention of "simple" febrile convulsions. *Arch Dis Child*. 1980;55(3):171–174

22. Camfield PR, Camfield CS, Tibbles JA. Carbamazepine does not prevent febrile seizures in phenobarbital failures. *Neurology*. 1982;32(3):288–289

23. Bacon CJ, Hierons AM, Mucklow JC, Webb JK, Rawlins MD, Weightman D. Placebo-controlled study of phenobarbitone and phenytoin in the prophylaxis of febrile convulsions. *Lancet*. 1981;2(8247):600–604

24. Melchior JC, Buchthal F, Lennox Buchthal M. The ineffectiveness of diphenylhydantoin in preventing febrile convulsions in the age of greatest risk, under 3 years. *Epilepsia*. 1971;12(1): 55–62

25. Rosman NP, Colton T, Labazzo J, et al. A controlled trial of diazepam administered during febrile illnesses to prevent recurrence of febrile seizures. *N Engl J Med*. 1993;329(2):79–84

26. Verrotti A, Latini G, di Corcia G, et al. Intermittent oral diazepam prophylaxis in febrile convulsions: its effectiveness for febrile seizure recurrence. *Eur J Pediatr Neurol*. 2004;8(3): 131–134

27. Lahat E, Goldman M, Barr J, Bistritzer T, Berkovitch M. Comparison of intranasal midazolam with intravenous diazepam for treating febrile seizures in children: prospective randomized study. *BMJ*. 2000;321(7253):83–86

28. McIntyre J, Robertson S, Norris E, et al. Safety and efficacy of buccal midazolam versus rectal diazepam for emergency treatment of seizures in children: a randomized controlled trial. *Lancet*. 2005;366(9481):205–210

29. Knudsen FU, Paerregaard A, Andersen R, Andresen J. Long term outcome of prophylaxis for febrile convulsions. *Arch Dis Child*. 1996;74(1):13–18

30. Pellock JM, Shinnar S. Respiratory adverse events associated with diazepam rectal gel. *Neurology*. 2005;64(10):1768–1770

31. Schnaiderman D, Lahat E, Sheefer T, Aladjem M. Antipyretic effectiveness of acetaminophen in febrile seizures: ongoing prophylaxis versus sporadic usage. *Eur J Pediatr*. 1993;152(9): 747–749

32. Uhari M, Rantala H, Vainionpaa L, Kurttila R. Effect of acetaminophen and of low dose intermittent doses of diazepam on prevention of recurrences of febrile seizures. *J Pediatr*. 1995; 126(6):991–995

33. van Stuijvenberg M, Derksen-Lubsen G, Steyerberg EW, Habbema JDF, Moll HA. Randomized, controlled trial of ibuprofen syrup administered during febrile illnesses to prevent febrile seizure recurrences. *Pediatrics*. 1998;102(5). Available at: www.pediatrics.org/cgi/content/full/102/5/e51

34. van Esch A, Van Steensel-Moll HA, Steyerberg EW, Offringa M, Habbema JDF, Derksen-Lubsen G. Antipyretic efficacy of ibuprofen and acetaminophen in children with febrile seizures. *Arch Pediatr Adolesc Med*. 1995;149(6):632–637

35. van Esch A, Steyerberg EW, Moll HA, et al. A study of the efficacy of antipyretic drugs in the prevention of febrile seizure recurrence. *Ambul Child Health*. 2000;6(1):19–26

36. Easley RB, Altemeier WA. Central nervous system manifestations of an ibuprofen overdose reversed by naloxone. *Pediatr Emerg Care*. 2000;16(1):39–41

37. American Academy of Pediatrics, Committee on Drugs. Acetaminophen toxicity in children. *Pediatrics*. 2001;108(4): 1020–1024

Febrile Seizures: Guideline for the Neurodiagnostic Evaluation of the Child With a Simple Febrile Seizure

- *Clinical Practice Guideline*

Clinical Practice Guideline—Febrile Seizures: Guideline for the Neurodiagnostic Evaluation of the Child With a Simple Febrile Seizure

SUBCOMMITTEE ON FEBRILE SEIZURES

KEY WORD

seizure

ABBREVIATIONS

AAP—American Academy of Pediatrics
Hib—*Haemophilus influenzae* type b
EEG—electroencephalogram
CT—computed tomography

www.pediatrics.org/cgi/doi/10.1542/peds.2010-3318

doi:10.1542/peds.2010-3318

All clinical practice guidelines from the American Academy of Pediatrics automatically expire 5 years after publication unless reaffirmed, revised, or retired at or before that time.

PEDIATRICS (ISSN Numbers: Print, 0031-4005; Online, 1098-4275).

abstract

OBJECTIVE: To formulate evidence-based recommendations for health care professionals about the diagnosis and evaluation of a simple febrile seizure in infants and young children 6 through 60 months of age and to revise the practice guideline published by the American Academy of Pediatrics (AAP) in 1996.

METHODS: This review included search and analysis of the medical literature published since the last version of the guideline. Physicians with expertise and experience in the fields of neurology and epilepsy, pediatrics, epidemiology, and research methodologies constituted a subcommittee of the AAP Steering Committee on Quality Improvement and Management. The steering committee and other groups within the AAP and organizations outside the AAP reviewed the guideline. The subcommittee member who reviewed the literature for the 1996 AAP practice guidelines searched for articles published since the last guideline through 2009, supplemented by articles submitted by other committee members. Results from the literature search were provided to the subcommittee members for review. Interventions of direct interest included lumbar puncture, electroencephalography, blood studies, and neuroimaging. Multiple issues were raised and discussed iteratively until consensus was reached about recommendations. The strength of evidence supporting each recommendation and the strength of the recommendation were assessed by the committee member most experienced in informatics and epidemiology and graded according to AAP policy.

CONCLUSIONS: Clinicians evaluating infants or young children after a simple febrile seizure should direct their attention toward identifying the cause of the child's fever. Meningitis should be considered in the differential diagnosis for any febrile child, and lumbar puncture should be performed if there are clinical signs or symptoms of concern. For any infant between 6 and 12 months of age who presents with a seizure and fever, a lumbar puncture is an option when the child is considered deficient in *Haemophilus influenzae* type b (Hib) or *Streptococcus pneumoniae* immunizations (ie, has not received scheduled immunizations as recommended), or when immunization status cannot be determined, because of an increased risk of bacterial meningitis. A lumbar puncture is an option for children who are pretreated with antibiotics. In general, a simple febrile seizure does not usually require further evaluation, specifically electroencephalography, blood studies, or neuroimaging. *Pediatrics* 2011;127:389–394

DEFINITION OF THE PROBLEM

This practice guideline provides recommendations for the neurodiagnostic evaluation of neurologically healthy infants and children 6 through 60 months of age who have had a simple febrile seizure and present for evaluation within 12 hours of the event. It replaces the 1996 practice parameter.[1] This practice guideline is not intended for patients who have had complex febrile seizures (prolonged, focal, and/or recurrent), and it does not pertain to children with previous neurologic insults, known central nervous system abnormalities, or history of afebrile seizures.

TARGET AUDIENCE AND PRACTICE SETTING

This practice guideline is intended for use by pediatricians, family physicians, child neurologists, neurologists, emergency physicians, nurse practitioners, and other health care providers who evaluate children for febrile seizures.

BACKGROUND

A febrile seizure is a seizure accompanied by fever (temperature $\geq$ 100.4°F or 38°C[2] by any method), without central nervous system infection, that occurs in infants and children 6 through 60 months of age. Febrile seizures occur in 2% to 5% of all children and, as such, make up the most common convulsive event in children younger than 60 months. In 1976, Nelson and Ellenberg,[3] using data from the National Collaborative Perinatal Project, further defined febrile seizures as being either simple or complex. Simple febrile seizures were defined as primary generalized seizures that lasted for less than 15 minutes and did not recur within 24 hours. Complex febrile seizures were defined as focal, prolonged ($\geq$15 minutes), and/or recurrent within 24 hours. Children who had simple febrile seizures had no evidence of increased mortality, hemiplegia, or mental retardation. During follow-up evaluation, the risk of epilepsy after a

simple febrile seizure was shown to be only slightly higher than that of the general population, whereas the chief risk associated with simple febrile seizures was recurrence in one-third of the children. The authors concluded that simple febrile seizures are benign events with excellent prognoses, a conclusion reaffirmed in the 1980 consensus statement from the National Institutes of Health.[3,4]

The expected outcomes of this practice guideline include the following:

1. Optimize clinician understanding of the scientific basis for the neurodiagnostic evaluation of children with simple febrile seizures.

2. Aid the clinician in decision-making by using a structured framework.

3. Optimize evaluation of the child who has had a simple febrile seizure by detecting underlying diseases, minimizing morbidity, and reassuring anxious parents and children.

4. Reduce the costs of physician and emergency department visits, hospitalizations, and unnecessary testing.

5. Educate the clinician to understand that a simple febrile seizure usually does not require further evaluation, specifically electroencephalography, blood studies, or neuroimaging.

METHODOLOGY

To update the clinical practice guideline on the neurodiagnostic evaluation of children with simple febrile seizures,[1] the American Academy of Pediatrics (AAP) reconvened the Subcommittee on Febrile Seizures. The committee was chaired by a child neurologist and consisted of a neuroepidemiologist, 3 additional child neurologists, and a practicing pediatrician. All panel members reviewed and signed the AAP voluntary disclosure and conflict-of-interest form. No conflicts were reported. Participation in the guideline process was voluntary and not paid. The guideline was reviewed by members of the AAP Steering Commit-

tee on Quality Improvement and Management; members of the AAP Section on Administration and Practice Management, Section on Developmental and Behavioral Pediatrics, Section on Epidemiology, Section on Infectious Diseases, Section on Neurology, Section on Neurologic Surgery, Section on Pediatric Emergency Medicine, Committee on Pediatric Emergency Medicine, Committee on Practice and Ambulatory Medicine, Committee on Child Health Financing, Committee on Infectious Diseases, Committee on Medical Liability and Risk Management, Council on Children With Disabilities, and Council on Community Pediatrics; and members of outside organizations including the Child Neurology Society, the American Academy of Neurology, the American College of Emergency Physicians, and members of the Pediatric Committee of the Emergency Nurses Association.

A comprehensive review of the evidence-based literature published from 1996 to February 2009 was conducted to discover articles that addressed the diagnosis and evaluation of children with simple febrile seizures. Preference was given to population-based studies, but given the scarcity of such studies, data from hospital-based studies, groups of young children with febrile illness, and comparable groups were reviewed. Decisions were made on the basis of a systematic grading of the quality of evidence and strength of recommendations.

In the original practice parameter,[1] 203 medical journal articles were reviewed and abstracted. An additional 372 articles were reviewed and abstracted for this update. Emphasis was placed on articles that differentiated simple febrile seizures from other types of seizures. Tables were constructed from the 70 articles that best fit these criteria.

The evidence-based approach to guideline development requires that the evidence in support of a recommendation be identified, appraised, and summarized and that an explicit link between

Evidence Quality	Preponderance of Benefit or Harm	Balance of Benefit and Harm
A. Well-designed RCTs or diagnostic studies on relevant population	**Strong**	
B. RCTs or diagnostic studies with minor limitations; overwhelmingly consistent evidence from observational studies		**Option**
C. Observational studies (case-control and cohort design)	**Rec**	
D. Expert opinion, case reports, reasoning from first principles	**Option**	**No Rec**
X. Exceptional situations for which validating studies cannot be performed and there is a clear preponderance of benefit or harm	**Strong** **Rec**	

FIGURE 1

Integrating evidence quality appraisal with an assessment of the anticipated balance between benefits and harms if a policy is carried out leads to designation of a policy as a strong recommendation, recommendation, option, or no recommendation. RCT indicates randomized controlled trial; Rec, recommendation.

evidence and recommendations be defined. Evidence-based recommendations reflect the quality of evidence and the balance of benefit and harm that is anticipated when the recommendation is followed. The AAP policy statement "Classifying Recommendations for Clinical Practice Guidelines"[5] was followed in designating levels of recommendations (see Fig 1).

KEY ACTION STATEMENTS

Action Statement 1

Action Statement 1a

A lumbar puncture should be performed in any child who presents with a seizure and a fever and has meningeal signs and symptoms (eg, neck stiffness, Kernig and/or Brudzinski signs) or in any child whose history or examination suggests the presence of meningitis or intracranial infection.

- Aggregate evidence level: B (overwhelming evidence from observational studies).

- Benefits: Meningeal signs and symptoms strongly suggest meningitis, which, if bacterial in etiology, will likely be fatal if left untreated.

- Harms/risks/costs: Lumbar puncture is an invasive and often painful procedure and can be costly.

- Benefits/harms assessment: Preponderance of benefit over harm.

- Value judgments: Observational data and clinical principles were used in making this judgment.

- Role of patient preferences: Although parents may not wish to have their child undergo a lumbar puncture, health care providers should explain that if meningitis is not diagnosed and treated, it could be fatal.

- Exclusions: None.

- Intentional vagueness: None.

- Policy level: Strong recommendation.

Action Statement 1b

In any infant between 6 and 12 months of age who presents with a seizure and fever, a lumbar puncture is an option when the child is considered deficient in *Haemophilus influenzae* type b (Hib) or *Streptococcus pneumoniae* immunizations (ie, has not received scheduled immunizations as recommended) or when immunization status cannot be determined because of an increased risk of bacterial meningitis.

- Aggregate evidence level: D (expert opinion, case reports).

- Benefits: Meningeal signs and symptoms strongly suggest meningitis, which, if bacterial in etiology, will

likely be fatal or cause significant long-term disability if left untreated.

- Harms/risks/costs: Lumbar puncture is an invasive and often painful procedure and can be costly.

- Benefits/harms assessment: Preponderance of benefit over harm.

- Value judgments: Data on the incidence of bacterial meningitis from before and after the existence of immunizations against Hib and *S pneumoniae* were used in making this recommendation.

- Role of patient preferences: Although parents may not wish their child to undergo a lumbar puncture, health care providers should explain that in the absence of complete immunizations, their child may be at risk of having fatal bacterial meningitis.

- Exclusions: This recommendation applies only to children 6 to 12 months of age. The subcommittee felt that clinicians would recognize symptoms of meningitis in children older than 12 months.

- Intentional vagueness: None.

- Policy level: Option.

Action Statement 1c

A lumbar puncture is an option in the child who presents with a seizure and fever and is pretreated with antibiotics, because antibiotic treatment can mask the signs and symptoms of meningitis.

- Aggregate evidence level: D (reasoning from clinical experience, case series).

- Benefits: Antibiotics may mask meningeal signs and symptoms but may be insufficient to eradicate meningitis; a diagnosis of meningitis, if bacterial in etiology, will likely be fatal if left untreated.

- Harms/risks/costs: Lumbar puncture is an invasive and often painful procedure and can be costly.

- Benefits/harms assessment: Preponderance of benefit over harm.
- Value judgments: Clinical experience and case series were used in making this judgment while recognizing that extensive data from studies are lacking.
- Role of patient preferences: Although parents may not wish to have their child undergo a lumbar puncture, medical providers should explain that in the presence of pretreatment with antibiotics, the signs and symptoms of meningitis may be masked. Meningitis, if untreated, can be fatal.
- Exclusions: None.
- Intentional vagueness: Data are insufficient to define the specific treatment duration necessary to mask signs and symptoms. The committee determined that the decision to perform a lumbar puncture will depend on the type and duration of antibiotics administered before the seizure and should be left to the individual clinician.
- Policy level: Option.

The committee recognizes the diversity of past and present opinions regarding the need for lumbar punctures in children younger than 12 months with a simple febrile seizure. Since the publication of the previous practice parameter,[1] however, there has been widespread immunization in the United States for 2 of the most common causes of bacterial meningitis in this age range: Hib and *S pneumoniae*. Although compliance with all scheduled immunizations as recommended does not completely eliminate the possibility of bacterial meningitis from the differential diagnosis, current data no longer support routine lumbar puncture in well-appearing, fully immunized children who present with a simple febrile seizure.[6–8] Moreover, although approximately 25% of young children with meningitis have seizures as the presenting sign of the disease, some are either obtunded or comatose when evaluated by a physician for the seizure, and the remainder most often have obvious clinical signs of meningitis (focal seizures, recurrent seizures, petechial rash, or nuchal rigidity).[9–11] Once a decision has been made to perform a lumbar puncture, then blood culture and serum glucose testing should be performed concurrently to increase the sensitivity for detecting bacteria and to determine if there is hypoglycorrhachia characteristic of bacterial meningitis, respectively.

Recent studies that evaluated the outcome of children with simple febrile seizures have included populations with a high prevalence of immunization.[7,8] Data for unimmunized or partially immunized children are lacking. Therefore, lumbar puncture is an option for young children who are considered deficient in immunizations or those in whom immunization status cannot be determined. There are also no definitive data on the outcome of children who present with a simple febrile seizure while already on antibiotics. The authors were unable to find a definition of "pretreated" in the literature, so they consulted with the AAP Committee on Infectious Diseases. Although there is no formal definition, pretreatment can be considered to include systemic antibiotic therapy by any route given within the days before the seizure. Whether pretreatment will affect the presentation and course of bacterial meningitis cannot be predicted but will depend, in part, on the antibiotic administered, the dose, the route of administration, the drug's cerebrospinal fluid penetration, and the organism causing the meningitis. Lumbar puncture is an option in any child pretreated with antibiotics before a simple febrile seizure.

Action Statement 2

An electroencephalogram (EEG) should not be performed in the evaluation of a neurologically healthy child with a simple febrile seizure.

- Aggregate evidence level: B (overwhelming evidence from observational studies).
- Benefits: One study showed a possible association with paroxysmal EEGs and a higher rate of afebrile seizures.[12]
- Harms/risks/costs: EEGs are costly and may increase parental anxiety.
- Benefits/harms assessment: Preponderance of harm over benefit.
- Value judgments: Observational data were used for this judgment.
- Role of patient preferences: Although an EEG might have limited prognostic utility in this situation, parents should be educated that the study will not alter outcome.
- Exclusions: None.
- Intentional vagueness: None.
- Policy level: Strong recommendation.

There is no evidence that EEG readings performed either at the time of presentation after a simple febrile seizure or within the following month are predictive of either recurrence of febrile seizures or the development of afebrile seizures/epilepsy within the next 2 years.[13,14] There is a single study that found that a paroxysmal EEG was associated with a higher rate of afebrile seizures.[12] There is no evidence that interventions based on this test would alter outcome.

Action Statement 3

The following tests should not be performed routinely for the sole purpose of identifying the cause of a simple febrile seizure: measurement of serum electrolytes, calcium, phosphorus, magnesium, or blood glucose or complete blood cell count.

- Aggregate evidence level: B (overwhelming evidence from observational studies).
- Benefits: A complete blood cell count may identify children at risk for bacte-

remia; however, the incidence of bacteremia in febrile children younger than 24 months is the same with or without febrile seizures.

- Harms/risks/costs: Laboratory tests may be invasive and costly and provide no real benefit.
- Benefits/harms assessment: Preponderance of harm over benefit.
- Value judgments: Observational data were used for this judgment.
- Role of patient preferences: Although parents may want blood tests performed to explain the seizure, they should be reassured that blood tests should be directed toward identifying the source of their child's fever.
- Exclusions: None.
- Intentional vagueness: None.
- Policy level: Strong recommendation.

There is no evidence to suggest that routine blood studies are of benefit in the evaluation of the child with a simple febrile seizure.[15–18] Although some children with febrile seizures have abnormal serum electrolyte values, their condition should be identifiable by obtaining appropriate histories and performing careful physical examinations. It should be noted that as a group, children with febrile seizures have relatively low serum sodium concentrations. As such, physicians and caregivers should avoid overhydration with hypotonic fluids.[18] Complete blood cell counts may be useful as a means of identifying young children at risk of bacteremia. It should be noted, however, that the incidence of bacteremia in children younger than 24 months with or without febrile seizures is the same. When fever is present, the decision regarding the need for laboratory testing should be directed toward identifying the source of the fever rather

than as part of the routine evaluation of the seizure itself.

Action Statement 4

Neuroimaging should not be performed in the routine evaluation of the child with a simple febrile seizure.

- Aggregate evidence level: B (overwhelming evidence from observational studies).
- Benefits: Neuroimaging might provide earlier detection of fixed structural lesions, such as dysplasia, or very rarely, abscess or tumor.
- Harms/risks/costs: Neuroimaging tests are costly, computed tomography (CT) exposes children to radiation, and MRI may require sedation.
- Benefits/harms assessment: Preponderance of harm over benefit.
- Value judgments: Observational data were used for this judgment.
- Role of patient preferences: Although parents may want neuroimaging performed to explain the seizure, they should be reassured that the tests carry risks and will not alter outcome for their child.
- Exclusions: None.
- Intentional vagueness: None.
- Policy level: Strong recommendation.

The literature does not support the use of skull films in evaluation of the child with a febrile seizure.[15,19] No data have been published that either support or negate the need for CT or MRI in the evaluation of children with simple febrile seizures. Data, however, show that CT scanning is associated with radiation exposure that may escalate future cancer risk. MRI is associated with risks from required sedation and high cost.[20,21] Extrapolation of data from the

literature on the use of CT in neurologically healthy children who have generalized epilepsy has shown that clinically important intracranial structural abnormalities in this patient population are uncommon.[22,23]

CONCLUSIONS

Clinicians evaluating infants or young children after a simple febrile seizure should direct their attention toward identifying the cause of the child's fever. Meningitis should be considered in the differential diagnosis for any febrile child, and lumbar puncture should be performed if the child is ill-appearing or if there are clinical signs or symptoms of concern. A lumbar puncture is an option in a child 6 to 12 months of age who is deficient in Hib and *S pneumoniae* immunizations or for whom immunization status is unknown. A lumbar puncture is an option in children who have been pretreated with antibiotics. In general, a simple febrile seizure does not usually require further evaluation, specifically EEGs, blood studies, or neuroimaging.

SUBCOMMITTEE ON FEBRILE SEIZURES, 2002–2010
Patricia K. Duffner, MD (neurology, no conflicts)
Peter H. Berman, MD (neurology, no conflicts)
Robert J. Baumann, MD (neuroepidemiology, no conflicts)
Paul Graham Fisher, MD (neurology, no conflicts)
John L. Green, MD (general pediatrics, no conflicts)
Sanford Schneider, MD (neurology, no conflicts)

STAFF
Caryn Davidson, MA

OVERSIGHT BY THE STEERING COMMITTEE ON QUALITY IMPROVEMENT AND MANAGEMENT, 2009–2011

REFERENCES

1. American Academy of Pediatrics, Provisional Committee on Quality Improvement and Subcommittee on Febrile Seizures. Practice parameter: the neurodiagnostic evaluation of a child with a first simple febrile seizure. *Pediatrics.* 1996;97(5): 769–772; discussion 773–775

2. Michael Marcy S, Kohl KS, Dagan R, et al; Brighton Collaboration Fever Working Group. Fever as an adverse event following immunization: case definition and guidelines of data collection, analysis, and presentation. *Vaccine.* 2004;22(5–6):551–556

3. Nelson KB, Ellenberg JH. Predictors of epilepsy in children who have experienced febrile seizures. *N Engl J Med.* 1976;295(19): 1029–1033

4. Consensus statement: febrile seizures—long-term management of children with fever-associated seizures. *Pediatrics.* 1980; 66(6):1009–1012

5. American Academy of Pediatrics, Steering Committee on Quality Improvement and Management. Classifying recommendations for clinical practice guidelines. *Pediatrics.* 2004;114(3):874–877

6. Trainor JL, Hampers LC, Krug SE, Listernick R. Children with first-time simple febrile seizures are at low risk of serious bacterial illness. *Acad Emerg Med.* 2001;8(8):781–787

7. Shaked O, Peña BM, Linares MY, Baker RL. Simple febrile seizures: are the AAP guidelines regarding lumbar puncture being followed? *Pediatr Emerg Care.* 2009;25(1): 8–11

8. Kimia AA, Capraro AJ, Hummel D, Johnston P, Harper MB. Utility of lumbar puncture for first simple febrile seizure among children 6 to 18 months of age. *Pediatrics.* 2009; 123(1):6–12

9. Warden CR, Zibulewsky J, Mace S, Gold C, Gausche-Hill M. Evaluation and management of febrile seizures in the out-of-hospital and emergency department settings. *Ann Emerg Med.* 2003;41(2):215–222

10. Rutter N, Smales OR. Role of routine investigations in children presenting with their first febrile convulsion. *Arch Dis Child.* 1977; 52(3):188–191

11. Green SM, Rothrock SG, Clem KJ, Zurcher RF, Mellick L. Can seizures be the sole manifestation of meningitis in febrile children? *Pediatrics.* 1993;92(4):527–534

12. Kuturec M, Emoto SE, Sofijanov N, et al. Febrile seizures: is the EEG a useful predictor of recurrences? *Clin Pediatr (Phila).* 1997; 36(1):31–36

13. Frantzen E, Lennox-Buchthal M, Nygaard A. Longitudinal EEG and clinical study of children with febrile convulsions. *Electroencephalogr Clin Neurophysiol.* 1968;24(3): 197–212

14. Thorn I. The significance of electroencephalography in febrile convulsions. In: Akimoto H, Kazamatsuri H, Seino M, Ward A, eds. *Advances in Epileptology: XIIIth International Epilepsy Symposium.* New York, NY: Raven Press; 1982:93–95

15. Jaffe M, Bar-Joseph G, Tirosh E. Fever and convulsions: indications for laboratory investigations. *Pediatrics.* 1981;67(5): 729–731

16. Gerber MA, Berliner BC. The child with a "simple" febrile seizure: appropriate diagnostic evaluation. *Am J Dis Child.* 1981; 135(5):431–443

17. Heijbel J, Blom S, Bergfors PG. Simple febrile convulsions: a prospective incidence study and an evaluation of investigations initially needed. *Neuropadiatrie.* 1980;11(1): 45–56

18. Thoman JE, Duffner PK, Shucard JL. Do serum sodium levels predict febrile seizure recurrence within 24 hours? *Pediatr Neurol.* 2004;31(5):342–344

19. Nealis GT, McFadden SW, Ames RA, Ouellette EM. Routine skull roentgenograms in the management of simple febrile seizures. *J Pediatr.* 1977;90(4):595–596

20. Stein SC, Hurst RW, Sonnad SS. Meta-analysis of cranial CT scans in children: a mathematical model to predict radiation-induced tumors associated with radiation exposure that may escalate future cancer risk. *Pediatr Neurosurg.* 2008;44(6): 448–457

21. Brenner DJ, Hall EJ. Computed tomography: an increasing source of radiation exposure. *N Engl J Med.* 2007;357(22):2277–2284

22. Yang PJ, Berger PE, Cohen ME, Duffner PK. Computed tomography and childhood seizure disorders. *Neurology.* 1979;29(8): 1084–1088

23. Bachman DS, Hodges FJ, Freeman JM. Computerized axial tomography in chronic seizure disorders of childhood. *Pediatrics.* 1976;58(6):828–832

Febrile Seizures Clinical Practice Guidelines
Quick Reference Tools

- Recommendation Summaries
  — Febrile Seizures: Clinical Practice Guideline for the Long-term Management of the Child With Simple Febrile Seizures
  — Febrile Seizures: Guidelines for the Neurodiagnostic Evaluation of the Child With a Simple Febrile Seizure
- *ICD-9-CM/ICD-10-CM* Coding Quick Reference for Febrile Seizures
- AAP Patient Education Handout
  — *Febrile Seizures*

Recommendation Summaries

Febrile Seizures: Clinical Practice Guideline for the Long-term Management of the Child With Simple Febrile Seizures

On the basis of the risks and benefits of the effective therapies, neither continuous nor intermittent anticonvulsant therapy is recommended for children with 1 or more simple febrile seizures.

- Aggregate evidence quality: B (randomized, controlled trials and diagnostic studies with minor limitations).
- Benefit: prevention of recurrent febrile seizures, which are not harmful and do not significantly increase the risk for development of future epilepsy.
- Harm: adverse effects including rare fatal hepatotoxicity (especially in children younger than 2 years who are also at greatest risk of febrile seizures), thrombocytopenia, weight loss and gain, gastrointestinal disturbances, and pancreatitis with valproic acid and hyperactivity, irritability, lethargy, sleep disturbances, and hypersensitivity reactions with phenobarbital; lethargy, drowsiness, and ataxia for intermittent diazepam as well as the risk of masking an evolving central nervous system infection.
- Benefits/harms assessment: preponderance of harm over benefit.
- Policy level: recommendation.

Febrile Seizures: Guidelines for the Neurodiagnostic Evaluation of the Child With a Simple Febrile Seizure

Action Statement 1a

A lumbar puncture should be performed in any child who presents with a seizure and a fever and has meningeal signs and symptoms (eg, neck stiffness, Kernig and/or Brudzinski signs) or in any child whose history or examination suggests the presence of meningitis or intracranial infection.

Action Statement 1b

In any infant between 6 and 12 months of age who presents with a seizure and fever, a lumbar puncture is an option when the child is considered deficient in *Haemophilus influenzae* type b (Hib) or *Streptococcus pneumoniae* immunizations (ie, has not received scheduled immunizations as recommended) or when immunization status cannot be determined because of an increased risk of bacterial meningitis.

Action Statement 1c

A lumbar puncture is an option in the child who presents with a seizure and fever and is pretreated with antibiotics, because antibiotic treatment can mask the signs and symptoms of meningitis.

Action Statement 2

An electroencephalogram (EEG) should not be performed in the evaluation of a neurologically healthy child with a simple febrile seizure.

Action Statement 3

The following tests should not be performed routinely for the sole purpose of identifying the cause of a simple febrile seizure: measurement of serum electrolytes, calcium, phosphorus, magnesium, or blood glucose or complete blood cell count.

Action Statement 4

Neuroimaging should not be performed in the routine evaluation of the child with a simple febrile seizure.

Coding Quick Reference for Febrile Seizures	
ICD-9-CM	*ICD-10-CM*
780.31 Seizure, febrile, simple	**R56.00** Simple febrile convulsions
780.32 Seizure, febrile, complex	**R56.01** Complex febrile convulsions

Febrile Seizures

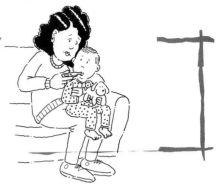

In some children, fevers can trigger seizures. Febrile seizures occur in 2% to 5% of all children between the ages of 6 months and 5 years. Seizures, sometimes called "fits" or "spells," are frightening, but they usually are harmless. Read on for information from the American Academy of Pediatrics that will help you understand febrile seizures and what happens if your child has one.

What is a febrile seizure?

A febrile seizure usually happens during the first few hours of a fever. The child may look strange for a few moments, then stiffen, twitch, and roll his eyes. He will be unresponsive for a short time, his breathing will be disturbed, and his skin may appear a little darker than usual. After the seizure, the child quickly returns to normal. Seizures usually last less than 1 minute but, although uncommon, can last for up to 15 minutes.

Febrile seizures rarely happen more than once within a 24-hour period. Other kinds of seizures (ones that are not caused by fever) last longer, can affect only one part of the body, and may occur repeatedly.

What do I do if my child has a febrile seizure?

If your child has a febrile seizure, act immediately to prevent injury.

- Place her on the floor or bed away from any hard or sharp objects.
- Turn her head to the side so that any saliva or vomit can drain from her mouth.
- Do not put anything into her mouth; she will not swallow her tongue.
- Call your child's doctor.
- If the seizure does not stop after 5 minutes, call 911 or your local emergency number.

Will my child have more seizures?

Febrile seizures tend to run in families. The risk of having seizures with other episodes of fever depends on the age of your child. Children younger than 1 year of age at the time of their first seizure have about a 50% chance of having another febrile seizure. Children older than 1 year of age at the time of their first seizure have only a 30% chance of having a second febrile seizure.

Will my child get epilepsy?

Epilepsy is a term used for multiple and recurrent seizures. Epileptic seizures are not caused by fever. Children with a history of febrile seizures are at only a slightly higher risk of developing epilepsy by age 7 than children who have not had febrile seizures.

Are febrile seizures dangerous?

While febrile seizures may be very scary, they are harmless to the child. Febrile seizures do not cause brain damage, nervous system problems, paralysis, intellectual disability (formerly called mental retardation), or death.

How are febrile seizures treated?

If your child has a febrile seizure, call your child's doctor right away. He or she will want to examine your child in order to determine the cause of your child's fever. It is more important to determine and treat the cause of the fever rather than the seizure. A spinal tap may be done to be sure your child does not have a serious infection like meningitis, especially if your child is younger than 1 year of age.

In general, doctors do not recommend treatment of a simple febrile seizure with preventive medicines. However, this should be discussed with your child's doctor. In cases of prolonged or repeated seizures, the recommendation may be different.

Medicines like acetaminophen and ibuprofen can help lower a fever, but they do not prevent febrile seizures. Your child's doctor will talk with you about the best ways to take care of your child's fever.

If your child has had a febrile seizure, do not fear the worst. These types of seizures are not dangerous to your child and do not cause long-term health problems. If you have concerns about this issue or anything related to your child's health, talk with your child's doctor.

The information contained in this publication should not be used as a substitute for the medical care and advice of your pediatrician. There may be variations in treatment that your pediatrician may recommend based on individual facts and circumstances.

From your doctor

American Academy
of Pediatrics

DEDICATED TO THE HEALTH OF ALL CHILDREN™

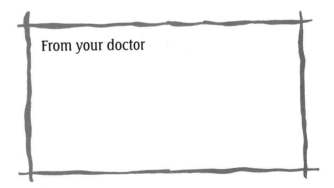

Management of Hyperbilirubinemia in the Newborn Infant 35 or More Weeks of Gestation

- *Clinical Practice Guideline*
- *Technical Report Summary*
- *Technical Report*
- *2009 Commentaries*

Readers of this clinical practice guideline are urged to review the technical reports to enhance the evidence-based decision-making process. The full technical reports are available on the companion CD-ROM.

AMERICAN ACADEMY OF PEDIATRICS

CLINICAL PRACTICE GUIDELINE

Subcommittee on Hyperbilirubinemia

Management of Hyperbilirubinemia in the Newborn Infant 35 or More Weeks of Gestation

ABSTRACT. Jaundice occurs in most newborn infants. Most jaundice is benign, but because of the potential toxicity of bilirubin, newborn infants must be monitored to identify those who might develop severe hyperbilirubinemia and, in rare cases, acute bilirubin encephalopathy or kernicterus. The focus of this guideline is to reduce the incidence of severe hyperbilirubinemia and bilirubin encephalopathy while minimizing the risks of unintended harm such as maternal anxiety, decreased breastfeeding, and unnecessary costs or treatment. Although kernicterus should almost always be preventable, cases continue to occur. These guidelines provide a framework for the prevention and management of hyperbilirubinemia in newborn infants of 35 or more weeks of gestation. In every infant, we recommend that clinicians 1) promote and support successful breastfeeding; 2) perform a systematic assessment before discharge for the risk of severe hyperbilirubinemia; 3) provide early and focused follow-up based on the risk assessment; and 4) when indicated, treat newborns with phototherapy or exchange transfusion to prevent the development of severe hyperbilirubinemia and, possibly, bilirubin encephalopathy (kernicterus). *Pediatrics* 2004; 114:297–316; *hyperbilirubinemia, newborn, kernicterus, bilirubin encephalopathy, phototherapy.*

ABBREVIATIONS. AAP, American Academy of Pediatrics; TSB, total serum bilirubin; TcB, transcutaneous bilirubin; G6PD, glucose-6-phosphate dehydrogenase; ETCO$_c$, end-tidal carbon monoxide corrected for ambient carbon monoxide; B/A, bilirubin/albumin; UB, unbound bilirubin.

BACKGROUND

In October 1994, the Provisional Committee for Quality Improvement and Subcommittee on Hyperbilirubinemia of the American Academy of Pediatrics (AAP) produced a practice parameter dealing with the management of hyperbilirubinemia in the healthy term newborn.[1] The current guideline represents a consensus of the committee charged by the AAP with reviewing and updating the existing guideline and is based on a careful review of the evidence, including a comprehensive literature review by the New England Medical Center Evidence-Based Practice Center.[2] (See "An Evidence-Based Review of Important Issues Concerning Neonatal Hyperbilirubinemia"[3] for a description of the methodology, questions addressed, and conclusions of this report.) This guideline is intended for use by hospitals and pediatricians, neonatologists, family physicians, physician assistants, and advanced practice nurses who treat newborn infants in the hospital and as outpatients. A list of frequently asked questions and answers for parents is available in English and Spanish at www.aap.org/family/jaundicefaq.htm.

DEFINITION OF RECOMMENDATIONS

The evidence-based approach to guideline development requires that the evidence in support of a policy be identified, appraised, and summarized and that an explicit link between evidence and recommendations be defined. Evidence-based recommendations are based on the quality of evidence and the balance of benefits and harms that is anticipated when the recommendation is followed. This guideline uses the definitions for quality of evidence and balance of benefits and harms established by the AAP Steering Committee on Quality Improvement Management.[4] See Appendix 1 for these definitions.

The draft practice guideline underwent extensive peer review by committees and sections within the AAP, outside organizations, and other individuals identified by the subcommittee as experts in the field. Liaison representatives to the subcommittee were invited to distribute the draft to other representatives and committees within their specialty organizations. The resulting comments were reviewed by the subcommittee and, when appropriate, incorporated into the guideline.

BILIRUBIN ENCEPHALOPATHY AND KERNICTERUS

Although originally a pathologic diagnosis characterized by bilirubin staining of the brainstem nuclei and cerebellum, the term "kernicterus" has come to be used interchangeably with both the acute and chronic findings of bilirubin encephalopathy. Bilirubin encephalopathy describes the clinical central nervous system findings caused by bilirubin toxicity to the basal ganglia and various brainstem nuclei. To avoid confusion and encourage greater consistency in the literature, the committee recommends that in infants the term "acute bilirubin encephalopathy" be used to describe the acute manifestations of bilirubin toxicity seen in the first weeks after birth and that the term "kernicterus" be reserved for the chronic and permanent clinical sequelae of bilirubin toxicity.

See Appendix 1 for the clinical manifestations of acute bilirubin encephalopathy and kernicterus.

FOCUS OF GUIDELINE

The overall aim of this guideline is to promote an approach that will reduce the frequency of severe neonatal hyperbilirubinemia and bilirubin encephalopathy and minimize the risk of unintended harm such as increased anxiety, decreased breastfeeding, or unnecessary treatment for the general population and excessive cost and waste. Recent reports of kernicterus indicate that this condition, although rare, is still occurring.[2,5–10]

Analysis of these reported cases of kernicterus suggests that if health care personnel follow the recommendations listed in this guideline, kernicterus would be largely preventable.

These guidelines emphasize the importance of universal systematic assessment for the risk of severe hyperbilirubinemia, close follow-up, and prompt intervention when indicated. The recommendations apply to the care of infants at 35 or more weeks of gestation. These recommendations seek to further the aims defined by the Institute of Medicine as appropriate for health care:[11] safety, effectiveness, efficiency, timeliness, patient-centeredness, and equity. They specifically emphasize the principles of patient safety and the key role of timeliness of interventions to prevent adverse outcomes resulting from neonatal hyperbilirubinemia.

The following are the key elements of the recommendations provided by this guideline. Clinicians should:

1. Promote and support successful breastfeeding.
2. Establish nursery protocols for the identification and evaluation of hyperbilirubinemia.
3. Measure the total serum bilirubin (TSB) or transcutaneous bilirubin (TcB) level on infants jaundiced in the first 24 hours.
4. Recognize that visual estimation of the degree of jaundice can lead to errors, particularly in darkly pigmented infants.
5. Interpret all bilirubin levels according to the infant's age in hours.
6. Recognize that infants at less than 38 weeks' gestation, particularly those who are breastfed, are at higher risk of developing hyperbilirubinemia and require closer surveillance and monitoring.
7. Perform a systematic assessment on all infants before discharge for the risk of severe hyperbilirubinemia.
8. Provide parents with written and verbal information about newborn jaundice.
9. Provide appropriate follow-up based on the time of discharge and the risk assessment.
10. Treat newborns, when indicated, with phototherapy or exchange transfusion.

PRIMARY PREVENTION

In numerous policy statements, the AAP recommends breastfeeding for all healthy term and near-term newborns. This guideline strongly supports this general recommendation.

RECOMMENDATION 1.0: Clinicians should advise mothers to nurse their infants at least 8 to 12 times per day for the first several days[12] *(evidence quality C: benefits exceed harms).*

Poor caloric intake and/or dehydration associated with inadequate breastfeeding may contribute to the development of hyperbilirubinemia.[6,13,14] Increasing the frequency of nursing decreases the likelihood of subsequent significant hyperbilirubinemia in breastfed infants.[15–17] Providing appropriate support and advice to breastfeeding mothers increases the likelihood that breastfeeding will be successful.

Additional information on how to assess the adequacy of intake in a breastfed newborn is provided in Appendix 1.

RECOMMENDATION 1.1: The AAP recommends against routine supplementation of nondehydrated breastfed infants with water or dextrose water (evidence quality B and C: harms exceed benefits).

Supplementation with water or dextrose water will not prevent hyperbilirubinemia or decrease TSB levels.[18,19]

SECONDARY PREVENTION

RECOMMENDATION 2.0: Clinicians should perform ongoing systematic assessments during the neonatal period for the risk of an infant developing severe hyperbilirubinemia.

Blood Typing

RECOMMENDATION 2.1: All pregnant women should be tested for ABO and Rh (D) blood types and have a serum screen for unusual isoimmune antibodies (evidence quality B: benefits exceed harms).

RECOMMENDATION 2.1.1: If a mother has not had prenatal blood grouping or is Rh-negative, a direct antibody test (or Coombs' test), blood type, and an Rh (D) type on the infant's (cord) blood are strongly recommended (evidence quality B: benefits exceed harms).

RECOMMENDATION 2.1.2: If the maternal blood is group O, Rh-positive, it is an option to test the cord blood for the infant's blood type and direct antibody test, but it is not required provided that there is appropriate surveillance, risk assessment before discharge, and follow-up[20] *(evidence quality C: benefits exceed harms).*

Clinical Assessment

RECOMMENDATION 2.2: Clinicians should ensure that all infants are routinely monitored for the development of jaundice, and nurseries should have established protocols for the assessment of jaundice. Jaundice should be assessed whenever the infant's vital signs are measured but no less than every 8 to 12 hours (evidence quality D: benefits versus harms exceptional).

In newborn infants, jaundice can be detected by blanching the skin with digital pressure, revealing the underlying color of the skin and subcutaneous tissue. The assessment of jaundice must be per-

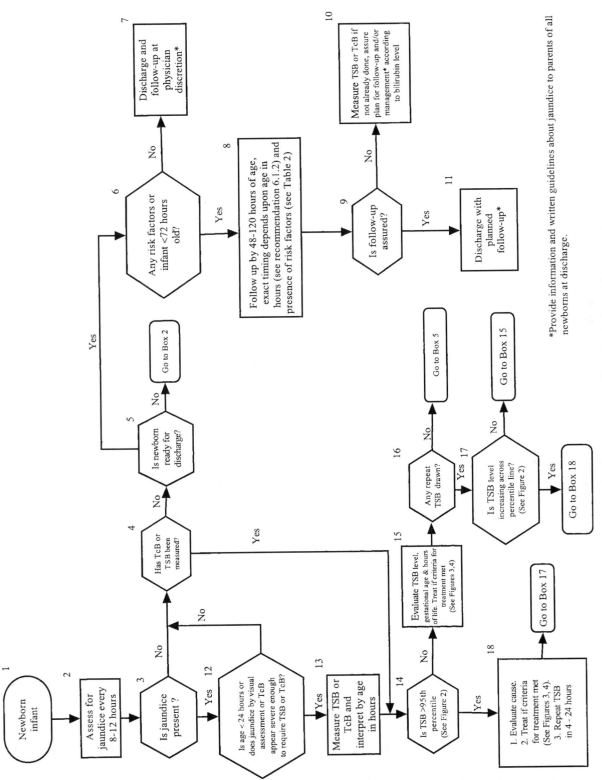

Fig 1. Algorithm for the management of jaundice in the newborn nursery.

*Provide information and written guidelines about jaundice to parents of all newborns at discharge.

formed in a well-lit room or, preferably, in daylight at a window. Jaundice is usually seen first in the face and progresses caudally to the trunk and extremities,[21] but visual estimation of bilirubin levels from the degree of jaundice can lead to errors.[22–24] In most infants with TSB levels of less than 15 mg/dL (257 μmol/L), noninvasive TcB-measurement devices can provide a valid estimate of the TSB level.[2,25–29] See Appendix 1 for additional information on the clinical evaluation of jaundice and the use of TcB measurements.

RECOMMENDATION 2.2.1: Protocols for the assessment of jaundice should include the circumstances in which nursing staff can obtain a TcB level or order a TSB measurement (evidence quality D: benefits versus harms exceptional).

Laboratory Evaluation

RECOMMENDATION 3.0: A TcB and/or TSB measurement should be performed on every infant who is jaundiced in the first 24 hours after birth (Fig 1 and Table 1)[30] (evidence quality C: benefits exceed harms). The need for and timing of a repeat TcB or TSB measurement will depend on the zone in which the TSB falls (Fig 2),[25,31] the age of the infant, and the evolution of the hyperbilirubinemia. Recommendations for TSB measurements after the age of 24 hours are provided in Fig 1 and Table 1.

See Appendix 1 for capillary versus venous bilirubin levels.

RECOMMENDATION 3.1: A TcB and/or TSB measurement should be performed if the jaundice appears excessive for the infant's age (evidence quality D: benefits versus harms exceptional). If there is any doubt about the degree of jaundice, the TSB or TcB should be measured. Visual estimation of bilirubin levels from the degree of jaundice can lead to errors, particularly in darkly pigmented infants (evidence quality C: benefits exceed harms).

RECOMMENDATION 3.2: All bilirubin levels should be interpreted according to the infant's age in hours (Fig 2) (evidence quality C: benefits exceed harms).

Cause of Jaundice

RECOMMENDATION 4.1: The possible cause of jaundice should be sought in an infant receiving phototherapy or whose TSB level is rising rapidly (ie, crossing percentiles [Fig 2]) and is not explained by the history and physical examination (evidence quality D: benefits versus harms exceptional).

RECOMMENDATION 4.1.1: Infants who have an elevation of direct-reacting or conjugated bilirubin should have a urinalysis and urine culture.[32] Additional laboratory evaluation for sepsis should be performed if indicated by history and physical examination (evidence quality C: benefits exceed harms).

See Appendix 1 for definitions of abnormal levels of direct-reacting and conjugated bilirubin.

RECOMMENDATION 4.1.2: Sick infants and those who are jaundiced at or beyond 3 weeks should have a measurement of total and direct or conjugated bilirubin to identify cholestasis (Table 1) (evidence quality D: benefit versus harms exceptional). The results of the newborn thyroid and galactosemia screen should also be checked in these infants (evidence quality D: benefits versus harms exceptional).

RECOMMENDATION 4.1.3: If the direct-reacting or conjugated bilirubin level is elevated, additional evaluation for the causes of cholestasis is recommended (evidence quality C: benefits exceed harms).

RECOMMENDATION 4.1.4: Measurement of the glucose-6-phosphate dehydrogenase (G6PD) level is recommended for a jaundiced infant who is receiving phototherapy and whose family history or ethnic or geographic origin suggest the likelihood of G6PD deficiency or for an infant in whom the response to phototherapy is poor (Fig 3) (evidence quality C: benefits exceed harms).

G6PD deficiency is widespread and frequently unrecognized, and although it is more common in the populations around the Mediterranean and in the Middle East, Arabian peninsula, Southeast Asia, and Africa, immigration and intermarriage have transformed G6PD deficiency into a global problem.[33,34]

TABLE 1. Laboratory Evaluation of the Jaundiced Infant of 35 or More Weeks' Gestation

Indications	Assessments
Jaundice in first 24 h	Measure TcB and/or TSB
Jaundice appears excessive for infant's age	Measure TcB and/or TSB
Infant receiving phototherapy or TSB rising rapidly (ie, crossing percentiles [Fig 2]) and unexplained by history and physical examination	Blood type and Coombs' test, if not obtained with cord blood
	Complete blood count and smear
	Measure direct or conjugated bilirubin
	It is an option to perform reticulocyte count, G6PD, and ETCO$_c$, if available
	Repeat TSB in 4–24 h depending on infant's age and TSB level
TSB concentration approaching exchange levels or not responding to phototherapy	Perform reticulocyte count, G6PD, albumin, ETCO$_c$, if available
Elevated direct (or conjugated) bilirubin level	Do urinalysis and urine culture. Evaluate for sepsis if indicated by history and physical examination
Jaundice present at or beyond age 3 wk, or sick infant	Total and direct (or conjugated) bilirubin level
	If direct bilirubin elevated, evaluate for causes of cholestasis
	Check results of newborn thyroid and galactosemia screen, and evaluate infant for signs or symptoms of hypothyroidism

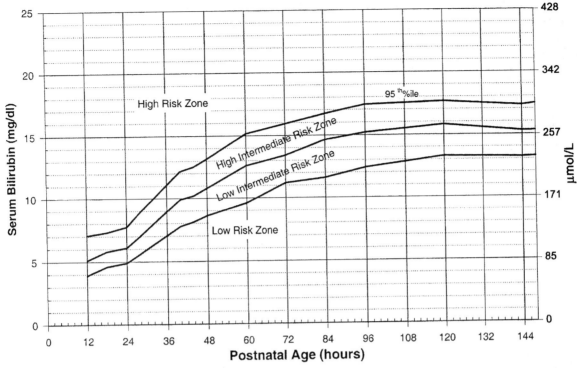

Fig 2. Nomogram for designation of risk in 2840 well newborns at 36 or more weeks' gestational age with birth weight of 2000 g or more or 35 or more weeks' gestational age and birth weight of 2500 g or more based on the hour-specific serum bilirubin values. The serum bilirubin level was obtained before discharge, and the zone in which the value fell predicted the likelihood of a subsequent bilirubin level exceeding the 95th percentile (high-risk zone) as shown in Appendix 1, Table 4. Used with permission from Bhutani et al.[31] See Appendix 1 for additional information about this nomogram, which should not be used to represent the natural history of neonatal hyperbilirubinemia.

Furthermore, G6PD deficiency occurs in 11% to 13% of African Americans, and kernicterus has occurred in some of these infants.[5,33] In a recent report, G6PD deficiency was considered to be the cause of hyperbilirubinemia in 19 of 61 (31.5%) infants who developed kernicterus.[5] (See Appendix 1 for additional information on G6PD deficiency.)

Risk Assessment Before Discharge

RECOMMENDATION 5.1: Before discharge, every newborn should be assessed for the risk of developing severe hyperbilirubinemia, and all nurseries should establish protocols for assessing this risk. Such assessment is particularly important in infants who are discharged before the age of 72 hours (evidence quality C: benefits exceed harms).

RECOMMENDATION 5.1.1: The AAP recommends 2 clinical options used individually or in combination for the systematic assessment of risk: predischarge measurement of the bilirubin level using TSB or TcB and/or assessment of clinical risk factors. Whether either or both options are used, appropriate follow-up after discharge is essential (evidence quality C: benefits exceed harms).

The best documented method for assessing the risk of subsequent hyperbilirubinemia is to measure the TSB or TcB level[25,31,35–38] and plot the results on a nomogram (Fig 2). A TSB level can be obtained at the time of the routine metabolic screen, thus obviating the need for an additional blood sample. Some authors have suggested that a TSB measurement should be part of the routine screening of all newborns.[5,31] An infant whose predischarge TSB is in the

low-risk zone (Fig 2) is at very low risk of developing severe hyperbilirubinemia.[5,38]

Table 2 lists those factors that are clinically signif-

TABLE 2. Risk Factors for Development of Severe Hyperbilirubinemia in Infants of 35 or More Weeks' Gestation (in Approximate Order of Importance)

Major risk factors
  Predischarge TSB or TcB level in the high-risk zone (Fig 2)[25,31]
  Jaundice observed in the first 24 h[30]
  Blood group incompatibility with positive direct antiglobulin test, other known hemolytic disease (eg, G6PD deficiency), elevated ETCO$_c$
  Gestational age 35–36 wk[39,40]
  Previous sibling received phototherapy[40,41]
  Cephalohematoma or significant bruising[39]
  Exclusive breastfeeding, particularly if nursing is not going well and weight loss is excessive[39,40]
  East Asian race[39]*
Minor risk factors
  Predischarge TSB or TcB level in the high intermediate-risk zone[25,31]
  Gestational age 37–38 wk[39,40]
  Jaundice observed before discharge[40]
  Previous sibling with jaundice[40,41]
  Macrosomic infant of a diabetic mother[42,43]
  Maternal age ≥25 y[39]
  Male gender[39,40]
Decreased risk (these factors are associated with decreased risk of significant jaundice, listed in order of decreasing importance)
  TSB or TcB level in the low-risk zone (Fig 2)[25,31]
  Gestational age ≥41 wk[39]
  Exclusive bottle feeding[39,40]
  Black race[38]*
  Discharge from hospital after 72 h[40,44]

* Race as defined by mother's description.

icant and most frequently associated with an increase in the risk of severe hyperbilirubinemia. But, because these risk factors are common and the risk of hyperbilirubinemia is small, individually the factors are of limited use as predictors of significant hyperbilirubinemia.[39] Nevertheless, if no risk factors are present, the risk of severe hyperbilirubinemia is extremely low, and the more risk factors present, the greater the risk of severe hyperbilirubinemia.[39] The important risk factors most frequently associated with severe hyperbilirubinemia are breastfeeding, gestation below 38 weeks, significant jaundice in a previous sibling, and jaundice noted before discharge.[39,40] A formula-fed infant of 40 or more weeks' gestation is at very low risk of developing severe hyperbilirubinemia.[39]

Hospital Policies and Procedures

RECOMMENDATION 6.1: All hospitals should provide written and verbal information for parents at the time of discharge, which should include an explanation of jaundice, the need to monitor infants for jaundice, and advice on how monitoring should be done (evidence quality D: benefits versus harms exceptional).

An example of a parent-information handout is available in English and Spanish at www.aap.org/family/jaundicefaq.htm.

Follow-up

RECOMMENDATION 6.1.1: All infants should be examined by a qualified health care professional in the first few days after discharge to assess infant well-being and the presence or absence of jaundice. The timing and location of this assessment will be determined by the length of stay in the nursery, presence or absence of risk factors for hyperbilirubinemia (Table 2 and Fig 2), and risk of other neonatal problems (evidence quality C: benefits exceed harms).

Timing of Follow-up

RECOMMENDATION 6.1.2: Follow-up should be provided as follows:

Infant Discharged	Should Be Seen by Age
Before age 24 h	72 h
Between 24 and 47.9 h	96 h
Between 48 and 72 h	120 h

For some newborns discharged before 48 hours, 2 follow-up visits may be required, the first visit between 24 and 72 hours and the second between 72 and 120 hours. Clinical judgment should be used in determining follow-up. Earlier or more frequent follow-up should be provided for those who have risk factors for hyperbilirubinemia (Table 2), whereas those discharged with few or no risk factors can be seen after longer intervals (evidence quality C: benefits exceed harms).

RECOMMENDATION 6.1.3: If appropriate follow-up cannot be ensured in the presence of elevated risk for developing severe hyperbilirubinemia, it may be necessary to delay discharge either until appropriate follow-up can be ensured or the period of greatest risk has passed (72-96 hours) (evidence quality D: benefits versus harms exceptional).

Follow-up Assessment

RECOMMENDATION 6.1.4: The follow-up assessment should include the infant's weight and percent change from birth weight, adequacy of intake, the pattern of voiding and stooling, and the presence or absence of jaundice (evidence quality C: benefits exceed harms). Clinical judgment should be used to determine the need for a bilirubin measurement. If there is any doubt about the degree of jaundice, the TSB or TcB level should be measured. Visual estimation of bilirubin levels can lead to errors, particularly in darkly pigmented infants (evidence quality C: benefits exceed harms).

See Appendix 1 for assessment of the adequacy of intake in breastfeeding infants.

TREATMENT

Phototherapy and Exchange Transfusion

RECOMMENDATION 7.1: Recommendations for treatment are given in Table 3 and Figs 3 and 4 (evidence quality C: benefits exceed harms). If the TSB does not fall or continues to rise despite intensive phototherapy, it is very likely that hemolysis is occurring. The committee's recommendations for discontinuing phototherapy can be found in Appendix 2.

RECOMMENDATION 7.1.1: In using the guidelines for phototherapy and exchange transfusion (Figs 3 and 4), the direct-reacting (or conjugated) bilirubin level should not be subtracted from the total (evidence quality D: benefits versus harms exceptional).

In unusual situations in which the direct bilirubin level is 50% or more of the total bilirubin, there are no good data to provide guidance for therapy, and consultation with an expert in the field is recommended.

RECOMMENDATION 7.1.2: If the TSB is at a level at which exchange transfusion is recommended (Fig 4) or if the TSB level is 25 mg/dL (428 μmol/L) or higher at any time, it is a medical emergency and the infant should be admitted immediately and directly to a hospital pediatric service for intensive phototherapy. These infants should not be referred to the emergency department, because it delays the initiation of treatment[54] (evidence quality C: benefits exceed harms).

RECOMMENDATION 7.1.3: Exchange transfusions should be performed only by trained personnel in a neonatal intensive care unit with full monitoring and resuscitation capabilities (evidence quality D: benefits versus harms exceptional).

RECOMMENDATION 7.1.4: In isoimmune hemolytic disease, administration of intravenous γ-globulin (0.5-1 g/kg over 2 hours) is recommended if the TSB is rising despite intensive phototherapy or the TSB level is within 2 to 3 mg/dL (34-51 μmol/L) of the exchange level (Fig 4).[55] If necessary, this dose can be repeated in 12 hours (evidence quality B: benefits exceed harms).

Intravenous γ-globulin has been shown to reduce the need for exchange transfusions in Rh and ABO hemolytic disease.[55–58] Although data are limited, it is reasonable to assume that intravenous γ-globulin will also be helpful in the other types of Rh hemolytic disease such as anti-C and anti-E.

TABLE 3. Example of a Clinical Pathway for Management of the Newborn Infant Readmitted for Phototherapy or Exchange Transfusion

Treatment
    Use intensive phototherapy and/or exchange transfusion as indicated in Figs 3 and 4 (see
        Appendix 2 for details of phototherapy use)
Laboratory tests
    TSB and direct bilirubin levels
    Blood type (ABO, Rh)
    Direct antibody test (Coombs')
    Serum albumin
    Complete blood cell count with differential and smear for red cell morphology
    Reticulocyte count
    $ETCO_c$ (if available)
    G6PD if suggested by ethnic or geographic origin or if poor response to phototherapy
    Urine for reducing substances
    If history and/or presentation suggest sepsis, perform blood culture, urine culture, and
        cerebrospinal fluid for protein, glucose, cell count, and culture
Interventions
    If TSB ≥25 mg/dL (428 μmol/L) or ≥20 mg/dL (342 μmol/L) in a sick infant or infant <38 wk
        gestation, obtain a type and crossmatch, and request blood in case an exchange transfusion is
        necessary
    In infants with isoimmune hemolytic disease and TSB level rising in spite of intensive
        phototherapy or within 2–3 mg/dL (34–51 μmol/L) of exchange level (Fig 4), administer
        intravenous immunoglobulin 0.5–1 g/kg over 2 h and repeat in 12 h if necessary
    If infant's weight loss from birth is >12% or there is clinical or biochemical evidence of
        dehydration, recommend formula or expressed breast milk. If oral intake is in question, give
        intravenous fluids.
For infants receiving intensive phototherapy
    Breastfeed or bottle-feed (formula or expressed breast milk) every 2–3 h
    If TSB ≥25 mg/dL (428 μmol/L), repeat TSB within 2–3 h
    If TSB 20–25 mg/dL (342–428 μmol/L), repeat within 3–4 h. If TSB <20 mg/dL (342 μmol/L),
        repeat in 4–6 h. If TSB continues to fall, repeat in 8–12 h
    If TSB is not decreasing or is moving closer to level for exchange transfusion or the
        TSB/albumin ratio exceeds levels shown in Fig 4, consider exchange transfusion (see Fig 4 for
        exchange transfusion recommendations)
    When TSB is <13–14 mg/dL (239 μmol/L), discontinue phototherapy
    Depending on the cause of the hyperbilirubinemia, it is an option to measure TSB 24 h after
        discharge to check for rebound

Serum Albumin Levels and the Bilirubin/Albumin Ratio

RECOMMENDATION 7.1.5: It is an option to measure the serum albumin level and consider an albumin level of less than 3.0 g/dL as one risk factor for lowering the threshold for phototherapy use (see Fig 3) (evidence quality D: benefits versus risks exceptional.).

RECOMMENDATION 7.1.6: If an exchange transfusion is being considered, the serum albumin level should be measured and the bilirubin/albumin (B/A) ratio used in conjunction with the TSB level and other factors in determining the need for exchange transfusion (see Fig 4) (evidence quality D: benefits versus harms exceptional).

The recommendations shown above for treating hyperbilirubinemia are based primarily on TSB levels and other factors that affect the risk of bilirubin encephalopathy. This risk might be increased by a prolonged (rather than a brief) exposure to a certain TSB level.[59,60] Because the published data that address this issue are limited, however, it is not possible to provide specific recommendations for intervention based on the duration of hyperbilirubinemia.

See Appendix 1 for the basis for recommendations 7.1 through 7.1.6 and for the recommendations provided in Figs 3 and 4. Appendix 1 also contains a discussion of the risks of exchange transfusion and the use of B/A binding.

Acute Bilirubin Encephalopathy

RECOMMENDATION 7.1.7: Immediate exchange transfusion is recommended in any infant who is jaun-

diced and manifests the signs of the intermediate to advanced stages of acute bilirubin encephalopathy[61,62] (hypertonia, arching, retrocollis, opisthotonos, fever, high-pitched cry) even if the TSB is falling (evidence quality D: benefits versus risks exceptional).

Phototherapy

RECOMMENDATION 7.2: All nurseries and services treating infants should have the necessary equipment to provide intensive phototherapy (see Appendix 2) (evidence quality D: benefits exceed risks).

Outpatient Management of the Jaundiced Breastfed Infant

RECOMMENDATION 7.3: In breastfed infants who require phototherapy (Fig 3), the AAP recommends that, if possible, breastfeeding should be continued (evidence quality C: benefits exceed harms). It is also an option to interrupt temporarily breastfeeding and substitute formula. This can reduce bilirubin levels and/or enhance the efficacy of phototherapy[63–65] (evidence quality B: benefits exceed harms). In breastfed infants receiving phototherapy, supplementation with expressed breast milk or formula is appropriate if the infant's intake seems inadequate, weight loss is excessive, or the infant seems dehydrated.

IMPLEMENTATION STRATEGIES

The Institute of Medicine[11] recommends a dramatic change in the way the US health care system

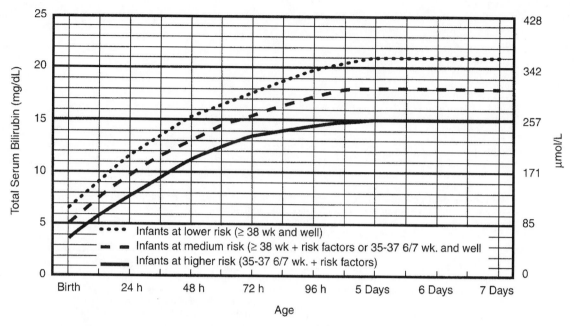

- Use total bilirubin. Do not subtract direct reacting or conjugated bilirubin.
- Risk factors = isoimmune hemolytic disease, G6PD deficiency, asphyxia, significant lethargy, temperature instability, sepsis, acidosis, or albumin < 3.0g/dL (if measured)
- For well infants 35-37 6/7 wk can adjust TSB levels for intervention around the medium risk line. It is an option to intervene at lower TSB levels for infants closer to 35 wks and at higher TSB levels for those closer to 37 6/7 wk.
- It is an option to provide conventional phototherapy in hospital or at home at TSB levels 2-3 mg/dL (35-50mmol/L) below those shown but home phototherapy should not be used in any infant with risk factors.

Fig 3. Guidelines for phototherapy in hospitalized infants of 35 or more weeks' gestation.
   Note: These guidelines are based on limited evidence and the levels shown are approximations. The guidelines refer to the use of intensive phototherapy which should be used when the TSB exceeds the line indicated for each category. Infants are designated as "higher risk" because of the potential negative effects of the conditions listed on albumin binding of bilirubin,[45–47] the blood-brain barrier,[48] and the susceptibility of the brain cells to damage by bilirubin.[48]
   "Intensive phototherapy" implies irradiance in the blue-green spectrum (wavelengths of approximately 430–490 nm) of at least 30 $\mu W/cm^2$ per nm (measured at the infant's skin directly below the center of the phototherapy unit) and delivered to as much of the infant's surface area as possible. Note that irradiance measured below the center of the light source is much greater than that measured at the periphery. Measurements should be made with a radiometer specified by the manufacturer of the phototherapy system.
   See Appendix 2 for additional information on measuring the dose of phototherapy, a description of intensive phototherapy, and of light sources used. If total serum bilirubin levels approach or exceed the exchange transfusion line (Fig 4), the sides of the bassinet, incubator, or warmer should be lined with aluminum foil or white material.[50] This will increase the surface area of the infant exposed and increase the efficacy of phototherapy.[51]
   If the total serum bilirubin does not decrease or continues to rise in an infant who is receiving intensive phototherapy, this strongly suggests the presence of hemolysis.
   Infants who receive phototherapy and have an elevated direct-reacting or conjugated bilirubin level (cholestatic jaundice) may develop the bronze-baby syndrome. See Appendix 2 for the use of phototherapy in these infants.

ensures the safety of patients. The perspective of safety as a purely individual responsibility must be replaced by the concept of safety as a property of systems. Safe systems are characterized by a shared knowledge of the goal, a culture emphasizing safety, the ability of each person within the system to act in a manner that promotes safety, minimizing the use of memory, and emphasizing the use of standard procedures (such as checklists), and the involvement of patients/families as partners in the process of care.
   These principles can be applied to the challenge of preventing severe hyperbilirubinemia and kernicterus. A systematic approach to the implementation of these guidelines should result in greater safety. Such approaches might include

- The establishment of standing protocols for nursing assessment of jaundice, including testing TcB and TSB levels, without requiring physician orders.

- Checklists or reminders associated with risk factors, age at discharge, and laboratory test results that provide guidance for appropriate follow-up.
- Explicit educational materials for parents (a key component of all AAP guidelines) concerning the identification of newborns with jaundice.

FUTURE RESEARCH

Epidemiology of Bilirubin-Induced Central Nervous System Damage

   There is a need for appropriate epidemiologic data to document the incidence of kernicterus in the newborn population, the incidence of other adverse effects attributable to hyperbilirubinemia and its management, and the number of infants whose TSB levels exceed 25 or 30 mg/dL (428-513 $\mu mol/L$). Organizations such as the Centers for Disease Control and Prevention should implement strategies for appropriate data gathering to identify the number of

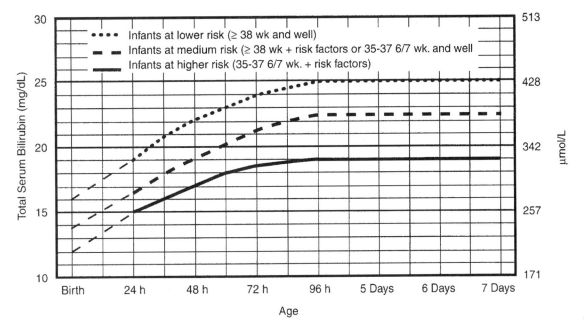

- The dashed lines for the first 24 hours indicate uncertainty due to a wide range of clinical circumstances and a range of responses to phototherapy.
- Immediate exchange transfusion is recommended if infant shows signs of acute bilirubin encephalopathy (hypertonia, arching, retrocollis, opisthotonos, fever, high pitched cry) or if TSB is ≥5 mg/dL (85 µmol/L) above these lines.
- Risk factors - isoimmune hemolytic disease, G6PD deficiency, asphyxia, significant lethargy, temperature instability, sepsis, acidosis.
- Measure serum albumin and calculate B/A ratio (See legend)
- Use total bilirubin. Do not subtract direct reacting or conjugated bilirubin
- If infant is well and 35-37 6/7 wk (median risk) can individualize TSB levels for exchange based on actual gestational age.

Fig 4. Guidelines for exchange transfusion in infants 35 or more weeks' gestation.

Note that these suggested levels represent a consensus of most of the committee but are based on limited evidence, and the levels shown are approximations. See ref. 3 for risks and complications of exchange transfusion. During birth hospitalization, exchange transfusion is recommended if the TSB rises to these levels despite intensive phototherapy. For readmitted infants, if the TSB level is above the exchange level, repeat TSB measurement every 2 to 3 hours and consider exchange if the TSB remains above the levels indicated after intensive phototherapy for 6 hours.

The following B/A ratios can be used together with but in not in lieu of the TSB level as an additional factor in determining the need for exchange transfusion[52]:

Risk Category	B/A Ratio at Which Exchange Transfusion Should be Considered	
	TSB mg/dL/Alb, g/dL	TSB µmol/L/Alb, µmol/L
Infants ≥38 0/7 wk	8.0	0.94
Infants 35 0/7–36 6/7 wk and well or ≥38 0/7 wk if higher risk or isoimmune hemolytic disease or G6PD deficiency	7.2	0.84
Infants 35 0/7–37 6/7 wk if higher risk or isoimmune hemolytic disease or G6PD deficiency	6.8	0.80

If the TSB is at or approaching the exchange level, send blood for immediate type and crossmatch. Blood for exchange transfusion is modified whole blood (red cells and plasma) crossmatched against the mother and compatible with the infant.[53]

infants who develop serum bilirubin levels above 25 or 30 mg/dL (428-513 µmol/L) and those who develop acute and chronic bilirubin encephalopathy. This information will help to identify the magnitude of the problem; the number of infants who need to be screened and treated to prevent 1 case of kernicterus; and the risks, costs, and benefits of different strategies for prevention and treatment of hyperbilirubinemia. In the absence of these data, recommendations for intervention cannot be considered definitive.

Effect of Bilirubin on the Central Nervous System

The serum bilirubin level by itself, except when it is extremely high and associated with bilirubin encephalopathy, is an imprecise indicator of long-term neurodevelopmental outcome.[2] Additional studies are needed on the relationship between central nervous system damage and the duration of hyperbilirubinemia, the binding of bilirubin to albumin, and changes seen in the brainstem auditory evoked response. These studies could help to better identify risk, clarify the effect of bilirubin on the central nervous system, and guide intervention.

Identification of Hemolysis

Because of their poor specificity and sensitivity, the standard laboratory tests for hemolysis (Table 1) are frequently unhelpful.[66,67] However, end-tidal carbon monoxide, corrected for ambient carbon monoxide (ETCO$_c$), levels can confirm the presence or absence of hemolysis, and measurement of ETCO$_c$ is the only clinical test that provides a direct measurement of the rate of heme catabolism and the rate of bilirubin production.[68,69] Thus, ETCO$_c$ may be helpful in determining the degree of surveillance needed and the timing of intervention. It is not yet known, however, how ETCO$_c$ measurements will affect management.

Nomograms and the Measurement of Serum and TcB

It would be useful to develop an age-specific (by hour) nomogram for TSB in populations of newborns that differ with regard to risk factors for hyperbilirubinemia. There is also an urgent need to improve the precision and accuracy of the measurement of TSB in the clinical laboratory.[70,71] Additional studies are also needed to develop and validate noninvasive (transcutaneous) measurements of serum bilirubin and to understand the factors that affect these measurements. These studies should also assess the cost-effectiveness and reproducibility of TcB measurements in clinical practice.[2]

Pharmacologic Therapy

There is now evidence that hyperbilirubinemia can be effectively prevented or treated with tin-mesoporphyrin,[72–75] a drug that inhibits the production of heme oxygenase. Tin-mesoporphyrin is not approved by the US Food and Drug Administration. If approved, tin-mesoporphyrin could find immediate application in preventing the need for exchange transfusion in infants who are not responding to phototherapy.[75]

Dissemination and Monitoring

Research should be directed toward methods for disseminating the information contained in this guideline to increase awareness on the part of physicians, residents, nurses, and parents concerning the issues of neonatal hyperbilirubinemia and strategies for its management. In addition, monitoring systems should be established to identify the impact of these guidelines on the incidence of acute bilirubin encephalopathy and kernicterus and the use of phototherapy and exchange transfusions.

CONCLUSIONS

Kernicterus is still occurring but should be largely preventable if health care personnel follow the recommendations listed in this guideline. These recommendations emphasize the importance of universal, systematic assessment for the risk of severe hyperbilirubinemia, close follow-up, and prompt intervention, when necessary.

SUBCOMMITTEE ON HYPERBILIRUBINEMIA
M. Jeffrey Maisels, MB, BCh, Chairperson
Richard D. Baltz, MD
Vinod K. Bhutani, MD
Thomas B. Newman, MD, MPH
Heather Palmer, MB, BCh
Warren Rosenfeld, MD
David K. Stevenson, MD
Howard B. Weinblatt, MD

CONSULTANT
Charles J. Homer, MD, MPH, Chairperson
   American Academy of Pediatrics Steering
   Committee on Quality Improvement and
   Management

STAFF
Carla T. Herrerias, MPH

ACKNOWLEDGMENTS

M.J.M. received grant support from Natus Medical, Inc, for multinational study of ambient carbon monoxide; WellSpring Pharmaceutical Corporation for study of Stannsoporfin (tin-mesoporphyrin); and Minolta, Inc, for study of the Minolta/Hill-Rom Air-Shields transcutaneous jaundice meter model JM-103. V.K.B. received grant support from WellSpring Pharmaceutical Corporation for study of Stannsoporfin (tin-mesoporphyrin) and Natus Medical, Inc, for multinational study of ambient carbon monoxide and is a consultant (volunteer) to SpectrX (BiliChek transcutaneous bilirubinometer). D.K.S. is a consultant to and holds stock options through Natus Medical, Inc.

The American Academy of Pediatrics Subcommittee on Hyperbilirubinemia gratefully acknowledges the help of the following organizations, committees, and individuals who reviewed drafts of this guideline and provided valuable criticisms and commentary: American Academy of Pediatrics Committee on Nutrition; American Academy of Pediatrics Committee on Practice and Ambulatory Medicine; American Academy of Pediatrics Committee on Child Health Financing; American Academy of Pediatrics Committee on Medical Liability; American Academy of Pediatrics Committee on Fetus and Newborn; American Academy of Pediatrics Section on Perinatal Pediatrics; Centers for Disease Control and Prevention; Parents of Infants and Children With Kernicterus (PICK); Charles Ahlfors, MD; Daniel Batton, MD; Thomas Bojko, MD; Sarah Clune, MD; Sudhakar Ezhuthachan, MD; Lawrence Gartner, MD; Cathy Hammerman, MD; Thor Hansen, MD; Lois Johnson, MD; Michael Kaplan, MB, ChB; Tony McDonagh, PhD; Gerald Merenstein, MD; Mary O'Shea, MD; Max Perlman, MD; Ronald Poland, MD; Alex Robertson, MD; Firmino Rubaltelli, MD; Steven Shapiro, MD; Stanford Singer, MD; Ann Stark, MD; Gautham Suresh, MD; Margot VandeBor, MD; Hank Vreman, PhD; Philip Walson, MD; Jon Watchko, MD; Richard Wennberg, MD; and Chap-Yung Yeung, MD.

REFERENCES

1. American Academy of Pediatrics, Provisional Committee for Quality Improvement and Subcommittee on Hyperbilirubinemia. Practice parameter: management of hyperbilirubinemia in the healthy term newborn. *Pediatrics.* 1994;94:558–562

2. Ip S, Glicken S, Kulig J, Obrien R, Sege R, Lau J. *Management of Neonatal Hyperbilirubinemia.* Rockville, MD: US Department of Health and Human Services, Agency for Healthcare Research and Quality; 2003. AHRQ Publication 03-E011

3. Ip S, Chung M, Kulig J. et al. An evidence-based review of important issues concerning neonatal hyperbilirubinemia. *Pediatrics.* 2004;113(6). Available at: www.pediatrics.org/cgi/content/full/113/6/e644

4. American Academy of Pediatrics, Steering Committee on Quality Improvement and Management. A taxonomy of recommendations. *Pediatrics.* 2004; In press

5. Johnson LH, Bhutani VK, Brown AK. System-based approach to management of neonatal jaundice and prevention of kernicterus. *J Pediatr.* 2002;140:396–403

6. Maisels MJ, Newman TB. Kernicterus in otherwise healthy, breast-fed term newborns. *Pediatrics.* 1995;96:730–733

7. MacDonald M. Hidden risks: early discharge and bilirubin toxicity due to glucose-6-phosphate dehydrogenase deficiency. *Pediatrics.* 1995;96:734–738

8. Penn AA, Enzman DR, Hahn JS, Stevenson DK. Kernicterus in a full term infant. *Pediatrics.* 1994;93:1003–1006

9. Washington EC, Ector W, Abboud M, Ohning B, Holden K. Hemolytic jaundice due to G6PD deficiency causing kernicterus in a female newborn. *South Med J.* 1995;88:776–779

10. Ebbesen F. Recurrence of kernicterus in term and near-term infants in Denmark. *Acta Paediatr.* 2000;89:1213–1217

11. Institue of Medicine. *Crossing the Quality Chasm: A New Health System for the 21st Century.* Washington, DC: National Academy Press; 2001

12. American Academy of Pediatrics, American College of Obstetricians and Gynecologists. *Guidelines for Perinatal Care.* 5th ed. Elk Grove Village, IL: American Academy of Pediatrics; 2002:220–224

13. Bertini G, Dani C, Trochin M, Rubaltelli F. Is breastfeeding really favoring early neonatal jaundice? *Pediatrics.* 2001;107(3). Available at: www.pediatrics.org/cgi/content/full/107/3/e41

14. Maisels MJ, Gifford K. Normal serum bilirubin levels in the newborn and the effect of breast-feeding. *Pediatrics.* 1986;78:837–843

15. Yamauchi Y, Yamanouchi I. Breast-feeding frequency during the first 24 hours after birth in full-term neonates. *Pediatrics.* 1990;86:171–175

16. De Carvalho M, Klaus MH, Merkatz RB. Frequency of breastfeeding and serum bilirubin concentration. *Am J Dis Child.* 1982;136:737–738

17. Varimo P, Similä S, Wendt L, Kolvisto M. Frequency of breast feeding and hyperbilirubinemia [letter]. *Clin Pediatr (Phila).* 1986;25:112

18. De Carvalho M, Holl M, Harvey D. Effects of water supplementation on physiological jaundice in breast-fed babies. *Arch Dis Child.* 1981;56:568–569

19. Nicoll A, Ginsburg R, Tripp JH. Supplementary feeding and jaundice in newborns. *Acta Paediatr Scand.* 1982;71:759–761

20. Madlon-Kay DJ. Identifying ABO incompatibility in newborns: selective vs automatic testing. *J Fam Pract.* 1992;35:278–280

21. Kramer LI. Advancement of dermal icterus in the jaundiced newborn. *Am J Dis Child.* 1969;118:454–458

22. Moyer VA, Ahn C, Sneed S. Accuracy of clinical judgment in neonatal jaundice. *Arch Pediatr Adolesc Med.* 2000;154:391–394

23. Davidson LT, Merritt KK, Weech AA. Hyperbilirubinemia in the newborn. *Am J Dis Child.* 1941;61:958–980

24. Tayaba R, Gribetz D, Gribetz I, Holzman IR. Noninvasive estimation of serum bilirubin. *Pediatrics.* 1998;102(3). Available at: www.pediatrics.org/cgi/content/full/102/3/e28

25. Bhutani V, Gourley GR, Adler S, Kreamer B, Dalman C, Johnson LH. Noninvasive measurement of total serum bilirubin in a multiracial predischarge newborn population to assess the risk of severe hyperbilirubinemia. *Pediatrics.* 2000;106(2). Available at: www.pediatrics.org/cgi/content/full/106/2/e17

26. Yasuda S, Itoh S, Isobe K, et al. New transcutaneous jaundice device with two optical paths. *J Perinat Med.* 2003;31:81–88

27. Maisels MJ, Ostrea EJ Jr, Touch S, et al. Evaluation of a new transcutaneous bilirubinometer. *Pediatrics.* 2004;113:1638–1645

28. Ebbesen F, Rasmussen LM, Wimberley PD. A new transcutaneous bilirubinometer, bilicheck, used in the neonatal intensive care unit and the maternity ward. *Acta Paediatr.* 2002;91:203–211

29. Rubaltelli FF, Gourley GR, Loskamp N, et al. Transcutaneous bilirubin measurement: a multicenter evaluation of a new device. *Pediatrics.* 2001;107:1264–1271

30. Newman TB, Liljestrand P, Escobar GJ. Jaundice noted in the first 24 hours after birth in a managed care organization. *Arch Pediatr Adolesc Med.* 2002;156:1244–1250

31. Bhutani VK, Johnson L, Sivieri EM. Predictive ability of a predischarge hour-specific serum bilirubin for subsequent significant hyperbilirubinemia in healthy term and near-term newborns. *Pediatrics.* 1999;103:6–14

32. Garcia FJ, Nager AL. Jaundice as an early diagnostic sign of urinary tract infection in infancy. *Pediatrics.* 2002;109:846–851

33. Kaplan M, Hammerman C. Severe neonatal hyperbilirubinemia: a potential complication of glucose-6-phosphate dehydrogenase deficiency. *Clin Perinatol.* 1998;25:575–590

34. Valaes T. Severe neonatal jaundice associated with glucose-6-phosphate dehydrogenase deficiency: pathogenesis and global epidemiology. *Acta Paediatr Suppl.* 1994;394:58–76

35. Alpay F, Sarici S, Tosuncuk HD, Serdar MA, Inanç N, Gökçay E. The value of first-day bilirubin measurement in predicting the development of significant hyperbilirubinemia in healthy term newborns. *Pediatrics.*

36. Carbonell X, Botet F, Figueras J, Riu-Godo A. Prediction of hyperbilirubinaemia in the healthy term newborn. *Acta Paediatr.* 2001;90:166–170

37. Kaplan M, Hammerman C, Feldman R, Brisk R. Predischarge bilirubin screening in glucose-6-phosphate dehydrogenase-deficient neonates. *Pediatrics.* 2000;105:533–537

38. Stevenson DK, Fanaroff AA, Maisels MJ, et al. Prediction of hyperbilirubinemia in near-term and term infants. *Pediatrics.* 2001;108:31–39

39. Newman TB, Xiong B, Gonzales VM, Escobar GJ. Prediction and prevention of extreme neonatal hyperbilirubinemia in a mature health maintenance organization. *Arch Pediatr Adolesc Med.* 2000;154:1140–1147

40. Maisels MJ, Kring EA. Length of stay, jaundice, and hospital readmission. *Pediatrics.* 1998;101:995–998

41. Gale R, Seidman DS, Dollberg S, Stevenson DK. Epidemiology of neonatal jaundice in the Jerusalem population. *J Pediatr Gastroenterol Nutr.* 1990;10:82–86

42. Berk MA, Mimouni F, Miodovnik M, Hertzberg V, Valuck J. Macrosomia in infants of insulin-dependent diabetic mothers. *Pediatrics.* 1989;83:1029–1034

43. Peevy KJ, Landaw SA, Gross SJ. Hyperbilirubinemia in infants of diabetic mothers. *Pediatrics.* 1980;66:417–419

44. Soskolne El, Schumacher R, Fyock C, Young ML, Schork A. The effect of early discharge and other factors on readmission rates of newborns. *Arch Pediatr Adolesc Med.* 1996;150:373–379

45. Ebbesen F, Brodersen R. Risk of bilirubin acid precipitation in preterm infants with respiratory distress syndrome: considerations of blood/brain bilirubin transfer equilibrium. *Early Hum Dev.* 1982;6:341–355

46. Cashore WJ, Oh W, Brodersen R. Reserve albumin and bilirubin toxicity index in infant serum. *Acta Paediatr Scand.* 1983;72:415–419

47. Cashore WJ. Free bilirubin concentrations and bilirubin-binding affinity in term and preterm infants. *J Pediatr.* 1980;96:521–527

48. Bratlid D. How bilirubin gets into the brain. *Clin Perinatol.* 1990;17:449–465

49. Wennberg RP. Cellular basis of bilirubin toxicity. *N Y State J Med.* 1991;91:493–496

50. Eggert P, Stick C, Schroder H. On the distribution of irradiation intensity in phototherapy. Measurements of effective irradiance in an incubator. *Eur J Pediatr.* 1984;142:58–61

51. Maisels MJ. Why use homeopathic doses of phototherapy? *Pediatrics.* 1996;98:283–287

52. Ahlfors CE. Criteria for exchange transfusion in jaundiced newborns. *Pediatrics.* 1994;93:488–494

53. American Association of Blood Banks Technical Manual Committee. Perinatal issues in transfusion practice. In: Brecher M, ed. *Technical Manual.* Bethesda, MD: American Association of Blood Banks; 2002:497–515

54. Garland JS, Alex C, Deacon JS, Raab K. Treatment of infants with indirect hyperbilirubinemia. Readmission to birth hospital vs nonbirth hospital. *Arch Pediatr Adolesc Med.* 1994;148:1317–1321

55. Gottstein R, Cooke R. Systematic review of intravenous immunoglobulin in haemolytic disease of the newborn. *Arch Dis Child Fetal Neonatal Ed.* 2003;88:F6–F10

56. Sato K, Hara T, Kondo T, Iwao H, Honda S, Ueda K. High-dose intravenous gammaglobulin therapy for neonatal immune haemolytic jaundice due to blood group incompatibility. *Acta Paediatr Scand.* 1991;80:163–166

57. Rubo J, Albrecht K, Lasch P, et al. High-dose intravenous immune globulin therapy for hyperbilirubinemia caused by Rh hemolytic disease. *J Pediatr.* 1992;121:93–97

58. Hammerman C, Kaplan M, Vreman HJ, Stevenson DK. Intravenous immune globulin in neonatal ABO isoimmunization: factors associated with clinical efficacy. *Biol Neonate.* 1996;70:69–74

59. Johnson L, Boggs TR. Bilirubin-dependent brain damage: incidence and indications for treatment. In: Odell GB, Schaffer R, Simopoulos AP, eds. *Phototherapy in the Newborn: An Overview.* Washington, DC: National Academy of Sciences; 1974:122–149

60. Ozmert E, Erdem G, Topcu M. Long-term follow-up of indirect hyperbilirubinemia in full-term Turkish infants. *Acta Paediatr.* 1996;85:1440–1444

61. Volpe JJ. *Neurology of the Newborn.* 4th ed. Philadelphia, PA: W. B. Saunders; 2001

62. Harris M, Bernbaum J, Polin J, Zimmerman R, Polin RA. Developmental follow-up of breastfed term and near-term infants with marked hyperbilirubinemia. *Pediatrics.* 2001;107:1075–1080

63. Osborn LM, Bolus R. Breast feeding and jaundice in the first week of life. *J Fam Pract.* 1985;20:475–480

64. Martinez JC, Maisels MJ, Otheguy L, et al. Hyperbilirubinemia in the breast-fed newborn: a controlled trial of four interventions. *Pediatrics.* 1993;91:470–473

65. Amato M, Howald H, von Muralt G. Interruption of breast-feeding versus phototherapy as treatment of hyperbilirubinemia in full-term infants. *Helv Paediatr Acta.* 1985;40:127–131

66. Maisels MJ, Gifford K, Antle CE, Leib GR. Jaundice in the healthy newborn infant: a new approach to an old problem. *Pediatrics.* 1988;81:505–511

67. Newman TB, Easterling MJ. Yield of reticulocyte counts and blood smears in term infants. *Clin Pediatr (Phila).* 1994;33:71–76

68. Herschel M, Karrison T, Wen M, Caldarelli L, Baron B. Evaluation of the direct antiglobulin (Coombs') test for identifying newborns at risk for hemolysis as determined by end-tidal carbon monoxide concentration (ETCOc); and comparison of the Coombs' test with ETCOc for detecting significant jaundice. *J Perinatol.* 2002;22:341–347

69. Stevenson DK, Vreman HJ. Carbon monoxide and bilirubin production in neonates. *Pediatrics.* 1997;100:252–254

70. Vreman HJ, Verter J, Oh W, et al. Interlaboratory variability of bilirubin measurements. *Clin Chem.* 1996;42:869–873

71. Lo S, Doumas BT, Ashwood E. Performance of bilirubin determinations in US laboratories—revisited. *Clin Chem.* 2004;50:190–194

72. Kappas A, Drummond GS, Henschke C, Valaes T. Direct comparison of Sn-mesoporphyrin, an inhibitor of bilirubin production, and phototherapy in controlling hyperbilirubinemia in term and near-term newborns. *Pediatrics.* 1995;95:468–474

73. Martinez JC, Garcia HO, Otheguy L, Drummond GS, Kappas A. Control of severe hyperbilirubinemia in full-term newborns with the inhibitor of bilirubin production Sn-mesoporphyrin. *Pediatrics.* 1999;103:1–5

74. Suresh G, Martin CL, Soll R. Metalloporphyrins for treatment of unconjugated hyperbilirubinemia in neonates. *Cochrane Database Syst Rev.* 2003;2:CD004207

75. Kappas A, Drummond GS, Munson DP, Marshall JR. Sn-mesoporphyrin interdiction of severe hyperbilirubinemia in Jehovah's Witness newborns as an alternative to exchange transfusion. *Pediatrics.* 2001;108:1374–1377

APPENDIX 1: Additional Notes

Definitions of Quality of Evidence and Balance of Benefits and Harms

The Steering Committee on Quality Improvement and Management categorizes evidence quality in 4 levels:

1. Well-designed, randomized, controlled trials or diagnostic studies on relevant populations
2. Randomized, controlled trials or diagnostic studies with minor limitations; overwhelming, consistent evidence from observational studies
3. Observational studies (case-control and cohort design)
4. Expert opinion, case reports, reasoning from first principles

The AAP defines evidence-based recommendations as follows:[1]

• Strong recommendation: the committee believes that the benefits of the recommended approach clearly exceed the harms of that approach and that the quality of the supporting evidence is either excellent or impossible to obtain. Clinicians should follow these recommendations unless a clear and compelling rationale for an alternative approach is present.

• Recommendation: the committee believes that the benefits exceed the harms, but the quality of evidence on which this recommendation is based is not as strong. Clinicians should also generally follow these recommendations but should be alert to new information and sensitive to patient prefer-

ences. In this guideline, the term "should" implies a recommendation by the committee.

• Option: either the quality of the evidence that exists is suspect or well-performed studies have shown little clear advantage to one approach over another. Patient preference should have a substantial role in influencing clinical decision-making when a policy is described as an option.

• No recommendation: there is a lack of pertinent evidence and the anticipated balance of benefits and harms is unclear.

Anticipated Balance Between Benefits and Harms

The presence of clear benefits or harms supports stronger statements for or against a course of action. In some cases, however, recommendations are made when analysis of the balance of benefits and harms provides an exceptional dysequilibrium and it would be unethical or impossible to perform clinical trials to "prove" the point. In these cases the balance of benefit and harm is termed "exceptional."

Clinical Manifestations of Acute Bilirubin Encephalopathy and Kernicterus

Acute Bilirubin Encephalopathy

In the early phase of acute bilirubin encephalopathy, severely jaundiced infants become lethargic and hypotonic and suck poorly.[2,3] The intermediate phase is characterized by moderate stupor, irritability, and hypertonia. The infant may develop a fever and high-pitched cry, which may alternate with drowsiness and hypotonia. The hypertonia is manifested by backward arching of the neck (retrocollis) and trunk (opisthotonos). There is anecdotal evidence that an emergent exchange transfusion at this stage, in some cases, might reverse the central nervous system changes.[4] The advanced phase, in which central nervous system damage is probably irreversible, is characterized by pronounced retrocollis-opisthotonos, shrill cry, no feeding, apnea, fever, deep stupor to coma, sometimes seizures, and death.[2,3,5]

Kernicterus

In the chronic form of bilirubin encephalopathy, surviving infants may develop a severe form of athetoid cerebral palsy, auditory dysfunction, dental-enamel dysplasia, paralysis of upward gaze, and, less often, intellectual and other handicaps. Most infants who develop kernicterus have manifested some or all of the signs listed above in the acute phase of bilirubin encephalopathy. However, occasionally there are infants who have developed very high bilirubin levels and, subsequently, the signs of kernicterus but have exhibited few, if any, antecedent clinical signs of acute bilirubin encephalopathy.[3,5,6]

Clinical Evaluation of Jaundice and TcB Measurements

Jaundice is usually seen in the face first and progresses caudally to the trunk and extremities,[7] but because visual estimation of bilirubin levels from the degree of jaundice can lead to errors,[8–10] a low threshold should be used for measuring the TSB.

Devices that provide a noninvasive TcB measurement have proven very useful as screening tools,[11] and newer instruments give measurements that provide a valid estimate of the TSB level.[12–17] Studies using the new TcB-measurement instruments are limited, but the data published thus far suggest that in most newborn populations, these instruments generally provide measurements within 2 to 3 mg/dL (34–51 μmol/L) of the TSB and can replace a measurement of serum bilirubin in many circumstances, particularly for TSB levels less than 15 mg/dL (257 μmol/L).[12–17] Because phototherapy "bleaches" the skin, both visual assessment of jaundice and TcB measurements in infants undergoing phototherapy are not reliable. In addition, the ability of transcutaneous instruments to provide accurate measurements in different racial groups requires additional study.[18,19] The limitations of the accuracy and reproducibility of TSB measurements in the clinical laboratory[20–22] must also be recognized and are discussed in the technical report.[23]

Capillary Versus Venous Serum Bilirubin Measurement

Almost all published data regarding the relationship of TSB levels to kernicterus or developmental outcome are based on capillary blood TSB levels. Data regarding the differences between capillary and venous TSB levels are conflicting.[24,25] In 1 study the capillary TSB levels were higher, but in another they were lower than venous TSB levels.[24,25] Thus, obtaining a venous sample to "confirm" an elevated capillary TSB level is not recommended, because it will delay the initiation of treatment.

Direct-Reacting and Conjugated Bilirubin

Although commonly used interchangeably, direct-reacting bilirubin is not the same as conjugated bilirubin. Direct-reacting bilirubin is the bilirubin that reacts directly (without the addition of an accelerating agent) with diazotized sulfanilic acid. Conjugated bilirubin is bilirubin made water soluble by binding with glucuronic acid in the liver. Depending on the technique used, the clinical laboratory will report total and direct-reacting or unconjugated and conjugated bilirubin levels. In this guideline and for clinical purposes, the terms may be used interchangeably.

Abnormal Direct and Conjugated Bilirubin Levels

Laboratory measurement of direct bilirubin is not precise,[26] and values between laboratories can vary widely. If the TSB is at or below 5 mg/dL (85 μmol/L), a direct or conjugated bilirubin of more than 1.0 mg/dL (17.1 μmol/L) is generally considered abnormal. For TSB values higher than 5 mg/dL (85 μmol/L), a direct bilirubin of more than 20% of the TSB is considered abnormal. If the hospital laboratory measures conjugated bilirubin using the Vitros (formerly Ektachem) system (Ortho-Clinical Diagnostics, Raritan, NJ), any value higher than 1 mg/dL is considered abnormal.

Assessment of Adequacy of Intake in Breastfeeding Infants

The data from a number of studies[27–34] indicate that unsupplemented, breastfed infants experience their maximum weight loss by day 3 and, on average, lose 6.1% ± 2.5% (SD) of their birth weight. Thus, ~5% to 10% of fully breastfed infants lose 10% or more of their birth weight by day 3, suggesting that adequacy of intake should be evaluated and the infant monitored if weight loss is more than 10%.[35] Evidence of adequate intake in breastfed infants also includes 4 to 6 thoroughly wet diapers in 24 hours and the passage of 3 to 4 stools per day by the fourth day. By the third to fourth day, the stools in adequately breastfed infants should have changed from meconium to a mustard yellow, mushy stool.[36] The above assessment will also help to identify breastfed infants who are at risk for dehydration because of inadequate intake.

Nomogram for Designation of Risk

Note that this nomogram (Fig 2) does not describe the natural history of neonatal hyperbilirubinemia, particularly after 48 to 72 hours, for which, because of sampling bias, the lower zones are spuriously elevated.[37] This bias, however, will have much less effect on the high-risk zone (95th percentile in the study).[38]

G6PD Dehydrogenase Deficiency

It is important to look for G6PD deficiency in infants with significant hyperbilirubinemia, because some may develop a sudden increase in the TSB. In addition, G6PD-deficient infants require intervention at lower TSB levels (Figs 3 and 4). It should be noted also that in the presence of hemolysis, G6PD levels can be elevated, which may obscure the diagnosis in the newborn period so that a normal level in a hemolyzing neonate does not rule out G6PD deficiency.[39] If G6PD deficiency is strongly suspected, a repeat level should be measured when the infant is 3 months old. It is also recognized that immediate laboratory determination of G6PD is generally not available in most US hospitals, and thus translating the above information into clinical practice is cur-

TABLE 4. Risk Zone as a Predictor of Hyperbilirubinemia[39]

TSB Before Discharge	Newborns (Total = 2840), n (%)	Newborns Who Subsequently Developed a TSB Level >95th Percentile, n (%)
High-risk zone (>95th percentile)	172 (6.0)	68 (39.5)
High intermediate-risk zone	356 (12.5)	46 (12.9)
Low intermediate-risk zone	556 (19.6)	12 (2.26)
Low-risk zone	1756 (61.8)	0

rently difficult. Nevertheless, practitioners are reminded to consider the diagnosis of G6PD deficiency in infants with severe hyperbilirubinemia, particularly if they belong to the population groups in which this condition is prevalent. This is important in the African American population, because these infants, as a group, have much lower TSB levels than white or Asian infants.[40,41] Thus, severe hyperbilirubinemia in an African American infant should always raise the possibility of G6PD deficiency.

Basis for the Recommendations 7.1.1 Through 7.1.6 and Provided in Figs 3 and 4

Ideally, recommendations for when to implement phototherapy and exchange transfusions should be based on estimates of when the benefits of these interventions exceed their risks and cost. The evidence for these estimates should come from randomized trials or systematic observational studies. Unfortunately, there is little such evidence on which to base these recommendations. As a result, treatment guidelines must necessarily rely on more uncertain estimates and extrapolations. For a detailed discussion of this question, please see "An Evidence-Based Review of Important Issues Concerning Neonatal Hyperbilirubinemia."[23]

The recommendations for phototherapy and exchange transfusion are based on the following principles:

- The main demonstrated value of phototherapy is that it reduces the risk that TSB levels will reach a level at which exchange transfusion is recommended.[42–44] Approximately 5 to 10 infants with TSB levels between 15 and 20 mg/dL (257–342 μmol/L) will receive phototherapy to prevent the TSB in 1 infant from reaching 20 mg/dL (the number needed to treat).[12] Thus, 8 to 9 of every 10 infants with these TSB levels will not reach 20 mg/dL (342 μmol/L) even if they are not treated. Phototherapy has proven to be a generally safe procedure, although rare complications can occur (see Appendix 2).
- Recommended TSB levels for exchange transfusion (Fig 4) are based largely on the goal of keeping TSB levels below those at which kernicterus has been reported.[12,45–48] In almost all cases, exchange transfusion is recommended only after phototherapy has failed to keep the TSB level below the exchange transfusion level (Fig 4).
- The recommendations to use phototherapy and exchange transfusion at lower TSB levels for infants of lower gestation and those who are sick are based on limited observations suggesting that sick infants (particularly those with the risk factors listed in Figs 3 and 4)[49–51] and those of lower gestation[51–54] are at greater risk for developing kernicterus at lower bilirubin levels than are well infants of more than 38 6/7 weeks' gestation. Nevertheless, other studies have not confirmed all of these associations.[52,55,56] There is no doubt, however, that infants at 35 to 37 6/7 weeks' gestation are at a much greater risk of developing very high

TSB levels.[57,58] Intervention for these infants is based on this risk as well as extrapolations from more premature, lower birth-weight infants who do have a higher risk of bilirubin toxicity.[52,53]
- For all newborns, treatment is recommended at lower TSB levels at younger ages because one of the primary goals of treatment is to prevent additional increases in the TSB level.

Subtle Neurologic Abnormalities Associated With Hyperbilirubinemia

There are several studies demonstrating measurable transient changes in brainstem-evoked potentials, behavioral patterns, and the infant's cry[59–63] associated with TSB levels of 15 to 25 mg/dL (257–428 μmol/L). In these studies, the abnormalities identified were transient and disappeared when the serum bilirubin levels returned to normal with or without treatment.[59,60,62,63]

A few cohort studies have found an association between hyperbilirubinemia and long-term adverse neurodevelopmental effects that are more subtle than kernicterus.[64–67] Current studies, however, suggest that although phototherapy lowers the TSB levels, it has no effect on these long-term neurodevelopmental outcomes.[68–70]

Risks of Exchange Transfusion

Because exchange transfusions are now rarely performed, the risks of morbidity and mortality associated with the procedure are difficult to quantify. In addition, the complication rates listed below may not be generalizable to the current era if, like most procedures, frequency of performance is an important determinant of risk. Death associated with exchange transfusion has been reported in approximately 3 in 1000 procedures,[71,72] although in otherwise well infants of 35 or more weeks' gestation, the risk is probably much lower.[71–73] Significant morbidity (apnea, bradycardia, cyanosis, vasospasm, thrombosis, necrotizing enterocolitis) occurs in as many as 5% of exchange transfusions,[71] and the risks associated with the use of blood products must always be considered.[74] Hypoxic-ischemic encephalopathy and acquired immunodeficiency syndrome have occurred in otherwise healthy infants receiving exchange transfusions.[73,75]

Serum Albumin Levels and the B/A Ratio

The legends to Figs 3 and 4 and recommendations 7.1.5 and 7.1.6 contain references to the serum albumin level and the B/A ratio as factors that can be considered in the decision to initiate phototherapy (Fig 3) or perform an exchange transfusion (Fig 4). Bilirubin is transported in the plasma tightly bound to albumin, and the portion that is unbound or loosely bound can more readily leave the intravascular space and cross the intact blood-brain barrier.[76] Elevations of unbound bilirubin (UB) have been associated with kernicterus in sick preterm newborns.[77,78] In addition, elevated UB concentrations are more closely associated than TSB levels with transient abnormalities in the audiometric brainstem response in term[79] and preterm[80] infants. Long-term studies relating B/A binding in infants to developmental outcome are limited and conflicting.[69,81,82] In addition, clinical laboratory measurement of UB is not currently available in the United States.

The ratio of bilirubin (mg/dL) to albumin (g/dL) does correlate with measured UB in newborns[83] and can be used as an approximate surrogate for the measurement of UB. It must be recognized, however, that both albumin levels and the ability of albumin to bind bilirubin vary significantly between newborns.[83,84] Albumin binding of bilirubin is impaired in sick infants,[84–86] and some studies show an increase in binding with increasing gestational[86,87] and postnatal[87,88] age, but others have not found a significant effect of gestational age on binding.[89] Furthermore, the risk of bilirubin encephalopathy is unlikely to be a simple function of the TSB level or the concentration of UB but is more likely a combination of both (ie, the total amount of bilirubin available [the miscible pool of bilirubin] as well as the tendency of bilirubin to enter the tissues [the UB concentration]).[83] An additional factor is the possible susceptibility of the cells of the central nervous system to damage by bilirubin.[90] It is therefore a clinical option to use the B/A ratio together with, but not in lieu of, the TSB level as an additional factor in determining the need for exchange transfusion[83] (Fig 4).

REFERENCES

1. American Academy of Pediatrics, Steering Committee on Quality Improvement and Management. Classification of recommendations for clinical practice guidelines. *Pediatrics*. 2004; In press
2. Johnson LH, Bhutani VK, Brown AK. System-based approach to management of neonatal jaundice and prevention of kernicterus. *J Pediatr*. 2002;140:396–403
3. Volpe JJ. *Neurology of the Newborn*. 4th ed. Philadelphia, PA: W. B. Saunders; 2001
4. Harris M, Bernbaum J, Polin J, Zimmerman R, Polin RA. Developmental follow-up of breastfed term and near-term infants with marked hyperbilirubinemia. *Pediatrics*. 2001;107:1075–1080
5. Van Praagh R. Diagnosis of kernicterus in the neonatal period. *Pediatrics*. 1961;28:870–876
6. Jones MH, Sands R, Hyman CB, Sturgeon P, Koch FP. Longitudinal study of incidence of central nervous system damage following erythroblastosis fetalis. *Pediatrics*. 1954;14:346–350
7. Kramer LI. Advancement of dermal icterus in the jaundiced newborn. *Am J Dis Child*. 1969;118:454–458
8. Moyer VA, Ahn C, Sneed S. Accuracy of clinical judgment in neonatal jaundice. *Arch Pediatr Adolesc Med*. 2000;154:391–394
9. Davidson LT, Merritt KK, Weech AA. Hyperbilirubinemia in the newborn. *Am J Dis Child*. 1941;61:958–980
10. Tayaba R, Gribetz D, Gribetz I, Holzman IR. Noninvasive estimation of serum bilirubin. *Pediatrics*. 1998;102(3). Available at: www.pediatrics.org/cgi/content/full/102/3/e28
11. Maisels MJ, Kring E. Transcutaneous bilirubinometry decreases the need for serum bilirubin measurements and saves money. *Pediatrics*. 1997;99:599–601
12. Ip S, Glicken S, Kulig J, Obrien R, Sege R, Lau J. *Management of Neonatal Hyperbilirubinemia*. Rockville, MD: US Department of Health and Human Services, Agency for Healthcare Research and Quality; 2003. AHRQ Publication 03-E011
13. Bhutani V, Gourley GR, Adler S, Kreamer B, Dalman C, Johnson LH. Noninvasive measurement of total serum bilirubin in a multiracial predischarge newborn population to assess the risk of severe hyperbilirubinemia. *Pediatrics*. 2000;106(2). Available at: www.pediatrics.org/cgi/content/full/106/2/e17
14. Yasuda S, Itoh S, Isobe K, et al. New transcutaneous jaundice device with two optical paths. *J Perinat Med*. 2003;31:81–88
15. Maisels MJ, Ostrea EJ Jr, Touch S, et al. Evaluation of a new transcutaneous bilirubinometer. *Pediatrics*. 2004;113:1638–1645
16. Ebbesen F, Rasmussen LM, Wimberley PD. A new transcutaneous bilirubinometer, bilicheck, used in the neonatal intensive care unit and the maternity ward. *Acta Paediatr*. 2002;91:203–211
17. Rubaltelli FF, Gourley GR, Loskamp N, et al. Transcutaneous bilirubin measurement: a multicenter evaluation of a new device. *Pediatrics*. 2001;107:1264–1271
18. Engle WD, Jackson GL, Sendelbach D, Manning D, Frawley W. Assessment of a transcutaneous device in the evaluation of neonatal hyperbilirubinemia in a primarily Hispanic population. *Pediatrics*. 2002;110:61–67
19. Schumacher R. Transcutaneous bilirubinometry and diagnostic tests: "the right job for the tool." *Pediatrics*. 2002;110:407–408
20. Vreman HJ, Verter J, Oh W, et al. Interlaboratory variability of bilirubin measurements. *Clin Chem*. 1996;42:869–873
21. Doumas BT, Eckfeldt JH. Errors in measurement of total bilirubin: a perennial problem. *Clin Chem*. 1996;42:845–848
22. Lo S, Doumas BT, Ashwood E. Performance of bilirubin determinations in US laboratories—revisited. *Clin Chem*. 2004;50:190–194
23. Ip S, Chung M, Kulig J. et al. An evidence-based review of important issues concerning neonatal hyperbilirubinemia. *Pediatrics*. 2004;113(6). Available at: www.pediatrics.org/cgi/content/full/113/6/e644
24. Leslie GI, Philips JB, Cassady G. Capillary and venous bilirubin values: are they really different? *Am J Dis Child*. 1987;141:1199–1200
25. Eidelman AI, Schimmel MS, Algur N, Eylath U. Capillary and venous bilirubin values: they are different—and how [letter]! *Am J Dis Child*. 1989;143:642
26. Watkinson LR, St John A, Penberthy LA. Investigation into paediatric bilirubin analyses in Australia and New Zealand. *J Clin Pathol*. 1982;35:52–58
27. Bertini G, Dani C, Trochin M, Rubaltelli F. Is breastfeeding really favoring early neonatal jaundice? *Pediatrics*. 2001;107(3). Available at: www.pediatrics.org/cgi/content/full/107/3/e41
28. De Carvalho M, Klaus MH, Merkatz RB. Frequency of breastfeeding and serum bilirubin concentration. *Am J Dis Child*. 1982;136:737–738
29. De Carvalho M, Holl M, Harvey D. Effects of water supplementation on physiological jaundice in breast-fed babies. *Arch Dis Child*. 1981;56:568–569
30. Nicoll A, Ginsburg R, Tripp JH. Supplementary feeding and jaundice in newborns. *Acta Paediatr Scand*. 1982;71:759–761
31. Butler DA, MacMillan JP. Relationship of breast feeding and weight loss to jaundice in the newborn period: review of the literature and results of a study. *Cleve Clin Q*. 1983;50:263–268
32. De Carvalho M, Robertson S, Klaus M. Fecal bilirubin excretion and serum bilirubin concentration in breast-fed and bottle-fed infants. *J Pediatr*. 1985;107:786–790
33. Gourley GR, Kreamer B, Arend R. The effect of diet on feces and jaundice during the first three weeks of life. *Gastroenterology*. 1992;103:660–667
34. Maisels MJ, Gifford K. Breast-feeding, weight loss, and jaundice. *J Pediatr*. 1983;102:117–118
35. Laing IA, Wong CM. Hypernatraemia in the first few days: is the incidence rising? *Arch Dis Child Fetal Neonatal Ed*. 2002;87:F158–F162
36. Lawrence RA. Management of the mother-infant nursing couple. In: *A Breastfeeding Guide for the Medical Profession*. 4th ed. St Louis, MO: Mosby-Year Book, Inc; 1994:215-277
37. Maisels MJ, Newman TB. Predicting hyperbilirubinemia in newborns: the importance of timing. *Pediatrics*. 1999;103:493–495
38. Bhutani VK, Johnson L, Sivieri EM. Predictive ability of a predischarge hour-specific serum bilirubin for subsequent significant hyperbilirubinemia in healthy term and near-term newborns. *Pediatrics*. 1999;103:6–14
39. Beutler E. Glucose-6-phosphate dehydrogenase deficiency. *Blood*. 1994;84:3613–3636
40. Linn S, Schoenbaum SC, Monson RR, Rosner B, Stubblefield PG, Ryan KJ. Epidemiology of neonatal hyperbilirubinemia. *Pediatrics*. 1985;75:770–774
41. Newman TB, Easterling MJ, Goldman ES, Stevenson DK. Laboratory evaluation of jaundiced newborns: frequency, cost and yield. *Am J Dis Child*. 1990;144:364–368
42. Martinez JC, Maisels MJ, Otheguy L, et al. Hyperbilirubinemia in the breast-fed newborn: a controlled trial of four interventions. *Pediatrics*. 1993;91:470–473
43. Maisels MJ. Phototherapy—traditional and nontraditional. *J Perinatol*. 2001;21(suppl 1):S93–S97
44. Brown AK, Kim MH, Wu PY, Bryla DA. Efficacy of phototherapy in prevention and management of neonatal hyperbilirubinemia. *Pediatrics*. 1985;75:393–400

45. Armitage P, Mollison PL. Further analysis of controlled trials of treatment of hemolytic disease of the newborn. *J Obstet Gynaecol Br Emp.* 1953;60:602–605

46. Mollison PL, Walker W. Controlled trials of the treatment of haemolytic disease of the newborn. *Lancet.* 1952;1:429–433

47. Hsia DYY, Allen FH, Gellis SS, Diamond LK. Erythroblastosis fetalis. VIII. Studies of serum bilirubin in relation to kernicterus. *N Engl J Med.* 1952;247:668–671

48. Newman TB, Maisels MJ. Does hyperbilirubinemia damage the brain of healthy full-term infants? *Clin Perinatol.* 1990;17:331–358

49. Ozmert E, Erdem G, Topcu M. Long-term follow-up of indirect hyperbilirubinemia in full-term Turkish infants. *Acta Paediatr.* 1996;85: 1440–1444

50. Perlman JM, Rogers B, Burns D. Kernicterus findings at autopsy in 2 sick near-term infants. *Pediatrics.* 1997;99:612–615

51. Gartner LM, Snyder RN, Chabon RS, Bernstein J. Kernicterus: high incidence in premature infants with low serum bilirubin concentration. *Pediatrics.* 1970;45:906–917

52. Watchko JF, Oski FA. Kernicterus in preterm newborns: past, present, and future. *Pediatrics.* 1992;90:707–715

53. Watchko J, Claassen D. Kernicterus in premature infants: current prevalence and relationship to NICHD Phototherapy Study exchange criteria. *Pediatrics.* 1994;93(6 Pt 1):996–999

54. Stern L, Denton RL. Kernicterus in small, premature infants. *Pediatrics.* 1965;35:486–485

55. Turkel SB, Guttenberg ME, Moynes DR, Hodgman JE. Lack of identifiable risk factors for kernicterus. *Pediatrics.* 1980;66:502–506

56. Kim MH, Yoon JJ, Sher J, Brown AK. Lack of predictive indices in kernicterus. A comparison of clinical and pathologic factors in infants with or without kernicterus. *Pediatrics.* 1980;66:852–858

57. Newman TB, Xiong B, Gonzales VM, Escobar GJ. Prediction and prevention of extreme neonatal hyperbilirubinemia in a mature health maintenance organization. *Arch Pediatr Adolesc Med.* 2000;154:1140–1147

58. Newman TB, Escobar GJ, Gonzales VM, Armstrong MA, Gardner MN, Folck BF. Frequency of neonatal bilirubin testing and hyperbilirubinemia in a large health maintenance organization. *Pediatrics.* 1999;104: 1198–1203

59. Vohr BR. New approaches to assessing the risks of hyperbilirubinemia. *Clin Perinatol.* 1990;17:293–306

60. Perlman M, Fainmesser P, Sohmer H, Tamari H, Wax Y, Pevsmer B. Auditory nerve-brainstem evoked responses in hyperbilirubinemic neonates. *Pediatrics.* 1983;72:658–664

61. Nakamura H, Takada S, Shimabuku R, Matsuo M, Matsuo T, Negishi H. Auditory and brainstem responses in newborn infants with hyperbilirubinemia. *Pediatrics.* 1985;75:703–708

62. Nwaesei CG, Van Aerde J, Boyden M, Perlman M. Changes in auditory brainstem responses in hyperbilirubinemic infants before and after exchange transfusion. *Pediatrics.* 1984;74:800–803

63. Wennberg RP, Ahlfors CE, Bickers R, McMurtry CA, Shetter JL. Abnormal auditory brainstem response in a newborn infant with hyperbilirubinemia: improvement with exchange transfusion. *J Pediatr.* 1982;100:624–626

64. Soorani-Lunsing I, Woltil H, Hadders-Algra M. Are moderate degrees of hyperbilirubinemia in healthy term neonates really safe for the brain? *Pediatr Res.* 2001;50:701–705

65. Grimmer I, Berger-Jones K, Buhrer C, Brandl U, Obladen M. Late neurological sequelae of non-hemolytic hyperbilirubinemia of healthy term neonates. *Acta Paediatr.* 1999;88:661–663

66. Seidman DS, Paz I, Stevenson DK, Laor A, Danon YL, Gale R. Neonatal hyperbilirubinemia and physical and cognitive performance at 17 years of age. *Pediatrics.* 1991;88:828–833

67. Newman TB, Klebanoff MA. Neonatal hyperbilirubinemia and long-term outcome: another look at the collaborative perinatal project. *Pediatrics.* 1993;92:651–657

68. Scheidt PC, Bryla DA, Nelson KB, Hirtz DG, Hoffman HJ. Phototherapy for neonatal hyperbilirubinemia: six-year follow-up of the National Institute of Child Health and Human Development clinical trial. *Pediatrics.* 1990;85:455–463

69. Scheidt PC, Graubard BI, Nelson KB, et al. Intelligence at six years in relation to neonatal bilirubin levels: follow-up of the National Institute of Child Health and Human Development Clinical Trial of Phototherapy. *Pediatrics.* 1991;87:797–805

70. Seidman DS, Paz I, Stevenson DK, Laor A, Danon YL, Gale R. Effect of phototherapy for neonatal jaundice on cognitive performance. *J Perinatol.* 1994;14:23–28

71. Keenan WJ, Novak KK, Sutherland JM, Bryla DA, Fetterly KL. Morbidity and mortality associated with exchange transfusion. *Pediatrics.* 1985; 75:417–421

72. Hovi L, Siimes MA. Exchange transfusion with fresh heparinized blood is a safe procedure: Experiences from 1069 newborns. *Acta Paediatr Scand.* 1985;74:360–365

73. Jackson JC. Adverse events associated with exchange transfusion in healthy and ill newborns. *Pediatrics.* 1997;99(5):e7. Available at: www.pediatrics.org/cgi/content/full/99/5/e7

74. Schreiber GB, Busch MP, Kleinman SH, Korelitz JJ. The risk of transfusion-transmitted viral infections. *N Engl J Med.* 1996;334:1685–1690

75. Maisels MJ, Newman TB. Kernicterus in otherwise healthy, breast-fed term newborns. *Pediatrics.* 1995;96:730–733

76. Bratlid D. How bilirubin gets into the brain. *Clin Perinatol.* 1990;17: 449–465

77. Cashore WJ, Oh W. Unbound bilirubin and kernicterus in low-birth-weight infants. *Pediatrics.* 1982;69:481–485

78. Nakamura H, Yonetani M, Uetani Y, Funato M, Lee Y. Determination of serum unbound bilirubin for prediction of kernicterus in low birth-weight infants. *Acta Paediatr Jpn.* 1992;34:642–647

79. Funato M, Tamai H, Shimada S, Nakamura H. Vigintiphobia, unbound bilirubin, and auditory brainstem responses. *Pediatrics.* 1994;93:50–53

80. Amin SB, Ahlfors CE, Orlando MS, Dalzell LE, Merle KS, Guillet R. Bilirubin and serial auditory brainstem responses in premature infants. *Pediatrics.* 2001;107:664–670

81. Johnson L, Boggs TR. Bilirubin-dependent brain damage: incidence and indications for treatment. In: Odell GB, Schaffer R, Simopoulos AP, eds. *Phototherapy in the Newborn: An Overview.* Washington, DC: National Academy of Sciences; 1974:122–149

82. Odell GB, Storey GNB, Rosenberg LA. Studies in kernicterus. 3. The saturation of serum proteins with bilirubin during neonatal life and its relationship to brain damage at five years. *J Pediatr.* 1970;76:12–21

83. Ahlfors CE. Criteria for exchange transfusion in jaundiced newborns. *Pediatrics.* 1994;93:488–494

84. Cashore WJ. Free bilirubin concentrations and bilirubin-binding affinity in term and preterm infants. *J Pediatr.* 1980;96:521–527

85. Ebbesen F, Brodersen R. Risk of bilirubin acid precipitation in preterm infants with respiratory distress syndrome: considerations of blood/brain bilirubin transfer equilibrium. *Early Hum Dev.* 1982;6:341–355

86. Cashore WJ, Oh W, Brodersen R. Reserve albumin and bilirubin toxicity index in infant serum. *Acta Paediatr Scand.* 1983;72:415–419

87. Ebbesen F, Nyboe J. Postnatal changes in the ability of plasma albumin to bind bilirubin. *Acta Paediatr Scand.* 1983;72:665–670

88. Esbjorner E. Albumin binding properties in relation to bilirubin and albumin concentrations during the first week of life. *Acta Paediatr Scand.* 1991;80:400–405

89. Robertson A, Sharp C, Karp W. The relationship of gestational age to reserve albumin concentration for binding of bilirubin. *J Perinatol.* 1988; 8:17–18

90. Wennberg RP. Cellular basis of bilirubin toxicity. *N Y State J Med.* 1991;91:493–496

APPENDIX 2: Phototherapy

There is no standardized method for delivering phototherapy. Phototherapy units vary widely, as do the types of lamps used in the units. The efficacy of phototherapy depends on the dose of phototherapy administered as well as a number of clinical factors (Table 5).[1]

Measuring the Dose of Phototherapy

Table 5 shows the radiometric quantities used in measuring the phototherapy dose. The quantity most commonly reported in the literature is the spectral irradiance. In the nursery, spectral irradiance can be measured by using commercially available radiometers. These instruments take a single measurement across a band of wavelengths, typically 425 to 475 or 400 to 480 nm. Unfortunately, there is no standardized method for reporting phototherapy dosages in the clinical literature, so it is difficult to compare published studies on the efficacy of phototherapy and manufacturers' data for the irradiance produced by different systems.[2] Measurements of irradiance from the same system, using different radiometers,

TABLE 5.   Factors That Affect the Dose and Efficacy of Phototherapy

Factor	Mechanism/Clinical Relevance	Implementation and Rationale	Clinical Application
Spectrum of light emitted	Blue-green spectrum is most effective. At these wavelengths, light penetrates skin well and is absorbed maximally by bilirubin.	Special blue fluorescent tubes or other light sources that have most output in the blue-green spectrum and are most effective in lowering TSB.	Use special blue tubes or LED light source with output in blue-green spectrum for intensive PT.
Spectral irradiance (irradiance in certain wavelength band) delivered to surface of infant	↑ irradiance → ↑ rate of decline in TSB	Irradiance is measured with a radiometer as μW/cm^2 per nm. Standard PT units deliver 8–10 μW/cm^2 per nm (Fig 6). Intensive PT requires >30 μW/cm^2 per nm.	If special blue fluorescent tubes are used, bring tubes as close to infant as possible to increase irradiance (Fig 6). Note: This cannot be done with halogen lamps because of the danger of burn. Special blue tubes 10–15 cm above the infant will produce an irradiance of at least 35 μW/cm^2 per nm.
Spectral power (average spectral irradiance across surface area)	↑ surface area exposed → ↑ rate of decline in TSB	For intensive PT, expose maximum surface area of infant to PT.	Place lights above and fiber-optic pad or special blue fluorescent tubes* below the infant. For maximum exposure, line sides of bassinet, warmer bed, or incubator with aluminum foil.
Cause of jaundice	PT is likely to be less effective if jaundice is due to hemolysis or if cholestasis is present. (↑ direct bilirubin)		When hemolysis is present, start PT at lower TSB levels. Use intensive PT. Failure of PT suggests that hemolysis is the cause of jaundice. If ↑ direct bilirubin, watch for bronze baby syndrome or blistering.
TSB level at start of PT	The higher the TSB, the more rapid the decline in TSB with PT.		Use intensive PT for higher TSB levels. Anticipate a more rapid decrease in TSB when TSB >20 mg/dL (342 μmol/L).

PT indicates phototherapy; LED, light-emitting diode.
* Available in the Olympic BiliBassinet (Olympic Medical, Seattle, WA).

can also produce significantly different results. The width of the phototherapy lamp's emissions spectrum (narrow versus broad) will affect the measured irradiance. Measurements under lights with a very focused emission spectrum (eg, blue light-emitting diode) will vary significantly from one radiometer to another, because the response spectra of the radiometers vary from manufacturer to manufacturer. Broader-spectrum lights (fluorescent and halogen) have fewer variations among radiometers. Manufacturers of phototherapy systems generally recommend the specific radiometer to be used in measuring the dose of phototherapy when their system is used.

It is important also to recognize that the measured irradiance will vary widely depending on where the measurement is taken. Irradiance measured below the center of the light source can be more than double that measured at the periphery, and this dropoff at the periphery will vary with different phototherapy units. Ideally, irradiance should be measured at multiple sites under the area illuminated by the unit and the measurements averaged. The International Electrotechnical Commission[3] defines the "effective surface area" as the intended treatment surface that is illuminated by the phototherapy light. The commission uses 60 × 30 cm as the standard-sized surface.

Is It Necessary to Measure Phototherapy Doses Routinely?

Although it is not necessary to measure spectral irradiance before each use of phototherapy, it is important to perform periodic checks of phototherapy units to make sure that an adequate irradiance is being delivered.

The Dose-Response Relationship of Phototherapy

Figure 5 shows that there is a direct relationship between the irradiance used and the rate at which the serum bilirubin declines under phototherapy.[4] The data in Fig 5 suggest that there is a saturation point beyond which an increase in the irradiance produces no added efficacy. We do not know, however, that a saturation point exists. Because the conversion of bilirubin to excretable photoproducts is partly irreversible and follows first-order kinetics, there may not be a saturation point, so we do not know the maximum effective dose of phototherapy.

Effect on Irradiance of the Light Spectrum and the Distance Between the Infant and the Light Source

Figure 6 shows that as the distance between the light source and the infant decreases, there is a corresponding increase in the spectral irradiance.[5] Fig 6 also demonstrates the dramatic difference in irradi-

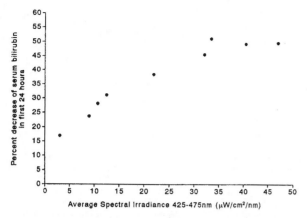

Fig 5. Relationship between average spectral irradiance and decrease in serum bilirubin concentration. Term infants with nonhemolytic hyperbilirubinemia were exposed to special blue lights (Phillips TL 52/20W) of different intensities. Spectral irradiance was measured as the average of readings at the head, trunk, and knees. Drawn from the data of Tan.[4] Source: *Pediatrics*. 1996;98: 283-287.

ance produced within the important 425- to 475-nm band by different types of fluorescent tubes.

What is Intensive Phototherapy?

Intensive phototherapy implies the use of high levels of irradiance in the 430- to 490-nm band (usually 30 μW/cm^2 per nm or higher) delivered to as much of the infant's surface area as possible. How this can be achieved is described below.

Using Photocorrect Effectively

Light Source

The spectrum of light delivered by a phototherapy unit is determined by the type of light source and

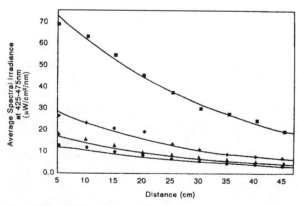

Fig 6. Effect of light source and distance from the light source to the infant on average spectral irradiance. Measurements were made across the 425- to 475-nm band by using a commercial radiometer (Olympic Bilimeter Mark II) and are the average of measurements taken at different locations at each distance (irradiance at the center of the light is much higher than at the periphery). The phototherapy unit was fitted with eight 24-in fluorescent tubes. ■ indicates special blue, General Electric 20-W F20T12/BB tube; ◆, blue, General Electric 20-W F20T12/B tube; ▲, daylight blue, 4 General Electric 20-W F20T12/B blue tubes and 4 Sylvania 20-W F20T12/D daylight tubes; •, daylight, Sylvania 20-W F20T12/D daylight tube. Curves were plotted by using linear curve fitting (True Epistat, Epistat Services, Richardson, TX). The best fit is described by the equation $y = Ae^{Bx}$. Source: *Pediatrics*. 1996;98:283-287.

any filters used. Commonly used phototherapy units contain daylight, cool white, blue, or "special blue" fluorescent tubes. Other units use tungsten-halogen lamps in different configurations, either free-standing or as part of a radiant warming device. Recently, a system using high-intensity gallium nitride light-emitting diodes has been introduced.[6] Fiber-optic systems deliver light from a high-intensity lamp to a fiber-optic blanket. Most of these devices deliver enough output in the blue-green region of the visible spectrum to be effective for standard phototherapy use. However, when bilirubin levels approach the range at which intensive phototherapy is recommended, maximal efficiency must be sought. The most effective light sources currently commercially available for phototherapy are those that use special blue fluorescent tubes[7] or a specially designed light-emitting diode light (Natus Inc, San Carlos, CA).[6] The special blue fluorescent tubes are labeled F20T12/BB (General Electric, Westinghouse, Sylvania) or TL52/20W (Phillips, Eindhoven, The Netherlands). It is important to note that special blue tubes provide much greater irradiance than regular blue tubes (labeled F20T12/B) (Fig 6). Special blue tubes are most effective because they provide light predominantly in the blue-green spectrum. At these wavelengths, light penetrates skin well and is absorbed maximally by bilirubin.[7]

There is a common misconception that ultraviolet light is used for phototherapy. The light systems used do not emit significant ultraviolet radiation, and the small amount of ultraviolet light that is emitted by fluorescent tubes and halogen bulbs is in longer wavelengths than those that cause erythema. In addition, almost all ultraviolet light is absorbed by the glass wall of the fluorescent tube and the Plexiglas cover of the phototherapy unit.

Distance From the Light

As can be seen in Fig 6, the distance of the light source from the infant has a dramatic effect on the spectral irradiance, and this effect is most significant when special blue tubes are used. To take advantage of this effect, the fluorescent tubes should be placed as close to the infant as possible. To do this, the infant should be in a bassinet, not an incubator, because the top of the incubator prevents the light from being brought sufficiently close to the infant. In a bassinet, it is possible to bring the fluorescent tubes within approximately 10 cm of the infant. Naked term infants do not become overheated under these lights. It is important to note, however, that the halogen spot phototherapy lamps cannot be positioned closer to the infant than recommended by the manufacturers without incurring the risk of a burn. When halogen lamps are used, manufacturers recommendations should be followed. The reflectors, light source, and transparent light filters (if any) should be kept clean.

Surface Area

A number of systems have been developed to provide phototherapy above and below the infant.[8,9] One commercially available system that does this is the BiliBassinet (Olympic Medical, Seattle, WA). This unit provides special blue fluorescent tubes above and below the infant. An alternative is to place fiber-optic pads below an infant with phototherapy lamps above. One disadvantage of fiber-optic pads is that they cover a relatively small surface area so that 2 or 3 pads may be needed.[5] When bilirubin levels are extremely high and must be lowered as rapidly as possible, it is essential to expose as much of the infant's surface area to phototherapy as possible. In these situations, additional surface-area exposure can be achieved by lining the sides of the bassinet with aluminum foil or a white cloth.[10]

In most circumstances, it is not necessary to remove the infant's diaper, but when bilirubin levels approach the exchange transfusion range, the diaper should be removed until there is clear evidence of a significant decline in the bilirubin level.

What Decline in the Serum Bilirubin Can You Expect?

The rate at which the bilirubin declines depends on the factors listed in Table 5, and different responses can be expected depending on the clinical circumstances. When bilirubin levels are extremely high (more than 30 mg/dL [513 μmol/L]), and intensive phototherapy is used, a decline of as much as 10 mg/dL (171 μmol/L) can occur within a few hours,[11] and a decrease of at least 0.5 to 1 mg/dL per hour can be expected in the first 4 to 8 hours.[12] On average, for infants of more than 35 weeks' gestation readmitted for phototherapy, intensive phototherapy can produce a decrement of 30% to 40% in the initial bilirubin level by 24 hours after initiation of phototherapy.[13] The most significant decline will occur in the first 4 to 6 hours. With standard phototherapy systems, a decrease of 6% to 20% of the initial bilirubin level can be expected in the first 24 hours.[8,14]

Intermittent Versus Continuous Phototherapy

Clinical studies comparing intermittent with continuous phototherapy have produced conflicting results.[15–17] Because all light exposure increases bilirubin excretion (compared with darkness), no plausible scientific rationale exists for using intermittent phototherapy. In most circumstances, however, phototherapy does not need to be continuous. Phototherapy may be interrupted during feeding or brief parental visits. Individual judgment should be exercised. If the infant's bilirubin level is approaching the exchange transfusion zone (Fig 4), phototherapy should be administered continuously until a satisfactory decline in the serum bilirubin level occurs or exchange transfusion is initiated.

Hydration

There is no evidence that excessive fluid administration affects the serum bilirubin concentration. Some infants who are admitted with high bilirubin levels are also mildly dehydrated and may need supplemental fluid intake to correct their dehydration. Because these infants are almost always breast-fed, the best fluid to use in these circumstances is a milk-based formula, because it inhibits the enterohepatic circulation of bilirubin and should help to lower the serum bilirubin level. Because the photo-products responsible for the decline in serum bilirubin are excreted in urine and bile,[18] maintaining adequate hydration and good urine output should help to improve the efficacy of phototherapy. Unless there is evidence of dehydration, however, routine intravenous fluid or other supplementation (eg, with dextrose water) of term and near-term infants receiving phototherapy is not necessary.

When Should Phototherapy Be Stopped?

There is no standard for discontinuing phototherapy. The TSB level for discontinuing phototherapy depends on the age at which phototherapy is initiated and the cause of the hyperbilirubinemia.[13] For infants who are readmitted after their birth hospitalization (usually for TSB levels of 18 mg/dL [308 μmol/L] or higher), phototherapy may be discontinued when the serum bilirubin level falls below 13 to 14 mg/dL (239-239 μmol/L). Discharge from the hospital need not be delayed to observe the infant for rebound.[13,19,20] If phototherapy is used for infants with hemolytic diseases or is initiated early and discontinued before the infant is 3 to 4 days old, a follow-up bilirubin measurement within 24 hours after discharge is recommended.[13] For infants who are readmitted with hyperbilirubinemia and then discharged, significant rebound is rare, but a repeat TSB measurement or clinical follow-up 24 hours after discharge is a clinical option.[13]

Home Phototherapy

Because the devices available for home phototherapy may not provide the same degree of irradiance or surface-area exposure as those available in the hospital, home phototherapy should be used only in infants whose bilirubin levels are in the "optional phototherapy" range (Fig 3); it is not appropriate for infants with higher bilirubin concentrations. As with hospitalized infants, it is essential that serum bilirubin levels be monitored regularly.

Sunlight Exposure

In their original description of phototherapy, Cremer et al[21] demonstrated that exposure of newborns to sunlight would lower the serum bilirubin level. Although sunlight provides sufficient irradiance in the 425- to 475-nm band to provide phototherapy, the practical difficulties involved in safely exposing a naked newborn to the sun either inside or outside (and avoiding sunburn) preclude the use of sunlight as a reliable therapeutic tool, and it therefore is not recommended.

Complications

Phototherapy has been used in millions of infants for more than 30 years, and reports of significant toxicity are exceptionally rare. Nevertheless, phototherapy in hospital separates mother and infant, and eye patching is disturbing to parents. The most important, but uncommon, clinical complication occurs in infants with cholestatic jaundice. When these infants are exposed to phototherapy, they may develop a dark, grayish-brown discoloration of the skin, serum, and urine (the bronze infant syndrome).[22] The pathogenesis of this syndrome is unknown, but it may be related to an accumulation of porphyrins and other metabolites in the plasma of infants who develop cholestasis.[22,23] Although it occurs exclusively in infants with cholestasis, not all infants with cholestatic jaundice develop the syndrome.

This syndrome generally has had few deleterious consequences, and if there is a need for phototherapy, the presence of direct hyperbilirubinemia should not be considered a contraindication to its use. This is particularly important in sick neonates. Because the products of phototherapy are excreted in the bile, the presence of cholestasis will decrease the efficacy of phototherapy. Nevertheless, infants with direct hyperbilirubinemia often show some response to phototherapy. In infants receiving phototherapy who develop the bronze infant syndrome, exchange transfusion should be considered if the TSB is in the intensive phototherapy range and phototherapy does not promptly lower the TSB. Because of the paucity of data, firm recommendations cannot be made. Note, however, that the direct serum bilirubin should not be subtracted from the TSB concentration in making decisions about exchange transfusions (see Fig 4).

Rarely, purpura and bullous eruptions have been described in infants with severe cholestatic jaundice receiving phototherapy,[24,25] and severe blistering and photosensitivity during phototherapy have occurred in infants with congenital erythropoietic porphyria.[26,27] Congenital porphyria or a family history of porphyria is an absolute contraindication to the use of phototherapy, as is the concomitant use of drugs or agents that are photosensitizers.[28]

REFERENCES

1. Maisels MJ. Phototherapy—traditional and nontraditional. *J Perinatol.* 2001;21(suppl 1):S93–S97
2. Fiberoptic phototherapy systems. *Health Devices.* 1995;24:132–153
3. International Electrotechnical Commission. Medical electrical equipment—part 2-50: particular requirements for the safety of infant phototherapy equipment. 2000. IEC 60601-2-50. Available at www.iec.ch. Accessed June 7, 2004
4. Tan KL. The pattern of bilirubin response to phototherapy for neonatal hyperbilirubinemia. *Pediatr Res.* 1982;16:670–674
5. Maisels MJ. Why use homeopathic doses of phototherapy? *Pediatrics.* 1996;98:283–287
6. Seidman DS, Moise J, Ergaz Z, et al. A new blue light-emitting phototherapy device: a prospective randomized controlled study. *J Pediatr.* 2000;136:771–774
7. Ennever JF. Blue light, green light, white light, more light: treatment of neonatal jaundice. *Clin Perinatol.* 1990;17:467–481
8. Garg AK, Prasad RS, Hifzi IA. A controlled trial of high-intensity double-surface phototherapy on a fluid bed versus conventional phototherapy in neonatal jaundice. *Pediatrics.* 1995;95:914–916
9. Tan KL. Phototherapy for neonatal jaundice. *Clin Perinatol.* 1991;18:423–439
10. Eggert P, Stick C, Schroder H. On the distribution of irradiation intensity in phototherapy. Measurements of effective irradiance in an incubator. *Eur J Pediatr.* 1984;142:58–61
11. Hansen TW. Acute management of extreme neonatal jaundice—the potential benefits of intensified phototherapy and interruption of enterohepatic bilirubin circulation. *Acta Paediatr.* 1997;86:843–846
12. Newman TB, Liljestrand P, Escobar GJ. Infants with bilirubin levels of 30 mg/dL or more in a large managed care organization. *Pediatrics.* 2003;111(6 Pt 1):1303–1311
13. Maisels MJ, Kring E. Bilirubin rebound following intensive phototherapy. *Arch Pediatr Adolesc Med.* 2002;156:669–672
14. Tan KL. Comparison of the efficacy of fiberoptic and conventional phototherapy for neonatal hyperbilirubinemia. *J Pediatr.* 1994;125:607–612
15. Rubaltelli FF, Zanardo V, Granati B. Effect of various phototherapy regimens on bilirubin decrement. *Pediatrics.* 1978;61:838–841
16. Maurer HM, Shumway CN, Draper DA, Hossaini AA. Controlled trial comparing agar, intermittent phototherapy, and continuous phototherapy for reducing neonatal hyperbilirubinemia. *J Pediatr.* 1973;82:73–76
17. Lau SP, Fung KP. Serum bilirubin kinetics in intermittent phototherapy of physiological jaundice. *Arch Dis Child.* 1984;59:892–894
18. McDonagh AF, Lightner DA. 'Like a shrivelled blood orange'—bilirubin, jaundice, and phototherapy. *Pediatrics.* 1985;75:443–455
19. Yetman RJ, Parks DK, Huseby V, Mistry K, Garcia J. Rebound bilirubin levels in infants receiving phototherapy. *J Pediatr.* 1998;133:705–707
20. Lazar L, Litwin A, Merlob P. Phototherapy for neonatal nonhemolytic hyperbilirubinemia. Analysis of rebound and indications for discontinuing therapy. *Clin Pediatr (Phila).* 1993;32:264–267
21. Cremer RJ, Perryman PW, Richards DH. Influence of light on the hyperbilirubinemia of infants. *Lancet.* 1958;1(7030):1094–1097
22. Rubaltelli FF, Jori G, Reddi E. Bronze baby syndrome: a new porphyrin-related disorder. *Pediatr Res.* 1983;17:327–330
23. Meisel P, Jahrig D, Theel L, Ordt A, Jahrig K. The bronze baby syndrome: consequence of impaired excretion of photobilirubin? *Photobiochem Photobiophys.* 1982;3:345–352
24. Mallon E, Wojnarowska F, Hope P, Elder G. Neonatal bullous eruption as a result of transient porphyrinemia in a premature infant with hemolytic disease of the newborn. *J Am Acad Dermatol.* 1995;33:333–336
25. Paller AS, Eramo LR, Farrell EE, Millard DD, Honig PJ, Cunningham BB. Purpuric phototherapy-induced eruption in transfused neonates: relation to transient porphyrinemia. *Pediatrics.* 1997;100:360–364
26. Tonz O, Vogt J, Filippini L, Simmler F, Wachsmuth ED, Winterhalter KH. Severe light dermatosis following phototherapy in a newborn infant with congenital erythropoietic urophyria [in German]. *Helv Paediatr Acta.* 1975;30:47–56
27. Soylu A, Kavukcu S, Turkmen M. Phototherapy sequela in a child with congenital erythropoietic porphyria. *Eur J Pediatr.* 1999;158:526–527
28. Kearns GL, Williams BJ, Timmons OD. Fluorescein phototoxicity in a premature infant. *J Pediatr.* 1985;107:796–798

ERRATUM

Two errors appeared in the American Academy of Pediatrics clinical practice guideline, titled "Management of Hyperbilirubinemia in the Newborn Infant 35 or More Weeks of Gestation," that was published in the July 2004 issue of *Pediatrics* (2004;114:297–316). On page 107, Background section, first paragraph, the second sentence should read: "The current guideline represents a consensus of the committee charged by the AAP with reviewing and updating the existing guideline and is based on a careful review of the evidence, including a comprehensive literature review by the Agency for Healthcare Research and Quality and the New England Medical Center Evidence-Based Practice Center.[2]" On page 118, Appendix 1, first paragraph, the 4 levels of evidence quality should have been labeled A, B, C, and D rather than 1, 2, 3, and 4, respectively. The American Academy of Pediatrics regrets these errors.

Technical Report Summary:
An Evidence-Based Review of Important Issues Concerning Neonatal Hyperbilirubinemia

Authors:

Stanley Ip, MD; Mei Chung, MPH; John Kulig, MD, MPH; Rebecca O'Brien, MD; Robert Sege, MD, PhD; Stephan Glicken, MD; M. Jeffrey Maisels, MB, BCh; and Joseph Lau, MD, and the Subcommittee on Hyperbilirubinemia

American Academy of Pediatrics
PO Box 927, 141 Northwest Point Blvd
Elk Grove Village, IL 60009-0927

For the complete technical report, including tables, figures, and references, please see the companion CD-ROM.

ABSTRACT. This article is adapted from a published evidence report concerning neonatal hyperbilirubinemia with an added section on the risk of blood exchange transfusion (BET). Based on a summary of multiple case reports that spanned more than 30 years, we conclude that kernicterus, although infrequent, has at least 10% mortality and at least 70% long-term morbidity. It is evident that the preponderance of kernicterus cases occurred in infants with a bilirubin level higher than 20 mg/dL. Given the diversity of conclusions on the relationship between peak bilirubin levels and behavioral and neurodevelopmental outcomes, it is apparent that the use of a single total serum bilirubin level to predict long-term outcomes is inadequate and will lead to conflicting results. Evidence for efficacy of treatments for neonatal hyperbilirubinemia was limited. Overall, the 4 qualifying studies showed that phototherapy had an absolute risk-reduction rate of 10% to 17% for prevention of serum bilirubin levels higher than 20 mg/dL in healthy infants with jaundice. There is no evidence to suggest that phototherapy for neonatal hyperbilirubinemia has any long-term adverse neurodevelopmental effects. Transcutaneous measurements of bilirubin have a linear correlation to total serum bilirubin and may be useful as screening devices to detect clinically significant jaundice and decrease the need for serum bilirubin determinations. Based on our review of the risks associated with BETs from 15 studies consisting mainly of infants born before 1970, we conclude that the mortality within 6 hours of BET ranged from 3 per 1000 to 4 per 1000 exchanged infants who were term and without serious hemolytic diseases. Regardless of the definitions and rates of BET-associated morbidity and the various pre-exchange clinical states of the exchanged infants, in many cases the morbidity was minor (eg, postexchange anemia). Based on the results from the most recent study to report BET morbidity, the overall risk of permanent sequelae in 25 sick infants who survived BET was from 5% to 10%.

The American Academy of Pediatrics (AAP) requested an evidence report from the Agency for Healthcare Research and Quality (AHRQ) that would critically examine the available evidence regarding the effect of high levels of bilirubin on behavioral and neurodevelopmental outcomes, role of various comorbid effect modifiers (eg, sepsis and hemolysis) on neurodevelopment, efficacy of phototherapy, reliability of various strategies in predicting significant hyperbilirubinemia, and accuracy of transcutaneous bilirubin (TcB) measurements. The report was used by the AAP to update the 1994 AAP guidelines for the management of neonatal hyperbilirubinemia. This review focuses on otherwise healthy term or near-term (at least 34 weeks' estimated gestational age [EGA] or at least 2500 g birth weight) infants with hyperbilirubinemia. This article is adapted from that published report with an added section on the risk of blood exchange transfusion (BET).

Neither hyperbilirubinemia nor kernicterus are reportable diseases, and there are no reliable sources of information providing national annual estimates. Since the advent of effective prevention of rhesus (Rh) incompatibility and treatment of elevated bilirubin levels with phototherapy, kernicterus has become uncommon. When laboratory records of a 1995–1996 birth cohort of more than 50 000 California infants were examined, Newman et al reported that 2% had total serum bilirubin (TSB) levels higher than 20 mg/dL, 0.15% had levels higher than 25 mg/dL, and only 0.01% had levels higher than 30 mg/dL. (These data were from infants with clinically identified hyperbilirubinemia and, as such, represent a minimum estimate of the true incidence of extreme hyperbilirubinemia.) This is undoubtedly the result of successful prevention of hemolytic anemia and the application of effective treatment of elevated serum bilirubin levels in accordance with currently accepted medical practice. Projecting the California estimates to the national birth rate of 4 million per year, one can predict 80 000, 6000, and 400 newborns per year with bilirubin levels of more than 20, 25, and 30 mg/dL, respectively.

Recently, concern has been expressed that the increase in early hospital discharges, coupled with a rise in breast-feeding rates, has led to a rise in the rate of preventable kernicterus resulting from "unattended to" hyperbilirubinemia. However, a report published in 2002, based on a national registry established since 1992, reported only 90 cases of kernicterus, although the efficiency of case ascertainment is not clear. Thus, there are no data to establish incidence trends reliably for either hyperbilirubinemia or kernicterus.

Despite these constraints, there has been substantial research on the neurodevelopmental outcomes of hyperbilirubinemia and its prediction and treatment. Subsequent sections of this review describe in more detail the precise study questions and the existing published work in this area.

METHODOLOGY

This evidence report is based on a systematic review of the medical literature. Our Evidence-Based Practice Center formed a review team consisting of pediatricians and Evidence-Based Practice Center methodologic staff to review the literature and perform data abstraction and analysis. For details regarding methodology, please see the original AHRQ report.

Key Questions

Question 1: What is the relationship between peak bilirubin levels and/or duration of hyperbilirubinemia and neurodevelopmental outcome?
Question 2: What is the evidence for effect modification of the results in question 1 by GA, hemolysis, serum albumin, and other factors? Question 3: What are the quantitative estimates of efficacy of treatment for 1) reducing peak bilirubin levels (eg, number needed to treat [NNT] at 20 mg/dL to keep TSB from rising); 2) reducing the duration of hyperbilirubinemia (eg, average number of hours by which time TSB is higher than 20 mg/dL may be shortened by treatment); and 3) improving neurodevelopmental outcomes?
Question 4: What is the efficacy of various strategies for predicting hyperbilirubinemia, including hour-specific bilirubin percentiles? Question 5: What is the accuracy of TcB measurements?

Search Strategies

We searched the Medline database on September 25, 2001, for publications from 1966 to the present using relevant medical subject heading terms ("hyperbilirubinemia"; "hyperbilirubinemia, hereditary"; "bilirubin"; "jaundice, neonatal"; and "kernicterus") and text words ("bilirubin,""hyperbilirubinemia,""jaundice," "kernicterus,"and "neonatal"). The abstracts were limited to human subjects and English-language studies focusing on newborns between birth and 1 month of age. In addition, the same text words used for the Medline search were used to search the Pre-Medline database. The strategy yielded 4280 Medline and 45 Pre-Medline abstracts. We consulted domain experts and examined relevant review articles for additional studies. A supplemental search for case reports of kernicterus in reference lists of relevant articles and reviews was performed also.

Screening and Selection Process

In our preliminary screening of abstracts, we identified more than 600 potentially relevant articles in total for questions 1, 2, and 3. To handle this large number of articles, we devised the following scheme to address the key questions and ensure that the report was completed within the time and resource constraints. We included only studies that measured neurodevelopmental or behavioral outcomes (except for question 3, part 1, for which we evaluated all studies addressing the efficacy of treatment). For the specific question of quantitative estimates of efficacy of treatment, all studies concerning therapies designed to prevent hyperbilirubinemia (generally bilirubin greater than or equal to 20 mg/dL) were included in the review.

Inclusion Criteria

The target population of this review was healthy, term infants. For the purpose of this review, we included articles concerning infants who were at least 34 weeks' EGA at the time of birth. From studies that reported birth weight rather than age, infants whose birth weight was greater than or equal to 2500 g were included. This cutoff was derived from findings of the National Institute of Child Health and Human Development (NICHD) hyperbilirubinemia study, in which none of the 1339 infants weighing greater than or equal to 2500 g were less than 34 weeks' EGA. Articles were selected for inclusion in the systematic review based on the following additional criteria:

Question 1 or 2 (Risk Association)

- Population: infants greater than or equal to 34 weeks' EGA or birth weight greater than or equal to 2500 g.
- Sample size: more than 5 subjects per arm
- Predictors: jaundice or hyperbilirubinemia
- Outcomes: at least 1 behavioral/neurodevelopmental outcome reported in the article
- Study design: prospective cohorts (more than 2 arms), prospective cross-sectional study, prospective longitudinal study, prospective single-arm study, or retrospective cohorts (more than 2 arms)

Case Reports of Kernicterus

- Population: kernicterus case
- Study design: case reports with kernicterus as a predictor or an outcome

Kernicterus, as defined by authors, included any of the following: acute phase of kernicterus (poor feeding, lethargy, high-pitched cry, increased tone, opisthotonos, or seizures), kernicterus sequelae (motor delay, sensorineural hearing loss, gaze palsy, dental dysplasia, cerebral palsy, or mental retardation), necropsy finding of yellow staining in the brain nuclei.

Question 3 (Efficacy of Treatment at Reducing Serum Bilirubin)

- Population: infants greater than or equal to 34 weeks' EGA or birth weight greater than or equal to 2500 g
- Sample size: more than 10 subjects per arm
- Treatments: any treatment for neonatal hyperbilirubinemia
- Outcomes: serum bilirubin level higher than or equal to 20 mg/dL or frequency of BET specifically for bilirubin level higher than or equal to 20 mg/dL
- Study design: randomized or nonrandomized, controlled trials

For All Other Issues

- Population: infants greater than or equal to 34 weeks' EGA or birth weight greater than or equal to 2500 g
- Sample size: more than 10 subjects per arm for phototherapy; any sample size for other treatments
- Treatments: any treatment for neonatal hyperbilirubinemia
- Outcomes: at least 1 neurodevelopmental outcome was reported in the article

Question 4 or 5 (Diagnosis)

- Population: infants greater than or equal to 34 weeks' EGA or birth weight greater than or equal to 2500 g
- Sample size: more than 10 subjects
- Reference standard: laboratory-based TSB

Exclusion Criteria

Case reports of kernicterus were excluded if they did not report serum bilirubin level or GA and birth weight.

Results of Screening of Titles and Abstracts

There were 158, 174, 99, 153, and 79 abstracts for questions 1, 2, 3, 4, and 5, respectively. Some articles were relevant to more than 1 question.

Results of Screening of Full-Text Articles

After full-text screening (according to the inclusion and exclusion criteria described previously), 138 retrieved articles were included in this report. There were 35 articles in the correlation section (questions 1 and 2), 28 articles of kernicterus case reports, 21 articles in the treatment section (question 3), and 54 articles in the diagnosis section (questions 4 and 5). There were inevitable overlaps, because treatment effects and assessment of neurodevelopmental outcomes were inherent in many study designs.

Reporting the Results

Articles that passed the full-text screening were grouped according to topic and analyzed in their entirety. Extracted data were synthesized into evidence tables.

Summarizing the Evidence of Individual Studies

Grading of the evidence can be useful for indicating the overall methodologic quality of a study. The evidence-grading scheme used here assesses 4 dimensions that are important for the proper interpretation of the evidence: study size, applicability, summary of results, and methodologic quality.

Definitions of Terminology

- Confounders (for question 1 only): 1) An ideal study design to answer question 1 would follow 2 groups, jaundiced and normal infants, without treating any infant for a current or consequent jaundice condition and observe their neurodevelopmental outcomes. Therefore, any treatment received by the subjects in the study was defined as a confounder. 2) If subjects had known risk factors for jaundice such as prematurity, breastfeeding, or low birth weight, the risk factors were defined as confounders. 3) Any disease condition other than jaundice was defined as a confounder. 4) Because bilirubin level is the essential predictor, if the study did not report or measure bilirubin levels for the subjects, lack of bilirubin measurements was defined as a confounder.
- Acute phase of kernicterus: poor feeding, lethargy, high-pitched cry, increased tone, opisthotonos, or seizures.
- Chronic kernicterus sequelae: motor delay, sensorineural hearing loss, gaze palsy, dental dysplasia, cerebral palsy, or mental retardation.

Statistical Analyses

In this report, 2 statistical analyses were performed in which there were sufficient data: the NNT and receiver operating characteristics (ROC) curve.

NNT

The NNT can be a clinically meaningful metric to assess the benefits of clinical trials. It is calculated by taking the inverse of the absolute risk difference. The absolute risk difference is the difference between the event rates between the treatment and control groups. For example, if the event rate is 15% in the control group and 10% in the treatment group, the absolute risk difference is 5% (an absolute risk reduction of 5%). The NNT then would be 20 (1 divided by 0.05), meaning that 20 patients will need to be treated to see 1 fewer event. In the setting of neonatal hyperbilirubinemia, NNT might be interpreted as the number of newborns needed to be treated (with phototherapy) at 13 to 15 mg/dL to prevent 1 newborn from reaching 20 mg/dL.

ROC Curve

ROC curves were developed for individual studies in question 4 if multiple thresholds of a diagnostic technology were reported. The areas under the curves (AUCs) were calculated to provide an assessment of the overall accuracy of the tests.

Meta-analyses of Diagnostic Test Performance

Meta-analyses were performed to quantify the TcB measurements for which the data were sufficient. We used 3 complementary methods for assessing diagnostic test performance: summary ROC analysis, independently combined sensitivity and specificity values, and meta-analysis of correlation coefficients.

RESULTS

Question 1. What Is the Relationship Between Peak Bilirubin Levels and/or Duration of Hyperbilirubinemia and Neurodevelopmental Outcome?

The first part of the results for this question deals with kernicterus; the second part deals with otherwise healthy term or near-term infants who had hyperbilirubinemia.

Case Reports of Kernicterus

Our literature search identified 28 case-report articles of infants with kernicterus that reported sufficient data for analysis. (The largest case series of 90 healthy term and near-term infants with kernicterus was reported by Johnson et al in 2002, but no individual data were available and therefore were not included in this analysis.

Those cases with available individual data previously reported were included in this analysis.) Most of the articles were identified in Medline and published since 1966. We retrieved additional articles published before 1966 based on review of references in articles published since 1966. Our report focuses on term and near-term infants (greater than or equal to 34 weeks' EGA). Only infants with measured peak bilirubin level and known GA or birth weight or with clinical or autop-sy-diagnosed kernicterus were included in the analysis. It is important to note that some of these peak levels were obtained more than 7 days after birth and therefore may not have represented true peak levels. Similarly, some of the diagnoses of kernicterus were made only at autopsies, and the measured bilirubin levels were obtained more than 24 hours before the infants died, and therefore the reported bilirubin levels may not have reported the true peak levels. Because of the small number of subjects, none of the following comparisons are statistically significant. Furthermore, because case reports in this section represent highly selected cases, interpreting these data must be done cautiously.

Demographics of Kernicterus Cases

Articles identified through the search strategy span from 1955 to 2001 with a total of 123 cases of kernicterus. Twelve cases in 2 studies were reported before 1960; however, some studies reported cases that spanned almost 2 decades. Data on subjects' birth years were reported in only 55 cases. Feeding status, gender, racial background, and ethnicity were not noted in most of the reports. Of those that were reported, almost all the subjects were breastfed and most were males.

Geographic Distribution of Reported Kernicterus Cases

The 28 case reports with a total of 123 cases are from 14 different countries. They are the United States, Singapore, Turkey, Greece, Taiwan, Denmark, Canada, Japan, United Kingdom, France, Jamaica, Norway, Scotland, and Germany. The number of kernicterus cases in each study ranged from 1 to 12.

Kernicterus has been defined by pathologic findings, acute clinical findings, and chronic sequelae (such as deafness or athetoid cerebral palsy). Because of the small number of subjects, all definitions of kernicterus have been included in the analysis. Exceptions will be noted in the following discussion.

Kernicterus Cases With Unknown Etiology

Among infants at greater than or equal to 34 weeks' GA or who weighed 2500 g or more at birth and had no known explanation for kernicterus, there were 35 infants with peak bilirubin ranging from 22.5 to 54 mg/dL. Fifteen had no information on gender, 14 were males, and 6 were females. Fourteen had no information on feeding,

20 were breastfed, and 1 was formula-fed. More than 90% of the infants with kernicterus had bilirubin higher than 25 mg/dL: 25% of the kernicterus cases had peak TSB levels up to 29.9 mg/dL, and 50% had peak TSB levels up to 34.9 mg/dL (Fig 2). There was no association between bilirubin level and birth weight.

Four infants died. Four infants who had acute clinical kernicterus had normal follow-up at 3 to 6 years by telephone. One infant with a peak bilirubin level of 44 mg/dL had a flat brainstem auditory evoked response (BAER) initially but normalized at 2 months of age; this infant had normal neurologic and developmental examinations at 6 months of age. Ten infants had chronic sequelae of kernicterus when followed up between 6 months and 7 years of age. Seven infants were noted to have neurologic findings consistent with kernicterus; however, the age at diagnosis was not provided. Nine infants had a diagnosis of kernicterus with no follow-up information provided. To summarize, 11% of this group of infants died, 14% survived with no sequelae, and at least 46% had chronic sequelae. The distribution of peak TSB levels was higher when only infants who died or had chronic sequelae were included.

Kernicterus Cases With Comorbid Factors

In the 88 term and near-term infants diagnosed with kernicterus and who had hemolysis, sepsis, and other neonatal complications, bilirubin levels ranged from 4.0 to 51.0 mg/dL (as previously mentioned, these may not represent true peak levels; the bilirubin level of 4 mg/dL was measured more than 24 hours before the infant died, the diagnosis of kernicterus was made by autopsy). Forty-two cases provided no information on gender, 25 were males, and 21 were females. Seventy-two cases had no information on feeding, 15 were breastfed, and 1 was formula-fed. Most infants with kernicterus had bilirubin levels higher than 20 mg/dL: 25% of the kernicterus cases had peak TSB levels up to 24.9 mg/dL, and 50% had peak TSB levels up to 29.9 mg/dL (Fig 4). In this group, there was no association between the bilirubin levels and birth weight.

Five infants without clinical signs of kernicterus were diagnosed with kernicterus by autopsy. Eight infants died of kernicterus. One infant was found to have a normal neurologic examination at 4 months of age. Another infant with galactosemia and a bilirubin level of 43.6 mg/dL who had acute kernicterus was normal at 5 months of age. Forty-nine patients had chronic sequelae ranging from hearing loss to athetoid cerebral palsy; the follow-up age reported ranged from 4 months to 14 years. Twenty-one patients were diagnosed with kernicterus, with no fol-low-up information. Not including the autopsy-diagnosed kernicterus, 10% of these infants died (8/82), 2% were found to be normal at 4 to 5 months of age, and

at least 60% had chronic sequelae. The distribution of peak TSB levels was slightly higher when only infants who died or had chronic sequelae were included.

Evidence Associating Bilirubin Exposures With Neurodevelopmental Outcomes in Healthy Term or Near-Term Infants

This section examines the evidence associating bilirubin exposures with neurodevelopmental outcomes primarily in subjects without kernicterus. Studies that were designed specifically to address the behavioral and neurodevelopmental outcomes in healthy infants at more than or equal to 34 weeks' GA will be discussed first. With the exception of the results from the Collaborative Perinatal Project (CPP) (CPP, with 54 795 subjects, has generated many follow-up studies with a smaller number of subjects, and those studies were discussed together in a separate section in the AHRQ summary report), the remainder of the studies that include mixed subjects (preterm and term, diseased and nondiseased) were categorized and discussed by outcome measures. These measures include behavioral and neurologic outcomes; hearing impairment, including sensorineural hearing loss; and intelligence measurements.

The CPP, with 54 795 live births between 1959 and 1966 from 12 centers in the United States, produced the largest database for the study of hyperbilirubinemia. Newman and Klebanoff, focusing only on black and white infants weighing 2500 g or more at birth, did a comprehensive analysis of 7-year outcome in 33 272 subjects. All causes of jaundice were included in the analysis. The study found no consistent association between peak bilirubin level and intelligence quotient (IQ). Sensorineural hearing loss was not related to bilirubin level. Only the frequency of abnormal or suspicious neurologic examinations was associated with bilirubin level. The specific neurologic examination items most associated with bilirubin levels were mild and nonspecific motor abnormalities.

In other studies stemming from the CPP population, there was no consistent evidence to suggest neurologic abnormalities in children with neonatal bilirubin higher than 20 mg/dL when followed up to 7 years of age.

A question that has concerned pediatricians for many years is whether moderate hyperbilirubinemia is associated with abnormalities in neurodevelopmental outcome in term healthy infants without perinatal or neonatal problems. Only 4 prospective studies and 1 retrospective study have the requisite subject characteristics to address this issue. Although there were some short-term (less than 12 months) abnormal neurologic or behavioral characteristics noted in infants with high bilirubin, the studies had methodologic problems and did not show consistent results.

Evidence Associating Bilirubin Exposures With Neurodevelopmental Outcomes in All Infants

These studies consist of subjects who, in addition to healthy term newborns, might include newborns less than 34 weeks' GA and neonatal complications such as sepsis, respiratory distress, hemolytic disorders, and other factors. Nevertheless, some of the conclusions drawn might be applicable to a healthy term population. In these studies, greater emphasis will be placed on the reported results for the group of infants who were at greater than or equal to 34 weeks' EGA or weighed 2500 g or more at birth.

Studies Measuring Behavioral and Neurologic Outcomes in Infants With Hyperbilirubinemia

A total of 9 studies in 11 publications examined primarily behavioral and neurologic outcomes in patients with hyperbilirubinemia. Of these 9 studies, 3 were of high methodologic quality. One short-term study showed a correlation between bilirubin level and decreased scores on newborn behavioral measurements. One study found no difference in prevalence of central nervous system abnormalities at 4 years old if bilirubin levels were less than 20 mg/dL, but infants with bilirubin levels higher than 20 mg/dL had a higher prevalence of central nervous system abnormalities. Another study that followed infants with bilirubin levels higher than 16 mg/dL found no relationship between bilirubin and neurovisuomotor testing at 61 to 82 months of age. Although data reported in the remainder of the studies are of lower methodologic quality, there is a suggestion of abnormalities in neurodevelopmental screening tests in infants with bilirubin levels higher than 20 mg/dL, at least by the Denver Developmental Screening Test, when infants were followed up at 1 year of age. It seems that bilirubin levels higher than 20 mg/dL may have short-term (up to 1 year of age) adverse effects at least by the Denver Developmental Screening Test, but there is no strong evidence to suggest neurologic abnormalities in children with neonatal bilirubin levels higher than 20 mg/dL when followed up to 7 years of age.

Effect of Bilirubin on Brainstem Auditory Evoked Potential (BAEP)

The following group of studies, in 14 publications, primarily examined the effect of bilirubin on BAEP or hearing impairment. Eight high-quality studies showed a significant relationship between abnormalities in BAEP and high bilirubin levels. Most reported resolution of abnormalities with treatment. Three studies reported hearing impairment associated with elevated bilirubin (higher than 16–20 mg/dL).

Effect of Bilirubin on Intelligence Outcomes

Eight studies looked primarily at the effect of bilirubin on intelligence outcomes. Four high-quality studies with follow-up ranging from 6.5 to 17 years reported no association between IQ and bilirubin level.

Question 2. What Is the Evidence for Effect Modification of the Results in Question 1 by GA, Hemolysis, Serum Albumin, and Other Factors?

There is only 1 article that directly addressed this question. Naeye, using the CPP population, found that at 4 years old the frequency of low IQ with increasing bilirubin levels increased more rapidly in infants with infected amniotic fluid. At 7 years old, neurologic abnormalities also were more prevalent in that subgroup of infants.

When comparing the group of term and near-term infants with comorbid factors who had kernicterus to the group of infants with idiopathic hyperbilirubinemia and kernicterus, the overall mean bilirubin was 31.6 ± 9 mg/dL in the former, versus 35.4 ± 8 mg/dL in the latter (difference not significant). Infants with glucose-6-phosphate dehydrogenase deficiency, sepsis, ABO incompatibility, or Rh incompatibility had similar mean bilirubin levels. Infants with more than 1 comorbid factor had a slightly lower mean bilirubin level of 29.1 ± 16.1 mg/dL.

Eighteen of 23 (78%) term infants with idiopathic hyperbilirubinemia and who developed acute kernicterus survived the neonatal period with chronic sequelae. Thirty-nine of 41 (95%) term infants with kernicterus and ABO or Rh incompatibility had chronic sequelae. Four of 5 (80%) infants with sepsis and kernicterus had chronic sequelae. All 4 infants with multiple comorbid factors had sequelae.

No firm conclusions can be drawn regarding co-morbid factors and kernicterus, because this is a small number of patients from a variety of case reports.

There was no direct study concerning serum albumin level as an effect modifier of neurodevelopmental outcome in infants with hyperbilirubinemia. One report found a significant association between reserve albumin concentration and latency to wave V in BAEP studies.

In addition, Ozmert et al noted that exchange transfusion and the duration that the infant's serum indirect bilirubin level remained higher than 20 mg/dL were important risk factors for prominent neurologic abnormalities.

Question 3. What Are the Quantitative Estimates of Efficacy of Treatment at 1) Reducing Peak Bilirubin Levels (eg, NNT at 20 mg/dL to Keep TSB From Rising); 2) Reducing the Duration of Hyperbilirubinemia (eg, Average Number of Hours by Which Time TSB Levels Higher Than 20 mg/dL May Be Shortened by Treatment); and 3) Improving Neurodevelopmental Outcomes?

Studies on phototherapy efficacy in terms of preventing TSB rising to the level that would require BET (and therefore would be considered "failure of phototherapy") were reviewed for the quantitative estimates of efficacy of phototherapy. Because trials evaluating the efficacy of phototherapy at improving neurodevelopmental outcomes by comparing 1 group of infants with treatment to an untreated group do not exist, the effects of treatment on neurodevelopmental outcomes could only be reviewed descriptively. Furthermore, all the reports primarily examined the efficacy of treatment at 15 mg/dL to prevent TSB from exceeding 20 mg/dL. There is no study to examine the efficacy of treatment at 20 mg/dL to prevent the TSB from rising.

Efficacy of Phototherapy for Prevention of TSB Levels Higher Than 20 mg/dL

Four publications examined the clinical efficacy of phototherapy for prevention of TSB levels higher than 20 mg/dL.

Two studies evaluated the same sample of infants. Both reports were derived from a randomized, controlled trial of phototherapy for neonatal hyperbilirubinemia commissioned by the NICHD between 1974 and 1976.

Because the phototherapy protocols differed significantly in the remaining studies, their results could not be statistically combined and are reported here separately. A total of 893 term or near-term jaundiced infants (325 in the treatment group and 568 in the control group) were evaluated in the current review.

The development, design, and sample composition of NICHD phototherapy trial were reported in detail elsewhere. The NICHD controlled trial of phototherapy for neonatal hyperbilirubinemia consisted of 672 infants who received phototherapy and 667 control infants. Brown et al evaluated the efficacy of phototherapy for prevention of the need for BET in the NICHD study population. For the purpose of current review, only the subgroup of 140 infants in the treatment groups and 136 in the control groups with birth weights 2500 g or more and greater than or equal to 34 weeks' GA were evaluated. The serum bilirubin level as criterion for BET in infants with birth weights of 2500 g or more was 20 mg/dL at standard risk and 18 mg/dL at high risk. It was found that infants with hyperbilirubinemia secondary to nonhemolytic causes who received phototherapy had a 14.3% risk reduction of BET than infants in no treatment group. NNT for prevention of the need for BET or for TSB levels higher than 20 mg/dL was 7 (95% confidence interval [CI]: 6–8). However, phototherapy did not reduce the need for BET for infants with hemolytic diseases or in the high-risk group. No therapeutic effect on reducing the BET rate in infants at greater than or equal to 34 weeks' GA with hemolytic disease was observed.

The same group of infants, 140 subjects in the treatment group and 136 controls with birth weights 2500 g or more and greater than or equal to 34 weeks' GA, were evaluated for the effect of phototherapy on the hyperbilirubinemia of Coombs' positive hemolytic disease in the study of Maurer et al. Of the 276 infants whose birth weights were 2500 g or more, 64 (23%) had positive Coombs' tests: 58 secondary to ABO incompatibility and 6 secondary to Rh incompatibility. Thirty-four of 64 in this group received phototherapy. The other 30 were placed in the control group. Of the 212 subjects who had negative Coombs' tests, 106 were in the treatment group and the same number was in the control group. No therapeutic effect on reducing the BET rate was observed in infants with Coombs' positive hemolytic disease, but there was a 9.4% absolute risk reduction in infants who had negative Coombs' tests. In this group of infants, the NNT for prevention of the need for BET, or a TSB higher than 20 mg/dL, was 11 (95% CI: 10–12).

A more recent randomized, controlled trial compared the effect of 4 different interventions on hyperbilirubinemia (serum bilirubin concentration greater than or equal to 291 μmol/L or 17 mg/dL) in 125 term breastfed infants. Infants with any congenital anomalies, neonatal complications, hematocrit more than 65%, significant bruising or large cephalohematomas, or hemolytic disease were excluded. The 4 interventions in the study were 1) continue breastfeeding and observe ($N = 25$); 2) discontinue breastfeeding and substitute formula ($N = 26$); 3) discontinue breastfeeding, substitute formula, and administer phototherapy ($N = 38$); and 4) continue breastfeeding and administer phototherapy ($N = 36$). The interventions were considered failures if serum bilirubin levels reached 324 μmol/L or 20 mg/dL. For the purpose of the current review, we regrouped the subjects into treatment group or phototherapy group and control group or no-phototherapy group. Therefore, the original groups 4 and 3 became the treatment groups I and II, and the original groups 1 and 2 were the corresponding control groups I and II. It was found that treatment I, phototherapy with continuation of breastfeeding, had a 10% absolute risk-reduction rate, and the NNT for prevention of a serum bilirubin level higher than 20 mg/dL was 10 (95% CI: 9–12). Compared with treatment I, treatment II (phototherapy with discontinuation of breastfeeding) was significantly more efficacious. The absolute risk-reduction rate was 17%, and the NNT for prevention of a serum bilirubin level exceeding 20 mg/dL was 6 (95% CI: 5–7).

John reported the effect of phototherapy in 492 term neonates born during 1971 and 1972 who developed unexplained jaundice with bilirubin levels higher than 15 mg/dL. One hundred eleven infants received phototherapy, and 381 did not. The author stated: "The choice of therapy was, in effect, random since two pediatricians approved of the treatment and two did not." The results showed that phototherapy had an 11% risk reduction of BET, performed in treatment and control groups when serum bilirubin levels exceeded 20 mg/dL. Therefore, the NNT for prevention of a serum bilirubin level higher than 20 mg/dL was 9 (95% CI: 8–10).

Regardless of different protocols for phototherapy, the NNT for prevention of serum bilirubin levels higher than 20 mg/dL ranged from 6 to 10 in healthy term or near-term infants. Evidence for the efficacy of treatments for neonatal hyperbilirubinemia was limited. Overall, the 4 qualifying studies showed that phototherapy had an absolute risk-reduction rate of 10% to 17% for prevention of serum bilirubin exceeding 20 mg/dL in healthy and jaundiced infants (TSB levels higher than or equal to 13 mg/dL) born at greater than or equal to 34 weeks' GA. Phototherapy combined with cessation of breastfeeding and substitution with formula was found to be the most efficient treatment protocol for healthy term or near-term infants with jaundice.

Effectiveness of Reduction in Bilirubin Level on BAER in Jaundiced Infants With Greater Than or Equal to 34 Weeks' EGA

Eight studies that compared BAER before and after treatments for neonatal hyperbilirubinemia are discussed in this section. Of the 8 studies, 3 studies treated jaundiced infants by administering phototherapy followed by BET according to different guidelines, 4 studies treated jaundiced infants with BET only, and 1 study did not specify what treatments jaundiced infants received. All the studies consistently showed that treatments for neonatal hyperbilirubinemia significantly improved abnormal BAERs in healthy jaundiced infants and jaundiced infants with hemolytic disease.

Effect of Phototherapy on Behavioral and Neurologic Outcomes and IQ

Five studies looked at the effect of hyperbilirubinemia and phototherapy on behavior. Of the 5 studies, 4 used the Brazelton Neonatal Behavioral Assessment Scale and 1 used the Vineland Social Maturity Scale. Three studies reported lower scores in the orientation cluster of the Brazelton Neonatal Behavioral Assessment Scale in the infants treated with phototherapy. The other 2 studies did not find behavioral changes in the phototherapy group. One study evaluated IQ at the age of 17 years. In 42 term infants with severe hyperbilirubinemia who were treated with phototherapy, 31 were also treated with BET. Forty-two infants who did not receive phototherapy were selected as controls. No significant difference in IQ between the 2 groups was found.

Effect of Phototherapy on Visual Outcomes

Three studies were identified that studied the effect of serum bilirubin and treatment on visual outcomes. All showed no short-or long-term (up to 36 months) effect on vision as a result of phototherapy when infants' eyes are protected properly during treatment.

Question 4. What Is the Accuracy of Various Strategies for Predicting Hyperbilirubinemia, Including Hour-Specific Bilirubin Percentiles?

Ten qualifying studies published from 1977 to 2001 examining 5 prediction methods of neonatal hyperbilirubinemia were included. A total of 8167 neonates, most healthy near-term or term infants, were subjects. These studies were conducted among multiple racial groups in multiple countries including China, Denmark, India, Israel, Japan, Spain, and the United States. Some studies included subjects with ABO incompatibility, and some did not. Four studies examined the accuracy of cord bilirubin level as a test for predicting the development of clinically significant neonatal jaundice. Four studies investigated the test performance of serum bilirubin levels before 48 hours of life to predict hyperbilirubinemia. Two studies further compared the test performances of cord bilirubin with that of early serum bilirubin levels. The accuracy of end-tidal carbon monoxide concentration as a predictor of the development of hyperbilirubinemia was examined in Okuyama et al and Stevenson et al. The study by Stevenson et al also examined the test performance of a combined strategy of end-tidal carbon monoxide concentration and early serum bilirubin levels. Finally, 2 studies tested the efficacy of predischarge risk assessment, determined by a risk index model and hour-specific bilirubin percentile, respectively, for predicting neonatal hyperbilirubinemia.

ROC curves were developed for 3 of the predictive strategies. The AUCs were calculated to provide an assessment of the overall accuracy of the tests. Hour-specific bilirubin percentiles had an AUC of 0.93, cord bilirubin levels had an AUC of 0.74, and predischarge risk index had an AUC of 0.80. These numbers should not be compared directly with each other, because the studies had different population characteristics and different defining parameters for hyperbilirubinemia.

Question 5. What Is the Accuracy of TcB Measurements?

A total of 47 qualifying studies in 50 publications examining the test performance of TcB measurements and/or the correlation of TcB measurements to serum bilirubin levels was reviewed in this section. Of the 47 studies, the Minolta Air-Shields jaundice meter (Air-Shields, Hatboro, PA) was used in 41 studies, the BiliCheck (SpectRx Inc, Norcross, GA) was used in 3 studies, the Ingram icterometer (Thomas A. Ingram and Co, Birmingham, England; distributed in the United States by Cascade Health Care Products, Salem, OR) was used in 4 studies, and the ColorMate III (Chromatics Color Sciences International Inc, New York, NY) was used in 1 study.

Based on the evidence from the systematic review, TcB measurements by each of the 4 devices described in the literature (the Minolta Air-Shields jaundice meter, Ingram icterometer, BiliCheck, and Chromatics ColorMate

III) have a linear correlation to TSB and may be useful as screening devices to detect clinically significant jaundice and decrease the need for serum bilirubin determinations.

Minolta Air-Shields Jaundice Meter

Generally, TcB readings from the forehead or sternum have correlated well with TSB but with a wide range of correlation coefficients, from a low of 0.52 for subgroup of infants less than 37 weeks' GA to as high as 0.96. Comparison of correlations across studies is difficult because of differences in study design and selection procedures. TcB indices that correspond to various TSB levels vary from institution to institution but seem to be internally consistent. Different TSB threshold levels were used across studies; therefore, there is limited ability to combine data across the studies. Most of the studies used TcB measurements taken at the forehead, several studies used multiple sites and combined results, 1 study used only the midsternum site, and 3 studies took the TcB measurement at multiple sites.

The Minolta Air-Shields jaundice meter seems to perform less well in black infants, compared with white infants, performs best when measurements are made at the sternum, and performs less well when infants have been exposed to phototherapy. This instrument requires daily calibration, and each institution must develop its own correlation curves of TcB to TSB. Eleven studies of the test performance of the Minolta Air-Shields jaundice meter measuring at forehead to predict a serum bilirubin threshold of higher than or equal to 13 mg/dL were included in the following analysis. A total of 1560 paired TcB and serum bilirubin measurements were evaluated. The cutoff points of Minolta AirShields TcB measurements (TcB index) ranged from 13 to 24 for predicting a serum bilirubin level higher than or equal to 13 mg/dL. As a screening test, it does not perform consistently across studies, as evidenced by the heterogeneity in the summary ROC curves not explained by threshold effect. The overall unweighted pooled estimates of sensitivity and specificity were 0.85 (0.77–0.91) and 0.77 (0.66–0.85).

Ingram Icterometer

The Ingram icterometer consists of a strip of transparent Plexiglas on which 5 yellow transverse stripes of precise and graded hue are painted. The correlation coefficients (r) in the 4 studies ranged from 0.63 to 0.97. The icterometer has the added limitation of lacking the objectivity of the other methods, because it depends on observer visualization of depth of yellow color of the skin.

BiliCheck

The recently introduced BiliCheck device, which uses reflectance data from multiple wavelengths, seems to be a significant improvement over the older devices (the Ingram icterometer and the Minolta Air-Shields jaundice meter) because of its ability to determine correction factors

for the effect of melanin and hemoglobin. Three studies examined the accuracy of the BiliCheck TcB measurements to predict TSB ("gold standard"). All studies were rated as high quality. The correlation coefficient ranged from 0.83 to 0.91. In 1 study, the BiliCheck was shown to be as accurate as the laboratory measurement of TSB when compared with the reference gold-standard high-performance liquid chromatography (HPLC) measurement of TSB. Analysis of covariance found no differences in test performance by postnatal age, GA, birth weight, or race; however, 66.7% were white and only 4.3% were black.

Chromatics ColorMate III

One study that evaluated the performance of the ColorMate III transcutaneous bilirubinometer was reviewed. The correlation coefficient for the whole study group was 0.9563, and accuracy was not affected by race, weight, or phototherapy. The accuracy of the device is increased by the determination of an infant's underlying skin type before the onset of visual jaundice; thus, a drawback to the method when used as a screening device is that all infants would require an initial baseline measurement.

CONCLUSIONS AND DISCUSSION

Summarizing case reports of kernicterus from different investigators in different countries from different periods is problematic. First, definitions of kernicterus used in these reports varied greatly. They included gross yellow staining of the brain, microscopic neuronal degeneration, acute clinical neuromotor impairment, neuroauditory impairment, and chronic neuromotor impairment. In some cases, the diagnoses were not established until months or years after birth. Second, case reports without controls makes interpretation difficult, especially in infants with comorbid factors, and could very well lead to misinterpretation of the role of bilirubin in neurodevelopmental outcomes. Third, different reports used different outcome measures. "Normal at follow-up" may be based on parental reporting, physician assessment, or formal neuropsychologic testing. Fourth, time of reported follow-up ranged from days to years. Fifth, cases were reported from different countries at different periods and with different standards of practice managing hyperbilirubinemia. Some countries have a high prevalence of glucose-6-phosphate dehydrogenase deficiency. Some have cultural practices that predispose their infants to agents that cause hyperbilirubinemia (such as clothing stored in dressers with naphthalene moth balls). The effect of the differences on outcomes cannot be known for certain. Finally, it is difficult to infer from case reports the true incidence of this uncommon disorder.

To recap our findings, based on a summary of multiple case reports that spanned more than 30 years, we conclude that kernicterus, although infrequent, has significant mortality (at least 10%) and long-term morbidity (at least

70%). It is evident that the preponderance of kernicterus cases occurred in infants with high bilirubin (more than 20 mg/dL).

Of 26 (19%) term or near-term infants with acute manifestations of kernicterus and reported follow-up data, 5 survived without sequelae, whereas only 3 of 63 (5%) infants with acute kernicterus and comorbid factors were reported to be normal at follow-up. This result suggests the importance of comorbid factors in determining long-term outcome in infants initially diagnosed with kernicterus.

For future research, reaching a national consensus in defining this entity, as in the model suggested by Johnson et al, will help in formulating a valid comparison of different databases. It is also apparent that, without good prevalence and incidence data on hyperbilirubinemia and kernicterus, one would not be able to estimate the risk of kernicterus at a given bilirubin level. Making severe hyperbilirubinemia (eg, greater than or equal to 25 mg/dL) and kernicterus reportable conditions would be a first step in that direction. Also, because kernicterus is infrequent, doing a multicenter case-control study with kernicterus may help to delineate the role of bilirubin in the development of kernicterus.

Hyperbilirubinemia, in most cases, is a necessary but not sufficient condition to explain kernicterus. Factors acting in concert with bilirubin must be studied to seek a satisfactory explanation. Information from duration of exposure to bilirubin and albumin binding of bilirubin may yield a more useful profile of the risk of kernicterus.

Only a few prospective controlled studies looked specifically at behavioral and neurodevelopmental outcomes in healthy term infants with hyperbilirubinemia. Most of these studies have a small number of subjects. Two short-term studies with well-defined measurement of newborn behavioral organization and physiologic measurement of cry are of high methodologic quality; however, the significance of long-term abnormalities in newborn behavior scales and variations in cry formant frequencies are unknown. There remains little information on the long-term effects of hyperbilirubinemia in healthy term infants.

Among the mixed studies (combined term and preterm, nonhemolytic and hemolytic, nondiseased and diseased), the following observations can be made:

- Nine of 15 studies (excluding the CPP) addressing neuroauditory development and bilirubin level were of high quality. Six of them showed BAER abnormalities correlated with high bilirubin levels. Most reported resolution with treatment. Three studies reported hearing impairment associated with elevated bilirubin (more than 16 to more than 20 mg/dL). We conclude that a high bilirubin level does have an adverse effect on neuroauditory function, but the adverse effect on BAER is reversible.

- Of the 8 studies reporting intelligence outcomes in subjects with hyperbilirubinemia, 4 studies were considered high quality. These 4 studies reported no association between IQ and bilirubin level, with follow-up ranging from 6.5 to 17 years. We conclude that there is no evidence to suggest a linear association of bilirubin level and IQ.

- The analysis of the CPP population found no consistent association between peak bilirubin level and IQ. Sensorineural hearing loss was not related to bilirubin level. Only the frequency of abnormal or suspicious neurologic examinations was associated with bilirubin level. In the rest of the studies from the CPP population, there was no consistent evidence to suggest neurologic abnormalities in children with neonatal bilirubin levels more than 20 mg/dL when followed up to 7 years of age.

A large prospective study comprising healthy infants greater than or equal to 34 weeks' GA with hyperbilirubinemia, specifically looking at long-term neurodevelopmental outcomes, has yet to be done. The report of Newman and Klebanoff came closest to that ideal because of the large number of subjects and the study's analytic approach. However, a population born from 1959 to 1966 is no longer representative of present-day newborns: 1) there is now increased ethnic diversity in our newborn population; 2) breast milk jaundice has become more common than hemolytic jaundice; 3) phototherapy for hyperbilirubinemia has become standard therapy; and 4) hospital stays are shorter. These changes in biologic, cultural, and health care characteristics make it difficult to apply the conclusions from the CPP population to present-day newborns.

Although short-term studies, in general, have good methodologic quality, they use tools that have unknown long-term predictive abilities. Long-term studies suffer from high attrition rates of the study population and a nonuniform approach to defining "normal neurodevelopmental outcomes." The total bilirubin levels reported in all the studies mentioned were measured anywhere from the first day of life to more than 2 weeks of life. Definitions of significant hyperbilirubinemia ranged from greater than or equal to 12 mg/dL to greater than or equal to 20 mg/dL.

Given the diversity of conclusions reported, except in cases of kernicterus with sequelae, it is evident that the use of a single TSB level (within the range described in this review) to predict long-term behavioral or neurodevelopmental outcomes is inadequate and will lead to conflicting results.

Evidence for the efficacy of treatments for neonatal hyperbilirubinemia was limited. Overall, the 4 qualifying studies showed that phototherapy had an absolute risk-reduction rate of 10% to 17% for prevention of serum bilirubin exceeding 20 mg/dL in healthy jaundiced infants

(TSB higher than or equal to 13 mg/dL) of greater than or equal to 34 weeks' GA. Phototherapy combined with cessation of breastfeeding and substitution with formula was found to be the most efficient treatment protocol for healthy term or near-term infants with jaundice. There is no evidence to suggest that phototherapy for neonatal hyperbilirubinemia has any long-term adverse neuro-developmental effects in either healthy jaundiced infants or infants with hemolytic disease. It is also noted that in all the studies listed, none of the infants received what is currently known as "intensive phototherapy." Although phototherapy did not reduce the need for BET in infants with hemolytic disease in the NICHD phototherapy trial, it could be attributable to the low dose of phototherapy used. Proper application of "intensive phototherapy" should decrease the need for BET further.

It is difficult to draw conclusions regarding the accuracy of various strategies for prediction of neonatal hyperbilirubinemia. The first challenge is the lack of consistency in defining clinically significant neonatal hyperbilirubinemia. Not only did multiple studies use different levels of TSB to define neonatal hyperbilirubinemia, but the levels of TSB defined as significant also varied by age, but age at TSB determination varied by study as well. For example, significant levels of TSB were defined as more than 11.7, more than or equal to 15, more than 15, more than 16, more than 17, and more than or equal to 25 mg/dL.

A second challenge is the heterogeneity of the study populations. The studies were conducted in many racial groups in different countries including China, Denmark, India, Israel, Japan, Spain, and the United States. Although infants were defined as healthy term and near-term newborns, these studies included neonates with potential for hemolysis from ABO-incompatible pregnancies as well as breastfed and bottle-fed infants (often not specified). Therefore, it is not possible to directly compare the different predicting strategies. However, all the strategies provided strong evidence that early jaundice predicts late jaundice.

Hour-specific bilirubin percentiles had an AUC of 0.93, implying great accuracy of this strategy. In that study, 2976 of 13 003 eligible infants had a postdischarge TSB measurement, as discussed by Maisels and Newman. Because of the large number of infants who did not have a postdischarge TSB, the actual study sample would be deficient in study participants with low predischarge bilirubin levels, leading to false high-sensitivity estimates and false low-specificity estimates. Moreover, the population in the study is not representative of the entire US population. The strategy of using early hour-specific bilirubin percentiles to predict late jaundice looks promising, but a large multicenter study (with evaluation of potential differences by race and ethnicity as well as prenatal, natal, and postnatal factors) may need to be undertaken to produce more applicable data.

TcB measurements by each of the 3 devices described in the literature, the Minolta Air-Shields jaundice meter, the Ingram icterometer, and the Bili-Check, have a linear correlation to TSB and may be useful as screening devices to detect clinically significant jaundice and decrease the need for serum bilirubin determinations.

The recently introduced BiliCheck device, which uses reflectance data from multiple wavelengths, seems to be a significant improvement over the older devices (the Ingram icterometer and the Minolta Air-Shields jaundice meter) because of its ability to determine correction factors for the effect of melanin and hemoglobin. In 1 study, the BiliCheck was shown to be as accurate as laboratory measures of TSB when compared with the reference gold-standard HPLC measurement of TSB.

Future research should confirm these findings in larger samples of diverse populations and address issues that might affect performance, such as race, GA, age at measurement, phototherapy, sunlight exposure, feeding and accuracy as screening instruments, performance at higher levels of bilirubin, and ongoing monitoring of jaundice. Additionally, studies should address cost-effectiveness and reproducibility in actual clinical practice. Given the interlaboratory variability of measurements of TSB, future studies of noninvasive measures of bilirubin should use HPLC and routine laboratory methods of TSB as reference standards, because the transcutaneous measures may prove to be as accurate as the laboratory measurement when compared with HPLC as the gold standard.

Using correlation coefficients to determine the accuracy of TcB measurements should be interpreted carefully because of several limitations:

- The correlation coefficient does not provide any information about the clinical utility of the diagnostic test.
- Although correlation coefficients measure the association between TcB and "standard" serum bilirubin measurements, the correlation coefficient is highly dependent on the distribution of serum bilirubin in the study population selected.
- Correlation measures ignore bias and measure relative rather than absolute agreement.

ADDENDUM: THE RISK OF BET

At the suggestion of AAP technical experts, a review of the risks associated with BET was also undertaken after the original AHRQ report was published. Articles were obtained from an informal survey of studies published since 1960 dealing with large populations that permitted calculations of the risks of morbidity and mortality. Of 15 studies, 8 consisted of subjects born before 1970. One article published in 1997 consisted of subjects born in 1994 and 1995.

Fifteen studies that reported data on BET-related mortality and/or morbidity were included in this review. Three categories were created to describe the percentage of subjects who met the criteria of the target population of our evidence report (ie, term idiopathic jaundice infants). Category I indicates that more than 50% of the study subjects were term infants whose pre-exchange clinical state was vigorous or stable and without disease conditions other than jaundice. Category II indicates that between 10% and 50% of the study subjects had category I characteristics. Category III indicates that more than 90% of the study subjects were preterm infants and/or term infants whose pre-exchange clinical state was not stable or was critically ill and with other disease conditions.

BET Subject and Study Characteristics

Because BET is no longer the mainstay of treatment for hyperbilirubinemia, most infants who underwent BETs were born in the 1950s to 1970s. Two recent studies reported BET-related mortality and morbidity for infants born from 1981 to 1995. After 1970, there were more infants who were premature, low birth weight or very low birth weight, and/or had a clinical condition(s) other than jaundice who received BETs than those born in earlier years. Not all infants in this review received BETs for hyperbilirubinemia. Because of limited data on subjects' bilirubin levels when the BETs were performed, we could not exclude those nonjaundiced infants.

BET-Associated Mortality

For all infants, the reported BET-related mortality ranged from 0% to 7%. There were no consistent definitions for BET-related mortality in the studies. An infant who died within 6 hours after the BET was the first used to define a BET-related death by Boggs and Westphal in 1960. Including the study from Boggs and Westphal, there were 3 studies reporting the 6-hour mortality, and they ranged from 0% to 1.9%. It is difficult to isolate BET as the sole factor in explaining mortality, because most of the subjects have significant associated pre-exchange disease morbidities. Most of the infants who died from BET had blood incompatibility and sepsis or were premature, had kernicterus, and/or were critically ill before undergoing BET. When only term infants were counted, the 6-hour mortality ranged from 3 to 19 per 1000 exchanged. When those term infants with serious hemolytic diseases (such as Rh incompatibility) were excluded, the 6-hour mortality ranged from 3 to 4 per 1000 exchanged infants. All these infants were born before 1970, and their jaundice was primarily due to ABO incompatibility.

BET-Associated Morbidity

There is an extensive list of complications that have been associated with BETs. Complications include those related to the use of blood products (infection, hemolysis of transfused blood, thromboembolization, graft versus host reactions), metabolic derangements (acidosis and perturbation of the serum concentrations of potassium, sodium, glucose, and calcium), cardiorespiratory reactions (including arrhythmias, apnea, and cardiac arrest), complications related to umbilical venous and arterial catheterization, and other miscellaneous complications. As noted previously, the pre-exchange clinical state of the infants studied varied widely, as did the definitions and rates of BET-associated morbidity. In many cases, however, the morbidity was minor (eg, postexchange anemia).

In the NICHD cooperative phototherapy study, morbidity (apnea, bradycardia, cyanosis, vasospasm, thrombosis) was observed in 22 of 328 (6.7%) patients in whom BETs were performed (no data available in 3 BETs). Of the 22 adverse events, 6 were mild episodes of bradycardia associated with calcium infusion. If those infants are excluded, as well as 2 who experienced transient arterial spasm, the incidence of "serious morbidity" associated with the procedure itself was 5.22%.

The most recent study to report BET morbidity in the era of contemporary neonatal care provides data on infants cared for from 1980 to 1995 at the Children's Hospital and University of Washington Medical Center in Seattle. Of 106 infants receiving BET, 81 were healthy and there were no deaths; however, 1 healthy infant developed severe necrotizing enterocolitis requiring surgery. Of 25 sick infants (12 required mechanical ventilation), there were 5 deaths, and 3 developed permanent sequelae, including chronic aortic obstruction from BET via the umbilical artery, intraventricular hemorrhage with subsequent developmental delay, and sudden respiratory deterioration from a pulmonary hemorrhage and subsequent global developmental delay. The author classified the deaths as "possibly" ($n = 3$) or "probably" ($n = 2$) and the complications as "possibly" ($n = 2$) or "probably" ($n = 1$) resulting from the BET. Thus in 25 sick infants, the overall risk of death or permanent sequelae ranged from 3 of 25 to 8 of 25 (12%–32%) and of permanent sequelae in survivors from 1 of 20 to 2 of 20 (5%–10%).

Most of the mortality and morbidity rates reported date from a time at which BET was a common procedure in nurseries. This is no longer the case, and newer phototherapy techniques are likely to reduce the need for BETs even further. Because the frequency of performance of any procedure is an important determinant of risk, the fact that BET is so rarely performed today could result in higher mortality and morbidity rates. However, none of the reports before 1986 included contemporary monitoring capabilities such as pulse oximetry, which should provide earlier identification of potential problems and might decrease morbidity and mortality. In addition, current standards for the monitoring of transfused blood products has significantly reduced the risk of transfusion-transmitted viral infections.

TECHNICAL REPORT

Phototherapy to Prevent Severe Neonatal Hyperbilirubinemia in the Newborn Infant 35 or More Weeks of Gestation

abstract

OBJECTIVE: To standardize the use of phototherapy consistent with the American Academy of Pediatrics clinical practice guideline for the management of hyperbilirubinemia in the newborn infant 35 or more weeks of gestation.

METHODS: Relevant literature was reviewed. Phototherapy devices currently marketed in the United States that incorporate fluorescent, halogen, fiber-optic, or blue light-emitting diode light sources were assessed in the laboratory.

RESULTS: The efficacy of phototherapy units varies widely because of differences in light source and configuration. The following characteristics of a device contribute to its effectiveness: (1) emission of light in the blue-to-green range that overlaps the in vivo plasma bilirubin absorption spectrum ($\sim$460–490 nm); (2) irradiance of at least 30 μW·cm^{-2}·nm^{-1} (confirmed with an appropriate irradiance meter calibrated over the appropriate wavelength range); (3) illumination of maximal body surface; and (4) demonstration of a decrease in total bilirubin concentrations during the first 4 to 6 hours of exposure.

RECOMMENDATIONS (SEE APPENDIX FOR GRADING DEFINITION): The intensity and spectral output of phototherapy devices is useful in predicting potential effectiveness in treating hyperbilirubinemia (group B recommendation). Clinical effectiveness should be evaluated before and monitored during use (group B recommendation). Blocking the light source or reducing exposed body surface should be avoided (group B recommendation). Standardization of irradiance meters, improvements in device design, and lower-upper limits of light intensity for phototherapy units merit further study. Comparing the in vivo performance of devices is not practical, in general, and alternative procedures need to be explored. *Pediatrics* 2011;128:e1046–e1052

Vinod K. Bhutani, MD, and THE COMMITTEE ON FETUS AND NEWBORN

KEY WORDS
phototherapy, newborn jaundice, hyperbilirubinemia, light treatment

ABBREVIATION
LED—light-emitting diode

This document is copyrighted and is property of the American Academy of Pediatrics and its Board of Directors. All authors have filed conflict of interest statements with the American Academy of Pediatrics. Any conflicts have been resolved through a process approved by the Board of Directors. The American Academy of Pediatrics has neither solicited nor accepted any commercial involvement in the development of the content of this publication.

The guidance in this report does not indicate an exclusive course of treatment or serve as a standard of medical care. Variations, taking into account individual circumstances, may be appropriate.

www.pediatrics.org/cgi/doi/10.1542/peds.2011-1494

doi:10.1542/peds.2011-1494

All technical reports from the American Academy of Pediatrics automatically expire 5 years after publication unless reaffirmed, revised, or retired at or before that time.

PEDIATRICS (ISSN Numbers: Print, 0031-4005; Online, 1098-4275).

INTRODUCTION

Clinical trials have validated the efficacy of phototherapy in reducing excessive unconjugated hyperbilirubinemia, and its implementation has drastically curtailed the use of exchange transfusions.[1] The initiation and duration of phototherapy is defined by a specific range of total bilirubin values based on an infant's postnatal age and the potential risk for bilirubin neurotoxicity.[1] Clinical response to phototherapy depends on the efficacy of the phototherapy device as well as the balance between an infant's rates of bilirubin production and elimination. The active agent in phototherapy is light delivered in measurable doses, which makes phototherapy conceptually similar to pharmacotherapy. This report standardizes the use of phototherapy consistent with the American Academy of Pediatrics clinical practice guideline for the management of hyperbilirubinemia in the newborn infant 35 or more weeks of gestation.

I. COMMERCIAL LIGHT SOURCES

A wide selection of commercial phototherapy devices is available in the United States. A complete discussion of devices is beyond the scope of this review; some are described in Tables 1 and 2. Phototherapy devices can be categorized according to their light source as follows: (1) fluorescent-tube devices that emit different colors (cool white daylight, blue [B], special blue [BB], turquoise, and green) and are straight (F20 T12, 60 cm, 20 W), U-shaped, or spiral-shaped; (2) metal halide bulbs, used in spotlights and incubator lights; (3) light-emitting diodes (LEDs) or metal halide bulbs, used with fiber-optic light guides in pads, blankets, or spotlights; and (4) high-intensity LEDs, used as over- and under-the-body devices.

TABLE 1 Phototherapy Devices Commonly Used in the United States and Their Performance Characteristics

Device	Manufacturer	Distance to Patient (cm)	Footprint Area (Length × Width, cm²)	% Treatable BSA	Spectrum, Total (nm)	Bandwidth* (nm)	Peak (nm)	Footprint Irradiance (μW/cm²/nm)		
								Min	Max	Mean ± SD
Light Emitting Diodes [LED]										
neoBLUE	Natus Medical, San Carlos, CA	30	1152 (48 × 24)	100	420–540	20	462	12	37	30 ± 7
PortaBed	Stanford University, Stanford, CA	≥5	1740 (30 × 58)	100	425–540	27	463	40	76	67 ± 8
Fluorescent										
BiliLite CW/BB	Olympic Medical, San Carlos, CA	45	2928 (48 × 61)	100	380–720	69	578	6	10	8 ± 1
BiliLite BB	Olympic Medical, San Carlos, CA	45	2928 (48 × 61)	100	400–550	35	445	11	22	17 ± 2
BiliLite TL52	Olympic Medical, San Carlos, CA	45	2928 (48 × 61)	100	400–626	69	437	13	23	19 ± 3
BiliBed	Medela, McHenry, IL	0	693 (21 × 33)	71	400–560	80	450	14	59	36 ± 2
Halogen										
MinBiliLite	Olympic Medical, San Carlos, CA	45	490 (25 diam)	54	350–800	190	580	<1	19	7 ± 5
Phototherapy Lite	Philips Inc, Andover, MA	45	490 (25 diam)	54	370–850	200	590	<1	17	5 ± 5
Halogen fiberoptic										
BiliBlanket	Ohmeda, Fairfield, CT	0	150 (10 × 15)	24	390–600	70	533	9	31	20 ± 6
Wallaby II Preterm	Philips, Inc, Andover, MA	0	117 (9 × 13)	19	400–560	45	513	8	30	16 ± 6
Wallaby II Term	Philips, Inc, Andover, MA	0	280 (8 × 35)	53	400–560	45	513	6	11	8 ± 1
SpotLight 1000	Philips, Inc, Andover, MA	45	490 (25 diam)	54	400–560	45	513	1	11	6 ± 3
PEP Model 2000	PEP, Fryeburg, ME	23	1530 (30 × 51)	100	400–717	63	445	12	49	28 ± 11
Bili Soft	GE Healthcare, Laurel, MD	71	825 (25 × 33)	71	400–670	40	453	1	52	25 ± 16

Data in Table 1 are expanded and updated from that previously reported by Vreman et al.[3] The definitions and standards for device assessment are explained below.

EMISSION SPECTRAL QUALITIES: Measured data of the light delivered by each of the light sources are presented as the minimum, maximum and range. Light source emission spectra within the range of 300–700 nm were recorded after the device had reached stable light emission, using a miniature fiberoptic radiometer (IRRAD2000, Ocean Optics, Inc, Dunedin, FL). For precision based device assessment, the spectral bandwidth (*), which is defined as the width of the emission spectrum in nm at 50% of peak light intensity, is the preferred method to distinguish and compare the total range emission spectrum (data usually provided by manufacturers). Emission peak values are also used to characterize the quality of light emitted by a given light source.

IRRADIANCE: Measured data are presented as mean ± standard deviation (SD), representing the irradiance of blue light (including spectral bandwidth), for each device's light footprint at the manufacturer-recommended distance. To compare diverse devices, the spectral irradiance (μW/cm2/nm) measurements were made using calibrated BiliBlanket Meters I and II (Ohmeda, GE Healthcare, Fairfield, CT), which were found to yield identical results with stable output phototherapy devices. This type of meter was selected from the several devices with different photonic characteristics that are commercially available, because it has a wide sensitivity range (400–520 nm with peak sensitivity at 450 nm), which overlaps the bilirubin absorption spectrum and which renders it suitable for the evaluation of narrow and broad wavelength band light sources. The devices have been found exceptionally stable during several years of use and agree closely after each annual calibration.

FOOTPRINT: The minimum and maximum irradiance measured (at the intervals provided or defined) in the given irradiance footprint of the device (length × width). The footprint of a device is that area which is occupied by a patient to receive phototherapy. The irradiance footprint has greater dimensions than the emission surface, which is measured at the point where the light exits a phototherapy device. The minimum and maximum values are shown to indicate the range of irradiances encountered with a device and can be used as an indication of the uniformity of the emitted light. Most devices conform to an international standard to deliver a minimum/maximum footprint light ratio of no lower than 0.4.

BSA: BODY SURFACE AREA refers to percent (%) exposure of either the ventral or dorsal planar surface exposed to light and irradiance measurements are accurate to ±0.5.

All of the reported devices are marketed in the United States except the PortaBed, which is a non-licensed Stanford-developed research device and the Dutch Crigler-Najjar Association (used by Crigler-Najjar patients).

TABLE 2 Maximum Spectral Irradiance of Phototherapy Devices (Using Commercial Light Meters at Manufacturer Recommended Distances) Compared to Clear-Sky Sunlight

Light Meter [Range, Peak]	Footprint Irradiance, (μW/cm^2/nm^a)							
	Halogen/Fiberoptic			Fluorescent		LED		Sunlight
	BiliBlanket	Wallaby (Neo)		PEP Bed	Martin/Philips BB	neoBLUE	PortaBed	@ Zenith on 8/31/05
		II	III					
	@ Contact	@ Contact		@ 10 cm	@ 25 cm	@ 30 cm	@ 10 cm	Level Ground
BiliBlanket Meter II [400–520, 450 nm]	34	28	34	40	69	34	76	144
Bili-Meter, Model 22 [425–475, 460 nm]	29	16	32	49	100	25	86	65**
Joey Dosimeter, JD-100 [420–550, 470 nm]	53	51	60	88	174	84	195	304**
PMA-2123 Bilirubin Detector^a (400–520, 460 nm)	24	24	37	35	70	38	73	81
GoldiLux UVA Photometer, GRP-1^b [315–400, 365 nm]	<0.04	<0.04	<0.04	<0.04	<0.04	<0.04	<0.04	2489

Data in Table 2 were tested and compiled by Hendrik J. Vreman (June 2007 and reverified December 2010).

** Irradiance presented to this meter exceeded its range. Measurement was made through a stainless-steel screen that attenuated the measured irradiance to 57%, which was subsequently corrected by this factor.

^{a} Solar Light Company, Inc., Glenside, PA 19038.

^{b} Oriel Instruments, Stratford, CT 06615 and SmartMeter GRP-1 with UV-A probe. GRP-1 measures UV-A light as μW/cm^2. No artificial light source delivered significant (<0.04 μW/cm^2) UV-A radiation at the distances measured.

II. STANDARDS FOR PHOTOTHERAPY DEVICES

Methods for reporting and measuring phototherapy doses are not standardized. Comparisons of commercially available phototherapy devices that use in vitro photodegradation techniques may not accurately predict clinical efficacy.[2] A recent report explored an approach to standardizing and quantifying the magnitude of phototherapy delivered by various devices.[3] Table 1 lists technical data for some of the devices marketed in the United States.[3] Factors to consider in prescribing and implementing phototherapy are (1) emission range of the light source, (2) the light intensity (irradiance), (3) the exposed ("treatable") body surface area illuminated, and (4) the decrease in total bilirubin concentration. A measure of the effectiveness of phototherapy to rapidly configure the bilirubin molecule to less toxic photoisomers (measured in seconds) is not yet clinically available.

A. Light Wavelength

The visible white light spectrum ranges from approximately 350 to 800 nm. Bilirubin absorbs visible light most strongly in the blue region of the spectrum (~460 nm). Absorption of light transforms unconjugated bilirubin molecules bound to human serum albumin in solution into bilirubin photoproducts (predominantly isomers of bilirubin).[2,4,5] Because of the photophysical properties of skin, the most effective light in vivo is probably in the blue-to-green region (~460–490 nm).[2] The first prototype phototherapy device to result in a clinically significant rate of bilirubin decrease used a blue (B) fluorescent-tube light source with 420- to 480-nm emission.[6,7] More effective narrow-band special blue bulbs (F20T12/BB [General Electric, Westinghouse, Sylvania] or TL52/20W [Phillips]) were subsequently used.[8,9] Most recently, commercial compact fluorescent-tube light sources and devices that use LEDs of narrow spectral bandwidth have been used.[9–14] Unless specified otherwise, plastic covers or optical filters need to be used to remove potentially harmful ultraviolet light.

Clinical Context

Devices with maximum emission within the 460- to 490-nm (blue-green) region of the visible spectrum are probably the most effective for treating hyperbilirubinemia.[2,4] Lights with broader emission also will work, although not as effectively. Special blue (BB) fluorescent lights are effective but should not be confused with white lights painted blue or covered with blue plastic sheaths, which should not be used. Devices that contain high-intensity gallium nitride LEDs with emission within the 460- to 490-nm regions are also effective and have a longer lifetime (>20 000 hours), lower heat output, low infrared emission, and no ultraviolet emission.

B. Measuring Light Irradiance

Light intensity or energy output is defined by irradiance and refers to the number of photons (spectral energy) that are delivered per unit area (cm^2) of exposed skin.[1] The dose of phototherapy is a measure of the irradiance delivered for a specific duration and adjusted to the exposed body surface area. Determination of an in vivo dose-response relationship is confounded by the optical properties of skin and the rates of bilirubin production and elimination.[1] Irradiance is measured with a radiometer (W·cm^{-2}) or spectroradiometer (μW·cm^{-2}·nm^{-1}) over a given wavelength band. Table 2 compares the spectral irradiance of some of the devices in the US market, as measured with different brands of meters. Often, radiometers measure wavelengths that do not penetrate skin well or that are far from optimal for phototherapy and, therefore, may be of little value for predicting the clinical efficacy of phototherapy units. A direct relationship between irradiance and the rate of in vivo total bilirubin concentration decrease was described in the report of a study of term "healthy" infants with nonhemolytic hyperbilirubinemia (peak values: 15–18 mg/dL) using fluorescent Philips daylight (TL20W/54, TL20W/52) and special blue (TLAK 40W/03) lamps.[15,16] The American Academy of Pediatrics has recommended that the irradiance for intensive phototherapy be at least 30 μW·cm^{-2}·nm^{-1} over the waveband interval 460 to 490 nm.[1] Devices that emit lower irradiance may be supplemented with auxiliary devices. Much higher doses (>65 μW·cm^{-2}·nm^{-1}) might have (as-yet-unidentified) adverse effects. Currently, no single method is in general use for measuring phototherapy dosages. In addition, the calibration methods, wavelength responses, and geometries of instruments are not standardized. Consequently, different radiometers may show different values for the same light source.[2]

Clinical Context

For routine measurements, clinicians are limited by reliance on irradiance meters supplied or recommended by the manufacturer. Visual estimations of brightness and use of ordinary photometric or colorimetric light meters are inappropriate.[1,2] Maximal irradiance can be achieved by bringing the light source close to the infant[1]; however, this should not be done with halogen or tungsten lights, because the heat generated can cause a burn. Furthermore, with some fixtures, increasing the proximity may reduce the exposed body surface area. Irradiance distribution in the illuminated area

(footprint) is rarely uniform; measurements at the center of the footprint may greatly exceed those at the periphery and are variable among phototherapy devices.[1] Thus, irradiance should be measured at several sites on the infant's body surface. The ideal distance and orientation of the light source should be maintained according to the manufacturer's recommendations. The irradiance of all lamps decreases with use; manufacturers may provide useful-lifetime estimates, which should not be exceeded.

C. Optimal Body Surface Area

An infant's total body surface area[17] can be influenced by the disproportionate head size, especially in the more preterm infant. Complete (100%) exposure of the total body surface to light is impractical and limited by use of eye masks and diapers. Circumferential illumination (total body surface exposure from multiple directions) achieves exposure of approximately 80% of the total body surface. In clinical practice, exposure is usually planar: ventral with overhead light sources and dorsal with lighted mattresses. Approximately 35% of the total body surface (ventral or dorsal) is exposed with either method. Changing the infant's posture every 2 to 3 hours may maximize the area exposed to light. Exposed body surface area treated rather than the number of devices (double, triple, etc) used is clinically more important. Maximal skin surface illumination allows for a more intensive exposure and may require combined use of more than 1 phototherapy device.[1]

Clinical Context

Physical obstruction of light by equipment, such as radiant warmers, head covers, large diapers, eye masks that enclose large areas of the scalp, tape, electrode patches, and insulating plastic covers, decrease the exposed skin

surface area. Circumferential phototherapy maximizes the exposed area. Combining several devices, such as fluorescent tubes with fiber-optic pads or LED mattresses placed below the infant or bassinet, will increase the surface area exposed. If the infant is in an incubator, the light rays should be perpendicular to the surface of the incubator to minimize reflectance and loss of efficacy.[1,2]

D. Rate of Response Measured by Decrease in Serum Bilirubin Concentration

The clinical impact of phototherapy should be evident within 4 to 6 hours of initiation with an anticipated decrease of more than 2 mg/dL (34 μmol/L) in serum bilirubin concentration.[1] The clinical response depends on the rates of bilirubin production, enterohepatic circulation, and bilirubin elimination; the degree of tissue bilirubin deposition[15,16,18]; and the rates of the photochemical reactions of bilirubin. Aggressive implementation of phototherapy for excessive hyperbilirubinemia, sometimes referred to as the "crash-cart" approach,[19,20] has been reported to reduce the need for exchange transfusion and possibly reduce the severity of bilirubin neurotoxicity.

Clinical Context

Serial measurements of bilirubin concentration are used to monitor the effectiveness of phototherapy, but the value of these measurements can be confounded by changes in bilirubin production or elimination and by a sudden increase in bilirubin concentration (rebound) if phototherapy is stopped. Periodicity of serial measurements is based on clinical judgment.

III. EVIDENCE FOR EFFECTIVE PHOTOTHERAPY

Light-emission characteristics of phototherapy devices help in predicting

TABLE 3 Practice Considerations for Optimal Administration of Phototherapy

Checklist	Recommendation	Implementation
Light source (nm)	Wavelength spectrum in ~460- 490-nm blue-green light region	Know the spectral output of the light source
Light irradiance ($\mu W \cdot cm^{-2} \cdot nm^{-1}$)	Use optimal irradiance: >30 $\mu W \cdot cm^{-2} \cdot nm^{-1}$ within the 460- to 490-nm waveband	Ensure uniformity over the light footprint area
Body surface area (cm^2)	Expose maximal skin area	Reduce blocking of light
Timeliness of implementation	Urgent or "crash-cart" intervention for excessive hyperbilirubinemia	May conduct procedures while infant is on phototherapy
Continuity of therapy	Briefly interrupt for feeding, parental bonding, nursing care	After confirmation of adequate bilirubin concentration decrease
Efficacy of intervention	Periodically measure rate of response in bilirubin load reduction	Degree of total serum/plasma bilirubin concentration decrease
Duration of therapy	Discontinue at desired bilirubin threshold; be aware of possible rebound increase	Serial bilirubin measurements based on rate of decrease

their effectiveness (group B recommendation) (see Appendix). The clinical effectiveness of the device should be known before and monitored during clinical application (group B recommendation). Local guidelines (instructions) for routine clinical use should be available. Important factors that need to be considered are listed in Table 3. Obstructing the light source and reducing the exposed body surface area must be avoided (group B recommendation).

These recommendations are appropriate for clinical care in high-resource settings. In low-resource settings the use of improvised technologies and affordable phototherapy device choices need to meet minimum efficacy and safety standards.

IV. SAFETY AND PROTECTIVE MEASURES

A clinician skilled in newborn care should assess the neonate's clinical status during phototherapy to ensure adequate hydration, nutrition, and temperature control. Clinical improvement or progression of jaundice should also be assessed, including signs suggestive of early bilirubin encephalopathy such as changes in sleeping pattern, deteriorating feeding pattern, or inability to be consoled while crying.[1] Staff should be educated regarding the importance of safely minimizing the distance of the phototherapy device from the infant. They should be aware that the intensity of light decreases at the outer perimeter of the light footprint and recognize the effects of physical factors that could impede or obstruct light exposure. Staff should be aware that phototherapy does not use ultraviolet light and that exposure to the lights is mostly harmless. Four decades of neonatal phototherapy use has revealed no serious adverse clinical effects in newborn infants 35 or more weeks of gestation. For more preterm infants, who are usually treated with prophylactic rather than therapeutic phototherapy, this may not be true. Informed staff should educate parents regarding the care of their newborn infant undergoing phototherapy. Devices must comply with general safety standards listed by the International Electrotechnical Commission.[21] Other clinical considerations include:

a. Interruption of phototherapy: After a documented decrease in bilirubin concentration, continuous exposure to the light source may be interrupted and the eye mask removed to allow for feeding and maternal-infant bonding.[1]

b. Use of eye masks: Eye masks to prevent retinal damage are used routinely, although there is no evidence to support this recommendation. Retinal damage has been documented in the unpatched eyes of newborn monkeys exposed to phototherapy, but there are no similar data available from human newborns, because eye patches have always been used.[22–24] Purulent eye discharge and conjunctivitis in term infants have been reported with prolonged use of eye patches.[25,26]

c. Use of diapers: Concerns for the long-term effects of continuous phototherapy exposure of the reproductive system have been raised but not substantiated.[27–29] Diapers may be used for hygiene but are not essential.

d. Other protective considerations: Devices used in environments with high humidity and oxygen must meet electrical and fire hazard safety standards.[21] Phototherapy is contraindicated in infants with congenital porphyria or those treated with photosensitizing drugs.[1] Prolonged phototherapy has been associated with increased oxidant stress and lipid peroxidation[30] and riboflavin deficiency.[31] Recent clinical reports of other adverse outcomes (eg, malignant melanoma, DNA damage, and skin changes) have yet to be validated.[1,2,32,33] Phototherapy does not exacerbate hemolysis.[34]

V. RESEARCH NEEDS

Among the gaps in knowledge that remain regarding the use of phototherapy to prevent severe neonatal hyperbilirubinemia, the following are among the most important:

1. The ability to measure the actual wavelength and irradiance delivered by a phototherapy device is urgently needed to assess the efficiency of

phototherapy in reducing total serum bilirubin concentrations.

2. The safety and efficacy of home phototherapy remains a research priority.

3. Further delineation of the short- and long-term consequences of exposing infants with conjugated and unconjugated hyperbilirubinemia to phototherapy is needed.

4. Whether use of phototherapy reduces the risk of bilirubin neurotoxicity in a timely and effective manner needs further exploration.

SUMMARY

Clinicians and hospitals should ensure that the phototherapy devices they use fully illuminate the patient's body surface area, have an irradiance level of $\geq 30 \ \mu W \cdot cm^{-2} \cdot nm^{-1}$ (confirmed with accuracy with an appropriate spectral radiometer) over the waveband of approximately 460 to 490 nm, and are implemented in a timely manner. Standard procedures should be documented for their safe deployment.

LEAD AUTHOR

Vinod K. Bhutani, MD

COMMITTEE ON FETUS AND NEWBORN, 2010–2011

Lu-Ann Papile, MD, Chairperson
Jill E. Baley, MD
Vinod K. Bhutani, MD
Waldemar A. Carlo, MD
James J. Cummings, MD
Praveen Kumar, MD
Richard A. Polin, MD
Rosemarie C. Tan, MD, PhD
Kristi L. Watterberg, MD

FORMER COMMITTEE MEMBER

David H. Adamkin, MD

LIAISONS

CAPT Wanda Denise Barfield, MD, MPH – *Centers for Disease Control and Prevention*
William H. Barth Jr, MD – *American College of Obstetricians and Gynecologists*
Ann L. Jefferies, MD – *Canadian Paediatric Society*
Rosalie O. Mainous, PhD, RNC, NNP – *National Association of Neonatal Nurses*
Tonse N. K. Raju, MD, DCH – *National Institutes of Health*
Kasper S. Wang – *AAP Section on Surgery*

CONSULTANTS

M. Jeffrey Maisels, MBBCh, DSc
Antony F. McDonagh, PhD
David K. Stevenson, MD
Hendrik J. Vreman, PhD

STAFF

Jim Couto, MA

REFERENCES

1. American Academy of Pediatrics, Subcommittee on Hyperbilirubinemia. Management of hyperbilirubinemia in the newborn infant 35 or more weeks of gestation [published correction appears in *Pediatrics*. 2004;114(4):1138]. *Pediatrics*. 2004;114(1):297–316

2. McDonagh AF, Agati G, Fusi F, Pratesi R. Quantum yields for laser photocyclization of bilirubin in the presence of human serum albumin: dependence of quantum yield on excitation wavelength. *Photochem Photobiol*. 1989;50(3):305–319

3. Vreman HJ, Wong RJ, Murdock JR, Stevenson DK. Standardized bench method for evaluating the efficacy of phototherapy devices. *Acta Paediatr*. 2008;97(3):308–316

4. Maisels MJ, McDonagh AF. Phototherapy for neonatal jaundice. *N Engl J Med*. 2008;358(9):920–928

5. McDonagh AF, Lightner DA. Phototherapy and the photobiology of bilirubin. *Semin Liver Dis*. 1988;8(3):272–283

6. Cremer RJ, Perryman PW, Richards DH. Influence of light on the hyperbilirubinaemia of infants. *Lancet*. 1958;1(7030):1094–1097

7. Ennever JF, McDonagh AF, Speck WT. Phototherapy for neonatal jaundice: optimal wavelengths of light. *J Pediatr*. 1983;103(2):295–299

8. Ennever JF, Sobel M, McDonagh AF, Speck WT. Phototherapy for neonatal jaundice: in vitro comparison of light sources. *Pediatr Res*. 1984;18(7):667–670

9. Nakamura S, Fasol G. InGaN single-quantum-well LEDs. In: *The Blue Laser Diode*. Berlin, Germany: Springer-Verlag; 1997:201–221

10. Vreman HJ, Wong RJ, Stevenson DK, et al. Light-emitting diodes: a novel light source for phototherapy. *Pediatr Res*. 1998;44(5):804–809

11. Maisels MJ, Kring EA, DeRidder J. Randomized controlled trial of light-emitting diode phototherapy. *J Perinatol*. 2007;27(9):565–567

12. Seidman DS, Moise J, Ergaz Z, et al. A new blue light-emitting phototherapy device: a prospective randomized controlled study. *J Pediatr*. 2000;136(6):771–774

13. Martins BM, de Carvalho M, Moreira ME, Lopes JM. Efficacy of new microprocessed phototherapy system with five high intensity light emitting diodes (Super LED) [in Portuguese]. *J Pediatr (Rio J)*. 2007;83(3):253–258

14. Kumar P, Murki S, Malik GK, et al. Light-emitting diodes versus compact fluorescent tubes for phototherapy in neonatal jaundice: a multi-center randomized controlled trial. *Indian Pediatr*. 2010;47(2):131–137

15. Tan KL. The nature of the dose-response relationship of phototherapy for neonatal hyperbilirubinemia. *J Pediatr*. 1977;90(3):448–452

16. Tan KL. The pattern of bilirubin response to phototherapy for neonatal hyperbilirubinaemia. *Pediatr Res*. 1982;16(8):670–674

17. Mosteller RD. Simplified calculation of body-surface area. *N Engl J Med*. 1987;317(17):1098

18. Jährig K, Jährig D, Meisel P. Dependence of the efficiency of phototherapy on plasma bilirubin concentration. *Acta Paediatr Scand*. 1982;71(2):293–299

19. Johnson L, Bhutani VK, Karp K, Sivieri EM, Shapiro SM. Clinical report from the pilot USA Kernicterus Registry (1992 to 2004). *J Perinatol*. 2009;29(suppl 1):S25–S45

20. Hansen TW, Nietsch L, Norman E, et al. Reversibility of acute intermediate phase bilirubin encephalopathy. *Acta Paediatr*. 2009;98(10):1689–1694

21. International Electrotechnical Commission. International standard: medical electrical equipment part 2-50—particular requirements for the safety of infant phototherapy equipment 60601-2-50, ed2.0. (2009-03-24). Available at: http://webstore.iec.ch/webstore/webstore.nsf/Artnum_PK/42737. Accessed December 21, 2010

22. Ente G, Klein SW. Hazards of phototherapy. *N Engl J Med*. 1970;283(10):544–545

23. Messner KH, Maisels MJ, Leure-DuPree AE. Phototoxicity to the newborn primate retina. *Invest Ophthalmol Vis Sci*. 1978;17(2):178–182

24. Patz A, Souri EN. Phototherapy and other ocular risks to the newborn. *Sight Sav Rev*. 1972;42(1):29–33

25. Paludetto R, Mansi G, Rinaldi P, Saporito M, De Curtis M, Ciccimarra F. Effects of

different ways of covering the eyes on behavior of jaundiced infants treated with phototherapy. *Biol Neonate*. 1985;47(1): 1–8

26. Fok TF, Wong W, Cheung KL. Eye protection for newborns under phototherapy: comparison between a modified headbox and the conventional eyepatches. *Ann Trop Paediatr*. 1997;17(4):349–354

27. Koç H, Altunhan H, Dilsiz A, et al. Testicular changes in newborn rats exposed to phototherapy. *Pediatr Dev Pathol*. 1999;2(4): 333–336

28. Wurtman RJ. The effects of light on the human body. *Sci Am*. 1975;233(1):69–77

29. Cetinkursun S, Demirbag S, Cincik M, Baykal B, Gunal A. Effects of phototherapy on newborn rat testicles. *Arch Androl*. 2006;52(1): 61–70

30. Lightner DA, Linnane WP, Ahlfors CE. Bilirubin photooxidation products in the urine of jaundiced neonates receiving phototherapy. *Pediatr Res*. 1984;18(8):696–700

31. Sisson TR. Photodegradation of riboflavin in neonates. *Fed Proc*. 1987;46(5): 1883–1885

32. Bauer J, Büttner P, Luther H, Wiecker TS, Möhrle M, Garbe C. Blue light phototherapy of neonatal jaundice does not increase the risk for melanocytic nevus development. *Arch Dermatol*. 2004;140(4):493–494

33. Tatli MM, Minnet C, Kocyigit A, Karadag A. Phototherapy increases DNA damage in lymphocytes of hyperbilirubinemic neonates. *Mutat Res*. 2008;654(1):93–95

34. Maisels MJ, Kring EA. Does intensive phototherapy produce hemolysis in newborns of 35 or more weeks gestation? *J Perinatol*. 2006;26(8):498–500

APPENDIX Definition of Grades for Recommendation and Suggestion for Practice

Grade	Definition	Suggestion for Practice
A	This intervention is recommended. There is a high certainty that the net benefit is substantial	Offer and administer this intervention
B	This intervention is recommended. There is a moderate certainty that the net benefit is moderate to substantial	Offer and administer this intervention
C	This intervention is recommended. There may be considerations that support the use of this intervention in an individual patient. There is a moderate to high certainty that the net benefit is small	Offer and administer this intervention only if other considerations support this intervention in an individual patient
D	This intervention is not recommended. There is a moderate to high certainty that the intervention has no net benefit and that the harms outweigh the benefits	Discourage use of this intervention
I	The current evidence is insufficient to assess the balance of benefits against and harms of this intervention. There is a moderate to high certainty that the intervention has no net benefit and that the harms outweigh the benefits. Evidence is lacking, of poor quality, or conflicting, and the balance of benefits and harms cannot be determined	If this intervention is conducted, the patient should understand the uncertainty about the balance of benefits and harms

US Preventive Services Task Force Grade definitions, May, 2008 (available at www.uspreventiveservicestaskforce.org/3rduspstf/ratings.htm).

Hyperbilirubinemia in the Newborn Infant ≥35 Weeks' Gestation: An Update With Clarifications

AUTHORS: M. Jeffrey Maisels, MB, BCh, DSc,[a] Vinod K. Bhutani, MD,[b] Debra Bogen, MD,[c] Thomas B. Newman, MD, MPH,[d] Ann R. Stark, MD,[e] and Jon F. Watchko, MD[f]

[a]Department of Pediatrics, Oakland University William Beaumont School of Medicine and Division of Neonatology, Beaumont Children's Hospital, Royal Oak, Michigan; [b]Department of Neonatal and Developmental Medicine, Lucile Salter Packard Children's Hospital, Stanford University, Palo Alto, California; [c]Division of General Academic Pediatrics, Department of Pediatrics, University of Pittsburgh School of Medicine, Children's Hospital of Pittsburgh, Pittsburgh, Pennsylvania; [d]Department of Epidemiology and Biostatistics, Department of Pediatrics, University of California, San Francisco, California; [e]Department of Pediatrics and Section of Neonatology, Baylor College of Medicine and Texas Children's Hospital, Houston, Texas; and [f]Division of Newborn Medicine, Department of Pediatrics, University of Pittsburgh School of Medicine, Pittsburgh, Pennsylvania

ABBREVIATIONS

AAP—American Academy of Pediatrics
G6PD—glucose-6-phosphate dehydrogenase
TSB—total serum bilirubin
TcB—transcutaneous bilirubin

Opinions expressed in this commentary are those of the author and not necessarily those of the American Academy of Pediatrics or its Committees.

www.pediatrics.org/cgi/doi/10.1542/peds.2009-0329

doi:10.1542/peds.2009-0329

Accepted for publication Jun 3, 2009

Address correspondence to M. Jeffrey Maisels, MB, BCh, DSc, Beaumont Children's Hospital, 3601 W. 13 Mile Rd, Royal Oak, MI 48073. E-mail: JMaisels@beaumont.edu

PEDIATRICS (ISSN Numbers: Print, 0031-4005; Online, 1098-4275).

FINANCIAL DISCLOSURE: Dr Maisels is a consultant to and has received grant support from Draeger Medical Inc; the other authors have no financial relationships relevant to this article to disclose.

In July 2004, the Subcommittee on Hyperbilirubinemia of the American Academy of Pediatrics (AAP) published its clinical practice guideline on the management of hyperbilirubinemia in the newborn infant ≥35 weeks of gestation,[1] and a similar guideline was published in 2007 by the Canadian Paediatric Society.[2] Experience with implementation of the AAP guideline suggests that some areas require clarification. The 2004 AAP guideline also expressed hope that its implementation would "reduce the incidence of severe hyperbilirubinemia and bilirubin encephalopathy. . . ." We do not know how many practitioners are following the guideline, nor do we know the current incidence of bilirubin encephalopathy in the United States. We do know, however, that kernicterus is still occurring in the United States, Canada, and Western Europe.[3–7] In 2002, the National Quality Forum suggested that kernicterus should be classified as a "serious reportable event,"[8] sometimes termed a "never event,"[9] implying that with appropriate monitoring, surveillance, and intervention, this devastating condition can, or should, be eliminated. Although this is certainly a desirable objective, it is highly unlikely that it can be achieved given our current state of knowledge and practice.[10] In certain circumstances (notably, glucose-6-phosphate dehydrogenase [G6PD] deficiency, sepsis, genetic predisposition, or other unknown stressors), acute, severe hyperbilirubinemia can occur and can produce brain damage despite appropriate monitoring and intervention.

In addition to clarifying certain items in the 2004 AAP guideline, we recommend universal predischarge bilirubin screening using total serum bilirubin (TSB) or transcutaneous bilirubin (TcB) measurements, which help to assess the risk of subsequent severe hyperbilirubinemia. We also recommend a more structured approach to management and follow-up according to the predischarge TSB/TcB, gestational age, and other risk factors for hyperbilirubinemia. These recommendations represent a consensus of expert opinion based on the available evidence, and they are supported by several independent reviewers. Nevertheless, their efficacy in preventing kernicterus and their cost-effectiveness are unknown.

METHODS

We reviewed the report on screening for neonatal hyperbilirubinemia published by the Agency for Healthcare Research and Quality and prepared by the Tufts-New England Medical Center Evidence-Based Practice Center,[11] the current report by the US Preventive Services Task Force,[12] and other relevant literature.[1,3–10,13–26]

TABLE 1 Important Risk Factors for Severe Hyperbilirubinemia

Predischarge TSB or TcB measurement in the high-risk or high-intermediate–risk zone
Lower gestational age
Exclusive breastfeeding, particularly if nursing is not going well and weight loss is excessive
Jaundice observed in the first 24 h
Isoimmune or other hemolytic disease (eg, G6PD deficiency)
Previous sibling with jaundice
Cephalohematoma or significant bruising
East Asian race

TABLE 2 Hyperbilirubinemia Neurotoxicity Risk Factors

Isoimmune hemolytic disease
G6PD deficiency
Asphyxia
Sepsis
Acidosis
Albumin <3.0 mg/dL

RISK FACTORS

The 2004 AAP guideline includes 2 categories of risk factors, but the distinction between these 2 categories has not been clear to all users of the guideline.

Laboratory and Clinical Factors That Help to Assess the Risk of Subsequent Severe Hyperbilirubinemia

These "risk factors for hyperbilirubinemia" are listed in Table 1. Understanding the predisposition to subsequent hyperbilirubinemia provides guidance for timely follow-up as well as the need for additional clinical and laboratory evaluation.

Laboratory and Clinical Factors That Might Increase the Risk of Brain Damage in an Infant Who Has Hyperbilirubinemia

These risk factors for bilirubin neurotoxicity are listed in the figures of the 2004 AAP guideline that provide recommendations for the use of phototherapy and exchange transfusion. These "neurotoxicity risk factors" encompass those that might increase the risk of brain damage in an infant who has severe hyperbilirubinemia[1] (see Fig 1 and Table 2). The neurotoxicity risk factors are used in making the decision to initiate phototherapy or perform an exchange transfusion. These interventions are recommended at a lower bilirubin level when any of the neurotoxicity risk factors is present. Some conditions are found in both risk-factor categories. For example, lower gestational age and isoimmune hemolytic disease increase the likelihood of subsequent severe hyperbilirubinemia as well as the risk of brain damage by bilirubin.

PREDISCHARGE RISK ASSESSMENT FOR SUBSEQUENT SEVERE HYPERBILIRUBINEMIA

The 2004 AAP guideline recommends a predischarge bilirubin measurement and/or assessment of clinical risk factors to evaluate the risk of subsequent severe hyperbilirubinemia.[1] New evidence suggests that combining a predischarge measurement of TSB or TcB with clinical risk factors might improve the prediction of the risk of subsequent hyperbilirubinemia.[13,14,23] In addition, when interpreted by using the hour-specific nomogram (Fig 2), measurement of TSB or TcB also provides a quantitative assessment of the degree of hyperbilirubinemia. This provides guidance regarding the need (or lack of need) for additional testing to identify a cause of the hyperbilirubinemia and for additional TSB measurements.[1]

The TSB can be measured from the same sample that is drawn for the

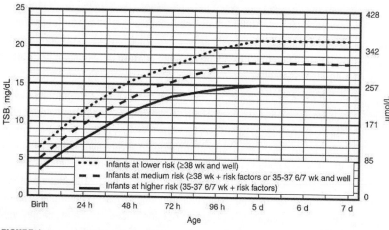

FIGURE 1

Guidelines for phototherapy in hospitalized infants ≥35 weeks' gestation. Note that these guidelines are based on limited evidence and that the levels shown are approximations. The guidelines refer to the use of intensive phototherapy, which should be used when the TSB level exceeds the line indicated for each category.

- Use total bilirubin. Do not subtract direct-reacting or conjugated bilirubin.
- Risk factors are isoimmune hemolytic disease, G6PD deficiency, asphyxia, significant lethargy, temperature instability, sepsis, acidosis, or an albumin level of <3.0 g/dL (if measured).
- For well infants at 35 to 37⁶⁄₇ weeks' gestation, one can adjust TSB levels for intervention around the medium-risk line. It is an option to intervene at lower TSB levels for infants closer to 35 weeks' gestation and at higher TSB levels for those closer to 37⁶⁄₇ weeks' gestation.
- It is an option to provide conventional phototherapy in the hospital or at home at TSB levels of 2 to 3 mg/dL (35–50 μmol/L) below those shown, but home phototherapy should not be used in any infant with risk factors.

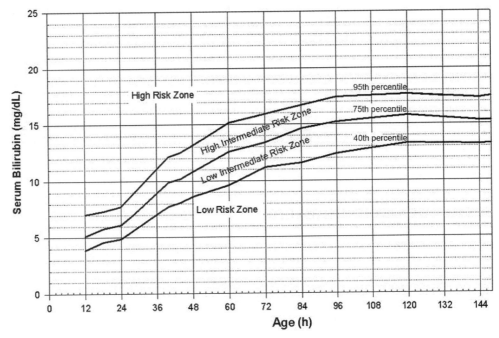

FIGURE 2
Nomogram for designation of risk in 2840 well newborns at ≥36 weeks' gestational age with birth weight of ≥2000 g or ≥35 weeks' gestational age and birth weight of ≥2500 g based on the hour-specific serum bilirubin values. (Reproduced with permission from Bhutani VK, Johnson L, Sivieri EM. *Pediatrics*. 1999;103[1]:6–14.)

metabolic screen. The risk zone (Fig 2) and the other clinical risk factors (Table 3) are then combined to assess the risk of subsequent hyperbilirubinemia and to formulate a plan for management and follow-up (Fig 3). When combined with the risk zone, the factors that are most predictive of hyperbilirubinemia risk are lower gestational age and exclusive breastfeeding.[13,14,23] The lower the gestational age, the greater the risk of developing hyperbilirubinemia.[13,14,23] For those infants from whom ≥2 successive TSB or TcB measurements are obtained, it is helpful to plot the data on the nomogram[15] to assess the rate of rise. Hemolysis is likely if the TSB/TcB is crossing percentiles on the nomogram and suggests the need for further testing and follow-up (see Table 1 in the 2004 AAP guideline).

Therefore, we recommend that a predischarge measurement of TSB or TcB be performed and the risk zone for hyperbilirubinemia determined[15] on the basis of the infant's age in hours and the TSB or TcB measurement.

It should be noted that, even with a low predischarge TSB or TcB level, the risk of subsequent hyperbilirubinemia is not zero,[13,17] so appropriate follow-up should always be provided (Fig 3).

RESPONSE TO PREDISCHARGE TSB MEASUREMENTS

Figure 3 provides our recommendations for management and follow-up, according to predischarge screening. Note that this algorithm represents a consensus of the authors and is based on interpretation of limited evidence (see below).

FOLLOW-UP AFTER DISCHARGE

Most infants discharged at <72 hours should be seen within 2 days of discharge.

Earlier follow-up might be necessary for infants who have risk factors for severe hyperbilirubinemia,[1,13,14,23] whereas those in the lower risk zones with few or no risk factors can be seen later (Fig 3). Figure 3 also provides additional suggestions for evaluation and management at the first follow-up visit.

TcB MEASUREMENTS

TcB measurements are being used with increasing frequency in hospi-

TABLE 3 Other Risk Factors for Severe Hyperbilirubinemia to be Considered with the Gestational Age and the Pre-discharge TSB or TcB level (see Figure 3)

Exclusive breastfeeding, particularly if nursing is not going well and/or weight loss is excessive (>8 – 10%)
Isoimmune or other hemolytic disease (eg, G6PD deficiency, hereditary spherocytosis)
Previous sibling with jaundice
Cephalohematoma or significant bruising
East Asian race

The gestational age and the predischarge TSB or TcB level are the most important factors that help to predict the risk of hyperbilirubinemia. The risk increases with each decreasing week of gestation from 42–35 weeks (see Figure 3)

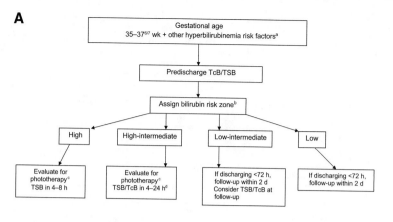

A

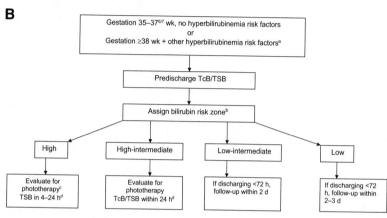

B

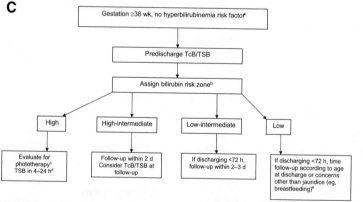

C

FIGURE 3
Algorithm providing recommendations for management and follow-up according to predischarge bilirubin measurements, gestation, and risk factors for subsequent hyperbilirubinemia.

- Provide lactation evaluation and support for all breastfeeding mothers.
- Recommendation for timing of repeat TSB measurement depends on age at measurement and how far the TSB level is above the 95th percentile (Fig 2). Higher and earlier initial TSB levels require an earlier repeat TSB measurement.
- Perform standard clinical evaluation at all follow-up visits.
- For evaluation of jaundice see 2004 AAP guideline.[1]
- [a] Table 3. [b] Fig 2. [c] Fig 1. [d] In hospital or as outpatient. [e] Follow-up recommendations can be modified according to level of risk for hyperbilirubinemia; depending on the circumstances in infants at low risk, later follow-up can be considered.

tal nurseries and in some outpatient settings. They have the advantage of providing instantaneous information and probably reduce the likelihood of missing a clinically significant TSB, making them particularly useful in outpatient practice. TcB measurements can significantly reduce the number of TSB measurements that are required, but as with any point-of-care test, regular monitoring for appropriate quality assurance by comparison with TSB measurements is necessary. Significant variation can occur among instruments, and the use of a new instrument should be compared with hospital laboratory measurements to ensure that the instrument is working properly; such checks should be performed periodically. TcB is a measurement of the yellow color of the blanched skin and subcutaneous tissue, not the serum, and should be used as a screening tool to help determine whether the TSB should be measured. Although TcB measurements provide a good estimate of the TSB level, they are not a substitute for TSB values, and a TSB level should always be obtained when therapeutic intervention is being considered.

Most studies in term and late-preterm infants have indicated that the TcB tends to underestimate the TSB, particularly at higher TSB levels.[18] Thus, investigators have adopted various techniques to avoid missing a high TSB level (ie, a false-negative TcB measurement). These techniques include measuring the TSB if

- the TcB value is at 70% of the TSB level recommended for the use of phototherapy[19];
- the TcB value is above the 75th percentile on the Bhutani nomogram (Fig 1)[15] or the 95th percentile on a TcB nomogram[16] (in 1 study, if the TcB was <75th percentile on the Bhutani nomogram, 0 of 349 infants

had a TSB level above the 95th percentile [a negative predictive value of 100%][20]; or

- at follow-up after discharge, the TcB value is >13 mg/dL (222 μmol/L)[21] (in this outpatient study, no infant who had a TcB value of ≤13 mg/dL had a TSB level of >17 mg/dL [291 μmol/L]).[21]

COSTS

The introduction of universal predischarge bilirubin screening, follow-up visits, and TSB/TcB measurements might increase costs. Ideally, a cost/benefit analysis should include the cost to prevent 1 case of kernicterus. The cost per case, however, highly depends on the incidence of kernicterus as well as its potential reduction resulting from the intervention. By using a strategy similar to that suggested in this guideline, and assuming an incidence of kernicterus of 1 in 100 000 live births and a relative risk reduction of 70%, the cost to prevent 1 case of kernicterus has been estimated as approximately $5.7 million.[22] Because we do not know the current incidence of kernicterus in the United States or the actual relative risk reduction (if these guidelines were implemented universally), we cannot calculate the true cost/benefit ratio. Taking into account the lifetime cost of an infant with kernicterus, it is possible that there could be savings.[22]

DISCUSSION

While endeavoring to clarify some areas addressed in the 2004 AAP guideline, we have also introduced new recommendations, both for the predischarge assessment of the risk of subsequent hyperbilirubinemia and for follow-up testing. We recognize that the quality of evidence for recommending universal predischarge screening and for the suggested management and follow-up (Fig 3) is limited and, in the absence of higher levels of evidence, our recommendations must, therefore, be based on expert opinion. As indicated in the reviews by the US Preventive Services Task Force[12] and Trikalinos et al[11] in this issue of *Pediatrics*, there are currently no good data to indicate that the implementation of these recommendations will reduce the risk of kernicterus, although published data suggest that predischarge screening can reduce the incidence of a TSB level of ≥25 mg/dL,[24,25] perhaps by increasing the use of phototherapy.[24] Nevertheless, because kernicterus is a devastating condition that leads to serious and permanent neurologic damage, and because published reports and our own review of cases in the medicolegal setting suggest that many of these cases could have been prevented, a reasonable argument can be made for implementing the suggested recommendations in the absence of better evidence. Because kernicterus is a rare condition, it is unlikely that we will be able to obtain adequate evidence in the short-term to support our recommendations. In their elegant polemic, Auerbach et al[26] discussed "the tension between needing to improve care and knowing how to do it." They noted that, in the absence of appropriate evidence, "bold efforts at improvement can consume tremendous resources yet confer only a small benefit."[26] We

also recognize that although predischarge testing is relatively inexpensive and convenient, measuring the TSB after discharge is more difficult. TcB measurement is quite easy but is not currently available in most primary care settings. In addition, more evidence is needed to support the cost and efficacy of these recommendations. There is certainly a risk that these recommendations could lead to additional testing and an increase in both appropriate and inappropriate use of phototherapy.[1,24] Nevertheless, it is our opinion that universal screening, when combined with the clinical risk factors (of which gestational age and exclusive breastfeeding are most important) and targeted follow-up, is a systems approach that is easy to implement and understand, and it provides a method of identifying infants who are at high or low risk for the development of severe hyperbilirubinemia. In addition to risk assessment, the measurement of TSB or TcB when interpreted by using the hour-specific nomogram provides the caregiver with an immediate and quantitative mechanism for assessing the degree of hyperbilirubinemia and the need for additional surveillance and testing. As such, it could play an important role in preventing acute bilirubin encephalopathy, although this has yet to be demonstrated.

ACKNOWLEDGMENTS

We are grateful for reviews and critiques of this commentary by neonatologists, bilirubinologists, pediatricians, and pediatric residents.

REFERENCES

1. American Academy of Pediatrics, Subcommittee on Hyperbilirubinemia. Management of hyperbilirubinemia in the newborn infant 35 or more weeks of gestation [published correction appears in *Pediatrics*. 2004;114(4):1138]. *Pediatrics*. 2004;114(1):297–316
2. Canadian Paediatric Society, Fetus and Newborn Committee. Guidelines for detection, manage-

ment and prevention of hyperbilirubinemia in term and late preterm newborn infants (35 or more weeks' gestation). *Paediatr Child Health*. 2007;12(5):1B–12B

3. Sgro M, Campbell DM, Fallah S, Shah V. Kernicterus, January 2007 to December 2009. Canadian Paediatric Surveillance Program 2008 Results. Available at: www.cps.ca/english/surveillance/CPSP/index.htm. Accessed July 30, 2009

4. Manning D, Todd P, Maxwell M, Platt MJ. Prospective surveillance study of severe hyperbilirubinaemia in the newborn in the UK and Ireland. *Arch Dis Child Fetal Neonatal Ed*. 2007;92(5): F342–F346

5. Bartmann P, Schaaff F. Kernicterus in Germany 2003–2005. *E-PAS*. 2007;617936.23

6. Ebbesen F. Recurrence of kernicterus in term and near-term infants in Denmark. *Acta Paediatr*. 2000;89(10):1213–1217

7. Ebbesen F, Andersson C, Verder H, et al. Extreme hyperbilirubinaemia in term and near-term infants in Denmark. *Acta Paediatr*. 2005;94(1):59–64

8. National Quality Forum. *Serious Reportable Events in Healthcare: A Consensus Report*. Washington, DC: National Quality Forum; 2002

9. Davidson L, Thilo EH. How to make kernicterus a "never event." *Neoreviews*. 2003;4(11):308–314

10. Watchko JF. Vigintiphobia revisited. *Pediatrics*. 2005;115(6):1747–1753

11. Trikalinos T, Chung M, Lau J, Ip S. Systematic review of screening for bilirubin encephalopathy in neonates. *Pediatrics*. 2009;124(4):1162–1171

12. US Preventive Services Task Force. Screening of infants for hyperbilirubinemia to prevent chronic bilirubin encephalopathy: recommendation statement. *Pediatrics*. 2009;124(4):1172–1177

13. Keren R, Luan X, Friedman S, Saddlemire S, Cnaan A, Bhutani V. A comparison of alternative risk-assessment strategies for predicting significant neonatal hyperbilirubinemia in term and near-term infants. *Pediatrics*. 2008;121(1). Available at: www.pediatrics.org/cgi/content/full/121/1/e170

14. Newman T, Liljestrand P, Escobar G. Combining clinical risk factors with bilirubin levels to predict hyperbilirubinemia in newborns. *Arch Pediatr Adolesc Med*. 2005;159(2):113–119

15. Bhutani VK, Johnson L, Sivieri EM. Predictive ability of a predischarge hour-specific serum bilirubin for subsequent significant hyperbilirubinemia in healthy-term and near-term newborns. *Pediatrics*. 1999;103(1):6–14

16. Maisels MJ, Kring E. Transcutaneous bilirubin levels in the first 96 hours in a normal newborn population of ≥35 weeks' of gestation. *Pediatrics*. 2006;117(4):1169–1173

17. Stevenson DK, Fanaroff AA, Maisels MJ, et al. Prediction of hyperbilirubinemia in near-term and term infants. *Pediatrics*. 2001;108(1):31–39

18. Maisels MJ. Transcutaneous bilirubinometry. *Neoreviews*. 2006;7(5):e217–e225

19. Ebbesen F, Rasmussen LM, Wimberley PD. A new transcutaneous bilirubinometer, BiliCheck, used in the neonatal intensive care unit and the maternity ward. *Acta Paediatr*. 2002;91(2):203–211

20. Bhutani V, Gourley GR, Adler S, Kreamer B, Dalman C, Johnson LH. Noninvasive measurement of total serum bilirubin in a multiracial predischarge newborn population to assess the risk of severe hyperbilirubinemia. *Pediatrics*. 2000;106(2). Available at: www.pediatrics.org/cgi/content/full/106/2/e17

21. Engle W, Jackson GC, Stehel EK, Sendelbach D, Manning MD. Evaluation of a transcutaneous jaundice meter following hospital discharge in term and near-term neonates. *J Perinatol*. 2005; 25(7):486–490

22. Suresh G, Clark R. Cost-effectiveness of strategies that are intended to prevent kernicterus in newborn infants. *Pediatrics*. 2004;114(4):917–924

23. Maisels MJ, Deridder JM, Kring EA, Balasubramaniam M. Routine transcutaneous bilirubin measurements combined with clinical risk factors improve the prediction of subsequent hyperbilirubinemia. *J Perinatol*. 2009; In press

24. Kuzniewicz MW, Escobar GJ, Newman TB. The impact of universal bilirubin screening on severe hyperbilirubinemia and phototherapy use in a managed care organization. *Pediatrics*. 2009; 124(4):1031–1039

25. Eggert L, Wiedmeier SE, Wilson J, Christensen R. The effect of instituting a prehospital-discharge newborn bilirubin screening program in an 18-hospital health system. *Pediatrics*. 2006;117(5). Available at: www.pediatrics.org/cgi/content/full/117/5/e855

26. Auerbach AD, Landefeld CS, Shojania K. The tension between needing to improve care and knowing how to do it. *N Engl J Med*. 2007;357(6):608–613

Universal Bilirubin Screening, Guidelines, and Evidence

AUTHOR: Thomas B. Newman, MD, MPH

Division of Clinical Epidemiology, Department of Epidemiology and Biostatistics, and Division of General Pediatrics, Department of Pediatrics, University of California, San Francisco, California; and Division of Research, Kaiser Permanente Medical Care Program, Oakland, California

ABBREVIATIONS

AAP—American Academy of Pediatrics
USPSTF—US Preventive Services Task Force
TSB—total serum bilirubin

www.pediatrics.org/cgi/doi/10.1542/peds.2009-0412

doi:10.1542/peds.2009-0412

Accepted for publication Feb 17, 2009

Address correspondence to Thomas B. Newman, MD, MPH, University of California, Department of Epidemiology and Biostatistics, Box 0560, San Francisco, CA 94143. E-mail newman@epi.ucsf.edu

PEDIATRICS (ISSN Numbers: Print, 0031-4005; Online, 1098-4275).

FINANCIAL DISCLOSURE: *The author has indicated he has no financial relationships relevant to this article to disclose.*

In a commentary[1] and update of the 2004 American Academy of Pediatrics (AAP) guideline "Management of Hyperbilirubinemia in the Newborn Infant 35 or More Weeks of Gestation"[2] in this issue of *Pediatrics*, Maisels et al recommend that all newborns have a bilirubin measurement before discharge from their birth hospitalization. In contrast, a recommendation statement from the US Preventive Services Task Force (USPSTF),[3] supported by a systematic review,[4] concludes that evidence is insufficient to make that recommendation. As an author of the commentary[1] and the 2004 AAP jaundice guideline[2] who also has been critical of guidelines based on insufficient evidence,[5–11] I have felt particularly torn about this recommendation.

Perhaps partly because I have served as an expert consultant on dozens of heartbreaking kernicterus legal cases,[12] I find the argument in favor of universal bilirubin screening and systematic follow-up persuasive. We know kernicterus is devastating and that, although rare, cases are continuing to occur. Furthermore, anecdotal evidence suggests that many cases could have been prevented by earlier measurement of bilirubin levels, leading to closer follow-up and earlier initiation of appropriate therapy.[13,14] We have not had randomized trials to show that universal screening and systematic follow-up will lead to a reduction in kernicterus, but considerable research in the area of optimizing patient safety suggests that there is room for improvement in the 2004 guidelines. Specifically, we know that in the absence of universal screening, detection and management of clinically significant hyperbilirubinemia during the birth hospitalization relies on several imperfect steps: (1) nurses and doctors need to remember to examine the infant for jaundice; (2) they need to distinguish visually between jaundice that is and is not clinically significant for the infant's age in hours; and (3) they need to combine information from this visual assessment of jaundice and/or a total serum bilirubin (TSB) level with knowledge of the newborn's other risk factors to determine the need for and timing of bilirubin measurements, follow-up visits, and treatments. We also know that nurseries are busy places and that sometimes people may not do things that they should[15] or might do them under suboptimal conditions, such as assessing jaundice in the dim light found in many hospital rooms. Finally, compared with the devastating effects of kernicterus, the costs and risks of screening seem low, particularly with a transcutaneous bilirubinometer, which may actually decrease the number of serum bilirubin measurements obtained.[16]

On the other hand, as a proponent of evidence-based medicine, I recognize the insufficiency of the data to support the recommendation.[3,4] The rationale outlined above would apply whether the incidence of kernicterus were 1 in 10 000 or 1 in 1 million, but surely the potential benefits of screening depend on how much kernicterus there is to prevent, and this is not known. Even if we knew the incidence of kernicterus, the proportion that might be preventable by screening and systematic follow-up is unclear. Although plaintiffs in malpractice cases commonly assert that infants with bilirubin levels in the 40s at 4 or 5 days must have had proportionately high levels at the time of discharge (even if no or minimal jaundice was noted at that time), there is little evidence to support this assertion. Studies of the predictive value of early bilirubin levels have had much lower levels of hyperbilirubinemia (TSB of 17–20 mg/dL).[3] Because they may have different causes, such as glucose-6-phosphate dehydrogenase deficiency and infection, the very high levels that lead to kernicterus may be less predictable. Moreover, several studies have revealed that in the absence of any jaundice, a TSB level of $\geq$12 mg/dL is extremely unlikely.[17–20] As an experienced generalist who believes he can recognize at least some newborns who definitely are not jaundiced, I sympathize with colleagues who may question the cost-efficacy of measuring bilirubin (particularly if it involves an additional poke or trying to squeeze more blood out of a recalcitrant heel) in a light-skinned 2-day-old who has no hint of jaundice. Requiring a bilirubin measurement for every such infant because some clinicians may forget or be careless feels like keeping the whole class after school for the transgressions of a few.

After doing my best to reconcile these opposing viewpoints, I believe that universal predischarge bilirubin screening is a good idea but that the evidence is not sufficient to recommend it in an AAP guideline. This is consistent with AAP policy. In a 2004 statement, the Steering Committee on Quality Improvement and Management outlined levels of evidence and strengths of AAP guidelines.[21] The policy stated that ex-

cept in "exceptional situations where validating studies cannot be performed and there is a clear preponderance of benefit or harm," if the level of evidence is "expert opinion, case reports, and reasoning from first principles," a course of action should be designated an option rather than a recommendation. Because, as is explicitly acknowledged in the commentary, expert opinion, case reports, and reasoning from first principles are exactly the level of evidence that supports the recommendation for universal bilirubin screening, and because we wanted to make that recommendation, it needed to be published as a commentary rather than a guideline.

Is this AAP policy on evidence and guideline recommendations a good one? I believe it is. Practicing clinicians need and appreciate guidance from experts, but they also recognize the impossibility of following every guideline that an expert committee might recommend for them and need protection from well-meaning but sometimes paternalistic committees with their own agendas.[22] Guideline committees tend to be dominated by academics and subspecialists with special interest, expertise, and even emotional investment in the diseases for which they are producing guidelines.[23] Most of us authors of the hyperbilirubinemia commentary are no exception.[12,24] Although interest and expertise are invaluable, the career focus on a particular disease, with resulting close relationships with funders, patients, advocacy groups, industry, and each other, may lead to a narrow perspective in which heroic efforts at preventing or treating the target disease feel justified, even when a favorable balance of benefits over risks and costs is uncertain.[23] And, although slavishly adhering to evidence standards could lead to failure to recommend beneficial treatments[25,26] even what seem

like obvious, common-sense interventions can have unintended adverse consequences.[27,28]

The USPSTF uses a different model for producing guidelines, in which expertise at appraising and synthesizing evidence trumps disease-specific expertise.[29] Recommendations of the USPSTF are typically based on the results of systematic reviews of evidence, often performed by one of the Agency for Healthcare Research and Quality's evidence-based practice centers. Such thorough reviews are not within time, expertise, and budget constraints of most guideline committees. Ironically, however, the recommendation to measure a bilirubin level for every infant before discharge was the subject of just such a review,[4] which concluded that the evidence is insufficient to make a recommendation for or against universal bilirubin screening ("I" rating).[3]

The USPSTF statement comments not only on the lack of evidence that universal bilirubin screening will prevent bilirubin encephalopathy but also on the insufficiency of evidence regarding risks and efficacy of phototherapy.[3] This is important, because an unintended consequence of institution of universal bilirubin screening might be a greater focus on the danger of hyperbilirubinemia, leading to excessive use of phototherapy. There is evidence that this has occurred in the Northern California Kaiser Permanente Medical Care Program, in which increased bilirubin testing was associated with a decrease in bilirubin levels of >25 mg/dL and also an increase in use of phototherapy at levels lower than those recommended in the 2004 AAP guideline.[30] Thus, it is worth stressing that the recommendation for bilirubin screening should not be misinterpreted as suggesting the need for phototherapy at lower bilirubin levels.

The Maisels et al commentary on hyperbilirubinemia published in this issue came about because of a need to clarify the 2004 guideline and because the AAP had been asked for a statement that either recommended universal bilirubin screening or explained why not. I suspect that having the recommendation for universal screening come in the form of a commentary, rather than a guideline, will be disappointing to both advocates and opponents of universal screening. However, I believe it is the right decision. For now, it represents what some bilirubin experts believe is reasonable on the basis of limited evidence. With additional research, we hope to be able to make a stronger recommendation in the future.

ACKNOWLEDGMENT

This work was partially supported by National Institute of Child Health and Human Development grant R01 HD047557.

REFERENCES

1. Maisels MJ, Bhutani VK, Bogen D, Newman TB, Stark AR, Watchko JF. Management of hyperbilirubinemia in the newborn infant ≥35 weeks' gestation: an update with clarifications. *Pediatrics.* 2009;124(4):1193–1198

2. American Academy of Pediatrics, Subcommittee on Hyperbilirubinemia. Management of hyperbilirubinemia in the newborn infant 35 or more weeks of gestation [published correction appears in *Pediatrics.* 2004;114(4):1138]. *Pediatrics.* 2004;114(1):297–316

3. US Preventive Services Task Force. Screening of infants for hyperbilirubinemia to prevent chronic bilirubin encephalopathy: recommendation statement. *Pediatrics.* 2009;124(4):1172–1177

4. Trikalinos T, Chung M, Lau J, Ip S. Systematic review of screening for bilirubin encephalopathy in neonates. *Pediatrics.* 2009;124(4):1162–1171

5. Newman TB, Garber AM, Holtzman NA, Hulley SB. Problems with the report of the expert panel on blood cholesterol levels in children and adolescents. *Arch Pediatr Adolesc Med.* 1995;149(3):241–247

6. Newman TB, Garber AM. Cholesterol screening in children and adolescents. *Pediatrics.* 2000;105(3 pt 1):637–638

7. Newman TB, Johnston BD, Grossman DC. Effects and costs of requiring child-restraint systems for young children traveling on commercial airplanes. *Arch Pediatr Adolesc Med.* 2003;157(10):969–974

8. Newman TB. Evidence does not support American Academy of Pediatrics recommendation for routine imaging after a first urinary tract infection. *Pediatrics.* 2005;116(6):1613–1614

9. Newman TB. If it's not worth doing, it's not worth doing well. *Pediatrics.* 2005;115(1):196; author reply 196–197

10. Newman TB. Much pain, little gain from voiding cystourethrograms after urinary tract infection. *Pediatrics.* 2006;118(5):2251; author reply 2251–2252

11. Newman TB. Industry-sponsored "expert committee recommendations for acne management" promote expensive drugs on the basis of weak evidence. *Pediatrics.* 2007;119(3):650; author reply 650–651

12. Newman TB. The power of stories over statistics. *BMJ.* 2003;327(7429):1424–1427

13. Maisels MJ, Baltz RD, Bhutani VK, et al. Neonatal jaundice and kernicterus. *Pediatrics.* 2001;108(3):763–765

14. Johnson LH, Bhutani VK, Brown AK. System-based approach to management of neonatal jaundice and prevention of kernicterus. *J Pediatr.* 2002;140(4):396–403

15. Newman TB, Liljestrand P, Escobar GJ. Jaundice noted in the first 24 hours after birth in a managed care organization. *Arch Pediatr Adolesc Med.* 2002;156(12):1244–1250

16. Maisels MJ, Kring E. Transcutaneous bilirubinometry decreases the need for serum bilirubin measurements and saves money. *Pediatrics.* 1997;99(4):599–601

17. Davidson L, Merritt K, Weech A. Hyperbilirubinemia in the newborn. *Am J Dis Child.* 1941;61(5):958–980

18. Madlon-Kay DJ. Recognition of the presence and severity of newborn jaundice by parents, nurses, physicians, and icterometer. *Pediatrics.* 1997;100(3). Available at: www.pediatrics.org/cgi/content/full/100/3/e3

19. Moyer VA, Ahn C, Sneed S. Accuracy of clinical judgment in neonatal jaundice. *Arch Pediatr Adolesc Med.* 2000;154(4):391–394

20. Riskin A, Kuglman A, Abend-Weinger M, Green M, Hemo M, Bader D. In the eye of the beholder: how accurate is clinical estimation of jaundice in newborns? *Acta Paediatr.* 2003;92(5):574–576

21. American Academy of Pediatrics, Steering Committee on Quality Improvement and Management. Classifying recommendations for clinical practice guidelines. *Pediatrics.* 2004;114(3):874–877

22. Sanghavi D. Plenty of guidelines, but where's the evidence? *The New York Times*. December 9, 2008:D6

23. Hayward RA. Access to clinically-detailed patient information: a fundamental element for improving the efficiency and quality of healthcare. *Med Care*. 2008;46(3):229–231

24. Newman TB, Maisels MJ. Less aggressive treatment of neonatal jaundice and reports of kernicterus: lessons about practice guidelines. *Pediatrics*. 2000;105(1 pt 3):242–245

25. Smith GC, Pell JP. Parachute use to prevent death and major trauma related to gravitational challenge: systematic review of randomised controlled trials. *BMJ*. 2003;327(7429):1459–1461

26. Potts M, Prata N, Walsh J, Grossman A. Parachute approach to evidence based medicine. *BMJ*. 2006;333(7570):701–703

27. Auerbach AD, Landefeld CS, Shojania KG. The tension between needing to improve care and knowing how to do it. *N Engl J Med*. 2007;357(6):608–613

28. Shojania KG, Duncan BW, McDonald KM, Wachter RM. Safe but sound: patient safety meets evidence-based medicine. *JAMA*. 2002;288(4):508–513

29. Moyer VA, Nelson D; US Preventive Services Task Force. Pediatricians and the US Preventive Services Task Force: a natural partnership to enhance the health of children. *Pediatrics*. 2008;122(1):174–176

30. Kuzniewicz MW, Escobar GJ, Newman TB. The impact of universal bilirubin screening on severe hyperbilirubinemia and phototherapy use in a managed care organization. *Pediatrics*. 2009;124(4):1031–1039

Hyperbilirubinemia Clinical Practice Guideline Quick Reference Tools

- Recommendation Summary
  — Management of Hyperbilirubinemia in the Newborn Infant 35 or More Weeks of Gestation
- *ICD-9-CM/ICD-10-CM* Coding Quick Reference for Hyperbilirubinemia
- AAP Patient Education Handout
  — *Jaundice and Your Newborn*

Recommendation Summary

Management of Hyperbilirubinemia in the Newborn Infant 35 or More Weeks of Gestation

The following are the key elements of the recommendations provided by this guideline. Clinicians should:

1. Promote and support successful breastfeeding.
2. Establish nursery protocols for the identification and evaluation of hyperbilirubinemia.
3. Measure the total serum bilirubin (TSB) or transcutaneous bilirubin (TcB) level on infants jaundiced in the first 24 hours.
4. Recognize that visual estimation of the degree of jaundice can lead to errors, particularly in darkly pigmented infants.
5. Interpret all bilirubin levels according to the infant's age in hours.
6. Recognize that infants at less than 38 weeks' gestation, particularly those who are breastfed, are at higher risk of developing hyperbilirubinemia and require closer surveillance and monitoring.
7. Perform a systematic assessment on all infants before discharge for the risk of severe hyperbilirubinemia.
8. Provide parents with written and verbal information about newborn jaundice.
9. Provide appropriate follow-up based on the time of discharge and the risk assessment.
10. Treat newborns, when indicated, with phototherapy or exchange transfusion.

<table>
<tr><th colspan="2">Coding Quick Reference for Hyperbilirubinemia</th></tr>
<tr><th colspan="1">ICD-9-CM</th><th colspan="1">ICD-10-CM</th></tr>
<tr><td>774.2 Jaundice of prematurity</td><td>P59.0 Neonatal jaundice associated with preterm delivery</td></tr>
<tr><td>774.39 Jaundice, newborn, breast milk</td><td>P59.3 Neonatal jaundice from breast milk inhibitor</td></tr>
<tr><td>774.6 Jaundice, newborn, physiologic jaundice</td><td>P59.9 Neonatal jaundice, unspecified</td></tr>
<tr><td>782.4 Jaundice, unspecified, not newborn</td><td>R17 Unspecified jaundice</td></tr>
</table>

Jaundice and Your Newborn

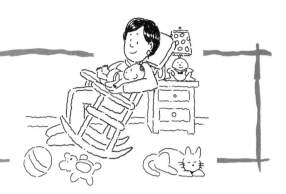

Congratulations on the birth of your new baby!

To make sure your baby's first week is safe and healthy, it is important that

1. You find a pediatrician you are comfortable with for your baby's ongoing care.
2. Your baby is checked for jaundice in the hospital.
3. If you are breastfeeding, you get the help you need to make sure it is going well.
4. Make sure your baby is seen by a doctor or nurse at 3 to 5 days of age.
5. If your baby is discharged before age 72 hours, your baby should be seen by a doctor or nurse within 2 days of discharge from the hospital.

Q: What is jaundice?

A: Jaundice is the yellow color seen in the skin of many newborns. It happens when a chemical called *bilirubin* builds up in the baby's blood. Jaundice can occur in babies of any race or color.

Q: Why is jaundice common in newborns?

A: Everyone's blood contains bilirubin, which is removed by the liver. Before birth, the mother's liver does this for the baby. Most babies develop jaundice in the first few days after birth because it takes a few days for the baby's liver to get better at removing bilirubin.

Q: How can I tell if my baby is jaundiced?

A: The skin of a baby with jaundice usually appears yellow. The best way to see jaundice is in good light, such as daylight or under fluorescent lights. Jaundice usually appears first in the face and then moves to the chest, abdomen, arms, and legs as the bilirubin level increases. The whites of the eyes may also be yellow. Jaundice may be harder to see in babies with darker skin color.

Q: Can jaundice hurt my baby?

A: Most babies have mild jaundice that is harmless, but in unusual situations the bilirubin level can get very high and might cause brain damage. This is why newborns should be checked carefully for jaundice and treated to prevent a high bilirubin level.

Q: How should my baby be checked for jaundice?

A: If your baby looks jaundiced in the first few days after birth, your baby's doctor or nurse may use a skin or blood test to check your baby's bilirubin level. However, because estimating the bilirubin level based on the baby's appearance can be difficult, some experts recommend that a skin or blood test be done even if your baby does not appear jaundiced. A bilirubin level is always needed if jaundice develops before the baby is 24 hours old. Whether a test is needed after that depends on the baby's age, the amount of jaundice, and whether the baby has other factors that make jaundice more likely or harder to see.

Q: Does breastfeeding affect jaundice?

A: Jaundice is more common in babies who are breastfed than babies who are formula-fed, but this occurs mainly in newborns who are not nursing well. If you are breastfeeding, you should nurse your baby at least 8 to 12 times a day for the first few days. This will help you produce enough milk and will help to keep the baby's bilirubin level down. If you are having trouble breastfeeding, ask your baby's doctor or nurse or a lactation specialist for help. Breast milk is the ideal food for your baby.

Q: When should my newborn get checked after leaving the hospital?

A: It is important for your baby to be seen by a nurse or doctor when the baby is between 3 and 5 days old, because this is usually when a baby's bilirubin level is highest. This is why, if your baby is discharged before age 72 hours, your baby should be seen within 2 days of discharge. The timing of this visit may vary depending on your baby's age when released from the hospital and other factors.

Q: Which babies require more attention for jaundice?

A: Some babies have a greater risk for high levels of bilirubin and may need to be seen sooner after discharge from the hospital. Ask your doctor about an early follow-up visit if your baby has any of the following:

- A high bilirubin level before leaving the hospital
- Early birth (more than 2 weeks before the due date)
- Jaundice in the first 24 hours after birth
- Breastfeeding that is not going well
- A lot of bruising or bleeding under the scalp related to labor and delivery
- A parent, brother, or sister who had high bilirubin and received light therapy

Q: When should I call my baby's doctor?

A: Call your baby's doctor if

- Your baby's skin turns more yellow.
- Your baby's abdomen, arms, or legs are yellow.
- The whites of your baby's eyes are yellow.
- Your baby is jaundiced and is hard to wake, fussy, or not nursing or taking formula well.

Q: How is harmful jaundice prevented?

A: Most jaundice requires no treatment. When treatment is necessary, placing your baby under special lights while he or she is undressed will lower the bilirubin level. Depending on your baby's bilirubin level, this can be done in the hospital or at home. Jaundice is treated at levels that are much lower than those at which brain damage is a concern. Treatment can prevent the harmful effects of jaundice. Putting your baby in sunlight is not recommended as a safe way of treating jaundice. Exposing your baby to sunlight might help lower the bilirubin level, but this will only work if the baby is completely undressed. This cannot be done safely inside your home because your baby will get cold, and newborns should never be put in direct sunlight outside because they might get sunburned.

Q: When does jaundice go away?

A: In breastfed babies, jaundice often lasts for more than 2 to 3 weeks. In formula-fed babies, most jaundice goes away by 2 weeks. If your baby is jaundiced for more than 3 weeks, see your baby's doctor.

The information contained in this publication should not be used as a substitute for the medical care and advice of your pediatrician. There may be variations in treatment that your pediatrician may recommend based on individual facts and circumstances.

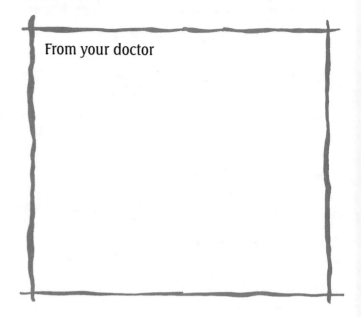

From your doctor

American Academy
of Pediatrics

DEDICATED TO THE HEALTH OF ALL CHILDREN™

The American Academy of Pediatrics is an organization of 60,000 primary care pediatricians, pediatric medical subspecialists, and pediatric surgical specialists dedicated to the health, safety, and well-being of infants, children, adolescents, and young adults.

American Academy of Pediatrics
Web site—www.aap.org

The Diagnosis and Management of Acute Otitis Media

- *Clinical Practice Guideline*

CLINICAL PRACTICE GUIDELINE

The Diagnosis and Management of Acute Otitis Media

abstract

This evidence-based clinical practice guideline is a revision of the 2004 acute otitis media (AOM) guideline from the American Academy of Pediatrics (AAP) and American Academy of Family Physicians. It provides recommendations to primary care clinicians for the management of children from 6 months through 12 years of age with uncomplicated AOM.

In 2009, the AAP convened a committee composed of primary care physicians and experts in the fields of pediatrics, family practice, otolaryngology, epidemiology, infectious disease, emergency medicine, and guideline methodology. The subcommittee partnered with the Agency for Healthcare Research and Quality and the Southern California Evidence-Based Practice Center to develop a comprehensive review of the new literature related to AOM since the initial evidence report of 2000. The resulting evidence report and other sources of data were used to formulate the practice guideline recommendations.

The focus of this practice guideline is the appropriate diagnosis and initial treatment of a child presenting with AOM. The guideline provides a specific, stringent definition of AOM. It addresses pain management, initial observation versus antibiotic treatment, appropriate choices of antibiotic agents, and preventive measures. It also addresses recurrent AOM, which was not included in the 2004 guideline. Decisions were made on the basis of a systematic grading of the quality of evidence and benefit-harm relationships.

The practice guideline underwent comprehensive peer review before formal approval by the AAP.

This clinical practice guideline is not intended as a sole source of guidance in the management of children with AOM. Rather, it is intended to assist primary care clinicians by providing a framework for clinical decision-making. It is not intended to replace clinical judgment or establish a protocol for all children with this condition. These recommendations may not provide the only appropriate approach to the management of this problem. *Pediatrics* 2013;131:e964–e999

Allan S. Lieberthal, MD, FAAP, Aaron E. Carroll, MD, MS, FAAP, Tasnee Chonmaitree, MD, FAAP, Theodore G. Ganiats, MD, Alejandro Hoberman, MD, FAAP, Mary Anne Jackson, MD, FAAP, Mark D. Joffe, MD, FAAP, Donald T. Miller, MD, MPH, FAAP, Richard M. Rosenfeld, MD, MPH, FAAP, Xavier D. Sevilla, MD, FAAP, Richard H. Schwartz, MD, FAAP, Pauline A. Thomas, MD, FAAP, and David E. Tunkel, MD, FAAP, FACS

KEY WORDS
acute otitis media, otitis media, otoscopy, otitis media with effusion, watchful waiting, antibiotics, antibiotic prophylaxis, tympanostomy tube insertion, immunization, breastfeeding

ABBREVIATIONS
AAFP—American Academy of Family Physicians
AAP—American Academy of Pediatrics
AHRQ—Agency for Healthcare Research and Quality
AOM—acute otitis media
CI—confidence interval
FDA—US Food and Drug Administration
LAIV—live-attenuated intranasal influenza vaccine
MEE—middle ear effusion
MIC—minimum inhibitory concentration
NNT—number needed to treat
OM—otitis media
OME—otitis media with effusion
OR—odds ratio
PCV7—heptavalent pneumococcal conjugate vaccine
PCV13—13-valent pneumococcal conjugate vaccine
RD—rate difference
SNAP—safety-net antibiotic prescription
TIV—trivalent inactivated influenza vaccine
TM—tympanic membrane
WASP—wait-and-see prescription

(Continued on last page)

Key Action Statement 1A: Clinicians should diagnose acute otitis media (AOM) in children who present with moderate to severe bulging of the tympanic membrane (TM) *or* new onset of otorrhea not due to acute otitis externa. Evidence Quality: Grade B. Strength: Recommendation.

Key Action Statement 1B: Clinicians should diagnose AOM in children who present with mild bulging of the TM *and* recent (less than 48 hours) onset of ear pain (holding, tugging, rubbing of the ear in a nonverbal child) or intense erythema of the TM. Evidence Quality: Grade C. Strength: Recommendation.

Key Action Statement 1C: Clinicians should not diagnose AOM in children who do not have middle ear effusion (MEE) (based on pneumatic otoscopy and/or tympanometry). Evidence Quality: Grade B. Strength: Recommendation.

Key Action Statement 2: The management of AOM should include an assessment of pain. If pain is present, the clinician should recommend treatment to reduce pain. Evidence Quality: Grade B. Strength: Strong Recommendation.

Key Action Statement 3A: Severe AOM: The clinician should prescribe antibiotic therapy for AOM (bilateral or unilateral) in children 6 months and older with severe signs or symptoms (ie, moderate or severe otalgia or otalgia for at least 48 hours or temperature 39°C [102.2°F] or higher). Evidence Quality: Grade B. Strength: Strong Recommendation.

Key Action Statement 3B: Non-severe bilateral AOM in young children: The clinician should prescribe antibiotic therapy for bilateral AOM in children 6 months through 23 months of age without severe signs or symptoms (ie, mild otalgia for less than 48 hours and temperature less than 39°C [102.2°F]). Evidence Quality: Grade B. Strength: Recommendation.

Key Action Statement 3C: Non-severe unilateral AOM in young children: The clinician should either prescribe antibiotic therapy *or* offer observation with close follow-up based on joint decision-making with the parent(s)/caregiver for unilateral AOM in children 6 months to 23 months of age without severe signs or symptoms (ie, mild otalgia for less than 48 hours and temperature less than 39°C [102.2°F]). When observation is used, a mechanism must be in place to ensure follow-up and begin antibiotic therapy if the child worsens or fails to improve within 48 to 72 hours of onset of symptoms. Evidence Quality: Grade B. Strength: Recommendation.

Key Action Statement 3D: Nonsevere AOM in older children: The clinician should either prescribe antibiotic therapy *or* offer observation with close follow-up based on joint decision-making with the parent(s)/caregiver for AOM (bilateral or unilateral) in children 24 months or older without severe signs or symptoms (ie, mild otalgia for less than 48 hours and temperature less than 39°C [102.2°F]). When observation is used, a mechanism must be in place to ensure follow-up and begin antibiotic therapy if the child worsens or fails to improve within 48 to 72 hours of onset of symptoms. Evidence Quality: Grade B. Strength: Recommendation.

Key Action Statement 4A: Clinicians should prescribe amoxicillin for AOM when a decision to treat with antibiotics has been made *and* the child has not received amoxicillin in the past 30 days *or* the child does not have concurrent purulent conjunctivitis *or* the child is not allergic to penicillin. Evidence Quality: Grade B. Strength: Recommendation.

Key Action Statement 4B: Clinicians should prescribe an antibiotic with additional β-lactamase coverage for AOM when a decision to treat with antibiotics has been made, *and* the child has received amoxicillin in the last 30 days *or* has concurrent purulent conjunctivitis, *or* has a history of recurrent AOM unresponsive to amoxicillin. Evidence Quality: Grade C. Strength: Recommendation.

Key Action Statement 4C: Clinicians should reassess the patient if the caregiver reports that the child's symptoms have worsened or failed to respond to the initial antibiotic treatment within 48 to 72 hours and determine whether a change in therapy is needed. Evidence Quality: Grade B. Strength: Recommendation.

Key Action Statement 5A: Clinicians should not prescribe prophylactic antibiotics to reduce the frequency of episodes of AOM in children with recurrent AOM. Evidence Quality: Grade B. Strength: Recommendation.

Key Action Statement 5B: Clinicians may offer tympanostomy tubes for recurrent AOM (3 episodes in 6 months or 4 episodes in 1 year with 1 episode in the preceding 6 months). Evidence Quality: Grade B. Strength: Option.

Key Action Statement 6A: Clinicians should recommend pneumococcal conjugate vaccine to all children according to the schedule of the Advisory Committee on Immunization Practices of the Centers for Disease Control and Prevention, American Academy of Pediatrics (AAP), and American Academy of Family Physicians (AAFP). Evidence Quality: Grade B. Strength: Strong Recommendation.

Key Action Statement 6B: Clinicians should recommend annual influenza vaccine to all children according to the schedule of the Advisory Committee on Immunization Practices, AAP, and AAFP. Evidence Quality: Grade B. Strength: Recommendation.

2Key Action Statement 6C: Clinicians should encourage exclusive breastfeeding for at least 6 months. Evidence Quality: Grade B. Strength: Recommendation.

Key Action Statement 6D: Clinicians should encourage avoidance of tobacco smoke exposure. Evidence Quality: Grade C. Strength: Recommendation.

INTRODUCTION

In May 2004, the AAP and AAFP published the "Clinical Practice Guideline: Diagnosis and Management of Acute Otitis Media".[1] The guideline offered 8 recommendations ranked according to level of evidence and benefit-harm relationship. Three of the recommendations—diagnostic criteria, observation, and choice of antibiotics—led to significant discussion, especially among experts in the field of otitis media (OM). Also, at the time the guideline was written, information regarding the heptavalent pneumococcal conjugate vaccine (PCV7) was not yet published. Since completion of the guideline in November 2003 and its publication in May 2004, there has been a significant body of additional literature on AOM.

Although OM remains the most common condition for which antibacterial agents are prescribed for children in the United States[2,3] clinician visits for OM decreased from 950 per 1000 children in 1995–1996 to 634 per 1000 children in 2005–2006. There has been a proportional decrease in antibiotic prescriptions for OM from 760 per 1000 in 1995–1996 to 484 per 1000 in 2005–2006. The percentage of OM visits

resulting in antibiotic prescriptions remained relatively stable (80% in 1995–1996; 76% in 2005–2006).[2] Many factors may have contributed to the decrease in visits for OM, including financial issues relating to insurance, such as copayments, that may limit doctor visits, public education campaigns regarding the viral nature of most infectious diseases, use of the PCV7 pneumococcal vaccine, and increased use of the influenza vaccine. Clinicians may also be more attentive to differentiating AOM from OM with effusion (OME), resulting in fewer visits coded for AOM and fewer antibiotic prescriptions written.

Despite significant publicity and awareness of the 2004 AOM guideline, evidence shows that clinicians are hesitant to follow the guideline recommendations. Vernacchio et al[4] surveyed 489 primary care physicians as to their management of 4 AOM scenarios addressed in the 2004 guideline. No significant changes in practice were noted on this survey, compared with a survey administered before the 2004 AOM guideline. Coco[5] used the National Ambulatory Medical Care Survey from 2002 through 2006 to determine the frequency of AOM visits without antibiotics before and after publication of the 2004 guideline. There was no difference in prescribing rates. A similar response to otitis guidelines was found in Italy as in the United States.[6,7] These findings parallel results of other investigations regarding clinician awareness and adherence to guideline recommendations in all specialties, including pediatrics.[8] Clearly, for clinical practice guidelines to be effective, more must be done to improve their dissemination and implementation.

This revision and update of the AAP/AAFP 2004 AOM guideline[1] will evaluate published evidence on the diagnosis and management of uncomplicated AOM and make recommendations based on that evidence. The guideline is intended

for primary care clinicians including pediatricians and family physicians, emergency department physicians, otolaryngologists, physician assistants, and nurse practitioners. The scope of the guideline is the diagnosis and management of AOM, including recurrent AOM, in children 6 months through 12 years of age. It applies only to an otherwise healthy child without underlying conditions that may alter the natural course of AOM, including but not limited to the presence of tympanostomy tubes; anatomic abnormalities, including cleft palate; genetic conditions with craniofacial abnormalities, such as Down syndrome; immune deficiencies; and the presence of cochlear implants. Children with OME without AOM are also excluded.

Glossary of Terms

AOM—the rapid onset of signs and symptoms of inflammation in the middle ear[9,10]

Uncomplicated AOM—AOM without otorrhea[1]

Severe AOM—AOM with the presence of moderate to severe otalgia or fever equal to or higher than 39°C[9,10]

Nonsevere AOM—AOM with the presence of mild otalgia and a temperature below 39°C[9,10]

Recurrent AOM—3 or more well-documented and separate AOM episodes in the preceding 6 months or 4 or more episodes in the preceding 12 months with at least 1 episode in the past 6 months[11,12]

OME—inflammation of the middle ear with liquid collected in the middle ear; the signs and symptoms of acute infection are absent[9]

MEE—liquid in the middle ear without reference to etiology, pathogenesis, pathology, or duration[9]

Otorrhea—discharge from the ear, originating at 1 or more of the following sites: the external auditory canal, middle ear, mastoid, inner ear, or intracranial cavity

Otitis externa—an infection of the external auditory canal

Tympanometry—measuring acoustic immittance (transfer of acoustic energy) of the ear as a function of ear canal air pressure[13,14]

Number needed to treat (NNT)—the number of patients who need to be treated to prevent 1 additional bad outcome[15]

Initial antibiotic therapy—treatment of AOM with antibiotics that are prescribed at the time of diagnosis with the intent of starting antibiotic therapy as soon as possible after the encounter

Initial observation—initial management of AOM limited to symptomatic relief, with commencement of antibiotic therapy only if the child's condition worsens at any time or does not show clinical improvement within 48 to 72 hours of diagnosis; a mechanism must be in place to ensure follow-up and initiation of antibiotics if the child fails observation

METHODS

Guideline development using an evidence-based approach requires that all evidence related to the guideline is gathered in a systematic fashion, objectively assessed, and then described so readers can easily see the links between the evidence and recommendations made. An evidence-based approach leads to recommendations that are guided by both the quality of the available evidence and the benefit-to-harm ratio that results from following the recommendation. Figure 1 shows the relationship of evidence quality and benefit-harm balance in determining the level of recommendation. Table 1 presents the AAP definitions and implications of different levels of evidence-based recommendations.[16]

In preparing for the 2004 AAP guidelines, the Agency for Healthcare Research and Quality (AHRQ) funded and conducted an exhaustive review of the literature on diagnosis and management of AOM.[17–19] In 2008, the AHRQ and the Southern California Evidence-Based Practice Center began a similar process of reviewing the literature published since the 2001 AHRQ report. The AAP again partnered with AHRQ and the Southern California Evidence-Based Practice Center to develop the evidence report, which served as a major source of data for these practice guideline recommendations.[20,21] New key questions were determined by a technical expert panel. The scope of the new report went beyond the 2001 AHRQ report to include recurrent AOM.

The key questions addressed by AHRQ in the 2010 report were as follows:

1. Diagnosis of AOM: What are the operating characteristics (sensitivity, specificity, and likelihood ratios) of clinical symptoms and otoscopic findings (such as bulging TM) to diagnose uncomplicated AOM and to distinguish it from OME?

2. What has been the effect of the use of heptavalent PCV7 on AOM microbial epidemiology, what organisms (bacterial and viral) are associated with AOM since the introduction of PCV7, and what are the patterns of antimicrobial resistance in AOM since the introduction of PCV7?

3. What is the comparative effectiveness of various treatment options for treating uncomplicated AOM in average risk children?

4. What is the comparative effectiveness of different management options for recurrent OM (uncomplicated) and persistent OM or relapse of AOM?

5. Do treatment outcomes in Questions 3 and 4 differ by characteristics of the condition (AOM), patient, environment, and/or health care delivery system?

6. What adverse effects have been observed for treatments for which outcomes are addressed in Questions 3 and 4?

For the 2010 review, searches of PubMed and the Cochrane Database of Systematic Reviews, Cochrane Central Register of Controlled Trials, and Education Resources Information Center were conducted by using the same search strategies used for the 2001 report for publications from 1998 through June 2010. Additional terms or conditions not considered in the 2001 review (recurrent OM, new drugs, and heptavalent pneumococcal vaccine) were also included. The Web of Science was also used to search for citations of the 2001 report and its peer-reviewed publications. Titles were screened independently by 2

Evidence Quality	Preponderance of Benefit or Harm	Balance of Benefit and Harm
A. Well designed RCTs* or diagnostic studies on relevant population	Strong Recommendation	Option
B. RCTs or diagnostic studies with minor limitations; overwhelmingly consistent evidence from observational studies		
C. Observational studies (case-control and cohort design)	Recommendation	
D. Expert opinion, case reports, reasoning from first principles	Option	No Rec
X. Exceptional situations in which validating studies cannot be performed and there is a clear preponderance of benefit or harm	Strong Recommendation / Recommendation	

FIGURE 1

Relationship of evidence quality and benefit-harm balance in determining the level of recommendation. RCT, randomized controlled trial.

TABLE 1 Guideline Definitions for Evidence-Based Statements

Statement	Definition	Implication
Strong Recommendation	A strong recommendation in favor of a particular action is made when the anticipated benefits of the recommended intervention clearly exceed the harms (as a strong recommendation against an action is made when the anticipated harms clearly exceed the benefits) and the quality of the supporting evidence is excellent. In some clearly identified circumstances, strong recommendations may be made when high-quality evidence is impossible to obtain and the anticipated benefits strongly outweigh the harms.	Clinicians should follow a strong recommendation unless a clear and compelling rationale for an alternative approach is present.
Recommendation	A recommendation in favor of a particular action is made when the anticipated benefits exceed the harms, but the quality of evidence is not as strong. Again, in some clearly identified circumstances, recommendations may be made when high-quality evidence is impossible to obtain but the anticipated benefits outweigh the harms.	Clinicians would be prudent to follow a recommendation but should remain alert to new information and sensitive to patient preferences.
Option	Options define courses that may be taken when either the quality of evidence is suspect or carefully performed studies have shown little clear advantage to 1 approach over another.	Clinicians should consider the option in their decision-making, and patient preference may have a substantial role.
No Recommendation	No recommendation indicates that there is a lack of pertinent published evidence and that the anticipated balance of benefits and harms is presently unclear.	Clinicians should be alert to new published evidence that clarifies the balance of benefit versus harm.

pediatricians with experience in conducting systematic reviews.

For the question pertaining to diagnosis, efficacy, and safety, the search was primarily for clinical trials. For the question pertaining to the effect of PCV7 on epidemiology and microbiology, the group searched for trials that compared microbiology in the same populations before and after introduction of the vaccine or observational studies that compared microbiology across vaccinated and unvaccinated populations.

In total, the reviewers examined 7646 titles, of which 686 titles were identified for further review. Of those, 72 articles that met the predetermined inclusion and exclusion criteria were reviewed in detail. Investigators abstracted data into standard evidence tables, with accuracy checked by a second investigator. Studies were quality-rated by 2 investigators by using established criteria. For randomized controlled trials, the Jadad criteria were used.[22] QUADAS criteria[23] were used to evaluate the studies that pertained to diagnosis. GRADE criteria were applied to pooled analyses.[24] Data abstracted

included parameters necessary to define study groups, inclusion/exclusion criteria, influencing factors, and outcome measures. Some of the data for analysis were abstracted by a biostatistician and checked by a physician reviewer. A sequential resolution strategy was used to match and resolve the screening and review results of the 2 pediatrician reviewers.

For the assessment of treatment efficacy, pooled analyses were performed for comparisons for which 3 or more trials could be identified. Studies eligible for analyses of questions pertaining to treatment efficacy were grouped for comparisons by treatment options. Each comparison consisted of studies that were considered homogeneous across clinical practice. Because some of the key questions were addressed in the 2001 evidence report,[17] studies identified in that report were included with newly identified articles in the 2010 evidence report.[20]

Decisions were made on the basis of a systematic grading of the quality of evidence and strength of recommendations as well as expert consensus when

definitive data were not available. Results of the literature review were presented in evidence tables and published in the final evidence report.[20]

In June 2009, the AAP convened a new subcommittee to review and revise the May 2004 AOM guideline.[1] The subcommittee comprised primary care physicians and experts in the fields of pediatrics, family practice, otolaryngology, epidemiology, infectious disease, emergency medicine, and guideline methodology. All panel members reviewed the AAP policy on conflict of interest and voluntary disclosure and were given an opportunity to present any potential conflicts with the subcommittee's work. All potential conflicts of interest are listed at the end of this document. The project was funded by the AAP. New literature on OM is continually being published. Although the systematic review performed by AHRQ could not be replicated with new literature, members of the Subcommittee on Diagnosis and Management of Acute Otitis Media reviewed additional articles. PubMed was searched by using the single search term "acute otitis media," approximately every 6 months from June 2009 through October 2011 to obtain new articles. Subcommittee members evaluated pertinent articles for quality of methodology and importance of results. Selected articles used in the AHRQ review were also reevaluated for their quality. Conclusions were based on the consensus of the subcommittee after the review of newer literature and reevaluation of the AHRQ evidence. Key action statements were generated using BRIDGE-Wiz (Building Recommendations in a Developers Guideline Editor), an interactive software tool that leads guideline development through a series of questions that are intended to create a more actionable set of key action statements.[25] BRIDGE-Wiz also incorporates the quality of available evidence into the final determination of the strength of each recommendation.

After thorough review by the subcommittee for this guideline, a draft was reviewed by other AAP committees and sections, selected outside organizations, and individuals identified by the subcommittee as experts in the field. Additionally, members of the subcommittee were encouraged to distribute the draft to interested parties in their respective specialties. All comments were reviewed by the writing group and incorporated into the final guideline when appropriate.

This clinical practice guideline is not intended as a sole source of guidance in the management of children with AOM. Rather, it is intended to assist clinicians in decision-making. It is not intended to replace clinical judgment or establish a protocol for the care of all children with this condition. These recommendations may not provide the only appropriate approach to the management of children with AOM.

It is AAP policy to review and update evidence-based guidelines every 5 years.

KEY ACTION STATEMENTS
Key Action Statement 1A

Clinicians should diagnose AOM in children who present with moderate to severe bulging of the TM *or* new onset of otorrhea not due to acute otitis externa. (Evidence Quality: Grade B, Rec. Strength: Recommendation)

Key Action Statement Profile: KAS 1A

Aggregate evidence quality	Grade B
Benefits	• Identify a population of children most likely to benefit from intervention. • Avoid unnecessary treatment of those without highly certain AOM. • Promote consistency in diagnosis.
Risks, harms, cost	May miss AOM that presents with a combination of mild bulging, intense erythema, or otalgia that may not necessarily represent less severe disease and may also benefit from intervention.
Benefits-harms assessment	Preponderance of benefit.
Value judgments	Identification of a population of children with highly certain AOM is beneficial. Accurate, specific diagnosis is helpful to the individual patient. Modification of current behavior of overdiagnosis is a goal. Increased specificity is preferred even as sensitivity is lowered.
Intentional vagueness	By using stringent diagnostic criteria, the TM appearance of less severe illness that might be early AOM has not been addressed.
Role of patient preferences	None
Exclusions	None
Strength	**Recommendation**
Notes	Tympanocentesis studies confirm that using these diagnostic findings leads to high levels of isolation of pathogenic bacteria. Evidence is extrapolated from treatment studies that included tympanocentesis.

Key Action Statement 1B

Clinicians should diagnose AOM in children who present with mild bulging of the TM *and* recent (less than 48 hours) onset of ear pain (holding, tugging, rubbing of the ear in a nonverbal child) or intense erythema of the TM. (Evidence Quality: Grade C, Rec. Strength: Recommendation)

Key Action Statement Profile: KAS 1B

Aggregate evidence quality	Grade C
Benefits	Identify AOM in children when the diagnosis is not highly certain.
Risks, harms, cost	Overdiagnosis of AOM. Reduced precision in diagnosis.
Benefits-harms assessment	Benefits greater than harms.
Value judgments	None.
Intentional vagueness	Criteria may be more subjective.
Role of patient preferences	None
Exclusions	None
Strength	**Recommendation**
Notes	Recent onset of ear pain means within the past 48 hours.

Key Action Statement 1C

Clinicians should not diagnose AOM in children who do not have MEE (based on pneumatic otoscopy and/or tympanometry). (Evidence Quality: Grade B, Rec. Strength: Recommendation)

Key Action Statement Profile: KAS 1C

Aggregate evidence quality	Grade B
Benefits	Reduces overdiagnosis and unnecessary treatment. Increases correct diagnosis of other conditions with symptoms that otherwise might be attributed to AOM. Promotes the use of pneumatic otoscopy and tympanometry to improve diagnostic accuracy.
Risks, harms, cost	Cost of tympanometry. Need to acquire or reacquire skills in pneumatic otoscopy and tympanometry for some clinicians.
Benefits-harms assessment	Preponderance of benefit.
Value judgments	AOM is overdiagnosed, often without adequate visualization of the TM. Early AOM without effusion occurs, but the risk of overdiagnosis supersedes that concern.
Intentional vagueness	None
Role of patient preferences	None
Exclusions	Early AOM evidenced by intense erythema of the TM.
Strength	**Recommendation**

Purpose of This Section

There is no gold standard for the diagnosis of AOM. In fact, AOM has a spectrum of signs as the disease develops.[26] Therefore, the purpose of this section is to provide clinicians and researchers with a working clinical definition of AOM and to differentiate AOM from OME. The criteria were chosen to achieve high specificity recognizing that the resulting decreased sensitivity may exclude less severe presentations of AOM.

Changes From AAP/AAFP 2004 AOM Guideline

Accurate diagnosis of AOM is critical to sound clinical decision-making and high-quality research. The 2004 "Clinical Practice Guideline: Diagnosis and Management of AOM"[1] used a 3-part definition for AOM: (1) acute onset of symptoms, (2) presence of MEE, and (3) signs of acute middle ear inflammation. This definition generated extensive discussion and reanalysis of the AOM diagnostic evidence. The 2004 definition lacked precision to exclude cases of OME, and diagnoses of AOM could be made in children with acute onset of symptoms, including severe otalgia and MEE, without other otoscopic findings of inflammation.[27] Furthermore, the use of "uncertain diagnosis" in the 2004 AOM guideline may have permitted diagnoses of AOM without clear visualization of the TM. Earlier studies may have enrolled children who had OME rather than AOM, resulting in the possible classification of such children as improved because their nonspecific symptoms would have abated regardless of therapy.[28–30] Two studies, published in 2011, used stringent diagnostic criteria for diagnosing AOM with much less risk of conclusions based on data from mixed patients.[31,32]

Since publication of the 2004 AOM guideline, a number of studies have been conducted evaluating scales for the presence of symptoms. These studies did not show a consistent correlation of symptoms with the initial diagnosis of AOM, especially in preverbal children.[33–35]

Recent research has used precisely stated stringent criteria of AOM for purposes of the studies.[31,32] The current guideline endorses stringent otoscopic diagnostic criteria as a basis for management decisions (described later). As clinicians use the proposed stringent criteria to diagnose AOM, they should be aware that children with AOM may also present with recent onset of ear pain and intense erythema of the TM as the only otoscopic finding.

Symptoms

Older children with AOM usually present with a history of rapid onset of ear pain. However, in young preverbal children, otalgia as suggested by tugging/rubbing/holding of the ear, excessive crying, fever, or changes in the child's sleep or behavior pattern as noted by the parent are often relatively nonspecific symptoms. A number of studies have attempted to correlate symptom scores with diagnoses of AOM.

A systematic review[36] identified 4 articles that evaluated the accuracy of symptoms.[37–40] Ear pain appeared useful in diagnosing AOM (combined positive likelihood ratio 3.0–7.3, negative likelihood ratio 0.4–0.6); however, it was only present in 50% to 60% of children with AOM. Conclusions from these studies may be limited, because they (1) enrolled children seen by specialists, not likely to represent the whole spectrum of severity of illness; (2) used a clinical diagnosis of AOM based more on symptomatology rather than on tympanocentesis; and (3) included relatively older children.[37,40]

Laine et al[34] used a questionnaire administered to 469 parents who suspected their children, aged 6 to 35 months, had AOM. Of the children, 237 had AOM using strict otoscopic criteria, and 232 had upper respiratory tract infection without AOM. Restless sleep, ear rubbing, fever, and nonspecific respiratory or gastrointestinal tract symptoms did not differentiate children with or without AOM.

McCormick et al[30] used 2 symptom scores—a 3-item score (OM-3), consisting of symptoms of physical suffering such as ear pain or fever, emotional distress (irritability, poor appetite), and limitation in activity; and a 5-item score (Ear Treatment Group Symptom Questionnaire, 5 Items [ETG-5]), including fever, earache, irritability, decreased appetite, and sleep disturbance—to assess AOM symptoms at the time of diagnosis and daily during the 10-day treatment or observation period. They found both to be a responsive measure of changes in clinical symptoms. The same group[35] also tested a visual scale, Acute Otitis Media-Faces Scale (AOM-FS), with faces similar to the Wong-Baker pain scale.[41] None of the scales were adequately sensitive for making the diagnosis of AOM based on symptoms. The AOM-FS combined with an otoscopy score, OS-8,[30] were presented as a double-sided pocket card. The combination of AOM-FS and OS-8 was more responsive to change than either instrument alone.

Shaikh et al[33,42] validated a 7-item parent-reported symptom score (Acute Otitis Media Severity of Symptom Scale [AOM-SOS]) for children with AOM, following stringent guidance of the US Food and Drug Administration (FDA) on the development of patient-reported outcome scales. Symptoms included ear tugging/rubbing/holding, excessive crying, irritability, difficulty sleeping, decreased activity or appetite, and fever. AOM-SOS was correlated with otoscopic diagnoses (AOM, OME, and normal middle ear status). AOM-SOS changed appropriately in response to clinical change. Its day-to-day responsiveness supports its usefulness in following AOM symptoms over time.

Signs of AOM

Few studies have evaluated the relationship of otoscopic findings in AOM

and tympanocentesis. A study by Karma et al[43] is often cited as the best single study of otoscopic findings in AOM. However, the study uses only a symptom-based diagnosis of AOM plus the presence of MEE. Thus, children with acute upper respiratory tract infection symptoms and OME would have been considered to have AOM. There also were significant differences in findings at the 2 centers that participated in the study.

The investigators correlated TM color, mobility, and position with the presence of middle ear fluid obtained by tympanocentesis. At 2 sites in Finland (Tampere and Oulu), 2911 children were followed from 6 months to 2.5 years of age. A single otolaryngologist at Tampere and a single pediatrician at Oulu examined subjects. Color, position, and mobility were recorded. Myringotomy and aspiration were performed if MEE was suspected. AOM was diagnosed if MEE was found and the child had fever, earache, irritability, ear rubbing or tugging, simultaneous other acute respiratory tract symptoms, vomiting, or diarrhea. The presence or absence of MEE was noted, but no analyses of the fluid, including culture, were performed. Pneumatic otoscopic findings were classified as follows: color—hemorrhagic, strongly red, moderately red, cloudy or dull, slightly red, or normal; position—bulging, retracted, or normal; and mobility—distinctly impaired, slightly impaired, or normal.

For this analysis, 11 804 visits were available. For visits with acute symptoms, MEE was found in 84.9% and 81.8% at the 2 sites at which the study was performed. There were significant differences among the results at the 2 centers involved in the study. Table 2 shows specific data for each finding.

The combination of a "cloudy," bulging TM with impaired mobility was the

TABLE 2 Otoscopic Findings in Children With Acute Symptoms and MEE[a]

TM Finding in Acute Visits With MEE	Group I (Tampere, Finland), %	Group II (Oulu, Finland), %
Color		
Distinctly red	69.8	65.6
Hemorrhagic	81.3	62.9
Strongly red	87.7	68.1
Moderately red	59.8	66.0
Slightly red	39.4	16.7
Cloudy	95.7	80.0
Normal	1.7	4.9
Position		
Bulging	96.0	89
Retracted	46.8	48.6
Normal	32.1	22.2
Mobility		
Distinctly impaired	94.0	78.5
Slightly impaired	59.7	32.8
Normal	2.7	4.8

[a] Totals are greater than 100%, because each ear may have had different findings.[43]

best predictor of AOM using the symptom-based diagnosis in this study. Impaired mobility had the highest sensitivity and specificity (approximately 95% and 85%, respectively). Cloudiness had the next best combination of high sensitivity (~74%) and high specificity (~93%) in this study. Bulging had high specificity (~97%) but lower sensitivity (~51%). A TM that was hemorrhagic, strongly red, or moderately red also correlated with the presence of AOM, and a TM that was only "slightly red" was not helpful diagnostically.

McCormick et al reported that a bulging TM was highly associated with the presence of a bacterial pathogen, with or without a concomitant viral pathogen.[44] In a small study, 31 children (40 ears) underwent myringotomy.[45] Bulging TMs had positive bacterial cultures 75% of the time. The percentage of positive cultures for a pathogen increased to 80% if the color of the TM was yellow. The conclusion is that moderate to severe bulging of the TM represents the most important characteristic in the diagnosis of AOM—a finding that has implications for clinical care, research, and education.

The committee recognized that there is a progression from the presence of MEE to the bulging of the TM, and it is often difficult to differentiate this equivocal appearance from the highly certain AOM criteria advocated in this guideline.[26] As such, there is a role for individualized diagnosis and management decisions. Examples of normal, mild bulging, moderate bulging, and severe bulging can be seen in Fig 2.

Distinguishing AOM From OME

OME may occur either as the aftermath of an episode of AOM or as a consequence of eustachian tube dysfunction attributable to an upper respiratory tract infection.[46] However, OME may also precede and predispose to the development of AOM. These 2 forms of OM may be considered segments of a disease continuum.[47] However, because OME does not represent an acute infectious process that benefits from antibiotics, it is of utmost importance for clinicians to become proficient in distinguishing normal middle ear status from OME or AOM. Doing so will avoid unnecessary use of antibiotics, which leads to increased adverse effects of medication and facilitates the development of antimicrobial resistance.

Examination of the TM

Accurate diagnosis of AOM in infants and young children may be difficult.

Symptoms may be mild or overlap with those of an upper respiratory tract illness. The TM may be obscured by cerumen, and subtle changes in the TM may be difficult to discern. Additional factors complicating diagnosis may include lack of cooperation from the child; less than optimal diagnostic equipment, including lack of a pneumatic bulb; inadequate instruments for clearing cerumen from the external auditory canal; inadequate assistance for restraining the child; and lack of experience in removing cerumen and performing pneumatic otoscopy.

The pneumatic otoscope is the standard tool used in diagnosing OM. Valuable also is a surgical head, which greatly facilitates cleaning cerumen from an infant's external auditory canal. Cerumen may be removed by using a curette, gentle suction, or irrigation.[48] The pneumatic otoscope should have a light source of sufficient brightness and an air-tight seal that permits application of positive and negative pressure. In general, nondisposable specula achieve a better seal with less pain because of a thicker, smoother edge and better light transmission properties. The speculum size should be chosen to gently seal at the outer portion of the external auditory canal.

Pneumatic otoscopy permits assessment of the contour of the TM (normal, retracted, full, bulging), its color (gray, yellow, pink, amber, white, red, blue), its translucency (translucent,

semiopaque, opaque), and its mobility (normal, increased, decreased, absent). The normal TM is translucent, pearly gray, and has a ground-glass appearance (Fig 2A). Specific landmarks can be visualized. They include the short process and the manubrium of the malleus and the pars flaccida, located superiorly. These are easily observed and help to identify the position of the TM. Inward movement of the TM on positive pressure in the external canal and outward movement on negative pressure should occur, especially in the superior posterior quadrant. When the TM is retracted, the short process of the malleus becomes more prominent, and the manubrium appears shortened because of its change in position within the middle ear. Inward motion occurring with positive pressure is restricted or absent, because the TM is frequently as far inward as its range of motion allows. However, outward mobility can be visualized when negative pressure is applied. If the TM does not move perceptibly with applications of gentle positive or negative pressure, MEE is likely. Sometimes, the application of pressure will make an air-fluid interface behind the TM (which is diagnostic of MEE) more evident.[49]

Instruction in the proper evaluation of the child's middle ear status should begin with the first pediatric rotation in medical school and continue throughout postgraduate training.[50]

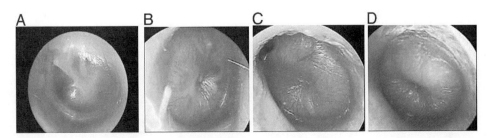

FIGURE 2

A, Normal TM. B, TM with mild bulging. C, TM with moderate bulging. D, TM with severe bulging. Courtesy of Alejandro Hoberman, MD.

Continuing medical education should reinforce the importance of, and retrain the clinician in, the use of pneumatic otoscopy.[51] Training tools include the use of a video-otoscope in residency programs, the use of Web-based educational resources,[49,52] as well as simultaneous or sequential examination of TMs with an expert otoscopist to validate findings by using a double headed or video otoscope. Tools for learning the ear examination can be found in a CD distributed by the Johns Hopkins University School of Medicine and the Institute for Johns Hopkins Nursing,[53] also available at http://www2.aap.org/sections/infectdis/video.cfm,[54] and through a Web-based program, ePROM: Enhancing Proficiency in Otitis Media.[52]

Key Action Statement 2

The management of AOM should include an assessment of pain. If pain is present, the clinician should recommend treatment to reduce pain. (Evidence Quality: Grade B, Rec. Strength: Strong Recommendation)

Key Action Statement Profile: KAS 2

Aggregate evidence quality	Grade B
Benefits	Relieves the major symptom of AOM.
Risks, harms, cost	Potential medication adverse effects. Variable efficacy of some modes of treatment.
Benefits-harms assessment	Preponderance of benefit.
Value judgments	Treating pain is essential whether or not antibiotics are prescribed.
Intentional vagueness	Choice of analgesic is not specified.
Role of patient preferences	Parents may assist in the decision as to what means of pain relief they prefer.
Exclusions	Topical analgesics in the presence of a perforated TM.
Strength	**Strong Recommendation**

Purpose of This Section

Pain is the major symptom of AOM. This section addresses and updates the literature on treating otalgia.

Changes From AAP/AAFP 2004 AOM Guideline

Only 2 new articles directly address the treatment of otalgia. Both address topical treatment. The 2 new articles are consistent with the 2004 guideline statement. The text of the 2004 guideline is, therefore, reproduced here, with the addition of discussion of the 2 new articles. Table 3 has been updated to include the new references.

Treatment of Otalgia

Many episodes of AOM are associated with pain.[55] Some children with OME also have ear pain. Although pain is a common symptom in these illnesses, clinicians often see otalgia as a peripheral concern not requiring direct attention.[56] Pain associated with AOM can be substantial in the first few days of illness and often persists longer in young children.[57] Antibiotic therapy of AOM does not provide symptomatic relief in the first 24 hours[58–61] and even after 3 to 7 days, there may be persistent pain, fever, or both in 30% of children younger than 2 years.[62] In contrast, analgesics do relieve pain associated with AOM within 24 hours[63] and should be used whether antibiotic therapy is or is not prescribed; they should be continued as long as needed. The AAP published the policy statement "The Assessment and Management of Acute Pain in Infants, Children, and Adolescents"[64] to assist the clinician in addressing pain in the context of illness. The management of pain, especially during the first 24 hours of an episode of AOM, should be addressed regardless of the use of antibiotics.

Various treatments of otalgia have been used, but none has been well studied. The clinician should select a treatment on the basis of a consideration of benefits and risks and, wherever possible, incorporate parent/caregiver and patient preference (Table 3).

TABLE 3 Treatments for Otalgia in AOM

Treatment Modality	Comments
Acetaminophen, ibuprofen[63]	Effective analgesia for mild to moderate pain. Readily available. Mainstay of pain management for AOM.
Home remedies (no controlled studies that directly address effectiveness) Distraction External application of heat or cold Oil drops in external auditory canal	May have limited effectiveness.
Topical agents	
Benzocaine, procaine, lidocaine[65,67,70]	Additional, but brief, benefit over acetaminophen in patients older than 5 y.
Naturopathic agents[68]	Comparable to amethocaine/phenazone drops in patients older than 6 y.
Homeopathic agents[71,72]	No controlled studies that directly address pain.
Narcotic analgesia with codeine or analogs	Effective for moderate or severe pain. Requires prescription; risk of respiratory depression, altered mental status, gastrointestinal tract upset, and constipation.
Tympanostomy/myringotomy[73]	Requires skill and entails potential risk.

Since the 2004 guideline was published, there have been only 2 significant new articles.

Bolt et al reported in 2008 on a double-blind placebo-controlled trial at the Australia Children's Hospital emergency department conducted in 2003–2004.[65] They used a convenience sample of children 3 to 17 years of age diagnosed with AOM in the ED. They excluded children with perforation of the TM, pressure-equalizing tube, allergy to local anesthetic or paracetamol, epilepsy, or liver, renal, or cardiac disease. Sixty-three eligible children were randomized to receive aqueous lidocaine or normal saline ear drops up to 3 times in 24 hours. They demonstrated a statistically significant 50% reduction in reported pain at 10 and 30 minutes but not at 20 minutes after application of topical lidocaine, compared with normal saline. Complications were minimal: 3 children reported some dizziness the next day, and none reported tinnitus. A limitation was that some children had received oral acetaminophen before administration of ear drops.

A Cochrane review of topical analgesia for AOM[66] searched the Cochrane register of controlled trials, randomized controlled trials, or quasi-randomized controlled trials that compared otic preparations to placebo or that compared 2 otic preparations. It included studies of adults and children, without TM perforation.

It identified 5 trials in children 3 to 18 years of age. Two (including Bolt et al,[65] discussed above) compared anesthetic drops and placebo at diagnosis of AOM. In both studies, some children also received oral analgesics. Three studies compared anesthetic ear drops with naturopathic herbal drops. Naturopathic drops were favored 15 to 30 minutes after installation, and 1 to 3 days after diagnosis, but the difference was not statistically significant. The Cochrane group concluded that there is limited evidence that ear drops are effective at 30 minutes and unclear if results from these studies are a result of the natural course of illness, placebo effect of receiving treatment, soothing effect of any liquid in the ear, or the drops themselves. Three of the studies included in this review were cited in the 2004 AAP guideline[67–69] and the 1 new paper by Bolt et al.[65]

Key Action Statement 3A

Severe AOM

The clinician should prescribe antibiotic therapy for AOM (bilateral or unilateral) in children 6 months and older with severe signs or symptoms (ie, moderate or severe otalgia or otalgia for at least 48 hours, or temperature 39°C [102.2°F] or higher). (Evidence Quality: Grade B, Rec. Strength: Strong Recommendation)

Key Action Statement Profile: KAS 3A

Aggregate evidence quality	Grade B
Benefits	Increased likelihood of more rapid resolution of symptoms. Increased likelihood of resolution of AOM.
Risks, harms, cost	Adverse events attributable to antibiotics, such as diarrhea, diaper dermatitis, and allergic reactions. Overuse of antibiotics leads to increased bacterial resistance. Cost of antibiotics.
Benefits-harms assessment	Preponderance of benefit over harm.
Value judgments	None
Role of patient preference	None
Intentional vagueness	None
Exclusions	None
Strength	**Strong Recommendation**

Key Action Statement 3B

Nonsevere Bilateral AOM in Young Children

The clinician should prescribe antibiotic therapy for bilateral AOM in children younger than 24 months without severe signs or symptoms (ie, mild otalgia for less than 48 hours, temperature less than 39°C [102.2°F]). (Evidence Quality: Grade B, Rec. Strength: Recommendation)

Key Action Statement Profile: KAS 3B

Aggregate evidence quality	Grade B
Benefits	Increased likelihood of more rapid resolution of symptoms. Increased likelihood of resolution of AOM.
Risks, harms, cost	Adverse events attributable to antibiotics, such as diarrhea, diaper dermatitis, and allergic reactions. Overuse of antibiotics leads to increased bacterial resistance. Cost of antibiotics.
Benefits-harms assessment	Preponderance of benefit over harm.
Value judgments	None
Role of patient preference	None
Intentional vagueness	None
Exclusions	None
Strength	**Recommendation**

Key Action Statement 3C

Nonsevere Unilateral AOM in Young Children

The clinician should either prescribe antibiotic therapy *or* offer observation with close follow-up based on joint decision-making with the parent(s)/caregiver for unilateral AOM in children 6 months to 23 months of age without severe signs or symptoms (ie, mild otalgia for less than 48 hours, temperature less than 39°C [102.2°F]). When observation is used, a mechanism must be in place to ensure

follow-up and begin antibiotic therapy if the child worsens or fails to improve within 48 to 72 hours of onset of symptoms. (Evidence Quality: Grade B, Rec. Strength: Recommendation)

Key Action Statement Profile: KAS 3C

Aggregate evidence quality	Grade B
Benefits	Moderately increased likelihood of more rapid resolution of symptoms with initial antibiotics. Moderately increased likelihood of resolution of AOM with initial antibiotics.
Risks, harms, cost	Adverse events attributable to antibiotics, such as diarrhea, diaper dermatitis, and allergic reactions. Overuse of antibiotics leads to increased bacterial resistance. Cost of antibiotics.
Benefits-harms assessment	Moderate degree of benefit over harm.
Value judgments	Observation becomes an alternative as the benefits and harms approach balance.
Role of patient preference	Joint decision-making with the family is essential before choosing observation.
Intentional vagueness	Joint decision-making is highly variable from family to family
Exclusions	None
Strength	**Recommendation**
Note	In the judgment of 1 Subcommittee member (AH), antimicrobial treatment of these children is preferred because of a preponderance of benefit over harm. AH did not endorse Key Action Statement 3C

Key Action Statement 3D

Nonsevere AOM in Older Children

The clinician should either prescribe antibiotic therapy *or* offer observation with close follow-up based on joint decision-making with the parent(s)/caregiver for AOM (bilateral or unilateral) in children 24 months or older without severe signs or symptoms (ie, mild otalgia for less than 48 hours, temperature less than 39°C [102.2°F]). When observation is used, a mechanism must be in place to ensure follow-up and begin antibiotic therapy if the child worsens or fails to improve within 48 to 72 hours of onset of symptoms. (Evidence Quality: Grade B, Rec Strength: Recommendation)

Key Action Statement Profile: KAS 3D

Aggregate evidence quality	Grade B
Benefits	*Initial antibiotic treatment:* Slightly increased likelihood of more rapid resolution of symptoms; slightly increased likelihood of resolution of AOM. *Initial observation:* Decreased use of antibiotics; decreased adverse effects of antibiotics; decreased potential for development of bacterial resistance.
Risks, harms, cost	*Initial antibiotic treatment:* Adverse events attributable to antibiotics such as diarrhea, rashes, and allergic reactions. Overuse of antibiotics leads to increased bacterial resistance. *Initial observation:* Possibility of needing to start antibiotics in 48 to 72 h if the patient continues to have symptoms. Minimal risk of adverse consequences of delayed antibiotic treatment. Potential increased phone calls and doctor visits.
Benefits-harms assessment	Slight degree of benefit of initial antibiotics over harm.
Value judgments	Observation is an option as the benefits and harms approach balance.
Role of patient preference	Joint decision-making with the family is essential before choosing observation.
Intentional vagueness	Joint decision-making is highly variable from family to family.
Exclusions	None
Strength	**Recommendation.**

Purpose of This Section

The purpose of this section is to offer guidance on the initial management of AOM by helping clinicians choose between the following 2 strategies:

1. *Initial antibiotic therapy,* defined as treatment of AOM with antibiotics that are prescribed at the time of diagnosis with the intent of starting antibiotic therapy as soon as possible after the encounter.

2. *Initial observation,* defined as initial management of AOM limited to symptomatic relief, with commencement of antibiotic therapy only if the child's condition worsens at any time or does not show clinical improvement within 48 to 72 hours of diagnosis. A mechanism must be in place to ensure follow-up and initiation of antibiotics if the child fails observation.

This section assumes that the clinician has made an accurate diagnosis of AOM by using the criteria and strategies outlined earlier in this guideline. Another assumption is that a clear distinction is made between the role of analgesics and antibiotics in providing symptomatic relief for children with AOM.

Changes From Previous AOM Guideline

The AOM guideline published by the AAP and AAFP in 2004 proposed, for the first time in North America, an "observation option" for selected children with AOM, building on successful implementation of a similar policy in the state of New York[74] and the use of a similar paradigm in many countries in Europe. A common feature of both approaches was to prioritize initial antibiotic therapy according to diagnostic certainty, with greater reliance on observation when the diagnosis was uncertain. In response to criticism that allowing an "uncertain diagnosis" might condone incomplete visualization of the TM or allow inappropriate antibiotic use, this category has been eliminated with greater emphasis now placed on maximizing diagnostic accuracy for AOM.

Since the earlier AOM guideline was published, there has been substantial new research on initial management of AOM, including randomized controlled trials of antibiotic therapy versus placebo or no therapy,[31,32,75] immediate versus delayed antibiotic therapy,[30,76,77] or delayed antibiotic with or without a concurrent prescription.[78] The Hoberman and Tähtinen articles are especially important as they used stringent criteria for diagnosing AOM.[31,32] Systematic reviews have been published on delayed antibiotic therapy,[79] the natural history of AOM in untreated children,[57] predictive factors for antibiotic benefits,[62] and the effect of antibiotics on asymptomatic MEE after therapy.[80] Observational studies provide additional data on outcomes of initial observation with delayed antibiotic therapy, if needed,[81] and on the relationship of previous antibiotic therapy for AOM to subsequent acute mastoiditis.[82,83]

In contrast to the earlier AOM guideline,[1] which recommended antibiotic therapy for all children 6 months to 2 years of age with a certain diagnosis,

the current guideline indicates a choice between initial antibiotic therapy or initial observation in this age group for children with unilateral AOM and mild symptoms but only after joint decision-making with the parent(s)/caregiver (Table 4). This change is supported by evidence on the safety of observation or delayed prescribing in young children.[30,31,32,75,76,81] A mechanism must be in place to ensure follow-up and begin antibiotics if the child fails observation.

Importance of Accurate Diagnosis

The recommendations for management of AOM assume an accurate diagnosis on the basis of criteria outlined in the diagnosis section of this guideline. Many of the studies since the 2004 AAP/AAFP AOM guideline[1] used more stringent and well-defined AOM diagnostic definitions than were previously used. Bulging of the TM was required for diagnosis of AOM for most of the children enrolled in the most recent studies.[31,32] By using the criteria in this guideline, clinicians will more accurately distinguish AOM from OME. The management of OME can be found in guidelines written by the AAP, AAFP, and American Academy of Otolaryngology-Head and Neck Surgery.[84,85]

Age, Severity of Symptoms, Otorrhea, and Laterality

Rovers et al[62] performed a systematic search for AOM trials that (1) used random allocation of children, (2) included children 0 to 12 years of age with AOM, (3) compared antibiotics with placebo or no treatment, and (4) had pain or fever as an outcome. The original investigators were asked for their original data.

Primary outcome was pain and/or fever ($>38°C$) at 3 to 7 days. The adverse effects of antibiotics were also analyzed. Baseline predictors were age <2 years versus ≥ 2 years, bilateral AOM versus unilateral AOM, and the presence versus absence of otorrhea. Statistical methods were used to assess heterogeneity and to analyze the data.

Of the 10 eligible studies, the investigators of 6 studies[30,75,86–89] provided the original data requested, and 4 did not. A total of 1642 patients were included in the 6 studies from which data were obtained. Of the cases submitted, the average age was 3 to 4 years, with 35% of children younger than 2 years. Bilateral AOM was present in 34% of children, and 42% of children had a bulging TM. Otorrhea was present in 21% of children. The antibiotic and control groups were comparable for all characteristics.

The rate difference (RD) for pain, fever, or both between antibiotic and control groups was 13% (NNT = 8). For children younger than 2 years, the RD was 15% (NNT = 7); for those ≥ 2 years, RD was 11% (NNT = 10). For unilateral AOM, the RD was 6% (NNT = 17); for bilateral AOM, the RD was 20% (NNT = 5). When unilateral AOM was broken into age groups, among those younger than 2 years, the RD was 5% (NNT = 20), and among those ≥ 2 years, the RD was 7% (NNT = 15). For bilateral AOM in children younger than 2 years, the RD was 25% (NNT = 4); for

TABLE 4 Recommendations for Initial Management for Uncomplicated AOM[a]

Age	Otorrhea With AOM[a]	Unilateral or Bilateral AOM[a] With Severe Symptoms[b]	Bilateral AOM[a] Without Otorrhea	Unilateral AOM[a] Without Otorrhea
6 mo to 2 y	Antibiotic therapy	Antibiotic therapy	Antibiotic therapy	Antibiotic therapy or additional observation
≥ 2 y	Antibiotic therapy	Antibiotic therapy	Antibiotic therapy or additional observation	Antibiotic therapy or additional observation[c]

[a] Applies only to children with well-documented AOM with high certainty of diagnosis (see Diagnosis section).

[b] A toxic-appearing child, persistent otalgia more than 48 h, temperature $\geq 39°C$ (102.2°F) in the past 48 h, or if there is uncertain access to follow-up after the visit.

[c] This plan of initial management provides an opportunity for shared decision-making with the child's family for those categories appropriate for additional observation. If observation is offered, a mechanism must be in place to ensure follow-up and begin antibiotics if the child worsens or fails to improve within 48 to 72 h of AOM onset.

bilateral AOM in children ≥2 years, the RD was 12% (NNT = 9). For otorrhea, the RD was 36% (NNT = 3). One child in the control group who developed meningitis had received antibiotics beginning on day 2 because of worsening status. There were no cases of mastoiditis.

In a Cochrane Review, Sanders et al[59] identified 10 studies that met the following criteria: (1) randomized controlled trial, (2) compared antibiotic versus placebo or antibiotic versus observation, (3) age 1 month to 15 years, (4) reported severity and duration of pain, (5) reported adverse events, and (6) reported serious complications of AOM, recurrent attacks, and hearing problems. Studies were analyzed for risk of bias and assessment of heterogeneity. The studies were the same as analyzed by Rovers et al[62] but included the 4 studies for which primary data were not available to Rovers.[60,61,90,91]

The authors' conclusions were that antibiotics produced a small reduction in the number of children with pain 2 to 7 days after diagnosis. They also concluded that most cases spontaneously remitted with no complications (NNT = 16). Antibiotics were most beneficial in children younger than 2 years with bilateral AOM and in children with otorrhea.

Two recent studies only included children younger than 3 years[32] or younger than 2 years.[31] Both included only subjects in whom the diagnosis of AOM was certain. Both studies used improvement of symptoms and improvement in the appearance of the TM in their definitions of clinical success or failure.

Hoberman et al[31] conducted a randomized, double-blind, placebo-controlled study of the efficacy of antimicrobial treatment on AOM. The criteria for AOM were acute symptoms with a score of at least 3 on the AOM-SOS,

a validated symptom scale[33,92]; MEE; and moderate or marked bulging of the TM or slight bulging accompanied by either otalgia or marked erythema of the TM. They chose to use high-dose amoxicillin-clavulanate (90 mg/kg/day) as active treatment, because it has the best oral antibiotic coverage for organisms causing AOM. Included in the study were 291 patients 6 to 23 months of age: 144 in the antibiotic group and 147 in the placebo group. The primary outcome measures were the time to resolution of symptoms and the symptom burden over time. The initial resolution of symptoms (ie, the first recording of an AOM-SOS score of 0 or 1) was recorded among the children who received amoxicillin-clavulanate in 35% by day 2, 61% by day 4, and 80% by day 7. Among children who received placebo, an AOM-SOS score of 0 or 1 was recorded in 28% by day 2, 54% by day 4, and 74% by day 7 (P = .14 for the overall comparison). For sustained resolution of symptoms (ie, the time to the second of 2 successive recordings of an AOM-SOS score of 0 or 1), the corresponding values were 20% at day 2, 41% at day 4, and 67% at day 7 with amoxicillin-clavulanate, compared with 14%, 36%, and 53% with placebo (P = .04 for the overall comparison). The symptom burden (ie, mean AOM-SOS scores) over the first 7 days were lower for the children treated with amoxicillin-clavulanate than for those who received placebo (P = .02). Clinical failure at or before the 4- to 5-day visit was defined as "either a lack of substantial improvement in symptoms, a worsening of signs on otoscopic examination, or both," and clinical failure at the 10- to 12-day visit was defined as "the failure to achieve complete or nearly complete resolution of symptoms and of otoscopic signs, without regard to the persistence or resolution of middle ear

effusion." Treatment failure occurred by day 4 to 5 in 4% of the antimicrobial treatment group versus 23% in the placebo group (P < .001) and at day 10 to 12 in 16% of the antimicrobial treatment group versus 51% in the placebo group (NNT = 2.9, P < .001). In a comparison of outcome in unilateral versus bilateral AOM, clinical failure rates by day 10 to 12 in children with unilateral AOM were 9% in those treated with amoxicillin-clavulanate versus 41% in those treated with placebo (RD, 32%; NNT = 3) and 23% vs 60% (RD, 37%; NNT = 3) in those with bilateral AOM. Most common adverse events were diarrhea (25% vs 15% in the treatment versus placebo groups, respectively; P = .05) and diaper dermatitis (51% vs 35% in the treatment versus placebo groups, respectively; P = .008). One placebo recipient developed mastoiditis. According to these results, antimicrobial treatment of AOM was more beneficial than in previous studies that used less stringent diagnostic criteria.

Tähtinen et al[32] conducted a randomized, double-blind, placebo-controlled, intention-to-treat study of amoxicillin-clavulanate (40 mg/kg/day) versus placebo. Three hundred nineteen patients from 6 to 35 months of age were studied: 161 in the antibiotic group and 158 in the placebo group. AOM definition was the presence of MEE, distinct erythema over a bulging or yellow TM, and acute symptoms such as ear pain, fever, or respiratory symptoms. Compliance was measured by using daily patient diaries and number of capsules remaining at the end of the study. Primary outcome was time to treatment failure defined as a composite of 6 independent components: no improvement in overall condition by day 3, worsening of the child's condition at any time, no improvement in otoscopic signs by day 8, perforation of the TM, development of severe infection (eg, pneumonia, mastoiditis), and any other reason for stopping the study drug/placebo.

Groups were comparable on multiple parameters. In the treatment group, 135 of 161 patients (84%) were younger than 24 months, and in the placebo group, 124 of 158 patients (78%) were younger than 24 months. Treatment failure occurred in 18.6% of the treatment group and 44.9% in the placebo group (NNT = 3.8, $P < .001$). Rescue treatment was needed in 6.8% of the treatment group and 33.5% of placebo patients ($P < .001$). Contralateral AOM developed in 8.2% and 18.6% of treatment and placebo groups, respectively ($P = .007$). There was no significant difference in use of analgesic or antipyretic medicine, which was used in 84.2% of the amoxicillin-clavulanate group and 85.9% of the placebo group.

Parents of child care attendees on placebo missed more days of work ($P = .005$). Clinical failure rates in children with unilateral AOM were 17.2% in those treated with amoxicillin-clavulanate versus 42.7% in those treated with placebo; for bilateral AOM, clinical failure rates were 21.7% for those treated with amoxicillin-clavulanate versus 46.3% in the placebo group. Reported rates of treatment failure by day 8 were 17.2% in the amoxicillin-clavulanate group versus 42.7% in the placebo group in children with unilateral AOM and 21.7% vs 46.3% among those with bilateral disease.

Adverse events, primarily diarrhea and/or rash, occurred in 52.8% of the treatment group and 36.1% of the placebo group ($P = .003$). Overall condition as evaluated by the parents and otoscopic appearance of the TM showed a benefit of antibiotics over placebo at the end of treatment visit ($P < .001$). Two placebo recipients

developed a severe infection; 1 developed pneumococcal bacteremia, and 1 developed radiographically confirmed pneumonia.

Most studies have excluded children with severe illness and all exclude those with bacterial disease other than AOM (pneumonia, mastoiditis, meningitis, streptococcal pharyngitis). Kaleida et al[91] compared myringotomy alone with myringotomy plus antibiotics. Severe AOM was defined as temperature >39°C (102.2°F) or the presence of severe otalgia. Patients with severe AOM in the group that received only myringotomy (without initial antibiotics) had much worse outcomes.

Initial Antibiotic Therapy

The rationale for antibiotic therapy in children with AOM is based on a high prevalence of bacteria in the accompanying MEE.[93] Bacterial and viral cultures of middle ear fluid collected by tympanocentesis from children with AOM showed 55% with bacteria only and 15% with bacteria and viruses. A beneficial effect of antibiotics on AOM was first demonstrated in 1968,[94] followed by additional randomized trials and a meta-analysis[95] showing a 14% increase in absolute rates of clinical improvement. Systematic reviews of the literature published before 2011[21,59,62] revealed increases of clinical improvement with initial antibiotics of 6% to 12%.

Randomized clinical trials using stringent diagnostic criteria for AOM in young children[31,32] show differences in clinical improvement of 26% to 35% favoring initial antibiotic treatment as compared with placebo. Greater benefit of immediate antibiotic therapy was observed for bilateral AOM[62,96] or AOM associated with otorrhea.[62] In most randomized trials,[30,75,77,88,89] antibiotic therapy also decreased the duration of pain, analgesic use, or

school absence and parent days missed from work.

Children younger than 2 years with AOM may take longer to improve clinically than older children,[57] and although they are more likely to benefit from antibiotics,[31,32] AOM in many children will resolve without antibiotics.[62] A clinically significant benefit of immediate antibiotic therapy is observed for bilateral AOM,[62,96] *Streptococcus pneumoniae* infection, or AOM associated with otorrhea.[62]

Initial Observation for AOM

In systematic reviews of studies that compare antibiotic therapy for AOM with placebo, a consistent finding has been the overall favorable natural history in control groups (NNT = 8–16).[12,59,62,95] However, randomized trials in these reviews had varying diagnostic criteria that would have permitted inclusion of some children with OME, viral upper respiratory infections, or myringitis, thereby limiting the ability to apply these findings to children with a highly certain AOM diagnosis. In more recent AOM studies[31,32] using stringent diagnostic criteria, approximately half of young children (younger than 2–3 years) experienced clinical success when given placebo, but the effect of antibiotic therapy was substantially greater than suggested by studies without precise diagnosis (NNT = 3–4).

Observation as initial management for AOM in properly selected children does not increase suppurative complications, provided that follow-up is ensured and a rescue antibiotic is given for persistent or worsening symptoms.[17] In contrast, withholding of antibiotics in all children with AOM, regardless of clinical course, would risk a return to the suppurative complications observed in the preantibiotic era. At the population level, antibiotics halve the risk of mastoiditis after AOM, but the high NNT of approximately 4800 patients to prevent 1 case of mastoiditis precludes a strategy of universal antibiotic therapy as a means to prevent mastoiditis.[83]

The favorable natural history of AOM makes it difficult to demonstrate significant differences in efficacy between antibiotic and placebo when a successful outcome is defined by relief or improvement of presenting signs and symptoms. In contrast, when otoscopic improvement (resolution of TM bulging, intense erythema, or both) is also required for a positive outcome,[31,32] the NNT is 3 to 4, compared with 8 to 16 for symptom improvement alone in older studies that used less precise diagnostic criteria. MEE, however, may persist for weeks or months after an AOM episode and is not a criterion for otoscopic failure.

National guidelines for initial observation of AOM in select children were first implemented in the Netherlands[97] and subsequently in Sweden,[98] Scotland,[99] the United States,[1] the United Kingdom,[100] and Italy.[101] All included observation as an initial treatment option under specified circumstances.

In numerous studies, only approximately one-third of children initially observed received a rescue antibiotic for persistent or worsening AOM,[30,32,76,81,89,102] suggesting that antibiotic use could potentially be reduced by 65% in eligible children. Given the high incidence of AOM, this reduction could help substantially in curtailing antibiotic-related adverse events.

McCormick et al[30] reported on 233 patients randomly assigned to receive immediate antibiotics (amoxicillin, 90 mg/kg/day) or to undergo watchful waiting. Criteria for inclusion were symptoms of ear infection, otoscopic evidence of AOM, and nonsevere AOM

based on a 3-item symptom score (OM-3) and TM appearance based on an 8-item scale (OS-8). Primary outcomes were parent satisfaction with AOM care, resolution of AOM symptoms after initial treatment, AOM failure and recurrence, and nasopharyngeal carriage of S pneumoniae strains resistant to antibiotics after treatment. The study was confounded by including patients who had received antibiotics in the previous 30 days.

In the watchful waiting group, 66% of children completed the study without antibiotics. There was no difference in parent satisfaction scores at day 12. A 5-item symptom score (ETG-5) was assessed at days 0 to 10 by using patient diaries. Subjects receiving immediate antibiotics resolved their symptoms faster than did subjects who underwent watchful waiting ($P = .004$). For children younger than 2 years, the difference was greater ($P = .008$). Otoscopic and tympanogram scores were also lower in the antibiotic group as opposed to the watchful waiting group ($P = .02$ for otoscopic score, $P = .004$ for tympanogram). Combining all ages, failure and recurrence rates were lower for the antibiotic group (5%) than for the watchful waiting group (21%) at 12 days. By day 30, there was no difference in failure or recurrence for the antibiotic and watchful waiting groups (23% and 24%, respectively). The association between clinical outcome and intervention group was not significantly different between age groups. Immediate antibiotics resulted in eradication of S pneumoniae carriage in the majority of children, but S pneumoniae strains cultured from children in the antibiotic group at day 12 were more likely to be multidrug resistant than were strains cultured from children in the watchful waiting group.

The decision not to give initial antibiotic treatment and observe should be

a joint decision of the clinician and the parents. In such cases, a system for close follow-up and a means of beginning antibiotics must be in place if symptoms worsen or no improvement is seen in 48 to 72 hours.

Initial observation of AOM should be part of a larger management strategy that includes analgesics, parent information, and provisions for a rescue antibiotic. Education of parents should include an explanation about the self-limited nature of most episodes of AOM, especially in children 2 years and older; the importance of pain management early in the course; and the potential adverse effects of antibiotics. Such an approach can substantially reduce prescription fill rates for rescue antibiotics.[103]

A critical component of any strategy involving initial observation for AOM is the ability to provide a rescue antibiotic if needed. This is often done by using a "safety net" or a "wait-and-see prescription,"[76,102] in which the parent/caregiver is given an antibiotic prescription during the clinical encounter but is instructed to fill the prescription only if the child fails to improve within 2 to 3 days or if symptoms worsen at any time. An alternative approach is not to provide a written prescription but to instruct the parent/caregiver to call or return if the child fails to improve within 2 to 3 days or if symptoms worsen.

In one of the first major studies of observation with a safety-net antibiotic prescription (SNAP), Siegel et al[102] enrolled 194 patients with protocol defined AOM, of whom 175 completed the study. Eligible patients were given a SNAP with instructions to fill the prescription only if symptoms worsened or did not improve in 48 hours. The SNAP was valid for 5 days. Pain medicine was recommended to be taken as needed. A phone interview was conducted 5 to 10 days after diagnosis.

One hundred twenty of 175 families did not fill the prescription. Reasons for filling the prescription (more than 1 reason per patient was acceptable) were as follows: continued pain, 23%; continued fever, 11%; sleep disruption, 6%; missed days of work, 3%; missed days of child care, 3%; and no reason given, 5%. One 16-month-old boy completed observation successfully but 6 weeks later developed AOM in the opposite ear, was treated with antibiotics, and developed postauricular cellulitis.

In a similar study of a "wait-and-see prescription" (WASP) in the emergency department, Spiro et al[76] randomly assigned 283 patients to either a WASP or standard prescription. Clinicians were educated on the 2004 AAP diagnostic criteria and initial treatment options for AOM; however, diagnosis was made at the discretion of the clinician. Patients were excluded if they did not qualify for observation per the 2004 guidelines. The primary outcome was whether the prescription was filled within 3 days of diagnosis. Prescriptions were not filled for 62% and 13% of the WASP and standard prescription patients, respectively ($P < .001$). Reasons for filling the prescription in the WASP group were fever (60%), ear pain (34%), or fussy behavior (6%). No serious adverse events were reported.

Strategies to observe children with AOM who are likely to improve on their own without initial antibiotic therapy reduces common adverse effects of antibiotics, such as diarrhea and diaper dermatitis. In 2 trials, antibiotic therapy significantly increased the absolute rates of diarrhea by 10% to 20% and of diaper rash or dermatitis by 6% to 16%.[31,32] Reduced antibiotic use may also reduce the prevalence of resistant bacterial pathogens. Multidrug-resistant *S pneumoniae* continues to be a significant concern for AOM, despite universal immunization of children in the United States with heptavalent pneumococcal conjugate vaccine.[104,105] In contrast, countries with low antibiotic use for AOM have a low prevalence of resistant nasopharyngeal pathogens in children.[106]

Key Action Statement 4A

Clinicians should prescribe amoxicillin for AOM when a decision to treat with antibiotics has been made *and* the child has not received amoxicillin in the past 30 days *or* the child does not have concurrent purulent conjunctivitis *or* the child is not allergic to penicillin. (Evidence Quality: Grade B, Rec. Strength: Recommendation)

Key Action Statement Profile: KAS 4A

Aggregate evidence quality	Grade B
Benefits	Effective antibiotic for most children with AOM. Inexpensive, safe, acceptable taste, narrow antimicrobial spectrum.
Risks, harms, cost	Ineffective against β-lactamase–producing organisms. Adverse effects of amoxicillin.
Benefits-harms assessment	Preponderance of benefit.
Value judgments	Better to use a drug that has reasonable cost, has an acceptable taste, and has a narrow antibacterial spectrum.
Intentional vagueness	The clinician must determine whether the patient is truly penicillin allergic.
Role of patient preferences	Should be considered if previous bad experience with amoxicillin.
Exclusions	Patients with known penicillin allergy.
Strength	**Recommendation.**

Key Action Statement 4B

Clinicians should prescribe an antibiotic with additional β-lactamase coverage for AOM when a decision to treat with antibiotics has been made *and* the child has received amoxicillin in the past 30 days *or* has concurrent purulent conjunctivitis *or* has a history of recurrent AOM unresponsive to amoxicillin. (Evidence Quality: Grade C, Rec. Strength: Recommendation)

Key Action Statement Profile: KAS 4B

Aggregate evidence quality	Grade C
Benefits	Successful treatment of β-lactamase–producing organisms.
Risks, harms, cost	Cost of antibiotic. Increased adverse effects.
Benefits-harms assessment	Preponderance of benefit.
Value judgments	Efficacy is more important than taste.
Intentional vagueness	None.
Role of patient preferences	Concern regarding side effects and taste.
Exclusions	Patients with known penicillin allergy.
Strength	**Recommendation**

Key Action Statement 4C

Clinicians should reassess the patient if the caregiver reports that the child's symptoms have worsened or failed to respond to the initial antibiotic treatment within 48 to 72 hours and determine whether a change in therapy is needed. (Evidence Quality: Grade B, Rec. Strength: Recommendation)

Key Action Statement Profile: KAS 4C

Aggregate evidence quality	Grade B
Benefits	Identify children who may have AOM caused by pathogens resistant to previous antibiotics.
Risks, harms, cost	Cost. Time for patient and clinician to make change. Potential need for parenteral medication.
Benefit-harm assessment	Preponderance of benefit.
Value judgments	None.
Intentional vagueness	"Reassess" is not defined. The clinician may determine the method of assessment.
Role of patient preferences	Limited.
Exclusions	Appearance of TM improved.
Strength	**Recommendation**

Purpose of This Section

If an antibiotic will be used for treatment of a child with AOM, whether as initial management or after a period of observation, the clinician must choose an antibiotic that will have a high likelihood of being effective against the most likely etiologic bacterial pathogens with considerations of cost, taste, convenience, and adverse effects. This section proposes first- and second-line antibiotics that best meet these criteria while balancing potential benefits and harms.

Changes From AAP/AAFP 2004 AOM Guideline

Despite new data on the effect of PCV7 and updated data on the in vitro susceptibility of bacterial pathogens most likely to cause AOM, the recommendations for the first-line antibiotic remains unchanged from 2004. The current guideline contains revised recommendations regarding penicillin allergy based on new data. The increase of multidrug-resistant strains of pneumococci is noted.

Microbiology

Microorganisms detected in the middle ear during AOM include pathogenic bacteria, as well as respiratory viruses.[107–110] AOM occurs most frequently as a consequence of viral upper respiratory tract infection,[111–113] which leads to eustachian tube inflammation/dysfunction, negative middle ear pressure, and movement of secretions containing the upper respiratory tract infection causative virus and pathogenic bacteria in the nasopharynx into the middle ear cleft. By using comprehensive and sensitive microbiologic testing, bacteria and/or viruses can be detected in the middle ear fluid in up to 96% of AOM cases (eg, 66% bacteria and viruses together, 27% bacteria alone, and 4% virus alone).[114] Studies using less sensitive or less comprehensive microbiologic assays have yielded less positive results for bacteria and much less positive results for viruses.[115–117] The 3 most common bacterial pathogens in AOM are *S pneumoniae*, nontypeable *Haemophilus influenzae*, and *Moraxella catarrhalis*.[111] *Streptococcus pyogenes* (group A β-hemolytic streptococci) accounts for less than 5% of AOM cases. The proportion of AOM cases with pathogenic bacteria isolated from the middle ear fluids varies depending on bacteriologic techniques, transport issues, and stringency of AOM definition. In series of reports from the United States and Europe from 1952–1981 and 1985–1992, the mean percentage of cases with bacterial pathogens isolated from the middle ear fluids was 69% and 72%, respectively.[118] A large series from the University of Pittsburgh Otitis Media Study Group reported bacterial pathogens in 84% of the middle ear fluids from 2807 cases of AOM.[118] Studies that applied more stringent otoscopic criteria and/or use of bedside specimen plating on solid agar in addition to liquid transport media have a reported rate of recovery of pathogenic bacteria from middle ear exudates ranging from 85% to 90%.[119–121] When using appropriate stringent diagnostic criteria, careful specimen handling, and sensitive microbiologic techniques, the vast majority of cases of AOM will involve pathogenic bacteria either alone or in concert with viral pathogens.

Among AOM bacterial pathogens, *S pneumoniae* was the most frequently cultured in earlier reports. Since the debut and routine use of PCV7 in 2000, the ordinal frequency of these 3 major middle ear pathogens has evolved.[105] In the first few years after PCV7 introduction, *H influenzae* became the most frequently isolated middle ear pathogen, replacing *S pneumoniae*.[122,123] Shortly thereafter, a shift to non-PCV7 serotypes of *S pneumoniae* was described.[124] Pichichero et al[104] later reported that 44% of 212 AOM cases seen in 2003–2006 were caused by *H influenzae*, and 28% were caused by *S pneumoniae*, with a high proportion of highly resistant *S pneumoniae*. In that study, a majority (77%) of cases involved recurrent disease or initial treatment failure. A later report[125] with data from 2007 to 2009, 6 to 8 years after the introduction of PCV7 in the United States, showed that PCV7 strains of *S pneumoniae* virtually disappeared from the middle ear fluid of children with AOM who had been vaccinated. However, the frequency of isolation of non-PCV7 serotypes of *S pneumoniae* from the middle ear fluid overall was increased; this has made isolation of *S pneumoniae* and *H influenzae* of children with AOM nearly equal.

In a study of tympanocentesis over 4 respiratory tract illness seasons in a private practice, the percentage of

S pneumoniae initially decreased relative to *H influenzae*. In 2005–2006 (*N* = 33), 48% of bacteria were *S pneumoniae*, and 42% were *H influenzae*. For 2006–2007 (*N* = 37), the percentages were equal at 41%. In 2007–2008 (*N* = 34), 35% were *S pneumoniae*, and 59% were *H influenzae*. In 2008–2009 (*N* = 24), the percentages were 54% and 38%, respectively, with an increase in intermediate and nonsusceptible *S pneumoniae*.[126] Data on nasopharyngeal colonization from PCV7-immunized children with AOM have shown continued presence of *S pneumoniae* colonization. Revai et al[127] showed no difference in *S pneumoniae* colonization rate among children with AOM who have been unimmunized, underimmunized, or fully immunized with PCV7. In a study during a viral upper respiratory tract infection, including mostly PCV7-immunized children (6 months to 3 years of age), *S pneumoniae* was detected in 45.5% of 968 nasopharyngeal swabs, *H influenzae* was detected in 32.4%, and *M catarrhalis* was detected in 63.1%.[128] Data show that nasopharyngeal colonization of children vaccinated with PCV7 increasingly is caused by *S pneumoniae* serotypes not contained in the vaccine.[129–132] With the use of the recently licensed 13-valent pneumococcal conjugate vaccine (PCV13),[133] the patterns of nasopharyngeal colonization and infection with these common AOM bacterial pathogens will continue to evolve.

Investigators have attempted to predict the type of AOM pathogenic bacteria on the basis of clinical severity, but results have not been promising. *S pyogenes* has been shown to occur more commonly in older children[134] and to cause a greater degree of inflammation of the middle ear and TM, a greater frequency of spontaneous rupture of the TM, and more frequent progression to acute mastoiditis

compared with other bacterial pathogens.[134–136] As for clinical findings in cases with *S pneumoniae* and nontypeable *H influenzae*, some studies suggest that signs and symptoms of AOM caused by *S pneumoniae* may be more severe (fever, severe earache, bulging TM) than those caused by other pathogens.[44,121,137] These findings were refuted by results of the studies that found AOM caused by nontypeable *H influenzae* to be associated with bilateral AOM and more severe inflammation of the TM.[96,138] Leibovitz et al[139] concluded, in a study of 372 children with AOM caused by *H influenzae* (*N* = 138), *S pneumoniae* (*N* = 64), and mixed *H influenzae* and *S pneumoniae* (*N* = 64), that clinical/otologic scores could not discriminate among various bacterial etiologies of AOM. However, there were significantly different clinical/otologic scores between bacterial culture negative and culture positive cases. A study of middle ear exudates of 82 cases of bullous myringitis has shown a 97% bacteria positive rate, primarily *S pneumoniae*. In contrast to the previous belief, mycoplasma is rarely the causative agent in this condition.[140] Accurate prediction of the bacterial cause of AOM on the basis of clinical presentation, without bacterial culture of the middle ear exudates, is not possible, but specific etiologies may be predicted in some situations. Published evidence has suggested that AOM associated with conjunctivitis (otitis-conjunctivitis syndrome) is more likely caused by nontypeable *H influenzae* than by other bacteria.[141–143]

Bacterial Susceptibility to Antibiotics

Selection of antibiotic to treat AOM is based on the suspected type of bacteria and antibiotic susceptibility pattern, although clinical pharmacology

and clinical and microbiologic results and predicted compliance with the drug are also taken into account. Early studies of AOM patients show that 19% of children with *S pneumoniae* and 48% with *H influenzae* cultured on initial tympanocentesis who were not treated with antibiotic cleared the bacteria at the time of a second tympanocentesis 2 to 7 days later.[144] Approximately 75% of children infected with *M catarrhalis* experienced bacteriologic cure even after treatment with amoxicillin, an antibiotic to which it is not susceptible.[145,146]

Antibiotic susceptibility of major AOM bacterial pathogens continues to change, but data on middle ear pathogens have become scanty because tympanocentesis is not generally performed in studies of children with uncomplicated AOM. Most available data come from cases of persistent or recurrent AOM. Current US data from a number of centers indicates that approximately 83% and 87% of isolates of *S pneumoniae* from all age groups are susceptible to regular (40 mg/kg/day) and high-dose amoxicillin (80–90 mg/kg/day divided twice daily), respectively.[130,147–150] Pediatric isolates are smaller in number and include mostly ear isolates collected from recurrent and persistent AOM cases with a high percentage of multidrug-resistant *S pneumoniae*, most frequently nonvaccine serotypes that have recently increased in frequency and importance.[104]

High-dose amoxicillin will yield middle ear fluid levels that exceed the minimum inhibitory concentration (MIC) of all *S pneumoniae* serotypes that are intermediately resistant to penicillin (penicillin MICs, 0.12–1.0 µg/mL), and many but not all highly resistant serotypes (penicillin MICs, ≥2 µg/mL) for a longer period of the dosing interval and has been shown to improve bacteriologic and clinical efficacy compared with the regular dose.[151–153] Hoberman et al[154] reported superior efficacy of high-dose amoxicillin-clavulanate in eradication of *S pneumoniae* (96%) from the middle ear at days 4 to 6 of therapy compared with azithromycin.

The antibiotic susceptibility pattern for *S pneumoniae* is expected to continue to evolve with the use of PCV13, a conjugate vaccine containing 13 serotypes of *S pneumoniae*.[133,155,156] Widespread use of PCV13 could potentially reduce diseases caused by multidrug-resistant pneumococcal serotypes and diminish the need for the use of higher dose of amoxicillin or amoxicillin-clavulanate for AOM.

Some *H influenzae* isolates produce β-lactamase enzyme, causing the isolate to become resistant to penicillins. Current data from different studies with non-AOM sources and geographic locations that may not be comparable show that 58% to 82% of *H influenzae* isolates are susceptible to regular- and high-dose amoxicillin.[130,147,148,157,158] These data represented a significant decrease in β-lactamase–producing *H*

influenzae, compared with data reported in the 2004 AOM guideline.

Nationwide data suggest that 100% of *M catarrhalis* derived from the upper respiratory tract are β-lactamase–positive but remain susceptible to amoxicillin-clavulanate.[159] However, the high rate of spontaneous clinical resolution occurring in children with AOM attributable to *M catarrhalis* treated with amoxicillin reduces the concern for the first-line coverage for this microorganism.[145,146] AOM attributable to *M catarrhalis* rarely progresses to acute mastoiditis or intracranial infections.[102,160,161]

Antibiotic Therapy

High-dose amoxicillin is recommended as the first-line treatment in most patients, although there are a number of medications that are clinically effective (Table 5). The justification for the use of amoxicillin relates to its effectiveness against common AOM bacterial pathogens as well as its safety, low cost, acceptable taste, and narrow microbiologic spectrum.[145,151] In children who have taken amoxicillin in the previous 30 days, those with concurrent conjunctivitis, or those

for whom coverage for β-lactamase–positive *H influenzae* and *M catarrhalis* is desired, therapy should be initiated with high-dose amoxicillin-clavulanate (90 mg/kg/day of amoxicillin, with 6.4 mg/kg/day of clavulanate, a ratio of amoxicillin to clavulanate of 14:1, given in 2 divided doses, which is less likely to cause diarrhea than other amoxicillin-clavulanate preparations).[162]

Alternative initial antibiotics include cefdinir (14 mg/kg per day in 1 or 2 doses), cefuroxime (30 mg/kg per day in 2 divided doses), cefpodoxime (10 mg/kg per day in 2 divided doses), or ceftriaxone (50 mg/kg, administered intramuscularly). It is important to note that alternative antibiotics vary in their efficacy against AOM pathogens. For example, recent US data on in vitro susceptibility of *S pneumoniae* to cefdinir and cefuroxime are 70% to 80%, compared with 84% to 92% amoxicillin efficacy.[130,147–149] In vitro efficacy of cefdinir and cefuroxime against *H influenzae* is approximately 98%, compared with 58% efficacy of amoxicillin and nearly 100% efficacy of amoxicillin-clavulanate.[158] A multicenter double tympanocentesis open-label study of

TABLE 5 Recommended Antibiotics for (Initial or Delayed) Treatment and for Patients Who Have Failed Initial Antibiotic Treatment

Initial Immediate or Delayed Antibiotic Treatment		Antibiotic Treatment After 48–72 h of Failure of Initial Antibiotic Treatment	
Recommended First-line Treatment	Alternative Treatment (if Penicillin Allergy)	Recommended First-line Treatment	Alternative Treatment
Amoxicillin (80–90 mg/ kg per day in 2 divided doses)	Cefdinir (14 mg/kg per day in 1 or 2 doses)	Amoxicillin-clavulanate[a] (90 mg/kg per day of amoxicillin, with 6.4 mg/kg per day of clavulanate in 2 divided doses)	Ceftriaxone, 3 d Clindamycin (30–40 mg/kg per day in 3 divided doses), with or without third-generation cephalosporin
or	Cefuroxime (30 mg/kg per day in 2 divided doses)	or	Failure of second antibiotic
Amoxicillin-clavulanate[a] (90 mg/kg per day of amoxicillin, with 6.4 mg/kg per day of clavulanate [amoxicillin to clavulanate ratio, 14:1] in 2 divided doses)	Cefpodoxime (10 mg/kg per day in 2 divided doses)	Ceftriaxone (50 mg IM or IV for 3 d)	Clindamycin (30–40 mg/kg per day in 3 divided doses) plus third-generation cephalosporin Tympanocentesis[b]
	Ceftriaxone (50 mg IM or IV per day for 1 or 3 d)		Consult specialist[b]

IM, intramuscular; IV, intravenous.

[a] May be considered in patients who have received amoxicillin in the previous 30 d or who have the otitis-conjunctivitis syndrome.

[b] Perform tympanocentesis/drainage if skilled in the procedure, or seek a consultation from an otolaryngologist for tympanocentesis/drainage. If the tympanocentesis reveals multidrug-resistant bacteria, seek an infectious disease specialist consultation.

[c] Cefdinir, cefuroxime, cefpodoxime, and ceftriaxone are highly unlikely to be associated with cross-reactivity with penicillin allergy on the basis of their distinct chemical structures. See text for more information.

cefdinir in recurrent AOM attributable to H influenzae showed eradication of the organism in 72% of patients.[163]

For penicillin-allergic children, recent data suggest that cross-reactivity among penicillins and cephalosporins is lower than historically reported.[164–167] The previously cited rate of cross-sensitivity to cephalosporins among penicillin-allergic patients (approximately 10%) is likely an overestimate. The rate was based on data collected and reviewed during the 1960s and 1970s. A study analyzing pooled data of 23 studies, including 2400 patients with reported history of penicillin allergy and 39 000 with no penicillin allergic history concluded that many patients who present with a history of penicillin allergy do not have an immunologic reaction to penicillin.[166] The chemical structure of the cephalosporin determines the risk of cross-reactivity between specific agents.[165,168] The degree of cross-reactivity is higher between penicillins and first-generation cephalosporins but is negligible with the second- and third-generation cephalosporins. Because of the differences in the chemical structures, cefdinir, cefuroxime, cefpodoxime, and ceftriaxone are highly unlikely to be associated with cross-reactivity with penicillin.[165] Despite this, the Joint Task Force on Practice Parameters; American Academy of Allergy, Asthma and Immunology; American College of Allergy, Asthma and Immunology; and Joint Council of Allergy, Asthma and Immunology[169] stated that "cephalosporin treatment of patients with a history of penicillin allergy, selecting out those with severe reaction histories, show a reaction rate of 0.1%." They recommend a cephalosporin in cases without severe and/or recent penicillin allergy reaction history when skin test is not available.

Macrolides, such as erythromycin and azithromycin, have limited efficacy against both H influenzae and S pneumoniae.[130,147–149] Clindamycin lacks efficacy against H influenzae. Clindamycin alone (30–40 mg/kg per day in 3 divided doses) may be used for suspected penicillin-resistant S pneumoniae; however, the drug will likely not be effective for the multidrug-resistant serotypes.[130,158,166]

Several of these choices of antibiotic suspensions are barely palatable or frankly offensive and may lead to avoidance behaviors or active rejection by spitting out the suspension. Palatability of antibiotic suspensions has been compared in many studies.[170–172] Specific antibiotic suspensions such as cefuroxime, cefpodoxime, and clindamycin may benefit from adding taste-masking products, such as chocolate or strawberry flavoring agents, to obscure the initial bitter taste and the unpleasant aftertaste.[172,173] In the patient who is persistently vomiting or cannot otherwise tolerate oral medication, even when the taste is masked, ceftriaxone (50 mg/kg, administered intramuscularly in 1 or 2 sites in the anterior thigh, or intravenously) has been demonstrated to be effective for the initial or repeat antibiotic treatment of AOM.[174,175] Although a single injection of ceftriaxone is approved by the US FDA for the treatment of AOM, results of a double tympanocentesis study (before and 3 days after single dose ceftriaxone) by Leibovitz et al[175] suggest that more than 1 ceftriaxone dose may be required to prevent recurrence of the middle ear infection within 5 to 7 days after the initial dose.

Initial Antibiotic Treatment Failure

When antibiotics are prescribed for AOM, clinical improvement should be noted within 48 to 72 hours. During the 24 hours after the diagnosis of AOM,

the child's symptoms may worsen slightly. In the next 24 hours, the patient's symptoms should begin to improve. If initially febrile, the temperature should decline within 48 to 72 hours. Irritability and fussiness should lessen or disappear, and sleeping and drinking patterns should normalize.[176,177] If the patient is not improved by 48 to 72 hours, another disease or concomitant viral infection may be present, or the causative bacteria may be resistant to the chosen therapy.

Some children with AOM and persistent symptoms after 48 to 72 hours of initial antibacterial treatment may have combined bacterial and viral infection, which would explain the persistence of ongoing symptoms despite appropriate antibiotic therapy.[109,178,179] Literature is conflicting on the correlation between clinical and bacteriologic outcomes. Some studies report good correlation ranging from 86% to 91%,[180,181] suggesting continued presence of bacteria in the middle ear in a high proportion of cases with persistent symptoms. Others report that middle ear fluid from children with AOM in whom symptoms are persistent is sterile in 42% to 49% of cases.[123,182] A change in antibiotic may not be required in some children with mild persistent symptoms.

In children with persistent, severe symptoms of AOM and unimproved otologic findings after initial treatment, the clinician may consider changing the antibiotic (Table 5). If the child was initially treated with amoxicillin and failed to improve, amoxicillin-clavulanate should be used. Patients who were given amoxicillin-clavulanate or oral third-generation cephalosporins may receive intramuscular ceftriaxone (50 mg/kg). In the treatment of AOM unresponsive to initial antibiotics, a 3-day course of ceftriaxone has been shown to be better than a 1-day regimen.[175]

Although trimethoprim-sulfamethoxazole and erythromycin-sulfisoxazole had been useful as therapy for patients with AOM, pneumococcal surveillance studies have indicated that resistance to these 2 combination agents is substantial.[130,149,183] Therefore, when patients fail to improve while receiving amoxicillin, neither trimethoprim-sulfamethoxazole[184] nor erythromycin-sulfisoxazole is appropriate therapy.

Tympanocentesis should be considered, and culture of middle ear fluid should be performed for bacteriologic diagnosis and susceptibility testing when a series of antibiotic drugs have failed to improve the clinical condition. If tympanocentesis is not available, a course of clindamycin may be used, with or without an antibiotic that covers nontypeable *H influenzae* and *M catarrhalis*, such as cefdinir, cefixime, or cefuroxime.

Because *S pneumoniae* serotype 19A is usually multidrug-resistant and may not be responsive to clindamycin,[104,149] newer antibiotics that are not approved by the FDA for treatment of AOM, such as levofloxacin or linezolid, may be indicated.[185–187] Levofloxacin is a quinolone antibiotic that is not approved by the FDA for use in children. Linezolid is effective against resistant Gram-positive bacteria. It is not approved by the FDA for AOM treatment and is expensive. In children with repeated treatment failures, every effort should be made for bacteriologic diagnosis by tympanocentesis with Gram stain, culture, and antibiotic susceptibility testing of the organism(s) present. The clinician may consider consulting with pediatric medical subspecialists, such as an otolaryngologist for possible tympanocentesis, drainage, and culture and an infectious disease expert, before use of unconventional drugs such as levofloxacin or linezolid.

When tympanocentesis is not available, 1 possible way to obtain information on the middle ear pathogens and their antimicrobial susceptibility is to obtain a nasopharyngeal specimen for bacterial culture. Almost all middle ear pathogens derive from the pathogens colonizing the nasopharynx, but not all nasopharyngeal pathogens enter the middle ear to cause AOM. The positive predictive value of nasopharyngeal culture during AOM (likelihood that bacteria cultured from the nasopharynx is the middle ear pathogen) ranges from 22% to 44% for *S pneumoniae*, 50% to 71% for nontypeable *H influenzae*, and 17% to 19% for *M catarrhalis*. The negative predictive value (likelihood that bacteria not found in the nasopharynx are not AOM pathogens) ranges from 95% to 99% for all 3 bacteria.[188,189] Therefore, if nasopharyngeal culture is negative for specific bacteria, that organism is likely not the AOM pathogen. A negative culture for *S pneumoniae*, for example, will help eliminate the concern for multidrug-resistant bacteria and the need for unconventional therapies, such as levofloxacin or linezolid. On the other hand, if *S pneumoniae* is cultured from the nasopharynx, the antimicrobial susceptibility pattern can help guide treatment.

Duration of Therapy

The optimal duration of therapy for patients with AOM is uncertain; the usual 10-day course of therapy was derived from the duration of treatment of streptococcal pharyngotonsillitis. Several studies favor standard 10-day therapy over shorter courses for children younger than 2 years.[162,190–194] Thus, for children younger than 2 years and children with severe symptoms, a standard 10-day course is recommended. A 7-day course of oral antibiotic appears to be equally effective in children 2 to 5 years of age with mild or moderate AOM. For children 6 years and older with mild to moderate

symptoms, a 5- to 7-day course is adequate treatment.

Follow-up of the Patient With AOM

Once the child has shown clinical improvement, follow-up is based on the usual clinical course of AOM. There is little scientific evidence for a routine 10- to 14-day reevaluation visit for all children with an episode of AOM. The physician may choose to reassess some children, such as young children with severe symptoms or recurrent AOM or when specifically requested by the child's parent.

Persistent MEE is common and can be detected by pneumatic otoscopy (with or without verification by tympanometry) after resolution of acute symptoms. Two weeks after successful antibiotic treatment of AOM, 60% to 70% of children have MEE, decreasing to 40% at 1 month and 10% to 25% at 3 months after successful antibiotic treatment.[177,195] The presence of MEE without clinical symptoms is defined as OME. OME must be differentiated clinically from AOM and requires infrequent additional monitoring but not antibiotic therapy. Assurance that OME resolves is particularly important for parents of children with cognitive or developmental delays that may be affected adversely by transient hearing loss associated with MEE. Detailed recommendations for the management of the child with OME can be found in the evidence-based guideline from the AAP/AAFP/American Academy of Otolaryngology-Head and Neck Surgery published in 2004.[84,85]

Key Action Statement 5A

Clinicians should *NOT* prescribe prophylactic antibiotics to reduce the frequency of episodes of AOM in children with recurrent AOM. (Evidence Quality: Grade B, Rec. Strength: Recommendation)

Key Action Statement Profile: KAS 5A

Aggregate evidence quality	Grade B
Benefits	No adverse effects from antibiotic. Reduces potential for development of bacterial resistance. Reduced costs.
Risks, harms, cost	Small increase in episodes of AOM.
Benefit-harm assessment	Preponderance of benefit.
Value judgments	Potential harm outweighs the potential benefit.
Intentional vagueness	None.
Role of patient preferences	Limited.
Exclusions	Young children whose only alternative would be tympanostomy tubes.
Strength	**Recommendation**

Key Action Statement 5B

Clinicians may offer tympanostomy tubes for recurrent AOM (3 episodes in 6 months or 4 episodes in 1 year, with 1 episode in the preceding 6 months). (Evidence Quality: Grade B, Rec. Strength: Option)

Key Action Statement Profile: KAS 5B

Aggregate evidence quality	Grade B
Benefits	Decreased frequency of AOM. Ability to treat AOM with topical antibiotic therapy.
Risks, harms, cost	Risks of anesthesia or surgery. Cost. Scarring of TM, chronic perforation, cholesteatoma. Otorrhea.
Benefits-harms assessment	Equilibrium of benefit and harm.
Value judgments	None.
Intentional vagueness	Option based on limited evidence.
Role of patient preferences	Joint decision of parent and clinician.
Exclusions	Any contraindication to anesthesia and surgery.
Strength	**Option**

Purpose of This Section

Recurrent AOM has been defined as the occurrence of 3 or more episodes of AOM in a 6-month period or the occurrence of 4 or more episodes of AOM in a 12-month period that includes at least 1 episode in the preceding 6 months.[20] These episodes should be well documented and separate acute infections.[11]

Winter season, male gender, and passive exposure to smoking have been associated with an increased likelihood of recurrence. Half of children younger than 2 years treated for AOM will experience a recurrence within 6 months. Symptoms that last more than 10 days may also predict recurrence.[196]

Changes From AAP/AAFP 2004 AOM Guideline

Recurrent AOM was not addressed in the 2004 AOM guideline. This section addresses the literature on recurrent AOM.

Antibiotic Prophylaxis

Long-term, low-dose antibiotic use, referred to as antibiotic prophylaxis or chemoprophylaxis, has been used to treat children with recurrent AOM to prevent subsequent episodes.[85] A 2006 Cochrane review analyzed 16 studies of long-term antibiotic use for AOM and found such use prevented 1.5 episodes of AOM per year, reducing in half the number of AOM episodes during the period of treatment.[197] Randomized placebo-controlled trials of prophylaxis reported a decrease of 0.09 episodes per month in the frequency of AOM attributable to therapy (approximately 0.5 to 1.5 AOM episodes per year for 95% of children). An estimated 5 children would need to be treated for 1 year to prevent 1 episode of OM. The effect may be more substantial for children with 6 or more AOM episodes in the preceding year.[12]

This decrease in episodes of AOM occurred only while the prophylactic antibiotic was being given. The modest benefit afforded by a 6-month course of antibiotic prophylaxis does not have longer-lasting benefit after cessation of therapy. Teele showed no differences between children who received prophylactic antibiotics compared with those who received placebo in AOM recurrences or persistence of OME.[198]

Antibiotic prophylaxis is not appropriate for children with long-term MEE or for children with infrequent episodes of AOM. The small reduction in frequency of AOM with long-term antibiotic prophylaxis must be weighed against the cost of such therapy; the potential adverse effects of antibiotics, principally allergic reaction and gastrointestinal tract consequences, such as diarrhea; and their contribution to the emergence of bacterial resistance.

Surgery for Recurrent AOM

The use of tympanostomy tubes for treatment of ear disease in general, and for AOM in particular, has been controversial.[199] Most published studies of surgical intervention for OM focus on children with persistent MEE with or without AOM. The literature on surgery for recurrent AOM as defined here is scant. A lack of consensus among otolaryngologists regarding the role of surgery for recurrent AOM was reported in a survey of Canadian otolaryngologists in which 40% reported they would "never," 30% reported they would "sometimes," and 30% reported they would "often or always" place tympanostomy tubes for a hypothetical 2-year-old child with frequent OM without persistent MEE or hearing loss.[200]

Tympanostomy tubes, however, remain widely used in clinical practice for both OME and recurrent OM.[201] Recurrent

AOM remains a common indication for referral to an otolaryngologist.

Three randomized controlled trials have compared the number of episodes of AOM after tympanostomy tube placement or no surgery.[202] Two found significant improvement in mean number of AOM episodes after tympanostomy tubes during a 6-month follow-up period.[203,204] One study randomly assigned children with recurrent AOM to groups receiving placebo, amoxicillin prophylaxis, or tympanostomy tubes and followed them for 2 years.[205] Although prophylactic antibiotics reduced the rate of AOM, no difference in number of episodes of AOM was noted between the tympanostomy tube group and the placebo group over 2 years. A Cochrane review of studies of tympanostomy tubes for recurrent AOM analyzed 2 studies[204,206] that met inclusion criteria and found that tympanostomy tubes reduced the number of episodes of AOM by 1.5 episodes in the 6 months after surgery.[207] Tympanostomy tube insertion has been shown to improve disease-specific quality-of-life measures in children with OM.[208] One multicenter, nonrandomized observational study showed large improvements in a disease-specific quality-of-life instrument that measured psychosocial domains of physical suffering, hearing loss, speech impairment, emotional distress, activity limitations, and caregiver concerns that are associated with ear infections.[209] These benefits of tympanostomy tubes have been demonstrated in mixed populations of children that include children with OME as well as recurrent AOM.

Beyond the cost, insertion of tympanostomy tubes is associated with a small but finite surgical and anesthetic risk. A recent review looking at protocols to minimize operative risk reported no major complications, such as sensorineural hearing loss, vascular injury, or ossicular chain disruption, in 10 000 tube insertions performed primarily by residents, although minor complications such as TM tears or displaced tubes in the middle ear were seen in 0.016% of ears.[210] Long-term sequelae of tympanostomy tubes include TM structural changes including focal atrophy, tympanosclerosis, retraction pockets, and chronic perforation. One meta-analysis found tympanosclerosis in 32% of patients after placement of tympanostomy tubes and chronic perforations in 2.2% of patients who had short-term tubes and 16.6% of patients with long-term tubes.[211]

Adenoidectomy, without myringotomy and/or tympanostomy tubes, did not reduce the number of episodes of AOM when compared with chemoprophylaxis or placebo.[212] Adenoidectomy alone should not be used for prevention of AOM but may have benefit when performed with placement of tympanostomy tubes or in children with previous tympanostomy tube placement in OME.[213]

Prevention of AOM: Key Action Statement 6A

Pneumococcal Vaccine

Clinicians should recommend pneumococcal conjugate vaccine to all children according to the schedule of the Advisory Committee on Immunization Practices, AAP, and AAFP. (Evidence Quality: Grade B, Rec. Strength: Strong Recommendation)

Key Action Statement Profile: KAS 6A

Aggregate evidence quality	Grade B
Benefits	Reduced frequency of AOM attributable to vaccine serotypes. Reduced risk of serious pneumococcal systemic disease.
Risks, harms, cost	Potential vaccine side effects. Cost of vaccine.
Benefits-harms assessment	Preponderance of benefit.
Value judgments	Potential vaccine adverse effects are minimal.
Intentional vagueness	None.
Role of patient preferences	Some parents may choose to refuse the vaccine.
Exclusions	Severe allergic reaction (eg, anaphylaxis) to any component of pneumococcal vaccine or any diphtheria toxoid-containing vaccine.
Strength	**Strong Recommendation**

Key Action Statement 6B

Influenza Vaccine: Clinicians should recommend annual influenza vaccine to all children according to the schedule of the Advisory Committee on Immunization Practices, AAP, and AAFP. (Evidence Quality: Grade B, Rec. Strength: Recommendation)

Key Action Statement Profile: KAS 6B

Aggregate evidence quality	Grade B
Benefits	Reduced risk of influenza infection. Reduction in frequency of AOM associated with influenza.
Risks, harms, cost	Potential vaccine adverse effects. Cost of vaccine. Requires annual immunization.
Benefits-harms assessment	Preponderance of benefit.
Value judgments	Potential vaccine adverse effects are minimal.
Intentional vagueness	None
Role of patient preferences	Some parents may choose to refuse the vaccine.
Exclusions	See CDC guideline on contraindications (http://www.cdc.gov/flu/professionals/acip/shouldnot.htm).
Strength	**Recommendation**

Key Action Statement 6C

Breastfeeding: Clinicians should encourage exclusive breastfeeding for at least 6 months. (Evidence Quality: Grade B, Rec. Strength: Recommendation)

Key Action Statement Profile: KAS 6C

Aggregate evidence quality	Grade B
Benefits	May reduce the risk of early AOM. Multiple benefits of breastfeeding unrelated to AOM.
Risk, harm, cost	None
Benefit-harm assessment	Preponderance of benefit.
Value judgments	The intervention has value unrelated to AOM prevention.
Intentional vagueness	None
Role of patient preferences	Some parents choose to feed formula.
Exclusions	None
Strength	**Recommendation**

Key Action Statement 6D

Clinicians should encourage avoidance of tobacco smoke exposure. (Evidence Quality: Grade C, Rec. Strength: Recommendation)

Key Action Statement Profile: KAS 6D

Aggregate evidence quality	Grade C
Benefits	May reduce the risk of AOM.
Risks, harms, cost	None
Benefits-harms assessment	Preponderance of benefit.
Value judgments	Avoidance of tobacco exposure has inherent value unrelated to AOM.
Intentional vagueness	None
Role of patient preferences	Many parents/caregivers choose not to stop smoking. Some also remain addicted, and are unable to quit smoking.
Exclusions	None
Strength	**Recommendation**

Purpose of This Section

The 2004 AOM guideline noted data on immunizations, breastfeeding, and lifestyle changes that would reduce the risk of acquiring AOM. This section addresses new data published since 2004.

Changes From AAP/AAFP 2004 AOM Guideline

PCV7 has been in use in the United States since 2000. PCV13 was introduced in the United States in 2010. The 10-valent pneumococcal nontypeable *H influenzae* protein D-conjugate vaccine was recently licensed in Europe for prevention of diseases attributable to *S pneumoniae* and nontypeable *H influenzae*. Annual influenza immunization is now recommended for all children 6 months of age and older in the United States.[214,215] Updated information regarding these vaccines and their effect on the incidence of AOM is reviewed.

The AAP issued a new breastfeeding policy statement in February 2012.[216] This guideline also includes a recommendation regarding tobacco smoke exposure. Bottle propping, pacifier use, and child care are discussed, but no recommendations are made because of limited evidence. The use of xylitol, a possible adjunct to AOM prevention, is discussed; however, no recommendations are made.

Pneumococcal Vaccine

Pneumococcal conjugate vaccines have proven effective in preventing OM caused by pneumococcal serotypes contained in the vaccines. A meta-analysis of 5 studies with AOM as an outcome determined that there is a 29% reduction in AOM caused by all pneumococcal serotypes among children who received PCV7 before 24 months of age.[217] Although the overall benefit seen in clinical trials for all causes of AOM is small (6%–7%),[218–221] observational studies have shown that medical office visits for otitis were reduced by up to 40% comparing years before and after introduction of PCV7.[222–224] Grijvala[223] reported no effect, however, among children first vaccinated at older ages. Poehling et al[225] reported reductions of frequent AOM and PE tube use after introduction of PCV7. The observations by some of greater benefit observed in the community than in clinical trials is not fully understood but may be related to effects of herd immunity or may be attributed to secular trends or changes in AOM diagnosis patterns over time.[223,226–229] In a 2009 Cochrane review,[221] Jansen et al found that the overall reduction in AOM incidence may only be 6% to 7% but noted that even that small rate may have public health relevance. O'Brien et al concurred and noted in addition the potential for cost savings.[230] There is evidence that serotype replacement may reduce the long-term efficacy of pneumococcal conjugate vaccines against AOM,[231] but it is possible that new pneumococcal conjugate vaccines may demonstrate an increased effect on reduction in AOM.[232–234] Data on AOM reduction secondary to the PCV13 licensed in the United States in 2010 are not yet available.

The *H influenzae* protein D-conjugate vaccine recently licensed in Europe has potential benefit of protection against 10 serotypes of *S pneumoniae* and nontypeable *H influenzae*.[221,234]

Influenza Vaccine

Most cases of AOM follow upper respiratory tract infections caused by viruses, including influenza viruses. As many as two-thirds of young children with influenza may have AOM.[235] Investigators have studied the efficacy of trivalent inactivated influenza vaccine (TIV) and live-attenuated intranasal influenza vaccine (LAIV) in preventing AOM. Many studies have demonstrated 30% to 55% efficacy of influenza vaccine in prevention of AOM during the respiratory illness season.[6,235–239] One study reported no benefit of TIV in reducing AOM burden; however, 1 of the 2 respiratory illness seasons during which this study was conducted had a relatively low influenza activity. A pooled analysis[240] of 8 studies comparing LAIV versus TIV or placebo[241–248] showed a higher efficacy of LAIV compared with both placebo and with TIV. Influenza vaccination is now recommended for all children 6 months of age and older in the United States.[214,215]

Breastfeeding

Multiple studies provide evidence that breastfeeding for at least 4 to 6 months reduces episodes of AOM and recurrent AOM.[249–253] Two cohort studies, 1 retrospective study[250] and 1 prospective study,[253] suggest a dose response, with some protection from partial breastfeeding and the greatest protection from exclusive breastfeeding through 6 months of age. In multivariate analysis controlling for exposure to child care settings, the risk of nonrecurrent otitis is 0.61 (95% confidence interval [CI]: 0.4–0.92) comparing exclusive breastfeeding through 6 months of age with no breastfeeding or breastfeeding less than 4 months. In a prospective cohort, Scariatti[253] found a significant dose-response effect. In this study, OM was self-reported by parents. In a systematic review, McNiel et al[254] found that when exclusive breastfeeding was set as the normative standard, the recalculated odds ratios (ORs) revealed the risks of any formula use. For example, any formula use in the first 6 months of age was significantly associated with increased incidence of OM (OR: 1.78; 95% CI: 1.19–2.70; OR: 4.55; 95% CI: 1.64–12.50 in the available studies; pooled OR for any formula in the first 3 months of age, 2.00; 95% CI: 1.40–2.78). A number of studies[255–259] addressed the association of AOM and other infectious illness in infants with duration and exclusivity of breastfeeding, but all had limitations and none had a randomized controlled design. However, taken together, they continue to show a protective effect of exclusive breastfeeding. In all studies, there has been a predominance of white subjects, and child care attendance and smoking exposure may not have been completely controlled. Also, feeding methods were self-reported.

The consistent finding of a lower incidence of AOM and recurrent AOM with increased breastfeeding supports the AAP recommendation to encourage exclusive breastfeeding for the first 6 months of life and to continue for at least the first year and beyond for as long as mutually desired by mother and child.[216]

Lifestyle Changes

In addition to its many other benefits,[260] eliminating exposure to passive tobacco smoke has been postulated to reduce the incidence of AOM in infancy.[252,261–264] Bottles and pacifiers have been associated with AOM. Avoiding supine bottle feeding ("bottle propping") and reducing or eliminating pacifier use in the second 6 months of life may reduce AOM incidence.[265–267] In a recent cohort study, pacifier use was associated with AOM recurrence.[268]

During infancy and early childhood, reducing the incidence of upper respiratory tract infections by altering child care-center attendance patterns can reduce the incidence of recurrent AOM significantly.[249,269]

Xylitol

Xylitol, or birch sugar, is chemically a pentitol or 5-carbon polyol sugar alcohol. It is available as chewing gum, syrup, or lozenges. A 2011 Cochrane review[270] examined the evidence for the use of xylitol in preventing recurrent AOM. A statistically significant 25% reduction in the risk of occurrence of AOM among healthy children at child care centers in the xylitol group compared with the control group (relative risk: 0.75; 95% CI: 0.65 to 0.88; RD: −0.07; 95% CI: −0.12 to −0.03) in the 4 studies met criteria for analysis.[271–274] Chewing gum and lozenges containing xylitol appeared to be more effective than syrup. Children younger than 2 years, those at the greatest risk of having AOM, cannot safely use lozenges or chewing gum. Also, xylitol needs to be given 3 to 5 times a day to be effective. It is not effective for treating AOM and it must be taken daily throughout the respiratory illness season to have an effect. Sporadic or as-needed use is not effective.

Future Research

Despite advances in research partially stimulated by the 2004 AOM guideline, there are still many unanswered clinical questions in the field. Following are possible clinical research questions that still need to be resolved.

Diagnosis

There will probably never be a gold standard for diagnosis of AOM because of the continuum from OME to AOM. Conceivably, new techniques that could be used on the small amount of fluid obtained during tympanocentesis could identify inflammatory markers in addition to the presence of bacteria or viruses. However, performing tympanocentesis studies on children with uncomplicated otitis is likely not feasible because of ethical and other considerations.

Devices that more accurately identify the presence of MEE and bulging that are easier to use than tympanometry during office visits would be welcome, especially in the difficult-to-examine infant. Additional development of inexpensive, easy-to-use video pneumatic otoscopes is still a goal.

Initial Treatment

The recent studies of Hoberman[31] and Tähtinen[32] have addressed clinical and TM appearance by using stringent diagnostic criteria of AOM. However, the outcomes for less stringent diagnostic criteria, a combination of symptoms, MEE, and TM appearance not completely consistent with OME can only be inferred from earlier studies that used less stringent criteria but did not specify outcomes for various grades of findings. Randomized controlled trials on these less certain TM appearances using scales similar to the OS-8 scale[35] could clarify the benefit of initial antibiotics and initial observation for these less certain diagnoses. Such studies must also specify severity of illness, laterality, and otorrhea.

Appropriate end points must be established. Specifically is the appearance of the TM in patients without clinical symptoms at the end of a study significant for relapse, recurrence, or persistent MEE. Such a study would require randomization of patients with unimproved TM appearance to continued observation and antibiotic groups.

The most efficient and acceptable methods of initial observation should continue to be studied balancing the convenience and benefits with the potential risks to the patient.

Antibiotics

Amoxicillin-clavulanate has a broader spectrum than amoxicillin and may be a better initial antibiotic. However, because of cost and adverse effects, the subcommittee has chosen amoxicillin as first-line AOM treatment. Randomized controlled trials comparing the 2 with adequate power to differentiate clinical efficacy would clarify this choice. Stringent diagnostic criteria should be the standard for these studies. Antibiotic comparisons for AOM should now include an observation arm for patients with nonsevere illness to ensure a clinical benefit over placebo. Studies should also have enough patients to show small but meaningful differences.

Although there have been studies on the likelihood of resistant *S pneumoniae* or *H influenzae* in children in child care settings and with siblings younger than 5 years, studies are still needed to determine whether these and other risk factors would indicate a need for different initial treatment than noted in the guideline.

New antibiotics that are safe and effective are needed for use in AOM because of the development of multidrug-resistant organisms. Such new antibiotics must be tested against the currently available medications.

Randomized controlled trials using different durations of antibiotic therapy in different age groups are needed to optimize therapy with the possibility of decreasing duration of antibiotic use. These would need to be performed initially with amoxicillin and amoxicillin-clavulanate but should also be performed for any antibiotic used in AOM. Again, an observation arm should be included in nonsevere illness.

Recurrent AOM

There have been adequate studies regarding prophylactic antibiotic use in recurrent AOM. More and better controlled studies of tympanostomy tube placement would help determine its benefit versus harm.

Prevention

There should be additional development of vaccines targeted at common organisms associated with AOM.[275] Focused epidemiologic studies on the benefit of breastfeeding, specifically addressing AOM prevention, including duration of breastfeeding and partial versus exclusive breastfeeding, would clarify what is now a more general database. Likewise, more focused studies of the effects of lifestyle changes would help clarify their effect on AOM.

Complementary and Alternative Medicine

There are no well-designed randomized controlled trials of the usefulness of complementary and alternative medicine in AOM, yet a large number of families turn to these methods. Although most alternative therapies are relatively inexpensive, some may be costly. Such studies should compare the alternative therapy to observation rather than antibiotics and only use an antibiotic arm if the alternative therapy is shown to be better than observation. Such studies should focus on children with less stringent criteria of AOM but using the same descriptive criteria for the patients as noted above.

DISSEMINATION OF GUIDELINES

An Institute of Medicine Report notes that "Effective multifaceted implementation strategies targeting both individuals and healthcare systems should be employed by implementers to promote adherence to trustworthy [clinical practice guidelines]."[230]

Many studies of the effect of clinical practice guidelines have been performed. In general, the studies show little overt change in practice after a guideline is published. However, as was seen after the 2004 AOM guideline, the number of visits for AOM and the number of prescriptions for antibiotics for AOM had decreased publication. Studies of educational and dissemination methods both at the practicing physician level and especially at the resident level need to be examined.

SUBCOMMITTEE ON DIAGNOSIS AND MANAGEMENT OF ACUTE OTITIS MEDIA

Allan S. Lieberthal, MD, FAAP (Chair, general pediatrician, no conflicts)

Aaron E. Carroll, MD, MS, FAAP (Partnership for Policy Implementation [PPI] Informatician, general academic pediatrician, no conflicts)

Tasnee Chonmaitree, MD, FAAP (pediatric infectious disease physician, no financial conflicts; published research related to AOM)

Theodore G. Ganiats, MD (family physician, American Academy of Family Physicians, no conflicts)

Alejandro Hoberman, MD, FAAP (general academic pediatrician, no financial conflicts; published research related to AOM)

Mary Anne Jackson, MD, FAAP (pediatric infectious disease physician, AAP Committee on Infectious Disease, no conflicts)

Mark D. Joffe, MD, FAAP (pediatric emergency medicine physician, AAP Committee/Section on Pediatric Emergency Medicine, no conflicts)

Donald T. Miller, MD, MPH, FAAP (general pediatrician, no conflicts)

Richard M. Rosenfeld, MD, MPH, FAAP (otolaryngologist, AAP Section on Otolaryngology, Head and Neck Surgery, American Academy of Otolaryngology-Head and Neck Surgery, no financial conflicts; published research related to AOM)

Xavier D. Sevilla, MD, FAAP (general pediatrics, Quality Improvement Innovation Network, no conflicts)

Richard H. Schwartz, MD, FAAP (general pediatrician, no financial conflicts; published research related to AOM)

Pauline A. Thomas, MD, FAAP (epidemiologist, general pediatrician, no conflicts)

David E. Tunkel, MD, FAAP, FACS (otolaryngologist, AAP Section on Otolaryngology, Head and Neck Surgery, periodic consultant to Medtronic ENT)

CONSULTANT

Richard N. Shiffman, MD, FAAP, FACMI (informatician, guideline methodologist, general academic pediatrician, no conflicts)

STAFF

Caryn Davidson, MA
Oversight by the Steering Committee on Quality Improvement and Management, 2009–2012

REFERENCES

1. American Academy of Pediatrics Subcommittee on Management of Acute Otitis Media. Diagnosis and management of acute otitis media. *Pediatrics.* 2004;113(5): 1451–1465

2. Grijalva CG, Nuorti JP, Griffin MR. Antibiotic prescription rates for acute respiratory tract infections in US ambulatory settings. *JAMA.* 2009;302(7): 758–766

3. McCaig LF, Besser RE, Hughes JM. Trends in antimicrobial prescribing rates for children and adolescents. *JAMA.* 2002;287 (23):3096–3102

4. Vernacchio L, Vezina RM, Mitchell AA. Management of acute otitis media by primary care physicians: trends since the release of the 2004 American Academy of Pediatrics/American Academy of Family Physicians clinical practice guideline. *Pediatrics.* 2007;120(2):281–287

5. Coco A, Vernacchio L, Horst M, Anderson A. Management of acute otitis media after publication of the 2004 AAP and AAFP clinical practice guideline. *Pediatrics.* 2010;125(2):214–220

6. Marchisio P, Mira E, Klersy C, et al. Medical education and attitudes about acute otitis media guidelines: a survey of Italian pediatricians and otolaryngologists. *Pediatr Infect Dis J.* 2009;28(1): 1–4

7. Arkins ER, Koehler JM. Use of the observation option and compliance with guidelines in treatment of acute otitis media. *Ann Pharmacother.* 2008;42(5): 726–727

8. Flores G, Lee M, Bauchner H, Kastner B. Pediatricians' attitudes, beliefs, and practices regarding clinical practice guidelines: a national survey. *Pediatrics.* 2000;105(3 pt 1):496–501

9. Bluestone CD. Definitions, terminology, and classification. In: Rosenfeld RM, Bluestone CD, eds. *Evidence-Based Otitis Media.* Hamilton, Canada: BC Decker; 2003:120–135

10. Bluestone CD, Klein JO. Definitions, terminology, and classification. In: Bluestone CD, Klein JO, eds. *Otitis Media in Infants and Children.* 4th ed. Hamilton, Canada: BC Decker; 2007:1–19

11. Dowell SF, Marcy MS, Phillips WR, et al. Otitis media: principles of judicious use of antimicrobial agents. *Pediatrics.* 1998;101 (suppl):165–171

12. Rosenfeld RM. Clinical pathway for acute otitis media. In: Rosenfeld RM, Bluestone CD, eds. *Evidence-Based Otitis Media.* 2nd ed. Hamilton, Canada: BC Decker; 2003: 280–302

13. Carlson LH, Carlson RD. Diagnosis. In: Rosenfeld RM, Bluestone CD, eds. *Evidence-Based Otitis Media.* Hamilton, Canada: BC Decker; 2003: 136–146

14. Bluestone CD, Klein JO. Diagnosis. In: *Otitis Media in Infants and Children.* 4th ed. Hamilton, Canada: BC Decker; 2007:147–212

15. University of Oxford, Centre for Evidence Based Medicine. Available at: www.cebm.net/index.aspx?o=1044. Accessed July 17, 2012

16. American Academy of Pediatrics Steering Committee on Quality Improvement and Management. Classifying recommendations for clinical practice guidelines. *Pediatrics.* 2004;114(3):874–877

17. Marcy M, Takata G, Shekelle P, et al. *Management of Acute Otitis Media.* Evidence Report/Technology Assessment No. 15. Rockville, MD: Agency for Healthcare Research and Quality; 2000

18. Chan LS, Takata GS, Shekelle P, Morton SC, Mason W, Marcy SM. Evidence assessment of management of acute otitis media: II. Research gaps and priorities for future research. *Pediatrics*. 2001;108(2): 248–254

19. Takata GS, Chan LS, Shekelle P, Morton SC, Mason W, Marcy SM. Evidence assessment of management of acute otitis media: I. The role of antibiotics in treatment of uncomplicated acute otitis media. *Pediatrics*. 2001;108(2):239–247

20. Shekelle PG, Takata G, Newberry SJ, et al. *Management of Acute Otitis Media: Update*. Evidence Report/Technology Assessment No. 198. Rockville, MD: Agency for Healthcare Research and Quality; 2010

21. Coker TR, Chan LS, Newberry SJ, et al. Diagnosis, microbial epidemiology, and antibiotic treatment of acute otitis media in children: a systematic review. *JAMA*. 2010;304(19):2161–2169

22. Jadad AR, Moore RA, Carroll D, et al. Assessing the quality of reports of randomized clinical trials: is blinding necessary? *Control Clin Trials*. 1996;17(1):1–12

23. Whiting P, Rutjes AW, Reitsma JB, Bossuyt PM, Kleijnen J. The development of QUADAS: a tool for the quality assessment of studies of diagnostic accuracy included in systematic reviews. *BMC Med Res Methodol*. 2003;3:25

24. Guyatt GH, Oxman AD, Vist GE, et al; GRADE Working Group. GRADE: an emerging consensus on rating quality of evidence and strength of recommendations. *BMJ*. 2008; 336(7650):924–926

25. Hoffman RN, Michel G, Rosenfeld RM, Davidson C. Building better guidelines with BRIDGE-Wiz: development and evaluation of a software assistant to promote clarity, transparency, and implementability. *J Am Med Inform Assoc*. 2012;19 (1):94–101

26. Kalu SU, Ataya RS, McCormick DP, Patel JA, Revai K, Chonmaitree T. Clinical spectrum of acute otitis media complicating upper respiratory tract viral infection. *Pediatr Infect Dis J*. 2011;30(2):95–99

27. Block SL, Harrison CJ. *Diagnosis and Management of Acute Otitis Media*. 3rd ed. Caddo, OK: Professional Communications; 2005:48–50

28. Wald ER. Acute otitis media: more trouble with the evidence. *Pediatr Infect Dis J*. 2003;22(2):103–104

29. Paradise JL, Rockette HE, Colborn DK, et al. Otitis media in 2253 Pittsburgh-area infants: prevalence and risk factors during the first two years of life. *Pediatrics*. 1997;99(3):318–333

30. McCormick DP, Chonmaitree T, Pittman C, et al. Nonsevere acute otitis media: a clinical trial comparing outcomes of watchful waiting versus immediate antibiotic treatment. *Pediatrics*. 2005;115(6): 1455–1465

31. Hoberman A, Paradise JL, Rockette HE, et al. Treatment of acute otitis media in children under 2 years of age. *N Engl J Med*. 2011;364(2):105–115

32. Tähtinen PA, Laine MK, Huovinen P, Jalava J, Ruuskanen O, Ruohola A. A placebo-controlled trial of antimicrobial treatment for acute otitis media. *N Engl J Med*. 2011;364(2):116–126

33. Shaikh N, Hoberman A, Paradise JL, et al. Development and preliminary evaluation of a parent-reported outcome instrument for clinical trials in acute otitis media. *Pediatr Infect Dis J*. 2009;28(1):5–8

34. Laine MK, Tähtinen PA, Ruuskanen O, Huovinen P, Ruohola A. Symptoms or symptom-based scores cannot predict acute otitis media at otitis-prone age. *Pediatrics*. 2010;125(5). Available at: www.pediatrics.org/cgi/content/full/125/5/e1154

35. Friedman NR, McCormick DP, Pittman C, et al. Development of a practical tool for assessing the severity of acute otitis media. *Pediatr Infect Dis J*. 2006;25(2):101–107

36. Rothman R, Owens T, Simel DL. Does this child have acute otitis media? *JAMA*. 2003; 290(12):1633–1640

37. Niemela M, Uhari M, Jounio-Ervasti K, Luotonen J, Alho OP, Vierimaa E. Lack of specific symptomatology in children with acute otitis media. *Pediatr Infect Dis J*. 1994;13(9):765–768

38. Heikkinen T, Ruuskanen O. Signs and symptoms predicting acute otitis media. *Arch Pediatr Adolesc Med*. 1995;149(1): 26–29

39. Ingvarsson L. Acute otalgia in children—findings and diagnosis. *Acta Paediatr Scand*. 1982;71(5):705–710

40. Kontiokari T, Koivunen P, Niemelä M, Pokka T, Uhari M. Symptoms of acute otitis media. *Pediatr Infect Dis J*. 1998;17(8):676–679

41. Wong DL, Baker CM. Pain in children: comparison of assessment scales. *Pediatr Nurs*. 1988;14(1):9–17

42. Shaikh N, Hoberman A, Paradise JL, et al. Responsiveness and construct validity of a symptom scale for acute otitis media. *Pediatr Infect Dis J*. 2009;28(1):9–12

43. Karma PH, Penttilä MA, Sipilä MM, Kataja MJ. Otoscopic diagnosis of middle ear effusion in acute and non-acute otitis media. I. The value of different otoscopic findings. *Int J Pediatr Otorhinolaryngol*. 1989;17(1):37–49

44. McCormick DP, Lim-Melia E, Saeed K, Baldwin CD, Chonmaitree T. Otitis media: can clinical findings predict bacterial or viral etiology? *Pediatr Infect Dis J*. 2000; 19(3):256–258

45. Schwartz RH, Stool SE, Rodriguez WJ, Grundfast KM. Acute otitis media: toward a more precise definition. *Clin Pediatr (Phila)*. 1981;20(9):549–554

46. Rosenfeld RM. Antibiotic prophylaxis for recurrent acute otitis media. In: Alper CM, Bluestone CD, eds. *Advanced Therapy of Otitis Media*. Hamilton, Canada: BC Decker; 2004

47. Paradise J, Bernard B, Colborn D, Smith C, Rockette H; Pittsburgh-area Child Development/Otitis Media Study Group. Otitis media with effusion: highly prevalent and often the forerunner of acute otitis media during the first year of life [abstract]. *Pediatr Res*. 1993;33:121A

48. Roland PS, Smith TL, Schwartz SR, et al. Clinical practice guideline: cerumen impaction. *Otolaryngol Head Neck Surg*. 2008;139(3 suppl 2):S1–S21

49. Shaikh N, Hoberman A, Kaleida PH, Ploof DL, Paradise JL. Videos in clinical medicine. Diagnosing otitis media—otoscopy and cerumen removal. *N Engl J Med*. 2010; 362(20):e62

50. Pichichero ME. Diagnostic accuracy, tympanocentesis training performance, and antibiotic selection by pediatric residents in management of otitis media. *Pediatrics*. 2002;110(6):1064–1070

51. Kaleida PH, Ploof DL, Kurs-Lasky M, et al. Mastering diagnostic skills: Enhancing Proficiency in Otitis Media, a model for diagnostic skills training. *Pediatrics*. 2009; 124(4). Available at: www.pediatrics.org/cgi/content/full/124/4/e714

52. Kaleida PH, Ploof D. ePROM: Enhancing Proficiency in Otitis Media. Pittsburgh, PA: University of Pittsburgh School of Medicine. Available at: http://pedsed.pitt.edu. Accessed December 31, 2011

53. Innovative Medical Education. *A View Through the Otoscope: Distinguishing Acute Otitis Media from Otitis Media with Effusion*. Paramus, NJ: Innovative Medical Education; 2000

54. American Academy of Pediatrics. Section on Infectious Diseases. A view through the otoscope: distinguishing acute otitis media from otitis media with effusion [video]. Available at: http://www2.aap.org/sections/infectdis/video.cfm. Accessed January 20, 2012

55. Hayden GF, Schwartz RH. Characteristics of earache among children with acute

otitis media. *Am J Dis Child.* 1985;139(7): 721–723

56. Schechter NL. Management of pain associated with acute medical illness. In: Schechter NL, Berde CB, Yaster M, eds. *Pain in Infants, Children, and Adolescents.* Baltimore, MD: Williams & Wilkins; 1993: 537–538

57. Rovers MM, Glasziou P, Appelman CL, et al. Predictors of pain and/or fever at 3 to 7 days for children with acute otitis media not treated initially with antibiotics: a meta-analysis of individual patient data. *Pediatrics.* 2007;119(3):579–585

58. Burke P, Bain J, Robinson D, Dunleavey J. Acute red ear in children: controlled trial of nonantibiotic treatment in children: controlled trial of nonantibiotic treatment in general practice. *BMJ.* 1991;303(6802): 558–562

59. Sanders S, Glasziou PP, DelMar C, Rovers M. Antibiotics for acute otitis media in children [review]. *Cochrane Database Syst Rev.* 2009;(2):1–43

60. van Buchem FL, Dunk JH, van't Hof MA. Therapy of acute otitis media: myringotomy, antibiotics, or neither? A double-blind study in children. *Lancet.* 1981;2(8252): 883–887

61. Thalin A, Densert O, Larsson A, et al. Is penicillin necessary in the treatment of acute otitis media? In: *Proceedings of the International Conference on Acute and Secretory Otitis Media. Part 1.* Amsterdam, Netherlands: Kugler Publications; 1986:441–446

62. Rovers MM, Glasziou P, Appelman CL, et al. Antibiotics for acute otitis media: an individual patient data meta-analysis. *Lancet.* 2006;368(9545):1429–1435

63. Bertin L, Pons G, d'Athis P, et al. A randomized, double-blind, multicentre controlled trial of ibuprofen versus acetaminophen and placebo for symptoms of acute otitis media in children. *Fundam Clin Pharmacol.* 1996;10(4):387–392

64. American Academy of Pediatrics. Committee on Psychosocial Aspects of Child and Family Health; Task Force on Pain in Infants, Children, and Adolescents. The assessment and management of acute pain in infants, children, and adolescents. *Pediatrics.* 2001;108(3): 793–797

65. Bolt P, Barnett P, Babl FE, Sharwood LN. Topical lignocaine for pain relief in acute otitis media: results of a double-blind placebo-controlled randomised trial. *Arch Dis Child.* 2008;93(1):40–44

66. Foxlee R, Johansson AC, Wejfalk J, Dawkins J, Dooley L, Del Mar C. Topical analgesia for

acute otitis media. *Cochrane Database Syst Rev.* 2006;(3):CD005657

67. Hoberman A, Paradise JL, Reynolds EA, Urkin J. Efficacy of Auralgan for treating ear pain in children with acute otitis media. *Arch Pediatr Adolesc Med.* 1997; 151(7):675–678

68. Sarrell EM, Mandelberg A, Cohen HA. Efficacy of naturopathic extracts in the management of ear pain associated with acute otitis media. *Arch Pediatr Adolesc Med.* 2001;155(7):796–799

69. Sarrell EM, Cohen HA, Kahan E. Naturopathic treatment for ear pain in children. *Pediatrics.* 2003;111(5 pt 1):e574–e579

70. Adam D, Federspil P, Lukes M, Petrowicz O. Therapeutic properties and tolerance of procaine and phenazone containing ear drops in infants and very young children. *Arzneimittelforschung.* 2009;59(10):504–512

71. Barnett ED, Levatin JL, Chapman EH, et al. Challenges of evaluating homeopathic treatment of acute otitis media. *Pediatr Infect Dis J.* 2000;19(4):273–275

72. Jacobs J, Springer DA, Crothers D. Homeopathic treatment of acute otitis media in children: a preliminary randomized placebo-controlled trial. *Pediatr Infect Dis J.* 2001;20(2):177–183

73. Rosenfeld RM, Bluestone CD. Clinical efficacy of surgical therapy. In: Rosenfeld RM, Bluestone CD, eds. *Evidence-Based Otitis Media. 2003.* Hamilton, Canada: BC Decker; 2003:227–240

74. Rosenfeld RM. Observation option toolkit for acute otitis media. *Int J Pediatr Otorhinolaryngol.* 2001;58(1):1–8

75. Le Saux N, Gaboury I, Baird M, et al. A randomized, double-blind, placebo-controlled noninferiority trial of amoxicillin for clinically diagnosed acute otitis media in children 6 months to 5 years of age. *CMAJ.* 2005;172(3):335–341

76. Spiro DM, Tay KY, Arnold DH, Dziura JD, Baker MD, Shapiro ED. Wait-and-see prescription for the treatment of acute otitis media: a randomized controlled trial. *JAMA.* 2006;296(10):1235–1241

77. Neumark T, Mölstad S, Rosén C, et al. Evaluation of phenoxymethylpenicillin treatment of acute otitis media in children aged 2–16. *Scand J Prim Health Care.* 2007;25(3):166–171

78. Chao JH, Kunkov S, Reyes LB, Lichten S, Crain EF. Comparison of two approaches to observation therapy for acute otitis media in the emergency department. *Pediatrics.* 2008;121(5). Available at: www.pediatrics.org/cgi/content/full/121/5/e1352

79. Spurling GK, Del Mar CB, Dooley L, Foxlee R. Delayed antibiotics for respiratory infections. *Cochrane Database Syst Rev.* 2007;(3):CD004417

80. Koopman L, Hoes AW, Glasziou PP, et al. Antibiotic therapy to prevent the development of asymptomatic middle ear effusion in children with acute otitis media: a meta-analysis of individual patient data. *Arch Otolaryngol Head Neck Surg.* 2008;134(2):128–132

81. Marchetti F, Ronfani L, Nibali SC, Tamburlini G; Italian Study Group on Acute Otitis Media. Delayed prescription may reduce the use of antibiotics for acute otitis media: a prospective observational study in primary care. *Arch Pediatr Adolesc Med.* 2005; 159(7):679–684

82. Ho D, Rotenberg BW, Berkowitz RG. The relationship between acute mastoiditis and antibiotic use for acute otitis media in children. *Arch Otolaryngol Head Neck Surg.* 2008;34(1):45–48

83. Thompson PL, Gilbert RE, Long PF, Saxena S, Sharland M, Wong IC. Effect of antibiotics for otitis media on mastoiditis in children: a retrospective cohort study using the United Kingdom general practice research database. *Pediatrics.* 2009; 123(2):424–430

84. American Academy of Family Physicians; American Academy of Otolaryngology-Head and Neck Surgery; American Academy of Pediatrics Subcommittee on Otitis Media With Effusion. Otitis media with effusion. *Pediatrics.* 2004;113(5):1412–1429

85. Rosenfeld RM, Culpepper L, Doyle KJ, et al; American Academy of Pediatrics Subcommittee on Otitis Media with Effusion; American Academy of Family Physicians; American Academy of Otolaryngology—Head and Neck Surgery. Clinical practice guideline: otitis media with effusion. *Otolaryngol Head Neck Surg.* 2004;130(suppl 5): S95–S118

86. Appelman CL, Claessen JQ, Touw-Otten FW, Hordijk GJ, de Melker RA. Co-amoxiclav in recurrent acute otitis media: placebo controlled study. *BMJ.* 1991;303(6815): 1450–1452

87. Burke P, Bain J, Robinson D, Dunleavey J. Acute red ear in children: controlled trial of nonantibiotic treatment in children: controlled trial of nonantibiotic treatment in general practice. *BMJ.* 1991;303(6802): 558–562

88. van Balen FA, Hoes AW, Verheij TJ, de Melker RA. Primary care based randomized, double blind trial of amoxicillin versus placebo in children aged under 2 years. *BMJ.* 2000;320(7231):350–354

89. Little P, Gould C, Williamson I, Moore M, Warner G, Dunleavey J. Pragmatic randomised controlled trial of two prescribing strategies for childhood acute otitis media. *BMJ*. 2001;322(7282):336–342

90. Mygind N, Meistrup-Larsen K-I, Thomsen J, Thomsen VF, Josefsson K, Sørensen H. Penicillin in acute otitis media: a double-blind placebo-controlled trial. *Clin Otolaryngol Allied Sci*. 1981;6(1):5–13

91. Kaleida PH, Casselbrant ML, Rockette HE, et al. Amoxicillin or myringotomy or both for acute otitis media: results of a randomized clinical trial. *Pediatrics*. 1991;87(4):466–474

92. Shaikh N, Hoberman A, Paradise JL, et al. Responsiveness and construct validity of a symptom scale for acute otitis media. *Pediatr Infect Dis J*. 2009;28(1):9–12

93. Heikkinen T, Chonmaitree T. Importance of respiratory viruses in acute otitis media. *Clin Microbiol Rev*. 2003;16(2):230–241

94. Halsted C, Lepow ML, Balassanian N, Emmerich J, Wolinsky E. Otitis media. Clinical observations, microbiology, and evaluation of therapy. *Am J Dis Child*. 1968;115(5):542–551

95. Rosenfeld RM, Vertrees J, Carr J, et al. Clinical efficacy of antimicrobials for acute otitis media: meta-analysis of 5,400 children from 33 randomized trials. *J Pediatr*. 1994;124(3):355–367

96. McCormick DP, Chandler SM, Chonmaitree T. Laterality of acute otitis media: different clinical and microbiologic characteristics. *Pediatr Infect Dis J*. 2007;26(7):583–588

97. Appelman CLM, Bossen PC, Dunk JHM, Lisdonk EH, de Melker RA, van Weert HCPM. NHG Standard Otitis Media Acuta (Guideline on acute otitis media of the Dutch College of General Practitioners). *Huisarts Wet*. 1990;33:242–245

98. Swedish Medical Research Council. Treatment for acute inflammation of the middle ear: consensus statement. Stockholm, Sweden: Swedish Medical Research Council; 2000. Available at: http://soapimg.icecube.snowfall.se/strama/Konsensut_ora_eng.pdf. Accessed July 18, 2012

99. Scottish Intercollegiate Guideline Network. Diagnosis and management of childhood otitis media in primary care. Edinburgh, Scotland: Scottish Intercollegiate Guideline Network; 2000. Available at: www.sign.ac.uk/guidelines/fulltext/66/index.html. Accessed July 18, 2012

100. National Institute for Health and Clinical Excellence, Centre for Clinical Practice. Respiratory tract infections—antibiotic prescribing: prescribing of antibiotics for self-limiting respiratory tract infections in adults and children in primary care. NICE Clinical Guideline 69. London, United Kingdom: National Institute for Health and Clinical Excellence; July 2008. Available at: www.nice.org.uk/CG069. Accessed July 18, 2012

101. Marchisio P, Bellussi L, Di Mauro G, et al. Acute otitis media: from diagnosis to prevention. Summary of the Italian guideline. *Int J Pediatr Otorhinolaryngol*. 2010;74(11):1209–1216

102. Siegel RM, Kiely M, Bien JP, et al. Treatment of otitis media with observation and a safety-net antibiotic prescription. *Pediatrics*. 2003;112(3 pt 1):527–531

103. Pshetizky Y, Naimer S, Shvartzman P. Acute otitis media—a brief explanation to parents and antibiotic use. *Fam Pract*. 2003;20(4):417–419

104. Pichichero ME, Casey JR. Emergence of a multiresistant serotype 19A pneumococcal strain not included in the 7-valent conjugate vaccine as an otopathogen in children. *JAMA*. 2007;298(15):1772–1778

105. Pichichero ME, Casey JR. Evolving microbiology and molecular epidemiology of acute otitis media in the pneumococcal conjugate vaccine era. *Pediatr Infect Dis J*. 2007;26(suppl 10):S12–S16

106. Nielsen HUK, Konradsen HB, Lous J, Frimodt-Møller N. Nasopharyngeal pathogens in children with acute otitis media in a low-antibiotic use country. *Int J Pediatr Otorhinolaryngol*. 2004;68(9):1149–1155

107. Pitkäranta A, Virolainen A, Jero J, Arruda E, Hayden FG. Detection of rhinovirus, respiratory syncytial virus, and coronavirus infections in acute otitis media by reverse transcriptase polymerase chain reaction. *Pediatrics*. 1998;102(2 pt 1):291–295

108. Heikkinen T, Thint M, Chonmaitree T. Prevalence of various respiratory viruses in the middle ear during acute otitis media. *N Engl J Med*. 1999;340(4):260–264

109. Chonmaitree T. Acute otitis media is not a pure bacterial disease. *Clin Infect Dis*. 2006;43(11):1423–1425

110. Williams JV, Tollefson SJ, Nair S, Chonmaitree T. Association of human metapneumovirus with acute otitis media. *Int J Pediatr Otorhinolaryngol*. 2006;70(7):1189–1193

111. Chonmaitree T, Heikkinen T. Role of viruses in middle-ear disease. *Ann N Y Acad Sci*. 1997;830:143–157

112. Klein JO, Bluestone CD. Otitis media. In: Feigin RD, Cherry JD, Demmler-Harrison GJ, Kaplan SL, eds. *Textbook of Pediatric Infectious Diseases*. 6th ed. Philadelphia, PA: Saunders; 2009:216–237

113. Chonmaitree T, Revai K, Grady JJ, et al. Viral upper respiratory tract infection and otitis media complication in young children. *Clin Infect Dis*. 2008;46(6):815–823

114. Ruohola A, Meurman O, Nikkari S, et al. Microbiology of acute otitis media in children with tympanostomy tubes: prevalences of bacteria and viruses. *Clin Infect Dis*. 2006;43(11):1417–1422

115. Ruuskanen O, Arola M, Heikkinen T, Ziegler T. Viruses in acute otitis media: increasing evidence for clinical significance. *Pediatr Infect Dis J*. 1991;10(6):425–427

116. Chonmaitree T. Viral and bacterial interaction in acute otitis media. *Pediatr Infect Dis J*. 2000;19(suppl 5):S24–S30

117. Nokso-Koivisto J, Räty R, Blomqvist S, et al. Presence of specific viruses in the middle ear fluids and respiratory secretions of young children with acute otitis media. *J Med Virol*. 2004;72(2):241–248

118. Bluestone CD, Klein JO. Microbiology. In: Bluestone CD, Klein JO, eds. *Otitis Media in Infants and Children*. 4th ed. Hamilton, Canada: BC Decker; 2007:101–126

119. Del Beccaro MA, Mendelman PM, Inglis AF, et al. Bacteriology of acute otitis media: a new perspective. *J Pediatr*. 1992;120(1):81–84

120. Block SL, Harrison CJ, Hedrick JA, et al. Penicillin-resistant *Streptococcus pneumoniae* in acute otitis media: risk factors, susceptibility patterns and antimicrobial management. *Pediatr Infect Dis J*. 1995;14(9):751–759

121. Rodriguez WJ, Schwartz RH. *Streptococcus pneumoniae* causes otitis media with higher fever and more redness of tympanic membranes than *Haemophilus influenzae* or *Moraxella catarrhalis*. *Pediatr Infect Dis J*. 1999;18(10):942–944

122. Block SL, Hedrick J, Harrison CJ, et al. Community-wide vaccination with the heptavalent pneumococcal conjugate significantly alters the microbiology of acute otitis media. *Pediatr Infect Dis J*. 2004;23(9):829–833

123. Casey JR, Pichichero ME. Changes in frequency and pathogens causing acute otitis media in 1995–2003. *Pediatr Infect Dis J*. 2004;23(9):824–828

124. McEllistrem MC, Adams JM, Patel K, et al. Acute otitis media due to penicillin-nonsusceptible *Streptococcus pneumoniae* before and after the introduction of the pneumococcal conjugate vaccine. *Clin Infect Dis*. 2005;40(12):1738–1744

125. Casey JR, Adlowitz DG, Pichichero ME. New patterns in the otopathogens causing acute otitis media six to eight years after introduction of pneumococcal conjugate vaccine. *Pediatr Infect Dis J*. 2010;29(4):304–309

126. Grubb MS, Spaugh DC. Microbiology of acute otitis media, Puget Sound region, 2005–2009. *Clin Pediatr (Phila)*. 2010;49(8):727–730

127. Revai K, McCormick DP, Patel J, Grady JJ, Saeed K, Chonmaitree T. Effect of pneumococcal conjugate vaccine on nasopharyngeal bacterial colonization during acute otitis media. *Pediatrics*. 2006;117(5):1823–1829

128. Pettigrew MM, Gent JF, Revai K, Patel JA, Chonmaitree T. Microbial interactions during upper respiratory tract infections. *Emerg Infect Dis*. 2008;14(10):1584–1591

129. O'Brien KL, Millar EV, Zell ER, et al. Effect of pneumococcal conjugate vaccine on nasopharyngeal colonization among immunized and unimmunized children in a community-randomized trial. *J Infect Dis*. 2007;196(8):1211–1220

130. Jacobs MR, Bajaksouzian S, Windau A, Good C. Continued emergence of non-vaccine serotypes of *Streptococcus pneumoniae* in Cleveland. *Proceedings of the 49th Interscience Conference on Antimicrobial Agents and Chemotherapy*; 2009:G1-G1556

131. Hoberman A, Paradise JL, Shaikh N, et al. Pneumococcal resistance and serotype 19A in Pittsburgh-area children with acute otitis media before and after introduction of 7-valent pneumococcal polysaccharide vaccine. *Clin Pediatr (Phila)*. 2011;50(2):114–120

132. Huang SS, Hinrichsen VL, Stevenson AE, et al. Continued impact of pneumococcal conjugate vaccine on carriage in young children. *Pediatrics*. 2009;124(1). Available at: www.pediatrics.org/cgi/content/full/124/1/e1

133. Centers for Disease Control and Prevention (CDC). Licensure of a 13-valent pneumococcal conjugate vaccine (PCV13) and recommendations for use among children—Advisory Committee on Immunization Practices (ACIP), 2010. *MMWR Morb Mortal Wkly Rep*. 2010;59(9):258–261

134. Segal N, Givon-Lavi N, Leibovitz E, Yagupsky P, Leiberman A, Dagan R. Acute otitis media caused by *Streptococcus pyogenes* in children. *Clin Infect Dis*. 2005;41(1):35–41

135. Luntz M, Brodsky A, Nusem S, et al. Acute mastoiditis—the antibiotic era: a multicenter study. *Int J Pediatr Otorhinolaryngol*. 2001;57(1):1–9

136. Nielsen JC. *Studies on the Aetiology of Acute Otitis Media*. Copenhagen, Denmark: Ejnar Mundsgaard Forlag; 1945

137. Palmu AA, Herva E, Savolainen H, Karma P, Mäkelä PH, Kilpi TM. Association of clinical signs and symptoms with bacterial findings in acute otitis media. *Clin Infect Dis*. 2004;38(2):234–242

138. Leibovitz E, Asher E, Piglansky L, et al. Is bilateral acute otitis media clinically different than unilateral acute otitis media? *Pediatr Infect Dis J*. 2007;26(7):589–592

139. Leibovitz E, Satran R, Piglansky L, et al. Can acute otitis media caused by *Haemophilus influenzae* be distinguished from that caused by *Streptococcus pneumoniae*? *Pediatr Infect Dis J*. 2003;22(6):509–515

140. Palmu AA, Kotikoski MJ, Kaijalainen TH, Puhakka HJ. Bacterial etiology of acute myringitis in children less than two years of age. *Pediatr Infect Dis J*. 2001;20(6):607–611

141. Bodor FF. Systemic antibiotics for treatment of the conjunctivitis-otitis media syndrome. *Pediatr Infect Dis J*. 1989;8(5):287–290

142. Bingen E, Cohen R, Jourenkova N, Gehanno P. Epidemiologic study of conjunctivitis-otitis syndrome. *Pediatr Infect Dis J*. 2005;24(8):731–732

143. Barkai G, Leibovitz E, Givon-Lavi N, Dagan R. Potential contribution by nontypable *Haemophilus influenzae* in protracted and recurrent acute otitis media. *Pediatr Infect Dis J*. 2009;28(6):466–471

144. Howie VM, Ploussard JH. Efficacy of fixed combination antibiotics versus separate components in otitis media. Effectiveness of erythromycin estrolate, triple sulfonamide, ampicillin, erythromycin estolate-triple sulfonamide, and placebo in 280 patients with acute otitis media under two and one-half years of age. *Clin Pediatr (Phila)*. 1972;11(4):205–214

145. Klein JO. Microbiologic efficacy of antibacterial drugs for acute otitis media. *Pediatr Infect Dis J*. 1993;12(12):973–975

146. Barnett ED, Klein JO. The problem of resistant bacteria for the management of acute otitis media. *Pediatr Clin North Am*. 1995;42(3):509–517

147. Tristram S, Jacobs MR, Appelbaum PC. Antimicrobial resistance in *Haemophilus influenzae*. *Clin Microbiol Rev*. 2007;20(2):368–389

148. Critchley IA, Jacobs MR, Brown SD, Traczewski MM, Tillotson GS, Janjic N. Prevalence of serotype 19A *Streptococcus pneumoniae* among isolates from U.S. children in 2005≠2006 and activity of faropenem. *Antimicrob Agents Chemother*. 2008;52(7):2639–2643

149. Jacobs MR, Good CE, Windau AR, et al. Activity of ceftaroline against emerging serotypes of Streptococcus pneumoniae. *Antimicrob Agents Chemother*. 2010;54(6):2716–2719

150. Jacobs MR. Antimicrobial-resistant *Streptococcus pneumoniae*: trends and management. *Expert Rev Anti Infect Ther*. 2008;6(5):619–635

151. Piglansky L, Leibovitz E, Raiz S, et al. Bacteriologic and clinical efficacy of high dose amoxicillin for therapy of acute otitis media in children. *Pediatr Infect Dis J*. 2003;22(5):405–413

152. Dagan R, Johnson CE, McLinn S, et al. Bacteriologic and clinical efficacy of amoxicillin/clavulanate vs. azithromycin in acute otitis media. *Pediatr Infect Dis J*. 2000;19(2):95–104

153. Dagan R, Hoberman A, Johnson C, et al. Bacteriologic and clinical efficacy of high dose amoxicillin/clavulanate in children with acute otitis media. *Pediatr Infect Dis J*. 2001;20(9):829–837

154. Hoberman A, Dagan R, Leibovitz E, et al. Large dosage amoxicillin/clavulanate, compared with azithromycin, for the treatment of bacterial acute otitis media in children. *Pediatr Infect Dis J*. 2005;24(6):525–532

155. De Wals P, Erickson L, Poirier B, Pépin J, Pichichero ME. How to compare the efficacy of conjugate vaccines to prevent acute otitis media? *Vaccine*. 2009;27(21):2877–2883

156. Shouval DS, Greenberg D, Givon-Lavi N, Porat N, Dagan R. Serotype coverage of invasive and mucosal pneumococcal disease in Israeli children younger than 3 years by various pneumococcal conjugate vaccines. *Pediatr Infect Dis J*. 2009;28(4):277–282

157. Jones RN, Farrell DJ, Mendes RE, Sader HS. Comparative ceftaroline activity tested against pathogens associated with community-acquired pneumonia: results from an international surveillance study. *J Antimicrob Chemother*. 2011;66(suppl 3):iii69–iii80

158. Harrison CJ, Woods C, Stout G, Martin B, Selvarangan R. Susceptibilities of Haemophilus influenzae, Streptococcus pneumoniae, including serotype 19A, and Moraxella catarrhalis paediatric isolates from 2005 to 2007 to commonly used antibiotics. *J Antimicrob Chemother*. 2009;63(3):511–519

159. Doern GV, Jones RN, Pfaller MA, Kugler K. *Haemophilus influenzae* and *Moraxella catarrhalis* from patients with community-acquired respiratory tract infections: antimicrobial susceptibility patterns from the SENTRY antimicrobial Surveillance Program (United States and Canada, 1997).

Antimicrob Agents Chemother. 1999;43(2): 385–389

160. Nussinovitch M, Yoeli R, Elishkevitz K, Varsano I. Acute mastoiditis in children: epidemiologic, clinical, microbiologic, and therapeutic aspects over past years. *Clin Pediatr (Phila).* 2004;43(3):261–267

161. Roddy MG, Glazier SS, Agrawal D. Pediatric mastoiditis in the pneumococcal conjugate vaccine era: symptom duration guides empiric antimicrobial therapy. *Pediatr Emerg Care.* 2007;23(11):779–784

162. Hoberman A, Paradise JL, Burch DJ, et al. Equivalent efficacy and reduced occurrence of diarrhea from a new formulation of amoxicillin/clavulanate potassium (Augmentin) for treatment of acute otitis media in children. *Pediatr Infect Dis J.* 1997;16(5):463–470

163. Arguedas A, Dagan R, Leibovitz E, Hoberman A, Pichichero M, Paris M. A multicenter, open label, double tympanocentesis study of high dose cefdinir in children with acute otitis media at high risk of persistent or recurrent infection. *Pediatr Infect Dis J.* 2006;25(3):211–218

164. Atanasković-Marković M, Velicković TC, Gavrović-Jankulović M, Vucković O, Nestorović B. Immediate allergic reactions to cephalosporins and penicillins and their cross-reactivity in children. *Pediatr Allergy Immunol.* 2005;16(4):341–347

165. Pichichero ME. Use of selected cephalosporins in penicillin-allergic patients: a paradigm shift. *Diagn Microbiol Infect Dis.* 2007;57(suppl 3):13S–18S

166. Pichichero ME, Casey JR. Safe use of selected cephalosporins in penicillin-allergic patients: a meta-analysis. *Otolaryngol Head Neck Surg.* 2007;136(3):340–347

167. DePestel DD, Benninger MS, Danziger L, et al. Cephalosporin use in treatment of patients with penicillin allergies. *J Am Pharm Assoc (2003).* 2008;48(4):530–540

168. Fonacier L, Hirschberg R, Gerson S. Adverse drug reactions to a cephalosporins in hospitalized patients with a history of penicillin allergy. *Allergy Asthma Proc.* 2005;26(2):135–141

169. Joint Task Force on Practice Parameters; American Academy of Allergy, Asthma and Immunology; American College of Allergy, Asthma and Immunology; Joint Council of Allergy, Asthma and Immunology. Drug allergy: an updated practice parameter. *Ann Allergy Asthma Immunol.* 2010;105(4): 259–273

170. Powers JL, Gooch WM, III, Oddo LP. Comparison of the palatability of the oral suspension of cefdinir vs. amoxicillin/clavulanate potassium, cefprozil and azithromycin in

pediatric patients. *Pediatr Infect Dis J.* 2000; 19(suppl 12):S174–S180

171. Steele RW, Thomas MP, Bégué RE. Compliance issues related to the selection of antibiotic suspensions for children. *Pediatr Infect Dis J.* 2001;20(1):1–5

172. Steele RW, Russo TM, Thomas MP. Adherence issues related to the selection of antistaphylococcal or antifungal antibiotic suspensions for children. *Clin Pediatr (Phila).* 2006;45(3):245–250

173. Schwartz RH. Enhancing children's satisfaction with antibiotic therapy: a taste study of several antibiotic suspensions. *Curr Ther Res.* 2000;61(8):570–581

174. Green SM, Rothrock SG. Single-dose intramuscular ceftriaxone for acute otitis media in children. *Pediatrics.* 1993;91(1): 23–30

175. Leibovitz E, Piglansky L, Raiz S, Press J, Leiberman A, Dagan R. Bacteriologic and clinical efficacy of one day vs. three day intramuscular ceftriaxone for treatment of nonresponsive acute otitis media in children. *Pediatr Infect Dis J.* 2000;19(11): 1040–1045

176. Rosenfeld RM, Kay D. Natural history of untreated otitis media. *Laryngoscope.* 2003;113(10):1645–1657

177. Rosenfeld RM, Kay D. Natural history of untreated otitis media. In: Rosenfeld RM, Bluestone CD, eds. *Evidence-Based Otitis Media.* 2nd ed. Hamilton, Canada: BC Decker; 2003:180–198

178. Arola M, Ziegler T, Ruuskanen O. Respiratory virus infection as a cause of prolonged symptoms in acute otitis media. *J Pediatr.* 1990;116(5):697–701

179. Chonmaitree T, Owen MJ, Howie VM. Respiratory viruses interfere with bacteriologic response to antibiotic in children with acute otitis media. *J Infect Dis.* 1990; 162(2):546–549

180. Dagan R, Leibovitz E, Greenberg D, Yagupsky P, Fliss DM, Leiberman A. Early eradication of pathogens from middle ear fluid during antibiotic treatment of acute otitis media is associated with improved clinical outcome. *Pediatr Infect Dis J.* 1998;17(9):776–782

181. Carlin SA, Marchant CD, Shurin PA, Johnson CE, Super DM, Rehmus JM. Host factors and early therapeutic response in acute otitis media. *J Pediatr.* 1991;118(2):178–183

182. Teele DW, Pelton SI, Klein JO. Bacteriology of acute otitis media unresponsive to initial antimicrobial therapy. *J Pediatr.* 1981; 98(4):537–539

183. Doern GV, Pfaller MA, Kugler K, Freeman J, Jones RN. Prevalence of antimicrobial re-

sistance among respiratory tract isolates of *Streptococcus pneumoniae* in North America: 1997 results from the SENTRY antimicrobial surveillance program. *Clin Infect Dis.* 1998;27(4):764–770

184. Leiberman A, Leibovitz E, Piglansky L, et al. Bacteriologic and clinical efficacy of trimethoprim-sulfamethoxazole for treatment of acute otitis media. *Pediatr Infect Dis J.* 2001;20(3):260–264

185. Humphrey WR, Shattuck MH, Zielinski RJ, et al. Pharmacokinetics and efficacy of linezolid in a gerbil model of *Streptococcus pneumoniae*-induced acute otitis media. *Antimicrob Agents Chemother.* 2003; 47(4):1355–1363

186. Arguedas A, Dagan R, Pichichero M, et al. An open-label, double tympanocentesis study of levofloxacin therapy in children with, or at high risk for, recurrent or persistent acute otitis media. *Pediatr Infect Dis J.* 2006;25(12):1102–1109

187. Noel GJ, Blumer JL, Pichichero ME, et al. A randomized comparative study of levofloxacin versus amoxicillin/clavulanate for treatment of infants and young children with recurrent or persistent acute otitis media. *Pediatr Infect Dis J.* 2008;27(6): 483–489

188. Howie VM, Ploussard JH. Simultaneous nasopharyngeal and middle ear exudate culture in otitis media. *Pediatr Digest.* 1971;13:31–35

189. Gehanno P, Lenoir G, Barry B, Bons J, Boucot I, Berche P. Evaluation of nasopharyngeal cultures for bacteriologic assessment of acute otitis media in children. *Pediatr Infect Dis J.* 1996;15(4): 329–332

190. Cohen R, Levy C, Boucherat M, Langue J, de La Rocque F. A multicenter, randomized, double-blind trial of 5 versus 10 days of antibiotic therapy for acute otitis media in young children. *J Pediatr.* 1998;133(5): 634–639

191. Pessey JJ, Gehanno P, Thoroddsen E, et al. Short course therapy with cefuroxime axetil for acute otitis media: results of a randomized multicenter comparison with amoxicillin/clavulanate. *Pediatr Infect Dis J.* 1999;18(10):854–859

192. Cohen R, Levy C, Boucherat M, et al. Five vs. ten days of antibiotic therapy for acute otitis media in young children. *Pediatr Infect Dis J.* 2000;19(5):458–463

193. Pichichero ME, Marsocci SM, Murphy ML, Hoeger W, Francis AB, Green JL. A prospective observational study of 5-, 7-, and 10-day antibiotic treatment for acute otitis media. *Otolaryngol Head Neck Surg.* 2001; 124(4):381–387

194. Kozyrskyj AL, Klassen TP, Moffatt M, Harvey K. Short-course antibiotics for acute otitis media. *Cochrane Database Syst Rev.* 2010; (9):CD001095

195. Shurin PA, Pelton SI, Donner A, Klein JO. Persistence of middle-ear effusion after acute otitis media in children. *N Engl J Med.* 1979;300(20):1121–1123

196. Damoiseaux RA, Rovers MM, Van Balen FA, Hoes AW, de Melker RA. Long-term prognosis of acute otitis media in infancy: determinants of recurrent acute otitis media and persistent middle ear effusion. *Fam Pract.* 2006;23(1):40–45

197. Leach AJ, Morris PS. Antibiotics for the prevention of acute and chronic suppurative otitis media in children. *Cochrane Database Syst Rev.* 2006;(4):CD004401

198. Teele DW, Klein JO, Word BM, et al; Greater Boston Otitis Media Study Group. Antimicrobial prophylaxis for infants at risk for recurrent acute otitis media. *Vaccine.* 2000;19(suppl 1):S140–S143

199. Paradise JL. On tympanostomy tubes: rationale, results, reservations, and recommendations. *Pediatrics.* 1977;60(1):86–90

200. McIsaac WJ, Coyte PC, Croxford R, Asche CV, Friedberg J, Feldman W. Otolaryngologists' perceptions of the indications for tympanostomy tube insertion in children. *CMAJ.* 2000;162(9):1285–1288

201. Casselbrandt ML. Ventilation tubes for recurrent acute otitis media. In: Alper CM, Bluestone CD, eds. *Advanced Therapy of Otitis Media.* Hamilton, Canada: BC Decker; 2004:113–115

202. Shin JJ, Stinnett SS, Hartnick CJ. Pediatric recurrent acute otitis media. In: Shin JJ, Hartnick CJ, Randolph GW, eds. *Evidence-Based Otolaryngology.* New York, NY: Springer; 2008:91–95

203. Gonzalez C, Arnold JE, Woody EA, et al. Prevention of recurrent acute otitis media: chemoprophylaxis versus tympanostomy tubes. *Laryngoscope.* 1986;96(12): 1330–1334

204. Gebhart DE. Tympanostomy tubes in the otitis media prone child. *Laryngoscope.* 1981;91(6):849–866

205. Casselbrant ML, Kaleida PH, Rockette HE, et al. Efficacy of antimicrobial prophylaxis and of tympanostomy tube insertion for prevention of recurrent acute otitis media: results of a randomized clinical trial. *Pediatr Infect Dis J.* 1992;11(4):278–286

206. El-Sayed Y. Treatment of recurrent acute otitis media chemoprophylaxis versus ventilation tubes. *Aust J Otolaryngol.* 1996; 2(4):352–355

207. McDonald S, Langton Hewer CD, Nunez DA. Grommets (ventilation tubes) for recurrent acute otitis media in children. *Cochrane Database Syst Rev.* 2008;(4): CD004741

208. Rosenfeld RM, Bhaya MH, Bower CM, et al. Impact of tympanostomy tubes on child quality of life. *Arch Otolaryngol Head Neck Surg.* 2000;126(5):585–592

209. Witsell DL, Stewart MG, Monsell EM, et al. The Cooperative Outcomes Group for ENT: a multicenter prospective cohort study on the outcomes of tympanostomy tubes for children with otitis media. *Otolaryngol Head Neck Surg.* 2005;132(2):180–188

210. Isaacson G. Six Sigma tympanostomy tube insertion: achieving the highest safety levels during residency training. *Otolaryngol Head Neck Surg.* 2008;139(3):353–357

211. Kay DJ, Nelson M, Rosenfeld RM. Meta-analysis of tympanostomy tube sequelae. *Otolaryngol Head Neck Surg.* 2001;124(4): 374–380

212. Koivunen P, Uhari M, Luotonen J, et al. Adenoidectomy versus chemoprophylaxis and placebo for recurrent acute otitis media in children aged under 2 years: randomised controlled trial. *BMJ.* 2004; 328(7438):487

213. Rosenfeld RM. Surgical prevention of otitis media. *Vaccine.* 2000;19(suppl 1):S134–S139

214. Centers for Disease Control and Prevention (CDC). Prevention and control of influenza with vaccines: recommendations of the Advisory Committee on Immunization Practices (ACIP), 2011. *MMWR Morb Mortal Wkly Rep.* 2011;60(33):1128–1132

215. American Academy of Pediatrics Committee on Infectious Diseases. Recommendations for prevention and control of influenza in children, 2011–2012. *Pediatrics.* 2011;128(4):813–825

216. Section on Breastfeeding. Breastfeeding and the use of human milk. *Pediatrics.* 2012;129(3). Available at: www.pediatrics.org/cgi/content/full/129/3/e827

217. Pavia M, Bianco A, Nobile CG, Marinelli P, Angelillo IF. Efficacy of pneumococcal vaccination in children younger than 24 months: a meta-analysis. *Pediatrics.* 2009; 123(6). Available at: www.pediatrics.org/cgi/content/full/123/6/e1103

218. Eskola J, Kilpi T, Palmu A, et al; Finnish Otitis Media Study Group. Efficacy of a pneumococcal conjugate vaccine against acute otitis media. *N Engl J Med.* 2001;344(6):403–409

219. Black S, Shinefield H, Fireman B, et al; Northern California Kaiser Permanente Vaccine Study Center Group. Efficacy, safety and immunogenicity of heptavalent pneumococcal conjugate vaccine in children. *Pediatr Infect Dis J.* 2000;19(3): 187–195

220. Jacobs MR. Prevention of otitis media: role of pneumococcal conjugate vaccines in reducing incidence and antibiotic resistance. *J Pediatr.* 2002;141(2):287–293

221. Jansen AG, Hak E, Veenhoven RH, Damoiseaux RA, Schilder AG, Sanders EA. Pneumococcal conjugate vaccines for preventing otitis media. *Cochrane Database Syst Rev.* 2009;(2):CD001480

222. Fireman B, Black SB, Shinefield HR, Lee J, Lewis E, Ray P. Impact of the pneumococcal conjugate vaccine on otitis media. *Pediatr Infect Dis J.* 2003;22(1):10–16

223. Grijalva CG, Poehling KA, Nuorti JP, et al. National impact of universal childhood immunization with pneumococcal conjugate vaccine on otitis media. *Pediatr Infect Dis J.* 2006;118(3):865–873

224. Zhou F, Shefer A, Kong Y, Nuorti JP. Trends in acute otitis media-related health care utilization by privately insured young children in the United States, 1997–2004. *Pediatrics.* 2008;121(2):253–260

225. Poehling KA, Szilagyi PG, Grijalva CG, et al. Reduction of frequent otitis media and pressure-equalizing tube insertions in children after introduction of pneumococcal conjugate vaccine. *Pediatrics.* 2007; 119(4):707–715

226. Pelton SI. Prospects for prevention of otitis media. *Pediatr Infect Dis J.* 2007;26 (suppl 10):S20–S22

227. Pelton SI, Leibovitz E. Recent advances in otitis media. *Pediatr Infect Dis J.* 2009;28 (suppl 10):S133–S137

228. De Wals P, Erickson L, Poirier B, Pépin J, Pichichero ME. How to compare the efficacy of conjugate vaccines to prevent acute otitis media? *Vaccine.* 2009;27(21): 2877–2883

229. Plasschaert AI, Rovers MM, Schilder AG, Verheij TJ, Hak E. Trends in doctor consultations, antibiotic prescription, and specialist referrals for otitis media in children: 1995–2003. *Pediatrics.* 2006;117(6): 1879–1886

230. O'Brien MA, Prosser LA, Paradise JL, et al. New vaccines against otitis media: projected benefits and cost-effectiveness. *Pediatrics.* 2009;123(6):1452–1463

231. Hanage WP, Auranen K, Syrjänen R, et al. Ability of pneumococcal serotypes and clones to cause acute otitis media: implications for the prevention of otitis media by conjugate vaccines. *Infect Immun.* 2004; 72(1):76–81

232. Prymula R, Peeters P, Chrobok V, et al. Pneumococcal capsular polysaccharides

conjugated to protein D for prevention of acute otitis media caused by both Streptococcus pneumoniae and non-typable *Haemophilus influenzae*: a randomised double-blind efficacy study. *Lancet*. 2006; 367(9512):740–748

233. Prymula R, Schuerman L. 10-valent pneumococcal nontypeable *Haemophilus influenzae* PD conjugate vaccine: Synflorix. *Expert Rev Vaccines*. 2009;8(11):1479–1500

234. Schuerman L, Borys D, Hoet B, Forsgren A, Prymula R. Prevention of otitis media: now a reality? *Vaccine*. 2009;27(42):5748–5754

235. Heikkinen T, Ruuskanen O, Waris M, Ziegler T, Arola M, Halonen P. Influenza vaccination in the prevention of acute otitis media in children. *Am J Dis Child*. 1991;145(4):445–448

236. Clements DA, Langdon L, Bland C, Walter E. Influenza A vaccine decreases the incidence of otitis media in 6- to 30-month-old children in day care. *Arch Pediatr Adolesc Med*. 1995;149(10):1113–1117

237. Belshe RB, Gruber WC. Prevention of otitis media in children with live attenuated influenza vaccine given intranasally. *Pediatr Infect Dis J*. 2000;19(suppl 5):S66–S71

238. Marchisio P, Cavagna R, Maspes B, et al. Efficacy of intranasal virosomal influenza vaccine in the prevention of recurrent acute otitis media in children. *Clin Infect Dis*. 2002;35(2):168–174

239. Ozgur SK, Beyazova U, Kemaloglu YK, et al. Effectiveness of inactivated influenza vaccine for prevention of otitis media in children. *Pediatr Infect Dis J*. 2006;25(5): 401–404

240. Block SL, Heikkinen T, Toback SL, Zheng W, Ambrose CS. The efficacy of live attenuated influenza vaccine against influenza-associated acute otitis media in children. *Pediatr Infect Dis J*. 2011;30(3):203–207

241. Ashkenazi S, Vertruyen A, Arístegui J, et al; CAIV-T Study Group. Superior relative efficacy of live attenuated influenza vaccine compared with inactivated influenza vaccine in young children with recurrent respiratory tract infections. *Pediatr Infect Dis J*. 2006;25(10):870–879

242. Belshe RB, Edwards KM, Vesikari T, et al; CAIV-T Comparative Efficacy Study Group. Live attenuated versus inactivated influenza vaccine in infants and young children [published correction appears in *N Engl J Med*. 2007;356(12):1283]. *N Engl J Med*. 2007;356(7):685–696

243. Bracco Neto H, Farhat CK, Tregnaghi MW, et al; D153-P504 LAIV Study Group. Efficacy and safety of 1 and 2 doses of live attenuated influenza vaccine in vaccine-naive children. *Pediatr Infect Dis J*. 2009;28(5): 365–371

244. Tam JS, Capeding MR, Lum LC, et al; Pan-Asian CAIV-T Pediatric Efficacy Trial Network. Efficacy and safety of a live attenuated, cold-adapted influenza vaccine, trivalent against culture-confirmed influenza in young children in Asia. *Pediatr Infect Dis J*. 2007;26(7):619–628

245. Vesikari T, Fleming DM, Aristegui JF, et al; CAIV-T Pediatric Day Care Clinical Trial Network. Safety, efficacy, and effectiveness of cold-adapted influenza vaccine-trivalent against community-acquired, culture-confirmed influenza in young children attending day care. *Pediatrics*. 2006;118(6):2298–2312

246. Forrest BD, Pride MW, Dunning AJ, et al. Correlation of cellular immune responses with protection against culture-confirmed influenza virus in young children. *Clin Vaccine Immunol*. 2008;15(7): 1042–1053

247. Lum LC, Borja-Tabora CF, Breiman RF, et al. Influenza vaccine concurrently administered with a combination measles, mumps, and rubella vaccine to young children. *Vaccine*. 2010;28(6):1566–1574

248. Belshe RB, Mendelman PM, Treanor J, et al. The efficacy of live attenuated, cold-adapted, trivalent, intranasal influenzavirus vaccine in children. *N Engl J Med*. 1998;338(20): 1405–1412

249. Daly KA, Giebink GS. Clinical epidemiology of otitis media. *Pediatr Infect Dis J*. 2000; 19(suppl 5):S31–S36

250. Duncan B, Ey J, Holberg CJ, Wright AL, Martinez FD, Taussig LM. Exclusive breastfeeding for at least 4 months protects against otitis media. *Pediatrics*. 1993;91(5): 867–872

251. Duffy LC, Faden H, Wasielewski R, Wolf J, Krystofik D. Exclusive breastfeeding protects against bacterial colonization and day care exposure to otitis media. *Pediatrics*. 1997;100(4). Available at: www.pediatrics.org/cgi/content/full/100/4/e7

252. Paradise JL. Short-course antimicrobial treatment for acute otitis media: not best for infants and young children. *JAMA*. 1997;278(20):1640–1642

253. Scariati PD, Grummer-Strawn LM, Fein SB. A longitudinal analysis of infant morbidity and the extent of breastfeeding in the United States. *Pediatrics*. 1997;99(6). Available at: www.pediatrics.org/cgi/content/full/99/6/e5

254. McNiel ME, Labbok MH, Abrahams SW. What are the risks associated with formula feeding? A re-analysis and review. *Breastfeed Rev*. 2010;18(2):25–32

255. Chantry CJ, Howard CR, Auinger P. Full breastfeeding duration and associated decrease in respiratory tract infection in US children. *Pediatrics*. 2006;117(2):425–432

256. Hatakka K, Piirainen L, Pohjavuori S, Poussa T, Savilahti E, Korpela R. Factors associated with acute respiratory illness in day care children. *Scand J Infect Dis*. 2010;42(9):704–711

257. Ladomenou F, Kafatos A, Tselentis Y, Galanakis E. Predisposing factors for acute otitis media in infancy. *J Infect*. 2010;61(1):49–53

258. Ladomenou F, Moschandreas J, Kafatos A, Tselentis Y, Galanakis E. Protective effect of exclusive breastfeeding against infections during infancy: a prospective study. *Arch Dis Child*. 2010;95(12):1004–1008

259. Duijts L, Jaddoe VW, Hofman A, Moll HA. Prolonged and exclusive breastfeeding reduces the risk of infectious diseases in infancy. *Pediatrics*. 2010;126(1). Available at: www.pediatrics.org/cgi/content/full/126/1/e18

260. Best D; Committee on Environmental Health; Committee on Native American Child Health; Committee on Adolescence. From the American Academy of Pediatrics: technical report—secondhand and prenatal tobacco smoke exposure. *Pediatrics*. 2009;124(5). Available at: www.pediatrics.org/cgi/content/full/124/5/e1017

261. Etzel RA, Pattishall EN, Haley NJ, Fletcher RH, Henderson FW. Passive smoking and middle ear effusion among children in day care. *Pediatrics*. 1992;90(2 pt 1): 228–232

262. Ilicali OC, Keleş N, Değer K, Savaş I. Relationship of passive cigarette smoking to otitis media. *Arch Otolaryngol Head Neck Surg*. 1999;125(7):758–762

263. Wellington M, Hall CB. Pacifier as a risk factor for acute otitis media [letter]. *Pediatrics*. 2002;109(2):351–352, author reply 353

264. Kerstein R. Otitis media: prevention instead of prescription. *Br J Gen Pract*. 2008;58(550):364–365

265. Brown CE, Magnuson B. On the physics of the infant feeding bottle and middle ear sequela: ear disease in infants can be associated with bottle feeding. *Int J Pediatr Otorhinolaryngol*. 2000;54(1):13–20

266. Niemelä M, Pihakari O, Pokka T, Uhari M. Pacifier as a risk factor for acute otitis media: a randomized, controlled trial of parental counseling. *Pediatrics*. 2000;106(3): 483–488

267. Tully SB, Bar-Haim Y, Bradley RL. Abnormal tympanography after supine bottle feeding. *J Pediatr.* 1995;126(6):S105–S111

268. Rovers MM, Numans ME, Langenbach E, Grobbee DE, Verheij TJ, Schilder AG. Is pacifier use a risk factor for acute otitis media? A dynamic cohort study. *Fam Pract.* 2008;25(4):233–236

269. Adderson EE. Preventing otitis media: medical approaches. *Pediatr Ann.* 1998;27(2):101–107

270. Azarpazhooh A, Limeback H, Lawrence HP, Shah PS. Xylitol for preventing acute otitis media in children up to 12 years of age. *Cochrane Database Syst Rev.* 2011;(11): CD007095

271. Hautalahti O, Renko M, Tapiainen T, Kontiokari T, Pokka T, Uhari M. Failure of xylitol given three times a day for preventing acute otitis media. *Pediatr Infect Dis J.* 2007;26(5):423–427

272. Tapiainen T, Luotonen L, Kontiokari T, Renko M, Uhari M. Xylitol administered only during respiratory infections failed to prevent acute otitis media. *Pediatrics.* 2002;109(2). Available at: www.pediatrics.org/cgi/content/full/109/2/e19

273. Uhari M, Kontiokari T, Koskela M, Niemelä M. Xylitol chewing gum in prevention of acute otitis media: double blind randomised trial. *BMJ.* 1996;313(7066):1180–1184

274. Uhari M, Kontiokari T, Niemelä M. A novel use of xylitol sugar in preventing acute otitis media. *Pediatrics.* 1998;102(4 pt 1): 879–884

275. O'Brien MA, Prosser LA, Paradise JL, et al. New vaccines against otitis media: projected benefits and cost-effectiveness. *Pediatrics.* 2009;123(6):1452–1463

(Continued from first page)

All clinical practice guidelines from the American Academy of Pediatrics automatically expire 5 years after publication unless reaffirmed, revised, or retired at or before that time.

www.pediatrics.org/cgi/doi/10.1542/peds.2012-3488

doi:10.1542/peds.2012-3488

PEDIATRICS (ISSN Numbers: Print, 0031-4005; Online, 1098-4275).

Otitis Media With Effusion

- *Clinical Practice Guideline*

AMERICAN ACADEMY OF PEDIATRICS

CLINICAL PRACTICE GUIDELINE

American Academy of Family Physicians, American Academy of Otolaryngology-Head and Neck Surgery, and American Academy of Pediatrics Subcommittee on Otitis Media With Effusion

Otitis Media With Effusion

ABSTRACT. The clinical practice guideline on otitis media with effusion (OME) provides evidence-based recommendations on diagnosing and managing OME in children. This is an update of the 1994 clinical practice guideline "Otitis Media With Effusion in Young Children," which was developed by the Agency for Healthcare Policy and Research (now the Agency for Healthcare Research and Quality). In contrast to the earlier guideline, which was limited to children 1 to 3 years old with no craniofacial or neurologic abnormalities or sensory deficits, the updated guideline applies to children aged 2 months through 12 years with or without developmental disabilities or underlying conditions that predispose to OME and its sequelae. The American Academy of Pediatrics, American Academy of Family Physicians, and American Academy of Otolaryngology-Head and Neck Surgery selected a subcommittee composed of experts in the fields of primary care, otolaryngology, infectious diseases, epidemiology, hearing, speech and language, and advanced-practice nursing to revise the OME guideline.

The subcommittee made a strong recommendation that clinicians use pneumatic otoscopy as the primary diagnostic method and distinguish OME from acute otitis media.

The subcommittee made recommendations that clinicians should 1) document the laterality, duration of effusion, and presence and severity of associated symptoms at each assessment of the child with OME, 2) distinguish the child with OME who is at risk for speech, language, or learning problems from other children with OME and more promptly evaluate hearing, speech, language, and need for intervention in children at risk, and 3) manage the child with OME who is not at risk with watchful waiting for 3 months from the date of effusion onset (if known) or diagnosis (if onset is unknown).

The subcommittee also made recommendations that 4) hearing testing be conducted when OME persists for 3 months or longer or at any time that language delay, learning problems, or a significant hearing loss is suspected in a child with OME, 5) children with persistent OME who are not at risk should be reexamined at 3- to 6-month intervals until the effusion is no longer present, significant hearing loss is identified, or structural abnormalities of the eardrum or middle ear are suspected, and 6) when a child becomes a surgical candidate (tympanostomy tube insertion is the preferred initial procedure). Adenoidectomy should not be performed unless a distinct indication exists (nasal obstruction, chronic adenoiditis); repeat surgery consists of adenoidectomy plus myringotomy with or without tubeinsertion. Tonsillectomy alone or myringotomy alone should not be used to treat OME.

The subcommittee made negative recommendations that 1) population-based screening programs for OME not be performed in healthy, asymptomatic children, and 2) because antihistamines and decongestants are ineffective for OME, they should not be used for treatment; antimicrobials and corticosteroids do not have long-term efficacy and should not be used for routine management.

The subcommittee gave as options that 1) tympanometry can be used to confirm the diagnosis of OME and 2) when children with OME are referred by the primary clinician for evaluation by an otolaryngologist, audiologist, or speech-language pathologist, the referring clinician should document the effusion duration and specific reason for referral (evaluation, surgery) and provide additional relevant information such as history of acute otitis media and developmental status of the child. The subcommittee made no recommendations for 1) complementary and alternative medicine as a treatment for OME, based on a lack of scientific evidence documenting efficacy, or 2) allergy management as a treatment for OME, based on insufficient evidence of therapeutic efficacy or a causal relationship between allergy and OME. Last, the panel compiled a list of research needs based on limitations of the evidence reviewed.

The purpose of this guideline is to inform clinicians of evidence-based methods to identify, monitor, and manage OME in children aged 2 months through 12 years. The guideline may not apply to children more than 12 years old, because OME is uncommon and the natural history is likely to differ from younger children who experience rapid developmental change. The target population includes children with or without developmental disabilities or underlying conditions that predispose to OME and its sequelae. The guideline is intended for use by providers of health care to children, including primary care and specialist physicians, nurses and nurse practitioners, physician assistants, audiologists, speech-language pathologists, and child-development specialists. The guideline is applicable to any setting in which children with OME would be identified, monitored, or managed.

This guideline is not intended as a sole source of guidance in evaluating children with OME. Rather, it is designed to assist primary care and other clinicians by providing an evidence-based framework for decision-making strategies. It is not intended to replace clinical judgment or establish a protocol for all children with this condition and may not provide the only appropriate approach to diagnosing and managing this problem. *Pediatrics* 2004;113:1412–1429; *acute otitis media, antibacterial, antibiotic.*

This document was approved by the American Academy of Otolaryngology–Head and Neck Surgery Foundation, Inc and the American Academy of Pediatrics, and is published in the May 2004 issue of *Otolaryngology–Head and Neck Surgery* and the May 2004 issue of *Pediatrics*.
PEDIATRICS (ISSN 0031 4005). Copyright © 2004 by the American Academy of Otolaryngology–Head and Neck Surgery Foundation, Inc and the American Academy of Pediatrics.

ABBREVIATIONS. OME, otitis media with effusion; AOM, acute otitis media; AAP, American Academy of Pediatrics; AHRQ, Agency for Healthcare Research and Quality; EPC, Southern California Evidence-Based Practice Center; CAM, complementary and alternative medicine; HL, hearing level.

Otitis media with effusion (OME) as discussed in this guideline is defined as the presence of fluid in the middle ear without signs or symptoms of acute ear infection.[1,2] OME is considered distinct from acute otitis media (AOM), which is defined as a history of acute onset of signs and symptoms, the presence of middle-ear effusion, and signs and symptoms of middle-ear inflammation. Persistent middle-ear fluid from OME results in decreased mobility of the tympanic membrane and serves as a barrier to sound conduction.[3] Approximately 2.2 million diagnosed episodes of OME occur annually in the United States, yielding a combined direct and indirect annual cost estimate of $4.0 billion.[2]

OME may occur spontaneously because of poor eustachian tube function or as an inflammatory response following AOM. Approximately 90% of children (80% of individual ears) have OME at some time before school age,[4] most often between ages 6 months and 4 years.[5] In the first year of life, >50% of children will experience OME, increasing to >60% by 2 years.[6] Many episodes resolve spontaneously within 3 months, but ~30% to 40% of children have recurrent OME, and 5% to 10% of episodes last 1 year or longer.[1,4,7]

The primary outcomes considered in the guideline include hearing loss; effects on speech, language, and learning; physiologic sequelae; health care utilization (medical, surgical); and quality of life.[1,2] The high prevalence of OME, difficulties in diagnosis and assessing duration, increased risk of conductive hearing loss, potential impact on language and cognition, and significant practice variations in management[8] make OME an important condition for the use of up-to-date evidence-based practice guidelines.

METHODS

General Methods and Literature Search

In developing an evidence-based clinical practice guideline on managing OME, the American Academy of Pediatrics (AAP), American Academy of Family Physicians, and American Academy of Otolaryngology-Head and Neck Surgery worked with the Agency for Healthcare Research and Quality (AHRQ) and other organizations. This effort included representatives from each partnering organization along with liaisons from audiology, speech-language pathology, informatics, and advanced-practice nursing. The most current literature on managing children with OME was reviewed, and research questions were developed to guide the evidence-review process.

The AHRQ report on OME from the Southern California Evidence-Based Practice Center (EPC) focused on key questions of natural history, diagnostic methods, and long-term speech, language, and hearing outcomes.[2] Searches were conducted through January 2000 in Medline, Embase, and the Cochrane Library. Additional articles were identified by review of reference listings in proceedings, reports, and other guidelines. The EPC accepted 970 articles for full review after screening 3200 abstracts. The EPC reviewed articles by using established quality criteria[9,10] and included randomized trials, prospective cohorts, and validations of diagnostic tests (validating cohort studies).

The AAP subcommittee on OME updated the AHRQ review with articles identified by an electronic Medline search through April 2003 and with additional material identified manually by subcommittee members. Copies of relevant articles were distributed to the subcommittee for consideration. A specific search for articles relevant to complementary and alternative medicine (CAM) was performed by using Medline and the Allied and Complementary Medicine Database through April 2003. Articles relevant to allergy and OME were identified by using Medline through April 2003. The subcommittee met 3 times over a 1-year period, ending in May 2003, with interval electronic review and feedback on each guideline draft to ensure accuracy of content and consistency with standardized criteria for reporting clinical practice guidelines.[11]

In May 2003, the Guidelines Review Group of the Yale Center for Medical Informatics used the Guideline Elements Model[12] to categorize content of the present draft guideline. Policy statements were parsed into component decision variables and actions and then assessed for decidability and executability. Quality appraisal using established criteria[13] was performed with Guideline Elements Model-Q Online.[14,15] Implementation issues were predicted by using the Implementability Rating Profile, an instrument under development by the Yale Guidelines Review Group (R. Shiffman, MD, written communication, May 2003). OME subcommittee members received summary results and modified an advanced draft of the guideline.

The final draft practice guideline underwent extensive peer review by numerous entities identified by the subcommittee. Comments were compiled and reviewed by the subcommittee cochairpersons. The recommendations contained in the practice guideline are based on the best available published data through April 2003. Where data are lacking, a combination of clinical experience and expert consensus was used. A scheduled review process will occur 5 years from publication or sooner if new compelling evidence warrants earlier consideration.

Classification of Evidence-Based Statements

Guidelines are intended to reduce inappropriate variations in clinical care, produce optimal health outcomes for patients, and minimize harm. The evidence-based approach to guideline development requires that the evidence supporting a policy be identified, appraised, and summarized and that an explicit link between evidence and statements be defined. Evidence-based statements reflect the quality of evidence and the balance of benefit and harm that is anticipated when the statement is followed. The AAP definitions for evidence-based statements[16] are listed in Tables 1 and 2.

Guidelines are never intended to overrule professional judgment; rather, they may be viewed as a relative constraint on individual clinician discretion in a particular clinical circumstance. Less frequent variation in practice is expected for a strong recommendation than might be expected with a recommendation. Options offer the most opportunity for practice variability.[17] All clinicians should always act and decide in a way that they believe will best serve their patients' interests and needs regardless of guideline recommendations. Guidelines represent the best judgment of a team of experienced clinicians and methodologists addressing the scientific evidence for a particular topic.[16]

Making recommendations about best practices involves value judgments on the desirability of various outcomes associated with management options. Value judgments applied by the OME subcommittee were made in an effort to minimize harm and diminish unnecessary therapy. Emphasis was placed on promptly identifying and managing children at risk for speech, language, or learning problems to maximize opportunities for beneficial outcomes. Direct costs also were considered in the statements concerning diagnosis and screening and to a lesser extent in other statements.

1A. PNEUMATIC OTOSCOPY: CLINICIANS SHOULD USE PNEUMATIC OTOSCOPY AS THE PRIMARY DIAGNOSTIC METHOD FOR OME, AND OME SHOULD BE DISTINGUISHED FROM AOM

This is a strong recommendation based on systematic review of cohort studies and the preponderance of benefit over harm.

TABLE 1. Guideline Definitions for Evidence-Based Statements

Statement	Definition	Implication
Strong Recommendation	A strong recommendation means that the subcommittee believes that the benefits of the recommended approach clearly exceed the harms (or that the harms clearly exceed the benefits in the case of a strong negative recommendation) and that the quality of the supporting evidence is excellent (grade A or B).* In some clearly identified circumstances, strong recommendations may be made based on lesser evidence when high-quality evidence is impossible to obtain and the anticipated benefits strongly outweigh the harms.	Clinicians should follow a strong recommendation unless a clear and compelling rationale for an alternative approach is present.
Recommendation	A recommendation means that the subcommittee believes that the benefits exceed the harms (or that the harms exceed the benefits in the case of a negative recommendation), but the quality of evidence is not as strong (grade B or C).* In some clearly identified circumstances, recommendations may be made based on lesser evidence when high-quality evidence is impossible to obtain and the anticipated benefits outweigh the harms.	Clinicians also should generally follow a recommendation but should remain alert to new information and sensitive to patient preferences.
Option	An option means that either the quality of evidence that exists is suspect (grade D)* or that well-done studies (grade A, B, or C)* show little clear advantage to one approach versus another.	Clinicians should be flexible in their decision-making regarding appropriate practice, although they may set boundaries on alternatives; patient preference should have a substantial influencing role.
No Recommendation	No recommendation means that there is both a lack of pertinent evidence (grade D)* and an unclear balance between benefits and harms.	Clinicians should feel little constraint in their decision-making and be alert to new published evidence that clarifies the balance of benefit versus harm; patient preference should have a substantial influencing role.

* See Table 2 for the definitions of evidence grades.

TABLE 2. Evidence Quality for Grades of Evidence

Grade	Evidence Quality
A	Well-designed, randomized, controlled trials or diagnostic studies performed on a population similar to the guideline's target population
B	Randomized, controlled trials or diagnostic studies with minor limitations; overwhelmingly consistent evidence from observational studies
C	Observational studies (case-control and cohort design)
D	Expert opinion, case reports, or reasoning from first principles (bench research or animal studies)

1B. TYMPANOMETRY: TYMPANOMETRY CAN BE USED TO CONFIRM THE DIAGNOSIS OF OME

This option is based on cohort studies and a balance of benefit and harm.

Diagnosing OME correctly is fundamental to proper management. Moreover, OME must be differentiated from AOM to avoid unnecessary antimicrobial use.[18,19]

OME is defined as fluid in the middle ear without signs or symptoms of acute ear infection.[2] The tympanic membrane is often cloudy with distinctly impaired mobility,[20] and an air-fluid level or bubble may be visible in the middle ear. Conversely, diagnosing AOM requires a history of acute onset of signs and symptoms, the presence of middle-ear effusion, and signs and symptoms of middle-ear inflammation. The critical distinguishing feature is that only AOM has acute signs and symptoms. Distinct redness of the tympanic membrane should not be a criterion for prescribing antibiotics, because it has poor predictive value for AOM and is present in ~5% of ears with OME.[20]

The AHRQ evidence report[2] systematically reviewed the sensitivity, specificity, and predictive values of 9 diagnostic methods for OME. Pneumatic otoscopy had the best balance of sensitivity and specificity, consistent with the 1994 guideline.[1] Meta-analysis revealed a pooled sensitivity of 94% (95% confidence interval: 91%–96%) and specificity of 80% (95% confidence interval: 75%–86%) for validated observers using pneumatic otoscopy versus myringotomy as the gold standard. Pneumatic otoscopy therefore should remain the primary method of OME diagnosis, because the instrument is readily available in practice settings, cost-effective, and accurate in experienced hands. Non–pneumatic otoscopy is not advised for primary diagnosis.

The accuracy of pneumatic otoscopy in routine clinical practice may be less than that shown in published results, because clinicians have varying training and experience.[21,22] When the diagnosis of OME is uncertain, tympanometry or acoustic reflectometry should be considered as an adjunct to pneumatic otoscopy. Tympanometry with a standard 226-Hz probe tone is reliable for infants 4 months old or older and has good interobserver agreement of curve patterns in routine clinical practice.[23,24] Younger infants require specialized equipment with a higher probe tone frequency. Tympanometry generates costs related to instrument purchase, annual calibration, and test administration. Acoustic reflectometry with spectral gradient analysis is a low-cost alternative to tympanometry that does not require an airtight seal in the ear canal; however, validation studies primarily have used children 2 years old or older with a high prevalence of OME.[25–27]

Although no research studies have examined whether pneumatic otoscopy causes discomfort, expert consensus suggests that the procedure does not have to be painful, especially when symptoms of acute infection (AOM) are absent. A nontraumatic examination is facilitated by using a gentle touch, restraining the child properly when necessary, and inserting the speculum only into the outer one third (cartilaginous portion) of the ear canal.[28] The pneumatic bulb should be compressed slightly before insertion, because OME often is associated with a negative middle-ear pressure, which can be assessed more accurately by releasing the already compressed bulb. The otoscope must be fully charged, the bulb (halogen or xenon) bright and luminescent,[29] and the insufflator bulb attached tightly to the head to avoid the loss of an air seal. The window must also be sealed.

Evidence Profile: Pneumatic Otoscopy

- Aggregate evidence quality: A, diagnostic studies in relevant populations.
- Benefit: improved diagnostic accuracy; inexpensive equipment.
- Harm: cost of training clinicians in pneumatic otoscopy.
- Benefits-harms assessment: preponderance of benefit over harm.
- Policy level: strong recommendation.

Evidence Profile: Tympanometry

- Aggregate evidence quality: B, diagnostic studies with minor limitations.
- Benefit: increased diagnostic accuracy beyond pneumatic otoscopy; documentation.
- Harm: acquisition cost, administrative burden, and recalibration.
- Benefits-harms assessment: balance of benefit and harm.
- Policy level: option.

1C. SCREENING: POPULATION-BASED SCREENING PROGRAMS FOR OME ARE NOT RECOMMENDED IN HEALTHY, ASYMPTOMATIC CHILDREN

This recommendation is based on randomized, controlled trials and cohort studies, with a preponderance of harm over benefit.

This recommendation concerns population-based screening programs of all children in a community or a school without regard to any preexisting symptoms or history of disease. This recommendation does not address hearing screening or monitoring of specific children with previous or recurrent OME.

OME is highly prevalent in young children. Screening surveys of healthy children ranging in age from infancy to 5 years old show a 15% to 40% point prevalence of middle-ear effusion.[5,7,30–36] Among children examined at regular intervals for a year, ~50% to 60% of child care center attendees[32] and 25% of school-aged children[37] were found to have a middle-ear effusion at some time during the examination period, with peak incidence during the winter months.

Population-based screening has not been found to influence short-term language outcomes,[33] and its long-term effects have not been evaluated in a randomized, clinical trial. Therefore, the recommendation against screening is based not only on the ability to identify OME but more importantly on a lack of demonstrable benefits from treating children so identified that exceed the favorable natural history of the disease. The New Zealand Health Technology Assessment[38] could not determine whether preschool screening for OME was effective. More recently, the Canadian Task Force on Preventive Health Care[39] reported that insufficient evidence was available to recommend including or excluding routine early screening for OME. Although screening for OME is not inherently harmful, potential risks include inaccurate diagnoses, overtreating self-limited disease, parental anxiety, and the costs of screening and unnecessary treatment.

Population-based screening is appropriate for conditions that are common, can be detected by a sensitive and specific test, and benefit from early detection and treatment.[40] The first 2 requirements are fulfilled by OME, which affects up to 80% of children by school entry[2,5,7] and can be screened easily with tympanometry (see recommendation 1B). Early detection and treatment of OME identified by screening, however, have not been shown to improve intelligence, receptive language, or expressive language.[2,39,41,42] Therefore, population-based screening for early detection of OME in asymptomatic children has not been shown to improve outcomes and is not recommended.

Evidence Profile: Screening

- Aggregate evidence quality: B, randomized, controlled trials with minor limitations and consistent evidence from observational studies.
- Benefit: potentially improved developmental outcomes, which have not been demonstrated in the best current evidence.

- Harm: inaccurate diagnosis (false-positive or false-negative), overtreating self-limited disease, parental anxiety, cost of screening, and/or unnecessary treatment.
- Benefits-harms assessment: preponderance of harm over benefit.
- Policy level: recommendation against.

2. DOCUMENTATION: CLINICIANS SHOULD DOCUMENT THE LATERALITY, DURATION OF EFFUSION, AND PRESENCE AND SEVERITY OF ASSOCIATED SYMPTOMS AT EACH ASSESSMENT OF THE CHILD WITH OME

This recommendation is based on observational studies and strong preponderance of benefit over harm.

Documentation in the medical record facilitates diagnosis and treatment and communicates pertinent information to other clinicians to ensure patient safety and reduce medical errors.[43] Management decisions in children with OME depend on effusion duration and laterality plus the nature and severity of associated symptoms. Therefore, these features should be documented at every medical encounter for OME. Although no studies have addressed documentation for OME specifically, there is room for improvement in documentation of ambulatory care medical records.[44]

Ideally, the time of onset and laterality of OME can be defined through diagnosis of an antecedent AOM, a history of acute onset of signs or symptoms directly referable to fluid in the middle ear, or the presence of an abnormal audiogram or tympanogram closely after a previously normal test. Unfortunately, these conditions are often lacking, and the clinician is forced to speculate on the onset and duration of fluid in the middle ear(s) in a child found to have OME at a routine office visit or school screening audiometry.

In ~40% to 50% of cases of OME, neither the affected children nor their parents or caregivers describe significant complaints referable to a middle-ear effusion.[45,46] In some children, however, OME may have associated signs and symptoms caused by inflammation or the presence of effusion (not acute infection) that should be documented, such as

- Mild intermittent ear pain, fullness, or "popping"
- Secondary manifestations of ear pain in infants, which may include ear rubbing, excessive irritability, and sleep disturbances
- Failure of infants to respond appropriately to voices or environmental sounds, such as not turning accurately toward the sound source
- Hearing loss, even when not specifically described by the child, suggested by seeming lack of attentiveness, behavioral changes, failure to respond to normal conversational-level speech, or the need for excessively high sound levels when using audio equipment or viewing television
- Recurrent episodes of AOM with persistent OME between episodes
- Problems with school performance
- Balance problems, unexplained clumsiness, or delayed gross motor development[47–50]
- Delayed speech or language development

The laterality (unilateral versus bilateral), duration of effusion, and presence and severity of associated symptoms should be documented in the medical record at each assessment of the child with OME. When OME duration is uncertain, the clinician must take whatever evidence is at hand and make a reasonable estimate.

Evidence Profile: Documentation

- Aggregate evidence quality: C, observational studies.
- Benefits: defines severity, duration has prognostic value, facilitates future communication with other clinicians, supports appropriate timing of intervention, and, if consistently unilateral, may identify a problem with specific ear other than OME (eg, retraction pocket or cholesteatoma).
- Harm: administrative burden.
- Benefits-harms assessment: preponderance of benefit over harm.
- Policy level: recommendation.

3. CHILD AT RISK: CLINICIANS SHOULD DISTINGUISH THE CHILD WITH OME WHO IS AT RISK FOR SPEECH, LANGUAGE, OR LEARNING PROBLEMS FROM OTHER CHILDREN WITH OME AND SHOULD EVALUATE HEARING, SPEECH, LANGUAGE, AND NEED FOR INTERVENTION MORE PROMPTLY

This recommendation is based on case series, the preponderance of benefit over harm, and ethical limitations in studying children with OME who are at risk.

The panel defines the child at risk as one who is at increased risk for developmental difficulties (delay or disorder) because of sensory, physical, cognitive, or behavioral factors listed in Table 3. These factors are not caused by OME but can make the child less tolerant of hearing loss or vestibular problems secondary to middle-ear effusion. In contrast the child with OME who is not at risk is otherwise healthy and does not have any of the factors shown in Table 3.

Earlier guidelines for managing OME have applied only to young children who are healthy and exhibit no developmental delays.[1] Studies of the relationship between OME and hearing loss or speech/language development typically exclude children with craniofacial anomalies, genetic syndromes, and other developmental disorders. Therefore, the available literature mainly applies to otherwise healthy children who meet inclusion criteria for randomized,

TABLE 3. Risk Factors for Developmental Difficulties*

Permanent hearing loss independent of OME
Suspected or diagnosed speech and language delay or disorder
Autism-spectrum disorder and other pervasive developmental disorders
Syndromes (eg, Down) or craniofacial disorders that include cognitive, speech, and language delays
Blindness or uncorrectable visual impairment
Cleft palate with or without associated syndrome
Developmental delay

* Sensory, physical, cognitive, or behavioral factors that place children who have OME at an increased risk for developmental difficulties (delay or disorder).

controlled trials. Few, if any, existing studies dealing with developmental sequelae caused by hearing loss from OME can be generalized to children who are at risk.

Children who are at risk for speech or language delay would likely be affected additionally by hearing problems from OME,[51] although definitive studies are lacking. For example, small comparative studies of children or adolescents with Down syndrome[52] or cerebral palsy[53] show poorer articulation and receptive language associated with a history of early otitis media. Large studies are unlikely to be forthcoming because of methodologic and ethical difficulties inherent in studying children who are delayed or at risk for further delays. Therefore, clinicians who manage children with OME should determine whether other conditions coexist that put a child at risk for developmental delay (Table 3) and then take these conditions into consideration when planning assessment and management.

Children with craniofacial anomalies (eg, cleft palate; Down syndrome; Robin sequence; coloboma, heart defect, choanal atresia, retarded growth and development, genital anomaly, and ear defect with deafness [CHARGE] association) have a higher prevalence of chronic OME, hearing loss (conductive and sensorineural), and speech or language delay than do children without these anomalies.[54–57] Other children may not be more prone to OME but are likely to have speech and language disorders, such as those children with permanent hearing loss independent of OME,[58,59] specific language impairment,[60] autism-spectrum disorders,[61] or syndromes that adversely affect cognitive and linguistic development. Some retrospective studies[52,62,63] have found that hearing loss caused by OME in children with cognitive delays, such as Down syndrome, has been associated with lower language levels. Children with language delays or disorders with OME histories perform more poorly on speech-perception tasks than do children with OME histories alone.[64,65]

Children with severe visual impairments may be more susceptible to the effects of OME, because they depend on hearing more than children with normal vision.[51] Any decrease in their most important remaining sensory input for language (hearing) may significantly compromise language development and their ability to interact and communicate with others. All children with severe visual impairments should be considered more vulnerable to OME sequelae, especially in the areas of balance, sound localization, and communication.

Management of the child with OME who is at increased risk for developmental delays should include hearing testing and speech and language evaluation and may include speech and language therapy concurrent with managing OME, hearing aids or other amplification devices for hearing loss independent of OME, tympanostomy tube insertion,[54,63,66,67] and hearing testing after OME resolves to document improvement, because OME can mask a permanent underlying hearing loss and delay detection.[59,68,69]

Evidence Profile: Child at Risk

- Aggregate evidence quality: C, observational studies of children at risk; D, expert opinion on the ability of prompt assessment and management to alter outcomes.
- Benefits: optimizing conditions for hearing, speech, and language; enabling children with special needs to reach their potential; avoiding limitations on the benefits of educational interventions because of hearing problems from OME.
- Harm: cost, time, and specific risks of medications or surgery.
- Benefits-harms assessment: exceptional preponderance of benefits over harm based on subcommittee consensus because of circumstances to date precluding randomized trials.
- Policy level: recommendation.

4. WATCHFUL WAITING: CLINICIANS SHOULD MANAGE THE CHILD WITH OME WHO IS NOT AT RISK WITH WATCHFUL WAITING FOR 3 MONTHS FROM THE DATE OF EFFUSION ONSET (IF KNOWN) OR DIAGNOSIS (IF ONSET IS UNKNOWN)

This recommendation is based on systematic review of cohort studies and the preponderance of benefit over harm.

This recommendation is based on the self-limited nature of most OME, which has been well documented in cohort studies and in control groups of randomized trials.[2,70]

The likelihood of spontaneous resolution of OME is determined by the cause and duration of effusion.[70] For example, ~75% to 90% of residual OME after an AOM episode resolves spontaneously by 3 months.[71–73] Similar outcomes of defined onset during a period of surveillance in a cohort study are observed for OME.[32,37] Another favorable situation involves improvement (not resolution) of newly detected OME defined as change in tympanogram from type B (flat curve) to non-B (anything other than a flat curve). Approximately 55% of children so defined improve by 3 months,[70] but one third will have OME relapse within the next 3 months.[4] Although a type B tympanogram is an imperfect measure of OME (81% sensitivity and 74% specificity versus myringotomy), it is the most widely reported measure suitable for deriving pooled resolution rates.[2,70]

Approximately 25% of newly detected OME of unknown prior duration in children 2 to 4 years old resolves by 3 months when resolution is defined as a change in tympanogram from type B to type A/C1 (peak pressure >200 daPa).[2,70,74–77] Resolution rates may be higher for infants and young children in whom the preexisting duration of effusion is generally shorter, and particularly for those observed prospectively in studies or in the course of well-child care. Documented bilateral OME of 3 months' duration or longer resolves spontaneously after 6 to 12 months in ~30% of children primarily 2 years old or older, with only marginal benefits if observed longer.[70]

Any intervention for OME (medical or surgical) other than observation carries some inherent harm. There is little harm associated with a specified period of observation in the child who is not at risk for speech, language, or learning problems. When observing children with OME, clinicians should inform the parent or caregiver that the child may experience reduced hearing until the effusion resolves, especially if it is bilateral. Clinicians may discuss strategies for optimizing the listening and learning environment until the effusion resolves. These strategies include speaking in close proximity to the child, facing the child and speaking clearly, repeating phrases when misunderstood, and providing preferential classroom seating.[78,79]

The recommendation for a 3-month period of observation is based on a clear preponderance of benefit over harm and is consistent with the original OME guideline intent of avoiding unnecessary surgery.[1] At the discretion of the clinician, this 3-month period of watchful waiting may include interval visits at which OME is monitored by using pneumatic otoscopy, tympanometry, or both. Factors to consider in determining the optimal interval(s) for follow-up include clinical judgment, parental comfort level, unique characteristics of the child and/or his environment, access to a health care system, and hearing levels (HLs) if known.

After documented resolution of OME in all affected ears, additional follow-up is unnecessary.

Evidence Profile: Watchful Waiting

- Aggregate evidence quality: B, systematic review of cohort studies.
- Benefit: avoid unnecessary interventions, take advantage of favorable natural history, and avoid unnecessary referrals and evaluations.
- Harm: delays in therapy for OME that will not resolve with observation; prolongation of hearing loss.
- Benefits-harms assessment: preponderance of benefit over harm.
- Policy level: recommendation.

5. MEDICATION: ANTIHISTAMINES AND DECONGESTANTS ARE INEFFECTIVE FOR OME AND ARE NOT RECOMMENDED FOR TREATMENT; ANTIMICROBIALS AND CORTICOSTEROIDS DO NOT HAVE LONG-TERM EFFICACY AND ARE NOT RECOMMENDED FOR ROUTINE MANAGEMENT

This recommendation is based on systematic review of randomized, controlled trials and the preponderance of harm over benefit.

Therapy for OME is appropriate only if persistent and clinically significant benefits can be achieved beyond spontaneous resolution. Although statistically significant benefits have been demonstrated for some medications, they are short-term and relatively small in magnitude. Moreover, significant adverse events may occur with all medical therapies.

The prior OME guideline[1] found no data supporting antihistamine-decongestant combinations in treating OME. Meta-analysis of 4 randomized trials showed no significant benefit for antihistamines or decongestants versus placebo. No additional studies have been published since 1994 to change this recommendation. Adverse effects of antihistamines and decongestants include insomnia, hyperactivity, drowsiness, behavioral change, and blood-pressure variability.

Long-term benefits of antimicrobial therapy for OME are unproved despite a modest short-term benefit for 2 to 8 weeks in randomized trials.[1,80,81] Initial benefits, however, can become nonsignificant within 2 weeks of stopping the medication.[82] Moreover, ~7 children would need to be treated with antimicrobials to achieve one short-term response.[1] Adverse effects of antimicrobials are significant and may include rashes, vomiting, diarrhea, allergic reactions, alteration of the child's nasopharyngeal flora, development of bacterial resistance,[83] and cost. Societal consequences include direct transmission of resistant bacterial pathogens in homes and child care centers.[84]

The prior OME guideline[1] did not recommend oral steroids for treating OME in children. A later meta-analysis[85] showed no benefit for oral steroid versus placebo within 2 weeks but did show a short-term benefit for oral steroid plus antimicrobial versus antimicrobial alone in 1 of 3 children treated. This benefit became nonsignificant after several weeks in a prior meta-analysis[1] and in a large, randomized trial.[86] Oral steroids can produce behavioral changes, increased appetite, and weight gain.[1] Additional adverse effects may include adrenal suppression, fatal varicella infection, and avascular necrosis of the femoral head.[3] Although intranasal steroids have fewer adverse effects, one randomized trial[87] showed statistically equivalent outcomes at 12 weeks for intranasal beclomethasone plus antimicrobials versus antimicrobials alone for OME.

Antimicrobial therapy with or without steroids has not been demonstrated to be effective in long-term resolution of OME, but in some cases this therapy can be considered an option because of short-term benefit in randomized trials, when the parent or caregiver expresses a strong aversion to impending surgery. In this circumstance, a single course of therapy for 10 to 14 days may be used. The likelihood that the OME will resolve long-term with these regimens is small, and prolonged or repetitive courses of antimicrobials or steroids are strongly not recommended.

Other nonsurgical therapies that are discussed in the OME literature include autoinflation of the eustachian tube, oral or intratympanic use of mucolytics, and systemic use of pharmacologic agents other than antimicrobials, steroids, and antihistamine-decongestants. Insufficient data exist for any of these therapies to be recommended in treating OME.[3]

Evidence Profile: Medication

- Aggregate evidence quality: A, systematic review of well-designed, randomized, controlled trials.

- Benefit: avoid side effects and reduce cost by not administering medications; avoid delays in definitive therapy caused by short-term improvement then relapse.
- Harm: adverse effects of specific medications as listed previously; societal impact of antimicrobial therapy on bacterial resistance and transmission of resistant pathogens.
- Benefits-harms assessment: preponderance of harm over benefit.
- Policy level: recommendation against.

6. HEARING AND LANGUAGE: HEARING TESTING IS RECOMMENDED WHEN OME PERSISTS FOR 3 MONTHS OR LONGER OR AT ANY TIME THAT LANGUAGE DELAY, LEARNING PROBLEMS, OR A SIGNIFICANT HEARING LOSS IS SUSPECTED IN A CHILD WITH OME; LANGUAGE TESTING SHOULD BE CONDUCTED FOR CHILDREN WITH HEARING LOSS

This recommendation is based on cohort studies and the preponderance of benefit over risk.

Hearing Testing

Hearing testing is recommended when OME persists for 3 months or longer or at any time that language delay, learning problems, or a significant hearing loss is suspected. Conductive hearing loss often accompanies OME[1,88] and may adversely affect binaural processing,[89] sound localization,[90] and speech perception in noise.[91–94] Hearing loss caused by OME may impair early language acquisition,[95–97] but the child's home environment has a greater impact on outcomes[98]; recent randomized trials[41,99,100] suggest no impact on children with OME who are not at risk as identified by screening or surveillance.

Studies examining hearing sensitivity in children with OME report that average pure-tone hearing loss at 4 frequencies (500, 1000, 2000, and 4000 Hz) ranges from normal hearing to moderate hearing loss (0–55 dB). The 50th percentile is an ~25-dB HL, and ~20% of ears exceed 35-dB HL.[101,102] Unilateral OME with hearing loss results in overall poorer binaural hearing than in infants with normal middle-ear function bilaterally.[103,104] However, based on limited research, there is evidence that children experiencing the greatest conductive hearing loss for the longest periods may be more likely to exhibit developmental and academic sequelae.[1,95,105]

Initial hearing testing for children 4 years old or older can be done in the primary care setting.[106] Testing should be performed in a quiet environment, preferably in a separate closed or sound-proofed area set aside specifically for that purpose. Conventional audiometry with earphones is performed with a fail criterion of more than 20-dB HL at 1 or more frequencies (500, 1000, 2000, and 4000 Hz) in either ear.[106,107] Methods not recommended as substitutes for primary care hearing testing include tympanometry and pneumatic otoscopy,[102] caregiver judgment regarding hearing loss,[108,109] speech audiometry, and tuning forks, acoustic reflectometry, and behavioral observation.[1]

Comprehensive audiologic evaluation is recommended for children who fail primary care testing, are less than 4 years old, or cannot be tested in the primary care setting. Audiologic assessment includes evaluating air-conduction and bone-conduction thresholds for pure tones, speech-detection or speech-recognition thresholds,[102] and measuring speech understanding if possible.[94] The method of assessment depends on the developmental age of the child and might include visual reinforcement or conditioned orienting-response audiometry for infants 6 to 24 months old, play audiometry for children 24 to 48 months old, or conventional screening audiometry for children 4 years old and older.[106] The auditory brainstem response and otoacoustic emission are tests of auditory pathway structural integrity, not hearing, and should not substitute for behavioral pure-tone audiometry.[106]

Language Testing

Language testing should be conducted for children with hearing loss (pure-tone average more than 20-dB HL on comprehensive audiometric evaluation). Testing for language delays is important, because communication is integral to all aspects of human functioning. Young children with speech and language delays during the preschool years are at risk for continued communication problems and later delays in reading and writing.[110–112] In one study, 6% to 8% of children 3 years old and 2% to 13% of kindergartners had language impairment.[113] Language intervention can improve communication and other functional outcomes for children with histories of OME.[114]

Children who experience repeated and persistent episodes of OME and associated hearing loss during early childhood may be at a disadvantage for learning speech and language.[79,115] Although Shekelle et al[2] concluded that there was no evidence to support the concern that OME during the first 3 years of life was related to later receptive or expressive language, this meta-analysis should be interpreted cautiously, because it did not examine specific language domains such as vocabulary and the independent variable was OME and not hearing loss. Other meta-analyses[79,115] have suggested at most a small negative association of OME and hearing loss on children's receptive and expressive language through the elementary school years. The clinical significance of these effects for language and learning is unclear for the child not at risk. For example, in one randomized trial,[100] prompt insertion of tympanostomy tubes for OME did not improve developmental outcomes at 3 years old regardless of baseline hearing. In another randomized trial,[116] however, prompt tube insertion achieved small benefits for children with bilateral OME and hearing loss.

Clinicians should ask the parent or caregiver about specific concerns regarding their child's language development. Children's speech and language can be tested at ages 6 to 36 months by direct engagement of a child and interviewing the parent using the Early Language Milestone Scale.[117] Other approaches require interviewing only the child's parent or caregiver, such as the MacArthur Communicative Development Inventory[118] and the Language Development Survey.[119] For older children, the Denver Developmental Screening Test II[120] can be used to screen general development including speech and language. Comprehensive speech and language evaluation is recommended for children who fail testing or whenever the child's parent or caregiver expresses concern.[121]

Evidence Profile: Hearing and Language

- Aggregate evidence quality: B, diagnostic studies with minor limitations; C, observational studies.
- Benefit: to detect hearing loss and language delay and identify strategies or interventions to improve developmental outcomes.
- Harm: parental anxiety, direct and indirect costs of assessment, and/or false-positive results.
- Balance of benefit and harm: preponderance of benefit over harm.
- Policy level: recommendation.

7. SURVEILLANCE: CHILDREN WITH PERSISTENT OME WHO ARE NOT AT RISK SHOULD BE REEXAMINED AT 3- TO 6-MONTH INTERVALS UNTIL THE EFFUSION IS NO LONGER PRESENT, SIGNIFICANT HEARING LOSS IS IDENTIFIED, OR STRUCTURAL ABNORMALITIES OF THE EARDRUM OR MIDDLE EAR ARE SUSPECTED

This recommendation is based on randomized, controlled trials and observational studies with a preponderance of benefit over harm.

If OME is asymptomatic and is likely to resolve spontaneously, intervention is unnecessary even if OME persists for more than 3 months. The clinician should determine whether risk factors exist that would predispose the child to undesirable sequelae or predict nonresolution of the effusion. As long as OME persists, the child is at risk for sequelae and must be reevaluated periodically for factors that would prompt intervention.

The 1994 OME guideline[1] recommended surgery for OME persisting 4 to 6 months with hearing loss but requires reconsideration because of later data on tubes and developmental sequelae.[122] For example, selecting surgical candidates using duration-based criteria (eg, OME >3 months or exceeding a cumulative threshold) does not improve developmental outcomes in infants and toddlers who are not at risk.[41,42,99,100] Additionally, the 1994 OME guideline did not specifically address managing effusion without significant hearing loss persisting more than 6 months.

Asymptomatic OME usually resolves spontaneously, but resolution rates decrease the longer the effusion has been present,[36,76,77] and relapse is common.[123] Risk factors that make spontaneous resolution less likely include[124,125]:

- Onset of OME in the summer or fall season
- Hearing loss more than 30-dB HL in the better-hearing ear

- History of prior tympanostomy tubes
- Not having had an adenoidectomy

Children with chronic OME are at risk for structural damage of the tympanic membrane[126] because the effusion contains leukotrienes, prostaglandins, and arachidonic acid metabolites that invoke a local inflammatory response.[127] Reactive changes may occur in the adjacent tympanic membrane and mucosal linings. A relative underventilation of the middle ear produces a negative pressure that predisposes to focal retraction pockets, generalized atelectasis of the tympanic membrane, and cholesteatoma.

Structural integrity is assessed by carefully examining the entire tympanic membrane, which, in many cases, can be accomplished by the primary care clinician using a handheld pneumatic otoscope. A search should be made for retraction pockets, ossicular erosion, and areas of atelectasis or atrophy. If there is any uncertainty that all observed structures are normal, the patient should be examined by using an otomicroscope. All children with these tympanic membrane conditions, regardless of OME duration, should have a comprehensive audiologic evaluation.

Conditions of the tympanic membrane that generally mandate inserting a tympanostomy tube are posterosuperior retraction pockets, ossicular erosion, adhesive atelectasis, and retraction pockets that accumulate keratin debris. Ongoing surveillance is mandatory, because the incidence of structural damage increases with effusion duration.[128]

As noted in recommendation 6, children with persistent OME for 3 months or longer should have their hearing tested. Based on these results, clinicians can identify 3 levels of action based on HLs obtained for the better-hearing ear using earphones or in sound field using speakers if the child is too young for ear-specific testing.

1. HLs of ≥40 dB (at least a moderate hearing loss): A comprehensive audiologic evaluation is indicated if not previously performed. If moderate hearing loss is documented and persists at this level, surgery is recommended, because persistent hearing loss of this magnitude that is permanent in nature has been shown to impact speech, language, and academic performance.[129–131]
2. HLs of 21 to 39 dB (mild hearing loss): A comprehensive audiologic evaluation is indicated if not previously performed. Mild sensorineural hearing loss has been associated with difficulties in speech, language, and academic performance in school,[129,132] and persistent mild conductive hearing loss from OME may have a similar impact. Further management should be individualized based on effusion duration, severity of hearing loss, and parent or caregiver preference and may include strategies to optimize the listening and learning environment (Table 4) or surgery. Repeat hearing testing should be performed in 3 to 6 months if OME persists at follow-up evaluation or tympanostomy tubes have not been placed.
3. HLs of ≤20 dB (normal hearing): A repeat hearing test should be performed in 3 to 6 months if OME persists at follow-up evaluation.

TABLE 4.   Strategies for Optimizing the Listening-Learning Environment for Children With OME and Hearing Loss*

Get within 3 feet of the child before speaking.
Turn off competing audio signals such as unnecessary music and television in the background.
Face the child and speak clearly, using visual clues (hands, pictures) in addition to speech.
Slow the rate, raise the level, and enunciate speech directed at the child.
Read to or with the child, explaining pictures and asking questions.
Repeat words, phrases, and questions when misunderstood.
Assign preferential seating in the classroom near the teacher.
Use a frequency-modulated personal- or sound-field-amplification system in the classroom.

* Modified with permission from Roberts et al.[78,79]

In addition to hearing loss and speech or language delay, other factors may influence the decision to intervene for persistent OME. Roberts et al[98,133] showed that the caregiving environment is more strongly related to school outcome than was OME or hearing loss. Risk factors for delays in speech and language development caused by a poor caregiving environment included low maternal educational level, unfavorable child care environment, and low socioeconomic status. In such cases, these factors may be additive to the hearing loss in affecting lower school performance and classroom behavior problems.

Persistent OME may be associated with physical or behavioral symptoms including hyperactivity, poor attention, and behavioral problems in some studies[134–136] and reduced child quality of life.[46] Conversely, young children randomized to early versus late tube insertion for persistent OME showed no behavioral benefits from early surgery.[41,100] Children with chronic OME also have significantly poorer vestibular function and gross motor proficiency when compared with non-OME controls.[48–50] Moreover, vestibular function, behavior, and quality of life can improve after tympanostomy tube insertion.[47,137,138] Other physical symptoms of OME that, if present and persistent, may warrant surgery include otalgia, unexplained sleep disturbance, and coexisting recurrent AOM. Tubes reduce the absolute incidence of recurrent AOM by ~1 episode per child per year, but the relative risk reduction is 56%.[139]

The risks of continued observation of children with OME must be balanced against the risks of surgery. Children with persistent OME examined regularly at 3- to 6-month intervals, or sooner if OME-related symptoms develop, are most likely at low risk for physical, behavioral, or developmental sequelae of OME. Conversely, prolonged watchful waiting of OME is not appropriate when regular surveillance is impossible or when the child is at risk for developmental sequelae of OME because of comorbidities (Table 3). For these children, the risks of anesthesia and surgery (see recommendation 9) may be less than those of continued observation.

Evidence Profile: Surveillance

- Aggregate evidence quality: C, observational studies and some randomized trials.

- Benefit: avoiding interventions that do not improve outcomes.
- Harm: allowing structural abnormalities to develop in the tympanic membrane, underestimating the impact of hearing loss on a child, and/or failing to detect significant signs or symptoms that require intervention.
- Balance of benefit and harm: preponderance of benefit over harm.
- Policy level: recommendation.

8. REFERRAL: WHEN CHILDREN WITH OME ARE REFERRED BY THE PRIMARY CARE CLINICIAN FOR EVALUATION BY AN OTOLARYNGOLOGIST, AUDIOLOGIST, OR SPEECH-LANGUAGE PATHOLOGIST, THE REFERRING CLINICIAN SHOULD DOCUMENT THE EFFUSION DURATION AND SPECIFIC REASON FOR REFERRAL (EVALUATION, SURGERY) AND PROVIDE ADDITIONAL RELEVANT INFORMATION SUCH AS HISTORY OF AOM AND DEVELOPMENTAL STATUS OF THE CHILD

This option is based on panel consensus and a preponderance of benefit over harm.

This recommendation emphasizes the importance of communication between the referring primary care clinician and the otolaryngologist, audiologist, and speech-language pathologist. Parents and caregivers may be confused and frustrated when a recommendation for surgery is made for their child because of conflicting information about alternative management strategies. Choosing among management options is facilitated when primary care physicians and advanced-practice nurses who best know the patient's history of ear problems and general medical status provide the specialist with accurate information. Although there are no studies showing improved outcomes from better documentation of OME histories, there is a clear need for better mechanisms to convey information and expectations from primary care clinicians to consultants and subspecialists.[140–142]

When referring a child for evaluation to an otolaryngologist, the primary care physician should explain the following to the parent or caregiver of the patient:

- Reason for referral: Explain that the child is seeing an otolaryngologist for evaluation, which is likely to include ear examination and audiologic testing, and not necessarily simply to be scheduled for surgery.
- What to expect: Explain that surgery may be recommended, and let the parent know that the otolaryngologist will explain the options, benefits, and risks further.
- Decision-making process: Explain that there are many alternatives for management and that surgical decisions are elective; the parent or caregiver should be encouraged to express to the surgeon any concerns he or she may have about the recommendations made.

When referring a child to an otolaryngologist, audiologist, or speech-language pathologist, the minimum information that should be conveyed in writing includes:

- Duration of OME: State how long fluid has been present.
- Laterality of OME: State whether one or both ears have been affected.
- Results of prior hearing testing or tympanometry.
- Suspected speech or language problems: State whether there had been a delay in speech and language development or whether the parent or a caregiver has expressed concerns about the child's communication abilities, school achievement, or attentiveness.
- Conditions that might exacerbate the deleterious effects of OME: State whether the child has conditions such as permanent hearing loss, impaired cognition, developmental delays, cleft lip or palate, or an unstable or nonsupportive family or home environment.
- AOM history: State whether the child has a history of recurrent AOM.

Additional medical information that should be provided to the otolaryngologist by the primary care clinician includes:

- Parental attitude toward surgery: State whether the parents have expressed a strong preference for or against surgery as a management option.
- Related conditions that might require concomitant surgery: State whether there have been other conditions that might warrant surgery if the child is going to have general anesthesia (eg, nasal obstruction and snoring that might be an indication for adenoidectomy or obstructive breathing during sleep that might mean tonsillectomy is indicated).
- General health status: State whether there are any conditions that might present problems for surgery or administering general anesthesia, such as congenital heart abnormality, bleeding disorder, asthma or reactive airway disease, or family history of malignant hyperthermia.

After evaluating the child, the otolaryngologist, audiologist, or speech-language pathologist should inform the referring physician regarding his or her diagnostic impression, plans for additional assessment, and recommendations for ongoing monitoring and management.

Evidence Profile: Referral

- Aggregate evidence quality: C, observational studies.
- Benefit: better communication and improved decision-making.
- Harm: confidentiality concerns, administrative burden, and/or increased parent or caregiver anxiety.
- Benefits-harms assessment: balance of benefit and harm.
- Policy level: option.

9. SURGERY: WHEN A CHILD BECOMES A SURGICAL CANDIDATE, TYMPANOSTOMY TUBE INSERTION IS THE PREFERRED INITIAL PROCEDURE; ADENOIDECTOMY SHOULD NOT BE PERFORMED UNLESS A DISTINCT INDICATION EXISTS (NASAL OBSTRUCTION, CHRONIC ADENOIDITIS). REPEAT SURGERY CONSISTS OF ADENOIDECTOMY PLUS MYRINGOTOMY, WITH OR WITHOUT TUBE INSERTION. TONSILLECTOMY ALONE OR MYRINGOTOMY ALONE SHOULD NOT BE USED TO TREAT OME

This recommendation is based on randomized, controlled trials with a preponderance of benefit over harm.

Surgical candidacy for OME largely depends on hearing status, associated symptoms, the child's developmental risk (Table 3), and the anticipated chance of timely spontaneous resolution of the effusion. Candidates for surgery include children with OME lasting 4 months or longer with persistent hearing loss or other signs and symptoms, recurrent or persistent OME in children at risk regardless of hearing status, and OME and structural damage to the tympanic membrane or middle ear. Ultimately, the recommendation for surgery must be individualized based on consensus between the primary care physician, otolaryngologist, and parent or caregiver that a particular child would benefit from intervention. Children with OME of any duration who are at risk are candidates for earlier surgery.

Tympanostomy tubes are recommended for initial surgery because randomized trials show a mean 62% relative decrease in effusion prevalence and an absolute decrease of 128 effusion days per child during the next year.[139,143–145] HLs improve by a mean of 6 to 12 dB while the tubes remain patent.[146,147] Adenoidectomy plus myringotomy (without tube insertion) has comparable efficacy in children 4 years old or older[143] but is more invasive, with additional surgical and anesthetic risks. Similarly, the added risk of adenoidectomy outweighs the limited, short-term benefit for children 3 years old or older without prior tubes.[148] Consequently, adenoidectomy is not recommended for initial OME surgery unless a distinct indication exists, such as adenoiditis, postnasal obstruction, or chronic sinusitis.

Approximately 20% to 50% of children who have had tympanostomy tubes have OME relapse after tube extrusion that may require additional surgery.[144,145,149] When a child needs repeat surgery for OME, adenoidectomy is recommended (unless the child has an overt or submucous cleft palate), because it confers a 50% reduction in the need for future operations.[143,150,151] The benefit of adenoidectomy is apparent at 2 years old,[150] greatest for children 3 years old or older, and independent of adenoid size.[143,151,152] Myringotomy is performed concurrent with adenoidectomy. Myringotomy plus adenoidectomy is effective for children 4 years old or older,[143] but tube insertion is advised for younger children, when potential relapse of effusion must be minimized (eg, children at risk) or pronounced inflammation of the tympanic membrane and middle-ear mucosa is present.

Tonsillectomy or myringotomy alone (without adenoidectomy) is not recommended to treat OME. Although tonsillectomy is either ineffective[152] or of limited efficacy,[148,150] the risks of hemorrhage (~2%) and additional hospitalization outweigh any potential benefits unless a distinct indication for tonsillectomy exists. Myringotomy alone, without tube placement or adenoidectomy, is ineffective for chronic OME,[144,145] because the incision closes within several days. Laser-assisted myringotomy extends the ventilation period several weeks,[153] but randomized trials with concurrent controls have not been conducted to establish efficacy. In contrast, tympanostomy tubes ventilate the middle ear for an average of 12 to 14 months.[144,145]

Anesthesia mortality has been reported to be ~1: 50 000 for ambulatory surgery,[154] but the current fatality rate may be lower.[155] Laryngospasm and bronchospasm occur more often in children receiving anesthesia than adults. Tympanostomy tube sequelae are common[156] but are generally transient (otorrhea) or do not affect function (tympanosclerosis, focal atrophy, or shallow retraction pocket). Tympanic membrane perforations, which may require repair, are seen in 2% of children after placement of short-term (grommet-type) tubes and 17% after long-term tubes.[156] Adenoidectomy has a 0.2% to 0.5% incidence of hemorrhage[150,157] and 2% incidence of transient velopharyngeal insufficiency.[148] Other potential risks of adenoidectomy, such as nasopharyngeal stenosis and persistent velopharyngeal insufficiency, can be minimized with appropriate patient selection and surgical technique.

There is a clear preponderance of benefit over harm when considering the impact of surgery for OME on effusion prevalence, HLs, subsequent incidence of AOM, and the need for reoperation after adenoidectomy. Information about adenoidectomy in children less than 4 years old, however, remains limited. Although the cost of surgery and anesthesia is nontrivial, it is offset by reduced OME and AOM after tube placement and by reduced need for reoperation after adenoidectomy. Approximately 8 adenoidectomies are needed to avoid a single instance of tube reinsertion; however, each avoided surgery probably represents a larger reduction in the number of AOM and OME episodes, including those in children who did not require additional surgery.[150]

Evidence Profile: Surgery

- Aggregate evidence quality: B, randomized, controlled trials with minor limitations.
- Benefit: improved hearing, reduced prevalence of OME, reduced incidence of AOM, and less need for additional tube insertion (after adenoidectomy).
- Harm: risks of anesthesia and specific surgical procedures; sequelae of tympanostomy tubes.
- Benefits-harms assessment: preponderance of benefit over harm.
- Policy level: recommendation.

10. CAM: NO RECOMMENDATION IS MADE REGARDING CAM AS A TREATMENT FOR OME

There is no recommendation based on lack of scientific evidence documenting efficacy and an uncertain balance of harm and benefit.

The 1994 OME guideline[1] made no recommendation regarding CAM as a treatment for OME, and no subsequent controlled studies have been published to change this conclusion. The current statement of "no recommendation" is based on the lack of scientific evidence documenting efficacy plus the balance of benefit and harm.

Evidence concerning CAM is insufficient to determine whether the outcomes achieved for OME differ from those achieved by watchful waiting and spontaneous resolution. There are no randomized, controlled trials with adequate sample sizes on the efficacy of CAM for OME. Although many case reports and subjective reviews on CAM treatment of AOM were found, little is published on OME treatment or prevention. Homeopathy[158] and chiropractic treatments[159] were assessed in pilot studies with small numbers of patients that failed to show clinically or statistically significant benefits. Consequently, there is no research base on which to develop a recommendation concerning CAM for OME.

The natural history of OME in childhood (discussed previously) is such that almost any intervention can be "shown" to have helped in an anecdotal, uncontrolled report or case series. The efficacy of CAM or any other intervention for OME can only be shown with parallel-group, randomized, controlled trials with valid diagnostic methods and adequate sample sizes. Unproved modalities that have been claimed to provide benefit in middle-ear disease include osteopathic and chiropractic manipulation, dietary exclusions (such as dairy), herbal and other dietary supplements, acupuncture, traditional Chinese medicine, and homeopathy. None of these modalities, however, have been subjected yet to a published, peer-reviewed, clinical trial.

The absence of any published clinical trials also means that all reports of CAM adverse effects are anecdotal. A systematic review of recent evidence[160] found significant serious adverse effects of unconventional therapies for children, most of which were associated with inadequately regulated herbal medicines. One report on malpractice liability associated with CAM therapies[161] did not address childhood issues specifically. Allergic reactions to echinacea occur but seem to be rare in children.[162] A general concern about herbal products is the lack of any governmental oversight into product quality or purity.[160,163,164] Additionally, herbal products may alter blood levels of allopathic medications, including anticoagulants. A possible concern with homeopathy is the worsening of symptoms, which is viewed as a positive, early sign of homeopathic efficacy. The adverse effects of manipulative therapies (such as chiropractic treatments and osteopathy) in children are difficult to assess because of scant evidence, but a case series of 332 children treated for AOM or OME with chiropractic manipulation did not mention any side effects.[165] Quadriplegia has been reported, however, after spinal manipulation in an infant with torticollis.[166]

Evidence Profile: CAM

- Aggregate evidence quality: D, case series without controls.
- Benefit: not established.
- Harm: potentially significant depending on the intervention.
- Benefits-harms assessment: uncertain balance of benefit and harm.
- Policy level: no recommendation.

11. ALLERGY MANAGEMENT: NO RECOMMENDATION IS MADE REGARDING ALLERGY MANAGEMENT AS A TREATMENT FOR OME

There is no recommendation based on insufficient evidence of therapeutic efficacy or a causal relationship between allergy and OME.

The 1994 OME guideline[1] made no recommendation regarding allergy management as a treatment for OME, and no subsequent controlled studies have been published to change this conclusion. The current statement of "no recommendation" is based on insufficient evidence of therapeutic efficacy or a causal relationship between allergy and OME plus the balance of benefit and harm.

A linkage between allergy and OME has long been speculated but to date remains unquantified. The prevalence of allergy among OME patients has been reported to range from less than 10% to more than 80%.[167] Allergy has long been postulated to cause OME through its contribution to eustachian tube dysfunction.[168] The cellular response of respiratory mucosa to allergens has been well studied. Therefore, similar to other parts of respiratory mucosa, the mucosa lining the middle-ear cleft is capable of an allergic response.[169,170] Sensitivity to allergens varies among individuals, and atopy may involve neutrophils in type I allergic reactions that enhance the inflammatory response.[171]

The correlation between OME and allergy has been widely reported, but no prospective studies have examined the effects of immunotherapy compared with observation alone or other management options. Reports of OME cure after immunotherapy or food-elimination diets[172] are impossible to interpret without concurrent control groups because of the favorable natural history of most untreated OME. The documentation of allergy in published reports has been defined inconsistently (medical history, physical examination, skin-prick testing, nasal smears, serum immunoglobulin E and eosinophil counts, inflammatory mediators in effusions). Study groups have been drawn primarily from specialist offices, likely lack heterogeneity, and are not representative of general medical practice.

Evidence Profile: Allergy Management

- Aggregate evidence quality: D, case series without controls.

- Benefit: not established.
- Harm: adverse effects and cost of medication, physician evaluation, elimination diets, and desensitization.
- Benefits-harms assessment: balance of benefit and harm.
- Policy level: no recommendation.

RESEARCH NEEDS

Diagnosis

- Further standardize the definition of OME.
- Assess the performance characteristics of pneumatic otoscopy as a diagnostic test for OME when performed by primary care physicians and advanced-practice nurses in the routine office setting.
- Determine the optimal methods for teaching pneumatic otoscopy to residents and clinicians.
- Develop a brief, reliable, objective method for diagnosing OME.
- Develop a classification method for identifying the presence of OME for practical use by clinicians that is based on quantifiable tympanometric characteristics.
- Assess the usefulness of algorithms combining pneumatic otoscopy and tympanometry for detecting OME in clinical practice.
- Conduct additional validating cohort studies of acoustic reflectometry as a diagnostic method for OME, particularly in children less than 2 years old.

Child At Risk

- Better define the child with OME who is at risk for speech, language, and learning problems.
- Conduct large, multicenter, observational cohort studies to identify the child at risk who is most susceptible to potential adverse sequelae of OME.
- Conduct large, multicenter, observational cohort studies to analyze outcomes achieved with alternative management strategies for OME in children at risk.

Watchful Waiting

- Define the spontaneous resolution of OME in infants and young children (existing data are limited primarily to children 2 years old or older).
- Conduct large-scale, prospective cohort studies to obtain current data on the spontaneous resolution of newly diagnosed OME of unknown prior duration (existing data are primarily from the late 1970s and early 1980s).
- Develop prognostic indicators to identify the best candidates for watchful waiting.
- Determine whether the lack of impact from prompt insertion of tympanostomy tubes on speech and language outcomes seen in asymptomatic young children with OME identified by screening or intense surveillance can be generalized to older children with OME or to symptomatic children with OME referred for evaluation.

Medication

- Clarify which children, if any, should receive antimicrobials, steroids, or both for OME.
- Conduct a randomized, placebo-controlled trial on the efficacy of antimicrobial therapy, with or without concurrent oral steroid, in avoiding surgery in children with OME who are surgical candidates and have not received recent antimicrobials.
- Investigate the role of mucosal surface biofilms in refractory or recurrent OME and develop targeted interventions.

Hearing and Language

- Conduct longitudinal studies on the natural history of hearing loss accompanying OME.
- Develop improved methods for describing and quantifying the fluctuations in hearing of children with OME over time.
- Conduct prospective controlled studies on the relation of hearing loss associated with OME to later auditory, speech, language, behavioral, and academic sequelae.
- Develop reliable, brief, objective methods for estimating hearing loss associated with OME.
- Develop reliable, brief, objective methods for estimating speech or language delay associated with OME.
- Evaluate the benefits and administrative burden of language testing by primary care clinicians.
- Agree on the aspects of language that are vulnerable to or affected by hearing loss caused by OME, and reach a consensus on the best tools for measurement.
- Determine whether OME and associated hearing loss place children from special populations at greater risk for speech and language delays.

Surveillance

- Develop better tools for monitoring children with OME that are suitable for routine clinical care.
- Assess the value of new strategies for monitoring OME, such as acoustic reflectometry performed at home by the parent or caregiver, in optimizing surveillance.
- Improve our ability to identify children who would benefit from early surgery instead of prolonged surveillance.
- Promote early detection of structural abnormalities in the tympanic membrane associated with OME that may require surgery to prevent complications.
- Clarify and quantify the role of parent or caregiver education, socioeconomic status, and quality of the caregiving environment as modifiers of OME developmental outcomes.
- Develop methods for minimizing loss to follow-up during OME surveillance.

Surgery

- Define the role of adenoidectomy in children 3 years old or younger as a specific OME therapy.
- Conduct controlled trials on the efficacy of tympanostomy tubes for developmental outcomes in children with hearing loss, other symptoms, or speech and language delay.
- Conduct randomized, controlled trials of surgery versus no surgery that emphasize patient-based outcome measures (quality of life, functional health status) in addition to objective measures (effusion prevalence, HLs, AOM incidence, reoperation).
- Identify the optimal ways to incorporate parent or caregiver preference into surgical decision-making.

CAM

- Conduct randomized, controlled trials on the efficacy of CAM modalities for OME.
- Develop strategies to identify parents or caregivers who use CAM therapies for their child's OME, and encourage surveillance by the primary care clinician.

Allergy Management

- Evaluate the causal role of atopy in OME.
- Conduct randomized, controlled trials on the efficacy of allergy therapy for OME that are generalizable to the primary care setting.

CONCLUSIONS

This evidence-based practice guideline offers recommendations for identifying, monitoring, and managing the child with OME. The guideline emphasizes appropriate diagnosis and provides options for various management strategies including observation, medical intervention, and referral for surgical intervention. These recommendations should provide primary care physicians and other health care providers with assistance in managing children with OME.

SUBCOMMITTEE ON OTITIS MEDIA WITH EFFUSION
Richard M. Rosenfeld, MD, MPH, Cochairperson
 American Academy of Pediatrics
 American Academy of Otolaryngology-Head and Neck Surgery
Larry Culpepper, MD, MPH, Cochairperson
 American Academy of Family Physicians
Karen J. Doyle, MD, PhD
 American Academy of Otolaryngology-Head and Neck Surgery
Kenneth M. Grundfast, MD
 American Academy of Otolaryngology-Head and Neck Surgery
Alejandro Hoberman, MD
 American Academy of Pediatrics
Margaret A. Kenna, MD
 American Academy of Otolaryngology-Head and Neck Surgery
Allan S. Lieberthal, MD
 American Academy of Pediatrics
Martin Mahoney, MD, PhD
 American Academy of Family Physicians
Richard A. Wahl, MD
 American Academy of Pediatrics
Charles R. Woods, Jr, MD, MS
 American Academy of Pediatrics

Barbara Yawn, MD, MSc
American Academy of Family Physicians

CONSULTANTS
S. Michael Marcy, MD
Richard N. Shiffman, MD

LIAISONS
Linda Carlson, MS, CPNP
National Association of Pediatric Nurse
Practitioners
Judith Gravel, PhD
American Academy of Audiology
Joanne Roberts, PhD
American Speech-Language-Hearing Association
STAFF
Maureen Hannley, PhD
American Academy of Otolaryngology-Head and
Neck Surgery
Carla T. Herrerias, MPH
American Academy of Pediatrics
Bellinda K. Schoof, MHA, CPHQ
American Academy of Family Physicians

ACKNOWLEDGMENTS

Dr Marcy serves as a consultant to Abbott Laboratories Glaxo-SmithKline (vaccines).

REFERENCES

1. Stool SE, Berg AO, Berman S, et al. *Otitis Media With Effusion in Young Children. Clinical Practice Guideline, Number 12.* AHCPR Publication No. 94-0622. Rockville, MD: Agency for Health Care Policy and Research, Public Health Service, US Department of Health and Human Services; 1994

2. Shekelle P, Takata G, Chan LS, et al. *Diagnosis, Natural History, and Late Effects of Otitis Media With Effusion. Evidence Report/Technology Assessment No. 55.* AHRQ Publication No. 03-E023. Rockville, MD: Agency for Healthcare Research and Quality; 2003

3. Williamson I. Otitis media with effusion. *Clin Evid.* 2002;7:469–476

4. Tos M. Epidemiology and natural history of secretory otitis. *Am J Otol.* 1984;5:459–462

5. Paradise JL, Rockette HE, Colborn DK, et al. Otitis media in 2253 Pittsburgh area infants: prevalence and risk factors during the first two years of life. *Pediatrics.* 1997;99:318–333

6. Casselbrant ML, Mandel EM. Epidemiology. In: Rosenfeld RM, Bluestone CD, eds. *Evidence-Based Otitis Media.* 2nd ed. Hamilton, Ontario: BC Decker; 2003:147–162

7. Williamson IG, Dunleavy J, Baine J, Robinson D. The natural history of otitis media with effusion—a three-year study of the incidence and prevalence of abnormal tympanograms in four South West Hampshire infant and first schools. *J Laryngol Otol.* 1994;108:930–934

8. Coyte PC, Croxford R, Asche CV, To T, Feldman W, Friedberg J. Physician and population determinants of rates of middle-ear surgery in Ontario. *JAMA.* 2001;286:2128–2135

9. Tugwell P. How to read clinical journals: III. To learn the clinical course and prognosis of disease. *Can Med Assoc J.* 1981;124:869–872

10. Jaeschke R, Guyatt G, Sackett DL. Users' guides to the medical literature. III. How to use an article about a diagnostic test. A. Are the results of the study valid? Evidence-Based Medicine Working Group. *JAMA.* 1994;271:389–391

11. Shiffman RN, Shekelle P, Overhage JM, Slutsky J, Grimshaw J, Deshpande AM. Standardized reporting of clinical practice guidelines: a proposal from the Conference on Guideline Standardization. *Ann Intern Med.* 2003;139:493–498

12. Shiffman RN, Karras BT, Agrawal A, Chen R, Marenco L, Nath S. GEM: a proposal for a more comprehensive guideline document model using XML. *J Am Med Inform Assoc.* 2000;7:488–498

13. Shaneyfelt TM, Mayo-Smith MF, Rothwangl J. Are guidelines following guidelines? The methodological quality of clinical practice guidelines in the peer-reviewed medical literature. *JAMA.* 1999;281:1900–1905

14. Agrawal A, Shiffman RN. Evaluation of guideline quality using GEM-Q. *Medinfo.* 2001;10:1097–1101

15. Yale Center for Medical Informatics. GEM: The Guideline Elements Model. Available at: http://ycmi.med.yale.edu/GEM/. Accessed December 8, 2003

16. American Academy of Pediatrics, Steering Committee on Quality Improvement and Management. A taxonomy of recommendations for clinical practice guidelines. *Pediatrics.* 2004; In press

17. Eddy DM. *A Manual for Assessing Health Practices and Designing Practice Policies: The Explicit Approach.* Philadelphia, PA: American College of Physicians; 1992

18. Dowell SF, Marcy MS, Phillips WR, Gerber MA, Schwartz B. Otitis media—principles of judicious use of antimicrobial agents. *Pediatrics.* 1998;101:165–171

19. Dowell SF, Butler JC, Giebink GS, et al. Acute otitis media: management and surveillance in an era of pneumococcal resistance—a report from the Drug-Resistant *Streptococcus pneumoniae* Therapeutic Working Group. *Pediatr Infect Dis J.* 1999;18:1–9

20. Karma PH, Penttila MA, Sipila MM, Kataja MJ. Otoscopic diagnosis of middle ear effusion in acute and non-acute otitis media. I. The value of different otoscopic findings. *Int J Pediatr Otorhinolaryngol.* 1989;17:37–49

21. Pichichero ME, Poole MD. Assessing diagnostic accuracy and tympanocentesis skills in the management of otitis media. *Arch Pediatr Adolesc Med.* 2001;155:1137–1142

22. Steinbach WJ, Sectish TC. Pediatric resident training in the diagnosis and treatment of acute otitis media. *Pediatrics.* 2002;109:404–408

23. Palmu A, Puhakka H, Rahko T, Takala AK. Diagnostic value of tympanometry in infants in clinical practice. *Int J Pediatr Otorhinolaryngol.* 1999;49:207–213

24. van Balen FA, Aarts AM, De Melker RA. Tympanometry by general practitioners: reliable? *Int J Pediatr Otorhinolaryngol.* 1999;48:117–123

25. Block SL, Mandel E, McLinn S, et al. Spectral gradient acoustic reflectometry for the detection of middle ear effusion by pediatricians and parents. *Pediatr Infect Dis J.* 1998;17:560–564, 580

26. Barnett ED, Klein JO, Hawkins KA, Cabral HJ, Kenna M, Healy G. Comparison of spectral gradient acoustic reflectometry and other diagnostic techniques for detection of middle ear effusion in children with middle ear disease. *Pediatr Infect Dis J.* 1998;17:556–559, 580

27. Block SL, Pichichero ME, McLinn S, Aronovitz G, Kimball S. Spectral gradient acoustic reflectometry: detection of middle ear effusion by pediatricians in suppurative acute otitis media. *Pediatr Infect Dis J.* 1999;18:741–744

28. Schwartz RH. A practical approach to the otitis prone child. *Contemp Pediatr.* 1987;4:30–54

29. Barriga F, Schwartz RH, Hayden GF. Adequate illumination for otoscopy. Variations due to power source, bulb, and head and speculum design. *Am J Dis Child.* 1986;140:1237–1240

30. Sorenson CH, Jensen SH, Tos M. The post-winter prevalence of middle-ear effusion in four-year-old children, judged by tympanometry. *Int J Pediatr Otorhinolaryngol.* 1981;3:119–128

31. Fiellau-Nikolajsen M. Epidemiology of secretory otitis media. A descriptive cohort study. *Ann Otol Rhinol Laryngol.* 1983;92:172–177

32. Casselbrant ML, Brostoff LM, Cantekin EI, et al. Otitis media with effusion in preschool children. *Laryngoscope.* 1985;95:428–436

33. Zielhuis GA, Rach GH, van den Broek P. Screening for otitis media with effusion in preschool children. *Lancet.* 1989;1:311–314

34. Poulsen G, Tos M. Repetitive tympanometric screenings of two-year-old children. *Scand Audiol.* 1980;9:21–28

35. Tos M, Holm-Jensen S, Sorensen CH. Changes in prevalence of secretory otitis from summer to winter in four-year-old children. *Am J Otol.* 1981;2:324–327

36. Thomsen J, Tos M. Spontaneous improvement of secretory otitis. A long-term study. *Acta Otolaryngol.* 1981;92:493–499

37. Lous J, Fiellau-Nikolajsen M. Epidemiology of middle ear effusion and tubal dysfunction. A one-year prospective study comprising monthly tympanometry in 387 non-selected seven-year-old children. *Int J Pediatr Otorhinolaryngol.* 1981;3:303–317

38. New Zealand Health Technology Assessment. *Screening Programmes for the Detection of Otitis Media With Effusion and Conductive Hearing Loss in Pre-School and New Entrant School Children: A Critical Appraisal of the Literature.* Christchurch, New Zealand: New Zealand Health Technology Assessment; 1998:61

39. Canadian Task Force on Preventive Health Care. Screening for otitis media with effusion: recommendation statement from the Canadian Task Force on Preventive Health Care. *CMAJ.* 2001;165:1092–1093

40. US Preventive Services Task Force. *Guide to Clinical Preventive Services.* 2nd ed. Baltimore, MD: Williams & Wilkins; 1995

41. Paradise JL, Feldman HM, Campbell TF, et al. Effect of early or delayed insertion of tympanostomy tubes for persistent otitis media on

developmental outcomes at the age of three years. *N Engl J Med.* 2001;344:1179–1187

42. Rovers MM, Krabble PF, Straatman H, Ingels K, van der Wilt GJ, Zielhuis GA. Randomized controlled trial of the effect of ventilation tubes (grommets) on quality of life at age 1–2 years. *Arch Dis Child.* 2001;84:45–49

43. Wood DL. Documentation guidelines: evolution, future direction, and compliance. *Am J Med.* 2001;110:332–334

44. Soto CM, Kleinman KP, Simon SR. Quality and correlates of medical record documentation in the ambulatory care setting. *BMC Health Serv Res.* 2002;2:22–35

45. Marchant CD, Shurin PA, Turczyk VA, Wasikowski DE, Tutihasi MA, Kinney SE. Course and outcome of otitis media in early infancy: a prospective study. *J Pediatr.* 1984;104:826–831

46. Rosenfeld RM, Goldsmith AJ, Tetlus L, Balzano A. Quality of life for children with otitis media. *Arch Otolaryngol Head Neck Surg.* 1997;123:1049–1054

47. Casselbrant ML, Furman JM, Rubenstein E, Mandel EM. Effect of otitis media on the vestibular system in children. *Ann Otol Rhinol Laryngol.* 1995;104:620–624

48. Orlin MN, Effgen SK, Handler SD. Effect of otitis media with effusion on gross motor ability in preschool-aged children: preliminary findings. *Pediatrics.* 1997;99:334–337

49. Golz A, Angel-Yeger B, Parush S. Evaluation of balance disturbances in children with middle ear effusion. *Int J Pediatr Otorhinolaryngol.* 1998;43:21–26

50. Casselbrant ML, Redfern MS, Furman JM, Fall PA, Mandel EM. Visual-induced postural sway in children with and without otitis media. *Ann Otol Rhinol Laryngol.* 1998;107:401–405

51. Ruben R. Host susceptibility to otitis media sequelae. In: Rosenfeld RM, Bluestone CD, eds. *Evidence-Based Otitis Media.* 2nd ed. Hamilton, ON, Canada: BC Decker; 2003:505–514

52. Whiteman BC, Simpson GB, Compton WC. Relationship of otitis media and language impairment on adolescents with Down syndrome. *Ment Retard.* 1986;24:353–356

53. van der Vyver M, van der Merwe A, Tesner HE. The effects of otitis media on articulation in children with cerebral palsy. *Int J Rehabil Res.* 1988;11:386–389

54. Paradise JL, Bluestone CD. Early treatment of the universal otitis media of infants with cleft palate. *Pediatrics.* 1974;53:48–54

55. Schwartz DM, Schwartz RH. Acoustic impedance and otoscopic findings in young children with Down's syndrome. *Arch Otolaryngol.* 1978;104:652–656

56. Corey JP, Caldarelli DD, Gould HJ. Otopathology in cranial facial dysostosis. *Am J Otol.* 1987;8:14–17

57. Schonweiler R, Schonweiler B, Schmelzeisen R. Hearing capacity and speech production in 417 children with facial cleft abnormalities [in German]. *HNO.* 1994;42:691–696

58. Ruben RJ, Math R. Serous otitis media associated with sensorineural hearing loss in children. *Laryngoscope.* 1978;88:1139–1154

59. Brookhouser PE, Worthington DW, Kelly WJ. Middle ear disease in young children with sensorineural hearing loss. *Laryngoscope.* 1993;103:371–378

60. Rice ML. Specific language impairments: in search of diagnostic markers and genetic contributions. *Ment Retard Dev Disabil Res Rev.* 1997;3:350–357

61. Rosenhall U, Nordin V, Sandstrom M, Ahlsen G, Gillberg C. Autism and hearing loss. *J Autism Dev Disord.* 1999;29:349–357

62. Cunningham C, McArthur K. Hearing loss and treatment in young Down's syndrome children. *Child Care Health Dev.* 1981;7:357–374

63. Shott SR, Joseph A, Heithaus D. Hearing loss in children with Down syndrome. *Int J Pediatr Otorhinolaryngol.* 2001;61:199–205

64. Clarkson RL, Eimas PD, Marean GC. Speech perception in children with histories of recurrent otitis media. *J Acoust Soc Am.* 1989;85:926–933

65. Groenen P, Crul T, Maassen B, van Bon W. Perception of voicing cues by children with early otitis media with and without language impairment. *J Speech Hear Res.* 1996;39:43–54

66. Hubbard TW, Paradise JL, McWilliams BJ, Elster BA, Taylor FH. Consequences of unremitting middle-ear disease in early life. Otologic, audiologic, and developmental findings in children with cleft palate. *N Engl J Med.* 1985;312:1529–1534

67. Nunn DR, Derkay CS, Darrow DH, Magee W, Strasnick B. The effect of very early cleft palate closure on the need for ventilation tubes in the first years of life. *Laryngoscope.* 1995;105:905–908

68. Pappas DG, Flexer C, Shackelford L. Otological and habilitative management of children with Down syndrome. *Laryngoscope.* 1994;104:1065–1070

69. Vartiainen E. Otitis media with effusion in children with congenital or early-onset hearing impairment. *J Otolaryngol.* 2000;29:221–223

70. Rosenfeld RM, Kay D. Natural history of untreated otitis media. *Laryngoscope.* 2003;113:1645–1657

71. Teele DW, Klein JO, Rosner BA. Epidemiology of otitis media in children. *Ann Otol Rhinol Laryngol Suppl.* 1980;89:5–6

72. Mygind N, Meistrup-Larsen KI, Thomsen J, Thomsen VF, Josefsson K, Sorensen H. Penicillin in acute otitis media: a double-blind, placebo-controlled trial. *Clin Otolaryngol.* 1981;6:5–13

73. Burke P, Bain J, Robinson D, Dunleavey J. Acute red ear in children: controlled trial of nonantibiotic treatment in general practice. *BMJ.* 1991;303:558–562

74. Fiellau-Nikolajsen M, Lous J. Prospective tympanometry in 3-year-old children. A study of the spontaneous course of tympanometry types in a nonselected population. *Arch Otolaryngol.* 1979;105:461–466

75. Fiellau-Nikolajsen M. Tympanometry in 3-year-old children. Type of care as an epidemiological factor in secretory otitis media and tubal dysfunction in unselected populations of 3-year-old children. *ORL J Otorhinolaryngol Relat Spec.* 1979;41:193–205

76. Tos M. Spontaneous improvement of secretory otitis and impedance screening. *Arch Otolaryngol.* 1980;106:345–349

77. Tos M, Holm-Jensen S, Sorensen CH, Mogensen C. Spontaneous course and frequency of secretory otitis in 4-year-old children. *Arch Otolaryngol.* 1982;108:4–10

78. Roberts JE, Zeisel SA. *Ear Infections and Language Development.* Rockville, MD: American Speech-Language-Hearing Association and the National Center for Early Development and Learning; 2000

79. Roberts JE, Rosenfeld RM, Zeisel SA. Otitis media and speech and language: a meta-analysis of prospective studies. *Pediatrics.* 2004;113(3). Available at: www.pediatrics.org/cgi/content/full/113/3/e238

80. Williams RL, Chalmers TC, Stange KC, Chalmers FT, Bowlin SJ. Use of antibiotics in preventing recurrent otitis media and in treating otitis media with effusion. A meta-analytic attempt to resolve the brouhaha. *JAMA.* 1993;270:1344–1351

81. Rosenfeld RM, Post JC. Meta-analysis of antibiotics for the treatment of otitis media with effusion. *Otolaryngol Head Neck Surg.* 1992;106:378–386

82. Mandel EM, Rockette HE, Bluestone CD, Paradise JL, Nozza RJ. Efficacy of amoxicillin with and without decongestant-antihistamine for otitis media with effusion in children. Results of a double-blind, randomized trial. *N Engl J Med.* 1987;316:432–437

83. McCormick AW, Whitney CG, Farley MM, et al. Geographic diversity and temporal trends of antimicrobial resistance in *Streptococcus pneumoniae* in the United States. *Nat Med.* 2003;9:424–430

84. Levy SB. *The Antibiotic Paradox. How the Misuse of Antibiotic Destroys Their Curative Powers.* Cambridge, MA: Perseus Publishing; 2002

85. Butler CC, van der Voort JH. Oral or topical nasal steroids for hearing loss associated with otitis media with effusion in children. *Cochrane Database Syst Rev.* 2002;4:CD001935

86. Mandel EM, Casselbrant ML, Rockette HE, Fireman P, Kurs-Lasky M, Bluestone CD. Systemic steroid for chronic otitis media with effusion in children. *Pediatrics.* 2002;110:1071–1080

87. Tracy JM, Demain JG, Hoffman KM, Goetz DW. Intranasal beclomethasone as an adjunct to treatment of chronic middle ear effusion. *Ann Allergy Asthma Immunol.* 1998;80:198–206

88. Joint Committee on Infant Hearing. Year 2000 position statement: principles and guidelines for early hearing detection and intervention programs. *Am J Audiol.* 2000;9:9–29

89. Pillsbury HC, Grose JH, Hall JW III. Otitis media with effusion in children. Binaural hearing before and after corrective surgery. *Arch Otolaryngol Head Neck Surg.* 1991;117:718–723

90. Besing J, Koehnke J A test of virtual auditory localization. *Ear Hear.* 1995;16:220–229

91. Jerger S, Jerger J, Alford BR, Abrams S. Development of speech intelligibility in children with recurrent otitis media. *Ear Hear.* 1983;4:138–145

92. Gravel JS, Wallace IF. Listening and language at 4 years of age: effects of early otitis media. *J Speech Hear Res.* 1992;35:588–595

93. Schilder AG, Snik AF, Straatman H, van den Broek P. The effect of otitis media with effusion at preschool age on some aspects of auditory perception at school age. *Ear Hear.* 1994;15:224–231

94. Rosenfeld RM, Madell JR, McMahon A. Auditory function in normal-hearing children with middle ear effusion. In: Lim DJ, Bluestone CD, Casselbrant M, Klein JO, Ogra PL, eds. *Recent Advances in Otitis Media: Proceedings of the 6th International Symposium.* Hamilton, ON, Canada: BC Decker; 1996:354–356

95. Friel-Patti S, Finitzo T. Language learning in a prospective study of otitis media with effusion in the first two years of life. *J Speech Hear Res.* 1990;33:188–194

96. Wallace IF, Gravel JS, McCarton CM, Stapells DR, Bernstein RS, Ruben RJ. Otitis media, auditory sensitivity, and language outcomes at one year. *Laryngoscope.* 1988;98:64–70

97. Roberts JE, Burchinal MR, Medley LP, et al. Otitis media, hearing sensitivity, and maternal responsiveness in relation to language during infancy. *J Pediatr.* 1995;126:481–489

98. Roberts JE, Burchinal MR, Zeisel SA. Otitis media in early childhood in relation to children's school-age language and academic skills. *Pediatrics.* 2002;110:696–706

99. Rovers MM, Straatman H, Ingels K, van der Wilt GJ, van den Broek P, Zielhuis GA. The effect of ventilation tubes on language development in infants with otitis media with effusion: a randomized trial. *Pediatrics.* 2000;106(3). Available at: www.pediatrics.org/cgi/content/full/106/3/e42

100. Paradise JL, Feldman HM, Campbell TF, et al. Early versus delayed insertion of tympanostomy tubes for persistent otitis media: developmental outcomes at the age of three years in relation to prerandomization illness patterns and hearing levels. *Pediatr Infect Dis J.* 2003;22:309–314

101. Kokko E. Chronic secretory otitis media in children. A clinical study. *Acta Otolaryngol Suppl.* 1974;327:1–44

102. Fria TJ, Cantekin EI, Eichler JA. Hearing acuity of children with otitis media with effusion. *Arch Otolaryngol.* 1985;111:10–16

103. Gravel JS, Wallace IF. Effects of otitis media with effusion on hearing in the first three years of life. *J Speech Lang Hear Res.* 2000;43:631–644

104. Roberts JE, Burchinal MR, Zeisel S, et al. Otitis media, the caregiving environment, and language and cognitive outcomes at 2 years. *Pediatrics.* 1998;102:346–354

105. Gravel JS, Wallace IF, Ruben RJ. Early otitis media and later educational risk. *Acta Otolaryngol.* 1995;115:279–281

106. Cunningham M, Cox EO; American Academy of Pediatrics, Committee on Practice and Ambulatory Medicine, Section on Otolaryngology and Bronchoesophagology. Hearing assessment in infants and children: recommendations beyond neonatal screening. *Pediatrics.* 2003;111:436–440

107. American Speech-Language-Hearing Association Panel on Audiologic Assessment. *Guidelines for Audiologic Screening.* Rockville, MD: American Speech-Language-Hearing Association; 1996

108. Rosenfeld RM, Goldsmith AJ, Madell JR. How accurate is parent rating of hearing for children with otitis media? *Arch Otolaryngol Head Neck Surg.* 1998;124:989–992

109. Brody R, Rosenfeld RM, Goldsmith AJ, Madell JR. Parents cannot detect mild hearing loss in children. *Otolaryngol Head Neck Surg.* 1999;121:681–686

110. Catts HW, Fey ME, Zhang X, Tomblin JB. Language basis of reading and reading disabilities: evidence from a longitudinal investigation. *Sci Stud Read.* 1999;3:331–362

111. Johnson CJ, Beitchman JH, Young A, et al. Fourteen-year follow-up of children with and without speech/language impairments: speech/language stability and outcomes. *J Speech Lang Hear Res.* 1999;42:744–760

112. Scarborough H, Dobrich W. Development of children with early language delay. *J Speech Hear Res.* 1990;33:70–83

113. Tomblin JB, Records NL, Buckwalter P, Zhang X, Smith E, O'Brien M. Prevalence of specific language impairment in kindergarten children. *J Speech Lang Hear Res.* 1997;40:1245–1260

114. Glade MJ. *Diagnostic and Therapeutic Technology Assessment: Speech Therapy in Patients With a Prior History of Recurrent Acute or Chronic Otitis Media With Effusion.* Chicago, IL: American Medical Association; 1996:1–14

115. Casby MW. Otitis media and language development: a meta-analysis. *Am J Speech Lang Pathol.* 2001;10:65–80

116. Maw R, Wilks J, Harvey I, Peters TJ, Golding J. Early surgery compared with watchful waiting for glue ear and effect on language development in preschool children: a randomised trial. *Lancet.* 1999;353:960–963

117. Coplan J. *Early Language Milestone Scale.* 2nd ed. Austin, TX: PRO-ED; 1983

118. Fenson L, Dale PS, Reznick JS, et al. *MacArthur Communicative Development Inventories. User's Guide and Technical Manual.* San Diego, CA: Singular Publishing Group; 1993

119. Rescoria L. The Language Development Survey: a screening tool for delayed language in toddlers. *J Speech Hear Dis.* 1989;54:587–599

120. Frankenburg WK, Dodds JA, Faucal A, et al. *Denver Developmental Screening Test II.* Denver, CO: University of Colorado Press; 1990

121. Klee T, Pearce K, Carson DK. Improving the positive predictive value of screening for developmental language disorder. *J Speech Lang Hear Res.* 2000;43:821–833

122. Shekelle PG, Ortiz E, Rhodes S, et al. Validity of the Agency for Healthcare Research and Quality clinical practice guidelines: how quickly do guidelines become outdated? *JAMA.* 2001;286:1461–1467

123. Zielhuis GA, Straatman H, Rach GH, van den Broek P. Analysis and presentation of data on the natural course of otitis media with effusion in children. *Int J Epidemiol.* 1990;19:1037–1044

124. MRC Multi-centre Otitis Media Study Group. Risk factors for persistence of bilateral otitis media with effusion. *Clin Otolaryngol.* 2001;26:147–156

125. van Balen FA, De Melker RA. Persistent otitis media with effusion: can it be predicted? A family practice follow-up study in children aged 6 months to 6 years. *J Fam Pract.* 2000;49:605–611

126. Sano S, Kamide Y, Schachern PA, Paparella MM. Micropathologic changes of pars tensa in children with otitis media with effusion. *Arch Otolaryngol Head Neck Surg.* 1994;120:815–819

127. Yellon RF, Doyle WJ, Whiteside TL, Diven WF, March AR, Fireman P. Cytokines, immunoglobulins, and bacterial pathogens in middle ear effusions. *Arch Otolaryngol Head Neck Surg.* 1995;121:865–869

128. Maw RA, Bawden R. Tympanic membrane atrophy, scarring, atelectasis and attic retraction in persistent, untreated otitis media with effusion and following ventilation tube insertion. *Int J Pediatr Otorhinolaryngol.* 1994;30:189–204

129. Davis JM, Elfenbein J, Schum R, Bentler RA. Effects of mild and moderate hearing impairment on language, educational, and psychosocial behavior of children. *J Speech Hear Disord.* 1986;51:53–62

130. Carney AE, Moeller MP. Treatment efficacy: hearing loss in children. *J Speech Lang Hear Res.* 1998;41:S61–S84

131. Karchmer MA, Allen TE. The functional assessment of deaf and hard of hearing students. *Am Ann Deaf.* 1999;144:68–77

132. Bess FH, Dodd-Murphy J, Parker RA. Children with minimal sensorineural hearing loss: prevalence, educational performance, and functional status. *Ear Hear.* 1998;19:339–354

133. Roberts JE, Burchinal MR, Jackson SC, et al. Otitis media in early childhood in relation to preschool language and school readiness skills among black children. *Pediatrics.* 2000;106:725–735

134. Haggard MP, Birkin JA, Browning GG, Gatehouse S, Lewis S. Behavior problems in otitis media. *Pediatr Infect Dis J.* 1994;13:S43–S50

135. Bennett KE, Haggard MP. Behaviour and cognitive outcomes from middle ear disease. *Arch Dis Child.* 1999;80:28–35

136. Bennett KE, Haggard MP, Silva PA, Stewart IA. Behaviour and developmental effects of otitis media with effusion into the teens. *Arch Dis Child.* 2001;85:91–95

137. Wilks J, Maw R, Peters TJ, Harvey I, Golding J. Randomised controlled trial of early surgery versus watchful waiting for glue ear: the effect on behavioural problems in pre-school children. *Clin Otolaryngol.* 2000;25:209–214

138. Rosenfeld RM, Bhaya MH, Bower CM, et al. Impact of tympanostomy tubes on child quality of life. *Arch Otolaryngol Head Neck Surg.* 2000;126:585–592

139. Rosenfeld RM, Bluestone CD. Clinical efficacy of surgical therapy. In: Rosenfeld RM, Bluestone CD, eds. *Evidence-Based Otitis Media.* 2nd ed. Hamilton, ON, Canada: BC Decker; 2003:227–240

140. Kuyvenhoven MM, De Melker RA. Referrals to specialists. An exploratory investigation of referrals by 13 general practitioners to medical and surgical departments. *Scand J Prim Health Care.* 1990;8:53–57

141. Haldis TA, Blankenship JC. Telephone reporting in the consultant-generalist relationship. *J Eval Clin Pract.* 2002;8:31–35

142. Reichman S. The generalist's patient and the subspecialist. *Am J Manag Care.* 2002;8:79–82

143. Gates GA, Avery CA, Prihoda TJ, Cooper JC Jr. Effectiveness of adenoidectomy and tympanostomy tubes in the treatment of chronic otitis media with effusion. *N Engl J Med.* 1987;317:1444–1451

144. Mandel EM, Rockette HE, Bluestone CD, Paradise JL, Nozza RJ. Myringotomy with and without tympanostomy tubes for chronic otitis media with effusion. *Arch Otolaryngol Head Neck Surg.* 1989;115:1217–1224

145. Mandel EM, Rockette HE, Bluestone CD, Paradise JL, Nozza RJ. Efficacy of myringotomy with and without tympanostomy tubes for chronic otitis media with effusion. *Pediatr Infect Dis J.* 1992;11:270–277

146. University of York Centre for Reviews and Dissemination. The treatment of persistent glue ear in children. *Eff Health Care.* 1992;4:1–16

147. Rovers MM, Straatman H, Ingels K, van der Wilt GJ, van den Broek P, Zielhuis GA. The effect of short-term ventilation tubes versus watchful waiting on hearing in young children with persistent otitis media with effusion: a randomized trial. *Ear Hear.* 2001;22:191–199

148. Paradise JL, Bluestone CD, Colborn DK, et al. Adenoidectomy and adenotonsillectomy for recurrent acute otitis media: parallel randomized clinical trials in children not previously treated with tympanostomy tubes. *JAMA.* 1999;282:945–953

149. Boston M, McCook J, Burke B, Derkay C. Incidence of and risk factors for additional tympanostomy tube insertion in children. *Arch Otolaryngol Head Neck Surg.* 2003;129:293–296

150. Coyte PC, Croxford R, McIsaac W, Feldman W, Friedberg J. The role of adjuvant adenoidectomy and tonsillectomy in the outcome of insertion of tympanostomy tubes. *N Engl J Med.* 2001;344:1188–1195

151. Paradise JL, Bluestone CD, Rogers KD, et al. Efficacy of adenoidectomy for recurrent otitis media in children previously treated with tympanostomy-tube placement. Results of parallel randomized and nonrandomized trials. *JAMA.* 1990;263:2066–2073

152. Maw AR. Chronic otitis media with effusion (glue ear) and adenotonsillectomy: prospective randomised controlled study. *Br Med J (Clin Res Ed).* 1983;287:1586–1588

153. Cohen D, Schechter Y, Slatkine M, Gatt N, Perez R. Laser myringotomy in different age groups. *Arch Otolaryngol Head Neck Surg.* 2001;127: 260–264

154. Holzman RS. Morbidity and mortality in pediatric anesthesia. *Pediatr Clin North Am.* 1994;41:239–256

155. Cottrell JE, Golden S. *Under the Mask: A Guide to Feeling Secure and Comfortable During Anesthesia and Surgery.* New Brunswick, NJ: Rutgers University Press; 2001

156. Kay DJ, Nelson M, Rosenfeld RM. Meta-analysis of tympanostomy tube sequelae. *Otolaryngol Head Neck Surg.* 2001;124:374–380

157. Crysdale WS, Russel D. Complications of tonsillectomy and adenoidectomy in 9409 children observed overnight. *CMAJ.* 1986;135: 1139–1142

158. Harrison H, Fixsen A, Vickers A. A randomized comparison of homeopathic and standard care for the treatment of glue ear in children. *Complement Ther Med.* 1999;7:132–135

159. Sawyer CE, Evans RL, Boline PD, Branson R, Spicer A. A feasibility study of chiropractic spinal manipulation versus sham spinal manipulation for chronic otitis media with effusion in children. *J Manipulative Physiol Ther.* 1999;22:292–298

160. Ernst E. Serious adverse effects of unconventional therapies for children and adolescents: a systematic review of recent evidence. *Eur J Pediatr.* 2003;162:72–80

161. Cohen MH, Eisenberg DM. Potential physician malpractice liability associated with complementary and integrative medical therapies. *Ann Intern Med.* 2002;136:596–603

162. Mullins RJ, Heddle R. Adverse reactions associated with echinacea: the Australian experience. *Ann Allergy Asthma Immunol.* 2002;88:42–51

163. Miller LG, Hume A, Harris IM, et al. White paper on herbal products. American College of Clinical Pharmacy. *Pharmacotherapy.* 2000;20: 877–891

164. Angell M, Kassirer JP. Alternative medicine—the risks of untested and unregulated remedies. *N Engl J Med.* 1998;339:839–841

165. Fallon JM. The role of chiropractic adjustment in the care and treatment of 332 children with otitis media. *J Clin Chiropractic Pediatr.* 1997;2:167–183

166. Shafrir Y, Kaufman BA. Quadriplegia after chiropractic manipulation in an infant with congenital torticollis caused by a spinal cord astrocytoma. *J Pediatr.* 1992;120:266–269

167. Corey JP, Adham RE, Abbass AH, Seligman I. The role of IgE-mediated hypersensitivity in otitis media with effusion. *Am J Otolaryngol.* 1994;15:138–144

168. Bernstein JM. Role of allergy in eustachian tube blockage and otitis media with effusion: a review. *Otolaryngol Head Neck Surg.* 1996;114: 562–568

169. Ishii TM, Toriyama M, Suzuki JI. Histopathological study of otitis media with effusion. *Ann Otol Rhinol Laryngol.* 1980;89(suppl):83–86

170. Hurst DS, Venge P. Evidence of eosinophil, neutrophil, and mast-cell mediators in the effusion of OME patients with and without atopy. *Allergy.* 2000;55:435–441

171. Hurst DS, Venge P. The impact of atopy on neutrophil activity in middle ear effusion from children and adults with chronic otitis media. *Arch Otolaryngol Head Neck Surg.* 2002;128:561–566

172. Hurst DS. Allergy management of refractory serous otitis media. *Otolaryngol Head Neck Surg.* 1990;102:664–669

Otitis Media Clinical Practice Guidelines
Quick Reference Tools

- Action Statement Summary
  — The Diagnosis and Management of Acute Otitis Media
  — Otitis Media With Effusion
- *ICD-9-CM/ICD-10-CM* Coding Quick Reference for Otitis Media
- Bonus Feature
  — Continuum Model for Otitis Media
- AAP Patient Education Handouts
  — *Acute Ear Infections and Your Child*
  — *Middle Ear Fluid and Your Child*

Action Statement Summary

The Diagnosis and Management of Acute Otitis Media

Key Action Statement 1A
Clinicians should diagnose acute otitis media (AOM) in children who present with moderate to severe bulging of the tympanic membrane (TM) *or* new onset of otorrhea not due to acute otitis externa. Evidence Quality: Grade B. Strength: Recommendation.

Key Action Statement 1B
Clinicians should diagnose AOM in children who present with mild bulging of the TM *and* recent (less than 48 hours) onset of ear pain (holding, tugging, rubbing of the ear in a nonverbal child) or intense erythema of the TM. Evidence Quality: Grade C. Strength: Recommendation.

Key Action Statement 1C
Clinicians should not diagnose AOM in children who do not have middle ear effusion (MEE) (based on pneumatic otoscopy and/or tympanometry). Evidence Quality: Grade B. Strength: Recommendation.

Key Action Statement 2
The management of AOM should include an assessment of pain. If pain is present, the clinician should recommend treatment to reduce pain. Evidence Quality: Grade B. Strength: Strong Recommendation.

Key Action Statement 3A
Severe AOM: The clinician should prescribe antibiotic therapy for AOM (bilateral or unilateral) in children 6 months and older with severe signs or symptoms (ie, moderate or severe otalgia or otalgia for at least 48 hours or temperature 39°C [102.2°F] or higher). Evidence Quality: Grade B. Strength: Strong Recommendation.

Key Action Statement 3B
Nonsevere bilateral AOM in young children: The clinician should prescribe antibiotic therapy for bilateral AOM in children 6 months through 23 months of age without severe signs or symptoms (ie, mild otalgia for less than 48 hours and temperature less than 39°C [102.2°F]). Evidence Quality: Grade B. Strength: Recommendation.

Key Action Statement 3C
Nonsevere unilateral AOM in young children: The clinician should either prescribe antibiotic therapy *or* offer observa-tion with close follow-up based on joint decision-making with the parent(s)/caregiver for unilateral AOM in children 6 months to 23 months of age without severe signs or symptoms (ie, mild otalgia for less than 48 hours and temperature less than 39°C [102.2°F]). When observation is used, a mechanism must be in place to ensure follow-up and begin antibiotic therapy if the child worsens or fails to improve within 48 to 72 hours of onset of symptoms. Evidence Quality: Grade B. Strength: Recommendation.

Key Action Statement 3D
Nonsevere AOM in older children: The clinician should either prescribe antibiotic therapy *or* offer observation with close follow-up based on joint decision-making with the parent(s)/caregiver for AOM (bilateral or unilateral) in children 24 months or older without severe signs or symptoms (ie, mild otalgia for less than 48 hours and temperature less than 39°C [102.2°F]). When observation is used, a mechanism must be in place to ensure follow-up and begin antibiotic therapy if the child worsens or fails to improve within 48 to 72 hours of onset of symptoms. Evidence Quality: Grade B. Strength: Recommendation.

Key Action Statement 4A
Clinicians should prescribe amoxicillin for AOM when a decision to treat with antibiotics has been made *and* the child has not received amoxicillin in the past 30 days *or* the child does not have concurrent purulent conjunctivitis *or* the child is not allergic to penicillin. Evidence Quality: Grade B. Strength: Recommendation.

Key Action Statement 4B
Clinicians should prescribe an antibiotic with additional β-lactamase coverage for AOM when a decision to treat with antibiotics has been made, *and* the child has received amoxicillin in the last 30 days *or* has concurrent purulent conjunctivitis, *or* has a history of recurrent AOM unresponsive to amoxicillin. Evidence Quality: Grade C. Strength: Recommendation.

Key Action Statement 4C
Clinicians should reassess the patient if the caregiver reports that the child's symptoms have worsened or failed to respond to the initial antibiotic treatment within 48 to 72 hours and determine whether a change in therapy is needed. Evidence Quality: Grade B. Strength: Recommendation.

Key Action Statement 5A

Clinicians should not prescribe prophylactic antibiotics to reduce the frequency of episodes of AOM in children with recurrent AOM. Evidence Quality: Grade B. Strength: Recommendation.

Key Action Statement 5B

Clinicians may offer tympanostomy tubes for recurrent AOM (3 episodes in 6 months or 4 episodes in 1 year with 1 episode in the preceding 6 months). Evidence Quality: Grade B. Strength: Option.

Key Action Statement 6A

Clinicians should recommend pneumococcal conjugate vaccine to all children according to the schedule of the Advisory Committee on Immunization Practices of the Centers for Disease Control and prevention, American Academy of Pediatrics (AAP), and American Academy of Family Physicians (AAFP). Evidence Quality: Grade B. Strength: Strong Recommendation.

Otitis Media With Effusion

1A. Pneumatic Otoscopy

Clinicians should use pneumatic otoscopy as the primary diagnostic method for OME, and OME should be distinguished from AOM.

This is a strong recommendation based on systematic review of cohort studies and the preponderance of benefit over harm.

1B. Tympanometry

Tympanometry can be used to confirm the diagnosis a of OME.

This option is based on cohort studies and a balance of benefit and harm.

1C. Screening

Population-based screening programs for OME are not recommended in healthy, asymptomatic children.

This recommendation is based on randomized, controlled trials and cohort studies, with a preponderance of harm over benefit.

2. Documentation

Clinicians should document the laterality, duration of effusion, and presence and severity of associated symptoms at each assessment of the child with OME.

This recommendation is based on observational studies and strong preponderance of benefit over harm.

3. Child at Risk

Clinicians should distinguish the child with OME who is at risk for speech, language, or learning problems from other children with OME and should evaluate hearing, speech, language, and need for intervention more promptly.

This recommendation is based on case series, the preponderance of benefit over harm, and ethical limitations in studying children with OME who are at risk.

4. Watchful Waiting

Clinicians should manage the child with OME who is not at risk with watchful waiting for 3 months from the date of effusion onset (if known) or diagnosis (if onset is unknown).

This recommendation is based on systematic review of cohort studies and the preponderance of benefit over harm.

5. Medication

Antihistamines and decongestants are ineffective for OME and are not recommended for treatment; antimicrobials and corticosteroids do not have long-term efficacy and are not recommended for routine management.

This recommendation is based on systematic review of randomized, controlled trials and the preponderance of harm over benefit.

6. Hearing and Language

Hearing testing is recommended when OME persists for 3 months or longer or at any time that language delay, learning problems, or a significant hearing loss is suspected in a child with OME; language testing should be conducted for children with hearing loss.

This recommendation is based on cohort studies and the preponderance of benefit over risk.

7. Surveillance

Children with persistent OME who are not at risk should be reexamined at 3- to 6-month intervals until the effusion is no longer present, significant hearing loss is identified, or structural abnormalities of the eardrum or middle ear are suspected.

This recommendation is based on randomized, controlled trials and observational studies with a preponderance of benefit over harm.

8. Referral

When children with OME are referred by the primary care clinician for evaluation by an otolaryngologist, audiologist, or speech-language pathologist, the referring clinician should document the effusion duration and specific reason for referral (evaluation, surgery) and provide additional relevant information such as history of AOM and developmental status of the child.

This option is based on panel consensus and a preponderance of benefit over harm.

9. Surgery

When a child becomes a surgical candidate, tympanostomy tube insertion is the preferred initial procedure; adenoidectomy should not be performed unless a distinct indication exists (nasal obstruction, chronic adenoiditis). Repeat surgery consists of adenoidectomy plus myringotomy, with or without tube insertion. tonsillectomy alone or myringotomy alone should not be used to treat OME.

This recommendation is based on randomized, controlled trials with a preponderance of benefit over harm.

10. CAM

No recommendation is made regarding CAM as a treatment for OME.

There is no recommendation based on lack of scientific evidence documenting efficacy and an uncertain balance of harm and benefit.

11. Allergy Management

No recommendation is made regarding allergy management as a treatment for OME.

There is no recommendation based on insufficient evidence of therapeutic efficacy or a causal relationship between allergy and OME.

Coding Quick Reference for Otitis Media

ICD-9-CM	ICD-10-CM	
381.01　Otitis media, acute, serous	H65.00	Acute serous otitis media, unspecified ear
	H65.01	Right ear
	H65.02	Left ear
	H65.03	Bilateral
	H65.04	Recurrent, right ear
	H65.05	Recurrent, left ear
	H65.06	Recurrent, bilateral
	H65.07	Recurrent, unspecified ear
381.10　Otitis media, chronic, serous	H65.20	Chronic serous otitis media, unspecified ear
	H65.21	Right ear
	H65.22	Left ear
	H65.23	Bilateral
381.4　Otitis media with effusion	H65.90	Unspecified nonsuppurative otitis media, unspecified ear
	H65.91	Right ear
	H65.92	Left ear
	H65.93	Bilateral
382.00　Otitis media, acute, purulent	H66.001	Acute suppurative otitis media without spontaneous rupture of ear drum, right ear
	H66.002	Left ear
	H66.003	Bilateral
	H66.004	Recurrent, right ear
	H66.005	Recurrent, left ear
	H66.006	Recurrent, bilateral
	H66.007	Recurrent, unspecified ear
	H66.009	Unspecified ear
382.01　Otitis media, acute, purulent, with rupture	H66.011	Acute suppurative otitis media with spontaneous rupture of ear drum, right ear
	H66.012	Left ear
	H66.013	Bilateral
	H66.014	Recurrent, right ear
	H66.015	Recurrent, left ear
	H66.016	Recurrent, bilateral
	H66.017	Recurrent, unspecified ear
	H66.019	Unspecified ear
382.02　Otitis media, acute, purulent with associated condition (code underlying condition first)	H67.1	Otitis media in diseases classified elsewhere, right ear
	H67.2	Left ear
	H67.3	Bilateral
	H67.9	Unspecified ear
382.3　Otitis media, chronic, purulent	H66.3X1	Other chronic suppurative otitis media, right ear
	H66.3X2	Left ear
	H66.3X3	Bilateral
	H66.3X9	Unspecified ear

Continuum Model for Otitis Media

The following continuum model from *Coding for Pediatrics 2014* has been devised to express the various levels of service for otitis media. This model demonstrates the cumulative effect of the key criteria for each level of service using a single diagnosis as the common denominator. It also shows the importance of other variables, such as patient age, duration and severity of illness, social contexts, and comorbid conditions that often have key roles in pediatric cases.

Quick Reference for Codes Used in Continuum for Otitis Media				
E/M Code Level	**History**	**Examination**	**MDM**	**Time**
99211[a]	NA	NA	NA	5 minutes
99212	Problem-focused	Problem-focused	Straightforward	10 minutes
99213	Expanded problem-focused	Expanded problem-focused	Low	15 minutes
99214	Detailed	Detailed	Moderate	25 minutes
99215	Comprehensive	Comprehensive	High	40 minutes

Abbreviations: E/M, evaluation and management; MDM; medical decision-making; NA, not applicable.

[a] Low level E/M service that may not require the presence of a physician.

Adapted from American Academy of Pediatrics. *Coding for Pediatrics 2014: A Manual for Pediatric Documentation and Payment.* 19th ed. Elk Grove Village, IL: American Academy of Pediatrics; 2014.

Current Procedural Terminology (CPT®) 5-digit codes, nomenclature, and other data are copyright 2013 American Medical Association (AMA). All Rights Reserved.

Continuum Model for Otitis Media

CPT Code Vignette	History	Physical Examination	Medical Decision-making
99211* Nursing evaluations Follow-up on serous fluid or hearing loss with tympanogram (Be sure to code tympanogram [92567] and/or audiogram [92551 series] in addition to 99211.) *There are no required key components; however, the nurse must document his or her history, physical examination, and assessment to support medical necessity.*	1. Chief complaint 2. History of treatment		1. Completion of medication 2. No need for further therapy 3. No need for further follow-up
99212 Follow-up otitis media, uncomplicated with primary examination being limited to ears	Problem focused 1. Chief complaint 2. History of treatment 3. Difficulties with medication 4. Hearing status	Problem focused 1. Ears	Straightforward 1. Completion of medication 2. No need for further therapy 3. No need for further follow-up
99213 2-year-old presents with pinkeye and recent upper respiratory infection	Problem focused 1. Chief complaint 2. Brief history of present illness (HPI) plus pertinent review of systems (ROS) a. Symptoms b. Duration of illness c. Home management, including over-the-counter medications, and response d. Additional symptoms from ROS	Expanded problem focused 1. Ears 2. Nose 3. Throat 4. Conjunctiva 5. Overall appearance	Moderate or low complexity 1. Observation and nonprescription analgesics

Continuum Model for Otitis Media, continued

CPT Code Vignette	History	Physical Examination	Medical Decision-making

99214
An infant presents for suspected third episode within 2–3 months
Infant presents with fever and cough
	Detailed
	1. Chief complaint
	2. Detailed HPI plus pertinent ROS and pertinent past, family, and social history (PFSH)
	  a. Symptoms of illness
	  b. Fever, other signs
	  c. Any other medications
	  d. Allergies
	  e. Frequency of similar infection in past and response to treatment
	  f. Environmental factors (eg, tobacco exposure, child care)
	  g. Immunization status
	  h. Feeding history
		Detailed
		1. Overall appearance
		2. Hydration status
		3. Eyes
		4. Ears
		5. Nose
		6. Throat
		7. Lungs
		8. Skin
			Moderate complexity
			1. Treatment including antibiotics and supportive care.
			2. Consider/discuss tympano-centesis (**69420** or **69421**).
			3. Hearing evaluation planned.
			4. Discuss possible referral to an allergist or otolaryngologist for tympanostomy.
			5. Discuss contributing environmental factors and supportive treatment.

99215
3-month-old presents with high fever, vomiting, irritability
	Detailed
	1. Chief complaint
	2. Detailed HPI plus pertinent ROS and pertinent PFSH
	  a. Symptoms of illness
	  b. Fever, other signs
	  c. Any other medications
	  d. Allergies
	  e. Frequency of similar infection in past and response to treatment
	  f. Environmental factors (eg, tobacco exposure, child care)
	  g. Immunization status
	  h. Feeding history
		Detailed
		1. Overall appearance
		2. Hydration status
		3. Eyes
		4. Ears
		5. Nose
		6. Throat
		7. Lungs
		8. Skin
			High complexity
			1. Laboratory tests: Consider a complete blood cell count with differential, blood culture, blood urea nitrogen, creatinine, electrolytes, urinalysis with culture, chest x-ray, and possible lumbar puncture based on history and clinical findings.
			2. Antibiotic therapy: Consider parenteral antibiotics.
			3. Consider hospitalization based on history, physical findings, and laboratory studies.
			4. Determine need for follow-up (eg, reassess later in same day by phone or follow-up visit as well as later follow-up).
			5. Attempt oral rehydration in office.

Continuum Model for Otitis Media, continued

CPT Code Vignette	History	Physical Examination	Medical Decision-making
99214 or 99215 NOTE: Depending on the variables (ie, time), this example could be reported as 99214 or 99215. Extended evaluation of child with chronic or recurrent otitis media NOTE: Time is the key factor when counseling and/or coordination of care are more than 50% of the face-to-face time with the patient. For 99214, the total visit time would be 25 minutes; for 99215, the total time is 40 minutes. You must document time spent on counseling and/or coordination of care and list the areas discussed.	Detailed History with extended HPI as in 99214, but complete ROS and PFSH	Detailed or comprehensive General or single organ system (ears, nose, mouth, and throat)	Moderate or high complexity Tests: audiometry and/or tympanometry Extensive discussion of treatment options including but not limited to 1. Continued episodic treatment with antibiotics 2. Myringotomy and tube placement 3. Adenoidectomy 4. Allergy evaluation 5. Steroid therapy with weighing of risk-benefit ratio of various therapies

Acute Ear Infections and Your Child

Next to the common cold, an ear infection is the most common childhood illness. In fact, most children have at least one ear infection by the time they are 3 years old. Many ear infections clear up without causing any lasting problems.

The following is information from the American Academy of Pediatrics about the symptoms, treatments, and possible complications of acute *otitis media*, a common infection of the middle ear.

How do ear infections develop?

The ear has 3 parts—the outer ear, middle ear, and inner ear. A narrow channel (eustachian tube) connects the middle ear to the back of the nose. When a child has a cold, nose or throat infection, or allergy, the mucus and fluid can enter the eustachian tube causing a buildup of fluid in the middle ear. If bacteria or a virus infects this fluid, it can cause swelling and pain in the ear. This type of ear infection is called *acute otitis media* (*middle ear inflammation*).

Often after the symptoms of acute otitis media clear up, fluid remains in the ear, creating another kind of ear problem called *otitis media with effusion* (*middle ear fluid*). This condition is harder to detect than acute otitis media because except for the fluid and usually some mild hearing loss, there is often no pain or other symptoms present. This fluid may last several months and, in most cases, disappears on its own. The child's hearing then returns to normal.

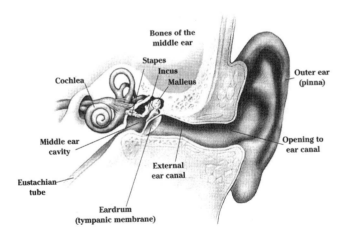

Cross-Section of the Ear

Is my child at risk for developing an ear infection?

Risk factors for developing childhood ear infections include

- **Age.** Infants and young children are more likely to get ear infections than older children. The size and shape of an infant's eustachian tube makes it easier for an infection to develop. Ear infections occur most often in children between 6 months and 3 years of age. Also, the younger a child is at the time of the first ear infection, the greater the chance he will have repeated infections.
- **Family history.** Ear infections can run in families. Children are more likely to have repeated middle ear infections if a parent or sibling also had repeated ear infections.
- **Colds.** Colds often lead to ear infections. Children in group child care settings have a higher chance of passing their colds to each other because they are exposed to more viruses from the other children.
- **Tobacco smoke.** Children who breathe in someone else's tobacco smoke have a higher risk of developing health problems, including ear infections.

How can I reduce the risk of an ear infection?

Some things you can do to help reduce your child's risk of getting an ear infection are

- Breastfeed instead of bottle-feed. Breastfeeding may decrease the risk of frequent colds and ear infections.
- Keep your child away from tobacco smoke, especially in your home or car.
- Throw away pacifiers or limit to daytime use, *if your child is older than 1 year.*
- Keep vaccinations up to date. Vaccines against bacteria (such as pneumococcal vaccine) and viruses (such as influenza vaccine) reduce the number of ear infections in children with frequent infections.

What are the symptoms of an ear infection?

Your child may have many symptoms during an ear infection. Talk with your pediatrician about the best way to treat your child's symptoms.

- **Pain.** The most common symptom of an ear infection is pain. Older children can tell you that their ears hurt. Younger children may only seem irritable and cry. You may notice this more during feedings because sucking and swallowing may cause painful pressure changes in the middle ear.
- **Loss of appetite.** Your child may have less of an appetite because of the ear pain.
- **Trouble sleeping.** Your child may have trouble sleeping because of the ear pain.
- **Fever.** Your child may have a temperature ranging from 100°F (normal) to 104°F.

- **Ear drainage.** You might notice yellow or white fluid, possibly blood-tinged, draining from your child's ear. The fluid may have a foul odor and will look different from normal earwax (which is orange-yellow or reddish-brown). Pain and pressure often decrease after this drainage begins, but this doesn't always mean that the infection is going away. If this happens it's not an emergency, but your child will need to see your pediatrician.
- **Trouble hearing.** During and after an ear infection, your child may have trouble hearing for several weeks. This occurs because the fluid behind the eardrum gets in the way of sound transmission. This is usually temporary and clears up after the fluid from the middle ear drains away.

Important: Your doctor *cannot* diagnose an ear infection over the phone; your child's eardrum must be examined by your doctor to confirm fluid buildup and signs of inflammation.

What causes ear pain?

There are other reasons why your child's ears may hurt besides an ear infection. The following can cause ear pain:

- An infection of the skin of the ear canal, often called "swimmer's ear"
- Reduced pressure in the middle ear from colds or allergies
- A sore throat
- Teething or sore gums
- Inflammation of the eardrum alone during a cold (without fluid buildup)

How are ear infections treated?

Because pain is often the first and most uncomfortable symptom of an ear infection, it's important to help comfort your child by giving her pain medicine. Acetaminophen and ibuprofen are over-the-counter (OTC) pain medicines that may help decrease much of the pain. Be sure to use the right dosage for your child's age and size. *Don't give aspirin to your child.* It has been associated with Reye syndrome, a disease that affects the liver and brain. There are also ear drops that may relieve ear pain for a short time. Ask your pediatrician whether these drops should be used. There is no need to use OTC cold medicines (decongestants and antihistamines), because they don't help clear up ear infections.

Not all ear infections require antibiotics. Some children who don't have a high fever and aren't severely ill may be observed without antibiotics. In most cases, pain and fever will improve in the first 1 to 2 days.

If your child is younger than 2 years, has drainage from the ear, has a fever higher than 102.5°F, seems to be in a lot of pain, is unable to sleep, isn't eating, or is acting ill, it's important to call your pediatrician. If your child is older than 2 years and your child's symptoms are mild, you may wait a couple of days to see if she improves.

Your child's ear pain and fever should improve or go away within 3 days of their onset. If your child's condition doesn't improve within 3 days, or worsens at any time, call your pediatrician. Your pediatrician may wish to see your child and may prescribe an antibiotic to take by mouth, if one wasn't given initially. If an antibiotic was already started, your child may need a different antibiotic. Be sure to follow your pediatrician's instructions closely.

If an antibiotic was prescribed, make sure your child finishes the entire prescription. If you stop the medicine too soon, some of the bacteria that caused the ear infection may still be present and cause an infection to start all over again.

As the infection starts to clear up, your child might feel a "popping" in the ears. This is a normal sign of healing. Children with ear infections don't need to stay home if they are feeling well, as long as a child care provider or someone at school can give them their medicine properly, if needed. If your child needs to travel in an airplane, or wants to swim, contact your pediatrician for specific instructions.

What are signs of hearing problems?

Because your child can have trouble hearing without other symptoms of an ear infection, watch for the following changes in behavior (especially during or after a cold):

- Talking more loudly or softly than usual
- Saying "huh?" or "what?" more than usual
- Not responding to sounds
- Having trouble understanding speech in noisy rooms
- Listening with the TV or radio turned up louder than usual

If you think your child may have difficulty hearing, call your pediatrician. Being able to hear and listen to others talk helps a child learn speech and language. This is especially important during the first few years of life.

Are there complications from ear infections?

Although it's very rare, complications from ear infections can develop, including the following:

- An infection of the inner ear that causes dizziness and imbalance (labyrinthitis)
- An infection of the skull behind the ear (mastoiditis)
- Scarring or thickening of the eardrum
- Loss of feeling or movement in the face (facial paralysis)
- Permanent hearing loss

It's normal for children to have several ear infections when they are young—even as many as 2 separate infections within a few months. Most ear infections that develop in children are minor. Recurring ear infections may be a nuisance, but they usually clear up without any lasting problems. With proper care and treatment, ear infections can usually be managed successfully. But, if your child has one ear infection after another for several months, you may want to talk about other treatment options with your pediatrician.

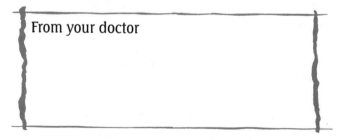

From your doctor

American Academy
of Pediatrics

DEDICATED TO THE HEALTH OF ALL CHILDREN™

The American Academy of Pediatrics is an organization of 60,000 primary care pediatricians, pediatric medical subspecialists, and pediatric surgical specialists dedicated to the health, safety, and well-being of infants, children, adolescents, and young adults.

American Academy of Pediatrics
Web site—www.HealthyChildren.org

Middle Ear Fluid and Your Child

The *middle* ear is the space behind the eardrum that is usually filled with air. When a child has middle ear fluid (otitis media with effusion), it means that a watery or mucus-like fluid has collected in the middle ear. *Otitis media* means *middle ear inflammation*, and *effusion* means *fluid*.

Middle ear fluid is **not** the same as an ear infection. An ear infection occurs when middle ear fluid is infected with viruses, bacteria, or both, often during a cold. Children with middle ear fluid have no signs or symptoms of infection. Most children don't have fever or severe pain, but may have mild discomfort or trouble hearing. About 90% of children get middle ear fluid at some time before age 5.

The following is information from the American Academy of Pediatrics about the causes, symptoms, risk reduction, testing, and treatments for middle ear fluid, as well as how middle ear fluid may affect your child's learning.

What causes middle ear fluid?

There is no one cause for middle ear fluid. Often your child's doctor may not know the cause. Middle ear fluid could be caused by
- A past ear infection
- A cold or flu
- Blockage of the eustachian tube (a narrow channel that connects the middle ear to the back of the nose)

What are the symptoms of middle ear fluid?

Many healthy children with middle ear fluid have little or no problems. They usually get better on their own. Often middle ear fluid is found at a regular checkup. Ear discomfort, if present, is usually mild. Your child may be irritable, rub his ears, or have trouble sleeping. Other symptoms include hearing loss, irritability, sleep problems, clumsiness, speech or language problems, and poor school performance. You may notice your child sitting closer to the TV or turning the sound up louder than usual. Sometimes it may seem like your child isn't paying attention to you, especially when at the playground or in a noisy environment.

Talk with your child's doctor if you are concerned about your child's hearing. Keep a record of your child's ear problems. Write down your child's name, child's doctor's name and number, date and type of ear problem or infection, treatment, and results. This may help your child's doctor find the cause of the middle ear fluid.

Can middle ear fluid affect my child's learning?

Some children with middle ear fluid are at risk for delays in speaking or may have problems with learning or schoolwork, especially children with
- Permanent hearing loss not caused by middle ear fluid
- Speech and language delays or disorders
- Developmental delay of social and communication skills disorders (for example, autism spectrum disorders)
- Syndromes that affect cognitive, speech, and language delays (for example, Down syndrome)
- Craniofacial disorders that affect cognitive, speech, and language delays (for example, cleft palate)
- Blindness or visual loss that can't be corrected

If your child is at risk and has ongoing middle ear fluid, her hearing, speech, and language should be checked.

How can I reduce the risk of middle ear fluid?

Children who live with smokers, attend group child care, or use pacifiers have more ear infections. Because some children who have middle ear infections later get middle ear fluid, you may want to
- Keep your child away from tobacco smoke.
- Keep your child away from children who are sick.
- Throw away pacifiers or limit to daytime use, *if your child is older than 1 year*.

Are there special tests to check for middle ear fluid?

Two tests that can check for middle ear fluid are *pneumatic otoscopy* and *tympanometry*. A pneumatic otoscope is the recommended test for middle ear fluid. With this tool, the doctor looks at the eardrum and uses air to see how well the eardrum moves. Tympanometry is another test for middle ear fluid that uses sound to see how well the eardrum moves. An eardrum with fluid behind it doesn't move as well as a normal eardrum. Your child must sit still for both tests; the tests are painless.

Because these tests don't check hearing level, a hearing test may be given, if needed. Hearing tests measure how well your child hears. Although hearing tests don't test for middle ear fluid, they can measure if the fluid is affecting your child's hearing level. The type of hearing test given depends on your child's age and ability to participate.

How can middle ear fluid be treated?

Middle ear fluid can be treated in several ways. Treatment options include observation and tube surgery or adenoid surgery. Because a treatment that works for one child may not work for another, your child's doctor can help you decide which treatment is best for your child and when you should see an ear, nose, and throat (ENT) specialist. If one treatment doesn't work, another treatment can be tried. Ask your child's doctor or ENT specialist about the costs, advantages, and disadvantages of each treatment.

When should middle ear fluid be treated?

Your child is more likely to need treatment for middle ear fluid if she has any of the following:

- Conditions placing her at risk for developmental delays (see "Can middle ear fluid affect my child's learning?")
- Fluid in both ears, especially if present more than 3 months
- Hearing loss or other significant symptoms (see "What are the symptoms of middle ear fluid?")

What treatments are not recommended?

A number of treatments are **not** recommended for young children with middle ear fluid.

- **Medicines** not recommended include antibiotics, decongestants, antihistamines, and steroids (by mouth or in nasal sprays). All of these have side effects and do not cure middle ear fluid.
- **Surgical treatments** not recommended include myringotomy (draining of fluid without placing a tube) and tonsillectomy (removal of the tonsils). If your child's doctor or ENT specialist suggests one of these surgeries, it may be for another medical reason. Ask your doctor why your child needs the surgery.

What about other treatment options?

There is no evidence that complementary and alternative medicine treatments or that treatment for allergies works to decrease middle ear fluid. Some of these treatments may be harmful and many are expensive.

The information contained in this publication should not be used as a substitute for the medical care and advice of your pediatrician. There may be variations in treatment that your pediatrician may recommend based on individual facts and circumstances.

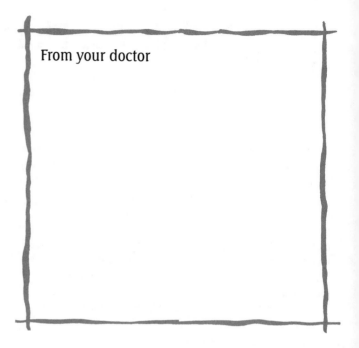

From your doctor

American Academy of Pediatrics

DEDICATED TO THE HEALTH OF ALL CHILDREN™

The American Academy of Pediatrics is an organization of 60,000 primary care pediatricians, pediatric medical subspecialists, and pediatric surgical specialists dedicated to the health, safety, and well-being of infants, children, adolescents, and young adults.

American Academy of Pediatrics
Web site — www.healthychildren.org

Clinical Practice Guideline for the Diagnosis and Management of Acute Bacterial Sinusitis in Children Aged 1 to 18 Years

- *Clinical Practice Guideline*
  - *PPI: AAP Partnership for Policy Implementation*
    See Appendix 2 for more information.

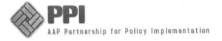

- *Technical Report*

Readers of this clinical practice guideline are urged to review the technical report to enhance the evidence-based decision-making process. The full technical report is available following the clinical practice guideline and on the companion CD-ROM.

CLINICAL PRACTICE GUIDELINE

Clinical Practice Guideline for the Diagnosis and Management of Acute Bacterial Sinusitis in Children Aged 1 to 18 Years

abstract

OBJECTIVE: To update the American Academy of Pediatrics clinical practice guideline regarding the diagnosis and management of acute bacterial sinusitis in children and adolescents.

METHODS: Analysis of the medical literature published since the last version of the guideline (2001).

RESULTS: The diagnosis of acute bacterial sinusitis is made when a child with an acute upper respiratory tract infection (URI) presents with (1) persistent illness (nasal discharge [of any quality] or daytime cough or both lasting more than 10 days without improvement), (2) a worsening course (worsening or new onset of nasal discharge, daytime cough, or fever after initial improvement), or (3) severe onset (concurrent fever [temperature ≥39°C/102.2°F] and purulent nasal discharge for at least 3 consecutive days). Clinicians should not obtain imaging studies of any kind to distinguish acute bacterial sinusitis from viral URI, because they do not contribute to the diagnosis; however, a contrast-enhanced computed tomography scan of the paranasal sinuses should be obtained whenever a child is suspected of having orbital or central nervous system complications. The clinician should prescribe antibiotic therapy for acute bacterial sinusitis in children with severe onset or worsening course. The clinician should either prescribe antibiotic therapy or offer additional observation for 3 days to children with persistent illness. Amoxicillin with or without clavulanate is the first-line treatment of acute bacterial sinusitis. Clinicians should reassess initial management if there is either a caregiver report of worsening (progression of initial signs/symptoms or appearance of new signs/symptoms) or failure to improve within 72 hours of initial management. If the diagnosis of acute bacterial sinusitis is confirmed in a child with worsening symptoms or failure to improve, then clinicians may change the antibiotic therapy for the child initially managed with antibiotic or initiate antibiotic treatment of the child initially managed with observation.

CONCLUSIONS: Changes in this revision include the addition of a clinical presentation designated as "worsening course," an option to treat immediately or observe children with persistent symptoms for 3 days before treating, and a review of evidence indicating that imaging is not necessary in children with uncomplicated acute bacterial sinusitis. *Pediatrics* 2013;132:e262–e280

Ellen R. Wald, MD, FAAP, Kimberly E. Applegate, MD, MS, FAAP, Clay Bordley, MD, FAAP, David H. Darrow, MD, DDS, FAAP, Mary P. Glode, MD, FAAP, S. Michael Marcy, MD, FAAP, Carrie E. Nelson, MD, MS, Richard M. Rosenfeld, MD, FAAP, Nader Shaikh, MD, MPH, FAAP, Michael J. Smith, MD, MSCE, FAAP, Paul V. Williams, MD, FAAP, and Stuart T. Weinberg, MD, FAAP

KEY WORDS
acute bacterial sinusitis, sinusitis, antibiotics, imaging, sinus aspiration

ABBREVIATIONS
AAP—American Academy of Pediatrics
AOM—acute otitis media
CT—computed tomography
PCV-13—13-valent pneumococcal conjugate vaccine
RABS—recurrent acute bacterial sinusitis
RCT—randomized controlled trial
URI—upper respiratory tract infection

www.pediatrics.org/cgi/doi/10.1542/peds.2013-1071

doi:10.1542/peds.2013-1071

PEDIATRICS (ISSN Numbers: Print, 0031-4005; Online, 1098-4275).

INTRODUCTION

Acute bacterial sinusitis is a common complication of viral upper respiratory infection (URI) or allergic inflammation. Using stringent criteria to define acute sinusitis, it has been observed that between 6% and 7% of children seeking care for respiratory symptoms has an illness consistent with this definition.[1-4]

This clinical practice guideline is a revision of the clinical practice guideline published by the American Academy of Pediatrics (AAP) in 2001.[5] It has been developed by a subcommittee of the Steering Committee on Quality Improvement and Management that included physicians with expertise in the fields of primary care pediatrics, academic general pediatrics, family practice, allergy, epidemiology and informatics, pediatric infectious diseases, pediatric otolaryngology, radiology, and pediatric emergency medicine. None of the participants had financial conflicts of interest, and only money from the AAP was used to fund the development of the guideline. The guideline will be reviewed in 5 years unless new evidence emerges that warrants revision sooner.

The guideline is intended for use in a variety of clinical settings (eg, office, emergency department, hospital) by clinicians who treat pediatric patients. The data on which the recommendations are based are included in a companion technical report, published in the electronic pages.[6] The Partnership for Policy Implementation has developed a series of definitions using accepted health information technology standards to assist in the implementation of this guideline in computer systems and quality measurement efforts. This document is available at: http://www2.aap.org/informatics/PPI.html.

This revision focuses on the diagnosis and management of acute sinusitis in children between 1 and 18 years of age. It does not apply to children with subacute or chronic sinusitis. Similar to the previous guideline, this document does not consider neonates and children younger than 1 year or children with anatomic abnormalities of the sinuses, immunodeficiencies, cystic fibrosis, or primary ciliary dyskinesia. The most significant areas of change from the 2001 guideline are in the addition of a clinical presentation designated as "worsening course," inclusion of new data on the effectiveness of antibiotics in children with acute sinusitis,[4] and a review of evidence indicating that imaging is not necessary to identify those children who will benefit from antimicrobial therapy.

METHODS

The Subcommittee on Management of Sinusitis met in June 2009 to identify research questions relevant to guideline revision. The primary goal was to update the 2001 report by identifying and reviewing additional studies of pediatric acute sinusitis that have been performed over the past decade.

Searches of PubMed were performed by using the same search term as in the 2001 report. All searches were limited to English-language and human studies. Three separate searches were performed to maximize retrieval of the most recent and highest-quality evidence for pediatric sinusitis. The first limited results to all randomized controlled trials (RCTs) from 1966 to 2009, the second to all meta-analyses from 1966 to 2009, and the third to all pediatric studies (limited to ages <18 years) published since the last technical report (1999–2009). Additionally, the Web of Science was queried to identify studies that cited the original AAP guidelines. This literature search was replicated in July 2010

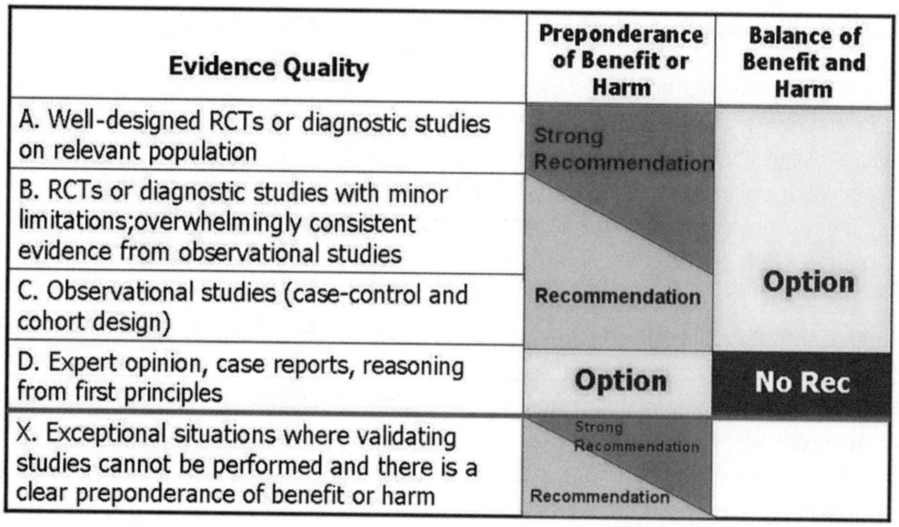

Evidence Quality	Preponderance of Benefit or Harm	Balance of Benefit and Harm
A. Well-designed RCTs or diagnostic studies on relevant population	Strong Recommendation	Option
B. RCTs or diagnostic studies with minor limitations; overwhelmingly consistent evidence from observational studies		
C. Observational studies (case-control and cohort design)	Recommendation	
D. Expert opinion, case reports, reasoning from first principles	Option	No Rec
X. Exceptional situations where validating studies cannot be performed and there is a clear preponderance of benefit or harm	Strong Recommendation / Recommendation	

FIGURE 1
Levels of recommendations. Rec, recommendation.

and November 2012 to capture recently published studies. The complete results of the literature review are published separately in the technical report.[6] In summary, 17 randomized studies of sinusitis in children were identified and reviewed. Only 3 trials met inclusion criteria. Because of significant heterogeneity among these studies, formal meta-analyses were not pursued.

The results from the literature review were used to guide development of the key action statements included in this document. These action statements were generated by using BRIDGE-Wiz (Building Recommendations in a Developers Guideline Editor, Yale School of Medicine, New Haven, CT), an interactive software tool that leads guideline development through a series of questions that are intended to create a more actionable set of key action statements.[7] BRIDGE-Wiz also incorporates the quality of available evidence into the final determination of the strength of each recommendation.

The AAP policy statement "Classifying Recommendations for Clinical Practice Guidelines" was followed in designating levels of recommendations (Fig 1).[8] Definitions of evidence-based statements are provided in Table 1. This guideline was reviewed by multiple groups in the AAP and 2 external organizations. Comments were compiled and reviewed by the subcommittee, and relevant changes were incorporated into the guideline.

KEY ACTION STATEMENTS

Key Action Statement 1

Clinicians should make a presumptive diagnosis of acute bacterial sinusitis when a child with an acute URI presents with the following:

- **Persistent illness, ie, nasal discharge (of any quality) or daytime cough or both lasting more than 10 days without improvement;**

OR

- **Worsening course, ie, worsening or new onset of nasal discharge, daytime cough, or fever after initial improvement;**

OR

- **Severe onset, ie, concurrent fever (temperature $\geq$39°C/102.2°F) and purulent nasal discharge for at least 3 consecutive days (Evidence Quality: B; Recommendation).**

KAS Profile 1

Aggregate evidence quality: B	
Benefit	Diagnosis allows decisions regarding management to be made. Children likely to benefit from antimicrobial therapy will be identified.
Harm	Inappropriate diagnosis may lead to unnecessary treatment. A missed diagnosis may lead to persistent infection or complications
Cost	Inappropriate diagnosis may lead to unnecessary cost of antibiotics. A missed diagnosis leads to cost of persistent illness (loss of time from school and work) or cost of caring for complications.
Benefits-harm assessment	Preponderance of benefit.
Value judgments	None.
Role of patient preference	Limited.
Intentional vagueness	None.
Exclusions	Children aged <1 year or older than 18 years and with underlying conditions.
Strength	Recommendation.

TABLE 1 Guideline Definitions for Evidence-Based Statements

Statement	Definition	Implication
Strong recommendation	A strong recommendation in favor of a particular action is made when the anticipated benefits of the recommended intervention clearly exceed the harms (as a strong recommendation against an action is made when the anticipated harms clearly exceed the benefits) and the quality of the supporting evidence is excellent. In some clearly identified circumstances, strong recommendations may be made when high-quality evidence is impossible to obtain and the anticipated benefits strongly outweigh the harms.	Clinicians should follow a strong recommendation unless a clear and compelling rationale for an alternative approach is present.
Recommendation	A recommendation in favor of a particular action is made when the anticipated benefits exceed the harms but the quality of evidence is not as strong. Again, in some clearly identified circumstances, recommendations may be made when high-quality evidence is impossible to obtain but the anticipated benefits outweigh the harms.	Clinicians would be prudent to follow a recommendation, but should remain alert to new information and sensitive to patient preferences.
Option	Options define courses that may be taken when either the quality of evidence is suspect or carefully performed studies have shown little clear advantage to one approach over another.	Clinicians should consider the option in their decision-making, and patient preference may have a substantial role.
No recommendation	No recommendation indicates that there is a lack of pertinent published evidence and that the anticipated balance of benefits and harms is presently unclear.	Clinicians should be alert to new published evidence that clarifies the balance of benefit versus harm.

The purpose of this action statement is to guide the practitioner in making a diagnosis of acute bacterial sinusitis on the basis of stringent clinical criteria. To develop criteria to be used in distinguishing episodes of acute bacterial sinusitis from other common respiratory infections, it is helpful to describe the features of an uncomplicated viral URI. Viral URIs are usually characterized by nasal symptoms (discharge and congestion/obstruction) or cough or both. Most often, the nasal discharge begins as clear and watery. Often, however, the quality of nasal discharge changes during the course of the illness. Typically, the nasal discharge becomes thicker and more mucoid and may become purulent (thick, colored, and opaque) for several days. Then the situation reverses, with the purulent discharge becoming mucoid and then clear again or simply resolving. The transition from clear to purulent to clear again occurs in uncomplicated viral URIs without the use of antimicrobial therapy.

Fever, when present in uncomplicated viral URI, tends to occur early in the illness, often in concert with other constitutional symptoms such as headache and myalgias. Typically, the fever and constitutional symptoms disappear in the first 24 to 48 hours, and the respiratory symptoms become more prominent (Fig 2).

The course of most uncomplicated viral URIs is 5 to 7 days.[9–12] As shown in Fig 2, respiratory symptoms usually peak in severity by days 3 to 6 and then begin to improve; however, resolving symptoms and signs may persist in some patients after day 10.[9,10]

Symptoms of acute bacterial sinusitis and uncomplicated viral URI overlap considerably, and therefore it is their persistence without improvement that suggests a diagnosis of acute sinusitis.[9,10,13] Such symptoms include

nasal discharge (of any quality: thick or thin, serous, mucoid, or purulent) or daytime cough (which may be worse at night) or both. Bad breath, fatigue, headache, and decreased appetite, although common, are not specific indicators of acute sinusitis.[14] Physical examination findings are also not particularly helpful in distinguishing sinusitis from uncomplicated URIs. Erythema and swelling of the nasal turbinates are nonspecific findings.[14] Percussion of the sinuses is not useful. Transillumination of the sinuses is difficult to perform correctly in children and has been shown to be unreliable.[15,16] Nasopharyngeal cultures do not reliably predict the etiology of acute bacterial sinusitis.[14,16]

Only a minority (~6%–7%) of children presenting with symptoms of URI will meet criteria for persistence.[3,4,11] As a result, before diagnosing acute bacterial sinusitis, it is important for the practitioner to attempt to (1) differentiate between sequential episodes of uncomplicated viral URI (which may seem to coalesce in the mind of the patient or parent) from the onset of acute bacterial sinusitis with persistent symptoms and (2) establish whether the symptoms are clearly not improving.

A worsening course of signs and symptoms, termed "double sickening," in the context of a viral URI is another presentation of acute bacterial sinusitis.[13,17] Affected children experience substantial and acute worsening of

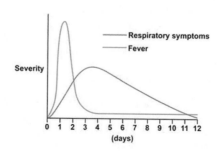

FIGURE 2
Uncomplicated viral URI.

respiratory symptoms (nasal discharge or nasal congestion or daytime cough) or a new fever, often on the sixth or seventh day of illness, after initial signs of recovery from an uncomplicated viral URI. Support for this definition comes from studies in children and adults, for whom antibiotic treatment of worsening symptoms after a period of apparent improvement was associated with better outcomes.[4]

Finally, some children with acute bacterial sinusitis may present with severe onset, ie, concurrent high fever (temperature >39°C) and purulent nasal discharge. These children usually are ill appearing and need to be distinguished from children with uncomplicated viral infections that are unusually severe. If fever is present in uncomplicated viral URIs, it tends to be present early in the illness, usually accompanied by other constitutional symptoms, such as headache and myalgia.[9,13,18] Generally, the constitutional symptoms resolve in the first 48 hours and then the respiratory symptoms become prominent. In most uncomplicated viral infections, including influenza, purulent nasal discharge does not appear for several days. Accordingly, it is the concurrent presentation of high fever and purulent nasal discharge for the first 3 to 4 days of an acute URI that helps to define the severe onset of acute bacterial sinusitis.[13,16,18] This presentation in children is the corollary to acute onset of headache, fever, and facial pain in adults with acute sinusitis.

Allergic and nonallergic rhinitis are predisposing causes of some cases of acute bacterial sinusitis in childhood. In addition, at their onset, these conditions may be mistaken for acute bacterial sinusitis. A family history of atopic conditions, seasonal occurrences, or occurrences with exposure to common allergens and other allergic diatheses in the index patient (eczema, atopic dermatitis, asthma) may suggest the presence of non-infectious rhinitis. The patient may have complaints of pruritic eyes and nasal mucosa, which will provide a clue to the likely etiology of the condition. On physical examination, there may be a prominent nasal crease, allergic shiners, cobblestoning of the conjunctiva or pharyngeal wall, or pale nasal mucosa as other indicators of the diagnosis.

Key Action Statement 2A

Clinicians should not obtain imaging studies (plain films, contrast-enhanced computed tomography [CT], MRI, or ultrasonography) to distinguish acute bacterial sinusitis from viral URI (Evidence Quality: B; Strong Recommendation).

KAS Profile 2A

Aggregate evidence quality: B; overwhelmingly consistent evidence from observational studies.

Benefit	Avoids exposure to radiation and costs of studies. Avoids unnecessary therapy for false-positive diagnoses.
Harm	None.
Cost	Avoids cost of imaging.
Benefits-harm assessment	Exclusive benefit.
Value judgments	Concern for unnecessary radiation and costs.
Role of patient preference	Limited. Parents may value a negative study and avoidance of antibiotics as worthy of radiation but panel disagrees.
Intentional vagueness	None.
Exclusions	Patients with complications of sinusitis.
Strength	Strong recommendation.

The purpose of this key action statement is to discourage the practitioner from obtaining imaging studies in children with uncomplicated acute bacterial sinusitis. As emphasized in Key Action Statement 1, acute bacterial sinusitis in children is a diagnosis that is made on the basis of stringent clinical criteria that describe signs, symptoms, and temporal patterns of a URI. Although historically imaging has been used as a confirmatory or diagnostic modality in children

suspected to have acute bacterial sinusitis, it is no longer recommended.

The membranes that line the nose are continuous with the membranes (mucosa) that line the sinus cavities, the middle ear, the nasopharynx, and the oropharynx. When an individual experiences a viral URI, there is inflammation of the nasal mucosa and, often, the mucosa of the middle ear and paranasal sinuses as well. The continuity of the mucosa of the upper respiratory tract is responsible for the controversy regarding the usefulness of images of the paranasal sinuses in contributing to a diagnosis of acute bacterial sinusitis.

As early as the 1940s, observations were made regarding the frequency of abnormal sinus radiographs in healthy children without signs or symptoms of current respiratory disease.[19] In addition, several investigators in the 1970s and 1980s observed that children with uncomplicated viral URI had frequent abnormalities of the paranasal sinuses on plain radiographs.[20–22] These abnormalities were the same as those considered to be diagnostic of acute bacterial sinusitis (diffuse opacification, mucosal swelling of at least 4 mm, or an air-fluid level).[16]

As technology advanced and CT scanning of the central nervous system and

skull became prevalent, several studies reported on incidental abnormalities of the paranasal sinuses that were observed in children.[23,24] Gwaltney et al[25] showed striking abnormalities (including air-fluid levels) in sinus CT scans of young adults with uncomplicated colds. Manning et al[26] evaluated children undergoing either CT or MRI of the head for indications other than respiratory complaints or suspected sinusitis. Each patient underwent rhinoscopy and otoscopy before imaging and each patient's parent was asked to fill out a questionnaire regarding recent symptoms of URI. Sixty-two percent of patients overall had physical findings or history consistent with an upper respiratory inflammatory process, and 55% of the total group showed some abnormalities on sinus imaging; 33% showed pronounced mucosal thickening or an air-fluid level. Gordts et al[27] made similar observations in children undergoing MRI. Finally, Kristo et al[28] performed MRI in children with URIs and confirmed the high frequency (68%) of major abnormalities seen in the paranasal sinuses.

In summary, when the paranasal sinuses are imaged, either with plain radiographs, contrast-enhanced CT, or MRI in children with uncomplicated URI, the majority of studies will be significantly abnormal with the same kind of findings that are associated with bacterial infection of the sinuses. Accordingly, although normal radiographs or CT or MRI results can ensure that a patient with respiratory symptoms does not have acute bacterial sinusitis, an abnormal image cannot confirm the diagnosis. Therefore, it is not necessary to perform imaging in children with uncomplicated episodes of clinical sinusitis. Similarly, the high likelihood of an abnormal imaging result in a child with an uncomplicated URI indicates that radiographic studies not be performed in an attempt to eliminate the diagnosis of sinusitis.

Key Action Statement 2B

Clinicians should obtain a contrast-enhanced CT scan of the paranasal sinuses and/or an MRI with contrast whenever a child is suspected of having orbital or central nervous system complications of acute bacterial sinusitis (Evidence Quality: B; Strong Recommendation).

KAS Profile 2B

Aggregate evidence quality: B; overwhelmingly consistent evidence from observational studies.

Benefit	Determine presence of abscesses, which may require surgical intervention; avoid sequelae because of appropriate aggressive management.
Harm	Exposure to ionizing radiation for CT scans; need for sedation for MRI.
Cost	Direct cost of studies.
Benefits-harm assessment	Preponderance of benefit.
Value judgments	Concern for significant complication that may be unrecognized and, therefore, not treated appropriately.
Role of patient preference	Limited.
Intentional vagueness	None.
Exclusions	None.
Strength	Strong recommendation.

The purpose of this key action statement is to have the clinician obtain contrast-enhanced CT images when children are suspected of having serious complications of acute bacterial sinusitis. The most common complication of acute sinusitis involves the orbit in children with ethmoid sinusitis who are younger than 5 years.[29–31] Orbital complications should be suspected when the child presents with a swollen eye, especially if accompanied by proptosis or impaired function of the extraocular muscles. Orbital complications of acute sinusitis have been divided into 5 categories: sympathetic effusion, subperiosteal abscess, orbital cellulitis, orbital abscess, and cavernous sinus thrombosis.[32] Although sympathetic effusion (inflammatory edema) is categorized as an

orbital complication, the site of infection remains confined to the sinus cavities; eye swelling is attributable to the impedance of venous drainage secondary to congestion within the ethmoid sinuses. Alternative terms for sympathetic effusion (inflammatory edema) are preseptal or periorbital cellulitis. The remaining "true" orbital complications are best visualized by contrast-enhanced CT scanning.

Intracranial complications of acute sinusitis, which are substantially less common than orbital complications, are more serious, with higher morbidity and mortality than those involving the orbit. Intracranial complications should be suspected in the patient who presents with a very severe headache, photophobia, seizures, or other focal neurologic findings. Intracranial complications include subdural empyema, epidural empyema, venous thrombosis, brain abscess, and meningitis.[29] Typically, patients with intracranial complications of acute bacterial sinusitis are previously healthy adolescent males with frontal sinusitis.[33,34]

There have been no head-to-head comparisons of the diagnostic accuracy of contrast-enhanced CT scanning to MRI with contrast in the evaluation

of orbital and intracranial complications of sinusitis in children. In general, the contrast-enhanced CT scan has been the preferred imaging study when complications of sinusitis are suspected.[35,36] However, there are documented cases in which a contrast-enhanced CT scan has not revealed the abnormality responsible for the clinical presentation and the MRI with contrast has, especially for intracranial complications and rarely for orbital complications.[37,38] Accordingly, the most recent appropriateness criteria from the American College of Radiology endorse both MRI with contrast and contrast-enhanced CT as complementary examinations when evaluating potential complications of sinusitis.[35] The availability and speed of obtaining the contrast-enhanced CT are desirable; however, there is increasing concern regarding exposure to radiation. The MRI, although very sensitive, takes longer than the contrast-enhanced CT and often requires sedation in young children (which carries its own risks). In older children and adolescents who may not require sedation, MRI with contrast, if available, may be preferred when intracranial complications are likely. Furthermore, MRI with contrast should be performed when there is persistent clinical concern or incomplete information has been provided by the contrast-enhanced CT scan.

Key Action Statement 3

Initial Management of Acute Bacterial Sinusitis

3A: "Severe onset and worsening course" acute bacterial sinusitis. The clinician should prescribe antibiotic therapy for acute bacterial sinusitis in children with severe onset or worsening course (signs, symptoms, or both) (Evidence Quality: B; Strong Recommendation).

KAS Profile 3A

Aggregate evidence quality: B; randomized controlled trials with limitations.	
Benefit	Increase clinical cures, shorten illness duration, and may prevent suppurative complications in a high-risk patient population.
Harm	Adverse effects of antibiotics.
Cost	Direct cost of therapy.
Benefits-harm assessment	Preponderance of benefit.
Value judgments	Concern for morbidity and possible complications if untreated.
Role of patient preference	Limited.
Intentional vagueness	None.
Exclusions	None.
Strength	Strong recommendation.

3B: "Persistent illness." The clinician should either prescribe antibiotic therapy OR offer additional outpatient observation for 3 days to children with persistent illness (nasal discharge of any quality or cough or both for at least 10 days without evidence of improvement) (Evidence Quality: B; Recommendation).

The purpose of this section is to offer guidance on initial management of persistent illness sinusitis by helping clinicians choose between the following 2 strategies:

1. Antibiotic therapy, defined as initial treatment of acute bacterial sinusitis with antibiotics, with the intent of starting antibiotic therapy as soon as possible after the encounter.

2. Additional outpatient observation, defined as initial management of acute bacterial sinusitis limited to continued observation for 3 days, with commencement of antibiotic therapy if either the child does not improve clinically within several days of diagnosis or if there is clinical worsening of the child's condition at any time.

In contrast to the 2001 AAP guideline,[5] which recommended antibiotic therapy for all children diagnosed with acute bacterial sinusitis, this guideline allows for additional observation of children presenting with persistent illness (nasal discharge of any quality or daytime cough or both for at least 10 days without evidence of improvement). In both guidelines, however, children presenting with severe or worsening illness (which was not defined explicitly in the 2001 guideline[5]) are to receive antibiotic therapy. The rationale for this approach (Table 2) is discussed below.

Antibiotic Therapy for Acute Bacterial Sinusitis

In the United States, antibiotics are prescribed for 82% of children with acute sinusitis.[39] The rationale for antibiotic therapy of acute bacterial sinusitis is based on the recovery of bacteria in high density ($\geq 10^4$ colony-forming units/mL) in 70% of maxillary sinus aspirates obtained from children with a clinical syndrome characterized by persistent nasal discharge, daytime cough, or both.[16,40] Children who present with severe-onset acute bacterial sinusitis are presumed to have bacterial infection, because a temperature of at least 39°C/102.2°F coexisting for at least 3 consecutive days with purulent nasal discharge is not consistent with the well-documented pattern of acute viral URI. Similarly, children with worsening-course acute bacterial sinusitis have a clinical course that is also not consistent with the steady improvement that characterizes an uncomplicated viral URI.[9,10]

KAS Profile 3B

Aggregate evidence quality: B; randomized controlled trials with limitations.	
Benefit	Antibiotics increase the chance of improvement or cure at 10 to 14 days (number needed to treat, 3–5); additional observation may avoid the use of antibiotics with attendant cost and adverse effects.
Harm	Antibiotics have adverse effects (number needed to harm, 3) and may increase bacterial resistance. Observation may prolong illness and delay start of needed antibiotic therapy.
Cost	Direct cost of antibiotics as well as cost of adverse reactions; indirect costs of delayed recovery when observation is used.
Benefits-harm assessment	Preponderance of benefit (because both antibiotic therapy and additional observation with rescue antibiotic, if needed, are appropriate management).
Value judgments	Role for additional brief observation period for selected children with persistent illness sinusitis, similar to what is recommended for acute otitis media, despite the lack of randomized trials specifically comparing additional observation with immediate antibiotic therapy and longer duration of illness before presentation.
Role of patient preference	Substantial role in shared decision-making that should incorporate illness severity, child's quality of life, and caregiver values and concerns.
Intentional vagueness	None.
Exclusions	Children who are excluded from randomized clinical trials of acute bacterial sinusitis, as defined in the text.
Strength	Recommendation.

Three RCTs have compared antibiotic therapy with placebo for the initial management of acute bacterial sinusitis in children. Two trials by Wald et al[4,41] found an increase in cure or improvement after antibiotic therapy compared with placebo with a number needed to treat of 3 to 5 children. Most children in these studies had persistent acute bacterial sinusitis, but children with severe or worsening illness were also included. Conversely, Garbutt et al,[42] who studied only children with persistent acute bacterial sinusitis, found no difference in outcomes for antibiotic versus placebo. Another RCT by Kristo et al,[43] often cited as showing no benefit from antibiotics for acute bacterial sinusitis, will not be considered further because of methodologic flaws, including weak entry criteria and inadequate dosing of antibiotic treatment.

The guideline recommends antibiotic therapy for severe or worsening acute bacterial sinusitis because of the benefits revealed in RCTs[4,41] and a theoretically higher risk of suppurative complications than for children who present with persistent symptoms. Orbital and intracranial complications of acute bacterial sinusitis have not been observed in RCTs, even when placebo was administered; however, sample sizes have inadequate power to preclude an increased risk. This risk, however, has caused some investigators to exclude children with severe acute bacterial sinusitis from trial entry.[42]

Additional Observation for Persistent Onset Acute Bacterial Sinusitis

The guideline recommends either antibiotic therapy or an additional brief period of observation as initial management strategies for children with persistent acute bacterial sinusitis because, although there are benefits to antibiotic therapy (number needed to treat, 3–5), some children improve on their own, and the risk of suppurative complications is low.[4,41] Symptoms of persistent acute bacterial sinusitis may be mild and have varying effects on a given child's quality of life, ranging from slight (mild cough, nasal discharge) to significant (sleep disturbance, behavioral changes, school or child care absenteeism). The benefits of antibiotic therapy in some trials[4,41] must also be balanced against an increased risk of adverse events (number need to harm, 3), most often self-limited diarrhea, but also including occasional rash.[4]

Choosing between antibiotic therapy or additional observation for initial management of persistent illness sinusitis presents an opportunity for shared decision-making with families (Table 2). Factors that might influence this decision include symptom severity, the child's quality of life, recent antibiotic use, previous experience or outcomes with acute bacterial sinusitis, cost of antibiotics, ease of administration, caregiver concerns about potential adverse effects of antibiotics, persistence of respiratory symptoms, or development of complications. Values and preferences expressed by the caregiver should be taken into consideration (Table 3).

Children with persistent acute bacterial sinusitis who received antibiotic therapy in the previous 4 weeks, those with concurrent bacterial infection (eg, pneumonia, suppurative cervical adenitis, group A streptococcal pharyngitis, or acute otitis media), those with actual or suspected complications of acute bacterial sinusitis, or those with underlying conditions should generally be managed with antibiotic therapy. The latter group includes children with asthma, cystic fibrosis, immunodeficiency, previous sinus surgery, or anatomic abnormalities of the upper respiratory tract.

Limiting antibiotic use in children with persistent acute bacterial sinusitis who may improve on their own reduces common antibiotic-related adverse events, such as diarrhea, diaper dermatitis, and skin rash. The most recent RCT of acute bacterial sinusitis in children[4] found adverse events of 44% with antibiotic and 14% with placebo.

Limiting antibiotics may also reduce the prevalence of resistant bacterial pathogens. Although this is always a desirable goal, no increase in resistant bacterial species was observed within the group of children treated with a single course of antimicrobial agents (compared with those receiving placebo) in 2 recent large studies of antibiotic versus placebo for children with acute otitis media.[44,45]

Key Action Statement 4

Clinicians should prescribe amoxicillin with or without clavulanate as first-line treatment when a decision has been made to initiate antibiotic treatment of acute bacterial sinusitis (Evidence Quality: B; Recommendation).

KAS Profile 4

Aggregate evidence quality: B; randomized controlled trials with limitations.

Benefit	Increase clinical cures with narrowest spectrum drug; stepwise increase in broadening spectrum as risk factors for resistance increase.
Harm	Adverse effects of antibiotics including development of hypersensitivity.
Cost	Direct cost of antibiotic therapy.
Benefits-harm assessment	Preponderance of benefit.
Value judgments	Concerns for not encouraging resistance if possible.
Role of patient preference	Potential for shared decision-making that should incorporate the caregiver's experiences and values.
Intentional vagueness	None.
Exclusions	May include allergy or intolerance.
Strength	Recommendation.

TABLE 2 Recommendations for Initial Use of Antibiotics for Acute Bacterial Sinusitis

Clinical Presentation	Severe Acute Bacterial Sinusitis[a]	Worsening Acute Bacterial Sinusitis[b]	Persistent Acute Bacterial Sinusitis[c]
Uncomplicated acute bacterial sinusitis without coexisting illness	Antibiotic therapy	Antibiotic therapy	Antibiotic therapy or additional observation for 3 days[d]
Acute bacterial sinusitis with orbital or intracranial complications	Antibiotic therapy	Antibiotic therapy	Antibiotic therapy
Acute bacterial sinusitis with coexisting acute otitis media, pneumonia, adenitis, or streptococcal pharyngitis	Antibiotic therapy	Antibiotic therapy	Antibiotic therapy

[a] Defined as temperature ≥39°C and purulent (thick, colored, and opaque) nasal discharge present concurrently for at least 3 consecutive days.

[b] Defined as nasal discharge or daytime cough with sudden worsening of symptoms (manifested by new-onset fever ≥38°C/100.4°F or substantial increase in nasal discharge or cough) after having experienced transient improvement of symptoms.

[c] Defined as nasal discharge (of any quality), daytime cough (which may be worse at night), or both, persisting for >10 days without improvement.

[d] Opportunity for shared decision-making with the child's family; if observation is offered, a mechanism must be in place to ensure follow-up and begin antibiotics if the child worsens at any time or fails to improve within 3 days of observation.

The purpose of this key action statement is to guide the selection of antimicrobial therapy once the diagnosis of acute bacterial sinusitis has been made. The microbiology of acute bacterial sinusitis was determined nearly 30 years ago through direct maxillary sinus aspiration in children with compatible signs and symptoms. The major bacterial pathogens recovered at that time were *Streptococcus pneumoniae* in approximately 30% of children and nontypeable *Haemophilus influenzae* and *Moraxella catarrhalis* in approximately 20% each.[16,40] Aspirates from the remaining 25% to 30% of children were sterile.

Maxillary sinus aspiration is rarely performed at the present time unless the course of the infection is unusually prolonged or severe. Although some authorities have recommended obtaining cultures from the middle meatus to determine the cause of a maxillary sinus infection, there are no data in children with acute bacterial sinusitis that have compared such cultures with cultures of a maxillary sinus aspirate. Furthermore, there are data indicating that the middle meatus in healthy children is commonly colonized with *S pneumoniae*, *H influenzae*, and *M catarrhalis*.[46]

Recent estimates of the microbiology of acute sinusitis have, of necessity, been based primarily on that of acute otitis media (AOM), a condition with relatively easy access to infective fluid through performance of tympanocentesis and one with a similar pathogenesis to acute bacterial sinusitis.[47,48] The 3 most common bacterial pathogens recovered from the middle ear fluid of children with AOM are the same as those that have been associated with acute bacterial sinusitis: *S pneumoniae*, nontypeable *H influenzae*, and *M catarrhalis*.[49] The proportion of each has varied from study to study depending on criteria used for diagnosis of AOM, patient characteristics, and bacteriologic techniques. Recommendations since the year 2000 for the routine use in infants of 7-valent and, more recently, 13-valent pneumococcal conjugate vaccine (PCV-13) have been associated with a decrease in recovery of *S pneumoniae* from ear fluid of children with AOM and a relative increase in the incidence of infections attributable to *H influenzae*.[50] Thus, on the basis of the proportions of bacteria found in middle ear infections, it is estimated that *S pneumoniae* and *H influenzae* are currently each responsible for approximately 30% of cases of acute bacterial sinusitis in children, and *M catarrhalis* is responsible for approximately 10%. These percentages are contingent on the assumption that approximately one-quarter of aspirates of maxillary sinusitis would still be sterile, as reported in earlier studies. *Staphylococcus aureus* is rarely isolated from sinus aspirates in children with acute bacterial sinusitis, and with the exception of acute maxillary sinusitis associated with infections of dental origin,[51] respiratory anaerobes are also rarely recovered.[40,52] Although *S aureus* is a very infrequent cause of acute bacterial sinusitis in children, it is a significant pathogen in the orbital and intracranial complications of sinusitis. The reasons for this discrepancy are unknown.

Antimicrobial susceptibility patterns for *S pneumoniae* vary considerably from community to community. Isolates obtained from surveillance centers nationwide indicate that, at the present time, 10% to 15% of upper respiratory tract isolates of *S pneumoniae* are nonsusceptible to penicillin[53,54]; however, values for penicillin nonsusceptibility as high as 50% to 60% have been reported in some areas.[55,56] Of the organisms that are resistant, approximately half are highly resistant to penicillin and the remaining half are intermediate in resistance.[53,54,56–59] Between 10% and 42% of *H influenzae*[56–59] and close to 100% of *M catarrhalis* are likely to be β-lactamase positive and nonsusceptible to amoxicillin. Because of dramatic geographic variability in the prevalence of β-lactamase–positive *H influenzae*, it is extremely desirable for the practitioner to be familiar with local patterns of susceptibility. Risk factors for the presence of organisms likely to be resistant to amoxicillin include attendance at child care, receipt of antimicrobial treatment within the previous 30 days, and age younger than 2 years.[50,55,60]

Amoxicillin remains the antimicrobial agent of choice for first-line treatment of uncomplicated acute bacterial sinusitis in situations in which antimicrobial resistance is not suspected. This recommendation is based on amoxicillin's effectiveness, safety, acceptable taste, low cost, and relatively narrow microbiologic spectrum. For children aged 2 years or older with uncomplicated acute bacterial sinusitis that is mild to moderate in degree of severity who do not attend child care and who have not been treated with an antimicrobial agent within the last 4 weeks, amoxicillin is recommended at a standard dose of 45 mg/kg per day in 2 divided doses. In communities with a high prevalence of nonsusceptible S pneumoniae (>10%, including intermediate- and high-level resistance), treatment may be initiated at 80 to 90 mg/kg per day in 2 divided doses, with a maximum of 2 g per dose.[55] This high-dose amoxicillin therapy is likely to achieve sinus fluid concentrations that are adequate to overcome the resistance of S pneumoniae, which is attributable to alteration in penicillin-binding proteins on the basis of data derived from patients with AOM.[61] If, within the next several years after licensure of PCV-13, a continuing decrease in isolates of S pneumoniae (including a decrease in isolates of nonsusceptible S pneumoniae) and an increase in β-lactamase–producing H influenzae are observed, standard-dose amoxicillin-clavulanate (45 mg/kg per day) may be most appropriate.

Patients presenting with moderate to severe illness as well as those younger than 2 years, attending child care, or who have recently been treated with

an antimicrobial may receive high-dose amoxicillin-clavulanate (80–90 mg/kg per day of the amoxicillin component with 6.4 mg/kg per day of clavulanate in 2 divided doses with a maximum of 2 g per dose). The potassium clavulanate levels are adequate to inhibit all β-lactamase–producing H influenzae and M catarrhalis.[56,59]

A single 50-mg/kg dose of ceftriaxone, given either intravenously or intramuscularly, can be used for children who are vomiting, unable to tolerate oral medication, or unlikely to be adherent to the initial doses of antibiotic.[62–64] The 3 major bacterial pathogens involved in acute bacterial sinusitis are susceptible to ceftriaxone in 95% to 100% of cases.[56,58,59] If clinical improvement is observed at 24 hours, an oral antibiotic can be substituted to complete the course of therapy. Children who are still significantly febrile or symptomatic at 24 hours may require additional parenteral doses before switching to oral therapy.

The treatment of patients with presumed allergy to penicillin has been controversial. However, recent publications indicate that the risk of a serious allergic reaction to second- and third-generation cephalosporins in patients with penicillin or amoxicillin allergy appears to be almost nil and no greater than the risk among patients without such allergy.[65–67] Thus, patients allergic to amoxicillin with a non–type 1 (late or delayed, >72 hours) hypersensitivity reaction can safely be treated with cefdinir, cefuroxime, or cefpodoxime.[66–68] Patients with a history of a serious type 1 immediate or accelerated (anaphylactoid) reaction to amoxicillin can also safely be treated with cefdinir, cefuroxime, or cefpodoxime. In both circumstances, clinicians may wish to determine individual tolerance by referral to an allergist for penicillin

and/or cephalosporin skin-testing before initiation of therapy.[66–68] The susceptibility of S pneumoniae to cefdinir, cefpodoxime, and cefuroxime varies from 60% to 75%,[56–59] and the susceptibility of H influenzae to these agents varies from 85% to 100%.[56,58] In young children (<2 years) with a serious type 1 hypersensitivity to penicillin and moderate or more severe sinusitis, it may be prudent to use a combination of clindamycin (or linezolid) and cefixime to achieve the most comprehensive coverage against both resistant S pneumoniae and H influenzae. Linezolid has excellent activity against all S pneumoniae, including penicillin-resistant strains, but lacks activity against H influenzae and M catarrhalis. Alternatively, a quinolone, such as levofloxacin, which has a high level of activity against both S pneumoniae and H influenzae, may be prescribed.[57,58] Although the use of quinolones is usually restricted because of concerns for toxicity, cost, and emerging resistance, their use in this circumstance can be justified.

Pneumococcal and H influenzae surveillance studies have indicated that resistance of these organisms to trimethoprim-sulfamethoxazole and azithromycin is sufficient to preclude their use for treatment of acute bacterial sinusitis in patients with penicillin hypersensitivity.[56,58,59,69]

The optimal duration of antimicrobial therapy for patients with acute bacterial sinusitis has not received systematic study. Recommendations based on clinical observations have varied widely, from 10 to 28 days of treatment. An alternative suggestion has been made that antibiotic therapy be continued for 7 days after the patient becomes free of signs and symptoms.[5] This strategy has the advantage of individualizing the treatment of each patient, results in a minimum course of 10 days, and avoids prolonged antimicrobial therapy in patients who are asymptomatic and therefore unlikely to adhere to the full course of treatment.[5]

Patients who are acutely ill and appear toxic when first seen (see below) can be managed with 1 of 2 options. Consultation can be requested from an otolaryngologist for consideration of maxillary sinus aspiration (with appropriate analgesia/anesthesia) to obtain a sample of sinus secretions for Gram stain, culture, and susceptibility testing so that antimicrobial therapy can be adjusted precisely. Alternatively, inpatient therapy can be initiated with intravenous cefotaxime or ceftriaxone, with referral to an otolaryngologist if the patient's condition worsens or fails to show improvement within 48 hours. If a complication is suspected, management will differ depending on the site and severity.

A recent guideline was published by the Infectious Diseases Society of America for acute bacterial rhinosinusitis in children and adults.[70] Their recommendation for initial empirical antimicrobial therapy for acute bacterial sinusitis in children was amoxicillin-clavulanate based on the concern that there is an increasing prevalence of *H influenzae* as a cause of sinusitis since introduction of the pneumococcal conjugate vaccines and an increasing prevalence of β-lactamase production among these strains. In contrast, this guideline from the AAP allows either amoxicillin or amoxicillin-clavulanate as first-line empirical therapy and is therefore inclusive of the Infectious Diseases Society of America's recommendation. Unfortunately, there are scant data available regarding the precise microbiology of acute bacterial sinusitis in the post–PCV-13 era. Prospective surveillance of nasopharyngeal cultures may be helpful in completely

aligning these recommendations in the future.

Key Action Statement 5A

Clinicians should reassess initial management if there is either a caregiver report of worsening (progression of initial signs/symptoms or appearance of new signs/symptoms) OR failure to improve (lack of reduction in all presenting signs/symptoms) within 72 hours of initial management (Evidence Quality: C; Recommendation).

KAS Profile 5A

Aggregate evidence quality: C; observational studies

Benefits	Identification of patients who may have been misdiagnosed, those at risk of complications, and those who require a change in management.
Harm	Delay of up to 72 hours in changing therapy if patient fails to improve.
Cost	Additional provider and caregiver time and resources.
Benefits-harm assessment	Preponderance of benefit.
Value judgments	Use of 72 hours to assess progress may result in excessive classification as treatment failures if premature; emphasis on importance of worsening illness in defining treatment failures.
Role of patient preferences	Caregivers determine whether the severity of the patient's illness justifies the report to clinician of the patient's worsening or failure to improve.
Intentional vagueness	None.
Exclusions	Patients with severe illness, poor general health, complicated sinusitis, immune deficiency, previous sinus surgery, or coexisting bacterial illness.
Strength	Recommendation.

The purpose of this key action statement is to ensure that patients with acute bacterial sinusitis who fail to improve symptomatically after initial management are reassessed to be certain that they have been correctly diagnosed and to consider initiation of alternate therapy to hasten resolution of symptoms and avoid complications. "Worsening" is defined as progression of presenting signs or symptoms of acute bacterial sinusitis or onset of new signs or symptoms. "Failure to improve" is lack of reduction in presenting signs or symptoms of acute

bacterial sinusitis by 72 hours after diagnosis and initial management; patients with persistent but improving symptoms do not meet this definition.

The rationale for using 72 hours as the time to assess treatment failure for acute bacterial sinusitis is based on clinical outcomes in RCTs. Wald et al[41] found that 18 of 35 patients (51%) receiving placebo demonstrated symptomatic improvement within 3 days of initiation of treatment; only an additional 3 patients receiving placebo (9%) improved between days 3 and 10. In the same study, 48 of 58 patients (83%) receiving antibiotics were cured or improved within 3 days; at 10 days, the overall rate of improvement was 79%, suggesting that no additional patients improved between days 3 and 10. In a more recent study, 17 of 19 children who ultimately failed initial therapy with either antibiotic or placebo demonstrated failure to improve within 72 hours.[4] Although Garbutt et al[42] did not report the percentage of patients who improved by day 3, they did demonstrate that the majority of improvement in symptoms occurred within the first 3 days of study entry whether they received active treatment or placebo.

Reporting of either worsening or failure to improve implies a shared responsibility between clinician and caregiver. Although the clinician should educate the caregiver regarding the anticipated reduction in symptoms within 3 days, it is incumbent on the caregiver to appropriately notify the clinician of concerns regarding worsening or failure to improve. Clinicians should emphasize the importance of reassessing those children whose symptoms are worsening whether or not antibiotic therapy was prescribed. Reassessment may be indicated before the 72-hour

process by which such reporting occurs should be discussed at the time the initial management strategy is determined.

Key Action Statement 5B

If the diagnosis of acute bacterial sinusitis is confirmed in a child with worsening symptoms or failure to improve in 72 hours, then clinicians may change the antibiotic therapy for the child initially managed with antibiotic OR initiate antibiotic treatment of the child initially managed with observation (Evidence Quality: D; Option based on expert opinion, case reports, and reasoning from first principles).

corresponds to the patient's pattern of illness, as defined in Key Action Statement 1. If caregivers report worsening of symptoms at any time in a patient for whom observation was the initial intervention, the clinician should begin treatment as discussed in Key Action Statement 4. For patients whose symptoms are mild and who have failed to improve but have not worsened, initiation of antimicrobial agents or continued observation (for up to 3 days) is reasonable.

If caregivers report worsening of symptoms after 3 days in a patient initially treated with antimicrobial agents, current signs and symptoms should be reviewed to determine whether acute bacterial sinusitis is still the best diagnosis. If sinusitis is still the best diagnosis, infection with drug-resistant bacteria is probable, and an alternate antimicrobial agent may be administered. Face-to-face reevaluation of the patient is desirable. Once the decision is made to change medications, the clinician should consider the limitations of the initial antibiotic coverage, the anticipated susceptibility of residual bacterial pathogens, and the ability of antibiotics to adequately penetrate the site of infection. Cultures of sinus or nasopharyngeal secretions in patients with initial antibiotic failure have identified a large percentage of bacteria with resistance to the original antibiotic.[71,72] Furthermore, multidrug-resistant *S pneumoniae* and β-lactamase–positive *H influenzae* and *M catarrhalis* are more commonly isolated after previous antibiotic exposure.[73–78] Unfortunately, there are no studies in children that have investigated the microbiology of treatment failure in acute bacterial sinusitis or cure rates using second-line antimicrobial agents. As a result, the likelihood of adequate antibiotic coverage for resistant organisms must be

KAS Profile 5B

Aggregate evidence quality: D; expert opinion and reasoning from first principles.	
Benefit	Prevention of complications, administration of effective therapy.
Harm	Adverse effects of secondary antibiotic therapy.
Cost	Direct cost of medications, often substantial for second-line agents.
Benefits-harm assessment	Preponderance of benefit.
Value judgments	Clinician must determine whether cost and adverse effects associated with change in antibiotic is justified given the severity of illness.
Role of patient preferences	Limited in patients whose symptoms are severe or worsening, but caregivers of mildly affected children who are failing to improve may reasonably defer change in antibiotic.
Intentional vagueness	None.
Exclusions	None.
Strength	Option.

mark if the patient is substantially worse, because it may indicate the development of complications or a need for parenteral therapy. Conversely, in some cases, caregivers may think that symptoms are not severe enough to justify a change to an antibiotic with a less desirable safety profile or even the time, effort, and resources required for reassessment. Accordingly, the circumstances under which caregivers report back to the clinician and the

The purpose of this key action statement is to ensure optimal antimicrobial treatment of children with acute bacterial sinusitis whose symptoms worsen or fail to respond to the initial intervention to prevent complications and reduce symptom severity and duration (see Table 4).

Clinicians who are notified by a caregiver that a child's symptoms are worsening or failing to improve should confirm that the clinical diagnosis of acute bacterial sinusitis addressed by extrapolations from studies of acute otitis media in children and sinusitis in adults and by using the results of data generated in vitro. A general guide to management of the child who worsens in 72 hours is shown in Table 4.

NO RECOMMENDATION

Adjuvant Therapy

Potential adjuvant therapy for acute sinusitis might include intranasal corticosteroids, saline nasal irrigation or lavage, topical or oral decongestants, mucolytics, and topical or oral antihistamines. A recent Cochrane review on decongestants, antihistamines, and nasal irrigation for acute sinusitis in children found no appropriately designed studies to determine the effectiveness of these interventions.[79]

Intranasal Steroids

The rationale for the use of intranasal corticosteroids in acute bacterial sinusitis is that an antiinflammatory agent may reduce the swelling around the sinus ostia and encourage drainage, thereby hastening recovery. However, there are limited data on how much inflammation is present, whether the inflammation is responsive to steroids, and whether there are differences in responsivity according to age. Nonetheless, there are several RCTs in adolescents and adults, most of which do show significant differences compared with placebo or active comparator that favor intranasal steroids in the reduction of symptoms and the patient's global assessment of overall improvement.[80–85] Several studies in adults with acute bacterial sinusitis provide data supporting the use of intranasal steroids as either monotherapy or adjuvant therapy to antibiotics.[81,86] Only one study did not show efficacy.[85]

There have been 2 trials of intranasal steroids performed exclusively in children: one comparing intranasal corticosteroids versus an oral decongestant[87] and the other comparing intranasal corticosteroids with placebo.[88] These studies showed a greater rate of complete resolution[87] or greater reduction in symptoms in patients receiving the steroid preparation, although the effects were modest.[88] It is important to note that nearly all of these studies (both those reported in children and adults) suffered from substantial methodologic problems. Examples of these methodologic problems are as follows: (1) variable inclusion criteria for sinusitis, (2) mixed populations of allergic and nonallergic subjects, and (3) different outcome criteria. All of these factors make deriving a clear conclusion difficult. Furthermore, the lack of stringent criteria in selecting the subject population increases the chance that the subjects had viral URIs or even persistent allergies rather than acute bacterial sinusitis.

The intranasal steroids studied to date include budesonide, flunisolide, fluticasone, and mometasone. There is no reason to believe that one steroid would be more effective than another, provided equivalent doses are used.

Potential harm in using nasal steroids in children with acute sinusitis includes the increased cost of therapy, difficulty in effectively administering nasal sprays in young children, nasal irritation and epistaxis, and potential systemic adverse effects of steroid use. Fortunately, no clinically significant steroid adverse effects have been discovered in studies in children.[89–96]

Saline Irrigation

Saline nasal irrigation or lavage (not saline nasal spray) has been used to remove debris from the nasal cavity and temporarily reduce tissue edema (hypertonic saline) to promote drainage from the sinuses. There have been very few RCTs using saline nasal irrigation or lavage in acute sinusitis, and these have had mixed results.[97,98] The 1 study in children showed greater improvement in nasal airflow and quality of life as well as a better rate of improvement in total symptom score when compared with placebo in patients treated with antibiotics and decongestants.[98] There are 2 Cochrane reviews published on the use of saline nasal irrigation in acute sinusitis in adults that showed variable results. One review published in 2007[99] concluded that it is a beneficial adjunct, but the other, published in 2010,[100] concluded that most trials were too small or contained too high a risk of bias to be confident about benefits.

Nasal Decongestants, Mucolytics, and Antihistamines

Data are insufficient to make any recommendations about the use of oral or topical nasal decongestants, mucolytics, or oral or nasal spray antihistamines as adjuvant therapy for acute bacterial sinusitis in children.[79] It is the opinion of the expert panel that antihistamines should not be used for the primary indication of acute bacterial sinusitis in any child, although such therapy might be helpful in reducing typical allergic symptoms in patients with atopy who also have acute sinusitis.

OTHER RELATED CONDITIONS

Recurrence of Acute Bacterial Sinusitis

Recurrent acute bacterial sinusitis (RABS) is an uncommon occurrence in healthy children and must be distinguished from recurrent URIs, exacerbations of allergic rhinitis, and chronic sinusitis. The former is defined by episodes of bacterial infection of the paranasal sinuses lasting fewer than 30 days and separated by intervals of

TABLE 3 Parent Information Regarding Initial Management of Acute Bacterial Sinusitis

How common are sinus infections in children?	Thick, colored, or cloudy mucus from your child's nose frequently occurs with a common cold or viral infection and does not by itself mean your child has sinusitis. In fact, fewer than 1 in 15 children get a true bacterial sinus infection during or after a common cold.
How can I tell if my child has bacterial sinusitis or simply a common cold?	Most colds have a runny nose with mucus that typically starts out clear, becomes cloudy or colored, and improves by about 10 d. Some colds will also include fever (temperature >38°C [100.4°F]) for 1 to 2 days. In contrast, acute bacterial sinusitis is likely when the pattern of illness is persistent, severe, or worsening.
	1. *Persistent* sinusitis is the most common type, defined as runny nose (of any quality), daytime cough (which may be worse at night), or both for at least 10 days without improvement.
	2. *Severe* sinusitis is present when fever (temperature ≥39°C [102.2°F]) lasts for at least 3 days in a row and is accompanied by nasal mucus that is thick, colored, or cloudy.
	3. *Worsening* sinusitis starts with a viral cold, which begins to improve but then worsens when bacteria take over and cause new-onset fever (temperature ≥38°C [100.4°F]) or a substantial increase in daytime cough or runny nose.
If my child has sinusitis, should he or she take an antibiotic?	Children with *persistent* sinusitis may be managed with either an antibiotic or with an additional brief period of observation, allowing the child up to another 3 days to fight the infection and improve on his or her own. The choice to treat or observe should be discussed with your doctor and may be based on your child's quality of life and how much of a problem the sinusitis is causing. In contrast, all children diagnosed with *severe* or *worsening* sinusitis should start antibiotic treatment to help them recover faster and more often.
Why not give all children with acute bacterial sinusitis an immediate antibiotic?	Some episodes of *persistent* sinusitis include relatively mild symptoms that may improve on their own in a few days. In addition, antibiotics can have adverse effects, which may include vomiting, diarrhea, upset stomach, skin rash, allergic reactions, yeast infections, and development of resistant bacteria (that make future infections more difficult to treat).

at least 10 days during which the patient is asymptomatic. Some experts require at least 4 episodes in a calendar year to fulfill the criteria for this condition. Chronic sinusitis is manifest as 90 or more uninterrupted days of respiratory symptoms, such as cough, nasal discharge, or nasal obstruction.

Children with RABS should be evaluated for underlying allergies, particularly allergic rhinitis; quantitative and functional immunologic defect(s),

chiefly immunoglobulin A and immunoglobulin G deficiency; cystic fibrosis; gastroesophageal reflux disease; or dysmotile cilia syndrome.[101] Anatomic abnormalities obstructing one or more sinus ostia may be present. These include septal deviation, nasal polyps, or concha bullosa (pneumatization of the middle turbinate); atypical ethmoid cells with compromised drainage; a lateralized middle turbinate; and intrinsic ostiomeatal anomalies.[102]

Contrast-enhanced CT, MRI, or endoscopy or all 3 should be performed for detection of obstructive conditions, particularly in children with genetic or acquired craniofacial abnormalities.

The microbiology of RABS is similar to that of isolated episodes of acute bacterial sinusitis and warrants the same treatment.[72] It should be recognized that closely spaced sequential courses of antimicrobial therapy may foster the emergence of antibiotic-resistant bacterial species as the causative agent in recurrent episodes. There are no systematically evaluated options for prevention of RABS in children. In general, the use of prolonged prophylactic antimicrobial therapy should be avoided and is not usually recommended for children with recurrent acute otitis media. However, when there are no recognizable predisposing conditions to remedy in children with RABS, prophylactic antimicrobial agents may be used for several months during the respiratory season. Enthusiasm for this strategy is tempered by concerns regarding the encouragement of bacterial resistance. Accordingly, prophylaxis should only be considered in carefully selected children whose infections have been thoroughly documented.

Influenza vaccine should be administered annually, and PCV-13 should be administered at the recommended ages for all children, including those with RABS. Intranasal steroids and nonsedating antihistamines can be helpful for children with allergic rhinitis, as can antireflux medications for those with gastroesophageal reflux disease. Children with anatomic abnormalities may require endoscopic surgery for removal of or reduction in ostiomeatal obstruction.

The pathogenesis of chronic sinusitis is poorly understood and appears to be multifactorial; however, many of the conditions associated with RABS

TABLE 4 Management of Worsening or Lack of Improvement at 72 Hours

Initial Management	Worse in 72 Hours	Lack of Improvement in 72 Hours
Observation	Initiate amoxicillin with or without clavulanate	Additional observation or initiate antibiotic based on shared decision-making
Amoxicillin	High-dose amoxicillin-clavulanate	Additional observation or high-dose amoxicillin-clavulanate based on shared decision-making
High-dose amoxicillin-clavulanate	Clindamycin[a] and cefixime OR linezolid and cefixime OR levofloxacin	Continued high-dose amoxicillin-clavulanate OR clindamycin[a] and cefixime OR linezolid and cefixime OR levofloxacin

[a] Clindamycin is recommended to cover penicillin-resistant S pneumoniae. Some communities have high levels of clindamycin-resistant S pneumoniae. In these communities, linezolid is preferred.

have also been implicated in chronic sinusitis, and it is clear that there is an overlap between the 2 syndromes.[101,102] In some cases, there may be episodes of acute bacterial sinusitis superimposed on a chronic sinusitis, warranting antimicrobial therapy to hasten resolution of the acute infection.

Complications of Acute Bacterial Sinusitis

Complications of acute bacterial sinusitis should be diagnosed when the patient develops signs or symptoms of orbital and/or central nervous system (intracranial) involvement. Rarely, complicated acute bacterial sinusitis can result in permanent blindness, other neurologic sequelae, or death if not treated promptly and appropriately. Orbital complications have been classified by Chandler et al.[32] Intracranial complications include epidural or subdural abscess, brain abscess, venous thrombosis, and meningitis.

Periorbital and intraorbital inflammation and infection are the most common complications of acute sinusitis and most often are secondary to acute ethmoiditis in otherwise healthy young children. These disorders are commonly classified in relation to the orbital septum; periorbital or preseptal inflammation involves only the eyelid, whereas postseptal (intraorbital) inflammation involves structures of the orbit. Mild cases of preseptal cellulitis (eyelid <50% closed) may be treated on an outpatient basis with appropriate

oral antibiotic therapy (high-dose amoxicillin-clavulanate for comprehensive coverage) for acute bacterial sinusitis and daily follow-up until definite improvement is noted. If the patient does not improve within 24 to 48 hours or if the infection is progressive, it is appropriate to admit the patient to the hospital for antimicrobial therapy. Similarly, if proptosis, impaired visual acuity, or impaired and/or painful extraocular mobility is present on examination, the patient should be hospitalized, and a contrast-enhanced CT should be performed. Consultation with an otolaryngologist, an ophthalmologist, and an infectious disease expert is appropriate for guidance regarding the need for surgical intervention and the selection of antimicrobial agents.

Intracranial complications are most frequently encountered in previously healthy adolescent males with frontal sinusitis.[33,34] In patients with altered mental status, severe headache, or Pott's puffy tumor (osteomyelitis of the frontal bone), neurosurgical consultation should be obtained. A contrast-enhanced CT scan (preferably coronal thin cut) of the head, orbits, and sinuses is essential to confirm intracranial or intraorbital suppurative complications; in such cases, intravenous antibiotics should be started immediately. Alternatively, an MRI may also be desirable in some cases of intracranial abnormality. Appropriate antimicrobial therapy for intraorbital complications include vancomycin (to cover possible methicillin-resistant

S aureus or penicillin-resistant S pneumoniae) and either ceftriaxone, ampicillin-sulbactam, or piperacillin-tazobactam.[103] Given the polymicrobial nature of sinogenic abscesses, coverage for anaerobes (ie, metronidazole) should also be considered for intraorbital complications and should be started in all cases of intracranial complications if ceftriaxone is prescribed.

Patients with small orbital, subperiosteal, or epidural abscesses and minimal ocular and neurologic abnormalities may be managed with intravenous antibiotic treatment for 24 to 48 hours while performing frequent visual and mental status checks.[104] In patients who develop progressive signs and symptoms, such as impaired visual acuity, ophthalmoplegia, elevated intraocular pressure (>20 mm), severe proptosis (>5 mm), altered mental status, headache, or vomiting, as well as those who fail to improve within 24 to 48 hours while receiving antibiotics, prompt surgical intervention and drainage of the abscess should be undertaken.[104] Antibiotics can be tailored to the results of culture and sensitivity studies when they become available.

AREAS FOR FUTURE RESEARCH

Since the publication of the original guideline in 2001, only a small number of high-quality studies of the diagnosis and treatment of acute bacterial sinusitis in children have been published.[5] Ironically, the number of published guidelines on the topic (5) exceeds the number of prospective, placebo-controlled clinical trials of either antibiotics or ancillary treatments of acute bacterial sinusitis. Thus, as was the case in 2001, there are scant data on which to base recommendations. Accordingly, areas for future research include the following:

Etiology

1. Reexamine the microbiology of acute sinusitis in children in the postpneumococcal conjugate vaccine era and determine the value of using newer polymerase chain reaction–based respiratory testing to document viral, bacterial, and polymicrobial disease.

2. Correlate cultures obtained from the middle meatus of the maxillary sinus of infected children with cultures obtained from the maxillary sinus by puncture of the antrum.

3. Conduct more and larger studies to more clearly define and correlate the clinical findings with the various available diagnostic criteria of acute bacterial sinusitis (eg, sinus aspiration and treatment outcome).

4. Develop noninvasive strategies to accurately diagnose acute bacterial sinusitis in children.

5. Develop imaging technology that differentiates bacterial infection from viral infection or allergic inflammation, preferably without radiation.

Treatment

1. Determine the optimal duration of antimicrobial therapy for children with acute bacterial sinusitis.

2. Evaluate a "wait-and-see prescription" strategy for children with persistent symptom presentation of acute sinusitis.

3. Determine the optimal antimicrobial agent for children with acute bacterial sinusitis, balancing the incentives of choosing narrow-spectrum agents against the known microbiology of the disease and resistance patterns of likely pathogens.

4. Determine the causes and treatment of subacute, recurrent acute, and chronic bacterial sinusitis.

5. Determine the efficacy of prophylaxis with antimicrobial agents to prevent RABS.

6. Determine the effects of bacterial resistance among S pneumoniae, H influenzae, and M catarrhalis on outcome of treatment with antibiotics by the performance of randomized, double-blind, placebo-controlled studies in well-defined populations of patients.

7. Determine the role of adjuvant therapies (antihistamines, nasal corticosteroids, mucolytics, decongestants, nasal irrigation, etc) in patients with acute bacterial sinusitis by the performance of prospective, randomized clinical trials.

8. Determine whether early treatment of acute bacterial sinusitis prevents orbital or central nervous system complications.

9. Determine the role of complementary and alternative medicine strategies in patients with acute bacterial sinusitis by performing systematic, prospective, randomized clinical trials.

10. Develop new bacterial and viral vaccines to reduce the incidence of acute bacterial sinusitis.

SUBCOMMITTEE ON ACUTE SINUSITIS

Ellen R. Wald, MD, FAAP (Chair, Pediatric Infectious Disease Physician: no financial conflicts; published research related to sinusitis)

Kimberly E. Applegate, MD, MS, FAAP (Radiologist, AAP Section on Radiology: no conflicts)

Clay Bordley, MD, MPH, FAAP (Pediatric Emergency and Hospitalist Medicine physician: no conflicts)

David H. Darrow, MD, FAAP (Otolaryngologist, AAP Section on Otolaryngology–Head and Neck Surgery: no conflicts)

Mary P. Glode, MD, FAAP (Pediatric Infectious Disease Physician, AAP Committee on Infectious Disease: no conflicts)

S. Michael Marcy, MD, FAAP (General Pediatrician with Infectious Disease Expertise, AAP Section on Infectious Diseases: no conflicts)

Nader Shaikh, MD, FAAP (General Academic Pediatrician: no financial conflicts; published research related to sinusitis)

Michael J. Smith, MD, MSCE, FAAP (Epidemiologist, Pediatric Infectious Disease Physician: research funding for vaccine clinical trials from Sanofi Pasteur and Novartis)

Paul V. Williams, MD, FAAP (Allergist, AAP Section on Allergy, Asthma, and Immunology: no conflicts)

Stuart T. Weinberg, MD, FAAP (PPI Informatician, General Academic Pediatrician: no conflicts)

Carrie E. Nelson, MD, MS (Family Physician, American Academy of Family Physicians: employed by McKesson Health Solutions)

Richard M. Rosenfeld, MD, MPH, FAAP (Otolaryngologist, AAP Section on Otolaryngology–Head and Neck Surgery, American Academy of Otolaryngology–Head and Neck Surgery: no financial conflicts; published research related to sinusitis)

CONSULTANT

Richard N. Shiffman, MD, FAAP (Informatician, Guideline Methodologist, General Academic Pediatrician: no conflicts)

STAFF

Caryn Davidson, MA

REFERENCES

1. Aitken M, Taylor JA. Prevalence of clinical sinusitis in young children followed up by primary care pediatricians. *Arch Pediatr Adolesc Med.* 1998;152(3):244–248

2. Kakish KS, Mahafza T, Batieha A, Ekteish F, Daoud A. Clinical sinusitis in children attending primary care centers. *Pediatr Infect Dis J.* 2000;19(11):1071–1074

3. Ueda D, Yoto Y. The ten-day mark as a practical diagnostic approach for acute paranasal sinusitis in children. *Pediatr Infect Dis J.* 1996;15(7):576–579

4. Wald ER, Nash D, Eickhoff J. Effectiveness of amoxicillin/clavulanate potassium in the treatment of acute bacterial sinusitis in children. *Pediatrics.* 2009;124(1):9–15

5. American Academy of Pediatrics, Subcommittee on Management of Sinusitis and Committee on Quality Improvement. Clinical practice guideline: management of sinusitis. *Pediatrics.* 2001;108(3):798–808

6. Smith MJ. AAP technical report: evidence for the diagnosis and treatment of acute uncomplicated sinusitis in children: a systematic review. 2013, In press.

7. Shiffman RN, Michel G, Rosenfeld RM, Davidson C. Building better guidelines with BRIDGE-Wiz: development and evaluation of a software assistant to promote clarity, transparency, and implementability. *J Am Med Inform Assoc.* 2012;19(1):94–101

8. American Academy of Pediatrics, Steering Committee on Quality Improvement and Management. Classifying recommendations for clinical practice guidelines. *Pediatrics.* 2004;114(3):874–877

9. Gwaltney JM, Jr, Hendley JO, Simon G, Jordan WS Jr. Rhinovirus infections in an industrial population. II. Characteristics of illness and antibody response. *JAMA.* 1967;202(6):494–500

10. Pappas DE, Hendley JO, Hayden FG, Winther B. Symptom profile of common colds in school-aged children. *Pediatr Infect Dis J.* 2008;27(1):8–11

11. Wald ER, Guerra N, Byers C. Frequency and severity of infections in day care: three-year follow-up. *J Pediatr.* 1991;118(4 pt 1):509–514

12. Wald ER, Guerra N, Byers C. Upper respiratory tract infections in young children: duration of and frequency of complications. *Pediatrics.* 1991;87(2):129–133

13. Meltzer EO, Hamilos DL, Hadley JA, et al. Rhinosinusitis: establishing definitions for clinical research and patient care. *J Allergy Clin Immunol.* 2004;114(6 suppl):155–212

14. Shaikh N, Wald ER. Signs and symptoms of acute sinusitis in children. *Pediatr Infect Dis J.* 2013; in press

15. Wald ER. The diagnosis and management of sinusitis in children: diagnostic considerations. *Pediatr Infect Dis.* 1985;4(6 suppl):S61–S64

16. Wald ER, Milmoe GJ, Bowen A, Ledesma-Medina J, Salamon N, Bluestone CD. Acute maxillary sinusitis in children. *N Engl J Med.* 1981;304(13):749–754

17. Lindbaek M, Hjortdahl P, Johnsen UL. Use of symptoms, signs, and blood tests to diagnose acute sinus infections in primary care: comparison with computed tomography. *Fam Med.* 1996;28(3):183–188

18. Wald ER. Beginning antibiotics for acute rhinosinusitis and choosing the right treatment. *Clin Rev Allergy Immunol.* 2006;30(3):143–152

19. Maresh MM, Washburn AH. Paranasal sinuses from birth to late adolescence. II. Clinical and roentgenographic evidence of infection. *Am J Dis Child.* 1940;60:841–861

20. Glasier CM, Mallory GB, Jr, Steele RW. Significance of opacification of the maxillary and ethmoid sinuses in infants. *J Pediatr.* 1989;114(1):45–50

21. Kovatch AL, Wald ER, Ledesma-Medina J, Chiponis DM, Bedingfield B. Maxillary sinus radiographs in children with non-respiratory complaints. *Pediatrics.* 1984;73(3):306–308

22. Shopfner CE, Rossi JO. Roentgen evaluation of the paranasal sinuses in children. *Am J Roentgenol Radium Ther Nucl Med.* 1973;118(1):176–186

23. Diament MJ, Senac MO, Jr, Gilsanz V, Baker S, Gillespie T, Larsson S. Prevalence of incidental paranasal sinuses opacification in pediatric patients: a CT study. *J Comput Assist Tomogr.* 1987;11(3):426–431

24. Glasier CM, Ascher DP, Williams KD. Incidental paranasal sinus abnormalities on CT of children: clinical correlation. *AJNR Am J Neuroradiol.* 1986;7(5):861–864

25. Gwaltney JM, Jr, Phillips CD, Miller RD, Riker DK. Computed tomographic study of the common cold. *N Engl J Med.* 1994;330(1):25–30

26. Manning SC, Biavati MJ, Phillips DL. Correlation of clinical sinusitis signs and symptoms to imaging findings in pediatric patients. *Int J Pediatr Otorhinolaryngol.* 1996;37(1):65–74

27. Gordts F, Clement PA, Destryker A, Desprechins B, Kaufman L. Prevalence of sinusitis signs on MRI in a non-ENT paediatric population. *Rhinology.* 1997;35(4):154–157

28. Kristo A, Uhari M, Luotonen J, et al. Paranasal sinus findings in children during respiratory infection evaluated with magnetic resonance imaging. *Pediatrics.* 2003;111(5 pt 1):e586–e589

29. Brook I. Microbiology and antimicrobial treatment of orbital and intracranial complications of sinusitis in children and their management. *Int J Pediatr Otorhinolaryngol.* 2009;73(9):1183–1186

30. Sultesz M, Csakanyi Z, Majoros T, Farkas Z, Katona G. Acute bacterial rhinosinusitis and its complications in our pediatric otolaryngological department between 1997 and 2006. *Int J Pediatr Otorhinolaryngol.* 2009;73(11):1507–1512

31. Wald ER. Periorbital and orbital infections. *Infect Dis Clin North Am.* 2007;21(2):393–408

32. Chandler JR, Langenbrunner DJ, Stevens ER. The pathogenesis of orbital complications in acute sinusitis. *Laryngoscope.* 1970;80(9):1414–1428

33. Kombogiorgas D, Seth R, Modha J, Singh J. Suppurative intracranial complications of sinusitis in adolescence. Single institute experience and review of the literature. *Br J Neurosurg.* 2007;21(6):603–609

34. Rosenfeld EA, Rowley AH. Infectious intracranial complications of sinusitis, other than meningitis in children: 12 year review. *Clin Infect Dis.* 1994;18(5):750–754

35. American College of Radiology. Appropriateness criteria for sinonasal disease. 2009. Available at: www.acr.org/~/media/8172B4DE503149248E64856857674BB5.pdf. Accessed November 6, 2012

36. Triulzi F, Zirpoli S. Imaging techniques in the diagnosis and management of rhinosinusitis in children. *Pediatr Allergy Immunol.* 2007;18(suppl 18):46–49

37. McIntosh D, Mahadevan M. Failure of contrast enhanced computed tomography scans to identify an orbital abscess. The benefit of magnetic resonance imaging. *J Laryngol Otol.* 2008;122(6):639–640

38. Younis RT, Anand VK, Davidson B. The role of computed tomography and magnetic resonance imaging in patients with sinusitis with complications. *Laryngoscope.* 2002;112(2):224–229

39. Shapiro DJ, Gonzales R, Cabana MD, Hersh AL. National trends in visit rates and antibiotic prescribing for children with acute sinusitis. *Pediatrics.* 2011;127(1):28–34

40. Wald ER, Reilly JS, Casselbrant M, et al. Treatment of acute maxillary sinusitis in childhood: a comparative study of amoxicillin and cefaclor. *J Pediatr.* 1984;104(2):297–302

41. Wald ER, Chiponis D, Ledesma-Medina J. Comparative effectiveness of amoxicillin and amoxicillin-clavulanate potassium in acute paranasal sinus infections in children: a double-blind, placebo-controlled trial. *Pediatrics.* 1986;77(6):795–800

42. Garbutt JM, Goldstein M, Gellman E, Shannon W, Littenberg B. A randomized, placebo-controlled trial of antimicrobial treatment for children with clinically diagnosed acute sinusitis. *Pediatrics.* 2001;107(4):619–625

43. Kristo A, Uhari M, Luotonen J, Ilkko E, Koivunen P, Alho OP. Cefuroxime axetil versus placebo for children with acute respiratory infection and imaging evidence of sinusitis: a randomized, controlled trial. *Acta Paediatr.* 2005;94(9): 1208–1213

44. Hoberman A, Paradise JL, Rockette HE, et al. Treatment of acute otitis media in children under 2 years of age. *N Engl J Med.* 2011;364(2):105–115

45. Tahtinen PA, Laine MK, Huovinen P, Jalava J, Ruuskanen O, Ruohola A. A placebo-controlled trial of antimicrobial treatment for acute otitis media. *N Engl J Med.* 2011;364(2):116–126

46. Gordts F, Abu Nasser I, Clement PA, Pierard D, Kaufman L. Bacteriology of the middle meatus in children. *Int J Pediatr Otorhinolaryngol.* 1999;48(2):163–167

47. Parsons DS, Wald ER. Otitis media and sinusitis: similar diseases. *Otolaryngol Clin North Am.* 1996;29(1):11–25

48. Revai K, Dobbs LA, Nair S, Patel JA, Grady JJ, Chonmaitree T. Incidence of acute otitis media and sinusitis complicating upper respiratory tract infection: the effect of age. *Pediatrics.* 2007;119(6). Available at: www.pediatrics.org/cgi/content/full/119/6/e1408

49. Klein JO, Bluestone CD. *Textbook of Pediatric Infectious Diseases.* 6th ed. Philadelphia, PA: Saunders; 2009

50. Casey JR, Adlowitz DG, Pichichero ME. New patterns in the otopathogens causing acute otitis media six to eight years after introduction of pneumococcal conjugate vaccine. *Pediatr Infect Dis J.* 2010;29(4): 304–309

51. Brook I, Gober AE. Frequency of recovery of pathogens from the nasopharynx of children with acute maxillary sinusitis before and after the introduction of vaccination with the 7-valent pneumococcal vaccine. *Int J Pediatr Otorhinolaryngol.* 2007;71(4):575–579

52. Wald ER. Microbiology of acute and chronic sinusitis in children. *J Allergy Clin Immunol.* 1992;90(3 pt 2):452–456

53. Centers for Disease Control and Prevention. Effects of new penicillin susceptibility breakpoints for *Streptococcus pneumoniae*—United States, 2006-2007. *MMWR Morb Mortal Wkly Rep.* 2008;57 (50):1353–1355

54. Centers for Disease Control and Prevention. Active Bacterial Core Surveillance (ABCs): Emerging Infections Program Network. 2011. Available at: www.cdc.gov/abcs/reports-findings/survreports/spneu09.html. Accessed November 6, 2012

55. Garbutt J, St Geme JW, III, May A, Storch GA, Shackelford PG. Developing community-specific recommendations for first-line treatment of acute otitis media: is high-dose amoxicillin necessary? *Pediatrics.* 2004;114(2):342–347

56. Harrison CJ, Woods C, Stout G, Martin B, Selvarangan R. Susceptibilities of *Haemophilus influenzae, Streptococcus pneumoniae,* including serotype 19A, and *Moraxella catarrhalis* paediatric isolates from 2005 to 2007 to commonly used antibiotics. *J Antimicrob Chemother.* 2009; 63(3):511–519

57. Critchley IA, Jacobs MR, Brown SD, Traczewski MM, Tillotson GS, Janjic N. Prevalence of serotype 19A Streptococcus pneumoniae among isolates from U.S. children in 2005-2006 and activity of faropenem. *Antimicrob Agents Chemother.* 2008;52(7):2639–2643

58. Jacobs MR, Good CE, Windau AR, et al. Activity of ceftaroline against recent emerging serotypes of *Streptococcus pneumoniae* in the United States. *Antimicrob Agents Chemother.* 2010;54(6):2716–2719

59. Tristram S, Jacobs MR, Appelbaum PC. Antimicrobial resistance in *Haemophilus influenzae. Clin Microbiol Rev.* 2007;20(2): 368–389

60. Levine OS, Farley M, Harrison LH, Lefkowitz L, McGeer A, Schwartz B. Risk factors for invasive pneumococcal disease in children: a population-based case-control study in North America. *Pediatrics.* 1999; 103(3). Available at: www.pediatrics.org/cgi/content/full/103/3/e28

61. Seikel K, Shelton S, McCracken GH Jr. Middle ear fluid concentrations of amoxicillin after large dosages in children with acute otitis media. *Pediatr Infect Dis J.* 1997;16(7):710–711

62. Cohen R, Navel M, Grunberg J, et al. One dose ceftriaxone vs. ten days of amoxicillin/clavulanate therapy for acute otitis media: clinical efficacy and change in nasopharyngeal flora. *Pediatr Infect Dis J.* 1999;18(5):403–409

63. Green SM, Rothrock SG. Single-dose intramuscular ceftriaxone for acute otitis media in children. *Pediatrics.* 1993;91(1): 23–30

64. Leibovitz E, Piglansky L, Raiz S, Press J, Leiberman A, Dagan R. Bacteriologic and clinical efficacy of one day vs. three day intramuscular ceftriaxone for treatment of nonresponsive acute otitis media in children. *Pediatr Infect Dis J.* 2000;19(11): 1040–1045

65. DePestel DD, Benninger MS, Danziger L, et al. Cephalosporin use in treatment of patients with penicillin allergies. *J Am Pharm Assoc.* 2008;48(4):530–540

66. Pichichero ME. A review of evidence supporting the American Academy of Pediatrics recommendation for prescribing cephalosporin antibiotics for penicillin-allergic patients. *Pediatrics.* 2005;115(4): 1048–1057

67. Pichichero ME, Casey JR. Safe use of selected cephalosporins in penicillin-allergic patients: a meta-analysis. *Otolaryngol Head Neck Surg.* 2007;136(3): 340–347

68. Park MA, Koch CA, Klemawesch P, Joshi A, Li JT. Increased adverse drug reactions to cephalosporins in penicillin allergy patients with positive penicillin skin test. *Int Arch Allergy Immunol.* 2010;153(3): 268–273

69. Jacobs MR. Antimicrobial-resistant Streptococcus pneumoniae: trends and management. *Expert Rev Anti Infect Ther.* 2008; 6(5):619–635

70. Chow AW, Benninger MS, Brook I, et al; Infectious Diseases Society of America. IDSA clinical practice guideline for acute bacterial rhinosinusitis in children and adults. *Clin Infect Dis.* 2012;54(8):e72–e112

71. Brook I, Gober AE. Resistance to antimicrobials used for therapy of otitis media and sinusitis: effect of previous antimicrobial therapy and smoking. *Ann Otol Rhinol Laryngol.* 1999;108(7 pt 1):645–647

72. Brook I, Gober AE. Antimicrobial resistance in the nasopharyngeal flora of children with acute maxillary sinusitis and maxillary sinusitis recurring after amoxicillin therapy. *J Antimicrob Chemother.* 2004;53(2):399–402

73. Dohar J, Canton R, Cohen R, Farrell DJ, Felmingham D. Activity of telithromycin and comparators against bacterial pathogens isolated from 1,336 patients with clinically diagnosed acute sinusitis. *Ann Clin Microbiol Antimicrob.* 2004;3(3): 15–21

74. Jacobs MR, Bajaksouzian S, Zilles A, Lin G, Pankuch GA, Appelbaum PC. Susceptibilities of *Streptococcus pneumoniae* and *Haemophilus influenzae* to 10 oral antimicrobial agents based on pharmacodynamic parameters: 1997 U.S. surveillance study. *Antimicrob Agents Chemother.* 1999;43(8):1901–1908

75. Jacobs MR, Felmingham D, Appelbaum PC, Gruneberg RN. The Alexander Project 1998-2000: susceptibility of pathogens isolated from community-acquired respiratory tract infection to commonly used antimicrobial agents. *J Antimicrob Chemother.* 2003;52(2):229–246

76. Lynch JP, III, Zhanel GG. *Streptococcus pneumoniae*: epidemiology and risk factors, evolution of antimicrobial resistance, and impact of vaccines. *Curr Opin Pulm Med.* 2010;16(3):217–225

77. Sahm DF, Jones ME, Hickey ML, Diakun DR, Mani SV, Thornsberry C. Resistance surveillance of *Streptococcus pneumoniae*, *Haemophilus influenzae* and *Moraxella catarrhalis* isolated in Asia and Europe, 1997-1998. *J Antimicrob Chemother.* 2000; 45(4):457–466

78. Sokol W. Epidemiology of sinusitis in the primary care setting: results from the 1999-2000 respiratory surveillance program. *Am J Med.* 2001;111(suppl 9A):19S–24S

79. Shaikh N, Wald ER, Pi M. Decongestants, antihistamines and nasal irrigation for acute sinusitis in children. *Cochrane Database Syst Rev.* 2010;(12):CD007909

80. Dolor RJ, Witsell DL, Hellkamp AS, Williams JW, Jr, Califf RM, Simel DL. Comparison of cefuroxime with or without intranasal fluticasone for the treatment of rhinosinusitis. The CAFFS Trial: a randomized controlled trial. *JAMA.* 2001;286(24):3097–3105

81. Meltzer EO, Bachert C, Staudinger H. Treating acute rhinosinusitis: comparing efficacy and safety of mometasone furoate nasal spray, amoxicillin, and placebo. *J Allergy Clin Immunol.* 2005;116(6):1289–1295

82. Meltzer EO, Charous BL, Busse WW, Zinreich SJ, Lorber RR, Danzig MR. Added relief in the treatment of acute recurrent sinusitis with adjunctive mometasone furoate nasal spray. The Nasonex Sinusitis Group. *J Allergy Clin Immunol.* 2000;106 (4):630–637

83. Meltzer EO, Orgel HA, Backhaus JW, et al. Intranasal flunisolide spray as an adjunct to oral antibiotic therapy for sinusitis. *J Allergy Clin Immunol.* 1993;92(6):812–823

84. Nayak AS, Settipane GA, Pedinoff A, et al. Effective dose range of mometasone furoate nasal spray in the treatment of acute rhinosinusitis. *Ann Allergy Asthma Immunol.* 2002;89(3):271–278

85. Williamson IG, Rumsby K, Benge S, et al. Antibiotics and topical nasal steroid for treatment of acute maxillary sinusitis: a randomized controlled trial. *JAMA.* 2007; 298(21):2487–2496

86. Zalmanovici A, Yaphe J. Intranasal steroids for acute sinusitis. *Cochrane Database Syst Rev.* 2009;(4):CD005149

87. Yilmaz G, Varan B, Yilmaz T, Gurakan B. Intranasal budesonide spray as an adjunct to oral antibiotic therapy for acute sinusitis in children. *Eur Arch Otorhinolaryngol.* 2000;257(5):256–259

88. Barlan IB, Erkan E, Bakir M, Berrak S, Basaran MM. Intranasal budesonide spray as an adjunct to oral antibiotic therapy for acute sinusitis in children. *Ann Allergy Asthma Immunol.* 1997;78(6):598–601

89. Bruni FM, De Luca G, Venturoli V, Boner AL. Intranasal corticosteroids and adrenal suppression. *Neuroimmunomodulation.* 2009;16 (5):353–362

90. Kim KT, Rabinovitch N, Uryniak T, Simpson B, O'Dowd L, Casty F. Effect of budesonide aqueous nasal spray on hypothalamic-pituitary-adrenal axis function in children with allergic rhinitis. *Ann Allergy Asthma Immunol.* 2004;93(1):61–67

91. Meltzer EO, Tripathy I, Maspero JF, Wu W, Philpot E. Safety and tolerability of fluticasone furoate nasal spray once daily in paediatric patients aged 6-11 years with allergic rhinitis: subanalysis of three randomized, double-blind, placebo-controlled, multicentre studies. *Clin Drug Investig.* 2009;29(2):79–86

92. Murphy K, Uryniak T, Simpson B, O'Dowd L. Growth velocity in children with perennial allergic rhinitis treated with budesonide aqueous nasal spray. *Ann Allergy Asthma Immunol.* 2006;96(5):723–730

93. Ratner PH, Meltzer EO, Teper A. Mometasone furoate nasal spray is safe and effective for 1-year treatment of children with perennial allergic rhinitis. *Int J Pediatr Otorhinolaryngol.* 2009;73(5):651–657

94. Skoner DP, Gentile DA, Doyle WJ. Effect on growth of long-term treatment with intranasal triamcinolone acetonide aqueous in children with allergic rhinitis. *Ann*

Allergy Asthma Immunol. 2008;101(4): 431–436

95. Weinstein S, Qaqundah P, Georges G, Nayak A. Efficacy and safety of triamcinolone acetonide aqueous nasal spray in children aged 2 to 5 years with perennial allergic rhinitis: a randomized, double-blind, placebo-controlled study with an open-label extension. *Ann Allergy Asthma Immunol.* 2009;102(4):339–347

96. Zitt M, Kosoglou T, Hubbell J. Mometasone furoate nasal spray: a review of safety and systemic effects. *Drug Saf.* 2007;30(4): 317–326

97. Adam P, Stiffman M, Blake RL Jr. A clinical trial of hypertonic saline nasal spray in subjects with the common cold or rhinosinusitis. *Arch Fam Med.* 1998;7(1):39–43

98. Wang YH, Yang CP, Ku MS, Sun HL, Lue KH. Efficacy of nasal irrigation in the treatment of acute sinusitis in children. *Int J Pediatr Otorhinolaryngol.* 2009;73(12): 1696–1701

99. Harvey R, Hannan SA, Badia L, Scadding G. Nasal saline irrigations for the symptoms of chronic rhinosinusitis. *Cochrane Database Syst Rev.* 2007;(3):CD006394

100. Kassel JC, King D, Spurling GK. Saline nasal irrigation for acute upper respiratory tract infections. *Cochrane Database Syst Rev.* 2010;(3):CD006821

101. Shapiro GG, Virant FS, Furukawa CT, Pierson WE, Bierman CW. Immunologic defects in patients with refractory sinusitis. *Pediatrics.* 1991;87(3):311–316

102. Wood AJ, Douglas RG. Pathogenesis and treatment of chronic rhinosinusitis. *Postgrad Med J.* 2010;86(1016):359–364

103. Liao S, Durand ML, Cunningham MJ. Sinogenic orbital and subperiosteal abscesses: microbiology and methicillin-resistant *Staphylococcus aureus* incidence. *Otolaryngol Head Neck Surg.* 2010;143(3):392–396

104. Oxford LE, McClay J. Medical and surgical management of subperiosteal orbital abscess secondary to acute sinusitis in children. *Int J Pediatr Otorhinolaryngol.* 2006;70(11):1853–1861

TECHNICAL REPORT

Evidence for the Diagnosis and Treatment of Acute Uncomplicated Sinusitis in Children: A Systematic Review

abstract

In 2001, the American Academy of Pediatrics published clinical practice guidelines for the management of acute bacterial sinusitis (ABS) in children. The technical report accompanying those guidelines included 21 studies that assessed the diagnosis and management of ABS in children. This update to that report incorporates studies of pediatric ABS that have been performed since 2001. Overall, 17 randomized controlled trials of the treatment of sinusitis in children were identified and analyzed. Four randomized, double-blind, placebo-controlled trials of antimicrobial therapy have been published. The results of these studies varied, likely due to differences in inclusion and exclusion criteria. Because of this heterogeneity, formal meta-analyses were not performed. However, qualitative analysis of these studies suggests that children with greater severity of illness at presentation are more likely to benefit from antimicrobial therapy. An additional 5 trials compared different antimicrobial therapies but did not include placebo groups. Six trials assessed a variety of ancillary treatments for ABS in children, and 3 focused on subacute sinusitis. Although the number of pediatric trials has increased since 2001, there are still limited data to guide the diagnosis and management of ABS in children. Diagnostic and treatment guidelines focusing on severity of illness at the time of presentation have the potential to identify those children most likely to benefit from antimicrobial therapy and at the same time minimize unnecessary use of antibiotics. *Pediatrics* 2013;132:e284–e296

Michael J. Smith, MD, MSCE

KEY WORDS
acute bacterial sinusitis, antibiotics, ancillary treatment, diagnosis, systematic review

ABBREVIATIONS
AAP—American Academy of Pediatrics
CT—computed tomography

www.pediatrics.org/cgi/doi/10.1542/peds.2013-1072

doi:10.1542/peds.2013-1072

PEDIATRICS (ISSN Numbers: Print, 0031-4005; Online, 1098-4275).

INTRODUCTION

Acute bacterial sinusitis is reported as a complication of 5% to 10% of upper respiratory tract infections in children[1,2] and is 1 of the more common indications for antibiotic use in the United States. In 2001, the American Academy of Pediatrics (AAP) published clinical practice guidelines for the management of sinusitis in children.[3] The 2001 technical report that accompanied those guidelines included an analysis of 21 studies published from January 1966 through March 1999 which assessed the diagnosis and therapeutic management of acute sinusitis in children.[4] These included 5 randomized controlled trials involving 255 children and 8 case series involving 418 children. The primary goal of the current analysis was to update the 2001 technical report by identifying and reviewing additional studies of pediatric acute sinusitis that have been performed in the last decade to aid the revision of the AAP practice guidelines.

This technical report revisits the same questions as the original report: (1) What is the efficacy of various types of antimicrobial therapy in children with acute sinusitis? (2) What is the efficacy of nonantimicrobial ancillary treatments in children with acute sinusitis? (3) What is the concordance of various clinical, laboratory, and radiographic findings in the diagnosis of acute sinusitis? In addition, the Subcommittee on Management of Sinusitis met before the initial literature search for the current report and raised additional questions:

1. What is the incidence of adverse events in the treatment of sinusitis?

2. Are there data to support the clinical definitions of acute, subacute, and recurrent acute sinusitis?

3. Are there data to recommend a specific duration of symptoms that distinguishes bacterial from viral sinusitis?

4. How have the epidemiology and bacteriology of acute sinusitis changed in the pneumococcal conjugate vaccine era?

5. Is there evidence to support antimicrobial prophylaxis in children with recurrent sinusitis?

6. What other guidelines for the management of acute sinusitis in children exist?

METHODS

Searches of PubMed were performed by using the same search term as in the 2001 report ("sinusitis"). All searches were limited to English language and human studies. Three separate searches were performed to maximize retrieval of the most recent and highest-quality evidence for pediatric sinusitis. The first search limited results to all randomized controlled trials from 1966 to 2009, the second to all meta-analyses from 1966 to 2009, and the third to all pediatric studies (age limit <18 years) published since the last technical report (1999–2009). In addition, Web of Science was used to search for additional studies that cited the 2001 technical report and guidelines as well as citations of each double-blind, randomized controlled pediatric trial identified. The Cochrane Database of Systematic Reviews was also reviewed. Finally, ClinicalTrials.gov was searched to identify results of unpublished and ongoing studies. The Jadad scale (Table 1) was used to assess the quality of randomized trials included in this analysis.[5] Additional literature updates using the same search strategies were performed in July 2010 and November 2012.

Whenever possible, data from randomized controlled trials (preferably placebo controlled) were used to answer the questions raised by the committee. When no such data were available, separate literature searches were performed.

TABLE 1 Criteria for Assessing Randomized Trials

Give 1 point for each of the following:
a. The study is described as randomized
b. The study is described as double-blind
c. There was a description of withdrawals and dropouts
Given 1 additional point if:
a. For randomized studies, the method of randomization was described and is appropriate
b. For double-blind studies, the method of blinding was described and is appropriate
Deduct 1 point if:
c. For randomized studies, the method of randomization was described and is inappropriate
d. For double-blind studies, the method of blinding was described and is inappropriate

Adapted from Jadad et al.[5]

RESULTS

In the initial search, 183 randomized trials were identified, 98 of which were published since 1998. Of these 98, a total of 62 were eliminated on the basis of titles indicating a focus on adults, chronic sinusitis, or post-surgical management. Inclusion criteria and results of the remaining 36 studies were reviewed. Seven studies included adolescents as young as 12 years, but they represented <2% of the study population, and no age-specific results were reported. Twenty-one additional studies included teenagers but did not report how many were included; average ages for these studies were in the third to fourth decade of life. The updated literature search in July 2010 identified 2 additional randomized controlled trials that focused on ancillary treatment of sinusitis in children. A final search performed in November 2012 did not identify any additional controlled trials.

Overall, 17 randomized studies of sinusitis in children were identified and included in the current analysis. The meta-analysis search identified 1 study that focused exclusively on children and 2 others that focused primarily on adults but also assessed and separately reported results of pediatric studies. A review of ClinicalTrials.gov identified 28 sinusitis studies including children aged <18 years, only 3 of which were limited exclusively to children. One of these (Wald et al[6]) has recently been published and is included in the analysis; the other 2 studies are not yet recruiting patients.

TREATMENT

Efficacy of Antimicrobial Therapy

Randomized Placebo-Controlled Trials

Four randomized, double-blind, placebo-controlled trials involving 392 children were identified (Table 2).[6–9] An additional study[10] that was included in the previous technical report was excluded because it included patients with chronic and subacute sinusitis. The results of these 4 studies varied. Two studies favored treatment, and the other 2 found no significant difference in clinical cure between the treatment and control groups.

Clinical improvement in children receiving placebo ranged from 14% to 79% across the 4 studies, suggesting significant heterogeneity. The outcomes in the treatment groups were less varied, ranging from 50% to 81%. However, the efficacies of specific treatments are difficult to compare directly because the studies were performed over a 25-year period, during which a universal conjugate pneumococcal vaccination program was introduced and the prevalence of penicillin-resistant *Streptococcus pneumoniae* and β-lactamase–producing *Moraxella* and *Haemophilus* species increased.

The disparity in outcomes in the placebo groups is likely explained by the different methods used in each study. Notably, the inclusion criteria differed between each of the 4 studies. For instance, the minimal duration of symptoms required for entry into the study by Kristo et al[9] was not specified and averaged between 8 and 9 days for the treatment and control groups, respectively. Furthermore, only 32% of subjects had symptoms lasting at least 10 days. Therefore, the results of this study are not generalizable to the AAP definition of sinusitis, which is 10 days of symptoms, and should not be considered in the revised guidelines. Inclusion criteria for persistent symptoms in the other 3 studies were similar. Each specified respiratory symptoms that persisted for at least 10 days but <30 days. Only the 1986 study by Wald et al[7] required an abnormal radiograph for study entry.

Another study by Wald et al (in 2009)[6] was the only trial to include a subgroup of children who met criteria for worsening (on or after day 6 with fever or increase in symptoms) or severe (temperature ≥102°F with purulent discharge for at least 3 consecutive days) symptoms of sinusitis.

Exclusion criteria for each of these 3 studies had some similarities. Allergy to study drug, recent receipt of antibiotics, and concurrent bacterial infection requiring treatment were exclusion criteria in all of the studies. Complications of sinusitis were also listed as exclusion criteria, although the definitions of this factor differed between the studies. For instance, Garbutt et al[8] excluded children with "fulminant sinusitis," including children with fever ≥39°C (102.2°F); this condition was a specific inclusion criterion for the severe group in the 2009 study by Wald et al.[6] In addition, underlying medical conditions were used to exclude children, but the specific diagnoses differed in the 3 studies. Wald et al[7] excluded children with a variety of underlying medical conditions, including history of asthma and allergic rhinitis. Garbutt et al[8] only excluded children with cystic fibrosis; children with asthma and allergic rhinitis were included. Wald et al[6] only excluded children with immunodeficiency or anatomic abnormality of the upper respiratory tract.

The 3 studies used similar randomization schemes: patients were stratified according to age group and clinical severity before randomization. However, the metrics of clinical severity differed. The 2 studies by Wald et al[6,7] used a 10-point questionnaire (Table 3), and the study by Garbutt et al[8] used the S5 score (Table 4), previously validated by the same author.[11] Although each of these 3 studies stratified patients according to clinical severity before randomization,

separate results stratified by severity are not reported. This information may be helpful in the identification of patients (on the basis of clinical grounds) who might benefit from antimicrobial therapy.

Another key methodologic difference is that the study by Wald et al (1986)[7] did not use intention-to-treat analysis. Fifteen (14%) of 108 children were excluded because of lack of compliance or drug toxicity, which may have introduced bias.

Because of these significant differences in study design, formal meta-analyses were not performed. However, qualitative analysis of these results suggests that there may be certain clinical characteristics that identify patients who benefit from antimicrobial therapy.

Randomized Controlled Comparison Trials

In addition to the 4 placebo-controlled studies described previously, there have been other randomized studies of acute sinusitis in children comparing different antimicrobial treatment courses (Table 5).[12–16] Three of these were included in the previous report, and 2 additional studies have been published since 1998. None of these studies demonstrated a clear advantage of 1 therapy over another, and rates of cure or improvement were well above 80%. Although these studies offer some insight into the relative efficacies of different treatments, they do not include a placebo group. This factor is important given that many of the children included in these studies may have improved spontaneously without any specific antimicrobial therapy. In addition, none of these studies was designed as noninferiority or equivalence studies and, therefore, may have been underpowered to detect true differences between competing treatments.

TABLE 2 Randomized, Placebo-Controlled Trials of Antimicrobial Treatment of Acute Sinusitis in Children

Variable	Wald et al[7]	Garbutt et al[8]	Kristo et al[9]	Wald et al[6]
Inclusion criteria	Nasal discharge of any quality	"Persistent upper respiratory symptoms"	Acute respiratory symptoms suggestive of sinusitis that were "not improving"	Persistent: nasal discharge of any quality and/or daytime cough persisting for >10 d without improvement
	and/or		Nasal discharge and obstruction, sneezing, cough	Worsening: worsening on or after day 6 with fever or increase in symptoms
	Cough			Severe: temperature ≥102°F with purulent nasal discharge for at least 3 consecutive days
	Symptoms present for 10–30 d	Symptoms present for 10–28 d	Symptoms present <3 wk, no lower bound	Symptoms present <30 d, lower bound per definitions above
	Age: 2–16 y	Age: 1–18 y	Age: 4–10 y	Age: 1–10 y
Exclusion criteria	Abnormal radiograph results	NA	Abnormal US	NA
	Penicillin allergy	Allergy	Allergy	Allergy
	Previous Rx within 3 d	Previous Rx within 2 wk	Previous Rx within 4 wk	Previous Rx within 15 d
	Underlying conditions (asthma, allergic rhinitis, CF, sickle cell anemia, congenital heart disease, immunodeficiency)	CF only	Previous sinus surgery	Underlying conditions (immunodeficiency or anatomic abnormality of upper respiratory tract)
	Otitis media, pneumonia, GAS pharyngitis (throat/NP culture performed at study enrollment)	"Fulminant sinusitis"	Current antimicrobial Rx	Concurrent bacterial infection
	Severe headache or periorbital swelling	(fever >39°C, facial swelling, facial pain)	"Complications of sinus disease"	Complication of sinusitis requiring hospitalization, IV antibiotics, or subspecialty evaluation.
	Normal radiograph of paranasal sinuses	NA	NA	NA
Source of patients	Primary or secondary care patients at an academic children's hospital	3 suburban primary care practices	1 private health care center	2 private practices, 1 hospital-based clinic
Randomization			Block randomization	Assigned to persistent or nonpersistent group then
	Stratified by age: (<6 and ≥6 y)	Stratified by age: (<7 and ≥7 y)		Stratified by age: (<6 and ≥6 y)
	And clinical severity	And clinical severity		And clinical severity
	Then randomized	Then randomized		Then randomized
Metric for severity	Clinical severity score: <8 is mild and ≥8 is severe	Clinical severity score using S5 score	8 acute symptoms, rated 0–4	Same as Wald et al[7]
Telephone follow-up	1, 2, 3, 5, and 7 d	3, 7, 10, 14, 21, 28, and 60 d	NA	1, 2, 3, 5, 7, 10, 20, and 30 d
Clinical visit	Day 10	Day 14	Day 14	Day 14
Primary outcome	Clinical outcome at 3 and 10 d	Change in sinus symptoms at day 14	% complete cure at 2 wk	Cure at day 14
Secondary outcomes	Not specified	Adverse events	Adverse effects	Adverse events
		Relapse	Improvement without complications	Proportion with treatment failure
		Change in functional status		
		Parental satisfaction with treatment	Days when analgesics, nasal decongestants or cough mixtures were given	
N placebo	35	55	41	28
N treatment group	30 amoxicillin (40 mg/kg per day) divided 3 times/d for 10 d	58 amoxicillin (40 mg/kg per day) divided 3 times/d for 14 d	41 cefuroxime 125 mg 2 times/d for 10 d	28 amoxicillin/clavulanate (90 mg/kg amoxicillin + 6.4 mg clavulanate) divided 2 times/d for 14 days
	28 amoxicillin/clavulanate	48 amoxicillin/clavulanate (45 mg/kg per day amoxicillin) divided 2 times/d for 14 d		
Adjuvant therapy	None were prescribed. Not formally studied	Prescription or over-the-counter symptomatic treatments allowed. Use recorded	Analgesics, nose drops, and cough mixtures allowed. Use recorded in diary	Use "discouraged"—not formally studied
Compliance	History and remaining medications at follow-up visit	Self-report at day 14	Residual drugs collected at day 14	History and remaining medications at follow-up visit

TABLE 2 Continued

Variable	Wald et al[7]	Garbutt et al[8]	Kristo et al[9]	Wald et al[6]
Adverse events	Children who developed rash and diarrhea were excluded from analysis	Assessed at day 14	Assessed at day 14	Assessed at day 14
Loss to follow-up	15 children excluded because of adverse events (8) and noncompliance (7)	None (typographic error in original manuscript)	3 children (2 placebo, 1 treatment) lost to follow-up	6 lost to follow-up in treatment group
Primary outcome	Cure at 10 d: Amoxicillin: 20/30 (67%); Amoxicillin/ clavulanate: 18/28 (64%); Placebo: 15/35 (43%) Total: Antibiotic: 38/58; Placebo: 15/35 (66% vs 43%; $P < .05$) Failure at 10 d: Amoxicillin: 5/30; Amoxicillin/clavulanate: 7/28; Placebo: 14/35 Total: Antibiotic: 12/58; Placebo: 15/35 (21% vs 43%; $P < .05$)	Improvement at 14 d: Amoxicillin: 79% (46/58; Amoxicillin/clavulanate: 81% (39/48); Placebo: 79% (43/55)	Cure at 14 d: 22/35 in experimental group vs 21/37 in placebo (63% vs 57%; $P = .64$)	Cure at 14 d: 14/28 in experimental group vs 4/28 in placebo (50% vs 14%' $P = .01$) Failure at 14 d: 4/28 in experimental group vs 19/28 in placebo (14% vs 68%; $P < .001$) If all subjects lost to follow-up were considered failures, therapy is still effective (35% vs 68%; $P = .032$)
Jadad score	3	5	4	4

CF, cystic fibrosis; GAS, group A streptococcal; IV, intravenous; NA, not applicable; NP, nasopharyngeal; Rx, prescription; US, ultrasonography.

In addition to these randomized comparator studies, Garbutt et al[8] and Wald et al[7] used amoxicillin and amoxicillin/clavulanic acid treatments arms in their placebo-controlled studies. No significant differences between these 2 treatments were detected.

Adverse Events Associated With Antimicrobial Therapy

Randomized Placebo-Controlled Trials

Adverse effects of treatment were described in all 3 studies. In the first study by Wald et al,[7] rash developed in 1 child in the amoxicillin group and 1 in the placebo group. Diarrhea, requiring cessation of therapy, developed in 6 children in the amoxicillin/clavulanic acid group and 1 child in the placebo group. In the study by Garbutt et al,[8] one-half of all study participants reported an adverse effect; these events were equally distributed across the study groups. Diarrhea was reported by 20% to 22% of participants ($P = .97$ between the 3 groups). The only reported adverse effect that reached statistical significance was abdominal pain, which occurred in 29% of children in the amoxicillin group but only 15% and 9% of children in the amoxicillin/clavulanate and placebo groups, respectively ($P = .02$). In the most recent study by Wald et al,[6] 44% of children in the experimental group experienced an adverse event compared with 14% in the control group ($P = .014$). The incidences of specific adverse events were not described, but diarrhea was reportedly the most common. Although efficacy data from the study by Kristo et al[9] should not be considered in the guidelines, data can be used to compare adverse events associated with antimicrobial therapy compared with placebo. In this study, 3 children developed self-limited diarrhea (1 in the cefuroxime group and 2 in the placebo group).

Randomized Controlled Comparison Trials

Adverse events were reported in 4 of these studies.[12,14–16] The incidence of

TABLE 3 Scale Used in Studies by Wald et al[6,7]

Symptoms or Signs	Points
Abnormal nasal or postnasal discharge	
Minimal	1
Severe	2
Nasal congestion	1
Cough	2
Malodorous breath	1
Facial tenderness	3
Erythematous nasal mucosa	1
Fever	
<38.5°C	1
≥38.5°C	2
Headache (retro-orbital)	
Severe	3
Mild	1

Interpretation: <8 = mild, ≥8 = severe.

TABLE 4 Scale Used by Garbutt et al[11]

Symptom	Points			
	1	2	3	0
Blocked up or stuffy nose	Small	Medium	Large	Not a problem or do not know
Headaches or face pain	Small	Medium	Large	Not a problem or do not know
Coughing during the day	Small	Medium	Large	Not a problem or do not know
Coughing at night	Small	Medium	Large	Not a problem or do not know
Color of child's mucus			Yellow or green	None or clear

S5 score is obtained by averaging the scores for each symptom. In the clinical trial,[8] children were stratified into 2 groups before randomization: S5 score <2 or S5 score ≥2.

TABLE 5 Randomized Controlled Trials Comparing Different Antimicrobial Treatments for Acute Sinusitis

Author (Year)	Age (y)	Antimicrobial Agents	Duration	N	Cured (%)	Improved (%)	Failed (%)	Relapsed (%)	Recurred (%)	Jadad Score
Poachanukoon and Kitcharoensakkul (2008)[12]	1–15	Amoxicillin-clavulanate (80–90 mg/kg per day)	14 d	72	ND	85	ND	11	6	3
		Cefditoren (4–6 mg/kg) 2 times/d	14 d	66	ND	79	ND	9	3	
Simon (1999)[13]	0.5–17	Erythromycin (40 mg/kg per day)	14 d	50	96	ND	4	ND	10	1
		Ceftibuten (9 mg/kg per day)	10 d	50	92	ND	8	ND	12	
		Ceftibuten (9 mg/kg per day)	15 d	50	92	ND	8	ND	8	
		Ceftibuten (9 mg/kg per day)	20 d	50	100	ND	0	ND	8	
Ficnar et al (1997)[14]	0.5–12	Azithromycin (10 mg/kg per day)	3 d	27	96	ND	0	4	ND	1
		Azithromycin (10 mg/kg on day 1, then 5 mg/kg on days 2–5)	5 d	18	100	ND	0	0	ND	
Careddu et al (1993)[15]	2–14	Brodimoprim (10 mg/kg on day 1, then 5 mg/kg per day)	8 d	25	96	ND	4	ND	ND	1
		Amoxicillin-clavulanate (50 mg/kg per day)	NS	27	85	ND	15	ND	ND	
Wald et al (1984)[16]	1–16	Amoxicillin (40 mg/kg per day)	10 d	27	81	4	11	4	4	3
		Cefaclor (40 mg/kg per day)	10 d	23	78	9	4	11	17	

ND, not determined; NS, not specified.

adverse events did not differ between study groups for 3 of these studies. Poachanukoon and Kitcharoensakkul[12] reported a higher rate of diarrhea (18.1%) in children receiving amoxicillin/clavulanate compared with those receiving cefditoren (4.5% [P = .02]). However, diarrhea was self-limited and did not require termination of medication or study withdrawal.

ANCILLARY TREATMENTS

Six randomized-controlled trials have assessed a variety of ancillary treatments for acute sinusitis (Table 6)[17–20] and are summarized here.

Steroids

The 2001 technical report described 1 study that assessed the efficacy of intranasal steroids in children.[17] In that study, 89 children received amoxicillin/clavulanate (40 mg/kg per day) and were randomized to receive either budesonide nasal spray (n = 43) or placebo (n = 46) for 3 weeks. Although no difference in symptom improvement was noted between the groups at the end of therapy (3 weeks), children in the budesonide group had improved cough and nasal discharge at 2 weeks,

whereas children in the placebo group did not, suggesting that corticosteroids may lead to more rapid resolution of symptoms. Since then, there has been 1 other randomized controlled trial in children studying the efficacy of intranasal budesonide.[18] In this study, 52 children (mean age: 8 years; age range: 6–16 years) with acute maxillary sinusitis received cefaclor (40 mg/kg) for 10 days with either pseudoephedrine (2 × 30 mg daily) or intranasal budesonide (2 × 100 μg daily) for 10 days. There was no placebo group. Children with underlying allergy were excluded. Children in the budesonide group had statistically significantly better resolution of headache, cough, nasal stuffiness, and nasal drainage. There were no adverse events reported. However, these authors defined acute sinusitis as an infection that could take up to 12 weeks for complete resolution, and the results may therefore not be generalizable to AAP guidelines.

Decongestant-Antihistamine

No randomized controlled studies have been performed since a study cited in the 2001 report.[19] All children in that

study received 14 days of amoxicillin (37.5–50 mg/kg per day, divided 3 times per day). They were then randomized to receive either placebo or the combination of oxymetazoline nasal spray and an oral decongestant-antihistamine. Both groups had marked clinical improvement in symptoms 3 days into treatment. In addition, there were no significant differences in clinical or radiographic findings between the 2 groups at the end of treatment.

Nasal Spray

One randomized controlled trial compared the use of 14 days of treatment with Ems mineral salts versus xylometazoline (0.05% solution) nasal spray in children with acute sinusitis.[20] There was no placebo group, and antibiotic use was not permitted. The primary outcome was mucosal inflammation (rubescence, swelling, and discharge) at baseline, day 7, and day 14. There were no significant differences between the 2 groups at day 14. However, at day 7, the mineral salt group had less nasal discharge than the xylometazoline group (P = .0163), suggesting that the spray may lead to more

TABLE 6 Randomized Controlled Trials of Ancillary Therapies for Acute Sinusitis

Author (Year)	Age (y)	Inclusion Criteria	Primary Therapy	LOT	Other Treatments	N	Main Outcome	Jadad Score
Barlan et al (1997)[17]	1–15	2 major, or 1 major and 2 minor criteria. Duration >7 d; Major criteria: purulent nasal discharge, purulent pharyngeal drainage, cough; Minor criteria: periorbital edema, facial pain, tooth pain, earache, sore throat, wheeze, headache, foul breath, fever	Intranasal budesonide (50 µg each nostril) 2 times/ day; Intranasal placebo bid	21 / 21	All received amoxicillin/ clavulanate (40 mg/kg per day)	43 / 46	No difference in cough or nasal discharge scores at weeks 1 or 3. Budesonide scores statistically lower (less symptomatic) at week 2 for both outcomes	2
Yilmaz et al (2000)[18]	6–16	Specific symptoms not specified. Duration: infection that could take up to 12 wk to resolve	Intranasal budesonide (2 × 100 µg) / Oral pseudoephedrine (2 × 30 mg)	10 / 10	All received cefaclor (40 mg/kg per day)	26 / 26	Budesonide group statistically better improvement in headache, cough, nasal stuffiness, and nasal drainage at day 10	1
McCormick et al (1996)[19]	1–18	8–29 d of sinusitis symptoms	Oxymetazoline nasal spray (0.05%) plus syrup with decongestant- antihistamine / Placebo nasal spray and syrup	14 / 14	All children received amoxicillin by age/weight: 10–12 kg, 150 mg tid; 12.1–15 kg, 200 mg tid; >15 kg, 250 mg tid; Teenagers: 40 mg/kg per day (maximum: 500 tid)	34 / 34	No difference between groups in mean symptom score at enrollment, day 3, or day 14	4
Michel et al (2005)[20]	2–6	"Definition give[n] by the AAP"	Intranasal isotonic Ems mineral salts / Intranasal xylometazoline (0.05%)	14 / 14	No additional treatment (including antibiotics) allowed	66[a]	No difference in symptoms at day 14. Ems group had statistically significant less inflammation at day 7	2
Wang et al (2009)[21]	3–12	(1) URI with purulent nasal discharge and/ or cough >7 d (2) Abnormal findings of 1 or both maxillary sinuses by Water's projection	Standard therapy plus normal saline nasal irrigation, 15–20 mL per nostril 1–3 times/day / Standard therapy alone	21 / 21	"Standard therapy" defined as systemic antibiotics, mucolytics, and nasal decongestants	30 / 39	Saline group had better scores for daytime rhinorrhea and nighttime nasal congestion. No statistically significant differences in quality of life score, nasal smear, or Water's projection	1
Unuvar et al (2010)[22]	3–12	(1) 10–30 d of URTI symptoms (2) Presence of severe symptoms of rhinosinusitis	Erdosteine syrup (5–8 mg/kg/day orally divided bid) / Placebo	14 / 14	None	49 / 43	No significant difference in clinical improvement at 14 d between the 2 groups	4

bid, 2 times per day; LOT, length of therapy; tid, 3 times per day; URTI, upper respiratory tract infection.

[a] Sixty-six patients in trial; numbers in each treatment arm not specified.

rapid resolution of symptoms. Wang et al[21] randomized 69 children to receive standard therapy (systemic antibiotics, mucolytic agents, and nasal decongestants) or standard therapy plus nasal irrigation (15–20 mL of normal saline administered via syringe to each nostril 1–3 times per day). Outcomes included a daily nasal symptom score (summarized weekly), pediatric rhinoconjunctivitis quality of life questionnaire (at baseline and 3 weeks), weekly nasal peak expiratory flow rate, weekly nasal smear, and Water's projection (baseline and 3 weeks). The irrigation group had significantly better symptom scores for daytime (but not nighttime) rhinorrhea at weeks 1, 2, and 3 and nighttime (but not daytime) nasal congestion at weeks 1, 2, and 3. Children in the irrigation group also had better nasal peak expiratory flow rates and slightly better quality of life scores at 3 weeks. There were no statistically significant differences in nasal smear or Water's projections between the 2 groups after 3 weeks of treatment.

Mucolytic Agents

One randomized controlled trial assessed S5 scores in 49 children receiving the mucolytic erdosteine compared with 43 children who received placebo.[22] After 14 days of treatment, there was no significant difference in S5 scores between the 2 groups.

In addition to these studies, which were specifically designed to assess the efficacy of nonantimicrobial therapy, use of ancillary measures was measured and reported for 2 of the randomized trials of antimicrobial use. In the study by Garbutt et al,[8] there were no significant differences in the overall use of ancillary therapies between the treatment and placebo groups (52% vs 48% vs 49%; $P = .92$). Although individual-level data were not presented, this finding makes it unlikely that unbalanced use of adjuvant therapies contributed to the study outcomes. Among individual therapies, only use of combination products was reported more frequently in 1 group (10% of amoxicillin/clavulanate vs 0% and 2% of amoxicillin and placebo, respectively; $P = .01$). In the study by Poachanukoon and Kitcharoensakkul,[12] use of concomitant intranasal corticosteroids (52%) and oral decongestants (22%) was common but did not differ between the study groups.

DIAGNOSIS

Although sinus aspiration remains the gold standard for diagnosis of acute sinusitis, it is rarely practiced outside of the research setting. Furthermore, few recent studies have used aspiration as a criterion for study entry or used bacteriologic cure as an outcome. Despite these microbiologic limitations, evidence from the trials summarized previously can answer a slightly different question: which (if any) clinical, laboratory, and/or radiologic findings are able to discriminate between children who are likely to benefit from antimicrobial therapy and those who are not?

CLINICAL FINDINGS

Duration of Symptoms

The most commonly used diagnostic criterion for acute bacterial sinusitis is persistent or prolonged duration of symptoms for 10 to 14 days.[23] This criterion is based on the observation that most viral upper respiratory tract infections last 5 to 7 days.[3] However, the study by Garbutt et al[8] demonstrated that duration of symptoms alone was not sufficient to warrant antimicrobial therapy. A minimum of 10 days of symptoms was required for study entry, and all 3 groups had a mean duration of symptoms greater than 2 weeks (amoxicillin: 15.8 days; amoxicillin/clavulanate: 18.5 days; placebo: 15.4 days).

Signs and Symptoms

Purulent rhinorrhea, nasal congestion, and headache are other common findings used to diagnose sinusitis.[23] The various clinical trials used different combinations of these findings in their inclusion criteria. The 3 placebo-controlled studies limited to children with at least 10 days of symptoms also used clinical severity scores based on these signs and symptoms

Tables 2 and 3 stratify study participants before randomization. Because this stratification occurred before randomization, severity-specific results might help clarify which children are likely to benefit from antimicrobial therapy.

Imaging Studies

The 2001 guidelines recommended that radiologic studies should not be used to diagnose sinusitis in children 6 years or younger and that computed tomography (CT) should be considered only for children requiring surgery.[3] Ultrasonography has also been suggested as a potential diagnostic tool for acute sinusitis. The 2001 technical

report cited 1 study that demonstrated good concordance between ultrasonographic findings and retrieval of fluid on sinus aspiration.[24] On the basis of that study, ultrasonographic findings (either mucosal thickening of ≥ 5 mm or fluid in at least 1 maxillary sinus) were used as entry criteria in the study by Kristo et al.[9] In that study, children also underwent occipitomental radiography, and the film results were defined as positive for sinusitis if there was mucosal thickening of at least 4 mm, an air-fluid level, or total opacification of at least 1 maxillary sinus. Eighty-nine percent of children in the treatment group and 92% of those in the placebo group met this criterion, suggesting good concordance between plain films and ultrasonography. However, these findings were not predictive of which children would benefit from antimicrobial therapy. Radiographic studies were not used in the other 2 recent placebo-controlled studies.[6,8]

Laboratory Studies

None of the studies required routine laboratory studies for study entry. Microbiologic samples were only obtained in 2 placebo-controlled studies and did not include direct sinus sampling. Wald et al[7] used results of throat and nasopharyngeal cultures to exclude patients with group A streptococcal pharyngitis from their study. Kristo et al[9] obtained nasopharyngeal cultures on all patients but only reported those with results positive for *Streptococcus pneumoniae* and *Haemophilus influenzae*, which occurred in 12.5% of study participants.

SUBACUTE SINUSITIS

Subacute sinusitis has been defined as infection that lasts between 30 and 90 days.[3] Three small randomized controlled trials assessing the efficacy of different treatment strategies for subacute sinusitis were identified (Table 7).[25–27] None of these studies included a placebo group. One compared empirical amoxicillin/clavulanate with culture-based (from nasal mucosa) antimicrobial treatment.[25] Culture of nasal specimens was not performed on the children in the empirical antibiotic group. Five (18.5%) of 27 culture results in the experimental group were positive for amoxicillin/clavulanate-resistant organisms (1 *Pseudomonas* species, 2 resistant to *S pneumoniae,* and 2 anaerobic streptococci), and appropriate therapy was initiated. Nasal obstruction at day 14 was unchanged or worse for 9 children (36%) in the empirical arm but only 4 children (15%) in the culture-based arm ($P = .037$, per authors). Another study compared azithromycin versus amoxicillin/clavulanate.[26] The third compared amoxicillin, amoxicillin/clavulanic acid, trimethoprim/sulfamethoxazole, and no antimicrobial therapy.[27] In these 2 studies, no advantage was detected in any treatment arm compared with others. However, the studies were small and were likely not powered to detect true differences.

CLINICAL QUESTIONS FOR WHICH HIGH-QUALITY DATA ARE LACKING

Definitions of Acute, Subacute, and Recurrent Acute Sinusitis

The definitions of acute, subacute, and recurrent acute sinusitis are outlined in the 2001 AAP guidelines.[3] Although logical and based on the presumed pathogenesis of these distinct clinical entities, there are few clinical or laboratory data to confirm these definitions in children. One study of subacute sinusitis included 52 sinus aspirations of 40 children with subacute (30–120 days of symptoms) sinusitis and found similar pathogens as in acute sinusitis.[28] The definition of subacute sinusitis used in this study and in the study be Ng et al[26] were derived from an expert consensus panel.[29] The study by El-Hennawi et al[23] cites the 2001 AAP guidelines, and the study by Dohlman et al[25] does not provide a reference for the study definition of subacute sinusitis.

Epidemiology of Sinusitis in the Pneumococcal Conjugate Vaccine Era

A separate literature search was performed to identify studies of sinusitis in the era of the pneumococcal conjugate vaccine. Although there are substantial data regarding the epidemiology of invasive pneumococcal disease and acute otitis media since implementation of pneumococcal immunization, no recent pediatric sinusitis studies that included microbiologic data were identified. Brook et al[30] compared culture results from sinuses of adults before and after introduction of the pneumococcal conjugate vaccine. There was a statistically significant decrease in the prevalence of *S pneumoniae* and a significant increase in the prevalence of *H influenzae.* In addition, there was a 12% decrease in penicillin resistance observed in pneumococcal

TABLE 7 Randomized Controlled Trials of Antimicrobial Therapy for Subacute Sinusitis

Author (Year)	Age (y)	Inclusion Criteria	Antimicrobial Agents	Length	Other Treatments	N	Better (%)	Worse or Same (%)	Jadad Score
El-Hennawi et al (2006)[25]	<2	Persistent nasal discharge and nasal obstruction for 30–90 d	Amoxicillin-clavulanate (40 mg/kg per day)	14 d	All had therapeutic nasal suction every third day	30	64	36	2
			Culture-based (nasal suction)			30			
			Amoxicillin/clavulanate (40 mg/kg per day)			12	83	17	
			Amoxicillin/clavulanate (90 mg/kg per day)	14 d		6	100	0	
			Other antibiotics			5	100	0	
			No antibiotics (negative culture result)			4	50	50	
Ng et al (2000)[26]	5–16	Nasal discharge or blockage for 30–120 d and abnormal sinus radiograph	Azithromycin (10 mg/kg per day)	3 d	All received budesonide nasal spray 50 µg/nostril 2 times/day for 91 d	20	ND[a]	30	3
			Amoxicillin/clavulanate (312 mg 3 times/day if aged ≤12 y or 375 mg 3 times/day if aged >12 y)	14 d		21	ND[a]	24	
Dohlman et al (1993)[27]	2–16	Mucoid nasal drainage, cough, or poorly controlled asthma for 3 wk–3 mo and abnormal sinus radiograph	Amoxicillin (30-40 mg/kg per day)	21 d	All received oral phenylephrine, phenylpropanolamine, and guaifenesin; all received saline nasal spray	25	72	28	3
			Amoxicillin-clavulanate (30-40 mg/kg per day)	21 d		26	73	27	
			TMP/SMX (8 mg/kg per day)	21 d		26	69	31	
			None			19	63	37	

ND, not determined; TMP/SMX, trimethoprim/sulfamethoxazole.

[a] This study only reported "failures."

isolates and a 6% increase in β-lactamase–producing *H influenzae,* but these findings did not reach statistical significance. The same authors also compared nasopharyngeal (but not sinus) cultures in children before and after licensure of the pneumococcal conjugate vaccine and found similar results.[31]

Antimicrobial Prophylaxis

One small, nonrandomized study of antimicrobial prophylaxis in children with chronic sinusitis was identified.[32] Twenty-six of 86 children with chronic sinusitis received prophylaxis for 1 year. There was a 50% reduction in the number of episodes of sinusitis in 19 (73%) subjects. Nearly 25% of the children in the cohort had an underlying immunologic defect, but this discovery did not predict efficacy of prophylaxis. A randomized controlled study of azithromycin prophylaxis for acute recurrent sinusitis in children was identified on ClinicalTrials.gov and began recruiting patients in August 2009.

Duration of Symptoms

As presented previously, data from randomized trials suggest that duration of symptoms alone is not predictive of necessity of antimicrobial therapy. A small case series of complications of rhinosinusitis (almost exclusively orbital cellulitis) in children was recently published.[33] The authors noted that only 3 of 20 children admitted to a single institution over a 10-year period had symptoms of sinusitis for >10 days before hospitalization. On the basis of these data, they concluded that prevention of complications should not be a justification for initiating treatment after 10 days of symptoms.

Imaging

Since publication of the guidelines, there have been additional studies of children undergoing CT of the head that have confirmed the poor specificity of CT for acute sinusitis.[34,35] In addition, several small observational studies have assessed the use of MRI to diagnose acute sinusitis.[36–38] In the first, MRI was performed on a group of children 4 to 7 years of age presenting to a primary care center with any sign of respiratory infection.[36] Forty-one (68%) of 60 children had a major abnormality on imaging. Twenty-six children underwent follow-up 2 weeks later. Of these, 18 (69%) still had abnormal MRI findings, although this finding did not correlate with clinical symptoms. Another study by the same authors compared MRI findings in a convenience sample of children without respiratory complaints. Eight of 19 asymptomatic children had abnormal MRI findings.[37] A similar study found abnormal sinuses in 14 (31%) of 45 asymptomatic children.[38]

OTHER PEDIATRIC SINUSITIS GUIDELINES

Published guidelines were identified during the primary literature search. In addition, the Guidelines International Network (www.g-i-n.net) database was searched but yielded no results. Recently published pediatric guidelines for acute bacterial sinusitis are presented in Table 8.[39–42] These include English-language, pediatric-specific guidelines and other English-language guidelines that included separate recommendations for children. These guidelines were in near-complete concordance with the 2001 AAP guidelines in terms of clinical diagnosis, choice of antimicrobial agents, avoidance of radiographic studies, and avoidance of adjuvant therapies. One exception was that the European position paper recommended topical corticosteroids (in addition to oral antibiotics) as a grade A recommendation.[39]

The American College of Radiology Appropriateness Criteria, last updated in 2009, are another set of professional recommendations relevant to the diagnosis of sinusitis in children.[43] In summary, no radiologic studies are recommended by the American College of Radiology for acute uncomplicated sinusitis. Coronal CT of the paranasal sinuses is recommended for children with symptoms that persist after 10 days of appropriate therapy. Cranial CT with contrast, including the sinuses and orbits, is recommended for suspected complications of sinusitis.

DISCUSSION

The 2001 technical report noted a paucity of high-quality evidence for establishing the diagnosis and management of acute sinusitis in children. Nearly a decade later, data are still limited. Overall, 17 randomized controlled trials of pediatric acute sinusitis were identified. Of these, only 10 studies scored 3 points or higher on the Jadad scale, which is considered indicative of good study design.[5] These findings are consistent with other recent systematic reviews of pediatric acute sinusitis. A 2002 Cochrane review included data from 6 randomized controlled trials involving 562 children.[44] However, 2 studies focused on chronic sinusitis and 1 focused on subacute sinusitis. In addition, a recently published meta-analysis of studies comparing antimicrobial therapy versus placebo in all age groups identified only 3 studies that included children, all of which were included in the current review.[45] The publication of another placebo-controlled trial in 2009 is a significant contribution; however, only 310 children with acute sinusitis (392 if the Kristo study is included) have been studied in placebo-controlled fashion, with inconsistent results. Although meta-analysis techniques are designed to increase sample size and power,

TABLE 8 Summary of Other Published Guidelines for the Management of Acute Sinusitis in Children

Guideline	Antimicrobial Guidelines for Acute Bacterial Sinusitis (Sinus and Allergy Health Partnership, 2004)[39]	Cincinnati Children's Hospital Evidence-Based Guideline (2006)[40]	European Position Paper on Primary Care Diagnosis and Management of Rhinosinusitis and Nasal Polyps (2007)[41]	Guidelines for Treatment of Acute and Subacute Rhinosinusitis in Children (Italy, 2008)[42]
Diagnosis	No resolution after 10 d or worsens after 5–7 d with any of the following: nasal drainage, nasal congestion, facial pressure/pain, postnasal drainage, hyposmia/anosmia, fever, cough, fatigue, maxillary dental pain, and ear pressure/fullness	Clinical: at least 10 d without improvement Specific note: character of nasal discharge is not useful	(1) Cold with nasal discharge, daytime cough worsening at night >10 d (2) Cold that seems more severe than usual (3) Cold that was improving but suddenly worsens	(1) URTI without improvement within 10 d (2) URTI with severe symptoms (high fever, purulent rhinorrhea, headache, facial pain) (3) URTI that completely recedes within 3–4 d but recurs within 10 d
Imaging	Not recommended routinely	Not routinely recommended. For children with persistent findings or complications, imaging decisions should be made in consultation with consulting subspecialists	Not recommended	Not recommended. CT when surgery being considered
Antimicrobials	Mild disease, no recent antibiotics: amoxicillin/clavulanate, amoxicillin, cefpodoxime, cefuroxime, cefdinir. For allergies: TMP/SMX, macrolides Moderate disease or mild disease with recent antibiotics: amoxicillin/clavulanate (high-dose), ceftriaxone For allergies, same as above, plus clindamycin	First-line: high-dose amoxicillin or amoxicillin/clavulanate for 10–14 d Second-line: cefuroxime, cefpodoxime, cefdinir. For allergies: second-line antibiotics if non-type I reaction Clarithromycin or azithromycin for type I reaction	Recommended: specific agents not discussed	Amoxicillin 50 mg/kg per day If recent antibiotic exposure, school-attendance, or suspicion of antibiotic-resistant pathogens: Amoxicillin/clavulanate (80-90 mg/kg per day), cefuroxime (30 mg/kg per day), or cefaclor (50 mg/kg per day)
Adjuvant therapies	NA	Not recommended (antitussives, mucolytics, inhaled steroids, β_2- agonists, antihistamines, decongestants)	Topical steroids (in addition to systemic antibiotics) listed as a level lb recommendation (from at least 1 RCT)	Antihistamines, corticosteroids, decongestants, expectorants, mucolytics, and vasoconstrictors not recommended. Antibiotic prophylaxis not recommended
Complications	NA	Consult otolaryngologist and/or ophthalmologist	Immediate referral/hospitalization	Prompt, aggressive, multidisciplinary intervention

This table incorporates pediatric-specific guidelines (Cincinnati, Italy) as well as general guidelines with pediatric-specific recommendations (Sinus and Allergy Health Partnership, European Position Paper). CT, computed tomography; NA; not applicable; RCT, randomized controlled trial; TMP/SMX, trimethoprim/sulfamethoxazole; URTI, upper respiratory tract infection.

these were not pursued given the significant heterogeneity between the studies.

There are no reliable diagnostic criteria to distinguish between children with acute viral and bacterial sinusitis. However, the inclusion and exclusion criteria used in the 2 randomized studies that demonstrated a benefit of antimicrobial therapy compared with placebo offer insight into criteria that may identify children who are likely to benefit from antimicrobial therapy. Qualitatively, greater severity of illness at the time of presentation seems to be associated with increased likelihood of antimicrobial efficacy.

No studies of the microbiology of acute sinusitis in children have been published since the introduction of the conjugate pneumococcal vaccine. It is reasonable to assume that the same pathogen shifts observed in acute otitis media are found in acute bacterial sinusitis. However, this assumption would not necessarily imply that the treatment outcomes for otitis and sinusitis are the same.

Although the need for and choice of antimicrobial therapy remains controversial, the short-term adverse effect profiles for common antibacterial agents used in the management of sinusitis seem to be fairly benign. Two studies found no significant differences in adverse events between placebo and antimicrobial therapy.[8,9] A third reported that, although adverse effects were more common in the treatment group, those events occuring in children who received high-dose amoxicillin/clavulanate were mostly mild and self-limited.[6] However, the long-term effects of antimicrobial use on resistance patterns at the population level remain unmeasured and need to be considered in the revised guidelines.

Evidence to support the use of ancillary measures in the management of acute sinusitis in children is limited. Two small, randomized controlled studies demonstrated that children treated with intranasal steroids had better outcomes compared with children treated with systemic decongestants plus antibiotics[18] or antibiotics alone.[17] One of these studies demonstrated that corticosteroids hastened resolution of symptoms, but cure at the end of the study was equivalent. The other

defined acute sinusitis as an infection lasting up to 12 weeks, which may not be applicable to the definition of acute sinusitis used in the AAP guidelines. The efficacy of decongestants and antihistamines for sinusitis has not been proven. Given recent concerns regarding their safety profile in young children, the use of these agents should be avoided.

CONCLUSIONS

There are limited data to guide the diagnosis and management of acute

bacterial sinusitis in children. Although there have been 4 placebo-controlled studies of antimicrobial therapy in children with acute sinusitis, the results of these studies varied. It is clear that some children with sinusitis benefit from antibiotic use and some do not. Diagnostic and treatment guidelines focusing on severity of illness at the time of presentation have the potential to identify children who will benefit from therapy and at the same time minimize unnecessary use of antibiotics.

REFERENCES

1. Aitken M, Taylor JA. Prevalence of clinical sinusitis in young children followed up by primary care pediatricians. *Arch Pediatr Adolesc Med*. 1998;152(3):244–248

2. Revai K, Dobbs LA, Nair S, Patel JA, Grady JJ, Chonmaitree T. Incidence of acute otitis media and sinusitis complicating upper respiratory tract infection: the effect of age. *Pediatrics*. 2007;119(6). Available at: www.pediatrics.org/cgi/content/full/119/6/e1408

3. Wald ER, Bordley WC, Darrow DH, et al. Clinical practice guideline: management of sinusitis. *Pediatrics*. 2001;108(3):798–808

4. Ioannidis JP, Lau J. Technical report: evidence for the diagnosis and treatment of acute uncomplicated sinusitis in children: a systematic overview. *Pediatrics*. 2001;108 (3). Available at: www.pediatrics.org/cgi/content/full/108/3/e57

5. Jadad AR, Moore RA, Carroll D, et al. Assessing the quality of reports of randomized clinical trials: is blinding necessary? *Control Clin Trials*. 1996;17(1):1–12

6. Wald ER, Nash D, Eickhoff J. Effectiveness of amoxicillin/clavulanate potassium in the treatment of acute bacterial sinusitis in children. *Pediatrics*. 2009;124(1):9–15

7. Wald ER, Chiponis D, Ledesmamedina J. Comparative effectiveness of amoxicillin and amoxicillin-clavulanate potassium in acute para-nasal sinus infections in children: a double-blind, placebo-controlled trial. *Pediatrics*. 1986;77(6):795–800

8. Garbutt JM, Goldstein M, Gellman E, Shannon W, Littenberg B. A randomized, placebo-

controlled trial of antimicrobial treatment for children with clinically diagnosed acute sinusitis. *Pediatrics*. 2001;107(4):619–625

9. Kristo A, Uhari M, Luotonen J, Ilkko E, Koivunen P, Alho OP. Cefuroxime axetil versus placebo for children with acute respiratory infection and imaging evidence of sinusitis: a randomized, controlled trial. *Acta Paediatr*. 2005;94(9):1208–1213

10. Jeppesen F, Illum P. Pivampicillin (Pondocillin) in treatment of maxillary sinusitis. *Acta Otolaryngol*. 1972;74(5):375–382

11. Garbutt JM, Gellman EF, Littenberg B. The development and validation of an instrument to assess acute sinus disease in children. *Qual Life Res*. 1999;8(3):225–233

12. Poachanukoon O, Kitcharoensakkul M. Efficacy of cefditoren pivoxil and amoxicillin/clavulanate in the treatment of pediatric patients with acute bacterial rhinosinusitis in Thailand: a randomized, investigator-blinded, controlled trial. *Clin Ther*. 2008;30 (10):1870–1879

13. Simon MW. Treatment of acute sinusitis in childhood with ceftibuten. *Clin Pediatr (Phila)*. 1999;38(5):269–272

14. Ficnar B, Huzjak N, Oreskovic K, Matrapazovski M, Klinar I. Azithromycin: 3-day versus 5-day course in the treatment of respiratory tract infections in children. *J Chemother*. 1997;9(1):38–43

15. Careddu P, Bellosta C, Tonelli P, Boccazzi A. Efficacy and tolerability of brodimoprim in pediatric infections. *J Chemother*. 1993;5 (6):543–545

16. Wald ER, Reilly JS, Casselbrant M, et al. Treatment of acute maxillary sinusitis in childhood: a comparative study of amoxicillin and cefaclor. *J Pediatr*. 1984;104(2):297–302

17. Barlan IB, Erkan E, Bakir M, Berrak S, Basaran MM. Intranasal budesonide spray as an adjunct to oral antibiotic therapy for acute sinusitis in children. *Ann Allergy Asthma Immunol*. 1997;78(6):598–601

18. Yilmaz G, Varan B, Yilmaz T, Gurakan B. Intranasal budesonide spray as an adjunct to oral antibiotic therapy for acute sinusitis in children. *Eur Arch Otorhinolaryngol*. 2000; 257(5):256–259

19. McCormick DP, John SD, Swischuk LE, Uchida T. A double-blind, placebo-controlled trial of decongestant-antihistamine for the treatment of sinusitis in children. *Clin Pediatr (Phila)*. 1996;35(9):457–460

20. Michel O, Essers S, Heppt WJ, Johannssen V, Reuter W, Hommel G. The value of Ems mineral salts in the treatment of rhinosinusitis in children: prospective study on the efficacy of mineral salts versus xylometazoline in the topical nasal treatment of children. *Int J Pediatr Otorhinolaryngol*. 2005;69(10):1359–1365

21. Wang YH, Yang CP, Ku MS, Sun HL, Lue KH. Efficacy of nasal irrigation in the treatment of acute sinusitis in children. *Int J Pediatr Otorhinolaryngol*. 2009;73:1696–1701

22. Unuvar E, Tamay Z, Yildiz I, et al. Effectiveness of erdosteine, a second generation mucolytic agent, in children with acute rhinosinusitis: a randomized, placebo

controlled, double-blinded clinical study. *Acta Paediatr.* 2010;99(4):585–589

23. McQuillan L, Crane LA, Kempe A. Diagnosis and management of acute sinusitis by pediatricians. *Pediatrics.* 2009;123(2). Available at: www.pediatrics.org/cgi/content/full/123/2/e193

24. Revonta M, Suonpaa J. Diagnosis and follow-up of ultrasonographical sinus changes in children. *Int J Pediatr Otorhinolaryngol.* 1982;4(4):301–308

25. El-Hennawi DM, Abou-Halawa AS, Zaher SR. Management of clinically diagnosed subacute rhinosinusitis in children under the age of two years: a randomized, controlled study. *J Laryngol Otol.* 2006;120(10):845–848

26. Ng DK, Chow PY, Leung LC, Chau KW, Chan E, Ho JC. A randomized controlled trial of azithromycin and amoxycillin/clavulanate in the management of subacute childhood rhinosinusitis. *J Paediatr Child Health.* 2000;36(4):378–381

27. Dohlman AW, Hemstreet MPB, Odrezin GT, Bartolucci AA. Subacute sinusitis: are antimicrobials necessary? *J Allergy Clin Immunol.* 1993;91(5):1015–1023

28. Wald ER, Byers C, Guerra N, Casselbrant M, Beste D. Subacute sinusitis in children. *J Pediatr.* 1989;115(1):28–32

29. The diagnosis and management of sinusitis in children: proceedings of a closed conference. *Pediatr Infect Dis.* 1985;4(suppl 6):S49–S81

30. Brook I, Foote PA, Hausfeld JN. Frequency of recovery of pathogens causing acute maxillary sinusitis in adults before and after introduction of vaccination of children with the 7-valent pneumococcal vaccine. *J Med Microbiol.* 2006;55(7):943–946

31. Brook I, Gober AE. Frequency of recovery of pathogens from the nasopharynx of children with acute maxillary sinusitis before and after the introduction of vaccination with the 7-valent pneumococcal vaccine. *Int J Pediatr Otorhinolaryngol.* 2007;71(4):575–579

32. Gandhi A, Brodsky L, Ballow M. Benefits of antibiotic-prophylaxis in children with chronic sinusitis: assessment of outcome predictors. *Allergy Proc.* 1993;14(1):37–43

33. Kristo A, Uhari M. Timing of rhinosinusitis complications in children. *Pediatr Infect Dis J.* 2009;28(9):769–771

34. Cotter CS, Stringer S, Rust KR, Mancuso A. The role of computed tomography scans in evaluating sinus disease in pediatric patients. *Int J Pediatr Otorhinolaryngol.* 1999;50(1):63–68

35. Schwartz RH, Pitkaranta A, Winther B. Computed tomography imaging of the maxillary and ethmoid sinuses in children with short-duration purulent rhinorrhea. *Otolaryngol Head Neck Surg.* 2001;124(2):160–163

36. Kristo A, Uhari M, Luotonen J, et al. Paranasal sinus findings in children during respiratory infection evaluated with magnetic resonance imaging. *Pediatrics.* 2003;111(5). Available at: www.pediatrics.org/cgi/content/full/111/5/e586

37. Kristo A, Alho OP, Luotonen J, Koivunen P, Tervonen O, Uhari M. Cross-sectional survey of paranasal sinus magnetic resonance imaging findings in schoolchildren. *Acta Paediatr.* 2003;92(1):34–36

38. Lim WK, Ram B, Fasulakis S, Kane KJ. Incidental magnetic resonance image sinus abnormalities in asymptomatic Australian children. *J Laryngol Otol.* 2003;117(12):969–972

39. Anon JB, Jacobs MR, Roche R, et al. Antimicrobial treatment guidelines for acute bacterial rhinosinusitis: executive summary. *Otolaryngol Head Neck Surg.* 2004;130(1):1–45

40. Acute Bacterial Sinusitis Guideline Team, Cincinnati Children's Hospital Medical Center. Evidence-based care guideline for medical management of acute bacterial sinusitis in children 1 through 17 years of age. Available at: www.cincinnatichildrens.org/svc/alpha/h/health-policy/ev-based/sinus.htm. Accessed November 6, 2012

41. Fokkens W, Lund V, Mullol J. European position paper on rhinosinusitis and nasal polyps 2007. *Rhinol Suppl.* 2007; (20):1–136

42. Esposito S, Principi N. Guidelines for the diagnosis and treatment of acute and subacute rhinosinusitis in children. *J Chemother.* 2008;20(2):147–157

43. American College of Radiology. Appropriateness criteria for sinonasal disease. Available at: www.acr.org/~/media/8172B4DE503149248E64856857674BB5.pdf. Accessed November 6, 2012

44. Morris P, Leach A. Antibiotics for persistent nasal discharge (rhinosinusitis) in children. *Cochrane Database Syst Rev.* 2002; (4):CD001094

45. Falagas ME, Giannopoulou KP, Vardakas KZ, Dimopoulos G, Karageorgopoulos DE. Comparison of antibiotics with placebo for treatment of acute sinusitis: a meta-analysis of randomised controlled trials. *Lancet Infect Dis.* 2008;8(9):543–552

Sinusitis Clinical Practice Guideline Quick Reference Tools

- Action Statement Summary
  — Clinical Practice Guideline for the Diagnosis and Management of Acute Bacterial Sinusitis in Children Aged 1 to 18 Years
- *ICD-9-CM/ICD-10-CM* Coding Quick Reference for Sinusitis
- AAP Patient Education Handout
  — *Sinusitis and Your Child*

Action Statement Summary

Clinical Practice Guideline for the Diagnosis and Management of Acute Bacterial Sinusitis in Children Aged 1 to 18 Years

Key Action Statement 1

Clinicians should make a presumptive diagnosis of acute bacterial sinusitis when a child with an acute URI presents with the following:

- Persistent illness, ie, nasal discharge (of any quality) or daytime cough or both lasting more than 10 days without improvement;

OR

- Worsening course, ie, worsening or new onset of nasal discharge, daytime cough, or fever after initial improvement;

OR

- Severe onset, ie, concurrent fever (temperature ≥39°C/102.2°F) and purulent nasal discharge for at least 3 consecutive days (Evidence Quality: B; Recommendation).

Key Action Statement 2A

Clinicians should not obtain imaging studies (plain films, contrast-enhanced computed tomography [CT], MRI, or ultrasonography) to distinguish acute bacterial sinusitis from viral URI (Evidence Quality: B; Strong Recommendation).

Key Action Statement 2B

Clinicians should obtain a contrast-enhanced CT scan of the paranasal sinuses and/or an MRI with contrast whenever a child is suspected of having orbital or central nervous system complications of acute bacterial sinusitis (Evidence Quality: B; Strong Recommendation).

Key Action Statement 3

Initial Management of Acute Bacterial Sinusitis

3A: "Severe onset and worsening course" acute bacterial sinusitis. The clinician should prescribe antibiotic therapy for acute bacterial sinusitis in children with severe onset or worsening course (signs, symptoms, or both) (Evidence Quality: B; Strong Recommendation).

3B: "Persistent illness." The clinician should either prescribe antibiotic therapy OR offer additional outpatient observation for 3 days to children with persistent illness (nasal discharge of any quality or cough or both for at least 10 days without evidence of improvement) (Evidence Quality: B; Recommendation).

Key Action Statement 4

Clinicians should prescribe amoxicillin with or without clavulanate as first-line treatment when a decision has been made to initiate antibiotic treatment of acute bacterial sinusitis (Evidence Quality: B; Recommendation).

Key Action Statement 5A

Clinicians should reassess initial management if there is either a caregiver report of worsening (progression of initial signs/symptoms or appearance of new signs/symptoms) OR failure to improve (lack of reduction in all presenting signs/symptoms) within 72 hours of initial management (Evidence Quality: C; Recommendation).

Key Action Statement 5B

If the diagnosis of acute bacterial sinusitis is confirmed in a child with worsening symptoms or failure to improve in 72 hours, then clinicians may change the antibiotic therapy for the child initially managed with antibiotic OR initiate antibiotic treatment of the child initially managed with observation (Evidence Quality: D; Option based on expert opinion, case reports, and reasoning from first principles).

Coding Quick Reference for Sinusitis	
ICD-9-CM	*ICD-10-CM*
461.9 Sinusitis, acute, unspecified	**J01.90** Acute sinusitis, unspecified **J01.91** Acute recurrent sinusitis, unspecified

Sinusitis and Your Child

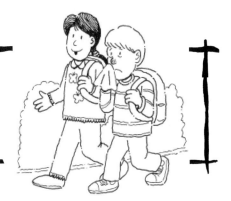

Sinusitis is an inflammation of the lining of the nose and sinuses. It is a very common infection in children.

Viral sinusitis usually accompanies a cold. Allergic sinusitis may accompany allergies such as hay fever. Bacterial sinusitis is a secondary infection caused by the trapping of bacteria in the sinuses during the course of a cold or allergy.

Fluid inside the sinuses

When your child has a viral cold or hay fever, the linings of the nose and sinus cavities swell up and produce more fluid than usual. This is why the nose gets congested and is "runny" during a cold.

Most of the time the swelling disappears by itself as the cold or allergy goes away. However, if the swelling does not go away, the openings that normally allow the sinuses to drain into the back of the nose get blocked and the sinuses fill with fluid. Because the sinuses are blocked and cannot drain properly, bacteria are trapped inside and grow there, causing a secondary infection. Although nose blowing and sniffing may be natural responses to this blockage, when excessive they can make the situation worse by pushing bacteria from the back of the nose into the sinuses.

Is it a cold or bacterial sinusitis?

It is often difficult to tell if an illness is just a viral cold or if it is complicated by a bacterial infection of the sinuses.

Generally viral colds have the following characteristics:

- Colds usually last only 5 to 10 days.
- Colds typically start with clear, watery nasal discharge. After a day or 2, it is normal for the nasal discharge to become thicker and white, yellow, or green. After several days, the discharge becomes clear again and dries.
- Colds include a daytime cough that often gets worse at night.
- If a fever is present, it is usually at the beginning of the cold and is generally low grade, lasting for 1 or 2 days.
- Cold symptoms usually peak in severity at 3 or 5 days, then improve and disappear over the next 7 to 10 days.

Signs and symptoms that your child may have bacterial sinusitis include:

- Cold symptoms (nasal discharge, daytime cough, or both) lasting more than 10 days *without improving*
- Thick yellow nasal discharge *and* a fever for at least 3 or 4 days in a row
- A severe headache behind or around the eyes that gets worse when bending over
- Swelling and dark circles around the eyes, especially in the morning
- Persistent bad breath along with cold symptoms (However, this also could be from a sore throat or a sign that your child is not brushing his teeth!)

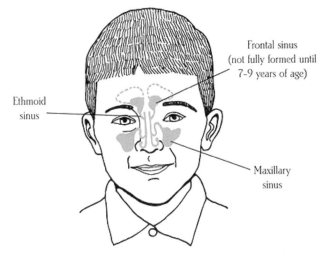

The linings of the sinuses and the nose always produce some fluid (secretions). This fluid keeps the nose and sinus cavities from becoming too dry and adds moisture to the air that you breathe.

In very rare cases, a bacterial sinus infection may spread to the eye or the central nervous system (the brain). If your child has the following symptoms, call your pediatrician immediately:

- Swelling and/or redness around the eyes, not just in the morning but all day
- Severe headache and/or pain in the back of the neck
- Persistent vomiting
- Sensitivity to light
- Increasing irritability

Diagnosing bacterial sinusitis

It may be difficult to tell a sinus infection from an uncomplicated cold, especially in the first few days of the illness. Your pediatrician will most likely be able to tell if your child has bacterial sinusitis after examining your child and hearing about the progression of symptoms. In older children, when the diagnosis is uncertain, your pediatrician may order computed tomographic (CT) scans to confirm the diagnosis.

Treating bacterial sinusitis

If your child has bacterial sinusitis, your pediatrician may prescribe an antibiotic for at least 10 days. Once your child is on the medication, symptoms should start to go away over the next 2 to 3 days—the nasal discharge will clear and the cough will improve. *Even though your child may seem better, continue to give the antibiotics for the prescribed length of time. Ending the medications too early could cause the infection to return.*

When a diagnosis of sinusitis is made in children with cold symptoms lasting more than 10 days without improving, some doctors may choose to continue observation for another few days. If your child's symptoms worsen during this time or do not improve after 3 days, antibiotics should be started.

If your child's symptoms show no improvement 2 to 3 days after starting the antibiotics, talk with your pediatrician. Your child might need a different medication or need to be re-examined.

Treating related symptoms of bacterial sinusitis

Headache or sinus pain. To treat headache or sinus pain, try placing a warm washcloth on your child's face for a few minutes at a time. Pain medications such as acetaminophen or ibuprofen may also help. (However, do not give your child aspirin. It has been associated with a rare but potentially fatal disease called Reye syndrome.)

Nasal congestion. If the secretions in your child's nose are especially thick, your pediatrician may recommend that you help drain them with saline nose drops. These are available without a prescription or can be made at home by adding 1⁄4 teaspoon of table salt to an 8-ounce cup of water. Unless advised by your pediatrician, do not use nose drops that contain medications because they can be absorbed in amounts that can cause side effects.

Placing a cool-mist humidifier in your child's room may help keep your child more comfortable. Clean and dry the humidifier daily to prevent bacteria or mold from growing in it (follow the instructions that came with the humidifier). Hot water vaporizers are not recommended because they can cause scalds or burns.

Remember

If your child has symptoms of a bacterial sinus infection, see your pediatrician. Your pediatrician can properly diagnose and treat the infection and recommend ways to help alleviate the discomfort from some of the symptoms.

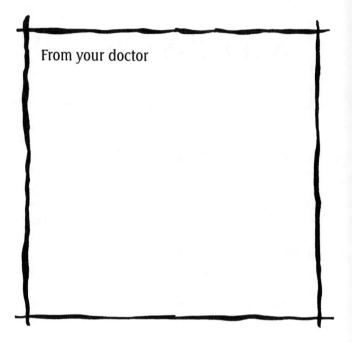

From your doctor

American Academy of Pediatrics

DEDICATED TO THE HEALTH OF ALL CHILDREN™

The American Academy of Pediatrics is an organization of 60,000 primary care pediatricians, pediatric medical subspecialists, and pediatric surgical specialists dedicated to the health, safety, and well-being of infants, children, adolescents, and young adults.

American Academy of Pediatrics
Web site — www.HealthyChildren.org

Diagnosis and Management of Childhood Obstructive Sleep Apnea Syndrome

- *Clinical Practice Guideline*
- *Technical Report*
  - *PPI: AAP Partnership for Policy Implementation*
    See Appendix 2 for more information.

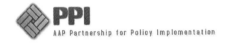

Readers of this clinical practice guideline are urged to review the technical report to enhance the evidence-based decision-making process. The full technical report is available following the clinical practice guideline and on the companion CD-ROM.

CLINICAL PRACTICE GUIDELINE

Diagnosis and Management of Childhood Obstructive Sleep Apnea Syndrome

abstract

OBJECTIVES: This revised clinical practice guideline, intended for use by primary care clinicians, provides recommendations for the diagnosis and management of the obstructive sleep apnea syndrome (OSAS) in children and adolescents. This practice guideline focuses on uncomplicated childhood OSAS, that is, OSAS associated with adenotonsillar hypertrophy and/or obesity in an otherwise healthy child who is being treated in the primary care setting.

METHODS: Of 3166 articles from 1999–2010, 350 provided relevant data. Most articles were level II–IV. The resulting evidence report was used to formulate recommendations.

RESULTS AND CONCLUSIONS: The following recommendations are made. (1) All children/adolescents should be screened for snoring. (2) Polysomnography should be performed in children/adolescents with snoring and symptoms/signs of OSAS; if polysomnography is not available, then alternative diagnostic tests or referral to a specialist for more extensive evaluation may be considered. (3) Adenotonsillectomy is recommended as the first-line treatment of patients with adenotonsillar hypertrophy. (4) High-risk patients should be monitored as inpatients postoperatively. (5) Patients should be reevaluated postoperatively to determine whether further treatment is required. Objective testing should be performed in patients who are high risk or have persistent symptoms/signs of OSAS after therapy. (6) Continuous positive airway pressure is recommended as treatment if adenotonsillectomy is not performed or if OSAS persists postoperatively. (7) Weight loss is recommended in addition to other therapy in patients who are overweight or obese. (8) Intranasal corticosteroids are an option for children with mild OSAS in whom adenotonsillectomy is contraindicated or for mild postoperative OSAS. *Pediatrics* 2012;130:576–584

Carole L. Marcus, MBBCh, Lee Jay Brooks, MD, Kari A. Draper, MD, David Gozal, MD, Ann Carol Halbower, MD, Jacqueline Jones, MD, Michael S. Schechter, MD, MPH, Stephen Howard Sheldon, DO, Karen Spruyt, PhD, Sally Davidson Ward, MD, Christopher Lehmann, MD, Richard N. Shiffman, MD

KEY WORDS
snoring, sleep-disordered breathing, adenotonsillectomy, continuous positive airway pressure

ABBREVIATIONS
AAP—American Academy of Pediatrics
AHI—apnea hypopnea index
CPAP—continuous positive airway pressure
OSAS—obstructive sleep apnea syndrome

This document is copyrighted and is property of the American Academy of Pediatrics and its Board of Directors. All authors have filed conflict of interest statements with the American Academy of Pediatrics. Any conflicts have been resolved through a process approved by the Board of Directors. The American Academy of Pediatrics has neither solicited nor accepted any commercial involvement in the development of the content of this publication.

The recommendations in this report do not indicate an exclusive course of treatment or serve as a standard of medical care. Variations, taking into account individual circumstances, may be appropriate.

All clinical practice guidelines from the American Academy of Pediatrics automatically expire 5 years after publication unless reaffirmed, revised, or retired at or before that time.

www.pediatrics.org/cgi/doi/10.1542/peds.2012-1671

doi:10.1542/peds.2012-1671

PEDIATRICS (ISSN Numbers: Print, 0031-4005; Online, 1098-4275).

INTRODUCTION

Obstructive sleep apnea syndrome (OSAS) is a common condition in childhood and can result in severe complications if left untreated. In 2002, the American Academy of Pediatrics (AAP) published a practice guideline for the diagnosis and management of childhood OSAS.[1] Since that time, there has been a considerable increase in publications and research on the topic; thus, the guidelines have been revised.

The purposes of this revised clinical practice guideline are to (1) increase the recognition of OSAS by primary care clinicians to minimize delay in diagnosis and avoid serious sequelae of OSAS; (2) evaluate diagnostic techniques; (3) describe treatment options; (4) provide guidelines for follow-up; and (5) discuss areas requiring further research. The recommendations in this statement do not indicate an exclusive course of treatment. Variations, taking into account individual circumstances, may be appropriate.

This practice guideline focuses on uncomplicated childhood OSAS—that is, the OSAS associated with adenotonsillar hypertrophy and/or obesity in an otherwise healthy child who is being treated in the primary care setting. This guideline specifically excludes infants younger than 1 year of age, patients with central apnea or hypoventilation syndromes, and patients with OSAS associated with other medical disorders, including but not limited to Down syndrome, craniofacial anomalies, neuromuscular disease (including cerebral palsy), chronic lung disease, sickle cell disease, metabolic disease, or laryngomalacia. These important patient populations are too complex to discuss within the scope of this article and require consultation with a pediatric subspecialist.

Additional information providing justification for the key action statements and a detailed review of the literature are provided in the accompanying technical report available online.[2]

METHODS OF GUIDELINE DEVELOPMENT

Details of the methods of guideline development are included in the accompanying technical report.[2] The AAP selected a subcommittee composed of pediatricians and other experts in the fields of sleep medicine, pulmonology, and otolaryngology, as well as experts from epidemiology and pediatric practice to develop an evidence base of literature on this topic. The committee included liaison members from the AAP Section on Otolaryngology-Head and Neck Surgery, American Thoracic Society, American Academy of Sleep Medicine, American College of Chest Physicians, and the National Sleep Foundation. Committee members signed forms disclosing conflicts of interest.

An automated search of the literature on childhood OSAS from 1999 to 2008 was performed by using 5 scientific literature search engines.[2] The medical subject heading terms that were used in all fields were snoring, apnea, sleep-disordered breathing, sleep-related breathing disorders, upper airway resistance, polysomnography, sleep study, adenoidectomy, tonsillectomy, continuous positive airway pressure, obesity, adiposity, hypopnea, hypoventilation, cognition, behavior, and neuropsychology. Reviews, case reports, letters to the editor, and abstracts were not included. Non–English-language articles, animal studies, and studies relating to infants younger than 1 year and to special populations (eg, children with craniofacial anomalies or sickle cell disease) were excluded. In several steps, a total of 3166 hits was reduced to 350 articles, which underwent detailed review.[2] Committee members selectively updated this literature search for articles published from 2008 to 2011 specific to guideline categories. Details of the literature grading system are available in the accompanying technical report.

Since publication of the previous guidelines, there has been an improvement in the quality of OSAS studies in the literature; however, there remain few randomized, blinded, controlled studies. Most studies were questionnaire or polysomnography based. Many studies used standard definitions for pediatric polysomnography scoring, but the interpretation of polysomnography (eg, the apnea hypopnea index [AHI] criterion used for diagnosis or to determine treatment) varied widely. The guideline notes the quality of evidence for each key action statement. Additional details are available in the technical report.

The evidence-based approach to guideline development requires that the evidence in support of each key action statement be identified, appraised, and summarized and that an explicit link between evidence and recommendations be defined. Evidence-based recommendations reflect the quality of evidence and the balance of benefit and harm that is anticipated when the recommendation is followed. The AAP policy statement, "Classifying Recommendations for Clinical Practice Guidelines,"[3] was followed in designating levels of recommendation (see Fig 1 and Table 1).

DEFINITION

This guideline defines OSAS in children as a "disorder of breathing during sleep characterized by prolonged partial upper airway obstruction and/or intermittent complete obstruction (obstructive apnea) that disrupts normal ventilation during sleep and normal sleep patterns,"[4] accompanied by symptoms or signs, as listed in Table 2. Prevalence rates based on level I and II studies range from 1.2% to 5.7%.[5–7] Symptoms include habitual snoring (often with intermittent pauses, snorts, or gasps), disturbed sleep, and daytime neurobehavioral problems. Daytime sleepiness may occur, but is uncommon in young children. OSAS is associated with neurocognitive impairment, behavioral problems, failure to thrive, hypertension, cardiac dysfunction, and systemic inflammation. Risk factors include adenotonsillar hypertrophy, obesity, craniofacial anomalies, and neuromuscular disorders. Only the first 2 risk factors are

Evidence Quality	Preponderance of Benefit or Harm	Balance of Benefit and Harm
A. Well designed RCTs or diagnostic studies on relevant population	Strong Recommendation	
B. RCTs or diagnostic studies with minor limitations;overwhelmingly consistent evidence from observational studies	Recommendation	Option
C. Observational studies (case-control and cohort design)		
D. Expert opinion, case reports, reasoning from first principles	Option	No Rec
X. Exceptional situations where validating studies cannot be performed and there is a clear preponderance of benefit or harm	Strong Recommendation / Recommendation	

FIGURE 1
Evidence quality. Integrating evidence quality appraisal with an assessment of the anticipated balance between benefits and harms if a policy is carried out leads to designation of a policy as a strong recommendation, recommendation, option, or no recommendation. RCT, randomized controlled trial; Rec, recommendation.

discussed in this guideline. In this guideline, obesity is defined as a BMI >95th percentile for age and gender.[8]

KEY ACTION STATEMENTS

Key Action Statement 1: Screening for OSAS

As part of routine health maintenance visits, clinicians should inquire whether the child or adolescent snores. If the answer is affirmative or if a child or adolescent presents with signs or symptoms of OSAS (Table 2), clinicians should perform a more focused evaluation. (Evidence Quality: Grade B, Recommendation Strength: Recommendation.)

Evidence Profile KAS 1

- Aggregate evidence quality: B

- Benefit: Early identification of OSAS is desirable, because it is a high-prevalence condition, and identification and treatment can result in alleviation of current symptoms, improved quality of life, prevention of sequelae, education of parents, and decreased health care utilization.

- Harm: Provider time, patient and parent time.

- Benefits-harms assessment: Preponderance of benefit over harm.

- Value judgments: Panelists believe that identification of a serious medical condition outweighs the time expenditure necessary for screening.

- Role of patient preferences: None.

- Exclusions: None.

- Intentional vagueness: None.

- Strength: Recommendation.

Almost all children with OSAS snore,[9–11] although caregivers frequently do not volunteer this information at medical visits.[12] Thus, asking about snoring at each health maintenance visit (as well as at other appropriate times, such as when evaluating for tonsillitis) is a sensitive, albeit nonspecific, screening measure that is quick and easy to perform. Snoring is common in children and adolescents; however, OSAS is less common. Therefore, an affirmative answer should be followed by a detailed history and examination to determine whether further evaluation for OSAS is needed (Table 2); this clinical evaluation alone

TABLE 1 Definitions and Recommendation Implications

Statement	Definition	Implication
Strong recommendation	A strong recommendation in favor of a particular action is made when the anticipated benefits of the recommended intervention clearly exceed the harms (as a strong recommendation against an action is made when the anticipated harms clearly exceed the benefits) and the quality of the supporting evidence is excellent. In some clearly identified circumstances, strong recommendations may be made when high-quality evidence is impossible to obtain and the anticipated benefits strongly outweigh the harms.	Clinicians should follow a strong recommendation unless a clear and compelling rationale for an alternative approach is present.
Recommendation	A recommendation in favor of a particular action is made when the anticipated benefits exceed the harms but the quality of evidence is not as strong. Again, in some clearly identified circumstances, recommendations may be made when high-quality evidence is impossible to obtain but the anticipated benefits outweigh the harms.	It would be prudent for clinicians to follow a recommendation, but they should remain alert to new information and sensitive to patient preferences.
Option	Options define courses that may be taken when either the quality of evidence is suspect or carefully performed studies have shown little clear advantage to one approach over another.	Clinicians should consider the option in their decision-making, and patient preference may have a substantial role.
No recommendation	No recommendation indicates that there is a lack of pertinent published evidence and that the anticipated balance of benefits and harms is presently unclear.	Clinicians should be alert to new published evidence that clarifies the balance of benefit versus harm.

TABLE 2 Symptoms and Signs of OSAS

History
  Frequent snoring (≥3 nights/wk)
  Labored breathing during sleep
  Gasps/snorting noises/observed
    episodes of apnea
  Sleep enuresis (especially secondary enuresis)[a]
  Sleeping in a seated position or with the neck
    hyperextended
  Cyanosis
  Headaches on awakening
  Daytime sleepiness
  Attention-deficit/hyperactivity disorder
  Learning problems
Physical examination
  Underweight or overweight
  Tonsillar hypertrophy
  Adenoidal facies
  Micrognathia/retrognathia
  High-arched palate
  Failure to thrive
  Hypertension

[a] Enuresis after at least 6 mo of continence.

does not establish the diagnosis (see technical report). Occasional snoring, for example, with an upper respiratory tract infection, is less of a concern than snoring that occurs at least 3 times a week and is associated with any of the symptoms or signs listed in Table 2.

Key Action Statement 2A: Polysomnography

If a child or adolescent snores on a regular basis and has any of the complaints or findings shown in Table 2, clinicians should either (1) obtain a polysomnogram (Evidence Quality A, Key Action strength: Recommendation) OR (2) refer the patient to a sleep specialist or otolaryngologist for a more extensive evaluation (Evidence quality D, Key Action strength: Option). (Evidence Quality: Grade A for polysomnography; Grade D for specialist referral, Recommendation Strength: Recommendation.)

Evidence Profile KAS 2A: Polysomnography

- Aggregate evidence quality: A
- Benefits: Establish diagnosis and determine severity of OSAS.

- Harm: Expense, time, anxiety/discomfort.
- Benefits-harms assessment: Preponderance of benefit over harm.
- Value judgments: Panelists weighed the value of establishing a diagnosis as more important than the minor potential harms listed.
- Role of patient preferences: Small because of preponderance of evidence that polysomnography is the most accurate way to make a diagnosis.
- Exclusions: See Key Action Statement 2B regarding lack of availability.
- Intentional vagueness: None.
- Strength: Recommendation.

Evidence Profile KAS 2A: Referral

- Aggregate evidence quality: D
- Benefits: Subspecialist may be better able to establish diagnosis and determine severity of OSAS.
- Harm: Expense, time, anxiety/discomfort.
- Benefits-harms assessment: Preponderance of benefit over harm.
- Value judgments: Panelists weighed the value of establishing a diagnosis as more important than the minor potential harms listed.
- Role of patient preferences: Large.
- Exclusions: None.
- Intentional vagueness: None.
- Strength: Option.

Although history and physical examination are useful to screen patients and determine which patients need further investigation for OSAS, the sensitivity and specificity of the history and physical examination are poor (see accompanying technical report). Physical examination when the child is awake may be normal, and the size of the tonsils cannot be used to predict the presence of OSAS in an individual child. Thus, objective testing is required. The gold standard test

is overnight, attended, in-laboratory polysomnography (sleep study). This is a noninvasive test involving the measurement of a number of physiologic functions overnight, typically including EEG; pulse oximetry; oronasal airflow, abdominal and chest wall movements, partial pressure of carbon dioxide (P_{CO_2}); and video recording.[13] Specific pediatric measuring and scoring criteria should be used.[13] Polysomnography will demonstrate the presence or absence of OSAS. Polysomnography also demonstrates the severity of OSAS, which is helpful in planning treatment and in postoperative short- and long-term management.

Key Action Statement 2B: Alternative Testing

If polysomnography is not available, then clinicians may order alternative diagnostic tests, such as nocturnal video recording, nocturnal oximetry, daytime nap polysomnography, or ambulatory polysomnography. (Evidence Quality: Grade C, Recommendation Strength: Option.)

Evidence Profile KAS 2B

- Aggregate evidence quality: C
- Benefit: Varying positive and negative predictive values for establishing diagnosis.
- Harm: False-negative and false-positive results may underestimate or overestimate severity, expense, time, anxiety/discomfort.
- Benefits-harms assessment: Equilibrium of benefits and harms.
- Value judgments: Opinion of the panel that some objective testing is better than none. Pragmatic decision based on current shortage of pediatric polysomnography facilities (this may change over time).
- Role of patient preferences: Small, if choices are limited by availability;

families may choose to travel to centers where more extensive facilities are available.

- Exclusions: None.
- Intentional vagueness: None.
- Strength: Option.

Although polysomnography is the gold standard for diagnosis of OSAS, there is a shortage of sleep laboratories with pediatric expertise. Hence, polysomnography may not be readily available in certain regions of the country. Alternative diagnostic tests have been shown to have weaker positive and negative predictive values than polysomnography, but nevertheless, objective testing is preferable to clinical evaluation alone. If an alternative test fails to demonstrate OSAS in a patient with a high pretest probability, full polysomnography should be sought.

Key Action Statement 3: Adenotonsillectomy

If a child is determined to have OSAS, has a clinical examination consistent with adenotonsillar hypertrophy, and does not have a contraindication to surgery (see Table 3), the clinician should recommend adenotonsillectomy as the first line of treatment. If the child has OSAS but does not have adenotonsillar hypertrophy, other treatment should be considered (see Key Action Statement 6). Clinical judgment is required to determine the benefits of adenotonsillectomy compared with other treatments in obese children with varying degrees of adenotonsillar hypertrophy. (Evidence Quality: Grade B, Recommendation Strength: Recommendation.)

Evidence Profile KAS 3

- Aggregate evidence quality: B
- Benefit: Improve OSAS and accompanying symptoms and sequelae.

- Harm: Pain, anxiety, dehydration, anesthetic complications, hemorrhage, infection, postoperative respiratory difficulties, velopharyngeal incompetence, nasopharyngeal stenosis, death.
- Benefits-harms assessment: Preponderance of benefit over harm.
- Value judgments: The panel sees the benefits of treating OSAS as more beneficial than the low risk of serious consequences.
- Role of patient preferences: Low; continuous positive airway pressure (CPAP) is an option but involves prolonged, long-term treatment as compared with a single, relatively low-risk surgical procedure.
- Exclusions: See Table 3.
- Intentional vagueness: None.
- Strength: Recommendation.

Adenotonsillectomy is very effective in treating OSAS. Adenoidectomy or tonsillectomy alone may not be sufficient, because residual lymphoid tissue may contribute to persistent obstruction. In otherwise healthy children with adenotonsillar hypertrophy, adenotonsillectomy is associated with improvements in symptoms and sequelae of OSAS. Postoperative polysomnography typically shows a major decrease in the number of obstructive events, although some obstructions may still be present. Although obese children may have less satisfactory results, many will be adequately treated with

adenotonsillectomy; however, further research is needed to determine which obese children are most likely to benefit from surgery. In this population, the benefits of a 1-time surgical procedure, with a small but real risk of complications, need to be weighed against long-term treatment with CPAP, which is associated with discomfort, disruption of family lifestyle, and risks of poor adherence. Potential complications of adenotonsillectomy are shown in Table 4. Although serious complications (including death) may occur, the rate of these complications is low, and the risks of complications need to be weighed against the consequences of untreated OSAS. In general, a 1-time only procedure with a relatively low morbidity is preferable to lifelong treatment with CPAP; furthermore, the efficacy of CPAP is limited by generally suboptimal adherence. Other treatment options, such as anti-inflammatory medications, weight loss, or tracheostomy, are less effective, are difficult to achieve, or have higher morbidity, respectively.

Key Action Statement 4: High-Risk Patients Undergoing Adenotonsillectomy

Clinicians should monitor high-risk patients (Table 5) undergoing adenotonsillectomy as inpatients postoperatively. (Evidence Quality: Grade B, Recommendation Strength: Recommendation.)

TABLE 3 Contraindications for Adenotonsillectomy

Absolute contraindications
No adenotonsillar tissue (tissue has been surgically removed)
Relative contraindications
Very small tonsils/adenoid
Morbid obesity and small tonsils/adenoid
Bleeding disorder refractory to treatment
Submucus cleft palate
Other medical conditions making patient medically unstable for surgery

TABLE 4 Risks of Adenotonsillectomy

Minor
Pain
Dehydration attributable to postoperative nausea/vomiting and poor oral intake
Major
Anesthetic complications
Acute upper airway obstruction during induction or emergence from anesthesia
Postoperative respiratory compromise
Hemorrhage
Velopharyngeal incompetence
Nasopharyngeal stenosis
Death

TABLE 5 Risk Factors for Postoperative Respiratory Complications in Children With OSAS Undergoing Adenotonsillectomy

Younger than 3 y of age
Severe OSAS on polysomnography[a]
Cardiac complications of OSAS
Failure to thrive
Obesity
Craniofacial anomalies[b]
Neuromuscular disorders[b]
Current respiratory infection

[a] It is difficult to provide exact polysomnographic criteria for severity, because these criteria will vary depending on the age of the child; additional comorbidities, such as obesity, asthma, or cardiac complications of OSAS; and other polysomnographic criteria that have not been evaluated in the literature, such as the level of hypercapnia and the frequency of desaturation (as compared with lowest oxygen saturation). Nevertheless, on the basis of published studies (primarily Level III, see Technical Report), it is recommended that all patients with a lowest oxygen saturation <80% (either on preoperative polysomnography or during observation in the recovery room postoperatively) or an AHI ≥24/h be observed as inpatients postoperatively as they are at increased risk for postoperative respiratory compromise. Additionally, on the basis of expert consensus, it is recommended that patients with significant hypercapnia on polysomnography (peak P_{CO_2} ≥60 mm Hg) be admitted postoperatively. The committee noted that most published studies were retrospective and not comprehensive, and therefore these recommendations may change if higher-level studies are published. Clinicians may decide to admit patients with less severe polysomnographic abnormalities based on a constellation of risk factors (age, comorbidities, and additional polysomnographic factors) for a particular individual.
[b] Not discussed in these guidelines.

Evidence Profile KAS 4

- Aggregate evidence quality: B
- Benefit: Effectively manage severe respiratory compromise and avoid death.
- Harm: Expense, time, anxiety.
- Benefits-harms assessment: Preponderance of benefit over harm.
- Value judgments: The panel believes that early recognition of any serious adverse events is critically important.
- Role of patient preferences: Minimal; this is an important safety issue.
- Exclusions: None.
- Intentional vagueness: None.
- Strength: Recommendation.

Patients with OSAS may develop respiratory complications, such as worsening of OSAS or pulmonary edema, in the immediate postoperative period. Death attributable to respiratory complications in the immediate postoperative period has been reported in patients with severe OSAS. Identified risk factors are shown in Table 5. High-risk patients should undergo surgery in a center capable of treating complex pediatric patients. They should be hospitalized overnight for close monitoring postoperatively. Children with an acute respiratory infection on the day of surgery, as documented by fever, cough, and/or wheezing, are at increased risk of postoperative complications and, therefore, should be rescheduled or monitored closely postoperatively. Clinicians should decide on an individual basis whether these patients should be rescheduled, taking into consideration the severity of OSAS in the particular patient and keeping in mind that many children with adenotonsillar hypertrophy have chronic rhinorrhea and nasal congestion, even in the absence of viral infections.

Key Action Statement 5: Reevaluation

Clinicians should clinically reassess all patients with OSAS for persisting signs and symptoms after therapy to determine whether further treatment is required. (Evidence Quality: Grade B, Recommendation Strength: Recommendation.)

Evidence Profile KAS 5A

- Aggregate evidence quality: B
- Benefit: Determine effects of treatment.
- Harm: Expense, time.
- Benefits-harms assessment: Preponderance of benefit over harm.
- Value judgments: Data show that a significant proportion of children continue to have abnormalities postoperatively; therefore, the panel deter-

mined that the benefits of follow-up outweigh the minor inconveniences.
- Role of patient preferences: Minimal; follow-up is good clinical practice.
- Exclusions: None.
- Intentional vagueness: None.
- Strength: Recommendation.

Clinicians should reassess OSAS-related symptoms and signs (Table 2) after 6 to 8 weeks of therapy to determine whether further evaluation and treatment are indicated. Objective data regarding the timing of the postoperative evaluation are not available. Most clinicians recommend reevaluation 6 to 8 weeks after treatment to allow for healing of the operative site and to allow time for upper airway, cardiac, and central nervous system recovery. Patients who remain symptomatic should undergo objective testing (see Key Action Statement 2) or be referred to a sleep specialist for further evaluation.

Key Action Statement 5B: Reevaluation of High-Risk Patients

Clinicians should reevaluate high-risk patients for persistent OSAS after adenotonsillectomy, including those who had a significantly abnormal baseline polysomnogram, have sequelae of OSAS, are obese, or remain symptomatic after treatment, with an objective test (see Key Action Statement 2) or refer such patients to a sleep specialist. (Evidence Quality: Grade B, Recommendation Strength: Recommendation.)

Evidence Profile KAS 5B

- Aggregate evidence quality: B
- Benefit: Determine effects of treatment.
- Harm: Expense, time, anxiety/discomfort.
- Benefits-harms assessment: Preponderance of benefit over harm.

- Value judgments: Given the panel's concerns about the consequences of OSAS and the frequency of postoperative persistence in high-risk groups, the panel believes that the follow-up costs are outweighed by benefits of recognition of persistent OSAS. A minority of panelists believed that all children with OSAS should have follow-up polysomnography because of the high prevalence of persistent postoperative abnormalities on polysomnography, but most panelists believed that persistent polysomnographic abnormalities in uncomplicated children with mild OSAS were usually mild in patients who were asymptomatic after surgery.

- Role of patient preferences: Minimal. Further evaluation is needed to determine the need for further treatment.

- Exclusions: None.

- Intentional vagueness: None.

- Strength: Recommendation.

Numerous studies have shown that a large proportion of children at high risk continue to have some degree of OSAS postoperatively[10,13,14]; thus, objective evidence is required to determine whether further treatment is necessary.

Key Action Statement 6: CPAP

Clinicians should refer patients for CPAP management if symptoms/signs (Table 2) or objective evidence of OSAS persists after adenotonsillectomy or if adenotonsillectomy is not performed. (Evidence Quality: Grade B, Recommendation Strength: Recommendation.)

Evidence Profile KAS 6

- Aggregate evidence quality: B
- Benefit: Improve OSAS and accompanying symptoms and sequelae.

- Harm: Expense, time, anxiety; parental sleep disruption; nasal and skin adverse effects; possible midface remodeling; extremely rare serious pressure-related complications, such as pneumothorax; poor adherence.

- Benefits-harms assessment: Preponderance of benefit over harm.

- Value judgments: Panelists believe that CPAP is the most effective treatment of OSAS that persists postoperatively and that the benefits of treatment outweigh the adverse effects. Other treatments (eg, rapid maxillary expansion) may be effective in specially selected patients.

- Role of patient preferences: Other treatments may be effective in specially selected patients.

- Exclusions: Rare patients at increased risk of severe pressure complications.

- Intentional vagueness: None.

- Policy level: Recommendation.

CPAP therapy is delivered by using an electronic device that delivers air at positive pressure via a nasal mask, leading to mechanical stenting of the airway and improved functional residual capacity in the lungs. There is no clear advantage of using bilevel pressure over CPAP.[15] CPAP should be managed by an experienced and skilled clinician with expertise in its use in children. CPAP pressure requirements vary among individuals and change over time; thus, CPAP must be titrated in the sleep laboratory before prescribing the device and periodically readjusted thereafter. Behavioral modification therapy may be required, especially for young children or those with developmental delays. Objective monitoring of adherence, by using the equipment software, is important. If adherence is suboptimal, the clinician should institute measures to improve adherence (such as behavioral modification, or treating side effects of

CPAP) and institute alternative treatments if these measures are ineffective.

Key Action Statement 7: Weight Loss

Clinicians should recommend weight loss in addition to other therapy if a child/adolescent with OSAS is overweight or obese. (Evidence Quality: Grade C, Recommendation Strength: Recommendation.)

Evidence Profile KAS 7

- Aggregate evidence quality: C

- Benefit: Improve OSAS and accompanying symptoms and sequelae; non–OSAS-related benefits of weight loss.

- Harm: Hard to achieve and maintain weight loss.

- Benefits-harms assessment: Preponderance of benefit over harm.

- Value judgments: The panel agreed that weight loss is beneficial for both OSAS and other health issues, but clinical experience suggests that weight loss is difficult to achieve and maintain, and even effective weight loss regimens take time; therefore, additional treatment is required in the interim.

- Role of patient preferences: Strong role for patient and family preference regarding nutrition and exercise.

- Exclusions: None.

- Intentional vagueness: None.

- Strength: Recommendation.

Weight loss has been shown to improve OSAS,[16,17] although the degree of weight loss required has not been determined. Because weight loss is a slow and unreliable process, other treatment modalities (such as adenotonsillectomy or CPAP therapy) should be instituted until sufficient weight loss has been achieved and maintained.

Key Action Statement 8: Intranasal Corticosteroids

Clinicians may prescribe topical intranasal corticosteroids for children with mild OSAS in whom adenotonsillectomy is contraindicated or for children with mild postoperative OSAS. (Evidence Quality: Grade B, Recommendation Strength: Option.)

Evidence Profile KAS 8

- Aggregate evidence quality: B

- Benefit: Improves mild OSAS and accompanying symptoms and sequelae.

- Harm: Some subjects may not have an adequate response. It is not known whether therapeutic effect persists long-term; therefore, long-term observation is required. Low risk of steroid-related adverse effects.

- Benefits-harms assessment: Preponderance of benefit over harm.

- Value judgments: The panel agreed that intranasal steroids provide a less invasive treatment than surgery or CPAP and, therefore, may be preferred in some cases despite lower efficacy and lack of data on long-term efficacy.

- Role of patient preferences: Moderate role for patient and family preference if OSAS is mild.

- Exclusions: None.

- Intentional vagueness: None.

- Strength: Option.

Mild OSAS is defined, for this indication, as an AHI <5 per hour, on the basis of studies on intranasal corticosteroids described in the accompanying technical report.[2] Several studies have shown that the use of intranasal steroids decreases the degree of OSAS; however, although OSAS improves, residual OSAS may remain. Furthermore, there is individual variability in response to treatment, and long-term studies have not been performed to determine the duration of improvement. Therefore, nasal steroids are not recommended as a first-line therapy. The response to treatment should be measured objectively after a course of treatment of approximately 6 weeks. Because the long-term effect of this treatment is unknown, the clinician should continue to observe the patient for symptoms of recurrence and adverse effects of corticosteroids.

AREAS FOR FUTURE RESEARCH

A detailed list of research recommendations is provided in the accompanying technical report.[2] There is a great need for further research into the prevalence of OSAS, sequelae of OSAS, best treatment methods, and the role of obesity. In particular, well-controlled, blinded studies, including randomized controlled trials of treatment, are needed to determine the best care for children and adolescents with OSAS.

SUBCOMMITTEE ON OBSTRUCTIVE SLEEP APNEA SYNDROME*

Carole L. Marcus, MBBCh, Chairperson (Sleep Medicine, Pediatric Pulmonologist; Liaison, American Academy of Sleep Medicine; Research Support from Philips Respironics; Affiliated with an academic sleep center; Published research related to OSAS)

Lee J. Brooks, MD (Sleep Medicine, Pediatric Pulmonologist; Liaison, American College of Chest Physicians; No financial conflicts; Affiliated with an academic sleep center; Published research related to OSAS)

Sally Davidson Ward, MD (Sleep Medicine, Pediatric Pulmonologist; No financial conflicts; Affiliated with an academic sleep center; Published research related to OSAS)

Kari A. Draper, MD (General Pediatrician; No conflicts)

David Gozal, MD (Sleep Medicine, Pediatric Pulmonologist; Research support from AstraZeneca; Speaker for Merck Company; Affiliated with an academic sleep center; Published research related to OSAS)

Ann C. Halbower, MD (Sleep Medicine, Pediatric Pulmonologist; Liaison, American Thoracic Society; Research Funding from Resmed; Affiliated with an academic sleep center; Published research related to OSAS)

Jacqueline Jones, MD (Pediatric Otolaryngologist; AAP Section on Otolaryngology-Head and Neck Surgery; Liaison, American Academy of Otolaryngology-Head and Neck Surgery; No financial conflicts; Affiliated with an academic otolaryngologic practice)

Christopher Lehman, MD (Neonatologist, Informatician; No conflicts)

Michael S. Schechter, MD, MPH (Pediatric Pulmonologist; AAP Section on Pediatric Pulmonology; Consultant to Genentech, Inc and Gilead, Inc, not related to Obstructive Sleep Apnea; Research Support from Mpex Pharmaceuticals, Inc, Vertex Pharmaceuticals Incorporated, PTC Therapeutics, Bayer Healthcare, not related to Obstructive Sleep Apnea)

Stephen Sheldon, MD (Sleep Medicine, General Pediatrician; Liaison, National Sleep Foundation; No financial conflicts; Affiliated with an academic sleep center; Published research related to OSAS)

Richard N. Shiffman, MD, MCIS (General pediatrics, Informatician; No conflicts)

Karen Spruyt, PhD (Clinical Psychologist, Child Neuropsychologist, and Biostatistician/Epidemiologist; No financial conflicts; Affiliated with an academic sleep center)

Oversight from the Steering Committee on Quality Improvement and Management, 2009–2012

STAFF

Caryn Davidson, MA

*Areas of expertise are shown in parentheses after each name.

ACKNOWLEDGMENTS

The committee thanks Jason Caboot, June Chan, Mary Currie, Fiona Healy, Maureen Josephson, Sofia Konstantinopoulou, H. Madan Kumar, Roberta Leu, Darius Loghmanee, Rajeev Bhatia, Argyri Petrocheilou, Harsha Vardhan, and Colleen Walsh for assisting with evidence extraction.

REFERENCES

1. Section on Pediatric Pulmonology, Subcommittee on Obstructive Sleep Apnea Syndrome. American Academy of Pediatrics. Clinical practice guideline: diagnosis and management of childhood obstructive sleep apnea syndrome. *Pediatrics.* 2002;109(4):704–712

2. Marcus CL, Brooks LJ, Davidson C, et al; American Academy of Pediatrics, Subcommittee on Obstructive Sleep Apnea

Syndrome. Technical report: diagnosis and management of childhood obstructive sleep apnea syndrome. *Pediatrics.* 2012; 130(3):In press

3. American Academy of Pediatrics Steering Committee on Quality Improvement and Management. Classifying recommendations for clinical practice guidelines. *Pediatrics.* 2004;114(3):874–877

4. American Thoracic Society. Standards and indications for cardiopulmonary sleep studies in children. *Am J Respir Crit Care Med.* 1996;153(2):866–878

5. Bixler EO, Vgontzas AN, Lin HM, et al. Sleep disordered breathing in children in a general population sample: prevalence and risk factors. *Sleep.* 2009;32(6):731–736

6. Li AM, So HK, Au CT, et al. Epidemiology of obstructive sleep apnoea syndrome in Chinese children: a two-phase community study. *Thorax.* 2010;65(11):991–997

7. O'Brien LM, Holbrook CR, Mervis CB, et al. Sleep and neurobehavioral characteristics of 5- to 7-year-old children with parentally reported symptoms of attention-deficit/hyperactivity disorder. *Pediatrics.* 2003; 111(3):554–563

8. Himes JH, Dietz WH; The Expert Committee on Clinical Guidelines for Overweight in Adolescent Preventive Services. Guidelines for overweight in adolescent preventive services: recommendations from an expert committee. *Am J Clin Nutr.* 1994;59(2):307–316

9. Mitchell RB. Adenotonsillectomy for obstructive sleep apnea in children: outcome evaluated by pre- and postoperative polysomnography. *Laryngoscope.* 2007;117(10):1844–1854

10. Suen JS, Arnold JE, Brooks LJ. Adenotonsillectomy for treatment of obstructive sleep apnea in children. *Arch Otolaryngol Head Neck Surg.* 1995;121(5):525–530

11. Nieminen P, Tolonen U, Löppönen H. Snoring and obstructive sleep apnea in children: a 6-month follow-up study. *Arch Otolaryngol Head Neck Surg.* 2000;126(4):481–486

12. Blunden S, Lushington K, Lorenzen B, Wong J, Balendran R, Kennedy D. Symptoms of sleep breathing disorders in children are underreported by parents at general practice visits. *Sleep Breath.* 2003;7(4):167–176

13. Apostolidou MT, Alexopoulos EI, Chaidas K, et al. Obesity and persisting sleep apnea after adenotonsillectomy in Greek children. *Chest.* 2008;134(6):1149–1155

14. Mitchell RB, Kelly J. Outcome of adenotonsillectomy for severe obstructive sleep apnea in children. *Int J Pediatr Otorhinolaryngol.* 2004;68(11):1375–1379

15. Marcus CL, Rosen G, Ward SL, et al. Adherence to and effectiveness of positive airway pressure therapy in children with obstructive sleep apnea. *Pediatrics.* 2006; 117(3). Available at: www.pediatrics.org/cgi/content/full/117/3/e442

16. Verhulst SL, Franckx H, Van Gaal L, De Backer W, Desager K. The effect of weight loss on sleep-disordered breathing in obese teenagers. *Obesity (Silver Spring).* 2009;17(6):1178–1183

17. Kalra M, Inge T. Effect of bariatric surgery on obstructive sleep apnoea in adolescents. *Paediatr Respir Rev.* 2006;7(4):260–267

TECHNICAL REPORT

Diagnosis and Management of Childhood Obstructive Sleep Apnea Syndrome

abstract

OBJECTIVE: This technical report describes the procedures involved in developing recommendations on the management of childhood obstructive sleep apnea syndrome (OSAS).

METHODS: The literature from 1999 through 2011 was evaluated.

RESULTS AND CONCLUSIONS: A total of 3166 titles were reviewed, of which 350 provided relevant data. Most articles were level II through IV. The prevalence of OSAS ranged from 0% to 5.7%, with obesity being an independent risk factor. OSAS was associated with cardiovascular, growth, and neurobehavioral abnormalities and possibly inflammation. Most diagnostic screening tests had low sensitivity and specificity. Treatment of OSAS resulted in improvements in behavior and attention and likely improvement in cognitive abilities. Primary treatment is adenotonsillectomy (AT). Data were insufficient to recommend specific surgical techniques; however, children undergoing partial tonsillectomy should be monitored for possible recurrence of OSAS. Although OSAS improved postoperatively, the proportion of patients who had residual OSAS ranged from 13% to 29% in low-risk populations to 73% when obese children were included and stricter polysomnographic criteria were used. Nevertheless, OSAS may improve after AT even in obese children, thus supporting surgery as a reasonable initial treatment. A significant number of obese patients required intubation or continuous positive airway pressure (CPAP) postoperatively, which reinforces the need for inpatient observation. CPAP was effective in the treatment of OSAS, but adherence is a major barrier. For this reason, CPAP is not recommended as first-line therapy for OSAS when AT is an option. Intranasal steroids may ameliorate mild OSAS, but follow-up is needed. Data were insufficient to recommend rapid maxillary expansion. *Pediatrics* 2012;130:e714–e755

Carole L. Marcus, MBBCh, Lee J. Brooks, MD, Sally Davidson Ward, MD, Kari A. Draper, MD, David Gozal, MD, Ann C. Halbower, MD, Jacqueline Jones, MD, Christopher Lehmann, MD, Michael S. Schechter, MD, MPH, Stephen Sheldon, MD, Richard N. Shiffman, MD, MCIS, and Karen Spruyt, PhD

KEY WORDS
adenotonsillectomy, continuous positive airway pressure, sleep-disordered breathing, snoring

ABBREVIATIONS
AAP—American Academy of Pediatrics
ADHD—attention-deficit/hyperactivity disorder
AHI—apnea hypopnea index
AT—adenotonsillectomy
BP—blood pressure
BPAP—bilevel positive airway pressure
CBCL—Child Behavior Checklist
CPAP—continuous positive airway pressure
CRP—C-reactive protein
ECG—electrocardiography
HOMA—homeostatic model assessment
HS—habitual snoring
IL—interleukin
OSAS—obstructive sleep apnea syndrome
PAP—positive airway pressure
PSG—polysomnography
PT—partial tonsillectomy
QoL—quality of life
RDI—respiratory distress index
SDB—sleep-disordered breathing
SES—socioeconomic status
SpO$_2$—oxygen saturation
URI—upper respiratory tract infection

(Continued on last page)

INTRODUCTION

This technical report describes in detail the procedures involved in developing the recommendations for the updated clinical practice guideline on childhood obstructive sleep apnea syndrome (OSAS).[1]

The clinical practice guideline is primarily aimed at pediatricians and other primary care clinicians (family physicians, nurse practitioners, and physician assistants) who treat children. The secondary audience for the guideline includes sleep medicine specialists, pediatric pulmonologists, neurologists, otolaryngologists, and developmental/behavioral pediatricians.

The primary focus of the committee was on OSAS in childhood.[2] The committee focused on otherwise healthy children who had adenotonsillar hypertrophy or obesity as underlying risk factors. Complex populations, including infants <1 year of age and children who had other medical conditions (eg, craniofacial anomalies, genetic or metabolic syndromes, neuromuscular disease, laryngomalacia, sickle cell disease), were excluded because these patients will typically require subspecialty referral.

Two professional studies recently published related guidelines: the American Academy of Otolaryngology–Head and Neck Surgery[3] and the American Academy of Sleep Medicine.[4] These guidelines have similar recommendations to many of the recommendations in the American Academy of Pediatrics (AAP) guideline.

The recommendations in this statement do not indicate an exclusive course of treatment. Variations, taking into account individual circumstances, may be appropriate.

METHODS

Literature Search

A literature search was performed that included English-language articles, children and adolescents aged 1 through 17.9 years, and publication between 1999 and 2008. Animal studies, abstracts, letters, case reports, and reviews were excluded. The Medical Subject Heading terms that were used in all fields were snoring, apnea, sleep-disordered breathing (SDB), sleep-related breathing disorders, upper

airway resistance, polysomnography (PSG), sleep study, adenoidectomy, tonsillectomy, continuous positive airway pressure (CPAP), obesity, adiposity, hypopnea, hypoventilation, cognition, behavior, and neuropsychology. Search engines used were PubMed, Scopus, Ovid, PsycINFO, EBSCO (including Health Source [Nursing], Child Development and Adolescent Studies), and CINAHL. Articles covering special populations (eg, infants aged <1 year, those with craniofacial anomalies or syndromes) were excluded during the title and abstract reviews.

Titles and available abstracts of articles found by the literature search were reviewed by the committee members in several rounds (see Results). In the first round, duplicates and erroneous hits from the literature search were excluded. In the second round, titles were reviewed for relevancy by 2 committee members. Articles with relevant titles were then reviewed by 2 reviewers each, on the basis of the abstract. Because of the large number of remaining articles, text-mining (Statistica, StatSoft version 9; StatSoft, Inc, Tulsa, OK) was performed on the method section of the articles to reduce the large amount of articles for the final step of quality assessment. Text-mining is the combined, automated process of analyzing unstructured, natural language text to discover information and knowledge that are typically difficult to retrieve.[5]

Unfortunately, text-mining revealed that few articles reported research methods, such as the study design (eg, clinical case series, retrospective, observational, clinical experiment), blinding of the assessment, and recruitment and/or scoring, that could have been applied for further selection. A manual screening of the questionable articles after text-mining resulted in a pool of 605 articles. The committee decided on a final round of title selection; that is, each

member was assigned a random batch of articles and selected titles based on relevance with respect to the guideline categories. These remaining articles were each reviewed and graded by a committee member, as detailed here. Because of the large volume of articles requiring detailed evaluation, some committee members recruited trainees and colleagues to assist them in the performance of these reviews, under their supervision. Jason Caboot, June Chan, Mary Currie, Fiona Healy, Maureen Josephson, Sofia Konstantinopoulou, H. Madan Kumar, Roberta Leu, Darius Loghmanee, Rajeev Bhatia, Argyri Petrocheilou, Harsha Vardhan, and Colleen Walsh participated. A literature search of more recent articles (2008–2011) was performed by individual committee members, per guideline category, and discussed during the committee meeting.

As would be expected from any panel of experts in a field, some of the citations were the work of the panel members. For this reason, a varied panel, including general pediatricians, pulmonologists, otolaryngologists, and sleep medicine physicians, was arranged to provide balance. For initial guideline drafts, committee members were assigned sections of the report that were not directly in their area of research, and the evidence, search results, and conclusions thereof were discussed by all committee members at a face-to-face meeting. Subsequent drafts of the guidelines and technical report were reviewed by all committee members.

Quality Assessment

The previous literature review form[6] was modified to include the evidence grading system developed by the American Academy of Neurology for the assessment of clinical utility of diagnostic tests (Table 1).[7] A specific customized software (OSA Taskforce;

TABLE 1 Evidence Grading System[7]

Level	Description
I	Evidence provided by a prospective study in a broad spectrum of persons who have the suspected condition, by using a reference (gold) standard for case definition, in which the test is applied in a blinded fashion, and enabling the assessment of appropriate test of diagnostic accuracy. All persons undergoing the diagnostic test have the presence or absence of the disease determined. Level I studies are judged to have a low risk of bias.
II	Evidence provided by a prospective study of a narrow spectrum of persons who have the suspected condition, or a well-designed retrospective study of a broad spectrum of persons who have an established condition (by gold standard) compared with a broad spectrum of controls, in which the test is applied in a blinded evaluation, and enabling the assessment of appropriate tests of diagnostic accuracy. Level II studies are judged to have a moderate risk of bias.
III	Evidence provided by a retrospective study in which either persons who have the established condition or controls are of a narrow spectrum, and in which the reference standard, if not objective, is applied by someone other than the person who performed (interpreted) the test. Level III studies are judged to have a moderate to high risk of bias.
IV	Any study design where the test is not applied in an independent evaluation or evidence is provided by expert opinion alone or in descriptive case series without controls. There is no blinding or there may be inadequate blinding. The spectrum of persons tested may be broad or narrow. Level IV studies are judged to have a very high risk of bias.

copyright Francesco Rundo and Karen Spruyt) was developed for the literature review form to standardize this part of the process. Of note, the quality assessment levels were comparable to the grading levels applied previously.[8,9] The quality assessment applied involved 4 tiers of evidence, with level I studies being judged to have a low risk of bias and level IV studies judged to have a very high level of bias. A weaker level of evidence indicates the need to integrate greater clinical judgment when applying results to clinical decision-making. The committee's quality assessment of data took into account not only the levels of evidence in relevant articles but also the number of articles identified, the magnitude and direction of various findings, and whether articles demonstrated convergent or divergent conclusions.

The evidence-based approach to guideline development requires that the evidence in support of each key action statement be identified, appraised, and summarized and that an explicit link between evidence and recommendations be defined. Evidence-based recommendations reflect the quality of evidence and the balance of benefit

and harm that is anticipated when the recommendation is followed. The AAP policy statement "Classifying Recommendations for Clinical Practice Guidelines"[10] was followed in designating levels of recommendations (Fig 1, Table 2).

RESULTS OF LITERATURE SEARCH

The automated Medical Subject Heading search resulted in 3166 hits. After duplicates and erroneous hits were excluded, 2395 hits fulfilled the criteria. After title review, 1091 articles were accepted, with a 0.70 interrater agreement between the 2 reviewers. These remaining articles were reviewed on the basis of the abstract, which resulted in 757 articles remaining, with a 0.60 agreement rate between reviewers. A final decision on those without agreement was made by the chairperson of the committee. Text-mining, although not helpful in reducing the number of articles for further evaluation, illustrated the spectrum of topics covered by the articles (Table 3). A manual screening of the questionable articles after text-mining resulted in a pool of 605 articles. The final round of title selection resulted in 397 articles for

detailed review. An additional 47 articles were found to not meet criteria during the detailed review. Thus, a total of 350 articles were included.

On the basis of the final 350 articles, one-third were epidemiologic studies, 26% were diagnostic studies, and 23% were treatment studies. Table 4 lists the type of study design; 34% of studies were descriptive and 32% were nonrandomized concurrent cohort series. PSG was the diagnostic method used for 57% of the articles, whereas 45% used questionnaires. The sample size varied from 9 to 6742 subjects. Figure 2 shows the level of evidence of the articles; 76% of studies were level III or IV. The majority of studies did not include a control group, which degraded the studies to level III or IV. Few studies applied any form of blinding.

Conclusion

There has been a large increase in the number of published studies since the initial guideline was published. However, there are few randomized, blinded, controlled studies. Most articles evaluated were level III or IV, and many studies were hampered by the lack of a control group. In most studies, blinding was not present or not reported. From a methodologic standpoint, a clear need for randomized clinical trials with blinding is evident.

TERMINOLOGY

OSAS in children is defined as a "disorder of breathing during sleep characterized by prolonged partial upper airway obstruction and/or intermittent complete obstruction (obstructive apnea) that disrupts normal ventilation during sleep and normal sleep patterns,"[2] accompanied by symptoms or signs as listed in Table 2 of the accompanying guideline. In this document, the term SDB is used to encompass both snoring and OSAS when studies did not distinguish between these entities.

PREVALENCE OF OSAS

The original clinical practice guideline found a prevalence of OSAS of 2% (3 studies) and a prevalence of habitual snoring (HS) of 3% to 12% (7 studies). Since publication of the original guideline, 10 studies (in 12 separate articles) used the gold standard of conventional overnight laboratory PSG to diagnose OSAS (Table 5). These studies were all levels I through IV, depending on the size and characteristics of the sample population, and represented many countries and age groups. They used various criteria, not all of which are standard, to diagnose OSAS. Many of the studies had a small sample size and/or studied only a selected high-risk sample of the population. Despite these limitations, the 10 studies found a prevalence of OSAS in the general pediatric population of 0% to 5.7%. Three studies to note were those of Bixler et al[11] from the United States, Li et al[12] from China, and O'Brien et al[13] from the United States. These 3 studies (levels I–II) had large sample sizes from the general pediatric population and reported OSAS prevalence rates of 1.2% to 5.7%. Six studies investigated the prevalence of OSAS by using various ambulatory studies rather than full, laboratory-based PSG (Table 6). Although the sample sizes were generally larger, home studies are not considered the gold standard of diagnosis and were thus level III. These studies found an OSAS prevalence of 0.8% to 24%. The 2 outliers (at 12% and 24%)[14,15] used more liberal criteria to diagnose OSAS. Excluding those studies, the OSAS prevalence was 0.8% to 2.8%.

Several studies attempted to discern variables associated with the presence of OSAS. Three studies found an equal prevalence between males and females,[16–18] and 2 studies found an increased prevalence in males.[12,15] Two studies reported an increased risk in children of ethnic minorities,[11,19] supporting older data.[20] Four studies found an increased risk in obese patients,[12,17,21,22] but 3 studies did

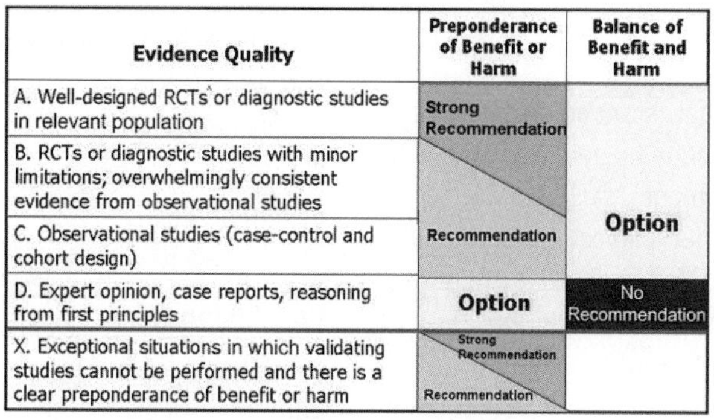

FIGURE 1

Evidence quality. Integrating evidence quality appraisal with an assessment of the anticipated balance between benefits and harms if a policy is carried out leads to designation of a policy as a strong recommendation, recommendation, option, or no recommendation. RCT, randomized controlled trial.

TABLE 2 Definitions and Recommendation Implications

Statement	Definition	Implication
Strong recommendation	A strong recommendation in favor of a particular action is made when the anticipated benefits of the recommended intervention clearly exceed the harms (as a strong recommendation against an action is made when the anticipated harms clearly exceed the benefits) and the quality of the supporting evidence is excellent. In some clearly identified circumstances, strong recommendations may be made when high-quality evidence is impossible to obtain and the anticipated benefits strongly outweigh the harms.	Clinicians should follow a strong recommendation unless a clear and compelling rationale for an alternative approach is present.
Recommendation	A recommendation in favor of a particular action is made when the anticipated benefits exceed the harms but the quality of evidence is not as strong. Again, in some clearly identified circumstances, recommendations may be made when high-quality evidence is impossible to obtain but the anticipated benefits outweigh the harms.	Clinicians would be prudent to follow a recommendation but should remain alert to new information and sensitive to patient preferences.
Option	Options define courses that may be taken when either the quality of evidence is suspect or carefully performed studies have shown little clear advantage to 1 approach over another.	Clinicians should consider the option in their decision-making, and patient preference may have a substantial role.
No recommendation	No recommendation indicates that there is a lack of pertinent published evidence and that the anticipated balance of benefits and harms is presently unclear.	Clinicians should be alert to new published evidence that clarifies the balance of benefit versus harm.

TABLE 3 Results of Text-Mining of the Methods Section of 757 Papers

Term Used for Text-Mining	Percentage of Papers
Snore/snoring	58.3
Polysomnography	53.6
Diagnosis	53.4
Medical management	51.6
Survey/questionnaire	38.8
Psychological	37.0
Surgery/surgical	35.9
Treatment	32.1
Design	27.8
Obese/obesity	25.0
BMI	24.6
Randomize	20.2
Blinding	16.4
Sampling	11.7
Control group	8.8
Actigraphy	2.6
Mortality	0.5

TABLE 4 Types of Studies in the Literature Based on 350 Articles

Type of Study	Percentage
Descriptive study	33.7
Nonrandomized concurrent cohort series	32.0
Descriptive study + other	10.8
Nonrandomized historical cohort series	7.8
Randomized clinical trial	4.6
Retrospective	3.6
Case-control study	1.3
Prospective consecutive cohort series	1.3
Cross-sectional population-based survey	1.0
Nonrandomized historical cohort series + other	1.0
Randomized + other	1.0
Undetermined	1.0
Nonrandomized concurrent cohort series + other	0.7
Experimental study	0.3

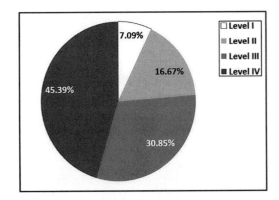

FIGURE 2
Levels of evidence of articles used for this report.

not.[15,16,23] Another study reported an increased risk of OSAS with increased waist circumference, a marker for obesity.[11] One study found an increased risk with nasal abnormalities,[11] 1 study found an increased risk with prematurity,[19] and 2 studies found increased risk with adenotonsillar hypertrophy.[12,22]

Multiple studies (levels II–IV) investigated the prevalence of HS, which is one of the most prominent manifestations of OSAS (Table 7). The presence of snoring was based on parental or personal questionnaires. Not all of the questionnaires used have been validated, and the data relied on subjective responses rather than objective clinical evaluations. The reported prevalence of HS varied widely, depending on the study and definition used, from 1.5% to 27.6%.

In summary, studies of OSAS and HS show varied prevalence rates, depending on the population studied, the methods used to measure breathing during sleep, and the definitions used for diagnosis. Nevertheless, the preponderance of evidence suggests a prevalence of OSAS in the range of 1% to 5%, making this a relatively common disease that would be encountered by most clinicians in primary practice.

Areas for Future Research

● Population-based studies on the gender and race distribution of OSAS among different age groups.

SEQUELAE OF OSAS

Neuropsychological and Cognitive Problems Associated With OSAS

Of the 350 articles related to this search over the last 10 years, 61 articles directly explored the relationship between SDB and cognitive or neuropsychological deficits. In total, 29 658 subjects were studied, including 2 level I studies[24,25] with a total of 174 subjects and 5 level II studies.[26–30] The diagnosis of SDB was based on clinical symptoms in 29 articles and on PSG in 32 articles.

Cognitive Deficits

All but 1 study (level IV)[31] demonstrated deficits in cognition or neuropsychological function in association with symptoms, signs, or diagnosis of SDB. The 1 exception examined children who had mild OSAS over a wide age range and did not include behavioral assessments. In this study, the mean IQ in the OSAS population was significantly above the standard mean. Some[32–34] but not all studies showed a correlation between the severity of obstructive apnea as measured on PSG and increasing neuropsychological morbidity. There are several reasons why correlations were not found for all studies. Standard PSG was developed to detect cardiorespiratory variations and may not be an adequate tool for detection of sleep changes that affect neuropsychological function. Another possibility is that any degree of SDB is associated with abnormal neuropsychological outcomes and might be affected variably by social, medical, environmental, or socioeconomic factors not measured by using PSG. This

TABLE 5 Prevalence of OSAS on the Basis of Laboratory PSG

Source	Year	No.	No. Undergoing PSG	Country	Age, y	OSAS Prevalence	HS Prevalence	OSAS Criteria/Comments
Anuntaseree et al[201]	2001	1005	8	Thailand	6–13	0.69%	8.5%	AHI ≥1
Anuntaseree et al[202]	2005	755	Unclear, possibly 10			1.3%	6.9%	Note: 2 studies used same cohort
							"most nights"	
Beebe et al[21]	2007	60 obese, 22 control	All	United States	10–16.9	0% normal, 13% obese		AHI >5; ↑ in obese
Bixler et al[11]	2009	5740	700	United States	5–12	1.2%		AHI ≥5; ↑ in ↑ waist circumference; ↑ with nasal abnormalities; ↑ in minority race
Brunetti et al[203]	2001	895	34 home monitoring, 12 PSG	Italy	3–11	1%–1.8%	4.9%	AHI >3
Brunetti et al[23]	2010						5.4%	Not ↑ in obese; Note: 2 studies used same cohort
							"always"	
Li et al[172]	2010	6447	619	China	5–13	4.8%	7.2%	Using ICSD-II criteria 4.8%; ↑ in boys
Li et al[12]	2010						"frequently"	↑ in obese; ↑ in ↑ tonsil size
Ng et al[204]	2002	200	16	Hong Kong	6.4 ± 4	1%	14.5%	AHI >1
O'Brien et al[13]	2003	5728	110	United States	5–7	5.7%	11.7%	AHI >5
Sogut et al[16]	2005	1198 total	28	Turkey	3–11	0.9%–1.3%	"frequent and loud" 3.3%, >3 times/week	Used AHI >3; Boys = girls; Not ↑ in obese
Wing et al[17]	2003	46 obese, 44 control	All	China	7–15	2.3%–4.5% control; 26% to 32.6% obese		OAI ≥1 or RDI ≥5; Boys = girls; ↑ in obese
Xu et al[22]	2008	99 obese, 99 control	All	China	Elementary school	0 if not obese and no ATH		AHI >5 or OAI >1; ↑ obese; ↑ in ATH

ATH, adenotonsillar hypertrophy; ICSD, International Classification of Sleep Disorders; OAI, obstructive apnea index.

possibility is confirmed by a recent level I study showing that obesity, OSAS, and neurocognitive outcomes are all interdependent.[35] Furthermore, most studies were not controlled for socioeconomic status (SES), which is important because SES strongly affects the results of neurocognitive testing and because OSAS is associated with low SES.[36] Although some studies have shown abnormalities in snorers compared with nonsnoring controls, in many of these studies, data in snorers still fell within the normal range.[24] In addition, cutoffs for OSAS used in some studies resulted in a blurring of boundaries between the OSAS and snoring groups. For example, Chervin et al used an obstructive apnea index cutoff of only ≥0.5/hour to define OSAS, and the mean apnea index for the OSAS group was 2.9 events/hour, indicating that the study group had mild OSAS, which was not that different from the snorers.[37,38] A study with a wider spectrum of severity may have attained different results. Finally, most studies have not controlled for obesity, which has been associated with neurobehavioral and cognitive abnormalities.

Although most studies simply compared groups, others have looked at the correlation between polysomnographic indices and neurocognitive/behavioral outcomes and have shown a correlation between different polysomnographic factors and cognitive outcomes, behavioral outcomes, and sleepiness.[32–34,39]

Cognitive deficits associated with pediatric SDB include general intelligence level as well as processes measured by using IQ subtests (Table 8). Specific functions objectively measured by using neuropsychological assessments and included in the research studies include:

- Learning, memory, and visuospatial skills

TABLE 6 Prevalence of OSAS on the Basis of Ambulatory Monitoring

Source	Year	No.	No. Undergoing Ambulatory Monitoring	Country	Age, y	OSAS Prevalence, %	HS Prevalence	OSAS Criteria and Comments
Castronovo et al[14]	2003	595	265	Italy	3–6	12	34.5% "Often" or "Always"	OAI ≥5
Goodwin et al[15]	2005	480	All	United States	6–11	24	10.5% "Frequently"	RDI ≥1 ↑ in male Not ↑ in obese
Hultcrantz and Löfstrand Tideström[205]	2009	393	26	Sweden	12	0.8	6.9% "Regularly"	AHI ≥1 and/ or OAI ≥1
Rosen et al[19]	2003	850	All	United States	8–11	2.2		AHI ≥5 or OAI ≥1 ↑ in AA ↑ in premature infants
Sánchez-Armengol et al[18]	2001	101	All	Spain	12–16	1.9	14.8%	Based on RDI ≥10 and snoring, witnessed apneas, and/or excessive daytime sleepiness.
Urschitz et al[206]	2010	1144	183	Germany	7.3–12.4	2.8	"Often"	Girls = boys AHI ≥1

OAI, obstructive apnea index; AA, African American.

TABLE 7 Prevalence of HS

Source	Year	No.	Country	Age, y	HS Prevalence, %	HS Criteria
Akcay et al[207]	2006	1784	Turkey	4–17	4.1	"Often"
Alexopoulos et al[208]	2006	1821	Greece	5–14	7.4	>3 times/wk
Archbold et al[209]	2002	1038	United States	2–13.9	17.1	"More than half of the time"
Bidad et al[167]	2006	2900	Iran	11–17	7.9	≥3 times/wk
Chng et al[210]	2004	11 114	Singapore	4–7	6.0	>3 times/wk
Corbo et al[166]	2001	2209	Italy	10–15	5.6	"Often"
Ersu et al[211]	2004	2147	Turkey	5–13	7.0	"Often"
Goodwin et al[212]	2003	1494	United States	4–11	10.5	"Snoring frequently or almost always"
Gottlieb et al[213]	2003	3019	United States	5	12	≥3 times/week
Johnson and Roth[45]	2006	1014	United States	13–16	6	"Every or nearly every night"
Kuehni et al[214]	2008	6811	United Kingdom	1–4	7.9	"Almost always"
Liu et al[215]	2005	517 in China 494 in USA	China United States	Grade school	1.5 (China) 9.9 (United States)	Snoring loudly 5–7 times/wk
Liu et al[215]	2005	5979	China	2–12	5.6	"Frequent"
Löfstrand-Tideström and Hultcrantz[216]	2007	509	Sweden	4–6	5.3–6.9	"Snoring every night"
Lu et al[217]	2003	974	Australia	2–5	10.5	≥4 times/week
Montgomery–Downs et al[44]	2003	1010	United States	Preschool	HS and risk of SDB, 22	≥3 times/week
Nelson and Kulnis[218]	2001	405	United States	6–17	17	"Often"
Ng et al[219]	2005	3047	China	6–12	10.9	6–7 times/wk
Perez-Chada et al[220]	2007	2210	Argentina	9–17	9	"Frequent"
Petry et al[221]	2008	998	Brazil	9–14	27.6	"Frequently" or "always"
Sahin et al[222]	2009	1164	Turkey	7–13	3.5	"Frequently" or "almost every day"
Sogut et al[16]	2005	1030	Turkey	12–17	4.0	"Often" or "always"
Tafur et al[223]	2009	806	Ecuador	6–12	15.1	"Often" or "always"
Urschitz et al[164]	2004	1144	Germany	Primary school	9.6	"Always" or "frequently"
Zhang et al[224]	2004	996	Australia	4–12	15.2	>4 times/wk

- Language, verbal fluency, and phonological skills
- Concept formation, analytic thinking, and verbal and nonverbal comprehension
- School performance and mathematical abilities
- Executive functions

Executive functions were measured by using both objective testing and parent questionnaires. Executive functions are a network of skills and higher order functions that control and regulate other cognitive processes. These skills require mental flexibility, impulse control,

TABLE 8 Cognitive Deficits Associated With Pediatric SDB

Type of Deficit	Source	Level	No.	Findings/Comments
Cognition, general intelligence	Beebe et al[225] Blunden et al[226] Kaemingk et al[33] Kennedy et al[34] Kurnatowski et al[227]	IV	895	Deficits of general intelligence, sensorimotor integration by objective measurement; behavioral abnormalities included as well
	Carvalho et al[228] Montgomery-Downs et al[50] Suratt et al[43]	III	1332	Objective measures of general intelligence, verbal skills affected by SDB
	Friedman et al[26] Halbower et al[28] O'Brien et al[29] Kohler et al[30]	II	473	General intelligence, executive function, language all affected by SDB and measured objectively
	O'Brien et al[24] Suratt et al[25]	I	174	General conceptual ability, verbal and nonverbal reasoning, vocabulary affected by SDB (and time in bed[25])
Poor school performance	Chervin et al[42] Johnson and Roth[45] Kaemingk et al[33] Ng et al[219] Perez-Chada et al[220] Shin et al[47] Urschitz et al[229]	IV	11 110	Academic achievement measured either by parent or school grades Additive factors were SES and ethnicity[42-45] or BMI,[42-45-47] which contributed to findings of poor school performance in SDB
	Montgomery-Downs et al[44]	III	1010	Snoring associates with ethnicity, school performance in SES-challenged preschool-aged children
Executive function	Beebe et al[225] LeBourgeois et al[230] Karpinski et al[231]	IV	179	Mental flexibility, impulse control Objective testing performed
	Halbower et al[28] Kohler et al[30]	II	123	Response preparation, working memory, fluid and quantitative reasoning; objective testing performed by blinded tester
Learning, information processing, memory, visuospatial skills	Goodwin et al[212] Hamasaki Uema et al[232] Kaemingk et al[33] Kennedy et al[34] Kurnatowski et al[227] O'Brien et al[233] Spruyt et al[234] Giordani et al[38]	IV	1838	Objective testing performed in all but Goodwin et al[212] (questionnaire)
	Halbower et al[28] Tauman et al[46]	II	112	Race[28] and BMI may play an additive role in inflammation[46] and cognitive dysfunction in SDB
	O'Brien et al[24]	I	118	Primary snoring without gas exchange abnormalities associates with significantly lower learning and memory
Language/verbal skills	Kurnatowski et al[227] O'Brien et al[233] Perez-Chada et al[220] Honaker et al[235] Lundeborg et al[51]	IV	3304	Deficits of language or verbal skills in SDB Objective testing performed in all studies
	Suratt et al[43] Montgomery-Downs et al[50]	III	114	Race and time in bed may contribute to abnormal language associated with SDB
	O'Brien et al[24] Suratt et al[25]	I	118	Primary snoring without gas exchange abnormalities associated with significantly lower verbal skills; deficits of language or verbal skills in SDB
Attention	Beebe et al[225] Chervin et al[236] Galland et al[237] Gottlieb et al[213] Hamasaki Uema et al[232] Kaemingk et al[33] Li et al[238] Mulvaney et al[32] Urschitz et al[229]	IV	6411	Objective testing performed for attention except in refs 32,33,213,229, and 236 in which parent or teacher questionnaires were used
	Chervin et al[37]	I	105	
	O'Brien et al[24]	I	118	Visual and auditory attention

and working memory. Executive functions are required for optimal school performance and are acquired through adolescence in developing children.

Behavioral Abnormalities

The investigations on the cognitive effects of SDB in the 61 studies often included measures of neurobehavioral outcomes (Table 9). Hyperactivity was the most commonly studied and/or reported behavioral abnormality associated with SDB. It was reported as a frequent symptom of SDB in younger children, and in fact, in 1 study, snoring was found to be strongly predictive of a future diagnosis of hyperactivity over the long-term (level IV).[40] Attention-deficit/hyperactivity disorder (ADHD) or ADHD symptoms, hypersomnolence, somatization, depression, atypicality, aggression, and abnormal social behaviors were the other most frequently reported behavioral abnormalities associated with SDB in children. Most behavioral difficulties were defined by using parent or teacher questionnaires in unblinded level IV studies.

Sleepiness

Two studies (levels I–II) have shown a relationship between polysomnographic measures and objective measurement of daytime sleepiness on multiple sleep latency testing.[27,39]

Exacerbation of Neuropsychological Deficits by Other Factors Underlying Childhood SDB

Abnormal behavioral alterations associated with SDB might be modified or directly caused by other sleep disorders, such as coexistent periodic limb movement disorder.[41] In children with SDB displaying deficits of cognition, school performance, or behavioral functioning, there may be additive roles played by race,[28,42–44] decreased time in bed,[25,43] and low SES,[28,42,44,45] at least in part because of

the association between obesity and low SES.[42] Markers of inflammation and increased cardiovascular risk may point to 1 mechanism related to decreased cognitive function associated with OSAS,[46] seen also in children who are obese. BMI correlated with abnormal cognitive function in pediatric SDB,[42,45,47] although OSAS was found to be an independent risk factor for cognitive deficits. Finally, in 2 studies examining brain function, neuronal injury of the brain[28] and altered cerebral blood flow[48] were found in children who had SDB compared with normal controls and were associated with behavior and cognitive problems. These findings indicate the possibility of preexisting medical problems causing the development of OSAS or, alternatively, OSAS causing brain injury. Therefore, studies showing improved cognition and behavior after treatment of SDB are 1 key in the determination of causality (see the following discussion).

Neuropsychological and Cognitive Deficits in Children Who Have SDB Improve After Treatment

In the previous guideline, there were few before-and-after treatment studies of pediatric SDB focusing on objectively measured cognitive problems. In the last 10 years, 19 studies have examined changes in behavior and/or cognition after surgical treatment of OSAS. The majority of investigations demonstrated agreement about posttreatment improvement of behavior, quality of life (QoL), hyperactivity, ADHD, and impulsivity (Table 10). The exception was 1 study of exercise treatment (level IV),[49] in which snoring improved in obese children but behavior and sleepiness did not. Most studies used subjective questionnaire reports. Excessive daytime sleepiness improved in 1 study that measured this factor, as did depression, sleep quality, and aggressive behavior. Since

publication of the last guideline, 3 additional studies have demonstrated improved cognitive function (by using objective measurement) after treatment of OSAS, including measures of general intelligence, attention, memory, and analytic thinking, including level II,[26] level III,[50] and level IV[37] studies (Table 10). Of concern, however, is that some recent articles suggest that certain deficits of cognition measured by using objective testing may not improve to a large extent after treatment of childhood OSAS. Language, IQ, and executive function did not improve significantly in a well-designed, controlled study of 92 children (level II).[30] General intelligence in at-risk populations improved in 1 study (level III),[50] but phonologic processes and verbal fluency did not improve to normal (level III[50] and level IV[51]). QoL increases after treatment.[37,52–58] Three studies demonstrated long-term (≥1 year) behavioral or QoL improvements.[37,52,53] The majority of these studies suggest that in developing children who are dependent on executive function, cognition, and behavioral skills for daily function and school performance, treatment of childhood SDB has benefits.

Conclusion

In summary, these studies suggest that, in developing children, early diagnosis and treatment of pediatric OSAS may improve a child's long-term cognitive and social potential and school performance. These findings imply that the earlier a child is treated for OSAS, the higher the trajectory for academic and, therefore, economic success, but research is needed to support that implication. There is demonstrated benefit in terms of behavior, attention, and social interactions, as well as likely improvement in cognitive abilities with

TABLE 9 Behavioral Abnormalities Associated With Pediatric SDB

Type of Deficit	Source	Level	No.	Test Conditions
Hyperactivity and/or ADHD	Chervin et al[236]	IV	8101	Hyperactivity generally measured by using parent questionnaire
	Chervin et al[40]			
	Galland et al[237]			
	Golan et al[239]			
	Gottlieb et al[213]			
	Johnson and Roth[45]			
	LeBourgeois et al[230]			
	Mitchell and Kelly[240]			
	Owens et al[189]			
	Roemmich et al[191]			
	Urschitz et al[229]			
	Montgomery-Downs et al[44]	III	1010	Survey data
	Chervin et al[37]	I	105	ADHD assessed by using psychiatric interview and validated instrument
Somatization, depression	Galland et al[237]	IV	205	
	Mitchell and Kelly[240]			
	Mitchell and Kelly[241]			
	Rudnick and Mitchell[242]			
	Suratt et al[43]	III	114	
	O'Brien et al[24]	I	118	
Behavior problems, general	Goldstein et al[55]	IV	1946	Behavior generally measured by using parent questionnaire
	Goldstein et al[243]			
	Hogan et al[48]			
	Li et al[238]			
	Mitchell and Kelly[241]			
	Mulvaney et al[32]			
	Owens et al[189]			
	Roemmich et al[191]			
	Rosen et al[244]			
	Rudnick and Mitchell[242]			
	Tran et al[58]			
	Wei et al[245]			
Aggression, oppositional and social problems	Chervin et al[246]	IV	4407	
	Gottlieb et al[213]			
	Galland et al[237]			
	Mitchell and Kelly[240]			
	Mulvaney et al[32]			
	O'Brien et al[24]	I	118	
Excessive daytime sleepiness	Goodwin et al[212]	IV	9729	Sleepiness measured by using questionnaire
	Perez-Chada et al[220]			
	Shin et al[47]			
	Urschitz et al[229]			
	Johnson and Roth[45]			
	Gozal et al[27]	II	92	Sleepiness measured objectively by multiple sleep latency testing on PSG
	Chervin et al[37]	I	105	Sleepiness measured objectively by multiple sleep latency testing on PSG
Anxiety	O'Brien et al[24]	I	118	

the treatment of pediatric OSAS. However, more long-term studies are needed. The risks of treatment depend on the type of treatment but include risk of surgery, risk of medication, nonadherence to therapy, and cost.

The risks of not treating children who have OSAS include potentially affecting the child's trajectory of developmental gains dependent on intelligence, executive function, and proper social interactions, ultimately lowering lifetime academic and social achievements. Therefore, the benefit of treating childhood OSAS outweighs the risk where treatment is feasible.

Areas for Future Research

- Further research is required to determine which domains of cognitive function will improve with treatment of OSAS. Reversibility of cognitive deficits associated with OSAS must be adjusted for the confounding effects of age, length of symptoms, SES, BMI, sleep duration, environment, and race and ethnicity.

Cardiovascular Effects of OSAS

A total of 24 studies related to cardiovascular effects of OSAS in childhood were identified since the last review. The levels of evidence were III and IV.

In a retrospective, level IV study of 271 clinical cases, only 1 child, who had congenital heart disease, had signs of cardiac failure preoperatively, and other cases had no evidence of left or right ventricular hypertrophy.[59] However, studies using more sophisticated, prospective techniques have found subclinical evidence of cardiac dysfunction. These studies are described in Table 11. Although postoperative adenotonsillectomy (AT) cardiac complications are rare (level IV),[59] left and right ventricular hypertrophy is significantly associated with postoperative respiratory complications (level III),[60] supporting the recommendation in the current and the previous guidelines that children who have cardiac abnormalities be monitored as inpatients postoperatively.

Blood pressure (BP) has also been shown to be affected by OSAS in children. There were 9 recent level III or IV studies, most of which showed a correlation between the presence/

TABLE 10 Cognitive, Behavioral, and QoL Abnormalities Improved After Treatment of Pediatric SBD

Deficit Measured	Source	Level	No.	Abnormalities Improved After SDB Treatment
Cognition/IQ	Chervin et al[37]	I	105	Attention measured on continuous performance test improved significantly after treatment
	Montgomery-Downs et al[50]	III	38	General conceptual ability improved (verbal fluency did not improve)
	Friedman et al[26]	II	59	Auditory-visual integration, auditory-motor memory, short-term memory, retention, analytic thinking, IQ/mental processing, attention all improved
Hyperactivity and/or ADHD	Galland et al[237] Li et al[238] Mitchell and Kelly[240] Mitchell and Kelly[241] Roemmich et al[191]	IV	247	Hyperactivity and/or diagnosis of ADHD improved
	Chervin et al[37]	I	105	Long-term improvement in hyperactivity
Somatization, depression	Galland et al[237] Mitchell and Kelly[240] Mitchell and Kelly[241]	IV	153	All showed improvement in depression and/or somatization
Behavior problems, general	Goldstein et al[55] Goldstein et al[243] Hogan et al[48] Li et al[238] Roemmich et al[191] Tran et al[58] Wei et al[245] Mitchell et al[53] Davis et al[49]	IV	450	All showed behavior improvement except Davis et al[49] Long-term behavior improvement in Mitchell et al[53]
Aggression, oppositional, and social problems	Galland et al[237] Mitchell and Kelly[240]	IV	113	Improvement in abnormal social behavior and aggression
Excessive daytime sleepiness	Chervin et al[37]	I	105	Sleepiness improved by 1 min, as measured by using multiple sleep latency testing on PSG
QoL	Colen et al[52] Constantin et al[54] Goldstein et al[55] Sohn et al[56] Silva and Leite[57] Tran et al[58]	IV	787	Includes disease-specific and emotional QoL[58] Long-term improvements ≥1 y[52-53]
	Chervin et al[37]	I	105	Long-term improvements at 1 y
Sleep quality	Constantin et al[54] Wei et al[245]	IV	590	Improved in both studies

severity of OSAS and indices of elevated BP (Table 12).

In a study by Kaditis et al,[61] overnight changes in brain natriuretic peptide levels were large in children who had an apnea hypopnea index (AHI) ≥5/hour when compared with those with milder OSAS and with controls (level III). This finding suggests the presence of nocturnal cardiac strain in children who have moderate to severe OSAS.

Two studies evaluated brain oxygenation and cerebral artery blood flow. Khadra et al[62] reported that male gender, arousal index, and amount of non–rapid eye movement sleep were associated with diminished cerebral oxygenation, whereas increasing mean arterial pressure, age, oxygen saturation (SpO_2), and amount of rapid eye movement sleep were associated with augmented cerebral oxygenation (level III). Hogan et al[48] found

a decrease in middle cerebral artery velocity postoperatively in patients treated for OSAS, whereas control subjects showed a slight increase over time (level IV).

Three studies evaluated autonomic variability in children who have OSAS. Constantin et al[63] reported resolution of tachycardia and diminished pulse rate variability after AT in children who had OSAS (diagnosis of OSAS based on oximetry plus questionnaire data) (level IV). Deng et al[64] studied heart rate variability and determined that heart rate chaos was modulated by OSAS as well as by sleep state (level IV). In a study of 28 children who had OSAS, O'Brien and Gozal[65] found evidence of altered autonomic nervous system regulation, as evidenced by increased sympathetic vascular reactivity, during wakefulness in these children (level III). These studies all suggest that OSAS places stress on the autonomic system.

In summary, a large number of studies, albeit primarily level III, found that cardiac changes occur in the presence of OSAS, with an effect on both the right and left ventricles. OSAS in childhood also has an effect on both systolic and diastolic BP. In addition, several studies suggest that childhood OSAS can affect autonomic regulation, brain oxygenation, and cerebral blood flow. These studies suggest that childhood OSAS may jeopardize long-term cardiovascular health.[66]

The association between left ventricular remodeling and 24-hour BP highlighted the role of SDB in increasing cardiovascular morbidity.

Areas for Future Research

- How reversible, after treatment, are cardiovascular changes in children who have OSAS?

- What are the long-term effects of OSAS on the cardiovascular system?

TABLE 11 Structural and Functional Cardiac Abnormalities in Children Who Have OSAS

Source	Level	No.	Findings
Left-sided cardiac dysfunction			
Amin et al[247]	III	28 OSAS 19 PS	Abnormalities of LV geometry in 39% of OSAS vs 15% of PS; OSAS associated with increased LV mass
Amin et al[248]	III	48 OSAS 15 PS	Dose-dependent decrease in LV diastolic function with increased severity of SDB
Right-sided cardiac dysfunction			
Duman et al[249]	III	21 children, ATH; 21 controls	Higher RV myocardial performance index in patient with adenotonsillar hypertrophy than in controls; this decreased significantly after AT, along with symptoms of OSAS
Ugur et al[250]	III	29 OSAS 26 PS	Improved RV diastolic function after AT, with postoperative values similar to controls
Biventricular cardiac dysfunction			
James et al[59]	IV	271	Case review of ECG and chest radiography results found only 1 case of cardiac failure, which occurred in a child who had congenital heart disease; most other cases showed no abnormalities
Weber et al[251]	III	30 OSAS 10 controls	Increased RV diameter and area during both systole and diastole; reduced LV diastolic diameter and ejection fraction

ATH, adenotonsillar hypertrophy; LV, left ventricle; PS, primary snoring; RV, right ventricle.

TABLE 12 BP in Children Who Have OSAS

Source	Level	No.	Findings
Kohyama et al[175]	IV	23 suspected OSAS	REM diastolic BP index correlated with AHI Age, BMI, and AHI were significant predictors of systolic BP index during REM
Kwok et al[66]	III	30 PS	Children with PS had increased daytime BP and reduced arterial distensibility
Leung et al[252]	III	96 suspected OSAS	Children with a higher AHI had higher wake systolic BP and sleep systolic and diastolic BP BMI, age, and desaturation index contributed to elevation of the diastolic BP during sleep, but only BMI contributed to the wake and sleeping systolic BP
Guilleminault et al[253]	III	Retrospective component: 301 suspected OSAS Prospective component: 78 OSAS	Some children who have OSAS have orthostatic hypotension
Li et al[176]	III	306 community sample	OSAS was associated with elevated daytime and nocturnal BP
Amin et al[177]	III	140 suspected OSAS	OSAS associated with an increase in morning BP surge, BP load, and 24-h BP. BP parameters predicted changes in left ventricular wall thickness
Amin et al[254]	III	39 OSAS 21 PS	OSAS was associated with 24-h BP dysregulation AHI, Spo2, and arousal contribute to abnormal BP control independent of obesity
Enright et al[255]	III	239 community sample	Obesity, sleep efficiency, and RDI were independently associated with elevated systolic BP
Kaditis et al[174]	IV	760 community sample	No difference in morning BP between habitual snorers and nonhabitual snorers

PS, primary snoring; REM, rapid eye movement.

Growth

The section on obesity contains a detailed review of obesity and OSAS, including the relationship between OSAS and the metabolic syndrome. The previous guideline documented many studies showing a relationship between OSAS and growth, and an increase in growth parameters after treatment of SDB by AT; this outcome has been confirmed by a number of more recent studies (as discussed in the recent meta-analysis by Bonuck et al[67]). In a confirmation of previous reports,[68,69] Selimoğlu et al[70] found a decreased level of serum insulin-like growth factor-I in children who have OSAS, which increased significantly 6 months after AT (level III).

Inflammation

Since the publication of the 2002 AAP guideline, there has been growing research on the role of OSAS in systemic inflammation. It has been postulated that OSAS results in intermittent hypoxemia, leading to production of reactive oxygen species. In addition, the hypoxemia and arousals from sleep lead to sympathetic activation. These factors may trigger inflammation or exacerbate obesity-related inflammation. However, the data on OSAS and markers of systemic inflammation in children are scarce and contradictory.

Eight studies (level II–III) measured levels of C-reactive protein (CRP) in children who had OSAS. Four studies (including 2 from the same center) showed no relationship between CRP and OSAS,[71–74] whereas 4 studies (2 from the same center) did show a relationship.[46,75–77] Part of the discrepancy between studies may be attributable to the varying proportions of obese subjects (because obesity is associated with high CRP levels) and varied age of subjects and definitions of OSAS in the different studies. Some studies controlled for obesity and degree of OSAS, whereas others did not. The studies showing a positive relationship indicated that OSAS was associated with elevated

CRP levels only above a certain threshold of severity. Thus, the relationship between OSAS and CRP seems to be complex and is affected by obesity and severity of OSAS.

A few level II and III studies have evaluated other circulating markers of inflammation in children who have OSAS. Two studies showed no difference in circulating intercellular adhesion molecule-1 between patients with OSAS and controls.[71,73] A single study found elevated p-selectin (a measure of platelet activation) in children who had OSAS compared with controls.[73] A single study showed elevated levels of interferon-γ in children who had OSAS.[74] One study showed increased interleukin (IL)-6 and lower IL-10 in those with OSAS,[78] whereas another study did not.[74] Another study reported no difference in cytokines IL-1β, IL-2, IL-4, IL-8, IL-12, and granulocyte macrophage colony-stimulating factor levels between children who had OSAS and controls.[74] Data on tumor necrosis factor-α are conflicting,[74,79] and differences in levels may be related to tumor necrosis factor-α gene polymorphisms.[80]

A pathology-based study found increased glucocorticoid receptors in adenotonsillar tissue from children who had OSAS compared with tissue from children who experienced chronic throat infections (level III)[81]; another study from the same group found elevated leukotriene receptors (level IV).[82] These findings provide a theoretical construct for the potential utility of antiinflammatory drugs as treatment of children who have OSAS, although possibly not for those who have already undergone AT.

In summary, the data on CRP are conflicting, but it may be that CRP levels increase above a certain threshold of severity of OSAS. Further research involving large samples of subjects who have varying degrees of OSAS severity,

with results controlled for BMI and age, are needed. There are too few data on other circulating markers of systemic inflammation to enable any recommendations.

Areas for Future Research

- Larger studies, stratified for the severity of OSAS and controlled for obesity, are required to determine whether OSAS is associated with systemic inflammation. If so, what are the long-term sequelae of this inflammation? Are inflammatory biomarkers potential good outcome measurements for OSAS treatment studies? Do they correlate with clinical outcomes or long-term prognosis?

METHODS OF DIAGNOSIS

The previous guideline discussed the diagnosis of OSAS in great detail. On the basis of published evidence at the time, it was concluded that the positive and predictive value of history and physical examination for the diagnosis of OSAS was 65% and 46%, respectively; that is, no better than chance. It was therefore recommended that objective testing be used for the diagnosis of OSAS. An evaluation of the literature regarding nocturnal pulse oximetry, video recording, nap PSG, and ambulatory PSG suggested that these methods tended to be helpful if results were positive but had a poor predictive value if results were negative. Thus, children who had negative study results should be referred for more comprehensive testing. These recommendations were based on only a few studies, most of which had a low level of evidence. Furthermore, it was recognized that these techniques were of limited use in evaluating the severity of OSAS (which is important in determining management, such as whether outpatient surgery can be performed safely). In

addition, the cost efficacy of these screening techniques had not been evaluated and would depend, in part, on how many patients eventually required full PSG. Since the publication of the initial guideline, there have been a number of new studies, but few are level I or II. Because few of the studies cited here included data that would enable calculation of overall sensitivity and specificity or positive and negative predictive values, an overall table could not be provided. For this section, PSG was considered the gold standard for diagnosis of OSAS.

Utility of History Alone for the Diagnosis of OSAS

Several level IV studies evaluated the use of history alone for the diagnosis of OSAS. Preutthipan et al[83] found overall poor sensitivity and specificity when evaluating various historical factors. The Pediatric Sleep Questionnaire published by Chervin et al[84] performed slightly better than other published questionnaires, with a sensitivity of 0.85 and a specificity of 0.87 by using a set cutoff. A follow-up study by the same group showed a sensitivity of 78% and a specificity of 72% for PSG-defined OSAS.[85] However, this is still a relatively low sensitivity and specificity for clinical purposes. By using this instrument, the same group also found that negative answers to only 2 questions on the Pediatric Sleep Questionnaire were helpful in identifying patients who had normal PSG results.[86] Taken together, the overall performance of questionnaire tools seems to support their use more as a screening tool than as a diagnostic tool, such that a negative score would be unlikely to mislabel a child with OSAS as being healthy, but a positive score would be unlikely to accurately diagnose a particular child with certainty.

Utility of Clinical Evaluation for the Diagnosis of OSAS

Similar to the data presented in the previous guideline, most studies found that clinical evaluation was not predictive of OSAS on PSG. Godwin et al[15] performed a large (N = 480), population-based study of 6- to 11-year-old children. The study included use of a standardized history, some clinical parameters, and ambulatory, full PSG (level II). They concluded that the sensitivity of any individual or combined clinical symptoms was poor. Certain parameters, such as snoring, excessive daytime sleepiness, and learning problems, had a high specificity.

In a level III study, van Someren et al[87] compared history and clinical examination by a pediatrician or otolaryngologist with abbreviated PSG (video recording, oximetry, and measurement of snoring). Both the sensitivity and specificity of the clinician's impression of moderate/severe OSAS were low (59% and 73%, respectively). In a similar number of cases, the clinicians underestimated (17%) and overestimated (16%) study results.

In a level III study, it was shown that waist circumference z score had a statistically significant but clinically poor correlation with symptoms of OSAS (R = 0.32, P = .006); BMI z score did not correlate with symptoms.[88]

Radiologic Studies

Several studies, all level III or IV, evaluated the utility of radiologic examinations in addition to clinical factors in establishing the diagnosis of OSAS (Table 13). Overall, these studies showed that the presence of airway narrowing on a lateral neck radiograph increased the probability of predicting OSAS on PSG. Cephalometric studies tended to show a small mandible in patients who had OSAS

compared with controls, although a study using an MRI did not confirm this.[89] None of the cephalometric studies provided sensitivity and specificity or positive and negative predictive values. Table 13 simplifies the cephalometric findings for the purpose of presentation. A level I study indicated that acoustic pharyngometry may be a useful screening technique for OSAS in older children, but approximately one-half of the children could not cooperate well with the testing.[90] One uncontrolled study (level IV) showed that nasal resistance, as measured by using rhinometry, had a high sensitivity and specificity for predicting polysomnographic OSAS.[91] This technique warrants further study and validation.

Snoring Evaluation

Two level IV studies found a weak association between objective snoring characteristics and the presence/severity of OSAS that was insufficient to assist in clinical diagnosis.[92,93]

Cardiovascular Parameters

Studies have evaluated the utility of screening tests based on heart rate or other vascular factors in predicting OSAS (Table 14). These studies ranged from studies of pulse rate alone to more sophisticated (and, hence, more expensive or time-consuming) studies, such as analyses of heart rate variability, pulse transit time, and peripheral arterial tonometry. Studies were level II through IV. Overall, the studies found changes in cardiovascular variables in children who had OSAS but with varying sensitivities and specificities. Thus, some of these measures may potentially be useful screening tests in the future if combined with other modalities that would increase the sensitivity and specificity but cannot

be recommended for clinical use at this point.

Nocturnal Oximetry

The previous AAP guideline, on the basis of a single study by Brouillette et al,[94] indicated that nocturnal pulse oximetry could provide an accurate screen for OSAS if the result was positive but that full PSG was needed if the oximetry result was negative. A need for further research in this area was indicated. Four additional studies were identified for the current report. Two of these did not compare oximetry versus PSG and therefore will not be discussed further.[95,96]

A follow-up study (level II) from the same group as the previous report by Brouillette et al[94] used overnight oximetry, primarily obtained in the home, to develop a scoring algorithm.[97] The subjects' median age was 4 years. The oximetry score correlated with the AHI obtained from PSG as well as with the presence of postoperative complications. However, the positive predictive value of oximetry for major postoperative respiratory compromise was only 13%. Of note, 80% of the 223 children had normal, inconclusive, or technically unsatisfactory oximetry results and were therefore referred for either repeat oximetry or PSG. In contrast, Kirk et al[98] compared overnight home oximetry (by using a system with an automated oximetry analysis algorithm that provided a desaturation index) with laboratory PSG in 58 children aged ≥4 years who had suspected OSAS (level III). They found poor agreement between the desaturation index on the basis of oximetry and the PSG-determined AHI. The sensitivity of oximetry for the identification of moderate OSAS (AHI >5/hour) was 67%, and specificity was 60%. The oximetry algorithm tended to overestimate the AHI at low levels and underestimate at high

TABLE 13 Relationship Between Airway Measurements and OSAS

Clinical Evaluation	Sleep Evaluation	Airway Evaluation	Source	Level	No.	Findings
Standardized history, clinical examination	PSG	Lateral neck radiography	Xu et al[256]	IV	50	Combinations of different predictor variables resulted in positive and negative predictor values ranging from 70% to 80%
Clinical examination	PSG	Lateral neck radiography	Jain and Sahni[257]	IV	40	Degree of OSAS correlated with adenoid size on radiography but not with tonsillar size on clinical examination
Clinical examination	PSG	Lateral neck radiography	Li et al[258]	IV	35	Tonsillar–pharyngeal ratio on radiography correlated with AHI but not clinical tonsil size. Clinical tonsil size did not correlate with AHI. For a ratio of 0.479, the sensitivity and specificity in predicting moderately severe OSAS (AHI >10/h) was 96% and 82%, respectively
NA	PSG	Cephalometry	Kawashima et al[259]	III	15 OSAS 30 controls	Evidence of retrognathia in OSAS group
Clinical examination	Ambulatory abbreviated recordings	Cephalometry	Kawashima et al[260]	III	38 OSAS 31 controls	OSAS: retrognathia, long facies in those OSAS subjects who had large tonsils
NA	None	Cephalometry	Kikuchi et al[261]	IV	29 suspected OSAS 41 controls	OSAS: long facies
Questionnaire	None	Cephalometry	Kulnis et al[262]	IV	28 snorers 28 controls	Snorers: retrognathia, shorter maxilla and cranial base
Standardized history	Nap PSG	Cephalometry	Zucconi et al[263]	III	26 snorers 26 controls	Snorers: retrognathia, decreased nasopharyngeal space
NA	PSG	MRI	Schiffman et al[89]	III	24 OSAS 24 controls	No difference in mandibular size between OSAS and controls
Clinical assessment of tonsillar size	Ambulatory cardiorespiratory recordings	Acoustic pharyngometry Cephalometry	Monahan et al[90]	I	203	Degree of OSAS correlated with airway size on pharyngometry but not with tonsillar size. Pharyngometric measures also correlated with mandibular length on cephalometry, only 78% of 8- to 11-y-old children could produce minimally acceptable data, and only 54% could produce high-quality data
Questionnaire, clinical examination	PSG	Rhinometry	Rizzi et al[91]	IV	73	Nasal resistance of 0.59 Pa/cm^3/s had a positive predictive value of 97% and a negative predictive value of 86%

levels. The authors concluded that oximetry alone was not adequate for the diagnosis of OSAS. On the basis of these limited studies, it seems as if oximetry alone is insufficient for the diagnosis of OSAS because of the high rate of inconclusive test results and the poor sensitivity and specificity compared with PSG, probably, in part, because children may have OSAS that results in arousals and sleep fragmentation but little desaturation. In addition, children tend to move a lot during sleep, which can result in movement artifact.

Ambulatory PSG

The term "ambulatory PSG" is used for unattended sleep studies conducted in the home. Frequently, ambulatory PSG consists of cardiorespiratory recordings alone. Although the use of ambulatory PSG is considered appropriate under certain circumstances in adults,[99] there is a paucity of studies evaluating ambulatory PSG in children. Zucconi et al[100] evaluated a home portable system comprising measurements of airflow (by using thermistry), snoring, chest and abdominal wall movements, electrocardiography (ECG), position, and oximetry (level II). However, the portable system was used in the sleep laboratory for the purpose of the study. A small sample of 12 children, 3 to 6 years of age, underwent routine PSG and in-laboratory portable testing on a consecutive night with the portable system. The portable system had good sensitivity for detecting a respiratory distress index (RDI) >5/hour (78% with automated scoring; 89% with human scoring) but a specificity of zero. Rosen et al[19] reported on a study of 664 children aged 8 to 11 years who underwent abbreviated ambulatory study (by using inductance plethysmography, oximetry, heart rate, and position) (level III). Of these home studies, 94% were considered technically adequate. A subsample of 55 children also underwent full laboratory PSG. Few details were given regarding this subsample. However, it was reported that the ambulatory studies had a sensitivity

TABLE 14 Utility of Cardiovascular Parameters in Predicting OSAS

Measure	Sleep Evaluation	Source	Level	No.	Findings
Pulse rate	Oximetry	Constantin et al[63]	IV	25 OSAS	Pulse rate decreases in children who have OSAS after AT
Pulse rate	Home cardiorespiratory studies	Noehren et al[264]	III	5 OSAS 20 controls	Pulse rate changes poor at detecting differences between respiratory events and movements, and between central and obstructive apneas
Heart rate variability	PSG	Deng et al[64]	IV	34 OSAS 18 controls	Heart rate chaos intensity had sensitivity of 72% and specificity of 81% for OSAS
Pulse transit time	PSG	Katz et al[265]	III	24 SDB 10 controls	Depending on the severity of the event, 80%–91% of obstructive respiratory events were associated with pulse transit time changes. However, pulse transit time changes also occurred with spontaneous arousals from sleep
Heart rate, pulse transit time	PSG	Foo et al[266] (similar data published in Foo and Lim[267])	III	15 suspected OSAS	Pulse rate had 70% sensitivity and 89% specificity, and pulse transit time had 75% sensitivity and 92% specificity in identifying obstructive events
Peripheral arterial tonometry	PSG	Tauman et al[268]	II	40 OSAS 20 controls	Peripheral arterial tonometry had sensitivity of 95% and specificity of 35% in identifying EEG arousals

of 88% and specificity of 98% in diagnosing a laboratory PSG–based AHI >5/hour. It is not clear why the results of this study were so different from that of Zucconi et al but may possibly be related to the older age of the subjects. Goodwin et al[101] used a full PSG system, including EEG measurements, in the unattended home environment in 157 children aged 5 to 12 years (level IV). Adequate data were obtained from 91% of subjects on the first attempt and 97% when the test was repeated if needed. Data were reported as excellent in 61% of cases and good in 36%. In a small subsample of 5 subjects, data were similar to those with laboratory PSG. This study shows the feasibility of performing unattended full ambulatory PSG in older children, but results may not be the same for young children. In summary, ambulatory PSG seems to be technically feasible in school-aged children, although data are not available for younger children. Studies of differing levels, and studying different age groups, found widely discrepant specificities for diagnosing moderate OSAS. Clearly, additional studies are needed.

Nocturnal PSG

Nocturnal, attended, laboratory PSG is considered the gold standard for diagnosis of OSAS because it provides an objective, quantitative evaluation of disturbances in respiratory and sleep patterns. A recent review describes some of the relationships between PSG and sequelae of OSAS (see "Pediatric Issues" section in Redline et al[102]). PSG allows patients to be stratified in terms of severity, which helps determine which children are at risk for sequelae (thus alerting pediatricians to screen for complications of OSAS); which children are at risk for postoperative complications and would, therefore, benefit from inpatient observation postoperatively; and which children are at high risk of persistence of OSAS postoperatively, who may then need postoperative PSG to assess the need for further treatment (eg, CPAP).

Adult patients may sleep poorly the first time they are in a sleep laboratory because of anxiety, the unfamiliar environment, and the attached sensors. This "first night effect" can lead to altered sleep architecture and possible underestimation of the severity of OSAS. Five studies (levels I–IV) evaluated the night-to-night variability of PSG in children[101,103–106]; in one of these articles,[101] only a small subsample had night-to-night variability evaluated (Table 15). The time difference between PSGs varied from 24

hours to 4 weeks. Although some of the studies showed minor differences in respiratory parameters from night to night, the studies suggest that few children would have been clinically misclassified on the basis of a single night's PSG. Thus, 1 night of PSG seems to be adequate to establish the diagnosis of OSAS. All studies showed significant differences in sleep architecture from night to night. Therefore, research studies evaluating sleep architecture would require >1 night of PSG. For consistency, it is recommended that PSG be performed and scored by using the pediatric criteria from the American Academy of Sleep Medicine scoring manual.[107]

Other Tests

The shape of the maximal flow-volume loop on pulmonary function testing has been used to attempt to screen for OSAS in adults. Young children cannot perform standard maximal flow-volume loops. One small study of 10 subjects evaluated the relationship between tidal breathing flow-volume loops and PSG (level III).[108] The sensitivity was 37.5% and specificity was 100%, indicating that this method is of limited utility in screening for OSAS.

Two studies by the same group evaluated whether urinary/serum

TABLE 15 Night-to-Night Variability in Polysomnographic Respiratory Parameters

Time Between Evaluations	Source	Level	No.	Findings
1–4 wk	Katz et al[103]	I	30 suspected OSAS	No significant group difference in the AHI between nights. Those with the highest AHI had the most variability. However, no patient was reclassified as primary snoring versus OSAS on the basis of the second study
7–50 d	Goodwin et al[101]	IV	12	Used unattended home PSG. Studies were successful in 10. No difference in AHI between nights in this small sample
Consecutive nights	Scholle et al[105]	III	131 OSAS	No difference in AHI between nights
Consecutive nights	Li et al[104]	III	46 obese 44 controls	AHI was greater on night 2 The first night would have correctly identified 11 (85%) of the 13 cases of OSAS if the worst obstructive apnea index over any single night was used as the criterion. However, the 2 cases that would have been missed by the single PSG had only borderline OSAS
Consecutive nights	Verhulst et al [106]	I	70 suspected OSAS	First night classified OSAS correctly in 91% of subjects, if the worst AHI over any night was used as the diagnostic criterion. All but 1 of those who were missed had an AHI <5/h

proteinomic analysis could be used to screen for the presence of OSAS. In a level I study of urinary proteinomics, the investigators found that a combination of urinary proteins could predict OSAS with a sensitivity of 95% and a specificity of 100%.[109] Similarly, in a level III study from the same group, the investigators found that a different set of proteins could be used to identify 15 of 20 children who had OSAS and 18 of 20 children who were snorers.[110] The authors note that they studied a highly selected population matched for age, gender, ethnicity, BMI, and inflammatory respiratory disorders, such as allergic rhinitis or asthma. Thus, this technique, although promising, requires further validation in typical clinical cohorts and duplication in another laboratory.

Summary

In summary, few of the screening techniques mentioned here have a sensitivity and specificity high enough to be relied on for clinical diagnosis. In addition, it should be noted that many of the studies used an AHI >5/hour when determining

sensitivity and specificity, although an AHI >1.5/hour is considered statistically abnormal in children.[111–113] Few studies used large study samples, and few were blinded. As a result, some of the studies of screening techniques resulted in contradictory evidence. On a pragmatic level, however, it is realized that current infrastructure is inadequate to provide PSG for all children with suspected OSAS. Therefore, the use of screening tests may be better than no objective testing at all. However, clinicians using these tests should familiarize themselves with the sensitivity and specificity of the test used and consider proceeding to full PSG if the test result is inconclusive.

Areas for Future Research

- Well-designed, large, controlled, blinded, multicenter, prospective studies are required to provide more definitive answers regarding the utility of screening tests for the diagnosis of OSAS. In particular, additional studies of ambulatory PSG in children of varying ages are needed.

TREATMENT OF OSAS

AT

Adenotonsillar hypertrophy is the most common cause of OSAS, and AT continues to be the primary treatment for this issue. Adenoidectomy alone may not be sufficient for children who have OSAS because it does not address oropharyngeal obstruction secondary to tonsillar hyperplasia. The previous guideline stated the importance of AT as the primary treatment for OSAS in children. No new literature is available to suggest a change to these recommendations. Table 3 in the guideline lists relative contraindications to AT. Note that whereas a submucus cleft palate is a relative contraindication to adenoidectomy, a partial adenoidectomy may be performed in such patients. However, postoperative PSG should be performed to ensure that OSAS has resolved.

AT in most children is associated with a low complication rate. Minor complications include pain and poor oral intake. More severe complications may include bleeding, infection, anesthetic complications, respiratory decompensation, velopharyngeal incompetence, subglottic stenosis, and, rarely, death.

Tarasiuk et al found that health care utilization costs were 226% higher in children with OSAS before diagnosis compared with control children[114] and that health care costs decreased by one-third in children who underwent AT, whereas there was no change in health care costs in control children or children who had untreated OSAS[115] (both studies were level IV).

Partial Tonsillectomy

Several newer techniques for tonsillectomy have gained increasing use since publication of the last guideline. The primary goal of these techniques is to decrease the morbidity associated with traditional tonsillectomy methods. One such technique is partial tonsillectomy (PT), in which a portion of tonsil tissue is left to cover the musculature of the tonsillar fossa. Multiple studies, ranging in level from II to IV, have evaluated recovery times and adverse effects from PT. However, only a few small, lower-level studies have specifically looked at the effect of PT on OSAS. In a level IV study, Tunkel et al[116] evaluated 14 children who underwent PSG before and after PT and found a cure rate (AHI $\leq$1/hour) of 93% postoperatively. In a retrospective study (level IV), Mangiardi et al[117] compared 15 children who underwent PT (of 45 eligible) with 15 children who underwent total tonsillectomy. This study had a number of technical limitations. A variety of techniques (overnight laboratory PSG, nap sleep studies, and limited-channel home sleep studies) were performed in subjects preoperatively, and limited-channel home sleep studies were performed in all patients postoperatively. These different monitoring techniques would be expected to provide varying results.[118,119] In both surgical groups, the authors found a higher rate of postoperative OSAS than typically reported in the literature, with a median (range) AHI of 7.5 $\pm$ 4.3/hour in the PT group and 8.8 $\pm$ 4.7/hour in the total tonsillectomy group (not significant).

PT carries an increased risk of regrowth of the tonsils, which occurred in 0.5% to 16% of patients in studies of varied duration. Celenk et al[120] performed a retrospective review of 42 children 1 to 10 years of age who underwent PT via radiofrequency ablation for symptoms of OSAS (level IV). Follow-up ranged from 6 to 32 months, with a mean follow-up of 14 months. They found tonsillar regrowth on physical examination in 7

(16.6%) patients; 5 of these were symptomatic and underwent completion tonsillectomy. The time frame for occurrence of regrowth ranged from 1 to 18 months. The authors noted that some episodes of regrowth occurred after episodes of tonsillitis. Zagólski[121] evaluated 374 children who underwent PT on the basis of clinical symptoms of OSAS (level IV). Patients underwent otolaryngology examinations annually for 4 years. Twenty-seven (7.2%) children had tonsillar regrowth; of those, 20 had clinical symptoms and, therefore, underwent completion tonsillectomy. Regrowth of the palatine tonsils was observed at a mean period of 3.8 years, suggesting the need for long-term follow-up. In a multicenter, retrospective case series of 870 children with a mean follow-up of 1.2 years, Solares et al[122] found an incidence of tonsillar regrowth of 0.5% (level III). The methods and criteria for assessing regrowth were not detailed in this article but may have been a clinical follow-up at 1 and 6 months postoperatively. The lower rate of regrowth in this study compared with the other studies may have been related to the shorter follow-up period. Eviatar et al[123] performed a long-term (10–14 years), retrospective, telephone survey comparing 33 children who had undergone PT for symptoms of OSAS versus 16 children who underwent tonsillectomy; children undergoing concomitant adenoidectomy were excluded (level III). They found similar rates of parent-reported snoring in the 2 groups (6.1% for PT, 12.5% for total tonsillectomy; not significant) but no cases of OSAS on the basis of symptoms.

PT for the treatment of adenotonsillar hypertrophy has shown some success in decreasing immediate postoperative pain. Derkay et al[124] prospectively evaluated 300 children undergoing

either PT or total tonsillectomy for adenotonsillar hypertrophy (level II). They found that children in the PT group had an earlier return to normal activity and were 3 times more likely not to need pain medication at 3 days compared with the total tonsillectomy group. There was no difference between groups in median return to a normal diet (3.0 vs 3.5 days). In a level III, retrospective study of 243 children undergoing PT versus 107 undergoing total tonsillectomy, Koltai et al[125] found less pain and quicker return to a normal diet in children undergoing PT. In a level II study, Sobol et al[126] prospectively evaluated 74 children who had adenotonsillar hypertrophy scheduled for AT. Their results showed a resumption to normal diet 1.7 days earlier in the PT group compared with children undergoing total tonsillectomy. There was no significant difference in the resolution of pain or return to normal activities between the 2 groups, but there was increased intraoperative blood loss in the PT group.

In summary, there are no level I studies comparing PT with total tonsillectomy in the pediatric population. Additional data are needed regarding the efficacy of PT for OSAS, by using objective outcome measurements. There is possibility of tonsillar regrowth after PT, with studies showing varied rates of regrowth. These studies are all limited by lack of blinding, lack of objective measures to quantitate tonsillar regrowth, and lack of polysomnographic data relating tonsillar regrowth to OSAS. Some studies found that patients who undergo PT have less pain and quicker recovery during the first few days compared with children undergoing total tonsillectomy. However, PT may be associated with greater intraoperative blood loss, and there is a risk of recurrent infections in the tonsillar remnants.[120,121,123] At this point, data are insufficient to recommend any particular surgical technique for tonsillectomy over another in terms of OSAS. However, children undergoing PT should be monitored carefully long-term to ensure that symptoms of OSAS related to tonsillar regrowth do not occur, and families should be warned about the possibility of recurrence of OSAS.

Postoperative Management After AT

Tonsillectomy and adenoidectomy can be safely performed in the vast majority of children on an outpatient basis. Risk factors that increase the risk of postoperative complications include age <3 years, severe OSAS, presence of cardiac complications, failure to thrive, obesity, and presence of upper respiratory tract infection (URI). Although there have been numerous publications regarding postoperative complications since publication of the last guideline, there have been no data to suggest a change in the previous recommendations. Children with medical comorbidities such as craniofacial anomalies, genetic syndromes, and neuromuscular disease are also high risk; these special populations are not covered by this guideline.

An important advantage of the objective documentation of the severity of OSAS by using PSG should be the ability to predict the need for overnight hospital stay after AT on the basis of a higher risk of postoperative complications. Severe OSAS has been proposed as a criterion for inpatient observation; the current evidence to define severe OSAS is derived primarily from level III retrospective studies. Although considerable physiologic information regarding the respiratory pattern and gas exchange during sleep is available from an overnight PSG, the available studies

have focused primarily on the AHI and, to a lesser degree, the nadir of the Sp_{O_2}. Relevant studies are listed in Table 16. Studies varied with regard to the type of patients included (proportion of obese patients; patients who had craniofacial and genetic syndromes) and severity of OSAS. Although the definition of postoperative respiratory compromise varied, most studies required that an intervention (eg, supplemental oxygen, nasopharyngeal tube, CPAP, intubation) be performed. Most studies found a high rate of postoperative respiratory complications. Different studies showed different PSG predictive factors for postoperative complications, and few studies developed receiver operating characteristic curves.[127] Nevertheless, studies were fairly consistent in indicating that an Sp_{O_2} <80% and an AHI >24/hour were predictive of postoperative respiratory compromise. These criteria are more conservative than the recently published clinical practice guidelines from the American Academy of Otolaryngology–Head and Neck Surgery, which recommend that children who have an AHI ≥10/hour and/or an Sp_{O_2} nadir <80% be admitted for overnight observation after AT.[3]

It is difficult to provide exact PSG criteria for OSAS severity because these criteria will vary depending on the age of the child; additional comorbidities, such as obesity, asthma, or cardiac complications of OSAS; and other PSG criteria that have not been evaluated in the literature, such as the level of hypercapnia and the frequency of desaturation (compared with Sp_{O_2} nadir). Therefore, on the basis of published studies (Table 16), it is recommended that patients who have an Sp_{O_2} nadir <80% (either on preoperative PSG or during observation in the recovery room postoperatively) or an AHI ≥24/hour be

observed as inpatients postoperatively because they are at increased risk of postoperative respiratory compromise. In addition, on the basis of expert consensus, it is recommended that patients with significant hypercapnia on PSG (peak P_{CO_2} ≥60 mm Hg) be admitted postoperatively. Clinicians may decide to admit patients who have less severe PSG abnormalities on the basis of a constellation of risk factors (age, comorbidities, and additional PSG factors) on an individual basis.

Data regarding URIs were based on studies of children undergoing general anesthesia for a variety of procedures. The committee could not identify any studies related specifically to URIs and AT. In a large, level III study, Tait et al[128] evaluated 1078 children 1 month to 18 years of age who were undergoing an elective surgical procedure. The presence of a URI was diagnosed by using a parental questionnaire. Data regarding perioperative respiratory events were recorded. There were no differences between children who had active URIs, recent URIs (within 4 weeks), and asymptomatic children with respect to the incidences of laryngospasm and bronchospasm. However, children who had active and recent URIs had significantly more episodes of breath-holding, desaturation <90%, and overall adverse respiratory events than children who had no URIs. Independent risk factors for the development of adverse respiratory events in children who had active URIs included use of an endotracheal tube (in those <5 years of age), preterm birth, history of reactive airway disease, paternal smoking, surgery involving the airway, the presence of copious secretions, and nasal congestion. In a large level III study of 831 children undergoing surgery with a laryngeal mask airway, von Ungern-Sternberg et al[129]

TABLE 16 Relationship Between PSG Parameters and Postoperative Respiratory Complications

Source	Level	Type of Study	No.	Study Group	Age, y	Special Populations Included[a]	Findings
Hill et al[269]	III	Retrospective	83	AHI >10	≤18	Yes	Major respiratory complication in 5%; minor in 20% Only age <2 y (P < .01) and AHI >24 (P < .05) significantly predicted postoperative airway complications Complication rate only 4% if special populations were excluded AHI >24 predicted 63% of complications
Jaryszak et al[270]	III	Retrospective	151	Any child who had a PSG	Not stated	Yes	Respiratory complication rate was 15% Children with complications had higher AHI (32 vs 14) and lower SpO_2 nadir (72% vs 84%) compared with those without complications
Koomson et al[271]	III	Retrospective	85	AHI >5	Not stated	Yes	Postoperative desaturation in 28% More likely to desaturate postoperatively if PSG SpO_2 nadir <80%
Ma et al[272]	III	Retrospective	86	Any child who had a PSG	1–16	Yes	Postoperative desaturation in 7% No difference in AHI between those with and without postoperative desaturation (11.6 ± 4.5 vs 14.7 ± 16.6)
Sanders et al[273]	I	Prospective	61	61 children who had OSAS vs 21 who had tonsillitis	2–16	No	Respiratory complication rate was 28% Subjects with RDI ≥30 were more likely to have laryngospasm and desaturation At an RDI ≥20, OSAS was more likely to have breath-holding on induction
Schroeder et al[274]	III	Retrospective	53	Severe OSAS (AHI >25)	Not stated	Yes	43% required oxygen or PAP Note: an additional 17 children were electively kept intubated postoperatively
Shine et al[196]	III	Retrospective	26	Obese OSAS	2–17	Obese; other comorbidities not stated	46% had respiratory complications Those requiring intervention for respiratory problems had a lower SpO_2 (68 ± 20% vs 87 ± 18%) but no difference in RDI (27 ± 44 vs 15 ± 28) than those who did not require intervention By using univariate analysis, a preoperative SpO_2 <70% was associated with postoperative respiratory compromise, but no threshold was found for RDI
Ye et al[127]	III	Retrospective	327	AHI ≥5	4–14	No	11% had respiratory complications An AHI of 26 had 74% sensitivity and 92% specificity for predicting postoperative respiratory complications

[a] Special populations include children with genetic syndromes and craniofacial abnormalities.

compared children who had a URI within 2 weeks of surgery versus those without a URI; 27% of children had a recent URI. They found a doubling of the incidence of laryngospasm, bronchospasm, and oxygen desaturation intraoperatively and in the recovery room in the children who had recent URIs, although the overall incidence of these events was low. The risk was highest in young children; those undergoing ear, nose, and throat surgery; and those in whom multiple attempts were made to insert the laryngeal mask airway. On the basis of data available regarding risk with general anesthesia,

the committee concluded that children who have an acute respiratory infection on the day of surgery, as documented by fever, cough, and/or wheezing, are at increased risk for postoperative complications and, therefore, should be rescheduled or monitored closely postoperatively. Clinicians should decide on an individual basis whether these patients should be rescheduled, taking into consideration the severity of OSAS in the particular patient and keeping in mind that many children who have adenotonsillar hypertrophy exhibit chronic rhinorrhea and nasal congestion even in the absence of viral infections.

Postoperative Persistence of OSAS After AT

Although the majority of children have a marked improvement in OSAS after AT, OSAS may persist postoperatively. OSAS is especially likely to persist in children who have underlying illnesses such as craniofacial anomalies, Down syndrome, and neuromuscular disease; these special populations are not included in this review.

Over the years since the committee's first consensus report, a number of studies have been published discussing the impact of surgery on childhood OSAS. Most of these studies were omitted from consideration for this review because of their lack of preoperative and postoperative PSGs. Many other studies reported changes in group averages for polysomnographic and other measures postoperatively. All published articles found that AT leads to significant improvement in polysomnographic parameters in the majority of patients (although not in all). Studies providing data that could be interpreted to provide an estimate of the proportion of patients who were cured of their OSAS are shown in Table 17. Twenty original articles on the topic have been published since 2002, including 2 meta-analyses[130,131] of other articles included in the review. The lack of uniform agreement regarding the polysomnographic criteria for diagnosis of OSAS complicates this analysis of postoperative persistence of OSAS, as it does other aspects of this review, in part because the preoperative PSG criteria for surgery are not uniform across the different articles, but more importantly, because the postoperative prevalence of OSAS is highly dependent on the stringency of diagnostic criteria. In some cases, articles helpfully provided data on residual prevalence of OSAS by using different polysomnographic criteria (eg, AHI >1/hour and AHI >5/hour). At this point, it is generally accepted that AT has a higher success rate than isolated adenoidectomy or tonsillectomy, so although a few of the articles included some patients undergoing only adenoidectomy, only tonsillectomy, or ancillary procedures such as nasal turbinectomy, most focused exclusively on the impact of AT.

As shown in Table 17, a total of 11 articles were published, describing 10 general population cohorts referred either to a pediatric sleep specialist or otolaryngologist for OSAS, and 1 meta-analysis of articles dating back to 1980. Most of these were case

series of patients, with significant methodologic flaws, including non-blinding and incomplete follow-up for a high proportion of patients, and these issues were present even in the methodologically strongest articles.[132–134] The polysomnographic criteria for OSAS in each article may or may not have been the same as those used as an indication for AT, and these varied from an AHI >1/hour to AHI >5/hour and RDI >2 to 5/hour. Surprisingly, the overall estimate of postoperative persistence of OSAS did not seem to vary greatly by polysomnographic criteria for surgery. Conversely, the estimates of residual OSAS were clearly related to which polysomnographic criteria for OSAS were applied to the postoperative PSGs. When using an AHI >1/hour as the criterion for residual OSAS, estimates of persistence ranged from 19%[135] to 73%,[133] whereas when using an AHI >5/hour as the criterion, the estimate of persistence of OSAS ranged from 13%[134] to 29%.[132] It is important to recognize that there are clearly recognizable risk factors for postoperative persistence of OSAS and that the prevalence of these risk factors in the populations studied had an important impact on their estimates of postoperative persistence of OSAS. For example, >50% of patients in the multicenter study of Bhattacharjee et al[133] were obese, whereas 21% of the patients in the series by Ye et al[134] were obese, defined as 95th percentile for the Chinese population. It should be emphasized that although many of these studies showed a high proportion of patients with residual OSAS after AT, most patients exhibited a marked decrease in AHI postoperatively.

Risk Factors for Postoperative OSAS

1. Obesity

Five studies focused attention on obese patients (defined as 95th percentile for weight or BMI for age), and 1

meta-analysis[131] combined 4 of these studies. The meta-analysis reported that 88% of obese patients still had a postoperative AHI >1/hour, 75% had a postoperative AHI >2/hour, and 51% had a postoperative AHI >5/hour. Preoperative obesity was found to be a significant risk factor for postoperative residual OSAS in several other studies[133–135] as well, even when multivariable modeling was used to control for other factors such as age and preoperative AHI. The odds ratios of persistent OSAS in obese patients ranged in these models from 3.2[134] to 4.7.[136] One study found that the relationship of BMI to risk of persistent OSAS was no longer significant when adjusted for preoperative AHI.[137] In contrast to all of the studies that looked at this factor, a study of obese Greek children found no difference in the prevalence of residual OSAS in obese versus nonobese children; part of the reason for this finding might be that this study used a slightly less stringent criterion for obesity (1.645 SDs weight for age, which is the 90th percentile).[138]

2. Baseline Severity of OSAS

All studies that evaluated baseline AHI as a potential risk factor for persistent postoperative OSAS found it to be a significant risk factor, even when adjusted for other comorbidities such as obesity.[132–134,136,139]

3. Age

A series limited to children aged <3 years reported a high incidence (65%) of treatment failures in these younger children, but this cohort included a large proportion of children who have other risk factors, such as severe OSAS and chromosomal and craniofacial abnormalities.[140] In contrast, 2 studies reported that increasing age (especially 7 years and older) is a risk factor for persistent

TABLE 17 Studies Providing an Estimate of the Proportion of Patients Who Were Cured of OSAS With Surgery

Source	Year	Level	No.	Age, y	Population	Polysomnographic Criterion for Surgery	Operation	Follow-up Period, mo	Subjects Who Had OSAS at Follow-up	Miscellaneous
General population studies										
Chervin et al[37] Dillon et al[275]	2006	I	39	5.0–12.9		AHI ≥1	AT	13 ± 1.4	21%	2 articles documented findings in the same population
Guilleminault et al[155]	2004	III	56	1.25–12.5		AHI ≥1 or RDI >2	AT: 36 (some of whom also had nasal turbinectomy and/or tonsillar wound suturing); A: 8; T: 11	3	AT: 19.4%; A: 100%; T: 100%	Half of AT failures were in obese patients
Guilleminault et al[141]	2007	III	199	1.5–14		AHI ≥1	AT in 183; A or T in 19; nasal turbinectomy in 17.4%	3–5	46.2%	Increased nasal turbinate score, presence of deviated nasal septum and increased Mallampati score of relationship of tongue to uvula and retro position of the mandible were all predictive of higher failure rate
Guilleminault et al[276]	2004	IV	284	2–12.1		AHI >1.5	AT in 228; A or T inferior turbinectomy in 73	3–4	8.8% of those with preoperative AHI <10 and AT; 64.7% of those with preoperative AHI ≥10. No breakdown provided regarding results of AT versus other surgery	An additional 99 children had RDI >1.5 and AHI <1.5. Of this group, 100% had normal RDI after AT and 9.2% had residual abnormal RDI after A or T. Difficult to interpret findings because of inconsistent reporting of data
Mitchell[152]	2007	III	79	3–14		AHI ≥5	AT	1–9.3	16% (AHI ≥5); 29% (AHI >1.5)	Severity of preoperative AHI predicted response: preoperative 5–10, 0% ≥5; preoperative 10–20, postoperative 12% ≥5; preoperative >20, postoperative 36% ≥5; 13/22 with postoperative snoring had AHI ≥5; 0/57 without postoperative snoring had AHI ≥5
Tal et al[277]	2003	IV	36	1.8–12.6		RDI >1	AT	4.6 (1–16)	11.11% had RDI >5	In logistic regression, AHI before surgery and family history of OSAS were significant predictors of AHI >5 postoperative
Tauman et al[137]	2006	III	110	6.4 ± 3.9		AHI ≥1	AT	1–15	46% AHI 1–5, 29% with AHI >5	
Walker et al[278]	2008	IV	34	0.93–5		RDI >5 in REM sleep	AT	9.8	35% with RDI >5	Treatment failures limited to those with preoperative RDI in REM >30
Bhattacharjee et al[133]	2010	III	578	6.9 ± 3.8		AHI ≥1	AT	1–24	72.8% with AHI ≥1; 21.6% >5	Large multicenter study. Age >7 y, increased BMI, presence of asthma, and high preoperative AHI were independent predictors of persistent postoperative OSAS

TABLE 17 Continued

Source	Year	Level	No.	Age, y	Population	Polysomnographic Criterion for Surgery	Operation	Follow-up Period, mo	Subjects Who Had OSAS at Follow-up	Miscellaneous
Brietzke and Gallagher[130]	2006	III	325	4.9	Various	AHI ≥1	AT	3.3	17.1% (depended on OSAS criteria for each study)	Meta-analysis of 11 case series published between 1980 and 2004
Ye et al[134]	2010	IV	84	7.1 ± 3.2	Chinese	AHI ≥5	AT	18–23	31% with AHI ≥1; 13.1% with AHI ≥5	Obesity and high preoperative AHI were significant independent predictors of treatment failure
Focus on obese populations										
Mitchell and Kelly[279]	2004	III	30	3.0–17.2	Obese (BMI > 95th percentile)	AHI >5	AT	5.6	54%	
Mitchell and Kelly[39]	2007	III	72	3–18	Comparison of obese (BMI >95th percentile) with nonobese	AHI ≥2: AHI 2–5 mild, AHI 5–15 moderate AHI ≥15 severe	AT	5–6	Obese: 76%: (46% mild; 15% moderate; 15% severe). Nonobese: 28%: (18% mild; 10% moderate).	Preoperative AHI and obesity were independent risk factors for postoperative OSAS. OR for persistent OSAS in obese, adjusted for preoperative AHI, was 3.7 (95% CI: 1.3–10.8)
O'Brien et al[136]	2006	III	69	7.1 ± 4.2	Obese (weight >2 SDs from mean for age)	RDI ≥5	AT	20.4 ± 16.8	Nonobese: 22.5%; Obese: 55%	Preoperative AHI and obesity were independent risk factors for postoperative OSAS. OR for persistent OSAS in obese, adjusted for preoperative AHI, was 4.7 (95% CI: 1.7–11.2)
Shine et al[194]	2006	IV	19	6.5 ± 4.4	Obese (BMI >95th percentile)	RDI>5	18 AT (1 with UPPP), 1 T	2–6	63%	Missing data
Costa and Mitchell[131]	2009	III	110	7.3–9.3	Obese	Various	AT	3–5.7	88% had postoperative AHI ≥1; 75% had postoperative AHI ≥2; 51% had postoperative AHI ≥5	Meta-analysis of 4 obesity studies included here
Apostolidou et al[138]	2008	IV	70	6.5 ± 2.2	Greek; obese defined as >1.645 SDs from mean weight for age	OAHI ≥1	AT	2–14	Overall: 75.7% with AHI ≥1 (77.3% obese, 75% nonobese). Among children with a preoperative OAHI ≥5: 9% with AHI ≥5 (8% obese, 10% nonobese)	
Focus on other special populations										
Mitchell and Kelly[140]	2005	III	20	1.1–3.0	Children <3 y	RDI >5	AT	4.1–20.4	65%: 25% RDI 5–10; 25% RDI 10–20; 15% RDI >20	Included comorbidities (Down syndrome, cardiac disease, cerebral palsy) excluded from this guideline. 60% of patients were severe, with RDI >20 at baseline
Mitchell and Kelly[280]	2004	III	29	1.4–17	Severe OSAS	RDI >5; severe: RDI ≥30	AT	6	69% with postoperative RDI >5	48% were obese

A, adenoidectomy; CI, confidence interval; OAHI, obstructive AHI; OR, odds ratio; T, tonsillectomy; REM, rapid eye movement; UPPP, uvulopharyngopalatoplasty.

OSAS, even when controlling for obesity.[132,133]

4. Other Potential Risk Factors

Individual studies have noted that nasal abnormalities or craniofacial disproportion,[141] family history of OSAS,[137] and presence of asthma[133] were all predictive of higher failure rate, but these findings were not substantiated by other studies. Of note, Mitchell[132] found that 13 of 22 patients in the cohort who had postoperative snoring had an AHI ≥5/hour, whereas none of the 57 patients who did not exhibit postoperative snoring had an AHI ≥5/hour. This supports the findings of older studies reviewed in the previous technical report that found absence of snoring to have a 100% negative predictive value for postoperative OSAS.[6] However, in the Chinese cohort, 2 of 11 patients who have persistent AHI ≥5/hour reportedly did not snore; it is unclear whether cultural considerations might have affected parental report of snoring.[134]

Summary

AT is the most effective surgical therapy for pediatric patients, leading to an improvement in polysomnographic parameters in the vast majority of patients. Despite this improvement, a significant proportion of patients are left with persistent OSAS after AT. The estimate of this proportion in a relatively low-risk population ranges from a low of 13% to 29% when using an AHI ≥5/hour as the criterion to a high of 73% when including obese children and adolescents and a conservative AHI ≥1/hour. Children at highest risk of persistent OSAS are those who are obese and those with a high preoperative AHI, especially those with an AHI ≥20/hour, as well as children >7 years of age. Absence of snoring postoperatively is

reassuring but may not be 100% specific; it may therefore be advisable to obtain a postoperative PSG in very-high-risk children even in the absence of reported persistent snoring.

Areas for Future Research

- What are the risks of persistence of OSAS and long-term recurrence of OSAS after PT versus total tonsillectomy? Large, prospective, randomized trials with objective outcome measures including PSG are needed.

- Better delineation of which patients would benefit from postoperative PSG.

- How well does resolution of OSAS correlate with resolution of complications of OSAS?

- Are some of the newer surgical techniques for AT equally effective in resolving OSAS?

- What are the risks of performing AT in a patient with a URI?

- What are the PSG parameters that predict postoperative respiratory compromise? Future research should focus on refining the AHI and Spo_2 nadir cutoffs for severe OSAS. In addition, it may be possible to glean other predictive information from the PSG, such as the extent of hypoventilation, the percent sleep time spent with Spo_2 <90%, the frequency of desaturation events, the length of apneas and hypopneas, and the presence of central apneas, to create formulae for risk scores.

CPAP

At the time of the previous report, there were few prospective studies on CPAP use in children, although several retrospective studies indicated that CPAP was efficacious in the treatment of pediatric OSAS. Since that time, there have been at least 7 recent

studies evaluating the use of positive airway pressure (PAP) in children and adolescents who have OSAS. One of these was a randomized trial with low power (level II),[142] and others were case series without controls (level IV). A descriptive study examined the use of behavioral intervention in improving CPAP adherence.[143] In addition, a level III study described use of a high-flow nasal cannula as an alternative to CPAP.[144] In contrast to the previous guidelines, several of the current studies obtained objective evaluation of CPAP adherence by downloading usage data from the CPAP device. In most studies, CPAP therapy was instituted for persistent OSAS after AT; in many cases, the patients had additional risk factors for OSAS, such as obesity or craniofacial anomalies.

A multicenter study (level II) evaluated PAP in 29 children who were randomly assigned either CPAP or bilevel positive airway pressure (BPAP).[142] Patients demonstrated significant improvement in sleepiness, snoring, AHI, and oxyhemoglobin saturation while using PAP during the 6-month follow-up period. However, approximately one-third of patients dropped out, and of those who used PAP, objective adherence was 5.3 ± 2.5 hours/night. Parents overestimated the hours of PAP use compared with the devices' actual objective recordings of use. There was no significant difference in adherence between the CPAP and BPAP groups. A retrospective chart review of 46 children started on PAP for OSAS that persisted after AT also showed significant improvement in symptoms of OSAS as well as in polysomnographic parameters (level IV).[145] Seventy percent of patients were considered adherent. Parental report of adherence was most divergent from the machines' recording in the least adherent patients. More than one-half of the children had complicating factors, such as Down syndrome and Prader-Willi syndrome.[145] Another study of a heterogeneous group of patients displayed varying CPAP adherence, with 31 of 79 children showing continued CPAP use (level IV).[146] A small, nonblinded retrospective study (level IV) suggested that adherence to CPAP could be improved with behavioral techniques if the family accepted the interventions.[143]

A retrospective review described 9 children who successfully used BPAP in the intensive care setting because of respiratory compromise after AT.[147] Another retrospective review described the successful use of CPAP in 9 patients of a heterogeneous group of 18 children aged <2 years.[148] A nonrandomized, prospective level III study of 12 children who had OSAS treated in the sleep laboratory with a high-flow open nasal cannula system as an alternative to formal CPAP demonstrated an improvement in oxyhemoglobin saturation and arousals, but not AHI, compared with baseline.[144] There was a decrease in sleep efficiency with the cannula compared with baseline. Long-term use and use in the home situation were not assessed.

In summary, several studies (levels II–IV) have confirmed earlier data demonstrating that nasal CPAP is effective in the treatment of both symptoms and polysomnographic evidence of OSAS, even in young children. However, adherence can be a major barrier to effective CPAP use. For this reason, CPAP is not recommended as first-line therapy for OSAS when AT is an option. However, it is useful in children who do not respond adequately to surgery or in whom surgery is contraindicated. Patient and family preference may also be a consideration (eg, in families with religious beliefs against surgery or blood transfusions). Objective assessment of CPAP adherence is important because parental estimates of use are often inaccurate. If the patient is nonadherent, then attempts should be made to improve adherence (eg, by addressing adverse effects, by using behavior modification techniques), or the patient should be treated with alternative methods. A study described in the previous report noted that CPAP pressures change over time in children, presumably because of growth and development.[149] Therefore, it is recommended that CPAP pressures be periodically reassessed in children.

At this time, data are insufficient to make a recommendation on the use of high-flow, open nasal cannula systems.

Areas for Future Research

- Efficacy of CPAP use as a first-line treatment of obese children.

- Determinants of CPAP adherence and ways to improve adherence.

- Long-term effects of CPAP, particularly on the development of the face, jaw, and teeth.

- Changes in CPAP pressure over time, and the frequency with which this needs to be monitored.

- Development of pediatric-specific devices and interfaces.

Medications

There have been several studies evaluating the use of corticosteroids and leukotriene antagonists in the treatment of OSAS. An older study showed no therapeutic effect of systemic steroids on OSAS.[150] Since then, 3 studies (1 level I, 1 level II, and 1 level III) have evaluated topical nasal steroids as treatment of OSAS, 1 level II study has evaluated montelukast, and 1 level IV study has evaluated a combination thereof. An additional level I study evaluated the effect of intranasal steroids on adenoidal size and symptoms related to adenoidal hypertrophy but did not include PSG in the evaluation.[151]

A small, level II, randomized, double-blind trial,[152] a level I, randomized, double-blind trial of 62 children,[153] and a nonrandomized, open-label level III study of intranasal steroids[154] all showed a moderate improvement in patients who had mild OSAS. However, significant residual OSAS remained in 2 of the studies. Berlucchi et al[151] reported an improvement in symptoms of adenoidal hypertrophy, including snoring and observed apnea, but did not obtain objective evidence of improvement in OSAS. Two studies showed shrinkage of adenoidal tissue.[151,153] All studies were short term (2–6 weeks), although 1 study showed persistent improvement 8 weeks after discontinuation of the steroids (Table 18).[153]

An open-label, nonrandomized, 16-week level IV study of montelukast in children who had mild OSAS found a statistically significant but small change in the AHI (AHI decreased from 3.0 ± 0.2 to 2.0 ± 0.3; $P = .017$).[82] Another small, open-label, nonrandomized, 12-week level IV study of combined montelukast and nasal steroids found a mild but statistically significant improvement in AHI in children who had mild OSAS (AHI decreased from 3.9 ± 1.2/hour to 0.3 ± 0.3/hour; $P < .001$).[155]

In summary, several small level I through IV studies suggest that topical steroids may ameliorate mild OSAS. However, the clinical effects are small. On the basis of these studies, intranasal steroids may be considered for treatment of mild OSAS (defined, for this indication, as an AHI <5/hour, on the basis of studies described in Table 18). Steroids should not be used as the primary treatment of moderate

TABLE 18 Studies of Antiinflammatory Medications for the Treatment of OSAS

Medication	Source	Level	No.	Duration, wk	Randomized	Placebo-Controlled	Baseline AHI (per h)	AHI on Treatment (per h)	P
Intranasal steroids	Brouillette et al[152]	II	13 OSAS 12 controls	6	Yes	Yes	10.7 ± 9.4	5.8 ± 7.9	.04
Intranasal steroids	Alexopoulos et al[154]	III	27 OSAS	4	No	No	5.2 ± 2.2	3.2 ± 1.5	<.001
Intranasal steroids	Kheirandish-Gozal and Gozal[153]	I	62 OSAS	6; crossover	Yes	Yes	3.7 ± 0.3	1.3 ± 0.2	<.001
Montelukast	Goldbart et al[82]	IV	24 OSAS 16 controls	16	No	No	3.0 ± 0.2	2.0 ± 0.3	.017
Intranasal steroids + montelukast	Kheirandish et al[155]	IV	22 OSAS 14 controls	12	No	No	3.9 ± 1.2	0.3 ± 0.3	<.001

or severe OSAS. Because the long-term effects of intranasal steroids are not known, follow-up evaluation is needed to ensure that the OSAS does not recur and to monitor for adverse effects. Of note, no studies specifically evaluated children who had atopy or chronic rhinitis, although 1 study mentioned that similar improvements were seen in children who had a history of allergic symptoms compared with those without.[153] Further study to determine whether children who have atopy are more likely to respond to this therapy is needed. Data are insufficient at this time to recommend treatment of OSAS with montelukast.

Areas for Future Research

- What is the optimal duration of intranasal steroid use? All trials have been short-term with a short-term follow-up. Does the OSAS recur on discontinuation of therapy? How often should objective assessment of treatment effects be performed?

- What is the efficacy of intranasal steroids in children who have chronic or atopic rhinitis?

- How do the benefits and adverse effects of long-term nasal steroids compare with surgery?

- Larger studies, stratified for severity of OSAS and controlled for obesity, to determine whether OSAS is associated with systemic inflammation

- Will these biomarkers be good outcome measurements for treatment studies? Do they correlate with clinical outcomes or long-term prognosis?

Rapid Maxillary Expansion

Rapid maxillary expansion has recently been used to treat OSAS in select pediatric populations. It is an orthodontic procedure designed to increase the transverse diameter of the hard palate by reopening the midpalatal suture. It does this by means of a fixed appliance with an expansion screw anchored on selected teeth. After 3 to 4 months of expansion, a normal mineralized suture is built up again. The procedure is typically used only in children with maxillary constriction and dental malocclusion. Two case series without controls (level IV) have evaluated this procedure as a treatment of OSAS in children. One study described 31 patients selected from an orthodontic clinic; 4 months after surgery, all patients had normalized AHI.[156] Another screened 260 patients in a sleep center to find 35 that were eligible; only 14 were studied.[157] There was a significant improvement in signs and symptoms of OSAS as well as polysomnographic parameters. In summary, rapid maxillary expansion is an orthodontic technique that holds promise as an alternative treatment of OSAS in children. However, data are insufficient to recommend its use at this time.

Areas for Future Research

- A randomized controlled trial to assess the efficacy of rapid maxillary expansion in the treatment of OSAS in children.

Positional Therapy

Several level IV, retrospective studies evaluated the effect of body position during sleep on OSAS. The studies had conflicting results. One study found that young children had an increased AHI in the supine position,[158] and another study found that young children did not have a positional change in AHI but older children did.[159] Another study found an increased obstructive apnea index but not AHI (except in the obese subgroup) in the supine position,[160] whereas a study of obese and nonobese children, which controlled for sleep stage in each position, found that AHI was lowest when children were prone.[161] No study evaluated the effect of changing body positions or the feasibility of maintaining a child in a certain position overnight. Therefore, at this point, no recommendations can be made with regard to positional therapy for OSAS in children.

Other Treatment Options

Specific craniofacial procedures, such as mandibular distraction osteogenesis, are appropriate for select children with craniofacial anomalies. However, a discussion of these children is beyond the scope of this guideline. Minimal experience is available regarding intraoral appliances in children.[162] A tracheotomy is extremely effective at treating OSAS but is associated with much morbidity and is typically a last resort if CPAP and other treatments fail to offer improvement for a child who has severe OSAS.

OBESITY AND OSAS

This section reviews the evidence regarding the relationships between obesity and SDB (this term is used to encompass both snoring and OSAS, especially in studies that did not distinguish between these entities) in the pediatric population. The prevalence of childhood obesity is increasing,[163] and many studies on obesity and OSAS have been published since the last guideline. Because childhood obesity has a major impact on OSAS, it is described in detail in this report. Obesity is defined as BMI >95th percentile for age and gender.

Epidemiology: Obesity as a Risk Factor for Snoring and OSAS

A number of large, cross-sectional, community-based studies including more than 21 500 children have examined the risk of SDB conferred by overweight and obesity (Table 19). The majority of these studies obtained information regarding potential SDB from questionnaires, but some included objective measurements such as oximetry or overnight PSG. Similarly, many studies based the determination of BMI on data from questionnaires. The ages ranged from 6 to 17 years, consistent with recruitment strategies using local schools. Countries from around the world are represented, including North America, Asia, Europe, and the Middle East. Taken together, these studies indicate that the risk of snoring in children is increased

twofold to fourfold with obesity (defined as BMI $\geq$90th or 95th percentile). When analyzed, BMI was found to be an independent risk factor for snoring.

Several studies based on surveys of thousands of children, in some cases supplemented by use of physical examinations, showed that overweight/obesity was associated with an increased prevalence of snoring (Table 19).[47,164–167] Fewer studies that included objective measurements to identify SDB were available. Two population-based studies using PSG demonstrated a relationship between overweight/obesity and OSAS.[11,12] In contrast to the findings of the majority of studies, Brunetti et al[23] found that although HS was more prevalent in obese children in a sample of schoolchildren, there was no difference in the incidence of OSAS on PSG among the subset of normal-weight, overweight, and obese children who have HS who had abnormal overnight oximetry results. Similar to the population-based studies, studies using case series or subjects recruited from sleep disorders programs (some of which use PSG and some of which use surveys) also showed a relationship between weight and SDB.[168,169]

From these studies, it can be concluded that obesity is an independent risk factor for snoring and OSAS. The range of evidence from individual studies was II to III (Table 19) and on the aggregate rise to level I. The studies reported on large numbers of children recruited from community-based samples, some of whom had face-to-face examinations and measurements. Data obtained in different settings yielded similar results. The impact of race, if any, is not yet clear. Population-based studies of Hispanic children, a group at high risk of obesity and related comorbidities, are not

yet available.[163] For the clinician, it is recommended that particular attention is needed for screening obese and overweight children for signs and symptoms of OSAS, with a low threshold for ordering diagnostic tests. Future research should focus on population-based studies, with objective measurements of both measures of adiposity and PSG, and should include larger numbers of African American and Hispanic youth.

Predictors of Obesity-Related SDB

A number of program-based studies provide information regarding the predictors for SDB in obese children. Carotenuto et al[88] reported via data gathered from parental questionnaires that in obese subjects referred for obesity evaluation and nonobese controls randomly selected from schools, the waist circumference z score correlated with symptoms of SDB ($R = 0.37$, $P < .006$) but BMI and subcutaneous fat did not (level III). Verhulst et al[170] examined 91 consecutive overweight or obese children referred for PSG and found that OSAS was not related to indices of obesity, including bioelectric impedance analysis fat mass (level III). Central apnea was significantly predicted by using BMI score, waist circumference, waist-to-hip circumference ratio, and percent fat mass. Tonsillar size was the only significant correlate in their model for moderate to severe OSAS. In a retrospective review of 482 Chinese children referred for PSG and evaluated by using BMI and a tonsillar grading scale, the group of 111 obese children had a significantly higher median AHI and percentage with AHI >1.5/hour than did the nonobese group (level III).[171] In a regression analysis of log AHI as dependent variable, BMI and tonsil grade were predictors, but age and gender were not. In a large study of schoolchildren in

TABLE 19 Risk of SDB Conferred by Overweight and Obesity

Source	Level	Type of Study	No.	Duration	Diagnostic Technique	Other Features	Findings	P for Obesity as a Risk Factor
Urschitz et al[164]	II	Community-based sample of third graders	1144	1 y	Parental report of snoring, BMI, SES, risk factors for rhinitis, asthma	Habitual snorers reassessed at 1 y, with 49% continuing to snore	BMI ≥90% conferred a 4 times higher risk of HS versus a BMI <75%; 25% of obese subjects had HS	
Corbo et al[166]	II	Community-based sample of 10- to 15-y-old children from 10 schools	2439	2 y	Parental questionnaire and nasal examination and BMI by physician		Snoring increased significantly with BMI >90% and was >2 times for BMI >95% vs <75%	.000
Shin et al[47]	IV	Cross-sectional community-based sample of high school students	3871	NA	Questionnaire (tested for reliability) completed by subject, caretakers, and sleep partner	Korean children; 8 % response rate to survey	Snoring frequency was significantly associated with increasing BMI	<.001
Bidad et al[167]	II	Cross-sectional study of 11- to 17-y-old children	3300	NA	Scripted face-to-face interview and measurements of BMI and tonsil size by physician	7.9% of sample with HS (≥3 nights per week when well)	>Twofold risk of snoring in overweight or obesity	
Stepanski et al[168]	III	Case series; mean age: 5.9 ± 3.7 y	190	NA	Clinical interview, PSG	68% with SDB (≥5 AHI, <90% SpO₂, sleep fragmentation, ECG changes)	BMI was higher in the SDB group	<.01
Rudnick et al[169]	III	Compared children scheduled for AT with control group from same urban setting	170 SDB 129 controls	NA	BMI, ethnicity		African American children who had SDB were more likely to be obese than African American children who did not have SDB	<.02
Li et al[12]	II	Cross-sectional study of 13 primary schools	6447 by questionnaire 410 high risk and 209 low risk with exam and PSG	NA	Questionnaire in all with PSG and examination in high-risk group and low-risk subset for comparison	Hong Kong 9172 sampled with 70% response rate	Male gender, BMI, and AT size were independently associated with OSA	
Li et al[172]	II	Cross-sectional study of 13 primary schools; same population as previous study	6349	NA	Questionnaire	Designed to determine prevalence of HS and associated symptoms.	Prevalence of HS was 7.2%; male gender, BMI, parental HS, nasal allergies, asthma were associated with snoring	<.0001
Brunetti et al[25]	II	Cross-sectional; mean age 7.3 y	1207 screened, 809 eligible	NA	Questionnaire in all followed by oximetry in the 44 who had HS; PSG in subset who had abnormal oximetry results	Southern Italy	HS more common in the obese group; no difference in OSA by PSG across weight groups	.02
Bixler et al[11]	II	Cross-sectional study of grades K–5	5740 had questionnaire 700 randomly selected for PSG, 490 completed	NA	Questionnaire followed by PSG in subset	Prevalence of AHI >5 1.2%. Strong linear relationship between waist circumference and BMI with SDB	Waist circumference associated with all levels of SDB; also nasal complaints and minority race	
Urschitz et al[165]	III	Cross-sectional community-based of primary schoolchildren	995	NA	Overnight oximetry		Overweight, smoke exposure, respiratory allergies were independent risk factors for sleep hypoxemia	

AT, adenotonsillar; K, kindergarten; NA, not available; OSA, obstructive sleep apnea.

Hong Kong, Li et al reported that male gender, BMI score, and tonsillar size were independently associated with OSAS (level II).[12,172] In 490 US school-children studied by using overnight PSG, Bixler et al[11] found waist circumference to be an independent risk factor for all levels of severity of OSAS (level II). Urschitz et al[165] studied 995 children in a cross-sectional, program-based study in Germany and divided those with SDB into mild (Spo_2 nadir 91%–93%), moderate (<90%), and recurrent hypoxemia (>3.9 episodes of desaturation per hour of sleep) groups (level III). Overweight (BMI >75th percentile) was found to be an independent risk factor for mild, moderate, and recurrent hypoxemia during sleep.

From these studies, it is observed that the distribution of body fat may be more important in predicting SDB than BMI alone. In addition, tonsillar size is important in predicting SDB, even in obese children. The authors of these articles comment that SDB is likely more complicated in obese children, with obesity contributing to gas exchange and respiratory pattern abnormalities. Obesity can result in decreased lung volumes, abnormal central nervous system ventilatory responses, decreased upper airway caliber, a potential impact of leptin on ventilation, and other factors. Taken together, the strength of the evidence for these study findings is level II. Findings are limited by the fact that controls were drawn from different populations than subjects and that the studies did not all reach the same conclusions regarding the importance of body fat distribution. The latter may have been affected by the use of different measurement techniques. Anthropomorphic measurement thresholds that indicate increased risk for SDB in children would be of use to clinicians. It is recommended that

clinicians consider fat distribution (eg, waist circumference) and not just BMI in their assessment of the risk of SDB.

Comorbidities: Interactions Between Obesity and SDB

Cardiovascular

Adults who have SDB and are obese are at increased risk of cardiovascular disease, including systemic hypertension and blunting of the normal decrease in BP during sleep (nocturnal dipping). This section deals with the evidence that children and adolescents who are obese and have SDB may be similarly at risk. Six studies evaluating SDB, obesity, and cardiovascular complications in children are available. Reade et al[173] retrospectively evaluated 130 patients referred for PSG and described 56 obese subjects (BMI >95th percentile), of whom 70% had hypertension and 54% had OSAS (level IV). Among the 34 nonobese subjects, only 8% (P < .0005) had hypertension and 29% had OSAS (P < .05). The authors concluded that BMI was a significant determinant of both SDB and diastolic BP, with the number of hypopneas predictive of diastolic BP in both weight categories. In a community-based sample of 760 Greek children evaluated by using morning BP measurements, BMI, and a questionnaire regarding sleep habits, Kaditis et al[174] identified 50 children who had HS (level IV). They found that 28% of the children in the HS group were obese versus 15% of nonsnoring children (significance not reported). They reported that HS had no impact on BP, but that age, gender, and BMI were significant covariates in predicting systolic BP; inclusion of HS in this analysis did not affect these relationships. Similar findings were identified for diastolic BP, with the exception that age had no effect. This study compared absolute BP

measurements rather than the variance from normal values on the basis of race, age, gender, and body size. Because children from 4 to 14 years of age were included, this may have affected the results and conclusions. Kohyama et al[175] examined 32 Asian subjects referred for PSG and measured overnight BP every 15 minutes. In this study, obstructive apneas and hypopneas were identified indirectly and, thus, could have been underestimated or overestimated compared with studies with more direct measurements of airflow (level IV). Subjects were divided into low (<10 obstructive events per hour; 16 subjects) and high AHI (>10 obstructive events per hour; 7 subjects). Of the total, 23 subjects tolerated the BP measurements. Three subjects were obese. BMI predicted the systolic BP during rapid eye movement sleep (P < .001) but did not predict any of the diastolic BP indices. Li et al[176] performed a population-based study of 306 Asian children 6 to 13 years of age who had overnight PSG and ambulatory day and night BP measurements (level III). Children who had primary snoring were excluded, and those who had OSAS were divided into normal, mild, and moderate (AHI >5) groups. Multiple linear regression analysis revealed significant associations for the severity of hypoxemia and AHI with day and night BP, respectively, independent of obesity. Although BP levels both awake and asleep increased with the severity of OSAS, obesity and waist circumference partially accounted for elevations in sleep systolic BP and sleep mean arterial pressure but not for diastolic BP measurements. Amin et al[177] studied 88 children who had OSAS ranging in severity from mild to severe and 52 controls matched for age and gender. They used PSG, ambulatory BP measurements, and actigraphy (level III). The obese SDB group, compared with the nonobese SDB group, had higher waking systolic BP ($P < .001$) and sleeping systolic BP ($P = .02$) after adjusting for severity of SDB. They concluded that there was no difference between the effects of SDB and obesity on waking systolic or diastolic BP or sleeping systolic BP but did find that SDB had a greater contribution to sleeping diastolic BP than did obesity.

In summary, this group of articles demonstrates that both obesity and SDB are associated with increased day and night BP in children, although hypertension per se is rare (aggregate evidence level III). It seems that after controlling for obesity, significant independent effects of SDB remain and that hypoxemia and the frequency of obstructive events, perhaps via sleep disruption or intrathoracic fluid shifts, are important. Practitioners should be aware that children and adolescents who have OSAS are at increased risk of elevated BP. Future studies would benefit from a treatment arm to determine whether BP improves with resolution of sleep apnea, as well as longitudinal studies to determine the impact of pediatric obesity related–SDB on adult hypertension.

Metabolic

Obesity is a risk factor for impaired glucose tolerance, liver disease, abnormal lipid profiles, and other metabolic derangements. OSAS has been explored as a possible contributor to these metabolic abnormalities. Ten articles were reviewed. Verhulst et al[178] studied 104 overweight/obese children and adolescents with Tanner staging, overnight PSG, oral glucose tolerance testing, lipid profile, and BP measurements (level IV). The subjects were divided into normal, mild, and moderate/severe SDB groups. Findings consistent with the metabolic syndrome were present in 37%. Those who had a moderate degree of SDB had a higher BMI z score than the

normal group, and the waist-to-hip circumference ratio increased across the 3 SDB groups. The severity of SDB was independently correlated with impaired glucose homeostasis and worse lipid profile. Mean Sp_{O_2} and Sp_{O_2} nadir during sleep were significant predictors of the metabolic syndrome ($P = .04$ for both). A community-based cohort of 270 adolescents was studied by Redline et al[179] using PSG, oral glucose tolerance testing, homeostatic model assessment (HOMA [a measure of insulin sensitivity]), BMI, waist circumference, BP measurements, Tanner stage, sleep diary, SES, and birth history (level II). Metabolic syndrome was defined as having at least 3 of the following 5 features: (1) waist circumference >75% of normal; (2) mean BP or diastolic BP >90% of normal or receiving current therapy for hypertension; (3) elevated triglycerides; (4) low high-density lipoprotein; or (5) abnormal oral glucose tolerance or fasting glucose test results. Twenty-five percent of the sample was overweight, and 19% were deemed to have metabolic syndrome. The authors found that children who had metabolic syndrome had more severe hypoxemia and decreased sleep efficiency and that as AHI severity increased, there was a progressive increase in the number of children who had metabolic syndrome ($P < .001$). Both overweight children and those who had metabolic syndrome were more prevalent in the SDB group ($P < .001$) and more were male. Age, race, birth history, and SES did not vary with SDB. With adjustment for BMI, the SDB group had higher BP, fasting insulin, and more abnormal HOMA and lipid profile. They concluded that adolescents who experience SDB are at a sevenfold increased risk of metabolic syndrome and that the relationship is not explained by gender, race, or SES and,

furthermore, persists with adjustment for BMI percentile.

A study by Kaditis et al[180] of 110 children (2–13 years of age) referred for snoring did not find an impact of SDB on glucose homeostasis in nonobese children. The subjects were divided into AHI ≥5/h and <5/h; the authors found no difference in HOMA, insulin, glucose, or lipid concentrations between the 2 groups (level III). There was no relationship identified between PSG indices and HOMA or fasting insulin. BMI, age, and gender were significant predictors for fasting insulin and HOMA in multiple linear regression analysis. They speculated that OSAS may have more detrimental effects in obese than in nonobese young subjects. Similarly, Tauman et al[181] studied 116 subjects referred for PSG, one-half of whom were obese, and 19 nonsnoring controls. The authors found no impact of SDB indices on metabolic parameters (level III). Only BMI and age were important, and there was no relationship between SDB and surrogate measures of insulin resistance. They concluded that obesity was the major determinant of insulin resistance and dyslipidemia. In obese children, data from de la Eva et al[182] demonstrated that the severity of OSAS correlated with fasting insulin levels, independent of BMI (level III). Of note, the study by Redline et al[179] included children older than those in the studies by Kaditis et al[180] and Tauman et al[181]; thus, the variation in the findings may be a function of the length of time SDB had been present or perhaps attributable to the strong influence puberty has on glucose homeostasis. Kelly et al[183] compared 37 prepubertal and 98 pubertal children in a study by using PSG, HOMA, adiponectin (an insulin-sensitizing hormone secreted by adipose tissue) measurements, as well as urinary catecholamine metabolites (level III).

Tanner stage was determined by self-attestation. In the prepubertal children, they found no association between polysomnographic parameters and metabolic measurements after correcting for BMI. Elevated fasting insulin (≥ 20 µU/mL) was significantly more common in the OSAS group ($P = .03$), even when corrected for BMI. When pubertal obese subjects were considered separately, the risk of elevated fasting insulin ($P = .04$) and impaired HOMA was greater in the OSAS group ($P = .05$). Pubertal children who had OSAS also had lower adiponectin and higher urinary catecholamine levels, even when controlled for BMI. Kelly et al concluded that OSAS further predisposes obese children to metabolic syndrome, likely through multiple mechanisms involving adipose tissue and the sympathetic nervous system.

In a study that included pretreatment and posttreatment measurements in 62 prepubertal children who had moderate to severe OSAS, Gozal et al[184] found that although nonobese children had no change in measures of glucose homeostasis after treatment of OSAS, obese children had a significant improvement even while BMI remained stable ($P < .001$) (level II). Similar effects were not seen in nonobese children. Treatment (AT) improved the lipid profile and inflammatory markers in both obese and nonobese children.

Other studies have examined different aspects of altered metabolism in obesity-related OSAS. Kheirandish-Gozal et al[185] found elevated alanine transaminase (a marker for fatty liver) in a large sample of obese children who had OSAS (level IV). Verhulst et al[186] found elevated serum uric acid (a marker of oxidative stress) in 62 overweight children who had OSAS, with a significant relationship between the severity of OSAS and

serum uric acid independent of abdominal adiposity ($P = .01$) (level IV). Verhulst et al[187] demonstrated that, in a group of 95 obese and overweight children, total white blood cell and neutrophil counts increased with hypoxemia, and they speculated that inflammation may contribute to cardiovascular morbidity in obesity-related SDB (level IV).

In summary, as expected, this group of studies confirms that obesity increases the risk of insulin resistance, dyslipidemia, and other metabolic abnormalities in children. The role that OSAS plays in altering glucose metabolism is still not entirely clear but is likely less important in younger children and in lean children. Conflicting studies exist regarding the independent effect of OSAS on metabolic measures when it coexists with obesity in children. Puberty has an important role in this relationship. Screening of obese children who have OSAS for markers of metabolic syndrome should be considered, especially in the adolescent age group. Individual studies were level II through IV, with an aggregate level of III.

Neurobehavioral

The neurobehavioral complications of OSAS are discussed in detail elsewhere in this technical report. However, 6 studies have explored the potential contribution of obesity to behavior and cognition in children with OSAS and will be discussed in this section. A subanalysis of the Tucson Children's Assessment of Sleep Apnea Study evaluating parent-rated behavioral problems in overweight children before and after controlling for OSAS was performed by Mulvaney et al (level II).[188] They analyzed data from 402 subjects, 15% of whom were overweight; data were derived from home overnight PSG, the Conners scale, and the Child Behavior Checklist

(CBCL). They found that, after controlling for OSAS, behaviors such as withdrawal and social problems were higher in obese children compared with nonobese children. This finding emphasizes the need to control for obesity when designing studies evaluating neurobehavioral issues in children with OSAS. Chervin et al[42] evaluated students in the second and fifth grades in 6 elementary schools (level IV). Only 146 of 806 surveys were returned. Parental survey of health, race, BMI, Pediatric Sleep Questionnaire, teacher-rated performance, and SES were collected. SDB was associated with African American race, SES, and poor teacher ratings ($P < .01$), but only SES was independently associated with school performance. Low SES was not associated with SDB when controlled for BMI. The authors concluded that future studies evaluating the relationship between school performance and SDB should incorporate direct measurements of SES and obesity. Owens et al[189] examined all children evaluated at a tertiary center for sleep problems between 1999 and 2005; they used PSG, BMI, the Children's Sleep Health Questionnaire, and a mental health history, including the CBCL (level IV). In this study of 235 participants, 56% had a BMI >85th percentile and were thus considered overweight. They found modest correlations between measures of SDB and both somatic complaints and social problems but not with other behavioral complaints. Increased BMI was associated with total CBCL score, internalizing, social, thought, withdrawn, anxious, somatic, and aggressive behavior domains in a dose-response fashion ($P = .03$), thus emphasizing the need to control for obesity in future studies. Short sleep also correlated with a number of subscales on the CBCL ($P < .001$). Additional sleep disorders added to the risk of behavior problems ($P < .001$). BMI predicted both total and internalizing CBCL scores, and sleep duration predicted externalizing scores. The presence of an additional sleep diagnosis was the strongest predictor of all 3 CBCL scores. They concluded that overweight, insufficient sleep, and other sleep disorders should be considered when evaluating and treating behavioral problems associated with SDB. Beebe et al[21] studied 60 obese subjects recruited from a weight-management program compared with 22 controls; tools used included BMI; parent- and self-reported validated sleep, behavior, and mood questionnaires; actigraphy; and PSG (level IV). They reported that the obese group had later bedtimes ($P < .05$), shorter ($P < .01$) and more disrupted sleep ($P < .05$), more symptoms of OSAS ($P < .001$), sleepiness ($P = .009$), parasomnias ($P = .007$), higher AHI ($P < .01$), and poorer school performance. Another study by Beebe et al[190] of 263 overweight subjects enrolled in a hospital-based weight-management program found a negative relationship between the severity of OSAS and school performance and parent- and teacher-reported behaviors that persisted with adjustment for gender, race, SES, sleep duration, and BMI (level IV). Interestingly, Roemmich et al[191] found a relationship between a decrease in motor activity and increasing weight in overweight children after surgical treatment of OSAS by using AT ($P = .03$) (level IV). They hypothesized that a decrease in physical activity and "fidgeting" energy expenditure were responsible for the weight gain. However, because obese controls without surgery were not studied, it is unclear whether the degree of weight gain was greater than typically seen in obese children.

In summary, these studies point to obesity as a potential important factor

in childhood performance, mood, and behavior (aggregate level III). Clinicians should be aware that children who are obese and have OSAS might continue to have difficulties in these domains after treatment of OSAS. It is recommended that sleep habits and nonrespiratory sleep complaints be included in the evaluation and treatment of obesity-related OSAS. The relationship between SES, obesity, and OSAS is complex and adds further emphasis to the premise that studies of behavior and cognition must be carefully designed and controlled.

QoL

Both obesity and OSAS can affect health-related QoL. Two studies have examined measures of QoL in children who are obese and have OSAS. In a study of 151 overweight children by Carno et al[192] that used surveys of QoL and SDB and PSG, overweight youth who have OSAS were found to have lower self- and parent-related QoL (level IV). Neither objective measures of OSAS by PSG nor BMI correlated with QoL, whereas reported symptoms of OSAS did ($P < .05$). Similarly, Crabtree et al[193] compared 85 children 8 to 12 years of age who had been referred for OSAS and who underwent PSG, BMI, QoL ascertainment, and the Children's Depression Inventory with a control group with previously documented normal PSG (level IV). They found that OSAS did not differ between obese and nonobese children and that there was no difference in QoL between children who snore and have OSAS. The referred SDB group had lower QoL scores than the control group ($P < .001$), but the authors found no difference between obese and nonobese SDB subjects or in those with OSAS versus snoring. They concluded that children who snore have a lower QoL than nonsnoring controls, and that this finding

was not related to obesity of the severity of SDB.

In summary, QoL is an important outcome measure that may be more related to perceived symptoms of OSAS than measured physiologic disturbances of sleep and breathing, even in the obese patient (aggregate level IV). The impact of obesity on QoL in children with SDB is yet to be determined by using population-based studies and is an important outcome measure to be included in longitudinal and treatment studies.

Surgical Treatment of OSAS in the Obese Child

Surgical treatment of OSAS in general is discussed in detail in the technical report, but 5 studies have examined this area in obesity-related OSAS and are discussed here. Shine et al[194] evaluated 19 obese patients treated with AT (level IV). Although OSAS improved significantly ($P < .01$), only 37% of patients were deemed cured (defined as a postoperative AHI <5/hour), and 10 (53%) subjects needed CPAP postoperatively. A level IV retrospective review by Spector et al[195] included 14 patients who were morbidly obese who were electively sent to the ICU after AT (per policy). One patient needed intubation, and 2 patients required BPAP. Another retrospective review of 26 morbidly obese patients, all of whom were sent to the ICU after AT as per routine, found that 14 patients (54%) had an uncomplicated postoperative course, and 12 (45%) required respiratory intervention, including 1 requiring intubation and 2 requiring BPAP.[196] Costa and Mitchell[131] evaluated the response to AT in a meta-analysis of 4 studies that included 110 obese children who had OSAS (level III). They found that OSAS improved but did not resolve after AT, with 88% of children having an AHI >1/hour and 51% of children having an AHI >5/hour postoperatively. Apostolidou et al[138] reported on 70 snoring children with a mean age of 5.8 ± 1.8 years who underwent AT; 22 (31%) were obese (level IV). PSG was performed both preoperatively and postoperatively. They found no difference in cure rates between obese and nonobese subjects who had OSAS, by using an AHI <1/hour as the definition of cure. However, there was an improvement in AHI in both groups, and approximately 90% of all subjects had an AHI <5/hour postoperatively.

In summary, few studies have evaluated the effects of AT in the obese child who has OSAS, and studies have been of a low level of evidence (aggregate level IV). Studies suggest that the AHI may improve significantly after AT, even in obese children, supporting the idea that surgery may be a reasonable first-line treatment, even in obese patients. However, better-level studies are needed to assess the effects of AT in obese children and adolescents, including evaluation of subgroups such as adolescents and the morbidly obese. A significant number of children required intubation or CPAP postoperatively, which reinforces the need for inpatient observation in obese children postoperatively. Studies have not been performed to determine whether children at high risk who are obese and have OSAS, such as those with pulmonary or systemic hypertension, waking hypoventilation, or pathologic daytime sleepiness, may benefit from stabilization with BPAP therapy before undergoing AT to decrease the risk of postoperative complications.

Weight Loss and Other Nonsurgical Treatments

There is a paucity of data regarding the effects of weight loss on OSAS in children and adolescents. Verhulst et al[197] found that weight loss was a successful treatment of OSAS in a group of 61 adolescents being cared for in a residential weight loss treatment program (level IV). Davis et al[49] studied the effects of exercise in 100 overweight children by administering the Pediatric Sleep Questionnaire before and after enrollment in a no-exercise group, a low-dose aerobic exercise program, or a high-dose aerobic exercise program for 3 months (level IV). They found no change in BMI, but 50% of children who screened positive for SDB improved to a negative screening result after intervention. They found their results to be consistent with a dose-response effect of exercise on improvement in SDB ($P < .001$). Academic achievement did not improve in concert with changes in the Pediatric Sleep Questionnaire. Kalra et al[198] showed a significant improvement in OSAS after bariatric surgery, in association with a mean weight loss of 58 kg (level IV). In summary, along with many other health-related benefits, achieving weight loss and increasing exercise seem to be beneficial for OSAS and should be recommended along with other interventions for OSAS in obese children and adolescents (aggregate level IV). However, it should be noted that the 2 weight loss studies involved treatment regimens that are not commonly available to the majority of obese children. The effects of more modest weight loss regimens require further evaluation.

Pulmonary Disease and Obesity-Related SDB

Two studies addressed the relationship between obesity-related SDB and pulmonary disease. This has been described in adults as the "overlap syndrome," when chronic obstructive pulmonary disease and OSAS are present in the same individual. As part of the Cleveland Children's Sleep and Health Study, Sulit et al[199] evaluated parent-reported wheeze and asthma, history of snoring, and PSG in 788 participants (level III). They found that children who experienced wheeze and asthma were more likely to be obese ($P = .0097$) and concluded that SDB may partially explain this finding. They speculated that obesity changes airway mechanics and that SDB may increase gastroesophageal reflux, leptin levels, and cytokines and, thus, increase lower airways inflammation. Dubern et al[200] studied 54 children who had BMI z scores >3, 74% of whom were pubertal, by using history, physical examination, assessment of body fat mass, Tanner stage, HOMA, lipid profile, leptin, pulmonary function tests, and PSG (level IV). They confirmed the presence of OSAS, lower functional residual capacity, increased airways resistance, lower airways obstruction, and insulin resistance in this group of morbidly obese children. Snoring and AHI correlated with BMI ($P = .01$) and neck/height ratio ($P = .03$) (adjusted for age, gender, Tanner stage, and ethnicity). Airways resistance correlated with snoring index and AHI after adjustment. These studies remind us that the upper airway is part of the respiratory system and that its function is affected by lung mechanics. Abnormalities of pulmonary mechanics related to obesity affect OSAS and may add to abnormalities of gas exchange during sleep. It is suggested that evaluation of the child who is obese and has OSAS should include a history and physical examination directed at the entire respiratory system, and pulmonary function testing may be indicated.

Areas for Future Research

● What threshold of easily obtained anthropomorphic measurements predicts a significant risk of OSAS?

Overweight as well as obese children should be included in future studies.

- Are there additive or multiplicative effects of OSAS and obesity on BP? How do these relationships evolve over time, and what is the impact of genetic and racial background? Does treatment of OSAS improve hypertension in obese children and adolescents?

- The effect of OSAS on metabolic syndrome in children and adolescents remains controversial. Future research should include treatment arms with careful measurements before and after interventions. Longitudinal studies that track changes during puberty and into adulthood would be of interest.

- Further research is needed to clarify the effects of AT on OSAS, including evaluation of subgroups such as adolescents and morbidly obese patients. There should also be studies evaluating the use of CPAP or BPAP before surgery in the obese population, as a way of stabilizing the cardiopulmonary system and reducing operative risk.

- What is the effect of modest weight loss on OSAS in children and adolescents? Research should be directed at identifying strategies to effectively implement weight loss and exercise programs in this population.

SUBCOMMITTEE ON OBSTRUCTIVE SLEEP APNEA SYNDROME*

Carole L. Marcus, MBBCh, Chairperson (sleep medicine, pediatric pulmonologist; liaison, American Academy of Sleep Medicine; research support from Philips Respironics; affiliated with an academic sleep center; published research related to OSAS)

Lee J. Brooks, MD (sleep medicine, pediatric pulmonologist; liaison, American College of Chest Physicians; no conflicts; affiliated with an academic sleep center; published research related to OSAS)

Sally Davidson Ward, MD (sleep medicine, pediatric pulmonologist; no conflicts; affiliated with an academic sleep center; published research related to OSAS)

Kari A. Draper, MD (general pediatrician; no conflicts)

David Gozal, MD (sleep medicine, pediatric pulmonologist; research support from Astra-Zeneca; speaker for Merck Company; affiliated with an academic sleep center; published research related to OSAS)

Ann C. Halbower, MD (sleep medicine, pediatric pulmonologist; liaison, American Thoracic Society; research funding from ResMed; affiliated with an academic sleep center; published research related to OSAS)

Jacqueline Jones, MD (pediatric otolaryngologist; AAP Section on Otolaryngology–Head and Neck Surgery; liaison, American Academy of Otolaryngology–Head and Neck Surgery; no conflicts; affiliated with an academic otolaryngologic practice)

Christopher Lehmann, MD (neonatologist, informatician; no conflicts)

Michael S. Schechter, MD, MPH (pediatric pulmonologist; AAP Section on Pediatric Pulmonology; consultant to Genentech, Inc and Gilead, Inc, not related to obstructive sleep apnea; research support from Mpex Pharmaceuticals, Inc, Vertex Pharmaceuticals Incorporated, PTC Therapeutics, and Bayer Healthcare, not related to obstructive sleep apnea)

Stephen Sheldon, MD (sleep medicine, general pediatrician; liaison, National Sleep Foundation; no conflicts; affiliated with an academic sleep center; published research related to OSAS)

Richard N. Shiffman, MD, MCIS (general pediatrics, informatician; no conflicts)

Karen Spruyt, PhD (clinical psychologist, child neuropsychologist, and biostatistician/epidemiologist; no conflicts; affiliated with an academic sleep center)

OVERSIGHT FROM THE STEERING COMMITTEE ON QUALITY IMPROVEMENT AND MANAGEMENT, 2009--2011

STAFF

Caryn Davidson, MA

*Areas of expertise are shown in parentheses after each name.

ACKNOWLEDGMENT

The Committee thanks Christopher Hickey for administrative assistance.

REFERENCES

1. American Academy of Pediatrics. Obstructive sleep apnea syndrome: clinical practice guideline for the diagnosis and management of childhood obstructive sleep apnea syndrome. *Pediatrics.* 2012; 130(3): In press

2. American Thoracic Society. Standards and indications for cardiopulmonary sleep studies in children. *Am J Respir Crit Care Med.* 1996;153(2):866–878

3. Roland PS, Rosenfeld RM, Brooks LJ, et al; American Academy of Otolaryngology–Head and Neck Surgery Foundation. Clinical practice guideline: Polysomnography for sleep-disordered breathing prior to tonsillectomy in children. *Otolaryngol Head Neck Surg.* 2011;145(suppl 1):S1–S15

4. Aurora RN, Zak RS, Karippot A, et al; American Academy of Sleep Medicine. Practice parameters for the respiratory indications for polysomnography in children. *Sleep.* 2011;34(3):379–388

5. Hearst MA. Untangling Text Data Mining. In: Proceedings of the 37th Annual Meeting of the Association for Computational Linguistics. Stroudsburg, PA: Association for Computational Linguistics; 1999:3–10

6. Schechter MS; Section on Pediatric Pulmonology, Subcommittee on Obstructive Sleep Apnea Syndrome. Technical report: diagnosis and management of childhood obstructive sleep apnea syndrome. *Pediatrics.* 2002;109(4). Available at: www.pediatrics.org/cgi/content/full/109/4/e69

7. Edlund W, Gronseth G, So Y, Franklin G. *Clinical Practice Guideline Process Manual.* 4th ed. St Paul, MN: American Academy of Neurology; 2005

8. Sackett DL. Rules of evidence and clinical recommendations for the management of patients. *Can J Cardiol.* 1993;9(6):487–489

9. Centre for Evidence-Based Medicine. *Levels of Evidence and Grades of Recommendations.* Oxford, United Kingdom: Headington; 2001

10. American Academy of Pediatrics Steering Committee on Quality Improvement and

Management. Classifying recommendations for clinical practice guidelines. *Pediatrics.* 2004;114(3):874–877

11. Bixler EO, Vgontzas AN, Lin HM, et al. Sleep disordered breathing in children in a general population sample: prevalence and risk factors. *Sleep.* 2009;32(6):731–736

12. Li AM, So HK, Au CT, et al. Epidemiology of obstructive sleep apnoea syndrome in Chinese children: a two-phase community study. *Thorax.* 2010;65(11):991–997

13. O'Brien LM, Holbrook CR, Mervis CB, et al. Sleep and neurobehavioral characteristics of 5- to 7-year-old children with parentally reported symptoms of attention-deficit/hyperactivity disorder. *Pediatrics.* 2003;111(3):554–563

14. Castronovo V, Zucconi M, Nosetti L, et al. Prevalence of habitual snoring and sleep-disordered breathing in preschool-aged children in an Italian community. *J Pediatr.* 2003;142(4):377–382

15. Goodwin JL, Kaemingk KL, Mulvaney SA, Morgan WJ, Quan SF. Clinical screening of school children for polysomnography to detect sleep-disordered breathing—the Tucson Children's Assessment of Sleep Apnea study (TuCASA). *J Clin Sleep Med.* 2005;1(3):247–254

16. Sogut A, Altin R, Uzun L, et al. Prevalence of obstructive sleep apnea syndrome and associated symptoms in 3–11-year-old Turkish children. *Pediatr Pulmonol.* 2005;39(3):251–256

17. Wing YK, Hui SH, Pak WM, et al. A controlled study of sleep related disordered breathing in obese children. *Arch Dis Child.* 2003;88(12):1043–1047

18. Sánchez-Armengol A, Fuentes-Pradera MA, Capote-Gil F, et al. Sleep-related breathing disorders in adolescents aged 12 to 16 years: clinical and polygraphic findings. *Chest.* 2001;119(5):1393–1400

19. Rosen CL, Larkin EK, Kirchner HL, et al. Prevalence and risk factors for sleep-disordered breathing in 8- to 11-year-old children: association with race and prematurity. *J Pediatr.* 2003;142(4):383–389

20. Redline S, Tishler PV, Schluchter M, Aylor J, Clark K, Graham G. Risk factors for sleep-disordered breathing in children. Associations with obesity, race, and respiratory problems. *Am J Respir Crit Care Med.* 1999;159(5 pt 1):1527–1532

21. Beebe DW, Lewin D, Zeller M, et al. Sleep in overweight adolescents: shorter sleep, poorer sleep quality, sleepiness, and sleep-disordered breathing. *J Pediatr Psychol.* 2007;32(1):69–79

22. Xu Z, Jiaqing A, Yuchuan L, Shen K. A case-control study of obstructive sleep apnea-hypopnea syndrome in obese and nonobese Chinese children. *Chest.* 2008;133(3):684–689

23. Brunetti L, Tesse R, Miniello VL, et al. Sleep-disordered breathing in obese children: the southern Italy experience. *Chest.* 2010;137(5):1085–1090

24. O'Brien LM, Mervis CB, Holbrook CR, et al. Neurobehavioral implications of habitual snoring in children. *Pediatrics.* 2004;114(1):44–49

25. Suratt PM, Barth JT, Diamond R, et al. Reduced time in bed and obstructive sleep-disordered breathing in children are associated with cognitive impairment. *Pediatrics.* 2007;119(2):320–329

26. Friedman BC, Hendeles-Amitai A, Kozminsky E, et al. Adenotonsillectomy improves neurocognitive function in children with obstructive sleep apnea syndrome. *Sleep.* 2003;26(8):999–1005

27. Gozal D, Wang M, Pope DW Jr. Objective sleepiness measures in pediatric obstructive sleep apnea. *Pediatrics.* 2001;108(3):693–697

28. Halbower AC, Degaonkar M, Barker PB, et al. Childhood obstructive sleep apnea associates with neuropsychological deficits and neuronal brain injury. *PLoS Med.* 2006;3(8):e301

29. O'Brien LM, Mervis CB, Holbrook CR, et al. Neurobehavioral correlates of sleep-disordered breathing in children. *J Sleep Res.* 2004;13(2):165–172

30. Kohler MJ, Lushington K, van den Heuvel CJ, Martin J, Pamula Y, Kennedy D. Adenotonsillectomy and neurocognitive deficits in children with sleep disordered breathing. *PLoS ONE.* 2009;4(10):e7343

31. Calhoun SL, Mayes SD, Vgontzas AN, Tsaoussoglou M, Shifflett LJ, Bixler EO. No relationship between neurocognitive functioning and mild sleep disordered breathing in a community sample of children. *J Clin Sleep Med.* 2009;5(3):228–234

32. Mulvaney SA, Goodwin JL, Morgan WJ, Rosen GR, Quan SF, Kaemingk KL. Behavior problems associated with sleep disordered breathing in school-aged children—the Tucson Children's Assessment of Sleep Apnea Study. *J Pediatr Psychol.* 2006;31(3):322–330

33. Kaemingk KL, Pasvogel AE, Goodwin JL, et al. Learning in children and sleep disordered breathing: findings of the Tucson Children's Assessment of Sleep Apnea (tuCASA) prospective cohort study. *J Int Neuropsychol Soc.* 2003;9(7):1016–1026

34. Kennedy JD, Blunden S, Hirte C, et al. Reduced neurocognition in children who snore. *Pediatr Pulmonol.* 2004;37(4):330–337

35. Spruyt K, Gozal D. A mediation model linking body weight, cognition, and sleep-disordered breathing. *Am J Respir Crit Care Med.* 2012;185(2):199–205

36. Spilsbury JC, Storfer-Isser A, Kirchner HL, et al. Neighborhood disadvantage as a risk factor for pediatric obstructive sleep apnea. *J Pediatr.* 2006;149(3):342–347

37. Chervin RD, Ruzicka DL, Giordani BJ, et al. Sleep-disordered breathing, behavior, and cognition in children before and after adenotonsillectomy. *Pediatrics.* 2006;117(4). Available at: www.pediatrics.org/cgi/content/full/117/4/e769

38. Giordani B, Hodges EK, Guire KE, et al. Neuropsychological and behavioral functioning in children with and without obstructive sleep apnea referred for tonsillectomy. *J Int Neuropsychol Soc.* 2008;14(4):571–581

39. Chervin RD, Weatherly RA, Ruzicka DL, et al. Subjective sleepiness and polysomnographic correlates in children scheduled for adenotonsillectomy vs other surgical care. *Sleep.* 2006;29(4):495–503

40. Chervin RD, Ruzicka DL, Archbold KH, Dillon JE. Snoring predicts hyperactivity four years later. *Sleep.* 2005;28(7):885–890

41. Chervin RD, Archbold KH. Hyperactivity and polysomnographic findings in children evaluated for sleep-disordered breathing. *Sleep.* 2001;24(3):313–320

42. Chervin RD, Clarke DF, Huffman JL, et al. School performance, race, and other correlates of sleep-disordered breathing in children. *Sleep Med.* 2003;4(1):21–27

43. Suratt PM, Peruggia M, D'Andrea L, et al. Cognitive function and behavior of children with adenotonsillar hypertrophy suspected of having obstructive sleep-disordered breathing. *Pediatrics.* 2006;118(3). Available at: www.pediatrics.org/cgi/content/full/118/3/e771

44. Montgomery-Downs HE, Jones VF, Molfese VJ, Gozal D. Snoring in preschoolers: associations with sleepiness, ethnicity, and learning. *Clin Pediatr (Phila).* 2003;42(8):719–726

45. Johnson EO, Roth T. An epidemiologic study of sleep-disordered breathing symptoms among adolescents. *Sleep.* 2006;29(9):1135–1142

46. Tauman R, Ivanenko A, O'Brien LM, Gozal D. Plasma C-reactive protein levels among children with sleep-disordered breathing. *Pediatrics.* 2004;113(6). Available at: www.pediatrics.org/cgi/content/full/113/6/e564

47. Shin C, Joo S, Kim J, Kim T. Prevalence and correlates of habitual snoring in high school students. *Chest.* 2003;124(5):1709–1715

48. Hogan AM, Hill CM, Harrison D, Kirkham FJ. Cerebral blood flow velocity and cognition in children before and after adenotonsillectomy. *Pediatrics.* 2008;122(1):75–82

49. Davis CL, Tkacz J, Gregoski M, Boyle CA, Lovrekovic G. Aerobic exercise and snoring in overweight children: a randomized controlled trial. *Obesity (Silver Spring).* 2006;14(11):1985–1991

50. Montgomery-Downs HE, Crabtree VM, Gozal D. Cognition, sleep and respiration in at-risk children treated for obstructive sleep apnoea. *Eur Respir J.* 2005;25(2):336–342

51. Lundeborg I, McAllister A, Samuelsson C, Ericsson E, Hultcrantz E. Phonological development in children with obstructive sleep-disordered breathing. *Clin Linguist Phon.* 2009;23(10):751–761

52. Colen TY, Seidman C, Weedon J, Goldstein NA. Effect of intracapsular tonsillectomy on quality of life for children with obstructive sleep-disordered breathing. *Arch Otolaryngol Head Neck Surg.* 2008;134(2):124–127

53. Mitchell RB, Kelly J, Call E, Yao N. Long-term changes in quality of life after surgery for pediatric obstructive sleep apnea. *Arch Otolaryngol Head Neck Surg.* 2004;130(4):409–412

54. Constantin E, Kermack A, Nixon GM, Tidmarsh L, Ducharme FM, Brouillette RT. Adenotonsillectomy improves sleep, breathing, and quality of life but not behavior. *J Pediatr.* 2007;150:540–546, 546.e1

55. Goldstein NA, Fatima M, Campbell TF, Rosenfeld RM. Child behavior and quality of life before and after tonsillectomy and adenoidectomy. *Arch Otolaryngol Head Neck Surg.* 2002;128(7):770–775

56. Sohn H, Rosenfeld RM. Evaluation of sleep-disordered breathing in children. *Otolaryngol Head Neck Surg.* 2003;128(3):344–352

57. Silva VC, Leite AJ. Quality of life in children with sleep-disordered breathing: evaluation by OSA-18. *Braz J Otorhinolaryngol.* 2006;72(6):747–756

58. Tran KD, Nguyen CD, Weedon J, Goldstein NA. Child behavior and quality of life in pediatric obstructive sleep apnea. *Arch Otolaryngol Head Neck Surg.* 2005;131(1):52–57

59. James AL, Runciman M, Burton MJ, Freeland AP. Investigation of cardiac function in children with suspected obstructive sleep apnea. *J Otolaryngol.* 2003;32(3):151–154

60. Kalra M, Kimball TR, Daniels SR, et al. Structural cardiac changes as a predictor of respiratory complications after adenotonsillectomy for obstructive breathing during sleep in children. *Sleep Med.* 2005;6(3):241–245

61. Kaditis AG, Alexopoulos EI, Hatzi F, et al. Overnight change in brain natriuretic peptide levels in children with sleep-disordered breathing. *Chest.* 2006;130(5):1377–1384

62. Khadra MA, McConnell K, VanDyke R, et al. Determinants of regional cerebral oxygenation in children with sleep-disordered breathing. *Am J Respir Crit Care Med.* 2008;178(8):870–875

63. Constantin E, McGregor CD, Cote V, Brouillette RT. Pulse rate and pulse rate variability decrease after adenotonsillectomy for obstructive sleep apnea. *Pediatr Pulmonol.* 2008;43(5):498–504

64. Deng ZD, Poon CS, Arzeno NM, Katz ES. Heart rate variability in pediatric obstructive sleep apnea. *Conf Proc IEEE Eng Med Biol Soc.* 2006;1:3565–3568

65. O'Brien LM, Gozal D. Autonomic dysfunction in children with sleep-disordered breathing. *Sleep.* 2005;28(6):747–752

66. Kwok KL, Ng DK, Cheung YF. BP and arterial distensibility in children with primary snoring. *Chest.* 2003;123(5):1561–1566

67. Bonuck KA, Freeman K, Henderson J. Growth and growth biomarker changes after adenotonsillectomy: systematic review and meta-analysis. *Arch Dis Child.* 2009;94(2):83–91

68. Bar A, Tarasiuk A, Segev Y, Phillip M, Tal A. The effect of adenotonsillectomy on serum insulin-like growth factor-I and growth in children with obstructive sleep apnea syndrome. *J Pediatr.* 1999;135(1):76–80

69. Nieminen P, Löppönen T, Tolonen U, Lanning P, Knip M, Löppönen H. Growth and biochemical markers of growth in children with snoring and obstructive sleep apnea. *Pediatrics.* 2002;109(4). Available at: www.pediatrics.org/cgi/content/full/109/4/e55

70. Selimoğlu E, Selimoğlu MA, Orbak Z. Does adenotonsillectomy improve growth in children with obstructive adenotonsillar hypertrophy? *J Int Med Res.* 2003;31(2):84–87

71. Apostolidou MT, Alexopoulos EI, Damani E, et al. Absence of blood pressure, metabolic, and inflammatory marker changes after adenotonsillectomy for sleep apnea in Greek children. *Pediatr Pulmonol.* 2008;43(6):550–560

72. Kaditis AG, Alexopoulos EI, Kalampouka E, et al. Morning levels of C-reactive protein in children with obstructive sleep-disordered breathing. *Am J Respir Crit Care Med.* 2005;171(3):282–286

73. O'Brien LM, Serpero LD, Tauman R, Gozal D. Plasma adhesion molecules in children with sleep-disordered breathing. *Chest.* 2006;129(4):947–953

74. Tam CS, Wong M, McBain R, Bailey S, Waters KA. Inflammatory measures in children with obstructive sleep apnoea. *J Paediatr Child Health.* 2006;42(5):277–282

75. Gozal D, Crabtree VM, Sans Capdevila O, Witcher LA, Kheirandish-Gozal L. C-reactive protein, obstructive sleep apnea, and cognitive dysfunction in school-aged children. *Am J Respir Crit Care Med.* 2007;176(2):188–193

76. Li AM, Chan MH, Yin J, et al. C-reactive protein in children with obstructive sleep apnea and the effects of treatment. *Pediatr Pulmonol.* 2008;43(1):34–40

77. Larkin EK, Rosen CL, Kirchner HL, et al. Variation of C-reactive protein levels in adolescents: association with sleep-disordered breathing and sleep duration. *Circulation.* 2005;111(15):1978–1984

78. Gozal D, Serpero LD, Sans Capdevila O, Kheirandish-Gozal L. Systemic inflammation in non-obese children with obstructive sleep apnea. *Sleep Med.* 2008;9(3):254–259

79. Gozal D, Serpero LD, Kheirandish-Gozal L, Capdevila OS, Khalyfa A, Tauman R. Sleep measures and morning plasma TNF-alpha levels in children with sleep-disordered breathing. *Sleep.* 2010;33(3):319–325

80. Khalyfa A, Serpero LD, Kheirandish-Gozal L, Capdevila OS, Gozal D. TNF-α gene polymorphisms and excessive daytime sleepiness in pediatric obstructive sleep apnea. *J Pediatr.* 2011;158(1):77–82

81. Goldbart AD, Veling MC, Goldman JL, Li RC, Brittian KR, Gozal D. Glucocorticoid receptor subunit expression in adenotonsillar tissue of children with obstructive sleep apnea. *Pediatr Res.* 2005;57(2):232–236

82. Goldbart AD, Goldman JL, Veling MC, Gozal D. Leukotriene modifier therapy for mild sleep-disordered breathing in children. *Am J Respir Crit Care Med.* 2005;172(3):364–370

83. Preutthipan A, Chantarojanasiri T, Suwanjutha S, Udomsubpayakul U. Can parents predict the severity of childhood obstructive sleep apnoea? *Acta Paediatr.* 2000;89(6):708–712

84. Chervin RD, Hedger K, Dillon JE, Pituch KJ. Pediatric sleep questionnaire (PSQ):

validity and reliability of scales for sleep-disordered breathing, snoring, sleepiness, and behavioral problems. *Sleep Med.* 2000;1(1):21–32

85. Chervin RD, Weatherly RA, Garetz SL, et al. Pediatric sleep questionnaire: prediction of sleep apnea and outcomes. *Arch Otolaryngol Head Neck Surg.* 2007;133(3): 216–222

86. Weatherly RA, Ruzicka DL, Marriott DJ, Chervin RD. Polysomnography in children scheduled for adenotonsillectomy. *Otolaryngol Head Neck Surg.* 2004;131(5): 727–731

87. van Someren V, Burmester M, Alusi G, Lane R. Are sleep studies worth doing? *Arch Dis Child.* 2000;83(1):76–81

88. Carotenuto M, Bruni O, Santoro N, Del Giudice EM, Perrone L, Pascotto A. Waist circumference predicts the occurrence of sleep-disordered breathing in obese children and adolescents: a questionnaire-based study. *Sleep Med.* 2006;7(4):357–361

89. Schiffman PH, Rubin NK, Dominguez T, et al. Mandibular dimensions in children with obstructive sleep apnea syndrome. *Sleep.* 2004;27(5):959–965

90. Monahan KJ, Larkin EK, Rosen CL, Graham G, Redline S. Utility of noninvasive pharyngometry in epidemiologic studies of childhood sleep-disordered breathing. *Am J Respir Crit Care Med.* 2002;165(11): 1499–1503

91. Rizzi M, Onorato J, Andreoli A, et al. Nasal resistances are useful in identifying children with severe obstructive sleep apnea before polysomnography. *Int J Pediatr Otorhinolaryngol.* 2002;65(1):7–13

92. Brietzke SE, Mair EA. Acoustical analysis of pediatric snoring: what can we learn? *Otolaryngol Head Neck Surg.* 2007;136(4): 644–648

93. Rembold CM, Suratt PM. Children with obstructive sleep-disordered breathing generate high-frequency inspiratory sounds during sleep. *Sleep.* 2004;27(6): 1154–1161

94. Brouillette RT, Morielli A, Leimanis A, Waters KA, Luciano R, Ducharme FM. Nocturnal pulse oximetry as an abbreviated testing modality for pediatric obstructive sleep apnea. *Pediatrics.* 2000; 105(2):405–412

95. Patel A, Watson M, Habibi P. Unattended home sleep studies for the evaluation of suspected obstructive sleep apnoea syndrome in children. *J Telemed Telecare.* 2005;11(suppl 1):100–102

96. Saito H, Araki K, Ozawa H, et al. Pulse-oximetry is useful in determining the indications for adeno-tonsillectomy in pediatric sleep-disordered breathing. *Int J Pediatr Otorhinolaryngol.* 2007;71(1):1–6

97. Nixon GM, Kermack AS, Davis GM, Manoukian JJ, Brown KA, Brouillette RT. Planning adenotonsillectomy in children with obstructive sleep apnea: the role of overnight oximetry. *Pediatrics.* 2004;113(1 pt 1):e19–e25

98. Kirk VG, Bohn SG, Flemons WW, Remmers JE. Comparison of home oximetry monitoring with laboratory polysomnography in children. *Chest.* 2003;124(5):1702–1708

99. Collop NA, Anderson WM, Boehlecke B, et al; Portable Monitoring Task Force of the American Academy of Sleep Medicine. Clinical guidelines for the use of unattended portable monitors in the diagnosis of obstructive sleep apnea in adult patients. *J Clin Sleep Med.* 2007;3(7): 737–747

100. Zucconi M, Calori G, Castronovo V, Ferini-Strambi L. Respiratory monitoring by means of an unattended device in children with suspected uncomplicated obstructive sleep apnea: a validation study. *Chest.* 2003;124(2):602–607

101. Goodwin JL, Enright PL, Kaemingk KL, et al. Feasibility of using unattended polysomnography in children for research—report of the Tucson Children's Assessment of Sleep Apnea study (TuCASA). *Sleep.* 2001;24(8):937–944

102. Redline S, Budhiraja R, Kapur V, et al. The scoring of respiratory events in sleep: reliability and validity. *J Clin Sleep Med.* 2007;3(2):169–200

103. Katz ES, Greene MG, Carson KA, et al. Night-to-night variability of polysomnography in children with suspected obstructive sleep apnea. *J Pediatr.* 2002;140(5):589–594

104. Li AM, Wing YK, Cheung A, et al. Is a 2-night polysomnographic study necessary in childhood sleep-related disordered breathing? *Chest.* 2004;126(5):1467–1472

105. Scholle S, Scholle HC, Kemper A, et al. First night effect in children and adolescents undergoing polysomnography for sleep-disordered breathing. *Clin Neurophysiol.* 2003;114(11):2138–2145

106. Verhulst SL, Schrauwen N, De Backer WA, Desager KN. First night effect for polysomnographic data in children and adolescents with suspected sleep disordered breathing. *Arch Dis Child.* 2006;91(3): 233–237

107. Iber C. *The AASM Manual for the Scoring of Sleep and Associated Events: Rules, Terminology and Technical Specification.* Westchester, FL: American Academy of Sleep Medicine; 2007

108. Sritippayawan S, Desudchit T, Prapphal N, Harnruthakorn C, Deerojanawong J, Samransamruajkit R. Validity of tidal breathing flow volume loops in diagnosing obstructive sleep apnea in young children with adenotonsillar hypertrophy: a preliminary study. *J Med Assoc Thai.* 2004;87(suppl 2):S45–S49

109. Gozal D, Jortani S, Snow AB, et al. Two-dimensional differential in-gel electrophoresis proteomic approaches reveal urine candidate biomarkers in pediatric obstructive sleep apnea. *Am J Respir Crit Care Med.* 2009;180(12):1253–1261

110. Shah ZA, Jortani SA, Tauman R, Valdes R, Jr;Gozal D. Serum proteomic patterns associated with sleep-disordered breathing in children. *Pediatr Res.* 2006;59(3): 466–470

111. Uliel S, Tauman R, Greenfeld M, Sivan Y. Normal polysomnographic respiratory values in children and adolescents. *Chest.* 2004;125(3):872–878

112. Traeger N, Schultz B, Pollock AN, Mason T, Marcus CL, Arens R. Polysomnographic values in children 2-9 years old: additional data and review of the literature. *Pediatr Pulmonol.* 2005;40(1):22–30

113. Witmans MB, Keens TG, Davidson Ward SL, Marcus CL. Obstructive hypopneas in children and adolescents: normal values. *Am J Respir Crit Care Med.* 2003;168(12): 1540

114. Reuveni H, Simon T, Tal A, Elhayany A, Tarasiuk A. Health care services utilization in children with obstructive sleep apnea syndrome. *Pediatrics.* 2002;110(1 pt 1):68–72

115. Tarasiuk A, Simon T, Tal A, Reuveni H. Adenotonsillectomy in children with obstructive sleep apnea syndrome reduces health care utilization. *Pediatrics.* 2004; 113(2):351–356

116. Tunkel DE, Hotchkiss KS, Carson KA, Sterni LM. Efficacy of powered intracapsular tonsillectomy and adenoidectomy. *Laryngoscope.* 2008;118(7):1295–1302

117. Mangiardi J, Graw-Panzer KD, Weedon J, Regis T, Lee H, Goldstein NA. Polysomnography outcomes for partial intracapsular versus total tonsillectomy. *Int J Pediatr Otorhinolaryngol.* 2010;74(12): 1361–1366

118. Marcus CL, Keens TG, Ward SL. Comparison of nap and overnight polysomnography in children. *Pediatr Pulmonol.* 1992;13(1): 16–21

119. Saeed MM, Keens TG, Stabile MW, Bolokowicz J, Davidson Ward SL. Should children with suspected obstructive sleep apnea syndrome and normal nap sleep studies have overnight sleep studies? *Chest.* 2000;118 (2):360–365

120. Celenk F, Bayazit YA, Yilmaz M, et al. Tonsillar regrowth following partial tonsillectomy with radiofrequency. *Int J Pediatr Otorhinolaryngol.* 2008;72(1):19–22

121. Zagólski O. Why do palatine tonsils grow back after partial tonsillectomy in children? *Eur Arch Otorhinolaryngol.* 2010;267 (10):1613–1617

122. Solares CA, Koempel JA, Hirose K, et al. Safety and efficacy of powered intracapsular tonsillectomy in children: a multicenter retrospective case series. *Int J Pediatr Otorhinolaryngol.* 2005;69(1):21–26

123. Eviatar E, Kessler A, Shlamkovitch N, Vaiman M, Zilber D, Gavriel H. Tonsillectomy vs. partial tonsillectomy for OSAS in children—10 years post-surgery follow-up. *Int J Pediatr Otorhinolaryngol.* 2009;73(5):637–640

124. Derkay CS, Darrow DH, Welch C, Sinacori JT. Post-tonsillectomy morbidity and quality of life in pediatric patients with obstructive tonsils and adenoid: microdebrider vs electrocautery. *Otolaryngol Head Neck Surg.* 2006;134(1):114–120

125. Koltai PJ, Solares CA, Koempel JA, et al. Intracapsular tonsillar reduction (partial tonsillectomy): reviving a historical procedure for obstructive sleep disordered breathing in children. *Otolaryngol Head Neck Surg.* 2003;129(5):532–538

126. Sobol SE, Wetmore RF, Marsh RR, Stow J, Jacobs IN. Postoperative recovery after microdebrider intracapsular or monopolar electrocautery tonsillectomy: a prospective, randomized, single-blinded study. *Arch Otolaryngol Head Neck Surg.* 2006;132(3): 270–274

127. Ye J, Liu H, Zhang G, Huang Z, Huang P, Li Y. Postoperative respiratory complications of adenotonsillectomy for obstructive sleep apnea syndrome in older children: prevalence, risk factors, and impact on clinical outcome. *J Otolaryngol Head Neck Surg.* 2009;38(1):49–58

128. Tait AR, Malviya S, Voepel-Lewis T, Munro HM, Seiwert M, Pandit UA. Risk factors for perioperative adverse respiratory events in children with upper respiratory tract infections. *Anesthesiology.* 2001;95(2): 299–306

129. von Ungern-Sternberg BS, Boda K, Schwab C, Sims C, Johnson C, Habre W. Laryngeal mask airway is associated with an increased incidence of adverse respiratory events in children with recent upper respiratory tract infections. *Anesthesiology.* 2007;107(5):714–719

130. Brietzke SE, Gallagher D. The effectiveness of tonsillectomy and adenoidectomy in the treatment of pediatric obstructive sleep apnea/hypopnea syndrome: a meta-analysis.

Otolaryngol Head Neck Surg. 2006;134(6): 979–984

131. Costa DJ, Mitchell R. Adenotonsillectomy for obstructive sleep apnea in obese children: a meta-analysis. *Otolaryngol Head Neck Surg.* 2009;140(4):455–460

132. Mitchell RB. Adenotonsillectomy for obstructive sleep apnea in children: outcome evaluated by pre- and postoperative polysomnography. *Laryngoscope.* 2007;117 (10):1844–1854

133. Bhattacharjee R, Kheirandish-Gozal L, Spruyt K, et al. Adenotonsillectomy outcomes in treatment of obstructive sleep apnea in children: a multicenter retrospective study. *Am J Respir Crit Care Med.* 2010;182(5):676–683

134. Ye J, Liu H, Zhang GH, et al. Outcome of adenotonsillectomy for obstructive sleep apnea syndrome in children. *Ann Otol Rhinol Laryngol.* 2010;119(8):506–513

135. Guilleminault C, Li K, Quo S, Inouye RN. A prospective study on the surgical outcomes of children with sleep-disordered breathing. *Sleep.* 2004;27(1):95–100

136. O'Brien LM, Sitha S, Baur LA, Waters KA. Obesity increases the risk for persisting obstructive sleep apnea after treatment in children. *Int J Pediatr Otorhinolaryngol.* 2006;70(9):1555–1560

137. Tauman R, Gulliver TE, Krishna J, et al. Persistence of obstructive sleep apnea syndrome in children after adenotonsillectomy. *J Pediatr.* 2006;149(6):803–808

138. Apostolidou MT, Alexopoulos EI, Chaidas K, et al. Obesity and persisting sleep apnea after adenotonsillectomy in Greek children. *Chest.* 2008;134(6):1149–1155

139. Mitchell RB, Kelly J. Outcome of adenotonsillectomy for obstructive sleep apnea in obese and normal-weight children. *Otolaryngol Head Neck Surg.* 2007;137(1): 43–48

140. Mitchell RB, Kelly J. Outcome of adenotonsillectomy for obstructive sleep apnea in children under 3 years. *Otolaryngol Head Neck Surg.* 2005;132(5):681–684

141. Guilleminault C, Huang YS, Glamann C, Li K, Chan A. Adenotonsillectomy and obstructive sleep apnea in children: a prospective survey. *Otolaryngol Head Neck Surg.* 2007; 136(2):169–175

142. Marcus CL, Rosen G, Ward SL, et al. Adherence to and effectiveness of positive airway pressure therapy in children with obstructive sleep apnea. *Pediatrics.* 2006; 117(3). Available at: www.pediatrics.org/ cgi/content/full/117/3/e442

143. Koontz KL, Slifer KJ, Cataldo MD, Marcus CL. Improving pediatric compliance with

positive airway pressure therapy: the impact of behavioral intervention. *Sleep.* 2003;26(8):1010–1015

144. McGinley B, Halbower A, Schwartz AR, Smith PL, Patil SP, Schneider H. Effect of a high-flow open nasal cannula system on obstructive sleep apnea in children. *Pediatrics.* 2009;124(1):179–188

145. Uong EC, Epperson M, Bathon SA, Jeffe DB. Adherence to nasal positive airway pressure therapy among school-aged children and adolescents with obstructive sleep apnea syndrome. *Pediatrics.* 2007;120(5). Available at: www.pediatrics.org/cgi/content/full/120/5/e1203

146. O'Donnell AR, Bjornson CL, Bohn SG, Kirk VG. Compliance rates in children using noninvasive continuous positive airway pressure. *Sleep.* 2006;29(5):651–658

147. Friedman O, Chidekel A, Lawless ST, Cook SP. Postoperative bilevel positive airway pressure ventilation after tonsillectomy and adenoidectomy in children—a preliminary report. *Int J Pediatr Otorhinolaryngol.* 1999;51(3):177–180

148. Downey R, III, Perkin RM, MacQuarrie J. Nasal continuous positive airway pressure use in children with obstructive sleep apnea younger than 2 years of age. *Chest.* 2000;117(6):1608–1612

149. Marcus CL, Ward SL, Mallory GB, et al. Use of nasal continuous positive airway pressure as treatment of childhood obstructive sleep apnea. *J Pediatr.* 1995;127(1): 88–94

150. Al-Ghamdi SA, Manoukian JJ, Morielli A, Oudjhane K, Ducharme FM, Brouillette RT. Do systemic corticosteroids effectively treat obstructive sleep apnea secondary to adenotonsillar hypertrophy? *Laryngoscope.* 1997;107(10):1382–1387

151. Berlucchi M, Salsi D, Valetti L, Parrinello G, Nicolai P. The role of mometasone furoate aqueous nasal spray in the treatment of adenoidal hypertrophy in the pediatric age group: preliminary results of a prospective, randomized study. *Pediatrics.* 2007;119(6). Available at: www.pediatrics. org/cgi/content/full/119/6/e1392

152. Brouillette RT, Manoukian JJ, Ducharme FM, et al. Efficacy of fluticasone nasal spray for pediatric obstructive sleep apnea. *J Pediatr.* 2001;138(6):838–844

153. Kheirandish-Gozal L, Gozal D. Intranasal budesonide treatment for children with mild obstructive sleep apnea syndrome. *Pediatrics.* 2008;122(1). Available at: www.pediatrics.org/cgi/content/full/122/ 1/e149

154. Alexopoulos EI, Kaditis AG, Kalampouka E, et al. Nasal corticosteroids for children

with snoring. *Pediatr Pulmonol.* 2004;38 (2):161–167

155. Kheirandish L, Goldbart AD, Gozal D. Intranasal steroids and oral leukotriene modifier therapy in residual sleep-disordered breathing after tonsillectomy and adenoidectomy in children. *Pediatrics.* 2006;117(1). Available at: www.pediatrics.org/cgi/content/full/117/1/e61

156. Pirelli P, Saponara M, Guilleminault C. Rapid maxillary expansion in children with obstructive sleep apnea syndrome. *Sleep.* 2004;27(4):761–766

157. Villa MP, Malagola C, Pagani J, et al. Rapid maxillary expansion in children with obstructive sleep apnea syndrome: 12-month follow-up. *Sleep Med.* 2007;8(2):128–134

158. Pereira KD, Roebuck JC, Howell L. The effect of body position on sleep apnea in children younger than 3 years. *Arch Otolaryngol Head Neck Surg.* 2005;131(11):1014–1016

159. Zhang XW, Li Y, Zhou F, Guo CK, Huang ZT. Association of body position with sleep architecture and respiratory disturbances in children with obstructive sleep apnea. *Acta Otolaryngol.* 2007;127(12):1321–1326

160. Dayyat E, Maarafeya MM, Capdevila OS, Kheirandish-Gozal L, Montgomery-Downs HE, Gozal D. Nocturnal body position in sleeping children with and without obstructive sleep apnea. *Pediatr Pulmonol.* 2007;42(4):374–379

161. Fernandes do Prado LB, Li X, Thompson R, Marcus CL. Body position and obstructive sleep apnea in children. *Sleep.* 2002;25(1):66–71

162. Villa MP, Bernkopf E, Pagani J, Broia V, Montesano M, Ronchetti R. Randomized controlled study of an oral jaw-positioning appliance for the treatment of obstructive sleep apnea in children with malocclusion. *Am J Respir Crit Care Med.* 2002;165 (1):123–127

163. Ogden CL, Carroll MD, Curtin LR, McDowell MA, Tabak CJ, Flegal KM. Prevalence of overweight and obesity in the United States, 1999-2004. *JAMA.* 2006;295(13):1549–1555

164. Urschitz MS, Guenther A, Eitner S, et al. Risk factors and natural history of habitual snoring. *Chest.* 2004;126(3):790–800

165. Urschitz MS, Eitner S, Wolff J, et al. Risk factors for sleep-related hypoxia in primary school children. *Pediatr Pulmonol.* 2007;42(9):805–812

166. Corbo GM, Forastiere F, Agabiti N, et al. Snoring in 9- to 15-year-old children: risk factors and clinical relevance. *Pediatrics.* 2001;108(5):1149–1154

167. Bidad K, Anari S, Aghamohamadi A, Gholami N, Zadhush S, Moaieri H. Prevalence and correlates of snoring in adolescents. *Iran J Allergy Asthma Immunol.* 2006;5(3):127–132

168. Stepanski E, Zayyad A, Nigro C, Lopata M, Basner R. Sleep-disordered breathing in a predominantly African-American pediatric population. *J Sleep Res.* 1999;8(1):65–70

169. Rudnick EF, Walsh JS, Hampton MC, Mitchell RB. Prevalence and ethnicity of sleep-disordered breathing and obesity in children. *Otolaryngol Head Neck Surg.* 2007;137(6):878–882

170. Verhulst SL, Schrauwen N, Haentjens D, et al. Sleep-disordered breathing in overweight and obese children and adolescents: prevalence, characteristics and the role of fat distribution. *Arch Dis Child.* 2007;92(3):205–208

171. Lam YY, Chan EY, Ng DK, et al. The correlation among obesity, apnea-hypopnea index, and tonsil size in children. *Chest.* 2006;130(6):1751–1756

172. Li AM, Au CT, So HK, Lau J, Ng PC, Wing YK. Prevalence and risk factors of habitual snoring in primary school children. *Chest.* 2010;138(3):519–527

173. Reade EP, Whaley C, Lin JJ, McKenney DW, Lee D, Perkin R. Hypopnea in pediatric patients with obesity hypertension. *Pediatr Nephrol.* 2004;19(9):1014–1020

174. Kaditis AG, Alexopoulos EI, Kostadima E, et al. Comparison of blood pressure measurements in children with and without habitual snoring. *Pediatr Pulmonol.* 2005;39(5):408–414

175. Kohyama J, Ohinata JS, Hasegawa T. Blood pressure in sleep disordered breathing. *Arch Dis Child.* 2003;88(2):139–142

176. Li AM, Au CT, Sung RY, et al. Ambulatory blood pressure in children with obstructive sleep apnoea: a community based study. *Thorax.* 2008;63(9):803–809

177. Amin R, Somers VK, McConnell K, et al. Activity-adjusted 24-hour ambulatory blood pressure and cardiac remodeling in children with sleep disordered breathing. *Hypertension.* 2008;51(1):84–91

178. Verhulst SL, Schrauwen N, Haentjens D, et al. Sleep-disordered breathing and the metabolic syndrome in overweight and obese children and adolescents. *J Pediatr.* 2007;150(6):608–612

179. Redline S, Storfer-Isser A, Rosen CL, et al. Association between metabolic syndrome and sleep-disordered breathing in adolescents. *Am J Respir Crit Care Med.* 2007;176(4):401–408

180. Kaditis AG, Alexopoulos EI, Damani E, et al. Obstructive sleep-disordered breathing and fasting insulin levels in nonobese children. *Pediatr Pulmonol.* 2005;40(6):515–523

181. Tauman R, O'Brien LM, Ivanenko A, Gozal D. Obesity rather than severity of sleep-disordered breathing as the major determinant of insulin resistance and altered lipidemia in snoring children. *Pediatrics.* 2005;116(1). Available at: www.pediatrics.org/cgi/content/full/116/1/e66

182. de la Eva RC, Baur LA, Donaghue KC, Waters KA. Metabolic correlates with obstructive sleep apnea in obese subjects. *J Pediatr.* 2002;140(6):654–659

183. Kelly A, Dougherty S, Cucchiara A, Marcus CL, Brooks LJ. Catecholamines, adiponectin, and insulin resistance as measured by HOMA in children with obstructive sleep apnea. *Sleep.* 2010;33(9):1185–1191

184. Gozal D, Capdevila OS, Kheirandish-Gozal L. Metabolic alterations and systemic inflammation in obstructive sleep apnea among nonobese and obese prepubertal children. *Am J Respir Crit Care Med.* 2008;177(10):1142–1149

185. Kheirandish-Gozal L, Sans Capdevila O, Kheirandish E, Gozal D. Elevated serum aminotransferase levels in children at risk for obstructive sleep apnea. *Chest.* 2008;133(1):92–99

186. Verhulst SL, Van Hoeck K, Schrauwen N, et al. Sleep-disordered breathing and uric acid in overweight and obese children and adolescents. *Chest.* 2007;132(1):76–80

187. Verhulst SL, Schrauwen N, Haentjens D, et al. Sleep-disordered breathing and systemic inflammation in overweight children and adolescents. *Int J Pediatr Obes.* 2008;3(4):234–239

188. Mulvaney SA, Kaemingk KL, Goodwin JL, Quan SF. Parent-rated behavior problems associated with overweight before and after controlling for sleep disordered breathing. *BMC Pediatr.* 2006;6:34

189. Owens JA, Mehlenbeck R, Lee J, King MM. Effect of weight, sleep duration, and comorbid sleep disorders on behavioral outcomes in children with sleep-disordered breathing. *Arch Pediatr Adolesc Med.* 2008;162(4):313–321

190. Beebe DW, Ris MD, Kramer ME, Long E, Amin R. The association between sleep disordered breathing, academic grades, and cognitive and behavioral functioning among overweight subjects during middle to late childhood. *Sleep.* 2010;33(11):1447–1456

191. Roemmich JN, Barkley JE, D'Andrea L, et al. Increases in overweight after

adenotonsillectomy in overweight children with obstructive sleep-disordered breathing are associated with decreases in motor activity and hyperactivity. *Pediatrics*. 2006;117(2). Available at: www.pediatrics.org/cgi/content/full/117/2/e200

192. Carno MA, Ellis E, Anson E, et al. Symptoms of sleep apnea and polysomnography as predictors of poor quality of life in overweight children and adolescents. *J Pediatr Psychol*. 2008;33(3):269–278

193. Crabtree VM, Varni JW, Gozal D. Health-related quality of life and depressive symptoms in children with suspected sleep-disordered breathing. *Sleep*. 2004;27(6):1131–1138

194. Shine NP, Lannigan FJ, Coates HL, Wilson A. Adenotonsillectomy for obstructive sleep apnea in obese children: effects on respiratory parameters and clinical outcome. *Arch Otolaryngol Head Neck Surg*. 2006;132(10):1123–1127

195. Spector A, Scheid S, Hassink S, Deutsch ES, Reilly JS, Cook SP. Adenotonsillectomy in the morbidly obese child. *Int J Pediatr Otorhinolaryngol*. 2003;67(4):359–364

196. Shine NP, Coates HL, Lannigan FJ, Duncan AW. Adenotonsillar surgery in morbidly obese children: routine elective admission of all patients to the intensive care unit is unnecessary. *Anaesth Intensive Care*. 2006;34(6):724–730

197. Verhulst SL, Franckx H, Van Gaal L, De Backer W, Desager K. The effect of weight loss on sleep-disordered breathing in obese teenagers. *Obesity (Silver Spring)*. 2009;17(6):1178–1183

198. Kalra M, Inge T, Garcia V, et al. Obstructive sleep apnea in extremely overweight adolescents undergoing bariatric surgery. *Obes Res*. 2005;13(7):1175–1179

199. Sulit LG, Storfer-Isser A, Rosen CL, Kirchner HL, Redline S. Associations of obesity, sleep-disordered breathing, and wheezing in children. *Am J Respir Crit Care Med*. 2005;171(6):659–664

200. Dubern B, Tounian P, Medjadhi N, Maingot L, Girardet JP, Boulé M. Pulmonary function and sleep-related breathing disorders in severely obese children. *Clin Nutr*. 2006;25(5):803–809

201. Anuntaseree W, Rookkapan K, Kuasirikul S, Thongsuksai P. Snoring and obstructive sleep apnea in Thai school-age children: prevalence and predisposing factors. *Pediatr Pulmonol*. 2001;32(3):222–227

202. Anuntaseree W, Kuasirikul S, Suntornlohanakul S. Natural history of snoring and obstructive sleep apnea in Thai school-age children. *Pediatr Pulmonol*. 2005;39(5):415–420

203. Brunetti L, Rana S, Lospalluti ML, et al. Prevalence of obstructive sleep apnea syndrome in a cohort of 1,207 children of southern Italy. *Chest*. 2001;120(6):1930–1935

204. Ng DK, Kwok KL, Poon G, Chau KW. Habitual snoring and sleep bruxism in a paediatric outpatient population in Hong Kong. *Singapore Med J*. 2002;43(11):554–556

205. Hultcrantz E, Löfstrand Tideström B. The development of sleep disordered breathing from 4 to 12 years and dental arch morphology. *Int J Pediatr Otorhinolaryngol*. 2009;73(9):1234–1241

206. Urschitz MS, Brockmann PE, Schlaud M, Poets CF. Population prevalence of obstructive sleep apnoea in a community of German third graders. *Eur Respir J*. 2010;36(3):556–568

207. Akcay A, Kara CO, Dagdeviren E, Zencir M. Variation in tonsil size in 4- to 17-year-old schoolchildren. *J Otolaryngol*. 2006;35(4):270–274

208. Alexopoulos EI, Kostadima E, Pagonari I, Zintzaras E, Gourgoulianis K, Kaditis AG. Association between primary nocturnal enuresis and habitual snoring in children. *Urology*. 2006;68(2):406–409

209. Archbold KH, Pituch KJ, Panahi P, Chervin RD. Symptoms of sleep disturbances among children at two general pediatric clinics. *J Pediatr*. 2002;140(1):97–102

210. Chng SY, Goh DY, Wang XS, Tan TN, Ong NB. Snoring and atopic disease: a strong association. *Pediatr Pulmonol*. 2004;38(3):210–216

211. Ersu R, Arman AR, Save D, et al. Prevalence of snoring and symptoms of sleep-disordered breathing in primary school children in Istanbul. *Chest*. 2004;126(1):19–24

212. Goodwin JL, Babar SI, Kaemingk KL, et al; Tucson Children's Assessment of Sleep Apnea Study. Symptoms related to sleep-disordered breathing in white and Hispanic children: the Tucson Children's Assessment of Sleep Apnea Study. *Chest*. 2003;124(1):196–203

213. Gottlieb DJ, Vezina RM, Chase C, et al. Symptoms of sleep-disordered breathing in 5-year-old children are associated with sleepiness and problem behaviors. *Pediatrics*. 2003;112(4):870–877

214. Kuehni CE, Strippoli MP, Chauliac ES, Silverman M. Snoring in preschool children: prevalence, severity and risk factors. *Eur Respir J*. 2008;31(2):326–333

215. Liu X, Liu L, Owens JA, Kaplan DL. Sleep patterns and sleep problems among schoolchildren in the United States and China. *Pediatrics*. 2005;115(suppl 1):241–249

216. Löfstrand-Tideström B, Hultcrantz E. The development of snoring and sleep related breathing distress from 4 to 6 years in a cohort of Swedish children. *Int J Pediatr Otorhinolaryngol*. 2007;71(7):1025–1033

217. Lu LR, Peat JK, Sullivan CE. Snoring in preschool children: prevalence and association with nocturnal cough and asthma. *Chest*. 2003;124(2):587–593

218. Nelson S, Kulnis R. Snoring and sleep disturbance among children from an orthodontic setting. *Sleep Breath*. 2001;5(2):63–70

219. Ng DK, Kwok KL, Cheung JM, et al. Prevalence of sleep problems in Hong Kong primary school children: a community-based telephone survey. *Chest*. 2005;128(3):1315–1323

220. Perez-Chada D, Perez-Lloret S, Videla AJ, et al. Sleep disordered breathing and daytime sleepiness are associated with poor academic performance in teenagers. A study using the Pediatric Daytime Sleepiness Scale (PDSS). *Sleep*. 2007;30(12):1698–1703

221. Petry C, Pereira MU, Pitrez PM, Jones MH, Stein RT. The prevalence of symptoms of sleep-disordered breathing in Brazilian schoolchildren. *J Pediatr (Rio J)*. 2008;84(2):123–129

222. Sahin U, Ozturk O, Ozturk M, Songur N, Bircan A, Akkaya A. Habitual snoring in primary school children: prevalence and association with sleep-related disorders and school performance. *Med Princ Pract*. 2009;18(6):458–465

223. Tafur A, Chérrez-Ojeda I, Patiño C, et al. Rhinitis symptoms and habitual snoring in Ecuadorian children. *Sleep Med*. 2009;10(9):1035–1039

224. Zhang G, Spickett J, Rumchev K, Lee AH, Stick S. Snoring in primary school children and domestic environment: a Perth school based study. *Respir Res*. 2004;5:19

225. Beebe DW, Wells CT, Jeffries J, Chini B, Kalra M, Amin R. Neuropsychological effects of pediatric obstructive sleep apnea. *J Int Neuropsychol Soc*. 2004;10(7):962–975

226. Blunden S, Lushington K, Lorenzen B, Martin J, Kennedy D. Neuropsychological and psychosocial function in children with a history of snoring or behavioral sleep problems. *J Pediatr*. 2005;146(6):780–786

227. Kurnatowski P, Putyński L, Lapienis M, Kowalska B. Neurocognitive abilities in children with adenotonsillar hypertrophy. *Int J Pediatr Otorhinolaryngol*. 2006;70(3):419–424

228. Carvalho LB, Prado LF, Silva L, et al. Cognitive dysfunction in children with sleep-disordered breathing. *J Child Neurol.* 2005;20(5):400–404

229. Urschitz MS, Eitner S, Guenther A, et al. Habitual snoring, intermittent hypoxia, and impaired behavior in primary school children. *Pediatrics.* 2004;114(4):1041–1048

230. LeBourgeois MK, Avis K, Mixon M, Olmi J, Harsh J. Snoring, sleep quality, and sleepiness across attention-deficit/hyperactivity disorder subtypes. *Sleep.* 2004;27(3):520–525

231. Karpinski AC, Scullin MH, Montgomery-Downs HE. Risk for sleep-disordered breathing and executive function in preschoolers. *Sleep Med.* 2008;9(4):418–424

232. Hamasaki Uema SF, Nagata Pignatari SS, Fujita RR, Moreira GA, Pradella-Hallinan M, Weckx L. Assessment of cognitive learning function in children with obstructive sleep breathing disorders. *Braz J Otorhinolaryngol.* 2007;73(3):315–320

233. O'Brien LM, Tauman R, Gozal D. Sleep pressure correlates of cognitive and behavioral morbidity in snoring children. *Sleep.* 2004;27(2):279–282

234. Spruyt K, Capdevila OS, Kheirandish-Gozal L, Gozal D. Inefficient or insufficient encoding as potential primary deficit in neurodevelopmental performance among children with OSA. *Dev Neuropsychol.* 2009;34(5):601–614

235. Honaker SM, Gozal D, Bennett J, Capdevila OS, Spruyt K. Sleep-disordered breathing and verbal skills in school-aged community children. *Dev Neuropsychol.* 2009;34(5):588–600

236. Chervin RD, Archbold KH, Dillon JE, et al. Inattention, hyperactivity, and symptoms of sleep-disordered breathing. *Pediatrics.* 2002;109(3):449–456

237. Galland BC, Dawes PJ, Tripp EG, Taylor BJ. Changes in behavior and attentional capacity after adenotonsillectomy. *Pediatr Res.* 2006;59(5):711–716

238. Li HY, Huang YS, Chen NH, Fang TJ, Lee LA. Impact of adenotonsillectomy on behavior in children with sleep-disordered breathing. *Laryngoscope.* 2006;116(7):1142–1147

239. Golan N, Shahar E, Ravid S, Pillar G. Sleep disorders and daytime sleepiness in children with attention-deficit/hyperactive disorder. *Sleep.* 2004;27(2):261–266

240. Mitchell RB, Kelly J. Child behavior after adenotonsillectomy for obstructive sleep apnea syndrome. *Laryngoscope.* 2005;115(11):2051–2055

241. Mitchell RB, Kelly J. Behavioral changes in children with mild sleep-disordered breathing or obstructive sleep apnea after adenotonsillectomy. *Laryngoscope.* 2007;117(9):1685–1688

242. Rudnick EF, Mitchell RB. Behavior and obstructive sleep apnea in children: is obesity a factor? *Laryngoscope.* 2007;117(8):1463–1466

243. Goldstein NA, Post JC, Rosenfeld RM, Campbell TF. Impact of tonsillectomy and adenoidectomy on child behavior. *Arch Otolaryngol Head Neck Surg.* 2000;126(4):494–498

244. Rosen CL, Storfer-Isser A, Taylor HG, Kirchner HL, Emancipator JL, Redline S. Increased behavioral morbidity in school-aged children with sleep-disordered breathing. *Pediatrics.* 2004;114(6):1640–1648

245. Wei JL, Mayo MS, Smith HJ, Reese M, Weatherly RA. Improved behavior and sleep after adenotonsillectomy in children with sleep-disordered breathing. *Arch Otolaryngol Head Neck Surg.* 2007;133(10):974–979

246. Chervin RD, Dillon JE, Archbold KH, Ruzicka DL. Conduct problems and symptoms of sleep disorders in children. *J Am Acad Child Adolesc Psychiatry.* 2003;42(2):201–208

247. Amin RS, Kimball TR, Bean JA, et al. Left ventricular hypertrophy and abnormal ventricular geometry in children and adolescents with obstructive sleep apnea. *Am J Respir Crit Care Med.* 2002;165(10):1395–1399

248. Amin RS, Kimball TR, Kalra M, et al. Left ventricular function in children with sleep-disordered breathing. *Am J Cardiol.* 2005;95(6):801–804

249. Duman D, Naiboglu B, Esen HS, Toros SZ, Demirtunc R. Impaired right ventricular function in adenotonsillar hypertrophy. *Int J Cardiovasc Imaging.* 2008;24(3):261–267

250. Ugur MB, Dogan SM, Sogut A, et al. Effect of adenoidectomy and/or tonsillectomy on cardiac functions in children with obstructive sleep apnea. *ORL J Otorhinolaryngol Relat Spec.* 2008;70(3):202–208

251. Weber SA, Montovani JC, Matsubara B, Fioretto JR. Echocardiographic abnormalities in children with obstructive breathing disorders during sleep. *J Pediatr (Rio J).* 2007;83(6):518–522

252. Leung LC, Ng DK, Lau MW, et al. Twenty-four-hour ambulatory BP in snoring children with obstructive sleep apnea syndrome. *Chest.* 2006;130(4):1009–1017

253. Guilleminault C, Khramsov A, Stoohs RA, et al. Abnormal blood pressure in prepubertal children with sleep-disordered breathing. *Pediatr Res.* 2004;55(1):76–84

254. Amin RS, Carroll JL, Jeffries JL, et al. Twenty-four-hour ambulatory blood pressure in children with sleep-disordered breathing. *Am J Respir Crit Care Med.* 2004;169(8):950–956

255. Enright PL, Goodwin JL, Sherrill DL, Quan JR, Quan SF; Tucson Children's Assessment of Sleep Apnea study. Blood pressure elevation associated with sleep-related breathing disorder in a community sample of white and Hispanic children: the Tucson Children's Assessment of Sleep Apnea study. *Arch Pediatr Adolesc Med.* 2003;157(9):901–904

256. Xu Z, Cheuk DK, Lee SL. Clinical evaluation in predicting childhood obstructive sleep apnea. *Chest.* 2006;130(6):1765–1771

257. Jain A, Sahni JK. Polysomnographic studies in children undergoing adenoidectomy and/or tonsillectomy. *J Laryngol Otol.* 2002;116(9):711–715

258. Li AM, Wong E, Kew J, Hui S, Fok TF. Use of tonsil size in the evaluation of obstructive sleep apnoea. *Arch Dis Child.* 2002;87(2):156–159

259. Kawashima S, Niikuni N, Chia-hung L, et al. Cephalometric comparisons of craniofacial and upper airway structures in young children with obstructive sleep apnea syndrome. *Ear Nose Throat J.* 2000;79(7):499–502, 505–506

260. Kawashima S, Peltomäki T, Sakata H, Mori K, Happonen RP, Rönning O. Craniofacial morphology in preschool children with sleep-related breathing disorder and hypertrophy of tonsils. *Acta Paediatr.* 2002;91(1):71–77

261. Kikuchi M, Higurashi N, Miyazaki S, Itasaka Y, Chiba S, Nezu H. Facial pattern categories of sleep breathing-disordered children using Ricketts analysis. *Psychiatry Clin Neurosci.* 2002;56(3):329–330

262. Kulnis R, Nelson S, Strohl K, Hans M. Cephalometric assessment of snoring and nonsnoring children. *Chest.* 2000;118(3):596–603

263. Zucconi M, Caprioglio A, Calori G, et al. Craniofacial modifications in children with habitual snoring and obstructive sleep apnoea: a case-control study. *Eur Respir J.* 1999;13(2):411–417

264. Noehren A, Brockmann PE, Urschitz MS, Sokollik C, Schlaud M, Poets CF. Detection of respiratory events using pulse rate in children with and without obstructive sleep apnea. *Pediatr Pulmonol.* 2010;45(5):459–468

265. Katz ES, Lutz J, Black C, Marcus CL. Pulse transit time as a measure of arousal and

respiratory effort in children with sleep-disordered breathing. *Pediatr Res.* 2003; 53(4):580–588

266. Foo JY, Bradley AP, Wilson SJ, Williams GR, Dakin C, Cooper DM. Screening of obstructive and central apnoea/hypopnoea in children using variability: a preliminary study. *Acta Paediatr.* 2006;95(5): 561–564

267. Foo JY, Lim CS. Development of a home screening system for pediatric respiratory sleep studies. *Telemed J E Health.* 2006; 12(6):698–701

268. Tauman R, O'Brien LM, Mast BT, Holbrook CR, Gozal D. Peripheral arterial tonometry events and electroencephalographic arousals in children. *Sleep.* 2004;27(3):502–506

269. Hill CA, Litvak A, Canapari C, et al. A pilot study to identify pre- and peri-operative risk factors for airway complications following adenotonsillectomy for treatment of severe pediatric OSA. *Int J Pediatr Otorhinolaryngol.* 2011;75(11):1385–1390

270. Jaryszak EM, Shah RK, Vanison CC, Lander L, Choi SS. Polysomnographic variables predictive of adverse respiratory events after pediatric adenotonsillectomy. *Arch Otolaryngol Head Neck Surg.* 2011;137(1): 15–18

271. Koomson A, Morin I, Brouillette R, Brown KA. Children with severe OSAS who have adenotonsillectomy in the morning are less likely to have postoperative desaturation than those operated in the afternoon. *Can J Anaesth.* 2004;51(1):62–67

272. Ma AL, Lam YY, Wong SF, Ng DK, Chan CH. Risk factors for post-operative complications in Chinese children with tonsillectomy and adenoidectomy for obstructive sleep apnea syndrome [published online ahead of print July 30, 2011]. *Sleep Breath.*

273. Sanders JC, King MA, Mitchell RB, Kelly JP. Perioperative complications of adenotonsillectomy in children with obstructive sleep apnea syndrome. *Anesth Analg.* 2006;103(5):1115–1121

274. Schroeder JW, Jr;Anstead AS, Wong H. Complications in children who electively remain intubated after adenotonsillectomy for severe obstructive sleep apnea. *Int J Pediatr Otorhinolaryngol.* 2009;73(8):1095–1099

275. Dillon JE, Blunden S, Ruzicka DL, et al. DSM-IV diagnoses and obstructive sleep apnea in children before and 1 year after adenotonsillectomy. *J Am Acad Child Adolesc Psychiatry.* 2007;46(11):1425–1436

276. Guilleminault C, Li KK, Khramtsov A, Pelayo R, Martinez S. Sleep disordered breathing: surgical outcomes in prepubertal children. *Laryngoscope.* 2004;114(1):132–137

277. Tal A, Bar A, Leiberman A, Tarasiuk A. Sleep characteristics following adenotonsillectomy in children with obstructive sleep apnea syndrome. *Chest.* 2003;124(3): 948–953

278. Walker P, Whitehead B, Gulliver T. Polysomnographic outcome of adenotonsillectomy for obstructive sleep apnea in children under 5 years old. *Otolaryngol Head Neck Surg.* 2008;139 (1):83–86

279. Mitchell RB, Kelly J. Adenotonsillectomy for obstructive sleep apnea in obese children. *Otolaryngol Head Neck Surg.* 2004;131(1):104–108

280. Mitchell RB, Kelly J. Outcome of adenotonsillectomy for severe obstructive sleep apnea in children. *Int J Pediatr Otorhinolaryngol.* 2004;68(11):1375–1379

(Continued from first page)

www.pediatrics.org/cgi/doi/10.1542/peds.2012-1672

doi:10.1542/peds.2012-1672

PEDIATRICS (ISSN Numbers: Print, 0031-4005; Online, 1098-4275).

Sleep Apnea Clinical Practice Guideline
Quick Reference Tools

- Action Statement Summary
  — Diagnosis and Management of Childhood Obstructive Sleep Apnea
- *ICD-9-CM/ICD-10-CM* Coding Quick Reference for Sleep Apnea
- AAP Patient Education Handout
  — *Sleep Apnea and Your Child*

Action Statement Summary

Diagnosis and Management of Childhood Obstructive Sleep Apnea

Key Action Statement 1: Screening for OSAS

As part of routine health maintenance visits, clinicians should inquire whether the child or adolescent snores. If the answer is affirmative or if a child or adolescent presents with signs or symptoms of OSAS (Table 2), clinicians should perform a more focused evaluation. (Evidence Quality: Grade B, Recommendation Strength: Recommendation.)

Key Action Statement 2A: Polysomnography

If a child or adolescent snores on a regular basis and has any of the complaints or findings shown in Table 2, clinicians should either (1) obtain a polysomnogram (Evidence Quality A, Key Action strength: Recommendation) OR (2) refer the patient to a sleep specialist or otolaryngologist for a more extensive evaluation (Evidence quality D, Key Action strength: Option). (Evidence Quality: Grade A for polysomnography; Grade D for specialist referral, Recommendation Strength: Recommendation.)

Key Action Statement 2B: Alternative Testing

If polysomnography is not available, then clinicians may order alternative diagnostic tests, such as nocturnal video recording, nocturnal oximetry, daytime nap polysomnography, or ambulatory polysomnography. (Evidence Quality: Grade C, Recommendation Strength: Option.)

Key Action Statement 3: Adenotonsillectomy

If a child is determined to have OSAS, has a clinical examination consistent with adenotonsillar hypertrophy, and does not have a contraindication to surgery (see Table 3), the clinician should recommend adenotonsillectomy as the first line of treatment. If the child has OSAS but does not have adenotonsillar hypertrophy, other treatment should be considered (see Key Action Statement 6). Clinical judgment is required to determine the benefits of adenotonsillectomy compared with other treatments in obese children with varying degrees of adenotonsillar hypertrophy. (Evidence Quality: Grade B, Recommendation Strength: Recommendation.)

Key Action Statement 4: High-Risk Patients Undergoing Adenotonsillectomy

Clinicians should monitor high-risk patients (Table 5) undergoing adenotonsillectomy as inpatients postoperatively. (Evidence Quality: Grade B, Recommendation Strength: Recommendation.)

Key Action Statement 5: Reevaluation

Clinicians should clinically reassess all patients with OSAS for persisting signs and symptoms after therapy to determine whether further treatment is required. (Evidence Quality: Grade B, Recommendation Strength: Recommendation.)

Key Action Statement 5B: Reevaluation of High-Risk Patients

Clinicians should reevaluate high-risk patients for persistent OSAS after adenotonsillectomy, including those who had a significantly abnormal baseline polysomnogram, have sequelae of OSAS, are obese, or remain symptomatic after treatment, with an objective test (see Key Action Statement 2) or refer such patients to a sleep specialist. (Evidence Quality: Grade B, Recommendation Strength: Recommendation.)

Key Action Statement 6: CPAP

Clinicians should refer patients for CPAP management if symptoms/signs (Table 2) or objective evidence of OSAS persists after adenotonsillectomy or if adenotonsillectomy is not performed. (Evidence Quality: Grade B, Recommendation Strength: Recommendation.)

Key Action Statement 7: Weight Loss

Clinicians should recommend weight loss in addition to other therapy if a child/adolescent with OSAS is overweight or obese. (Evidence Quality: Grade C, Recommendation Strength: Recommendation.)

Key Action Statement 8: Intranasal Corticosteroids

Clinicians may prescribe topical intranasal corticosteroids for children with mild OSAS in whom adenotonsillectomy is contraindicated or for children with mild postoperative OSAS. (Evidence Quality: Grade B, Recommendation Strength: Option.)

Coding Quick Reference for Sleep Apnea

ICD-9-CM	ICD-10-CM	
327.20 Sleep apnea, organic, unspecified	G47.30	Sleep apnea, unspecified
327.21 Sleep apnea, primary central	G47.31	Primary central sleep apnea
327.23 Sleep apnea, obstructive	G47.33	Obstructive sleep apnea (adult) (pediatric) (Code additional underlying conditions.)
	J35.3	Hypertrophy of tonsils with hypertrophy of adenoids
	E66.01	Morbid (severe) obesity due to excess calories
	E66.09	Other obesity due to excess calories
	E66.3	Overweight
	E66.8	Other obesity
	E66.9	Obesity, unspecified

Sleep Apnea and Your Child

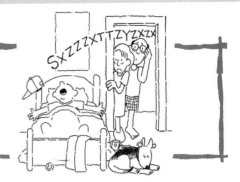

Does your child snore a lot? Does he sleep restlessly? Does he have difficulty breathing, or does he gasp or choke, while he sleeps?

If your child has these symptoms, he may have a condition known as sleep apnea.

Sleep apnea is a common problem that affects an estimated 2% of all children, including many who are undiagnosed.

If not treated, sleep apnea can lead to a variety of problems. These include heart, behavior, learning, and growth problems.

How do I know if my child has sleep apnea?

Symptoms of sleep apnea include

- Frequent snoring
- Problems breathing during the night
- Sleepiness during the day
- Difficulty paying attention
- Behavior problems

If you notice any of these symptoms, let your pediatrician know as soon as possible. Your pediatrician may recommend an overnight sleep study called a *polysomnogram*. Overnight polysomnograms are conducted at hospitals and major medical centers. During the study, medical staff will watch your child sleep. Several sensors will be attached to your child to monitor breathing, oxygenation, and brain waves. An electroencephalogram (EEG) is a test that measures brain waves.

The results of the study will show whether your child suffers from sleep apnea. Other specialists, such as pediatric pulmonologists, otolaryngologists, neurologists, and pediatricians with specialty training in sleep disorders, may help your pediatrician make the diagnosis.

What causes sleep apnea?

Many children with sleep apnea have larger tonsils and adenoids.

Tonsils are the round, reddish masses on each side of your child's throat. They help fight infections in the body. You can only see the adenoid with an x-ray or special mirror. It lies in the space between the nose and throat.

Large tonsils and adenoid may block a child's airway while she sleeps. This causes her to snore and wake up often during the night. However, not every child with large tonsils and adenoid has sleep

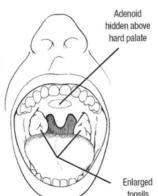

Adenoid hidden above hard palate

Enlarged tonsils

apnea. A sleep study can tell your doctor whether your child has sleep apnea or if she is simply snoring.

Children born with other medical conditions, such as Down syndrome, cerebral palsy, or craniofacial (skull and face) abnormalities, are at higher risk for sleep apnea. Overweight children are also more likely to suffer from sleep apnea.

How is sleep apnea treated?

The most common way to treat sleep apnea is to remove your child's tonsils and adenoid. This surgery is called a tonsillectomy and adenoidectomy. It is highly effective in treating sleep apnea.

Another effective treatment is nasal continuous positive airway pressure (CPAP), which requires the child to wear a mask while he sleeps. The mask delivers steady air pressure through the child's nose, allowing him to breathe comfortably. Continuous positive airway pressure is usually used in children who do not improve after tonsillectomy and adenoidectomy, or who are not candidates for tonsillectomy and adenoidectomy.

Children who may need additional treatment include children who are overweight or suffering from another complicating condition. Overweight children will improve if they lose weight, but may need to use CPAP until the weight is lost.

Remember

A good night's sleep is important to good health. If your child suffers from the symptoms of sleep apnea, talk with your pediatrician. A proper diagnosis and treatment can mean restful nights and restful days for your child and your family.

The information contained in this publication should not be used as a substitute for the medical care and advice of your pediatrician. There may be variations in treatment that your pediatrician may recommend based on individual facts and circumstances.

From your doctor

American Academy of Pediatrics

DEDICATED TO THE HEALTH OF ALL CHILDREN™

Urinary Tract Infection: Clinical Practice Guideline for the Diagnosis and Management of the Initial UTI in Febrile Infants and Children 2 to 24 Months

- *Clinical Practice Guideline*

  - *PPI: AAP Partnership for Policy Implementation*
    See Appendix 2 for more information.

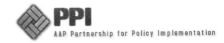

- *Technical Report*

  - *PPI: AAP Partnership for Policy Implementation*
    See Appendix 2 for more information.

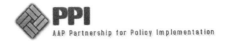

- *2011 Commentary*

Readers of this clinical practice guideline are urged to review the technical report to enhance the evidence-based decision-making process. The full technical report is available following the clinical practice guideline and on the companion CD-ROM.

CLINICAL PRACTICE GUIDELINE

Urinary Tract Infection: Clinical Practice Guideline for the Diagnosis and Management of the Initial UTI in Febrile Infants and Children 2 to 24 Months

SUBCOMMITTEE ON URINARY TRACT INFECTION, STEERING COMMITTEE ON QUALITY IMPROVEMENT AND MANAGEMENT

KEY WORDS
urinary tract infection, infants, children, vesicoureteral reflux, voiding cystourethrography

ABBREVIATIONS
SPA—suprapubic aspiration
AAP—American Academy of Pediatrics
UTI—urinary tract infection
RCT—randomized controlled trial
CFU—colony-forming unit
VUR—vesicoureteral reflux
WBC—white blood cell
RBUS—renal and bladder ultrasonography
VCUG—voiding cystourethrography

www.pediatrics.org/cgi/doi/10.1542/peds.2011-1330

doi:10.1542/peds.2011-1330

PEDIATRICS (ISSN Numbers: Print, 0031-4005; Online, 1098-4275).

Copyright © 2011 by the American Academy of Pediatrics

COMPANION PAPERS: Companions to this article can be found on pages 572 and e749, and online at www.pediatrics.org/cgi/doi/10.1542/peds.2011-1818 and www.pediatrics.org/cgi/doi/10.1542/peds.2011-1332.

abstract

OBJECTIVE: To revise the American Academy of Pediatrics practice parameter regarding the diagnosis and management of initial urinary tract infections (UTIs) in febrile infants and young children.

METHODS: Analysis of the medical literature published since the last version of the guideline was supplemented by analysis of data provided by authors of recent publications. The strength of evidence supporting each recommendation and the strength of the recommendation were assessed and graded.

RESULTS: Diagnosis is made on the basis of the presence of both pyuria and at least 50 000 colonies per mL of a single uropathogenic organism in an appropriately collected specimen of urine. After 7 to 14 days of antimicrobial treatment, close clinical follow-up monitoring should be maintained to permit prompt diagnosis and treatment of recurrent infections. Ultrasonography of the kidneys and bladder should be performed to detect anatomic abnormalities. Data from the most recent 6 studies do not support the use of antimicrobial prophylaxis to prevent febrile recurrent UTI in infants without vesicoureteral reflux (VUR) or with grade I to IV VUR. Therefore, a voiding cystourethrography (VCUG) is not recommended routinely after the first UTI; VCUG is indicated if renal and bladder ultrasonography reveals hydronephrosis, scarring, or other findings that would suggest either high-grade VUR or obstructive uropathy and in other atypical or complex clinical circumstances. VCUG should also be performed if there is a recurrence of a febrile UTI. The recommendations in this guideline do not indicate an exclusive course of treatment or serve as a standard of care; variations may be appropriate. Recommendations about antimicrobial prophylaxis and implications for performance of VCUG are based on currently available evidence. As with all American Academy of Pediatrics clinical guidelines, the recommendations will be reviewed routinely and incorporate new evidence, such as data from the Randomized Intervention for Children With Vesicoureteral Reflux (RIVUR) study.

CONCLUSIONS: Changes in this revision include criteria for the diagnosis of UTI and recommendations for imaging. *Pediatrics* 2011;128:595–610

INTRODUCTION

Since the early 1970s, occult bacteremia has been the major focus of concern for clinicians evaluating febrile infants who have no recognizable source of infection. With the introduction of effective conjugate vaccines against *Haemophilus influenzae* type b and *Streptococcus pneumoniae* (which have resulted in dramatic decreases in bacteremia and meningitis), there has been increasing appreciation of the urinary tract as the most frequent site of occult and serious bacterial infections. Because the clinical presentation tends to be nonspecific in infants and reliable urine specimens for culture cannot be obtained without invasive methods (urethral catheterization or suprapubic aspiration [SPA]), diagnosis and treatment may be delayed. Most experimental and clinical data support the concept that delays in the institution of appropriate treatment of pyelonephritis increase the risk of renal damage.[1,2]

This clinical practice guideline is a revision of the practice parameter published by the American Academy of Pediatrics (AAP) in 1999.[3] It was developed by a subcommittee of the Steering Committee on Quality Improvement and Management that included physicians with expertise in the fields of academic general pediatrics, epidemiology and informatics, pediatric infectious diseases, pediatric nephrology, pediatric practice, pediatric radiology, and pediatric urology. The AAP funded the development of this guideline; none of the participants had any financial conflicts of interest. The guideline was reviewed by multiple groups within the AAP (7 committees, 1 council, and 9 sections) and 5 external organizations in the United States and Canada. The guideline will be reviewed and/or revised in 5 years, unless new evidence emerges that warrants revision sooner. The guideline is intended

for use in a variety of clinical settings (eg, office, emergency department, or hospital) by clinicians who treat infants and young children. This text is a summary of the analysis. The data on which the recommendations are based are included in a companion technical report.[4]

Like the 1999 practice parameter, this revision focuses on the diagnosis and management of initial urinary tract infections (UTIs) in febrile infants and young children (2–24 months of age) who have no obvious neurologic or anatomic abnormalities known to be associated with recurrent UTI or renal damage. (For simplicity, in the remainder of this guideline the phrase "febrile infants" is used to indicate febrile infants and young children 2–24 months of age.) The lower and upper age limits were selected because studies on infants with unexplained fever generally have used these age limits and have documented that the prevalence of UTI is high (~5%) in this age group. In those studies, fever was defined as temperature of at least 38.0°C (≥100.4°F); accordingly, this definition of fever is used in this guideline. Neonates and infants less than 2 months of age are excluded, because there are special considerations in this age group that may limit the application of evidence derived from the studies of 2- to 24-month-old children. Data are insufficient to determine whether the evidence generated from studies of infants 2 to 24 months of age applies to children more than 24 months of age.

METHODS

To provide evidence for the guideline, 2 literature searches were conducted, that is, a surveillance of Medline-listed literature over the past 10 years for significant changes since the guideline was published and a systematic review of the literature on the effective-

ness of prophylactic antimicrobial therapy to prevent recurrence of febrile UTI/pyelonephritis in children with vesicoureteral reflux (VUR). The latter was based on the new and growing body of evidence questioning the effectiveness of antimicrobial prophylaxis to prevent recurrent febrile UTI in children with VUR. To explore this particular issue, the literature search was expanded to include trials published since 1993 in which antimicrobial prophylaxis was compared with no treatment or placebo treatment for children with VUR. Because all except 1 of the recent randomized controlled trials (RCTs) of the effectiveness of prophylaxis included children more than 24 months of age and some did not provide specific data according to grade of VUR, the authors of the 6 RCTs were contacted; all provided raw data from their studies specifically addressing infants 2 to 24 months of age, according to grade of VUR. Meta-analysis of these data was performed.

Results from the literature searches and meta-analyses were provided to committee members. Issues were raised and discussed until consensus was reached regarding recommendations. The quality of evidence supporting each recommendation and the strength of the recommendation were assessed by the committee member most experienced in informatics and epidemiology and were graded according to AAP policy[5] (Fig 1).

The subcommittee formulated 7 recommendations, which are presented in the text in the order in which a clinician would use them when evaluating and treating a febrile infant, as well as in algorithm form in the Appendix. This clinical practice guideline is not intended to be a sole source of guidance for the treatment of febrile infants with UTIs. Rather, it is intended to assist clinicians in decision-making. It is not intended to replace clinical judgment or to

Evidence Quality	Preponderance of Benefit or Harm	Balance of Benefit and Harm
A. Well designed RCTs or diagnostic studies on relevant population	Strong Recommendation	
B. RCTs or diagnostic studies with minor limitations;overwhelmingly consistent evidence from observational studies		Option
C. Observational studies (case-control and cohort design)	Recommendation	
D. Expert opinion, case reports, reasoning from first principles	Option	No Rec
X. Exceptional situations where validating studies cannot be performed and there is a clear preponderance of benefit or harm	Strong Recommendation / Recommendation	

FIGURE 1
AAP evidence strengths.

establish an exclusive protocol for the care of all children with this condition.

DIAGNOSIS

Action Statement 1

If a clinician decides that a febrile infant with no apparent source for the fever requires antimicrobial therapy to be administered because of ill appearance or another pressing reason, the clinician should ensure that a urine specimen is obtained for both culture and urinalysis before an antimicrobial agent is administered; the specimen needs to be obtained through catheterization or SPA, because the diagnosis of UTI cannot be established reliably through culture of urine collected in a bag (evidence quality: A; strong recommendation).

When evaluating febrile infants, clinicians make a subjective assessment of the degree of illness or toxicity, in addition to seeking an explanation for the fever. This clinical assessment determines whether antimicrobial therapy should be initiated promptly and affects the diagnostic process regarding UTI. If the clinician determines that the degree of illness warrants immediate antimicrobial therapy, then a urine specimen suitable for culture should be obtained through catheterization or SPA before antimicrobial agents are

administered, because the antimicrobial agents commonly prescribed in such situations would almost certainly obscure the diagnosis of UTI.

SPA has been considered the standard method for obtaining urine that is uncontaminated by perineal flora. Variable success rates for obtaining urine have been reported (23%–90%).[6–8] When ultrasonographic guidance is used, success rates improve.[9,10] The technique has limited risks, but technical expertise and experience are required, and many parents and physicians perceive the procedure as unacceptably invasive, compared with catheterization. However, there may be no acceptable alternative to SPA for boys with moderate or severe phimosis or girls with tight labial adhesions.

Urine obtained through catheterization for culture has a sensitivity of 95% and a specificity of 99%, compared with that obtained through SPA.[7,11,12] The techniques required for catheterization and SPA are well described.[13] When catheterization or SPA is being attempted, the clinician should have a sterile container ready to collect a urine specimen, because the preparation for the procedure may stimulate the child to void. Whether the urine is obtained through catheterization or is voided, the first few drops should be allowed to fall outside the sterile con-

tainer, because they may be contaminated by bacteria in the distal urethra.

Cultures of urine specimens collected in a bag applied to the perineum have an unacceptably high false-positive rate and are valid only when they yield negative results.[6,14–16] With a prevalence of UTI of 5% and a high rate of false-positive results (specificity: ~63%), a "positive" culture result for urine collected in a bag would be a false-positive result 88% of the time. For febrile boys, with a prevalence of UTI of 2%, the rate of false-positive results is 95%; for circumcised boys, with a prevalence of UTI of 0.2%, the rate of false-positive results is 99%. Therefore, in cases in which antimicrobial therapy will be initiated, catheterization or SPA is required to establish the diagnosis of UTI.

- Aggregate quality of evidence: A (diagnostic studies on relevant populations).

- Benefits: A missed diagnosis of UTI can lead to renal scarring if left untreated; overdiagnosis of UTI can lead to overtreatment and unnecessary and expensive imaging. Once antimicrobial therapy is initiated, the opportunity to make a definitive diagnosis is lost; multiple studies of antimicrobial therapy have shown that the urine may be rapidly sterilized.

- Harms/risks/costs: Catheterization is invasive.

- Benefit-harms assessment: Preponderance of benefit over harm.

- Value judgments: Once antimicrobial therapy has begun, the opportunity to make a definitive diagnosis is lost. Therefore, it is important to have the most-accurate test for UTI performed initially.

- Role of patient preferences: There is no evidence regarding patient preferences for bag versus catheterized urine. However, bladder tap has been shown to be more painful than urethral catheterization.

- Exclusions: None.

- Intentional vagueness: The basis of the determination that antimicrobial therapy is needed urgently is not specified, because variability in clinical judgment is expected; considerations for individual patients, such as availability of follow-up care, may enter into the decision, and the literature provides only general guidance.

- Policy level: Strong recommendation.

Action Statement 2

If a clinician assesses a febrile infant with no apparent source for the fever as not being so ill as to require immediate antimicrobial therapy, then the clinician should assess the likelihood of UTI (see below for how to assess likelihood).

Action Statement 2a

If the clinician determines the febrile infant to have a low likelihood of UTI (see text), then clinical follow-up monitoring without testing is sufficient (evidence quality: A; strong recommendation).

Action Statement 2b

If the clinician determines that the febrile infant is not in a low-risk group (see below), then there are 2 choices (evidence quality: A; strong recommendation). Option 1 is to obtain a urine specimen through catheterization or SPA for culture and urinalysis. Option 2 is to obtain a urine specimen through the most convenient means and to perform a urinalysis. If the urinalysis results suggest a UTI (positive leukocyte esterase test results or nitrite test or microscopic analysis results positive for leukocytes or bacteria), then a urine specimen should

Individual Risk Factors: Girls
White race
Age < 12 mo
Temperature ≥ 39°C
Fever ≥ 2 d
Absence of another source of infection

Probability of UTI	No. of Factors Present
≤1%	No more than 1
≤2%	No more than 2

Individual Risk Factors: Boys
Nonblack race
Temperature ≥ 39°C
Fever > 24 h
Absence of another source of infection

Probability of UTI	No. of Factors Present	
	Uncircumcised	Circumcised
≤1%	a	No more than 2
≤2%	None	No more than 3

FIGURE 2

Probability of UTI Among Febrile Infant Girls[28] and Infant Boys[30] According to Number of Findings Present. [a]Probability of UTI exceeds 1% even with no risk factors other than being uncircumcised.

be obtained through catheterization or SPA and cultured; if urinalysis of fresh (<1 hour since void) urine yields negative leukocyte esterase and nitrite test results, then it is reasonable to monitor the clinical course without initiating antimicrobial therapy, recognizing that negative urinalysis results do not rule out a UTI with certainty.

If the clinician determines that the degree of illness does not require immediate antimicrobial therapy, then the likelihood of UTI should be assessed. As noted previously, the overall prevalence of UTI in febrile infants who have no source for their fever evident on the basis of history or physical examination results is approximately 5%,[17,18] but it is possible to identify groups with higher-than-average likelihood and some with lower-than-average likelihood. The prevalence of UTI among febrile infant girls is more than twice that among febrile infant boys (relative risk: 2.27). The rate for uncircumcised boys is 4 to 20 times higher than that for circumcised boys, whose rate of UTI is only 0.2% to 0.4%.[19–24] The presence of another, clinically obvious source of infection reduces the likelihood of UTI by one-half.[25]

In a survey asking, "What yield is required to warrant urine culture in febrile infants?," the threshold was less than 1% for 10.4% of academicians and 11.7% for practitioners[26]; when the threshold was increased to 1% to 3%, 67.5% of academicians and 45.7% of practitioners considered the yield sufficiently high to warrant urine culture. Therefore, attempting to operationalize "low likelihood" (ie, below a threshold that warrants a urine culture) does not produce an absolute percentage; clinicians will choose a threshold depending on factors such as their confidence that contact will be maintained through the illness (so that a specimen can be obtained at a later time) and comfort with diagnostic uncertainty. Fig 2 indicates the number of risk factors associated with threshold probabilities of UTI of at least 1% and at least 2%.

In a series of studies, Gorelick, Shaw, and colleagues[27–29] derived and validated a prediction rule for febrile infant girls on the basis of 5 risk factors, namely, white race, age less than 12 months, temperature of at least 39°C, fever for at least 2 days, and absence of another source of infection. This prediction rule, with sensitivity of 88% and specificity of 30%, permits some infant girls to be considered in a low-likelihood group (Fig 2). For example, of girls with no identifiable source of infection, those who are non-white and more than 12 months of age with a recent onset (<2 days) of low-grade fever (<39°C) have less than a 1% probability of UTI; each additional risk factor increases the probability. It should be noted, however, that some of the factors (eg, duration of fever) may change during the course of the illness, excluding the infant from a low-likelihood designation and prompting testing as described in action statement 2a.

As demonstrated in Fig 2, the major risk factor for febrile infant boys is whether they are circumcised. The probability of UTI can be estimated on the basis of 4 risk factors, namely, nonblack race, temperature of at least 39°C, fever for more than 24 hours, and absence of another source of infection.[4,30]

If the clinician determines that the infant does not require immediate antimicrobial therapy and a urine specimen is desired, then often a urine collection bag affixed to the perineum is used. Many clinicians think that this collection technique has a low contamination rate under the following circumstances: the patient's perineum is properly cleansed and rinsed before application of the collection bag, the urine bag is removed promptly after urine is voided into the bag, and the specimen is refrigerated or processed immediately. Even if contamination from the perineal skin is minimized, however, there may be significant contamination from the vagina in girls or the prepuce in uncircumcised boys, the 2 groups at highest risk of UTI. A "positive" culture result from a specimen collected in a bag cannot be used to document a UTI; confirmation requires culture of a specimen collected through catheterization or SPA. Because there may be substantial delay waiting for the infant to void and a second specimen, obtained through catheterization, may be necessary if the urinalysis suggests the possibility of UTI, many clinicians prefer to obtain a

definitive urine specimen through catheterization initially.

- Aggregate quality of evidence: A (diagnostic studies on relevant populations).

- Benefits: Accurate diagnosis of UTI can prevent the spread of infection and renal scarring; avoiding overdiagnosis of UTI can prevent overtreatment and unnecessary and expensive imaging.

- Harms/risks/costs: A small proportion of febrile infants, considered at low likelihood of UTI, will not receive timely identification and treatment of their UTIs.

- Benefit-harms assessment: Preponderance of benefit over harm.

- Value judgments: There is a risk of UTI sufficiently low to forestall further evaluation.

- Role of patient preferences: The choice of option 1 or option 2 and the threshold risk of UTI warranting obtaining a urine specimen may be influenced by parents' preference to avoid urethral catheterization (if a bag urine sample yields negative urinalysis results) versus timely evaluation (obtaining a definitive specimen through catheterization).

- Exclusions: Because it depends on a range of patient- and physician-specific considerations, the precise threshold risk of UTI warranting obtaining a urine specimen is left to the clinician but is below 3%.

- Intentional vagueness: None.

- Policy level: Strong recommendation.

TABLE 1 Sensitivity and Specificity of Components of Urinalysis, Alone and in Combination

Test	Sensitivity (Range), %	Specificity (Range), %
Leukocyte esterase test	83 (67–94)	78 (64–92)
Nitrite test	53 (15–82)	98 (90–100)
Leukocyte esterase or nitrite test positive	93 (90–100)	72 (58–91)
Microscopy, WBCs	73 (32–100)	81 (45–98)
Microscopy, bacteria	81 (16–99)	83 (11–100)
Leukocyte esterase test, nitrite test, or microscopy positive	99.8 (99–100)	70 (60–92)

Action Statement 3

To establish the diagnosis of UTI, clinicians should require *both* urinalysis results that suggest infection (pyuria and/or bacteriuria) *and* the presence of at least 50 000 colony-forming units (CFUs) per mL of a uropathogen cultured from a urine specimen obtained through catheterization or SPA (evidence quality: C; recommendation).

Urinalysis

General Considerations

Urinalysis cannot substitute for urine culture to document the presence of UTI but needs to be used in conjunction with culture. Because urine culture results are not available for at least 24 hours, there is considerable interest in tests that may predict the results of the urine culture and enable presumptive therapy to be initiated at the first encounter. Urinalysis can be performed on any specimen, including one collected from a bag applied to the perineum. However, the specimen must be fresh (<1 hour after voiding with maintenance at room temperature or <4 hours after voiding with refrigeration), to ensure sensitivity and specificity of the urinalysis. The tests that have received the most attention are biochemical analyses of leukocyte esterase and nitrite through a rapid dipstick method and urine microscopic examination for white blood cells (WBCs) and bacteria (Table 1).

Urine dipsticks are appealing, because they provide rapid results, do not require microscopy, and are eligible for a waiver under the Clinical Laboratory Improvement Amendments. They indicate the presence of leukocyte esterase (as a surrogate marker for pyuria) and urinary nitrite (which is converted from dietary nitrates in the presence of most Gram-negative enteric bacteria in the urine). The conversion of dietary nitrates to nitrites by bacteria requires approximately 4 hours in the bladder.[31] The performance characteristics of both leukocyte esterase and nitrite tests vary according to the definition used for positive urine culture results, the age and symptoms of the population being studied, and the method of urine collection.

Nitrite Test

A nitrite test is not a sensitive marker for children, particularly infants, who empty their bladders frequently. Therefore, negative nitrite test results have little value in ruling out UTI. Moreover, not all urinary pathogens reduce nitrate to nitrite. The test is helpful when the result is positive, however, because it is highly specific (ie, there are few false-positive results).[32]

Leukocyte Esterase Test

The sensitivity of the leukocyte esterase test is 94% when it used in the context of clinically suspected UTI. Overall, the reported sensitivity in various studies is lower (83%), because the results of leukocyte esterase tests were related to culture results without exclusion of individuals with asymptomatic bacteriuria. The absence of leukocyte esterase in the urine of individuals with asymptomatic bacteriuria is an advantage of the test, rather than a limitation, because it distinguishes individuals with asymptomatic bacteriuria from those with true UTI.

The specificity of the leukocyte esterase test (average: 72% [range:

64%–92%]) generally is not as good as the sensitivity, which reflects the nonspecificity of pyuria in general. Accordingly, positive leukocyte esterase test results should be interpreted with caution, because false-positive results are common. With numerous conditions other than UTI, including fever resulting from other conditions (eg, streptococcal infections or Kawasaki disease), and after vigorous exercise, WBCs may be found in the urine. Therefore, a finding of pyuria by no means confirms that an infection of the urinary tract is present.

The absence of pyuria in children with true UTIs is rare, however. It is theoretically possible if a febrile child is assessed before the inflammatory response has developed, but the inflammatory response to a UTI produces both fever and pyuria; therefore, children who are being evaluated because of fever should already have WBCs in their urine. More likely explanations for significant bacteriuria in culture in the absence of pyuria include contaminated specimens, insensitive criteria for pyuria, and asymptomatic bacteriuria. In most cases, when true UTI has been reported to occur in the absence of pyuria, the definition of pyuria has been at fault. The standard method of assessing pyuria has been centrifugation of the urine and microscopic analysis, with a threshold of 5 WBCs per high-power field (~25 WBCs per μL). If a counting chamber is used, however, the finding of at least 10 WBCs per μL in uncentrifuged urine has been demonstrated to be more sensitive[33] and performs well in clinical situations in which the standard method does not, such as with very young infants.[34]

An important cause of bacteriuria in the absence of pyuria is asymptomatic bacteriuria. Asymptomatic bacteriuria often is associated with school-aged and older girls,[35] but it can be present

during infancy. In a study of infants 2 to 24 months of age, 0.7% of afebrile girls had 3 successive urine cultures with 10^5 CFUs per mL of a single uropathogen.[26] Asymptomatic bacteriuria can be easily confused with true UTI in a febrile infant but needs to be distinguished, because studies suggest that antimicrobial treatment may do more harm than good.[36] The key to distinguishing true UTI from asymptomatic bacteriuria is the presence of pyuria.

Microscopic Analysis for Bacteriuria

The presence of bacteria in a fresh, Gram-stained specimen of uncentrifuged urine correlates with 10^5 CFUs per mL in culture.[37] An "enhanced urinalysis," combining the counting chamber assessment of pyuria noted previously with Gram staining of drops of uncentrifuged urine, with a threshold of at least 1 Gram-negative rod in 10 oil immersion fields, has greater sensitivity, specificity, and positive predictive value than does the standard urinalysis[33] and is the preferred method of urinalysis when appropriate equipment and personnel are available.

Automated Urinalysis

Automated methods to perform urinalysis are now being used in many hospitals and laboratories. Image-based systems use flow imaging analysis technology and software to classify particles in uncentrifuged urine specimens rapidly.[38] Results correlate well with manual methods, especially for red blood cells, WBCs, and squamous epithelial cells. In the future, this may be the most common method by which urinalysis is performed in laboratories.

Culture

The diagnosis of UTI is made on the basis of quantitative urine culture results in addition to evidence of pyuria and/or bacteriuria. Urine specimens should be processed as expediently as possible. If the specimen is not processed promptly, then it should be refrigerated to prevent the growth of organisms that can occur in urine at room temperature; for the same reason, specimens that require transportation to another site for processing should be transported on ice. A properly collected urine specimen should be inoculated on culture medium that will allow identification of urinary tract pathogens.

Urine culture results are considered positive or negative on the basis of the number of CFUs that grow on the culture medium.[36] Definition of significant colony counts with regard to the method of collection considers that the distal urethra and periurethral area are commonly colonized by the same bacteria that may cause UTI; therefore, a low colony count may be present in a specimen obtained through voiding or catheterization when bacteria are not present in bladder urine. Definitions of positive and negative culture results are operational and not absolute. The time the urine resides in the bladder (bladder incubation time) is an important determinant of the magnitude of the colony count. The concept that more than 100 000 CFUs per mL indicates a UTI was based on morning collections of urine from adult women, with comparison of specimens from women without symptoms and women considered clinically to have pyelonephritis; the transition range, in which the proportion of women with pyelonephritis exceeded the proportion of women without symptoms, was 10 000 to 100 000 CFUs per mL.[39] In most instances, an appropriate threshold to consider bacteriuria "significant" in infants and children is the presence of at least 50 000 CFUs per mL of a single urinary pathogen.[40] (Organisms such as *Lactobacillus* spp, coagulase-negative staphylococci, and *Corynebacterium*

spp are not considered clinically relevant urine isolates for otherwise healthy, 2- to 24-month-old children.) Reducing the threshold from 100 000 CFUs per mL to 50 000 CFUs per mL would seem to increase the sensitivity of culture at the expense of decreased specificity; however, because the proposed criteria for UTI now include evidence of pyuria in addition to positive culture results, infants with "positive" culture results alone will be recognized as having asymptomatic bacteriuria rather than a true UTI. Some laboratories report growth only in the following categories: 0 to 1000, 1000 to 10 000, 10 000 to 100 000, and more than 100 000 CFUs per mL. In such cases, results in the 10 000 to 100 000 CFUs per mL range need to be evaluated in context, such as whether the urinalysis findings support the diagnosis of UTI and whether the organism is a recognized uropathogen.

Alternative culture methods, such as dipslides, may have a place in the office setting; sensitivity is reported to be in the range of 87% to 100%, and specificity is reported to be 92% to 98%, but dipslides cannot specify the organism or antimicrobial sensitivities.[41] Practices that use dipslides should do so in collaboration with a certified laboratory for identification and sensitivity testing or, in the absence of such results, may need to perform "test of cure" cultures after 24 hours of treatment.

- Aggregate quality of evidence: C (observational studies).
- Benefits: Accurate diagnosis of UTI can prevent the spread of infection and renal scarring; avoiding overdiagnosis of UTI can prevent overtreatment and unnecessary and expensive imaging. These criteria reduce the likelihood of overdiagnosis of UTI in infants with asymptomatic bacteriuria or contaminated specimens.

- Harms/risks/costs: Stringent diagnostic criteria may miss a small number of UTIs.
- Benefit-harms assessment: Preponderance of benefit over harm.
- Value judgments: Treatment of asymptomatic bacteriuria may be harmful.
- Role of patient preferences: We assume that parents prefer no action in the absence of a UTI (avoiding false-positive results) over a very small chance of missing a UTI.
- Exclusions: None.
- Intentional vagueness: None.
- Policy level: Recommendation.

MANAGEMENT

Action Statement 4

Action Statement 4a

When initiating treatment, the clinician should base the choice of route of administration on practical considerations. Initiating treatment orally or parenterally is equally efficacious. The clinician should base the choice of agent on local antimicrobial sensitivity patterns (if available) and should adjust the choice according to sensitivity testing of the isolated uropathogen (evidence quality: A; strong recommendation).

Action Statement 4b

The clinician should choose 7 to 14 days as the duration of antimicrobial therapy (evidence quality: B; recommendation).

The goals of treatment of acute UTI are to eliminate the acute infection, to prevent complications, and to reduce the likelihood of renal damage. Most children can be treated orally.[42–44] Patients whom clinicians judge to be "toxic" or who are unable to retain oral intake (including medications) should receive an antimicrobial agent parenter-

TABLE 2 Some Empiric Antimicrobial Agents for Parenteral Treatment of UTI

Antimicrobial Agent	Dosage
Ceftriaxone	75 mg/kg, every 24 h
Cefotaxime	150 mg/kg per d, divided every 6–8 h
Ceftazidime	100–150 mg/kg per d, divided every 8 h
Gentamicin	7.5 mg/kg per d, divided every 8 h
Tobramycin	5 mg/kg per d, divided every 8 h
Piperacillin	300 mg/kg per d, divided every 6–8 h

TABLE 3 Some Empiric Antimicrobial Agents for Oral Treatment of UTI

Antimicrobial Agent	Dosage
Amoxicillin-clavulanate	20–40 mg/kg per d in 3 doses
Sulfonamide	
Trimethoprim-sulfamethoxazole	6–12 mg/kg trimethoprim and 30-60 mg/kg sulfamethoxazole per d in 2 doses
Sulfisoxazole	120–150 mg/kg per d in 4 doses
Cephalosporin	
Cefixime	8 mg/kg per d in 1 dose
Cefpodoxime	10 mg/kg per d in 2 doses
Cefprozil	30 mg/kg per d in 2 doses
Cefuroxime axetil	20–30 mg/kg per d in 2 doses
Cephalexin	50–100 mg/kg per d in 4 doses

ally (Table 2) until they exhibit clinical improvement, generally within 24 to 48 hours, and are able to retain orally administered fluids and medications. In a study of 309 febrile infants with UTIs, only 3 (1%) were deemed too ill to be assigned randomly to either parenteral or oral treatment.[42] Parenteral administration of an antimicrobial agent also should be considered when compliance with obtaining an antimicrobial agent and/or administering it orally is uncertain. The usual choices for oral treatment of UTIs include a cephalosporin, amoxicillin plus clavulanic acid, or trimethoprim-sulfamethoxazole (Table 3). It is essential to know local patterns of susceptibility of coliforms to antimicrobial agents, particularly trimethoprim-sulfamethoxazole and cephalexin, because there is substantial geographic variability that needs to be taken into account during selection of an antimicrobial agent before sensitivity results are available. Agents that are excreted in the urine but do not achieve therapeutic concentrations in the bloodstream, such as nitrofurantoin, should not be used to treat febrile infants with UTIs, because parenchymal and serum antimicrobial concentrations may be insufficient to treat pyelonephritis or urosepsis.

Whether the initial route of administration of the antimicrobial agent is oral or parenteral (then changed to oral),

the total course of therapy should be 7 to 14 days. The committee attempted to identify a single, preferred, evidence-based duration, rather than a range, but data comparing 7, 10, and 14 days directly were not found. There is evidence that 1- to 3-day courses for febrile UTIs are inferior to courses in the recommended range; therefore, the minimal duration selected should be 7 days.

- Aggregate quality of evidence: A/B (RCTs).

- Benefits: Adequate treatment of UTI can prevent the spread of infection and renal scarring. Outcomes of short courses (1–3 d) are inferior to those of 7- to 14-d courses.

- Harms/risks/costs: There are minimal harm and minor cost effects of antimicrobial choice and duration of therapy.

- Benefit-harms assessment: Preponderance of benefit over harm.

- Value judgments: Adjusting antimicrobial choice on the basis of available data and treating according to best evidence will minimize cost and consequences of failed or unnecessary treatment.

- Role of patient preferences: It is assumed that parents prefer the most-effective treatment and the least amount of medication that ensures effective treatment.

- Exclusions: None.

- Intentional vagueness: No evidence

distinguishes the benefit of treating 7 vs 10 vs 14 days, and the range is allowable.

- Policy level: Strong recommendation/recommendation.

Action Statement 5

Febrile infants with UTIs should undergo renal and bladder ultrasonography (RBUS) (evidence quality: C; recommendation).

The purpose of RBUS is to detect anatomic abnormalities that require further evaluation, such as additional imaging or urologic consultation. RBUS also provides an evaluation of the renal parenchyma and an assessment of renal size that can be used to monitor renal growth. The yield of actionable findings is relatively low.[45,46] Widespread application of prenatal ultrasonography clearly has reduced the prevalence of previously unsuspected obstructive uropathy in infants, but the consequences of prenatal screening with respect to the risk of renal abnormalities in infants with UTIs have not yet been well defined. There is considerable variability in the timing and quality of prenatal ultrasonograms, and the report of "normal" ultrasonographic results cannot necessarily be relied on to dismiss completely the possibility of a structural abnormality unless the study was a detailed anatomic survey (with measurements), was performed during the third trimester, and was performed and interpreted by qualified individuals.[47]

The timing of RBUS depends on the clinical situation. RBUS is recommended during the first 2 days of treatment to identify serious complications, such as renal or perirenal abscesses or pyonephrosis associated with obstructive uropathy when the clinical illness is unusually severe or substantial clinical improvement is not occurring. For febrile infants with UTIs who demonstrate substantial clinical improvement, however, imaging does not need to occur early during the acute infection and can even be misleading; animal studies demonstrate that *Escherichia coli* endotoxin can produce dilation during acute infection, which could be confused with hydronephrosis, pyonephrosis, or obstruction.[48] Changes in the size and shape of the kidneys and the echogenicity of renal parenchyma attributable to edema also are common during acute infection. The presence of these abnormalities makes it inappropriate to consider RBUS performed early during acute infection to be a true baseline study for later comparisons in the assessment of renal growth.

Nuclear scanning with technetium-labeled dimercaptosuccinic acid has greater sensitivity for detection of acute pyelonephritis and later scarring than does either RBUS or voiding cystourethrography (VCUG). The scanning is useful in research, because it ensures that all subjects in a study have pyelonephritis to start with and it permits assessment of later renal scarring as an outcome measure. The findings on nuclear scans rarely affect acute clinical management, however, and are not recommended as part of routine evaluation of infants with their first febrile UTI. The radiation dose to the patient during dimercaptosuccinic acid scanning is generally low ($\sim$1 mSv),[49] although it may be increased in

children with reduced renal function. The radiation dose from dimercaptosuccinic acid is additive with that of VCUG when both studies are performed.[50] The radiation dose from VCUG depends on the equipment that is used (conventional versus pulsed digital fluoroscopy) and is related directly to the total fluoroscopy time. Moreover, the total exposure for the child will be increased when both acute and follow-up studies are obtained. The lack of exposure to radiation is a major advantage of RBUS, even with recognition of the limitations of this modality that were described previously.

- Aggregate quality of evidence: C (observational studies).

- Benefits: RBUS in this population will yield abnormal results in $\sim$15% of cases, and 1% to 2% will have abnormalities that would lead to action (eg, additional evaluation, referral, or surgery).

- Harms/risks/costs: Between 2% and 3% will be false-positive results, leading to unnecessary and invasive evaluations.

- Benefit-harms assessment: Preponderance of benefit over harm.

- Value judgments: The seriousness of the potentially correctable abnormalities in 1% to 2%, coupled with the absence of physical harm, was judged sufficiently important to tip the scales in favor of testing.

- Role of patient preferences: Because ultrasonography is noninvasive and poses minimal risk, we assume that parents will prefer RBUS over taking even a small risk of missing a serious and correctable condition.

- Exclusions: None.

- Intentional vagueness: None.

- Policy level: Recommendation.

Action Statement 6

Action Statement 6a

VCUG should not be performed routinely after the first febrile UTI; VCUG is indicated if RBUS reveals hydronephrosis, scarring, or other findings that would suggest either high-grade VUR or obstructive uropathy, as well as in other atypical or complex clinical circumstances (evidence quality B; recommendation).

Action Statement 6b

Further evaluation should be conducted if there is a recurrence of febrile UTI (evidence quality: X; recommendation).

For the past 4 decades, the strategy to protect the kidneys from further damage after an initial UTI has been to detect childhood genitourinary abnormalities in which recurrent UTI could increase renal damage. The most common of these is VUR, and VCUG is used to detect this. Management included continuous antimicrobial administration as prophylaxis and surgical intervention if VUR was persistent or recurrences of infection were not prevented with an antimicrobial prophylaxis regimen; some have advocated surgical intervention to correct high-grade reflux even when infection has not recurred. However, it is clear that there are a significant number of infants who develop pyelonephritis in whom VUR cannot be demonstrated, and the effectiveness of antimicrobial prophylaxis for patients who have VUR has been challenged in the past decade. Several studies have suggested that prophylaxis does not confer the desired benefit of preventing recurrent febrile UTI.[51–55] If prophylaxis is, in fact, not beneficial and VUR is not required for development of pyelonephritis, then the rationale for performing VCUG routinely after an initial febrile UTI must be questioned.

RCTs of the effectiveness of prophylaxis performed to date generally included children more than 24 months of age, and some did not provide complete data according to grade of VUR. These 2 factors have compromised meta-analyses. To ensure direct comparisons, the committee contacted the 6 researchers who had conducted the most recent RCTs and requested raw data from their studies.[51–56] All complied, which permitted the creation of a data set with data for 1091 infants 2 to 24 months of age according to grade of VUR. A χ^2 analysis (2-tailed) and a formal meta-analysis did not detect a statistically significant benefit of prophylaxis in preventing recurrence of febrile UTI/pyelonephritis in infants without reflux or those with grades I, II, III, or IV VUR (Table 4 and Fig 3). Only 5 infants with grade V VUR were included in the RCTs; therefore, data for those infants are not included in Table 4 or Fig 3.

The proportion of infants with high-grade VUR among all infants with febrile UTIs is small. Data adapted from current studies (Table 5) indicate that, of a hypothetical cohort of 100 infants with febrile UTIs, only 1 has grade V VUR; 99 do not. With a practice of waiting for a second UTI to perform VCUG, only 10 of the 100 would need to undergo the procedure and the 1 with grade V VUR would be identified. (It also is possible that the 1 infant with grade V VUR might have been identified after the first UTI on the basis of abnormal RBUS results that prompted VCUG to be performed.) Data to quantify additional potential harm to an infant who is not revealed to have high-grade VUR until a second UTI are not precise but suggest that the increment is insufficient to justify routinely subjecting all infants with an initial febrile UTI to VCUG (Fig 4). To minimize any harm incurred by that infant, attempts have been made to identify, at the time of

TABLE 4 Recurrences of Febrile UTI/Pyelonephritis in Infants 2 to 24 Months of Age With and Without Antimicrobial Prophylaxis, According to Grade of VUR

Reflux Grade	Prophylaxis		No Prophylaxis		P
	No. of Recurrences	Total N	No. of Recurrences	Total N	
None	7	210	11	163	.15
I	2	37	2	35	1.00
II	11	133	10	124	.95
III	31	140	40	145	.29
IV	16	55	21	49	.14

the initial UTI, those who have the greatest likelihood of having high-grade VUR. Unfortunately, there are no clinical or laboratory indicators that have been demonstrated to identify infants with high-grade VUR. Indications for VCUG have been proposed on the basis of consensus in the absence of data[57]; the predictive value of any of the indications for VCUG proposed in this manner is not known.

The level of evidence supporting routine imaging with VCUG was deemed insufficient at the time of the 1999 practice parameter to receive a recommendation, but the consensus of the subcommittee was to "strongly encourage" imaging studies. The position of the current subcommittee reflects the new evidence demonstrating antimicrobial prophylaxis not to be effective as presumed previously. Moreover, prompt diagnosis and effective treatment of a febrile UTI recurrence may be of greater importance regardless of whether VUR is present or the child is receiving antimicrobial prophylaxis. A national study (the Randomized Intervention for Children With Vesicoureteral Reflux study) is currently in progress to identify the effects of a prophylactic antimicrobial regimen for children 2 months to 6 years of age who have experienced a UTI, and it is anticipated to provide additional important data[58] (see Areas for Research).

Action Statement 6a

- Aggregate quality of evidence: B (RCTs).

- Benefits: This avoids, for the vast majority of febrile infants with UTIs, radiation exposure (of particular concern near the ovaries in girls), expense, and discomfort.

- Harms/risks/costs: Detection of a small number of cases of high-grade reflux and correctable abnormalities is delayed.

- Benefit-harms assessment: Preponderance of benefit over harm.

- Value judgments: The risks associated with radiation (plus the expense and discomfort of the procedure) for the vast majority of infants outweigh the risk of delaying the detection of the few with correctable abnormalities until their second UTI.

- Role of patient preferences: The judgment of parents may come into play, because VCUG is an uncomfortable procedure involving radiation exposure. In some cases, parents may prefer to subject their children to the procedure even when the chance of benefit is both small and uncertain. Antimicrobial prophylaxis seems to be ineffective in preventing recurrence of febrile UTI/pyelonephritis for the vast majority of infants. Some parents may want to avoid VCUG even after the second UTI. Because the benefit of identifying high-grade reflux is still in some doubt, these preferences should be considered. It is the judgment of the committee that VCUG is indicated after the second UTI.

- Exclusions: None.

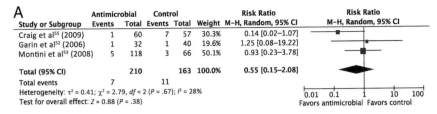

A

Study or Subgroup	Antimicrobial Events	Total	Control Events	Total	Weight	Risk Ratio M-H, Random, 95% CI
Craig et al[55] (2009)	1	60	7	57	30.3%	0.14 [0.02–1.07]
Garin et al[52] (2006)	1	32	1	40	19.6%	1.25 [0.08–19.22]
Montini et al[53] (2008)	5	118	3	66	50.1%	0.93 [0.23–3.78]
Total (95% CI)		**210**		**163**	**100.0%**	**0.55 [0.15–2.08]**
Total events	7		11			

Heterogeneity: $\tau^2 = 0.41$; $\chi^2 = 2.79$, $df = 2$ ($P = .67$); $I^2 = 28\%$
Test for overall effect: $Z = 0.88$ ($P = .38$)

B

Study or Subgroup	Antimicrobial Events	Total	Control Events	Total	Weight	Risk Ratio M-H, Random, 95% CI
Craig et al[55] (2009)	1	10	1	12	49.9%	1.20 [0.09–16.84]
Garin et al[52] (2006)	0	5	0	3		Not estimable
Montini et al[53] (2008)	1	15	1	8	50.1%	0.53 [0.04–7.44]
Roussey-Kesler et al[54] (2008)	0	7	0	12		Not estimable
Total (95% CI)		**37**		**35**	**100.0%**	**0.80 [0.12–5.16]**
Total events	2		2			

Heterogeneity: $\tau^2 = 0.00$; $\chi^2 = 0.18$, $df = 1$ ($P = .67$); $I^2 = 0\%$
Test for overall effect: $z = 0.24$ ($P = .81$)

C

Study or Subgroup	Antimicrobial Events	Total	Control Events	Total	Weight	Risk Ratio M-H, Random, 95% CI
Craig et al[55] (2009)	0	27	1	23	6.3%	0.29 [0.01–6.69]
Garin et al[52] (2006)	1	12	0	10	6.5%	2.54 [0.11–56.25]
Montini et al[53] (2008)	3	31	2	18	21.7%	0.87 [0.16–4.73]
Pennesi et al[51] (2008)	1	11	0	10	6.5%	2.75 [0.12–60.70]
Roussey-Kesler et al[54] (2008)	6	52	7	63	59.0%	1.04 [0.37–2.90]
Total (95% CI)		**133**		**124**	**100.0%**	**1.04 [0.47–2.29]**
Total events	11		10			

Heterogeneity: $\tau^2 = 0.00$; $\chi^2 = 1.38$, $df = 4$ ($P = .85$); $I^2 = 0\%$
Test for overall effect: $z = 0.10$ ($P = .92$)

D

Study or Subgroup	Antimicrobial Events	Total	Control Events	Total	Weight	Risk Ratio M-H, Random, 95% CI
Brandström et al[56] (2010)	5	41	14	43	20.9%	0.37 [0.15–0.95]
Craig et al[55] (2009)	1	24	4	29	7.1%	0.30 [0.04–2.53]
Garin et al[52] (2006)	4	8	0	12	4.5%	13.00 [0.79–212.80]
Montini et al[53] (2008)	6	22	6	13	21.5%	0.59 [0.24–1.45]
Pennesi et al[51] (2008)	9	22	7	24	23.6%	1.40 [0.63–3.12]
Roussey-Kesler et al[54] (2008)	6	23	9	24	22.3%	0.70 [0.29–1.64]
Total (95% CI)		**140**		**145**	**100.0%**	**0.75 [0.40–1.40]**
Total events	31		40			

Heterogeneity: $\tau^2 = 0.27$; $\chi^2 = 9.54$, $df = 5$ ($P = .09$); $I^2 = 48\%$
Test for overall effect: $z = 0.90$ ($P = .37$)

E

Study or Subgroup	Antimicrobial Events	Total	Control Events	Total	Weight	Risk Ratio M-H, Random, 95% CI
Brandström et al[56] (2010)	5	28	11	25	35.0%	0.41 [0.16–1.01]
Craig et al[55] (2009)	3	10	2	8	14.8%	1.20 [0.26–5.53]
Pennesi et al[51] (2008)	8	17	8	16	50.2%	0.94 [0.47–1.90]
Total (95% CI)		**55**		**49**	**100.0%**	**0.73 [0.39–1.35]**
Total events	16		21			

Heterogeneity: $\tau^2 = 0.07$; $\chi^2 = 2.57$, $df = 2$ ($P = .28$); $I^2 = 22\%$
Test for overall effect: $z = 1.01$ ($P = .31$)

FIGURE 3

A, Recurrences of febrile UTI/pyelonephritis in 373 infants 2 to 24 months of age without VUR, with and without antimicrobial prophylaxis (based on 3 studies; data provided by Drs Craig, Garin, and Montini). B, Recurrences of febrile UTI/pyelonephritis in 72 infants 2 to 24 months of age with grade I VUR, with and without antimicrobial prophylaxis (based on 4 studies; data provided by Drs Craig, Garin, Montini, and Roussey-Kesler). C, Recurrences of febrile UTI/pyelonephritis in 257 infants 2 to 24 months of age with grade II VUR, with and without antimicrobial prophylaxis (based on 5 studies; data provided by Drs Craig, Garin, Montini, Pennesi, and Roussey-Kesler). D, Recurrences of febrile UTI/ pyelonephritis in 285 infants 2 to 24 months of age with grade III VUR, with and without antimicrobial prophylaxis (based on 6 studies; data provided by Drs Brandström, Craig, Garin, Montini, Pennesi, and Roussey-Kesler). E, Recurrences of febrile UTI/pyelonephritis in 104 infants 2 to 24 months of age with grade IV VUR, with and without antimicrobial prophylaxis (based on 3 studies; data provided by Drs Brandström, Craig, and Pennesi). M-H indicates Mantel-Haenszel; CI, confidence interval.

TABLE 5 Rates of VUR According to Grade in Hypothetical Cohort of Infants After First UTI and After Recurrence

	Rate, %	
	After First UTI ($N = 100$)	After Recurrence ($N = 10$)
No VUR	65	26
Grades I–III VUR	29	56
Grade IV VUR	5	12
Grade V VUR	1	6

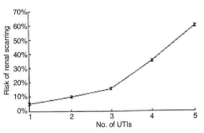

FIGURE 4
Relationship between renal scarring and number of bouts of pyelonephritis. Adapted from Jodal.[59]

- Intentional vagueness: None.

- Policy level: Recommendation.

Action Statement 6b

- Aggregate quality of evidence: X (exceptional situation).

- Benefits: VCUG after a second UTI should identify infants with very high-grade reflux.

- Harms/risks/costs: VCUG is an uncomfortable, costly procedure that involves radiation, including to the ovaries of girls.

- Benefit-harms assessment: Preponderance of benefit over harm.

- Value judgments: The committee judged that patients with high-grade reflux and other abnormalities may benefit from interventions to prevent further scarring. Further studies of treatment for grade V VUR are not underway and are unlikely in the near future, because the condition is uncommon and randomization of treatment in this group generally has been considered unethical.

- Role of patient preferences: As mentioned previously, the judgment of parents may come into play, because VCUG is an uncomfortable procedure involving radiation exposure. In some cases, parents may prefer to subject their children to the procedure even when the chance of benefit is both small and uncertain. The benefits of treatment of VUR remain unproven, but the point estimates suggest a small potential benefit. Similarly, parents may want to avoid VCUG even after the second UTI. Because the benefit of identifying high-grade reflux is still in some doubt, these preferences should be considered. It is the judgment of the committee that VCUG is indicated after the second UTI.

- Exclusions: None.

- Intentional vagueness: Further evaluation will likely start with VCUG but may entail additional studies depending on the findings. The details of further evaluation are beyond the scope of this guideline.

- Policy level: Recommendation.

Action Statement 7

After confirmation of UTI, the clinician should instruct parents or guardians to seek prompt medical evaluation (ideally within 48 hours) for future febrile illnesses, to ensure that recurrent infections can be detected and treated promptly (evidence quality: C; recommendation).

Early treatment limits renal damage better than late treatment,[1,2] and the risk of renal scarring increases as the number of recurrences increase (Fig 4).[59] For these reasons, all infants who have sustained a febrile UTI should have a urine specimen obtained at the onset of subsequent febrile illnesses, so that a UTI can be diagnosed and treated promptly.

- Aggregate quality of evidence: C (observational studies).

- Benefits: Studies suggest that early treatment of UTI reduces the risk of renal scarring.

- Harms/risks/costs: There may be additional costs and inconvenience to parents with more-frequent visits to the clinician for evaluation of fever.

- Benefit-harms assessment: Preponderance of benefit over harm.

- Value judgments: None.

- Role of patient preferences: Parents will ultimately make the judgment to seek medical care.

- Exclusions: None.

- Intentional vagueness: None.

- Policy level: Recommendation.

CONCLUSIONS

The committee formulated 7 key action statements for the diagnosis and treatment of infants and young children 2 to 24 months of age with UTI and unexplained fever. Strategies for diagnosis and treatment depend on whether the clinician determines that antimicrobial therapy is warranted immediately or can be delayed safely until urine culture and urinalysis results are available. Diagnosis is based on the presence of pyuria and at least 50 000 CFUs per mL of a single uropathogen in an appropriately collected specimen of urine; urinalysis alone does not provide a definitive diagnosis. After 7 to 14 days of antimicrobial treatment, close clinical follow-up monitoring should be maintained, with evaluation of the urine during subsequent febrile episodes to permit prompt diagnosis and treatment of recurrent infections. Ultrasonography of the kidneys and bladder should be performed to detect anatomic abnormalities that require further evaluation (eg, additional imaging or urologic consultation). Routine VCUG after the

first UTI is not recommended; VCUG is indicated if RBUS reveals hydronephrosis, scarring, or other findings that would suggest either high-grade VUR or obstructive uropathy, as well as in other atypical or complex clinical circumstances. VCUG also should be performed if there is a recurrence of febrile UTI.

AREAS FOR RESEARCH

One of the major values of a comprehensive literature review is the identification of areas in which evidence is lacking. The following 8 areas are presented in an order that parallels the previous discussion.

1. The relationship between UTIs in infants and young children and reduced renal function in adults has been established but is not well characterized in quantitative terms. The ideal prospective cohort study from birth to 40 to 50 years of age has not been conducted and is unlikely to be conducted. Therefore, estimates of undesirable outcomes in adulthood, such as hypertension and end-stage renal disease, are based on the mathematical product of probabilities at several steps, each of which is subject to bias and error. Other attempts at decision analysis and thoughtful literature review have recognized the same limitations. Until recently, imaging tools available for assessment of the effects of UTIs have been insensitive. With the imaging techniques now available, it may be possible to identify the relationship of scarring to renal impairment and hypertension.

2. The development of techniques that would permit an alternative to invasive sampling and culture would be valuable for general use. Special attention should be given to infant girls and uncircumcised boys, because urethral catheterization may

be difficult and can produce contaminated specimens and SPA now is not commonly performed. Incubation time, which is inherent in the culture process, results in delayed treatment or presumptive treatment on the basis of tests that lack the desired sensitivity and specificity to replace culture.

3. The role of VUR (and therefore of VCUG) is incompletely understood. It is recognized that pyelonephritis (defined through cortical scintigraphy) can occur in the absence of VUR (defined through VCUG) and that progressive renal scarring (defined through cortical scintigraphy) can occur in the absence of demonstrated VUR.[52,53] The presumption that antimicrobial prophylaxis is of benefit for individuals with VUR to prevent recurrences of UTI or the development of renal scars is not supported by the aggregate of data from recent studies and currently is the subject of the Randomized Intervention for Children With Vesicoureteral Reflux study.[58]

4. Although the effectiveness of antimicrobial prophylaxis for the prevention of UTI has not been demonstrated, the concept has biological plausibility. Virtually all antimicrobial agents used to treat or to prevent infections of the urinary tract are excreted in the urine in high concentrations. Barriers to the effectiveness of antimicrobial prophylaxis are adherence to a daily regimen, adverse effects associated with the various agents, and the potential for emergence of anti-

microbial resistance. To overcome these issues, evidence of effectiveness with a well-tolerated, safe product would be required, and parents would need sufficient education to understand the value and importance of adherence. A urinary antiseptic, rather than an antimicrobial agent, would be particularly desirable, because it could be taken indefinitely without concern that bacteria would develop resistance. Another possible strategy might be the use of probiotics.

5. Better understanding of the genome (human and bacterial) may provide insight into risk factors (VUR and others) that lead to increased scarring. Blood specimens will be retained from children enrolled in the Randomized Intervention for Children With Vesicoureteral Reflux study, for future examination of genetic determinants of VUR, recurrent UTI, and renal scarring.[58] VUR is recognized to "run in families,"[60,61] and multiple investigators are currently engaged in research to identify a genetic basis for VUR. Studies may also be able to distinguish the contribution of congenital dysplasia from acquired scarring attributable to UTI.

6. One of the factors used to assess the likelihood of UTI in febrile infants is race. Data regarding rates among Hispanic individuals are limited and would be useful for prediction rules.

7. This guideline is limited to the initial management of the first UTI in febrile infants 2 to 24 months of age. Some of

the infants will have recurrent UTIs; some will be identified as having VUR or other abnormalities. Further research addressing the optimal course of management in specific situations would be valuable.

8. The optimal duration of antimicrobial treatment has not been determined. RCTs of head-to-head comparisons of various duration would be valuable, enabling clinicians to limit antimicrobial exposure to what is needed to eradicate the offending uropathogen.

LEAD AUTHOR
Kenneth B. Roberts, MD

SUBCOMMITTEE ON URINARY TRACT INFECTION, 2009–2011
Kenneth B. Roberts, MD, Chair
Stephen M. Downs, MD, MS
S. Maria E. Finnell, MD, MS
Stanley Hellerstein, MD
Linda D. Shortliffe, MD
Ellen R. Wald, MD
J. Michael Zerin, MD

OVERSIGHT BY THE STEERING COMMITTEE ON QUALITY IMPROVEMENT AND MANAGEMENT, 2009–2011

STAFF
Caryn Davidson, MA

ACKNOWLEDGMENTS
The committee gratefully acknowledges the generosity of the researchers who graciously shared their data to permit the data set with data for 1091 infants aged 2 to 24 months according to grade of VUR to be compiled, that is, Drs Per Brandström, Jonathan Craig, Eduardo Garin, Giovanni Montini, Marco Pennesi, and Gwenaelle Roussey-Kesler.

REFERENCES

1. Winter AL, Hardy BE, Alton DJ, Arbus GS, Churchill BM. Acquired renal scars in children. *J Urol.* 1983;129(6):1190–1194

2. Smellie JM, Poulton A, Prescod NP. Retrospective study of children with renal scarring associated with reflux and urinary infection. *BMJ.* 1994;308(6938):1193–1196

3. American Academy of Pediatrics, Committee on Quality Improvement, Subcommittee on Urinary Tract Infection. Practice parameter: the diagnosis, treatment, and evaluation of the initial urinary tract infection in febrile infants and young children. *Pediatrics.* 1999;103(4):843–852

4. Finnell SM, Carroll AE, Downs SM, et al. Technical report: diagnosis and management of an initial urinary tract infection in febrile infants and young children. *Pediatrics.* 2011;128(3):e749

5. American Academy of Pediatrics, Steering Committee on Quality Improvement and Management. Classifying recommenda-

tions for clinical practice guidelines. *Pediatrics*. 2004;114(3):874–877

6. Leong YY, Tan KW. Bladder aspiration for diagnosis of urinary tract infection in infants and young children. *J Singapore Paediatr Soc*. 1976;18(1):43–47

7. Pryles CV, Atkin MD, Morse TS, Welch KJ. Comparative bacteriologic study of urine obtained from children by percutaneous suprapubic aspiration of the bladder and by catheter. *Pediatrics*. 1959;24(6):983–991

8. Djojohadipringgo S, Abdul Hamid RH, Thahir S, Karim A, Darsono I. Bladder puncture in newborns: a bacteriological study. *Paediatr Indones*. 1976;16(11–12):527–534

9. Gochman RF, Karasic RB, Heller MB. Use of portable ultrasound to assist urine collection by suprapubic aspiration. *Ann Emerg Med*. 1991;20(6):631–635

10. Buys H, Pead L, Hallett R, Maskell R. Suprapubic aspiration under ultrasound guidance in children with fever of undiagnosed cause. *BMJ*. 1994;308(6930):690–692

11. Kramer MS, Tange SM, Drummond KN, Mills EL. Urine testing in young febrile children: a risk-benefit analysis. *J Pediatr*. 1994;125(1):6–13

12. Bonadio WA. Urine culturing technique in febrile infants. *Pediatr Emerg Care*. 1987;3(2):75–78

13. Lohr J. *Pediatric Outpatient Procedures*. Philadelphia, PA: Lippincott; 1991

14. Taylor CM, White RH. The feasibility of screening preschool children for urinary tract infection using dipslides. *Int J Pediatr Nephrol*. 1983;4(2):113–114

15. Sørensen K, Lose G, Nathan E. Urinary tract infections and diurnal incontinence in girls. *Eur J Pediatr*. 1988;148(2):146–147

16. Shannon F, Sepp E, Rose G. The diagnosis of bacteriuria by bladder puncture in infancy and childhood. *Aust Pediatr J*. 1969;5(2):97–100

17. Hoberman A, Chao HP, Keller DM, Hickey R, Davis HW, Ellis D. Prevalence of urinary tract infection in febrile infants. *J Pediatr*. 1993;123(1):17–23

18. Haddon RA, Barnett PL, Grimwood K, Hogg GG. Bacteraemia in febrile children presenting to a paediatric emergency department. *Med J Aust*. 1999;170(10):475–478

19. Wiswell TE, Roscelli JD. Corroborative evidence for the decreased incidence of urinary tract infections in circumcised male infants. *Pediatrics*. 1986;78(1):96–99

20. To T, Agha M, Dick PT, Feldman W. Cohort study on circumcision of newborn boys and subsequent risk of urinary-tract infection. *Lancet*. 1998;352(9143):1813–1816

21. Wiswell TE, Hachey WE. Urinary tract infections and the uncircumcised state: an update. *Clin Pediatr (Phila)*. 1993;32(3):130–134

22. Wiswell TE, Smith FR, Bass JW. Decreased incidence of urinary tract infections in circumcised male infants. *Pediatrics*. 1985;75(5):901–903

23. Ginsburg CM, McCracken GH Jr. Urinary tract infections in young infants. *Pediatrics*. 1982;69(4):409–412

24. Craig JC, Knight JF, Sureshkumar P, Mantz E, Roy LP. Effect of circumcision on incidence of urinary tract infection in preschool boys. *J Pediatr*. 1996;128(1):23–27

25. Levine DA, Platt SL, Dayan PS, et al. Risk of serious bacterial infection in young febrile infants with respiratory syncytial virus infections. *Pediatrics*. 2004;113(6):1728–1734

26. Roberts KB, Charney E, Sweren RJ, et al. Urinary tract infection in infants with unexplained fever: a collaborative study. *J Pediatr*. 1983;103(6):864–867

27. Gorelick MH, Hoberman A, Kearney D, Wald E, Shaw KN. Validation of a decision rule identifying febrile young girls at high risk for urinary tract infection. *Pediatr Emerg Care*. 2003;19(3):162–164

28. Gorelick MH, Shaw KN. Clinical decision rule to identify febrile young girls at risk for urinary tract infection. *Arch Pediatr Adolesc Med*. 2000;154(4):386–390

29. Shaw KN, Gorelick M, McGowan KL, Yakscoe NM, Schwartz JS. Prevalence of urinary tract infection in febrile young children in the emergency department. *Pediatrics*. 1998;102(2). Available at: www.pediatrics.org/cgi/content/full/102/2/e16

30. Shaikh N, Morone NE, Lopez J, et al. Does this child have a urinary tract infection? *JAMA*. 2007;298(24):2895–2904

31. Powell HR, McCredie DA, Ritchie MA. Urinary nitrite in symptomatic and asymptomatic urinary infection. *Arch Dis Child*. 1987;62(2):138–140

32. Kunin CM, DeGroot JE. Sensitivity of a nitrite indicator strip method in detecting bacteriuria in preschool girls. *Pediatrics*. 1977;60(2):244–245

33. Hoberman A, Wald ER, Reynolds EA, Penchansky L, Charron M. Is urine culture necessary to rule out urinary tract infection in young febrile children? *Pediatr Infect Dis J*. 1996;15(4):304–309

34. Herr SM, Wald ER, Pitetti RD, Choi SS. Enhanced urinalysis improves identification of febrile infants ages 60 days and younger at low risk for serious bacterial illness. *Pediatrics*. 2001;108(4):866–871

35. Kunin C. A ten-year study of bacteriuria in schoolgirls: final report of bacteriologic, urologic, and epidemiologic findings. *J Infect Dis*. 1970;122(5):382–393

36. Kemper K, Avner E. The case against screening urinalyses for asymptomatic bacteriuria in children. *Am J Dis Child*. 1992;146(3):343–346

37. Wald E. Genitourinary tract infections: cystitis and pyelonephritis. In: Feigin R, Cherry JD, Demmler GJ, Kaplan SL, eds. *Textbook of Pediatric Infectious Diseases*. 5th ed. Philadelphia, PA: Saunders; 2004:541–555

38. Mayo S, Acevedo D, Quiñones-Torrelo C, Canós I, Sancho M. Clinical laboratory automated urinalysis: comparison among automated microscopy, flow cytometry, two test strips analyzers, and manual microscopic examination of the urine sediments. *J Clin Lab Anal*. 2008;22(4):262–270

39. Kass E. Asymptomatic infections of the urinary tract. *Trans Assoc Am Phys*. 1956;69:56–64

40. Hoberman A, Wald ER, Reynolds EA, Penchansky L, Charron M. Pyuria and bacteriuria in urine specimens obtained by catheter from young children with fever. *J Pediatr*. 1994;124(4):513–519

41. Downs SM. Technical report: urinary tract infections in febrile infants and young children. *Pediatrics*. 1999;103(4). Available at: www.pediatrics.org/cgi/content/full/103/4/e54

42. Hoberman A, Wald ER, Hickey RW, et al. Oral versus initial intravenous therapy for urinary tract infections in young febrile children. *Pediatrics*. 1999;104(1):79–86

43. Hodson EM, Willis NS, Craig JC. Antibiotics for acute pyelonephritis in children. *Cochrane Database Syst Rev*. 2007;(4):CD003772

44. Bloomfield P, Hodson EM, Craig JC. Antibiotics for acute pyelonephritis in children. *Cochrane Database Syst Rev*. 2005;(1):CD003772

45. Hoberman A, Charron M, Hickey RW, Baskin M, Kearney DH, Wald ER. Imaging studies after a first febrile urinary tract infection in young children. *N Engl J Med*. 2003;348(3):195–202

46. Jahnukainen T, Honkinen O, Ruuskanen O, Mertsola J. Ultrasonography after the first febrile urinary tract infection in children. *Eur J Pediatr*. 2006;165(8):556–559

47. Economou G, Egginton J, Brookfield D. The importance of late pregnancy scans for renal tract abnormalities. *Prenat Diagn*. 1994;14(3):177–180

48. Roberts J. Experimental pyelonephritis in the monkey, part III: pathophysiology of ure-

teral malfunction induced by bacteria. *Invest Urol.* 1975;13(2):117–120

49. Smith T, Evans K, Lythgoe MF, Anderson PJ, Gordon I. Radiation dosimetry of technetium-99m-DMSA in children. *J Nucl Med.* 1996;37(8):1336–1342

50. Ward VL. Patient dose reduction during voiding cystourethrography. *Pediatr Radiol.* 2006;36(suppl 2):168–172

51. Pennesi M, Travan L, Peratoner L, et al. Is antibiotic prophylaxis in children with vesicoureteral reflux effective in preventing pyelonephritis and renal scars? A randomized, controlled trial. *Pediatrics.* 2008; 121(6). Available at: www.pediatrics.org/cgi/content/full/121/6/e1489

52. Garin EH, Olavarria F, Garcia Nieto V, Valenciano B, Campos A, Young L. Clinical significance of primary vesicoureteral reflux and urinary antibiotic prophylaxis after acute pyelonephritis: a multicenter, randomized, controlled study. *Pediatrics.* 2006;117(3): 626–632

53. Montini G, Rigon L, Zucchetta P, et al. Prophylaxis after first febrile urinary tract infection in children? A multicenter, randomized, controlled, noninferiority trial. *Pediatrics.* 2008;122(5):1064–1071

54. Roussey-Kesler G, Gadjos V, Idres N, et al. Antibiotic prophylaxis for the prevention of recurrent urinary tract infection in children with low grade vesicoureteral reflux: results from a prospective randomized study. *J Urol.* 2008;179(2):674–679

55. Craig J, Simpson J, Williams G. Antibiotic prophylaxis and recurrent urinary tract infection in children. *N Engl J Med.* 2009; 361(18):1748–1759

56. Brandström P, Esbjorner E, Herthelius M, Swerkersson S, Jodal U, Hansson S. The Swedish Reflux Trial in Children, part III: urinary tract infection pattern. *J Urol.* 2010; 184(1):286–291

57. National Institute for Health and Clinical Excellence. *Urinary Tract Infection in Children: Diagnosis, Treatment, and Long-term Management: NICE Clinical Guideline 54.* London, England: National Institute for Health and Clinical Excellence; 2007. Available at: www.nice.org.uk/nicemedia/live/11819/36032/36032.pdf. Accessed March 14, 2011

58. Keren R, Carpenter MA, Hoberman A, et al. Rationale and design issues of the Randomized Intervention for Children With Vesicoureteral Reflux (RIVUR) study. *Pediatrics.* 2008;122(suppl 5):S240–S250

59. Jodal U. The natural history of bacteriuria in childhood. *Infect Dis Clin North Am.* 1987; 1(4):713–729

60. Eccles MR, Bailey RR, Abbott GD, Sullivan MJ. Unravelling the genetics of vesicoureteric reflux: a common familial disorder. *Hum Mol Genet.* 1996;5(Spec No.):1425–1429

61. Scott JE, Swallow V, Coulthard MG, Lambert HJ, Lee RE. Screening of newborn babies for familial ureteric reflux. *Lancet.* 1997; 350(9075):396–400

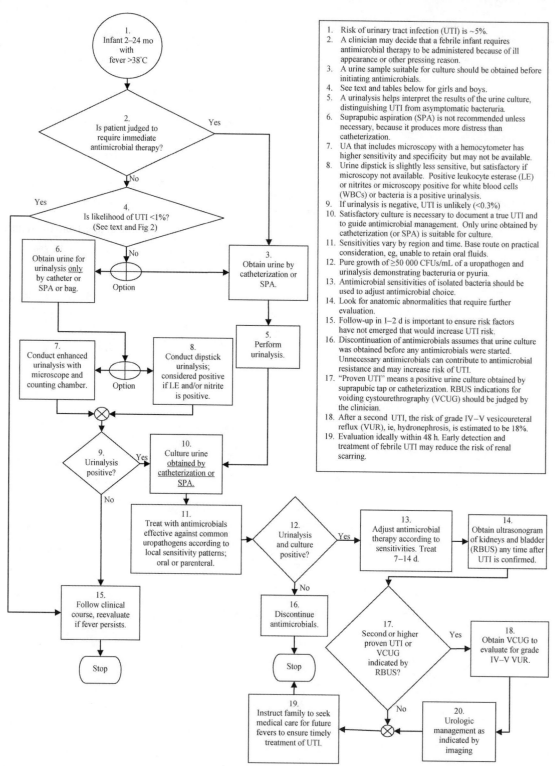

1. Risk of urinary tract infection (UTI) is ~5%.
2. A clinician may decide that a febrile infant requires antimicrobial therapy to be administered because of ill appearance or other pressing reason.
3. A urine sample suitable for culture should be obtained before initiating antimicrobials.
4. See text and tables below for girls and boys.
5. A urinalysis helps interpret the results of the urine culture, distinguishing UTI from asymptomatic bacteriuria.
6. Suprapubic aspiration (SPA) is not recommended unless necessary, because it produces more distress than catheterization.
7. UA that includes microscopy with a hemocytometer has higher sensitivity and specificity but may not be available.
8. Urine dipstick is slightly less sensitive, but satisfactory if microscopy not available. Positive leukocyte esterase (LE) or nitrites or microscopy positive for white blood cells (WBCs) or bacteria is a positive urinalysis.
9. If urinalysis is negative, UTI is unlikely (<0.3%)
10. Satisfactory culture is necessary to document a true UTI and to guide antimicrobial management. Only urine obtained by catheterization (or SPA) is suitable for culture.
11. Sensitivities vary by region and time. Base route on practical consideration, eg, unable to retain oral fluids.
12. Pure growth of ≥50 000 CFUs/mL of a uropathogen and urinalysis demonstrating bacteruria or pyuria.
13. Antimicrobial sensitivities of isolated bacteria should be used to adjust antimicrobial choice.
14. Look for anatomic abnormalities that require further evaluation.
15. Follow-up in 1–2 d is important to ensure risk factors have not emerged that would increase UTI risk.
16. Discontinuation of antimicrobials assumes that urine culture was obtained before any antimicrobials were started. Unnecessary antimicrobials can contribute to antimicrobial resistance and may increase risk of UTI.
17. "Proven UTI" means a positive urine culture obtained by suprapubic tap or catheterization. RBUS indications for voiding cystourethrography (VCUG) should be judged by the clinician.
18. After a second UTI, the risk of grade IV–V vesicoureteral reflux (VUR), ie, hydronephrosis, is estimated to be 18%.
19. Evaluation ideally within 48 h. Early detection and treatment of febrile UTI may reduce the risk of renal scarring.

APPENDIX
Clinical practice guideline algorithm.

Technical Report—Diagnosis and Management of an Initial UTI in Febrile Infants and Young Children

S. Maria E. Finnell, MD, MS, Aaron E. Carroll, MD, MS, Stephen M. Downs, MD, MS, and the Subcommittee on Urinary Tract Infection

KEY WORDS
urinary tract infection, infants, children, vesicoureteral reflux, voiding cystourethrography, antimicrobial, prophylaxis, antibiotic prophylaxis, pyelonephritis

ABBREVIATIONS
UTI—urinary tract infection
VUR—vesicoureteral reflux
VCUG—voiding cystourethrography
CI—confidence interval
RR—risk ratio
RCT—randomized controlled trial
LR—likelihood ratio
SPA—suprapubic aspiration

www.pediatrics.org/cgi/doi/10.1542/peds.2011-1332

doi:10.1542/peds.2011-1332

All technical reports from the American Academy of Pediatrics automatically expire 5 years after publication unless reaffirmed, revised, or retired at or before that time.

PEDIATRICS (ISSN Numbers: Print, 0031-4005; Online, 1098-4275).

Copyright © 2011 by the American Academy of Pediatrics

COMPANION PAPERS: Companions to this article can be found on pages 572 and 595, and online at www.pediatrics.org/cgi/doi/10.1542/peds.2011-1330, www.pediatrics.org/cgi/doi/10.1542/peds.2011-1818, and www.pediatrics.org/cgi/doi/10.1542/peds.2011-1330.

abstract

OBJECTIVES: The diagnosis and management of urinary tract infections (UTIs) in young children are clinically challenging. This report was developed to inform the revised, evidence-based, clinical guideline regarding the diagnosis and management of initial UTIs in febrile infants and young children, 2 to 24 months of age, from the American Academy of Pediatrics Subcommittee on Urinary Tract Infection.

METHODS: The conceptual model presented in the 1999 technical report was updated after a comprehensive review of published literature. Studies with potentially new information or with evidence that reinforced the 1999 technical report were retained. Meta-analyses on the effectiveness of antimicrobial prophylaxis to prevent recurrent UTI were performed.

RESULTS: Review of recent literature revealed new evidence in the following areas. Certain clinical findings and new urinalysis methods can help clinicians identify febrile children at very low risk of UTI. Oral antimicrobial therapy is as effective as parenteral therapy in treating UTI. Data from published, randomized controlled trials do not support antimicrobial prophylaxis to prevent febrile UTI when vesicoureteral reflux is found through voiding cystourethrography. Ultrasonography of the urinary tract after the first UTI has poor sensitivity. Early antimicrobial treatment may decrease the risk of renal damage from UTI.

CONCLUSIONS: Recent literature agrees with most of the evidence presented in the 1999 technical report, but meta-analyses of data from recent, randomized controlled trials do not support antimicrobial prophylaxis to prevent febrile UTI. This finding argues against voiding cystourethrography after the first UTI. *Pediatrics* 2011;128:e749–e770

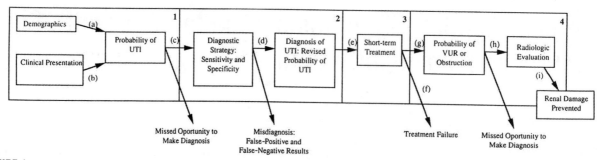

FIGURE 1
Evidence model from the 1999 technical report on the diagnosis and treatment of infants and children with UTIs.

In 1999, the Subcommittee on Urinary Tract Infection of the American Academy of Pediatrics released its guideline on detection, diagnosis, and management for children between 2 and 24 months of age with febrile urinary tract infections (UTIs).[1] The guideline was supported by a technical report[2] that included a critical review of the relevant literature and a cost-effectiveness analysis. Consistent with the policies of the American Academy of Pediatrics, the subcommittee has undertaken a revision of the guideline. This technical report was developed to support the guideline.[3]

The revised technical report was to be based on a selective review of the literature, focusing on changes in the evidence regarding detection, diagnosis, and management of UTIs in these children. The original technical report was designed around an evidence model (Fig 1). Each cell (numbered 1–4) corresponded to a stage in the recognition, diagnosis, or management of UTI. The boxes represented steps the clinician must follow, and the arrows represented the process of moving from one step to the next. Downward arrows represented undesirable consequences in management.[4]

In cell 1, the clinician must combine patient demographic data and other presenting clinical data to arrive at an assessment of the risk of UTI. Failure to do so results in a missed opportunity to make the diagnosis. In cell 2, the cli-

nician must undertake a diagnostic strategy, primarily involving laboratory testing, to arrive at a posterior (posttest) probability of UTI, ruling the diagnosis in or out. Poor test choices or interpretation of results can lead to misdiagnosis. In cell 3, the clinician must choose a treatment for acute UTI; in cell 4, the clinician must consider the possibility of structural or functional anomalies of the urinary tract and diagnose them appropriately to avoid ongoing renal damage.

Implicit in cell 4 is the idea that anomalies of the urinary tract, such as vesicoureteral reflux (VUR) and obstructions, may, if left untreated, lead to significant renal damage, resulting in hypertension or end-stage renal disease. Furthermore, it is assumed that treatment with medical or surgical therapies can prevent these consequences successfully.

The conclusions of the 1999 technical report were that there were high-quality data regarding the prevalence of UTI among febrile infants, the performance of standard diagnostic tests for UTI, and the prevalence of urinary tract abnormalities among children with UTI. The evidence indicating that certain patient characteristics (age, gender, and circumcision status) affected the probability of UTI was weaker. The evidence supporting the relationship between urinary tract abnormalities and future complications, such as hypertension or renal failure,

was considered very poor, and the effectiveness of treatments to prevent these complications was not addressed directly but was assumed.

The cost-effectiveness analysis using these data led to the conclusion that diagnosis and treatment of UTI and evaluation for urinary tract anomalies had borderline cost-effectiveness, costing approximately $700 000 per case of hypertension or end-stage renal disease prevented. On the basis of these results, the subcommittee recommended testing all children between 2 and 24 months of age with fever with no obvious source for UTI, by culturing urine obtained through bladder tap or catheterization. As an option for children who were not going to receive immediate antimicrobial treatment, the committee recommended ruling out UTI through urinalysis of urine obtained with any convenient method. The committee concluded that children found to have a UTI should undergo renal ultrasonography and voiding cystourethrography (VCUG) for evaluation for urinary tract abnormalities, most frequently VUR.

Ten years later, the subcommittee has undertaken a review of the technical analysis for a revised guideline. The strategy for this technical report was to survey the medical literature published in the past 10 years for studies of UTIs in young children. The literature was examined for any data that varied significantly from those analyzed in the first technical report. This survey found an emerging body of literature addressing the effectiveness of antimicrobial agents to prevent recurrent UTI. Therefore, the authors conducted a critical literature review and meta-analysis focused on that specific issue.

METHODS

Surveillance of Recent Literature

The authors searched Medline for articles published in the past 10 years with the medical subject headings "urinary tract infection" and "child (all)." The original search was conducted in 2007, but searches were repeated at intervals (approximately every 3 months) to identify new reports as the guideline was being developed. Titles were reviewed by 2 authors (Drs Downs and Carroll) to identify all articles that were potentially relevant and seemed to contain original data. All titles that were considered potentially relevant by either reviewer were retained. Abstracts of selected articles were reviewed, again to identify articles that were relevant to the guideline and that seemed to contain original data. Review articles that were relevant also were retained for review. Again, all abstracts that were considered potentially relevant by either reviewer were retained. In addition, members of the subcommittee submitted articles that they thought were relevant to be included in the review.

Selected articles were reviewed and summarized by 2 reviewers (Drs Finnell and Downs). The summaries were reviewed, and articles presenting potentially new information were retained. In addition, representative articles reinforcing evidence in the 1999 technical report were retained.

The most significant area of change in the UTI landscape was a new and growing body of evidence regarding the effectiveness of antimicrobial prophylaxis to prevent recurrent infections in

children with VUR. To explore this particular issue, a second, systematic, targeted literature search and formal meta-analysis were conducted to estimate the effectiveness of antimicrobial prophylaxis to prevent renal damage in children with VUR. In addition, 1 author (Dr Finnell) and the chairperson of the guideline committee (Dr Roberts) contacted the authors of those studies to obtain original data permitting subgroup analyses.

Targeted Literature Search and Meta-analysis

To examine specifically the effectiveness of antimicrobial prophylaxis to prevent recurrent UTI and pyelonephritis in children with VUR, a formal meta-analysis of randomized controlled trials (RCTs) was conducted. First, a systematic literature review focused on RCTs, including studies in press, was performed.

Inclusion Criteria

RCTs published in the past 15 years (1993–2009) that compared antimicrobial treatment versus no treatment or placebo treatment for the prevention of recurrent UTI and included a minimum of 6 months of follow-up monitoring were included. Published articles, articles in press, and published abstracts were included. There were no language restrictions. To be included, studies needed to enroll children who had undergone VCUG for determination of the presence and grade of VUR. Studies that examined antibiotic prophylaxis versus no treatment or placebo treatment were included.

Outcome Measures

The primary outcome was the number of episodes of pyelonephritis or febrile UTI diagnosed on the basis of the presence of fever and bacterial growth in urine cultures. A secondary outcome was an episode of any type of UTI, including cystitis, nonfebrile UTI, and

asymptomatic bacteriuria in addition to the cases of pyelonephritis or febrile UTI.

Search Methods

The initial literature search was conducted on June 24, 2008, and the search was repeated on April 14, 2009. Studies were obtained from the following databases: Medline (1993 to June 2008), Embase (1993 to June 2008), Cochrane Central Register for Controlled Trials, bibliographies of identified relevant articles and reviews, and the Web site www.ClinicalTrials.gov.

The search terms "vesico-ureteral reflux," "VUR," "vesicoureter*," "vesico ureter*," "vesicourethral," or "vesico urethral" and "antibiotic," "anti biotic," "antibacterial," "anti bacterial," "antimicrobial," "anti microbial," "antiinfective," or "anti infective" were used. The asterisk represents the truncation or wild card symbol, which indicates that all suffixes and variants were included. The search was limited to the publication types and subject headings for all clinical trials and included all keyword variants for "random" in Medline and Embase.[5] In addition, the Web site www.ClinicalTrials.gov was searched on May 20, 2010.

The search strategy and the screening of the titles for selection of potentially relevant abstracts were completed by 1 reviewer (Dr Finnell). Two reviewers (Drs Finnell and Downs) screened selected abstracts to identify appropriate articles. Published articles and abstracts that met the inclusion criteria were included in the meta-analysis. Additional information was sought from authors whose articles or abstracts did not contain the information needed for a decision regarding inclusion. The selection process is summarized in Fig 2.

Assessment of Studies

The quality of selected articles and abstracts was assessed with the scoring

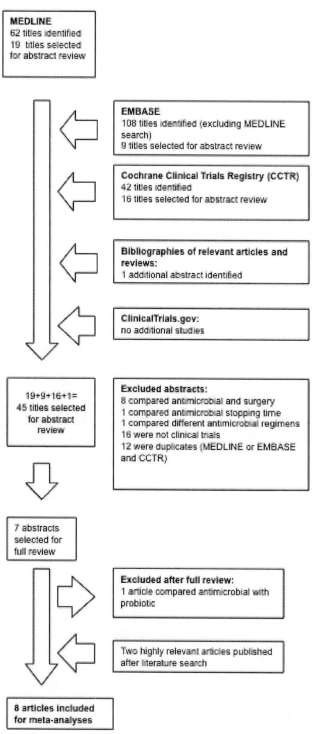

FIGURE 2
Study selection for meta-analyses.

Meta-analyses

All statistical tests were performed by using Review Manager 5.1 (Nordic Cochrane Centre, Copenhagen, Denmark). The following settings were used for the analyses: dichotomous outcome and Mantel-Haenzel statistical method. Data were analyzed with a random-effects model. When no statistically significant effect and no statistical heterogeneity were detected, data also were analyzed with a fixed-effects model, because that type of analysis is more likely to detect a difference. The effect measure was presented as a risk ratio (RR). The results for the primary outcome (pyelonephritis or febrile UTI) and the secondary outcome (any type of UTI, including cystitis, nonfebrile UTI, and asymptomatic bacteriuria) were calculated as point estimates with corresponding 95% confidence intervals (CIs). Heterogeneity was analyzed by using the Q statistic with a threshold of $P < .05$. The number of studies was insufficient for assessment of publication bias with a funnel plot.

Meta-analyses of Data According to VUR Grade and for Children 2 to 24 Months of Age

The published data on which the meta-analyses were based did not contain subgroup data relevant to the practice guideline. Specifically, some studies did not report outcomes according to the severity of VUR, and some did not report outcomes specific to the age range of interest (2–24 months). Therefore, the committee chairperson contacted the authors of the reports included in the meta-analysis, to obtain original data. Data on recurrence according to VUR grade and for the subgroup of children 2 to 24 months of age were received from the authors, and these data were analyzed in separate meta-analyses.

system described by Downs and Black in 1998.[6] Each study received scores (from 2 assessors) on a scale from 0 to 32. Six of the articles and abstracts were included in a first meta-analysis, which evaluated febrile UTI or pyelonephritis as the outcome. A second meta-analysis, which included all studies with the outcome "all UTI," also was conducted.

RESULTS

Surveillance of Recent Literature

The surveillance of recent literature yielded 1308 titles. Of those, 297 abstracts were selected for review. From among the abstracts, 159 articles were selected for full review. The results of this surveillance, as well as the full review and meta-analyses, are organized according to the evidence diagram in Fig 1.

Box 1: Prevalence and Risk Factors for UTI

The Presence of UTI Should Be Considered for Any Child 2 Months to 2 Years of Age With Unexplained Fever

The previous technical report described a very consistent UTI prevalence of 5% among children 2 to 24 months of age with a fever without obvious source. In 1996, Hoberman et al[7] conducted a study of urine diagnostic tests with a cohort of 4253 infants with fever and found a prevalence of 5%. Similarly, in a 1999 cohort study of 534 children 3 to 36 months of age with a temperature of more than 39°C and no apparent source of fever, UTI prevalence was determined to be 5%.[8] In a 1998 cohort study of 2411 children (boys and girls <12 months of age and girls 12–24 months of age) seen in the emergency department with a temperature of more than 38.5°C, Shaw et al[9] determined the prevalence of UTI to be 3.3%. Because 84% of those children were black, this estimate may be low for the general population (see below). In a meta-analysis of 14 studies, the pooled prevalence of UTI was 7% (95% CI: 5.5%–8.4%) among febrile children 0 to 24 months of age, of both genders, with or without additional symptoms of UTI.[10] In the 6- to 12-month age group, however, the prevalence was 5.4%; in the 12- to 24-month age group, the prevalence was 4.5%. Taken to-

gether, these estimates are consistent with a pooled prevalence of 5% determined in earlier studies.

The previous technical report examined the effects of age, gender, and circumcision status on the prevalence of UTI. The conclusion was that boys more than 1 year of age who had been circumcised were at sufficiently low risk of UTI (<1%) that evaluation of this subpopulation would not be cost-effective. New work confirms an approximately threefold to fourfold decreased risk of UTI among circumcised boys.[10] The difference seems to be greater for younger children.[11] Additional clinical characteristics were shown more recently to affect the risk of UTI among febrile infants and children. From a study by Shaikh et al,[12] a set of likelihood ratios (LRs) for various risk factors for UTI was derived (Table 1).

A simplified way to examine the data on boys from Shaikh et al[12] is first to ex-

clude boys with a history of UTI, because the guideline addresses only first-time UTIs, and to exclude those with ill appearance, because they are likely to require antimicrobial agents, in which case a urine specimen would be required. Finally, boys with and without circumcision should be considered separately. This leaves 4 risk factors for boys who present with fever, namely, temperature above 39°C, fever for more than 24 hours, no apparent fever source, and nonblack race. All 4 have similar LRs. If 2 assumptions are made, then the decision rule can be simplified. The first assumption is that, as a first approximation, each risk factor has a positive LR of 1.4 and a negative LR of 0.7. The second assumption is that the presence of each risk factor is conditionally independent of the others, given the presence or absence of UTI. With these reasonable assumptions, Table 2 applies to boys with no previous history of UTI

TABLE 1 LRs and Posttest Probabilities of UTI for Infant Boys According to Number of Findings Present

Finding	LR		Posttest Probability, %					
			All Boys		Circumcised Boys		Uncircumcised Boys	
	Positive	Negative	After Positive Results	After Negative Results	After Positive Results	After Negative Results	After Positive Results	After Negative Results
Uncircumcised	2.8	0.33	5.9	0.7	—	—	—	—
History of UTI	2.6	0.96	5.5	2.1	1.8	0.7	14.0	5.7
Temperature of >39°C	1.4	0.76	3.1	1.7	1.0	0.5	8.1	4.5
Fever without apparent source	1.4	0.69	3.1	1.5	1.0	0.5	8.1	4.1
Ill appearance	1.9	0.68	4.1	1.5	1.3	0.5	10.6	4.1
Fever for >24 h	2.0	0.9	4.3	2.0	1.4	0.6	11.1	5.3
Nonblack race	1.4	0.52	3.1	1.2	1.0	0.4	8.1	3.2

TABLE 2 LRs and Posttest Probabilities of UTI for Febrile Infant Boys According to Number of Findings Present

No. of Risk Factors	LR	Posttest Probability, %		
		All Boys	Uncircumcised	Circumcised
0	0.34	0.8	2.1	0.2
1	0.69	1.5	4.1	0.5
2	1.37	3.0	7.9	1.0
3	2.74	5.8	14.7	1.9
4	5.49	11.0	25.6	3.7

Risk factors: temperature above 39°C, fever for more than 24 hours, no apparent fever source, and nonblack race.

TABLE 3 LRs and Posttest Probabilities of UTI for Febrile Infant Girls According to Number of Findings Present (Prospective Original Study)

Cutoff Value, No. of Factors	LR		Posttest Probability, %	
	Positive	Negative (Approximate)	Below Cutoff Value	At or Above Cutoff Value
1	1.04	0.20	0.8	5.1
2	1.35	0.17	0.8	6.5
3	2.5	0.42	2.1	11.4
4	9.4	0.79	3.9	33.0
5	15.8	0.95	4.7	45.0

Risk factors: less than 12 months of age, white race, temperature > 39°C, fever for at least 2 days, and absence of another source of infection.

TABLE 4 LRs and Posttest Probabilities of UTI for Febrile Infant Girls According to Number of Findings Present (Retrospective Validation Study)

No. of Findings	LR	Posttest Probability, %
0 or 1	1.02	0.8
2	1.10	0.9
3	1.26	1.0
4	3.04	2.4
5	2.13	1.7

Risk factors: less than 12 months of age, white race, temperature > 39°C, fever for at least 2 days, and absence of another source of infection.

and do not appear ill. The LR is calculated as $LR = (1.4)^p \times (0.7)^n$, where p is the number of positive findings and n is the number of negative findings. This assumes that the clinician has assessed all 4 risk factors. It should be noted that, for uncircumcised boys, the risk of UTI never decreases below 2%. For circumcised boys, the probability exceeds 1% if there are 2 or more risk factors.

Other studies have shown that the presence of another, clinically obvious source of infection,[13] particularly documented viral infections,[14] such as respiratory syncytial virus infections,[15] reduces the risk of UTI by one-half. In a series of studies conducted by Gorelick, Shaw, and others,[9,16,17] male gender, black race, and no history of UTI were all found to reduce the risk. The authors derived a prediction rule specifically for girls, with 95% sensitivity and 31% specificity. In a subsequent validation study, they confirmed that these findings had predictive power, but the validation study used a weaker, retrospective, case-control design, compared with the more-robust, prospective, cohort design of the original derivation study. On the basis of the earlier cohort study and starting with a baseline risk of 5%, a child scoring low on the prediction rule would have a slightly less than 1% risk of UTI. To score this low on the prediction rule, a young girl would have to exhibit no more than 1 of the following features: less than 12 months of age, white race, temperature of more than 39°C, fever for at least 2 days, or absence of another source of infection.

However, those authors evaluated their decision rule with several different cutoff points, to determine the score below which the risk of UTI decreased below a test threshold of 1%. Unfortunately, the published article did not include the set of negative LRs needed to reproduce the posterior probabilities.[17] However, it was possible to approximate them through extrapolation from the receiver operating characteristic curve presented. On the basis of these estimated negative LRs and the positive LRs provided in the article,[17] Table 3 was derived. For each cutoff value in the number of risk factors, Table 3 shows the posterior probability for children with fewer than that number of risk factors (below the cutoff value) and for those with that number of risk factors *or more*. Therefore, the posttest probability is not the risk of UTI for children with exactly that

number of risk factors. Similar results could be derived from the validation study and are shown in Table 4. However, because the second study had a weaker design, the values in Table 3 are more reliable.

These studies provide criteria for practical decision rules that clinicians can use to select patients who need urine samples for analysis and/or culture. They do not establish a threshold or maximal risk of UTI above which a urine sample is needed. However, in surveys of pediatricians, Roberts et al[18] found that only 10% of clinicians thought that a urine culture is indicated if the probability of UTI is less than 1%. In addition, the cost-effectiveness analysis published in the 1999 technical report set a threshold of 1%. However, circumstances such as risk of loss to follow-up monitoring or other clinician concerns may shift this threshold up or down.

TABLE 5 List of Test Characteristics of Diagnostic Tests for UTI Reported in 1999 Technical Report[2]

Test	Sensitivity, %			Specificity, %		
	Range	Median	Mean	Range	Median	Mean
Leukocyte esterase test	67–94	84	83	64–92	77	78
Nitrite test	15–82	58	53	90–100	99	98
Blood assessment	25–64	53	47	60–89	85	78
Protein assessment	40–55	53	50	67–84	77	76
Microscopy, leukocytes	32–100	*78*	73	45–98	87	81
Microscopy, bacteria	16–99	88	81	11–100	93	83
Leukocyte esterase or nitrite test	90–100	92	93	58–91	70	72
Any positive test results in urinalysis	99–100	100	99.8	60–92	63	70

TABLE 6 Test Characteristics of Laboratory Tests for UTI in Children

Study	Test	Population	n	Sensitivity, %	Specificity, %
Lockhart et al[19] (1995)	Leukocyte esterase or nitrite test results positive	Prospective sample, <6 mo of age, ED	207	67	79
	Any bacteria with Gram-staining				
Hoberman et al[7] (1996)	>10 white blood cells per counting chamber or any bacteria per 10 oil emersion fields	<2 y of age, 95% febrile, ED	4253	96	93
Shaw et al[9] (1998)	Enhanced urinalysis	Infants <12 mo of age and girls <2 y of age, ≥38.5°C, ED	3873	94	84
	Dipslide or standard urinalysis			83	87
Lin et al[20] (2000)	Hemocytometer, ≥10 cells per μL	Systematic review, febrile infants hospitalized, febrile UTI	NA	83	89

ED indicates emergency department; NA, not applicable.

Box 2: Diagnostic Tests for UTI

The 1999 technical report reviewed a large number of studies that described diagnostic tests for UTI. The results are summarized in Table 5. This updated review of the literature largely reinforced the findings of the original technical report.

More-recent work compared microscopy, including the use of hemocytometers and counting chambers (enhanced urinalysis), with routine urinalysis or dipslide reagents (Table 6). Lockhart et al[19] found that the observation of any visible bacteria in an uncentrifuged, Gram-stained, urine sample had better sensitivity and specificity than did combined dipslide leukocyte esterase and nitrite test results. Hoberman et al[7] in 1996 and Shaw et al[20] in 1998 both evaluated enhanced urinalysis, consisting of more than 10 white blood cells in a counting chamber or any bacteria seen in 10 oil emersion fields; they found sensitivity of 94% to 96% and specificity of 84% to 93%. In 2000, Lin et al[21] found that a count of at least 10 white blood cells per μL in a hemocytometer was less sensitive (83%) but quite specific (89%). Given the sensitivity of enhanced urinalysis, the probability of UTI for a typical febrile infant with a previous likelihood of UTI of 5% would be reduced to 0.2% to 0.4% with negative enhanced urinalysis results.

Obtaining a Urine Sample

In the UTI practice parameters from 1999, the subcommittee defined the gold standard of a UTI to be growth of bacteria on a culture of urine obtained through suprapubic aspiration (SPA). In the previous technical report, SPA was reported to have success rates ranging from 23% to 90%,[22–24] although higher success rates have been achieved when SPA is conducted under ultrasonographic guidance.[25,26] SPA is considered more invasive than catheterization and, in RCTs from 2006[27] and 2010,[28] pain scores associated with SPA were significantly higher than those associated with catheterization. This result was found for both boys and girls. Similar to previous studies, these RCTs also revealed lower success rates for SPA (66% and 60%), compared with catheterization (83% and 78%).[27,28] In comparison with SPA results, cultures of urine specimens obtained through catheterization are 95% sensitive and 99% specific.[7,11,12]

Cultures of bag specimens are difficult to interpret. In the original technical report, sensitivity was assumed to be 100% but the specificity of bag cultures was shown to range between 14% and 84%.[2] Our updated surveillance of the literature did not show that these numbers have improved.[29–33] One article suggested that a new type of collection bag may result in improved specificity,[34] but that study was not controlled. With a prevalence of 5% and specificity of 70%,

the positive predictive value of a positive culture result for urine obtained in a bag would be 15%. This means that, of all positive culture results for urine obtained in a bag, 85% would be false-positive results.

Box 3: Short-term Treatment of UTIs

General Principles of Treatment

Published evidence regarding the short-term treatment of UTIs supports 4 main points. First, complications, such as bacteremia or renal scarring, are sufficiently common to necessitate early, thorough treatment of febrile UTIs in infants.[35] Second, treatment with orally administered antimicrobial agents is as effective as parenteral therapy.[36,37] Third, bacterial sensitivity to antimicrobial agents is highly variable across time and geographic areas, which suggests that therapy should be guided initially by local sensitivity patterns and should be adjusted on the basis of sensitivities of isolated pathogens.[38,39] Fourth, meta-analyses have suggested that shorter durations of oral therapy may not have a disadvantage over longer courses for UTIs. However, those studies largely excluded febrile UTI and pyelonephritis.[40]

Experimental and Clinical Data Support the Concept That Delays in the Institution of Appropriate Treatment for Pyelonephritis Increase the Risk of Renal Damage

The 1999 technical report cited evidence that febrile UTIs in children less

TABLE 7 Recent Studies Documenting the Prevalence of VUR Among Children With UTI

Study	Description	n	Prevalence, %
Sargent and Stringer[50] (1995)	Retrospective study of first VCUG for UTI in children 1 wk to 15 y of age	309	30
Craig et al[51] (1997)	Cross-sectional study of children <5 y of age with first UTI	272	28
McDonald et al[52] (2000)	Retrospective chart review of children with VCUG after UTI	176	19
Oostenbrink et al[53] (2000)	Cross-sectional study of children <5 y of age with first UTI	140	26
Mahant et al[54] (2001)	Retrospective chart review of children with VCUG after UTI	162	22
Mahant et al[55] (2002)	Retrospective review of VCUG in children <5 y of age admitted with first UTI	162	22
Chand et al[56] (2003)	Retrospective review of VCUG or radionuclide cystogram in children <7 y of age	15 504	35
Fernandez-Menendez et al[44] (2003)	Prospective cohort study of 158 children <5 y of age (85% < 2 y) with first UTI	158	22
Camacho et al[41] (2004)	Prospective cohort study of children 1 mo to 12 y of age (mean age: 20 mo) with first febrile UTI	152	21
Hansson et al[57] (2004)	Retrospective cross-sectional study of children <2 y of age with first UTI	303	26
Pinto[58] (2004)	Retrospective chart review of first VCUG for UTI in children 1 mo to 14 y of age	341	30
Zamir et al[59] (2004)	Cohort study of children 0–5 y of age hospitalized with first UTI	255	18

than 2 years of age are associated with bacterial sepsis in 10% of cases.[35] Furthermore, renal scarring is common among children who have febrile UTIs. The risk is higher among those with higher grades of VUR[41] but occurs with all grades, even when there is no VUR. Although it was not confirmed in all studies,[42,43] older work[2] and newer studies[44] demonstrated an increased risk of scarring with delayed treatment. Children whose treatment is delayed more than 48 hours after onset of fever may have a more than 50% higher risk of acquiring a renal scar.

Oral Versus Intravenous Therapy

In a RCT from 1999, Hoberman et al[36] studied children 1 to 24 months of age with febrile UTIs. They compared 14 days of oral cefixime treatment with 3 days of intravenous cefotaxime treatment followed by oral cefixime treatment to complete a 14-day course. The investigators found no difference in outcomes between children who were treated with an orally administered, third-generation cephalosporin alone and those who received intravenous treatment.

In a Cochrane review, Hodson et al[37] evaluated studies with children 0 to 18 years of age, examining oral versus intravenous therapy. No significant differences were found in duration of fever (2 studies; mean difference: 2.05 hours [95% CI: −0.84 to 4.94 hours]) or

renal parenchymal damage at 6 to 12 months (3 studies; RR: 0.80 [95% CI: 0.50−1.26]) between oral antimicrobial therapy (10−14 days) and intravenous antimicrobial treatment (3 days) followed by oral antimicrobial treatment (11 days).

Duration of Therapy

In the 1999 technical report, data slightly favoring longer-duration (7−10 days) over shorter-duration (1 dose to 3 days) antimicrobial therapy for pediatric patients with UTIs were presented.[2] Since then, several meta-analyses with different conclusions have been published on this topic.[40,45,46] A 2003 Cochrane review addressing the question analyzed studies that examined the difference in rates of recurrence for positive urine cultures after treatment.[40] It compared short (2−4 days) and standard (7−14 days) duration of treatment for UTIs and found no significant difference in the frequency of bacteriuria after completion of treatment (8 studies; RR: 1.06 [95% CI: 0.64−1.76]). Although the authors of the review did not exclude studies of children with febrile UTIs or pyelonephritis, each individual study included in the meta-analysis had already excluded such children. To date, there are no conclusive data on the duration of therapy for children with febrile UTIs or pyelonephritis.

Proof of Cure

Data supporting routine repeat cultures of urine during or after completion of antimicrobial therapy were not available for the 1999 technical report. Retrospective studies did not show "proof of bacteriologic cure" cultures to be beneficial.[47,48] Studies demonstrating that clinical response alone *ensures* bacteriologic cure are not available.

Box 4: Evaluation and Management of Urinary Tract Abnormalities

Prevalence of VUR

Several cohort studies published since the 1999 technical report provide estimates of the prevalence of VUR of various grades among infants and children with UTIs (Table 7). Overall, these estimates are reasonably consistent with those reported in earlier studies, although the grades of reflux are now reported more consistently, by using the international system of radiographic grading of VUR.[49]

The prevalence of VUR among children in these studies varies between 18% and 35%. The weighted average prevalence is 34%, but this is largely driven by the enormous retrospective study by Chand et al.[56] Most studies report a rate of 24% or less, which is less than the estimate of VUR prevalence in the 1999 technical report.

Data on the prevalence of VUR among children *without* a history of UTI do not

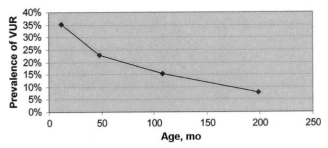

FIGURE 3
Prevalence of VUR as a function of the midpoint of each age stratum, as reported by Chand et al.[56]

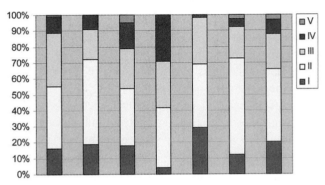

FIGURE 4
Distribution of reflux grades among children with VUR.[41,44,51,56,57,62,63]

exist. Using a retrospective approach and existing urine culture data, Hannula and Ventola and colleagues,[60,61] in 2 separate publications, found similar rates of prevalence of any grade of VUR among children with proven (37.4%) or certain (36%) UTI versus false (34.8%) or improbable (36%) UTI. These results suggest that VUR is prevalent even among children without a history of UTI.

The prevalence of VUR decreases with age. This was approximated by analysis across studies in the 1999 technical report. Since then, Chand et al[56] reported the prevalence VUR within age substrata of their cohort. Figure 3 shows the prevalence of VUR plotted as a function of the midpoint of each age stratum.

Seven studies reported the prevalence of different grades of reflux, by using the international grading system.[41,44,51,56,57,62,63] The distributions of different reflux grades among children who had VUR are shown in Fig 4. There is significant variability in the relative

predominance of each reflux grade, but grades II and III consistently are the most common. With the exception of the study by Camacho et al,[41] all studies showed grades IV and V to be the least frequent, and grade V accounted for 0% to 5% (weighted average: 3%) of reflux. With that value multiplied by the prevalence of VUR among young children with a first UTI, we

would expect grade V reflux to be present in <1% of children with a first UTI.

It has been suggested that the risk of VUR and, more specifically, high-grade VUR may be higher for children with recurrent UTI than for children with a first UTI. Although it was not tested directly in the studies reviewed, this idea can be tested and the magnitude of the effect can be estimated from the data found in the literature search for this meta-analysis.[64–70] These data clearly demonstrate that the risk of UTI recurrence is associated with VUR (Fig 5). Furthermore, this relationship allows the likelihood of each grade of reflux (given that a UTI recurrence has occurred) to be estimated by using Bayes' theorem, as follows:

$$p(VUR_i|UTI)$$

$$= \frac{p(UTI|VUR_i) \times p(VUR_i)}{\sum_{i=0}^{V} p(UTI|VUR_i) \times p(VUR_i)},$$

where $p(UTI|VUR_i)$ refers to the probability of VUR of grade i given the recurrence of UTI. If it is assumed that the conditional probabilities remain the same with second or third UTIs, then Bayes' theorem can be reapplied for a third UTI as well.

By using estimates of $p(UTI|VUR)$ (Fig 5) and the previously determined distri-

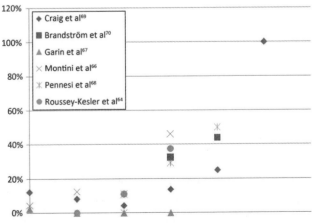

FIGURE 5
Probability of a recurrent febrile UTI as a function of VUR grade among infants 2 to 24 months of age in the control groups of the studies included in meta-analyses.[64,66–70]

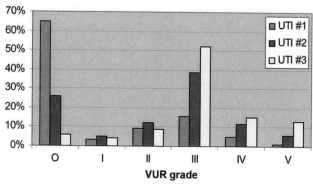

FIGURE 6
Distribution of VUR grades after different numbers of UTIs.

butions of VUR grades (Fig 4), a very approximate estimate of the distribution of VUR grades after the first, second, and third UTI can be made (Fig 6). The likelihood that there is no VUR decreases rapidly. Conversely, the likelihood of VUR grades III to V increases rapidly. The risk of grades I and II changes little.

Ultrasonography

Ultrasonography is used as a noninvasive technique to identify renal abnormalities in children after UTI. The sensitivity of the test varies greatly and has been reported to be as low as 5% for detection of renal scarring[71–73] and 10% for detection of VUR.[74] However, most studies report moderate specificity.

One possible reason for a decrease in specificity is that, in animal models, *Escherichia coli* endotoxin has been shown to produce temporary dilation of the urinary tract during acute infection.[75] Therefore, use of routine ultrasonography for children with UTIs during acute infection may increase the false-positive rate. However, no human data are available to confirm this hypothesis.

Ultrasonography is used during acute infection to identify renal or perirenal abscesses or pyonephrosis in children who fail to experience clinical improvement despite antimicrobial therapy. The sensitivity of ultrasonography for such complications is thought to be

very high, approaching 100%.[76] Therefore, ultrasonography in the case of a child with a UTI who is not responding to therapy as expected can be very helpful in ruling out these infectious complications.

Ultrasonography also is advocated for screening for renal abnormalities such as hydronephrosis, suggesting posterior urethral valves, ureteropelvic junction obstruction, or ureteroceles. The evidence model illustrates the expected outcomes from routine ultrasonography of the kidneys, ureters, and bladder after the first febrile UTI in infants and young children (Fig 7). The model is based on the study results documented in Tables 8 and 9 and a strategy of performing kidney and bladder ultrasonography for all infants with UTIs. The numbers are not exact for 2 reasons, namely, (1) study populations vary and do not always precisely meet the definitions of 2 to 24 months of age and febrile without an-

other fever source and, (2) even within similar populations, reported rates vary widely.

Ultrasonography yields ~15% positive results. However, it has a ~70% false-negative rate for reflux, scarring, and other abnormalities. Limited data exist regarding the false-negative rate for high-grade VUR (grade IV and V), but the studies reviewed presented 0% to 40% false-negative rates for detection of grade IV reflux through ultrasonography.[59,74] Among the 15% of results that are positive, between 1% and 24% are false-positive results. Of the true-positive results, ~40% represent some dilation of the collecting system, such as would be found on a VCUG; 10% represent abnormalities that are potentially surgically correctable (eg, ureteroceles or ureteropelvic junction obstruction). Approximately one-half represent findings such as horseshoe kidneys or renal scarring, for which there is no intervention but which might lead to further evaluations, such as technetium-99m–labeled dimercaptosuccinic acid renal scintigraphy. The 40% with dilation of the collecting system are problematic. This represents only a small fraction of children (15% × 88% × 40% = 5%) with first UTIs who would be expected to have VUR before ultrasonography. Ultrasonography does not seem to be enriching for this population (although ultrasonography might identify a population with higher-grade VUR).

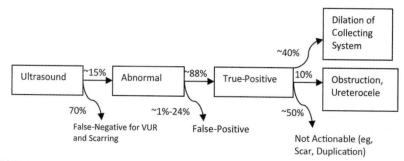

FIGURE 7
Evidence model for ultrasonography after a first UTI.

TABLE 8 Summary of Ultrasonography Literature

Study	n/N (%)	Comments
False-negative rate		
Scarring		
Smellie et al[73] (1995)	7/20 (35)	
Barry et al[77] (1998)	23/170 (14)	
Moorthy et al[71] (2004)	219/231 (95)	
Sinha et al[78] (2007)	61/79 (77)	Reported as renal units
Montini et al[79] (2009)	33/45 (73)	
VUR		
Smellie et al[73] (1995)	21/36 (58)	
Mahant et al[55] (2002)	14/35 (40)	
Hoberman et al[74] (2003)	104/117 (90)	
Zamir et al[59] (2004)	38/47 (81)	
Montini et al[79] (2009)	48/66 (73)	
Other		
Smellie et al[74] (1995)	5/5 (100)	Duplex kidney
False-positive rate		
Scarring		
Barry et al[77] (1998)	11/478 (2)	
Moorthy et al[71] (2004)	12/699 (1.7)	
Sinha et al[78] (2007)	9/870 (1)	
Monitini et al[79] (2009)	26/255 (10)	
VUR		
Smellie et al[73] (1995)	2/12 (17)	Normal VCUG, DMSA, and IVU results
Mahant et al[55] (2002)	30/127 (24)	
Hoberman et al[74] (2003)	17/185 (10)	
Zamir et al[59] (2004)	27/208 (13)	
Other		
Giorgi et al[80] (2005)	21/203 (10)	

IVU indicates intravenous urography; DMSA, dimercaptosuccinic acid.

Prenatal Ultrasonography

Urinary tract abnormalities also may be identified during prenatal ultrasonography,[85–87] which theoretically would decrease the number of new abnormalities found through later ultrasonography.[81] However, the extent to which normal prenatal ultrasonographic findings decrease the need for later studies remains in doubt.

Miron et al[88] studied 209 children who underwent ultrasonography prenatally and again after a UTI. They found that, among 9 children with abnormal ultrasonographic results after UTI, 7 had normal prenatal ultrasonographic results. These cases included 3 cases of hydronephrosis, 3 cases of moderate dilation, and 1 case of double collecting system. Similarly, in a study by Lakhoo et al[89] in 1996, 22 of 39 children with UTIs had normal prenatal ultrasonographic results but "abnormal" post-UTI ultrasonographic results; the abnormalities were not described. These studies suggest that normal prenatal ultrasonographic findings may not be sufficient to obviate the need for additional studies if a UTI occurs in infancy.

Results of Targeted Literature Review and Meta-analysis on Prophylaxis to Prevent Recurrent UTI

Study Identification

For the meta-analysis of studies on the effectiveness of antimicrobial agents to prevent recurrent UTI in children with VUR, we reviewed a total of 213 titles from our primary literature search. Of those, 45 were retained for abstract review on the basis of the title, of which 7 were selected for full review. Six of the studies met the inclusion criteria. Figure 2 summarizes the selection process.

Thirty-eight abstracts were excluded before full review (Fig 2). Eight of those studies were RCTs comparing prophylactic antimicrobial agent use with some type of surgical intervention. None of those studies included a placebo arm.[90–97] One study compared different lengths of antimicrobial prophylaxis.[98] Another study compared different antimicrobial regimens but did not include a placebo arm.[99] Sixteen studies were determined, on closer inspection, to be not clinical trials but prospective cohort studies, reviews, systematic reviews, or meta-analyses. Twelve studies were found twice, either in Medline or Embase and the Cochrane Clinical Trials Registry.

One article was excluded after full review (Fig 2). That study compared prophylactic antimicrobial agent use with probiotic use.[65] The study was not included in the meta-analysis, but the results are described separately.

There are RCTs of antimicrobial prophylaxis that are older than 15 years. In 4 studies from the 1970s, a total of 179 children were enrolled.[100–103] Less than 20% of those children had VUR. Because of limited reporting of results in that subgroup, those older studies were not included in the analyses.

Two additional RCTs comparing antimicrobial prophylaxis and placebo treatment for children were published in October 2009.[69,70] The first trial enrolled children 0 to 18 years of age after a first UTI, with 2% of enrolled children (12 of 576 children) being more than 10 years of age. The second trial enrolled children diagnosed as having VUR after a first UTI (194 [96%] of 203 children) or after prenatal ultrasonography (9 [4%] of 203 children), who were then assigned randomly to receive antimicrobial prophylaxis, surveillance, or endoscopic therapy, at 1 to 2 years of age. The majority of these children (132 children [65%]) had been diagnosed as having VUR before 1

TABLE 9 Distribution of Positive Ultrasonographic Findings

Study	n/N (%)
Alon and Ganapathy[62] (1999)	19/124 (15)
Minimal unilateral changes	
VUR	2 (1.6)
Normal VCUG findings	2 (1.6)
Resolved on repeat study	2 (1.6)
Not monitored further	3 (2.4)
Major changes	8 (6.5)
VUR	1 (1.6)
Normal findings	1 (1.6)
Posterior urethral valve	1 (1.6)
Hydroureternephrosis	1 (1.6)
Gelfand et al[81] (2000)	141/844 (16.7)
Bladder wall thickening	31 (3.7)
Hydroureter	6 (0.7)
Parenchymal abnormalities	42 (5.0)
Pelvocalyceal dilation	27 (3.2)
Renal calculus	1 (0.1)
Simple renal cyst	1 (0.1)
Urethelial thickening	31 (3.7)
Jothilakshmi et al[82] (2001)	42/262 (16)
Duplex kidney	3 (1)
Crossed renal ectopia	1 (0.38)
Horseshoe kidney	1 (0.38)
Hydronephrosis	5 (1.9)
Megaureter	6 (2.3)
Polycystic kidney	1 (0.38)
Pelviureteric junction obstruction	1 (0.38)
Posterior urethral valve	2 (0.76)
Renal calculus	3 (0.01)
Rotated kidney	2 (0.76)
Ureterocele	2 (0.76)
VUR	7 (2.7)
Hoberman et al[74] (2003)	37/309 (12)
Dilated pelvis	13 (4.2)
Pelvocaliectasis	12 (3.9)
Hydronephrosis	2 (0.6)
Dilated ureter	9 (2.9)
Double collecting system	3 (1.0)
Extrarenal pelvis	1 (0.3)
Calculus	1 (0.3)
Zamir et al[59] (2004)	36/255 (14.1)
Mild unilateral pelvis dilation	32 (12.5)
Moderate unilateral pelvis dilation	1 (0.04)
Enlargement kidney	1 (0.04)
Small renal cyst	1 (0.04)
Double collecting system and severe hydronephrosis	1 (0.04)
Jahnukainen et al[83] (2006)[a]	23/155 (14.8)
Hydronephrosis	8 (5)
Double collecting system	11 (7)
Multicystic dysplasia	1 (0.6)
Renal hypoplasia	1 (0.6)
Solitary kidney	1 (0.6)
Horseshoe kidney	1 (0.6)
Huang et al[84] (2008)	112/390 (28.7)
Nephromegaly	46 (11.8)
Isolated hydronephrosis	20 (5.1)
Intermittent hydronephrosis	3 (0.8)
Hydroureter	8 (2.1)
Hydroureter and hydronephrosis	3 (0.8)
Thickened bladder wall	11 (2.8)
Small kidneys	8 (2.1)
Simple ureterocele	5 (1.3)
Double collecting systems	4 (1.0)
Increased echogenicity	3 (0.8)
Horseshoe kidney	1 (0.3)
Montini et al[79] (2009)	38/300 (13)
Dilated pelvis, ureter, or pelvis and calyces	12 (4)
Renal swelling or local parenchymal changes	10 (3.3)
Increased bladder wall or pelvic mucosa, thickness	6 (2)
Other	10 (3.3)

[a] Hospitalized children with UTI.

year of age and thus had been receiving prophylaxis before random assignment. These studies were included in the meta-analysis.

Description of Included Studies

Table 10 presents characteristics of the 8 included studies.[64,66–70,104,105] Four studies enrolled children after diagnosis of a first episode of pyelonephritis.[64,66–68] In those 4 studies, pyelonephritis was described as fever of more than 38°C or 38.5°C and positive urine culture results. In 1 of those studies,[67] dimercaptosuccinic acid scanning results consistent with acute pyelonephritis represented an additional requirement for inclusion. The remaining studies had slightly different inclusion criteria. In the study by Craig et al[71] from 2009, symptoms consistent with UTI and positive urine culture results were required for inclusion. Fever was documented for 79% of enrolled children (454 of 576 children). In the study by Brandström et al,[70] 96% of enrolled children (194 of 203 children) had pyelonephritis, defined in a similar manner as in the 6 initial studies. The remaining patients were enrolled after prenatal diagnosis of VUR. The 2 included abstracts described studies that enrolled any child with VUR and not only children who had had pyelonephritis.[104,105] Seven of the 8 studies (all except the study by Reddy et al[108]) reported a gender ratio. Among those studies, there were 67% girls and 33% boys. Six studies compared antimicrobial treatment with no treatment. Only 2 studies were placebo controlled, and those 2 were the only blinded studies.[69,105] The grade of VUR among the enrolled children varied from 0 to V, but few of the children had grade V VUR.

The ages of children included in the initial meta-analyses were 0 to 18 years; therefore, some children were included who were outside the target

TABLE 10 Studies Included in Meta-analysis

Study	Study Sites	n		Age	VUR Grade	Antimicrobial Agents	Control	Follow-up Period, mo	Outcome
		VUR	No VUR						
Craig et al[105] (2002)	Australia	46	0	0–3 mo	I–V	TMP-SMX	Placebo	36	UTI and renal damage
Craig et al[69] (2009)	Australia	243	234	0–18 y	I–V	TMP-SMX	Placebo	12	Symptomatic UTI, febrile UTI, hospitalization, and renal scarring
Garin et al[67] (2006)	Chile, Spain, United States	113	105	3 mo to 18 y	0–III	TMP-SMX/ nitrofurantoin	No treatment	12	Asymptomatic UTI, cystitis, pyelonephritis, and renal scarring
Brandström et al[70] (2010)	Sweden	203	0	1–2 y	III–IV	TMP-SMX/cefadroxil, nitrofurantoin	No treatment	48	Febrile UTI, reflux status, and renal scarring
Montini et al[66] (2008)	Italy	128	210	2 mo to 7 y	0–III	TMP-SMX/amoxicillin- clavulanate	No treatment	12	Febrile UTI and renal scarring
Pennesi et al[68] (2008)	Italy	100	0	0–30 mo	II–IV	TMP-SMX	No treatment	48	UTI and renal scarring
Reddy et al[104] (1997)	United States	29	0	1–10 y	I–V	TMP-SMX/ nitrofurantoin	No treatment	24	UTI, progression of disease, need for surgery, parental compliance
Roussey-Kesler et al[64] (2008)	France	225	0	1–36 m	I–III	TMP-SMX	No treatment	18	Febrile and afebrile UTI

TMP-SMX indicates trimethoprim-sulfamethoxazole.

age range for this report and for whom other factors (eg, voiding and bowel habits) might have played a role. The median age of the included children, however, was not above 3 years in any of the included studies in which it was reported. Separate meta-analyses were subsequently performed for the subgroup of children who were 2 to 24 months of age. The duration of antimicrobial treatment and follow-up monitoring ranged from 12 to 48 months. The antimicrobial agents used were trimethoprim-sulfamethoxazole (1–2 or 5–10 mg/kg),[64,68,69,105] trimethoprim-sulfamethoxazole or amoxicillin-clavulanic acid (15 mg/kg),[66] trimethoprim-sulfamethoxazole or nitrofurantoin,[67,104] or trimethoprim-sulfamethoxazole, cefadroxil, or nitrofurantoin.[70] Urine collection methods differed among studies. Bag specimens were reported for 3 studies.[64,66,70] In an additional 4 studies, the description of the urine collection methods did not exclude the use of bag specimens.[67,68,104,105] Recurrent UTI was described as (1) asymptomatic bacteriuria (diagnosed through screening cultures), (2) cystitis, (3) febrile UTI, and (4) pyelonephritis (diagnosed on the basis of focal or diffuse uptake on di-mercaptosuccinic acid scans) in the different articles.

Quality Assessment

The included studies received scores (from 2 assessors) from 7 to 26 (scale range: 0–32) with the scoring system described by Downs and Black,[6] with a median score of 16. Score deductions resulted from lack of blinding of patients (all except 2 studies[69,105]), lack of blinding of assessors (all except 2 studies[69,105]), limited or no information about patients lost to follow-up monitoring (3 studies[64,67,104]), lack of reporting of adverse effects (all except 2 studies[66,69]), and small sample sizes. The lowest scores, 7 and 12, were received by the 2 abstracts because of lack of details in the descriptions of the methods.[104,105]

Antimicrobial Therapy Versus No Treatment

Overview of Findings

Described here are the results of several meta-analyses, subdivided according to type of recurrence (pyelonephritis versus UTI), degree of VUR (none to grade V), and patient age. In summary, antimicrobial prophylaxis does not seem to reduce significantly the rates of recurrence of pyelonephritis, regardless of age or degree of reflux. Although prophylaxis seems to reduce significantly but only slightly the risk of UTI when all forms are included, most of this effect is attributable to reductions in rates of cystitis or asymptomatic bacteriuria, which would not be expected to lead to ongoing renal damage.

Recurrence of Pyelonephritis/Febrile UTI Among All Studied Children With VUR of Any Grade

Recurrence of pyelonephritis was reported in 6 of the 8 studies. The study by Pennesi et al[68] presented the results as recurrence of pyelonephritis, but recurrence was defined as episodes of fever or "symptoms of UTI." When contacted, this author confirmed that all reported recurrences were characterized by fever above 38.5°C. Therefore, the article was included in the meta-analysis. With a random-effects model, there was no significant difference in rates of recurrence of pyelonephritis for children who received antimicrobial therapy and those who did not. This meta-analysis yielded a RR of 0.77 (95% CI: 0.47–1.24) (Fig 8). Heterogeneity test-

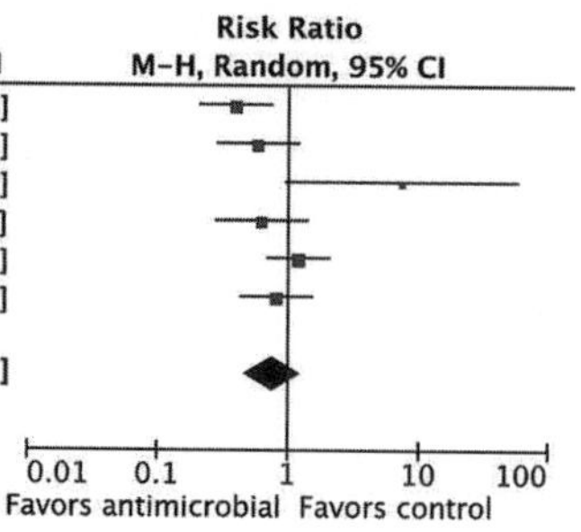

FIGURE 8

Combined estimates of the effect of antimicrobial prophylaxis on prevention of pyelonephritis in children with VUR, from random-effects modeling. RRs and 95% CIs are shown. M-H indicates Mantel-Haenszel.

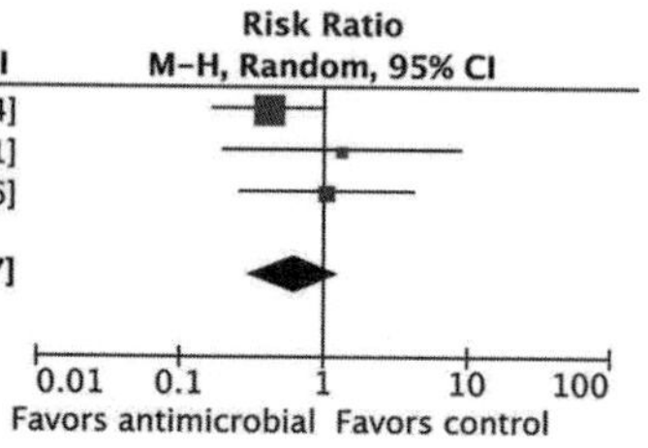

FIGURE 9

Combined estimates of the effect of antimicrobial prophylaxis on prevention of pyelonephritis in children without VUR, from random-effects modeling. RRs and 95% CIs are shown. M-H indicates Mantel-Haenszel.

ing results were significant ($P = .04$), which indicated statistical heterogeneity between studies.

Recurrence of Pyelonephritis/Febrile UTI Among Children of All Ages Without VUR

There was no significant difference in rates of recurrence of pyelonephritis for children without VUR who received antimicrobial therapy and those who did not. With random-effects modeling, the meta-analysis yielded a RR of 0.62 (95% CI: 0.30–1.27) (Fig 9). Heterogeneity testing results were not significant ($P = .39$). Because no difference was detected with a random-effects model and there was no statistical heterogeneity in this analysis, analysis also was conducted with a fixed-effects model. With fixed-effects modeling, the meta-analysis yielded a RR of 0.61 (95% CI: 0.31–1.23).

Recurrence of Pyelonephritis/Febrile UTI Among Children of All Ages With VUR, According to Grade

Table 11 summarizes the results of separate meta-analyses of subpopula-

TABLE 11 Combined Estimates of Effect of Antimicrobial Prophylaxis on Prevention of Pyelonephritis for All Children According to Grade of VUR

VUR Grade	No. of Children	No. of Studies	RR (95% CI)[a]
0	549	3	0.62 (0.30–1.27)
I–II	455	5	0.94 (0.49–1.80)
III	347	6	0.74 (0.42–1.29)
IV	122	3	0.69 (0.39–1.20)
V	5	1	0.40 (0.08–1.90)

[a] From random-effects model.

tions from each study with different grades of VUR. None of those analyses showed a statistically significant difference in rates of recurrence with random- or fixed-effects modeling. Random-effects modeling results are presented.

Recurrence of Pyelonephritis/Febrile UTI Among Children 2 to 24 Months of Age With VUR of Any Grade

There was no significant difference in rates of recurrence of pyelonephritis for children 2 to 24 months of age with VUR who received antimicrobial agents and those who did not. With random-effects modeling, the meta-analysis yielded a RR of 0.78

(95% CI: 0.48–1.26) (Fig 10). Heterogeneity testing results were not significant ($P = .07$). With fixed-effects modeling, the meta-analysis yielded a RR of 0.79 (95% CI: 0.58–1.07). Heterogeneity testing results were not significant ($P = .07$).

Recurrence of Pyelonephritis/Febrile UTI Among Children 2 to 24 Months of Age With No VUR

There was no significant difference in rates of recurrence of pyelonephritis for children 2 to 24 months of age without VUR who received antimicrobial agents and those who did not. With random-effects modeling, the meta-analysis yielded a RR of 0.55 (95% CI:

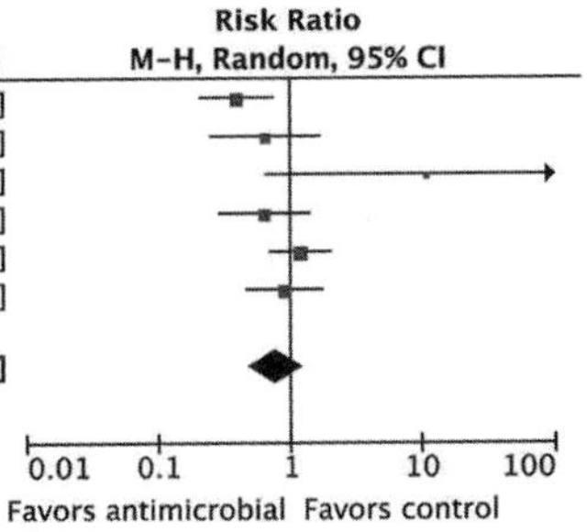

FIGURE 10
Combined estimates of the effect of antimicrobial prophylaxis on prevention of pyelonephritis in children 2 to 24 months of age with any grade of VUR, from random-effects modeling. RRs and 95% CIs are shown. M-H indicates Mantel-Haenszel.

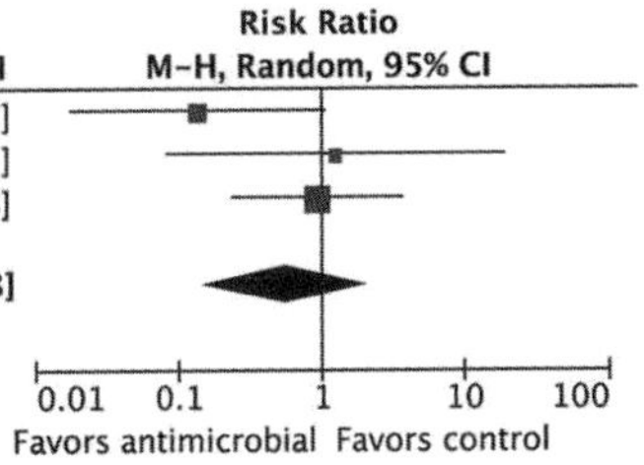

FIGURE 11
Combined estimates of the effect of antimicrobial prophylaxis on prevention of pyelonephritis in children 2 to 24 months of age without VUR, from random-effects modeling. RRs and 95% CIs are shown. M-H indicates Mantel-Haenszel.

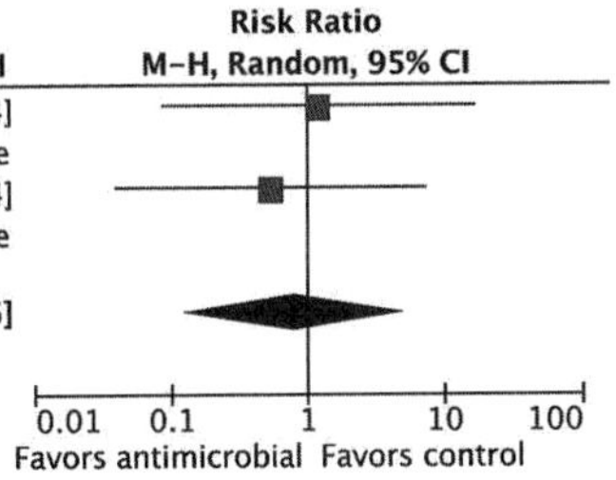

FIGURE 12
Combined estimates of the effect of antimicrobial prophylaxis on prevention of pyelonephritis in children 2 to 24 months of age with grade I VUR, from random-effects modeling. RRs and 95% CIs are shown. M-H indicates Mantel-Haenszel.

0.15–2.08) (Fig 11). Heterogeneity testing results were not significant ($P =$ .25). With fixed-effects modeling, the meta-analysis yielded a RR of 0.48 (95% CI: 0.18–1.27). Heterogeneity testing results were not significant ($P =$ .25).

Recurrence of Pyelonephritis/Febrile UTI Among Children 2 to 24 Months of Age According to Grade of VUR

When results were analyzed according to VUR grade, there was no significant difference in rates of recurrence of pyelonephritis for children 2 to 24 months of age who received antimicrobial agents and those who did not in any of the analyses, with

random- or fixed-effects modeling. Results of random-effects modeling are presented in Figs 12 through 16. Heterogeneity testing results were not significant in any of the analyses.

Recurrence of Any Type of UTI Among Children of All Ages With VUR of Any Grade

In this meta-analysis, in which the 2 published abstracts that never resulted in published articles were included, there was a statistically significant difference in rates of recurrence of any type of UTI for children with VUR who received antimicrobial agents and those who did not. With random-effects modeling, the meta-analysis yielded a

RR of 0.70 (95% CI: 0.51–0.96) (Fig 17). Heterogeneity testing results were not significant ($P =$ .20).

The inclusion of the published abstracts[104,105] in these meta-analyses can be criticized, because the investigators in those studies enrolled all children with VUR and not just those who had been diagnosed as having UTI; therefore, *recurrent* UTIs were not measured. With exclusion of the 2 abstracts from the meta-analyses for prevention of any UTI, the RR with random-effects modeling would be 0.73 (95% CI: 0.53–1.01). Heterogeneity testing results were not significant ($P =$ .16).

Study or Subgroup	Antimicrobial Events	Total	Control Events	Total	Weight	Risk Ratio M-H, Random, 95% CI
Craig et al[69] (2009)	0	27	1	23	6.3%	0.29 [0.01–6.69]
Garin et al[67] (2006)	1	12	0	10	6.5%	2.54 [0.11–56.25]
Montini et al[66] (2008)	3	31	2	18	21.7%	0.87 [0.16–4.73]
Pennesi et al[68] (2008)	1	11	0	10	6.5%	2.75 [0.12–60.70]
Roussey-Kesler et al[64] (2008)	6	52	7	63	59.0%	1.04 [0.37–2.90]
Total (95% CI)		**133**		**124**	**100.0%**	**1.04 [0.47–2.29]**
Total events	11		10			

Heterogeneity: $\tau^2 = 0.00$; $\chi^2 = 1.38$, $df = 4$ ($P = .85$); $I^2 = 0\%$
Test for overall effect: $z = 0.10$ ($P = .92$)

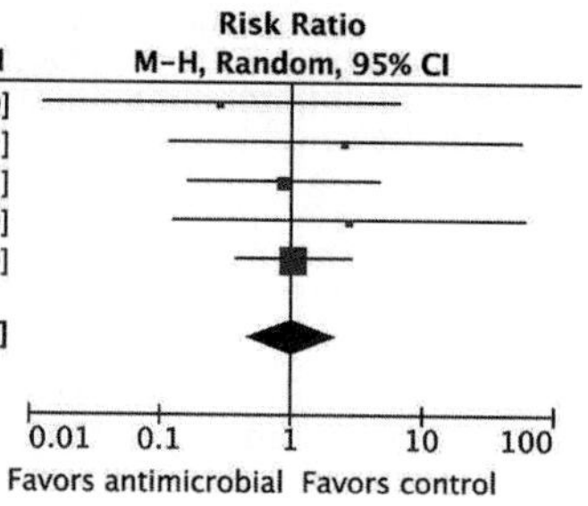

FIGURE 13

Combined estimates of the effect of antimicrobial prophylaxis on prevention of pyelonephritis in children 2 to 24 months of age with grade II VUR, from random-effects modeling. RRs and 95% CIs are shown. M-H indicates Mantel-Haenszel.

Study or Subgroup	Antimicrobial Events	Total	Control Events	Total	Weight	Risk Ratio M-H, Random, 95% CI
Brandström et al[70] (2010)	5	41	14	43	20.9%	0.37 [0.15–0.95]
Craig et al[69] (2009)	1	24	4	29	7.1%	0.30 [0.04–2.53]
Garin et al[67] (2006)	4	8	0	12	4.5%	13.00 [0.79–212.80]
Montini et al[66] (2008)	6	22	6	13	21.5%	0.59 [0.24–1.45]
Pennesi et al[68] (2008)	9	22	7	24	23.6%	1.40 [0.63–3.12]
Roussey-Kesler et al[64] (2008)	6	23	9	24	22.3%	0.70 [0.29–1.64]
Total (95% CI)		**140**		**145**	**100.0%**	**0.75 [0.40–1.40]**
Total events	31		40			

Heterogeneity: $\tau^2 = 0.27$; $\chi^2 = 9.54$, $df = 5$ ($P = .09$); $I^2 = 48\%$
Test for overall effect: $z = 0.90$ ($P = .37$)

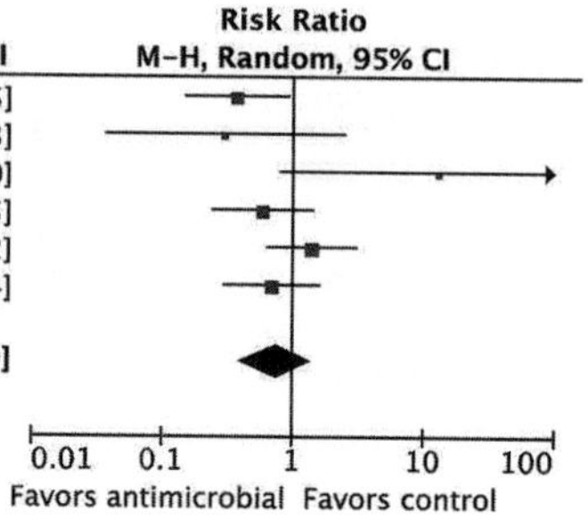

FIGURE 14

Combined estimates of the effect of antimicrobial prophylaxis on prevention of pyelonephritis in children 2 to 24 months of age with grade III VUR, from random-effects modeling. RRs and 95% CIs are shown. M-H indicates Mantel-Haenszel.

Study or Subgroup	Antimicrobial Events	Total	Control Events	Total	Weight	Risk Ratio M-H, Random, 95% CI
Brandström et al[70] (2010)	5	28	11	25	35.0%	0.41 [0.16–1.01]
Craig et al[69] (2009)	3	10	2	8	14.8%	1.20 [0.26–5.53]
Pennesi et al[68] (2008)	8	17	8	16	50.2%	0.94 [0.47–1.90]
Total (95% CI)		**55**		**49**	**100.0%**	**0.73 [0.39–1.35]**
Total events	16		21			

Heterogeneity: $\tau^2 = 0.07$; $\chi^2 = 2.57$, $df = 2$ ($P = .28$); $I^2 = 22\%$
Test for overall effect: $z = 1.01$ ($P = .31$)

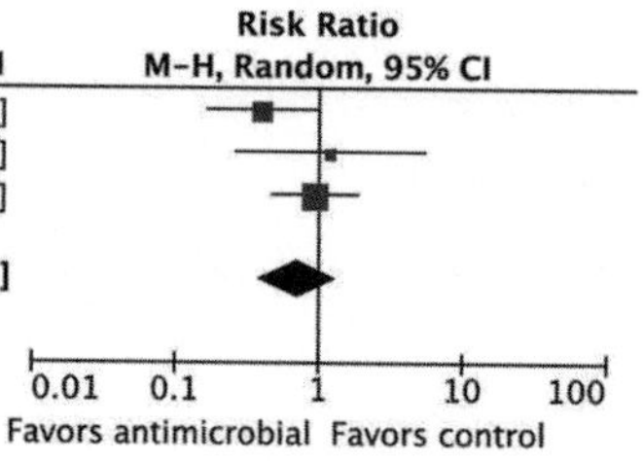

FIGURE 15

Combined estimates of the effect of antimicrobial prophylaxis on prevention of pyelonephritis in children 2 to 24 months of age with grade IV VUR, from random-effects modeling. RRs and 95% CIs are shown. M-H indicates Mantel-Haenszel.

Study or Subgroup	Antimicrobial Events	Total	Control Events	Total	Weight	Risk Ratio M-H, Random, 95% CI
Craig et al[69] (2009)	1	4	1	1	100.0%	0.40 [0.08–1.90]
Total (95% CI)		**4**		**1**	**100.0%**	**0.40 [0.08–1.90]**
Total events	1		1			

Heterogeneity: Not applicable
Test for overall effect: $z = 1.15$ ($P = .25$)

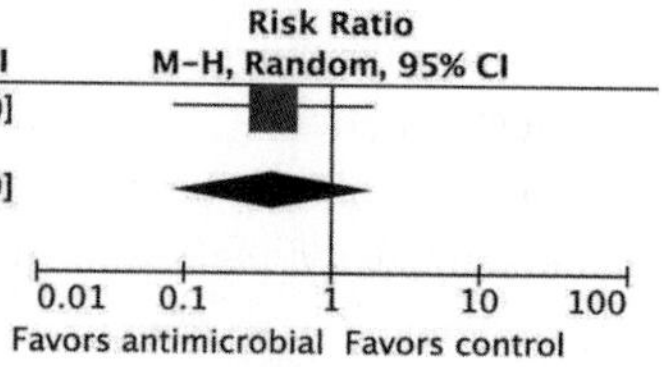

FIGURE 16

Estimate of the effect of antimicrobial prophylaxis on prevention of pyelonephritis in children 2 to 24 months of age with grade V VUR, from random-effects modeling. RRs and 95% CIs are shown. M-H indicates Mantel-Haenszel.

Recurrence of Any Type of UTI Among Children of All Ages Without VUR

There was no significant difference in rates of recurrence of any type of UTI for children without VUR who received antimicrobial agents and those who did not. With random-effects modeling, the meta-analysis yielded a RR of 0.72 (95% CI: 0.43–1.20) (Fig 18). Heterogeneity testing results were not significant ($P = .37$).

Effect on Studies of Inclusion of Bag Specimens

With the exception of the study by Craig et al,[69] no studies reported that bag urine specimens were excluded. The inclusion of such specimens might

Study or Subgroup	Antimicrobial Events	Total	Control Events	Total	Weight	Risk Ratio M-H, Random, 95% CI	Risk Ratio M-H, Random, 95% CI
Brandström et al[70] (2010)	10	69	25	68	15.4%	0.39 [0.21–0.76]	
Craig et al[105] (2002)	0	23	2	23	1.1%	0.20 [0.01–3.95]	
Craig et al[69] (2009)	14	122	21	121	16.2%	0.66 [0.35–1.24]	
Garin et al[67] (2006)	13	55	13	58	14.8%	1.05 [0.54–2.07]	
Montini et al[66] (2008)	10	82	9	46	11.1%	0.62 [0.27–1.42]	
Pennesi et al[68] (2008)	18	50	15	50	18.6%	1.20 [0.68–2.11]	
Reddy et al[104] (1997)	1	13	5	16	2.3%	0.25 [0.03–1.85]	
Roussey-Kesler et al[64] (2008)	18	103	32	121	20.6%	0.66 [0.40–1.11]	
Total (95% CI)		517		503	100.0%	0.70 [0.51–0.96]	
Total events	84		122				

Heterogeneity: $\tau^2 = 0.06$; $\chi^2 = 9.88$, $df = 7$ ($P = .20$); $I^2 = 29\%$
Test for overall effect: $z = 2.22$ ($P = .03$)

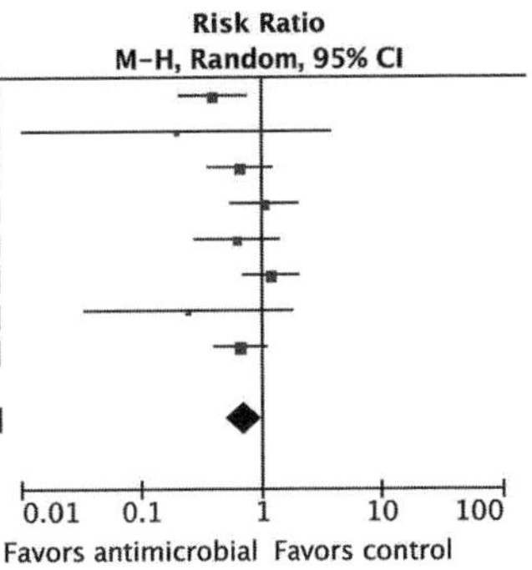

FIGURE 17

Combined estimates of the effect of antimicrobial prophylaxis on prevention of any UTI in children with any grade of VUR, from random-effects modeling. RRs and 95% CIs are shown. M-H indicates Mantel-Haenszel.

Study or Subgroup	Antimicrobial Events	Total	Control Events	Total	Weight	Risk Ratio M-H, Random, 95% CI	Risk Ratio M-H, Random, 95% CI
Craig et al[69] (2009)	15	119	17	115	62.7%	0.85 [0.45–1.63]	
Garin et al[67] (2006)	4	45	14	60	24.1%	0.38 [0.13–1.08]	
Montini et al[66] (2008)	5	129	3	81	13.2%	1.05 [0.26–4.26]	
Total (95% CI)		293		256	100.0%	0.72 [0.43–1.20]	
Total events	24		34				

Heterogeneity: $\tau^2 = 0.00$; $\chi^2 = 1.98$, $df = 2$ ($P = .37$); $I^2 = 0\%$
Test for overall effect: $z = 1.25$ ($P = .21$)

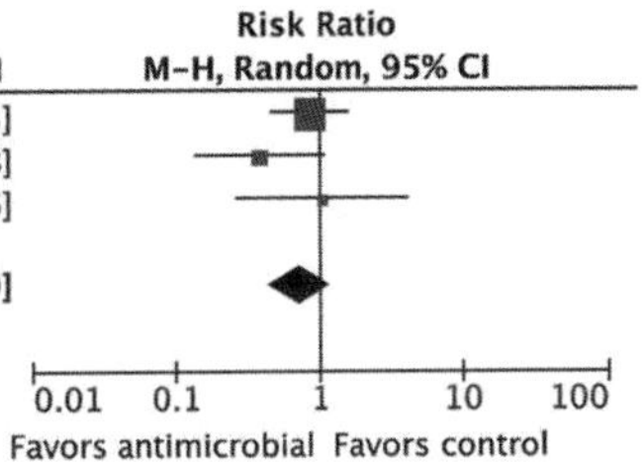

FIGURE 18

Combined estimates of the effect of antimicrobial prophylaxis on prevention of any UTI in children without VUR, from random-effects modeling. RRs and 95% CIs are shown. M-H indicates Mantel-Haenszel.

have resulted in increased numbers of false-positive urine culture results in both the antimicrobial prophylaxis and control groups, yielding a bias toward the null hypothesis in those studies.

Results of Excluded Study

The study by Lee et al[65] was excluded from the meta-analysis because it compared antimicrobial prophylaxis with probiotic treatment. A total of 120 children 13 to 36 months of age with a history of UTI and VUR of grade I to V who had been receiving trimethoprim-sulfamethoxazole once daily for 1 year were again assessed for VUR; if VUR persisted, then children were assigned randomly either to continue to receive trimethoprim-sulfamethoxazole or to receive *Lactobacillus acidophilus* twice daily for 1 additional year. The study showed no statistical difference in recurrent UTI rates between the 2 groups during the second year of follow-up monitoring.

Antimicrobial Prophylaxis and Antimicrobial Resistance

The antimicrobial resistance patterns of the pathogens isolated during UTI recurrences were assessed in 5 of the RCTs included in the meta-analyses.[64,66,68–70] All authors concluded that UTI recurrences with antimicrobial-resistant bacteria were more common in the groups of children assigned randomly to receive antimicrobial prophylaxis. In the placebo/surveillance groups, the proportions of resistant bacteria ranged from 0% to 39%; in the antimicrobial prophylaxis groups, the proportions of resistant bacteria ranged from 53% to 100%. These results are supported by other studies in which antimicrobial prophylaxis has been shown to promote resistant organisms.[106,107]

Surgical Intervention Versus Antimicrobial Prophylaxis

Data on the effectiveness of surgical interventions for VUR are quite limited.

To date, only 1 RCT has compared surgical intervention (only endoscopic therapy) for VUR with placebo treatment.[70] In that study, there was a statistically significant difference in the rates of recurrence of febrile UTI for girls treated with endoscopic therapy and those under surveillance (10 of 43 vs 24 of 42 girls; $P = .0014$). No such difference was noted among boys, for whom the results trended in the opposite direction (4 of 23 vs 1 of 26 boys). A meta-analysis examined the outcomes of UTIs and febrile UTIs in children assigned randomly to either reflux correction plus antimicrobial therapy or antimicrobial therapy alone.[108] By 2 years, the authors found no significant reduction in the risk of UTI in the surgery plus antimicrobial therapy group, compared with the antimicrobial therapy-only group (4 studies; RR: 1.07 [95% CI: 0.55–2.09]). The frequency of febrile UTIs was reported in only 2 studies. Children in the surgery plus antimicrobial therapy group had significantly fewer febrile UTIs than did children in the antimicrobial therapy-only group between 0 and 5 years after intervention (RR: 0.43 [95% CI: 0.27–0.70]). Although there may be some promise in endoscopic interventions for children with VUR, to date there are insufficient data to show whether and for whom such interventions may be helpful.

Long-term Consequences of VUR

The link between VUR discovered after the first UTI and subsequent hypertension and end-stage renal disease remains tenuous at best. There have been no longitudinal studies monitoring children long enough to quantify these outcomes. Retrospective studies evaluated highly selected populations, and their findings might not apply to otherwise healthy children with a first UTI.[109–112] Ecologic data from Australia demonstrated no changes in the rates of hypertension and renal failure since the widespread introduction of antimicrobial prophylaxis and ureteric reimplantation surgery for VUR in the 1960s.[113]

DISCUSSION

Review of the evidence regarding diagnosis and management of UTIs in 2- to 24-month-old children yields the following. First, the prevalence of UTI in febrile infants remains about the same, at ~5%. Studies have provided demographic features (age, race, and gender) and clinical characteristics (height and duration of fever, other causes of fever, and circumcision) that can help clinicians identify febrile infants whose low risk of UTI obviates the need for further evaluation.

Among children who do not receive immediate antimicrobial therapy, UTI can be ruled out on the basis of completely negative urinalysis results. For this purpose, enhanced urinalysis is preferable. However, facilities for urine microscopy with counting chambers and Gram staining may not be available in

all settings. A urine reagent strip with negative nitrite and leukocyte esterase reaction results is sufficient to rule out UTI if the pretest risk is moderate (~5%). Diagnosis of UTI is best achieved with a combination of culture and urinalysis. Cultures of urine collected through catheterization, compared with SPA, are nearly as sensitive and specific but have higher success rates and the process is less painful. Cultures of urine collected in bags have unacceptably high false-positive rates.

The previous guideline recommended VCUG after the first UTI for children between 2 and 24 months of age. The rationale for this recommendation was that antimicrobial prophylaxis among children with VUR could reduce subsequent episodes of pyelonephritis and additional renal scarring. However, evidence does not support antimicrobial prophylaxis to prevent UTI when VUR is found through VCUG. The only statistically significant effect of antimicrobial prophylaxis was in preventing UTI that included cystitis and asymptomatic bacteriuria. Statistically significant differences in the rates of febrile UTI or pyelonephritis were not seen. Moreover, VCUG is one of the most uncomfortable radiologic procedures performed with children.[114–116]

Even if additional studies were to show a statistically significant effect of prophylaxis in preventing pyelonephritis, our point estimates suggest that the RR would be ~0.80, corresponding to a reduction in RR of 20%. If we take into account the prevalence of VUR, the risk of recurrent UTI in those children, and this modest *potential* effect, we can determine that ~100 children would need to undergo VCUG for prevention of 1 UTI in the first year. Even more striking is the fact that the evidence of benefit is the same (or better) for children with *no* VUR, which makes the benefit of VCUG more dubious. Taken in light of the marginal cost-effectiveness of the procedure found under the more-optimistic as-

sumptions in the 1999 technical report, these data argue against VCUG after the first UTI. VCUG after a second or third UTI would have a higher yield of higher grades of reflux, but the optimal care for infants with higher-grade reflux is still not clear. Ultrasonography of the kidneys, ureters, and bladder after a first UTI has poor sensitivity and only a modest yield of "actionable" findings. However, the procedure is less invasive, less uncomfortable, and less risky (in terms of radiation) than is VCUG.

There is a significant risk of renal scarring among children with febrile UTI, and some evidence suggests that early antimicrobial treatment mitigates that risk. It seems prudent to recommend early evaluation (in the 24- to 48-hour time frame) of subsequent fevers and prompt treatment of UTI to minimize subsequent renal scarring.

LEAD AUTHORS

S. Maria E. Finnell, MD, MS
Aaron E. Carroll, MD, MS
Stephen M. Downs, MD, MS

SUBCOMMITTEE ON URINARY TRACT INFECTION, 2009–2011

Kenneth B. Roberts, MD, Chair
Stephen M. Downs, MD, MS
S. Maria E. Finnell, MD, MS
Stanley Hellerstein, MD
Linda D. Shortliffe, MD
Ellen R. Wald, MD
J. Michael Zerin, MD

OVERSIGHT BY THE STEERING COMMITTEE ON QUALITY IMPROVEMENT AND MANAGEMENT, 2009–2011

STAFF

Caryn Davidson, MA

ACKNOWLEDGMENTS

The committee gratefully acknowledges the generosity of the researchers who graciously shared their data to permit the data set with data for 1096 infants 2 to 24 months of age according to grade of VUR to be compiled, that is, Drs Per Brandström, Jonathan Craig, Eduardo Garin, Giovanni Montini, Marco Pennesi, and Gwenaelle Roussey-Kesler.

REFERENCES

1. American Academy of Pediatrics, Committee on Quality Improvement, Subcommittee on Urinary Tract Infection. Practice parameter: the diagnosis, treatment, and evaluation of the initial urinary tract infection in febrile infants and young children. *Pediatrics.* 1999;103(4):843–852

2. Downs SM. Technical report: urinary tract infections in febrile infants and young children. *Pediatrics.* 1999;103(4). Available at: www.pediatrics.org/cgi/content/full/103/4/e54

3. American Academy of Pediatrics, Committee on Quality Improvement, Subcommittee on Urinary Tract Infection. Urinary tract infection: clinical practice guideline for the diagnosis and management of initial urinary tract infections in febrile infants and children 2 to 24 months of age. *Pediatrics.* 2011;128(3):595–610

4. Eddy DM. Clinical decision making: from theory to practice: guidelines for policy statements: the explicit approach. *JAMA.* 1990;263(16):2239–2242

5. Haynes RB, McKibbon KA, Wilczynski NL, Walter SD, Werre SR; Hedge Team. Optimal search strategies for retrieving scientifically strong studies of treatment from Medline: analytical survey. *BMJ.* 2005; 330(7501):1179

6. Downs S, Black N. The feasibility of creating a checklist for the assessment of the methodological quality both of randomised and non-randomised studies of health care interventions. *J Epidemiol Community Health.* 1998;52(6):377–384

7. Hoberman A, Wald ER, Reynolds EA, Penchansky L, Charron M. Is urine culture necessary to rule out urinary tract infection in young febrile children? *Pediatr Infect Dis J.* 1996;15(4):304–309

8. Haddon RA, Barnett PL, Grimwood K, Hogg GG. Bacteraemia in febrile children presenting to a paediatric emergency department. *Med J Aust.* 1999;170(10):475–478

9. Shaw KN, Gorelick M, McGowan KL, Yakscoe NM, Schwartz JS. Prevalence of urinary tract infection in febrile young children in the emergency department. *Pediatrics.* 1998;102(2). Available at: www.pediatrics.org/cgi/content/full/102/2/e16

10. Shaikh N, Morone NE, Bost JE, Farrell MH. Prevalence of urinary tract infection in childhood: a meta-analysis. *Pediatr Infect Dis J.* 2008;27(4):302–308

11. To T, Agha M, Dick PT, Feldman W. Cohort study on circumcision of newborn boys and subsequent risk of urinary-tract infection. *Lancet.* 1998;352(9143):1813–1816

12. Shaikh N, Morone NE, Lopez J, et al. Does this child have a urinary tract infection? *JAMA.* 2007;298(24):2895–2904

13. Pantell RH, Newman TB, Bernzweig J, et al. Management and outcomes of care of fever in early infancy. *JAMA.* 2004;291(10):1203–1212

14. Byington CL, Enriquez FR, Hoff C, et al. Serious bacterial infections in febrile infants 1 to 90 days old with and without viral infections. *Pediatrics.* 2004;113(6):1662–1666

15. Levine DA, Platt SL, Dayan PS, et al. Risk of serious bacterial infection in young febrile infants with respiratory syncytial virus infections. *Pediatrics.* 2004;113(6):1728–1734

16. Gorelick MH, Hoberman A, Kearney D, Wald E, Shaw KN. Validation of a decision rule identifying febrile young girls at high risk for urinary tract infection. *Pediatr Emerg Care.* 2003;19(3):162–164

17. Gorelick MH, Shaw KN. Clinical decision rule to identify febrile young girls at risk for urinary tract infection. *Arch Pediatr Adolesc Med.* 2000;154(4):386–390

18. Roberts KB, Charney E, Sweren RJ, et al. Urinary tract infection in infants with unexplained fever: a collaborative study. *J Pediatr.* 1983;103(6):864–867

19. Lockhart GR, Lewander WJ, Cimini DM, Josephson SL, Linakis JG. Use of urinary Gram stain for detection of urinary tract infection in infants. *Ann Emerg Med.* 1995;25(1):31–35

20. Shaw KN, McGowan KL, Gorelick MH, Schwartz JS. Screening for urinary tract infection in infants in the emergency department: which test is best? *Pediatrics.* 1998;101(6). Available at: www.pediatrics.org/cgi/content/full/101/6/e1

21. Lin DS, Huang FY, Chiu NC, et al. Comparison of hemocytometer leukocyte counts and standard urinalyses for predicting urinary tract infections in febrile infants. *Pediatr Infect Dis J.* 2000;19(3):223–227

22. Leong YY, Tan KW. Bladder aspiration for diagnosis of urinary tract infection in infants and young children. *J Singapore Paediatr Soc.* 1976;18(1):43–47

23. Pryles CV, Atkin MD, Morse TS, Welch KJ. Comparative bacteriologic study of urine obtained from children by percutaneous suprapubic aspiration of the bladder and by catheter. *Pediatrics.* 1959;24(6):983–991

24. Djojohadipringgo S, Abdul Hamid RH, Thahir S, Karim A, Darsono I. Bladder puncture in newborns: a bacteriological study. *Paediatr Indones.* 1976;16(11–12):527–534

25. Gochman RF, Karasic RB, Heller MB. Use of portable ultrasound to assist urine collection by suprapubic aspiration. *Ann Emerg Med.* 1991;20(6):631–635

26. Buys H, Pead L, Hallett R, Maskell R. Suprapubic aspiration under ultrasound guidance in children with fever of undiagnosed cause. *BMJ.* 1994;308(6930):690–692

27. Kozer E, Rosenbloom E, Goldman D, Lavy G, Rosenfeld N, Goldman M. Pain in infants who are younger than 2 months during suprapubic aspiration and transurethral bladder catheterization: a randomized, controlled study. *Pediatrics.* 2006;118(1). Available at: www.pediatrics.org/cgi/content/full/118/1/e51

28. El-Naggar W, Yiu A, Mohamed A, et al. Comparison of pain during two methods of urine collection in preterm infants. *Pediatrics.* 2010;125(6):1224–1229

29. Al-Orifi F, McGillivray D, Tange S, Kramer MS. Urine culture from bag specimens in young children: are the risks too high? *J Pediatr.* 2000;137(2):221–226

30. Etoubleau C, Reveret M, Brouet D, et al. Moving from bag to catheter for urine collection in non-toilet-trained children suspected of having urinary tract infection: a paired comparison of urine cultures. *J Pediatr.* 2009;154(6):803–806

31. Alam M, Coulter J, Pacheco J, et al. Comparison of urine contamination rates using three different methods of collection: clean-catch, cotton wool pad and urine bag. *Ann Trop Paediatr.* 2005;25(1):29–34

32. Li PS, Ma LC, Wong SN. Is bag urine culture useful in monitoring urinary tract infection in infants? *J Paediatr Child Health.* 2002;38(4):377–381

33. Karacan C, Erkek N, Senel S, Akin Gunduz S, Catli G, Tavil B. Evaluation of urine collection methods for the diagnosis of urinary tract infection in children. *Med Princ Pract.* 2010;19(3):188–191

34. Perlhagen M, Forsberg T, Perlhagen J, Nivesjö M. Evaluating the specificity of a new type of urine collection bag for infants. *J Pediatr Urol.* 2007;3(5):378–381

35. Ginsburg CM, McCracken GH Jr. Urinary tract infections in young infants. *Pediatrics.* 1982;69(4):409–412

36. Hoberman A, Wald ER, Hickey RW, et al. Oral versus initial intravenous therapy for urinary tract infections in young febrile children. *Pediatrics.* 1999;104(1):79–86

37. Hodson EM, Willis NS, Craig JC. Antibiotics

for acute pyelonephritis in children. *Cochrane Database Syst Rev.* 2007;(4): CD003772

38. Zhanel GG, Hisanaga TL, Laing NM, et al. Antibiotic resistance in outpatient urinary isolates: final results from the North American Urinary Tract Infection Collaborative Alliance (NAUTICA). *Int J Antimicrob Agents.* 2005;26(5):380–388

39. Gaspari RJ, Dickson E, Karlowsky J, Doern G. Antibiotic resistance trends in paediatric uropathogens. *Int J Antimicrob Agents.* 2005;26(4):267–271

40. Michael M, Hodson EM, Craig JC, Martin S, Moyer VA. Short versus standard duration oral antibiotic therapy for acute urinary tract infection in children. *Cochrane Database Syst Rev.* 2003;(1):CD003966

41. Camacho V, Estorch M, Fraga G, et al. DMSA study performed during febrile urinary tract infection: a predictor of patient outcome? *Eur J Nucl Med Mol Imaging.* 2004; 31(6):862–866

42. Hewitt IK, Zucchetta P, Rigon L, et al. Early treatment of acute pyelonephritis in children fails to reduce renal scarring: data from the Italian Renal Infection Study Trials. *Pediatrics.* 2008;122(3):486–490

43. Doganis D, Siafas K, Mavrikou M, et al. Does early treatment of urinary tract infection prevent renal damage? *Pediatrics.* 2007; 120(4). Available at: www.pediatrics.org/cgi/content/full/120/4/e922

44. Fernández-Menéndez JM, Málaga S, Matesanz JL, SolíS G, Alonso S, Pérez-Méndez C. Risk factors in the development of early technetium-99m dimercaptosuccinic acid renal scintigraphy lesions during first urinary tract infection in children. *Acta Paediatr.* 2003;92(1):21–26

45. Keren R, Chan E. A meta-analysis of randomized, controlled trials comparing short- and long-course antibiotic therapy for urinary tract infections in children. *Pediatrics.* 2002;109(5). Available at: www.pediatrics.org/cgi/content/full/109/5/e70

46. Tran D, Muchant DG, Aronoff SC. Short-course versus conventional length antimicrobial therapy for uncomplicated lower urinary tract infections in children: a meta-analysis of 1279 patients. *J Pediatr.* 2001;139(1):93–99

47. Oreskovic NM, Sembrano EU. Repeat urine cultures in children who are admitted with urinary tract infections. *Pediatrics.* 2007; 119(2). Available at: www.pediatrics.org/cgi/content/full/119/2/e325

48. Currie ML, Mitz L, Raasch CS, Greenbaum LA. Follow-up urine cultures and fever in children with urinary tract infection. *Arch*

Pediatr Adolesc Med. 2003;157(12): 1237–1240

49. Lebowitz RL, Olbing H, Parkkulainen KV, Smellie JM, Tamminen-Mobius TE. International system of radiographic grading of vesicoureteric reflux. *Pediatr Radiol.* 1985; 15(2):105–109

50. Sargent MA, Stringer DA. Voiding cystourethrography in children with urinary tract infection: the frequency of vesicoureteric reflux is independent of the specialty of the physician requesting the study. *AJR.* 1995;164(5):1237–1241

51. Craig JC, Knight JF, Sureshkumar P, Lam A, Onikul E, Roy LP. Vesicoureteric reflux and timing of micturating cystourethrography after urinary tract infection. *Arch Dis Child.* 1997;76(3):275–277

52. McDonald A, Scranton M, Gillespie R, Mahajan V, Edwards GA. Voiding cystourethrograms and urinary tract infections: how long to wait? *Pediatrics.* 2000;105(4). Available at: www.pediatrics.org/cgi/content/full/105/4/e50

53. Oostenbrink R, van der Heijden AJ, Moons KG, Moll HA. Prediction of vesico-ureteric reflux in childhood urinary tract infection: a multivariate approach. *Acta Paediatr.* 2000;89(7):806–810

54. Mahant S, To T, Friedman J. Timing of voiding cystourethrogram in the investigation of urinary tract infections in children. *J Pediatr.* 2001;139(4):568–571

55. Mahant S, Friedman J, MacArthur C. Renal ultrasound findings and vesicoureteral reflux in children hospitalised with urinary tract infection. *Arch Dis Child.* 2002;86(6): 419–420

56. Chand DH, Rhoades T, Poe SA, Kraus S, Strife CF. Incidence and severity of vesicoureteral reflux in children related to age, gender, race and diagnosis. *J Urol.* 2003;170(4):1548–1550

57. Hansson S, Dhamey M, Sigström O, et al. Dimercapto-succinic acid scintigraphy instead of voiding cystourethrography for infants with urinary tract infection. *J Urol.* 2004;172(3):1071–1073

58. Pinto K. Vesicoureteral reflux in the Hispanic child with urinary tract infection. *J Urol.* 2004;171(3):1266–1267

59. Zamir G, Sakran W, Horowitz Y, Koren A, Miron D. Urinary tract infection: is there a need for routine renal ultrasonography? *Arch Dis Child.* 2004;89(5):466–468

60. Hannula A, Venhola M, Renko M, Pokka T, Huttunen NP, Uhari M. Vesicoureteral reflux in children with suspected and proven urinary tract infection. *Pediatr Nephrol.* 2010;25(8):1463–1469

61. Venhola M, Hannula A, Huttunen NP, Renko M, Pokka T, Uhari M. Occurrence of vesicoureteral reflux in children. *Acta Paediatr.* 2010;99(12):1875–1878

62. Alon US, Ganapathy S. Should renal ultrasonography be done routinely in children with first urinary tract infection? *Clin Pediatr (Phila).* 1999;38(1):21–25

63. Greenfield SP, Ng M, Wan J. Experience with vesicoureteral reflux in children: clinical characteristics. *J Urol.* 1997;158(2): 574–577

64. Roussey-Kesler G, Gadjos V, Idres N, et al. Antibiotic prophylaxis for the prevention of recurrent urinary tract infection in children with low grade vesicoureteral reflux: results from a prospective randomized study. *J Urol.* 2008;179(2):674–679

65. Lee SJ, Shim YH, Cho SJ, Lee JW. Probiotics prophylaxis in children with persistent primary vesicoureteral reflux. *Pediatr Nephrol.* 2007;22(9):1315–1320

66. Montini G, Rigon L, Zucchetta P, et al. Prophylaxis after first febrile urinary tract infection in children? A multicenter, randomized, controlled, noninferiority trial. *Pediatrics.* 2008;122(5):1064–1071

67. Garin EH, Olavarria F, Garcia Nieto V, Valenciano B, Campos A, Young L. Clinical significance of primary vesicoureteral reflux and urinary antibiotic prophylaxis after acute pyelonephritis: a multicenter, randomized, controlled study. *Pediatrics.* 2006;117(3):626–632

68. Pennesi M, Travan L, Peratoner L, et al. Is antibiotic prophylaxis in children with vesicoureteral reflux effective in preventing pyelonephritis and renal scars? A randomized, controlled trial. *Pediatrics.* 2008; 121(6). Available at: www.pediatrics.org/cgi/content/full/121/6/e1489

69. Craig J, Simpson J, Williams G. Antibiotic prophylaxis and recurrent urinary tract infection in children. *N Engl J Med.* 2009; 361(18):1748–1759

70. Brandström P, Esbjorner E, Herthelius M, Swerkersson S, Jodal U, Hansson S. The Swedish Reflux Trial in Children, part III: urinary tract infection pattern. *J Urol.* 2010;184(1):286–291

71. Moorthy I, Wheat D, Gordon I. Ultrasonography in the evaluation of renal scarring using DMSA scan as the gold standard. *Pediatr Nephrol.* 2004;19(2):153–156

72. Biggi A, Dardanelli L, Pomero G, et al. Acute renal cortical scintigraphy in children with a first urinary tract infection. *Pediatr Nephrol.* 2001;16(9):733–738

73. Smellie JM, Rigden SP, Prescod NP. Urinary tract infection: a comparison of four

methods of investigation. *Arch Dis Child.* 1995;72(3):247–260

74. Hoberman A, Charron M, Hickey RW, Baskin M, Kearney DH, Wald ER. Imaging studies after a first febrile urinary tract infection in young children. *N Engl J Med.* 2003;348(3):195–202

75. Roberts J. Experimental pyelonephritis in the monkey, part III: pathophysiology of ureteral malfunction induced by bacteria. *Invest Urol.* 1975;13(2):117–120

76. Wippermann CF, Schofer O, Beetz R, et al. Renal abscess in childhood: diagnostic and therapeutic progress. *Pediatr Infect Dis J.* 1991;10(6):446–450

77. Barry BP, Hall N, Cornford E, Broderick NJ, Somers JM, Rose DH. Improved ultrasound detection of renal scarring in children following urinary tract infection. *Clin Radiol.* 1998;53(10):747–751

78. Sinha MD, Gibson P, Kane T, Lewis MA. Accuracy of ultrasonic detection of renal scarring in different centres using DMSA as the gold standard. *Nephrol Dial Transplant.* 2007;22(8):2213–2216

79. Montini G, Zucchetta P, Tomasi L, et al. Value of imaging studies after a first febrile urinary tract infection in young children: data from Italian Renal Infection Study 1. *Pediatrics.* 2009;123(2). Available at: www.pediatrics.org/cgi/content/full/123/2/e239

80. Giorgi LJ Jr, Bratslavsky G, Kogan BA. Febrile urinary tract infections in infants: renal ultrasound remains necessary. *J Urol.* 2005;173(2):568–570

81. Gelfand MJ, Barr LL, Abunku O. The initial renal ultrasound examination in children with urinary tract infection: the prevalence of dilated uropathy has decreased. *Pediatr Radiol.* 2000;30(10):665–670

82. Jothilakshmi K, Vijayaraghavan B, Paul S, Matthai J. Radiological evaluation of the urinary tract in children with urinary infection. *Indian J Pediatr.* 2001;68(12):1131–1133

83. Jahnukainen T, Honkinen O, Ruuskanen O, Mertsola J. Ultrasonography after the first febrile urinary tract infection in children. *Eur J Pediatr.* 2006;165(8):556–559

84. Huang HP, Lai YC, Tsai IJ, Chen SY, Tsau YK. Renal ultrasonography should be done routinely in children with first urinary tract infections. *Urology.* 2008;71(3):439–443

85. Economou G, Egginton J, Brookfield D. The importance of late pregnancy scans for renal tract abnormalities. *Prenat Diagn.* 1994;14(3):177–180

86. Rosendahl H. Ultrasound screening for fetal urinary tract malformations: a prospective study in general population. *Eur J Obstet Gynecol Reprod Biol.* 1990;36(1–2):27–33

87. Paduano L, Giglio L, Bembi B, Peratoner L, Benussi, G. Clinical outcome of fetal uropathy, part II: sensitivity of echography for prenatal detection of obstructive pathology. *J Urol.* 1991;146(4):1097–1098

88. Miron D, Daas A, Sakran W, Lumelsky D, Koren A, Horovitz Y. Is omitting post urinary-tract-infection renal ultrasound safe after normal antenatal ultrasound? An observational study. *Arch Dis Child.* 2007;92(6):502–504

89. Lakhoo K, Thomas DF, Fuenfer M, D'Cruz AJ. Failure of pre-natal ultrasonography to prevent urinary infection associated with underlying urological abnormalities. *Br J Urol.* 1996;77(6):905–908

90. Scholtmeijer RJ. Treatment of vesicoureteric reflux: results of a prospective study. *Br J Urol.* 1993;71(3):346–349

91. Smellie JM, Barratt TM, Chantler C, et al. Medical versus surgical treatment in children with severe bilateral vesicoureteric reflux and bilateral nephropathy: a randomised trial. *Lancet.* 2001;357(9265):1329–1333

92. Jodal U, Smellie JM, Lax H, Hoyer PF. Ten-year results of randomized treatment of children with severe vesicoureteral reflux: final report of the International Reflux Study in Children. *Pediatr Nephrol.* 2006;21(6):785–792

93. Capozza N, Caione P. Dextranomer/hyaluronic acid copolymer implantation for vesico-ureteral reflux: a randomized comparison with antibiotic prophylaxis. *J Pediatr.* 2002;140(2):230–234

94. Wingen AM, Koskimies O, Olbing H, Seppanen J, Tamminen-Mobius T. Growth and weight gain in children with vesicoureteral reflux receiving medical versus surgical treatment: 10-year results of a prospective, randomized study. *Acta Paediatr.* 1999;88(1):56–61

95. Smellie JM, Tamminen-Möbius T, Olbing H, et al. Radiologic findings in the kidney of children with severe reflux: five-year comparative study of conservative and surgical treatment [in German]. *Urologe A.* 1993;32(1):22–29

96. Olbing H, Smellie JM, Jodal U, Lax H. New renal scars in children with severe VUR: a 10-year study of randomized treatment. *Pediatr Nephrol.* 2003;18(11):1128–1131

97. Olbing H, Hirche H, Koskimies O, et al. Renal growth in children with severe vesicoureteral reflux: 10-year prospective study of medical and surgical treatment. *Radiology.* 2000;216(3):731–737

98. Al-Sayyad AJ, Pike JG, Leonard MP. Can prophylactic antibiotics safely be discontinued in children with vesicoureteral reflux? *J Urol.* 2005;174(4):1587–1589

99. Kaneko K, Ohtomo Y, Shimizu T, Yamashiro Y, Yamataka A, Miyano T. Antibiotic prophylaxis by low-dose cefaclor in children with vesicoureteral reflux. *Pediatr Nephrol.* 2003;18(5):468–470

100. Lohr JA, Nunley DH, Howards SS, Ford RF. Prevention of recurrent urinary tract infections in girls. *Pediatrics.* 1977;59(4):562–565

101. Smellie JM, Katz G, Grüneberg RN. Controlled trial of prophylactic treatment in childhood urinary-tract infection. *Lancet.* 1978;2(8082):175–178

102. Savage DC, Howie G, Adler K, Wilson MI. Controlled trial of therapy in covert bacteriuria of childhood. *Lancet.* 1975;1(7903):358–361

103. Stansfeld JM. Duration of treatment for urinary tract infections in children. *Br Med J.* 1975;3(5975):65–66

104. Reddy PP, Evans MT, Hughes PA, et al. Antimicrobial prophylaxis in children with vesicoureteral reflux: a randomized prospective study of continuous therapy vs intermittent therapy vs surveillance. *Pediatrics.* 1997;100(3 suppl):555–556

105. Craig J, Roy L, Sureshkumar P, Burke J, Powell H. Long-term antibiotics to prevent urinary tract infection in children with isolated vesicoureteric reflux: a placebo-controlled randomized trial. *J Am Soc Nephrol.* 2002;13(3):3A

106. Bitsori M, Maraki S, Kalmanti M, Galanakis E. Resistance against broad-spectrum β-lactams among uropathogens in children. *Pediatr Nephrol.* 2009;24(12):2381–2386

107. Conway PH, Cnaan A, Zaoutis T, Henry BV, Grundmeier RW, Keren R. Recurrent urinary tract infections in children: risk factors and association with prophylactic antimicrobials. *JAMA.* 2007;298(2):179–186

108. Hodson EM, Wheeler DM, Vimalchandra D, Smith GH, Craig JC. Interventions for primary vesicoureteric reflux. *Cochrane Database Syst Rev.* 2007;(3):CD001532

109. xWilliams DI, Kenawi MM. The prognosis of pelviureteric obstruction in childhood: a review of 190 cases. *Eur Urol.* 1976;2(2):57–63

110. Mihindukulasuriya JC, Maskell R, Polak A. A study of fifty-eight patients with renal scarring associated with urinary tract infection. *Q J Med.* 1980;49(194):165–178

111. McKerrow W, Davidson-Lamb N, Jones PF. Urinary tract infection in children. *Br Med J (Clin Res Ed)*. 1984;289(6440):299–303

112. Jacobson SH, Eklof O, Lins LE, Wikstad I, Winberg J. Long-term prognosis of post-infectious renal scarring in relation to radiological findings in childhood: a 27-year follow-up. *Pediatr Nephrol*. 1992;6(1):19–24

113. Craig JC, Irwig LM, Knight JF, Roy LP. Does treatment of vesicoureteric reflux in childhood prevent end-stage renal disease attributable to reflux nephropathy? *Pediatrics*. 2000;105(6):1236–1241

114. Phillips D, Watson AR, Collier J. Distress and radiological investigations of the urinary tract in children. *Eur J Pediatr*. 1996;155(8):684–687

115. Phillips DA, Watson AR, MacKinlay D. Distress and the micturating cystourethrogram: does preparation help? *Acta Paediatr*. 1998;87(2):175–179

116. Robinson M, Savage J, Stewart M, Sweeney L. The diagnostic value, parental and patient acceptability of micturating cysto-urethrography in children. *Ir Med J*. 1999;92(5):366–368

The New American Academy of Pediatrics Urinary Tract Infection Guideline

This issue of *Pediatrics* includes a long-awaited update[1] of the American Academy of Pediatrics (AAP) 1999 urinary tract infection (UTI) practice parameter.[2] The new guideline is accompanied by a technical report[3] that provides a comprehensive literature review and also a new meta-analysis, for which the authors obtained individual-level data from investigators. The result is an exceptionally evidence-based guideline that differs in important ways from the 1999 guideline and sets a high standard for transparency and scholarship.

The guideline and technical report address a logical sequence of questions that arise clinically, including (1) Which children should have their urine tested? (2) How should the sample be obtained? (3) How should UTIs be treated? (4) What imaging and follow-up are recommended after a diagnosis of UTI? and (5) How should children be followed after a UTI has been diagnosed? I will follow that same sequence in this commentary. I will mention some important areas of agreement and make other suggestions when I believe alternative recommendations are supported by available evidence.

WHICH CHILDREN SHOULD HAVE THEIR URINE TESTED?

Unlike the 1999 practice parameter, which recommended urine testing for all children aged 2 months to 2 years with unexplained fever,[2] the new guideline recommends selective urine testing based on the prior probability of UTI, which is an important improvement. The guideline and technical report do an admirable job summarizing the main factors that determine that prior probability (summarized in Table 1 in the clinical report). This table will help clinicians estimate whether the probability of UTI is ≥1% or ≥2%, values that the authors suggest are reasonable thresholds for urine testing.

The guideline appropriately states that the threshold probability for urine testing is not known and that "clinicians will choose a threshold depending on factors such as their confidence that contact will be maintained through the illness. . . and comfort with diagnostic uncertainty." However, the authors assert that this threshold is below 3%, which indicates that it is worth performing urine tests on more than 33 febrile children to identify a single UTI. This is puzzling, because the only study cited to support a specific testing threshold found that 33% of academicians and 54% of practitioners had a urine culture threshold higher than 3%.[4]

An evidence-based urine-testing threshold probability would be based on the risks and costs of urine testing compared with the benefits of diagnosing a UTI. These benefits are not known and probably are not uniform; the younger and sicker an infant is and the longer he or she has been febrile, the greater the likely benefit of diagnosing and treating a UTI. Because acute symptoms of most UTIs seem to resolve un-

AUTHOR: Thomas B. Newman, MD, MPH

Division of Clinical Epidemiology, Department of Epidemiology and Biostatistics, and Division of General Pediatrics, Department of Pediatrics, University of California, San Francisco, California

ABBREVIATIONS
AAP—American Academy of Pediatrics
UTI—urinary tract infection
VCUG—voiding cystourethrogram
VUR—vesicoureteral reflux

Opinions expressed in these commentaries are those of the author and not necessarily those of the American Academy of Pediatrics or its Committees.

www.pediatrics.org/cgi/doi/10.1542/peds.2011-1818

doi:10.1542/peds.2011-1818

Accepted for publication Jun 28, 2011

Address correspondence to Thomas B. Newman, MD, MPH, Department of Epidemiology and Biostatistics, UCSF Box 0560, San Francisco, CA 94143. E-mail: newman@epi.ucsf.edu

PEDIATRICS (ISSN Numbers: Print, 0031-4005; Online, 1098-4275).

FINANCIAL DISCLOSURE: *The author has indicated he has no financial relationships relevant to this article to disclose.*

COMPANION PAPERS: Companions to this article can be found on pages 595 and e749, and online at www.pediatrics.org/cgi/doi/10.1542/peds.2011-1330 and www.pediatrics.org/cgi/doi/10.1542/peds.2011-1332.

eventfully, even without treatment,[5,6] some of the impetus for diagnosing UTIs rests on the belief that doing so will reduce the risk of renal scarring and associated sequelae.[7] This belief needs to be proven, and the benefit quantified, if a urine-testing threshold is to be evidence-based. Until then, rather than automatically testing urine on the basis of the risk factors and the 1% or 2% threshold suggested in Table 1, clinicians should continue to individualize. It seems reasonable, for example, to defer urine tests on the large number of febrile infants for whom, if their parents had called for advice, we would have estimated their probability of UTI or other serious illness to be low enough that they could be safely initially watched at home.

A potential source of confusion is that Table 1 lists "absence of another source of infection" as a risk factor, and the technical report indicates that this factor has a likelihood ratio of ~1.4 for UTI. However, the inclusion of this risk factor in the table is inconsistent with the text of the guideline, which directs clinicians to assess the likelihood of UTI in febrile infants with no apparent source for the fever. If children with an apparent source for their fever are included, the use of Table 1 could lead to excessive urine testing (eg, among infants with colds). For example, even using the 2% testing threshold, according to Table 1 all non-black uncircumcised boys younger than 24 months with any fever of any duration, even with an apparent source, would need their urine tested. I doubt that this level of urine testing is necessary or was intended by the authors of the guideline.

HOW SHOULD THE SAMPLE BE OBTAINED?

I am glad the new guideline continues to offer the option of obtaining urine for urinalyses noninvasively, but I am

not convinced that the bag urine can never be used for culture. If the urinalysis is used to select urine for culture, the prior probability may sometimes be in a range where the bag culture will be useful. For example, the technical report calculates that "with a prevalence of 5% and specificity of 70%, the positive predictive value of a positive culture obtained by bag would be 15%." However, with the same 5% pretest probability, a positive nitrite test would raise the probability of UTI to ~75% (using the median sensitivity [58%] and specificity [99%] in the technical report). This is high enough to make the positive culture on bag urine convincing (and perhaps unnecessary).

Although bag urine cultures can lead to errors, catheterized urine cultures are not perfect[1] and urethral catheterization is painful,[8] frightening,[9] and risks introducing infection.[10] Fortunately, if other recommendations in the guideline are followed (including the elimination of routine voiding cystourethrograms [VCUGs] and outpatient rather than inpatient antimicrobial therapy; see below), the adverse consequences of falsely positive bag cultures will be markedly attenuated.

HOW SHOULD UTIs BE TREATED?

The guideline recognizes regional variation in antimicrobial susceptibility patterns and appropriately suggests that they dictate the choice of initial treatment. However, I would adjust the choice on the basis of the clinical course rather than on sensitivity testing of the isolated uropathogen, as recommended in the guideline. At the University of California at San Francisco we have the option of a "screening" urine culture, which provides only the colony count and Gram-stain results for positive cultures (eg, "10⁵ Gram-negative rods"). We can later add identification and sensitivities of the organism in the rare instances in which

obtaining them is clinically indicated. Use of screening cultures can lead to considerable savings, because identification of organisms and antimicrobial susceptibility testing are expensive and unnecessary in the majority of cases in which patients are better within 24 hours of starting treatment.

The guideline and technical report cite good evidence that oral antimicrobial treatment is as effective as parenteral treatment and state that the choice of route of administration should be based on "practical considerations." However, the examples they cite for when parenteral antibiotics are reasonable (eg, toxic appearance and inability to retain oral medications) seem more like clinical than practical considerations. Given equivalent estimates of efficacy and the dramatic differences in cost, the guideline could have more forcefully recommended oral treatment in the absence of clinical contraindications.

WHAT IMAGING IS INDICATED AFTER UTI?

As in the 1999 AAP guideline, the current guideline recommends a renal/bladder ultrasound examination after a first febrile UTI to rule out anatomic abnormalities (particularly obstruction) that warrant further evaluation. Although the yield of this test is low, particularly if there has been a normal third-trimester prenatal ultrasound scan, the estimated 1% to 2% yield of actionable abnormalities was believed to be sufficient to justify this noninvasive test. This may be so, but it is important to note that it is not just the yield of abnormalities but also the evidence of an advantage of early detection and cost-effectiveness that must be considered when deciding whether an ultrasound scan is indicated after the first febrile UTI, and this evidence was not reviewed.

The recommendation most dramatically different from the 1999 guideline is that a VCUG not be routinely performed after a first febrile UTI. The main reason for this change is the accumulation of evidence casting doubt on the benefit of making a diagnosis of vesicoureteral reflux (VUR). To put these data in historical perspective, operative ureteral reimplantation was standard treatment for VUR until randomized trials found it to be no better than prophylactic antibiotics at preventing renal scarring.[11–13] Although, as one commentator put it, "It is psychologically difficult to accept results that suggest that time-honored methods that are generally recommended and applied are of no or doubtful value,"[14] ureteral reimplantation was gradually replaced with prophylactic antibiotics as standard treatment for VUR. This was not because of evidence of benefit of antibiotics but because their use was easier and less invasive than ureteral reimplantation. Finally, in the last few years, several randomized trials have investigated the efficacy of prophylactic antibiotics for children with reflux and have found little, if any, benefit.[1,3] Thus, the risks, costs, and discomfort of the VCUG are hard to justify, because there is no evidence that patients benefit from having their VUR diagnosed.[15–18]

The recommendation not to perform a VCUG after the first UTI is consistent with a guideline published by the United Kingdom's National Institute for Health and Clinical Excellence (NICE).[19] However, unlike the AAP, the NICE does not recommend that VCUGs be performed routinely for recurrent UTIs in infants older than 6 months, which makes sense; the arguments against VCUGs after a first UTI still hold after a second UTI. The AAP recommendation to perform a VCUG after the second UTI is based on the increasing likelihood of detecting higher grades of reflux in children with recurrent UTIs and the belief that detecting grade V reflux is beneficial. However, the guideline appropriately recognizes that grade V reflux is rare and that the benefits of diagnosing it are still in some doubt. Therefore, the guideline suggests that parent preferences be considered in making these imaging decisions.

HOW SHOULD CHILDREN BE FOLLOWED AFTER A UTI HAS BEEN DIAGNOSED?

The guideline recommends that parents or guardians of children with confirmed UTI "seek prompt (ideally within 48 hours) medical evaluation for future febrile illnesses to ensure that recurrent infections can be detected and treated promptly." As pointed out in the guideline, parents will ultimately make the judgment to seek medical care, and there is room for judgment here. After-hours or weekend visits would not generally be required for infants who appear well, and the necessity and urgency of the visit would be expected to increase with the discomfort of the child, the height and duration of the fever, the absence of an alternative source, and the number of previous UTIs.

It should be noted that the guideline does not recommend prophylactic antibiotics to prevent UTI recurrences. This was a good decision; meta-analyses[3,20] have revealed no significant reduction in symptomatic UTI from such prophylaxis regardless of whether VUR was present. Even in the study that showed a benefit,[21] the absolute risk reduction for symptomatic UTI over the 1-year follow-up period was only ~6%, and there was no reduction in hospitalizations for UTI or in renal scarring. Thus, as one colleague put it, if UTI prophylaxis worked, it would offer the opportunity to "treat 16 children with antibiotics for a year to prevent treating one child with antibiotics for a week." (A. R. Schroeder, MD, written communication, June 24, 2011).

CONCLUSIONS

I salute the authors of the new AAP UTI guideline and the accompanying technical report. Both publications represent a significant advance that should be helpful to clinicians and families dealing with this common problem.

REFERENCES

1. American Academy of Pediatrics, Subcommittee on Urinary Tract Infection, Steering Committee on Quality Improvement and Management. Diagnosis and management of initial UTIs in febrile infants and children aged 2 to 24 months. *Pediatrics.* 2011;128(3):595–610

2. American Academy of Pediatrics, Committee on Quality Improvement, Subcommittee on Urinary Tract Infection. Practice parameter: the diagnosis, treatment, and evaluation of the initial urinary tract infection in febrile infants and young children [published corrections appear in *Pediatrics.* 1999;103(5 pt 1):1052 and *Pediatrics.*

1999;104(1 pt 1):118]. *Pediatrics.* 1999; 103(4 pt 1):843–852

3. American Academy of Pediatrics, Subcommittee on Urinary Tract Infection, Steering Committee on Quality Improvement and Management. The diagnosis and management of the initial urinary tract infection in febrile infants and young children. *Pediatrics.* 2011;128(3). Available at: www.pediatrics.org/cgi/content/full/128/3/e749

4. Roberts KB, Charney E, Sweren RJ, et al. Urinary tract infection in infants with unexplained fever: a collaborative study. *J Pediatr.* 1983;103(6):864–867

5. Newman TB, Bernzweig JA, Takayama JI, Finch SA, Wasserman RC, Pantell RH. Urine testing and urinary tract infections in febrile infants seen in office settings: the Pediatric Research in Office Settings' Febrile Infant Study. *Arch Pediatr Adolesc Med.* 2002;156(1):44–54

6. Craig JC, Williams GJ, Jones M, et al. The accuracy of clinical symptoms and signs for the diagnosis of serious bacterial infection in young febrile children: prospective cohort study of 15 781 febrile illnesses. *BMJ.* 2010;340:c1594

7. Roberts KB. Urinary tract infections in

young febrile infants: is selective testing acceptable? *Arch Pediatr Adolesc Med.* 2002; 156(1):6–7

8. Mularoni PP, Cohen LL, DeGuzman M, Mennuti-Washburn J, Greenwald M, Simon HK. A randomized clinical trial of lidocaine gel for reducing infant distress during urethral catheterization. *Pediatr Emerg Care.* 2009;25(7):439–443

9. Merritt KA, Ornstein PA, Spicker B. Children's memory for a salient medical procedure: implications for testimony. *Pediatrics.* 1994;94(1):17–23

10. Lohr JA, Downs SM, Dudley S, Donowitz LG. Hospital-acquired urinary tract infections in the pediatric patient: a prospective study. *Pediatr Infect Dis J.* 1994;13(1):8–12

11. Birmingham Reflux Study Group. Prospective trial of operative versus non-operative treatment of severe vesicoureteric reflux in children: five years' observation. *Br Med J (Clin Res Ed).* 1987;295(6592):237–241

12. Weiss R, Duckett J, Spitzer A. Results of a randomized clinical trial of medical versus surgical management of infants and children with grades III and IV primary vesicoureteral reflux (United States). The International Reflux Study in Children. *J Urol.* 1992;148(5 pt 2):1667–1673

13. Smellie JM, Tamminen-Mobius T, Olbing H, et al. Five-year study of medical or surgical treatment in children with severe reflux: radiological renal findings. The International Reflux Study in Children. *Pediatr Nephrol.* 1992;6(3):223–230

14. Winberg J. Management of primary vesicoureteric reflux in children: operation ineffective in preventing progressive renal damage. *Infection.* 1994;22(suppl 1):S4–S7

15. Ortigas A, Cunningham A. Three facts to know before you order a VCUG. *Contemp Pediatr.* 1997;14(9):69–79

16. Craig JC, Irwig LM, Knight JF, Roy LP. Does treatment of vesicoureteric reflux in childhood prevent end-stage renal disease attributable to reflux nephropathy? *Pediatrics.* 2000;105(6):1236–1241

17. Verrier Jones K. Time to review the value of imaging after urinary tract infection in infants. *Arch Dis Child.* 2005;90(7):663–664

18. Newman TB. Much pain, little gain from voiding cystourethrograms after urinary tract infection. *Pediatrics.* 2006;118(5):2251

19. National Collaborating Centre for Women's and Children's Health. *Urinary Tract Infection in Children: Diagnosis, Treatment and Long-term Management.* National Institute for Health and Clinical Excellence Clinical Guideline. London, United Kingdom: RCOG Press; 2007

20. Dai B, Liu Y, Jia J, Mei C. Long-term antibiotics for the prevention of recurrent urinary tract infection in children: a systematic review and meta-analysis. *Arch Dis Child.* 2010;95(7):499–508

21. Craig JC, Simpson JM, Williams GJ, et al; Prevention of Recurrent Urinary Tract Infection in Children With Vesicoureteric Reflux and Normal Renal Tracts (PRIVENT) Investigators. Antibiotic prophylaxis and recurrent urinary tract infection in children. *N Engl J Med.* 2009;361(18):1748–1759

Urinary Tract Infection Clinical Practice Guideline Quick Reference Tools

- Action Statement Summary
  — Urinary Tract Infection: Clinical Practice Guideline for the Diagnosis and Management of the Initial UTI in Febrile Infants and Children 2 to 24 Months
- *ICD-9-CM/ICD-10-CM* Coding Quick Reference for Urinary Tract Infection
- AAP Patient Education Handout
  — *Urinary Tract Infections in Young Children*

Action Statement Summary

Urinary Tract Infection: Clinical Practice Guideline for the Diagnosis and Management of the Initial UTI in Febrile Infants and Children 2 to 24 Months

Action Statement 1

If a clinician decides that a febrile infant with no apparent source for the fever requires antimicrobial therapy to be administered because of ill appearance or another pressing reason, the clinician should ensure that a urine specimen is obtained for both culture and urinalysis before an antimicrobial agent is administered; the specimen needs to be obtained through catheterization or SPA, because the diagnosis of UTI cannot be established reliably through culture of urine collected in a bag (evidence quality: A; strong recommendation).

Action Statement 2

If a clinician assesses a febrile infant with no apparent source for the fever as not being so ill as to require immediate antimicrobial therapy, then the clinician should assess the likelihood of UTI (see below for how to assess likelihood).

Action Statement 2a

If the clinician determines the febrile infant to have a low likelihood of UTI (see text), then clinical follow-up monitoring without testing is sufficient (evidence quality: A; strong recommendation).

Action Statement 2b

If the clinician determines that the febrile infant is not in a low-risk group (see below), then there are 2 choices (evidence quality: A; strong recommendation). Option 1 is to obtain a urine specimen through catheterization or SPA for culture and urinalysis. Option 2 is to obtain a urine specimen through the most convenient means and to perform a urinalysis. If the urinalysis results suggest a UTI (positive leukocyte esterase test results or nitrite test or microscopic analysis results positive for leukocytes or bacteria), then a urine specimen should be obtained through catheterization or SPA and cultured; if urinalysis of fresh (<1 hour since void) urine yields negative leukocyte esterase and nitrite test results, then it is reasonable to monitor the clinical course without initiating antimicrobial therapy, recognizing that negative urinalysis results do not rule out a UTI with certainty.

Action Statement 3

To establish the diagnosis of UTI, clinicians should require *both* urinalysis results that suggest infection (pyuria and/or bacteriuria) *and* the presence of at least 50 000 colony-forming units (CFUs) per mL of a uropathogen cultured from a urine specimen obtained through catheterization or SPA (evidence quality: C; recommendation).

Action Statement 4a

When initiating treatment, the clinician should base the choice of route of administration on practical considerations. Initiating treatment orally or parenterally is equally efficacious. The clinician should base the choice of agent on local antimicrobial sensitivity patterns (if available) and should adjust the choice according to sensitivity testing of the isolated uropathogen (evidence quality: A; strong recommendation).

Action Statement 4b

The clinician should choose 7 to 14 days as the duration of antimicrobial therapy (evidence quality: B; recommendation).

Action Statement 5

Febrile infants with UTIs should undergo renal and bladder ultrasonography (RBUS) (evidence quality: C; recommendation).

Action Statement 6a

VCUG should not be performed routinely after the first febrile UTI; VCUG is indicated if RBUS reveals hydronephrosis, scarring, or other findings that would suggest either high-grade VUR or obstructive uropathy, as well as in other atypical or complex clinical circumstances (evidence quality B; recommendation).

Action Statement 6b

Further evaluation should be conducted if there is a recurrence of febrile UTI (evidence quality: X; recommendation).

Action Statement 7

After confirmation of UTI, the clinician should instruct parents or guardians to seek prompt medical evaluation (ideally within 48 hours) for future febrile illnesses, to ensure that recurrent infections can be detected and treated promptly (evidence quality: C; recommendation).

Coding Quick Reference for Urinary Tract Infection	
ICD-9-CM	*ICD-10-CM*
599.0 Urinary tract infection, site not specified	**N39.0** Urinary tract infection, site not specified
771.82 Urinary tract infection, newborn	**P39.3** Neonatal urinary tract infection

Urinary Tract Infections in Young Children

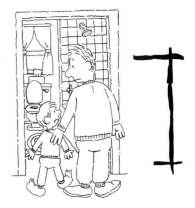

Urinary tract infections (UTIs) are common in young children. These infections can lead to serious health problems. UTIs may go untreated because the symptoms may not be obvious to the child or the parents. The following is information from the American Academy of Pediatrics about UTIs—what they are, how children get them, and how they are treated.

The urinary tract

The urinary tract makes and stores urine. It is made up of the kidneys, ureters, bladder, and urethra (see illustration on the next page). The kidneys produce urine. Urine travels from the kidneys down 2 narrow tubes called the ureters to the bladder. The bladder is a thin muscular bag that stores urine until it is time to empty urine out of the body. When it is time to empty the bladder, a muscle at the bottom of the bladder relaxes. Urine then flows out of the body through a tube called the urethra. The opening of the urethra is at the end of the penis in boys and above the vaginal opening in girls.

Urinary tract infections

Normal urine has no germs (bacteria). However, bacteria can get into the urinary tract from 2 sources: (1) the skin around the rectum and genitals and (2) the bloodstream from other parts of the body. Bacteria may cause infections in any or all parts of the urinary tract, including the following:

- Urethra (called urethritis)
- Bladder (called cystitis)
- Kidneys (called pyelonephritis)

UTIs are common in infants and young children. The frequency of UTIs in girls is much greater than in boys. About 3% of girls and 1% of boys will have a UTI by 11 years of age. A young child with a high fever and no other symptoms has a 1 in 20 chance of having a UTI. Uncircumcised boys have more UTIs than those who have been circumcised.

Symptoms

Symptoms of UTIs may include the following:

- Fever
- Pain or burning during urination
- Need to urinate more often, or difficulty getting urine out
- Urgent need to urinate, or wetting of underwear or bedding by a child who knows how to use the toilet
- Vomiting, refusal to eat
- Abdominal pain
- Side or back pain
- Foul-smelling urine
- Cloudy or bloody urine
- Unexplained and persistent irritability in an infant
- Poor growth in an infant

Diagnosis

If your child has symptoms of a UTI, your child's doctor will do the following:

- Ask about your child's symptoms.
- Ask about any family history of urinary tract problems.
- Ask about what your child has been eating and drinking.
- Examine your child.
- Get a urine sample from your child.

Your child's doctor will need to test your child's urine to see if there are bacteria or other abnormalities.

Ways urine is collected

Urine must be collected and analyzed to determine if there is a bacterial infection. Older children are asked to urinate into a container.

There are 3 ways to collect urine from a young child:

1. The preferred method is to place a small tube, called a catheter, through the urethra into the bladder. Urine flows through the tube into a special urine container.
2. Another method is to insert a needle through the skin of the lower abdomen to draw urine from the bladder. This is called needle aspiration.
3. If your child is very young or not yet toilet trained, the child's doctor may place a plastic bag over the genitals to collect the urine. Since bacteria on the skin can contaminate the urine and give a false test result, this method is used only to screen for infection. If an infection seems to be present, the doctor will need to collect urine through 1 of the first 2 methods in order to determine if bacteria are present.

Your child's doctor will discuss with you the best way to collect your child's urine.

Treatment

UTIs are treated with antibiotics. The way your child receives the antibiotic depends on the severity and type of infection. Antibiotics are usually given by mouth, as liquid or pills. If your child has a fever or is vomiting and is unable to keep fluids down, the antibiotics may be put directly into a vein or injected into a muscle.

UTIs need to be treated right away to

- Get rid of the infection.
- Prevent the spread of the infection outside of the urinary tract.
- Reduce the chances of kidney damage.

Infants and young children with UTIs usually need to take antibiotics for 7 to 14 days, sometimes longer. Make sure your child takes all the medicine your child's doctor prescribes. Do not stop giving your child the medicine until the child's doctor says the treatment is finished, even if your child feels better. UTIs can return if not fully treated.

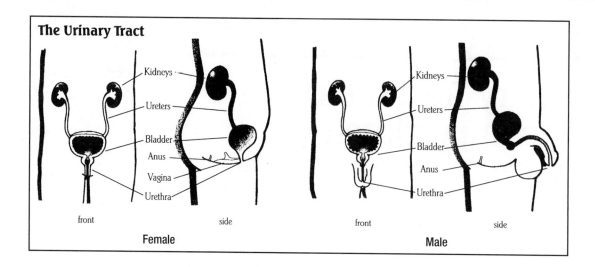

The Urinary Tract

Female

Male

Follow-up

If the UTI occurs early in life, your child's doctor will probably want to make sure the urinary tract is normal with a kidney and bladder ultrasound. This test uses sound waves to examine the bladder and kidneys.

In addition, your child's doctor may want to make sure that the urinary tract is functioning normally and is free of any damage. Several tests are available to do this, including the following:

Voiding cystourethrogram (VCUG). A catheter is placed into the urethra and the bladder is filled with a liquid that can be seen on x-rays. This test shows whether the urine is flowing back from the bladder toward the kidneys instead of all of it coming out through the urethra as it should.

Nuclear scans. Radioactive material is injected into a vein to see if the kidneys are normal. There are many kinds of nuclear scans, each giving different information about the kidneys and bladder. The radioactive material gives no more radiation than any other kind of x-ray.

Remember

UTIs are common and most are easy to treat. Early diagnosis and prompt treatment are important because untreated or repeated infections can cause long-term medical problems. Children who have had one UTI are more likely to have another. Be sure to see your child's doctor early if your child has had a UTI in the past and has fever. Talk with your child's doctor if you suspect that your child might have a UTI.

The information contained in this publication should not be used as a substitute for the medical care and advice of your pediatrician. There may be variations in treatment that your pediatrician may recommend based on individual facts and circumstances.

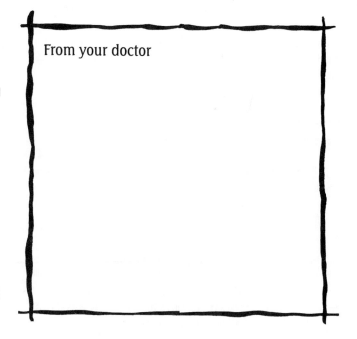

From your doctor

American Academy
of Pediatrics

DEDICATED TO THE HEALTH OF ALL CHILDREN™

The American Academy of Pediatrics is an organization of 60,000 primary care pediatricians, pediatric medical subspecialists, and pediatric surgical specialists dedicated to the health, safety, and well-being of infants, children, adolescents, and young adults.

American Academy of Pediatrics
Web site — www.aap.org

Endorsed Clinical Practice Guidelines

. . . .

The American Academy of Pediatrics endorses and accepts as its policy the following guidelines from other organizations.

AUTISM

Screening and Diagnosis of Autism
Quality Standards Subcommittee of the American Academy of Neurology and the Child Neurology Society

ABSTRACT. Autism is a common disorder of childhood, affecting 1 in 500 children. Yet, it often remains unrecognized and undiagnosed until or after late preschool age because appropriate tools for routine developmental screening and screening specifically for autism have not been available. Early identification of children with autism and intensive, early intervention during the toddler and preschool years improves outcome for most young children with autism. This practice parameter reviews the available empirical evidence and gives specific recommendations for the identification of children with autism. This approach requires a dual process: 1) routine developmental surveillance and screening specifically for autism to be performed on all children to first identify those at risk for any type of atypical development, and to identify those specifically at risk for autism; and 2) to diagnose and evaluate autism, to differentiate autism from other developmental disorders. (8/00)

CEREBRAL PALSY

Diagnostic Assessment of the Child With Cerebral Palsy
Quality Standards Subcommittee of the American Academy of Neurology and the Practice Committee of the Child Neurology Society

ABSTRACT. *Objective.* The Quality Standards Subcommittee of the American Academy of Neurology and the Practice Committee of the Child Neurology Society develop practice parameters as strategies for patient management based on analysis of evidence. For this parameter the authors reviewed available evidence on the assessment of a child suspected of having cerebral palsy (CP), a nonprogressive disorder of posture or movement due to a lesion of the developing brain.

Methods. Relevant literature was reviewed, abstracted, and classified. Recommendations were based on a four-tiered scheme of evidence classification.

Results. CP is a common problem, occurring in about 2 to 2.5 per 1,000 live births. In order to establish that a brain abnormality exists in children with CP that may, in turn, suggest an etiology and prognosis, neuroimaging is recommended with MRI preferred to CT (Level A). Metabolic and genetic studies should not be routinely obtained in the evaluation of the child with CP (Level B). If the clinical history or findings on neuroimaging do not determine a specific structural abnormality or if there are additional and atypical features in the history or clinical examination, metabolic and genetic testing should be considered (Level C). Detection of a brain malformation in a child with CP warrants consideration of an underlying genetic or metabolic etiology. Because the incidence of cerebral infarction is high in children with hemiplegic CP, diagnostic testing for coagulation disorders should be considered (Level B). However, there is insufficient evidence at present to be precise as to what studies should be ordered. An EEG is not recommended unless there are features suggestive of epilepsy or a specific epileptic syndrome (Level A). Because children with CP may have associated deficits of mental retardation, ophthalmologic and hearing impairments, speech and language disorders, and oral-motor dysfunction, screening for these conditions should be part of the initial assessment (Level A).

Conclusions. Neuroimaging results in children with CP are commonly abnormal and may help determine the etiology. Screening for associated conditions is warranted as part of the initial evaluation. (3/04)

COMMUNITY-ACQUIRED PNEUMONIA

The Management of Community-Acquired Pneumonia (CAP) in Infants and Children Older Than 3 Months of Age
Pediatric Infectious Diseases Society and Infectious Diseases Society of America

ABSTRACT. Evidenced-based guidelines for management of infants and children with community-acquired pneumonia (CAP) were prepared by an expert panel comprising clinicians and investigators representing community pediatrics, public health, and the pediatric specialties of critical care, emergency medicine, hospital medicine, infectious diseases, pulmonology, and surgery. These guidelines are intended for use by primary care and subspecialty providers responsible for the management of otherwise healthy infants and children with CAP in both outpatient and inpatient settings. Site-of-care management, diagnosis, antimicrobial and adjunctive surgical therapy, and prevention are discussed. Areas that warrant future investigations are also highlighted. (10/11)

CONGENITAL ADRENAL HYPERPLASIA

Congenital Adrenal Hyperplasia Due to Steroid 21-hydroxylase Deficiency: An Endocrine Society Clinical Practice Guideline
The Endocrine Society

CONCLUSIONS. We recommend universal newborn screening for severe steroid 21-hydroxylase deficiency followed by confirmatory tests. We recommend that prenatal treatment of CAH continue to be regarded as experimental. The diagnosis rests on clinical and hormonal data; genotyping is reserved for equivocal cases and genetic counseling. Glucocorticoid dosage should be minimized to avoid iatrogenic Cushing's syndrome. Mineralocorticoids and, in infants, supplemental sodium are recommended in classic CAH patients. We recommend against the routine use of experimental therapies to promote growth and delay puberty; we suggest patients avoid adrenalectomy. Surgical guidelines emphasize early single-stage genital repair for severely virilized girls, performed by experienced surgeons. Clinicians should consider patients' quality of life, consulting mental health professionals as appropriate. At the transition to adulthood, we recommend monitoring for potential complications of CAH. Finally, we recommend judicious use of medication during pregnancy and in symptomatic patients with nonclassic CAH. (9/10)

DEPRESSION

Guidelines for Adolescent Depression in Primary Care (GLAD-PC): I. Identification, Assessment, and Initial Management

Rachel A. Zuckerbrot, MD; Amy H. Cheung, MD; Peter S. Jensen, MD; Ruth E. K. Stein, MD; Danielle Laraque, MD; and the GLAD-PC Steering Group

ABSTRACT. **Objectives.** To develop clinical practice guidelines to assist primary care clinicians in the management of adolescent depression. This first part of the guidelines addresses identification, assessment, and initial management of adolescent depression in primary care settings.

Methods. By using a combination of evidence- and consensus-based methodologies, guidelines were developed by an expert steering committee in 5 phases, as informed by (1) current scientific evidence (published and unpublished), (2) a series of focus groups, (3) a formal survey, (4) an expert consensus workshop, and (5) draft revision and iteration among members of the steering committee.

Results. Guidelines were developed for youth aged 10 to 21 years and correspond to initial phases of adolescent depression management in primary care, including identification of at-risk youth, assessment and diagnosis, and initial management. The strength of each recommendation and its evidence base are summarized. The identification, assessment, and initial management section of the guidelines includes recommendations for (1) identification of depression in youth at high risk, (2) systematic assessment procedures using reliable depression scales, patient and caregiver interviews, and Diagnostic and Statistical Manual of Mental Disorders, Fourth Edition criteria, (3) patient and family psychoeducation, (4) establishing relevant links in the community, and (5) the establishment of a safety plan.

Conclusions. This part of the guidelines is intended to assist primary care clinicians in the identification and initial management of depressed adolescents in an era of great clinical need and a shortage of mental health specialists but cannot replace clinical judgment; these guidelines are not meant to be the sole source of guidance for adolescent depression management. Additional research that addresses the identification and initial management of depressed youth in primary care is needed, including empirical testing of these guidelines. (11/07)

Guidelines for Adolescent Depression in Primary Care (GLAD-PC): II. Treatment and Ongoing Management

Amy H. Cheung, MD; Rachel A. Zuckerbrot, MD; Peter S. Jensen, MD; Kareem Ghalib, MD; Danielle Laraque, MD; Ruth E. K. Stein, MD; and the GLAD-PC Steering Group

ABSTRACT. **Objectives.** To develop clinical practice guidelines to assist primary care clinicians in the management of adolescent depression. This second part of the guidelines addresses treatment and ongoing management of adolescent depression in the primary care setting.

Methods. Using a combination of evidence- and consensus-based methodologies, guidelines were developed in 5 phases as informed by (1) current scientific evidence (published and unpublished), (2) a series of focus groups, (3) a formal survey, (4) an expert consensus workshop, and (5) revision and iteration among members of the steering committee.

Results. These guidelines are targeted for youth aged 10 to 21 years and offer recommendations for the management of adolescent depression in primary care, including (1) active monitoring of mildly depressed youth, (2) details for the specific application of evidence-based medication and psychotherapeutic approaches in cases of moderate-to-severe depression, (3) careful monitoring of adverse effects, (4) consultation and coordination of care with mental health specialists, (5) ongoing tracking of outcomes, and (6) specific steps to be taken in instances of partial or no improvement after an initial treatment has begun. The strength of each recommendation and its evidence base are summarized.

Conclusions. These guidelines cannot replace clinical judgment, and they should not be the sole source of guidance for adolescent depression management. Nonetheless, the guidelines may assist primary care clinicians in the management of depressed adolescents in an era of great clinical need and a shortage of mental health specialists. Additional research concerning the management of youth with depression in primary care is needed, including the usability, feasibility, and sustainability of guidelines and determination of the extent to which the guidelines actually improve outcomes of youth with depression. (11/07)

DIALYSIS

Shared Decision-Making in the Appropriate Initiation of and Withdrawal from Dialysis, 2nd Edition
Renal Physicians Association (10/10)

ENDOCARDITIS

Prevention of Infective Endocarditis: Guidelines From the American Heart Association

Walter Wilson, MD, Chair; Kathryn A. Taubert, PhD, FAHA; Michael Gewitz, MD, FAHA; Peter B. Lockhart, DDS; Larry M. Baddour, MD; Matthew Levison, MD; Ann Bolger, MD, FAHA; Christopher H. Cabell, MD, MHS; Masato Takahashi, MD, FAHA; Robert S. Baltimore, MD; Jane W. Newburger, MD, MPH, FAHA; Brian L. Strom, MD; Lloyd Y. Tani, MD; Michael Gerber, MD; Robert O. Bonow, MD, FAHA; Thomas Pallasch, DDS, MS; Stanford T. Shulman, MD, FAHA; Anne H. Rowley, MD; Jane C. Burns, MD; Patricia Ferrieri, MD; Timothy Gardner, MD, FAHA; David Goff, MD, PhD, FAHA; David T. Durack, MD, PhD

ABSTRACT. **Background.** The purpose of this statement is to update the recommendations by the American Heart Association (AHA) for the prevention of infective endocarditis that were last published in 1997.

Methods and Results. A writing group was appointed by the AHA for their expertise in prevention and treatment of infective endocarditis, with liaison members representing the American Dental Association, the Infectious Diseases Society of America, and the American Academy of Pediatrics. The writing group reviewed input from national and international experts on infective endocarditis. The recommendations in this document reflect analyses of relevant literature regarding procedure-related bacteremia and infective endocarditis, in vitro susceptibility data of the most common microorganisms that cause infective endocarditis, results of prophylactic studies in animal models of experimental endocarditis, and retrospective and prospective studies of prevention of infective endocarditis. MEDLINE database searches from 1950 to 2006 were done for English-language papers using the following search terms: endocarditis, infective endocarditis, prophylaxis, prevention, antibiotic, antimicrobial, pathogens, organisms, dental, gastrointestinal, genitourinary, streptococcus, enterococcus, staphylococcus, respiratory, dental surgery, pathogenesis, vaccine, immunization, and bacteremia. The reference lists of the identified papers were also searched. We also searched the AHA online library. The American College of Cardiology/AHA classification of recommendations and levels of evidence for practice guidelines were used. The paper was subsequently reviewed by outside experts not affiliated with the writing group and by the AHA Science Advisory and Coordinating Committee.

Conclusions. The major changes in the updated recommendations include the following: (1) The Committee concluded that only an extremely small number of cases of infective endocarditis might be prevented by antibiotic prophylaxis for dental procedures even if such prophylactic therapy were 100% effective. (2) Infective endocarditis prophylaxis for dental procedures should be recommended only for patients with underlying cardiac conditions associated with the highest risk of adverse outcome from infective endocarditis. (3) For patients with these underlying cardiac conditions, prophylaxis is recommended for all dental procedures that involve manipulation of gingival tissue or the periapical region of teeth or perforation of the oral mucosa. (4) Prophylaxis is not recommended based solely on an increased lifetime risk of acquisition of infective endocarditis. (5) Administration of antibiotics solely to prevent endocarditis is not recommended for patients who undergo a genitourinary or gastrointestinal tract procedure. These changes are intended to define more clearly when infective endocarditis prophylaxis is or is not recommended and to provide more uniform and consistent global recommendations. (*Circulation.* 2007;116:1736–1754.) (5/07)

FLUORIDE
Recommendations for Using Fluoride to Prevent and Control Dental Caries in the United States
Centers for Disease Control and Prevention (8/01)

FOOD ALLERGY
Guidelines for the Diagnosis and Management of Food Allergy in the United States: Report of the NIAID-Sponsored Expert Panel
National Institute of Allergy and Infectious Diseases

ABSTRACT. Food allergy is an important public health problem that affects children and adults and may be increasing in prevalence. Despite the risk of severe allergic reactions and even death, there is no current treatment for food allergy: the disease can only be managed by allergen avoidance or treatment of symptoms. The diagnosis and management of food allergy also may vary from one clinical practice setting to another. Finally, because patients frequently confuse nonallergic food reactions, such as food intolerance, with food allergies, there is an unfounded belief among the public that food allergy prevalence is higher than it truly is. In response to these concerns, the National Institute of Allergy and Infectious Diseases, working with 34 professional organizations, federal agencies, and patient advocacy groups, led the development of clinical guidelines for the diagnosis and management of food allergy. These Guidelines are intended for use by a wide variety of health care professionals, including family practice physicians, clinical specialists, and nurse practitioners. The Guidelines include a consensus definition for food allergy, discuss comorbid conditions often associated with food allergy, and focus on both IgE-mediated and non-IgE-mediated reactions to food. Topics addressed include the epidemiology, natural history, diagnosis, and management of food allergy, as well as the management of severe symptoms and anaphylaxis. These Guidelines provide 43 concise clinical recommendations and additional guidance on points of current controversy in patient management. They also identify gaps in the current scientific knowledge to be addressed through future research. (12/10)

GASTROENTERITIS
Managing Acute Gastroenteritis Among Children: Oral Rehydration, Maintenance, and Nutritional Therapy
Centers for Disease Control and Prevention (11/03)

GASTROESOPHAGEAL REFLUX
Guidelines for Evaluation and Treatment of Gastroesophageal Reflux in Infants and Children
North American Society for Pediatric Gastroenterology, Hepatology, and Nutrition

ABSTRACT. Gastroesophageal reflux (GER), defined as passage of gastric contents into the esophagus, and GER disease (GERD), defined as symptoms or complications of GER, are common pediatric problems encountered by both primary and specialty medical providers. Clinical manifestations of GERD in children include vomiting, poor weight gain, dysphagia, abdominal or substernal pain, esophagitis and respiratory disorders. The GER Guideline Committee of the North American Society for Pediatric Gastroenterology and Nutrition has formulated a clinical practice guideline for the management of pediatric GER. The GER Guideline Committee, consisting of a primary care pediatrician, two clinical epidemiologists (who also practice primary care pediatrics) and five pediatric gastroenterologists, based its recommendations on an integration of a comprehensive and systematic review of the medical literature combined with expert opinion. Consensus was achieved through Nominal Group Technique, a structured quantitative method.

The Committee examined the value of diagnostic tests and treatment modalities commonly used for the management of GERD, and how those interventions can be applied to clinical situations in the infant and older child.

The guideline provides recommendations for management by the primary care provider, including evaluation, initial treatment, follow-up management and indications for consultation by a specialist. The guideline also provides recommendations for management by the pediatric gastroenterologist.

This document represents the official recommendations of the North American Society for Pediatric Gastroenterology and Nutrition on the evaluation and treatment of gastroesophageal reflux in infants and children. The American Academy of Pediatrics has also endorsed these recommendations. The recommendations are summarized in a synopsis within the article. This review and recommendations are a general guideline and are not intended as a substitute for clinical judgment or as a protocol for the management of all patients with this problem. (2001)

GROUP B STREPTOCOCCAL DISEASE
Prevention of Perinatal Group B Streptococcal Disease: Revised Guidelines from CDC, 2010
Centers for Disease Control and Prevention

SUMMARY. Despite substantial progress in prevention of perinatal group B streptococcal (GBS) disease since the 1990s, GBS remains the leading cause of early-onset neonatal sepsis in the United States. In 1996, CDC, in collaboration with relevant professional societies, published guidelines for the prevention of perinatal group B streptococcal disease (CDC. Prevention of perinatal group B streptococcal disease: a public health perspective. *MMWR* 1996;45[No. RR-7]); those guidelines were updated and republished in 2002 (CDC. Prevention of perinatal group B streptococcal disease: revised guidelines from CDC. *MMWR* 2002;51[No. RR-11]). In June 2009, a meeting of clinical and public health representatives was held to reevaluate prevention strategies on the basis of data collected after the issuance of the 2002 guidelines. This report presents CDC's updated guidelines, which have been endorsed by the American College of Obstetricians and Gynecologists, the American Academy of Pediatrics, the American College of Nurse-Midwives, the American Academy of Family Physicians, and the American Society for Microbiology. The recommendations were made on the basis of available evidence when such evidence was sufficient and on expert opinion when available evidence was insufficient. The key changes in the 2010 guidelines include the following:

- expanded recommendations on laboratory methods for the identification of GBS,
- clarification of the colony-count threshold required for reporting GBS detected in the urine of pregnant women,
- updated algorithms for GBS screening and intrapartum chemoprophylaxis for women with preterm labor or preterm premature rupture of membranes,
- a change in the recommended dose of penicillin-G for chemoprophylaxis,
- updated prophylaxis regimens for women with penicillin allergy, and
- a revised algorithm for management of newborns with respect to risk for early-onset GBS disease.

Universal screening at 35–37 weeks' gestation for maternal GBS colonization and use of intrapartum antibiotic prophylaxis has resulted in substantial reductions in the burden of early-onset GBS disease among newborns. Although early-onset GBS disease has become relatively uncommon in recent years, the rates of maternal GBS colonization (and therefore the risk for early-onset GBS disease in the absence of intrapartum antibiotic prophylaxis) remain unchanged since the 1970s. Continued efforts are needed to sustain and improve on the progress achieved in the prevention of GBS disease. There also is a need to monitor for potential adverse consequences of intrapartum antibiotic prophylaxis (e.g., emergence of bacterial antimicrobial resistance or increased incidence or severity of non-GBS neonatal pathogens). In the absence of a licensed GBS vaccine, universal screening and intrapartum antibiotic prophylaxis continue to be the cornerstones of early-onset GBS disease prevention. (11/10)

HELICOBACTER PYLORI INFECTION
Helicobacter pylori Infection in Children: Recommendations for Diagnosis and Treatment
North American Society for Pediatric Gastroenterology, Hepatology, and Nutrition (11/00)

HEMATOPOIETIC STEM CELL TRANSPLANT
Guidelines for Preventing Opportunistic Infections Among Hematopoietic Stem Cell Transplant Recipients
Centers for Disease Control and Prevention, Infectious Diseases Society of America, and the American Society of Blood and Marrow Transplantation (10/00)

HUMAN IMMUNODEFICIENCY VIRUS
Guidelines for the Prevention and Treatment of Opportunistic Infections in HIV-Exposed and HIV-Infected Children
US Department of Health and Human Services

SUMMARY. This report updates the last version of the Guidelines for the Prevention and Treatment of Opportunistic Infections (OIs) in HIV-Exposed and HIV-Infected Children, published in 2009. These guidelines are intended for use by clinicians and other health-care workers providing medical care for HIV-exposed and HIV-infected children in the United States. The guidelines discuss opportunistic pathogens that occur in the United States and ones that might be acquired during international travel, such as malaria. Topic areas covered for each OI include a brief description of the epidemiology, clinical presentation, and diagnosis of the OI in children; prevention of exposure; prevention of first episode of disease; discontinuation of primary prophylaxis after immune reconstitution; treatment of disease; monitoring for adverse effects during treatment, including immune reconstitution inflammatory syndrome (IRIS); management of treatment failure; prevention of disease recurrence; and discontinuation of secondary prophylaxis after immune reconstitution. A separate document providing recommendations for prevention and treatment of OIs among HIV-infected adults and post-pubertal adolescents (*Guidelines for the Prevention and Treatment of Opportunistic*

Infections in HIV-Infected Adults and Adolescents) was prepared by a panel of adult HIV and infectious disease specialists (see http://aidsinfo.nih.gov/guidelines).

These guidelines were developed by a panel of specialists in pediatric HIV infection and infectious diseases (the Panel on Opportunistic Infections in HIV-Exposed and HIV-Infected Children) from the U.S. government and academic institutions. For each OI, one or more pediatric specialists with subject-matter expertise reviewed the literature for new information since the last guidelines were published and then proposed revised recommendations for review by the full Panel. After these reviews and discussions, the guidelines underwent further revision, with review and approval by the Panel, and final endorsement by the National Institutes of Health (NIH), Centers for Disease Control and Prevention (CDC), the HIV Medicine Association (HIVMA) of the Infectious Diseases Society of America (IDSA), the Pediatric Infectious Disease Society (PIDS), and the American Academy of Pediatrics (AAP). So that readers can ascertain how best to apply the recommendations in their practice environments, the recommendations are rated by a letter that indicates the strength of the recommendation, a Roman numeral that indicates the quality of the evidence supporting the recommendation, and where applicable, a * notation that signifies a hybrid of higher-quality adult study evidence and consistent but lower-quality pediatric study evidence.

More detailed methodologic considerations are listed in Appendix 1 (Important Guidelines Considerations), including a description of the make-up and organizational structure of the Panel, definition of financial disclosure and management of conflict of interest, funding sources for the guidelines, methods of collecting and synthesizing evidence and formulating recommendations, public commentary, and plans for updating the guidelines. The names and financial disclosures for each of the Panel members are listed in Appendices 2 and 3, respectively.

An important mode of childhood acquisition of OIs and HIV infection is from infected mothers. HIV-infected women may be more likely to have coinfections with opportunistic pathogens (e.g., hepatitis C) and more likely than women who are not HIV-infected to transmit these infections to their infants. In addition, HIV-infected women or HIV-infected family members coinfected with certain opportunistic pathogens may be more likely to transmit these infections horizontally to their children, resulting in increased likelihood of primary acquisition of such infections in young children. Furthermore, transplacental transfer of antibodies that protect infants against serious infections may be lower in HIV-infected women than in women who are HIV-uninfected. Therefore, infections with opportunistic pathogens may affect not just HIV-infected infants but also HIV-exposed, uninfected infants. These guidelines for treating OIs in children, therefore, consider treatment of infections in all children—HIV-infected and HIV-uninfected—born to HIV-infected women.

In addition, HIV infection increasingly is seen in adolescents with perinatal infection who are now surviving into their teens and in youth with behaviorally acquired HIV infection. Guidelines for postpubertal adolescents can be found in the adult OI guidelines, but drug pharmacokinetics (PK) and response to treatment may differ in younger prepubertal or pubertal adolescents. Therefore, these guidelines also apply to treatment of HIV-infected youth who have not yet completed pubertal development.

Major changes in the guidelines from the previous version in 2009 include:

- Greater emphasis on the importance of antiretroviral therapy (ART) for prevention and treatment of OIs, especially those OIs for which no specific therapy exists;
- Increased information about diagnosis and management of IRIS;
- Information about managing ART in children with OIs, including potential drug-drug interactions;
- Updated immunization recommendations for HIV-exposed and HIV-infected children, including pneumococcal, human papillomavirus, meningococcal, and rotavirus vaccines;
- Addition of sections on influenza, giardiasis, and isosporiasis;
- Elimination of sections on aspergillosis, bartonellosis, and HHV-6 and HHV-7 infections; and
- Updated recommendations on discontinuation of OI prophylaxis after immune reconstitution in children.

The most important recommendations are highlighted in boxed major recommendations preceding each section, and a table of dosing recommendations appears at the end of each section. The guidelines conclude with summary tables that display dosing recommendations for all of the conditions, drug toxicities and drug interactions, and 2 figures describing immunization recommendations for children aged 0 to 6 years and 7 to 18 years.

The terminology for describing use of antiretroviral (ARV) drugs for treatment of HIV infection has been standardized to ensure consistency within the sections of these guidelines and with the *Guidelines for the Use of Antiretroviral Agents in Pediatric HIV Infection*. Combination antiretroviral therapy (cART) indicates use of multiple (generally 3 or more) ARV drugs as part of an HIV treatment regimen that is designed to achieve virologic suppression; highly active antiretroviral therapy (HAART), synonymous with cART, is no longer used and has been replaced by cART; the term ART has been used when referring to use of ARV drugs for HIV treatment more generally, including (mostly historical) use of one- or two-agent ARV regimens that do not meet criteria for cART.

Because treatment of OIs is an evolving science, and availability of new agents or clinical data on existing agents may change therapeutic options and preferences, these recommendations will be periodically updated and will be available at http://AIDSinfo.nih.gov. (11/13)

INFLUENZA

Seasonal Influenza in Adults and Children—Diagnosis, Treatment, Chemoprophylaxis, and Institutional Outbreak Management: Clinical Practice Guidelines of the Infectious Diseases Society of America

Infectious Diseases Society of America

EXECUTIVE SUMMARY. *Background.* Influenza virus infection causes significant morbidity and mortality in the United States each year. The majority of persons infected with influenza virus exhibit self-limited, uncomplicated, acute febrile respiratory symptoms or are asymptomatic. However, severe disease and complications due to infection, including hospitalization and death, may occur in elderly persons, in very young persons, in persons with underlying medical conditions (including pulmonary and cardiac disease, diabetes, and immunosuppression), and in previously healthy persons. Early treatment with antiviral medications may reduce the severity and duration of symptoms, hospitalizations, and complications (otitis media, bronchitis, pneumonia), and may reduce the use of outpatient services and antibiotics, extent and quantity of viral shedding, and possibly mortality in certain populations. Vaccination is the best method for preventing influenza, but antivirals may also be used as primary or secondary means of preventing influenza transmission in certain settings.

The Centers for Disease Control and Prevention's (CDC's) Advisory Committee on Immunization Practices and the American Academy of Pediatrics provide recommendations on the appropriate use of trivalent inactivated and live, attenuated influenza vaccines, as well as information on diagnostics and antiviral use for treatment and chemoprophylaxis. The CDC's influenza Web site (http://www.cdc.gov/flu) also summarizes up-to-date information on current recommendations for influenza diagnostic testing and antiviral use. The Infectious Diseases Society of America's (IDSA's) influenza guideline provides an evidence-based set of recommendations and background on influenza with contributions from many sources, including the CDC, the American Academy of Pediatrics, the American College of Physicians, the American Academy of Family Physicians, the Pediatric Infectious Diseases Society, the Society for Healthcare Epidemiology of America, practicing clinicians, and the IDSA, to guide decision-making on these issues. The current guideline development process included a systematic weighting of the quality of the evidence and the grade of recommendation (table 1). These guidelines apply to seasonal (interpandemic) influenza and not to avian or pandemic disease. Clinical management guidelines for sporadic human infections due to avian A (H5N1) viruses have been published by the World Health Organization. (4/09)

INTRAVASCULAR CATHETER-RELATED INFECTIONS

Guidelines for the Prevention of Intravascular Catheter-Related Infections

Society of Critical Care Medicine, Infectious Diseases Society of America, Society for Healthcare Epidemiology of America, Surgical Infection Society, American College of Chest Physicians, American Thoracic Society, American Society of Critical Care Anesthesiologists, Association for Professionals in Infection Control and Epidemiology, Infusion Nurses Society, Oncology Nursing Society, Society of Cardiovascular and Interventional Radiology, American Academy of Pediatrics, and the Healthcare Infection Control Practices Advisory Committee of the Centers for Disease Control and Prevention

ABSTRACT. These guidelines have been developed for practitioners who insert catheters and for persons responsible for surveillance and control of infections in hospital, outpatient, and home health-care settings. This report was prepared by a working group comprising members from professional organizations representing the disciplines of critical care medicine, infectious diseases, health-care infection control, surgery, anesthesiology, interventional radiology, pulmonary medicine, pediatric medicine, and nursing. The working group was led by the Society of Critical Care Medicine (SCCM), in collaboration with the Infectious Disease Society of America (IDSA), Society for Healthcare Epidemiology of America (SHEA), Surgical Infection Society (SIS), American College of Chest Physicians (ACCP), American Thoracic Society (ATS), American Society of Critical Care Anesthesiologists (ASCCA), Association for Professionals in Infection Control and Epidemiology (APIC), Infusion Nurses Society (INS), Oncology Nursing Society (ONS), Society of Cardiovascular and Interventional Radiology (SCVIR), American Academy of Pediatrics (AAP), and the Healthcare Infection Control Practices Advisory Committee (HICPAC) of the Centers for Disease Control and Prevention (CDC) and is intended to replace the *Guideline for Prevention of Intravascular Device-Related Infections* published in 1996. These guidelines are intended to provide evidence-based recommendations for preventing catheter-related infections. Major areas of emphasis include 1) educating and training health-care providers who insert and maintain catheters; 2) using maximal sterile barrier precautions during central venous catheter insertion; 3) using a 2% chlorhexidine preparation for skin antisepsis; 4) avoiding routine replacement of central venous catheters as a strategy to prevent infection; and 5) using antiseptic/antibiotic impregnated short-term central venous catheters if the rate of infection is high despite adherence to other strategies (ie, education and training, maximal sterile barrier precautions, and 2% chlorhexidine for skin antisepsis). These guidelines also identify performance indicators that can be used locally by health-care institutions or organizations to monitor their success in implementing these evidence-based recommendations. (11/02)

JAUNDICE

Guideline for the Evaluation of Cholestatic Jaundice in Infants

North American Society for Pediatric Gastroenterology, Hepatology, and Nutrition

ABSTRACT. For the primary care provider, cholestatic jaundice in infancy, defined as jaundice caused by an elevated conjugated bilirubin, is an uncommon but potentially serious problem that indicates hepatobiliary dysfunction. Early detection of cholestatic jaundice by the primary care physician and timely, accurate diagnosis by the pediatric gastroenterologist are important for successful treatment and a favorable prognosis. The Cholestasis Guideline Committee of the North American Society for Pediatric Gastroenterology, Hepatology and Nutrition has formulated a clinical practice guideline for the diagnostic evaluation of cholestatic jaundice in the infant. The Cholestasis Guideline Committee, consisting of a primary care pediatrician, a clinical epidemiologist (who also practices primary care pediatrics), and five pediatric gastroenterologists, based its recommendations on a comprehensive and systematic review of the medical literature integrated with expert opinion. Consensus was achieved through the Nominal Group Technique, a structured quantitative method.

The Committee examined the value of diagnostic tests commonly used for the evaluation of cholestatic jaundice and how those interventions can be applied to clinical situations in the infant. The guideline provides recommendations for management by the primary care provider, indications for consultation by a pediatric gastroenterologist, and recommendations for management by the pediatric gastroenterologist.

The Cholestasis Guideline Committee recommends that any infant noted to be jaundiced at 2 weeks of age be evaluated for cholestasis with measurement of total and direct serum bilirubin. However, breast-fed infants who can be reliably monitored and who have an otherwise normal history (no dark urine or light stools) and physical examination may be asked to return at 3 weeks of age and, if jaundice persists, have measurement of total and direct serum bilirubin at that time.

This document represents the official recommendations of the North American Society for Pediatric Gastroenterology, Hepatology and Nutrition on the evaluation of cholestatic jaundice in infants. The American Academy of Pediatrics has also endorsed these recommendations. These recommendations are a general guideline and are not intended as a substitute for clinical judgment or as a protocol for the care of all patients with this problem. (8/04)

METHICILLIN-RESISTANT *STAPHYLOCOCCUS AUREUS*

Clinical Practice Guidelines by the Infectious Diseases Society of America for the Treatment of Methicillin-Resistant *Staphylococcus aureus* Infections in Adults and Children

Infectious Diseases Society of America

ABSTRACT. Evidence-based guidelines for the management of patients with methicillin-resistant Staphylococcus aureus (MRSA) infections were prepared by an Expert Panel of the Infectious Diseases Society of America (IDSA). The guidelines are intended for use by health care providers who care for adult and pediatric patients with MRSA infections. The guidelines discuss the management of a variety of clinical syndromes associated with MRSA disease, including skin and soft tissue infections (SSTI), bacteremia and endocarditis, pneumonia, bone and joint infections, and central nervous system (CNS) infections. Recommendations are provided regarding vancomycin dosing and monitoring, management of infections due to MRSA strains with reduced susceptibility to vancomycin, and vancomycin treatment failures. (2/11)

MIGRAINE HEADACHE

Pharmacological Treatment of Migraine Headache in Children and Adolescents

Quality Standards Subcommittee of the American Academy of Neurology and the Practice Committee of the Child Neurology Society (12/04)

RADIOLOGY

Neuroimaging of the Neonate

Quality Standards Subcommittee of the American Academy of Neurology and the Practice Committee of the Child Neurology Society

ABSTRACT. *Objective.* The authors reviewed available evidence on neonatal neuroimaging strategies for evaluating both very low birth weight preterm infants and encephalopathic term neonates.

Imaging for the preterm neonate. Routine screening cranial ultrasonography (US) should be performed on all infants of <30 weeks' gestation once between 7 and 14 days of age and should be optimally repeated between 36 and 40 weeks' postmenstrual age. This strategy detects lesions such as intraventricular hemorrhage, which influences clinical care, and those such as periventricular leukomalacia and low-pressure ventriculomegaly, which provide information about long-term neurodevelopmental outcome. There is insufficient evidence for routine MRI of all very low birth weight preterm infants with abnormal results of cranial US.

Imaging for the term infant. Noncontrast CT should be performed to detect hemorrhagic lesions in the encephalopathic term infant with a history of birth trauma, low hematocrit, or coagulopathy. If CT findings are inconclusive, MRI should be performed between days 2 and 8 to assess the location and extent of injury. The pattern of injury identified with conventional MRI may provide diagnostic and prognostic information for term infants with evidence of encephalopathy. In particular, basal ganglia and thalamic lesions detected by conventional MRI are associated with poor neurodevelopmental outcome. Diffusion-weighted imaging may allow earlier detection of these cerebral injuries.

Recommendations. US plays an established role in the management of preterm neonates of <30 weeks' gestation. US also provides valuable prognostic information when the infant reaches 40 weeks' postmenstrual age. For encephalopathic term infants, early CT should be used to exclude hemorrhage; MRI should be performed later in the first postnatal week to establish the pattern of injury and predict neurologic outcome. (6/02)

SEDATION AND ANALGESIA
Clinical Policy: Evidence-Based Approach to Pharmacologic Agents Used in Pediatric Sedation and Analgesia in the Emergency Department
American College of Emergency Physicians (10/04)

SEIZURE
Evaluating a First Nonfebrile Seizure in Children
Quality Standards Subcommittee of the American Academy of Neurology, the Child Neurology Society, and the American Epilepsy Society

ABSTRACT. **Objective.** The Quality Standards Subcommittee of the American Academy of Neurology develops practice parameters as strategies for patient management based on analysis of evidence. For this practice parameter, the authors reviewed available evidence on evaluation of the first nonfebrile seizure in children in order to make practice recommendations based on this available evidence. Methods: Multiple searches revealed relevant literature and each article was reviewed, abstracted, and classified. Recommendations were based on a three-tiered scheme of classification of the evidence. Results: Routine EEG as part of the diagnostic evaluation was recommended; other studies such as laboratory evaluations and neuroimaging studies were recommended as based on specific clinical circumstances. Conclusions: Further studies are needed using large, well-characterized samples and standardized data collection instruments. Collection of data regarding appropriate timing of evaluations would be important. (8/00)

Treatment of the Child With a First Unprovoked Seizure
Quality Standards Subcommittee of the American Academy of Neurology and the Practice Committee of the Child Neurology Society

ABSTRACT. The Quality Standards Subcommittee of the American Academy of Neurology and the Practice Committee of the Child Neurology Society develop practice parameters as strategies for patient management based on analysis of evidence regarding risks and benefits. This parameter reviews published literature relevant to the decision to begin treatment after a child or adolescent experiences a first unprovoked seizure and presents evidence-based practice recommendations. Reasons why treatment may be considered are discussed. Evidence is reviewed concerning risk of recurrence as well as effect of treatment on prevention of recurrence and development of chronic epilepsy. Studies of side effects of anticonvulsants commonly used to treat seizures in children are also reviewed. Relevant articles are classified according to the Quality Standards Subcommittee classification scheme. Treatment after a first unprovoked seizure appears to decrease the risk of a second seizure, but there are few data from studies involving only children. There appears to be no benefit of treatment with regard to the prognosis for long-term seizure remission. Antiepileptic drugs (AED) carry risks of side effects that are particularly important in children. The decision as to whether or not to treat children and adolescents who have experienced a first unprovoked seizure must be based on a risk–benefit assessment that weighs the risk of having another seizure against the risk of chronic AED therapy. The decision should be individualized and take into account both medical issues and patient and family preference. (1/03)

STATUS EPILEPTICUS
Diagnostic Assessment of the Child With Status Epilepticus (An Evidence-based Review)
Quality Standards Subcommittee of the American Academy of Neurology and the Practice Committee of the Child Neurology Society

ABSTRACT. **Objective.** To review evidence on the assessment of the child with status epilepticus (SE).

Methods. Relevant literature were reviewed, abstracted, and classified. When data were missing, a minimum diagnostic yield was calculated. Recommendations were based on a four-tiered scheme of evidence classification.

Results. Laboratory studies (Na^{++} or other electrolytes, Ca^{++}, glucose) were abnormal in approximately 6% and are generally ordered as routine practice. When blood or spinal fluid cultures were done on these children, blood cultures were abnormal in at least 2.5% and a CNS infection was found in at least 12.8%. When antiepileptic drug (AED) levels were ordered in known epileptic children already taking AEDs, the levels were low in 32%. A total of 3.6% of children had evidence of ingestion. When studies for inborn errors of metabolism were done, an abnormality was found in 4.2%. Epileptiform abnormalities occurred in 43% of EEGs of children with SE and helped determine the nature and location of precipitating electroconvulsive events (8% generalized, 16% focal, and 19% both). Abnormalities on neuroimaging studies that may explain the etiology of SE were found in at least 8% of children.

Recommendations. Although common clinical practice is that blood cultures and lumbar puncture are obtained if there is a clinical suspicion of a systemic or CNS infection, there are insufficient data to support or refute recommendations as to whether blood cultures or lumbar puncture should be done on a routine basis in children in whom there is no clinical suspicion of a systemic or CNS infection (Level U). AED levels should be considered when a child with treated epilepsy develops SE (Level B). Toxicology studies and metabolic studies for inborn errors of metabolism may be considered in children with SE when there are clinical indicators for concern or when the initial evaluation reveals no etiology (Level C). An EEG may be considered in a child with SE as it may be helpful in determining whether there are focal or generalized epileptiform abnormalities that may guide further testing for the etiology of SE, when there is a suspicion of pseudostatus epilepticus (nonepileptic SE), or nonconvulsive SE, and may guide treatment (Level C). Neuroimaging may be considered after the child with SE has been stabilized if there are clinical indications or if the etiology is unknown (Level C). There is insufficient evidence to support or refute routine neuroimaging in a child presenting with SE (Level U). (11/06)

TOBACCO USE

Treating Tobacco Use and Dependence: 2008 Update
US Department of Health and Human Services

ABSTRACT. *Treating Tobacco Use and Dependence: 2008 Update*, a Public Health Service-sponsored Clinical Practice Guideline, is a product of the Tobacco Use and Dependence Guideline Panel ("the Panel"), consortium representatives, consultants, and staff. These 37 individuals were charged with the responsibility of identifying effective, experimentally validated tobacco dependence treatments and practices. The updated Guideline was sponsored by a consortium of eight Federal Government and nonprofit organizations: the Agency for Healthcare Research and Quality (AHRQ); Centers for Disease Control and Prevention (CDC); National Cancer Institute (NCI); National Heart, Lung, and Blood Institute (NHLBI); National Institute on Drug Abuse (NIDA); American Legacy Foundation; Robert Wood Johnson Foundation (RWJF); and University of Wisconsin School of Medicine and Public Health's Center for Tobacco Research and Intervention (UW-CTRI). This Guideline is an updated version of the 2000 *Treating Tobacco Use and Dependence: Clinical Practice Guideline* that was sponsored by the U.S. Public Health Service, U. S. Department of Health and Human Services.

An impetus for this Guideline update was the expanding literature on tobacco dependence and its treatment. The original 1996 Guideline was based on some 3,000 articles on tobacco treatment published between 1975 and 1994. The 2000 Guideline entailed the collection and screening of an additional 3,000 articles published between 1995 and 1999. The 2008 Guideline update screened an additional 2,700 articles; thus, the present Guideline update reflects the distillation of a literature base of more than 8,700 research articles. Of course, this body of research was further reviewed to identify a much smaller group of articles that served as the basis for focused Guideline data analyses and review.

This Guideline contains strategies and recommendations designed to assist clinicians; tobacco dependence treatment specialists; and health care administrators, insurers, and purchasers in delivering and supporting effective treatments for tobacco use and dependence. The recommendations were made as a result of a systematic review and meta-analysis of 11 specific topics identified by the Panel (proactive quitlines; combining counseling and medication relative to either counseling or medication alone; varenicline; various medication combinations; long-term medications; cessation interventions for individuals with low socioeconomic status/limited formal education; cessation interventions for adolescent smokers; cessation interventions for pregnant smokers; cessation interventions for individuals with psychiatric disorders, including substance use disorders; providing cessation interventions as a health benefit; and systems interventions, including provider training and the combination of training and systems interventions). The strength of evidence that served as the basis for each recommendation is indicated clearly in the Guideline update. A draft of the Guideline update was peer reviewed prior to publication,

and the input of 81 external reviewers was considered by the Panel prior to preparing the final document. In addition, the public had an opportunity to comment through a *Federal Register* review process. The key recommendations of the updated Guideline, *Treating Tobacco Use and Dependence: 2008 Update*, based on the literature review and expert Panel opinion, are as follows:

Ten Key Guideline Recommendations

The overarching goal of these recommendations is that clinicians strongly recommend the use of effective tobacco dependence counseling and medication treatments to their patients who use tobacco, and that health systems, insurers, and purchasers assist clinicians in making such effective treatments available.

1. Tobacco dependence is a chronic disease that often requires repeated intervention and multiple attempts to quit. Effective treatments exist, however, that can significantly increase rates of long-term abstinence.

2. It is essential that clinicians and health care delivery systems consistently identify and document tobacco use status and treat every tobacco user seen in a health care setting.

3. Tobacco dependence treatments are effective across a broad range of populations. Clinicians should encourage every patient willing to make a quit attempt to use the counseling treatments and medications recommended in this Guideline.

4. Brief tobacco dependence treatment is effective. Clinicians should offer every patient who uses tobacco at least the brief treatments shown to be effective in this Guideline.

5. Individual, group, and telephone counseling are effective, and their effectiveness increases with treatment intensity. Two components of counseling are especially effective, and clinicians should use these when counseling patients making a quit attempt:

   • Practical counseling (problemsolving/skills training)

   • Social support delivered as part of treatment

6. Numerous effective medications are available for tobacco dependence, and clinicians should encourage their use by all patients attempting to quit smoking—except when medically contraindicated or with specific populations for which there is insufficient evidence of effectiveness (i.e., pregnant women, smokeless tobacco users, light smokers, and adolescents).

   • Seven first-line medications (5 nicotine and 2 non-nicotine) reliably increase long-term smoking abstinence rates:

     – Bupropion SR

     – Nicotine gum

     – Nicotine inhaler

     – Nicotine lozenge

     – Nicotine nasal spray

     – Nicotine patch

     – Varenicline

- Clinicians also should consider the use of certain combinations of medications identified as effective in this Guideline.

7. Counseling and medication are effective when used by themselves for treating tobacco dependence. The combination of counseling and medication, however, is more effective than either alone. Thus, clinicians should encourage all individuals making a quit attempt to use both counseling and medication.

8. Telephone quitline counseling is effective with diverse populations and has broad reach. Therefore, both clinicians and health care delivery systems should ensure patient access to quitlines and promote quitline use.

9. If a tobacco user currently is unwilling to make a quit attempt, clinicians should use the motivational treatments shown in this Guideline to be effective in increasing future quit attempts.

10. Tobacco dependence treatments are both clinically effective and highly cost-effective relative to interventions for other clinical disorders. Providing coverage for these treatments increases quit rates. Insurers and purchasers should ensure that all insurance plans include the counseling and medication identified as effective in this Guideline as covered benefits.

The updated Guideline is divided into seven chapters that provide an overview, including methods (Chapter 1); information on the assessment of tobacco use (Chapter 2); clinical interventions, both for patients willing and unwilling to make a quit attempt at this time (Chapter 3); intensive interventions (Chapter 4); systems interventions for health care administrators, insurers, and purchasers (Chapter 5); the scientific evidence supporting the Guideline recommendations (Chapter 6); and information relevant to specific populations and other topics (Chapter 7).

A comparison of the findings of the updated Guideline with the 2000 Guideline reveals the considerable progress made in tobacco research over the brief period separating these two publications. Tobacco dependence increasingly is recognized as a chronic disease, one that typically requires ongoing assessment and repeated intervention. In addition, the updated Guideline offers the clinician many more effective treatment strategies than were identified in the original Guideline. There now are seven different first-line effective agents in the smoking cessation pharmacopoeia, allowing the clinician and patient many different medication options. In addition, recent evidence provides even stronger support for counseling (both when used alone and with other treatments) as an effective tobacco cessation strategy; counseling adds to the effectiveness of tobacco cessation medications, quitline counseling is an effective intervention with a broad reach, and counseling increases tobacco cessation among adolescent smokers.

Finally, there is increasing evidence that the success of any tobacco dependence treatment strategy cannot be divorced from the health care system in which it is embedded. The updated Guideline contains new evidence that health care policies significantly affect the likelihood that smokers will receive effective tobacco dependence treatment and successfully stop tobacco use. For instance, making tobacco dependence treatment a covered benefit of insurance plans increases the likelihood that a tobacco user will receive treatment and quit successfully. Data strongly indicate that effective tobacco interventions require coordinated interventions. Just as the clinician must intervene with his or her patient, so must the health care administrator, insurer, and purchaser foster and support tobacco intervention as an integral element of health care delivery. Health care administrators and insurers should ensure that clinicians have the training and support to deliver consistent, effective intervention to tobacco users.

One important conclusion of this Guideline update is that the most effective way to move clinicians to intervene is to provide them with information regarding multiple effective treatment options and to ensure that they have ample institutional support to use these options. Joint actions by clinicians, administrators, insurers, and purchasers can encourage a culture of health care in which failure to intervene with a tobacco user is inconsistent with standards of care. (5/08)

VESICOURETERAL REFLUX
Report on the Management of Primary Vesicoureteral Reflux in Children
American Urological Association (5/97)

Affirmation of Value
Clinical Practice Guidelines

. . . .

These guidelines are not endorsed as policy of the American Academy of Pediatrics (AAP). Documents that lack a clear description of the process for identifying, assessing, and incorporating research evidence are not eligible for AAP endorsement as practice guidelines. However, such documents may be of educational value to members of the AAP.

ASTHMA
Environmental Management of Pediatric Asthma:
Guidelines for Health Care Providers
National Environmental Education Foundation

INTRODUCTION (EXCERPT). These guidelines are the product of a new Pediatric Asthma Initiative aimed at integrating environmental management of asthma into pediatric health care. This document outlines competencies in environmental health relevant to pediatric asthma that should be mastered by primary health care providers, and outlines the environmental interventions that should be communicated to patients.

These environmental management guidelines were developed for pediatricians, family physicians, internists, pediatric nurse practitioners, pediatric nurses, and physician assistants. In addition, these guidelines should be integrated into respiratory therapists' and licensed case/care (LICSW) management professionals' education and training.

The guidelines contain three components:

- Competencies: An outline of the knowledge and skills that health care providers and health professional students should master and demonstrate in order to incorporate management of environmental asthma triggers into pediatric practice.

- Environmental History Form: A quick, easy, user-friendly document that can be utilized as an intake tool by the health care provider to help determine pediatric patients' environmental asthma triggers.

- Environmental Intervention Guidelines: Follow-up questions and intervention solutions to environmental asthma triggers. (8/05)

PALLIATIVE CARE AND HOSPICE
Standards of Practice for Pediatric Palliative Care and Hospice
National Hospice and Palliative Care Organization (2/09)

SLEEP APNEA
Practice Guidelines for the Perioperative Management of Patients with Obstructive Sleep Apnea
American Society of Anesthesiologists (5/06)

TURNER SYNDROME
Care of Girls and Women With Turner Syndrome:
A Guideline of the Turner Syndrome Study Group
Turner Syndrome Consensus Study Group

ABSTRACT. *Objectives.* The objective of this work is to provide updated guidelines for the evaluation and treatment of girls and women with Turner syndrome (TS).

Participants. The Turner Syndrome Consensus Study Group is a multidisciplinary panel of experts with relevant clinical and research experience with TS that met in Bethesda, Maryland, April 2006. The meeting was supported by the National Institute of Child Health and unrestricted educational grants from pharmaceutical companies.

Evidence. The study group used peer-reviewed published information to form its principal recommendations. Expert opinion was used where good evidence was lacking.

Consensus. The study group met for 3 d to discuss key issues. Breakout groups focused on genetic, cardiological, auxological, psychological, gynecological, and general medical concerns and drafted recommendations for presentation to the whole group. Draft reports were available for additional comment on the meeting web site. Synthesis of the section reports and final revisions were reviewed by e-mail and approved by whole-group consensus.

Conclusions. We suggest that parents receiving a prenatal diagnosis of TS be advised of the broad phenotypic spectrum and the good quality of life observed in TS in recent years. We recommend that magnetic resonance angiography be used in addition to echocardiography to evaluate the cardiovascular system and suggest that patients with defined cardiovascular defects be cautioned in regard to pregnancy and certain types of exercise. We recommend that puberty should not be delayed to promote statural growth. We suggest a comprehensive educational evaluation in early childhood to identify potential attention-deficit or nonverbal learning disorders. We suggest that caregivers address the prospect of premature ovarian failure in an open and sensitive manner and emphasize the critical importance of estrogen treatment for feminization and for bone health during the adult years. All individuals with TS require continued monitoring of hearing and thyroid function throughout the lifespan. We suggest that adults with TS be monitored for aortic enlargement, hypertension, diabetes, and dyslipidemia. (1/07)

2013 Policies

From the American Academy of Pediatrics

• •

- *Policy Statements*
  ORGANIZATIONAL PRINCIPLES TO GUIDE AND DEFINE THE CHILD HEALTH CARE SYSTEM
  AND TO IMPROVE THE HEALTH OF ALL CHILDREN

- *Clinical Reports*
  GUIDANCE FOR THE CLINICIAN IN RENDERING PEDIATRIC CARE

- *Technical Reports*
  BACKGROUND INFORMATION TO SUPPORT AMERICAN ACADEMY OF PEDIATRICS POLICY

Includes policy statements, clinical reports, and technical reports published between January 1, 2013, and January 1, 2014.

INTRODUCTION

This section of the *Pediatric Clinical Practice Guidelines & Policies: A Compendium of Evidence-based Research for Pediatric Practice* manual is composed of policy statements, clinical reports, and technical reports issued by the American Academy of Pediatrics (AAP) and is designed as a quick reference tool for AAP members, staff, and other interested parties. Section 4 includes the full text of all AAP policies published in 2013. Section 5 is a compilation of all active AAP statements (through January 1, 2014) arranged alphabetically, with abstracts where applicable. A committee index (Appendix 1) and subject index are also available. The companion CD-ROM contains the full text of all current policy statements, clinical reports, and technical reports (through January 1, 2014). These materials should help answer questions that arise about the AAP position on child health care issues. **However, it should be remembered that AAP policy statements, clinical reports, and technical reports do not indicate an exclusive course of treatment or serve as a standard of medical care. Variations, taking into account individual circumstances, may be appropriate.**

The policy statements have been written by AAP committees, councils, task forces, or sections and approved by the AAP Board of Directors. Most of these statements have appeared previously in *Pediatrics*, *AAP News*, or *News & Comments* (the forerunner of *AAP News*).

This section does not contain all AAP policies. It does not include

- Press releases.
- Motions and resolutions that were approved by the Board of Directors. These can be found in the Board of Directors' minutes.
- Policies in manuals, pamphlets, booklets, or other AAP publications. These items can be ordered through the AAP. To order, visit our online Bookstore at www.aap.org/bookstore or call toll-free 888/227-1770.
- Testimony before Congress or government agencies.

All policy statements, clinical reports, and technical reports from the American Academy of Pediatrics automatically expire 5 years after publication unless reaffirmed, revised, or retired at or before that time. Please check the American Academy of Pediatrics Web site at www.aap.org for up-to-date reaffirmations, revisions, and retirements.

Calcium and Vitamin D Requirements of Enterally Fed Preterm Infants

- *Clinical Report*

CLINICAL REPORT

Calcium and Vitamin D Requirements of Enterally Fed Preterm Infants

abstract

Bone health is a critical concern in managing preterm infants. Key nutrients of importance are calcium, vitamin D, and phosphorus. Although human milk is critical for the health of preterm infants, it is low in these nutrients relative to the needs of the infants during growth. Strategies should be in place to fortify human milk for preterm infants with birth weight <1800 to 2000 g and to ensure adequate mineral intake during hospitalization and after hospital discharge. Biochemical monitoring of very low birth weight infants should be performed during their hospitalization. Vitamin D should be provided at 200 to 400 IU/day both during hospitalization and after discharge from the hospital. Infants with radiologic evidence of rickets should have efforts made to maximize calcium and phosphorus intake by using available commercial products and, if needed, direct supplementation with these minerals. *Pediatrics* 2013;131:e1676–e1683

Steven A. Abrams, MD and the COMMITTEE ON NUTRITION

KEY WORDS
preterm infants, human milk, vitamin D, calcium, phosphorous, nutrient intake

ABBREVIATIONS
25-OH-D—25-hydroxyvitamin D
APA—alkaline phosphatase activity
IOM—Institute of Medicine
VLBW—very low birth weight

www.pediatrics.org/cgi/doi/10.1542/peds.2013-0420

doi:10.1542/peds.2013-0420

All clinical reports from the American Academy of Pediatrics automatically expire 5 years after publication unless reaffirmed, revised, or retired at or before that time.

PEDIATRICS (ISSN Numbers: Print, 0031-4005; Online, 1098-4275).

In 2011, the Institute of Medicine (IOM) released dietary guidelines for calcium and vitamin D intakes for all age groups.[1] However, no intake recommendations were made specifically for preterm infants, because they were considered a special population and did not fit within the guidelines for dietary reference intakes developed by the IOM. Preterm infants have unique bone mineral requirements that may not be assumed to be similar to those of full-term newborn infants. Previous statements in the United States have limited their recommendations to full-term infants.[2,3] However, The European Society for Pediatric Gastroenterology, Hepatology, and Nutrition has recently described enteral nutrition recommendations for preterm infants.[4,5]

Data on in utero bone mineralization rates are limited. Cadaver studies, beginning with the classic work of Widdowson et al,[6] generally support an in utero accretion of calcium during the third trimester of 100 to 130 mg/kg per day, peaking between 32 and 36 weeks' gestation. Phosphorus accretion is approximately half the accretion of calcium throughout gestation. Remarkably, more recent reevaluation of these data by using modern body composition techniques[7] provided values similar to those developed by Widdowson et al.[6]

In full-term infants, there is a strong correlation between maternal and infant cord blood 25-hydroxyvitamin D (25-OH-D) concentrations, although the cord blood concentration is less than the maternal concentration.[8] A substantial proportion of pregnant women, especially

African American and Hispanic women in the United States and Europe, have 25-OH-D concentrations <20 ng/mL (50 nmol/L),[9] a value set for the basis of the Recommended Dietary Allowance.[1] However, in utero, skeletal mineralization is primarily independent of maternal vitamin D status, making the clinical significance of 25-OH-D concentrations during pregnancy unclear.[10,11]

EFFECTS OF PRETERM BIRTH ON MINERAL METABOLISM

Population-based studies of rickets among preterm infants are lacking; therefore, the frequency is not known or reliably estimated. Approximately 10% to 20% of hospitalized infants with birth weight <1000 g have radiographically defined rickets (metaphyseal changes) despite current nutritional practices.[12] This frequency is much lower than the 50% incidence in this population described before fortification of human milk and the use of preterm high mineral containing formulas were routine.[13] One challenge in identifying the prevalence of rickets is the confusion related to terminology. Rickets is defined by radiographic findings, not by any biochemical findings. Standard radiographic definitions of rickets are used. Poorly defined terms, such as osteopenia or biochemical rickets, are often used in the literature interchangeably with radiographically defined rickets. Rickets is not widely reported in preterm infants with birth weight >1500 g unless there are health issues severely limiting enteral nutrition.

Limited long-term studies of bone mineralization exist in former preterm infants. In general, these studies do not demonstrate significant long-term negative effects on bone health in preterm infants who demonstrate catch-up growth occurring during the

first 2 years after birth.[14] A single study demonstrated a small decrease in young adolescent height when the alkaline phosphatase concentration exceeded 1200 IU/L.[15] That study was limited because of the use of formulas containing relatively low amounts of energy and protein. The preterm infants had reduced adult height and low lumbar spine bone mineral density compared with population reference data, and the deficits were greatest in those with birth weight <1200 g and those born small for gestational age.[16]

One study indicated a significant decrease in height during the prepubertal years of former very low birth weight (VLBW) infants exposed to dexamethasone for the treatment of bronchopulmonary dysplasia.[17] In addition, Dalziel et al[18] demonstrated that prenatal steroid use did not affect peak bone mass. It appeared that slower fetal growth, rather than preterm birth, predicted lower peak bone mass. The lower peak bone mass in those born small for gestational age was appropriate for their adult height.

IN-HOSPITAL ASSESSMENT AND MANAGEMENT

A summary of high-risk factors for the development of rickets is shown in Table 1. It is common medical practice to assess VLBW infants biochemically for evidence of abnormalities of bone-related parameters, especially the serum alkaline phosphatase activity (APA) and serum phosphorus concentration, and subsequently to evaluate them

radiographically if these evaluations suggest a high risk of developing rickets. No absolute values for a low serum phosphorus concentration exist, with values below ~4 mg/dL often, but not always, being considered associated with low phosphorus status. On the other hand, there is little, if any, evidence supporting measuring bone mineral-related laboratory values in infants with birth weight >1500 g unless infants are unable to achieve full feeds or have other conditions, such as severe cholestasis or renal disease, placing them at risk for bone loss.

Typically, a very high serum APA (>1000 IU/L) is suggestive, but not proof, of rickets. In 1 study, values >1000 IU/L were associated with an incidence of radiologic rickets of ~50% to 60%,[12] although some cases were also seen with serum APA in the range of 800 to 1000 IU/L. Elevations of serum APA and clinical rickets are uncommon in the first 4 weeks after birth at any gestational age. Therefore, screening the serum APA and serum phosphorus at 4 to 6 weeks after birth in VLBW infants followed by biweekly monitoring is appropriate. Typically, the APA will peak at 400 to 800 IU/L and then decrease in VLBW infants who do not develop rickets. In this circumstance, clinical experience indicates that if the infant has APA values in this range and has achieved full feeds of human milk with a mineral-containing fortifier or formula designed for preterm infants, there is minimal, if any, risk of developing rickets, and measurement of APA can usually be stopped.

TABLE 1 High-Risk Criteria for Rickets in Preterm Infants

Born at <27 weeks' gestation
Birth weight <1000 g
Long-term parenteral nutrition (eg, >4 to 5 weeks)
Severe bronchopulmonary dysplasia with use of loop diuretics (eg, furosemide) and fluid restriction
Long-term steroid use
History of necrotizing enterocolitis
Failure to tolerate formulas or human milk fortifiers with high mineral content

Other markers of bone status include serum osteocalcin concentration and bone-specific APA; the latter has been considered of value in cases of cholestasis to help identify the bone-related fraction from total APA. At present, there are no data demonstrating clinical utility of measuring serum osteocalcin concentration and bone-specific APA in neonates, and normal values do not exist for preterm infants. Backstrom et al[19] found no additional information gained from measurement of bone-specific APA compared with total APA in preterm infants. It is, therefore, unlikely that these laboratory values, which are poorly standardized in neonates and expensive to obtain, will be a substantial aspect of clinical decision-making in an individual infant.

The ultimate diagnosis of rickets requires a radiographic evaluation, usually of either the wrist or the knee. Chest radiographs revealing abnormalities of the ribs may be suggestive of rickets, but a confirmatory long-bone film of the wrist or knee should be obtained to confirm the diagnosis. The radiologist should categorize the infant as likely having or not having rickets. Nonspecific terms, such as "osteopenia" or "washed out bones," have little clinical meaning. Rickets in preterm infants appears radiographically similar to rickets in older infants and should be characterized as such. The use of either bone ultrasonography or, before discharge, dual energy radiographic absorptiometry to evaluate bone status may be considered. However, the lack of data related to normal values in former preterm infants indicate that these are performed primarily for research purposes. Current data do not support routine use of any of these techniques for preterm infants, including those with abnormal radiographic findings.

CALCIUM AND PHOSPHORUS INTAKE AND ABSORPTION

Rickets in preterm infants is almost always attributable to decreased total absorbed calcium and phosphorus. Decreases in absorption can result from either low intake or low absorption efficiency.[20] Several studies have revealed that, in healthy preterm infants, calcium absorption averages ~50% to 60% of intake,[21–24] which is similar to that of breastfed full-term infants.[1] In contrast, phosphorus absorption is typically 80% to 90% of dietary intake.[23]

Unfortified human milk, parenteral nutrition, and infant formulas designed for full-term infants, including amino acid-based and soy-based formulas, do not contain enough calcium and phosphorus to fully meet the needs for bone mineralization in preterm infants. Even at very high rates of absorption (eg, 80% or more), the calcium and phosphorus intakes from unfortified human milk or formulas not intended for preterm infants would be a limiting factor in bone growth.[20] Table 2 provides sample numbers for the intake, absorption, and retention of calcium in a VLBW infant fed fortified human milk or a formula for preterm infants typically used in the United States compared with unfortified human milk.

Although most attention is focused on calcium intake, the very high urinary calcium concentrations found in preterm infants fed unfortified human milk suggests that phosphorus deficiency is at least as important, if not more important, than calcium deficiency in the etiology of this disease.[4,25,26] Some cases of hypercalcemia have been reported in preterm infants fed unfortified human milk as a result of the very low phosphorus content and resultant relative excess of calcium.[27]

VITAMIN D IN PRETERM INFANTS

Vitamin D enhances the absorption of calcium, and in general, calcium absorption efficiency is greater in people whose calcium intake is low and in whom vitamin D-dependent absorption increases. However, in preterm infants, the calcium absorption fraction appears to be relatively constant across a wide range of intakes. It has been suggested[21] that most calcium absorption may not be vitamin D dependent in preterm infants in the first month after birth but rather occurs primarily via a passive, paracellular absorption. This hypothesis is unproven, however, and the exact timing and proportion of vitamin D-dependent absorption of calcium and phosphorus in preterm infants is unknown. Some older data suggest an effect of high-dose vitamin D on calcium absorption, but these data have not been verified by using isotopic techniques nor performed on groups of infants using currently available high mineral-containing diets.[5]

TABLE 2 Approximate Calcium Balance in a Typical Infant Receiving 120 kcal/kg Per Day Intake

	Calcium Concentration (mg/dL)	Intake (mg/kg per day)	Absorption %	Total Absorption (mg/kg per day)	Approximate Retention (mg/kg per day)
Human milk[a]	25	38	60	25	15–20
Preterm formula/fortified human milk	145	220	50–60	120–130	100–120

[a] Human milk assumed to be 20 kcal/oz, and preterm formula and fortified human milk assumed to be 24 kcal/oz.

TABLE 3 Intakes of Calcium, Phosphorus, and Vitamin D From Various Enteral Nutrition Feedings at 160 mL/kg Per Day Used in the United States

	Unfortified Human Milk[a] (20 kcal/oz)	Fortified Human Milk[a] (24 kcal/oz)	Preterm Formula (24 kcal/oz)	Transitional Formula (22 kcal/oz)
Calcium (mg/kg)	37	184–218	210–234	125–144
Phosphorus (mg/kg)	21	102–125	107–130	74–80
Vitamin D (IU/day)[b]	2.4	283–379	290–468	125–127

[a] Human milk data based on mature human milk.[38]
[b] Based on an infant weighing 1500 g.

It is accepted that the best available marker of vitamin D exposure and vitamin D status is the serum 25-OH-D concentration.[1] Although the active form of vitamin D is 1,25 dihydroxyvitamin D, its serum value is not closely associated with overall outcomes or vitamin D exposure.[1] Therefore, excluding rare cases of severe renal disease or suspicion of vitamin D-resistant rickets, vitamin D status in preterm infants as well as older infants should be monitored exclusively by measuring the serum 25-OH-D concentration, not the 1,25 dihydroxyvitamin D concentration.

Data on the relationship between vitamin D intake and serum 25-OH-D in preterm infants are extremely limited. Backstrom et al[28] found that an intake of 200 IU/kg in the first 6 weeks after birth led to mean 25-OH-D concentrations of ~50 nmol/L and 80 nmol/L by 12 weeks of age (to convert from nmol/L to ng/mL, divide by 2.5). Similar results were found by Koo et al.[29] Most full-term infants achieve 25-OH-D concentrations of more than 50 nmol/L with vitamin D intakes of 400 IU/day.[1] However, it is difficult to extrapolate data from full-term infants to preterm infants, especially those who are hospitalized, in whom UV B-mediated vitamin D formation is likely to be minimal and in whom fat mass, in which vitamin D and its metabolites are stored, is minimal. A recent study revealed a high incidence of very low 25-OH-D concentrations in the cord blood of Arab preterm infants in the Middle East, likely attributable to very low maternal vitamin D status.[30]

CARE OF VLBW INFANTS RELATED TO BONE HEALTH

Calcium, Phosphorus, and Vitamin D

The basic approach to prevention of rickets in preterm infants is the use of diets containing high amounts of minerals. In almost all infants with birth weight <1800 to 2000 g, regardless of gestational age, it is recommended to use formulas designed for preterm infants or human milk supplemented with fortifiers designed for use in this population. Bone mineral content is low in infants who are small for gestational age, leading to the recommendation to use these products on the basis of weight rather than gestational age.[31] Further research is needed, however, to clarify whether this is appropriate practice for all preterm infants with birth weight <2000 g.

In the United States, fortified human milk and formulas designed for preterm infants provide calcium intakes of ~180 to 220 mg/kg per day and approximately half that amount of phosphorus (Table 3). Two widely used sets of recommendations in the United States from Tsang et al[32] and Klein et al[33] (Table 4) are consistent with these intakes, and for calcium, it

is reasonable to adopt the lower value and the higher value of the 2 as a range for recommended intakes (ie, 150 to 220 mg/kg per day). For phosphorus, the lower value of 60 mg/kg per day would lead to a 2:1 ratio or higher with the recommended calcium intakes, and thus, a minimum lower intake level of 75 mg/kg per day is recommended to provide a calcium-to-phosphorous ratio less than 2:1. Although no optimal calcium-to-phosphorous ratio is identified, generally a 1.5 to 1.7:1 ratio may be optimal for preterm infants.[34] For an upper intake recommendation for phosphorous, the higher value of 140 mg/kg per day is suggested. As noted later, phosphorus deficiency may occur in some preterm infants, and thus, a higher upper level recommendation is provided.

Pending further research, using the full-term infant vitamin D intake recommendation of 400 IU/day is appropriate for preterm infants born with birth weight >1500 g. Potential risks related to high 25-OH-D concentrations are unknown, and the established upper tolerable intake of 1000 IU/day for healthy full-term infants may be considered an upper intake for preterm infants as well.

TABLE 4 Recommendations for Enteral Nutrition for VLBW Infants

	Calcium, mg/kg per day	Phosphorus, mg/kg per day	Vitamin D, IU/day
Tsang et al (2005)[32]	100–220	60–140	150–400[a]
Klein (2002)[33]	150–220	100–130	135–338[b]
Agostoni[c] (2010)[5]	120–140	65–90	800–1000
This AAP clinical report	150–220	75–140	200–400

[a] Text says "aim to deliver 400 IU/daily."
[b] 90–125 IU/kg (total amount shown is for 1.5-kg infant).
[c] Reflects European recommendations.

For VLBW infants, few data are available. Their smaller size may lead to a lower need for vitamin D to achieve adequate 25-OH-D concentrations,[28,29] but further data are needed on this relationship. On the basis of limited data, a vitamin D intake of 200 to 400 IU/day for VLBW infants is recommended. This intake should be increased to 400 IU/day when weight exceeds ~1500 g and the infant is tolerating full enteral nutrition. Because this would require supplemental vitamins being added in addition to available human milk fortifiers, some may wish to wait until weight is closer to 2000 g to provide a full 400 IU/day because of concern about the osmolarity of vitamin supplements. These intake recommendations should be subject to clinical trials with rickets and fractures as clinical outcomes.

Comparisons With Other Recommendations

In Europe, a considerably lower target for calcium and phosphorus intake is common (Table 4). European guidelines generally suggest higher intakes of vitamin D of 800 to 1000 IU/day,[4,5] but there is no direct comparison of this approach compared with the approach used in the United States. Although this vitamin D intake is likely safe and is within the tolerable upper intake limit of the IOM for full-term infants,[1] no data are available for groups of VLBW infants and especially infants with birth weight <1000 g to assess the safety of providing these vitamin D intakes, which, on a body-weight basis may be 5 to 10 times the amount recommended for full-term neonates.

As noted by the IOM report,[1] there are no clinical outcome data to support routine measurement of vitamin D concentrations in preterm infants. Infants with cholestasis, other malabsorptive disorders, or renal disease should be considered for assessment, targeting a 25-OH-D concentration >50 ng/mL.[1,3] Preterm infants with radiologic evidence of rickets or high APA (>800 IU/L) are often provided the tolerable upper intake total of 1000 IU/day of vitamin D; however, no evidence-based data are available to support any specific benefit to this practice.

Research in a small number of preterm infants has suggested improvement in bone mineral content with an exercise or physical therapy program for preterm infants. No studies have demonstrated a decrease in rickets or fractures with such a program. Care would need to be taken because of the fragile nature of the preterm infants' bones. At present, this therapy requires further clinical investigation before it can be recommended for routine use.[35]

OTHER MANAGEMENT ISSUES

Despite the use of feedings with high mineral content, some infants may develop rickets. The management of infants who have rickets and remain dependent on intravenous nutrition is beyond the scope of this review, but in general, maximizing calcium and phosphorus intake from intravenous nutrition while minimizing factors that lead to mineral loss (steroids, some diuretics) is advised. Management approaches for infants who are fed enterally are described in Table 5. These principles have not been tested in controlled trials but reflect expert opinion related to mineral intake and metabolism.

Whether minerals should be added directly to human milk separate from the use of human milk fortifiers is controversial. This practice has been advocated, combined with monitoring of urinary calcium and phosphorus.[36] Although shown to be effective in some small studies, adding minerals directly to human milk, especially in the absence of using human milk fortifiers, is not widely performed in the United States for routine management of VLWB infants, because individually supplementing these minerals does not also provide the extra protein and other nutrients needed for growth.

However, in some infants who have evidence of rickets, the need for fluid restriction or inability to tolerate formula designed for preterm infants or human milk fortifier may lead to the need to directly supplement calcium and phosphorus. Optimal or safest forms and doses of calcium and phosphorus to add directly to the diet of preterm infants are unknown. In general, most widely used is calcium glubionate, a liquid form of calcium

TABLE 5 Management Approach for Enterally Fed Preterm Infants With Radiologic Evidence of Rickets

1. Maximize nutrient intake. Consider increasing human milk fortifier and/or feeding volume of preterm formula, as clinically indicated. If unable to tolerate human milk fortifier or preterm formula, then will likely need elemental minerals added as described below.
2. If no further increases in these can be made, add elemental calcium and phosphorus as tolerated. Usually beginning at 20 mg/kg per day of elemental calcium and 10–20 mg/kg per day elemental phosphorus and increasing, as tolerated, usually to a maximum of 70–80 mg/kg per day of elemental calcium and 40–50 mg/kg per day elemental phosphorus.
3. Evaluate cholestasis and vitamin D status. May consider measuring 25-OH-D concentration, targeting serum 25-OH-D concentration of >20 ng/mL (50 nmol/L).
4. Follow serum phosphorus concentration and serum APA weekly or biweekly.
5. Recheck radiographs for evidence of rickets at 5- to 6-week intervals until resolved.
6. Advise caregiving team to be cautious in handling of infant.
7. Limit use of steroids and furosemide, as clinically feasible.

containing 23 mg/mL of elemental calcium for oral supplementation. When needed, starting doses of 20 mg/kg per day of elemental calcium may be used, increasing slowly to a maximum of approximately 60 to 70 mg/kg per day of elemental calcium. Data specific to the use of calcium carbonate are not available, but the high pH of the neonatal intestine may make calcium carbonate less than ideal. Calcium gluconate (9.3 mg/mL elemental calcium) may also be used. Salts that contain both calcium and phosphorus are also used.[23] For example, calcium tribasic phosphate contains 0.39 mg calcium and 0.28 mg of phosphorus per milligram of powder, although calcium tribasic phosphate must be compounded as a liquid for administration to infants.

A special population is older preterm infants who develop a low serum phosphorus concentration, often in conjunction with a serum APA <500 IU/L. The specific cause of this low serum phosphorus concentration is unknown, but it is likely partly related to the use of phosphorus in nonbone tissue, such as muscle. The exact serum phosphorus concentration for which evidence demonstrates a need to supplement phosphorus without calcium is not known, but a serum concentration below ~4.0 mg/dL, especially if present for more than 1 to 2 weeks, suggests consideration of adding phosphorus directly.

An ideal oral form of phosphorus for use in preterm infants does not exist. Administering the intravenous preparations orally can be considered, because they are lower in osmolarity than are commercially available phosphorus-containing liquids. For example, potassium phosphate provides 31 mg of elemental phosphorus per millimole, and a dose of 10 to 20 mg/kg per day of elemental phosphorus is reasonable and will likely resolve hypophosphatemia in most preterm infants.

Transitioning Off High-Mineral Containing Products

Decreasing mineral intake, by either using less human milk fortifier or discontinuing the use of formulas for preterm infants, is often begun at a body weight of ~2000 g. Delaying the switch to transitional formulas and continuing the use of formula designed for preterm infants or human milk fortifier should be considered for infants on fluid restriction, especially <150 mL/kg per day, or for infants with a prolonged course of parenteral nutrition and a persistent elevation of serum APA (ie, >800 IU/L). Use of formula designed for preterm infants would likely be safe until body weight of at least 3000 g is reached, after which some concern might be present about vitamins or minerals (especially vitamin A) exceeding the established tolerable upper intake levels.[37] No clinical evidence of vitamin A toxicity exists, although for intakes slightly above the upper level, a risk-benefit assessment may need to be performed regarding use of formulas designed for preterm infants in some larger infants.

Preterm infants who do not tolerate cow milk protein or lactose-containing products represent a special circumstance. Amino acid-based, soy-based, and other specialized infant formulas generally have higher levels of minerals than do routine infant formulas, but the bioavailability of these minerals, especially in high-risk infants such as those with a history of feeding intolerance or intestinal failure, is uncertain. As such, biochemical monitoring may need to be continued for an extended period of time, and in some cases, direct supplementation with added minerals should be considered.

POSTDISCHARGE MANAGEMENT OF PRETERM INFANTS

VLBW infants who are discharged exclusively breastfeeding will often do well from a bone mineral perspective; however, they may be at risk for a very high serum APA after discharge. No specific research or clinical studies have addressed this issue. A measurement of serum APA 2 to 4 weeks after discharge is appropriate in exclusively breastfed former VLBW infants, with careful follow-up for values >800 IU/L and consideration of direct mineral supplementation if serum APA exceeds 1000 IU/L. Parents may also choose to provide some feedings per day of a higher mineral-containing formula (such as transitional formulas at 22 kcal/oz) to infants with birth weight <1500 g after hospital discharge. Transitional formulas contain 22 kcal/oz, and their nutrient contents are between those used for full-term infants and those used for preterm infants.

No data are available to define the length of time exclusively breastfed infants receiving such formula supplements or transitional formula need to continue them. This decision is often driven by growth in weight, head circumference, and length, not by bone mineral concerns. Infants consuming less than ~800 mL of currently marketed transitional formula daily after discharge from the hospital will receive <400 IU/day of vitamin D for several weeks to several months. It is reasonable to supplement these infants with a small amount of vitamin D (often 200 to 400 IU/day) to ensure a total intake of at least 400 IU/day.

From a bone mineral perspective, infants with birth weight 1500 to 2000 g will generally do well with exclusive breastfeeding or routine infant formula after discharge from the hospital. Some pediatricians choose to use a transitional infant formula after infants reach ~34 weeks' postmenstrual age or ~1800 to 2000 g body weight.

There are no specific studies related to the bone mineral needs of infants who are "late preterm" (ie, 34–36 weeks' gestation and >2000 g at birth). However, there are no clinical reports of mineral deficiency or rickets in this population whether breastfed exclusively or fed formula designed for preterm infants, as long as long-term vitamin D status is adequate. Therefore, it is likely that late preterm infants do not generally need special management related to bone minerals after discharge from the hospital. Breastfed preterm infants who are at home should receive 400 IU/day of vitamin D. Formula-fed preterm infants receiving formulas designed for full-term infants would generally not achieve an intake of 400 IU/day of vitamin D until consuming ~800 mL of formula daily, depending on the formula. Providing these infants with an additional 200 to 400 IU/day may be considered, but there are no data indicating any clinical benefit to this practice.

Small-for-gestational-age infants at or near term, such as is common in many global settings, may usually be provided minerals in the same way as larger infants of the same gestational age. Such infants should be monitored carefully for growth, and an adequate intake of vitamin D should be ensured.

SUMMARY

1. Preterm infants, especially those <27 weeks' gestation or with birth weight <1000 g with a history of multiple medical problems, are at high-risk of rickets.

2. Routine evaluation of bone mineral status by using biochemical testing is indicated for infants with birth weight <1500 g but not those with birth weight >1500 g. Biochemical testing should usually be started 4 to 5 weeks after birth.

3. Serum APA >800 to 1000 IU/L or clinical evidence of fractures should lead to a radiographic evaluation for rickets and management focusing on maximizing calcium and phosphorus intake and minimizing factors leading to bone mineral loss.

4. A persistent serum phosphorus concentration less than ~4.0 mg/dL should be followed, and consideration should be given for phosphorus supplementation.

5. Routine management of preterm infants, especially those with birth weight <1800 to 2000 g, should include human milk fortified with minerals or formulas designed for preterm infants (see Table 4 for details).

6. At the time of discharge from the hospital, VLBW infants will often be provided higher intakes of minerals than are provided by human milk or formulas intended for term infants through the use of transitional formulas. If exclusively breastfed, a follow-up serum APA at 2 to 4 weeks after discharge from the hospital may be considered.

7. When infants reach a body weight >1500 g and tolerate full enteral feeds, vitamin D intake should generally be ~400 IU/day, up to a maximum of 1000 IU/day.

LEAD AUTHOR

Steven A. Abrams, MD

COMMITTEE ON NUTRITION, 2011–2012

Jatinder J. S. Bhatia, MD, Chairperson
Steven A. Abrams, MD
Mark R. Corkins, MD
Sarah D. de Ferranti, MD
Neville H. Golden, MD
Janet Silverstein, MD

LIAISONS

Laurence Grummer-Strawn, PhD – *Centers for Disease Control and Prevention*
Rear Admiral Van S. Hubbard, MD, PhD – *National Institutes of Health*
Valerie Marchand, MD – *Canadian Pediatric Society*
Benson M. Silverman, MD – *Food and Drug Administration*
Valery Soto, MS, RD, LD – *US Department of Agriculture*

STAFF

Debra L. Burrowes, MHA

REFERENCES

1. Institute of Medicine. *Dietary Reference Intakes for Vitamin D and Calcium*. Washington, DC: The National Academies Press; 2011

2. Wagner CL, Greer FR; American Academy of Pediatrics Section on Breastfeeding; American Academy of Pediatrics Committee on Nutrition. Prevention of rickets and vitamin D deficiency in infants, children, and adolescents. *Pediatrics*. 2008;122(5): 1142–1152

3. Misra M, Pacaud D, Petryk A, Collett-Solberg PF, Kappy M; Drug and Therapeutics Committee of the Lawson Wilkins Pediatric Endocrine Society. Vitamin D deficiency in children and its management: review of current knowledge and recommendations. *Pediatrics*. 2008;122(2):398–417

4. Rigo J, Pieltain C, Salle B, Senterre J. Enteral calcium, phosphate and vitamin D requirements and bone mineralization in preterm infants. *Acta Paediatr*. 2007;96(7):969–974

5. Agostoni C, Buonocore G, Carnielli VP, et al; ESPGHAN Committee on Nutrition. Enteral nutrient supply for preterm infants: commentary from the European Society of Paediatric Gastroenterology, Hepatology and Nutrition Committee on Nutrition. *J Pediatr Gastroenterol Nutr*. 2010;50(1):85–91

6. Widdowson EM, McCance RA, Spray CM. The chemical composition of the human body. *Clin Sci*. 1951;10:113–125

7. Ellis KJ, Shypailo RJ, Schanler RJ. Body composition of the preterm infant. *Ann Hum Biol.* 1994;21(6):533–545

8. Hollis RW, Johnson D, Hulsey TC, Ebcling M, Wagner CL. Vitamin D supplementation during pregnancy: double-blind, randomized clinical trial of safety and effectiveness. *J Bone Miner Res.* 2011;26(10):2341–2357

9. Nassar N, Halligan GH, Roberts CL, Morris JM, Ashton AW. Systematic review of first-trimester vitamin D normative levels and outcomes of pregnancy. *Am J Obstet Gynecol.* 2011;205(3):208.e1–208.e7

10. Abrams SA. In utero physiology: role in nutrient delivery and fetal development for calcium, phosphorus, and vitamin D. *Am J Clin Nutr.* 2007;85(2):604S–607S

11. Brannon PM, Picciano MF. Vitamin D in pregnancy and lactation in humans. *Annu Rev Nutr.* 2011;31:89–115

12. Mitchell SM, Rogers SP, Hicks PD, Hawthorne KM, Parker BR, Abrams SA. High frequencies of elevated alkaline phosphatase activity and rickets exist in extremely low birth weight infants despite current nutritional support. *BMC Pediatr.* 2009;9:47

13. Lyon AJ, McIntosh N, Wheeler K, Williams JE. Radiological rickets in extremely low birthweight infants. *Pediatr Radiol.* 1987;17(1):56–58

14. Schanler RJ, Burns PA, Abrams SA, Garza C. Bone mineralization outcomes in human milk-fed preterm infants. *Pediatr Res.* 1992;31(6):583–586

15. Lucas A, Brooke OG, Baker BA, Bishop N, Morley R. High alkaline phosphatase activity and growth in preterm neonates. *Arch Dis Child.* 1989;64(7 Spec No):902–909

16. Fewtrell MS, Williams JE, Singhal A, Murgatroyd PR, Fuller N, Lucas A. Early diet and peak bone mass: 20 year follow-up of a randomized trial of early diet in infants born preterm. *Bone.* 2009;45(1):142–149

17. Wang D, Vandermeulen J, Atkinson SA. Early life factors predict abnormal growth and bone accretion at prepuberty in former premature infants with/without neonatal dexamethasone exposure. *Pediatr. Res.* 2007;61(1):111–116

18. Dalziel SR, Fenwick S, Cundy T, et al. Peak bone mass after exposure to antenatal betamethasone and prematurity: follow-up of a randomized controlled trial. *J Bone Miner Res.* 2006;21(8):1175–1186

19. Backström MC, Kouri T, Kuusela AL, et al. Bone isoenzyme of serum alkaline phosphatase and serum inorganic phosphate in metabolic bone disease of prematurity. *Acta Paediatr.* 2000;89(7):867–873

20. Atkinson SA. Calcium, phosphorus and vitamin D needs of low birthweight infants on various feedings. *Acta Paediatr Scand Suppl.* 1989;351:104–108

21. Bronner F, Salle BL, Putet G, Riog J, Senterre J. Net calcium absorption in premature infants: results of 103 metabolic balance studies. *Am J Clin Nutr.* 1992;56(6):1037–1044

22. Hicks PD, Rogers SP, Hawthorne KM, Chen Z, Abrams SA. Calcium absorption in very low birth weight infants with and without bronchopulmonary dysplasia. *J Pediatr.* 2011;158(6):885–890, e1

23. Schanler RJ, Abrams SA, Garza C. Mineral balance studies in very low birth weight infants fed human milk. *J Pediatr.* 1988;113(1 pt 2):230–238

24. Abrams SA, Esteban NV, Vieira NE, Yergey AL. Dual tracer stable isotopic assessment of calcium absorption and endogenous fecal excretion in low birth weight infants. *Pediatr Res.* 1991;29(6):615–618

25. Rowe J, Rowe D, Horak E, et al. Hypophosphatemia and hypercalciuria in small premature infants fed human milk: evidence for inadequate dietary phosphorus. *J Pediatr.* 1984;104(1):112–117

26. Sann L, David L, Loras B, Lahet C, Frederich A, Bethenod M. Neonatal hypercalcemia in preterm infants fed with human milk. *Helv Paediatr Acta.* 1985;40(2–3):117–126

27. Sann L, Loras B, David L, et al. Effect of phosphate supplementation to breast fed very low birthweight infants on urinary calcium excretion, serum immunoreactive parathyroid hormone and plasma 1,25-dihydroxy-vitamin D concentration. *Acta Paediatr Scand.* 1985;74(5):664–668

28. Backström MC, Mäki R, Kuusela AL, et al. Randomised controlled trial of vitamin D supplementation on bone density and biochemical indices in preterm infants. *Arch Dis Child Fetal Neonatal Ed.* 1999;80(3):F161–F166

29. Koo WW, Krug-Wispe S, Neylan M, Succop P, Oestreich AE, Tsang RC. Effect of three levels of vitamin D intake in preterm infants receiving high mineral-containing milk. *J Pediatr Gastroenterol Nutr.* 1995;21(2):182–189

30. Dawodu A, Nath R. High prevalence of moderately severe vitamin D deficiency in preterm infants. *Pediatr Int.* 2011;53(2):207–210

31. Lapillonne A, Braillon P, Claris O, Chatelain PG, Delmas PD, Salle BL. Body composition in appropriate and in small for gestational age infants. *Acta Paediatr.* 1997;86(2):196–200

32. Tsang RC, Uauy R, Koletzko B, Zlotkin SH, eds. *Nutrition of the Preterm Infant: Scientific Basis and Practical Guidelines*, 2nd ed. Cincinnati, OH: Digital Educational Publishing Inc; 2005

33. Klein CJ. Nutrient requirements for preterm infant formulas. *J Nutr.* 2002;132(6 suppl 1):1395S–1577S

34. Rowe JC, Goetz CA, Carey DE, Horak E. Achievement of in utero retention of calcium and phosphorus accompanied by high calcium excretion in very low birth weight infants fed a fortified formula. *J Pediatr.* 1987;110(4):581–585

35. Schulzke SM, Trachsel D, Patole SK. Physical activity programs for promoting bone mineralization and growth in preterm infants. *Cochrane Database Syst Rev.* 2007;(2):CD005387

36. Trotter A, Pohlandt F. Calcium and phosphorus retention in extremely preterm infants supplemented individually. *Acta Paediatr.* 2002;91(6):680–683

37. Institute of Medicine. *Dietary Reference Intakes for Vitamin A, Vitamin K, Arsenic, Boron, Chromium, Copper, Iodine, Iron, Manganese, Molybdenum, Nickel, Silicon, Vanadium, and Zinc.* Washington, DC: National Academies Press; 2001

38. American Academy of Pediatrics, Committee on Nutrition. *Pediatric Nutrition Handbook.* Kleinman RE, ed. 6th ed. Elk Grove Village, IL: American Academy of Pediatrics; 2009

Caregiver-Fabricated Illness in a Child: A Manifestation of Child Maltreatment

- *Clinical Report*

CLINICAL REPORT

Caregiver-Fabricated Illness in a Child: A Manifestation of Child Maltreatment

abstract

Caregiver-fabricated illness in a child is a form of child maltreatment caused by a caregiver who falsifies and/or induces a child's illness, leading to unnecessary and potentially harmful medical investigations and/or treatment. This condition can result in significant morbidity and mortality. Although caregiver-fabricated illness in a child has been widely known as Munchausen syndrome by proxy, there is ongoing discussion about alternative names, including pediatric condition falsification, factitious disorder (illness) by proxy, child abuse in the medical setting, and medical child abuse. Because it is a relatively uncommon form of maltreatment, pediatricians need to have a high index of suspicion when faced with a persistent or recurrent illness that cannot be explained and that results in multiple medical procedures or when there are discrepancies between the history, physical examination, and health of a child. This report updates the previous clinical report "Beyond Munchausen Syndrome by Proxy: Identification and Treatment of Child Abuse in the Medical Setting." The authors discuss the need to agree on appropriate terminology, provide an update on published reports of new manifestations of fabricated medical conditions, and discuss approaches to assessment, diagnosis, and management, including how best to protect the child from further harm. *Pediatrics* 2013;132:590–597

Emalee G. Flaherty, MD, FAAP, and Harriet L. MacMillan, MD, and COMMITTEE ON CHILD ABUSE AND NEGLECT

KEY WORDS
Munchausen syndrome by proxy, pediatric condition falsification, factitious disorder by proxy, medical child abuse, child maltreatment, Child Protective Services, covert video surveillance, multidisciplinary child protection team, Munchausen syndrome

ABBREVIATION
CVS—covert video surveillance

This document is copyrighted and is property of the American Academy of Pediatrics and its Board of Directors. All authors have filed conflict of interest statements with the American Academy of Pediatrics. Any conflicts have been resolved through a process approved by the Board of Directors. The American Academy of Pediatrics has neither solicited nor accepted any commercial involvement in the development of the content of this publication.

The guidance in this report does not indicate an exclusive course of treatment or serve as a standard of medical care. Variations, taking into account individual circumstances, may be appropriate.

www.pediatrics.org/cgi/doi/10.1542/peds.2013-2045

doi:10.1542/peds.2013-2045

All clinical reports from the American Academy of Pediatrics automatically expire 5 years after publication unless reaffirmed, revised, or retired at or before that time.

PEDIATRICS (ISSN Numbers: Print, 0031-4005; Online, 1098-4275).

Copyright © 2013 by the American Academy of Pediatrics

INTRODUCTION

Few conditions are as difficult to diagnose and manage as illness induced or falsified by caregivers. Although this condition has been widely known as Munchausen syndrome by proxy, there is ongoing debate about alternative names, including pediatric condition falsification, factitious disorder (illness) by proxy, child abuse in the medical setting, and medical child abuse. The previous clinical report from the American Academy of Pediatrics called this form of maltreatment "child abuse in a medical setting," noting that it can include physical abuse, medical neglect, and psychological maltreatment.[1] This term was used to focus attention on the harm caused to the child. Roesler and Jenny[2] concurred that pediatricians should focus on the maltreatment that happened to the child rather than the offender's motivation. They coined the term "medical child abuse," which they defined as "a child receiving unnecessary and harmful or potentially harmful medical care at the instigation of a caretaker." Despite the variability in terms, there is general agreement that this condition causes serious harm and is associated with significant morbidity and mortality.[3] The sections that follow provide an overview of the spectrum of the condition, the epidemiology, and an approach to assessment, diagnosis, and management.

DESCRIPTION

The essential feature of the condition that will be referred to in this report as fabricated illness in a child is the caregiver's falsification and/or inducement of physical or psychological symptoms or signs in a child.[4] The term "fabricated illness in a child" has been used in this report to reflect the emphasis on the child as the victim of the abuse rather than on the mental status or motivation of the caregiver who has caused the signs and/or symptoms.

Just as the name has been under debate, the definition has been controversial, partly because early definitions often included the offender's motivation. To be consistent with the approach to diagnosing other forms of child maltreatment, the definition and diagnosis of caregiver-fabricated illness in a child should focus on the child's exposure to risk and harm and associated injuries or impairment rather than the motivation of the offender.[1,2,5,6] Caregiver-fabricated illness in a child is best defined as maltreatment that occurs when a child has received unnecessary and harmful or potentially harmful medical care because of the caregiver's fabricated claims or signs and symptoms induced by the caregiver.[2]

SPECTRUM OF PRESENTATIONS

This type of maltreatment has no typical presentation, but a broad range of manifestations has been described,

as shown in Table 1. In separate literature reviews, Rosenberg[7] and Feldman and Brown[8] determined that bleeding, seizures, central nervous system depression, apnea, diarrhea, vomiting, fever, and rash were the most common presentations. Approximately one-quarter of children present with renal and urologic manifestations, including urinary tract infections and hematuria.[9] Illnesses commonly are reported to involve multiple organs, and the children are frequently seen by numerous subspecialists. Apnea and anorexia/feeding problems are the 2 most commonly reported symptoms.[10] Emotional and behavioral conditions, such as attention-deficit/hyperactivity disorder, learning disabilities, dissociative disorders, and psychosis, have all been fabricated by caregivers.[11–13] Allegations of sexual abuse have also been fabricated.[14–16]

Some of the forms of fabricated illness reported in more recent literature include hypernatremic dehydration,[17]

immunodeficiency,[18] celiac disease,[19] and Gaucher disease.[20] A retrospective review of calls to the National Poison Data System from 2000 to 2008 for pharmaceutical exposures that were coded as "malicious" and occurred in a child younger than 7 years revealed 1437 cases (average of 160 cases/year).[21] Ethanol, laxatives, and benzodiazepines, in that order, were the most common pharmaceutical categories. The pharmaceutical exposure may have been an intentional poisoning, drug-facilitated sexual abuse, or fabricated illness. Eighteen children (1.2%) died, and 2.2% suffered some major signs or symptoms related to the exposure. Most of the deaths were related to exposure to a sedating agent, including antihistamines and opioids.

The offending caregiver may fabricate or invent a history of illness, exaggerate a real disease, or underreport signs and symptoms. The caregiver may actually produce the signs and symptoms of illness or may both fabricate the

TABLE 1 Symptoms and Signs by System Involved

Allergic: food allergy, rash
Dermatologic: erythema, vesiculations from burns, lacerations, scratches, puncture wounds, eczema
Developmental: learning disabilities, attention-deficit/ hyperactivity disorders, neuromotor dysfunctions, pervasive developmental delay, psychosis
Endocrine: polydipsia, polyuria, hypoglycemia, diabetes, glycosuria
Gastrointestinal: abdominal pain, anorexia, diarrhea, dehydration, esophageal burns, vomiting, weight loss, bowel obstruction, gut dyskinesias, bleeding including hematemesis and hematochezia or melena, bleeding from nasogastric tube, bleeding from ileostomy, disorders leading to a need for parenteral nutrition
Hematologic: bleeding, easy bruising, anemia
Infection: fever, leukopenia, sepsis, septic arthritis, osteomyelitis; failure to resolve infections with antibiotics to which bacteria are susceptible; onset of new infection while the child is receiving antibiotics to which the bacteria are susceptible; unusual bacteria from the site of infection or infection with multiple simultaneous organisms of low pathogenicity
Metabolic: mitochondrial disorders, without positive testing
Neurologic: seizures, headaches, weakness, disorder of consciousness
Oncologic: leukemia, other cancers
Ophthalmic: recurrent hemorrhagic conjunctivitis, keratitis, eyelid swelling, unequal pupils, nystagmus, periorbital cellulitis
Orthopedic: limping
Otic: otorrhea, recurrent infections
Renal: hematuria, proteinuria, renal calculi, bacteriuria, renal insufficiency, hypertension, nocturia, hypernatremia, hyponatremia, hypokalemia, pyuria, renal failure
Respiratory: presentation with an acute life-threatening event, apnea including sleep apnea, cystic fibrosis, bleeding from the upper respiratory tract, intractable asthma, hemoptysis, cyanosis, hypoxia
Rheumatologic: arthritis, arthralgia, morning stiffness

Data are from refs 2, 3, and 7.

clinical picture and cause the signs and symptoms. There is a spectrum of severity of fabricated illness, and 1 form may evolve into another: for example, a caregiver may begin by fabricating a history and move on to actually cause signs and symptoms of illness.

The caregiver's fabrications may lead physicians to cause chronic medical complications or disabilities through their treatments, for example, by inserting an unnecessary gastric tube for feeding. Caregivers' actions may induce emotional or psychiatric disease in their children. The caregiver may coach the victim or others into misrepresenting the victim as ill. The child and family members may be convinced of the child's illness. There is often a significant delay from months to years between when the child presents with initial symptoms to the time of diagnosis.[7,22]

EPIDEMIOLOGY

Although fabricated illness in a child is relatively rare, best estimates suggest that health professionals will likely encounter at least 1 case during their career.[23] This form of maltreatment often goes unrecognized and unreported even when it is recognized. The reported incidence is approximately 0.5 to 2.0 per 100 000 children younger than 16 years.[7,24,25] Inappropriate invasive investigations or treatments, including drug therapy, were inflicted on 93% of the children in the cases reported over 2 years in the United Kingdom.[24] In this prospective surveillance study conducted in the United Kingdom and the Republic of Ireland, 85% of the notifying pediatricians estimated the certainty of their diagnosis as greater than 90%. In this study, it appears that pediatricians needed to have a strong degree of certainty before reporting, suggesting that many cases go unreported when a physician is less sure of the diagnosis. A diagnosis of

fabricated illness in a child may also not be made because of the inconsistency in diagnostic criteria. Failure to consider the possibility in the differential diagnosis is the most common reason for the missed diagnosis.[7,26]

Males and females are victimized equally.[7,10] The median age at diagnosis is between 14 months and 2.7 years.[10] Most of the victims are infants and toddlers, although approximately 25% of cases occur in children older than 6 years.[10,22,24] Illness fabricated by a caregiver has been described in many other countries and cultures.[8] Siblings of children who are victims of fabricated illness are also frequently abused.[24,27,28] In 1 large series, 25% of the siblings had died and 61.3% of the siblings had illnesses similar to those of the victims of fabricated illness.[10]

Although mothers are most commonly the offenders, fathers, grandparents, boyfriends, and child care providers have been found responsible.[24,29] Cases in which parents have colluded to fabricate illness have been reported as well.[11] There are reports of children who appear to actively collude with the offender in producing the fabricated illness and who later independently fabricate their own illness as they become older.[30] In addition, older children have been reported to fabricate illness, both by falsifying symptoms and/or signs of illness, without adult collusion.[18,25,31,32]

Although a discussion of the etiology for such behavior by caregivers is beyond the scope of this report, it is important for clinicians to be aware of some of the caregiver risk indicators for fabricating illness in a child. These include caregivers who (1) appear to need or thrive on attention from physicians,[13] (2) insist that the child cannot cope without the parent's ongoing attention,[13] (3) are either directly involved in professions related

to health care[3] or at least are very knowledgeable medically and have a familiarity with medical terminology, and (4) have a history of factitious disorder or somatoform disorder.[33,34] Although such indicators are useful in raising awareness about the possibility of fabricated illness among children of otherwise apparently caring families, such features are quite nonspecific and should not be used to make the diagnosis.[35] These characteristics overlap considerably with those of caregivers who are advocates for their children with genuine illnesses, and some parents who fabricate illness in their children do not show such features.[35] It is important to underscore that there is no consistent psychological presentation or psychiatric diagnosis among caregivers who have fabricated illness in a child.[36]

Children who are victims of fabricated illness can suffer significant morbidity and mortality.[21,24,27,28,37] Mortality rates of 6% to 9% have been reported, and approximately the same percentage suffer long-term disability or permanent injury.[7,10,24] By definition, all victims suffer some short-term morbidity related to unnecessary procedures or treatments. The abuse often continues in the hospital[38] and has even occurred in the ICU.[17,39] Approximately 75% of the morbidity experienced by children has been precipitated by caregivers' behaviors while the children are hospitalized.[7]

DIAGNOSIS

The diagnosis of fabricated illness in a child can be especially difficult, because the signs and symptoms reported by a caregiver may not actually be present during the physician's evaluation. When illness is induced or fabricated, the signs and symptoms may fluctuate and be inconsistent with normal physiology. Indicators that should cause the pediatrician to consider fabricated illness in a child are shown in Table 2. A caregiver who seeks another medical opinion when told that the child does not have illness or who resists reassurance that the child is healthy should raise concern about possible fabricated illness. Other potential areas for concern include a caregiver who perseverates about borderline abnormal results of no clinical relevance, despite repeated reassurance, or who refutes the validity of normal results. In the previous clinical report, it was suggested that the physician consider the following 3 questions in the diagnostic assessment of suspected fabricated illness:

1. Are the history, signs, and symptoms of disease credible?

2. Is the child receiving unnecessary and harmful or potentially harmful medical care?

3. If so, who is instigating the evaluations and treatment?

A multidisciplinary evaluation involving medical, psychosocial, child protective services, and legal professionals is important.[40] Because of the complexity of the diagnosis of fabricated illness in a child, the physician may want to consult with a specialist in child abuse pediatrics. A physician with expertise in child abuse and fabricated illness in a child may be able to provide a more objective opinion than a physician more closely involved with the family.[41,42] A complete review of the medical record, although potentially daunting, is imperative.[35] Because medical records are generally extensive and usually involve multiple medical sites, identification of the condition as fabricated may be missed if the complete medical records are not reviewed. The complete medical record may not be readily available if care has been sought at different clinical settings.

It is important to understand that as many as 30% of children with fabricated illness have an underlying medical illness.[7] Eventually, most of the victims will have iatrogenic signs and symptoms of illness.

When reviewing medical records, it is useful to make a chronological summary of medical contacts. This summary may reveal one or more of the following: (1) use of multiple medical facilities; (2) excessive and/or inappropriate pattern of utilization, including procedures, medications, tests, hospitalizations, and surgeries; (3) a pattern of missed appointments and discharge of the child against medical advice; and (4) a history of the opinions of physicians about the child's medical problems, illnesses, and treatments being misrepresented to other physicians. It is essential to review the entire record, including daily notes by all health care professionals, rather than simply focusing on summary reports, such as discharge summaries. When a child is hospitalized, it is important that all staff attribute the source of medical information in their notes: for example, nurses should document whether they witnessed that a child was apneic or that the caregiver told them the child was apneic. As shown in Table 3, it is useful to create a table that includes the following elements for each health contact: name of patient, date, location, reason for contact, reported signs/symptoms as stated by the caregiver, objective observations documented by the physician, conclusions/diagnosis made, treatment provided, efficacy of treatment, and other comments or observations. The veracity of the claims made by the caregiver can then be assessed for each symptom and sign.[35] An important overall issue to consider is whether the medical history provided by the caregiver matches the history in the medical record and whether the diagnosis reported by the caregiver matches the diagnosis made by the physician. Because fabricating caregivers can misrepresent medical information provided by various medical professionals, it is helpful to have all involved physicians conference and develop a consensus management plan.

Because physicians may be reluctant to identify possible concerns about induced illness in the record, it is also important to contact the individual physicians to discuss whether they have any concerns about possible fabrication of illness. A physician directly involved in the ongoing assessment or treatment of a child who may be the victim of fabricated illness can legally contact other physicians involved in the current or past care of the patient to obtain information relevant to the ongoing assessment or treatment of the child. If there is any aspect of that physician contact

TABLE 2 Indicators of Possible Fabricated Illness in a Child

- Diagnosis does not match the objective findings
- Signs or symptoms are bizarre
- Caregiver or suspected offender does not express relief or pleasure when told that child is improving or that child does not have a particular illness
- Inconsistent histories of symptoms from different observers
- Caregiver insists on invasive or painful procedures and hospitalizations
- Caregiver's behavior does not match expressed distress or report of symptoms (eg, unusually calm)
- Signs and symptoms begin only in the presence of 1 caregiver
- Sibling has or had an unusual or unexplained illness or death
- Sensitivity to multiple environmental substances or medicines
- Failure of the child's illness to respond to its normal treatments or unusual intolerance to those treatments
- Caregiver publicly solicits sympathy or donations or benefits because of the child's rare illness
- Extensive unusual illness history in the caregiver or caregivers' family; caregiver's history of somatization disorders

TABLE 3 Sample Table for Chart Review

Date	Location	Reason for Contact	Reported Signs/Symptoms per Caregiver	Objective Observations by Physician	Conclusions/ Diagnosis Made	Treatment Provided	Efficacy of Treatments	Other Comments or Observations

that may be for forensic purposes or done in consultation with child protective services, consider obtaining the caregiver's consent and/or obtaining legal advice before making such contact. The medical record of the siblings should be reviewed in the same thorough fashion.

If a child with the possible fabricated illness is verbal, the child should be interviewed separately from the caregiver for his or her recollection of any symptoms, including where and when they occurred. It is also important to take a careful family and social history, including information about any unusual or frequent illnesses in the extended family and siblings.

Fabricated illness in a child, like other forms of child maltreatment, is not a diagnosis of exclusion. The pediatrician should evaluate the child for illness fabrication while simultaneously searching for other medical explanations for the illness: for example, unusual and rare medical problems, such as cyclic vomiting or mitochondrial disease. Some parents are overanxious or difficult, and others perceive their child as vulnerable because of some earlier traumatic event, such as extreme prematurity, and may "shop around" for a physician.[43] When parental behaviors result in harm to the child, the child has been maltreated, whatever the caregiver's motivation.[37]

The specific features of an evaluation for fabricated illness in a child depend on the type of fabrication suspected. The pediatrician may need to perform toxicology tests if poisoning is suspected or may need to request blood group typing or subtyping if blood contamination is a concern. If testing is needed to confirm the diagnosis, the child must be protected from any additional or ongoing harm while the evaluation is underway. Although the hospital is generally considered an appropriate setting to complete this testing, the offending caregiver often continues the illness fabrication in the hospital.[7] Consequently, the caregiver's contact with the child may need to be supervised to protect the child from further harm.

If there are concerns that a child may be a victim of fabricated illness, physicians should defer procedures and prescriptions. The physician's responsibility is to protect the child.

COVERT VIDEO SURVEILLANCE

Covert video surveillance (CVS) has been proposed as a method of ensuring the child's safety during the hospitalization, as well as to expose and document the offending caregiver's fabricating behavior toward the child while in the hospital.[44,45] The use of CVS has been controversial.[46] Some argue that it is an invasion of the parent's right to privacy or that it represents entrapment.[47] Others respond that privacy is not guaranteed in a hospital setting, because health care providers, such as nurses, may walk into patient rooms at any time unannounced. Also, for some conditions, monitors are attached to a child and sound at the nurses' station. Some consider CVS to be a diagnostic tool,[48] but others argue that the recordings can be difficult to interpret and that

a caregiver may be falsely accused of harm.[47] Because it can be difficult to prove to child protective services and in legal proceedings that illness has been fabricated, some children will not be protected from further harm without the use of CVS to document the abuse. Some of the disadvantages of the use of CVS include its cost, the need for real-time monitoring to interrupt any harm to a child, and the risk of additional harm to the child even with close monitoring.[44,45]

In 1 series, CVS was required to make the diagnosis of fabricated illness in a child in more than half of the cases. In 10% of the cases, however, it proved helpful because it showed that the child had a medical problem.[45] CVS has been used to detect caregivers suffocating infants, intentionally causing fractures, administering poison, and injecting harmful substances into intravenous lines. Some offending caregivers, who were previously thought to be very attentive to the child, were shown to ignore the child when no one was watching. CVS can also disprove a caregiver's falsified claim, such as showing that apnea did not occur when a caregiver has reported it. Furthermore, CVS has the potential to show that the abuse was premeditated and occurred without provocation.

If CVS is to be implemented, the hospital should develop protocols that guide its use. The protocols should include provision for continuous monitoring, training for the observers or monitors, and a plan that ensures rapid intervention if the child is observed to be at risk.

An approach that can be considered instead of CVS is separation of the child from the suspected offending caregiver and subsequent observation of the child's condition. The child must be separated for sufficient time to determine whether there is any change in the child's condition while, as much as possible, maintaining constant all other management, such as medication use. During this trial period, the suspected offending caregiver must not be allowed any contact with the child unless strict third-party supervision is maintained. Intervention by child protective services will likely be required to establish and maintain this separation. If symptoms do not disappear, this is strong indication that the symptoms were not fabricated, providing the child has been adequately protected during the separation. The association between the trial separation and any improvement in a child's condition may be difficult to prove in a legal setting, especially because improvement in a child's condition may be attributed to a spontaneous remission or resolution of the underlying medical problem.

MANAGEMENT AND PROGNOSIS

Reporting Suspected Maltreatment

Physicians should report any reasonable suspicions of child abuse promptly to child protective services authorities. All states have laws that mandate physicians report suspected child maltreatment if they have reasonable cause to suspect. In a review by Sheridan,[10] only approximately one-third of the cases of suspected fabricated illness in a child had been reported. Another study found that pediatricians do not report unless they are almost certain of the diagnosis of fabricated illness. In this study, the pediatricians estimated the probability that their diagnosis was correct as greater than 90%.[24] Although the laws do not require this

level of certainty for reporting, physicians may be concerned that a caregiver will escalate the illness induction to "prove" the child's illness. Also, pediatricians may be reluctant to report suspicions of illness fabrication because of previous experience with child protective services and the legal system failing to protect a child without additional corroborating evidence.

Many state child protective services systems do not list fabricated illness or any of its various names as a specific form of child maltreatment. When reporting suspected fabricated illness in these states, the pediatrician should focus on how the child was affected: for example, the pediatrician may report suspected physical abuse, emotional abuse, risk of harm, and all the categories that apply to the particular situation. Pediatricians should collaborate with child protective services and law enforcement to ensure the best outcome for the child.

Outcome if Reported

Even when fabricated illness is reported to child protective services, many children are not protected from further harm. In the 2-year surveillance study in the United Kingdom and the Republic of Ireland referred to previously,[24] approximately one-third of the children (46 of 119) were allowed to return home.[28] Approximately one-quarter of the children (27) still had signs or symptoms of abuse at follow-up. Only one-third of the children were placed in caregiving arrangements outside the control of the alleged offending parent. Child protective services and the courts were more likely to intervene and protect children who were young and who had been physically abused as opposed to older children who suffered other harm.

If children who have been victims of fabricated illness are returned home to the care of the offending caregiver,

reabuse is common.[28,49] Approximately 40% suffer further abuse, including other forms of maltreatment, such as physical and emotional abuse.[49] On the basis of Rosenberg's review,[7] in 20% of the fatal cases the child had been returned home after the parents had been confronted about the suspicion of fabricated illness, and the child subsequently died. In a study in 54 children with a diagnosis of fabricated illness followed for 1 to 14 years, many of the children manifested other problems, including emotional and behavioral conditions, such as conduct disorders. Criminal conviction of the offending caregiver was found in only 8% of the cases in the Rosenberg series.[7]

In a cohort study that had several methodologic limitations, including follow-up of only approximately 50% of the original sample identified, the factors associated with better outcomes for children who had been victimized included the following: (1) continuous positive input from the spouse and/or grandparents, (2) successful short-term foster care before returning to live with the offending caregiver, (3) the offender's long-term therapeutic relationship with a social worker, (4) successful remarriage for the offending caregiver, (5) early adoption of the victim, and (6) long-term foster care placement.[49] It was not possible to determine the relative benefits for children of remaining with the abusing caregiver versus being separated. Among those children who were with the fabricator of the illness at the time of this study, children placed away from their mother, even temporarily, appeared to have a better outcome than those who did not experience this separation.

Caregiver Treatment and Reunification

When confronted with the suspicion that the illness has been fabricated,

15% to 45% of offenders admitted to causing or fabricating the child's illness, although many denied any deception.[7,45] In general, the prognosis has been poor for offenders, but there are some reports of apparent successful treatment.[50] Identifying an offender's motivation may not be critical to making a diagnosis of fabricated illness in a child, but understanding the motivation is important for determining the course of treatment.[34,51] Schreier[11] outlines the following indicators of successful treatment: (1) the abuser admits to the abuse and has been able to describe specifically how he or she abused the child, (2) the abuser has experienced an appropriate emotional response to his or her behaviors and the harm he or she has caused the child, (3) the abuser has developed strategies to better identify and manage his or her needs to avoid abusing the child in the future, and (4) the abuser has demonstrated these skills, with monitoring, over a significant period of time. Schreier also asserts that the partners of offending caregivers should participate in treatment, because they have frequently colluded in the abuse of the child. The partner's lack of nurture for the offending caregiver may also be 1 motivation for the child's abuse.

SUMMARY

Caregiver-fabricated illness in a child is a relatively rare but very serious form of child maltreatment. The pediatrician who suspects that signs or symptoms of a disease are being fabricated should focus on the harm or potential harm to the child caused by the actions of that caregiver and by the efforts of medical personnel to diagnose and treat a nonexistent disease. Pediatricians need to have a high index of suspicion and be alert to the possibility when signs and symptoms do not fit a particular illness, when they appear resistant to treatment, or when they evolve into another or additional illnesses. Proper diagnosis of fabricated disease involves a thorough evaluation of medical records, clear communication among medical professionals, and often, a multidisciplinary approach. If the child protective services system's response seems inadequate, the pediatrician should ask a local specialist in child abuse pediatrics for advice and assistance. A focus on the motives of the caregiver, although useful in therapy, is not necessary for a diagnosis of this form of child maltreatment.

LEAD AUTHORS

Emalee G. Flaherty, MD, FAAP
Harriet L. MacMillan, MD

COMMITTEE ON CHILD ABUSE AND NEGLECT, 2012–2013

Cindy W. Christian, MD, FAAP, Chairperson
James E. Crawford-Jakubiak, MD, FAAP
Emalee G. Flaherty, MD, FAAP
John M. Leventhal, MD, FAAP
James L. Lukefahr, MD, FAAP
Robert D. Sege, MD, PhD, FAAP

LIAISONS

Harriet L. MacMillan, MD – *American Academy of Child and Adolescent Psychiatry*
Catherine M. Nolan, MSW, ACSW – *Administration for Children, Youth, and Families*
Janet Saul, PhD – *Centers for Disease Control and Prevention*

STAFF

Tammy Piazza Hurley

REFERENCES

1. Stirling J Jr; American Academy of Pediatrics Committee on Child Abuse and Neglect. Beyond Munchausen syndrome by proxy: identification and treatment of child abuse in a medical setting. *Pediatrics*. 2007;119(5):1026–1030

2. Roesler TA, Jenny C. *Medical Child Abuse: Beyond Munchausen Syndrome by Proxy*. Elk Grove Village, IL: American Academy of Pediatrics; 2009

3. Shaw RJ, Dayal S, Hartman JK, DeMaso DR. Factitious disorder by proxy: pediatric condition falsification. *Harv Rev Psychiatry*. 2008;16(4):215–224

4. American Psychiatric Association. Diagnostic and Statistical Manual of Mental Disorders. 4th ed, text revision. Washington, DC: American Psychiatric Association; 2000

5. Rosenberg DA. Munchausen syndrome by proxy: medical diagnostic criteria. *Child Abuse Negl*. 2003;27(4):421–430

6. Brown P, Tierney C. Munchausen syndrome by proxy. *Pediatr Rev*. 2009;30(10):414–415;, discussion 415

7. Rosenberg DA. Web of deceit: a literature review of Munchausen syndrome by proxy. *Child Abuse Negl*. 1987;11(4):547–563

8. Feldman MD, Brown RM. Munchausen by proxy in an international context. *Child Abuse Negl*. 2002;26(5):509–524

9. Feldman KW, Feldman MD, Grady R, Burns MW, McDonald R. Renal and urologic manifestations of pediatric condition falsification/Munchausen by proxy. *Pediatr Nephrol*. 2007;22(6):849–856

10. Sheridan MS. The deceit continues: an updated literature review of Munchausen syndrome by proxy. *Child Abuse Negl*. 2003;27(4):431–451

11. Schreier H. Munchausen by proxy. *Curr Probl Pediatr Adolesc Health Care*. 2004;34(3):126–143

12. Rittner L, Pulos S, Lennon R. Pediatric condition falsification in attention-deficit/hyperactivity disorder. *N Am J Psychol*. 2005;7(3):353–359

13. Ayoub CC, Schreier HA, Keller C. Munchausen by proxy: presentations in special education. *Child Maltreat*. 2002;7(2):149–159

14. Meadow R. False allegations of abuse and Munchausen syndrome by proxy. *Arch Dis Child*. 1993;68(4):444–447

15. Hornor G. Repeated sexual abuse allegations: a problem for primary care providers. *J Pediatr Health Care*. 2001;15(2):71–76

16. Schreier HA. Repeated false allegations of sexual abuse presenting to sheriffs: when is it Munchausen by proxy? *Child Abuse Negl*. 1996;20(10):985–991

17. Su E, Shoykhet M, Bell MJ. Severe hypernatremia in a hospitalized child: Munchausen by proxy. *Pediatr Neurol*. 2010;43(4):270–273

18. Awadallah N, Vaughan A, Franco K, Munir F, Sharaby N, Goldfarb J. Munchausen by proxy: a case, chart series, and literature review of older victims. *Child Abuse Negl.* 2005;29(8):931–941

19. Lasher LJ, Feldman MD. Celiac disease as a manifestation of Munchausen by proxy. *South Med J.* 2004;97(1):67–69

20. Al-Owain M, Al-Zaidan H, Al-Hashem A, Kattan H, Al-Dowaish A. Munchausen syndrome by proxy mimicking as Gaucher disease. *Eur J Pediatr.* 2010;169(8):1029–1032

21. Yin S. Malicious use of pharmaceuticals in children. *J Pediatr.* 2010;157(5):832–836

22. Denny SJ, Grant CC, Pinnock R. Epidemiology of Munchausen syndrome by proxy in New Zealand. *J Paediatr Child Health.* 2001;37(3):240–243

23. Fabricated or induced illness by carers: a complex conundrum. *Lancet.* 2010;375 (9713):433

24. McClure RJ, Davis PM, Meadow SR, Sibert JR. Epidemiology of Munchausen syndrome by proxy, non-accidental poisoning, and non-accidental suffocation. *Arch Dis Child.* 1996;75(1):57–61

25. Ehrlich S, Pfeiffer E, Salbach H, Lenz K, Lehmkuhl U. Factitious disorder in children and adolescents: a retrospective study. *Psychosomatics.* 2008;49(5):392–398

26. Squires JE, Squires RH Jr. Munchausen syndrome by proxy: ongoing clinical challenges. *J Pediatr Gastroenterol Nutr.* 2010; 51(3):248–253

27. Bools CN, Neale BA, Meadow SR. Comorbidity associated with fabricated illness (Munchausen syndrome by proxy). *Arch Dis Child.* 1992;67(1):77–79

28. Davis P, McClure RJ, Rolfe K, et al. Procedures, placement, and risks of further abuse after Munchausen syndrome by proxy, non-accidental poisoning, and non-accidental suffocation. *Arch Dis Child.* 1998;78(3):217–221

29. Meadow R. Munchausen syndrome by proxy abuse perpetrated by men. *Arch Dis Child.* 1998;78(3):210–216

30. Libow JA. Beyond collusion: active illness falsification. *Child Abuse Negl.* 2002;26(5):525–536

31. Libow JA. Child and adolescent illness falsification. *Pediatrics.* 2000;105(2):336–342

32. Shapiro M, Nguyen M. Psychological sequelae of Munchausen's syndrome by proxy. *Child Abuse Negl.* 2011;35(2):87–88

33. Bools C, Neale B, Meadow R. Munchausen syndrome by proxy: a study of psychopathology. *Child Abuse Negl.* 1994;18(9):773–788

34. Bass C, Jones D. Psychopathology of perpetrators of fabricated or induced illness in children: case series. *Br J Psychiatry.* 2011;199(2):113–118

35. Sanders MJ, Bursch B. Forensic assessment of illness falsification, Munchausen by proxy, and factitious disorder, NOS. *Child Maltreat.* 2002;7(2):112–124

36. Parnell TF. The use of psychological evaluation. In: Parnell TF, Day DO, eds. *Munchausen by Proxy Syndrome: Misunderstood Child Abuse.* Thousand Oaks, CA: Sage; 1998:129–150

37. Meadow R. Mothering to death. *Arch Dis Child.* 1999;80(4):359–362

38. Schreier H. On the importance of motivation in Munchausen by Proxy: the case of Kathy Bush. *Child Abuse Negl.* 2002;26(5):537–549

39. Carter KE, Izsak E, Marlow J. Munchausen syndrome by proxy caused by ipecac poisoning. *Pediatr Emerg Care.* 2006;22(9):655–656

40. Horwath J. Developing good practice in cases of fabricated and induced illness by carers: new guidance and the training implications. *Child Abuse Rev.* 2003;12(1):58–63

41. Schreier H, Ricci LR. Follow-up of a case of Munchausen by proxy syndrome. *J Am Acad Child Adolesc Psychiatry.* 2002;41(12):1395–1396

42. Siegel DM. Munchausen syndrome by proxy: a pediatrician's observations. *Fam Syst Health.* 2009;27(1):113–115

43. Thomasgard M, Metz WP. The vulnerable child syndrome revisited. *J Dev Behav Pediatr.* 1995;16(1):47–53

44. Southall DP, Plunkett MC, Banks MW, Falkov AF, Samuels MP. Covert video recordings of life-threatening child abuse: lessons for child protection. *Pediatrics.* 1997;100(5):735–760

45. Hall DE, Eubanks L, Meyyazhagan LS, Kenney RD, Johnson SC. Evaluation of covert video surveillance in the diagnosis of Munchausen syndrome by proxy: lessons from 41 cases. *Pediatrics.* 2000;105(6):1305–1312

46. Foreman DM. Detecting fabricated or induced illness in children. *BMJ.* 2005;331 (7523):978–979

47. Morley C. Concerns about using and interpreting covert video surveillance. *BMJ.* 1998;316(7144):1603–1605

48. Shinebourne EA. Covert video surveillance and the principle of double effect: a response to criticism. *J Med Ethics.* 1996;22(1):26–31

49. Bools CN, Neale BA, Meadow SR. Follow up of victims of fabricated illness (Munchausen syndrome by proxy). *Arch Dis Child.* 1993;69(6):625–630

50. Sanders MJ. Narrative family treatment of Munchausen by Proxy: a successful case. *Fam Syst Health.* 1996;14(3):315–329

51. Bursch B, Schreier HA, Ayoub CC, Libow JA, Sanders MJ, Yorker BC. Further thoughts on "Beyond Munchausen by proxy: identification and treatment of child abuse in a medical setting". *Pediatrics.* 2008;121(2):444–445; author reply 445

Children, Adolescents, and the Media

- *Policy Statement*

POLICY STATEMENT

Children, Adolescents, and the Media

abstract

Media, from television to the "new media" (including cell phones, iPads, and social media), are a dominant force in children's lives. Although television is still the predominant medium for children and adolescents, new technologies are increasingly popular. The American Academy of Pediatrics continues to be concerned by evidence about the potential harmful effects of media messages and images; however, important positive and prosocial effects of media use should also be recognized. Pediatricians are encouraged to take a media history and ask 2 media questions at every well-child visit: How much recreational screen time does your child or teenager consume daily? Is there a television set or Internet-connected device in the child's bedroom? Parents are encouraged to establish a family home use plan for all media. Media influences on children and teenagers should be recognized by schools, policymakers, product advertisers, and entertainment producers. *Pediatrics* 2013;132:958–961

COUNCIL ON COMMUNICATIONS AND MEDIA

KEY WORDS
media, television, new technology, family media use plan, media history, media education

ABBREVIATION
AAP—American Academy of Pediatrics

INTRODUCTION

Media, from traditional television to the "new media" (including cell phones, iPads, and social media), are a dominant force in children's lives. Although media are not the leading cause of any major health problem in the United States, the evidence is now clear that they can and do contribute substantially to many different risks and health problems and that children and teenagers learn from, and may be negatively influenced by, the media. However, media literacy and prosocial uses of media may enhance knowledge, connectedness, and health. The overwhelming penetration of media into children's and teenagers' lives necessitates a renewed commitment to changing the way pediatricians, parents, teachers, and society address the use of media to mitigate potential health risks and foster appropriate media use.

According to a recent study, the average 8- to 10-year-old spends nearly 8 hours a day with a variety of different media, and older children and teenagers spend >11 hours per day.[1] Presence of a television (TV) set in a child's bedroom increases these figures even more, and 71% of children and teenagers report having a TV in their bedroom.[1] Young people now spend more time with media than they do in school—it is the leading activity for children and teenagers other than sleeping.[1,2]

In addition to time spent with media, what has changed dramatically is the media landscape.[3,4] TV remains the predominant medium (>4 hours per day) but nearly one-third of TV programming is viewed on alternative platforms (computers, iPads, or cell phones). Nearly all children and teenagers have Internet access (84%), often high-speed, and one-third have

www.pediatrics.org/cgi/doi/10.1542/peds.2013-2656

doi:10.1542/peds.2013-2656

PEDIATRICS (ISSN Numbers: Print, 0031-4005; Online, 1098-4275).

Copyright © 2013 by the American Academy of Pediatrics

access in their own bedroom. Computer time accounts for up to 1.5 hours per day; half of this is spent in social networking, playing games, or viewing videos. New technology has arrived in a big way: some 75% of 12- to 17-year-olds now own cell phones, up from 45% in 2004. Nearly all teenagers (88%) use text messaging. Teenagers actually talk less on their phones than any other age group except for senior citizens,[5,6] but in the first 3 months of 2011, teenagers 13 through 17 years of age sent an average of 3364 texts per month.[5] Half of teenagers send 50 or more text messages per day, and one-third send more than 100 per day.[5] Teenagers access social media sites from cell phones,[6] and as reviewed in a recent clinical report from the American Academy of Pediatrics (AAP), social media, mainly Facebook, offers opportunities and potential risks to young wired users.[7] They are also avid multitaskers, often using several technologies simultaneously,[1] but multitasking teenagers are inefficient.[8] For example, using a mobile phone while driving may result in both poor communication and dangerous driving.[9]

Despite all of this media time and new technology, many parents seem to have few rules about use of media by their children and adolescents. In a recent study, two-thirds of children and teenagers report that their parents have "no rules" about time spent with media.[1] Many young children see PG-13 and R-rated movies—either online, on TV, or in movie theaters—that contain problematic content and are clearly inappropriate for them.[10,11] Few parents have rules about cell phone use for their children or adolescents. More than 60% of teenagers send and/or receive text messages after "lights out," and they report increased levels of tiredness, including at school.[12] One study found that 20% of adolescents either sent or received a sexually explicit image by cell phone or Internet.[13]

For nearly 3 decades, the AAP has expressed concerns about the amount of time that children and teenagers spend with media and about some of the content they view. In a series of policy statements, the AAP has delineated its concerns about media violence,[14] sex in the media,[10] substance use,[11] music and music videos,[15] obesity and the media,[16] and infant media use.[17] At the same time, existing AAP policy discusses the positive, prosocial uses of media and the need for media education in schools and at home.[18] Shows like "Sesame Street" can help children learn numbers and letters, and the media can also teach empathy, racial and ethnic tolerance, and a whole variety of interpersonal skills.[19] Prosocial media may also influence teenagers. Helping behaviors can increase after listening to prosocial (rather than neutral) song lyrics, and positive information about adolescent health is increasingly available through new media, including YouTube videos and campaigns that incorporate cell phone text messages.[20]

RECOMMENDATIONS FOR PEDIATRICIANS AND OTHER HEALTH CARE PROVIDERS

- Become educated about critical media topics (media use, violence, sex, obesity, substance use, new technology) via continuing medical education programs.

- Ask 2 media questions and provide age-appropriate counseling for families at every well-child visit: How much recreational screen time does your child or teenager consume daily? Is there a TV set or an Internet-connected electronic device (computer, iPad, cell phone) in the child's or teenager's bedroom? In a busy clinic or office, these 2 targeted questions are key. There is considerable evidence that a bedroom TV increases the risk for obesity, substance use, and exposure to sexual content.[1,21–26]

- Take a more detailed media history with children or teenagers who demonstrate aggressive behavior; are overweight or obese; use tobacco, alcohol, or other drugs; or have difficulties in school.

- Examine your own media use habits; pediatricians who watch more TV are less likely to advise families to follow AAP recommendations.[27]

PEDIATRICIANS SHOULD RECOMMEND THE FOLLOWING TO PARENTS

- Limit the amount of total entertainment screen time to <1 to 2 hours per day.

- Discourage screen media exposure for children <2 years of age.

- Keep the TV set and Internet-connected electronic devices out of the child's bedroom.

- Monitor what media their children are using and accessing, including any Web sites they are visiting and social media sites they may be using.

- Coview TV, movies, and videos with children and teenagers, and use this as a way of discussing important family values.

- Model active parenting by establishing a family home use plan for all media. As part of the plan, enforce a mealtime and bedtime "curfew" for media devices, including cell phones. Establish reasonable but firm rules about cell phones, texting, Internet, and social media use.

RECOMMENDATIONS FOR SCHOOLS

Community-based pediatricians, especially those serving in an advisory role to schools, are influential voices in school and neighborhood forums and can work to encourage a team approach among the medical home, the school home, and the family home. So pediatricians, especially those serving as school physicians or school medical advisors should:

- Educate school boards and school administrators about evidence-based health risks associated with unsupervised, unlimited media access and use by children and adolescents, as well as ways to mitigate those risks, such as violence prevention, sex education, and drug use-prevention programs.

- Encourage the continuation and expansion of media education programs, or initiate implementation of media education programs in settings where they are currently lacking.

- Encourage innovative use of technology where it is not already being used, such as online education programs for children with extended but medically justified school absences.

- Work collaboratively with parent-teacher associations to encourage parental guidance in limiting or monitoring age-appropriate screen times. In addition, schools that do use new technology like iPads need to have strict rules about what students can access.

PEDIATRICIANS SHOULD WORK WITH THE AAP AND LOCAL CHAPTERS TO CHALLENGE THE ENTERTAINMENT INDUSTRY TO DO THE FOLLOWING

- Establish an ongoing dialogue with health organizations like the AAP, the American Medical Association, the American Psychological Association, and the American Public Health Association to maximize prosocial content in media and minimize harmful effects (eg, portrayals of smoking, violence, etc).

- Make movies smoke-free, without characters smoking or product placement.[11]

PEDIATRICIANS SHOULD WORK WITH THE AAP AND LOCAL CHAPTERS TO CHALLENGE MANUFACTURERS OF PRODUCTS WITH PUBLIC HEALTH IMPLICATIONS (TOBACCO, ALCOHOL, FOOD) TO DO THE FOLLOWING

- Make socially responsible decisions on marketing products to youth; betterment of their health is the ultimate goal.

PEDIATRICIANS SHOULD WORK WITH THE AAP AND LOCAL CHAPTERS TO CHALLENGE THE FEDERAL GOVERNMENT TO DO THE FOLLOWING

- Advocate for a federal report within either the National Institutes of Health or the Institute of Medicine on the impact of media on children and adolescents that would establish a baseline of what is currently known and what new research needs to be conducted.

- Encourage the entertainment industry and the advertising industry to create more prosocial programming and to reassess the effects of their current programming.

- Issue strong regulations—self-regulation is not likely to work—that would restrict the advertising of junk food and fast food to children and adolescents.

- Establish an ongoing funding mechanism for new media research.

- Initiate legislation and rules that would ban alcohol advertising from television.[11]

- Work with the Department of Education to support the creation and implementation of media education curricula for schoolchildren and teenagers.

LEAD AUTHORS

Victor C. Strasburger, MD, FAAP
Marjorie J. Hogan, MD, FAAP

COUNCIL ON COMMUNICATIONS AND MEDIA EXECUTIVE COMMITTEE, 2013–2014

Deborah Ann Mulligan, MD, FAAP, Chairperson
Nusheen Ameenuddin, MD, MPH, FAAP
Dimitri A. Christakis, MD, MPH, FAAP
Corinn Cross, MD, FAAP
Daniel B. Fagbuyi, MD, FAAP
David L. Hill, MD, FAAP
Marjorie J. Hogan, MD, FAAP
Alanna Estin Levine, MD, FAAP
Claire McCarthy, MD, FAAP
Megan A. Moreno, MD, MSEd, MPH, FAAP
Wendy Sue Lewis Swanson, MD, MBE, FAAP

FORMER EXECUTIVE COMMITTEE MEMBERS

Tanya Remer Altmann, MD, FAAP
Ari Brown, MD, FAAP
Kathleen Clarke-Pearson, MD, FAAP
Holly Lee Falik, MD, FAAP
Gilbert L. Fuld, MD, FAAP, Immediate Past Chairperson
Kathleen G. Nelson, MD, FAAP
Gwenn S. O'Keeffe, MD, FAAP
Victor C. Strasburger, MD, FAAP

LIAISONS

Michael Brody, MD – *American Academy of Child and Adolescent Psychiatry*
Jennifer Pomeranz, JD, MPH – *American Public Health Association*
Brian Wilcox, PhD – *American Psychological Association*

STAFF

Veronica Laude Noland

REFERENCES

1. Rideout V. *Generation M2: Media in the Lives of 8- to 18-Year-Olds.* Menlo Park, CA: Kaiser Family Foundation; 2010

2. Strasburger VC, Jordan AB, Donnerstein E. Health effects of media on children and adolescents. *Pediatrics.* 2010;125(4):756–767

3. Lenhart A. Teens and sexting. Washington, DC: Pew Internet and American Life Project; December 15, 2009. Available at: www.

pewinternet.org/~/media//Files/Reports/2009/PIP_Teens_and_Sexting.pdf. Accessed February 29, 2012

4. Nielsen Company. *Television, Internet and Mobile Usage in the U.S.: A2/M2 Three Screen Report.* New York, NY: Nielsen Company; 2009

5. Lenhart A. *Teens, Smartphones & Texting.* Washington, DC: Pew Internet and American Life Project; March 19, 2012. Available at: http://pewinternet.org/~/media//Files/Reports/2012/PIP_Teens_Smartphones_and_Texting.pdf. Accessed August 26, 2013

6. Lenhart A, Ling R, Campbell S, Purcell K. Teens and mobile phones. Washington, DC: Pew Internet and American Life Project, Pew Research Center; April 20, 2010. Available at: www.pewinternet.org/Reports/2010/Teens-and-Mobile-Phones.aspx. Accessed February 29, 2012

7. O'Keeffe GS, Clarke-Pearson K; Council on Communications and Media. Clinical report: the impact of social media on children, adolescents, and families. *Pediatrics.* 2011;127(4):800–804

8. Rubinstein JS, Meyer DE, Evans JE. Executive control of cognitive processes in task switching. *J Exp Psychol Hum Percept Perform.* 2001;27(4):763–797

9. O'Malley Olsen E, Shults RA, Eaton DK. Texting while driving and other risky motor vehicle behaviors among US high school students. *Pediatrics.* 2013;131(6). Available at: www.pediatrics.org/cgi/content/full/131/6/e1708

10. American Academy of Pediatrics, Council on Communications and Media. Policy statement: sexuality, contraception, and the media. *Pediatrics.* 2010;126(3):576–582

11. American Academy of Pediatrics, Council on Communications and Media. Policy statement: children, adolescents, substance abuse, and the media. *Pediatrics.* 2010;126(4):791–799

12. Van den Bulck J. Adolescent use of mobile phones for calling and for sending text messages after lights out: results from a prospective cohort study with a one-year follow-up. *Sleep.* 2007;30(9):1220–1223

13. National Campaign to Prevent Teen and Unplanned Pregnancy. *Sex and Tech.* Washington, DC: National Campaign to Prevent Teen and Unplanned Pregnancy; 2008

14. American Academy of Pediatrics Council on Communications and Media. Policy statement: media violence. *Pediatrics.* 2009;124(5):1495–1503

15. American Academy of Pediatrics, Council on Communications and Media. Policy statement: impact of music, music lyrics, and music videos on children and youth. *Pediatrics.* 2009;124(5):1488–1494

16. American Academy of Pediatrics, Council on Communications and Media. Policy statement: children, adolescents, obesity, and the media. *Pediatrics.* 2011;128(1):201–208

17. American Academy of Pediatrics, Council on Communications and Media. Policy statement: media use by children younger than 2 years. *Pediatrics.* 2011;128(5):1040–1045

18. American Academy of Pediatrics, Council on Communications and Media. Policy statement: media education. *Pediatrics.* 2010;126(5):1012–1017

19. Hogan MJ, Strasburger VC. Media and prosocial behavior in children and adoles-cents. In: Nucci L, Narvaez D, eds. *Handbook of Moral and Character Education.* Mahwah, NJ: Lawrence Erlbaum; 2008:537–553

20. Hogan MJ. Prosocial effects of media. *Pediatr Clin North Am.* 2012;59(3):635–645

21. Staiano AE, Harrington DM, Broyles ST, Gupta AK, Katzmarzyk PT. Television, adiposity, and cardiometabolic risk in children and adolescents. *Am J Prev Med.* 2013;44(1):40–47

22. Hanewinkel R, Sargent JD. Longitudinal study of exposure to entertainment media and alcohol use among German adolescents. *Pediatrics.* 2009;123(3):989–995

23. Jackson C, Brown JD, Pardun CJ. A TV in the bedroom: implications for viewing habits and risk behaviors during early adolescence. *J Broadcast Electron Media.* 2008;52(3):349–367

24. Adachi-Mejia AM, Longacre MR, Gibson JJ, Beach ML, Titus-Ernstoff LT, Dalton MA. Children with a TV in their bedroom at higher risk for being overweight. *Int J Obes (Lond).* 2007;31(4):644–651

25. Kim JL, Collins RL, Kanouse DE, et al. Sexual readiness, household policies, and other predictors of adolescents' exposure to sexual content in mainstream entertainment television. *Media Psychol.* 2006;8(4):449–471

26. Gruber EL, Want PH, Christensen JS, Grube JW, Fisher DA. Private television viewing, parental supervision, and sexual and substance use risk behaviors in adolescents [abstract]. *J Adolesc Health.* 2005;36(2):107

27. Gentile DA, Oberg C, Sherwood NE, Story M, Walsh DA, Hogan M. Well-child visits in the video age: pediatricians and the American Academy of Pediatrics' guidelines for children's media use. *Pediatrics.* 2004;114(5):1235–1241

Community Pediatrics: Navigating the Intersection of Medicine, Public Health, and Social Determinants of Children's Health

- *Policy Statement*

POLICY STATEMENT

Community Pediatrics: Navigating the Intersection of Medicine, Public Health, and Social Determinants of Children's Health

COUNCIL ON COMMUNITY PEDIATRICS

KEY WORDS

community pediatrics, child advocacy, public health, social determinants of health

www.pediatrics.org/cgi/doi/10.1542/peds.2012-3933

doi:10.1542/peds.2012-3933

PEDIATRICS (ISSN Numbers: Print, 0031-4005; Online, 1098-4275).

abstract

This policy statement provides a framework for the pediatrician's role in promoting the health and well-being of all children in the context of their families and communities. It offers pediatricians a definition of community pediatrics, emphasizes the importance of recognizing social determinants of health, and delineates the need to partner with public health to address population-based child health issues. It also recognizes the importance of pediatric involvement in child advocacy at local, state, and federal levels to ensure all children have access to a high-quality medical home and to eliminate child health disparities. This statement provides a set of specific recommendations that underscore the critical nature of this dimension of pediatric practice, teaching, and research. *Pediatrics* 2013;131:623–628

Environmental and social factors contribute significantly to the health and well-being of children in the contexts of families, schools, and communities. Over the past decade, the Institute of Medicine recognized and quantified the effects of external factors on early brain development and the health of children in 2 seminal reports, *Neurons to Neighborhoods*[1] in 2000 and *Children's Health, the Nation's Wealth*[2] in 2004. As understanding of the mechanisms and impact of biological, behavioral, cultural, social, and physical environments on healthy development deepens and expands, the long-standing role of pediatricians in promoting the physical, mental, and social health and well-being of all children must also evolve.[3] The field of pediatrics must address the problems facing children in the 21st century by influencing these critical determinants of child health and well-being.[4] To do so, pediatricians must successfully merge their traditional clinical skills with public health, population-based approaches to practice, and advocacy.

DEFINITION OF COMMUNITY PEDIATRICS

The American Academy of Pediatrics (AAP) offers a definition of community pediatrics to remind all pediatricians, pediatric medical subspecialists, and pediatric surgical specialists alike of the profound importance of the community dimension in pediatric practice. Community pediatrics is the practice of promoting and integrating the positive social, cultural, and environmental influences on children's health as well as addressing potential negative effects that deter optimal child health and development within a community. Community pediatrics includes all of the following:

- A perspective that expands the pediatrician's focus from one child to the well-being of all children in the community;

- A recognition that family, educational, social, cultural, spiritual, economic, environmental, and political forces affect the health and functioning of children;

- A synthesis of clinical practice and public health principles to promote the health of all children within the context of the family, school, and community[5]; and

- A commitment to collaborate with community partners to advocate for and provide quality services equitably for all children.[6,7]

Participating in community activities to improve the health and welfare of all children is considered an integral part of the professional role and ethical obligation of all pediatricians. For many pediatricians, efforts to promote the health of children have been directed at attending to the needs of particular children in a practice setting, on an individual basis, and providing them with a medical home[8] in concert with pediatricians' own community interests and commitments. Increasingly, however, the major threats to the healthy development of America's children stem from problems that cannot be addressed adequately by the practice model alone.[9] These problems include infant mortality; preventable infectious diseases; dental caries; sedentary lifestyles; chronic health care needs; obesity, metabolic syndrome, and other historically adult-onset chronic diseases; high levels of intentional and unintentional injuries; exposure to violence in

all forms; risks of neurodevelopmental disabilities and illnesses from exposure to environmental tobacco smoke, lead, and other environmental hazards; substance abuse; mental health conditions; poor school readiness[10]; family dysfunction; sexual health, unwanted pregnancies, and sexually transmitted diseases; relatively low rates of breastfeeding; social, medical, behavioral, economic, and environmental effects of disasters[11]; and inequitable access to medical homes[12] and basic material resources and poverty.[13] Whether the pediatrician is communicating with patients and families or with a community, it is critical to remember that this must be done in a culturally and linguistically effective manner to be successful. On the part of pediatricians, culturally effective communication includes behaviors and attitudes that are appropriate to care for patients and families with a wide variety of cultural attributes.

SOCIAL DETERMINANTS OF HEALTH

In the past decade, increasing attention has been paid toward recognizing the social determinants of children's physical, mental, and behavioral health. Briefly, social determinants are the economic and social conditions that shape the health of individuals and communities. In 2005, the World Health Organization established a Commission on the Social Determinants of Health to examine the evidence of the effects of social determinants on health outcomes, specifically for the purpose of promoting health equity globally. With the description of the life course health development model[14] and the recognition of the life course health development perspective by agencies serving children and families, including the US Maternal and Child Health Bureau, the effects of poor social and economic factors in childhood on the quality of adult health have become increasingly clear. For example,

authors of studies have examined the link between childhood obesity and cardiovascular disease in adulthood, lack of adequate calcium and vitamin D intake in childhood on adult osteoporosis, and childhood maltreatment and family dysfunction on adult mental and physical health problems.[13,15,16]

Childhood obesity, dental caries, asthma, and early mental health issues are prevalent in today's child population and interact reciprocally with family dysfunction or school stress. Pediatricians must have the knowledge, skills, and willingness to address these issues in addition to more traditional clinical solutions. An integral approach to doing so incorporates interdisciplinary practice. As former AAP president Robert Haggerty, MD, reminded us in 1995, "we must become partners with others, or we will become increasingly irrelevant to the health of children."[17] Pediatricians should recognize that health care is merely 1 influential component of overall health and well-being for children and families, and children often move through other systems, such as education, child welfare, mental health/social services, and juvenile justice. Interdisciplinary communication and coordination are crucial for successfully addressing all factors that contribute to a child's health and well-being.

THE NATURAL AND BUILT ENVIRONMENTS

The physical environment is an important part of a community. Health hazards from toxic environmental exposures (such as mold, heavy metals, and fluorocarbons) are routinely recognized and brought to the attention of pediatricians. Less consideration has been given to the potential for adverse effects on health from "built environments," such as poor-quality housing, lack of access to opportunities for safe gross motor play, inadequate transportation, especially for children with limited mobility, and lack of coordinated community planning, although awareness has grown over the past decade of the effects of the built environment on the childhood obesity epidemic.[18] Accessible housing and transportation options that meet the needs of all children and families, including those with mobility, sensory, and health impairments, to travel safely and making all community and leisure environments accessible to all children, especially those with special needs, has the potential to decrease the risk of obesity and metabolic syndrome.

Because the design of a child's physical environment can cause or prevent illness or injury, a high-quality environment is essential for children to achieve optimal health and development. Community planning and building and land-use policies can either undermine or promote safety, health, and optimal development while simultaneously preserving future resources. Children in low-income families are more likely to be exposed to structural hazards in the home and are more likely to have diseases such as lead poisoning and asthma. Although environmental risks are more prevalent in low-income families, children from any income level may be exposed. For all children, examining the quality of a child's physical environment is crucial when assessing children's health. Pediatrician advocates are needed to speak out for children's needs in the physical environment.

PARTNERING WITH PUBLIC HEALTH

One could argue that pediatricians have always been a part of the public health system. As trusted sources of information for parents and front-line providers of preventive health care for children, pediatricians have fulfilled

the role of addressing the needs of populations of children, whether they are in an early education and child care setting, school, or local community. Pediatricians often contribute to the public health system by recognizing and reporting illnesses, hazards, and trends to public health departments.

Because of this responsibility, pediatricians should know where to get accurate information regarding the latest public and school health issues facing children in their communities, as well as how to communicate this information effectively either individually to families or to groups in public forums or through the media. The Institute of Medicine has recently provided a framework for primary care and public health professions to work together.[19] Pediatricians should partner with local health departments and school districts and child welfare agencies to be aware of programs for children and families that address certain needs, such as injury prevention, child maltreatment prevention, lead poisoning, environmental tobacco smoke control, breastfeeding promotion, overweight/obesity prevention, asthma, perinatal care, trauma, child abuse prevention, and disaster preparedness.[20–23] One example of a pediatric/public health approach would be to ensure that children's issues are addressed in disaster planning/response.

LOCAL, STATE, AND FEDERAL ADVOCACY

The passage of the Patient Protection and Affordable Care Act in 2010 was a milestone in health care in the United States that could not have been achieved without advocacy on multiple levels by many groups of people, including pediatricians. Pediatricians have always advocated on behalf of the nation's youngest citizens, whether on

the individual level for necessary services or more widely at the community, state, or federal level in legislative avenues. Because children do not have a voice in government, others must speak up on behalf of the nation's most vulnerable population of citizens.

In recent years, pediatric medical education has promoted the formal training of residents in legislative advocacy. The AAP Community Pediatrics Training Initiative has developed advocacy training modules for use in pediatric residency training programs and is supporting individual programs to implement advocacy rotations in their curricula. Statewide collaboratives, such as in California and more recently in New Jersey, have been established to serve as networks for residency programs to share advocacy curricula and support implementation of new curricular experiences in legislative advocacy. These efforts are in direct response to the recognition that, to influence policies and laws affecting children and families, pediatricians need specialized skill sets to be effective advocates on multiple levels.

With the passage of the 2010 Patient Protection and Affordable Care Act, pediatric leadership and advocacy will be crucial to ensure some just reward for the activities described in this policy statement. To counter the growing financial and productivity pressures on practicing pediatricians, some recognition of the importance of addressing the social determinants of children's health will be necessary in the financing models for accountable care organizations.[24]

RECOMMENDATIONS

With the shifting epidemiology of problems facing children and growing recognition that social determinants play a major role in children's health, pediatricians must have a second "bag of tools" in addition to the clinical "doctor's bag" that addresses more traditional agents of childhood disease. This second bag of tools includes skills such as being able to function in an interdisciplinary fashion; partnering with public health and child welfare entities; recognizing root sources of health and pathology from children's social, economic, physical, and educational environments; and advocating on multiple levels. The following recommendations offer guidelines for pediatricians to optimize their effectiveness as clinical practitioners and advocates in the community. To accomplish these recommendations, payment and financing systems must be appropriately aligned and recognize clinicians who provide population-based prevention.[25]

1. Pediatricians should use community data (epidemiologic, demographic, and economic) to increase their understanding of the effects that social determinants have on child health outcomes.

2. Pediatricians should work together with public health departments, school districts,[21–23] child welfare agencies, community and children's hospitals, and colleagues in related professions to identify and decrease barriers to the health and well-being of children in the communities they serve.[26,27] In addition, pediatricians should have access to information about community programs and resources that could affect the health and well-being of the children in their community.

3. Pediatricians should routinely, and in a culturally effective manner, promote preventive health strategies for common childhood issues (ie, immunization, injury prevention, oral health, sexual health, nutrition, obesity prevention, breastfeeding, positive parenting, and abuse and neglect) in both individual well-child visits as well as on a population level within a community. Pediatricians can play an important role in coordinating and focusing new and existing services to realize maximum benefit for all children.[28,29]

4. Pediatricians and other members of the community should interact with and advocate to improve all settings and organizations in which children spend time (eg, early education and child care facilities, schools, school-based health centers, family support and resource centers, youth programs, recreation venues, and transportation systems). Together with families, schools and community resources should be considered as primary assets in promoting children's health, safety, and development.

5. Pediatricians should advocate for universal access to health care in a medical home and for the social, economic, educational, and environmental resources essential for every child's healthy development, including those in foster care who may have no other natural advocates.

6. Pediatricians should be able to interface with the media and be able to be trusted sources of information for parents and the general public about public health issues pertaining to children, such as vaccine safety and emergency/disaster/crisis medical issues.

7. Pediatric medical education (both undergraduate and graduate) should include specific curricula on community and public health topics pertaining to child health, including social determinants of health, how to identify and access community resources, school

health, health care systems and financing, and child advocacy, including interactions with the public child welfare system and legislative advocacy skills.

8. Continuing medical education programs should consider and periodically review basic community pediatric competencies to be included in maintenance of certification efforts for pediatricians.[30] Maintenance of certification and quality improvement activities should include options to address child health issues in community settings.

9. AAP chapters and their members should provide leadership for further understanding of community pediatrics and encourage participation in creative, community-based, integrated models such as those supported through the Community Access to Child Health program and the Healthy Tomorrows Partnership for Children program.

10. The AAP is committed to continued recognition and provision of leadership and support to pediatricians to develop and exercise advocacy skills at the local, state, and national levels to ensure that children have access to care, to resources, and to conditions that promote healthy development. This includes support for the following:

- Federal and state programs that reduce the burden of debt on medical students in pediatric primary care and pediatric medical subspecialty and surgical specialty fellowships, including but not limited to the National Health Service Corps.

- Incorporation into the curricula for residency programs and for young physicians' discussion of different strategies for engaging in community activities no matter the practice setting.

- Expectation of community engagement as an explicit part of comprehensive clinical payment models currently under development, including the patient-centered medical home and accountable care organizations.

11. The AAP is committed to continuing to strategically address the lack of payment for the work pediatricians do in the community, which addresses social determinants of health and population-based health issues, much of which is currently uncompensated. Not only should these services be recognized as a crucial part of child health, but also, payment for these services should be at a reasonable and fair level so that pediatricians can afford to pursue these activities in their communities.

By caring for children in the context of their families and communities, pediatricians play an important role in promoting the health and well-being of the nation's youngest citizens. Pediatricians who work with schools, early education and child care programs, community agencies and organizations, and local public health departments and child welfare agencies equip themselves to be effective child advocates in the community. Pediatricians can also play a crucial role in public health by communicating important facts about issues facing children's health; ensuring children's issues are addressed in disaster planning and response efforts[11]; and advocating at the local, state, and federal legislative levels for universal access for all children to high-quality medical homes and for social policies that promote equal opportunities for the development of children, families, and communities. The recommendations in this policy statement are meant to provide a framework for guiding the development of relevant curricula in pediatric medical education and supporting the practice of high-quality and effective pediatric care.

LEAD AUTHORS

Peter A. Gorski, MD, MPA
Alice A. Kuo, MD, PhD

COUNCIL ON COMMUNITY PEDIATRICS, 2011–2012

Deise C. Granado-Villar, MD, MPH, Chairperson
Benjamin A. Gitterman, MD, Vice Chairperson
Jeffrey M. Brown, MD, MPH
Lance A. Chilton, MD
William H. Cotton, MD
Thresia B. Gambon, MD
Peter A. Gorski, MD, MPA
Colleen A. Kraft, MD
Alice A. Kuo, MD, PhD
Gonzalo J. Paz-Soldan, MD
Barbara Zind, MD

LIAISONS

Benjamin Hoffman, MD – *Chairperson, Indian Health Special Interest Group*
Melissa A. Briggs, MD – *Section on Medical Students, Residents, and Fellowship Trainees*
Frances J. Dunston, MD, MPH
Charles R. Feild, MD, MPH – *Chairperson, Prevention and Public Health Special Interest Group*
M. Edward Ivancic, MD – *Chairperson, Rural Health Special Interest Group*
David M. Keller, MD – *Chairperson, Community Pediatrics Education and Training Special Interest Group*

STAFF

Regina M. Shaefer, MPH

REFERENCES

1. Institute of Medicine, Committee on Integrating the Science of Early Childhood Development. In: Shonkoff JP, Phillips DA, eds. *From Neurons to Neighborhoods: The Science of Early Childhood Programs.* Washington, DC: National Academies Press; 2000

2. National Research Council and Institute of Medicine, Committee on Evaluation of Children's Health. *Children's Health, the Nation's Wealth: Assessing and Improving Child Health.* Washington, DC: National Academies Press; 2004

3. Garner AS, Shonkoff JP; Committee on Psychosocial Aspects of Child and Family Health; Committee on Early Childhood, Adoption, and Dependent Care; Section on Developmental and Behavioral Pediatrics. Early childhood adversity, toxic stress, and the role of the pediatrician: translating developmental science into lifelong health. *Pediatrics.* 2012;129(1). Available at: www.pediatrics.org/cgi/content/full/129/1/e224

4. Starmer AJ, Duby JC, Slaw KM, Edwards A, Leslie LK; Members of Vision of Pediatrics 2020 Task Force. Pediatrics in the year 2020 and beyond: preparing for plausible futures. *Pediatrics.* 2010;126(5):971–981

5. Haggerty RJ. Community pediatrics. *N Engl J Med.* 1968;278(1):15–21

6. Gruen RL, Pearson SD, Brennan TA. Physician-citizens—public roles and professional obligations. *JAMA.* 2004;291(1):94–98

7. Oberg CN. Pediatric advocacy: yesterday, today, and tomorrow. *Pediatrics.* 2003;112(2):406–409

8. American Academy of Pediatrics, Medical Home Initiatives for Children With Special Needs Project Advisory Committee. The medical home. *Pediatrics.* 2002;110(1 pt 1):184–186

9. Nazarian LF. A look at the private practice of the future. *Pediatrics.* 1995;96(4 pt 2):812–816

10. Dworkin PH. Ready to learn: a mandate for pediatrics. *J Dev Behav Pediatr.* 1993;14(3):192–196

11. National Commission on Children and Disasters. 2010 Report to the President and Congress. Available at: http://archive.ahrq.gov/prep/nccdreport/. Accessed October 12, 2011

12. Sia CC. Abraham Jacobi Award address, April 14, 1992 the medical home: pediatric practice and child advocacy in the 1990s. *Pediatrics.* 1992;90(3):419–423

13. Conroy K, Sandel M, Zuckerman B. Poverty grown up: how childhood socioeconomic status impacts adult health. *J Dev Behav Pediatr.* 2010;31(2):154–160

14. Halfon N, Hochstein M. Life course health development: an integrated framework for

developing health, policy, and research. *Milbank Q.* 2002;80(3):433–479, iii

15. Shonkoff JP, Boyce WT, McEwen BS. Neuroscience, molecular biology, and the childhood roots of health disparities: building a new framework for health promotion and disease prevention. *JAMA.* 2009;301(21):2252–2259

16. Felitti VJ, Anda RF, Nordenberg D, et al. Relationship of childhood abuse and household dysfunction to many of the leading causes of death in adults. The Adverse Childhood Experiences (ACE) Study. *Am J Prev Med.* 1998;14(4):245–258

17. Haggerty RJ. Child health 2000: new pediatrics in the changing environment of children's needs in the 21st century. *Pediatrics.* 1995;96(4 pt 2):804–812

18. Tester JM; Committee on Environmental Health. The built environment: designing communities to promote physical activity in children. *Pediatrics.* 2009;123(6):1591–1598

19. Institute of Medicine. *Primary Care and Public Health: Exploring Integration to Improve Population Health.* Washington, DC: National Academies Press; 2012

20. Magalnick H, Mazyck D; American Academy of Pediatrics Council on School Health. Role of the school nurse in providing school health services. *Pediatrics.* 2008;121(5):1052–1056

21. Nader P. A pediatrician's primer for school health activities. *Pediatr Rev.* 1982;4(3):82–92

22. Sicherer SH, Mahr T; American Academy of Pediatrics Section on Allergy and Immunology. Management of food allergy in the school setting. *Pediatrics.* 2010;126(6):1232–1239

23. Wheeler L, Buckley R, Gerald LB, Merkle S, Morrison TA. Working with schools to improve pediatric asthma management. *Pediatr Asthma Allergy Immunol.* 2009;22(4):197–208

24. Accountable Care Organization Work Group. Accountable care organizations (ACOs) and pediatricians: evaluation and engagement. *AAP News.* 2011;32(1):1

25. Libby R; Committee on Child Health Financing American Academy of Pediatrics. Principles of health care financing. *Pediatrics.* 2010;126(5):1018–1021

26. Werlieb D; American Academy of Pediatrics, Task Force on the Family. Converging trends in family research and pediatrics: recent findings for the American Academy of Pediatrics Task Force on the Family. *Pediatrics.* 2003;111(6 pt 2):1572–1587

27. Jacobi A. The best means of combating infant mortality. *JAMA.* 1912;58:1735–1744

28. Haggerty RJ. Community pediatrics: past and present. *Pediatr Ann.* 1994;23(12):657–658, 661–663

29. Zuckerman B, Parker S. Preventive pediatrics—new models of providing needed health services. *Pediatrics.* 1995;95(5):758–762

30. Mullan F. Sounding board. Community-oriented primary care: an agenda for the '80s. *N Engl J Med.* 1982;307(17):1076–1078

Condom Use by Adolescents

- *Policy Statement*

POLICY STATEMENT

Condom Use by Adolescents

COMMITTEE ON ADOLESCENCE

ABBREVIATIONS
CDC—Centers for Disease Control and Prevention
FC—female condom
FDA—Food and Drug Administration
HIV—human immunodeficiency virus
HPV—human papillomavirus
MSM—men who have sex with men
STI—sexually transmitted infection
YRBS—Youth Risk Behavior Survey

www.pediatrics.org/cgi/doi/10.1542/peds.2013-2821

doi:10.1542/peds.2013-2821

PEDIATRICS (ISSN Numbers: Print, 0031-4005; Online, 1098-4275).

Copyright © 2013 by the American Academy of Pediatrics

abstract

Rates of sexual activity, pregnancies, and births among adolescents have continued to decline during the past decade to historic lows. Despite these positive trends, many adolescents remain at risk for unintended pregnancy and sexually transmitted infections (STIs). This policy statement has been developed to assist the pediatrician in understanding and supporting the use of condoms by their patients to prevent unintended pregnancies and STIs and address barriers to their use. When used consistently and correctly, male latex condoms reduce the risk of pregnancy and many STIs, including HIV. Since the last policy statement published 12 years ago, there is an increased evidence base supporting the protection provided by condoms against STIs. Rates of acquisition of STIs/HIV among adolescents remain unacceptably high. Interventions that increase availability or accessibility to condoms are most efficacious when combined with additional individual, small-group, or community-level activities that include messages about safer sex. Continued research is needed to inform public health interventions for adolescents that increase the consistent and correct use of condoms and promote dual protection of condoms for STI prevention with other effective methods of contraception. *Pediatrics* 2013;132:973–981

INTRODUCTION

This policy statement updates a previous statement from the American Academy of Pediatrics published in 2001.[1] The medical and societal consequences of adolescent sexual activity, including sexually transmitted infections (STIs) and unintended pregnancies, remain a significant public health problem. Although abstinence of sexual activity is the most effective method for prevention of pregnancy and STIs, young people should be prepared for the time when they will become sexually active. Prevention of STIs in adolescents involves safer sexual practices by those who are sexually active or who no longer plan to be abstinent. Since publication of the previous statement, there has been increasing evidence supporting the effectiveness of condoms to prevent many STIs, including HIV. Increased availability of condoms has been shown to increase use, and widespread distribution programs have been recommended by the Centers for Disease Control and Prevention (CDC).[2]

In this policy statement, the use of condoms as a method of preventing STIs, including HIV and pregnancy will be reviewed including effectiveness, factors that influence use, and the roles that schools, communities, and parents can play in improving use of condoms and increased availability of condoms.

TRENDS IN ADOLESCENT SEXUAL ACTIVITY AND CONSEQUENCES

Despite recent data indicating that sexual activity has declined among adolescents, the current rates of sexual activity and health consequences of STIs and pregnancy remain a significant public health concern. The CDC, through its Youth Risk Behavior Survey (YRBS), reports sexual risk behaviors in a nationally representative sample of high school students surveyed biannually. In the most recently available YRBS (2011), 47.4% of students reported that they had ever had sexual intercourse, 33.7% reported that they were currently sexually active, and 15.3% had had sexual intercourse with four or more partners in their lifetime. Among sexually active students, 60.2% reported condom use during their last sexual encounter. Of additional concern, by 12th grade, nearly two-thirds (63.1%) of students reported ever being sexually active but reported lower use of condoms than did sexually active 9th- and 10th-graders.[3]

In 2011, approximately 330 000 teenagers gave birth,[4] and in 2008, the most recently available estimates are that 750 000 teenagers became pregnant.[5] Despite the fact that US teen birth rates are at the lowest level in the past 70 years,[6] the birth rate for US teenagers remains higher than other developed nations, and marked disparities by race/ethnicity and geographic area persist.[7]

Rates of STIs remain highest among adolescents and young adults, with estimates suggesting that 15- to 24-year-olds, who represent 25% of the sexually experienced population, acquire nearly half of all new STIs.[8] Rates of Chlamydia, gonorrhea, and syphilis

have all continued to increase in adolescent and young adults.[9] A study that examined the prevalence of STIs among female adolescents 14 to 19 years of age in the United States from the 2003–2004 NHANES reported a 24.1% prevalence of any of 5 STIs (Neisseria gonorrhea, Chlamydia trachomatis, Trichomonas vaginalis, herpes simplex virus type 2, and human papilloma virus [HPV] infections) among all female adolescents and a prevalence of 37.7% among sexually experienced females. Importantly, even among those whose sexual partner was the same age or 1 year older, the prevalence was high (25.6%), and among those with only 1 lifetime partner, the prevalence was 19.7%.[10]

For specific infections, in 2011 the highest Chlamydia rates were seen in 15- to 19-year-old (3.4%) and 20- to 24-year-old women (3.7%). Of concern, during 2010–2011, rates increased 4% for those aged 15 to 19 years and 11% for those aged 20 to 24 years. Reported rates of Chlamydia are lower among young men, likely because of decreased screening efforts, but have increased 6% for those 15 to 19 years of age and 12% for those 20 to 24 years of age between 2010 and 2011. In studies of higher-risk populations (for example, the National Job Training Program, an educational program for disadvantaged youth) at entry, rates of Chlamydia for women and men 16 to 24 years of age were 10.3% and 8%, respectively. Similarly, in juvenile correctional facilities, 13.5% of women and 6.5% of men screened positively for Chlamydia.[9]

Adolescent and young adult women also have the highest rates of gonorrhea compared with any other age and gender group and increased 1.4% in 15- to 19-year-old women during 2009–2010 (unchanged in 2011), and increased 5.4% in 20- to 24-year-old

women during 2010–2011. Adolescent and young adult men have also had increasing rates of gonorrhea, increasing 6% in those aged 20 to 24 years during 2010–2011.[9]

Syphilis rates in both men and women are highest in the 15- to 24-year old age group and increased most dramatically during 2010–2011 in 20- to 24-year-old men (5.2–21.9 cases/100 000), particularly in men who have sex with men (MSM).[9]

An estimated 10 065 young people aged 13 to 24 years received a diagnosis of HIV infection in 2011, accounting for 20% of all new infections in the United States. Among adolescent/young adult males living with and diagnosed with HIV, 77% acquired infection from MSM, 4% from heterosexual transmission, and 13% were perinatally acquired. Among females, 56% acquired infection by heterosexual transmission, and 34% were perinatally acquired.[11,12] Anonymous HIV screening in locations where youth 12 to 24 years of age congregate in communities surrounding the Adolescent Trials Network for HIV/AIDS interventions found a prevalence of HIV of 15.3% in 611 MSM tested, 60% of whom did not know they were infected.[13] In addition to patients with behaviorally acquired HIV infections, an estimated 9038 people with perinatally acquired HIV are now in adolescence and young adulthood. These youth are generally receiving highly active antiretroviral therapy, and concern exists for extensive drug-resistant strains.[14] In a prospective cohort study of the reproductive health of sexually active adolescent girls perinatally infected with HIV, the cumulative incidence of pregnancy at 19 years of age was 24%, and incidence of STIs was 26%, stressing the need for comprehensive HIV/STI-prevention strategies.[15]

CONDOM USE

Recent Trends in Adolescent Condom Use

The condom remains the most popularly used contraceptive method among teenagers.[3] An increased proportion of sexually active adolescents report using a condom at last intercourse, according to 2 CDC surveys. In the YRBS, condom use increased from 46.2% in 1991 to 60.2% in 2011.[3] The prevalence of condom use was higher among male (68.6%) than female (53.9%) students and higher among white (63.3%) and African American (62.4%) than Hispanic students (54.9%).[3] In the National Survey of Family Growth, condom use at last intercourse increased among females from 31% in 1988 to 52% in 2006–2010 and males from 53% to 75%.[16] Rates of actual condom use in both surveys may also be lower than thought because of the uncertain/questionable validity of self-report of this and other sexual behaviors that are prone to bias. For example, in a clinic-based sample of African American females 15 to 21 years of age in Atlanta, Georgia, 186 young women reported 100% condom use via an audio computer-assisted self-interviewing technique. In these young women, 34% had a positive biologic marker for unprotected vaginal sex in the past 14 days (a Y-chromosome polymerase chain reaction assay). As a possible explanation of these findings, condoms may have been used inconsistently or incorrectly, or youth might have provided socially desirable answers.[17]

Factors That Influence Condom Use

A number of factors, including individual, family, sociodemographic, attitude, education, relationship, and partner-related factors, influence condom use. For example, in a national study of adolescent males,[18] factors associated with greater consistency of condom use included African American race/ethnicity, more positive condom attitudes, and more discussion of health topics with parents. Adolescents who did not have formal sex education were half as likely to use a condom at first intercourse and even less likely to use condoms consistently. Lower condom use at first sex was associated with older age, an older or casual first sexual partner, and a partner using another method of contraception. These factors were also associated with lower condom use at last sex, except for having a casual sexual partner, which was associated with higher condom use.[18]

Higher rates of condom use are noted in youth who perceive their partners as wanting to use condoms and in those able to communicate their desire to use condoms with their partners.[19] Motivations for young people to have sex include the pursuit of fulfilling sexual experiences in addition to other motivations such as intimacy, procreation, or in response to peer or partner pressure. However, adolescents' lack of condom use is associated with perceptions that condoms reduce sexual pleasure and/or that partners disapprove of condom use.[20] Condom-promotion campaigns that include linking condom use to enhanced sensitivity and sensuality, and, thus, a more positive experience as a motivating factor, have found increased uptake of condoms and safer sex behaviors.[21–23]

The influence of social networks that encourage condom use is becoming increasingly recognized.[24,25] However, increased relationship intimacy and closeness to the partner's family can be associated with less condom use.[26] Condom use rates are higher in new relationships compared with established relationships.[27] Other factors associated with increased condom use include receiving comprehensive sex and HIV education programs,[28] attending schools where condoms are available,[29] and perceiving a risk of STIs.[30]

The effect of the media on adolescent sexual behavior has been reviewed in a recent American Academy of Pediatrics policy statement.[31] Adolescents are exposed to an increasing amount of sexual content in music, movies, magazines, television, and the Internet, and this exposure plays an important role in adolescent initiation of sexual activity. Despite the increasingly sexually explicit material in media and programming, there are rare messages promoting responsible sexual activity, such as contraception, including condom use.[31] On primetime television, 77% of programs have sexual content but only 14% reference risks or responsibility of sexual behavior.[32]

Adults, especially parents, play an important role in promoting the sexual health of adolescents. Bright Futures outlines how pediatricians and other health care providers can support parents in promoting healthy sexual development and sexuality, including the use of condoms to protect against STIs including HIV.[33] A number of studies have examined the role of parent-adolescent communication about sexual risk and association with increased adolescent use of condoms.[34–38] Parental communication about sexual risk and condom use are associated with increases in adolescents' use of condoms.[34–36,38] Timing of the discussion is important; in 1 study, the highest rates of condom use at first and last sex, as well as for regular use, were found among adolescent girls who communicated with their mothers about condom use before onset of sexual activity compared with after initiation.[34] In a recent longitudinal study of parents and their children regarding the timing of parent and child communication about sexual behaviors, more than 40% of the children had intercourse before there were discussions about STI symptoms, condom use, birth control, or partner condom refusal.[39] This suggests increased efforts are needed by pediatricians, educators, and those in public health to encourage parents to talk about these issues.

In a large study of African American and Puerto Rican teens aged 14 to 17 years, separate face-to-face interviews were conducted with 907 mother-adolescent pairs to examine factors that predicted mother-adolescent discussions about condoms. Those mothers who communicated effectively about condoms had greater knowledge of sexuality and HIV, perceived that they had enough information to discuss condoms, had received information from a health-related source, were comfortable in discussing condoms and sexuality, and believed that condom use prevents HIV. The implication for pediatricians is that providing parents with accurate information about adolescent sexual behavior, risks, and use and effectiveness of condoms can improve communication with their adolescents.[40]

Other opportunities for parents to become comfortable speaking with their adolescents about sexual health was demonstrated in a novel work site–based trial. In weekly small-group sessions, parent training with a standardized prevention curriculum, designed to help parents of 11- to 16-year-old children communicate about sexual health, found significant differences compared with a control group in discussions of these topics, including condom education. At baseline, 4% of adolescents reported that a parent had discussed with them how to use a condom, and by the 9-month follow-up survey, 36% reported receipt of instruction.[41]

EFFECTIVENESS OF CONDOM USE

Materials used for male condoms are of 3 types: most (>80%) are composed of latex (natural rubber), and a small proportion (<5%) are natural membrane (lamb cecum) or synthetic (eg, polyurethane; approximately 15%).[42] Only latex and synthetic condoms are recommended for prevention of STIs and HIV because natural membrane condoms contain small pores that may allow passage of viruses, including HIV, hepatitis B virus, and herpes simplex virus.[43,44] Synthetic condoms, when compared with latex condoms, are generally more resistant to deterioration and are compatible with both oil- and water-based lubricants. Synthetic condoms have similar failure rates to latex condoms in prevention of pregnancy.[45] Although not extensively studied, synthetic condoms are believed to provide STI protection similar to male latex condoms; however, US Food and Drug Administration (FDA) labeling currently restricts their recommended use for latex-sensitive or -allergic people.[42,45] Condoms lubricated with the spermicide nonoxynol-9 are no longer recommended, because they have a shorter shelf life, increased cost, and lack of added benefit compared with other lubricated condoms[46] and may increase likelihood of HIV transmission as a result of increased genital mucosal irritation.[47] In the United States, condoms are regulated as medical devices by the FDA, and stringent manufacturing standards exist such that each condom is tested for holes or weak spots before sale.[48]

Condoms can be highly effective against unintended pregnancy when used consistently and correctly. Method failure of the male condom for unintended pregnancy is estimated to be 2% in 12 months of use (ie, 2 pregnancies per 100 woman-years with perfect use), although with typical use, the failure rate (accounting for inconsistent and incorrect use) is 18%.[49] The most important non-contraceptive benefit of condom use is the additional protection against acquisition and transmission of STIs, including HIV. Evidence supporting the protection provided by condoms against acquisition of most STIs, including HIV, has increased markedly over the past decade.[50] If placed on the penis before genital contact and used throughout intercourse, condoms should prevent contact with semen, genital lesions, and infectious discharges in both males and females. Condoms greatly reduce the risk of STIs that are transmitted to or from the penile urethra, including gonorrhea, Chlamydia, trichomoniasis, hepatitis B virus, and HIV. Condoms also provide protection against STIs transmitted via skin-to-skin contact or contact with mucosal surfaces, including genital herpes simplex virus, HPV, syphilis, and chancroid in those affected areas covered by the condom.[51–54] Passage of the smallest sexually transmitted pathogen, hepatitis B virus, is effectively blocked by latex condoms, according to in vitro studies.[55–59] Most of the studies on condom effectiveness evaluate vaginal penile sexual activity. Latex and synthetic condoms also can be used during anogenital and orogenital intercourse to reduce the risk of STI.[42]

Well-designed epidemiologic studies and those of discordant couples have shown that condoms are highly effective against heterosexual transmission of HIV infection.[60] The most recent Cochrane review estimated the effectiveness of condom use at 80%.[61] Inconsistency of the estimates of the effectiveness of condoms against other STIs can be attributed to limitations in study design, because the quality of studies historically tended to be weaker than for studies of HIV.[54] Recent studies have empirically documented that the effectiveness of condom use against many STIs is underestimated because of limitations of study design.[62–68] Even with these limitations, these and more recent studies with improved methodologies have found that condoms provide protection against a variety of STIs, including gonorrhea, *Chlamydia*, trichomoniasis, genital herpes, and HPV.[53,54,65,69–74]

Given the coital-dependent nature of condoms, effectiveness against both unintended pregnancy and STIs is closely tied to the degree of consistency or correctness of use. Factors associated with decreased condom effectiveness include failure to use a condom with every act of intercourse; failure to use condoms throughout intercourse, such as placing condoms on after initiating intercourse or removing before ejaculation; condom breakage and slippage; and improper lubricant use with latex condoms (oil-based lubricants, such as petroleum jelly, baby oil, hand lotions, and some vaginal medications), which can reduce condom integrity and may result in breakage.[51]

Five key condom instructions reached by consensus at a World Health Organization Experts Meeting[51] are as follows:

1. Use a new condom for each act of sexual intercourse.

2. Before any genital contact, place the condom on the tip of the erect penis with the rolled side out.

3. Unroll the condom all the way to the base of the erect penis.

4. Immediately after ejaculation, hold the rim of the condom and withdraw the penis while it is still erect.

5. Throw away the used condom safely.

FEMALE CONDOM

The female condom 1 (FC1; Reality, Femy, Care Contraceptive Sheath, Femidom), a loose-fitting polyurethane sheath with 2 flexible polyurethane rings, introduced in 1994, was the first condom marketed to women but is no longer in production in the United States. The FC2 (similarly designed to the FC1 but made of nitrile and without a seam) was approved for use in 2009 by the US FDA and is the only female-initiated barrier method for STI prevention currently available in the United States. Data regarding contraceptive effectiveness of female condoms suggest estimated rates of pregnancy during the first 12 months of perfect use and typical use for FC1 were 5% and 21%; these pregnancy rates are slightly higher than those associated with use of the male condom.[75]

Although laboratory and clinical studies suggest that the female condom might be as effective as the male condom in preventing STIs, data are much more limited. Continued research is needed to evaluate the effectiveness and acceptability of female condoms, which currently account for less than 1% of US condom use overall.[75,76]

DUAL PROTECTION

Hormonal contraceptives and intrauterine devices offer pregnancy protection but no protection against STIs. Use of "dual methods" (the combined use of condoms and hormonal contraceptives or an intrauterine device) may be the optimal approach for protection against both pregnancy and STIs for adolescents. Although dual method use has been increasing over time, studies find that fewer than 25% of adolescents use dual methods[77–79] According to data from the National Survey of Family Growth, condom use is lower in women who use "highly effective user-independent methods of contraception" defined as injectables, intrauterine devices, and implants, even lower than those who use oral contraceptives.[80]

Adolescents with main and regular partners tend to discontinue condom use quickly, especially if other pregnancy prevention methods are used.[27] Studies that have examined dual method use among adolescents have found that increased use is associated with perceived risks of pregnancy and STIs, communication with parents about sexual risk, parental approval of birth control, positive attitudes toward condoms, increased use with casual partners versus main partners, partner support for condom use, and self-efficacy of condom negotiation.[77,78,81–84] In 1 clinic-based study of African American and Hispanic female adolescents who received counseling and watched a video incorporating themes of condom use and nonuse, researchers found that at 3-month follow-up, those who had the intervention were more than twice as likely to have used a condom at last intercourse than in the usual care group. However, differences did not persist at the 12-month follow-up.[85]

EFFORTS AIMED AT INCREASING CONDOM USE

Eighty-three studies of curriculum-based sex- and HIV-education programs among people younger than 25 years from all countries were reviewed, finding that two-thirds of the programs significantly improved one or more sexual behaviors. Of the 54 studies that evaluated effects on condom use, nearly half (48%) demonstrated an increase in condom use, and no studies found decreased condom use. Concern that these programs might hasten the initiation of sex appears unfounded. In the 52 studies that measured timing of initiation of sex, 42% found that sexual initiation was significantly delayed for at least 6 months, and 55% found no effect.[28]

Condom availability programs have been evaluated in a variety of settings. In a study of programs in Massachusetts high schools, adolescents in schools where condoms were available were more likely to receive condom use instruction and less likely to report lifetime or recent sexual intercourse, and adolescents who were sexually active were twice as likely to use condoms at most recent sexual encounter.[29] Likewise, clinic-based interventions have been shown to be effective in increasing condom use and decreasing STIs.[86,87] Clinic-based safer sex interventions are endorsed by the CDC.[88]

A recent meta-analysis of high-quality US and international studies of structural-level condom distribution interventions found significant effects on increased condom use, condom acquisition, condom carrying, delayed sexual initiation of youth, and reduced incidence of STIs. The interventions that increase availability or accessibility to condoms are most efficacious when combined with additional individual, small-group, or community-level activities. The intervention effects were significant across target participant characteristics (youth, adults, commercial sex workers, STI clinic populations, or males).[89]

RECOMMENDATIONS

1. Abstaining from sexual intercourse should be encouraged for adolescents as the most effective way to prevent STIs, including HIV infection, and unintended pregnancy.

2. Pediatricians and other clinicians should actively support and encourage the consistent and correct use of condoms as well as other reliable contraception as part of anticipatory guidance with adolescents

who are sexually active or contemplating sexual activity. The responsibility of males as well as females in preventing unintended pregnancies and STIs should be emphasized.

3. Pediatricians and other clinicians are encouraged to implement the recommendations in Bright Futures promoting communication between parents and adolescents about healthy sexual development and sexuality including the use and effectiveness of condoms.

4. Restrictions and barriers to condom availability should be removed, given the research that demonstrates that increased availability of condoms facilitates use. Beyond retail distribution of condoms, sexually active adolescents should have ready access to condoms at free or low cost where possible. Pediatricians and other clinicians are encouraged to provide condoms within their offices and to support availability within their communities.

5. Condom availability programs should be developed through a collaborative community process and accompanied by comprehensive sequential sexuality education to be most effective. This is ideally part of a K–12 health education program, with parental involvement, counseling, and positive peer support.

6. Schools should be considered appropriate sites for the availability of condoms because they contain large adolescent populations and may potentially provide a comprehensive array of related educational and health care resources. Training of youth to improve communication skills around condom negotiation with partners can occur in school-based settings.

7. Pediatricians and other clinicians should actively help raise awareness among parents and communities that

making condoms available to adolescents does not increase the onset or frequency of adolescent sexual activity and that use of condoms can help decrease rates of unintended pregnancy and acquisition of STIs.

8. Pediatricians and other clinicians should provide and support parental education programs that help parents develop communications skills with their adolescent children around prevention of STIs and proper use of condoms.

9. The American Academy of Pediatrics should encourage additional research to identify strategies to increase continued condom use in established relationships and strategies for use of dual protection with condoms aimed at prevention of STIs and a second contraceptive method for the most effective prevention of pregnancy.

LEAD AUTHOR

Rebecca F. O'Brien, MD

CONSULTANT

Lee Warner, PhD, Associate Director of Science
Centers for Disease Control and Prevention,
Division of Reproductive Health

COMMITTEE ON ADOLESCENCE 2010–2011

Margaret J. Blythe, MD, Chairperson
William P. Adelman, MD
Cora C. Breuner, MD, MPH
David A. Levine, MD
Arik V. Marcell, MD, MPH
Pamela J. Murray, MD, MPH
Rebecca F. O'Brien, MD, MD

LIAISONS

Loretta E. Gavin, PhD, MPH – *Centers for Disease Control and Prevention*
Rachel J. Miller, MD – *American College of Obstetricians and Gynecologists*
Jorge L. Pinzon, MD – *Canadian Pediatric Society*
Benjamin Shain, MD, PhD – *American Academy of Child and Adolescent Psychiatry*

STAFF

Karen S. Smith
Mark Del Monte, JD

REFERENCES

1. Kaplan DW, Feinstein RA, Fisher MM, et al; Committee on Adolescence. Condom use by adolescents. *Pediatrics*. 2001;107(6):1463–1469

2. Centers for Disease Control and Prevention. Condom Distribution as a Structural Level Intervention. Atlanta, GA: Centers for Disease Control and Prevention; 2010. Available at: www.cdc.gov/hiv/resources/factsheets/PDF/condom_distribution.pdf. Accessed April 25, 2012

3. Eaton DK, Kann L, Kinchen S, et al; Centers for Disease Control and Prevention (CDC). Youth risk behavior surveillance—United States, 2011. *MMWR Surveill Summ*. 2012;61(4 SS-4):1—162

4. Centers for Disease Control and Prevention. Births: final data 2011. *Natl Vital Stat Rep*. 2013;62(1). Available at: www.cdc.gov/nchs/data/nvsr/nvsr62/nvsr62_01.pdf. Accessed October 1, 2013

5. Ventura SJ, Curtin SC, Abma JC, Henshaw SK. Estimated pregnancy rates and rates of pregnancy outcomes for the United States, 1990–2008. *Natl Vital Stat Rep*. 2012;60(7):1—21

6. Centers for Disease Control and Prevention. U.S. teenage birth rate resumes decline. *NCHS Data Brief*. 2011;Feb(58):1–8

7. Santelli JS, Melnikas AJ. Teen fertility in transition: recent and historic trends in the United States. *Annu Rev Public Health*. 2010;31:371—383, 4, 383

8. Weinstock H, Berman S, Cates W Jr. Sexually transmitted diseases among American youth: incidence and prevalence estimates, 2000. *Perspect Sex Reprod Health*. 2004;36(1):6—10

9. Centers for Disease Control and Prevention. *Sexually Transmitted Disease Surveillance 2011*. Atlanta, GA: US Department of Health and Human Services; 2012

10. Forhan SE, Gottlieb SL, Sternberg MR, et al. Prevalence of sexually transmitted infections among female adolescents aged 14 to 19 in the United States. *Pediatrics*. 2009;124(6):1505—1512

11. Centers for Disease Control and Prevention. HIV Surveillance Report, 2011. February 2013. Vol. 23. Available at: www.cdc.gov/hiv/topics/surveillance/resources/reports. Accessed June 15, 2013

12. Centers for Disease and Prevention. HIV Surveillance in Adolescent and Young Adults (through 2011). Available at: www.cdc.gov/hiv/library/slideset. Accessed June 15, 2013

13. Barnes W, D'Angelo L, Yamazaki M, et al; Adolescent Trials Network for HIV/AIDS Interventions. Identification of HIV-infected 12- to 24-year-old men and women in 15 US cities through venue-based testing. *Arch Pediatr Adolesc Med*. 2010;164(3):273–276

14. Hazra R, Siberry GK, Mofenson LM. Growing up with HIV: children, adolescents, and young adults with perinatally acquired HIV infection. *Annu Rev Med*. 2010;61:169—185

15. Brogly SB, Watts DH, Ylitalo N, et al. Reproductive health of adolescent girls perinatally infected with HIV. *Am J Public Health*. 2007;97(6):1047—1052

16. Martinez G, Capen CE, Abma JC. Teenagers in the United States: sexual activity, contraceptive use and childbearing, 2006. National Survey of Family Growth. National Center for Health Statistics. *Vital Health Stat*. 2011;23(31)

17. Rose E, Diclemente RJ, Wingood GM, et al. The validity of teens' and young adults' self-reported condom use. *Arch Pediatr Adolesc Med*. 2009;163(1):61—64

18. Manlove J, Ikramullah E, Terry-Humen E. Condom use and consistency among male adolescents in the United States. *J Adolesc Health*. 2008;43(4):325—333

19. Tschann JM, Flores E, de Groat CL, Deardorff J, Wibbelsman CJ. Condom negotiation strategies and actual condom use among Latino youth. *J Adolesc Health*. 2010;47(3):254—262

20. Brown LK, DiClemente R, Crosby R, et al; Project Shield Study Group. Condom use among high-risk adolescents: anticipation of partner disapproval and less pleasure associated with not using condoms. *Public Health Rep*. 2008;123(5):601—607

21. Scott-Sheldon LA, Marsh KL, Johnson BT, Glasford DE. Condoms + pleasure = safer sex? A missing addend in the safer sex message. *AIDS Care*. 2006;18(7):750–754

22. Randolph ME, Pinkerton SD, Bogart LM, Cecil H, Abramson PR. Sexual pleasure and condom use. *Arch Sex Behav*. 2007;36(6):844–848

23. Crosby RA, Yarber WL, Graham CA, Sanders SA. Does it fit okay? Problems with condom use as a function of self-reported poor fit. *Sex Transm Infect*. 2010;86(1):36–38

24. Choi KH, Gregorich SE. Social network influences on male and female condom use among women attending family planning clinics in the United States. *Sex Transm Dis*. 2009;36(12):757–762

25. Rice E. The positive role of social networks and social networking technology in the condom-using behaviors of homeless young people. *Public Health Rep*. 2010;125(4):588–595

26. Aalsma MC, Fortenberry JD, Sayegh MA, Orr DP. Family and friend closeness to adolescent sexual partners in relationship to condom use. *J Adolesc Health*. 2006;38(3):173–178

27. Fortenberry JD, Tu W, Harezlak J, Katz BP, Orr DP. Condom use as a function of time in new and established adolescent sexual relationships. *Am J Public Health*. 2002;92(2):211–213

28. Kirby DB, Laris BA, Rolleri LA. Sex and HIV education programs: their impact on sexual behaviors of young people throughout the world. *J Adolesc Health*. 2007;40(3):206–217

29. Blake SM, Ledsky R, Goodenow C, Sawyer R, Lohrmann D, Windsor R. Condom availability programs in Massachusetts high schools: relationships with condom use and sexual behavior. *Am J Public Health*. 2003;93(6):955–962

30. Ellen JM, Adler N, Gurvey JE, Millstein SG, Tschann J. Adolescent condom use and perceptions of risk for sexually transmitted diseases: a prospective study. *Sex Transm Dis*. 2002;29(12):756–762

31. Council on Communications and Media. American Academy of Pediatrics. Policy statement—sexuality, contraception, and the media. *Pediatrics*. 2010;126(3):576–582

32. Kunkel D, Eyai K, Finnerty K, Biely E, Donnerstein E. *Sex on TV 4: A Biennial Report to the Kaiser Family Foundation*. Menlo Park, CA: Kaiser Family Foundation; 2005

33. Hagan JF, Shaw JS, Duncan PM, eds. *Bright Futures: Guidelines for Health Supervision of Infants, Children and Adolescents*. 3rd ed. Elk Grove Village, IL: Amercian Academy of Pediatrics; 2008

34. Miller KS, Levin ML, Whitaker DJ, Xu X. Patterns of condom use among adolescents: the impact of mother-adolescent communication. *Am J Public Health*. 1998;88(10):1542–1544

35. Whitaker DJ, Miller KS, May DC, Levin ML. Teenage partners' communication about sexual risk and condom use: the importance of parent-teenager discussions. *Fam Plann Perspect*. 1999;31(3):117–121

36. DiClemente RJ, Wingood GM, Crosby R, Cobb BK, Harrington K, Davies SL. Parent-adolescent communication and sexual risk behaviors among African American adolescent females. *J Pediatr*. 2001;139(3):407–412

37. Hutchinson MK, Jemmott JB, III, Jemmott LS, Braverman P, Fong GT. The role of mother-daughter sexual risk communication in reducing sexual risk behaviors among urban adolescent females: a prospective study. *J Adolesc Health.* 2003;33(2): 98–107

38. Hadley W, Brown LK, Lescano CM, et al; Project STYLE Study Group. Parent-adolescent sexual communication: associations of condom use with condom discussions. *AIDS Behav.* 2009;13(5):997–1004

39. Beckett MK, Elliott MN, Martino S, et al. Timing of parent and child communication about sexuality relative to children's sexual behaviors. *Pediatrics.* 2010;125(1):34–42

40. Miller KS, Whitaker DJ. Predictors of mother-adolescent discussions about condoms: implications for providers who serve youth. *Pediatrics.* 2001;108(2). Available at: www.pediatrics.org/cgi/content/full/108/2/e28

41. Schuster MA, Elliott MN, Kanouse DE. Evaluation of Talking Parents, Healthy Teens, a new worksite based parenting programme to promote parent-adolescent communication about sexual health: randomised controlled trial. *BMJ* 2008;337:308

42. Warner L, Steiner MJ. Male condoms. In: Hatcher RA, Guest F, Stewart F, et al. *Contraceptive Technology.* 20th ed. New York, NY: Ardent Media Inc

43. Carey RF, Lytle CD, Cyr WH. Implications of laboratory tests of condom integrity. *Sex Transm Dis.* 1999;26(4):216–220

44. Lytle CD, Routson LB, Seaborn GB, Dixon LG, Bushar HF, Cyr WH. An in vitro evaluation of condoms as barriers to a small virus. *Sex Transm Dis.* 1997;24(3):161–164

45. Gallo MF, Grimes DA, Lopez LM, Schulz KF. Non-latex versus latex male condoms for contraception. *Cochrane Database Syst Rev.* 2006; (1):CD003550

46. Centers for Disease Control and Prevention (CDC). Nonoxynol-9 spermicide contraception use—United States, 1999. *MMWR Morb Mortal Wkly Rep.* 2002;51(18):389–392

47. Wilkinson D, Tholandi M, Ramjee G, Rutherford GW. Nonoxynol-9 spermicide for prevention of vaginally acquired HIV and other sexually transmitted infections: systematic review and meta-analysis of randomised controlled trials including more than 5000 women. *Lancet Infect Dis.* 2002;2 (10):613–617

48. ASTM Committee F-16 on Fasteners. *Rubber Products; Standard Specifications for Rubber Contraceptives (Male Condoms-D3492). Selected ASTM Standards on Fastener-Related Materials, Coatings, and Testing.* West Conshohocken, PA: ASTM; 1996

49. Summary Table of Contraceptive Efficacy. Percentage of women experiencing an unintended pregnancy during the first year of typical use and the first year of perfect use of contraception and the percentage continuing use at the end of the first year. United States. Contraceptive efficacy. In: Hatcher RA, Trussell J, Nelson AL, Cates W, Stewart FH, Kowal D. *Contraceptive Technology.* 19th rev. ed. New York, NY: Ardent Media, 2007. Available at: www.contraceptivetechnology.org/table.html. Accessed April 25, 2012

50. Weller S, Davis K. Condom effectiveness in reducing heterosexual HIV transmission. *Cochrane Database Syst Rev.* 2001; (3): CD003255

51. Steiner MJ, Warner L, Stone KM, et al. Condoms and other barrier methods for prevention of STD/HIV infection, and pregnancy. In: Holmes KK, Sparling PF, Stamm WE, eds. *Sexually Transmitted Diseases,* 4th ed. New York, NY: MacGraw-Hill; 2008

52. Centers for Disease Control and Prevention. Sexually transmitted diseases treatment guidelines 2002. *MMWR Recomm Rep.* 2002;51(RR-6):1–78

53. Martin ET, Krantz E, Gottlieb SL, et al. A pooled analysis of the effect of condoms in preventing HSV-2 acquisition. *Arch Intern Med.* 2009;169(13):1233–1240

54. Warner L, Stone KM, Macaluso M, Buehler JW, Austin HD. Condom use and risk of gonorrhea and Chlamydia: a systematic review of design and measurement factors assessed in epidemiologic studies. *Sex Transm Dis.* 2006;33(1):36–51

55. Conant MA, Spicer DW, Smith CD. Herpes simplex virus transmission: condom studies. *Sex Transm Dis.* 1984;11(2):94–95

56. Katznelson S, Drew WL, Mintz L. Efficacy of the condom as a barrier to the transmission of cytomegalovirus. *J Infect Dis.* 1984;150(1):155–157

57. Rietmeijer CA, Krebs JW, Feorino PM, Judson FN. Condoms as physical and chemical barriers against human immunodeficiency virus. *JAMA.* 1988;259(12):1851–1853

58. Van de Perre P, Jacobs D, Sprecher-Goldberger S. The latex condom, an efficient barrier against sexual transmission of AIDS-related viruses. *AIDS.* 1987;1(1):49–52

59. Judson FN, Ehret JM, Bodin GF, Levin MJ, Rietmeijer CA. In vitro evaluations of condoms with and without nonoxynol 9 as physical and chemical barriers against Chlamydia trachomatis, herpes simplex virus type 2, and human immunodeficiency virus. *Sex Transm Dis.* 1989;16(2):51–56

60. Cates W Jr. The NIH condom report: the glass is 90% full. *Fam Plann Perspect.* 2001; 33(5):231–233

61. Pinkerton SD, Abramson PR. Effectiveness of condoms in preventing HIV transmission. *Soc Sci Med.* 1997;44(9):1303–1312

62. Devine OJ, Aral SO. The impact of inaccurate reporting of condom use and imperfect diagnosis of sexually transmitted disease infection in studies of condom effectiveness: a simulation-based assessment. *Sex Transm Dis.* 2004;31(10):588–595

63. Warner L, Macaluso M, Austin HD, et al. Application of the case-crossover design to reduce unmeasured confounding in studies of condom effectiveness. *Am J Epidemiol.* 2005;161(8):765–773

64. Warner L, Newman DR, Austin HD, et al; Project RESPECT Study Group. Condom effectiveness for reducing transmission of gonorrhea and chlamydia: the importance of assessing partner infection status. *Am J Epidemiol.* 2004;159(3):242–251

65. Niccolai LM, Rowhani-Rahbar A, Jenkins H, Green S, Dunne DW. Condom effectiveness for prevention of *Chlamydia trachomatis* infection. *Sex Transm Infect.* 2005;81(4): 323–325

66. Shlay JC, McClung MW, Patnaik JL, Douglas JM Jr. Comparison of sexually transmitted disease prevalence by reported condom use: errors among consistent condom users seen at an urban sexually transmitted disease clinic. *Sex Transm Dis.* 2004; 31(9):526–532

67. Shlay JC, McClung MW, Patnaik JL, Douglas JM Jr. Comparison of sexually transmitted disease prevalence by reported level of condom use among patients attending an urban sexually transmitted disease clinic. *Sex Transm Dis.* 2004;31(3):154–160

68. Paz-Bailey G, Koumans EH, Sternberg M, et al. The effect of correct and consistent condom use on chlamydial and gonococcal infection among urban adolescents. *Arch Pediatr Adolesc Med.* 2005;159(6):536–542

69. Gallo MF, Steiner MJ, Warner L, et al. Self-reported condom use is associated with reduced risk of chlamydia, gonorrhea, and trichomoniasis. *Sex Transm Dis.* 2007;34 (10):829–833

70. Winer RL, Hughes JP, Feng Q, et al. Condom use and the risk of genital human papillomavirus infection in young women. *N Engl J Med.* 2006;354(25):2645–2654

71. d'Oro LC, Parazzini F, Naldi L, La Vecchia C. Barrier methods of contraception, spermicides, and sexually transmitted diseases: a review. *Genitourin Med.* 1994;70(6):410–417

72. Manhart LE, Koutsky LA. Do condoms prevent genital HPV infection, external genital warts, or cervical neoplasia? A meta-analysis. *Sex Transm Dis.* 2002;29(11):725–735

73. Holmes KK, Levine R, Weaver M. Effectiveness of condoms in preventing sexually transmitted infections. *Bull World Health Organ.* 2004;82(6):454–461

74. Koss CA, Dunne EF, Warner L. A systematic review of epidemiologic studies assessing condom use and risk of syphilis. *Sex Transm Dis.* 2009;36(7):401–405

75. Vijayakumar G, Mabude Z, Smit J, Beksinska M, Lurie M. A review of female-condom effectiveness: patterns of use and impact on protected sex acts and STI incidence. *Int J STD AIDS.* 2006;17(10):652–659

76. Warner L, Gallo MF, Macaluso M. Condom use around the globe: how can we fulfil the prevention potential of male condoms? *Sex Health.* 2012;9(1):4–9

77. Bearinger LH, Resnick MD. Dual method use in adolescents: a review and framework for research on use of STD and pregnancy protection. *J Adolesc Health.* 2003;32(5):340–349

78. Santelli JS, Davis M, Celentano DD, Crump AD, Burwell LG. Combined use of condoms with other contraceptive methods among inner-city Baltimore women. *Fam Plann Perspect.* 1995;27(2):74–78

79. Anderson JE, Santelli J, Gilbert BC. Adolescent dual use of condoms and hormonal contraception: trends and correlates 1991–2001. *Sex Transm Dis.* 2003;30(9):719–722

80. Pazol K, Kramer MR, Hogue CJ. Condoms for dual protection: patterns of use with highly effective contraceptive methods. *Public Health Rep.* 2010;125(2):208–217

81. Ott MA, Adler NE, Millstein SG, Tschann JM, Ellen JM. The trade-off between hormonal contraceptives and condoms among adolescents. *Perspect Sex Reprod Health.* 2002;34(1):6–14

82. Sangi-Haghpeykar H, Posner SF, Poindexter AN III. Consistency of condom use among low-income hormonal contraceptive users. *Perspect Sex Reprod Health.* 2005;37(4):184–191

83. Sieving RE, Bearinger LH, Resnick MD, Pettingell S, Skay C. Adolescent dual method use: relevant attitudes, normative beliefs and self-efficacy. *J Adolesc Health.* 2007;40(3):275.e215–275.e222

84. de Visser R. Why do heterosexual young adults who use reliable contraception also use condoms? Results from a diary-based prospective longitudinal study. *Br J Health Psychol.* 2007;12(Pt 2):305–313

85. Roye C, Perlmutter Silverman P, Krauss B. A brief, low-cost, theory-based intervention to promote dual method use by black and Latina female adolescents: a randomized clinical trial. *Health Educ Behav.* 2007;34(4):608–621

86. Crosby R, DiClemente RJ, Charnigo R, Snow G, Troutman A. A brief, clinic-based, safer sex intervention for heterosexual African American men newly diagnosed with an STD: a randomized controlled trial. *Am J Public Health.* 2009;99(suppl 1):S96–S103

87. DiClemente RJ, Wingood GM, Rose ES, et al. Efficacy of sexually transmitted disease/human immunodeficiency virus sexual risk-reduction intervention for african american adolescent females seeking sexual health services: a randomized controlled trial. *Arch Pediatr Adolesc Med.* 2009;163(12):1112–1121

88. Centers for Disease Control and Prevention. *Compendium of HIV Prevention Interventions With Evidence of Effectiveness.* Atlanta, GA: Centers for Disease Control and Prevention; 1999, revised August 31, 2001

89. Charania MR, Crepaz N, Guenther-Gray C, et al. Efficacy of structural-level condom distribution interventions: a meta-analysis of U.S. and international studies, 1998–2007. *AIDS Behav.* 2011;15(7):1283–1297

Conflicts Between Religious or Spiritual Beliefs and Pediatric Care: Informed Refusal, Exemptions, and Public Funding

- *Policy Statement*

POLICY STATEMENT

Conflicts Between Religious or Spiritual Beliefs and Pediatric Care: Informed Refusal, Exemptions, and Public Funding

abstract

Although respect for parents' decision-making authority is an important principle, pediatricians should report suspected cases of medical neglect, and the state should, at times, intervene to require medical treatment of children. Some parents' reasons for refusing medical treatment are based on their religious or spiritual beliefs. In cases in which treatment is likely to prevent death or serious disability or relieve severe pain, children's health and future autonomy should be protected. Because religious exemptions to child abuse and neglect laws do not equally protect all children and may harm some children by causing confusion about the duty to provide medical treatment, these exemptions should be repealed. Furthermore, public health care funds should not cover alternative unproven religious or spiritual healing practices. Such payments may inappropriately legitimize these practices as appropriate medical treatment. *Pediatrics* 2013;132:962–965

INTRODUCTION

Religion plays an important role in the lives of many individuals. Fifty-eight percent of respondents to a recent poll reported that religion is very important in their lives, and 23% reported that it is fairly important.[1] The relationship between religion and medicine is complex. Some studies suggest "greater involvement in religion conveys more health-related benefits."[2] There are, however, times when religion and medicine conflict. The current policy statement addresses 3 related issues: (1) parents' refusal of medical treatment of their children; (2) religious exemptions to child abuse and neglect laws; and (3) public funding of alternative unproven religious or spiritual healing practices. The statement situates religious refusals within the scope of parental authority and argues that children's future autonomy should be protected. Religious exemption statutes do not protect all children equally and create uncertainty and, to protect children's health, should be repealed. Public health care funding should focus on established, effective therapies, and paying for spiritual healing practices may inadvertently engender medical neglect. The discussion of these specific topics should not be interpreted as a broader criticism of the interaction between religion and medicine.

COMMITTEE ON BIOETHICS

KEY WORDS
exemption, informed refusal, medical neglect, pediatrics, religion

ABBREVIATIONS
AAP—American Academy of Pediatrics
HHS—US Department of Health and Human Services

This document is copyrighted and is the property of the American Academy of Pediatrics and its Board of Directors. All authors have filed conflict of interest statements with the American Academy of Pediatrics. Any conflicts have been resolved through a process approved by the Board of Directors. The American Academy of Pediatrics has neither solicited nor accepted any commercial involvement in the development of the content of this publication.

The guidance in this statement does not indicate an exclusive course of treatment or serve as a standard of medical care. Variations, taking into account individual circumstances, may be appropriate.

All policy statements from the American Academy of Pediatrics automatically expire 5 years after publication unless reaffirmed, revised, or retired at or before that time.

www.pediatrics.org/cgi/doi/10.1542/peds.2013-2716

doi:10.1542/peds.2013-2716

PEDIATRICS (ISSN Numbers: Print, 0031-4005; Online, 1098-4275).

Copyright © 2013 by the American Academy of Pediatrics

RELIGIOUS OBJECTIONS TO MEDICAL CARE

Although parents have broad authority, they have less discretion in making medical decisions for their children than for themselves. On the basis of the ethical principles of autonomy and respect for persons, capacitated adults should have wide license in making medical decisions for themselves, including the refusal of potentially lifesaving medical treatment. Their liberty should only be limited in cases of direct harm to third parties, such as the risk of transmitting serious infectious diseases. Infants and children lack the ability to make autonomous medical decisions; therefore, the law generally authorizes their parents or guardians to make such decisions on their behalf. These decisions should primarily focus on the child's best interests.[3,4] Clinicians should afford parents and guardians significant discretion in their interpretation of these interests and collaborate with them to develop treatment plans that promote their children's health. Although family autonomy and privacy are important social values, parents' choices may be limited when they rise to the level of abuse or neglect.[5]

Failure to provide children with essential medical care has been increasingly recognized as a form of neglect. In 1983, the US Department of Health and Human Services (HHS) amended its definition of negligent treatment to include failure to provide adequate medical care.[6] A number of factors are relevant to the evaluation of suspected medical neglect, including likelihood and magnitude of the harm of foregoing medical treatment and the benefits, risks, and burdens of the proposed treatment.[7–9] For example, the risk of an individual unimmunized child contracting a communicable vaccine-preventable disease may be low if immunization rates in the community are high and disease prevalence

is low.[10] Serious harms include death, severe disability, or severe pain. The American Academy of Pediatrics (AAP) Committee on Child Abuse and Neglect identifies a variety of factors that can lead to children not receiving appropriate medical care and corresponding graduated management options for pediatricians. For example, lack of awareness, knowledge, or skills can be addressed by counseling and education.[7] Ethics consultation is an additional management option.[7,11] If less-restrictive alternatives are not available or successful, pediatricians should refer families to child protective services agencies. In emergencies, providers may be ethically justified in administering treatment immediately necessary to preserve life, prevent serious disability, or treat severe pain. They should notify child protective services as soon as possible.

The basis for some parents' rejection of medical treatment is religious or spiritual. Traditions vary in the scope of medical treatments they refuse. For example, members of the Followers of Christ refuse all medical treatment in favor of prayer, anointing with oil, and the laying on of hands.[12] Christian Scientists may use dentists and physicians for "mechanical" procedures, such as setting bones or childbirth, but consider most illnesses to be the result of the individual's mental attitude and seek healing through spiritual means, such as prayer. They consider these healing practices incompatible with concurrent medical treatment.[13] Other religious groups prohibit only specific medical interventions. On the basis of their interpretation of scripture, Jehovah's Witnesses only prohibit the use of blood and its major fractions.[14] Understanding these differences is important in identifying whether there are mutually acceptable alternatives.

Some religious refusals have, tragically, led to children's deaths from readily

treatable conditions, such as pneumonia, appendicitis, or diabetes.[12,15] Although the free exercise of religion, including parents teaching their children their religious beliefs, is an important societal value, it must be balanced against other important societal values, such as protecting children from serious harm.[16] In some situations, the issue is primarily an empirical one —the relative efficacy of medical and spiritual interventions. Although systematic empirical evidence of the efficacy of religious interventions is often lacking, the courts can judge efficacy by using criteria generally accepted by both parents and health care providers. In other situations, the issue involves differing conceptions of benefit and harm. Parents and guardians should have significant discretion in weighing the risks and benefits of a proposed treatment. At times, the primary benefit of refusing medical treatment or seeking alternative nonmedical treatment is religious or spiritual, such as the implications of the treatment on the patient's eternal salvation. In such cases, the potential benefit cannot be evaluated by using generally accepted criteria. In such situations, the child's future ability to decide this contested issue for himself or herself should be protected.[17] Some adolescents may possess adequate decision-making capacity to comprehend and evaluate the risks and benefits of medical treatment. The possibility of coercion should also be considered in the evaluation of whether a capacitated adolescent's dissent is autonomous.[18]

The courts have consistently ordered life-saving medical treatment over parental religious objections.[8,9] In passages frequently quoted in subsequent rulings, the US Supreme Court famously stated, "The right to practice religion freely does not include liberty to expose the community or the child to communicable disease or the latter to ill health or death" and "Parents may be free to become martyrs themselves. But it does not follow they are free, in identical circumstances, to make martyrs of their children before they have reached the age of full and legal discretion when they can make that choice for themselves."[19] There is less unanimity in judicial decisions if the condition is not life-threatening, the treatment has significant adverse effects, or the treatment has limited efficacy.[7–9] Courts may also consider the negative psychological effects of court-ordered treatment or medical foster care in their decisions.

RELIGIOUS EXEMPTIONS TO CHILD ABUSE AND NEGLECT LAWS

Most states have "religious exemptions" to their child abuse and neglect laws. These exemptions proliferated in response to the Child Abuse Prevention and Treatment Act of 1974. The act stated, "Provided, however, that a parent or guardian legitimately practicing his religious beliefs who thereby does not provide specified medical treatment for a child, for that reason alone shall not be considered a negligent parent or guardian."[20] Enacting exemptions was a condition for states to receive federal child abuse grants. More than 40 states adopted exemptions, which vary in their location within each state's code and wording.[8] Some apply to child protective services agencies' ability to intervene, and others apply to parents' criminal liability. The HHS revised its position, taking a neutral stance, when the act was reauthorized in 1983: "Nothing in this part should be construed as requiring or prohibiting a finding of negligent treatment or maltreatment when a parent practicing his or her religious beliefs does not, for that reason alone, provide medical treatment for a child."[21] After reauthorization of the act in 1987, HHS clarified that reports of medical neglect should

only be made if there is harm or a substantial risk of harm, and religious exemptions should be a matter of state discretion rather than federal imposition.[18] A number of states subsequently amended or repealed their religious exemption statutes.[8,16] Most recently, after the deaths of 2 children, Oregon repealed its exemption.[22]

The AAP believes that religious exemptions to state child abuse and neglect laws should be repealed. These exemptions fail to provide an equivalent level of protection to children whose parents practice spiritual healing and children whose parents do not.[16] In addition, they may create confusion that results in harm to children; parents may be unclear about their duty to provide medical treatment, child protective services agencies may falsely believe that they cannot intervene until after a child suffers serious injury or dies, and prosecutors and courts may be uncertain whether parents are subject to criminal liability if their child dies of medical neglect.[5,16] Although the exemptions could be revised to make it explicit that seeking medical care is required when a child is seriously ill,[5,8] repeal is preferable because it provides greater clarity.[16] For example, parents and spiritual healers who are members of groups that refuse all medical treatment may not be able to differentiate moderate from severe illnesses and, therefore, fail to seek medical attention in a timely manner.[14,16]

PUBLIC FUNDING OF SPIRITUAL HEALING PRACTICES

In addition to efforts to create religious exemptions, some churches and legislators have sought to provide public funds to pay for religious or spiritual healing practices. For example, Medicare and Medicaid cover care provided at Christian Science sanatoria and other religious nonmedical health care institutions and exempt these institutions

from medical oversight requirements.[23] In addition, there were unsuccessful efforts to include coverage of Christian Science practitioners in the 2009 federal health care reform bills[24] and ongoing efforts to include their services in the essential health benefits package. These efforts should be distinguished from both health care services provided by religious organizations, such as Roman Catholic and Seventh-day Adventist hospitals, and pastoral care provided as a bundled service.

Coverage for unproven care by unlicensed practitioners is poor public policy for several reasons. Fundamentally, public funds should be spent on established, effective therapies.[25] In addition, religious nonmedical health care institutions provide custodial rather than skilled nursing care, a benefit not covered in other institutions. Given patients' exemptions from undergoing medical examinations, it is not possible to determine whether patients of religious nonmedical health care institutions would otherwise qualify for benefits.[23,26] Because providing public funding for unproven alternative spiritual healing practices may be perceived as legitimating these services, parents may not believe that they have an obligation to seek medical treatment. Although the AAP recognizes the importance of addressing children's spiritual needs as part of the comprehensive care of children, it opposes public funding of religious or spiritual healing practices.

RECOMMENDATIONS

1. Pediatricians, pediatric medical subspecialists, and pediatric surgical specialists should respect families and their religious or spiritual beliefs and collaborate with them to develop treatment plans to promote their children's health.

2. Pediatricians, pediatric medical subspecialists, and pediatric surgical specialists should report

suspected cases of medical neglect to state child protective services agencies, regardless of whether the parents' decision is based on religious beliefs.

3. Pediatricians, pediatric medical subspecialists, pediatric surgical specialists, and the AAP and its chapters should work to repeal religious exemptions to child abuse and neglect laws and to prevent public payment for religious or spiritual healing practices.

LEAD AUTHORS

Armand H. Matheny Antommaria, MD, PhD
Kathryn L. Weise, MD

COMMITTEE ON BIOETHICS, 2011–2012

Mary E. Fallat, MD
Aviva L. Katz, MD
Mark R. Mercurio, MD
Margaret R. Moon, MD
Alexander L. Okun, MD
Sally A. Webb, MD
Kathryn L. Weise, MD

CONSULTANT

Jessica W. Berg, JD, MPH

PAST CONTRIBUTING COMMITTEE MEMBERS

Armand H. Matheny Antommaria, MD, PhD
Ian R. Holzman, MD
Lainie Friedman Ross, MD, PhD

LIAISONS

Douglas S. Diekema, MD, MPH – *American Board of Pediatrics*
Kevin W. Coughlin, MD – *Canadian Pediatric Society*
Steven J. Ralston, MD – *American College of Obstetricians and Gynecologists*

STAFF

Alison Baker, MS

REFERENCES

1. Gallup. Religion. Available at: www.gallup.com/poll/1690/religion.aspx. Accessed April 21, 2013

2. Krause N. Religion and health: making sense of a disheveled literature. *J Relig Health*. 2011;50(1):20–35

3. American Academy of Pediatrics, Committee on Bioethics. Informed consent, parental permission, and assent in pediatric practice. *Pediatrics*. 1995;95(2):314–317

4. Ross LF. *Children, Families, and Health Care Decision Making*. Oxford, UK: Clarendon Press; 1998

5. Gathings JT Jr. When rights clash: the conflict between a parent's right to free exercise of religion versus his child's right to life. *Cumberland Law Rev*. 1988–1989;19(3):585–616

6. Child Abuse and Neglect Prevention and Treatment, 45 CFR § 1340.2(d)(2)(i) (1983)

7. Jenny C; Committee on Child Abuse and Neglect, American Academy of Pediatrics. Recognizing and responding to medical neglect. *Pediatrics*. 2007;120(6):1385–1389

8. Malecha WF. Faith healing exemptions to child protection laws: keeping the faith versus medical care for children. *J Legis*. 1985;12(2):243–263

9. Trahan J. Constitutional law: parental denial of a child's medical treatment for religious reasons. *Annu Surv Am Law*. 1989; 1989(1):307–341

10. Diekema DS; American Academy of Pediatrics Committee on Bioethics. Responding to parental refusals of immunization of children. *Pediatrics*. 2005;115(5):1428–1431

11. American Academy of Pediatrics. Committee on Bioethics. Institutional ethics committees. *Pediatrics*. 2001;107(1):205–209

12. Mayes S. Another Followers of Christ couple indicted in death of a child. *The Oregonian*. July 31, 2010. Available at: www.oregonlive.com/oregon-city/index.ssf/2010/07/another_followers_of_christ_couple_indicted_in_death_of_a_child.html. Accessed August 15, 2012

13. Talbot NA. The position of the Christian Science church. *N Engl J Med*. 1983;309(26):1641–1644

14. Dixon JL, Smalley MG. Jehovah's Witnesses. The surgical/ethical challenge. *JAMA*. 1981;246(21):2471–2472

15. Asser SM, Swan R. Child fatalities from religion-motivated medical neglect. *Pediatrics*. 1998;101(4 pt 1):625–629

16. Monopoli PA. Allocating the costs of parental free exercise: striking a new balance between sincere religious belief and a child's right to medical treatment. *Pepperdine Law Rev*. 1991;18(2):319–352

17. Sheldon M. Ethical issues in the forced transfusion of Jehovah's Witness children. *J Emerg Med*. 1996;14(2):251–257

18. Guichon J, Mitchell I. Medical emergencies in children of orthodox Jehovah's Witness families: three recent legal cases, ethical issues and proposals for management. *Paediatr Child Health (Oxford)*. 2006;11(10):655–658

19. *Prince v Massachusetts*, 321 US 158, 170 (1944)

20. Child Abuse and Neglect Prevention and Treatment Act, 45 CFR § 1340.1-2(b) (1975)

21. Child Abuse and Neglect Prevention and Treatment Act, 45 CFR § 1340.2(d)(2)(ii) (1983)

22. Mayes S. Kitzhaber signs bill to eliminate religious defense for faith-healing parents. *The Oregonian*. June 16, 2011. Available at: www.oregonlive.com/oregon-city/index.ssf/2011/06/kitzhaber_signs_bill_to_eliminate_religious_defense_for_faith-healing_parents.html. Accessed August 15, 2012

23. Harris BR. Veiled in textual neutrality: is that enough? A candid reexamination of the constitutionality of Section 4454 of the Balanced Budget Act of 1997. *Alabama Law Rev*. 2010;61(2):393–423

24. Wan W. 'Spiritual health care' raises church-state concerns. *The Washington Post*. November 23, 2009. Available at: www.washingtonpost.com/wp-dyn/content/article/2009/11/22/AR2009112202216.html. Accessed August 15, 2012

25. Libby R; Committee on Child Health Financing American Academy of Pediatrics. Principles of health care financing. *Pediatrics*. 2010;126(5):1018–1021

26. *Children's Health Care Is a Legal Duty Inc v Min de Parle*, 212 F.3d 1084 (8th Cir. 2000), *cert. denied*, 532 US 957 (2001)

Consumption of Raw or Unpasteurized Milk and Milk Products by Pregnant Women and Children

- *Policy Statement*

POLICY STATEMENT

Consumption of Raw or Unpasteurized Milk and Milk Products by Pregnant Women and Children

COMMITTEE ON INFECTIOUS DISEASES and COMMITTEE ON NUTRITION

KEY WORDS
raw milk/milk products, unpasteurized milk/milk products, pregnant women, children

ABBREVIATIONS
AAP—American Academy of Pediatrics
FDA—Food and Drug Administration

www.pediatrics.org/cgi/doi/10.1542/peds.2013-3502

doi:10.1542/peds.2013-3502

PEDIATRICS (ISSN Numbers: Print, 0031-4005; Online, 1098-4275).

abstract

Sales of raw or unpasteurized milk and milk products are still legal in at least 30 states in the United States. Raw milk and milk products from cows, goats, and sheep continue to be a source of bacterial infections attributable to a number of virulent pathogens, including *Listeria monocytogenes, Campylobacter jejuni, Salmonella* species, *Brucella* species, and *Escherichia coli* 0157. These infections can occur in both healthy and immunocompromised individuals, including older adults, infants, young children, and pregnant women and their unborn fetuses, in whom life-threatening infections and fetal miscarriage can occur. Efforts to limit the sale of raw milk products have met with opposition from those who are proponents of the purported health benefits of consuming raw milk products, which contain natural or unprocessed factors not inactivated by pasteurization. However, the benefits of these natural factors have not been clearly demonstrated in evidence-based studies and, therefore, do not outweigh the risks of raw milk consumption. Substantial data suggest that pasteurized milk confers equivalent health benefits compared with raw milk, without the additional risk of bacterial infections. The purpose of this policy statement was to review the risks of raw milk consumption in the United States and to provide evidence of the risks of infectious complications associated with consumption of unpasteurized milk and milk products, especially among pregnant women, infants, and children. *Pediatrics* 2014;133:175–179

INTRODUCTION

Foodborne illness accounts for substantial morbidity and mortality in the United States. Estimates suggest that each year, as many as 48 million Americans experience foodborne illness, accounting for 128 000 hospitalizations and 3000 deaths.[1] In addition, surveillance estimates by the Centers for Disease Control and Prevention demonstrated no overall improvement in the incidence of foodborne illness in the United States from 2006 to 2009.[2] Among the most preventable of these foodborne illnesses are infections related to ingestion of raw or unpasteurized milk and milk products because of ubiquitous access to healthy, pasteurized milk and milk products, as well as legislation prohibiting the sale of raw dairy products in much of the United States. Reasons for the continued burden of disease related to raw or unpasteurized milk or milk products are primarily related to misinformation regarding the purported benefits of these raw dairy products. Consumption of raw dairy products is especially risky among populations such as pregnant women, infants, the elderly, and immunocompromised individuals, who are most susceptible to infection with pathogens ingested in raw milk or milk products. Evidence demonstrates the overwhelming benefits to food safety conferred by pasteurization and consumption of pasteurized dairy products.

EPIDEMIOLOGY OF DISEASES CAUSED BY RAW OR UNPASTEURIZED MILK AND MILK PRODUCTS IN THE UNITED STATES

Before pasteurization of milk began in the United States in the 1920s, consumption of raw dairy products accounted for a significant proportion of foodborne illnesses among Americans and resulted in hundreds of outbreaks of tuberculosis and infections caused by bacteria, such as *Brucella abortus*, streptococcal species, and enteric pathogens.[3] Although most milk and milk products consumed today in the United States are pasteurized, an estimated 1% to 3% of all dairy products consumed are not pasteurized. From 1998 through 2009 alone, consumption of raw milk or milk products in the United States resulted in 93 illness outbreaks, 1837 illnesses, 195 hospitalizations, and 2 deaths.[4] These foodborne illnesses were caused primarily by ingestion of raw milk or milk products contaminated with *Escherichia coli* O157, *Campylobacter* species, or *Salmonella* species. Seventy-nine percent of the outbreaks involved at least 1 person younger than 20 years.[4] In a second study, 121 dairy-associated foodborne illness outbreaks were identified in the United States from 1993 to 2006. Of these, 73 (60%) were associated with unpasteurized dairy products, resulting in 1571 cases, 202 hospitalizations, and

2 deaths; 60% of the patients were younger than 20 years. Thirteen percent of patients involved in raw milk or milk product foodborne illness outbreaks were hospitalized, compared with 1% of patients involved in outbreaks associated with pasteurized products. In addition, 55 (75%) of all 121 outbreaks occurred in 21 states that permitted the sale of unpasteurized dairy products.[5] Immigrant groups are another population at risk for illness from consumption of traditional foods made with raw milk.[6,7]

A number of pathogenic and opportunistic bacteria, parasites, and viruses (see Organisms Detected in Raw or Unpasteurized Milk or Milk Products) have been detected in raw milk or milk products.[4–22] In addition, patterns of dairy consumption appear to have affected the prevalence of illnesses associated with different dairy products. Among milk- or milk product–associated foodborne illness outbreaks reported to the Centers for Disease Control and Prevention between 1973 and 2009, 82% were attributable to raw milk or cheese. However, increasingly, recent illnesses associated with raw or unpasteurized cheese have been reported. This underscores the importance of all raw milk products as potential sources of illness.

Populations at highest risk of morbidity and mortality from foodborne illnesses include older adults, immunocompromised individuals, young infants, and children. The risks involved with infections attributable to consumption of raw milk and milk products are particularly high among pregnant women and their fetuses, as well as young children. For example, consumption of raw milk or milk products has been associated with a fivefold increase in toxoplasmosis among pregnant women[23]; listeriosis associated with high rates of stillbirths, preterm delivery, and neonatal infections, such as sepsis and meningitis[6];

and *E coli* O157–associated diarrheal disease and hemolytic-uremic syndrome, primarily among young children.[24] Between 17% and 33% of all cases of invasive disease attributable to *Listeria monocytogenes* in the United States occur among pregnant women, unborn fetuses, or newborn infants, a 13- to 17-fold increase compared with the general population.[25–27] Complications include a 20% risk of spontaneous abortion or stillbirth, with two-thirds of infants developing neonatal infection, including pneumonia, sepsis, or meningitis.[28]

GUIDELINES FOR SALES OF RAW OR UNPASTEURIZED MILK AND MILK PRODUCTS BY THE FOOD AND DRUG ADMINISTRATION AND INDIVIDUAL STATES

The modern pasteurization process consists of raising the temperature of milk to at least 161°F for more than 15 seconds, followed by rapid cooling. Since 1924, the Food and Drug Administration (FDA) has regulated the production, handling, transportation, processing, testing, and sale of milk in all 50 states in the United States. In 1987, the FDA prohibited the interstate shipment of raw milk for human consumption, effectively banning interstate commerce of raw milk or milk products. No federal agencies, however, including the FDA, have jurisdiction in the regulation and enforcement of milk sanitation within individual states. In 2011, the National Association of State Departments of Agriculture conducted a review demonstrating that 30 states allow raw milk sales, but only a few of these allow sales in grocery stores. In addition, the 1987 FDA ban on interstate raw dairy transport allows for an exception of cheese made from raw milk, provided the cheese has been aged a minimum of 60 days and is clearly labeled as unpasteurized. However, there is evidence that *E coli* can survive in cheese products even after a 60-day aging period,[29] and recent outbreaks of *E coli* 0157 illness associated with such unpasteurized, aged cheese have been documented in Arizona, California, Colorado, and New Mexico.[30]

RISKS AND BENEFITS OF RAW VERSUS PASTEURIZED MILK AND MILK PRODUCTS

Infections associated with consumption of raw and unpasteurized milk and milk products are related to contamination with pathogenic and opportunistic organisms from a variety of sources. Contamination of raw milk occurs by a number of mechanisms, including direct contact with bovine fecal matter; transmission of organisms from bovine skin or hide; clinical or subclinical mastitis; primary bovine diseases, such as tuberculosis; environmental contamination; and contact with insects, animals, and humans, for example, by contamination from soiled clothing.

Proponents of the health benefits of raw or unpasteurized milk and milk products claim that pasteurization destroys or neutralizes important nutrients in milks, such as proteins, carbohydrates, calcium, vitamins, and enzymes.[31–33] For example, claims that consumption of raw milk is not associated with lactose intolerance and that destruction of lactase by pasteurization of milk leads to lactose intolerance have not been substantiated by independent studies.[34–37] Other claims purporting links between pasteurized milk and autism, allergic reactions, and asthma have largely been based on testimonials or anecdotes and have not been demonstrated based on scientific data. In contrast, numerous scientific analyses have demonstrated that pasteurized milk and milk products contain equivalent levels of such nutrients compared with raw, unpasteurized milk and milk products.[31–39]

RECOMMENDATIONS FROM NATIONAL AND INTERNATIONAL ORGANIZATIONS REGARDING CONSUMPTION OF RAW OR UNPASTEURIZED MILK AND MILK PRODUCTS

Virtually all national and international advisory and regulatory committees related to food safety have strongly endorsed the principles of consuming only pasteurized milk and milk products. These include the American Medical Association, the American Veterinary Medical Association, the International Association for Food Protection, the National Environmental Health Association, the FDA, and the World Health Association. In January 2012, the US federal government denied a petition requesting federal-level legalization of all raw milk sales on the basis of its analysis of the scientific basis for the food safety benefits of pasteurization.[40]

The American Academy of Pediatrics (AAP) has strongly endorsed the use of pasteurized milk in its 2012 *Red Book*.[41]

CONCLUSIONS

In summary, the AAP strongly supports the position of the FDA and other national and international associations in endorsing the consumption of only pasteurized milk and milk products for pregnant women, infants, and children. The AAP also endorses a ban on the sale of raw or unpasteurized milk and milk products throughout the United States, including the sale of certain raw milk cheeses, such as fresh cheeses, soft cheeses, and soft-ripened cheeses. This recommendation is based on the multiplicity of data regarding the burden of illness associated with consumption of raw and unpasteurized milk and milk products, especially among pregnant women, fetuses and newborn infants, and infants and young children, as well as the strong scientific evidence that pasteurization does not alter the nutritional value of milk. The AAP also

encourages pediatricians to contact their state representatives to support a ban on sale of raw milk and milk products. Additional resources containing information regarding the safety of pasteurization and the risks of consuming raw or unpasteurized milk or milk products are provided in this statement.

ORGANISMS DETECTED IN RAW OR UNPASTEURIZED MILK OR MILK PRODUCTS

Bacteria
Brucella species
Campylobacter jejuni
Coxiella burnetii
Cryptosporidium species
Enterotoxigenic *Staphylococcus aureus*
Listeria monocytogenes
Mycobacterium bovis
Salmonella species
Escherichia coli
   Shiga toxin-producing *E coli* (STEC [eg, *E coli* 0157])
   Enterohemorrhagic *E coli* (EHEC)
   Enterotoxigenic *E coli* (ETEC)
   Shigella species
   Yersinia entercolitica

Parasites
Giardia species

Viruses
Norovirus
Rabies
Vaccinia

RESOURCES

- http://www.realrawmilkfacts.com/
- www.cdc.gov/foodsafety/rawmilk/raw-milk-index.html
- http://www.fda.gov/Food/FoodbornelllnessContaminants/BuyStoreServeSafeFood/ucm277854.htm
- FDA "Grade 'A' Pasteurized Milk Ordinance." 2011 Revision: http://www.fda.gov/downloads/Food/GuidanceRegulation/UCM291757.pdf
- FoodSafety.gov "Myths About Raw Milk": www.foodsafety.gov/keep/types/milk
- www.nationaldairycouncil.org/sitecollectiondocuments/research/dairy_council_digests/2011/dcd11-1w.pdf

REFERENCES

1. Centers for Disease Control and Prevention. Estimates of foodborne illness in the United States. Available at: www.cdc.gov/foodborneburden/. Accessed April 17, 2013

2. Centers for Disease Control and Prevention. Trends in foodborne illness in the United States. Available at: www.cdc.gov/foodborneburden/trends-in-foodborne-illness.html. Accessed April 17, 2013

3. Centers for Disease Control and Prevention. What is the history of the recommendation for pasteurization in the United States? Available at: http://www.cdc.gov/foodsafety/rawmilk/raw-milk-questions-and-answers.html#history. Accessed November 12, 2013

4. Centers for Disease Control and Prevention. How many outbreaks are related to raw milk? Available at: http://www.cdc.gov/foodsafety/rawmilk/raw-milk-questions-and-answers.html#related-outbreaks. Accessed November 12, 2013

5. Langer AJ, Ayers T, Grass J, Lynch M, Angulo FJ, Mahon BE; Centers for Disease Control and Prevention. Nonpasteurized dairy products, disease outbreaks, and state laws-United States, 1993–2006. Emerg Infect Dis. 2012;18(3):385–391

6. MacDonald PDM, Whitwam RE, Boggs JD, et al. Outbreak of listeriosis among Mexican immigrants as a result of consumption of illicitly produced Mexican-style cheese. Clin Infect Dis. 2005;40(5):677–682

7. Centers for Disease Control and Prevention (CDC). Outbreak of listeriosis associated with homemade Mexican-style cheese—North Carolina, October 2000-January 2001. MMWR Morb Mortal Wkly Rep. 2001;50(26): 560–562

8. D'Amico DJ, Donnelly CW. Microbiological quality of raw milk used for small-scale artisan cheese production in Vermont: effect of farm characteristics and practices. J Dairy Sci. 2010;93(1):134–147

9. Doyle MP, Roman DJ. Prevalence and survival of Campylobacter jejuni in unpasteurized milk. Appl Environ Microbiol. 1982;44(5):1154–1158

10. Gaya P, Medina M, Nuñez M. Enterobacteriaceae, coliforms, faecal coliforms and salmonellas in raw ewes' milk. J Appl Bacteriol. 1987;62(4):321–326

11. Houser BA, Donaldson SC, Kehoe SI, Heinrichs AJ, Jayarao BM. A survey of bacteriological quality and the occurrence of Salmonella in raw bovine colostrum. Foodborne Pathog Dis. 2008;5(6):853–858

12. Hussein HS, Sakuma T. Prevalence of shiga toxin-producing Escherichia coli in dairy cattle and their products. J Dairy Sci. 2005; 88(2):450–465

13. Jayarao BM, Donaldson SC, Straley BA, Sawant AA, Hegde NV, Brown JL. A survey of foodborne pathogens in bulk tank milk and raw milk consumption among farm families in Pennsylvania. J Dairy Sci. 2006;89(7): 2451–2458

14. Jayarao BM, Henning DR. Prevalence of foodborne pathogens in bulk tank milk. J Dairy Sci. 2001;84(10):2157–2162

15. Karns JS, Van Kessel JS, McCluskey BJ, Perdue ML. Prevalence of Salmonella enterica in bulk tank milk from US dairies

as determined by polymerase chain reaction. *J Dairy Sci.* 2005;88(10):3475–3479

16. Kim SG, Kim EH, Lafferty CJ, Dubovi E. *Coxiella burnetii* in bulk tank milk samples, United States. *Emerg Infect Dis.* 2005;11(4):619–621

17. Massa S, Goffredo E, Altieri C, Natola K. Fate of *Escherichia coli* O157:H7 in unpasteurized milk stored at 8 degrees C. *Lett Appl Microbiol.* 1999;28(1):89–92

18. Oliver SP, Jayarao BM, Almeida RA. Foodborne pathogens in milk and the dairy farm environment: food safety and public health implications. *Foodborne Pathog Dis.* 2005;2(2):115–129

19. Pitt WM, Harden TJ, Hull RR. Behavior of *Listeria* monocytogenes in pasteurized milk during fermentation with lactic acid bacteria. *J Food Prot.* 2000;63(7):916–920

20. Rea MC, Cogan TM, Tobin S. Incidence of pathogenic bacteria in raw milk in Ireland. *J Appl Bacteriol.* 1992;73(4):331–336

21. Van Kessel JS, Karns JS, Gorski L, McCluskey BJ, Perdue ML. Prevalence of *Salmonellae*, *Listeria* monocytogenes, and fecal coliforms in bulk tank milk on US dairies. *J Dairy Sci.* 2004;87(9):2822–2830

22. Wang G, Zhao T, Doyle MP. Survival and growth of *Escherichia coli* O157:H7 in unpasteurized and pasteurized milk. *J Food Prot.* 1997;60(6):610–613

23. Jones JL, Dargelas V, Roberts J, Press C, Remington JS, Montoya JG. Risk factors for *Toxoplasma gondii* infection in the United States. *Clin Infect Dis.* 2009;49(6):878–884

24. Guh A, Phan Q, Nelson R, et al. Outbreak of *Escherichia coli* O157 associated with raw milk, Connecticut, 2008. *Clin Infect Dis.* 2010;51(12):1411–1417

25. Silver HM. Listeriosis during pregnancy. *Obstet Gynecol Surv.* 1998;53(12):737–740

26. Voelker R. Listeriosis outbreak prompts action—finally. *JAMA.* 2002;288(21):2675–2676

27. Silk BJ, Date KA, Jackson KA, et al. Invasive listeriosis in the Foodborne Diseases Active Surveillance Network (FoodNet), 2004-2009: further targeted prevention needed for higher-risk groups. *Clin Infect Dis.* 2012;54 (suppl 5):S396–S404

28. Mylonakis E, Paliou M, Hohmann EL, Calderwood SB, Wing EJ. Listeriosis during pregnancy: a case series and review of 222 cases. *Medicine (Baltimore).* 2002;81(4):260–269

29. Schlesser JE, Gerdes R, Ravishankar S, Madsen K, Mowbray J, Teo AY. Survival of a five-strain cocktail of *Escherichia coli* O157:H7 during the 60-day aging period of cheddar cheese made from unpasteurized milk. *J Food Prot.* 2006;69(5):990–998

30. Centers for Disease Control and Prevention. Investigation update: multistate outbreak of *E. coli* O157:H7 infections associated with cheese. Available at: www.cdc.gov/ecoli/2010/cheese0157/index.html. Accessed April 17, 2013

31. Newkirk R, Hedberg C, Bender J. Establishing a milkborne disease outbreak profile: potential food defense implications. *Foodborne Pathog Dis.* 2011;8(3):433–437

32. Jay-Russell MT. Raw (unpasteurized) milk: are health-conscious consumers making an unhealthy choice? *Clin Infect Dis.* 2010; 51(12):1418–1419

33. Oliver SP, Boor KJ, Murphy SC, Murinda SE. Food safety hazards associated with consumption of raw milk. *Foodborne Pathog Dis.* 2009;6(7):793–806

34. Lin MY, Savaiano D, Harlander S. Influence of nonfermented dairy products containing bacterial starter cultures on lactose maldigestion in humans. *J Dairy Sci.* 1991;74 (1):87–95

35. McBean LD, Miller GD. Allaying fears and fallacies about lactose intolerance. *J Am Diet Assoc.* 1998;98(6):671–676

36. Onwulata CI, Rao DR, Vankineni P. Relative efficiency of yogurt, sweet acidophilus milk, hydrolyzed-lactose milk, and a commercial lactase tablet in alleviating lactose maldigestion. *Am J Clin Nutr.* 1989;49(6): 1233–1237

37. Savaiano DA, AbouElAnouar A, Smith DE, Levitt MD. Lactose malabsorption from yogurt, pasteurized yogurt, sweet acidophilus milk, and cultured milk in lactase-deficient individuals. *Am J Clin Nutr.* 1984;40(6): 1219–1223

38. Lejeune JT, Rajala-Schultz PJ. Food safety: unpasteurized milk: a continued public health threat. *Clin Infect Dis.* 2009;48(1):93–100

39. US Department of Health and Human Services, US Food and Drug Administration, Center for Food Safety and Applied Nutrition. Sale/consumption of raw milk-position statement (M-I-03-4). March 19, 2003. Available at: www.fda.gov/Food/GuidanceRegulation/GuidanceDocumentsRegulatoryInformation/Milk/ucm079103.htm. Accessed April 17, 2013

40. McKalip D. Official White House response to legalize raw milk sales on a federal level. Available at: https://petitions.whitehouse.gov/response/food-safety-and-raw-milk. Accessed April 17, 2013

41. American Academy of Pediatrics. Prevention of disease from potentially contaminated food products. In: Pickering LK, Baker CJ, Kimberlin DW, Long SS, eds. *Red Book: 2012 Report of the Committee on Infectious Diseases.* 28th ed. Elk Grove Village, IL: American Academy of Pediatrics; 2012:917–918

Early Intervention, IDEA Part C Services, and the Medical Home: Collaboration for Best Practice and Best Outcomes

• •

- *Clinical Report*

CLINICAL REPORT

Early Intervention, IDEA Part C Services, and the Medical Home: Collaboration for Best Practice and Best Outcomes

Richard C. Adams, MD, Carl Tapia, MD, and THE COUNCIL ON CHILDREN WITH DISABILITIES

KEY WORDS
Part C, IDEA, medical home, children with special health care needs, CSHCN, collaboration, comanagement, coaching, learning in the natural environment

ABBREVIATIONS
AAP—American Academy of Pediatrics
EI—early intervention
IDEA—Individuals With Disabilities Education Act

www.pediatrics.org/cgi/doi/10.1542/peds.2013-2305

doi:10.1542/peds.2013-2305

All clinical reports from the American Academy of Pediatrics automatically expire 5 years after publication unless reaffirmed, revised, or retired at or before that time.

PEDIATRICS (ISSN Numbers: Print, 0031-4005; Online, 1098-4275).

abstract

The medical home and the Individuals With Disabilities Education Act Part C Early Intervention Program share many common purposes for infants and children ages 0 to 3 years, not the least of which is a family-centered focus. Professionals in pediatric medical home practices see substantial numbers of infants and toddlers with developmental delays and/or complex chronic conditions. Economic, health, and family-focused data each underscore the critical role of timely referral for relationship-based, individualized, accessible early intervention services and the need for collaborative partnerships in care. The medical home process and Individuals With Disabilities Education Act Part C policy both support nurturing relationships and family-centered care; both offer clear value in terms of economic and health outcomes. Best practice models for early intervention services incorporate learning in the natural environment and coaching models. Proactive medical homes provide strategies for effective developmental surveillance, family-centered resources, and tools to support high-risk groups, and comanagement of infants with special health care needs, including the monitoring of services provided and outcomes achieved. *Pediatrics* 2013;132:e1073–e1088

In decades past, debate centered on the question: "does early childhood intervention work?" Time and extensive research clearly reveal an affirmative answer.[1] In the new millennium, the focus of discussion has turned to distinct conceptual matters and specific questions:

- What roles and actions are best assumed by collaborative professionals in providing a system of early intervention (EI) shared by pediatricians in the medical home and EI programs?

- What models of intervention are optimal when considering infants/toddlers, families, agencies, pediatricians, and best use of resources for optimal outcomes?

- What systematic barriers to optimal intervention are present and what supports are available to overcome them?

Given the ever-growing body of evidence demonstrating the value of EI services for infants with special needs and their families, there remains a necessity for close collaboration between the infants' medical home and their respective Individuals With Disabilities Education Act (IDEA) Part C state programs. This clinical report, reflecting the work of diverse stakeholders (clinicians, policy makers, academicians, family members, and governmental staffs), will:

1. Review the common core components of IDEA Part C and the medical home;

2. Review evidence of the value of medical home and EI programs for infants/toddlers with special needs;

3. Provide pediatricians with information on evidence-based best-practice models for effective EI;

4. Highlight systematic barriers to identification/integration of infants in EI services; and

5. Offer resources for medical home personnel and families to support this collaboration.

CORE COMPONENTS OF IDEA PART C AND THE MEDICAL HOME

IDEA Part C Programs

For more than half a century, the field of early childhood intervention has emphasized factors impacting an infant's overall function. These encompass both biologic (epigenetic, infectious, etc) and experiential variables (quality of relationships; exposure to, or lack of, opportunities for exploration and learning).[2] The importance of these early experiences was a compelling concept in the 1975 creation of the Education for All Handicapped Children Act (Pub L No. 94-142), which provided "special education" services for children 5 to 21 years of age. Eleven years later, the law was extended and broadened to incorporate the concept of support to infants 0 to 3 years old and their families. This 0 to 3 component, now called Part C of IDEA, addressed "an

urgent and substantial need" in several areas: (1) enhancing the development of infants and toddlers with special needs; (2) reducing downstream governmental costs of special education and/or institutionalization by intervening earlier; and (3) supporting the ability of families to interact with and meet the needs of the infant/toddler.[3–6]

The long-standing charge to each state's Part C program is to create and sustain a statewide, comprehensive, coordinated, family-centered, multidisciplinary, and interagency system of EI services for delivery in the local or regional area. In doing so, each state is required to establish eligibility criteria for serving, at a minimum, 2 cohorts of children: (1) those with a diagnosed physical or mental condition with a high likelihood of developmental delays; or (2) a developmental delay in 1 or more of 5 domains (cognitive, motor, communication, social/emotional, adaptive).[3,5] States may also elect to serve infants at risk for delay because of biological or environment risk factors and/or children who have been in Part C but are now eligible for preschool education (if the family desires to stay in the Part C system).

Because each state is charged with developing these eligibility criteria and is subject to legislative and budgetary constraints, notable variations in eligibility and services occur from state to state. Historically, federal monies for Part C are relatively small. Thus, states rely on systems of coordination with state, local, other public, and private funding sources, serving as payers of last resort rather than as primary payers for intervention services.

This model has demonstrated success on several levels. By 1992, 143 000 children and their families were receiving services via Part C. In 2009, that number had risen to 349 000, or

2.67% of the US population 3 years or younger. With variables related to eligibility criteria and budgets, the percentage of the 0- to 3-year-old population being served in 2009 ranged from 1.24% (Georgia) to 6.5% (Massachusetts). Despite fiscal challenges at the federal and state level, at the time of this publication, all 50 states continue to participate in the Part C program.[3,7]

The most recent reauthorization of IDEA Part C in 2004 placed increasing importance on quality measures of outcome, provision of services in the child's natural environment, and identification efforts for eligible infants ("child find"). There was also a strengthening of the relationship between EI and services being rendered in each state according to the Child Abuse Prevention and Treatment Act Reauthorization Act of 2010 (Pub L No. 111-320).[8]

Because of state-to-state variations regarding eligibility criteria, definitions of "developmental delay," and state budgetary priorities, the nature of EI services can seem heterogeneous when viewed through a national lens. Nonetheless, 2 core concepts remain stable across Part C programs across the country:

- Nurturing relationships are the fundamental elements for optimal early development; and

- IDEA Part C is dedicated to helping families better understand their infants and to coordinating the various regional systems and services available to the family and child.

The Medical Home

By definition, a "medical home" for children is a process of care. The American Academy of Pediatrics (AAP) has described the medical home as the provision of primary care to children that is accessible, family-centered, continuous, comprehensive, coordinated, compassionate, and culturally effective. Historically, the medical home was commonly discussed in the context of children with special health care needs, but increasingly, its value has been seen across the full spectrum of infants, children, and adolescents.[9–11]

Clearly, the core components of care that define a medical home match closely those specified legislatively in IDEA Part C. As child find is mandated in Part C, there is recognition that the pediatric medical home is an integral part of that process.[11] Emerging evidence supports the medical home process regarding its value to children's ultimate development and well-being.[12–18] The Healthy People 2020 goals and those of the Patient Protection and Affordable Care Act cite the promotion of the patient-centered medical home.[19,20] When considering the intersection of EI and the medical home, a key component of the medical home process is that of identifying infants and toddlers with developmental disorders.[21–25] A natural next step is timely and appropriate referral to EI services for coordinated, culturally effective, and family-centered developmental intervention.

Over the past decade, the medical home concept has extended beyond pediatric practices into those of family/community physicians and internal medicine. A recent workforce study by the AAP described a robust pediatric workforce for the population of US children but noted a significant problem of distribution (regional shortages and oversupplies).[26] Family physicians provide a medical home opportunity for approximately one-third of the US pediatric population. Historically, these services have been in rural communities; estimates suggest up to 5 million children/adolescents live in counties with no pediatrician. Supporting both family physician medical homes and Part C agencies serving rural and/or frontier areas of the country should be a focus at both the preservice and in-service levels.[27]

As the model of the pediatric medical home has gained support over recent years, the number of recommended or expected tasks/screening procedures for the primary pediatrician has also increased.[14] Acknowledging potential time and budgetary constraints within pediatric practices, methods to streamline identification of infant developmental delays have been developed and are critical to meeting family needs and successful referral to EI services for the child.[4,28]

EVIDENCE-BASED OUTCOMES AND BEST PRACTICE CONSIDERATIONS

Over the past half century, research in the neurosciences and in child development have placed an increasing priority on the support needed in the first few years of life as brain growth and function are being shaped for future "scaffolding" of skills and knowledge. Program development and methods of program evaluation have since been generated and demonstrated to assist in this neurodevelopmental process. From this body of work have emerged several global principles related to early childhood development and intervention for optimal development.[29] Brains are built over time and are modulated by the interactive influences of genes and experience that literally affect the architecture of the developing brain.

- Access to basic medical care (prenatal and during early childhood) prevents threats to healthy development through early diagnosis/identification of problems with subsequent EI and ongoing care management.

- When parents, community programs, and professionals who provide early childhood services (including the pediatrician in the medical home) promote supportive relationships and rich learning experiences for infants and young children, a stronger foundation is created for higher achievement in school and, eventually, the community.

- The economic cost of creating and applying supportive conditions for early childhood development is less than the alternative "down the road" costs of addressing problems later in childhood or adolescence.

- From a legislative and policy perspective, a strong investment in early childhood intervention is foundational for community and economic development on multiple levels.

Although these global incentives derive from studies across various medical and nonmedical fields, it is instructive to consider, more specifically, the benefits stemming from the 2 entities being considered: the medical home and EI services for infants and toddlers.

Benefits From Participation in a Medical Home

The primary care medical home, with core attributes including being family centered; community based; and accessible, coordinated, and continuous in support, has increasingly been endorsed by the AAP and other child-oriented agencies as highly valuable.[30] The core concepts of these processes of care seem intuitive for physicians charged with providing preventive and timely care to infants/toddlers.

The benefits of a medical home in providing efficient, high-quality, comprehensive primary care are well documented. For example, the medical home has been linked to improved health status, more timely care, increased family-centeredness, improved family functioning, and more appropriate health-care utilization.[9,10,13,17,31,32] The National Survey of Early Childhood Health reports that nearly half of parents have concerns about their child's development,[33] yet few parents report that their concerns are elicited during outpatient clinic visits.[34] In addition, children at high-risk of developmental delay have been associated with lower odds of having a medical home compared with children at low or no developmental risk.[35] Thus, a growing consensus recognizes the ability of a medical home process to provide developmental health services and promote a comprehensive system of community services for early childhood development,[33,36,37] a process altogether consistent with and supportive of the core elements of EI services under IDEA Part C.

Benefits From EI

When evaluating benefits derived from early identification and intervention, there are 2 major streams for measuring outcomes: (1) benefits to the child and the family; and (2) economic advantages derived from EI programs.[38]

An increasing number of well-constructed longitudinal studies have emerged over the past decade. The indicators measured reflect positive and sustainable outcomes. The Infant Health and Development Program tracked outcomes in low birth weight and preterm infants who received EI services. At 8 years of age, improvements were noted in verbal abilities, receptive language scores, and overall cognitive performance.[39] At the 18-year

follow-up, there were notable improvements in academic performance and endorsement of less risky behaviors, fewer arrests, and a lower dropout rate.[40] Other studies have generated similar positive data as long as 15 to 40 years beyond early childhood.[41,42]

Equally important to communities and agencies are the studies demonstrating the fiscal advantages of providing quality EI services. A 2003 report from the Federal Reserve Bank of Minneapolis reveals EI programs as "economic development initiatives" that should be at the top of economic lists for local and state governments. The authors found that 1 program demonstrated an $8 return for every dollar invested in EI and estimated that 80% of the benefits were directly applicable to society in general (because of more efficient use of school services and less use of criminal justice and other public systems).[43–46] In the 2008 study, The Economics of Early Childhood Policy,[47–49] Kilburn and Karoly provide the foundation for support of EI from strictly an economic

perspective and conclude: "The costs savings for government could be large enough to not only repay the initial costs of the program but also to possibly generate savings to government or society as a whole multiple times greater than the costs."

The benefits reflected in these studies and other studies expand the concept of EI from one of solely a social-service/educational policy to one of critical economic-development and conservative fiscal responsibility.[50] Availability of these data should support advocacy efforts of the medical home on behalf of infants (Fig 1).

MEDICAL HOMES, EI PROGRAMS, AND BEST PRACTICE MODELS

Given the evidence-based data regarding the value of medical homes and EI services, the continuing challenge is to identify which models of intervention are consistent with best practice consensus, and which demonstrate greatest outcomes with best stewardship of professional and fiscal resources. The medical home can be essential in helping families and

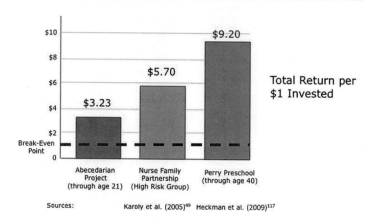

FIGURE 1

Cost/benefit analysis of benefits to society of early childhood programs. (Reprinted with permission from the Center on the Developing Child at Harvard University, www.developingchild.harvard.edu.).

diverse providers better understand the roles played by professionals involved in the infant's overall intervention program.

Two concepts are increasingly prioritized when translating evidence-based neuroscience into functional application for "best practice" provision of EI services:

1. Creating frequent opportunities that allow for "learning in the natural environment" rather than in simulated "treatment" situations; and

2. Utilizing methods of "coaching" as a model for families, medical homes, and EI programs providing services to infants.

The concept of providing intervention services within the context of a natural learning environment has been a legal and conceptual component of IDEA Part C intervention since its inception. Part C considers "natural environments" as meaning settings that are natural or typical for similarly aged and nondisabled peers. The broader concept of learning in the natural environment encompasses several key elements:

- There is base acknowledgment that learning takes place in the context of relationships, and as such, intervention strategies should enhance rather than disrupt typical activities unique to a family.

- There is endorsement of parents, siblings, extended family, and others as key agents for the infant's developmental learning.

- Thus, emphasis is on supporting those change agents and their abilities during everyday activities, rather than attempting to teach new skills outside of natural contexts.

- Focus is on function and development of personal-social skills in the infant while promoting awareness and confidence in parents to guide their infant with special needs.

Rather than a "medical model" wherein a specific treatment is applied directly to the child for a specific malady, the paradigm is shifted to a contextual and consultation-based delivery of supports and services to the family and the infant.[51,52] Similar to the concept of the medical home being a process, rather than an address, the concept of natural environment describes process rather than a physical address.[53] These concepts have been endorsed by national stakeholder organizations, including those of speech, physical, and occupational therapies.[54-56]

Increasingly, a best practice method, endorsed across diverse disciplines, provides coaching strategies to families for use in the child's natural learning environments. This method has been shown to build the capacities of a parent or other caretaker as new skills (both in the family member and the child) are acquired.[57,58] Coaching techniques to support parents are used by therapists in the natural learning environment and can be modified and applied by the pediatrician in the medical home process.[59-62] Key elements in the coaching process are shown in Table 1.

There is a more complex subset of infants who might benefit periodically from adjunctive traditional "hands-on" (direct) medical therapy. This is generally for specific goals and often for limited periods of time. These complex health care needs may include severe visual or hearing impairments, tracheotomies, and congenital malformations with inherent limitations to daily activities or needs, etc. Referrals for supportive direct services should be based on specific and measurable outcome goals. Preferably, such goals should be written in concert with the global goals of the family (also reflected in the individualized family service plan as a component of "care coordination").

Unfortunately, confusion is too often experienced by families when the infant is dually served by therapists applying direct medical therapy and professionals in the medical home and/or EI program by using transdisciplinary coaching within the natural learning environment. Unless these services are explained and

TABLE 1 Elements in the Coaching Process

Element	Examples for Application
Joint planning	Agreement by coach and parent on actions assumed by coach and subsequent opportunities for the parent to practice between coaching visits.
Observations	Consider the family's actions/practices/routines to better develop new skill sets, strategies, and ideas for use in the natural learning environment.
Action	Spontaneous or scheduled events, occurring in real-life situations, that allow the family member to practice, refine, or analyze new skills.
Reflections	The coach revisits the existing strategies to ensure they are in keeping with evidence-based practices and consider if/when modifications are needed.
Feedback	After the family member is allowed to reflect on strategies employed, actions being applied, and opportunities to practice new skills in the natural learning environment, the coach provides information affirming the parent's understanding or adds information to deepen the parent's understanding.

Modified from Rush DD, Shelden ML. *Evidence-Based Definition of Coaching Practices.* Morganton, NC: Center for the Advanced Study of Excellence in Early Childhood; 2005.[114]

closely coordinated, a mistrust of one professional or the other can develop.[57]

FOUR DEVELOPMENTALLY HIGH-RISK GROUPS COMMON TO MEDICAL HOMES AND EI PROGRAMS

Among all the children seen in the medical home, several subgroups involve particularly high risks, specific opportunities for EI services, and ongoing collaboration with the pediatrician:

Infants and Toddlers From Environments of Abuse or Neglect

Data from the US Department of Health and Human Services (2011) revealed ~825 000 substantiated cases of abuse/neglect resulting in 1770 child deaths.[63] Infants younger than 1 year remained the highest risk group for fatalities. Among children 0 to 3 years of age who are maltreated but survive, negative effects (social/emotional, cognitive, and/or physical) have been described in up to 47%.[64] Given the astounding cost of child protective services (provision of educational, judicial, and health-related services are estimated at $94 to $103 billion per year), the ability to identify and prevent conditions leading to maltreatment warrant serious consideration and action.[15]

A gap exists in the provision of EI services to maltreated infants and toddlers. Of the ~35% with a need, only 12.7% actually receive services.[65] The Child Abuse and Prevention Treatment Act of 2010 acknowledged this and sought to advance "effective practices and programs to improve activities that promote collaboration between the child protective services system and the medical community, including providers of mental health and developmental disability services,

and providers of early childhood intervention services."

Social and emotional development is most vulnerable to previous maltreatment, with attachment issues, severe feeding differences, and sleep disorders being especially prominent among infants.[66] Given research evidence that (1) early brain development affects lifelong capacity to regulate emotions and learn; (2) the "active ingredient" for brain development is the quality of relationships between the infant and those providing care and nurturing; and (3) infants/toddlers exposed to persistent multiple risk factors are in need of EI as early as possible, the close, collaborative interaction of the medical home and the regional Part C program is vital to infant outcome and community cost containment.[67,68]

Infants and Toddlers With Mental Health Issues

Closely related to the issues of maltreatment, but by no means limited to this group, are infants and toddlers experiencing mental health issues (either primary to the child or among their caregivers).[69] Coexisting conditions can act as "red flags" for developing infant mental health concerns (Table 2).[70,71] Likewise, mental health issues affecting the infant/toddler can result in additional developmental delay

or dysfunction.[15] As awareness of infant mental health issues increases and as more focus is placed on providing needed services for this group, the medical home and the Part C programs together remain at the forefront of identification, intervention, and surveillance over time.[72–75]

Elements of support for infant mental health include: (1) easy accessibility for diverse families; (2) a system for early identification of concerns and timely application of screening/referral; (3) provision of full access to an array of supportive resources; (4) promotion of family knowledge of conditions and of service delivery systems; and (5) ensuring family-centered care with family satisfaction as an outcome of interventions.[76,77] These elements are provided when the medical home process and the regional Part C program perform collaboratively. The focus of intervention to support infant mental health remains on the infant-caregiver relationship rather than on solely the child or adult.[78] Instruments such as the Ages and Stages, Third Edition,[79,80] the Ages and Stages: Social/Emotional screener,[81] Mental Health Screening Tool Zero to 5 Years,[82] and the AAP "Addressing Mental Health Concerns in Primary Care: A Clinician's Toolkit,"[83] among others, offer functional options for use with families.

TABLE 2 Risk Factors Potentially Impacting Infant Mental Health

Family and Associated Environmental Factors	Child Factors
Low socioeconomic status/poverty	Premature birth
Low maternal education	Low birth weight
History of domestic violence	"Difficult" temperament and/or poor "goodness of fit" with primary caregivers
Maternal/paternal depression	Exposure to "toxic stressors" (alcohol, illicit drugs, traumatic events, environmental exposures, such as lead, etc)
History of parental criminality	Cognitive dysfunction
Parental health problems	Genetic conditions with associated behavioral disorders
Parental mental health disorders	
Family history of mental health disorders	

Modified from Brauner CB, Stephens BC. Estimating the prevalence of early childhood serious emotional/behavioral disorders: challenges and recommendations. *Public Health Rep.* 2006;121(3):303–310.[70]

Infants and Toddlers From Culturally Diverse Backgrounds

Linguistic and/or cultural differences between families and professionals in the medical home or EI program create barriers to both appropriate screening and, potentially, to enrollment and provision of services. Families' beliefs and understanding of child development and differences in developmental progression reflect cultural perspectives. Their views of "community" and the child may differ from a professional's "deficit-oriented" interpretation of the child's functioning capacity.[84]

Numerous factors and variables affect the process of screening, referral, and service provision, including: socioeconomic status, religious differences, regional demographics, English proficiency or literacy, immigration status, family support systems, and access to services. When 1 or more of these potential barriers exist, the results may include families' feelings of being insulted or treated rudely, fear of the medical community in general, confusion about appointments/referrals, or being discounted in the decision process.[85–89]

The disparities noted previously can negatively affect the processes of care in the medical home and the regional Part C program.[90] Feinberg et al[91] discussed the effect of race on effective participation in EI programs. African American children with developmental delay(s) were 5 times less likely than were white children to receive EI services. Garcia and Ortiz[84] have described similar differences in the Latino population and have offered suggestions for prereferral interventions to support culturally and linguistically different populations. As medical home personnel consider quality improvement efforts, areas for consideration might include lack of awareness of racial privilege,

assumptions of the value of science over spirituality (in reference to developmental differences), importance of individual over the family group, and logistics required for higher frequency interactions with the developmental or medical community[91,92] (Table 3).

Infants and Toddlers From Economically Deprived Backgrounds

Robust data from economically at-risk populations describe (1) disparities in referral and provision of services for EI and developmental support; and (2) variations in policy commitment to low-income young children and families. Some of these disparities remain at the institutional/policy level within each state (eligibility criteria, coordination efforts, etc). For example, among states with narrow EI eligibility criteria, poor children are 18% less likely to receive EI services.[93] Some are the result of barriers discussed above relative to cultural differences and to mental health issues.[94–98]

The effects of poverty and comorbid conditions, such as food insecurity, have been linked not only to health and ultimate educational performance but also to mental health and behavior in

young children and their mothers.[99,100] It is critical for professionals in both medical homes and Part C programs to integrate quick and effective methods of surveillance for poverty-related issues, such as food insecurity, as a component of early childhood intervention[101] (Table 4).

TOOLS FOR THE MEDICAL HOME: MEETING THE CHALLENGES OF COLLABORATION

The medical home process is highly valued by families as they perceive "added value" benefits of more predictable care and less unplanned emergent care, especially among families of children with special needs.[12] As the value placed on the medical home continues to rise, so too are the seemingly unending expectations. But as screening procedures and protocols are encouraged, time and reimbursements remain significant limiting factors.[102,103] Thus, it is imperative that the professionals in the medical home have ready access to tools to provide efficient screening, surveillance, referral, and ongoing collaboration in support of infants/toddlers and EI services.[104]

In 2006, the AAP published a policy statement, "Identifying infants and

TABLE 3 Cultural Barriers to Medical Home Screening and Referral for EI Services

Families
    Limited proficiency in English (parent and/or child); differences in speech or dialect
    Limited reading skills
    Acculturation level and knowledge of/comfort with agencies
    Attitudes toward child development and disabilities
    Conflicts: work, child care, transportation, or financial
    Extended family expectations different from parents/professionals
Medical homes
    Sensitivity to cultural diversity within medical home staff
    Sensitivity to religious preferences and differing family traditions
    Paternalistic approaches to parents of infants from different cultures
    Use of medical jargon
EI programs
    Lack of language-appropriate information materials
    Shortage of available bilingual personnel
    Inflexible scheduling practices
    Sensitivity to cultural diversity among families served

Modified from Zhang C, Bennett T. Facilitating the meaningful participation of culturally and linguistically diverse families in the IFSP and IEP process. *Focus Autism Other Dev Disabil.* 2003;18(1):51–59.[115]

TABLE 4 Potential Questions for Social History in Families of Infants/Toddlers by Using the *IHELLP* Mnemonic

Area of Interest	Example Questions
Income	
General	Do you have fear of running short of money by the end of the month?
Food security	Do you or anyone in the family ever skip meals because there is not enough money for food?
	Do you receive assistance (food stamps, etc)?
Housing	Is housing or payment for housing a problem for you?
Associated utilities	Do you have trouble or concern about paying electric/gas/water bills?
Education and development	Do you have concerns about how your infant is developing?
Early childhood programs	Is your child in a program to assist you in supporting her development?
	Do you feel the need for such a program?
Legal status	Do you have questions about your immigration status or about benefits/services for you and your infant/toddler?
Literacy	Do you have trouble reading forms given from our office or agencies?
	Do have difficulty in reading generally?
	Do you read to your child each day? (Based on above answers)
Personal safety	Do you feel that you and your infant/toddler are safe in your present situation/relationship?
	Have you or your spouse ever been the subject of domestic violence?

Modified from Kenyon C, Sandel M, Silverstein M, Shakir A, Zuckerman B. Revisiting the social history for child health. *Pediatrics.* 2007;120(3). Available at: www.pediatrics.org/cgi/content/full/120/3/e734.[101]

young children with developmental disorders in the medical home: an algorithm for developmental surveillance and screening"[105] (http://pediatrics.aappublications.org/content/118/1/405.full.html), which offers a roadmap and valuable resources to the pediatrician seeking to identify and refer eligible infants for EI services. Since its publication, Earls et al[23] reported a longitudinal study of developmental and behavioral screening in a North Carolina project containing insightful ideas and suggestions for practical applications in practice.

King et al[24] conducted a quality improvement follow-up study on developmental screening and surveillance. Attempting to apply the algorithm suggested in the 2006 AAP policy statement, clear gains were made in identifying and referring young children to EI programs. But many practices described struggles in implementing the pro-

cesses in particularly busy seasons, with staff turnover, and regarding certain time-sensitive screens. Tracking of referrals made was difficult. King et al's[24] review (http://pediatrics.aappublications.org/content/125/2/350.full.html) offers insights for other medical homes attempting to optimize identification and referrals for EI.

Marks et al[106] in 2011 published suggestions for enhancing the algorithm for developmental and behavioral surveillance in children ages 0 to 5 years (http://cpj.sagepub.com/content/50/9/853). In addition to further data supporting the use of specific screening tools, the review offers practitioners specific guidance in the following components of care:

- Eliciting and addressing parents' concerns;

- Milestone and behavioral skill monitoring;

- Identifying developmental/behavioral risk and protective factors;

- Making accurate and informed observations about child-parent interactions; and

- Child referral resources.

Three other resources available to the medical home offer guidance and efficiency in approaching at-risk infants/toddler who have potential need for EI services. The 2006 clinical report from the AAP,[107] "Clinical genetic evaluation of the child with mental retardation or developmental delays," remains a useful tool for the practitioner in which decision trees, clinical guidelines, and resources for clinical application are outlined (http://pediatrics.aappublications.org/content/117/6/2304.full.html). Michaud's[108] overview of prescribing therapy services for children with motor disabilities (http://pediatrics.aappublications.org/content/113/6/1836.full.html) and Sneed et al's[109] review of the differences in prescribing therapies and medical equipment in medical versus educational settings (http://pediatrics.aappublications.org/content/114/5/e612.full.html) are both practical and insightful guides for the busy medical home.

Once the practitioner has identified an eligible infant/toddler in need of services, the family benefits from open and effective lines of collaboration between the medical home and the Part C program. A summary of suggestions for better communication between medical homes and EI programs is provided in Table 5.[110,111] A representative sample of the numerous resources available to the medical home and to families is outlined in Table 6.

Despite the barriers and challenges inherent to practitioners and programs, there remains strong potential for collaboration between medical homes and EI programs at the policy and programmatic levels.[89,112] Kozlowski et al[113] described an investigation comparing parents of toddlers with autism to those of children with other developmental disorders. The data, generated through the Louisiana Part C Program, described time delays between when parents first perceived differences in their children's communication styles and when referrals from physicians were made to the EI program. Collaborative model ventures such as this will continue to inform families, medical home professionals, EI service programs, and state agencies.

SUGGESTIONS FOR COLLABORATION BETWEEN THE MEDICAL HOME AND EI PROGRAMS

- Improving child-find and optimizing the referral process

Practitioners should incorporate the AAP recommendations for developmental surveillance, which allows for enhanced identification and timely referral for EI services.

The referral should set the stage for collaboration with EI programs. The AAP referral form is available (http://www.medicalhomeinfo.org/downloads/pdfs/EIReferralForm_1.pdf) and can help streamline the process, and individual states may have referral forms that are specific for the individual state Part C program. Such forms can be used in referrals to adjunctive service programs.

The referral provides an opportunity for education about appropriate developmental milestones, as well as eliciting family goals and expectations, which should inform supervision of the individualized family service plan and clinical approval for EI and other developmental services.

The medical home should incorporate a system for referral tracking. An example referral form (Appendix) provides a template to obtain family permission at the time of the referral so that EI programs can communicate the results of the initial evaluation with the medical home. Modifications for individual states/programs may be needed (Appendix).

- Efficient evaluation and coordination of services

Practitioners should not wait for a specific diagnosis before initiating an appropriate referral to EI. Early referral should request:

- assistance with multidisciplinary assessment;
- provision of support to parents in addition to the child;
- provision of knowledge about and integration with community resources; and
- a preferred mechanism for information return from the intervention program.

Various protocols are available to guide a stepwise developmental evaluation of infants and young children (see above). Included among

these resources is the AAP "Caring for Children With Autism Spectrum Disorders: A Resource Toolkit for Clinicians."

As practices enhance their capacity for care coordination, consideration should be given to develop mechanisms for identifying families who need assistance with the referral process or who have complex psychosocial or medical issues. These strategies might include:

- closer follow-up;
- linkage to a care coordinator; and
- incorporation of health information technology to assist in identification, clinical decision support, and tracking.

Families should be encouraged to partner with the professionals in the medical home to recognize and monitor appropriate consultation and service options. These may include:

- monitoring of the child's progress being made related to services being purchased;
- informing families of appropriate treatment models;
- being available to programs and school systems for clarification of medical issues that affect development and learning; and
- proactively planning the transition from Part C (birth to 3 years) to Part B of IDEA, and the 3- to 5-year-old programs in their local school system.
- Advocacy roles for physicians in the medical home

TABLE 5 Ideas for Communication/Collaboration Between Medical Homes and Part C

Channels for concise bidirectional, "minimum effort" communication needs to be in place and familiar to both the medical home and the regional Part C Program. Tools such as the AAP Referral Form for Early Intervention should be deemed acceptable (with modifications as needed) and readily available (http://www.medicalhomeinfo.org/downloads/pdfs/EIReferralForm_1.pdf).[113]

Professionals at both the medical home and the Part C program need continual update in medical records as the child is seen and changes are noted.

To best sustain the process of information sharing, the individuals at each program should know who one another are and how to contact directly when needed.

Information from the medical home should be available to the Part C assessment team before its evaluation and information, and recommendations on intervention should be forwarded to the medical home as the individualized family service plan is developed and modified.

When the child is seen by subspecialists, their input to both the medical home and the Part C program is valuable.

Timely and ongoing flow of information between the medical home and the Part C program reassures the family of coordinated, family-centered care; it relieves the family of the burden of having to interpret and transport the information.

Modified from Stille CJ. Communication, comanagement, and collaborative care for children and youth with special healthcare needs. *Pediatr Ann.* 2009;38(9):498–504.[110]

TABLE 6 Resources for Medical Homes and Families

Resource	Comments
American Academy of Pediatrics www.HealthyChildren.org	At the American Academy of Pediatrics Web site. Includes developmental milestones for infants/toddlers 0–5 y of age. Information about infants born preterm and about early childhood delays in all areas, including language and social skills, is available.
Zero To Three www.zerotothree.org	Includes information and resources on a number of topics, including early development, language, and behavior.
Learn the Sign, Act Early Center for Disease Control and Prevention, The National Center on Birth Defects and Developmental Disabilities www.cdc.gov/actearly	Provides an array of checklists, fact sheets, positive parenting tip sheets, and links to useful sites for specific issues.
National Dissemination Center for Children With Disabilities http://nichcy.org/babies 1-800-695-0285	Funded by the US Office of Special Education and Rehabilitative Services. This site provides information about services in one's state and local region. Information is guided for families, medical professionals, and school personnel.
Family Voices www.familyvoices.org	Family Voices aims to achieve family-centered care for all children and youth with special health care needs and/or disabilities. The site provides families with tools to make informed decisions, advocate for improved public and private policies, build partnerships among professionals and families, and serve as a partner in the child's health care. National and state sites and organizations are available.
Child and Family WebGuide: Expert Reviewed Sites on Children and Families www.cfw.tufts.edu	The WebGuide is a directory that evaluates, describes, and provides links to hundreds of sites containing information about child development research and practical advice for professionals and families.
Your Child: Development and Behavior Resources: A Guide to Information and Support for Parents www.med.umich.edu/yourchild/index. htm	The site provides: evidence-based information for families and professionals; links to support groups, agencies, and organizations; recommended books and other tools; links to sites for "timely topics"; and a guide for families on using the Internet to find reliable parenting information.
National Association for the Education of Young Children (NAEYC) http://www.naeyc.org/	Founded in 1926, NAEYC is the world's largest organization (80 000 members) working on behalf of young children. Resources and publications for medical homes, families, and agency programs for infants and toddlers are available.

Realize state-to-state differences in eligibility criteria, assessment policies, and services provided under Part C; be aware of updated changes in aspects of service for your state.

Be aware of potential costs to the family (public funding, private insurance, private pay).

Be cognizant of resources (fiscal and professional) available within the state and their local Part C programs and support efforts to optimize services to infants/toddlers. Maintain an updated resource list of local and regional services/resources, including both subspecialty consultants and supportive programs.

Assign time to meet with staff from local and regional programs (in office, over telephone, or through local continuing education or hospital staff meetings).

Work within AAP Chapter structures to monitor and encourage state governmental services to infants and children; interaction at the legislative and the agency levels is critical to support fiscal, policy, and quality assurances of outcomes. Fiscal considerations include both monies to operate quality programs and a system of proper reimbursements for primary physicians and specialists caring for children with special needs. Policy considerations include ensuring that families have timely access to primary and subspecialty services.

Explore opportunities to participate on statewide or regional boards tasked with oversight of the early childhood programs.

CONCLUSIONS

The positive economic effect of front-end EI services has been clearly demonstrated. Short-term and longitudinal data (even into young adulthood) demonstrate the value of early childhood intervention focusing on family-centered, coordinated services that support parent-child relationships as the core element of intervention. Likewise, the economic and health-related values (long-term) derived from being a child supported by the medical home process continue to emerge.

Seeking to enhance collaboration between the sister systems and to minimize systematic barriers is clearly in the best interest of infants, toddlers, their families, and the larger community. Such collaboration serves families in their critical roles as coaches to their children (living, playing, and growing in the infant's natural learning environment).

LEAD AUTHORS

Richard C. Adams, MD
Carl D. Tapia, MD

REFERENCES

1. Dreyer BP. Early childhood stimulation in the developing and developed world: if not now, when? *Pediatrics.* 2011;127(5): 975–977

2. Center on the Developing Child at Harvard University, National Forum on Early Childhood Program Evaluation, National Scientific Council on the Developing Child. *Young Children Develop in an Environment of Relationships.* Cambridge, MA: Center on the Developing Child, Harvard University; 2009. Available at: www.developingchild.harvard.edu. Accessed January 27, 2013

3. Hebbeler K, Greer M, Hutton B. From then to now: the evolution of Part C. *Zero Three.* 2011;3:4–10

4. Cole P, Oser C, Walsh S. Building on the foundations of Part C legislation. *Zero Three.* 2011;3:52–59

5. Childers DO, LaRosa AC. Early intervention. In: Voight RC, Macias MM, Myers SM, eds. *Developmental and Behavioral Pediatrics.* Elk Grove Village, IL: American Academy of Pediatrics; 2011:59–68

6. Council for Exceptional Children, Division for Early Childhood, and IDEA Infant and Toddler Coordinators Association. Individuals with Disabilities Education Act Part C: Early intervention program for infants and toddlers with disabilities: final regulations side by side comparison. Missoula, MT: Division for Early Childhood; October 2011. Available at: http://dec-sped.org/About_DEC/Whats_New?id=128. Accessed January 27, 2013

7. US Department of Education, Office of Special Education Programs, Data Analysis Systems. Infants and toddlers receiving early intervention services in accordance with Part C. 2009. Available at: www.ideadata.org/docs/CumulativeandPointintimebrief.pdf. Accessed January 27, 2013

8. US Department of Health and Human Services. About CAPTA: a legislative history. Washington, DC: Child Welfare Information Gateway; July 2011. Available at: www.childwelfare.gov/pubs/factsheets/about.pdf. Accessed January 27, 2013

9. Long WE, Bauchner H, Sege RD, Cabral HJ, Garg A. The value of the medical home for children without special health care needs. *Pediatrics.* 2012;129(1):87–98

10. Homer CJ, Klatka K, Romm D, et al. A review of the evidence for the medical home for children with special health care needs. *Pediatrics.* 2008;122(4). Available at: www.pediatrics.org/cgi/content/full/122/4/e922

11. Duby JC; American Academy of Pediatrics Council on Children With Disabilities. Role of the medical home in family-centered early intervention services. *Pediatrics.* 2007;120(5):1153–1158

12. Raphael JL, Mei M, Brousseau DC, Giordano TP. Associations between quality of primary care and health care use among children with special health care needs. *Arch Pediatr Adolesc Med.* 2011;165(5):399–404

13. Cooley WC, McAllister JW, Sherrieb K, Kuhlthau K. Improved outcomes associated with medical home implementation in pediatric primary care. *Pediatrics.* 2009;124(1):358–364

14. Romaire MA, Bell JF. The medical home, preventive care screenings, and counseling for children: evidence from the Medical Expenditure Panel Survey. *Acad Pediatr.* 2010;10(5):338–345

15. Ghandour RM, Perry DF, Kogan MD, Strickland BB. The medical home as a mediator of the relation between mental health symptoms and family burden among children with special health care needs. *Acad Pediatr.* 2011;11(2):161–169

16. Haggerty RJ. Caring for children with special needs: historical perspective. *Acad Pediatr.* 2011;11(2):107–109

17. Strickland BB, Jones JR, Ghandour RM, Kogan MD, Newacheck PW. The medical home: health care access and impact for children and youth in the United States. *Pediatrics.* 2011;127(4):604–611

18. Curry AE, Pfeiffer MR, Slopen ME, McVeigh KH. Rates of early intervention referral and significant developmental delay, by birthweight and gestational age. *Matern Child Health J.* 2012;16(5):989–996

19. Patient Protection and Affordable Care Act. Pub L No. 111-148 (2010). Available at: http://burgess.house.gov/UploadedFiles/hr3590_health_care_law_2010.pdf. Accessed January 27, 2013

20. Laraque D, Sia CC. Health care reform and the opportunity to implement a family-centered medical home for children. *JAMA.* 2010;303(23):2407–2408

21. Allen SG, Berry AD, Brewster JA, Chalasani RK, Mack PK. Enhancing developmentally oriented primary care: an Illinois initiative to increase developmental screening in medical homes. *Pediatrics.* 2010;126 (suppl 3):S160–S164

22. Earls MF, Hay SS. Setting the stage for success: implementation of developmental and behavioral screening and surveillance in primary care practice—the North Carolina Assuring Better Child Health and Development (ABCD) Project. *Pediatrics.* 2006; 118(1). Available at: www.pediatrics.org/cgi/content/full/118/1/e183

23. Earls MF, Andrews JE, Hay SS. A longitudinal study of developmental and behavioral screening and referral in North Carolina's Assuring Better Child Health and Development participating practices. *Clin Pediatr (Phila).* 2009;48(8):824–833

24. King TM, Tandon SD, Macias MM, et al. Implementing developmental screening and referrals: lessons learned from a national project. *Pediatrics.* 2010;125(2): 350–360

25. Kenney MK, Kogan MD. Special needs children with speech and hearing difficulties: prevalence and unmet needs. *Acad Pediatr.* 2011;11(2):152–160

26. American Academy of Pediatrics Committee on Pediatric Workforce. Pediatrician

workforce statement. *Pediatrics.* 2005;116 (1):263–269

27. Phillips RL, Jr, Bazemore AW, Dodoo MS, Shipman SA, Green LA. Family physicians in the child health care workforce: opportunities for collaboration in improving the health of children. *Pediatrics.* 2006; 118(3):1200–1206

28. Nelson HD, Nygren P, Walker M, Panoscha R. Screening for speech and language delay in preschool children: systematic evidence review for the US Preventive Services Task Force. *Pediatrics.* 2006;117 (2). Available at: www.pediatrics.org/cgi/content/full/117/2/e298

29. Center on the Developing Child at Harvard University, National Forum on Early Childhood Program Evaluation, and National Scientific Council on the Developing Child. *The Science of Early Childhood Development: Closing the Gap Between What We Know and What We Do.* Cambridge, MA: Center on the Developing Child, Harvard University, 2007. Available at: www.developingchild.harvard.edu. Accessed January 27, 2013

30. Guion WK, Mishoe S, Passmore GG, Witter P. Development of a concept map to convey understanding of patient and family-centered care. *J Healthc Qual.* 2010;32(6): 27–32

31. Livingood WC, Winterbauer NL, McCaskill Q, Wood D. Evaluating Medical Home constructs for children with special needs: integrating theory and logic models. *Fam Community Health.* 2007;30(4):E1–E15

32. Gordon JB, Colby HH, Bartelt T, Jablonski D, Krauthoefer ML, Havens P. A tertiary care-primary care partnership model for medically complex and fragile children and youth with special health care needs. *Arch Pediatr Adolesc Med.* 2007;161(10): 937–944

33. Halfon N, Inkelas M, Abrams M, Stevens G. *Quality of Preventive Health Care for Young Children, Strategies for Improvement.* New York, NY: The Commonwealth Fund; May 2005. Publication No. 822. Available at: www.healthychild.ucla.edu/publications/Documents/822_Halfon_quality_preventive_hlt_care_young_children.pdf. Accessed January 27, 2013

34. Winitzer RF, Bisgaier J, Grogan C, Rhodes K. "He only takes those type of patients on certain days": specialty care access for children with special health care needs. *Disabil Health J.* 2012;5(1):26–33

35. Coker TR, Shaikh Y, Chung PJ. Parent-reported quality of preventive care for children at-risk for developmental delay. *Acad Pediatr.* 2012;12(5):384–390

36. Federal Expert Work Group on Pediatric Subspecialty Capacity. *Promising State and Regional Approaches for Extending Access to Pediatric Subspecialty Care and Coordination With Primary Care.* Washington, DC. Maternal and Child Health Bureau; July 2011. Available at: www.googlesyndicatedsearch.com/u/medicalhome?q=subspecialty+and+medicl+home. Accessed January 27, 2013

37. Pinto-Martin JA, Dunkle M, Earls M, Fliedner D, Landes C. Developmental stages of developmental screening: steps to implementation of a successful program. *Am J Public Health.* 2005;95(11): 1928–1932

38. Perrin JM, Romm D, Bloom SR, et al. A family-centered, community-based system of services for children and youth with special health care needs. *Arch Pediatr Adolesc Med.* 2007;161(10):933–936

39. McCarton CM, Brooks-Gunn J, Wallace IF, et al. Results at age 8 years of early intervention for low-birth-weight premature infants. The Infant Health and Development Program. *JAMA.* 1997;277(2): 126–132

40. McCormick MC, Brooks-Gunn J, Buka SL, et al. Early intervention in low birth weight premature infants: results at 18 years of age for the Infant Health and Development Program. *Pediatrics.* 2006; 117(3):771–780

41. Herrod HG. Do first years really last a lifetime? *Clin Pediatr (Phila).* 2007;46(3): 199–205

42. Walker SP, Chang SM, Vera-Hernández M, Grantham-McGregor S. Early childhood stimulation benefits adult competence and reduces violent behavior. *Pediatrics.* 2011;127(5):849–857

43. Rolnick A, Grunewald R. Early intervention on a large scale. Available at: www.minneapolisfed.org/publications_papers/studies/earlychild/early_intervention.cfm. Accessed January 27, 2013

44. Reynolds AJ, Temple JA, Robertson DL, Mann EA. Long-term effects of an early childhood intervention on educational achievement and juvenile arrest: a 15-year follow-up of low-income children in public schools. *JAMA.* 2001;285(18):2339–2346

45. Bernanke BS. Early education. Presented at Children's Defense Fund National Conference; July 24, 2012; Cincinnati, OH. Available at: www.federalreserve.gov/newsevents/speech/bernanke20120724a.htm. Accessed January 27, 2013

46. Rydell MS, Chiesa J. *Investing in our children: what we know and don't know*

about the costs and benefits of early childhood interventions. Santa Monica, CA: RAND Corp; 1998. Available at: www.rand.org/pubs/monograph_reports/MR898/. Accessed January 27, 2013

47. Kilburn MR, Karoly LA. *The Economics of Early Childhood Policy.* Santa Monica, CA: RAND Corp; 2008

48. Karoly LA, Kilburn MR, Bigelow JH, Caulkins JP, Cannon JS. *Assessing Costs and Benefits of Early Childhood Intervention Programs: Overview and Applications to the Starting Early, Starting Smart Program.* Santa Monica, CA: RAND Corp; 2001. Publication No. MR-1336-CFP. Available at: www.rand.org/pubs/monograph_reports/MR1336/. Accessed January 27, 2013

49. Karoly LA, Kilburn MR, Cannon JS. *Early Childhood Interventions: Proven Results, Future Promise.* Santa Monica, CA: RAND Corp; 2005. Publication No. MG-341-PNC. Available at: www.rand.org/pubs/monographs/MG341.html. Accessed January 27, 2013

50. Chernoff J, Flanagan KD, McPhee C, Park J. *Preschool: First findings From the Third Follow-up of the Early Childhood Longitudinal Study, Birth Cohort (ECLS-B).* Washington, DC: National Center for Educational Statistics, Institute of Education Sciences, US Department of Education; 2007. Publication No. NCED 2008-025

51. Law MC, Darrah J, Pollock N, et al. Focus on function: a cluster, randomized controlled trial comparing child- versus context-focused intervention for young children with cerebral palsy. *Dev Med Child Neurol.* 2011;53(7):621–629

52. Darrah J, Law MC, Pollock N, et al. Context therapy: a new intervention approach for children with cerebral palsy. *Dev Med Child Neurol.* 2011;53(7):615–620

53. Center on the Developing Child at Harvard University, National Forum on Early Childhood Program Evaluation, and National Scientific Council on the Developing Child. *A Science-Based Framework for Early Childhood Policy: Using Evidence to Improve Outcomes in Learning, Behavior, and Health for Vulnerable Children.* Cambridge, MA: Center on the Developing Child, Harvard University; 2007

54. Pilkington K. Side-by side: transdisciplinary early intervention in natural environments. *OT Practice Online.* 2006;11(6): 12–17

55. Woods J. Providing early intervention services in natural environments. *The ASHA Leader.* 2008;13:14–17

56. American Physical Therapy Association. *Section on Pediatrics. Fact Sheet: Natural*

Environments in Early Intervention Services. Alexandria, VA: American Physical Therapy Association; 2012

57. Ideishi RI, O'Neil ME, Chiarello LA, Nixon-Cave K. Perspectives of therapist's role in care coordination between medical and early intervention services. *Phys Occup Ther Pediatr.* 2010;30(1):28–42

58. Friedman M, Woods J, Salisbury C. Caregiver coaching strategies for early intervention providers: moving toward operational definitions. *Infants Young Child.* 2012;25(1):62–82

59. Humphrey R, Wakeford L. Development of everyday activities: a model for occupation-centered therapy. *Infants Young Child.* 2008;21(3):230–240

60. Moore L, Koger D, Blomberg S, et al. Making best practice our practice: reflections on our journey into natural environments. *Infants Young Child.* 2012;25(1):95–105

61. Ray LD. Parenting and Childhood Chronicity: making visible the invisible work. *J Pediatr Nurs.* 2002;17(6):424–438

62. Campbell PH, Milbourne S, Wilcox MJ. Adaptation interventions to promote participation in natural settings. *Infants Young Child.* 2008;21(2):94–106

63. US Department of Health and Human Service, Administration for Children and Families, Children's Bureau. Child Maltreatment 2010. Available at: www.acf.hhs.gov/programs/cb/resource/child-maltreatment-2010. Accessed January 27, 2013

64. Ward H, Yoon A, Atkins J, Morries P, Oldham E, Wathen K. *Children at Risk in the Child Welfare System: Collaborations to Promote School Readiness.* University of Southern Maine, Catherine E Cutler Institute for Child and Family Policy; 2009. Available at: http://muskie.usm.maine.edu/schoolreadiness. Accessed January 27, 2013

65. Casanueva CE, Cross TP, Ringeisen H. Developmental needs and individualized family service plans among infants and toddlers in the child welfare system. *Child Maltreat.* 2008;13(3):245–258

66. Moxley KM, Squires J, Lindstrom L. Early intervention and maltreated children: a current look at the Child Abuse Prevention and Treatment Act and Part C. *Infants Young Child.* 2012;25(1):3–18

67. Knitzer J, Theberge S, Johnson K. *Reducing Maternal Depression and Its Impact on Young Children: Toward a Responsive Early Childhood Policy Framework.* Project Thrive: Issue Brief No. 2. New York, NY: National Center for Children in Poverty,

Columbia University; 2008. Available at: http://academiccommons.columbia.edu/catalog/ac:126465. Accessed January 27, 2013

68. Hibbard RA, Desch LW; American Academy of Pediatrics, Committee on Child Abuse and Neglect, Council on Children With Disabilities. Clinical report: maltreatment of children with disabilities [reaffirmed January 2011]. *Pediatrics.* 2007;119(5):1018–1025

69. Conroy S, Pariante CM, Marks MN, et al. Maternal psychopathology and infant development at 18 months: the impact of maternal personality disorder and depression. *J Am Acad Child Adolesc Psychiatry.* 2012;51(1):51–61

70. Brauner CB, Stephens CB. Estimating the prevalence of early childhood serious emotional/behavioral disorders: challenges and recommendations. *Public Health Rep.* 2006;121(3):303–310

71. Bonuck K, Grant R. Sleep problems and early developmental delay: implications for early intervention programs. *Intellect Dev Disabil.* 2012;50(1):41–52

72. Horwitz SM, Kelleher KJ, Stein RE, et al. Barriers to the identification and management of psychosocial issues in children and maternal depression. *Pediatrics.* 2007;119(1). Available at: www.pediatrics.org/cgi/content/full/119/1/e208

73. Ammerman RT, Putnam FW, Altaye M, et al. Changes in depressive symptoms in first time mothers in home visitation. *Child Abuse Negl.* 2009;33(3):127–138

74. Perry DF, Kaufman RK. *Integrating Early Childhood Mental Health Consultation With the Pyramid Model.* Washington, DC: The Technical Assistance Center on Social Emotional Intervention for Young Children, National Center for Effective Mental Health Consultation, Georgetown University Center for Child and Human Development; December 2009. Available at: www.challengingbehavior.org/do/resources/documents/brief_integrating.pdf. Accessed January 27, 2013

75. Sipes M, Matson JL, Turygin N. The use of the Battelle Developmental Inventory-Second Edition (BDI-2) as an early screener for autism spectrum disorders. *Dev Neurorehabil.* 2011;14(5):310–314

76. Baggett KM, Warlen L, Hamilton JL, Roberts JL, Staker M. Screening infant mental health indicators. *Infants Young Child.* 2007;20(4):300–310

77. Knapp PK, Ammen S, Arstein-Kerslake C, Poulsen MK, Mastergeorge A. Feasibility of expanding services for very young children in the public mental health setting.

J Am Acad Child Adolesc Psychiatry. 2007;46(2):152–161

78. Zeanah PD, Stafford B, Zeanah C. *Clinical Interventions to Enhance Infant Mental Health: A Selective Review.* Los Angeles, CA: National Center for Infant and Early Childhood Health Policy, University of Southern California; 2005

79. Ages & Stages Questionnaires. What is ASQ? Available at: www.agesandstages.com/asq/asqse.html. Accessed January 27, 2013

80. Squires J, Bricker D. Ages & Stages questionnaires, third edition (ASQ-3). Available at: http://products.brookespublishing.com/Ages-Stages-Questionnaires-Third-Edition-ASQ-3-Materials-Kit-P585.aspx. Accessed January 27, 2013

81. Squires J, Bricker D, Twombly E. Ages & Stages questionnaires: social-emotional (ASQ:SE), a parent-completed, child-monitoring system for social-emotional behaviors. Available at: http://products.brookespublishing.com/Ages-Stages-Questionnaires-Social-Emotional-ASQSE-P579.aspx. Accessed January 27, 2013

82. California Institute for Mental Health. Mental Health Screening Tool Zero to 5 Years (MHST 0-5). Sacramento, CA: California Institute for Mental Health. Available at: www.cimh.org/downloads/ScreeningTool0-5.pdf. Accessed January 27, 2013

83. American Academy of Pediatrics. *Addressing Mental Health Concerns in Primary Care: A Clinician's Toolkit.* Elk Grove Village, IL: American Academy of Pediatrics; 2010

84. García SB, Ortiz AB. Preventing disproportionate representation: culturally and responsive prereferral interventions. *Teach Except Child.* 2006;38(4):64–68

85. Bronheim S. *Cultural Competence: It All Starts at the Front Desk.* Washington, DC: National Center for Cultural Competence, Georgetown University Center for Child and Human Development; 2004. Available at: http://nccc.georgetown.edu/documents/FrontDeskArticle.pdf. Accessed January 27, 2013

86. Garcia SB, Mendez-Perez A. Mexican American mothers' beliefs about language disabilities: implications for early childhood intervention. *Remedial Spec Educ.* 2000;21:90–100

87. Hernandez D. *Young Hispanic Children in the US: A Demographic Portrait Based on Census 2000. Report to National Task Force on Early Childhood Education for Hispanics.* Tempe, AZ: Arizona State University; 2006. Available at: www.ecehispanic.

org/work/young_hispanic.pdf. Accessed January 27, 2013

88. National Center for Cultural Competence, Center for Child and Human Development, Georgetown University. Available at: http://www11.georgetown.edu/research/gucchd/nccc/features/CCHPA.html. Accessed August 23, 2013

89. Giannoni PP, Kass PH. Risk factors associated with children lost to care in a state early childhood intervention program. *Res Dev Disabil.* 2010;31(4):914–923

90. Feinberg E, Silverstein M, Donahue S, Bliss R. The impact of race on participation in Part C early intervention services. *J Dev Behav Pediatr.* 2011;32:284–291

91. Harry B. Collaboration with culturally and linguistically diverse families: ideal versus reality. *Except Child.* 2008;74(3):372–388

92. Okumura MJ, Van Cleave J, Gnanasekaran S, Houtrow A. Understanding factors associated with work loss for families caring for CSHCN. *Pediatrics.* 2009;124(suppl 4):S392–S398

93. McManus B, McCormick MC, Acevedo-Garcia D, Ganz M, Hauser-Cram P. The effect of state early intervention eligibility policy on participation among a cohort of young CSHCN. *Pediatrics.* 2009;124(suppl 4):S368–S374

94. Tamara H. *Disparities in Early Learning and Development: Lessons from the Early Childhood Longitudinal Study—Birth Cohort (ECLS-B).* Washington, DC: Child Trends; 2009

95. Cooper JL, Masi R, Vick J. *Social-Emotional Development in Early Childhood: What Every Policymaker Should Know.* New York, NY: National Center for Children in Poverty; August 2009. Available at: www.nccp.org. Accessed January 27, 2013

96. Stebbins H, Knitzer J. *United States Health and Nutrition: State Choices to Promote Quality. Improve the Odds: State Early Childhood Profiles.* 2007. Available at: www.nccp.org/publications/pdf/text_725.pdf. Accessed January 27, 2013

97. National Center for Children in Poverty. Improving the Odds for Young Children, State Profiles. Updated 2011. Available at: www.nccp.org/profiles/early_childhood.html. Accessed January 27, 2013

98. National Center for Children in Poverty. User's guide to the state early childhood profiles. Available at: www.nccp.org/profiles/early_childhood.html. Accessed January 27, 2013

99. Whitaker RC, Phillips SM, Orzol SM. Food insecurity and the risks of depression and anxiety in mothers and behavior problems in their preschool-aged children. *Pediatrics.* 2006;118(3). Available at: www.pediatrics.org/cgi/content/full/118/3/e859

100. Slopen N, Fitzmaurice G, Williams DR, Gilman SE. Poverty, food insecurity, and the behavior for childhood internalizing and externalizing disorders. *J Am Acad Child Adolesc Psychiatry.* 2010;49(5):444–452

101. Kenyon C, Sandel M, Silverstein M, Shakir A, Zuckerman B. Revisiting the social history for child health. *Pediatrics.* 2007;120(3). Available at: www.pediatrics.org/cgi/content/full/120/3/e734

102. Committee on Child Health Financing, American Academy of Pediatrics. Guiding principles for managed care arrangements for the health care of newborns, infants, children, adolescents, and young adults. Committee on Child Health Financing, American Academy of Pediatrics. *Pediatrics.* 2006;118(2):828–833

103. McManus M, Fox H, Limb S, et al. New workforce, practice, and payment reforms essential for improving access to pediatric subspecialty care within the medical home. *Arch Pediatr Adolesc Med.* 2009;163(3):200–202

104. Moeschler JB, Shevell M; American Academy of Pediatrics, Committee on Genetics. Clinical genetic evaluation of the child with mental retardation or developmental delays [reaffirmed May 2012]. *Pediatrics.* 2006;117(1):2304–2316

105. American Academy of Pediatrics, Council on Children With Disabilities. Policy statement: identifying infants and young children with developmental disorders in the medical home: an algorithm for developmental surveillance and screening [reaffirmed December 2009]. *Pediatrics.* 2006;118(1):405–420

106. Marks KP, Page Glascoe F, Macias MM. Enhancing the algorithm for developmental-behavioral surveillance and screening in children 0 to 5 years. *Clin Pediatr (Phila).* 2011;50(9):853–868

107. Moeschler JB, Shevell M; American Academy of Pediatrics, Committee on Genetics. Clinical genetic evaluation of the child with mental retardation or developmental delays. *Pediatrics.* 2006;117(6):2304–2316

108. Michaud LJ; American Academy of Pediatrics Committee on Children With Disabilities. Prescribing therapy services for children with motor disabilities. *Pediatrics.* 2004;113(6):1836–1838

109. Sneed RC, May WL, Stencel C. Policy versus practice: comparison of prescribing therapy and durable medical equipment in medical and educational settings. *Pediatrics.* 2004;114(5). Available at: www.pediatrics.org/cgi/content/full/114/5/e612

110. Stille CJ. Communication, comanagement, and collaborative care for children and youth with special healthcare needs. *Pediatr Ann.* 2009;38(9):498–504

111. Stille CJ, Frantz J, Vogel LC, Lighter D. Building communication between professionals at children's specialty hospitals and the medical home. *Clin Pediatr (Phila).* 2009;48(6):661–673

112. Houston KT, Behl DD, White KR, Forsman I. Federal privacy regulations and the provision of Early Hearing Detection and Intervention programs. *Pediatrics.* 2010;126(suppl 1):S28–S33

113. Kozlowski AM, Matson JL, Horovitz M, Worley JA, Neal D. Parents' first concerns of their child's development in toddlers with autism spectrum disorders. *Dev Neurorehabil.* 2011;14(2):72–78

114. Rush DD, Shelden ML. *Evidence-Based Definition of Coaching Practices.* Morganton, NC: Center for the Advanced Study of Excellence in Early Childhood; 2005

115. Zhang C, Bennett T. Facilitating the meaningful participation of culturally and linguistically diverse families in the IFSP and IEP process. *Focus Autism Other Dev Disabl.* 2003;18(1):51–59

116. American Academy of Pediatrics. Referral Form for Early Intervention Services. Elk Grove Village, IL: American Academy of Pediatrics; 2007. Available at: www.medicalhomeinfo.org/downloads/pdfs/EIReferralForm_1.pdf. Accessed January 27, 2013

117. Heckman JJ, Moon SH, et al. The Rate of Return to the High/Scope Perry Preschool Program. National Bureau of Economic Research. Working Paper No. 15471 Issued November 2009. Available at: www.nber.org/papers/w15471. Accessed August 23, 2013

Electronic Prescribing in Pediatrics: Toward Safer and More Effective Medication Management

- *Policy Statement*

POLICY STATEMENT

Electronic Prescribing in Pediatrics: Toward Safer and More Effective Medication Management

abstract

This policy statement identifies the potential value of electronic pre-scribing (e-prescribing) systems in improving quality and reducing harm in pediatric health care. On the basis of limited but positive pe-diatric data and on the basis of federal statutes that provide incentives for the use of e-prescribing systems, the American Academy of Pedi-atrics recommends the adoption of e-prescribing systems with pedi-atric functionality. The American Academy of Pediatrics also recommends a set of functions that technology vendors should provide when e-prescribing systems are used in environments in which chil-dren receive care. *Pediatrics* 2013;131:824–826

COUNCIL ON CLINICAL INFORMATION TECHNOLOGY EXECUTIVE COMMITTEE, 2011–2012

KEY WORDS
electronic prescribing, health information technology, medication, pediatrics, prescription, quality improvement

BACKGROUND

The American Academy of Pediatrics (AAP) is committed to providing the best and safest health care system possible for children.

Medication prescribing or ordering in pediatrics is an error-prone process that can lead to adverse medication events and patient harm.[1,2] Electronic prescribing (e-prescribing) is widely recognized as a component of the care process that improves quality and reduces costs by facilitating handoffs, improving clinical decision-making, and potentially improving medication adherence.

NEW INFORMATION

Prescribing error rates in children were estimated to be between 5% and 27% in a recent systematic review.[3] Prescribing errors are most prevalent with antibiotic agents but may occur even with medications that do not require weight-based dosing.[4] Medication errors in chil-dren may lead to more severe complications because of narrow therapeutic profiles and the inability of some children to communi-cate adverse effects. Many existing e-prescribing systems are not well designed for use in pediatric patients and lack the required features outlined in this statement. Parental health and English literacy have been shown to play important roles in the correct medication ad-ministration in children.[5,6]

From a legislative viewpoint, the past decade has been an active one for the national medication-prescribing landscape. In particular, 2 major statutes specifically addressed the goal of 100% adoption of e-prescribing through both time-dependent incentives and penalties.

www.pediatrics.org/cgi/doi/10.1542/peds.2013-0192

doi:10.1542/peds.2013-0192

PEDIATRICS (ISSN Numbers: Print, 0031-4005; Online, 1098-4275).

Copyright © 2013 by the American Academy of Pediatrics

The Medicare Improvements for Patients and Providers Act (Pub L No. 110-275 [2008]) provided for incentive payments to Medicare-participating providers that use e-prescribing software to generate prescriptions. The Health Information Technology for Economic and Clinical Health Act (Pub L No. 111-5 [2009]) established a program of incentive payments for Medicare and Medicaid providers who adopt, implement, and demonstrate meaningful use of health information technology. One of the key requirements of meaningful use is to generate and transmit prescriptions electronically to the pharmacy. The meaningful use requirements also encourage the routine use of medication lists, medication allergy lists, drug–drug interaction and drug-allergy checking, and drug formulary checking.

CONCLUSIONS

E-prescribing systems can improve the quality and safety of medication administration by reducing preventable adverse drug events,[7–9] reducing dosing errors,[10] improving communication,[11,12] avoiding adverse effects,[13,14] and improving efficiency.[15] The benefits of e-prescribing systems in pediatrics can only be achieved by systems with appropriate functionality and may be hampered by poorly developed systems[16] or implementation strategies.[17] At present, many e-prescribing systems fall short of providing expert-recommended functional characteristics.[18] Specific challenges in pediatric e-prescribing include age- and indication-specific, weight-based dosing requirements, rounding based on formulary (liquid or solid), the conversion of doses from an ingredient amount to a volume for liquids, the desire to provide easily administered home doses, and, when necessary, extemporaneously compounded dosage forms. Although these systems already confer numerous advantages over the paper-based

alternative, they will need to evolve to be an ideal platform for safe and effective pediatric medication prescribing. The features listed in Table 1, derived in part from previous work by the AAP,[19] will help address these challenges to safe and effective pediatric prescribing.

RECOMMENDATIONS

1. Because safety for children is paramount, e-prescribing systems used for the care of children should include, at a minimum, pediatric-specific medication catalogs; pediatric-specific decision support, such as weight-based dose calculations and individual and daily dose alerts; rounding; ingredient amount-to-volume conversions for liquid medications; metric-only labeling instructions; and pediatric drug information and formulation options. This recommendation may be implemented by sharing reports, such as the

accompanying technical report,[20] with standards development organizations and the Office of the National Coordinator for Health Information Technology—Authorized Testing and Certification Bodies to encourage the inclusion of minimum requirements into the development of standards and certification criteria.

2. When possible, e-prescribing systems should be implemented as part of a robust electronic health record and include drug–drug interaction and allergy checking. When implementing a stand-alone e-prescribing system, consideration should be given to a solid design (including correct field length and standard vocabulary) and the potential future need to generate reports with, transfer data to, or interface the e-prescribing system with an electronic health record. E-prescribing systems must be

TABLE 1 Pediatric Requirements for Safe and Effective e-Prescribing

Category	Pediatric Requirements
Patient information	Date of birth or age in units more specific than years
	Weight in kilograms
	Height in centimeters
	Any history of intolerable adverse effects or allergy to medications
Medication information	Indication-based dosing and individual and daily dose alerts, using a mg/kg per day or mg/m^2 per day formula, unless inappropriate
	Weight-based dosing calculations
	All available formulations, including liquid formulations that may be specific brands
	Common formulations requiring extemporaneous compounding or combinations of active ingredients
Cognitive support	Dose-range checking (minimum and maximum amount per dose, amount per day based on weight, surface area, and total dose)
	Automatic strength-to-volume conversions for liquid medications
	Adverse effect warnings specific to pediatric populations
	Alternative therapies based on ameliorable adverse effects
	Tall Man lettering to reduce medication selection errors
	Medication-specific indications to reduce ordering of sound-alike drugs
Pharmacy information	Pharmacies that will create extemporaneous compounds
Data transmission	Use of messaging standards for data transmission to pharmacies that include the patient's weight and notes pertaining to weight-based calculations
	Transmission of strength, concentration, and dose volume labeled in metric units for liquid medications

efficient for use in pediatric offices and must integrate well with existing office workflow. Recommendation 2 may be implemented by educating providers on the required elements of pediatric-appropriate e-prescribing systems through published reports, such as the accompanying technical report.[20]

3. E-prescribing systems should be able to provide patients and their parents with administration instructions based on their level of health literacy and their preferred language. Recommendation 3 may be implemented by educating e-prescribing vendors and providers of the need for this feature.

4. Pharmacies should work to enhance their technology infrastructure and workflows to enable efficient

acceptance and processing of electronic prescriptions generated and transmitted by certified health information technology. Furthermore, pharmacies should be capable of performing the dose-range checks to provide independent redundancy.

5. Private and public insurers and other third-party payers should offer financial incentives to health care providers and pharmacies to use e-prescribing systems with appropriate decision support.

6. States should work to harmonize their respective legislation to the US Drug Enforcement Agency's interim final rule on e-prescribing of controlled substances. Recommendations 4, 5, and 6 may be implemented by continued advocacy activities at the local, state, and national levels.

LEAD AUTHORS

Christoph U. Lehmann, MD
Kevin B. Johnson, MD, MS

COUNCIL ON CLINICAL INFORMATION TECHNOLOGY EXECUTIVE COMMITTEE, 2011–2012

Mark A. Del Beccaro, MD, Chairperson
Gregg Alexander, DO
Willa H. Drummond, MD, MS
Anne B. Francis, MD
Eric G. Handler, MD, MPH
Timothy D. Johnson, DO, MMM
George R. Kim, MD
Michael Leu, MD, MS, MHS
Eric Tham, MD, MS
Stuart T. Weinberg, MD
Alan E. Zuckerman, MD

CONSULTANTS

Christoph U. Lehmann, MD
Kevin B. Johnson, MD, MS

STAFF

Jennifer Mansour
Ielnaz Kashefipour, MPP

REFERENCES

1. Miller MR, Clark JS, Lehmann CU. Computer based medication error reporting: insights and implications. *Qual Saf Health Care.* 2006;15(3):208–213

2. Lehmann CU, Kim GR. Prevention of medication errors. *Clin Perinatol.* 2005;32(1):107–123

3. Miller MR, Robinson KA, Lubomski LH, Rinke ML, Pronovost PJ. Medication errors in paediatric care: a systematic review of epidemiology and an evaluation of evidence supporting reduction strategy recommendations. *Qual Saf Health Care.* 2007;16(2):116–126

4. Kaushal R, Goldmann DA, Keohane CA, et al. Medication errors in paediatric outpatients. *Qual Saf Health Care.* 2010;19(6):e30

5. Leyva M, Sharif I, Ozuah PO. Health literacy among Spanish-speaking Latino parents with limited English proficiency. *Ambul Pediatr.* 2005;5(1):56–59

6. Freedman RB, Jones SK, Lin A, Robin AL, Muir KW. Influence of parental health literacy and dosing responsibility on pediatric glaucoma medication adherence. *Arch Ophthalmol.* 2012;130(3):306–311

7. Ammenwerth E, Schnell-Inderst P, Machan C, Siebert U. The effect of electronic prescribing on medication errors and adverse drug events: a systematic review. *J Am Med Inform Assoc.* 2008;15(5):585–600

8. Jani YH, Ghaleb MA, Marks SD, Cope J, Barber N, Wong IC. Electronic prescribing reduced prescribing errors in a pediatric renal outpatient clinic. *J Pediatr.* 2008;152(2):214–218

9. Garg AX, Adhikari NK, McDonald H, et al. Effects of computerized clinical decision support systems on practitioner performance and patient outcomes: a systematic review. *JAMA.* 2005;293(10):1223–1238

10. Zimmer KP, Miller MR, Lee BH, Yaster M, Miller RE, Lehmann CU. Narcotic prescription writer: use in medical error reduction. *J Patient Saf.* 2008;4(2):98–105

11. Newby DA, Robertson J. Computerised prescribing: assessing the impact on prescription repeats and on generic substitution of some commonly used antibiotics. *Med J Aust.* 2010;192(4):192–195

12. Stenner SP, Chen Q, Johnson KB. Impact of generic substitution decision support on electronic prescribing behavior. *J Am Med Inform Assoc.* 2010;17(6):681–688

13. Classen DC, Pestotnik SL, Evans RS, Burke JP. Computerized surveillance of adverse drug events in hospitalized patients. *JAMA.* 1991;266(20):2847–2851

14. Evans RS, Classen DC, Pestotnik SL, Lundsgaarde HP, Burke JP. Improving empiric antibiotic selection using computer decision

support. *Arch Intern Med.* 1994;154(8):878–884

15. The Joint Commission. *A Guide to The Joint Commission's Medication Management Standards.* 2nd ed. Oakbrook Terrace, IL: The Joint Commission; 2009

16. Koppel R, Metlay J, Cohen A, et al. Role of computerized physician order entry systems in facilitating medication errors. *JAMA.* 2005;239(10):1197–1230

17. Han Y, Carcillo J, Venkataraman S, et al. Unexpected increased mortality after implementation of a commercially sold computerized physician order entry system. *Pediatrics.* 2005;116(6):1506–1512

18. Wang CJ, Marken RS, Meili RC, Straus JB, Landman AB, Bell DS. Functional characteristics of commercial ambulatory electronic prescribing systems: a field study. *J Am Med Inform Assoc.* 2005;12(3):346–356

19. Gerstle RS. Electronic prescribing systems in pediatrics: the rationale and functionality requirements. *Pediatrics.* 2007;119(6):1229–1231

20. American Academy of Pediatrics, Council on Clinical Information Technology. Technical report: electronic prescribing in pediatrics: toward safer and more effective medication management. *Pediatrics.* 2012, In press

ERRATA

An error occurred in this AAP Policy Statement titled "Electronic Prescribing in Pediatrics: Toward Safer and More Effective Medication Management" published in the April 2013 issue of *Pediatrics* (2013;131[4]:824–826; doi:10.1542/peds.2013-0192). The Policy Statement should have included a note that author Kevin Johnson's work was funded by the Agency for Healthcare Research and Quality.

doi:10.1542/peds.2013-1287

Electronic Prescribing in Pediatrics: Toward Safer and More Effective Medication Management

- *Technical Report*

TECHNICAL REPORT

Electronic Prescribing in Pediatrics: Toward Safer and More Effective Medication Management

abstract

This technical report discusses recent advances in electronic prescribing (e-prescribing) systems, including the evidence base supporting their limitations and potential benefits. Specifically, this report acknowledges that there are limited but positive pediatric data supporting the role of e-prescribing in mitigating medication errors, improving communication with dispensing pharmacists, and improving medication adherence. On the basis of these data and on the basis of federal statutes that provide incentives for the use of e-prescribing systems, the American Academy of Pediatrics recommends the adoption of e-prescribing systems with pediatric functionality. This report supports the accompanying policy statement from the American Academy of Pediatrics recommending the adoption of e-prescribing by pediatric health care providers. *Pediatrics* 2013;131:e1350–e1356

The US health care system has the distinction of being the world's most expensive delivery system while also having among the lowest levels of quality, as judged by many metrics, including infant mortality, life expectancy, and potential years of life lost.[1,2] More specifically, despite US leadership in establishing many standards of care that correlate with improved quality, the US health care system is able to deliver, at best, 60% of the recommended care in most practices.[3,4] Reasons for this inefficiency include the voluminous information resources to consult and the experts' parallel processing and modeling skills (including integrating considerations of the patient's other illnesses, lifestyle, and genome) required to make an optimal decision.[5] Other challenges include the health care system's existing methods of payment, which lead to fragmented care.[6] Difficult-to-resolve health disparities also occur when there are suboptimal interactions between a person's preferences, the regulatory/operational health care system, and internalized biases, stereotypes, or knowledge deficits. All of these challenges to information management affect the delivery of care.[7] For these reasons, health information technology (HIT) has become recognized as a set of tools that complement the provision of care.[8] Electronic prescribing (e-prescribing) is widely recognized as a component of the prescribing process that facilitates handoffs, improves clinical decision-making, and may improve medication adherence. E-prescribing was defined in 2008 by the Centers for Medicare and Medicaid Services as a system providing prescribers with

Kevin B. Johnson, MD, MS, Christoph U. Lehmann, MD, and the COUNCIL ON CLINICAL INFORMATION TECHNOLOGY

KEY WORDS
health information technology, electronic prescribing, quality improvement, pediatrics, medication, prescription

ABBREVIATIONS
CBO—Congressional Budget Office
EHR—electronic health record
HIT—health information technology
HITECH—Health Information Technology for Economic and Clinical Health
MIPPA—Medicare Improvements for Patients and Providers Act

The guidance in this report does not indicate an exclusive course of treatment or serve as a standard of medical care. Variations, taking into account individual circumstances, may be appropriate.

All technical reports from the American Academy of Pediatrics automatically expire 5 years after publication unless reaffirmed, revised, or retired at or before that time.

www.pediatrics.org/cgi/doi/10.1542/peds.2013-0193

doi:10.1542/peds.2013-0193

PEDIATRICS (ISSN Numbers: Print, 0031-4005; Online, 1098-4275).

the ability to generate and "electronically send an accurate, error-free and understandable prescription directly to a pharmacy from the point-of-care."

RATIONALE FOR ADOPTING E-PRESCRIBING

Adoption of e-prescribing has been strongly endorsed by a variety of professional societies and federal agencies for more than a decade.[9-13] The reason for almost unanimous support for e-prescribing tools is the mounting evidence in adult populations that e-prescribing can improve prescribing quality and provide better pharmacovigilance. Monitoring pharmaceuticals requires collecting, observing, researching, assessing, and evaluating data and derivative information related to safe, effective, and consistent medication use. Pharmacy data management successes reveal a path for transforming medication communication throughout the health care system. The Institute of Medicine summarized this literature in its publication *Preventing Medication Errors*[14] and recommended national mandates for this technology. There is less literature specific to pediatric populations; however, the literature that is specific to this population has been encouraging.

Quality Challenges for E-Prescribing in Pediatrics

By far, the strongest rationale for adopting e-prescribing recognizes the inherent challenges with pediatric prescribing, which are responsible for an error rate in children of between 5% and 27% in a recent systematic review.[15] Physiologic factors, such as the nearly universal need for weight or body surface area considerations in dosing, make medication ordering more prone to errors in children than in adults.[14,16,17] In addition to these physiologic factors, the therapeutic window for many drugs is smaller for children

than adults. Pharmacologic factors, including age-based variability in absorption, metabolism, and excretion of drugs in children as compared with adults, as well as the age-specific contraindications of certain medications, pose special vulnerabilities to the adverse effects of overdosing. The conversion of doses from ingredient amounts to volumes for liquids labeled for home use is also problematic.[18-20] Prescribing errors are most prevalent with antibiotic agents but may occur even in medications that do not require weight-based dosing or ingredient-to-volume conversion.[21] Medication errors in children may lead to more severe complications because of the inability of children to communicate some adverse effects.

Decreased Preventable Adverse Drug Events

Adverse drug events are defined as injuries "resulting from medical intervention related to a drug" and are the leading cause of iatrogenic harm to patients.[22] The Institute of Medicine conservatively estimated that each year, more than 1.5 million preventable adverse drug events occur in the United States.[14] In an ambulatory study in adults, 25% of patients experienced 1 or more adverse drug events (27 events per 100 patients).[23] Estimates in 1995 placed the cost of drug related morbidity and mortality between $20 billion and $130 billion, with most of the cost stemming from drug-related hospital admissions.[24]

The rate of adverse drug events attributable to ambulatory drug administration has been estimated at 3% to 4% in 1 study.[25] This rate is highest in children taking multiple prescription medications.[26] Pediatric patients, although less likely to suffer harm from an adverse event, are susceptible to more types of adverse events, but the quality of the evidence is variable.[27,28]

Studies evaluating e-prescribing systems reveal consistent reductions in potential adverse drug events in systems that organize and coherently report medication summaries.[29-31]

Reducing Dosing Errors

Dosing errors represent the most common medication error in pediatrics.[32] Although seemingly easy to catch, dosing error-checking is complicated by the fact that children's weights vary from as little as 500 g for micro premature infants to well over 100 kg for some obese adolescents, differing by a factor of more than 200. To illustrate the challenge, 2 patients (1 weighing 2 kg and the other 100 kg) discharged with a prescription for 5 mg/kg per day of ranitidine could receive a dose of between 10 mg and 300 mg a day and still not catch the attention of a pharmacist, because all doses between these amounts are reasonable for children, depending on their weight.

E-prescribing systems are able to present standardized dosing formulae, to use the patient's weight to calculate a dose, to convert that dose to a volume for liquids, and to present that dose in a format that is least likely to be confusing to the prescriber, pharmacist, nurse, or parent. Truly sophisticated prescribing systems use individual dose limits and total daily dose limits, compared with weight- or body surface area-based normal values.[33] Some particularly sophisticated systems write out the final dose (ie, "ten [10]") to further improve clarity and to reduce the risk of prescription tampering.[34] Finally, a recent article demonstrated the power of annotating electronic prescriptions with the actual calculation leading up to the dose.[35]

Improved Communication

After dosing errors, missing information and illegible prescriptions cause the majority of prescribing errors in children[36] and significantly impede the ability for these errors to be caught by pharmacists or other health care providers. Illegible handwriting may be at fault for at least 20% of all errors.[26,37] Groups such as the Pediatric Pharmacy Advocacy Group, the Institute for Safe Medication Practices, and the American Society of Health System Pharmacists[38] have espoused requirements for safe pediatric prescribing, recognizing that these prescriptions should include information about the child's age, weight, and indication for therapy and should adhere to a format (eg, no trailing zero) that minimizes miscommunication. The Institute for Safe Medication Practices, the American Academy of Pediatrics, and other groups support the labeling of all prescriptions for liquid medication with volume in milliliters (mL).[39-41]

Parental health and English literacy has been shown to play an important role in the correct medication administration in children.[42,43] E-prescribing systems may provide administration instructions that are appropriate for the parents' or child's health literacy and can be provided in the patient's or her family's primary language.

Software can default or force entry of specific information. For example, a date may be automatically populated, a weight may be pulled from an existing electronic health record (EHR), and a user may be prevented from completing the prescription until essential information has been completed. Pharmacists view the net effect of e-prescribing as positive in the areas of patient safety, effectiveness of care, and efficiency of care.[44,45] In pediatrics, e-prescribing can improve communication through both improving clarity of prescriptions and providing standardized information about indications for therapy, rationales for overriding allergy alerts, and the weight-based

calculations leading to a specific dose.[35] For all patients, e-prescribing systems can improve communication about provider willingness to allow generic substitution,[46-48] which, by avoiding higher copayments, can improve medication adherence.[49]

A study on prescriptions[35] demonstrated the value of including body weight and the process associated with calculating a dose. In this study, pharmacies stated that prescribing safety was improved by "showing your work" related to the cognitive processes associated with prescribing and found it especially beneficial in pediatric prescribing.

Avoiding Adverse Effects

Medication adverse effects may be related to interactions between a medication and the host (allergies or unintended effects) or may be related to other patient medications, dietary choices, or other diagnoses. These unintended consequences may be life-threatening or, more commonly, may lead to poor therapeutic adherence by children and families. Often, these consequences can be ameliorated by choosing an equally efficacious alternative therapy at the time of the initial prescription or after onset of the unintended effect. E-prescribing systems can display results of past therapy and help avoid prescribing medications that may not be tolerated. Systems that are more sophisticated warn about potential unintended effects, thereby decreasing the burden on the family and potentially having a beneficial effect on the economics of health care.[50,51]

Improving Efficiency

The process of prescribing and ensuring adherence is 1 of the most time consuming in practice settings. Both new and refilled prescriptions require attention to the 5 rights: making sure the right patient receives the right

medication in the right dose, using the right route, and at the right time. E-prescribing is able to help with many of these issues by providing early warnings for duplicate therapies, contraindications for use (such as in pregnancy or for lactating mothers), and other prescribing risks mentioned previously.

As a component of an efficient practice, e-prescribing may decrease delays in renewing chronic medications or in flagging renewals as inappropriate. In pediatrics, there is an additional challenge of modifying a dose for some medication refills as the child grows, which can be facilitated by information technology. Perhaps the most pervasive way that e-prescribing can boost practice efficiency is by recognizing the distributed nature of work in the ambulatory setting. For example, a well-designed e-prescribing system might allow a refill or new prescription to be drafted by 1 provider or designee and completed by an authorized prescriber either in the office or any location by using Web-enabled information technology.[34]

E-PRESCRIBING SYSTEM FUNCTIONAL REQUIREMENTS

The theoretical benefits of e-prescribing systems in pediatrics can only be achieved by systems with appropriate functionality and may be hampered by poorly developed systems[52] or implementation strategies.[49] At present, many e-prescribing systems fall short of providing expert recommended functional characteristics.[53] These features broadly cover patient identification and data access, current medication/medication history availability, medication selection, alerts and reminders, medication information, data transmission/storage, monitoring and renewals, prescribing practice feedback, and system security/confidentiality.

The use of e-prescribing systems in children will require overcoming some unique challenges inherent in pediatrics. Paramount among these challenges is the question about the relevance and sensitivity of drug interaction or adverse-effect alerts.[54,55] The existing insensitivity results in many false-positive alerts and subsequently in override rates ranging from 89% to 91%.[25,56-58] Although few studies have been published that assess this phenomenon in children, children tend to be on fewer chronic medications and, because of generally good renal and hepatic function, may be less at risk for severe adverse reactions,[59] thereby magnifying this concern in pediatrics.

Age- and indication-specific weight-based dosing requirements, coupled with the fact that home administration may be associated with a high potential for errors,[21] place additional requirements on the pediatric e-prescribing system (dose rounding, minimum/maximum dosing checks, etc) that may not be as important for adult prescribing. E-prescribing systems need to modify both dosing guidelines and dose-screening parameters to support pediatric dosing for every indication that warrants modified dosing regimens. Furthermore, they need to support the desire to provide easily administered home doses (in mL for liquids) and, when necessary, extemporaneously compounded dosage forms. In short, these systems will need to evolve to be an ideal platform for safe and effective pediatric medication prescribing, although they already confer numerous advantages over the paper-based alternative. The features listed in Table 1, derived in part from previous work by the American Academy of Pediatrics,[16] will help address these challenges to safe and effective pediatric e-prescribing.

TABLE 1 Pediatric Requirements for Safe and Effective Electronic Prescribing

Category	Pediatric Requirements
Patient information	Date of birth or age in units more specific than years
	Weight in kg
	Height in cm
	Any history of intolerable adverse effects or allergy to medications
Medication information	Indication-based dosing and individual and daily dose alerts, using mg/kg per day or mg/m² per day formula, unless inappropriate
	Weight-based dosing calculations
	All available formulations, including liquid formulations that may be specific brands
	Common formulations requiring extemporaneous compounding or combinations of active ingredients
Cognitive support	Dose range checking (minimum and maximum amount per dose, amount per day based on weight, surface area, and total dose)
	Automatic strength to volume conversions for liquid medications
	Adverse-effect warnings specific to pediatric populations
	Alternative therapies based on ameliorable adverse effects
	Tall-man lettering to reduce medication selection errors
	Medication-specific indications to reduce ordering of sound-alike drugs
Pharmacy information	Pharmacies that will create extemporaneous compounds
Data transmission	Use of messaging standards for data transmission to pharmacies that include the patient's weight and notes pertaining to weight-based calculations
	Transmission of strength, concentration, and dose volume labeled in metric units for liquid medications

FEDERAL INITIATIVES TO IMPROVE E-PRESCRIBING ADOPTION

The past decade has been an active one for the national medication prescribing landscape. In particular, 2 major statutes specifically address the goal of 100% e-prescribing adoption through both time-dependent incentives and penalties. Each of these statutes will be described below.

Medicare Improvements for Patients and Providers Act

The Medicare Improvements for Patients and Providers Act (MIPPA) became law on July 15, 2008 (Pub L No. 110-275). MIPPA was designed to avert a statutory Medicare reduction in payments for physicians and implement other changes. In addition to its effect on physician fees, MIPPA addressed the chasm between literature describing improved quality of care related to e-prescribing and the current state of poor adoption (especially among health care providers caring for older and sicker populations). It addressed this chasm by incentivizing the adoption of e-prescribing by authorized prescribers. MIPPA created new financial incentives to encourage physicians who provide services to Medicare patients to adopt technology that will allow them to order prescriptions electronically. Use of this technology is meant to reduce medical errors and help physicians consider cost issues as they make prescribing decisions. Under MIPPA, beginning in 2009, physicians received a 2% increase in payments, phasing down to 0.5% in 2013. However, in 2014 and afterward, physicians who have not implemented the technology will lose 2% of their payments. The incentives and penalties under MIPPA may have less of an effect on pediatric patients, because not all pediatricians see a sufficient number of Medicare-eligible patients.

The Health Information Technology for Economic and Clinical Health Act

The Health Information Technology for Economic and Clinical Health (HITECH) Act was incorporated as part of the American Recovery and Reinvestment Act of 2009 (H.R. 1), the economic stimulus bill signed into law on February 17, 2009 (Pub L No. 111-5). The HITECH Act is intended to promote the widespread adoption of HIT to support the electronic sharing of clinical data among hospitals, physicians, and other health care stakeholders. According to a 2009 report by Surescripts (http://www.surescripts.com/downloads/npr/national-progress-report.pdf), the number of prescribers sending prescriptions electronically more than doubled from 2008 to the end of 2009 to 156 000, which corresponds to only 25% of all office-based prescribers. The same report stated that 85% of community pharmacies, as well as the 6 largest mail-order pharmacies, were able to receive electronic prescriptions. Therefore, the infrastructure for e-prescribing is nearly ready, but prescribers have not yet fully adopted this technology. The HITECH Act builds on existing federal efforts to encourage e-prescribing/HIT adoption and use. The Congressional Budget Office (CBO) estimates that Medicare and Medicaid spending under the HITECH Act will total $32.7 billion over the 2009–2019 period. CBO hypothesizes, however, that widespread HIT adoption will reduce total spending on health care. Through 2019, CBO estimates that the HITECH Act will save the Medicare and Medicaid programs a total of approximately $12.5 billion. Under current law, CBO predicts that approximately 45% of hospitals and 65% of physicians will have adopted HIT by 2019. CBO estimates that the incentive mechanisms in the HITECH Act will boost those adoption rates to approximately 70% for hospitals and 90% for physicians.

The HITECH Act provides financial incentives for HIT use among health care practitioners. It establishes several grant programs to provide funding for investing in HIT infrastructure, purchasing certified EHRs, training, and the dissemination of best practices. E-prescribing functionality is a required component of these EHRs. Important to pediatricians, the legislation further authorizes a 100% federal match for payments to certain qualifying Medicaid service providers who acquire and use certified EHR technology.

E-Prescribing of Controlled Substances

In March 2010, the US Drug Enforcement Agency published the interim final rule on e-prescribing of controlled substances. Before the interim final rule, controlled substances were excluded from e-prescribing through a prohibition by the Drug Enforcement Agency. Even though this ruling will close the gap in e-prescribing, the rules require recertification of systems by outside auditors, new credentialing and auditing processes for prescribers, and a new level of authentication by prescribers before prescriptions are able to be routed electronically. Physicians must apply to federally approved credential service providers or certification authorities to verify their identity and obtain the necessary credentials to engage in e-prescribing of controlled substances. Once a provider is authorized by a third person in the practice to prescribe controlled substances, providers must provide 2 modes of identification, including a user identification/password, a token (like a smart card), or a biometric factor (like a thumbprint) (http://www.deadiversion.usdoj.gov/fed_regs/rules/2010/fr0331.htm). Because of the complexity required to prevent drug diversion (forgeries), vendor compliance and provider adoption is expected to take 1 to 2 years.

LEAD AUTHORS

Kevin B. Johnson, MD, MS
Christoph U. Lehmann, MD, MS

COUNCIL ON CLINICAL INFORMATION TECHNOLOGY EXECUTIVE COMMITTEE, 2011–2012

Mark A. Del Beccaro, MD, Chairperson
Gregg Alexander, DO
Willa H. Drummond, MD, MS
Anne B. Francis, MD
Eric G. Handler, MD, MPH
Timothy D. Johnson, DO, MMM
George R. Kim, MD
Michael Leu, MD, MS, MHS
Eric Tham, MD, MS
Stuart T. Weinberg, MD
Alan E. Zuckerman, MD

CONSULTANTS

Kevin B. Johnson, MD, MS
Christoph U. Lehmann, MD

STAFF

Jennifer Mansour
Ielnaz Kashefipour, MPP

REFERENCES

1. Stratos GA, Katz S, Bergen MR, Hallenbeck J. Faculty development in end-of-life care: evaluation of a national train-the-trainer program. *Acad Med.* 2006;81(11):1000–1007

2. US Department of Health. Health, United States. Rockville, MD. Washington, DC: US Department of Health, Education, and Welfare, Public Health Service, Health Resources Administration, National Center for Health Statistics; 1976. Available at: http://trove.nla.gov.au/work/3409744?selectedversion=NBD1081382. Accessed July 9, 2012

3. Mangione-Smith R, DeCristofaro AH, Setodji CM, et al. The quality of ambulatory care delivered to children in the United States. *N Engl J Med.* 2007;357(15):1515–1523

4. McGlynn EA, Asch SM, Adams J, et al. The quality of health care delivered to adults in the United States. *N Engl J Med.* 2003;348 (26):2635–2645

5. Ely JW, Osheroff JA, Maviglia SM, Rosenbaum ME. Patient-care questions that physicians are unable to answer. *J Am Med Inform Assoc.* 2007;14(4):407–414

6. O'Malley AS, Grossman JM, Cohen GR, Kemper NM, Pham HH. Are electronic medical records helpful for care coordination? Experiences of physician practices. *J Gen Intern Med.* 2010;25(3): 177–185

7. Institute of Medicine, Committee on Understanding and Eliminating Racial and Ethnic Disparities in Health Care. In: Smedley BD, Stith AY, Nelson AR, eds. *Unequal Treatment: Confronting Racial and Ethnic Disparities in Health Care.* Washington, DC: National Academies Press; 2003

8. Blumenthal D, Glaser JP. Information technology comes to medicine. *N Engl J Med.* 2007;356(24):2527–2534

9. AHIC endorses e-prescribing mandate. *Health Data Manag.* November 29, 2007. Available at: www.healthdatamanagement. com/news/mandate25246-1.html. Accessed June 26, 2012

10. Teich JM, Osheroff JA, Pifer EA, Sittig DF, Jenders RA; CDS Expert Review Panel. Clinical decision support in electronic prescribing: recommendations and an action plan: report of the joint clinical decision support workgroup. *J Am Med Inform Assoc.* 2005;12(4):365–376

11. US Department of Health and Human Services. HHS Broadband Fact Sheet. February 1, 2008. Available at: www.hhs.gov/ news/facts/eprescribing.html. Accessed June 26, 2012

12. Institute of Medicine. To err is human: building a safer health system. Washington, DC: National Academies Press; 2000. Available at: www.nap.edu/catalog.php?record_id=9728. Accessed June 26, 2012

13. Frederick J. Two more professional groups endorse e-prescribing initiative. June 8, 2008. Available at: www.drugstorenews. com/article/two-more-professional-groups-endorse-e-prescribing-initiative. Accessed June 26, 2012

14. Institute of Medicine, Committee on Identifying and Preventing Medication Errors. In: Aspden P, ed. *Preventing Medication Errors.* Washington, DC: National Academies Press; 2007

15. Miller MR, Robinson KA, Lubomski LH, Rinke ML, Pronovost PJ. Medication errors in paediatric care: a systematic review of epidemiology and an evaluation of evidence supporting reduction strategy recommendations. *Qual Saf Health Care.* 2007;16 (2):116–126

16. Gerstle RS, Lehmann CU; American Academy of Pediatrics Council on Clinical Information Technology. Electronic prescribing systems in pediatrics: the rationale and functionality requirements. *Pediatrics.* 2007; 119(6):1229–1231

17. Spooner SA; Council on Clinical Information Technology, American Academy of Pediatrics. Special requirements of electronic health record systems in pediatrics. *Pediatrics.* 2007;119(3):631–637

18. Lesar TS. Errors in the use of medication dosage equations. *Arch Pediatr Adolesc Med.* 1998;152(4):340–344

19. Lesar TS, Briceland L, Stein DS. Factors related to errors in medication prescribing. *JAMA.* 1997;277(4):312–317

20. Potts MJ, Phelan KW. Deficiencies in calculation and applied mathematics skills in pediatrics among primary care interns. *Arch Pediatr Adolesc Med.* 1996;150(7):748– 752

21. The Joint Commission. Sentinel event alert: preventing pediatric medication errors. *Jt Comm Perspect.* 2008;28(5):11–13, 15

22. Institute of Medicine, Committee on Quality in Healthcare in America. *To Err is Human: Building a Safer Health System. 1999.* Washington, DC: National Academies Press; 1999

23. Gandhi TK, Weingart SN, Borus J, et al. Adverse drug events in ambulatory care. *N Engl J Med.* 2003;348(16):1556–1564

24. Johnson JA, Bootman JL. Drug-related morbidity and mortality. A cost-of-illness model. *Arch Intern Med.* 1995;155(18): 1949–1956

25. Kaushal R, Goldmann DA, Keohane CA, et al. Adverse drug events in pediatric outpatients. *Ambul Pediatr.* 2007;7(5):383–389

26. Zandieh SO, Goldmann DA, Keohane CA, Yoon C, Bates DW, Kaushal R. Risk factors in preventable adverse drug events in pediatric outpatients. *J Pediatr.* 2008;152(2): 225–231

27. Miller GC, Britth HC, Valenti L. Adverse drug events in general practice patients in Australia. *Med J Aust.* 2006;184(7):321–324

28. Schedlbauer A, Prasad V, Mulvaney C, et al. What evidence supports the use of computerized alerts and prompts to improve clinicians' prescribing behavior? *J Am Med Inform Assoc.* 2009;16(4):531–538

29. Ammenwerth E, Schnell-Inderst P, Machan C, Siebert U. The effect of electronic prescribing on medication errors and adverse drug events: a systematic review. *J Am Med Inform Assoc.* 2008;15(5):585–600

30. Jani YH, Ghaleb MA, Marks SD, Cope J, Barber N, Wong IC. Electronic prescribing reduced prescribing errors in a pediatric renal outpatient clinic. *J Pediatr.* 2008;152 (2):214–218

31. Garg AX, Adhikari NK, McDonald H, et al. Effects of computerized clinical decision support systems on practitioner performance and patient outcomes: a systematic review. *JAMA.* 2005;293(10):1223–1238

32. Wong IC, Ghaleb MA, Franklin BD, Barber N. Incidence and nature of dosing errors in paediatric medications: a systematic review. *Drug Saf.* 2004;27(9):661–670

33. The Joint Commission. *A Guide to the Joint Commission's Medication Management Standards,* 2nd ed. Oakbrook Terrace, IL: The Joint Commission; 2009

34. Zimmer KP, Miller MR, Lee BH, Miller RE, Lehmann CU. Electronic narcotic prescription writer: use in medical error reduction. *J Patient Saf.* 2008;4(2):98–105

35. Johnson KB, Ho YX, Cala CM, Davison C. Showing Your Work: Impact of annotating electronic prescriptions with decision support results. *J Biomed Inform.* 2010;43 (2):321–325

36. Oshikoya KA, Ojo OI. Medication errors in paediatric outpatient prescriptions of a teaching hospital in Nigeria. *Nig Q J Hosp Med.* 2007;17(2):74–78

37. Kaushal R, Goldmann DA, Keohane CA, et al. Medication errors in paediatric outpatients. *Qual Saf Health Care.* 2010;19(6): e30

38. Levine SR, Cohen MR, Blanchard NR, et al. Guidelines for preventing medication errors in pediatrics. *J Pediatr Pharmacol Ther.* 2001;6:427–443

39. Falagas ME, Vouloumanou EK, Plessa E, Peppas G, Rafailidis PI. Inaccuracies in dosing drugs with teaspoons and tablespoons. *Int J Clin Pract.* 2010;64(9):1185– 1189

40. Institute for Safe Medicine Practices. Safety standards needed for expressing/ measuring doses of liquid medications. *ISMP Medication Safety Alert.* 2011;10:6

41. Yaffe SJ, Bierman CW, Cann HM, et al. Inaccuracies in administering liquid medication. *Pediatrics.* 1975;56(2):327–328

42. Leyva M, Sharif I, Ozuah PO. Health literacy among Spanish-speaking Latino parents with limited English proficiency. *Ambul Pediatr.* 2005;5(1):56–59

43. Freedman RB, Jones SK, Lin A, Robin AL, Muir KW. Influence of parental health literacy and dosing responsibility on pediatric glaucoma medication adherence. *Arch Ophthalmol.* 2012;130(3):306–311

44. Rupp MT, Warholak TL. Evaluation of e-prescribing in chain community pharmacy: best-practice recommendations. *J Am Pharm Assoc (2003).* 2008;48(3):364–370

45. Warholak TL, Rupp MT. Analysis of community chain pharmacists' interventions on electronic prescriptions. *J Am Pharm Assoc (2003).* 2009;49(1):59–64

46. Newby DA, Robertson J. Computerised prescribing: assessing the impact on prescription repeats and on generic substitution of some commonly used antibiotics. *Med J Aust.* 2010; 192(4):192–195

47. Stenner SP, Chen Q, Johnson KB. Impact of generic substitution decision support on electronic prescribing behavior. *J Am Med Inform Assoc.* 2010;17(6):681–688

48. Krueger KP, Berger BA, Felkey B. Medication adherence and persistence: a comprehensive review. *Adv Ther.* 2005;22(4):313–356

49. Han YY, Carcillo JA, Venkataraman ST, et al. Unexpected increased mortality after implementation of a commercially sold computerized physician order entry system. *Pediatrics.* 2005;116(6):1506–1512

50. Classen DC, Pestotnik SL, Evans RS, Burke JP. Computerized surveillance of adverse drug events in hospital patients. *JAMA.* 1991;266(20):2847–2851

51. Evans RS, Classen DC, Pestotnik SL, Lundsgaarde HP, Burke JP. Improving empiric antibiotic selection using computer decision support. *Arch Intern Med.* 1994; 154(8):878–884

52. Koppel R, Metlay JP, Cohen A, et al. Role of computerized physician order entry systems in facilitating medication errors. *JAMA.* 2005;293(10):1197–1203

53. Wang CJ, Marken RS, Meili RC, Straus JB, Landman AB, Bell DS. Functional characteristics of commercial ambulatory electronic prescribing systems: a field study. *J Am Med Inform Assoc.* 2005;12(3):346–356

54. Weingart SN, Massagli M, Cyrulik A, et al. Assessing the value of electronic prescribing in ambulatory care: a focus group study. *Int J Med Inform.* 2009;78(9):571–578

55. Lapane KL, Waring ME, Schneider KL, Dubé C, Quilliam BJ. A mixed method study of the merits of e-prescribing drug alerts in primary care. *J Gen Intern Med.* 2008;23(4):442–446

56. Weingart SN, Toth M, Sands DZ, Aronson MD, Davis RB, Phillips RS. Physicians' decisions to override computerized drug alerts in primary care. *Arch Intern Med.* 2003;163 (21):2625–2631

57. Rosenberg SN, Sullivan M, Juster IA, Jacques J. Overrides of medication alerts in ambulatory care. [lett] *Arch Intern Med.* 2009;169(14):1337–, author reply 1338

58. Shah NR, Seger AC, Seger DL, et al. Improving override rates for computerized prescribing alerts in ambulatory care. *AMIA Annu Symp Proc.* 2005;1110

59. Bourgeois FT, Mandl KD, Valim C, Shannon MW. Pediatric adverse drug events in the outpatient setting: an 11-year national analysis. *Pediatrics.* 2009;124(4). Available at: www.pediatrics.org/cgi/content/full/124/ 4/e744

ERRATA

An error occurred in this AAP Technical Report titled "Electronic Prescribing in Pediatrics: Toward Safer and More Effective Medication Management" published in the April 2013 issue of *Pediatrics* (2013;131[4]:e1350–e1356; originally published online March 25, 2013; doi:10.1542/peds.2013-0193). The Technical Report should have included a note that author Kevin Johnson's work was funded by the Agency for Healthcare Research and Quality.

doi:10.1542/peds.2013-1288

Enhancing Pediatric Workforce Diversity and Providing Culturally Effective Pediatric Care: Implications for Practice, Education, and Policy Making

- *Policy Statement*

POLICY STATEMENT

Enhancing Pediatric Workforce Diversity and Providing Culturally Effective Pediatric Care: Implications for Practice, Education, and Policy Making

COMMITTEE ON PEDIATRIC WORKFORCE

KEY WORDS
pediatrician, workforce, diversity, health disparities, culturally effective care, education

ABBREVIATIONS
AAP—American Academy of Pediatrics
CEHC—culturally effective health care
CME—continuing medical education
LGBT—lesbian, gay, bisexual, and transgender
URM—underrepresented in medicine

www.pediatrics.org/cgi/doi/10.1542/peds.2013-2268

doi:10.1542/peds.2013-2268

PEDIATRICS (ISSN Numbers: Print, 0031-4005; Online, 1098-4275).

Copyright © 2013 by the American Academy of Pediatrics

abstract

This policy statement serves to combine and update 2 previously independent but overlapping statements from the American Academy of Pediatrics (AAP) on culturally effective health care (CEHC) and workforce diversity. The AAP has long recognized that with the ever-increasing diversity of the pediatric population in the United States, the health of all children depends on the ability of all pediatricians to practice culturally effective care. CEHC can be defined as the delivery of care within the context of appropriate physician knowledge, understanding, and appreciation of all cultural distinctions, leading to optimal health outcomes. The AAP believes that CEHC is a critical social value and that the knowledge and skills necessary for providing CEHC can be taught and acquired through focused curricula across the spectrum of lifelong learning.

This statement also addresses workforce diversity, health disparities, and affirmative action. The discussion of diversity is broadened to include not only race, ethnicity, and language but also cultural attributes such as gender, religious beliefs, sexual orientation, and disability, which may affect the quality of health care. The AAP believes that efforts must be supported through health policy and advocacy initiatives to promote the delivery of CEHC and to overcome educational, organizational, and other barriers to improving workforce diversity. *Pediatrics* 2013;132:e1105–e1116

INTRODUCTION

This policy statement serves to combine and update 2 previous statements from the American Academy of Pediatrics (AAP) on culturally effective health care (CEHC)[1] and workforce diversity.[2] The impetus to combine these independent policy statements comes from the recognition that the provision of culturally effective care and enhancing the diversity of the pediatrician workforce represent parallel and often overlapping initiatives to improve care for pediatric patients. This policy statement provides guidance for policy makers, advocacy groups, medical educators, and physicians on the provision of CEHC and enhancing the diversity of the pediatrician workforce.

CEHC can be defined as the delivery of care within the context of appropriate physician knowledge, understanding, and appreciation of all cultural distinctions, leading to optimal health outcomes, quality of life, and family satisfaction.[1] For the purposes of this policy statement, the term "culture" is used to signify the full spectrum of values, behaviors, customs, language, race, ethnicity, gender, sexual orientation, religious beliefs, disabilities, and other distinct attributes of population groups. The AAP believes that "culturally effective care" is a more inclusive term than "cultural competence" because it encompasses the values of competence and, more important, focuses on the outcomes of the physician-patient or physician-family interaction.

The AAP has a distinguished history of promoting diversity within the pediatrician workforce. Of particular note is the 1994 *Report of the AAP Task Force on Minority Children's Access to Pediatric Care,*[3] which promulgated 66 recommendations covering a wide range of topics, from the health status of minority children, to barriers to accessing pediatric care, to workforce needs. Racial and ethnic diversity was also a major issue addressed by the report of the Task Force on the Future of Pediatric Education II,[4] which called for increases in the percentage of underrepresented in medicine (URM) pediatricians in practice and academic medicine to meet the needs of the ever-growing population of children from racial/ethnic minority groups.

Over the past decade, the discussion of patient diversity by the medical community has increasingly expanded beyond the traditional attributes of race and ethnicity to include cultural characteristics such as language, race, ethnicity, ancestry, national origin, immigration status, religion, age, marital status, gender, sexual orientation, gender identity or expression, and disability.[5] A broader and more inclusive definition of patient diversity consequently requires an expansion of diversity beyond race and ethnicity within the pediatrician workforce as

well. The AAP believes that it has an important leading role in applying this expanded definition of patient diversity to improve the provision of CEHC for all populations.

This statement makes the case for a diverse pediatrician workforce; explores the impact that patient attributes have on their health care; investigates CEHC education and training; and addresses health policy and implementation. These issues are complex and nuanced, and a forceful commitment from an educated leadership will be needed to fully achieve the statement's recommendations.

CASE FOR A DIVERSE WORKFORCE

The Association of American Medical Colleges' description of URM encompasses "those racial and ethnic populations that are underrepresented in the medical profession relative to their numbers in the general population."[6] URM groups in the United States currently include black and African American, American Indian and Alaska Native, Native Hawaiian and other Pacific Islander, Hispanic and Latino, as well as any Asian other than Chinese, Filipino, Japanese, Korean, Asian Indian, Thai, or Vietnamese/Southeast Asian.[7] Some of the most compelling evidence in support of increased workforce diversity is that physicians from URM groups disproportionately practice in underserved communities and treat a greater number of underrepresented minority, Medicaid, and uninsured patients.[5,8–10] Whatever the reason for these practice patterns, the contributions of the minority physician workforce to the care of these groups of patients are therefore significant.

Numerous studies have demonstrated that minority patients suffer from significant health disparities and experience more barriers to accessing health care services than do other nonminority patients, but access to

care for minority patients is improved when the physician and the patient are racially or ethnically consentient.[5,11,12] Such congruence between patient and physician is, however, relatively infrequent.[12] This is perhaps why a 2006 study by the Health Resources and Services Administration noted that "although studies in our review suggested that interpersonal care was on balance better in race concordant patient-practitioner relationships, and that patients tended to prefer practitioners of their own race, these findings did not apply to all patients and practitioners."[13]

A study examining patient-physician social concordance using 4 social characteristics (race, gender, age, and education) showed that lower patient-physician social correspondence was associated with less favorable patient perceptions of care and lower global satisfaction ratings; conversely, stepwise patient-physician similarities were shown to improve patient perceptions of care in an additive fashion.[14] A large study looking at patient-physician congruence in adult patients with diabetes mellitus who were at high risk of cardiovascular disease concluded that African American patients who received treatment from African American physicians were significantly more adherent to taking their medications and that Spanish-speaking patients were significantly more adherent to taking their medications when their physicians were linguistically concordant.[15] Consequently, there is an ongoing need to increase racial and ethnic diversity among the pediatrician workforce in part because minority pediatricians continue to be more likely to provide care to minority children and their families in a disproportionate manner.[2]

PATIENT ATTRIBUTES AND IMPACT ON HEALTH CARE

Data from the US Census Bureau project that by 2020, 44.5% of American children 0 to 19 years of age will belong to a racial or ethnic minority group.[16] Consideration of cultural attributes in addition to race and ethnicity would greatly increase this projection of diversity. For example, in 2010, there were 646 000 same-sex unmarried couple households in the United States, and a number of these households reported having children.[17] Data from 2008 indicate that 23% of US citizens were living in rural locations, 12% of US citizens who were living outside of residential facilities or nursing homes had a disability, and 4% identified themselves as lesbian, gay, bisexual, or transgender.[18]

According to the US Census Bureau, approximately 20% of the US population older than 5 years speaks a language other than English at home. Although the majority of these people report that they also speak English well, it is estimated that approximately 24.5 million people in the United States need some assistance with English. Approximately 62% of these people speak Spanish at home.[19]

Census data confirm the growing numbers of foreign-born immigrants residing in the United States. The US Census Bureau uses this term to refer to anyone who is not a US citizen at birth. This includes naturalized US citizens, lawful permanent residents (immigrants), temporary migrants (such as foreign students), humanitarian migrants (such as refugees and asylees), and persons illegally present in the United States.[16,20] However, obtaining accurate estimates of numbers of US foreign-born immigrants is difficult because of respondents' concerns regarding potential legal difficulties arising from participating in census activities. In addition, census data may not accurately provide information on migrant workers' children and the growing numbers of homeless children.

The pool of foreign-born immigrant children includes both legal and un-documented children as well as international adoptees. Foreign-born immigrant children often face multiple challenges, including language barriers, and in addition to the common illnesses typical of other US children, they may suffer from other diseases rarely diagnosed in the United States. Furthermore, the diversity of the US foreign-born immigrant population, manifested even in individuals from the same country of origin, is such that health needs and health literacy are extremely varied, making the delivery of care for this population still more challenging. Homeless children face higher rates of trauma-related injuries, developmental delays, neurologic problems, and asthma, among other conditions.[21] Migrant workers' children face similar health and linguistic challenges and, because of unstable living conditions, poverty, and other social constraints, are often unable to access comprehensive health care.[21]

Significant and pervasive racial and ethnic health and health care inequities persist among children with chronic health conditions, such as attention-deficit/hyperactivity disorder, asthma, autism spectrum disorder, Down syndrome, cerebral palsy, cystic fibrosis, diabetes, sickle cell anemia, obesity, traumatic brain injury, and HIV/AIDS.[22] Black and Hispanic parents of children with special health care needs report higher dissatisfaction with care and more difficulties navigating services for their children compared with their white counterparts.[23] Although Healthy People 2020 has listed "cultural sensitivity in health care provision" as 1 of 7 key determinants of health under the heading of health disparities,[18] addressing disparities in cultural attributes and attitudes between physicians and their patients, patients' families, and/or guardians requires educational interventions to ensure that pediatricians and other health care professionals are able to provide CEHC to a diverse patient population.[24] To better understand and overcome long-standing and minimally improving health care disparities, the Institute of Medicine in 2009 formed a Subcommittee on Standardized Collection of Race/Ethnicity Data for Healthcare Quality Improvement.[25]

Certain patient populations and communities suffer from poorer health compared with other populations. Reliable data have shown that patients who belong to racial, ethnic, linguistic, or other minority groups tend to have greater morbidity than do white, English-speaking patients.[12,26–32] Research has shown that early life events influence one's health over an entire lifetime and that there is a stepwise health gradient that is defined distinctly by socioeconomic status.[33,34] Healthy People 2020 has outlined much broader examples of health disparities beyond race and ethnicity, with disparate health outcomes noted to be associated with gender, sexual identity and orientation, age, disability, socioeconomic status, and geographic location.[18] Although some studies have suggested that, compared with heterosexual people, lesbian, gay, bisexual, and transgender (LGBT)*,[35] people face greater mental health challenges,[36] other studies have not found such mental health differences but instead simply disparities in accessing routine health care services.[37,38] LGBT patients may be reticent

*Some support groups, community organizations, and researchers are now using the acronym LGBTQ or GLBTQ instead of LGBT. The "Q" may represent questioning or queer (in a nonpejorative way) and includes individuals who are uncertain of their sexual orientation but may still be considered a sexual minority or who self-identify as queer. However, according to the Gay & Lesbian Alliance Against Defamation, the use of the term "queer" is not universally accepted within the LGBT community, and care should be taken to avoid its use unless quoting or describing someone who self-identifies as queer.

to disclose their sexual or gender identity in a medical encounter for fear of being judged and also may believe that their physician is unfamiliar with LGBT health concerns.[39] LGBT youth face additional challenges as they navigate middle school and high school, where they may experience varying degrees of harassment, discrimination, exclusion, and isolation,[40] which may lead to increased depressive symptomatology as well as increased risk of suicidal ideation and self-harm compared with their heterosexual peers.[41,42]

CEHC: EDUCATION AND TRAINING

The AAP maintains that CEHC should be promoted through health policy and education at all levels, from premedical education and medical school through residency training and continuing medical education (CME). This task is complex; multiple languages and dialects must be addressed, requiring significant resources ranging from translation services to community linkages as well as commitment from both the learner and the educator. Nevertheless, the AAP maintains that at every level of education, pediatricians must be able to interact effectively and respectfully with patients and their families regardless of the cultural differences that may exist between them. These educational efforts should enhance the knowledge and understanding of pediatricians and other child health care professionals about the cultures of their patients and their families and increase their ability to provide care in a manner that is responsive to the individual needs of each patient. Educational programs must focus on the enhancement of interpersonal and communication skills, which are essential to nurturing the pediatrician-patient or pediatrician-family relationship and optimizing the health status of patients.

In addition, programs to enhance student, trainee, and physician awareness

about their own preconceptions and cultural attributes will likely translate into more open communication with and greater appreciation of the cultural backgrounds of all patients.[43] Educational programs such as those developed through the National Center for Cultural Competence can be effective in training of students, house officers, and faculty.[44]

The literature pertaining to teaching multicultural issues to medical students is robust. Many medical educators believe that training physicians to provide CEHC should begin earlier, as part of undergraduate premedical curricula. Some medical educators have suggested that these educational endeavors should focus less on individual attitudes and the characteristics of minority groups and more on discussions pertaining to social barriers and inequities at the institutional or systems level.[45,46] Others have raised concerns about the model of addressing multiculturalism and cultural competence through lectures and occasional workshops and have argued for the incorporation of these topics as a continuum throughout medical school. Some medical schools, in an effort to better integrate these skills, have opted to identify space for these activities within existing courses on patient-physician relationships and medical interviewing and develop "thoughtfully prepared instructional material throughout the four-year curriculum."[46,47] Efforts to weave CEHC education into core pediatric clerkships in the third year of medical school have demonstrated success in increasing knowledge, enhancing attitudes, and improving clinical skills.[48]

Medical schools should choose to focus at least some of their recruitment efforts on encouraging students from underserved areas, including rural locations, to apply, and should also consider proficiency in a second language an asset in evaluating prospective

medical students. Educational endeavors that merit institutional and program support are instructional sessions for students and residents on how to use to their best advantage (and how to evaluate) professional medical interpreters and translation services. At a minimum, medical school curricula and pediatric residency education programs should include educational components that elucidate the impact of low English proficiency, low literacy, and low health literacy on pediatric health care and offer strategies for remediating these problems. Furthermore, increasing the number of bilingual educational opportunities in the US at all educational levels would increase the likelihood that future physicians would be more likely to speak the same language as their patients.

Program requirements for residency education in pediatrics developed by the Pediatric Residency Review Committee call for structured educational experiences that prepare residents for the role of child health advocate within the community and inclusion of the multicultural dimensions of health care in the curriculum.[49] The Residency Review and Redesign in Pediatrics (R^3P) Committee of the American Board of Pediatrics recognizes that there is a need for some flexibility in training to allow for a variety of career choices, acknowledging that residency education is merely a segment of an educational continuum that starts in medical school and is sustained throughout the years of clinical practice.[50] Immersion experiences for pediatric trainees have used community-academic partnerships to move CEHC training into underserved communities, enhancing educational experiences and creating classrooms without walls.[51,52] A curriculum designed to foster cultural humility asks physicians to engage in self-reflection and self-critique as lifelong learners and requires the physician to bring humility to the power balance in the physician-patient relationship.[53] This curriculum, piloted by 1 family practice program, resulted in increased patient engagement during the office visits as well as high levels of satisfaction reported by participating residents.[54] Such a curriculum could be adapted for appropriate pediatric resident outpatient practices.

Beyond residency training, pediatricians and other child health care professionals can benefit from CME to enhance the provision of CEHC. The AAP regularly incorporates CEHC into its CME programming. Other resources exist that may be helpful in identifying important components for educational activities. For example, the Culturally Effective Care Toolkit on the AAP Web site can provide guidance and resources for enhancing CEHC in practice.[55]

Educational programs may include a component that allows individual participants to analyze personal beliefs and values. Programs may focus on the communication aspects of providing CEHC by exploring how assumptions and stereotypes influence interactions between physicians and patients or their families, as well as between physicians and other clinicians. Because people are influenced by their own personal experiences and may or may not subscribe to group-assumed norms, people who share the same cultural background may think and act differently. For this reason, it is important that programs intended to address the cultural values and practices of specific groups not perpetuate stereotypes. Physicians must also be aware that the culture of medicine itself promotes certain attitudes and biases that may interfere at times with the physician-patient or physician-parent relationship.

Culture is not static; changes can and do occur over time. An appreciation of cultural change and the significance of intracultural diversity (variation among individuals within the same culture) can help to prevent cultural stereotyping.[56] Programs aimed at enhancing the provision of CEHC should be tailored to the demographics of the pediatric population or community where the pediatrician serves.

CEHC: BARRIERS AND OPPORTUNITIES

Cultural variations in verbal and nonverbal communication can be a major barrier to effective pediatric care. Although the role of culturally linked behaviors that may influence the physician-patient interaction, including eye contact, body language, and communication styles, has not been fully explored,[57] language barriers have been shown to have a major effect on health care. Parents and their children in the United States increasingly speak a language other than English at home and/or have limited English proficiency. When the pediatrician and his or her patient and the patient's family do not speak the same language with fluency, there is a potential for problems to occur, such as obtaining an inaccurate history, misunderstanding of therapies, and/or deferred medical visits.[58,59]

Pediatricians continue to struggle with recommendations to use trained interpreters and provision of appropriate language services.[60] These barriers could be addressed through the use of certified medical interpreters (or bilingual pediatricians and other pediatric health care professionals) to meet the needs of pediatric patients whose parents are not proficient enough in English to interact with members of the health care system.[61] These services, however, remain beyond the reach of many pediatricians because of their cost. In 2009, Medicaid or State Children's Health Insurance Programs in only 13 states and the District of Columbia provided reimbursement for language services, and many insurance carriers do not reimburse for such services because they expect medical practices to absorb the cost as part of their overall business expense.[62] Despite the difficulties associated with identifying and accessing appropriate language services, however, the AAP opposes the use of children and adolescents as medical interpreters for their parents and family members.

Another facet of the relationship between language and CEHC is health literacy. The Institute of Medicine defined health literacy as "the degree to which individuals have the capacity to obtain, process, and understand basic health information and services needed to make appropriate health decisions."[63] Although this is a particular problem for individuals with low or marginal literacy skills, health literacy can also affect patients and families with adequate language literacy. Many individuals, even those with high health literacy and for whom English is their native language, find the complex wording of insurance statements, benefits coverage, hospital admissions forms, prescription drug information sheets, and similar documents to be confusing. Low health literacy for pediatric patients and their families, similar to limited English proficiency, is a barrier to the provision of optimal pediatric health care. Whereas health literacy may not be a distinct cultural attribute, language and health literacy are greatly affected by cultural distinctions and, if low, directly contribute to unfavorable patient outcomes. A provision in the Patient Protection and Affordable Care Act of 2010 now requires that any summary of benefits and coverage be presented "in a culturally and linguistically appropriate manner."[64] Commonsense innovations such as these may alleviate some of the challenging implications of low health literacy across the patient population.

At the level of the individual pediatrician, CEHC requires acquisition of knowledge, development of skills, and demonstration of behaviors and attitudes that are appropriate to care for patients and families with a wide variety of cultural attributes. Physician demographics, gender, and religious beliefs are but a few of the factors that influence (often subconsciously) medical recommendations for patients from all backgrounds.[43] As such, physician self-reflection, self-knowledge, and self-critique have been identified as critical components of competence, which can be expanded further to encompass the concept of cultural humility. Practiced over time, these specific skills, in addition to conscious realignment of inherent imbalances in power that often undermine provider-patient communications and fostering of mutually respectful and dynamic partnerships within the community in which one practices, form the foundation for practicing with cultural humility.[53] Although using these knowledge bases, skills, behaviors, and attitudes is commonly referred to as cultural competence and cultural sensitivity, these terms focus on process. CEHC focuses on outcomes and emphasizes the need for continued monitoring and documentation.

Clearly, reasons for health disparities are numerous and may also include patients' cultural beliefs about health care and healing, dietary deficiencies, insufficient exercise, barriers to access to health care resources, financial indigence, inadequate insurance coverage, and inability to communicate with English-speaking physicians and other health care professionals. Trying to communicate effectively with parents who are deaf or hard of hearing also can pose significant barriers and may lead to suboptimal health care even when the child/patient is able to hear; this may direct the pediatrician to seek creative solutions to provide family-centered care.[65] One study evaluated 3 community-based, culturally and linguistically sensitive initiatives that demonstrated that it is possible to reduce or eliminate racial/ethnic disparities in the child health arena by engaging patients and reinforcing participant collaboration.[66] A paper on quality improvement initiatives highlighted how a patient-centered medical home serves to reduce disparities and demonstrated that family involvement and partnering with others in the community not directly involved in patient care are key components of a successful program.[67] The National Committee for Quality Assurance's Patient-Centered Medical Home 2011 Standards ask practices to assess the language needs and characteristics of their patient populations; the standards also expect practice-based care teams to be trained on effective patient communication, particularly with vulnerable populations.[68] The growing number of practices achieving Patient-Centered Medical Home recognition translates into a greater number of pediatricians who understand and appreciate the importance of CEHC.

Pediatricians should become knowledgeable about the resources available to their patients and families within their institutions (offices, hospitals), health maintenance organizations, and communities. Pediatricians who seek out opportunities to partner with institutions, such as third-party payers, hospitals, health departments, and education departments, will be better able to advocate for the specific cultural needs of their patients and thereby increase patient satisfaction and quality of health care.

WORKFORCE DIVERSITY: BARRIERS AND OPPORTUNITIES

The ethnic and racial gap between pediatricians (as well as other physicians) and their patients persists despite efforts to increase the diversity of the pediatrician workforce. Data from the AAP Annual Survey of Graduating Residents show that the percentage of underrepresented minorities (African American, Hispanic, and Native American) who graduated from US medical schools increased from 9% in 2003 to 15% in 2009, but this increase but was not statistically significant. Approximately a third of graduating residents report having grown up in a bilingual or multilingual family (34% in 2009; 29% in 2010).[69] Although these levels of URM pediatric trainees are encouraging, the percentages are far below the current estimates of the pediatric population, and these trends are unlikely to change drastically in the near future. Also, unlike most other medical specialties (except perhaps obstetrics and gynecology), the numbers of women entering pediatric training continue to increase and currently exceed the numbers of men in pediatric training.[70] Over time, it will be important to evaluate how this trend affects the availability of male pediatricians to treat patients who have this preference, which could, among other factors, be influenced by patient gender and specific cultural norms.

Literature in support of the Supreme Court decisions related to the University of Michigan's affirmative action policies has strongly stated the case for diversity at all levels of medical education. A more diverse faculty and student body is viewed as an indispensable component of quality medical education. Nevertheless, gains in enhancing diversity may be derailed by legislative actions, such as the passage of proposition 209 in 1996 in the state of California, which eliminated race-conscious admissions at public institutions. Since then, there has been a decline in the percentage of in-state minority students accepted to and matriculating in California medical schools, with no appreciable rebound over time.[71] Institutional diversity will increase the cultural exposure of all faculty and students, which will help to dispel stereotypes and improve cultural competence by virtue of everyday interactions. A more diverse workforce will likely lead to a more diverse medical research agenda for improving health and the delivery of health care services among racial, ethnic, and cultural minority patients. Creating such a workforce, it is argued, begins with the diversity of those admitted to doctor of medicine and doctor of philosophy educational programs. Indeed, in a modern multicultural society, promoting diversity within the medical profession to better reflect the diversity of the patient population while maintaining the high quality of the health care workforce is in keeping with the societal obligation of medical schools to produce well-trained professionals to meet the future health care needs of the country.[8,13,72] The Association of American Medical Colleges published its flagship statement in 2008 to serve as a tool for medical schools for the development of diversity-related policies and, in doing so, implored those in academic medicine to be "serious about creating and sustaining diversity in medical education, biomedical research, and the physician workforce."[73]

Financial incentives to encourage URM students to enter medical training continue to grow nationally through organizations such as the National Institute on Minority Health and Health Disparities, and through state and regional programs. These incentives, including loan forgiveness/repayment and tuition reimbursement, may help to address many financial barriers such as low family income and educational debt. Institutional programs, such as the Center of Excellence in

Diversity at Stanford University, reach out to promising premedical students to help prepare them for careers in medicine.[74] Diversity programs, along with educational institutions, acknowledge the importance of minority faculty concomitantly serving as mentors to minority students, serving on admissions committees, overseeing diversity initiatives, and serving in leadership positions at all levels. To support all of these activities, there must be a simultaneous commitment to increase diversity at the highest organizational and institutional levels.

Another approach to increasing the recruitment of minority students into the health professions is to focus on reaching out to individuals in earlier educational stages, such as elementary and high school. To maximize the effectiveness of these programs, appropriate support structures for these individuals within their communities, schools, postsecondary institutions, health care organizations, medical societies, and other entities need to be established. These support structures include financial incentives, mentoring and shadowing programs, adequate staffing for diversity programs, and educational and other initiatives related to cultural effectiveness and diversity. Holistic review of college and medical school applications may further bolster the numbers of URM students admitted to institutions of higher learning. Giving weight not only to the applicant's academic credentials but also to leadership potential, ability to work within a team, and interpersonal and communications skills, while taking into account personal circumstances, may provide more opportunities for outstanding students with essential nonacademic qualifications to succeed. There is clearly a need to pursue active recruitment of minority candidates for health-professions education programs. To increase the

small number of minority individuals entering pediatrics without negatively affecting the number entering other specialties, the total number of minority individuals entering medical school must first be increased.

Workforce diversity and CEHC may also be enhanced by increasing minority representation in hospital governance and leadership positions, which can heighten the institution's efforts to reduce health care disparities and promote diversity in management and leadership. For example, minorities comprise 29% of the patient population nationally, yet they represent only 14% of hospital board members, 14% of executive leadership positions, and 15% of first- and mid-level management positions.[75] Such data illustrate an opportunity to foster programs that promote minority representation in hospital decision-making roles.

HEALTH POLICY AND IMPLEMENTATION

Although mandates from government agencies and regulatory bodies have served as important policy leverage or motivation to promote the provision of CEHC, these mandates have been largely unfunded, implying that academic institutions, hospitals, pediatricians, and other physicians must defray the costs of their implementation.[76] Decreasing payment to physician practices for clinical care and decreasing hospital operating margins have rendered these mandates largely impractical. Additionally, financial and other incentives from insurers, government agencies, and other payers to reward physicians and hospitals for delivering CEHC have been meager and, hence, have not supplied the impetus and support to encourage fundamental systemic changes, which are often costly.

In an era when cost containment is an urgent priority for the health care community, research plays a pivotal role in changing the societal value of CEHC. The AAP regards CEHC as vital and a critical social value. However, many health care payers, employers, institutions, and others fear exacerbating current financial pressures and hardship when trying to provide such care. Many estimates of costs associated with poor child health do not take into account lifetime costs resulting from loss of productivity and earning potential; those who would contend that improving eligibility for health insurance will adequately address child health disparities need also to consider barriers such as insurance enrollment and access to care while recognizing the burden of certain chronic health conditions that disproportionately impact underserved children.[77] Reliable and timely data to demonstrate long-term decreases in health care costs, appropriate use of health care services, and improved patient health outcome measures would provide a solid foundation for addressing valid concerns about the financial implications of providing CEHC. To this end, culturally effective knowledge and skills need to be applied to research development and implementation. From a quality-of-care perspective, moreover, this research would allow policy makers to identify at-risk patient populations and to develop strategies to address health disparities on national, regional, state, and local levels.

Although Medicaid and other public insurers are placing increased emphasis on "cultural competence" and quality care,[78] few tools exist for health care payers to measure the outcomes of processes implemented to ensure CEHC. The use of patient-satisfaction scoring systems that assess shared decision-making, mutual respect, trust, and other culturally sensitive parameters should be encouraged. Survey

instruments should use quality measures that are within the scope of responsibility of the health care professional, and the results of these surveys should be used to identify priorities for continuing education. When carefully designed to reflect the health and wellness values of the specific community being surveyed, such outcomes-driven efforts will allow greater focus on the effectiveness of interventions designed to monitor and ensure quality care.

Sponsors of diversity initiatives must likewise be able to track their progress in reaching specific targets and goals through research and data-driven outcome measures. For instance, institutional goals and metrics that are established for the purpose of recruiting and retaining minority trainees and faculty could be used to assess effectiveness. It is difficult to improve what we cannot measure. Limited data on cultural minorities in medicine hamper the ability of the profession to evaluate the current status of diversity, implement activities to enhance it, and measure the outcomes of these activities. The AAP has begun to address this concern by compiling more data regarding better tracking of attributes other than race and ethnicity through research generated by its Annual Survey of Graduating Residents, its new Pediatrician Life and Career Experience Study, its membership surveys, and collaborations with external organizations. However, more must be done to measure progress in improving diversity within medicine and pediatrics.

CONCLUSIONS

Since adoption of the *Report of the AAP Task Force on Minority Children's Access to Pediatric Care,*[3] the AAP has strengthened its commitment to ensure that all infants, children, adolescents, and young adults have access to optimal CEHC, ideally through

a medical home.[80] Additionally, the AAP acknowledges that CEHC is multifaceted, complex, and often costly. The AAP believes that the education of pediatricians about cultural attributes and about the importance of implementing culturally effective practices and policies is essential. Because pediatricians are committed to lifelong learning, education that will enhance the provision of such care must be available at all levels, from premedical education and medical school through residency training and CME.

The medical community has made insufficient progress in diversifying its workforce. Improving diversity within the pediatrician workforce will require proactive leadership from the medical community in a number of areas, including recruitment, mentoring, education, organizational support systems, and financial incentives. Success will also depend on the collaboration and cooperation of many stakeholders, including the AAP, with respect to initiatives designed to promote diversity within the health professions. Pediatricians are not alone in seeking solutions to improve the delivery of pediatric health care to the neediest patients. Pediatricians, other health care professionals, hospitals, universities, community groups, health care payers and insurers, regulatory and accrediting bodies, legislators, and others have significant roles to play in ensuring CEHC and will have to participate in health policy deliberations on this topic. Broad-based participation will ensure that a pediatric focus and perspective are brought to bear on decisions that have a direct effect on the quality of care that is delivered to children. In particular, stakeholders will have to advocate for necessary financial, regulatory, and other support among decision-makers to implement appropriate changes to the US health care delivery system.

Individual pediatricians need educational tools; the pediatric community needs the results of outcomes research to bolster, validate, and sustain its effort; institutions need support and encouragement to provide appropriate and effective education and training; foundations and other organizations need to have a pediatric perspective in all health care and policy development considerations; and legislative bodies, including federal and state agencies, need to provide the funding and infrastructure necessary to implement and evaluate mandates. The AAP has played, and must continue to play, a pivotal role in all of these important health policy deliberations.

RECOMMENDATIONS

The AAP believes that increasing the diversity of the pediatrician workforce and enhancing the provision of culturally effective care to the pediatric population will help achieve the AAP mission of promoting optimal physical, mental, and social health and well-being for all infants, children, adolescents, and young adults. Thus, the AAP is committed to working in collaboration with AAP chapters and other groups, including but not limited to medical societies, hospitals, universities, health care payers and insurers, federal agencies, and policy makers, to achieve greater workforce diversity and promote the provision of culturally effective pediatric care and recommends the following:

1. Pediatricians should assume a leadership role in advocating for a diverse workforce. Diversity in this context includes a wide spectrum of racial, ethnic, and cultural attributes, which include values, behaviors, customs, language, sexual orientation, religious beliefs, socioeconomic status, and other distinct population attributes. Many individuals exhibiting such a broad range of perspectives and attributes are URM compared with their presence in the general population.

2. The AAP should support the development of sequentially staged programs that prepare URM students to pursue careers in health professions, including pediatrics. URM medical student, resident, or physician groups would encompass those individuals from ethnic and racial populations that are underrepresented in the medical profession relative to their numbers in the general population as a whole.

3. Medical student, resident, and faculty recruitment activities should support and advocate for the full spectrum of diversity as described in Recommendation 1.

4. Affirmative-action programs should be supported because they promote the entry of URM students into medical school.

5. Financial assistance should be broadened for URM students, including federal funding for diversity programs, Title VII funding, loan-forgiveness/repayment programs, and tuition reimbursement.

6. Educational and health care institutions and organizations must employ individuals who are primarily responsible for the implementation, management, and evaluation of diversity programs that address the full spectrum of diversity as described in Recommendation 1.

7. Institutional commitment to improve workforce diversity must include formal programs or mechanisms to ensure that individuals of diverse backgrounds can rise to leadership positions. Furthermore, commitment from a number of groups (including institutions, the AAP, AAP chapters, medical societies, federal agencies, and policy makers) is necessary to ensure the provision of CEHC.

8. Pediatricians should assume a leadership role in advocating for CEHC for all infants, children, adolescents, and young adults.

9. The AAP, along with health care organizations at all levels, should continue to participate in the development and assessment of effectiveness of educational programs that promote CEHC. The curricula should address issues including but not limited to the patient's and one's own cultural beliefs, values, behaviors, customs, language, sexual orientation, religious beliefs, disabilities, and other distinct attributes.

10. Pediatricians must continue to work locally with hospitals, offices, and managed care organizations as well as commercial and government insurance payers to develop policies and programs that address health care needs specific to their communities.

11. Mandates from both the government and insurers to improve the provision of CEHC must be accompanied by funding or payment to support the infrastructure necessary to implement these programs and assess their effectiveness.

12. Public and private incentive programs must be established to encourage the implementation of national, regional, state, and community-based initiatives to improve the delivery of CEHC.

LEAD AUTHORS
Beth A. Pletcher, MD, FAAP
Mary Ellen Rimsza, MD, FAAP

COMMITTEE ON PEDIATRIC WORKFORCE, 2011–2012

Mary Ellen Rimsza, MD, FAAP, Chairperson

William T. Basco, MD, MS, FAAP

Andrew J. Hotaling, MD, FAAP

Ted D. Sigrest, MD, FAAP

Frank A. Simon, MD, FAAP

FORMER COMMITTEE MEMBERS

Luisa I. Alvarado-Domenech, MD, FAAP

Beth A. Pletcher, MD, FAAP, Past Chairperson

Richard P. Shugerman, MD, FAAP

LIAISONS

Christopher E. Harris, MD, FAAP – *Section Forum Management Committee*

Gail A. McGuinness, MD, FAAP – *American Board of Pediatrics*

CONSULTANT

Kelly Towey, MEd

STAFF

Carrie L. Radabaugh, MPP

REFERENCES

1. Britton CV; American Academy of Pediatrics Committee on Pediatric Workforce. Ensuring culturally effective pediatric care: implications for education and health policy. *Pediatrics*. 2004;114(6):1677–1685

2. Friedman AL; American Academy of Pediatrics Committee on Pediatric Workforce. Enhancing the diversity of the pediatrician workforce. *Pediatrics*. 2007;119(4):833–837

3. American Academy of Pediatrics. *Report of the AAP Task Force on Minority Children's Access to Pediatric Care*. Elk Grove Village, IL: American Academy of Pediatrics; 1994

4. American Academy of Pediatrics, Task Force on the Future of Pediatric Education. The future of pediatric education II. Organizing pediatric education to meet the needs of infants, children, adolescents, and young adults in the 21st century. A collaborative project of the pediatric community. *Pediatrics*. 2000;105(1 pt 2):157–212

5. Cooper LA, Powe NR. *Disparities in Patient Experiences, Health Care Processes, and Outcomes: The Role of Patient-Provider Racial, Ethnic, and Language Concordance*. New York, NY: Commonwealth Fund; 2004

6. Association of American Medical Colleges. Definition of the term "underrepresented in medicine." Available at: https://www.aamc.org/initiatives/urm/. Accessed December 11, 2012

7. US Department of Health and Human Services, Health Resources and Services Administration. *Transforming the Face of Health Professions Through Cultural and Linguistic Competence Education: The Role of the HRSA Centers of Excellence*. Washington, DC: US Department of Health and Human Services, Health Resources and Services Administration. Available at: www.hrsa.gov/culturalcompetence/cultcompedu.pdf. Accessed December 11, 2012

8. Cohen JJ. The consequences of premature abandonment of affirmative action in medical school admissions. *JAMA*. 2003;289(9):1143–1149

9. Grumbach K, Hart LG, Mertz E, Coffman J, Palazzo L. Who is caring for the underserved? A comparison of primary care physicians and nonphysician clinicians in California and Washington. *Ann Fam Med*. 2003;1(2):97–104

10. Basco WT, Jr, Cull WL, O'Connor KG, Shipman SA. Assessing trends in practice demographics of underrepresented minority pediatricians, 1993–2007. *Pediatrics*. 2010;125(3):460–467

11. Toomey SL, Chien AT, Elliott MN, Ratner J, Schuster MA. Disparities in unmet need for care coordination: the national survey of children's health. *Pediatrics*. 2013;131(2):217–224

12. Collins KS, Hughes DL, Doty MM, Ives BL, Edwards JN, Tenney K. *Diverse Communities, Common Concerns: Assessing Health Care Quality for Minority Americans—Findings from the Commonwealth Fund 2001 Health Care Quality Survey*. New York, NY: Commonwealth Fund; 2002

13. US Department of Health and Human Services, Health Resources and Services Administration, Bureau of Health Professions. *The Rationale for Diversity in the Health Professions: A Review of the Evidence*. Rockville, MD: Bureau of Health Professions, Health Resources and Services Administration; 2006. Available at: http://bhpr.hrsa.gov/healthworkforce/reports/diversityreviewevidence.pdf. Accessed December 13, 2012

14. Thornton RL, Powe NR, Roter D, Cooper LA. Patient-physician social concordance, medical visit communication and patients' perceptions of health care quality. *Patient Educ Couns*. 2011;85(3):e201–e208

15. Traylor AH, Schmittdiel JA, Uratsu CS, Mangione CM, Subramanian U. Adherence to cardiovascular disease medications: does patient-provider race/ethnicity and language concordance matter? *J Gen Intern Med*. 2010;25(11):1172–1177

16. US Census Bureau. Projections of the total resident population by 5-year age groups, race, and Hispanic origin with special age categories: middle series, 2016 to 2020. Washington, DC: US Census Bureau; 2000. Available at: www.census.gov/population/projections/files/natproj/summary/np-t4-e.pdf. Accessed December 11, 2012

17. US Census Bureau. 2010 Census Briefs. Households and Families: 2010. Washington, DC: US Census Bureau; 2010. Available at: www.census.gov/prod/cen2010/briefs/c2010br-14.pdf. Accessed June 22, 2013

18. US Department of Health and Human Services, Office of Disease Prevention and Health Promotion. Healthy People 2020. Available at: http://wcww.healthypeople.gov/2020/about/default.aspx. Accessed June 20, 2012

19. US Census Bureau, American Community Survey Reports. Language use in the United States: 2007. Available at: www.census.gov/hhes/socdemo/language/data/acs/ACS-12.pdf. Accessed December 12, 2012

20. US Census Bureau. International migration. Frequently asked questions. Available at: www.census.gov/population/intmigration/about/faq.html. Accessed June 11, 2013

21. DuPlessis HM, Cora-Bramble D; American Academy of Pediatrics Committee on Community Health Services. Providing care for immigrant, homeless, and migrant children. *Pediatrics*. 2005;115(4):1095–1100

22. Berry JG, Bloom S, Foley S, Palfrey JS. Health inequity in children and youth with chronic health conditions. *Pediatrics*. 2010;126(suppl 3):S111–S119

23. Ngui EM, Flores G. Satisfaction with care and ease of using health care services among parents of children with special health care needs: the roles of race/ethnicity, insurance, language, and adequacy of family-centered care. *Pediatrics*. 2006;117(4):1184–1196

24. Stoddard JJ, Back MR, Brotherton SE. The respective racial and ethnic diversity of US pediatricians and American children. *Pediatrics*. 2000;105(1 pt 1):27–31

25. Ulmer C, McFadden B, Nerenz D, eds. *Race, Ethnicity, and Language Data: Standardization*

for Health Care Quality Improvement. Washington, DC: National Academies Press; 2009

26. Betancourt JR, Green AR, Carrillo JE. *Cultural Competence in Health Care: Emerging Frameworks and Practical Approaches.* New York, NY: The Commonwealth Fund; 2002

27. Collins KS, Tenney K, Hughes DL. *Quality of Health Care for African Americans.* New York, NY: The Commonwealth Fund; 2002

28. Doty MM. *Hispanic Patients' Double Burden: Lack of Health Insurance and Limited English.* New York, NY: The Commonwealth Fund; 2003

29. Doty MM, Ives BL. *Quality of Health Care for Hispanic Populations.* New York, NY: The Commonwealth Fund; 2002

30. Hughes DL. *Quality of Health Care for Asian Americans.* New York, NY: The Commonwealth Fund; 2002

31. Perot RT, Youdelman M. *Racial, Ethnic, and Primary Language Data Collection in the Health Care System: An Assessment of Federal Policies and Practices.* New York, NY: The Commonwealth Fund; 2001

32. Flores G; Committee On Pediatric Research. Technical report—racial and ethnic disparities in the health and health care of children. *Pediatrics.* 2010;125(4). Available at: www.pediatrics.org/cgi/content/full/125/4/e979

33. Braveman P, Barclay C. Health disparities beginning in childhood: a life-course perspective. *Pediatrics.* 2009;124(suppl 3): S163–S175

34. Guyer B, Ma S. Conceptualizing health disparities: panel reflections. *Pediatrics.* 2009; 124(suppl 3):S212–S213

35. Gay & Lesbian Alliance Against Defamation, Inc. *Media Reference Guide.* 8th ed. Available at: www.glaad.org/reference. Accessed June 20, 2012

36. Burgess D, Tran A, Lee R, van Ryn M. Effects of perceived discrimination on mental health and mental health services utilization among gay, lesbian, bisexual and transgender persons. *J LGBT Health Res.* 2007;3(4):1–14

37. Berg MB, Mimiaga MJ, Safren SA. Mental health concerns of gay and bisexual men seeking mental health services. *J Homosex.* 2008;54(3):293–306

38. Hiestand KR, Horne SG, Levitt HM. Effects of gender identity on experiences of healthcare for sexual minority women. *J LGBT Health Res.* 2007;3(4):15–27

39. Mayer KH, Bradford JB, Makadon HJ, Stall R, Goldhammer H, Landers S. Sexual and gender minority health: what we know and what needs to be done. *Am J Public Health.* 2008;98(6):989–995

40. Kosciw JG, Greytak EA, Diaz EM. Who, what, where, when, and why: demographic and ecological factors contributing to hostile school climate for lesbian, gay, bisexual, and transgender youth. *J Youth Adolesc.* 2009;38(7):976–988

41. Almeida J, Johnson RM, Corliss HL, Molnar BE, Azrael D. Emotional distress among LGBT youth: the influence of perceived discrimination based on sexual orientation. *J Youth Adolesc.* 2009;38(7):1001–1014

42. Russell ST, Ryan C, Toomey RB, Diaz RM, Sanchez J. Lesbian, gay, bisexual, and transgender adolescent school victimization: implications for young adult health and adjustment. *J Sch Health.* 2011;81(5): 223–230

43. Berger JT. The influence of physicians' demographic characteristics and their patients' demographic characteristics on physician practice: implications for education and research. *Acad Med.* 2008;83(1): 100–105

44. Georgetown University Center for Child and Human Development. National Center for Cultural Competence. Available at: http://www11.georgetown.edu/research/gucchd/nccc/. Accessed December 13, 2012

45. Green AR, Betancourt JR, Carrillo JE. Integrating social factors into cross-cultural medical education. *Acad Med.* 2002;77(3): 193–197

46. Wear D. Insurgent multiculturalism: rethinking how and why we teach culture in medical education. *Acad Med.* 2003;78(6): 549–554

47. Taylor JS. Confronting "culture" in medicine's "culture of no culture." *Acad Med.* 2003;78(6):555–559

48. Paul CR, Devries J, Fliegel J, Van Cleave J, Kish J. Evaluation of a culturally effective health care curriculum integrated into a core pediatric clerkship. *Ambul Pediatr.* 2008;8(3):195–199

49. Mulvey HJ, Ogle-Jewett EAB, Cheng TL, Johnson RL. Pediatric residency education. *Pediatrics.* 2000;106(2 pt 1):323–329

50. Jones MD, Jr, McGuinness GA, First LR, Leslie LK Residency Review and Redesign in Pediatrics Committee. Linking process to outcome: are we training pediatricians to meet evolving health care needs? *Pediatrics.* 2009;123(suppl 1):S1–S7

51. Sidelinger DE, Meyer D, Blaschke GS, et al. Communities as teachers: learning to deliver culturally effective care in pediatrics. *Pediatrics.* 2005;115(suppl 4):1160–1164

52. Zúñiga ML, Sidelinger DE, Blaschke GS, et al. Evaluation of residency training in the delivery of culturally effective care. *Med Educ.* 2006;40(12):1192–1200

53. Tervalon M, Murray-García J. Cultural humility versus cultural competence: a critical distinction in defining physician training outcomes in multicultural education. *J Health Care Poor Underserved.* 1998; 9(2):117–125

54. Juarez JA, Marvel K, Brezinski KL, Glazner C, Towbin MM, Lawton S. Bridging the gap: a curriculum to teach residents cultural humility. *Fam Med.* 2006;38(2):97–102

55. American Academy of Pediatrics. Culturally effective care toolkit. Available at: http://practice.aap.org/content.aspx?aid=2990. Accessed December 13, 2012

56. Pachter LM, Harwood RL. Culture and child behavior and psychosocial development. *J Dev Behav Pediatr.* 1996;17(3):191–198

57. Cooper-Patrick L, Gallo JJ, Gonzales JJ, et al. Race, gender, and partnership in the patient-physician relationship. *JAMA.* 1999; 282(6):583–589

58. Flores G, Laws MB, Mayo SJ, et al. Errors in medical interpretation and their potential clinical consequences in pediatric encounters. *Pediatrics.* 2003;111(1):6–14

59. Flores G, Abreu M, Olivar MA, Kastner B. Access barriers to health care for Latino children. *Arch Pediatr Adolesc Med.* 1998; 152(11):1119–1125

60. Kuo DZ, O'Connor KG, Flores G, Minkovitz CS. Pediatricians' use of language services for families with limited English proficiency. *Pediatrics.* 2007;119(4). Available at: www.pediatrics.org/cgi/content/full/119/4/e920

61. Weinick RM, Krauss NA. Racial/ethnic differences in children's access to care. *Am J Public Health.* 2000;90(11):1771–1774

62. Youdelman M. *Medicaid and SCHIP Reimbursement Models for Language Services (2009 Update).* Washington, DC: National Health Law Program; 2009

63. Institute of Medicine. In: Nielsen-Bohlman L, Panzer AM, Hamlin B, Kindig DA, eds. Health Literacy: A Prescription to End Confusion. Washington, DC: The National Academies Press; 2004

64. Patient Protection and Affordable Care Act Title I, Subtitle A, Part A, Subpart ii, Section 2715, Pub. L. 111-148, 124 (2010)

65. Swota AH, Hester DM. Ethics for the pediatrician: providing culturally effective health care. *Pediatr Rev.* 2011;32(3):e39–e43

66. Flores G. Devising, implementing, and evaluating interventions to eliminate health care disparities in minority children. *Pediatrics.* 2009;124(suppl 3): S214–S223

67. Chin MH, Alexander-Young M, Burnet DL. Health care quality-improvement approaches to reducing child health disparities. *Pediatrics.* 2009;124(suppl 3):S224–S236

68. National Committee for Quality Assurance. *Standards and Guidelines for NCQA's Patient-Centered Medical Home (PCMH)*. Washington, DC: National Committee for Quality Assurance; 2011

69. Frintner MP, Cull WL. Pediatric training and career intentions, 2003–2009. *Pediatrics*. 2012;129(3):522–528

70. American Academy of Pediatrics. AAP Graduating Resident Surveys, 1997–2012. Trends in the proportion of graduating pediatric residents who are women (1997–2012). Available at: www.aap.org/en-us/professional-resources/Research/pediatrician-surveys/Documents/Graduating_Residents_Survey_Trend_Data-Gender.pdf. Accessed May 20, 2013

71. Association of American Medical Colleges. *After Affirmative Action: Diversity at California Medical Schools*. Washington, DC: Association of American Medical Colleges; 2008

72. Smedley BD, Butler AS, Bristow LR, eds. *In the Nation's Compelling Interest: Ensuring Diversity in the Health Care Workforce*. Washington, DC: National Academies Press; 2004

73. Association of American Medical Colleges. *Roadmap to Diversity: Key Legal and Educational Policy Foundations for Medical Schools*. Washington, DC: Association of American Medical Colleges; 2008

74. Stanford School of Medicine. Center of Excellence in Diversity in Medical Education. Available at: http://coe.stanford.edu/. Accessed December 13, 2012

75. American Hospital Association and Institute for Diversity in Health Management. *Diversity & Disparities: A Benchmark Study of U.S. Hospitals*. Chicago, IL: American Hospital Association; 2012

76. US Department of Health and Human Services, Health Resources and Services Administration. *HRSA CAREAction. Mitigating Health Disparities Through Cultural Competence*. 2002. Available at: www.ask.hrsa.gov/detail_materials.cfm?ProdID=1655. Accessed December 13, 2012

77. Currie J. Policy interventions to address child health disparities: moving beyond health insurance. *Pediatrics*. 2009;124 (suppl 3):S246–S254

78. Federal Register. 42 CFR Part 400 et al. Medicaid program; Medicaid managed care; proposed rule. 1998;63(188):52022–52092. Available at: www.gpo.gov/fdsys/pkg/FR-1998-09-29/html/98-26068.htm. Accessed December 13, 2012

79. American Academy of Pediatrics, Medical Home Initiatives for Children with Special Needs Project Advisory Committee. The medical home [reaffirmed May 2008]. *Pediatrics*. 2002;110(1):184–186

Essential Contractual Language for Medical Necessity in Children

- *Policy Statement*

POLICY STATEMENT

Essential Contractual Language for Medical Necessity in Children

abstract

The previous policy statement from the American Academy of Pediatrics, "Model Language for Medical Necessity in Children," was published in July 2005. Since that time, there have been new and emerging delivery and payment models. The relationship established between health care providers and health plans should promote arrangements that are beneficial to all who are affected by these contractual arrangements. Pediatricians play an important role in ensuring that the needs of children are addressed in these emerging systems. It is important to recognize that health care plans designed for adults may not meet the needs of children. Language in health care contracts should reflect the health care needs of children and families. Informed pediatricians can make a difference in the care of children and influence the role of primary care physicians in the new paradigms. This policy highlights many of the important elements pediatricians should assess as providers develop a role in emerging care models. *Pediatrics* 2013;132:398–401

COMMITTEE ON CHILD HEALTH FINANCING

KEY WORDS
medical necessity, contractual language, pediatric care, children, insurance, health plans, payment

ABBREVIATIONS
AAP—American Academy of Pediatrics
ACA—Patient Protection and Affordable Care Act

This article was written by members of the American Academy of Pediatrics. It does not represent the views of the US government or any US government agency.

The recommendations in this statement do not indicate an exclusive course of treatment or serve as a standard of medical care. Variations, taking into account individual circumstances, may be appropriate.

The American Academy of Pediatrics (AAP) published the policy statement "Model Contractual Language for Medical Necessity in Children" in July 2005.[1] The chief principles articulated in that statement are still relevant, but given the structural shifts in the health care delivery system, they no longer adequately address the unique needs of children. This revised policy statement is an update of the 2005 statement.

In light of the passage and ongoing implementation of the Patient Protection and Affordable Care Act (ACA [Pub L No. 111-148]) in 2010, contractual obligations, as expressed in health plan-provider and health plan-beneficiary agreements, have a new significance with respect to the array of health care benefits made available to children and families. In particular, a much used term—"medical necessity"—is, in fact, generally ill defined. As stated in the previous policy statement, "The term 'medical necessity' is used by Medicaid and Medicare and in insurance contracts to refer to medical services that are generally recognized as appropriate for the diagnosis, prevention, or treatment of disease and injury." The term is found in insurance contractual language, and, as stated in the 2005 policy statement, "… an intervention will be covered if it is an otherwise covered category of service, not specifically excluded, and medically necessary." It

www.pediatrics.org/cgi/doi/10.1542/peds.2013-1637

doi:10.1542/peds.2013-1637

PEDIATRICS (ISSN Numbers: Print, 0031-4005; Online, 1098-4275).

Copyright © 2013 by the American Academy of Pediatrics

would appear that this statement provides a straightforward presentation of medical necessity. However, health insurance coverage is moderated by a host of federal regulations and statutes, state mandates, and other rules. Provider agreements are usually written to incorporate these rules and regulations. As the US Department of Health and Human Services moves to implement the provisions of the ACA, essential health care benefits are not guaranteed to be the same in every state. Consequently, benefits for children may vary from state to state or plan to plan and may contain specific exclusions. The AAP advocates for quality health care for children that promotes optimal growth and development with measures intended to prevent, diagnose, detect, ameliorate, or palliate the effects of physical, genetic, congenital, mental, or behavioral conditions, injuries, or disabilities.

Individuals with health insurance coverage, whether it be Medicaid, Medicare, or commercial insurance coverage, may be unaware of payment or benefit restrictions for the medical services they seek. In addition, services ordered by a physician might only be covered if conditions of medical necessity are met. Medical necessity means that a decision is needed about appropriateness for a specific treatment of a specific individual. The 2005 AAP statement drew on model language developed by Stanford University[2]; however, more specific considerations are needed for children because of their unique needs. Now, as the US Department of Health and Human Services is charged with implementation of the ACA, it is time to address medical necessity and the needs of children. Although Medicare has become the de facto standard of health care benefits and directly influences

commercial health care benefit plans, it is important to realize that health care standards designed for adult care often will not meet the needs of children. By and large, the Medicaid program provides coverage for a significant number of children, and it, too, can be influenced by health care standards designed for adults.

A definition of medical necessity for children must recognize that the needs of children differ from those of adults. The foundation for medical necessity for children should be based on the comprehensive, fully inclusive set of services provided by the Early and Periodic Screening, Diagnosis, and Treatment regimen embodied in Medicaid as well as the preventive care recommendations in *Bright Futures: Guidelines for Health Supervision of Infants, Children, and Adolescents,* as stipulated in Section 2713 of the ACA.[3] The language in the Stanford statement considered the scope of health problems, evidence of effectiveness, and value of the intervention. Medical necessity should be guided by these criteria, but health plan and even Medicare language generalizes across populations, as opposed to focusing on specific individuals or groups, including children, often in a manner that is blind to their particular needs. A definition of medical necessity is needed that is more functional or operational and specific to meet the needs of children. Informed pediatricians can help advance such a definition.

Variability in "Essential Health Benefits," as intended by the ACA, is also cause for concern. There are 10 categories of Essential Health Benefits, including item 10—pediatric services including vision and oral care. The states are allowed individually to define the benefits for each of these 10 categories. Therefore, there is a great likelihood of significant variation

in pediatric benefits throughout the nation. States are likely to use different methods of determining medical necessity.

Some examples may help to illustrate the unique needs of children. One such example is the nuance between rehabilitative and habilitative services. Rehabilitative and habilitative services and devices are specifically addressed as 1 of 10 necessary categories of Essential Health Benefits in the ACA. Currently, in many instances, health care coverage is limited to rehabilitative services, referring to the need to restore a lost function. Habilitation suggests a function or skill not yet acquired or attained. More specifically, the National Association of Insurance Commissioners defines habilitation as "health care services that help a person keep, *learn,* or improve skills and functioning for daily living." With today's medical knowledge, conditions poorly understood in the past may now be subject to significant improvement, even functions that have not yet been acquired. Habilitation and rehabilitation services are usually provided by the same professionals, the only difference being the indication for therapeutic intervention. The case is also illustrated when one considers speech therapy for a child with autism or physical therapy for a child with hypotonia—motor skills and developmental milestones not yet achieved. Every newborn infant is a well of unknown potential. The terms habilitative and rehabilitative should be interchangeable where children are concerned. Developmental milestones represent standards achieved by most children in a given time frame, but not all children follow the same trajectory. A primary focus needs to be on the potential for functional gain—hence, habilitative services.

Evidence of effectiveness is a cornerstone of medical necessity, yet such data for children may not be readily available. It would be beneficial if medical necessity was governed by traditional evidence grading, and if not available, a hierarchy or algorithm of standards should be applied. The AAP has published 2 policy statements to aid decision makers in classifying clinical recommendations and ensuring transparency in issuing clinical guidelines.[4,5] If patient-centered or scientific evidence for children is insufficient, then professional standards of care for children must be considered. The AAP, other pediatric medical specialty societies, and consensus expert pediatric opinion could serve as references for defining essential pediatric care in the context of medically necessary services. **Hence, the pediatric definition of medical necessity should be as follows: health care interventions that are evidence based, evidence informed, or based on consensus advisory opinion and that are recommended by recognized health care professionals, such as the AAP, to promote optimal growth and development in a child and to prevent, detect, diagnose, treat, ameliorate, or palliate the effects of physical, genetic, congenital, developmental, behavioral, or mental conditions, injuries, or disabilities.**

Value is another parameter in the consideration of medical necessity. Value is not simply a cost-benefit assumption. Value, in fact, may be a subjective consideration. The recipient may have an entirely different perception of value than the provider or payer. Value implies quality (ie, access to age-appropriate care, in an appropriate setting, by appropriate personnel) plus desired outcome at a reasonable cost. Pediatricians

recognize the so-called marginal effect of some services—extensive interventions for limited or no essential benefit. However, children deserve the intent embedded in the Medicaid provision of the Early and Periodic Screening, Diagnosis, and Treatment regimen, specifically treatment. Given a pediatric definition of medical necessity as mentioned previously, the value of services might also be considered. Examples in which this is particularly true include children with autism spectrum disorders, neurodevelopmental disorders, or expressive speech delay, conditions for which needs are unique and improvement may be slow. Similarly, services that have been provided for an appropriate period of time by an appropriate provider could be discontinued if there is no measureable benefit. In short, services should be provided to children, but continuity is only ensured if there is evidence of a significant measureable benefit. It may be that the only therapeutic benefit is maintenance at a given level of function. If this facilitates more manageable daily living, then the service has value. This might best be exemplified by the continuation of occupational or physical therapy for a child with neurologic damage if only to facilitate safe transfers or to minimize the usual contractures. The goal is to achieve value for both the recipient and the provider. Resources are limited, but every child, with or without disability, deserves the opportunity to declare his or her potential for improvement in his or her daily life. Difficult decisions are part of medical necessity. Cost should not be the basis for denial of services, but the delivery of care in a setting that demonstrates lower cost could be acceptable if quality is not compromised.

Transparency in today's health care delivery system is essential to credibility. Health plans need to be clear with respect to the evaluation and determinations of medical necessity. The decision pathway, authority credentials of decision makers, and timeliness in the process should feature identifiable criteria or benchmarks in rendering decisions relevant to medical necessity. The expectations of all health plans, including Medicaid and Medicare, should be clear in anticipation of medical necessity requirements, and similarly, the decision-making process should be equally transparent. Consideration might be given to the role of a family advocate or ombudsmen in protecting children and families and intervening to aid in solving their problems related to medical necessity decisions.

As health care reform advances, contracts between providers of care and health care organizations, whether they are medical group practices, accountable care organizations, or health plans, will define expectations and obligations. Essential language should exist to address the unique needs of children in the context of medical necessity. The right of a child to optimal growth and development should be a universal expectation limited only by the restraints of physical or genetic conditions. New and emerging health care delivery models, including accountable care organizations, bundled payments covering hospital and physician services, disease-management models, and others, will influence how health care services are managed for beneficiaries. There will also be contractual arrangements with providers of primary and specialty care, and federal and/or state regulations will influence these contractual relationships. This time of transition affords pediatricians an opportunity to affect not only overall health care benefits but also the medical necessity decisions that affect pediatric care. All of these agreements should feature essential language that recognizes the unique needs of children and ensures more equitable care for all children. The AAP and its member pediatricians are the informed advocates who can advance a better understanding of medical necessity decisions on behalf of children.

LEAD AUTHOR
Thomas F. Long, MD, FAAP

COMMITTEE ON CHILD HEALTH FINANCING, 2012–2013
Thomas F. Long, MD, FAAP, Chairperson
Mark Helm, MD, MBA, FAAP
Mark L. Hudak, MD, FAAP
Andrew D. Racine, MD, PhD, FAAP

Budd Shenkin, MD, FAAP
Iris Grace Snider, MD, FAAP
Patience Haydock White, MD, MA, FAAP
Norman Chip Harbaugh, MD, FAAP
Molly Droge, MD, FAAP

FORMER COMMITTEE MEMBERS
Thomas Chiu, MD, MBA, FAAP
Russell Clark Libby, MD, FAAP

STAFF
Edward Zimmerman, MS

REFERENCES

1. American Academy of Pediatrics Committee on Child Health Financing. Model contractual language for medical necessity for children. *Pediatrics.* 2005;116(1):261–262
2. Singer S, Berthold L, Vorhaus C, et al. *Decreasing Variation in Medical Necessity Decision-Making.* Stanford, CA: Center for Health Policy, Stanford University; 1999
3. Hagan J, Shaw J, Duncan P, eds. *Bright Futures: Guidelines for Health Supervision of Infants, Children, and Adolescents,* 3rd ed. Elk Grove Village, IL: American Academy of Pediatrics; 2008
4. American Academy of Pediatrics Steering Committee on Quality Improvement and Management. Classifying recommendations for clinical practice guidelines. *Pediatrics.* 2004;114(3):874–877
5. Shiffman RN, Marcuse EK, Moyer VA, et al; American Academy of Pediatrics Steering Committee on Quality Improvement and Management. Toward transparent clinical policies. *Pediatrics.* 2008;121(3):643–646

Ethical Controversies in Organ Donation After Circulatory Death

- *Policy Statement*

POLICY STATEMENT

Ethical Controversies in Organ Donation After Circulatory Death

COMMITTEE ON BIOETHICS

KEY WORDS
bioethics, children, circulatory death, ethics, organ donation, organ procurement

ABBREVIATIONS
DCD—donation after circulatory death
ECMO—extracorporeal membrane oxygenation

www.pediatrics.org/cgi/doi/10.1542/peds.2013-0672

doi:10.1542/peds.2013-0672

PEDIATRICS (ISSN Numbers: Print, 0031-4005; Online, 1098-4275).

Copyright © 2013 by the American Academy of Pediatrics

abstract

The persistent mismatch between the supply of and need for transplantable organs has led to efforts to increase the supply, including controlled donation after circulatory death (DCD). Controlled DCD involves organ recovery after the planned withdrawal of life-sustaining treatment and the declaration of death according to the cardiorespiratory criteria. Two central ethical issues in DCD are when organ recovery can begin and how to manage conflicts of interests. The "dead donor rule" should be maintained, and donors in cases of DCD should only be declared dead after the permanent cessation of circulatory function. Permanence is generally established by a 2- to 5-minute waiting period. Given ongoing controversy over whether the cessation must also be irreversible, physicians should not be required to participate in DCD. Because the preparation for organ recovery in DCD begins before the declaration of death, there are potential conflicts between the donor's and recipient's interests. These conflicts can be managed in a variety of ways, including informed consent and separating the various participants' roles. For example, informed consent should be sought for premortem interventions to improve organ viability, and organ procurement organization personnel and members of the transplant team should not be involved in the discontinuation of life-sustaining treatment or the declaration of death. It is also important to emphasize that potential donors in cases of DCD should receive integrated interdisciplinary palliative care, including sedation and analgesia. *Pediatrics* 2013;131:1021–1026

INTRODUCTION

The persistent mismatch between the supply of and need for transplantable organs and the resulting deaths of individuals on the waiting list have led to a variety of efforts to increase the supply. As of May 17, 2012, there were 878 individuals aged <18 years awaiting a kidney transplant and 513 awaiting a liver transplant. In 2011, 10 individuals aged <18 years died while waiting for a kidney transplant, and 20 children and adolescents died while waiting for a liver transplant.[1] One effort to increase the supply of transplantable organs has been renewed interest in donation after circulatory death (DCD), which is the retrieval of organs from individuals declared dead after the irreversible cessation of circulatory and respiratory functions. (This process was initially referred to as "nonheartbeating organ donation" and then as "donation after cardiac death." The most recent change in terminology emphasizes that the determination of death is based on the cessation of circulatory, not cardiac, functions.[2]) There are several forms of DCD, and the current statement focuses on "controlled" DCD: the recovery of organs after the planned withdrawal of life-sustaining medical treatment.[3]

Although DCD was the initial form of deceased organ donation, it was eclipsed by recovery of organs from individuals declared dead according to neurologic criteria after these criteria were established and evidence showed improved graft function from such donors. There was renewed interest in DCD in the 1990s, including the publication of the so-called Pittsburgh Protocol,[4,5] given the persistent shortage of transplantable organs. Recent estimates suggest that DCD could increase the supply of transplantable organs by 20%.[6] A number of subsequent reports and consensus statements have addressed points of controversy, such as the waiting period before the declaration of death and the use of premortem interventions to improve graft function.[7–10] More recent pediatric studies reporting similar graft survival in kidneys and livers from donors declared dead according to neurologic and cardiovascular criteria have further increased interest in DCD.[11]

Increased acceptance of DCD has resulted in regulatory oversight. The Joint Commission mandates that, although hospitals need not perform DCD, their policies must address it.[12] The United Network for Organ Sharing has articulated Model Elements for Controlled DCD Recovery Protocols[13] and requires its member hospitals that perform solid organ transplants

to develop protocols which address the required elements to facilitate the recovery of organs from donors in cases of DCD.[14] The Organ Donation Breakthrough Collaborative has also established the goal of having donors in DCD cases represent 10% of all organ donors.[15]

The current policy statement addresses the 2 major conceptual and ethical issues related to DCD: when can organ recovery begin, and how should conflicts of interests be managed? It provides greater detail than the American Academy of Pediatrics' policy statement "Pediatric Organ Donation and Transplantation,"[16] but it does not address general issues, such as medical examiner release of organs. Discussing these issues is particularly important given the variation among DCD policies at children's hospitals.[17] Standards must be met to maintain the integrity of and public confidence in the organ transplantation system.

DECLARATION OF DEATH

Whether and when donors in DCD cases are dead is important because cadaveric organ transplantation operates under the "dead donor rule." This rule can be characterized in 2 different ways, each with its own ethical justification. One version is that organ recovery must not cause the donor's death. This version is justified by the prohibition against the direct killing of innocent persons. The other version is that the donor must be dead before the recovery of vital organs. This version is based on preventing potential negative outcomes, such as the mistreatment of potential donors and the erosion of public confidence in transplantation.[18]

Some commentators have recommended abandoning the dead donor rule. Miller and Truog,[19] for example, argue that withdrawing life-sustaining

treatment causes patients' death and that there is no ethical bright line between withdrawing life-sustaining treatment and active euthanasia. They contend that patients or their surrogates, who have previously decided to have life-sustaining medical treatment withdrawn, should be permitted to consent to the premortem recovery of vital organs. Although they do not discuss the implications of their position for pediatrics, it would, in principle, extend to parents or guardians and capacitated adolescents or their proxies. Miller and Truog's arguments are not, however, compelling. For example, they conflate patients' right to refuse treatment with the distinction between killing and letting die. They also ignore well-developed arguments that the intentional killing of innocent persons is unethical and that the ethically relevant distinction is between different forms of letting die. The dead donor rule should, therefore, be retained, not only because the reasons supporting it are compelling but also because the reasons for abandoning it are insufficient.

The discussion of death commonly distinguishes definition, criteria, and tests. The predominant definition of death is "the cessation of functioning of the organism as a whole."[20] This definition focuses on the functions possessed by the whole organism, such as consciousness and control of circulation, respiration, and temperature, rather than the functions of its constituent parts. Although the definition states the necessary and jointly sufficient conditions for correctly applying the concept of death, the criteria specify measurable conditions, and physicians use the tests to evaluate the criteria at the bedside. The 2 criteria for death are the neurologic and the cardiorespiratory.

Drawing an analogy to the declaration of death in other clinical contexts, proponents of DCD argue that the cessation of circulatory function must be permanent but not irreversible. The cessation is permanent if it will not resume on its own through autoresuscitation or as a result of external action, such as cardiopulmonary resuscitation. Once sufficient time has elapsed to preclude the spontaneous recovery of circulatory function, it is permanent, because, as part of the decision to withdraw life-sustaining treatment, the parents or guardians previously decided to forego cardiopulmonary resuscitation. Irreversibility further requires that the function is incapable, within the limits of current technology, of being restored. Proponents of DCD contend that irreversibility is not necessary for the declaration of death.[21] Numerous professional organizations and consensus groups support this argument.[8–10]

Within this framework, how much time must elapse to preclude autoresuscitation sufficiently is a significant concern. Despite calls for additional research, data are limited on this topic. On the basis of narrative reviews, commentators have recommended waiting at least 2 minutes and not more than 5 minutes.[8–10] The authors of the most recent systematic review, noting the low quality and limited scope of reports, concluded there are no cases of autoresuscitation without cardiopulmonary resuscitation.[22] Until a large observational study that provides narrow confidence intervals around the duration of autoresuscitation is conducted, this timing remains a prudential judgment. Once death is declared, there is no need for an additional waiting period before the initiation of organ recovery efforts.

Declaring death requires tests in addition to definitions and criteria. It would be prudent to use more sensitive and/or objective tests when they are available. For example, using indwelling arterial catheters, Doppler ultrasonography, or echocardiography may be preferable to palpating pulses or auscultating heartbeats.[2]

There are, however, 2 significant criticisms of the proponents of DCD's arguments. One objection is that irreversibility is a necessary criterion for the declaration of death. Although permanence and irreversibility are causally related (ie, without intervention, permanent cessation will become irreversible), they are not contemporaneous. During the time between when circulatory function is permanently lost and when it is irreversibly lost, critics argue, individuals are dying but not yet dead.[23] This objection can also be stated in terms of the relationship between the cardiorespiratory and neurologic criteria of death. Rather than being independent criteria, the neurologic criteria are arguably fundamental. Although individuals who fulfill the cardiorespiratory criteria inevitably fulfill the neurologic criteria, if resuscitation is withheld, additional time must elapse.

A second criticism is that replacing irreversibility with permanence inappropriately makes the declaration of death contingent on the intent and action of others rather than an intrinsic condition of the organism.[23] Nevertheless, the criticism that retrieving vital organs from donors in DCD cases is the proximate cause of death is not sound. If sufficient time passes to preclude autoresuscitation, progressive hypoxia-ischemia of the central nervous system is the proximate cause of death.[24]

Although the need to increase the supply of transplantable organs is compelling and the arguments for the sufficiency of permanence for declaring death are widely accepted, the criticisms of these arguments are sufficient that physicians should not be required to retrieve organs from donors in cases of DCD.[25] Institutions have an obligation to provide patients and their families access to DCD. Whether institutions themselves should be able to refuse to perform DCD is ethically controversial because of burdens placed on patients and their families by alternatives, such as the transfer of patients to other institutions.[26] The American Academy of Pediatrics could not reach consensus on whether institutions may refuse to participate.

Recent publications have highlighted related conceptual and practical issues. In 2008, Boucek et al[27] reported successfully transplanting hearts from 3 infant donors in cases of DCD. Some criticized the waiting period of 75 seconds in 2 of the transplants as being too short. Shortening the waiting period is particularly problematic in infants because they were not part of the population in which autoresuscitation was studied, and their organs may be more resilient.[2] Others contended that the resumption of cardiac activity in the recipient negates the determination of death.[28] The current definition of death focuses on the loss of integrated functioning of the organism that is demonstrated by the absence of autoresuscitation. Residual function of individual organs and tissues is consistent with death of the organism as a whole.

Others have reported on the use of extracorporeal membrane oxygenation (ECMO) in donors to support organ perfusion between the declaration of death and organ recovery and, thereby, improve outcomes in the transplanted organs.[29,30] ECMO was originally designed to provide cardiorespiratory support to individuals with reversible cardiorespiratory failure. The use of ECMO in DCD is problematic because it artificially replaces circulatory function analogous to a ventilator in patients with severe brainstem or spinal cord injuries. The additional concern is that reperfusion of the brain could restore consciousness. A potential modification is to prevent perfusion of the brain or organs above the diaphragm.[2] It is not clear whether these measures are sufficient to permit donors to be declared dead according to the cardiorespiratory criteria or whether donors receiving ECMO should be evaluated by using the neurologic criteria.

CONFLICTS OF INTERESTS

In addition to conceptual and practical issues regarding the declaration of death, DCD involves a variety of conflicts of interests.[31] In contrast to donors declared dead according to the neurologic criteria, preparation for organ recovery efforts in DCD begins before the declaration of death. This preparation may include premortem interventions, such as placing lines or administering heparin, and modifications of the usual process of withdrawing life-sustaining treatment. These actions create the potential for conflicts between the interests of the donor and of the recipients.

These potential conflicts are exacerbated by the need to limit warm, and to a lesser extent cold, ischemic time. Organs tolerate oxygen deprivation better at colder temperatures than at warm ones. In "brain-dead" donors, the organs are relatively normally perfused before recovery and then rapidly cooled. In donors in cases of DCD, organs may experience hypoperfusion during the time between stopping life-sustaining treatment and recovering and cooling the organs. This hypoperfusion may damage the organs and impair their function. Premortem practices are altered in DCD to diminish warm ischemia times, and the maximum duration of organ recovery efforts is frequently stipulated.

(The fact that donation efforts will cease if the potential donor does not die within the specified time period should be disclosed as part of the informed consent process.)

The donor's informed consent is a potential way to manage the conflicts of interests. Capacitated adults can accept the risks involved in the donation process to benefit potential recipients. Informed consent by the donor is, however, unlikely in DCD. Most potential donors in cases of DCD have suffered serious, irreversible neurologic injuries and are incapacitated. Expressing one's interest in donation (eg, by signing a donor card) does not currently constitute informed consent for the modifications in premortem management required by DCD.[32]

Parents or guardians "consenting" for their children further complicate the issue. In contrast to surrogate decision makers for previously capacitated adults who should make decisions on the basis of substituted judgment, parents or guardians should make decisions based on their child's and family's interests. Giving permission for their child to become an organ donor may permit families to create meaning or value in a tragic circumstance. Changes in premortem treatment may create conflicts between the interests of the recipient and/or the family and the interests of the donor. Minimally, changes in premortem treatment should not be contrary to the donor's interests.

The potential for conflicts arises at multiple points in the donation process, including consent to organ donation, premortem interventions to promote organ viability, palliative care, and declaration of death.

- The decision to withdraw life-sustaining medical treatment should be separate or decoupled from the decision to attempt to donate organs.[7–10] The conceptual separation

of the issues can be reinforced by separating when the decisions are discussed and who participates in the discussions. This separation should be maintained, to the extent possible, if parents or guardians raise the issue of organ donation before deciding to withdraw life-sustaining medical treatment.

- Premortem interventions to improve organ viability should not harm the donor and require informed consent.[7,9,10] Premortem interventions may include medications, such as anticoagulants or vasodilators, and procedures, such as line placement. Most of these interventions are neutral to patients' interests. There is legitimate disagreement about whether anticoagulants may, in uncommon situations, contribute to the potential donor's death and whether the pain of line placement constitutes a relevant harm.[7] Parental permission is necessary for any premortem intervention to improve organ viability.

- Potential donors in cases of DCD should receive integrated interdisciplinary palliative care,[33] including sedation and analgesia.[8,9] In DCD, palliative care occurs concurrently with preliminary organ donation efforts. Efforts should be made to limit alterations in the process of withdrawing life-sustaining treatment, such as its location. Alterations in the process of withdrawing life-sustaining treatment to reduce warm ischemia times should also be disclosed as part of the informed consent process. Medications should not be used with the direct intention of controlling the time of death.[7,8,10]

- Although organ procurement organization personnel may be involved in evaluating potential donors and scheduling, they and members of the transplant team should not be involved in the decision to withdraw life-sustaining treatment or its actual discontinuation. Programs should consider whether physicians caring for potential recipients should also be excluded from involvement in premortem management. If there are no alternatives to members of the transplant team participating in premortem interventions, such as prepping and draping and/or line placement, they should physically leave the patient care area before the withdrawal of life-sustaining treatment.[7,10]

- As discussed previously, death should be declared by using relatively sensitive and objective tests. Organ procurement organization and transplant personnel should not be involved in the declaration of death. Programs should consider the appropriate role, if any, of those caring for potential recipients.[7–10]

Institutions should have policies regarding these issues and periodically review performance to promote adherence. Ethics committees can contribute to the development of policies and the resolution of dilemmas or conflicts in their implementation.

RECOMMENDATIONS

- The American Academy of Pediatrics considers DCD an ethically acceptable option when practiced within appropriate constraints, such as waiting a reasonable amount of time after the initial fulfillment of the cardiorespiratory criteria for death to preclude autoresuscitation before declaring death. On the basis of current evidence, the recommendation to wait between 2 and 5 minutes is reasonable.

- Additional research to better understand the phenomenon of autoresuscitation in infants and children should be conducted.

- Given legitimate ethical disagreement regarding the interpretation of the cardiorespiratory criteria for death, individual physicians should not be required to participate in DCD. Institutions should, nonetheless, provide access to DCD.

- Physicians should help institutions develop policies to manage the conflicts of interests inherent in the DCD process. Such policies should include:

  o the separation or decoupling of the decision to withdraw life-sustaining treatment from the decision to donate;

  o the prohibition of premortem interventions to improve organ viability that harm the patient;

  o the requirement of parental permission for acceptable premortem interventions;

  o the provision of integrated interdisciplinary palliative care; and

  o the prohibition of organ procurement organization staff and transplant team members from participating in the discontinuation of life-sustaining treatment or the declaration of death.

LEAD AUTHOR
Armand H. Matheny Antommaria, MD, PhD

COMMITTEE ON BIOETHICS, 2011–2012
Mary E. Fallat, MD
Aviva L. Katz, MD
Mark R. Mercurio, MD
Margaret R. Moon, MD
Alexander L. Okun, MD
Sally A. Webb, MD
Kathryn L. Weise, MD

CONSULTANT
Jessica W. Berg, JD, MPH

PAST CONTRIBUTING COMMITTEE MEMBERS
Armand H. Matheny Antommaria, MD, PhD
Ian R. Holzman, MD
Lainie Friedman Ross, MD, PhD

LIAISONS
Douglas S. Diekema, MD, MPH – *American Board of Pediatrics*
Kevin W. Coughlin, MD – *Canadian Pediatric Society*
Steven J. Ralston, MD – *American College of Obstetricians and Gynecologists*

STAFF
Alison Baker, MS

REFERENCES

1. US Department of Health and Human Services. Organ procurement and transplantation network. Available at: http://optn.transplant.hrsa.gov/latestData/step2.asp? Accessed May 31, 2012

2. Bernat JL, Capron AM, Bleck TP, et al. The circulatory-respiratory determination of death in organ donation. *Crit Care Med.* 2010;38(3):963–970

3. Daemen JW, Kootstra G, Wijnen RM, Yin M, Heineman E. Nonheart-beating donors: the Maastricht experience. *Clin Transpl.* 1994:303–316

4. University of Pittsburgh Medical Center policy and procedure manual. Management of terminally ill patients who may become organ donors after death. *Kennedy Inst Ethics J.* 1993;3(2):A1–A15

5. DeVita MA, Snyder JV. Development of the University of Pittsburgh Medical Center policy for the care of terminally ill patients who may become organ donors after death following the removal of life support. *Kennedy Inst Ethics J.* 1993;3(2):131–143

6. Pleacher KM, Roach ES, Van der Werf W, Antommaria AH, Bratton SL. Impact of a pediatric donation after cardiac death program. *Pediatr Crit Care Med.* 2009;10(2):166–170

7. Institute of Medicine. *Non-Heart-Beating Organ Transplantation: Medical and Ethical Issues in Procurement.* Washington, DC: National Academies Press; 1997

8. Ethics Committee, American College of Critical Care Medicine; Society of Critical Care Medicine. Recommendations for non-heartbeating organ donation. A position paper by the Ethics Committee, American College of Critical Care Medicine, Society of Critical Care Medicine. *Crit Care Med.* 2001; 29(9):1826–1831

9. Bernat JL, D'Alessandro AM, Port FK, et al. Report of a National Conference on Donation after cardiac death. *Am J Transplant.* 2006;6(2):281–291

10. Reich DJ, Mulligan DC, Abt PL, et al; ASTS Standards on Organ Transplantation Committee. ASTS recommended practice guidelines for controlled donation after cardiac death organ procurement and transplantation. *Am J Transplant.* 2009;9(9): 2004–2011

11. Abt P, Kashyap R, Orloff M, et al. Pediatric liver and kidney transplantation with allografts from DCD donors: a review of UNOS data. *Transplantation.* 2006;82(12):1708–1711

12. Joint Commission on Accreditation of Healthcare Organizations. Revisions to standard LD.3.110. *Jt Comm Perspect.* 2006;26(6):7

13. United Network for Organ Sharing (UNOS). Attachment III to Appendix B of the UNOS bylaws: model elements for controlled DCD recovery protocols. Richmond, VA: UNOS; 2007. Available at: www.unos.org/docs/Appendix_B_AttachIII.pdf. Accessed February 27, 2012

14. United Network for Organ Sharing (UNOS). Appendix B to bylaws: criteria for institutional memberships: transplant hospitals. Richmond, VA: UNOS; 2010. Available at: www.unos.org/docs/Appendix_B_II.pdf. Accessed February 27, 2012

15. US Department of Health and Human Services, Health Resources and Services Administration, Division of Transplantation. Donation and Transplantation Community of Practice (DTCP). Available at: www.organdonor.gov/grantProgramDtcp.asp. February 27, 2012

16. Committee on Hospital Care, Section on Surgery, and Section on Critical Care. Policy statement—pediatric organ donation and transplantation. *Pediatrics.* 2010;125 (4):822–828

17. Antommaria AH, Trotochaud K, Kinlaw K, Hopkins PN, Frader J. Policies on donation after cardiac death at children's hospitals: a mixed-methods analysis of variation. *JAMA.* 2009;301(18):1902–1908

18. Arnold RM, Youngner SJ. The dead donor rule: should we stretch it, bend it, or abandon it? *Kennedy Inst Ethics J.* 1993;3(2):263–278

19. Miller FG, Truog RD. *Death, Dying, and Organ Transplantation: Reconstructing Medical Ethics at the End of Life.* New York, NY: Oxford University Press; 2012

20. Bernat JL, Culver CM, Gert B. On the definition and criterion of death. *Ann Intern Med.* 1981;94(3):389–394

21. Bernat JL. Are organ donors after cardiac death really dead? *J Clin Ethics.* 2006;17(2): 122–132

22. Hornby K, Hornby L, Shemie SD. A systematic review of autoresuscitation after cardiac arrest. *Crit Care Med.* 2010;38(5): 1246–1253

23. Marquis D. Are DCD donors dead? *Hastings Cent Rep.* 2010;40(3):24–31

24. Menikoff J. Doubts about death: the silence of the Institute of Medicine. *J Law Med Ethics.* 1998;26(2):157–165

25. Committee on Bioethics. Policy statement—physician refusal to provide information or treatment on the basis of claims of conscience. *Pediatrics.* 2009;124(6):1689–1693

26. Wicclair MR. Pharmacies, pharmacists, and conscientious objection. *Kennedy Inst Ethics J.* 2006;16(3):225–250

27. Boucek MM, Mashburn C, Dunn SM, et al; Denver Children's Pediatric Heart Transplant Team. Pediatric heart transplantation after declaration of cardiocirculatory death. *N Engl J Med.* 2008;359(7):709–714

28. Veatch RM. Donating hearts after cardiac death—reversing the irreversible. *N Engl J Med.* 2008;359(7):672–673

29. Fondevila C, Hessheimer AJ, Ruiz A, et al. Liver transplant using donors after unexpected cardiac death: novel preservation protocol and acceptance criteria. *Am J Transplant.* 2007;7(7):1849–1855

30. Gravel MT, Arenas JD, Chenault R II, et al. Kidney transplantation from organ donors following cardiopulmonary death using extracorporeal membrane oxygenation support. *Ann Transplant.* 2004;9(1):57–58

31. Shaw BW Jr. Conflict of interest in the procurement of organs from cadavers following withdrawal of life support. *Kennedy Inst Ethics J.* 1993;3(2):179–187

32. Lawlor M, Kerridge I. Registering wishes about organ and tissue donation: personal discussion during licence renewal may be superior to online registration. *Intern Med J.* 2009;39(12):835–837

33. American Academy of Pediatrics. Committee on Bioethics and Committee on Hospital Care. Palliative care for children. *Pediatrics.* 2000;106(2 pt 1):351–357

Ethical and Policy Issues in Genetic Testing and Screening of Children

- *Policy Statement*

POLICY STATEMENT

Ethical and Policy Issues in Genetic Testing and Screening of Children

abstract

The genetic testing and genetic screening of children are common-place. Decisions about whether to offer genetic testing and screening should be driven by the best interest of the child. The growing literature on the psychosocial and clinical effects of such testing and screening can help inform best practices. This policy statement represents recommendations developed collaboratively by the American Academy of Pediatrics and the American College of Medical Genetics and Genomics with respect to many of the scenarios in which genetic testing and screening can occur. *Pediatrics* 2013;131:620–622

COMMITTEE ON BIOETHICS, COMMITTEE ON GENETICS, AND THE AMERICAN COLLEGE OF MEDICAL GENETICS AND GENOMICS SOCIAL, ETHICAL, AND LEGAL ISSUES COMMITTEE

KEY WORDS
genetic testing, genetic screening, newborn screening, predictive testing, disclosure, carrier identification

ABBREVIATIONS
AAP—American Academy of Pediatrics
ACMG—American College of Medical Genetics and Genomics

BACKGROUND

In 1953, Watson and Crick described the DNA double helix. Fifty years later, the full sequence of the human genome was published. Our knowledge of genetics grows rapidly, as does consumer interest in undergoing genetic testing. Statements about genetic testing of children in the United States written in the past 2 decades need to be updated to consider the ethical issues arising with new technologies and expanded uses of genetic testing and screening.[1,2] The growing literature on the psychosocial and clinical effects of such testing and screening can help inform us about best practices.

Genetic testing and screening of minors are commonplace. Every year, ~4 million infants in the United States undergo newborn screening for metabolic, hematologic, and endocrine abnormalities for which early treatment may prevent or reduce morbidity or mortality.

Outside of newborn screening, genetic testing of children is less commonly performed. Diagnostic genetic testing may be performed on a child with signs or symptoms of a potential genetic condition or for treatment decisions made on the basis of results of pharmacogenetic assays. Genetic testing may also be performed on an asymptomatic child with a positive family history for a specific genetic condition, particularly if early treatment may affect morbidity or mortality. The American Academy of Pediatrics (AAP) and the American College of Medical Genetics and Genomics (ACMG) provide the following recommendations regarding genetic testing and screening of minors. An accompanying technical report provides ethical explanations and empirical data in support of these recommendations (http://www.nature.com/gim/journal/vaop/ncurrent/full/gim2012176a.html).[3]

www.pediatrics.org/cgi/doi/10.1542/peds.2012-3680

doi:10.1542/peds.2012-3680

PEDIATRICS (ISSN Numbers: Print, 0031-4005; Online, 1098-4275).

Copyright © 2013 by the American Academy of Pediatrics

GENERAL RECOMMENDATIONS

1. Decisions about whether to offer genetic testing and screening should be driven by the best interest of the child.

2. Genetic testing is best offered in the context of genetic counseling. Genetic counseling can be performed by clinical geneticists, genetic counselors, or any other health care provider with appropriate training and expertise. The AAP and ACMG support the expansion of educational opportunities in human genomics and genetics for medical students, residents, and practicing pediatric primary care providers.

DIAGNOSTIC TESTING

3. In a child with symptoms of a genetic condition, the rationale for genetic testing is similar to that of other medical diagnostic evaluations. Parents or guardians should be informed about the risks and benefits of testing, and their permission should be obtained. Ideally and when appropriate, the assent of the child should be obtained.[4]

4. When performed for therapeutic purposes, pharmacogenetic testing of children is acceptable, with permission of parents or guardians and, when appropriate, the child's assent. If a pharmacogenetic test result carries implications beyond drug targeting or dose-responsiveness, the broader implications should be discussed before testing.

NEWBORN SCREENING

5. The AAP and ACMG support the mandatory offering of newborn screening for all children. After education and counseling about the substantial benefits of newborn screening, its remote risks, and the next steps in the event of a positive screening result, parents should have the option of refusing the procedure, and an informed refusal should be respected.

CARRIER TESTING

6. The AAP and ACMG do not support routine carrier testing in minors when such testing does not provide health benefits in childhood. The AAP and ACMG advise against school-based testing or screening programs, because the school environment is unlikely to be conducive to voluntary participation, thoughtful consent, privacy, confidentiality, or appropriate counseling about test results.

7. For pregnant adolescents or for adolescents considering reproduction, genetic testing and screening should be offered as clinically indicated, and the risks and benefits should be explained clearly.

PREDICTIVE GENETIC TESTING

8. Parents or guardians may authorize predictive genetic testing for asymptomatic children at risk of childhood-onset conditions. Ideally, the assent of the child should be obtained.

9. Predictive genetic testing for adult-onset conditions generally should be deferred unless an intervention initiated in childhood may reduce morbidity or mortality. An exception might be made for families for whom diagnostic uncertainty poses a significant psychosocial burden, particularly when an adolescent and his or her parents concur in their interest in predictive testing.

10. For ethical and legal reasons, health care providers should be cautious about providing predictive genetic testing to minors without the involvement of their parents or guardians, even if a minor is mature. Results of such tests may have significant medical, psychological, and social implications, not only for the minor but also for other family members.

HISTOCOMPATIBILITY TESTING

11. Tissue compatibility testing of minors of all ages is permissible to benefit immediate family members but should be conducted only after thorough exploration of the psychosocial, emotional, and physical implications of the minor serving as a potential stem cell donor. A donor advocate or similar mechanism should be in place from the outset to avert coercion and safeguard the interests of the child.[5]

ADOPTION

12. The rationale for genetic testing of children in biological families should apply for adopted children and children awaiting placement for adoption. If a child has a known genetic risk, prospective adoptive parents must be made aware of this possibility. In rare cases, it may be in a child's best interest to undergo predictive genetic testing for a known risk before adoption to ensure the child's placement with a family capable of and willing to accept the child's potential medical and developmental challenges. In the absence of such indications, genetic testing should not be performed as a condition of adoption.

DISCLOSURE

13. At the time of genetic testing, parents or guardians should be encouraged to inform their child of the test results at an appropriate age. Parents or guardians should be advised that, under most circumstances, a request by a mature adolescent for test results should be honored.

14. Results from genetic testing of a child may have implications for the parents and other family

members. Health care providers have an obligation to inform parents and the child, when appropriate, about these potential implications. Health care providers should encourage patients and families to share this information and offer to help explain the results to the extended family or refer them for genetic counseling.

15. Misattributed paternity, use of donor gametes, adoption, or other questions about family relationships may be uncovered "incidentally" whenever genetic testing is performed, particularly when testing multiple family members. This risk should be discussed, and a plan about disclosure or nondisclosure should be in place before testing.

DIRECT-TO-CONSUMER TESTING

16. The AAP and ACMG strongly discourage the use of direct-to-consumer and home kit genetic testing of children because of the lack of oversight on test content, accuracy, and interpretation.

LEAD AUTHORS

Lainie F. Ross MD, PhD (AAP Committee on Bioethics)
Howard M. Saal, MD (AAP Committee on Genetics)
Rebecca R. Anderson, JD, MS (ACMG Social, Ethical, and Legal Issues Committee)
Karen L. David, MD, MS (ACMG Social, Ethical, and Legal Issues Committee)

AAP COMMITTEE ON BIOETHICS, 2011–2012

Mary E. Fallat, MD, Chairperson
Aviva L. Katz, MD
Mark R. Mercurio, MD
Margaret R. Moon, MD
Alexander L. Okun, MD
Sally A. Webb, MD
Kathryn L. Weise, MD

PAST CONTRIBUTING COMMITTEE MEMBERS

Armand H. Matheny Antommaria, MD, PhD
Ian R. Holzman, MD
Lainie F. Ross, MD, PhD

LIAISONS

Douglas S. Diekema, MD, MPH – *American Board of Pediatrics*
Kevin W. Coughlin, MD – *Canadian Pediatric Society*
Steven J. Ralston, MD – *American College of Obstetricians and Gynecologists*

CONSULTANT

Jessica W. Berg, JD, MPH

STAFF

Alison Baker, MS

AAP COMMITTEE ON GENETICS, 2011–2012

Robert A. Saul, MD, Chairperson
Stephen R. Braddock, MD
Emily Chen, MD, PhD
Debra L. Freedenberg, MD
Marilyn C. Jones, MD
James M. Perrin, MD
Beth Anne Tarini, MD, MS

PAST CONTRIBUTING COMMITTEE MEMBERS

Howard M. Saal, MD

Gregory M. Enns, MB, ChB
Jeffrey R. Gruen, MD

LIAISONS

Katrina M. Dipple, MD, PhD – *American College of Medical Genetics*
Stuart K. Shapira, MD, PhD – *Centers for Disease Control and Prevention*
Sara M. Copeland, MD – *Health Resources and Services Administration*
Melissa A. Parisi, MD, PhD – *Eunice Kennedy Shriver National Institute of Child Health and Human Development*
W. Allen Hogge, MD – *American College of Obstetricians and Gynecologists*

STAFF

Paul Spire

ACMG SOCIAL, ETHICAL, AND LEGAL ISSUES COMMITTEE, 2011–2012

Karen L. David, MD, MS, Chair
Louis E. Bartoshesky, MD, MPH, Vice Chair
Rebecca R. Anderson, JD, MS
Robert G. Best, PhD
Jodi D. Hoffman, MD
Masamichi Ito, PhD*
Amy A. Lemke, MS, PhD
Mitzi L. Murray, MD
Richard R. Sharp, PhD
Vikas Bhambhani, MD

BOARD LIAISON

Lynn D. Fleisher, PhD, JD

PAST CONTRIBUTING COMMITTEE MEMBERS

Alexander Asamoah, MD, PhD
Gary S. Gottesman, MD
Lainie F. Ross, MD, PhD
* Dr Masamichi Ito works for Athena Diagnostics, a company that performs genetic testing in minors.

REFERENCES

1. American Society of Human Genetics Board of Directors; American College of Medical Genetics Board of Directors. Points to consider: ethical, legal, and psychosocial implications of genetic testing in children and adolescents. *Am J Hum Genet.* 1995;57(5): 1233–1241

2. American Academy of Pediatrics Committee on Bioethics. Ethical issues with genetic testing in pediatrics. *Pediatrics.* 2001;107(6): 1451–1455. Reaffirmed October 2004

3. American Academy of Pediatrics Committee on Bioethics, Committee on Genetics; American College of Medical Genetics Social, Ethical and Legal Issues Committee. Ethical and policy issues in genetic testing and screening of children. *Genetics in Medicine.* 2013;15(3): In press

4. American Academy of Pediatrics Committee on Bioethics. Informed consent, parental permission and assent in pediatric practice. *Pediatrics.* 1995;95(2):314–317. Reaffirmed October 2006

5. American Academy of Pediatrics Committee on Bioethics. Children as hematopoietic stem cell donors. *Pediatrics.* 2010;125(2): 392–404

Evaluating for Suspected Child Abuse: Conditions That Predispose to Bleeding

- *Technical Report*

TECHNICAL REPORT

Evaluating for Suspected Child Abuse: Conditions That Predispose to Bleeding

Shannon L. Carpenter, MD, MS, Thomas C. Abshire, MD, James D. Anderst, MD, MS and the SECTION ON HEMATOLOGY/ONCOLOGY AND COMMITTEE ON CHILD ABUSE AND NEGLECT

KEY WORDS
intracranial hemorrhage, inherited coagulation disorders, bruising, nonaccidental trauma

ABBREVIATIONS
AP—α-2 antiplasmin
aPTT—activated partial thromboplastin time
BSS—Bernard-Soulier syndrome
CNS—central nervous system
EDS—Ehlers-Danlos syndrome
FFP—fresh-frozen plasma
GT—Glanzmann thrombasthenia
ICH—intracranial hemorrhage
ITP—immune thrombocytopenia
NARBDR—North American Rare Bleeding Disorders Registry
OI—osteogenesis imperfecta
PAI-1—plasminogen activator inhibitor type 1
PFA-100—platelet function analyzer
PT—prothrombin time
VKDB—vitamin K deficiency bleeding
VWAg—von Willebrand antigen
VWD—von Willebrand disease
VWF—von Willebrand factor

www.pediatrics.org/cgi/doi/10.1542/peds.2013-0196

doi:10.1542/peds.2013-0196

PEDIATRICS (ISSN Numbers: Print, 0031-4005; Online, 1098-4275).

Copyright © 2013 by the American Academy of Pediatrics

abstract

Child abuse might be suspected when children present with cutaneous bruising, intracranial hemorrhage, or other manifestations of bleeding. In these cases, it is necessary to consider medical conditions that predispose to easy bleeding/bruising. When evaluating for the possibility of bleeding disorders and other conditions that predispose to hemorrhage, the pediatrician must consider the child's presenting history, medical history, and physical examination findings before initiating a laboratory investigation. Many medical conditions can predispose to easy bleeding. Before ordering laboratory tests for a disease, it is useful to understand the biochemical basis and clinical presentation of the disorder, condition prevalence, and test characteristics. This technical report reviews the major medical conditions that predispose to bruising/bleeding and should be considered when evaluating for abusive injury. *Pediatrics* 2013;131:e1357–e1373

INTRODUCTION

In the absence of known accidental mechanisms or medical causes, children with intracranial hemorrhage (ICH), cutaneous bruises, or other symptoms of bleeding might be suspected victims of child abuse. In such situations, physicians must often carefully evaluate for the possibility of a bleeding disorder or another medical condition as a possible cause. In addition, because of the legal proceedings associated with cases of potential abuse, physicians might feel compelled to rule out any theoretical possibility of a medical explanation for the child's findings despite clinical improbability. This can result in an expensive and, in the case of young children with limited total blood volume, potentially harmful laboratory investigation of diminished clinical value.

The list of congenital and acquired bleeding disorders that could potentially be confused with abusive injury is extensive: hemophilia, von Willebrand disease (VWD), disorders of fibrinogen, vitamin K deficiency, factor XIII and other factor deficiencies, thrombocytopenia, leukemia, aplastic anemia and other bone marrow infiltrative or failure syndromes, and platelet function abnormalities, among others. Most of these conditions can present with mucosal bleeding, such as epistaxis and cutaneous bruising, but some (especially factor deficiencies) have been noted to present with isolated ICH, or can increase susceptibility to severe ICH after minor trauma. Collagen disorders can also predispose to easy bruising/bleeding in some circumstances. This report reviews the rationale for the consideration of bleeding disorders and collagen disorders as a cause of or as contributing to ICH, bruising, or bleeding when child abuse is suspected, and addresses several unsupported hypotheses related to these issues.

CLINICAL APPROACH TO THE EVALUATION OF CONDITIONS THAT PREDISPOSE TO BLEEDING IN THE SETTING OF POSSIBLE ABUSE

In many children with bruising/ bleeding concerning for abuse, the evaluation for medical conditions causing or contributing to the findings noted on the physical examination can be completed by assessing the child's presenting symptoms, trauma history, medical history, family history, and medications. Before engaging in a laboratory evaluation, physicians should consider the following:

1. The specific clinical characteristics of the child's findings, along with a previous history of bleeding or bruising. Family history of bleeding or bruising or a history of specific coagulopathies and other conditions should be addressed.

2. The known presentations and prevalence of the various bleeding disorders, collagen disorders, or other medical conditions under consideration.

3. The medical probability that a specific medical condition might cause or contribute to the child's bleeding or bruising.

4. The statistical characteristics of the proposed laboratory testing.

5. The history of the use of blood products or other factor replacement products that might alter test results.

6. The associated costs of testing, both financial and medical, such as the blood volume needed for testing.

7. The anticipated benefit of identifying conditions that might cause bleeding or bruising.

CLINICAL CHARACTERISTICS

Nonintracranial Bleeding

The age and developmental capabilities of the child, history of trauma, and the location and pattern of bruising often provide significant evidence in determining the presence of abusive injury.[1–5] In many cases, the constellation of findings, taken in conjunction with the clinical history, can be so strongly consistent with abusive injury that a further laboratory investigation for medical conditions is not warranted. For instance, in a verbal child with a patterned slap mark who describes being hit with an open hand at the location of the slap mark, obtaining tests to rule out a bleeding disorder is unlikely to provide useful information. However, because few data exist comparing the specific clinical presentations of bleeding disorders and abuse, in some cases, a laboratory evaluation might be necessary to minimize the chances of a misdiagnosis. It also must be considered that the presence of a bleeding disorder or other medical condition does not rule out abuse as the etiology for bruising or bleeding.[6]

Other symptoms, such as hematemesis,[7] hematochezia,[8] and oronasal bleeding, can be caused by abuse or a bleeding disorder.[9–13] The relative frequencies of abuse or coagulopathies presenting with these symptoms should be considered, along with the patient's history and any other medical findings, such as fractures, neglect, and other manifestations of bleeding/ bruising, before ordering laboratory tests. An increasing number of findings unrelated to bleeding disorders and consistent with abuse decrease the overall likelihood of

a coagulopathy or other medical condition contributing to or causing bleeding or bruising. However, it is prudent to evaluate for bleeding disorders or other medical causes in children who have presenting symptoms that are not typical of inflicted injury.

ICH

Multiple studies have assessed the roles of history,[14] clinical and radiographic findings,[15–22] and outcomes[18,21,23,24] in making the diagnosis of abusive head trauma. In a recent study of ICH in bleeding disorders, ICH was the presenting event in 19.2%.[25] However, no studies have addressed how to differentiate whether patients who present with ICH in the absence of trauma or with a history of minimal trauma have a bleeding disorder either causing or contributing to the clinical findings. No studies have systematically compared the presentation, clinical findings, patterns of ICH, or presence of retinal hemorrhages between bleeding disorders and/or collagen disorders and abusive head trauma. Therefore, for children presenting with ICH but without other findings strongly suggestive of abuse, such as fractures,[26] significant abdominal trauma, burns, or patterned bruising, an evaluation for other medical conditions causing or contributing to the findings is necessary. Additionally, physicians must recognize that although evidence of old inflicted injury, such as healing fractures, could support the diagnosis of abuse, healing injuries may be unrelated to recent bruising or ICH. Physicians must assess their own comfort in making and supporting the diagnosis of abuse in the absence of an extensive laboratory evaluation.

REVIEW OF BLEEDING DISORDERS

This section describes the significant bleeding disorders that may require further evaluation in cases of suspected abuse, including their common presentations, incidence of ICH, and the method of diagnosis (Table 1).

Deficiency of Factor VIII or IX

Hemophilia A and B are attributable to deficiencies of factors VIII and IX, respectively. Factor VIII deficiency occurs in approximately 1 in 5000 live male births. Factor IX deficiency is rarer, occurring in 1 in 20 000 live male births. Because of the X-linked recessive inheritance pattern of these diseases, most patients affected with hemophilia are male. However, girls who are carriers can have low enough factor VIII or IX levels to present with bleeding as a result of homozygous mutations or extreme inactivation of the normal X chromosome. Rarely, a phenotypic female can have only 1 X chromosome and be affected with the disease (ie, testicular feminization, Turner syndrome).[27,28]

Major bleeding sequelae of hemophilia include bleeding into joints and soft tissues and ICH. The most common sites of the initial bleeding episode in one series were post-circumcision and intracranial.[29] ICH in a child with hemophilia can occur as a result of birth trauma, in response to mild head trauma, or spontaneously. ICH is estimated to occur in 5% to 12% of patients with hemophilia throughout their lives.[25,30,31] A review of 57 episodes of ICH in 52 patients with congenital factor deficiencies showed intraparenchymal and/or intraventricular bleeding in 39 patients, subdural in 15, subarachnoid in 2, and cerebellar in 1. Most of these patients (38) had severe hemophilia. The median age of presentation was 8 years (range, 1 month to 22 years). The overall prevalence of ICH in patients with hemophilia in this study was 9.1%.[25] The largest series to date of ICH in hemophilia reported a rate of 2.7% over 5 years in a cohort of 3629 patients with hemophilia, or 0.0054 cases per year. Most of the cases in this series were not the result of trauma (78.4%). Most (69%) occurred in patients with severe hemophilia, and 18% occurred in those with mild hemophilia. Sites of hemorrhage were intracerebral, subdural, subarachnoid, epidural, or unspecified. Trauma was implicated in all of the epidural hemorrhages, 36% of the subarachnoid hemorrhages, 10% of subdural hemorrhages, and 3% of intracerebral hemorrhages.[31] In a recent review of 97 patients with hemophilia who underwent a total of 295 computed tomography scans for head trauma, 9 (3%) were identified as having intracranial bleeding. The mean age of these patients was 3.7 ± 4.1 years. Most of the bleeding in these patients was subdural, although in 2 patients, bleeding was intraparenchymal.[32] A recent study of hemophilia in the first 2 years of life revealed 19.0% of first bleeding episodes ($n = 404$) were head bleeding, of which 36.4% were ICH. Seventy-five percent of the ICH occurred in infants younger than 1 month of age, and most of these were associated with delivery. In contrast to the aforementioned studies, the occurrence of ICH was distributed across all severities of the disease.[29]

Approximately two-thirds of patients who present with a diagnosis of hemophilia have a positive family history for the disease. The one-third of patients without a family history of hemophilia might represent new germ-line mutations.[29,33] Diagnosis of hemophilia requires measuring factor VIII or IX activity level. Hemophilia is categorized as severe if the factor level is <1%, moderate if the factor level is between 1% and 5%, and mild if the factor level is ≥5%. Spontaneous bleeding is more common in severe hemophilia. The activated partial thromboplastin time (aPTT) is prolonged in moderate and severe cases, but can be normal in patients with mild disease, depending on the laboratory's emphasis on detecting mild factor deficiencies. Factor VIII is also an acute phase reactant and can be elevated into the normal range in patients with mild disease in response to trauma or inflammation.[34]

VWD

VWD is the most common heritable bleeding disorder, and typically presents with mild to moderate mucocutaneous bleeding. Low von Willebrand factor (VWF) levels may occur in up to 1% of the population, but fewer people may present with symptoms (0.01% to 0.1%). The current prevalence of VWD can be difficult to ascertain because recent changes in consensus have resulted in more specific diagnostic criteria. The new criteria for diagnosis requires VWF <30% (normal range, 50% to 150%), resulting in fewer people with levels below the normal range meeting diagnostic criteria. Individuals with bleeding symptoms and VWF levels between 30% and 50% create a diagnostic dilemma.[35] In addition, because the bleeding symptoms of VWD are generally mild, there are likely to be patients who have not come to medical attention. On the basis of the number of symptomatic cases seen by hematology specialists, the prevalence has been estimated to be even lower than previously suggested (23 to 110 per million, or 0.0023% to 0.01%), meaning that many individuals with low VWF levels might never manifest bleeding symptoms.[36]

The laboratory evaluation for, and common presentations of, the various types of VWD are variable (Tables 2 and 3). Type 1 VWD is the most common form (approximately 80%) and is characterized by a normally

TABLE 1 Common Testing Strategies for Bleeding Disorders

Condition	Frequency	Inheritance	Screening Tests	Sn and Sp, %	PPV and NPV, %	Confirmatory Test
Factor abnormalities/deficiencies						
VWD type 1	1 per 1000	AD	PFA-100	Sn = 79–96[a] / Sp = 88–96[a]	PPV = 93.3 / NPV = 98.2	VWAg[b], VWF activity, VW multimer analysis, Factor VIII activity
VWD type 2A	Uncommon	AD or AR	PFA-100	Sn = 94–100[a] / Sp = 88–96[a]	PPV = 93.3 / NPV = 98.2	VWAg[b], VWF activity, VW multimer analysis, Factor VIII activity
VWD type 2B	Uncommon	AD	PFA-100	Sn = 93–96[a] / Sp = 88–96[a]	PPV = 93.3 / NPV = 98.2	VWAg[b], VWF activity, VW multimer analysis, Factor VIII activity
VWD type 2M	Uncommon	AD or AR	PFA-100	Sn = 94–97[a] / Sp = 88–96[a]	PPV = 93.3 / NPV = 98.2	VWAg[b], VWF activity, VW multimer analysis, Factor VIII activity
VWD type 2N	Uncommon	AR, or compound heterozygote	aPTT	NA	NA	VWF-Factor VIII binding assay
VWD type 3	1 per 300 000–1 000 000	AR, or compound heterozygote	PFA-100	Sn = 94–100[a] / Sp = 88–96[a]	PPV = 93.3 / NPV = 98.2	VWAg[b], Ristocetin cofactor, VWF multimer analysis, Factor VIII activity
Factor II deficiency (prothrombin)	26 reported cases, estimated 1 per 1–2 million		aPTT, PT (may be normal)	Sn = variable	NA	Factor II activity +/– antigen levels
Factor V deficiency	1 per 1 million	AR	aPTT, PT	Sn = variable	NA	Factor V activity
Combined factor V/factor VIII deficiency	1 per 1 million	AR	aPTT>PT	Sn = variable	NA	Factor V and factor VIII activities
Factor VII deficiency	1 per 300 000–500 000	AR	PT	Sn = variable	NA	Factor VII activity
Factor VIII deficiency	1 per 5000 male births	X-linked	aPTT	Sn = variable	NA	Factor VIII activity
Factor IX deficiency	1 per 20 000 male births	X-linked	aPTT	Sn = variable	NA	Factor IX activity
Factor X deficiency	1 per 1 million	AR	aPTT, PT, RVV	Sn = variable	NA	Factor X activity
Factor XI deficiency	1 per 100 000	AR	aPTT	Sn = variable	NA	Factor XI activity
Factor XIII deficiency	1 per 2–5 million	AR	Clot solubility	Sn = variable	NA	Factor XIII activity
Fibrinolytic defects						
AP deficiency	~40 reported cases	AR	Euglobin lysis test	Sn = variable	NA	AP activity
PAI-1 deficiency	Very rare	AR		Sn = variable	NA	PAI-1 antigen and activity
Defects of fibrinogen						
Afibrinogenemia	1 per 500 000	AR	PT, aPTT	Sn = high	NA	Fibrinogen level
Hypofibrinogenemia	Less than afibrinogenemia		PT, aPTT	Sn = variable	NA	Thrombin time, fibrinogen activity
Dysfibrinogenemia	1 per million		Thrombin time, fibrinogen level	Sn = variable	NA	Thrombin time, fibrinogen antigen and activity level comparison, reptilase time
Platelet disorders						
ITP	Age-related	NA	CBC	Sn = high	NA	Antiplatelet Ab (rarely needed)

TABLE 1 Continued

Condition	Frequency	Inheritance	Screening Tests	Sn and Sp, %	PPV and NPV, %	Confirmatory Test
GT	Very rare	AR	PFA-100	Sn = 97–100	NA	Platelet aggregation testing Flow cytometry
BSS	Rare	AR	PFA-100	Sn = 100	NA	Platelet aggregation testing Flow cytometry
Platelet release/storage disorders	Unknown, more common than other platelet function disorders	variable	PFA-100	Sn = 27–50	NA	Platelet aggregation and secretion Electron microscopy Molecular and cytogenetic testing

AD, autosomal dominant; AR, autosomal recessive; CBC, complete blood cell (count); NA, not available or not applicable; NPV, negative predictive value; PPV, positive predictive value; RVV, Russell viper venom (test); Sn, sensitivity; Sp, specificity; VW, von Willebrand; Ab, antibody.

a Values derived from data before 2008 National Institutes of Health Consensus guidelines. Sn and Sp using current diagnostic cutoffs unknown but would be expected to have higher Sp with lower Sn.

b May be reasonable to proceed directly to diagnostic testing depending on availability. See accompanying technical report for detailed discussion.[25]

functioning but decreased von Willebrand antigen (VWAg), resulting in low levels of both VWAg and VWF activity. Type 1 VWD has a wide range of bleeding severity and variable penetration among members of the same family. Type 2 VWD subtypes are characterized by abnormally functioning von Willebrand molecules and variable bleeding severity. Type 3 VWD presents with absence of VWF and a very low but detectable factor VIII level. The bleeding in type 3 VWD can be quite severe and can also include hemarthroses resulting from low factor VIII levels (Table 3).[35]

ICH has very rarely been reported in association with VWD. A single case series detailed 4 episodes of ICH thought to have occurred spontaneously in patients with no previous history of VWD. Patient ages ranged from 18 to 65 years of age.[37] There was an additional report of ICH in a newborn child with type 3 VWD and simultaneous sinovenous thrombosis.[38] One case report implicated type 1 VWD as a possible cause of subdural hematoma and retinal hemorrhages[39]; however, the laboratory findings in that case report did not meet the diagnostic criteria for definitive VWD,[40] and child abuse was not completely investigated, because no repeat skeletal survey was performed. Large mass-effect ICH associated with minor trauma in children with VWD outside of the typical age range for abusive head injury has been reported.[41,42] The extreme rarity of this presentation and the questions surrounding the validity of VWD causing ICH in some cases, indicate that VWD is not a typical cause of ICH.

The platelet function analyzer (PFA-100 [Siemens Healthcare Diagnostics, Tarrytown, NY]) has been proposed as a screening test for VWD, and results are often abnormal in patients who are known to have the disorder and have VWF levels <30%. It is superior to the bleeding time because of ease of testing but does not test for blood vessel integrity and is affected by medications, platelet count, and hematocrit. The bleeding time is not recommended for bleeding disorder screening because of poor test characteristics and the invasive nature of the test.[43] The utility of the PFA-100 as a screening tool for VWD has not been established with population studies. It can be a useful tool as a preliminary screen for VWD or a platelet function defect, but if the result is normal and clinical suspicion remains high, other specific testing for these disorders should be obtained. Abnormal results of the PFA-100 test should also prompt further testing as well.[35,40,44,45] It is important to realize that the PFA-100 is not a diagnostic test for bleeding disorders but rather acts as a quick screen in situations in which more specific testing is unavailable or will be delayed. If access to specific testing is available, it might be rational to skip the PFA-100. Specific testing consists of VWAg, VW activity (also referred to as ristocetin cofactor by some laboratories), factor VIII activity, and often, von Willebrand multimer analysis. Some practitioners also include ristocetin-induced platelet agglutination and/or a collagen-binding assay. Contributing to the difficulty of diagnosis, particularly for type 1 VWD, VWF levels increase in response to stress, pregnancy, and inflammation and exhibit significant variability within an individual. In addition, some patients' test results will fall below the lower limits of normal but above the current upper diagnostic cutoff (31% to 50%), creating a diagnostic dilemma.[35] Because of these issues and the lack of a single diagnostic test, the diagnosis of VWD might require repeated testing and is best accomplished by a pediatric hematologist.

TABLE 2 VWD Variants

Test	Type 1	Type 2A	Type 2B	PT-VWD	Type 2N	Type 2M	Type 3
VWF:Ag	Low	Low	Low	Low	Low	Low	Absent
VWF:Act	Low	VWF:Act/VWF:Ag <0.5	Low	Low	Low	VWF:Act/VWF:Ag <0.5	Absent
FVIII	Low	NI	NI	NI	Low	NI	Absent
RIPA	NI	Low	NI	NI	NI	Low	Absent
RIPA-LD	Absent	Absent	Increased	Increased	Absent	Absent	Absent
Frequency	70%–80%	10%–12%	3%–5%	0%–1%	1%–2%	1%–2%	1%–3%
Multimers	NI	Small	Small	Small	NI	NI	Absent

FVIII, factor VIII activity; NI, normal; PT-VWD, platelet-type pseudo VWD; RIPA, ristocetin-induced platelet aggregation; RIPA-LD, low-dose ristocetin-induced platelet aggregation; VWF:Act, VWF activity; VWF:Ag, VWF antigen. Reprinted with permission from Nichols WL, Hultin MB, James AH, et al. von Willebrand disease (VWD): evidence-based diagnosis and management guidelines, the National Heart, Lung, and Blood Institute (NHLBI) Expert Panel Reports (USA). *Haemophilia.* 2008;14(2):191.

TABLE 3 Common Bleeding Symptoms of Healthy Individuals and Patients With VWD

Symptoms	Healthy Individuals (n = 500; n = 341; n = 88; n = 60), %	All Types of VWD (n = 264; n = 1885),%	Type 1 VWD (n = 42; n = 671), %	Type 2 VWD (n = 497), %	Type 3 VWD (n = 66; n = 385), %
Epistaxis	4.6–22.7	38.1–62.5	53–61	63	66–77
Menorrhagia	23.0–68.4	47–60	32	32	56–69
Bleeding after dental extraction	4.8–41.9	28.6–51.5	17–31	39	53–70
Ecchymoses	11.8–50.0	49.2–50.4	50	NR	NR
Bleeding from minor cuts and abrasions	0.2–33.3	36	36	40	50
Gingival bleeding	7.4–47.1	26.1–34.8	29–31	35	56
Postoperative bleeding	1.4–28.2	19.5–28	20–47	23	41
Hemarthrosis	0–14.9	6.3–8.3	2–3	4	37–45
Gastrointestinal tract bleeding	0.6–27.7	14	5	8	20

NR, not reported. Reprinted with permission from Nichols WL, Hultin MB, James AH, et al. von Willebrand disease (VWD): evidence-based diagnosis and management guidelines, the National Heart, Lung, and Blood Institute (NHLBI) Expert Panel Reports (USA). *Haemophilia.* 2008;14(2):186.

Acquired von Willebrand syndrome is a rare phenomenon in pediatrics that can be associated with a number of clinical disorders, such as vascular anomalies, Wilms tumor and other cancers, cardiovascular lesions, hypothyroidism, lymphoproliferative or myeloproliferative disorders, storage disorders, autoimmune illnesses, monoclonal gammopathies, and certain medications. It has been estimated to occur at a prevalence of 0.04% to 0.13% in the general population, although the rate in pediatrics may be lower.[46] It is usually caused by autoimmune clearance or inhibition of VWF, increased shear stress causing consumption of VWF, or adsorption of VWF to cell surfaces. Laboratory tests used to diagnose acquired VWD are the same as those used to diagnose the congenital disorder. The addition of the von Willebrand propeptide can help to distinguish between the 2 entities.[46]

Factor VII Deficiency

Factor VII deficiency is the only plasma coagulation factor deficiency in which the prothrombin time (PT) alone is prolonged. The incidence is estimated as 1 in 300 000 to 1 in 500 000. To date, more than 150 cases have been reported. A quantitative factor VII determination by standard factor assay methods provides a definitive diagnosis. Homozygous patients usually have less than 10 U/dL of factor VII. Heterozygous patients have factor VII levels between 40 and 60 U/dL and might represent single or double heterozygous abnormalities. It is very important to use age and gestational-related normal ranges, because factor VII is naturally low at birth.[47]

ICH has been reported in 4.0% to 6.5% of patients with factor VII deficiency and usually occurs in those with severe disease (<1% factor activity), both spontaneously and as a result of

trauma.[48,49] Central nervous system (CNS) bleeding was reported in 4.4% of factor VII–deficient patients as a presenting symptom in 1 registry and was found to occur in subjects younger than 6 months.[49] Bleeding symptoms can be extremely variable, and individuals can have minimal bleeding despite very low levels of factor VII. Using the most recent severity grading system, all patients with CNS bleeding have severe disease by definition.[50] Intracranial bleeding in these patients has been recorded as intraparenchymal, intraventricular, subdural, and tentorial, often accompanied with overlying cephalohematoma and usually occurring soon after birth.[48,51,52]

It is also important to rule out acquired factor VII deficiency as a result of vitamin K deficiency, liver disease, or consumptive coagulopathy. Although in these conditions, one would expect more extensive coagulopathy, prolongation of the PT is often the only finding in the early stages of these disorders because of the short half-life of factor VII.

Factor XI Deficiency

Factor XI deficiency (also termed hemophilia C) has an estimated frequency in the general population of 1 in 100 000.[53,54] Factor XI deficiency occurs more frequently in the Ashkenazi Jewish population; approximately 0.2% of Ashkenazi Jewish people are homozygous and 11.0% are heterozygous for this disorder.[55]

Bleeding in factor XI deficiency tends to be mild and associated with trauma or surgery. Bleeding symptoms often cannot be predicted by the factor level. Serious spontaneous hemorrhage is uncommon, even in individuals with very low factor levels.[56] There was 1 report of subarachnoid hemorrhage in a 53-year-old man with previously undiagnosed factor XI deficiency. This patient was also found to have cerebral aneurysms.[57]

Laboratory screening tests reveal a prolonged aPTT and normal PT, though the aPTT can be normal in heterozygous patients with mild deficiency. Other screening test results are normal. The specific assay for factor XI is the definitive test for this deficiency. In homozygous individuals, factor XI activity ranges from <1 U/dL up to 10 U/dL. Severe deficiency is defined as <15 U/dL.[58] It is important to compare results with age-matched norms, because healthy ranges in infants are lower than those in adults.[59]

Factor XIII Deficiency

Factor XIII acts to covalently cross-link and stabilize fibrin. Because the PT and aPTT measure the production of fibrin from fibrinogen and the action of factor XIII is subsequent to the formation of fibrin, these tests are normal in factor XIII deficiency and therefore cannot be used to screen for this disorder. The clot solubility test, which is the most commonly used test to screen for factor XIII deficiency, is abnormal only in very severe deficiencies of factor XIII, typically with factor XIII activities <3% of normal. This is the level most experts believe is necessary to cause spontaneous bleeding. A quantitative test for factor XIII exists.[60,61]

Deficiency of factor XIII is rare, occurring in only approximately 1 in 2 to 5 million people. However, intracranial bleeding is a common manifestation of this disorder, occurring in up to one-third of those with the deficiency.[60,62] Bleeding has been reported in subdural, intraparenchymal, and epidural locations, although because most registries and case reports have not specified the location of ICH, it is likely that it has occurred in more disparate sites. ICH has been reported to occur occasionally in patients with factor levels >3%, and therefore, the diagnosis can be missed if only the clot solubility test is used.[63–65] Other manifestations of factor XIII deficiency are umbilical cord bleeding, muscle hematomas, and postoperative bleeding.[62]

Other Factor Deficiencies (Factors II, V, Combined V and VIII, and X)

Prothrombin (Factor II) Deficiency

Homozygous prothrombin deficiency occurs at an estimated prevalence of 1 in 1 to 2 million. The most common bleeding presentation in homozygous and heterozygous patients is bleeding involving the skin and mucous membranes. In the North American Rare Bleeding Disorders Registry (NARBDR), 11% of the subjects with factor II deficiency suffered a CNS complication (which included both ICH and ischemic stroke). In subjects with factor II levels <0.01 U/mL, the rate of ICH was 20%.[66]

Little description of these hemorrhages exists, although case reports have described subdural and epidural hematomas.[67–69] Homozygous patients can also present with surgical or trauma-induced bleeding.[70] Hemarthroses occurred in 42%, and gastrointestinal bleeding in 12% of homozygous subjects in one registry.[71] Acquired prothrombin deficiency can occur with vitamin K deficiency, liver disease, warfarin therapy, or overdose or in the setting of connective tissue disorders with accompanying lupus anticoagulant.[70]

The degree to which the PT and aPTT are prolonged varies from patient to patient, from a few seconds in some patients to more than 60 seconds in others, and occasionally, these screening results can be in the normal range.[47,71] The diagnosis is established with a factor assay for functional prothrombin (FII), along with immunologic tests for antigen levels if necessary.

Factor V Deficiency

Factor V deficiency is estimated to occur in 1 in 1 million people. Both homozygous and heterozygous patients with factor V deficiency typically have bleeding symptoms. Bleeding in homozygous patients tends to be spontaneous and occurs in the skin and mucous membranes, joints and muscles, genitourinary tract, gastrointestinal tract, and CNS. In the NARBDR, 8% of homozygous patients presented with intracranial bleeding.[66] Intrauterine subdural hematomas have been reported, as have spontaneous intraparenchymal hemorrhages.[72,73] Fifty-percent of heterozygous patients also had bleeding. Skin and mucous membrane bleeding were the most common manifestations, and none experienced ICH.[66]

Factor V can also be low in some platelet disorders, because it is also present in platelet α granules. In addition, acquired factor V deficiency can occur in patients with rheumatologic disorders or malignancies, patients using antimicrobial agents, or patients using topical bovine thrombin because of antibodies to factor V.[74]

In factor V deficiency, the PT and aPTT are both prolonged. Abnormal bleeding time or positive PFA-100 result is reported in approximately one-third of patients, perhaps related to a deficiency of factor V in platelet α granules.[53] Other screening test results are normal. Definitive diagnosis requires a factor V assay.

Combined Factor V and Factor VIII Deficiency

Combined deficiency of factor V and factor VIII is rare, occurring in 1 in 1 million people, with higher frequency in populations in which consanguinity is more common. In this syndrome, factor V and factor VIII levels (both antigen and activity) range from 5% to 30% of normal.[47,75] Bleeding is usually mild to moderate. Patients typically have easy bruising, epistaxis, and gum bleeding, as well as bleeding after trauma or surgery. Menorrhagia and postpartum bleeding in affected women have also been reported. Hemarthrosis can also occur. Intracranial bleeding is rare but has been reported in 1 patient of 46 reported in the 2 largest registries of this disorder (27 and 19 subjects, respectively).[76,77]

Combined deficiency of factor V and factor VIII is passed down in an autosomal-recessive fashion and is attributable to a mutation of a protein of the endoplasmic reticulum–Golgi intermediate compartment (ERGIC 53) encoded by the *LMAN1* gene. This protein has been shown to be important in facilitating protein transport from the endoplasmic reticulum to the Golgi apparatus. The decrease in factors V and VIII is, thus, attributable to defective intracellular transport and secretion unique to these 2 coagulation factors.[47] The PT and aPTT are prolonged in this disorder, with the prolongation of aPTT out of proportion to that of the PT.

Factor X Deficiency

The prevalence of factor X deficiency is 1 in 1 million in the general population and more common in populations with higher rates of consanguinity.[47] It is passed down in an autosomal-recessive pattern. As many as 1 in 500 people might be carriers of the disorder.[78] More severe deficiency would be expected to present earlier in life. Heterozygous cases might be identified incidentally by laboratory tests performed preoperatively or for another purpose.[79]

In the NARBDR, most bleeding symptoms in factor X deficiency were mucocutaneous, including easy bruising, followed by musculoskeletal bleeding. Intracranial bleeding occurred in 15% of the homozygous cohort, of which 54% had a factor X level <0.01 U/ mL. This cohort had the highest rate of ICH in the study, compared with other rare bleeding disorders. No heterozygous subjects experienced ICH.[66] Severely affected patients also present in the neonatal period with bleeding at circumcision, umbilical stump bleeding, or gastrointestinal hemorrhage.[78] The Greifswald factor X deficiency registry, which enrolls patients from Europe and Latin America, showed ICH in 21% of its cohort. ICH was reported only in patients who were homozygous and compound heterozygous.[80]

Severe liver disease can result in deficiency of all liver-produced factors, including factor X. Acquired factor X deficiency can also occur with amyloidosis, cancer, myeloma, infection, and use of sodium valproate. Acquired inhibitors to factor X have also been reported in association with upper respiratory infections and burns and usually present with active bleeding from multiple body sites.[78,80] Because of the frequency of the associated diseases, acquired factor X deficiency is actually fairly common. Although the overall rate is unknown, this disorder has been reported in up to 5% of patients with amyloidosis.[78] Therefore, diagnosis of inherited factor X deficiency in the face of concomitant medical diagnoses should be made carefully and ideally with the assistance of a pediatric hematologist.

Both the PT and aPTT are usually prolonged and correct with a 1:1 mix with normal plasma; however, with 2 types of mutations, the PT is prolonged and the aPTT is normal, whereas the opposite is true in another variant.[81] The Russell viper venom test is usually prolonged, although it can be normal in some variants.[53] A factor X assay is the definitive test, although it is important to compare results with normal levels for age and exclude vitamin K deficiency before confirming the diagnosis.

Vitamin K Deficiency

Vitamin K is required to complete the posttranslational alteration of factors II, VII, IX, and X and proteins C and S. In the absence of vitamin K, precursor proteins are synthesized by hepatic cells, but because γ-carboxyglutamic acid residues are absent, the calcium-binding sites are nonfunctional. Deficiency of vitamin K results in induced functional deficiencies of all of these proteins. If the level of functional proteins falls below 30 U/dL, bleeding symptoms can result, and the PT and/ or the aPTT will be prolonged.[82]

Vitamin K deficiency bleeding (VKDB) is most often seen in newborn infants in the first days of life (in infants who do not receive vitamin K at birth). Because their livers are still immature, synthesis of the vitamin K–dependent factors in newborn infants is 30% to 50% of adult levels. Almost all neonates are vitamin K deficient as a result of poor placental transmission of maternal vitamin K and the lack of colonization of the colon by vitamin K–producing bacteria in the neonate, although not all infants will go on to have VKDB without prophylaxis.

VKDB is divided into 3 subtypes: early, classic, and late. Early VKDB occurs primarily in infants of mothers who have been on a vitamin K–blocking medication, such as anticonvulsants, and usually occurs within hours to the first week of life. Classic-onset VKDB occurs between the first week and first month of life and is largely prevented by prophylactic vitamin K administration at birth. Late VKDB occurs from the first month to 3 months after birth.[83] This deficiency is more prevalent in breastfed babies, because human milk contains less vitamin K than does cow milk. It can be precipitated by acquired or inherited gastrointestinal tract disease. Infants with liver disease might also be susceptible.

Manifestations of VKDB are bleeding in the skin or from mucosal surfaces, bleeding from circumcision, generalized ecchymoses, large intramuscular hemorrhages, and ICH. Although VKDB is rare in countries that provide prophylaxis, more than 50% of infants with late VKDB will present with ICH.[82] VKDB is prevented in the United States by encouraging administration of vitamin K to all newborn infants. Although most states have laws that require administration, some do not. Administration of oral vitamin K prophylaxis reduces the incidence of late VKDB from 4.4 to 10.5/100 000 live births to 1.5 to 6.4/100 000 live births.[83] Intramuscular vitamin K prophylaxis

prevents almost all cases of late VKDB; however, these can still occur, particularly if there is an unrecognized underlying cause of vitamin K deficiency. Secondary VKDB can occur in the setting of hepatobiliary disease, antimicrobial therapy, coumarol poisoning/rat poison ingestion, biliary atresia, and chronic diarrhea. ICH in this setting is rare but does occur.[84]

Diagnosis of VKDB is the same regardless of underlying cause. Laboratory tests show prolonged PT and possibly aPTT for age. Specific factor assays for factors II, VII, IX, and X are markedly decreased. In patients who have already received vitamin K as treatment or transfusion of plasma, measurement of proteins induced by vitamin K absence can confirm the diagnosis.[82,84]

Inherited combined deficiencies of vitamin K–dependent proteins occur when there is a mutation in the γ-glutamyl carboxylase gene or the vitamin K epoxide reductase complex. Fewer than 30 cases have been reported. Bleeding symptoms range from mild to severe, and ICH has been reported. Some patients also have dysmorphic features or skeletal defects.[85]

Defects of Fibrinogen

Abnormalities of fibrinogen can result in complete lack of the protein (afibrinogenemia), decreased levels (hypofibrinogenemia), or an abnormally functioning molecule (dysfibrinogenemia). Clinical presentations range from mild to severe bleeding, and some patients have an increased risk of thrombosis as well, depending on the causative mutation.[86,87] Fibrinogen deficiencies can also be acquired in other medical disorders, such as liver disease or consumptive coagulopathy.[87]

Severe disorders of fibrinogen result in prolongation of PT and aPTT, but

milder disorders might be missed by these screening tests. Thrombin time tests conversion of fibrinogen to fibrin and is more sensitive to both deficiencies and abnormalities of fibrinogen than are PT and aPTT. Reptilase time is similar to thrombin time, except that it is not affected by heparin and might help distinguish hypofibrinogenemia from dysfibrinogenemia because of its slightly different mechanism of action. One can also measure the amount of fibrinogen antigen through a variety of methods.[87]

Most patients with dysfibrinogenemia are asymptomatic. Bleeding, when it is present, is typically mild and triggered by surgery or trauma, and thrombosis can occur. The presence of a bleeding or thrombotic phenotype is dependent on the underlying mutation.[88] One case report of ICH and cephalhematomas in a child with suspected dysfibrinogenemia has been published. The case in that report was unique in that the patient had a long history of bleeding and almost undetectable fibrinogen levels. In addition, the patient appeared to inherit his disease in a double heterozygous-recessive manner from consanguineous parents, in contrast to most cases, which are autosomal dominant in nature.[89]

Overall, bleeding symptoms in afibrinogenemia are variable and can range from mild to life threatening. ICH has been reported in patients with afibrinogenemia (5% to 10% of patients).[90,91] Up to 85% of patients present in the neonatal period with umbilical cord bleeding.[92]

Defects of Fibrinolysis

Fibrinolysis refers to the breakdown of the fibrin clot and is directed by plasmin. Plasmin is generated from plasminogen by the actions of plasminogen activators. The inhibitors of this action are α-2 antiplasmin (AP, also known as α-2 plasmin inhibitor and plasmin inhibitor), thrombin-activatable fibrinolysis inhibitor, and plasminogen activator inhibitor type 1 (PAI-1). Deficiencies in AP and PAI-1 have been described, although both are rare.[93,94]

Patients with PAI-1 deficiency have been described as having mild to moderate bleeding symptoms, such as epistaxis, menorrhagia, and delayed bleeding after surgery or trauma. Spontaneous bleeding is rare. Diagnosis of PAI-1 deficiency can be problematic in that the laboratory assay used for diagnosis is inaccurate at low levels. Normal ranges often are reported beginning at 0, creating a large crossover between those patients with an abnormality in PAI-1 and healthy individuals. Only 2 of the reported deficiencies of PAI-1 have been correlated with an underlying genetic defect.[94] In 1 large kindred in whom a null mutation was identified, ICH and bleeding into joints were reported after mild trauma.[95] ICH has been reported in 2 adults in whom the only underlying coagulation abnormality identified was a low PAI-1 level. One adult also had osteogenesis imperfecta (OI).[96,97]

There have been approximately 40 cases of AP deficiency reported in the literature. AP deficiency is inherited in an autosomal-recessive pattern, although heterozygous patients can also present with bleeding. Acquired deficiency has also been reported in patients with liver disease, disseminated intravascular coagulation, and acute promyelocytic leukemia. Homozygous patients tend to have severe bleeding similar to that seen in factor XIII deficiency, although ICH has not been reported. Heterozygous patients can have bleeding in response to trauma, surgery, or dental procedures or can be asymptomatic.[93,98] Intramedullary hematomas of long bones, which can occur without a history of trauma, are an unusual feature of homozygous AP deficiency.[99,100] Similar lesions have been seen in patients with afibrinogenemia. A shortened euglobulin lysis time can be used as a screening test for AP deficiency. Definitive diagnosis requires measurement of AP antigen and activity.[101]

Congenital Platelet Abnormalities

Platelets interact with VWF to adhere to sites of vessel wall injury. Subsequent activation and aggregation of platelets, which includes the release of granular contents, leads to formation of a platelet plug. Congenital platelet disorders can result in fewer platelets, abnormal function of platelets, or a combination of the two. There is a wide range in the presenting symptoms of these disorders, from mild mucocutaneous bleeding to severe life-threatening hemorrhage.[102]

The most severe and best-characterized platelet function disorders are also the rarest. These are the autosomal recessive disorders Bernard-Soulier syndrome (BSS) and Glanzmann thrombasthenia (GT). BSS results from absence or abnormal function of the GP Ib-IX-V receptor, which is responsible for platelet adhesion to VWF. Patients with BSS also commonly have mild thrombocytopenia with enlarged platelet size. In GT, the $\alpha IIb\beta 3$ platelet integrin is abnormal or missing, leading to impaired platelet aggregation, but the platelet count is normal. In both of these disorders, significant mucocutaneous bleeding and ICH have been reported, although ICH is rare, occurring in only 0.3% to 2.0% of patients with GT and even less in those with BSS.[103,104] The PFA-100 is a fairly reliable screening mechanism for these diagnoses (Table 1).[102,103]

Less well characterized but more common, the disorders of platelet signaling and secretion result from a variety of defects. Platelet activation leads to a conformational change in the platelet and normally results in secretion of platelet granule contents, which recruits other platelets to the site of injury. Without this response, platelets are unable to recruit other platelets. This group of disorders includes Quebec platelet disorder, the MYH9-related disorders, Scott syndrome, Hermansky-Pudlak syndrome, Chediak-Higashi syndrome, and Wiskott-Aldrich syndrome. Most bleeding with these disorders is mild and manifests as excessive bruising or menorrhagia. The PFA-100 does not reliably screen for these disorders.[105] More specific platelet aggregation and secretion testing is required, and occasionally, electron microscopic examination or genetic mutation testing is necessary to confirm the diagnosis.[102] All forms of genetic inheritance have been reported. Most patients with these disorders present with mucocutaneous bleeding manifestations or bleeding after surgery or trauma. Bleeding symptoms are variable and dependent on the specific defect. Joint bleeding can occur in some disorders. ICH has been reported after childbirth in neonates and trauma in older individuals. Some platelet function disorders are part of syndromes with associated physical findings. Individual review of these entities is outside of the scope of this report.[106,107] Of note, a variety of medications can lead to platelet dysfunction (eg, nonsteroidal antiinflammatory drugs, sodium valproate); therefore, a careful medication history should be obtained before diagnosing a congenital platelet abnormality.[108] Acquired thrombocytopenia, whether from medication, immune thrombocytopenia (ITP), maternal ITP, or neonatal alloimmune thrombocytopenia, should be readily diagnosed on the basis of a complete blood cell count. The rate of ICH in patients with idiopathic ITP is <1%.[109]

Vascular Disorders

Certain vascular disorders can present with bruising or bleeding. Two disorders that might be confused for abuse are outlined. Discussion of all vascular disorders is outside of the scope of this report but can be found elsewhere.[110]

Ehlers-Danlos

Ehlers-Danlos syndrome (EDS) consists of a group of genetically and clinically heterogeneous connective tissue diseases that might be mistaken for child abuse.[111,112] The exact prevalence of EDS is unknown but is estimated to be 1 in 5000.[113] There are 6 genetic subtypes, which differ in the underlying biochemical defect, inheritance pattern, and clinical symptoms[114]; however, prominent bruising and bleeding are seen in all subtypes.[115] Mutations in collagen type I, type III, type V, or the genes involved in processing type I collagen result in most EDS subtypes. The tendency to bleed and/or bruise in EDS is caused by an abnormal capillary structure with deficiency of normal perivascular collagen. Cutaneous blood vessels are poorly supported and can rupture when subject to shearing forces. Tests for bleeding disorders are generally normal, except for the Hess test, which can be abnormal, indicating capillary fragility.[115] Clinically, the disorder manifests itself with easy bruising, bleeding gums, prolonged bleeding after surgical procedures, and menorrhagia. When evaluating children with possible abusive findings, pediatricians should assess for the typical signs of EDS. Skin hyperextensibility describes skin that extends easily and snaps back after release and is best tested at the volar surface of the forearm.[115] Widened, thin scarring often occurs at knees, shins, elbows, and the forehead.[115] Joint hypermobility is also often seen.

The vascular type of EDS, also known as EDS type IV, particularly might be confused with child abuse.[111] The precise prevalence is not known but has been estimated to be 1 in 250 000.[116,117] Both autosomal-recessive and -dominant inheritance patterns, as well as sporadic mutations, have been described.[118] The clinical diagnosis is made on the basis of 4 criteria: easy bruising; skin with visible veins; characteristic facial features; and rupture of arteries, uterus, or intestines.[114] The diagnosis is confirmed by the demonstration that cultured fibroblasts synthesize abnormal type III procollagen molecules or by the identification of a mutation in the gene for type III procollagen (COL3A1).[119] Excessive bruising is the most common presentation, but other severe complications, such as spontaneous rupture of the bowel and hemorrhagic pneumothorax, can occur. Vascular ruptures, including renal or splenic arteries, aneurysmal rupture, or stroke can also occur. ICH, including subdural hemorrhage, has only very rarely been described, and findings would likely not be confused with those commonly seen in inflicted head injury.[118,120] Severe complications are rare in childhood.[116] Joint hypermobility is often limited to the small joints of the hands. Skin hypermobility is typically not present, but the skin is often translucent, showing a visible venous pattern.[121,122] The characteristic facial appearance includes prominent eyes, pinched nose, small lips, hollow cheeks, and lobeless ears.[117,121]

If clinical suspicion exists, the diagnosis of most subtypes of EDS can be evaluated with biochemical and molecular analysis. Cultured skin fibroblasts can be used for gel electrophoresis of collagen types I, III, and V. For the vascular subtype (EDS type IV), biochemical analysis of type III procollagen identifies more than 95% of patients, whereas molecular screening of the COL3A1 gene identifies up to 99% of mutations.[117,119]

OI

OI is a heterogeneous group of diseases characterized by bone fragility, dentinogenesis imperfecta, and adult hearing loss.[123] OI has been associated with easy bruising and ICH after minimal or no trauma.[124,125] Bleeding diathesis in OI is thought to occur as a result of platelet dysfunction and capillary fragility.[126,127]

Inheritance is generally autosomal-dominant, but autosomal-recessive inheritance and new mutations are known to occur. Most cases are the result of mutations in COL1A1 and COL1A2. At least 8 types of OI are known to exist, and the prevalence is approximated at 1 in 15 000 to 1 in 20 000.[128,129]

Testing for OI by using DNA sequencing or collagen analysis is available. Sensitivities and specificities vary depending on the type of OI, but approximately 90% of individuals with OI types I, II, III, and IV (but none with OI types V, VI, VII, or VIII) have an identifiable mutation in either COL1A1 or COL1A2.[125] Rare case reports have attributed multiple varieties of ICH, including subdural hematomas in children, to OI.[130–134] Additionally, 3 cases of relatively minor retinal hemorrhages coupled with subdural hematomas have been reported after trivial trauma in patients with OI type 1.[124] Despite these case reports, OI is a rare condition, and the occurrence of subdural hematomas and/or retinal hemorrhages attributable to OI is exceedingly rare.

Despite the reported associations of OI with easy bruising, no large-scale studies have characterized the frequency and nature of bruising in children with OI or compared these patterns to nonabused children without OI or abused children. In children with bruises only, in the absence of other clinical indicators of OI, such as short stature, blue sclera, wormian or demineralized bones, or family history, it is generally not necessary to rule out OI via collagen or DNA testing.

Unsupported Hypotheses

Many alternative hypotheses have been proposed to explain bruising or bleeding concerning for abuse that are not supported by scientific evidence. It is outside of the scope of this report to discuss all hypotheses of this nature. Two of the more common are intracranial findings concerning for abuse caused by the effects of vaccines or by intracranial thrombosis.

Vaccines Mimicking Abusive Head Trauma

Some have proposed that vaccines cause findings that might be confused with abusive head trauma.[135–137] The hypothesized mechanism is a combination of ascorbate (vitamin C) depletion and foreign protein in vaccines causing a high histamine level, which then leads to capillary fragility and venous bleeding. No scientific evidence exists to support the hypothesis that immunizations cause findings that might be confused with inflicted trauma.

Intracranial Venous Thrombosis Mimicking Abusive Head Trauma

The incidence of intracranial venous thrombosis in children is estimated to be 0.67 cases per 100 000 children per year.[138] Of these, approximately 28% involve hemorrhagic venous infarction; thus, the incidence of hemorrhagic venous infarction is 0.19 cases per 100 000 children per year.[138] Common congenital associations include factor V Leiden, prothrombin gene mutation, protein C or S

deficiency, and antithrombin deficiency. Other causes include infections (eg, otitis media, mastoiditis, sinusitis), dehydration, and trauma. Affected infants typically present with seizures and diffuse neurologic signs.[138] No studies have systematically compared characteristics of ICH resulting from intracranial thrombosis with characteristics of ICH resulting from trauma. A single study evaluating nontraumatic intracranial venous thrombosis detected no subdural hematoma in the study population (n = 36).[139] Additionally, bleeding from intracranial thrombosis has a typical appearance on magnetic resonance imaging, including localized bleeding near the thrombus, typically in an intraparenchymal distribution. This appearance is in contrast to the typical presenting features of deceleration head trauma, including thin-film subdural hemorrhages involving the interhemispheric region and the cerebral convexities.[22] If there is concern for intracranial thrombosis, magnetic resonance venography is the test of choice. Given the significant difference in appearance of ICH as a result of intracranial venous thrombosis in comparison with ICH from deceleration trauma, confusion between the 2 conditions should not exist.

INTERPRETATION OF TESTS

It should be noted that aPTT can be falsely prolonged in certain conditions, such as in the presence of a lupus anticoagulant, or can be prolonged and not indicate a true bleeding disorder, such as in factor XII deficiency or other contact factor deficiencies. In addition, patients who suffer a traumatic brain injury often have a transient coagulopathy that does not reflect an underlying congenital disorder.[140,141] It should also be noted that coagulation tests are very sensitive to specimen handling and should be performed in

laboratories experienced with these assays. Inappropriate handling commonly leads to false-positive results.

Patients who have sustained significant trauma also might receive transfusions of blood products. Fresh-frozen plasma (FFP) is prepared by separating the liquid portion of blood from the cellular portion after the collection of whole blood or by collecting the liquid portion of blood by using apheresis technique. By definition, each milliliter of FFP contains 1 unit of all normal coagulation factors and inhibitors of coagulation, but in general, 10 to 20 mL/kg will raise factor levels only by 15% to 25%.[142]

Cryoprecipitate is prepared by thawing FFP and refreezing the precipitate. It contains high concentrations of fibrinogen, factor VIII, VWF, and factor XIII. Each coagulation factor has a different half-life (Table 4). Therefore, the administration of FFP or cryoprecipitate will affect the investigation for a coagulation factor deficiency differently depending on the factor being measured.

FREQUENCY OF THE CONDITION AND MEDICAL PROBABILITY

Specific data regarding the prevalence of bleeding disorders within the population of children with ICH or subdural hemorrhage are not available; however, there are data on the frequency of ICH as a result of specific bleeding disorders. If the prevalence of a condition and the frequency of a particular presentation of that condition are known, a physician can construct the probability of that specific condition (bleeding disorder) resulting in the specific presentation (ICH):

$$P(B) = \text{Prev}(A) \times \text{Prev}(B|A),$$

where B is ICH attributable to condition A, P is probability, and Prev is prevalence. For example, factor XIII deficiency is extremely rare, occurring at an

TABLE 4 Half-Lives of Coagulation Factors

Factor	Half-Life Postinfusion, h
Fibrinogen	96–150
II	60
V	24
VII	4–6
VIII	11–12
IX	22
X	35
XI	60
XIII	144–300
VWF	8–12

Reprinted with permission from Goodnight S, Hathaway W. *Disorders of Hemostasis and Thrombosis: A Clinical Guide.* 2nd ed. New York, NY: McGraw-Hill Professional; 2001:497.

upper limit estimated population prevalence of 1 in 2 million; however, it can present with isolated intracranial bleeding in up to one-third of cases.[59] The estimated probability that factor XIII deficiency will cause an ICH in a person in the population at large is:

(Prevalence of factor XIII deficiency)

$\times$ (Prevalence of ICH in factor XIII deficiency)

$(1/2 \text{ million}) \times (1/3) = 1/6 \text{ million}$

Table 5 contains probabilities for congenital bleeding disorders to cause ICHs in the population at large.

No calculation was made in situations in which no reliable estimates of prevalence of the condition or frequency of ICH exist. The most liberal prevalence and frequency numbers were used, so as to provide the upper limits of probability.

CONCLUSIONS

In cases of suspected abuse involving bruising and/or bleeding, physicians must consider the possibility of coagulopathies causing or contributing to the findings. In many cases, the possible coagulopathies can be effectively evaluated by a thorough history and physical examination, and possibly by the specific nature of the child's findings; however, in some cases, a laboratory evaluation for coagulopathies might be necessary. The diagnosis of a bleeding disorder does not automatically rule out the presence of nonaccidental trauma. Because of the chronic nature of their disease, children with bleeding disorders may be at higher risk of abuse.[143]

Limited evidence exists comparing bruising and bleeding in children with coagulopathies with child victims of abuse. Conducting such studies would be difficult, given the overall rarity of coagulopathies; however, large databases exist for rare hematologic conditions, and modification of these databases to include factors, such as location of bruising or location/character of ICH, which would assist in discriminating between bleeding disorders and abuse, would be beneficial. In the absence of such data, physicians must use existing data, including epidemiologic and clinical factors, in their decision-making process.

LEAD AUTHORS

Shannon L. Carpenter, MD, MS
Thomas C. Abshire, MD
James D. Anderst, MD, MS

SECTION ON HEMATOLOGY/ONCOLOGY, 2012–2013

Jeffrey Hord, MD, Chairperson
Gary Crouch, MD
Gregory Hale, MD
Brigitta Mueller, MD
Zora Rogers, MD
Patricia Shearer, MD
Eric Werner, MD, Immediate Past Chairperson

FORMER EXECUTIVE COMMITTEE MEMBERS

Stephen Feig, MD
Eric Kodish, MD
Alan Gamis, MD

LIAISONS

Edwin Forman, MD–*Alliance for Childhood Cancer*

CONSULTANTS

Shannon L. Carpenter, MD, MS
Thomas C. Abshire, MD

STAFF

Suzanne Kirkwood, MS

COMMITTEE ON CHILD ABUSE AND NEGLECT, 2010-2011

Cindy W. Christian, MD, Chairperson
James Crawford-Jakubiak, MD
Emalee Flaherty, MD
John M. Leventhal, MD
James Lukefahr, MD
Robert Sege, MD, PhD

TABLE 5 Probabilities for Congenital Coagulopathies to Cause ICH[a]

Condition	Prevalence of Condition, Upper Limits	Prevalence of ICH, Upper Limits	Probability[b]
VWD	1/1000	Extremely rare	Low
Factor II deficiency	1/1 million	11%	1/10 million
Factor V deficiency	1/1 million	8% of homozygotes	1/10 million homozygotes
Combined factors V and VIII deficiency	1/1 million	2%	1/50 million
Factor VII deficiency	1/300 000	4%–6.5%	1/5 million
Factor VIII deficiency	1/5000 males	5%–12%	1/50 000 males
Factor IX deficiency	1/20 000 males	5%–12%	1/200 000 males
Factor X deficiency	1/1 million	21%	1/5 million
Factor XI deficiency	1/100 000	Extremely rare	Low
Factor XIII deficiency	1/2 million	33%	1/6 million
AP deficiency	40 cases reported	Not reported	Low
PAI-1 deficiency	Extremely rare	Common	Low
Afibrinogenemia	1/500 000	10%	1/5 million
Dysfibrinogenemia	1/1 million	Single case report	Low

[a] The probability of having a specific bleeding disorder increases in the setting of a family history of that specific named bleeding disorder or if the patient is from an ethnicity in which a specific bleeding disorder is more common (eg, Ashkenazi Jewish people and factor XI deficiency).

[b] "Probability" indicates the probability that an individual in the general population would have the following specific coagulopathy causing an ICH.

REFERENCES

1. Maguire S, Mann MK, Sibert J, Kemp A. Are there patterns of bruising in childhood which are diagnostic or suggestive of abuse? A systematic review. *Arch Dis Child.* 2005;90(2):182–186

2. Dunstan FD, Guildea ZE, Kontos K, Kemp AM, Sibert JR. A scoring system for bruise patterns: a tool for identifying abuse. *Arch Dis Child.* 2002;86(5):330–333

3. Sugar NF, Taylor JA, Feldman KW; Puget Sound Pediatric Research Network. Bruises in infants and toddlers: those who don't cruise rarely bruise. *Arch Pediatr Adolesc Med.* 1999;153(4):399–403

4. Carpenter RF. The prevalence and distribution of bruising in babies. *Arch Dis Child.* 1999;80(4):363–366

5. Feldman KW. Patterned abusive bruises of the buttocks and the pinnae. *Pediatrics.* 1992;90(4):633–636

6. O'Hare AE, Eden OB. Bleeding disorders and non-accidental injury. *Arch Dis Child.* 1984;59(9):860–864

7. Lieder HS, Irving SY, Mauricio R, Graf JM. Munchausen syndrome by proxy: a case report. *AACN Clin Issues.* 2005;16(2):178–184

8. Ulinski T, Lhopital C, Cloppet H, et al. Munchausen syndrome by proxy with massive proteinuria and gastrointestinal hemorrhage. *Pediatr Nephrol.* 2004;19(7):798–800

9. Stricker T, Lips U, Sennhauser FH. Oral bleeding: child abuse alert. *J Paediatr Child Health.* 2002;38(5):528–529

10. Walton LJ, Davies FC. Nasal bleeding and non-accidental injury in an infant. *Arch Dis Child.* 2010;95(1):53–54

11. Paranjothy S, Fone D, Mann M, et al. The incidence and aetiology of epistaxis in infants: a population-based study. *Arch Dis Child.* 2009;94(6):421–424

12. McIntosh N, Mok JY, Margerison A. Epidemiology of oronasal hemorrhage in the first 2 years of life: implications for child protection. *Pediatrics.* 2007;120(5):1074–1078

13. Evaluation of bleeding tendency in the outpatient child and adult. InGoodnight SH, Hathaway WE, eds. *Disorders of Hemostasis and Thrombosis.* 2nd ed. Lancaster, PA: McGraw-Hill; 2001:52–60

14. Hettler J, Greenes DS. Can the initial history predict whether a child with a head injury has been abused? *Pediatrics.* 2003;111(3):602–607

15. Maguire S, Pickerd N, Farewell D, Mann M, Tempest V, Kemp AM. Which clinical features distinguish inflicted from non-inflicted brain injury? A systematic review. *Arch Dis Child.* 2009;94(11):860–867

16. Vinchon M, Noule N, Tchofo PJ, Soto-Ares G, Fourier C, Dhellemmes P. Imaging of head injuries in infants: temporal correlates and forensic implications for the diagnosis of child abuse. *J Neurosurg Pediatr.* 2004;101(suppl 1):44–52

17. Vinchon M, de Foort-Dhellemmes S, Desurmont M, Delestret I. Confessed abuse versus witnessed accidents in infants: comparison of clinical, radiological, and ophthalmological data in corroborated cases. *Childs Nerv Syst.* 2010;26(5):637–645

18. Vinchon M, Defoort-Dhellemmes S, Desurmont M, Dhellemmes P. Accidental and nonaccidental head injuries in infants: a prospective study. *J Neurosurg.* 2005;102(suppl 4):380–384

19. Tung GA, Kumar M, Richardson RC, Jenny C, Brown WD. Comparison of accidental and nonaccidental traumatic head injury in children on noncontrast computed tomography. *Pediatrics.* 2006;118(2):626–633

20. Bechtel K, Stoessel K, Leventhal JM, et al. Characteristics that distinguish accidental from abusive injury in hospitalized young children with head trauma. *Pediatrics.* 2004;114(1):165–168

21. Ewing-Cobbs L, Kramer L, Prasad M, et al. Neuroimaging, physical, and developmental findings after inflicted and noninflicted traumatic brain injury in young children. *Pediatrics.* 1998;102(2 pt 1):300–307

22. Hymel KP, Makoroff KL, Laskey AL, Conaway MR, Blackman JA. Mechanisms, clinical presentations, injuries, and outcomes from inflicted versus noninflicted head trauma during infancy: results of a prospective, multicentered, comparative study. *Pediatrics.* 2007;119(5):922–929

23. Haviland J, Russell RI. Outcome after severe non-accidental head injury. *Arch Dis Child.* 1997;77(6):504–507

24. Hymel KP, Stoiko MA, Herman BE, et al. Head injury depth as an indicator of causes and mechanisms. *Pediatrics.* 2010;125(4):712–720

25. Mishra P, Naithani R, Dolai T, et al. Intracranial haemorrhage in patients with congenital haemostatic defects. *Haemophilia.* 2008;14(5):952–955

26. Offiah A, van Rijn RR, Perez-Rossello JM, Kleinman PK. Skeletal imaging of child abuse (non-accidental injury). *Pediatr Radiol.* 2009;39(5):461–470

27. Kasper CK, Buzin CH. Mosaics and haemophilia. *Haemophilia.* 2009;15(6):1181–1186

28. Di Michele DM. Hemophilia A (Factor VIII deficiency). In: Goodnight SH, Hathaway WE, eds. *Disorders of Hemostasis and Thrombosis,* 2nd ed. Lancaster, PA: McGraw-Hill; 2001:127–139

29. Kulkarni R, Soucie JM, Lusher J, et al; Haemophilia Treatment Center Network Investigators. Sites of initial bleeding episodes, mode of delivery and age of diagnosis in babies with haemophilia diagnosed before the age of 2 years: a report from The Centers for Disease Control and Prevention's (CDC) Universal Data Collection (UDC) project. *Haemophilia.* 2009;15(6):1281–1290

30. Nelson MD, Jr, Maeder MA, Usner D, et al. Prevalence and incidence of intracranial haemorrhage in a population of children with haemophilia. The Hemophilia Growth and Development Study. *Haemophilia.* 1999;5(5):306–312

31. Nuss R, Soucie JM, Evatt B; Hemophilia Surveillance System Project Investigators. Changes in the occurrence of and risk factors for hemophilia-associated intracranial hemorrhage. *Am J Hematol.* 2001;68(1):37–42

32. Witmer CM, Raffini LJ, Manno CS. Utility of computed tomography of the head following head trauma in boys with haemophilia. *Haemophilia.* 2007;13(5):560–566

33. Kasper CK, Lin JC. Prevalence of sporadic and familial haemophilia. *Haemophilia.* 2007;13(1):90–92

34. Franchini M, Favaloro EJ, Lippi G. Mild hemophilia A. *J Thromb Haemost.* 2010;8(3):421–432

35. Nichols WL, Hultin MB, James AH, et al. von Willebrand disease (VWD): evidence-based diagnosis and management guidelines, the National Heart, Lung, and Blood Institute (NHLBI) Expert Panel report (USA). *Haemophilia.* 2008;14(2):171–232

36. Sadler JE, Mannucci PM, Berntorp E, et al. Impact, diagnosis and treatment of von Willebrand disease. *Thromb Haemost.* 2000;84(2):160–174

37. Almaani WS, Awidi AS. Spontaneous intracranial hemorrhage secondary to von Willebrand's disease. *Surg Neurol.* 1986;26(5):457–460

38. Wetzstein V, Budde U, Oyen F, et al. Intracranial hemorrhage in a term newborn with severe von Willebrand disease type 3 associated with sinus venous thrombosis. *Haematologica.* 2006;91(suppl 12):ECR60

39. Stray-Pedersen A, Omland S, Nedregaard B, Klevberg S, Rognum TO. An infant with subdural hematoma and retinal hemorrhages: does von Willebrand disease explain the findings? *Forensic Sci Med Pathol.* 2011;7(1):37–41

40. National Heart Lung and Blood Institute. *The Diagnosis, Evaluation and Management of von Willebrand Disease.* Bethesda, MD: National Heart Lung and Blood Institute, National Institutes of Health, US Department of Health and Human Services; December, 2007. NIH Publication No. 08-5832

41. Ziv O, Ragni MV. Bleeding manifestations in males with von Willebrand disease. *Haemophilia.* 2004;10(2):162–168

42. Mizoi K, Onuma T, Mori K. Intracranial hemorrhage secondary to von Willebrand's disease and trauma. *Surg Neurol.* 1984;22(5):495–498

43. Harrison P, Mumford A. Screening tests of platelet function: update on their appropriate uses for diagnostic testing. *Semin Thromb Hemost.* 2009;35(2):150–157

44. Fressinaud E, Veyradier A, Truchaud F, et al. Screening for von Willebrand disease with a new analyzer using high shear stress: a study of 60 cases. *Blood.* 1998;91(4):1325–1331

45. Dean JA, Blanchette VS, Carcao MD, et al. von Willebrand disease in a pediatric-based population—comparison of type 1 diagnostic criteria and use of the PFA-100 and a von Willebrand factor/collagen-binding assay. *Thromb Haemost.* 2000;84(3):401–409

46. Kumar S, Pruthi RK, Nichols WL. Acquired von Willebrand disease. *Mayo Clin Proc.* 2002;77(2):181–187

47. Bolton-Maggs PHB, Perry DJ, Chalmers EA, et al. The rare coagulation disorders—review with guidelines for management from the United Kingdom Haemophilia Centre Doctors' Organisation. *Haemophilia.* 2004;10(5):593–628

48. Farah RA, Hamod D, Melick N, Giansily-Blaizot M, Sallah S. Successful prophylaxis against intracranial hemorrhage using weekly administration of activated recombinant factor VII in a newborn with severe factor VII deficiency. *J Thromb Haemost.* 2007;5(2):433–434

49. Mariani G, Herrmann FH, Dolce A, et al; International Factor VII Deficiency Study Group. Clinical phenotypes and factor VII genotype in congenital factor VII deficiency. *Thromb Haemost.* 2005;93(3):481–487

50. Lapecorella M, Mariani G; International Registry on Congenital Factor VII Deficiency. Factor VII deficiency: defining the clinical picture and optimizing therapeutic options. *Haemophilia.* 2008;14(6):1170–1175

51. Lee JH, Lee HJ, Bin JH, et al. A novel homozygous missense mutation in the factor VII gene of severe factor VII deficiency in a newborn baby. *Blood Coagul Fibrinolysis.* 2009;20(2):161–164

52. Wong WY, Huang WC, Miller R, McGinty K, Whisnant JK. Clinical efficacy and recovery levels of recombinant FVIIa (NovoSeven) in the treatment of intracranial haemorrhage in severe neonatal FVII deficiency. *Haemophilia.* 2000;6(1):50–54

53. Peyvandi F, Mannucci PM. Rare coagulation disorders. *Thromb Haemost.* 1999;82(4):1207–1214

54. Roberts HR, Hoffman M. Hemophilia and related conditions: inherited deficiencies of prothrombin (factor II), factor V, and factors VII to XII. In: Beutler E, Lichtman MA, Coller BS, Kipps TJ, eds. *William's Hematology.* 5th ed. New York, NY: McGraw-Hill; 1995:1413–1439

55. Bick RL. *Disorders of Thrombosis and Hemostasis: Clinical and Laboratory Practice.* Chicago, IL: American Society for Clinical Pathology Press; 1992

56. Gomez K, Bolton-Maggs P. Factor XI deficiency. *Haemophilia.* 2008;14(6):1183–1189

57. Vasileiadis I, El-Ali M, Nanas S, et al. First diagnosis of factor XI deficiency in a patient with subarachnoid haemorrhage. *Blood Coagul Fibrinolysis.* 2009;20(4):309–313

58. Duga S, Salomon O. Factor XI deficiency. *Semin Thromb Hemost.* 2009;35(4):416–425

59. Reverdiau-Moalic P, Delahousse B, Body G, Bardos P, Leroy J, Gruel Y. Evolution of blood coagulation activators and inhibitors in the healthy human fetus. *Blood.* 1996;88(3):900–906

60. Hsieh L, Nugent D. Factor XIII deficiency. *Haemophilia.* 2008;14(6):1190–1200

61. Karimi M, Bereczky Z, Cohan N, Muszbek L. Factor XIII deficiency. *Semin Thromb Hemost.* 2009;35(4):426–438

62. Ivaskevicius V, Seitz R, Kohler HP, et al; Study Group. International registry on factor XIII deficiency: a basis formed mostly on European data. *Thromb Haemost.* 2007;97(6):914–921

63. Newman RS, Jalili M, Kolls BJ, Dietrich R. Factor XIII deficiency mistaken for battered child syndrome: case of "correct" test ordering negated by a commonly accepted qualitative test with limited negative predictive value. *Am J Hematol.* 2002;71(4):328–330

64. Albanese A, Tuttolomondo A, Anile C, et al. Spontaneous chronic subdural hematomas in young adults with a deficiency in coagulation factor XIII. Report of three cases. *J Neurosurg.* 2005;102(6):1130–1132

65. Gordon M, Prakash N, Padmakumar B. Factor XIII deficiency: a differential diagnosis to be considered in suspected nonaccidental injury presenting with intracranial hemorrhage. *Clin Pediatr (Phila).* 2008;47(4):385–387

66. Acharya SS, Coughlin A, Dimichele DM; North American Rare Bleeding Disorder Study Group. Rare Bleeding Disorder Registry: deficiencies of factors II, V, VII, X, XIII, fibrinogen and dysfibrinogenemias. *J Thromb Haemost.* 2004;2(2):248–256

67. Strijks E, Poort SR, Renier WO, Gabreëls FJ, Bertina RM. Hereditary prothrombin deficiency presenting as intracranial haematoma in infancy. *Neuropediatrics.* 1999;30(6):320–324

68. Wong AYK, Hewitt J, Clarke BJ, et al. Severe prothrombin deficiency caused by prothrombin-Edmonton (R-4Q) combined with a previously undetected deletion. *J Thromb Haemost.* 2006;4(12):2623–2628

69. Akhavan S, Luciani M, Lavoretano S, Mannucci PM. Phenotypic and genetic analysis of a compound heterozygote for dys- and hypoprothrombinaemia. *Br J Haemol.* 2003;120(1):142–144

70. Meeks SL, Abshire TC. Abnormalities of prothrombin: a review of the pathophysiology, diagnosis, and treatment. *Haemophilia*. 2008;14(6):1159–1163

71. Lancellotti S, De Cristofaro R. Congenital prothrombin deficiency. *Semin Thromb Hemost*. 2009;35(4):367–381

72. Ellestad SC, Zimmerman SA, Thornburg C, Mitchell TE, Swamy GK, James AH. Severe factor V deficiency presenting with intracranial haemorrhage during gestation. *Haemophilia*. 2007;13(4):432–434

73. Salooja N, Martin P, Khair K, Liesner R, Hann I. Severe factor V deficiency and neonatal intracranial haemorrhage: a case report. *Haemophilia*. 2000;6(1):44–46

74. Huang JN, Koerper MA. Factor V deficiency: a concise review. *Haemophilia*. 2008;14(6):1164–1169

75. Spreafico M, Peyvandi F. Combined FV and FVIII deficiency. *Haemophilia*. 2008;14(6):1201–1208

76. Peyvandi F, Tuddenham EGD, Akhtari AM, Lak M, Mannucci PM. Bleeding symptoms in 27 Iranian patients with the combined deficiency of factor V and factor VIII. *Br J Haematol*. 1998;100(4):773–776

77. Mansouritorgabeh H, Rezaieyazdi Z, Pourfathollah AA, Rezai J, Esamaili H. Haemorrhagic symptoms in patients with combined factors V and VIII deficiency in north-eastern Iran. *Haemophilia*. 2004;10(3):271–275

78. Brown DL, Kouides PA. Diagnosis and treatment of inherited factor X deficiency. *Haemophilia*. 2008;14(6):1176–1182

79. Menegatti M, Peyvandi F. Factor X deficiency. *Semin Thromb Hemost*. 2009;35(4):407–415

80. Herrmann FH, Auerswald G, Ruiz-Saez A, et al; Greifswald Factor X Deficiency Study Group. Factor X deficiency: clinical manifestation of 102 subjects from Europe and Latin America with mutations in the factor 10 gene. *Haemophilia*. 2006;12(5):479–489

81. Millar DS, Elliston L, Deex P, et al. Molecular analysis of the genotype-phenotype relationship in factor X deficiency. *Hum Genet*. 2000;106(2):249–257

82. Shearer MJ. Vitamin K deficiency bleeding (VKDB) in early infancy. *Blood Rev*. 2009;23 (suppl 2):49–59

83. Zipursky A. Prevention of vitamin K deficiency bleeding in newborns. *Br J Haematol*. 1999;104(3):430–437

84. Miyasaka M, Nosaka S, Sakai H, et al. Vitamin K deficiency bleeding with intracranial hemorrhage: focus on secondary form. *Emerg Radiol*. 2007;14(5):323–329

85. Brenner B. Hereditary deficiency of vitamin K-dependent coagulation factors. *Thromb Haemost*. 2000;84(6):935–936

86. Girolami A, Ruzzon E, Tezza F, Scandellari R, Vettore S, Girolami B. Arterial and venous thrombosis in rare congenital bleeding disorders: a critical review. *Haemophilia*. 2006;12(4):345–351

87. Verhovsek M, Moffat KA, Hayward CPM. Laboratory testing for fibrinogen abnormalities. *Am J Hematol*. 2008;83(12):928–931

88. Hill M, Dolan G. Diagnosis, clinical features and molecular assessment of the dysfibrinogenaemias. *Haemophilia*. 2008;14(5):889–897

89. al-Fawaz IM, Gader AMA. Severe congenital dysfibrinogenemia (fibrinogen-Riyadh): a family study. *Acta Haematol*. 1992;88(4):194–197

90. Lak M, Keihani M, Elahi F, Peyvandi F, Mannucci PM. Bleeding and thrombosis in 55 patients with inherited afibrinogenaemia. *Br J Haematol*. 1999;107(1):204–206

91. Peyvandi F, Duga S, Akhavan S, Mannucci PM. Rare coagulation deficiencies. *Haemophilia*. 2002;8(3):308–321

92. Acharya SS, Dimichele DM. Rare inherited disorders of fibrinogen. *Haemophilia*. 2008;14(6):1151–1158

93. Favier R, Aoki N, de Moerloose P. Congenital alpha(2)-plasmin inhibitor deficiencies: a review. *Br J Haematol*. 2001;114(1):4–10

94. Mehta R, Shapiro AD. Plasminogen activator inhibitor type 1 deficiency. *Haemophilia*. 2008;14(6):1255–1260

95. Fay WP, Parker AC, Condrey LR, Shapiro AD. Human plasminogen activator inhibitor-1 (PAI-1) deficiency: characterization of a large kindred with a null mutation in the PAI-1 gene. *Blood*. 1997;90(1):204–208

96. Rughani AI, Holmes CE, Penar PL. A novel association between a chronic subdural hematoma and a fibrinolytic pathway defect: case report. *Neurosurgery*. 2009;64(6):E1192–, discussion E1192

97. Goddeau RP, Jr, Caplan LR, Alhazzani AA. Intraparenchymal hemorrhage in a patient with osteogenesis imperfecta and plasminogen activator inhibitor-1 deficiency. *Arch Neurol*. 2010;67(2):236–238

98. Carpenter SL, Mathew P. Alpha2-antiplasmin and its deficiency: fibrinolysis out of balance. *Haemophilia*. 2008;14(6):1250–1254

99. Devaussuzenet VMP, Ducou-le-Pointe HA, Doco AM, Mary PM, Montagne JR, Favier R. A case of intramedullary haematoma associated with congenital α_2-plasmin inhibitor deficiency. *Pediatr Radiol*. 1998;28(12):978–980

100. Takahashi Y, Tanaka T, Nakajima N, et al. Intramedullary multiple hematomas in siblings with congenital alpha-2-plasmin inhibitor deficiency: orthopedic surgery with protection by tranexamic acid. *Haemostasis*. 1991;21(5):321–327

101. Factor XIII, alpha-2-antiplasmin, and plasminogen activator inhibitor-1 deficiencies. InGoodnight SH, Hathaway WE, eds. *Disorders of Hemostasis and Thrombosis*. 2nd ed. Lancaster, PA: McGraw-Hill; 2001:184–191

102. Hayward CPM, Rao AK, Cattaneo M. Congenital platelet disorders: overview of their mechanisms, diagnostic evaluation and treatment. *Haemophilia*. 2006;12 (suppl 3):128–136

103. Alamelu J, Liesner R. Modern management of severe platelet function disorders. *Br J Haematol*. 2010;149(6):813–823

104. Di Minno G, Coppola A, Di Minno MND, Poon M-C. Glanzmann's thrombasthenia (defective platelet integrin alphaIIb-$\beta3$): proposals for management between evidence and open issues. *Thromb Haemost*. 2009;102(6):1157–1164

105. Favaloro EJ. Clinical utility of the PFA-100. *Semin Thromb Hemost*. 2008;34(8):709–733

106. McKay H, Derome F, Haq MA, et al. Bleeding risks associated with inheritance of the Quebec platelet disorder. *Blood*. 2004;104(1):159–165

107. Bolton-Maggs PHB, Chalmers EA, Collins PW, et al; UKHCDO. A review of inherited platelet disorders with guidelines for their management on behalf of the UKHCDO. *Br J Haematol*. 2006;135(5):603–633

108. Hassan AA, Kroll MH. Acquired disorders of platelet function. In: Berliner N, Lee SJ, Lineberger M, Vogelsang GB, eds. *American Society of Hematology Education Program Book*. Berkeley, CA: ASH; 2005:403–408

109. Neunert C, Lim W, Crowther M, Cohen A, Solberg L, Jr, Crowther MA American Society of Hematology. The American Society of Hematology 2011 evidence-based practice guideline for immune thrombocytopenia. *Blood*. 2011;117(16):4190–4207

110. Sirotnak AP. Medical disorders that mimic abusive head trauma. In: Frasier L, Rauth-Farley K, Alexander R, Parrish R, eds. *Abusive Head Trauma in Infants and Children*. 1st ed. St Louis, MO: GW Medical Publishing; 2006:191–214

111. Roberts DL, Pope FM, Nicholls AC, Narcisi P. Ehlers-Danlos syndrome type IV mimicking non-accidental injury in a child. *Br J Dermatol.* 1984;111(3):341–345

112. Owen SM, Durst RD. Ehlers-Danlos syndrome simulating child abuse. *Arch Dermatol.* 1984;120(1):97–101

113. Ehlers-Danlos National Foundation. Web Site. Available at: www.ednf.org/index. php?option=com_content&task=view&id= 1347&Itemid=88888968. Accessed April 19, 2012

114. Beighton P, De Paepe A, Steinmann B, Tsipouras P, Wenstrup RJ; Ehlers-Danlos National Foundation (USA) and Ehlers-Danlos Support Group (UK). Ehlers-Danlos syndromes: revised nosology, Villefranche, 1997. *Am J Med Genet.* 1998;77 (1):31–37

115. De Paepe A, Malfait F. Bleeding and bruising in patients with Ehlers-Danlos syndrome and other collagen vascular disorders. *Br J Haematol.* 2004;127(5):491–500

116. Pepin M, Schwarze U, Superti-Furga A, Byers PH. Clinical and genetic features of Ehlers-Danlos syndrome type IV, the vascular type. *N Engl J Med.* 2000;342(10): 673–680

117. Malfait F, De Paepe A. Bleeding in the heritable connective tissue disorders: mechanisms, diagnosis and treatment. *Blood Rev.* 2009;23(5):191–197

118. Schievink WI, Limburg M, Oorthuys JW, Fleury P, Pope FM. Cerebrovascular disease in Ehlers-Danlos syndrome type IV. *Stroke.* 1990;21(4):626–632

119. Pepin MG, Byers P. *Ehlers-Danlos Syndrome Type IV.* GeneReviews Web Site. Available at: www.ncbi.nlm.nih.gov/book-shelf/br.fcgi?book=gene&part=eds4. Accessed April 19, 2012

120. Ortiz Remacha PP, Candia J, Conde M. Recurrent subdural hemorrhage as the form of presentation of a type-IV Ehlers-Danlos syndrome [in Spanish]. *Rev Clin Esp.* 2000;200(3):181–182

121. Steinmann B, Royce P, Superti-Furga A. The Ehlers-Danlos syndrome. In: Royce B, Steinmann B, eds. *Connective Tissue and its Heritable Disorders.* 2nd ed. New York, NY: Wiley-Liss, Inc; 2002:431–523

122. Barabas GM, Barabas AP. The Ehlers-Danlos syndrome. A report of the oral and haematological findings in nine cases. *Br Dent J.* 1967;123(10):473–479

123. Jenny C; Committee on Child Abuse and Neglect. Evaluating infants and young children with multiple fractures. *Pediatrics.* 2006;118(3):1299–1303

124. Ganesh A, Jenny C, Geyer J, Shouldice M, Levin AV. Retinal hemorrhages in type I osteogenesis imperfecta after minor trauma. *Ophthalmology.* 2004;111(7):1428–1431

125. Steiner RD, Pepin MG, Byers P. Osteogenesis imperfecta. GeneReviews Web Site. Available at: www.ncbi.nlm.nih.gov/ bookshelf/br.fcgi?book=gene&part=oi. Accessed April 19, 2012

126. Evensen SA, Myhre L, Stormorken H. Haemostatic studies in osteogenesis imperfecta. *Scand J Haematol.* 1984;33 (2):177–179

127. Hathaway WE, Solomons CC, Ott JE. Platelet function and pyrophosphates in osteogenesis imperfecta. *Blood.* 1972;39 (4):500–509

128. Kuurila K, Kaitila I, Johansson R, Grénman R. Hearing loss in Finnish adults with osteogenesis imperfecta: a nationwide survey. *Ann Otol Rhinol Laryngol.* 2002;111 (10):939–946

129. Wynne-Davies R, Gormley J. Clinical and genetic patterns in osteogenesis imperfecta. *Clin Orthop Relat Res.* 1981; (159): 26–35

130. Parmar CD, Sinha AK, Hayhurst C, May PL, O'Brien DF. Epidural hematoma formation following trivial head trauma in a child with osteogenesis imperfecta. Case report. *J Neurosurg.* 2007;106(suppl 1):57–60

131. Pozzati E, Poppi M, Gaist G. Acute bilateral extradural hematomas in a case of osteogenesis imperfecta congenita. *Neurosurgery.* 1983;13(1):66–68

132. Sasaki-Adams D, Kulkarni A, Rutka J, Dirks P, Taylor M, Drake JM. Neurosurgical implications of osteogenesis imperfecta in children. Report of 4 cases. *J Neurosurg Pediatr.* 2008;1(3):229–236

133. Tokoro K, Nakajima F, Yamataki A. Infantile chronic subdural hematoma with local protrusion of the skull in a case of osteogenesis imperfecta. *Neurosurgery.* 1988;22(3):595–598

134. Groninger A, Schaper J, Messing-Juenger M, Mayatepek E, Rosenbaum T. Subdural hematoma as clinical presentation of osteogenesis imperfecta. *Pediatr Neurol.* 2005;32(2):140–142

135. Clemetson CAB. Is it "Shaken baby," or Barlow's disease variant? *J Am Phys Surg.* 2004;9(3):78–80

136. Clemetson CAB. Elevated blood histamine caused by vaccinations and Vitamin C deficiency may mimic the shaken baby syndrome. *Med Hypotheses.* 2004;62(4): 533–536

137. Gardner H. Immunizations, retinal, and subdural hemorrhage: are they related? *Med Hypotheses.* 2004;64(3):663

138. Brain and spine injuries in infancy and childhood. In: Barkovich AJ, ed. *Pediatric Neuroimaging.* 4th ed. Philadelphia, PA: Lippincott Williams & Wilkins; 2005:190–290

139. McLean LA, Frasier LD, Hedlund GL. Does intracranial venous thrombosis cause subdural hemorrhage in the pediatric population? *AJNR Am J Neuroradiol.* 2012; 33(7):1281–1284

140. Hymel KP, Abshire TC, Luckey DW, Jenny C. Coagulopathy in pediatric abusive head trauma. *Pediatrics.* 1997;99(3):371–375

141. Talving P, Lustenberger T, Lam L, et al. Coagulopathy after isolated severe traumatic brain injury in children. *J Trauma.* 2011;71(5):1205–1210

142. Boshkov LK. Plasma. In: Goodnight SH, Hathaway WE, eds. *Disorders of Hemostasis and Thrombosis,* 2nd ed. Lancaster, PA: McGraw-Hill; 2001:495–500

143. Sullivan PM, Knutson JF. Maltreatment and disabilities: a population-based epidemiological study. *Child Abuse Negl.* 2000;24 (10):1257–1273

Evaluation for Bleeding Disorders in Suspected Child Abuse

- *Clinical Report*

CLINICAL REPORT

Evaluation for Bleeding Disorders in Suspected Child Abuse

abstract

Bruising or bleeding in a child can raise the concern for child abuse. Assessing whether the findings are the result of trauma and/or whether the child has a bleeding disorder is critical. Many bleeding disorders are rare, and not every child with bruising/bleeding concerning for abuse requires an evaluation for bleeding disorders. In some instances, however, bleeding disorders can present in a manner similar to child abuse. The history and clinical evaluation can be used to determine the necessity of an evaluation for a possible bleeding disorder, and prevalence and known clinical presentations of individual bleeding disorders can be used to guide the extent of the laboratory testing. This clinical report provides guidance to pediatricians and other clinicians regarding the evaluation for bleeding disorders when child abuse is suspected. *Pediatrics* 2013;131:e1314–e1322

INTRODUCTION

Children often present for medical care with bleeding or bruising that can raise a concern for child abuse. Most commonly, this occurs with cutaneous bruises and intracranial hemorrhage (ICH), but other presentations, such as hematemesis,[1] hematochezia,[2] and oronasal bleeding can be caused by child abuse and/or bleeding disorders.[3–7] When bleeding or bruising is suspicious for child abuse, careful consideration of medical and other causes is warranted. The inappropriate diagnosis of child abuse could occur,[8–10] potentially resulting in the removal of a child from a home and/or the potential prosecution of an innocent person. Conversely, attributing an abusive injury to medical causes or accidental injury puts a child at risk for future abuse and possible death.[11] Laboratory evaluations should be conducted with the understanding that the presence of a bleeding disorder does not rule out abuse as the etiology for bruising or bleeding.[9] Similarly, the presence of a history of trauma (accidental or nonaccidental) does not exclude the presence of a bleeding disorder or other medical condition. This clinical report provides guidance to pediatricians and other clinicians regarding the evaluation for bleeding disorders when child abuse is suspected (Fig 1).

James D. Anderst, MD, MS, Shannon L. Carpenter, MD, MS, Thomas C. Abshire, MD and the SECTION ON HEMATOLOGY/ONCOLOGY and COMMITTEE ON CHILD ABUSE AND NEGLECT

KEY WORDS
intracranial hemorrhage, inherited coagulation disorders, bruising, nonaccidental trauma

ABBREVIATIONS
aPTT—activated partial thromboplastin time
DIC—disseminated intravascular coagulation
ICH—intracranial hemorrhage
ITP—immune thrombocytopenia
PFA-100—platelet function analyzer
PT—prothrombin time
VKDB—vitamin K deficiency bleeding
VWD—von Willebrand disease

The guidance in this report does not indicate an exclusive course of treatment or serve as a standard of medical care. Variations, taking into account individual circumstances, may be appropriate.

Accepted for publication Jan 23, 2013

www.pediatrics.org/cgi/doi/10.1542/peds.2013-0195

doi:10.1542/peds.2013-0195

All clinical reports from the American Academy of Pediatrics automatically expire 5 years after publication unless reaffirmed, revised, or retired at or before that time.

PEDIATRICS (ISSN Numbers: Print, 0031-4005; Online, 1098-4275).

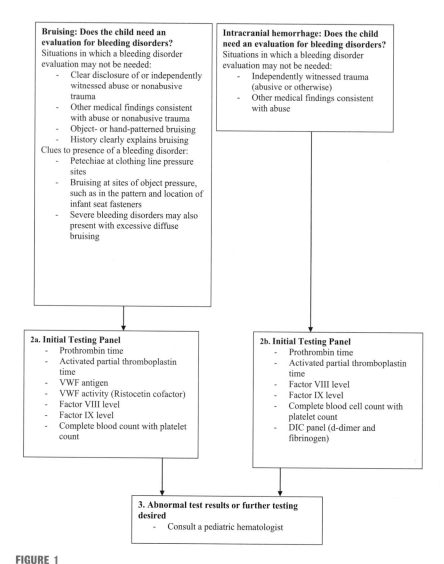

Bruising: Does the child need an evaluation for bleeding disorders?
Situations in which a bleeding disorder evaluation may not be needed:
- Clear disclosure of or independently witnessed abuse or nonabusive trauma
- Other medical findings consistent with abuse or nonabusive trauma
- Object- or hand-patterned bruising
- History clearly explains bruising

Clues to presence of a bleeding disorder:
- Petechiae at clothing line pressure sites
- Bruising at sites of object pressure, such as in the pattern and location of infant seat fasteners
- Severe bleeding disorders may also present with excessive diffuse bruising

Intracranial hemorrhage: Does the child need an evaluation for bleeding disorders?
Situations in which a bleeding disorder evaluation may not be needed:
- Independently witnessed trauma (abusive or otherwise)
- Other medical findings consistent with abuse

2a. Initial Testing Panel
- Prothrombin time
- Activated partial thromboplastin time
- VWF antigen
- VWF activity (Ristocetin cofactor)
- Factor VIII level
- Factor IX level
- Complete blood count with platelet count

2b. Initial Testing Panel
- Prothrombin time
- Activated partial thromboplastin time
- Factor VIII level
- Factor IX level
- Complete blood cell count with platelet count
- DIC panel (d-dimer and fibrinogen)

3. Abnormal test results or further testing desired
- Consult a pediatric hematologist

FIGURE 1
Recommended pathway for evaluation of possible bleeding disorders when child abuse is suspected. VWF, von Willebrand factor.

ASSESSING THE NEED FOR A LABORATORY EVALUATION FOR BLEEDING DISORDERS

The age and developmental capabilities of the child, history of trauma, the location and pattern of bruising, and, in the case of ICH, findings on neuroimaging should be considered when assessing children with bruising/bleeding for possible abuse.[12–18] Additionally, a medical history of symptoms suggestive of a bleeding disorder, such as significant bleeding after a circumcision or other surgery, epistaxis, bleeding from the umbilical stump, or excessive bleeding after dental procedures, increases the possibility of a bleeding disorder. Family history of a specific bleeding disorder or ethnicity of a population with higher rates of a certain bleeding disorder (eg, Amish) might necessitate testing for that condition. The child's medications should be documented, because certain drugs can affect the results of some tests that might be used to detect bleeding disorders, such as the platelet function analyzer (PFA-100; Siemens Healthcare Diagnostics, Tarrytown, NY) and platelet aggregation testing. Caregivers might state that their child "bruises easily." These statements are difficult to assess during an evaluation for possible abuse, as they can be a sign of a bleeding disorder, a reflection of the child's (fair) skin tone, or a fabrication to mask abuse. Children who are verbal and capable of providing a history should be interviewed away from potential offending caregivers, if possible. A thorough physical examination should include an evaluation of areas of bruising that have higher specificity for abuse,[14] such as the buttocks, ears, and genitals.

Any bleeding disorder can cause cutaneous bruising, and sometimes this bruising can be mild, can appear in locations that are considered suspicious for abuse,[19] and can appear at any age. Given the extreme rarity of some bleeding disorders, it is not reasonable to perform extensive laboratory testing for bleeding disorders in every child. In some cases, the constellation of findings, taken in conjunction with the clinical history and physical examination, can be so strongly consistent with an abusive injury that further laboratory investigation for medical conditions is not warranted. For instance, a child with a patterned slap mark who describes being hit with an open hand does not require a laboratory evaluation for a bleeding disorder.

In addition to bleeding disorders, the possibility of other medical causes of easy bruising or bleeding, such as Ehlers-Danlos syndrome, scurvy, cancer and other infiltrative disorders, glutaric aciduria, and arteriovenous malformations, should be assessed, as should a history of use of any medications or alternative therapies that may increase bleeding/bruising. Comprehensive descriptions of medical conditions that could be confused with child abuse and alternative therapies that may predispose to bleeding/bruising are beyond the scope of this report and can be found elsewhere.[20,21] Results of the history, review of systems, physical examination, and, in the case of ICH, neuroimaging are generally adequate to exclude these conditions. When there are concerns that a medical condition might be the cause of bruising or bleeding, the evaluation for the conditions in question should occur simultaneously with the evaluation for abuse.

Bruising

In the absence of independently witnessed accidental trauma or a known medical cause, any bruising in a nonmobile child is highly concerning for abuse and necessitates an evaluation for child abuse.[12–15] Additionally, bruising in a young infant could also be the first presentation of a bleeding disorder.[19] As such, a simultaneous evaluation for bleeding disorders is recommended in these cases. In mobile children, the locations and patterns of the bruising can be used to assess for the possibility of abuse (Table 1).

TABLE 1 Suspicion of Child Abuse in Ambulatory Children on the Basis of Characteristics of Bruises[14,15,17]

Less Suspicious for Child Abuse	More Suspicious for Child Abuse
Forehead	Location
Under chin	Face
Elbows	Ears
Lower arms	Neck
Hips	Upper arms
Shins	Trunk
Ankles	Hands
	Genitalia
	Buttocks
	Anterior, medial thighs
	Pattern
	Slap or hand marks
	Object marks
	Bite marks
	Bruises in clusters
	Multiple bruises of uniform shape
	Large cumulative size of bruising

In cases of bruising, the assessment of the need for an evaluation for bleeding disorders should focus on the following:

- the specific history offered to explain the bruising;
- the nature and location of bruising; and
- mobility and developmental status of the child.

The following factors generally exclude the need for an evaluation for a bleeding disorder:

- the caregivers' description of trauma sufficiently explains the bruising;
- the child or an independent witness is able to provide a history of abuse or nonabusive trauma that explains the bruising; or
- abusive object or hand-patterned bruising is present.

The injury history offered by caregivers might be purposefully misleading if the caregivers have caused the bruising by abusive means.

In nonmobile infants, bleeding disorders can present with bruising or petechiae in sites of normal handling or pressure. Examples of this include the following:

- petechiae at clothing line pressure sites;
- bruising at sites of object pressure, such as in the pattern and location of infant seat fasteners; and
- excessive diffuse bleeding if the child has a severe bleeding disorder.

Absence of these examples does not rule out a bleeding disorder; however, their presence might increase the probability of a bleeding disorder.

ICH

Excepting obvious known trauma, ICH in a nonmobile child is highly concerning for child abuse. Children can suffer ICH, such as a small subdural or an epidural hematoma underlying a site of impact, from a short fall; however, short falls rarely result in significant brain injury.[16] Birth trauma and some medical conditions can also result in ICH in infants. Consultation with a child abuse pediatrician should be considered in complex or concerning cases.

No studies have systematically compared the presentation, clinical findings, patterns of ICH, or presence of retinal hemorrhages found in children with bleeding disorders with those found in children in whom abusive head trauma is diagnosed. However, bleeding disorders can cause ICH in any part of the cranial contents, and up to 12% of children and young adults with bleeding disorders have had ICH at some time.[22,23] Children with ICH concerning for abuse require an evaluation for bleeding disorders. Exceptions to required evaluation can include the following:

- Independently witnessed or verifiable trauma (abusive or nonabusive),
- Other findings consistent with abuse, such as fractures, burns, or internal abdominal trauma.

Other Bleeding Symptoms

Children with conditions such as hematemesis, hematochezia, or oronasal bleeding as presenting symptoms should be evaluated on a case-by-case basis for possible abuse, particularly child abuse in a medical setting. Medical conditions and/or child abuse can cause these findings.

BLEEDING DISORDERS AND EXTENT OF EVALUATION

Bleeding disorders that can produce patterns of bruising or bleeding that mimic abuse include coagulation factor deficiencies/abnormalities, fibrinolytic defects, defects of fibrinogen, and platelet disorders. Table 2 contains a listing of the most common bleeding disorders in children and characteristics of potential testing strategies for each disorder. Most factor deficiencies can be detected by the prothrombin time (PT) and activated partial thromboplastin time (aPTT); however, von Willebrand disease (VWD) and factor XIII deficiency are not reliably detected by these screening tests. Additionally, mild deficiencies in factor VIII or factor IX (mild hemophilia) might not cause abnormalities in the aPTT but might still result in significant bleeding, including ICH, particularly after mild trauma. Fibrinolytic defects can cause significant bleeding/bruising but are extremely rare and require specific testing. Defects of fibrinogen are also rare and can be detected by the fibrinogen concentration and thrombin time.

The prevalence of mild platelet disorders is unknown, and testing for mild platelet disorders is challenging. The most common clinical presentations include bruising and mucocutaneous bleeding. The prevalence of ICH in mild platelet disorders is unknown but is likely to be low. Platelet aggregation testing, best performed by a pediatric hematologist, requires a relatively large volume of blood, and interpretation of the test result requires a specialist.[25] A PFA-100 can screen for many platelet function disorders, including more severe types, such as Bernard Soulier syndrome and Glanzmann thrombasthenia, as well as many types of VWD. However, the PFA-100 is not an effective screen for some types of VWD and milder platelet abnormalities. Individual patient characteristics, such as hematocrit, platelet count, pregnancy, age, multisystem trauma, sepsis, and medications, can affect the results of the PFA-100. Accurate

diagnosis often requires additional testing, such as specific von Willebrand testing or platelet aggregation; therefore, many centers have decreased or ceased use of the PFA-100.[25,26] Assessment of the results of a PFA-100 and the need for further testing are best accomplished in consultation with a pediatric hematologist.

Vitamin K Deficiency

Vitamin K deficiency in infants can result in bleeding in the skin or from mucosal surfaces from circumcision, generalized ecchymoses, large intramuscular hemorrhages, or ICH. Because of the widespread provision of vitamin K at birth, vitamin K deficiency bleeding (VKDB) is rare; however, not all states require vitamin K to be administered at birth, and some medical conditions predispose to VKDB.[24] In VKDB, there is a prolonged PT and possibly aPTT for age. In patients who have already received vitamin K, fresh-frozen plasma, or specific factor replacement as treatment, measurement of proteins induced by vitamin K absence can confirm the diagnosis.[27,28]

Coagulation Tests in Cases of Bruising

The initial screening panel in a patient who presents with bruising evaluates for conditions with a known prevalence more common than 1 per 500 000 people, including idiopathic thrombocytopenic purpura, all factor deficiencies (except factor XIII deficiency), and VWD (Fig 1). It does not evaluate for extremely rare conditions, including factor XIII deficiency, defects of fibrinogen, and fibrinolytic defects. This strategy also does not screen for extremely rare platelet disorders, such as Glanzmann thrombasthenia, and more common but relatively more difficult to detect

platelet disorders, such as platelet storage pool disorders. If test results are abnormal or expanded/detailed testing is necessary or preferred, consultation with a pediatric hematologist is recommended.

In many circumstances, children with bruising that is suspicious for abuse may be removed from a potentially dangerous setting where the abuse likely occurred. A thorough physical examination performed in the weeks after removal that reveals minimal bruising and/or bruising only in locations of common accidental bruises is supportive of abuse as the cause of the original suspicious bruising. Each case must be evaluated individually, however, considering the totality of findings, and with the understanding that the need for safety must be balanced with the emotional trauma of removing a child from his or her home. Bleeding disorders are generally permanent conditions that do not result in abatement after a change in caregivers. One exception to this is immune thrombocytopenia (ITP), which is a transient, often self-resolving bleeding disorder. Screening for ITP (platelet count) is necessary at the time of presentation with bruises.

Determining the Need for a Test: The Medical Probability

Specific data regarding the prevalence of bleeding disorders in the population of children with ICH or subdural hematoma is not available. However, there are data regarding the probability of specific bleeding disorders to cause ICH. If the prevalence of a condition and the frequency of a particular presentation of that condition are known, a physician can construct the probability of that specific condition (bleeding disorder) resulting in the specific presentation (ICH). The presence of "classic" bleeding symptoms, such as bleeding after circumcision,

TABLE 2 Common Testing Strategies for Bleeding Disorders

Condition	Frequency	Inheritance	Screening Tests	Sn and Sp, %	PPV and NPV,%	Confirmatory Test
Factor abnormalities/deficiencies						
VWD type 1	1/1000	AD	PFA-100	Sn = 79–96[a] / Sp = 88–96[a]	PPV = 93.3 / NPV = 98.2	VWAg[b], VWF activity, VW multimer analysis, Factor VIII activity
VWD type 2A	Uncommon	AD or AR	PFA-100	Sn = 94–100[a] / Sp = 88–96[a]	PPV = 93.3 / NPV = 98.2	VWAg[b], VWF activity, VW multimer analysis, Factor VIII activity
VWD type 2B	Uncommon	AD	PFA-100	Sn = 93–96[a] / Sp = 88–96[a]	PPV = 93.3 / NPV = 98.2	VWAg[b], VWF activity, VW multimer analysis, Factor VIII activity
VWD type 2M	Uncommon	AD or AR	PFA-100	Sn = 94–97[a] / Sp = 88–96[a]	PPV = 93.3 / NPV = 98.2	VWAg[b], VWF activity, VW multimer analysis, Factor VIII activity
VWD type 2N	Uncommon	AR, or compound heterozygote	aPTT	NA	NA	VWF-Factor VIII binding assay
VWD type 3	1/300 000–1 000 000	AR, or compound heterozygote	PFA-100	Sn = 94–100[a] / Sp = 88–96[a]	PPV = 93.3 / NPV = 98.2	VWAg[b], Ristocetin cofactor, VW multimer analysis, Factor VIII activity
Factor II deficiency (prothrombin)	26 reported cases, estimated 1/1–2 million		aPTT, PT (may be normal)	Sn = variable	NA	Factor II activity ± antigen levels
Factor V deficiency	1/1 million	AR	aPTT, PT	Sn = variable	NA	Factor V activity
Combined Factor V/Factor VIII deficiency	1/1 million	AR	aPTT>PT	Sn = variable	NA	Factor V and factor VIII activities
Factor VII deficiency	1/300 000–500 000	AR	PT	Sn = variable	NA	Factor VII activity
Factor VIII deficiency	1/5000 male births	X-linked	aPTT	Sn = variable	NA	Factor VIII activity
Factor IX deficiency	1/20 000 male births	X-linked	aPTT	Sn = variable	NA	Factor IX activity
Factor X deficiency	1/1 million	AR	aPTT, PT, RVV	Sn = variable	NA	Factor X activity
Factor XI deficiency	1/100 000	AR	aPTT	Sn = variable	NA	Factor XI activity
Factor XIII deficiency	1/2–5 million	AR	Clot solubility	Sn = variable	NA	Factor XIII activity
Fibrinolytic defects						
α-2 antiplasmin deficiency	~40 reported cases	AR	Euglobin lysis test	Sn = variable	NA	α-2 antiplasmin activity
PAI-1 deficiency	Very rare	AR		Sn = variable	NA	PAI -1 antigen and activity
Defects of fibrinogen						
Afibrinogenemia	1/500 000	AR	PT, aPTT	Sn = high	NA	Fibrinogen level
Hypofibrinogenemia	Less than afibrinogenemia		PT, aPTT	Sn = variable	NA	Thrombin time, fibrinogen activity
Dysfibrinogenemia	1/million		Thrombin time, fibrinogen level	Sn = variable	NA	Thrombin time, fibrinogen antigen and activity level comparison, reptilase time
Platelet disorders						
ITP	Age-related	NA	CBC	Sn = high	NA	Antiplatelet Ab (rarely needed)
Glanzmann thrombasthenia	Very rare	AR	PFA-100	Sn = 97–100	NA	Platelet aggregation testing Flow cytometry

TABLE 2 Continued

Condition	Frequency	Inheritance	Screening Tests	Sn and Sp, %	PPV and NPV,%	Confirmatory Test
Bernard Soulier syndrome	Rare	AR	PFA-100	Sn = 100	NA	Platelet aggregation testing Flow cytometry
Platelet release/storage disorders	Unknown, more common than other platelet function disorders	variable	PFA-100	Sn = 27–50	NA	Platelet aggregation and secretion Electron microscopy Molecular and cytogenetic testing

AD, autosomal dominant; AR, autosomal recessive; CBC, complete blood cell (count); NA, not available or not applicable; NPV, negative predictive value; PAI-1, plasminogen activator inhibitor-1; PPV, positive predictive value; RVV, Russell viper venom (test); Sn, sensitivity; Sp, specificity; VW, von Willebrand; VWAg, von Willebrand antigen; VWF, von Willebrand factor Ab, antibody.

a Values derived from data before 2008 National Institutes of Health Consensus guidelines. Sn and Sp using current diagnostic cutoffs unknown but would be expected to have higher Sp with lower Sn.

b May be reasonable to proceed directly to diagnostic testing depending on availability. See accompanying technical report for detailed discussion.[24]

umbilical stump bleeding, joint hemorrhage, and excessive soft tissue bleeding, increase the probability for a bleeding disorder; however, these findings are neither sensitive nor specific for bleeding disorders.

Coagulation Tests in the Setting of ICH

For bleeding disorders that cause ICH, the prevalence of the bleeding disorder and the prevalence of ICH in patients with each specific bleeding disorder can be used to construct the probability of the specific bleeding disorder to cause ICH (Table 3). Some probabilities are so low as to preclude calculation. Testing for these conditions is likely not useful. Mild hemophilia, which might be missed if only an aPTT test is ordered, can be detected by measuring specific levels of factor VIII and factor IX. Mild hemophilia can result in ICH, particularly after mild trauma, and because of the relatively high prevalence of the condition, the probability of mild factor VIII deficiency causing or contributing to ICH is 1 in 280 000 males. In populations with a high prevalence of factor XI deficiency, such as the Ashkenazi Jewish population, it might be reasonable to measure factor XI level.

Clinical and historical information can be used to determine the need for testing in children with isolated ICH concerning for abuse (Fig 1). The initial testing panel for ICH evaluates for conditions for which the probability for the condition resulting in ICH is greater than 1 per 5 million. The panel includes testing for most factor deficiencies and afibrinogenemia. This screening panel does not test for factor XIII deficiency, VWD, fibrinolytic defects, hypofibrinogenemia, and dysfibrinogenemia. These conditions either have not been associated with ICH or they are so rarely the cause of ICH that testing for the conditions is

not reasonable. Additionally, the initial screening panel evaluates for disseminated intravascular coagulation (DIC). Because DIC can cause any type of bruising/bleeding, including ICH, the finding of DIC in the context of suspected child abuse could significantly change the clinical approach to a patient. In children with DIC and bleeding symptoms as the only finding concerning for abuse, consideration must be given to the multitude of primary causes of DIC, including trauma, sepsis, and primary bleeding disorders, among many others.

Many children with ICH suspicious for abuse, if they survive, are placed in safe settings after hospital discharge. In these cases, testing for bleeding disorders can be deferred to a later date, with the exception of ITP. If blood products have been given to the patient, as can happen in severe ICH, the definitive evaluation for bleeding disorders should be postponed until the transfused blood components are no longer in the patient's system (Table 4). Assistance from a pediatric hematologist should be considered in addressing the possibility of factor deficiencies after a transfusion has occurred.

Many aspects of bleeding disorders are under investigation, and thus, changes in the understanding of the prevalence and severity of certain bleeding symptoms related to these disorders should be expected. For example, although hemophilia A and B are X-linked diseases and, therefore, typically thought to affect only male individuals, 25% to 50% of female carriers of hemophilia report excess bleeding; therefore, measurement of factor VIII and IX levels in female patients should be considered.[29] In addition, the population prevalence and/or clinical effects of mild platelet function disorders continue to be studied. In a patient with mucocutaneous symptoms, particularly if petechiae are

TABLE 3 Probabilities for Congenital Coagulopathies Causing ICH[a]

Condition	Prevalence of Condition, Upper Limits	Prevalence of ICH, Upper Limits	Probability[b]
VWD	1/1000	Extremely rare	Low
Factor II deficiency	1/1 million	11%	1/10 million
Factor V deficiency	1/1 million	8% of homozygotes	1/10 million homozygotes
Combined factors V and VIII deficiencies	1/1 million	2%	1/50 million
Factor VII deficiency	1/300 000	4%–6.5%	1/5 million
Factor VIII deficiency	1/5000 males	5%–12%	1/50 000 males
Factor IX deficiency	1/20 000 males	5%–12%	1/200 000 males
Factor X deficiency	1/1 million	21%	1/5 million
Factor XI deficiency	1/100 000	Extremely rare	Low
Factor XIII deficiency	1/2 million	33%	1/6 million
α-2 antiplasmin deficiency	40 cases reported	Not reported	Low
Plasminogen activator inhibitor-1 deficiency	Extremely rare	Common	Low
Afibrinogenemia	1/500 000	10%	1/5 million
Dysfibrinogenemia	1/1 million	Single case report	Low

[a] The probability of having a specific bleeding disorder increases in the setting of a family history of that specific named bleeding disorder or if the patient is from an ethnicity in which a specific bleeding disorder is more common (eg, Ashkenazi Jewish people and factor XI deficiency).
[b] "Probability" indicates the probability that an individual in the general population would have the following specific coagulopathy causing an ICH.

present, platelet aggregation testing should be considered.[25] Finally, because von Willebrand factor is an acute phase reactant, its levels can vary in response to clinical status, resulting in falsely elevated results. Many times, testing must be repeated up to 3 times to ensure reliable results.[30] If significant concern for VWD exists, consultation with a pediatric hematologist is suggested.

When Testing Indicates a Possible Bleeding Disorder in the Context of an Abuse Evaluation

Positive laboratory test results require further evaluation for the possibility of false-positive results and/or the ne-

TABLE 4 Half-Lives of Coagulation Factors

Factor	Half-Life Postinfusion, h
Fibrinogen	96–150
II	60
V	24
VII	4–6
VIII	11–12
IX	22
X	35
XI	60
XIII	144–300
VWF	8–12

VWF, von Willebrand factor.
Reprinted with permission from Goodnight S, Hathaway W. *Disorders of Hemostasis and Thrombosis: A Clinical Guide.* 2nd ed. New York, NY: McGraw-Hill Professional; 2001:497.

cessity for further testing. Prolongation of the PT and aPTT because of parenchymal damage has been noted in abusive head trauma and should not automatically be interpreted as evidence of a primary bleeding disorder.[31] Additionally, consideration must be given to the likelihood of a preexisting bleeding disorder as the primary cause of a child's bleeding/bruising. For example, given the relatively high prevalence of VWD, it is inevitable that some children with VWD will be abused and present with bleeding/bruising symptoms. Determining the causative factor in these situations is challenging. Bruising is a common finding in VWD. If a child has test results consistent with VWD and bruising concerning for abuse, a short-term change in home setting may be considered, understanding the cautions needed when using this approach. Only a few case reports have attributed ICH to VWD. Most reported ICH in children with VWD would not be confused with typical abusive ICH.[32–34] Given the rarity of ICH in VWD, particularly spontaneous ICH, testing consistent with VWD does not mean that ICH is definitively attributable to VWD, and abuse must still be considered.

Interpretation of Tests

It should be noted that the aPTT can be falsely prolonged in certain circumstances, such as in the presence of a lupus anticoagulant, or can be prolonged and might not indicate a true bleeding disorder, such as in factor XII deficiency or other contact factor deficiencies. In addition, patients who experience a traumatic brain injury often have a transient coagulopathy that does not reflect an underlying congenital disorder.[31,35] Coagulation tests are very sensitive to specimen handling and should be performed in laboratories experienced with these assays. Inappropriate handling commonly leads to false-positive results.

CONCLUSIONS

Children who present with bleeding and bruising symptoms that are concerning for abuse require careful evaluation for the potential of bleeding disorders as a cause. No single panel of tests rules out every possible bleeding disorder. Given the rarity of most bleeding disorders and the possible presence of specific clinical factors that decrease the likelihood of a bleeding disorder causing a child's findings, in many situations, extensive laboratory evaluation is not necessary. If a laboratory evaluation is conducted, tests should be chosen on the basis of the prevalence of the condition, patient and family history, ease of testing, blood volume required for testing, and, in the case of ICH, probability of a bleeding disorder causing ICH. Further consultation with a pediatric hematologist is recommended if specific, expanded testing is necessary, if preliminary testing suggests the presence of a bleeding disorder, if testing to rule out a specific bleeding disorder is needed, or if testing for very rare conditions is preferred.

GUIDANCE FOR PEDIATRICIANS

In children who have bruising or bleeding that is suspicious for abuse,

1. Complete medical, trauma, and family histories and a thorough physical examination are critical tools in evaluating for the possibility of abuse or medical conditions that predispose to bleeding/bruising.

2. In each case, careful consideration of the possibility of a medical condition causing the bleeding/ bruising is essential. Specific elements of the history and characteristics of the bleeding/bruising can be used to determine the need for a laboratory evaluation for bleeding disorders.

3. If the evaluation indicates a need for laboratory testing for bleeding disorders, initial testing is focused on the prevalence of the condition and potential of each specific condition to cause the specific findings in a given child (Fig 1).

4. Laboratory testing suggestive or indicating the presence of a bleeding disorder does not eliminate abuse from consideration. In children with bruising and laboratory testing suggestive of a bleeding disorder, a follow-up evaluation after a change in home setting can provide valuable information regarding the likelihood of a bleeding disorder causing the concerning findings.

5. Children with ICH often receive blood product transfusions. It is suggested that screening for bleeding disorders in these patients be delayed until elimination of the transfused blood clotting elements.

6. The discovery of new information regarding condition prevalence, laboratory testing, and clinical presentations of bleeding disorders is to be expected. Close collaboration with a pediatric hematologist is necessary to ensure the most current evaluation and testing methods.

LEAD AUTHORS

James D. Anderst, MD, MS
Shannon L. Carpenter, MD, MS
Thomas C. Abshire, MD

SECTION ON HEMATOLOGY/ONCOLOGY EXECUTIVE COMMITTEE, 2012–2013

Jeffrey Hord, MD, Chairperson
Gary Crouch, MD
Gregory Hale, MD
Brigitta Mueller, MD
Zora Rogers, MD
Patricia Shearer, MD
Eric Werner, MD, Immediate Past Chairperson

FORMER EXECUTIVE COMMITTEE MEMBERS

Stephen Feig, MD
Eric Kodish, MD
Alan Gamis, MD

LIAISONS

Edwin Forman, MD — *Alliance for Childhood Cancer*

CONSULTANT

Shannon Carpenter, MD, MS
Thomas Abshire, MD

STAFF

Suzanne Kirkwood, MS

COMMITTEE ON CHILD ABUSE AND NEGLECT, 2012–2013

Cindy W. Christian, MD, Chairperson
James Crawford-Jakubiak, MD
Emalee Flaherty, MD
John M. Leventhal, MD
James Lukefahr, MD
Robert Sege, MD PhD

LIAISONS

Harriet MacMillan, MD — *American Academy of Child and Adolescent Psychiatry*
Catherine Nolan, MSW — *ACSW, Administration for Children, Youth, and Families, Office on Child Abuse and Neglect*
Janet Saul, PhD — *Centers for Disease Control and Prevention*

CONSULTANT

James Anderst, MD, MS

STAFF

Tammy Piazza Hurley
Sonya Clay

REFERENCES

1. Lieder HS, Irving SY, Mauricio R, Graf JM. Munchausen syndrome by proxy: a case report. *AACN Clin Issues.* 2005;16(2):178–184

2. Ulinski T, Lhopital C, Cloppet H, et al. Munchausen syndrome by proxy with massive proteinuria and gastrointestinal hemorrhage. *Pediatr Nephrol.* 2004;19(7):798–800

3. Stricker T, Lips U, Sennhauser FH. Oral bleeding: Child abuse alert. *J Paediatr Child Health.* 2002;38(5):528–529

4. Walton LJ, Davies FC. Nasal bleeding and non-accidental injury in an infant. *Arch Dis Child.* 2010;95(1):53–54

5. Paranjothy S, Fone D, Mann M, et al. The incidence and aetiology of epistaxis in infants: a population-based study. *Arch Dis Child.* 2009;94(6):421–424

6. McIntosh N, Mok JY, Margerison A. Epidemiology of oronasal hemorrhage in the first 2 years of life: implications for child

protection. *Pediatrics*. 2007;120(5):1074–1078

7. Goodnight S, Hathaway W. *Disorders of Hemostasis and Thrombosis: A Clinical Guide*. 2nd ed. New York, NY: McGraw-Hill; 2001

8. Anderst JD, Kellogg N, Jung I. Is the diagnosis of physical abuse changed when Child Protective Services consults a Child Abuse Pediatrics subspecialty group as a second opinion? *Child Abuse Negl*. 2009; 33(8):481–489

9. O'Hare AE, Eden OB. Bleeding disorders and non-accidental injury. *Arch Dis Child*. 1984; 59(9):860–864

10. Scimeca PG, Cooper LB, Sahdev I. Suspicion of child abuse complicating the diagnosis of bleeding disorders. *Pediatr Hematol Oncol*. 1996;13(2):179–182

11. Jenny C, Hymel KP, Ritzen A, Reinert SE, Hay TC. Analysis of missed cases of abusive head trauma. *JAMA*. 1999;281(7):621–626

12. Sugar NF, Taylor JA, Feldman KW; Puget Sound Pediatric Research Network. Bruises in infants and toddlers: those who don't cruise rarely bruise. *Arch Pediatr Adolesc Med*. 1999;153(4):399–403

13. Carpenter RF. The prevalence and distribution of bruising in babies. *Arch Dis Child*. 1999;80(4):363–366

14. Maguire S, Mann MK, Sibert J, Kemp A. Are there patterns of bruising in childhood which are diagnostic or suggestive of abuse? A systematic review. *Arch Dis Child*. 2005;90(2):182–186

15. Jenny C, Reese R. Cutaneous manifestations of child abuse. In: Reese RM, Christian CW, eds. *Child Abuse Medical Diagnosis and Management*. 3rd ed. Chicago, IL: American Academy of Pediatrics; 2009:19–51

16. Chadwick DL, Bertocci G, Castillo E, et al. Annual risk of death resulting from short falls among young children: less than 1 in 1 million. *Pediatrics*. 2008;121(6):1213–1224

17. Dunstan FD, Guildea ZE, Kontos K, Kemp AM, Sibert JR. A scoring system for bruise patterns: a tool for identifying abuse. *Arch Dis Child*. 2002;86(5):330–333

18. Feldman KW. Patterned abusive bruises of the buttocks and the pinnae. *Pediatrics*. 1992;90(4):633–636

19. Jackson J, Carpenter SL, Anderst JD. Challenges in the evaluation for possible abuse: presentations of congenital bleeding disorders in childhood. *Child Abuse Negl*. 2012;36(2):127–134

20. Sirotnak AP. Medical disorders that mimic abusive head trauma. In: Frasier L, Rauth-Farley K, Alexander R, Parrish R, eds. *Abusive Head Trauma in Infants and Children*. St Louis, MO: G W Medical Publishing; 2006: 191–214

21. Dinehart SM, Henry L. Dietary supplements: altered coagulation and effects on bruising. *Dermatol Surg*. 2005;31(7 pt 2):819–826, discussion 826

22. Mishra P, Naithani R, Dolai T, et al. Intracranial haemorrhage in patients with congenital haemostatic defects. *Haemophilia*. 2008;14(5):952–955

23. Nelson MD, Jr, Maeder MA, Usner D, et al. Prevalence and incidence of intracranial haemorrhage in a population of children with haemophilia. The Hemophilia Growth and Development Study. *Haemophilia*. 1999; 5(5):306–312

24. Carpenter SL, Abshire T, Anderst JD; American Academy of Pediatrics, Section on Hematology/Oncology and Committee on Child Abuse and Neglect. Technical report: evaluation for conditions that predispose to bleeding when child abuse is suspected. *Pediatrics*. 2012; (in press)

25. Hayward CPM, Rao AK, Cattaneo M. Congenital platelet disorders: overview of their mechanisms, diagnostic evaluation and treatment. *Haemophilia*. 2006;12(suppl 3): 128–136

26. Nichols WL, Hultin MB, James AH, et al. von Willebrand disease (VWD): evidence-based diagnosis and management guidelines, the National Heart, Lung, and Blood Institute (NHLBI) Expert Panel report (USA). *Haemophilia*. 2008;14(2):171–232

27. Shearer MJ. Vitamin K deficiency bleeding (VKDB) in early infancy. *Blood Rev*. 2009;23 (2):49–59

28. Miyasaka M, Nosaka S, Sakai H, et al. Vitamin K deficiency bleeding with intracranial hemorrhage: focus on secondary form. *Emerg Radiol*. 2007;14(5):323–329

29. Plug I, Mauser-Bunschoten EP, Bröcker-Vriends AH, et al. Bleeding in carriers of hemophilia. *Blood*. 2006;108(1):52–56

30. National Heart, Lung, and Blood Institute. *The Diagnosis, Evaluation and Management of von Willebrand Disease*. Bethesda, MD: National Heart, Lung, and Blood Institute, National Institutes of Health, US Department of Health and Human Services; December 2007. NIH Publication No. 08-5832

31. Hymel KP, Abshire TC, Luckey DW, Jenny C. Coagulopathy in pediatric abusive head trauma. *Pediatrics*. 1997;99(3):371–375

32. Ragni MV, Bontempo FA, Hassett AC. von Willebrand disease and bleeding in women. *Haemophilia*. 1999;5(5):313–317

33. Ziv O, Ragni MV. Bleeding manifestations in males with von Willebrand disease. *Haemophilia*. 2004;10(2):162–168

34. Mizoi K, Onuma T, Mori K. Intracranial hemorrhage secondary to von Willebrand's disease and trauma. *Surg Neurol*. 1984;22 (5):495–498

35. Talving P, Lustenberger T, Lam L, et al. Coagulopathy after isolated severe traumatic brain injury in children. *J Trauma*. 2011;71(5):1205–1210

The Evaluation of Children in the Primary Care Setting When Sexual Abuse Is Suspected

- *Clinical Report*

CLINICAL REPORT

The Evaluation of Children in the Primary Care Setting When Sexual Abuse Is Suspected

abstract

This clinical report updates a 2005 report from the American Academy of Pediatrics on the evaluation of sexual abuse in children. The medical assessment of suspected child sexual abuse should include obtaining a history, performing a physical examination, and obtaining appropriate laboratory tests. The role of the physician includes determining the need to report suspected sexual abuse; assessing the physical, emotional, and behavioral consequences of sexual abuse; providing information to parents about how to support their child; and coordinating with other professionals to provide comprehensive treatment and follow-up of children exposed to child sexual abuse. *Pediatrics* 2013;132:e558–e567

Carole Jenny, MD, MBA, James E. Crawford-Jakubiak, MD, and COMMITTEE ON CHILD ABUSE AND NEGLECT

KEY WORD
sexual abuse

ABBREVIATIONS
AAP—American Academy of Pediatrics
HIV—human immunodeficiency virus
NAAT—nucleic acid amplification test
STI—sexually transmitted infection

This document is copyrighted and is property of the American Academy of Pediatrics and its Board of Directors. All authors have filed conflict of interest statements with the American Academy of Pediatrics. Any conflicts have been resolved through a process approved by the Board of Directors. The American Academy of Pediatrics has neither solicited nor accepted any commercial involvement in the development of the content of this publication.

The guidance in this report does not indicate an exclusive course of treatment or serve as a standard of medical care. Variations, taking into account individual circumstances, may be appropriate.

INTRODUCTION

Sexual abuse of children and adolescents is a common problem that is potentially damaging to their long-term physical and psychological health. The Fourth National Incidence Study on Child Abuse and Neglect[1] estimated that in 2006, 1.8 children per 1000 (or a total of 135 300 children) were victims of sexual abuse. Other national studies have found that 5% to 25% of adults reported being sexually abused as children, depending on the population studied and the methods used to define sexual abuse.[2–7] Pediatricians are likely to care for sexually abused children in their practices, even though many victims wait years before telling anyone about their abuse.[8,9] More than half of sexually abused children do not disclose their abuse until they are adults.[10]

A history of childhood sexual abuse can have lifelong deleterious effects on a child's physical and mental health. Sexual abuse increases the risk of developing posttraumatic stress disorder, anxiety disorder, depression,[11,12] low self-esteem,[13] and social phobias.[14] Children exposed to sexual abuse are more likely to need hospitalization for mental illness.[15] Adult survivors of child sexual abuse are more likely to become victims of intimate partner violence and sexual assault.[16,17] They are at higher risk of developing obesity,[18] sexual problems,[19] irritable bowel syndrome,[20] fibromyalgia,[21] and sexually transmitted infections (STIs), including infection with the human immunodeficiency virus (HIV).[22,23] They use more medical services as adults than those without a history of child sexual abuse[21,24] and are more likely to develop addictions to tobacco, drugs, and alcohol.[25–27]

www.pediatrics.org/cgi/doi/10.1542/peds.2013-1741

doi:10.1542/peds.2013-1741

All clinical reports from the American Academy of Pediatrics automatically expire 5 years after publication unless reaffirmed, revised, or retired at or before that time.

PEDIATRICS (ISSN Numbers: Print, 0031-4005; Online, 1098-4275).

In summary, child sexual abuse occurs commonly and can have lifelong effects on victims' physical and mental health. When the issue of possible sexual abuse is raised in the clinical setting, it is important for pediatricians to know how to respond to and evaluate the child, when to refer the child for evaluation by other professionals, when to report the case to the appropriate investigative agency, and how to counsel parents to decrease the long-term deleterious effects of the abuse. This clinical report updates an American Academy of Pediatrics (AAP) report from 2005 titled "The Evaluation of Sexual Abuse in Children."[28]

RESPONDING TO A PARENT'S CONCERN ABOUT POSSIBLE SEXUAL ABUSE

When a parent brings up the possibility of sexual abuse of his or her child, the pediatrician should immediately exclude the child from the discussion. Children (particularly young children) might be influenced by hearing their parents' concerns about abuse. Sometimes parents are overconcerned about normal childhood sexual behavior.[29] In those cases, reassuring and educating the parents will probably assuage their fears. Parents' overconcern could be related to their own adverse experiences in childhood, and in such cases, a more in-depth assessment to assist the parent is needed. Occasionally, parents might have concerns about possible sexual abuse because of relationship issues that arise between caregivers. Many of these concerns are raised in good faith but ultimately unfounded. Notwithstanding these caveats, every concern about possible sexual abuse should be approached objectively, thoughtfully, and with an open mind.

The pediatrician faces many challenges in evaluating possible sexual abuse to determine which cases warrant an immediate intervention in the office and which cases warrant reporting to investigative agencies or referral for evaluation by other professionals. In all these cases, the pediatrician should carefully document the parent's concerns, take a detailed history of the nature of the child's disclosure from the parents' perspective, ask what questions the parent used in eliciting the disclosure, and document a complete medical history, social history, and review of systems for urogenital and behavioral problems. It is important to note in the record the source of the information documented in the medical record. For example, be sure to say, "Mother tells me that the child said . . .," rather than writing, "The child said. . . ."

Often, a child will present to the pediatrician after direct disclosure to another person regarding sexual abuse. Less commonly, a child presents to the pediatrician with an abnormal genital or anal examination, pregnancy, an STI, or sexual abuse witnessed by a third party or by discovery of sexually graphic images or videos in the possession of a potential perpetrator. The general pediatrician's response depends on what resources are available in the community. Many communities and regions have specialized clinics or child advocacy centers where children can be referred when concerns of sexual abuse arise. In areas without these resources, the general pediatrician is often the most knowledgeable professional in the community regarding the evaluation and interviewing of children. If pediatricians find that their regions do not offer specialized abuse-related services (eg, child advocacy centers or hospital-based child protection programs), it is important for them to educate themselves about childhood genital and anal examinations and about how to interview children to get enough information to make appropriate decisions about reporting to child protective service agencies, referring to counseling facilities, or referring to pediatric clinics specializing in abuse evaluations. The AAP offers a variety of educational materials on child abuse to physicians, including a comprehensive CD-ROM,[30] textbooks on child abuse,[31,32] and educational offerings at the National Conference and Exhibition.

Whenever the issue of possible child sexual abuse arises in the office setting, 5 important issues should be addressed.

1. **The child's safety.** Is the child safe to go home? Is the child at imminent risk of additional harm if sent back to an environment where a possible perpetrator has access to the child? Is the child likely to be harmed or punished for disclosing abuse? Is there concern that the child might be coerced or intimidated to recant the disclosure? If any of these questions are answered "yes" or "maybe," this is a child protection emergency, and the appropriate authorities (child protective services or law enforcement) should be contacted immediately.

2. **Reporting to child protection authorities.** If the child is not at imminent risk, the pediatrician should decide whether child protective services should be contacted about the allegation. It is important to remember that in every state, and in all provinces and territories in Canada, it is mandated that professionals report *suspected* child abuse and neglect to the appropriate government agency (child protective services or police agencies, including tribal agencies). Studies have shown that some pediatricians are hesitant to involve outside agencies,

even if they strongly suspect abuse has occurred.[33] Pediatricians worry about the intrusion of agencies into family life, the risk of the child being separated from the parents, or the possibility that the family will leave the practice if reported to a child protection agency. Some pediatricians have experienced negative interactions with child protection agencies, which could make them distrustful of an agency's response and its effect on the family.[34] Some physicians might overestimate their ability to manage the situation within their practice. Physicians should not let these concerns act as barriers to protecting a child. In the United States, physicians are protected against liability for reporting a reasonable suspicion of child abuse and neglect if the report is made in good faith. This is also the case in many other jurisdictions, but because laws can vary, it is important for physicians to be familiar with the laws that pertain to their practice. Still, the safety of the child should take precedence over the physician's fear of lawsuits.

One problem lies in the definition of *suspected*. If a parent is going through a contentious divorce and the child is having symptoms of anxiety and depression, should abuse be suspected? If a child is sexually acting out with peers, should abuse be suspected? Each pediatrician will need to consider the facts of the individual case when making the decision to report suspected child abuse while bearing in mind the statutory requirements for reporting suspected abuse in his or her state. The threshold for reporting is low. The pediatrician should report when there is a reasonable suspicion that the child was abused. The child protective services agency then has the responsibility to conduct a thorough investigation to determine whether abuse has occurred.

3. **The child's mental health.** In every case, the patient should be assessed for possible mental health problems, and if any are identified, appropriate emergency mental health care should be sought. The initial disclosure of abuse can be extremely stressful for a young person. It is important to consider the possibility that symptoms of depression and posttraumatic stress disorder might already have developed. The family might be angry at the child because the disclosure has introduced stress into the family or because the threatened loss of a family member could result in financial insecurity. A disclosure of sexual abuse is perhaps one of the most explosive events that can occur in a family.

4. **The need for a physical examination.** If sexual abuse is suspected, a thorough examination should be performed to rule out injury, particularly if a child is reporting genital or anal pain or bleeding. If the abuse occurred in the distant past and the asymptomatic child is going to be referred to a specialty center for medical evaluation, examination might be deferred. If the child reports dysuria, a urinalysis is indicated. Rarely, acute sexual assault can cause severe genital or anal injury that can lead to excessive blood loss (a medical emergency).

5. **The need for forensic evidence collection.** Children who have had recent sexual contact involving the exchange of bodily fluids should be immediately referred to a specialized clinic or emergency department capable of collecting evidence using a forensic evidence kit.[35] Many states recommend that forensic evidence be collected if less than 72 hours have passed since the assault. Some states require evidence kits to be performed as late as 96 hours after assault. Some evidence supports limiting collection of forensic evidence in prepubertal children to those who present within 24 hours after assault.[36,37] As more laboratories use DNA testing to analyze forensic specimens, however, the time for collection of useful forensic evidence might be extended beyond the current 72-hour standard.[38,39] Pediatricians should familiarize themselves with the relevant policies of the jurisdiction in which they practice. The referral center also should be capable of evaluating the child for the appropriateness of antiretroviral HIV prophylaxis,[40] postexposure prophylaxis for STIs,[41] and pregnancy prophylaxis. HIV and pregnancy prophylaxis should be given as soon after the sexual contact as possible and are not recommended more than 72 hours after contact.

INTERVIEWING CHILDREN ABOUT POSSIBLE SEXUAL ABUSE

Depending on the community services available, the pediatrician should be prepared to conduct a basic interview with a verbal child about an abuse experience. Often, this is necessary to make the appropriate decision about referral to another facility or to report to child protective services. Several fundamental guidelines inform this process.

1. If the child spontaneously discloses abuse, it is important that the person hearing the disclosure respond by telling the child it is okay to talk about it with adults. If the child begins to make a disclosure and the physician says, "I'm

not the person you should tell this to," the child might be hesitant to disclose at another time.

2. The child should be separated from the parent for the interview if at all possible. Parents can subtly or not-so-subtly influence the child's statements. Separation from the parent is particularly important if the parent is a suspected perpetrator or is supportive of the suspected perpetrator, to prevent the child from feeling intimidated or threatened. The parent will later be present for the examination if that is the child's preference.

3. If the pediatrician has not already established a relationship with the patient, some time should be spent talking about nonthreatening issues, such as school, friends, or pets. It is difficult for a child to be asked painful or embarrassing questions without first feeling safe and supported by the adult asking the questions.

4. Pediatricians should tell children that it is their job as doctors to keep children healthy and that it is okay for children to talk about difficult or uncomfortable subjects with their doctors.

5. The pediatrician should not ask leading or suggestive questions. It is important to begin with open-ended, general questions about the child's likes and dislikes or about the people in the child's family. Then ask about things the child is worried or confused about, or about things that have happened to the child that have been unpleasant or stressful. A question should never suggest an answer. Examples of open-ended questions include the following:

"Is anything bothering you?"

"Tell me why you're here today."

"Do you think he would want you to tell me what happened?"

Examples of incorrect questions are as follows:

"Who touched your privates?"

"I know that Uncle Joe hurt you; tell me about it."

6. Developmentally appropriate language should be used with the child. The terms and concepts understood by a 12-year-old are very different from those understood by a 4-year-old. Be aware of the terms the child uses for the genitalia and anus. The parents should be asked in advance which terms the family uses for private parts and bathroom activities.

7. Any descriptions of abuse given by the child should be recorded word for word (using quotation marks) in the medical record, using the child's own language, and should be attributed to the child. When practical, the response should be recorded together with the question. For example, "When asked why she was not wearing underwear, the patient answered that . . ." or "Without my asking, the child stated that. . . ." Careful notes should be taken during the interview. Video or audio recording of the interview is not needed unless this is part of the pediatrician's regular practice.

8. The child should not be urged or coerced to talk about abuse. The child should be allowed to talk about it if he or she wants to, but there should never be an expectation that the child must disclose to the professional. The child should not be rewarded after a disclosure. (For example, "Tell me what happened with Uncle Joe, and then you can go back to your mom" is not an appropriate statement.) Forcing a child who has been abused to give a disclosure can be experienced by the

child as revictimization and loss of control and can make an already painful experience worse.

9. The pediatrician should remember that this is a *medical* interview and that he or she is obtaining information needed to make the appropriate diagnostic and treatment decisions. If the child makes an initial disclosure to the pediatrician, it is likely that the child will be interviewed again by another adult professional. Parents and children can be told this before the interview begins. Professionals with advanced training in forensic interviewing conduct a very different type of interview than the medical interview conducted in the clinical setting. Although it is important to avoid multiple interviews of the child, in many situations the interview will be a 2-stage process in which the initial evaluator obtains minimal facts to evaluate the need to report to the authorities, and a forensic evaluator conducts a more detailed interview.

10. The pediatrician should be supportive and empathic. Treat the patient with the same respect and caring given to all your patients. If the child tells you about abuse, show appropriate concern; do not act shocked, outraged, or dismissive.

11. Appropriate language should be used to interview children. Translators should be used if necessary, and the child's use of words to describe body parts should be understood.

12. If the pediatrician records his or her impression of the child's emotions during the examination or interview, these subjective impressions should be identified as such (eg, "It was my impression

that the child seemed agitated."). Similarly, if an observation is made that may bear on the truthfulness of the history, it should be clearly identified as separate from fact (eg, "I noted that the child and her mother used identical words when answering this same question. I therefore considered the possibility that the answers may have been rehearsed.").

THE PHYSICAL EXAMINATION WHEN SEXUAL ABUSE IS SUSPECTED

Studies have shown that pediatricians often have not been properly trained to examine the genitals and anuses of children when abuse is suspected.[42] Some of the most basic knowledge, such as the appropriate identification of anatomic structures, has not always been part of pediatric residencies or physicians' continuing education.[43,44] Appropriate techniques for evaluating children's anogenital regions are an important part of pediatric education.

When the question of sexual abuse arises in the medical setting, the pediatrician might want to consider whether the child should be triaged to another facility for evaluation, such as a child advocacy center or a specialized abuse assessment clinic at a children's hospital (after considering the safety questions discussed previously). If the pediatrician does not think that the situation constitutes an emergency, he or she should consider referring the child for evaluation if he or she is not confident that he or she has the necessary examination skills. Unnecessary multiple anogenital examinations should be avoided because they can be upsetting to a sexually abused child. On the other hand, routine examination of the genitals and anus (appropriately chaperoned)[45] during well child

examinations can help patients and parents understand that anogenital health is as important as the health of other parts of the body and will familiarize pediatricians with normal anatomic structures.

The anogenital examination should be preceded by a thorough general physical examination. Children who have experienced one type of abuse also are at risk for other types of abuse or neglect. In addition, the general physical examination establishes the physician's role and is likely to be an event the child has previously experienced at a physician's office.

The nature and process of the examination should be explained to the child in age-appropriate language before the examination takes place. An appropriate chaperone must be present. Most children will want a same-gender parent in the room during the examination. If a parent is not available, a second medical professional should be in the room to reassure the child, to assist the examining physician, and to act as a chaperone. A parent or caring professional at the head of the examination table can provide support for the child as well as reasonable assurance and distraction during the examination. Use of appropriate gowns and drapes can protect the child's modesty and make the child feel less vulnerable.

The examination of the genitalia and anus does not require the use of instruments in most cases. For girls, separation of the labia and gentle labial traction while the child is supine with the knees bent and hips abducted (frog-leg position) will adequately expose the genital structures. Speculum examinations are contraindicated in prepubertal children in the office setting. If intravaginal trauma is suspected, vaginoscopy should be performed under anesthesia.

In an adolescent, an examination for sexual abuse should follow the recommendations of the AAP regarding intravaginal examination using a speculum.[46] In many cases, a speculum examination is not needed in the absence of signs or symptoms of genital disease but is usually indicated after acute vaginal sexual assault to document injuries and to collect forensic specimens.[47] Girls should receive their first cervical cytologic examination (Papanicolaou test) at 21 years of age unless there are special circumstances, such as immune suppression or infection with HIV.[46,48]

For boys, the examination of the genitals consists of inspection of the penis and scrotum, documenting any noted trauma or scarring and any other abnormalities.

Examination of the anus is performed in most cases by external inspection with gentle traction of the buttocks to expose the anal sphincter while the child is supine with the knees pulled up to the chest (cannon-ball position). Anoscopy or a digital rectal examination is not routinely indicated.

Documenting the findings of the anogenital examination is important. In specialty centers, the examination is usually documented with photographs or videos. In the pediatric office, a detailed description of the structures will suffice. If photographs are taken, however, they should be treated as a confidential part of the medical record, and care should be taken to label them for proper identification.

An expert committee that has written practice standards for medical examinations in child advocacy centers recommends that all examinations be reviewed by an expert clinician.[49] This usually entails a secondary review of photographs or videos to verify the physical findings. If the examination findings are deemed to be abnormal or consistent with trauma, pediatricians also should have a secondary review of physical findings, either by having a clinician experienced in forensic anogenital examinations review the photographs or by referring the child to a center specializing in child abuse. Studies have shown there to be better agreement on interpretation of examination findings when clinicians have had extensive experience and education in the evaluation of child sexual abuse.[50]

All pediatricians should gain experience in the anogenital examination of children and adolescents. Many conditions can mimic trauma. It is important to recognize these findings and to distinguish them from lesions caused by child abuse.[51] The Supplemental Appendix reviews genital and anal conditions that can be confused with sexual abuse.

Most sexually abused children have normal anogenital examinations.[52,53] Many types of molestation (eg, oral genital contact or fondling) leave no permanent scars or marks. Even children who have been sexually penetrated often have normal examinations.[53,54] Anogenital tissues heal quickly and completely after many types of anal or genital trauma.[55,56] A normal examination of the genitals and anus neither confirms nor rules out sexual abuse. This fact should be mentioned in the assessment portion of the record. After the examination, it is important to reassure the child that he or she is healthy.

TESTING FOR STIs

STIs occur infrequently in prepubertal sexually abused children. A recent multisite prospective study of 536 children evaluated for suspected sexual abuse revealed that 8.2% of the female children younger than 14 years had an STI.[57] Chlamydia trachomatis

infections were found in 3.1% of the girls, and Neisseria gonorrhoeae infections were found in 3.3%. Only 1 girl tested positive for syphilis (0.3%), and none tested positive for HIV. Five of 12 girls with genital lesions tested positive for herpes simplex virus. Five of 85 symptomatic girls (5.9%) had Trichomonas vaginalis identified on a wet mount. Girls with vaginal discharge were more likely to have an STI.

Because STIs are not common in prepubertal children evaluated for abuse, culturing all sites for all organisms is not recommended if the child is asymptomatic. Each case should be evaluated individually for STI risk. Factors that should lead the physician to consider screening for STI include the following[41]:

1. Child has experienced penetration of the genitalia or anus.

2. Child has been abused by a stranger.

3. Child has been abused by a perpetrator known to be infected with an STI or at high risk of STIs (intravenous drug abusers, men who have sex with men, or people with multiple sexual partners).

4. Child has a sibling or other relative in the household with an STI.

5. Child lives in an area with a high rate of STI in the community.

6. Child has signs or symptoms of STIs.

7. Child has already been diagnosed with 1 STI.

Sexually abused adolescents are at higher risk of STIs and should be screened for all STIs, as would any sexually active adolescent presenting for routine care.

Genital and anal infections with N gonorrhoeae are rarely acquired perinatally, and outside the newborn period they are considered likely to be caused by sexual abuse.[58] C trachomatis infections in children older than

3 years also are likely to be sexually transmitted.[59] T vaginalis infection also should raise a concern of possible abuse.[60] Herpes simplex virus and genital warts (human papillomavirus) can be sexually transmitted in children, but these infections are not diagnostic of abuse by themselves.[61] HIV infections in children who have not been exposed to the virus perinatally, through blood products, or by needle sticks are also highly likely to be caused by abuse.[62] In any case of an STI in a child, a careful investigation into risk factors and contacts should be conducted, a thorough medical and social history should be obtained, and the child should be evaluated for possible sexual abuse.

The recommendations for laboratory methods best used to detect infection with C trachomatis and N gonorrhoeae in abused children are evolving. Current standards require these organisms to be confirmed by culture in cases of suspected sexual abuse that involve the legal system.[41] However, a recent multicenter study found that commercially available nucleic acid amplification tests (NAATs) are highly sensitive and specific for these organisms and that these tests provide "a better alternative than culture as a forensic standard."[63] The study also found that NAATs performed on urine specimens worked as well as vaginal swabs to detect infection in both prepubertal and postpubertal girls, obviating more invasive tests. All positive NAAT results in this study were confirmed by genotypic and sequence analysis tests, leading to a high positive predictive value for C trachomatis and N gonorrhoeae.

In medicolegal cases, culture-based tests have been preferred because of their high specificity (nearing 100%). This would make the possibility of a false-positive result highly unlikely. Unfortunately, culture-based tests for C trachomatis and N gonorrhoeae are very insensitive. In addition, many laboratories no longer offer culture-based tests, making it impossible to screen victims for infection using culture methods. If laboratories do maintain limited culture facilities, they would be more likely to provide false results, given limited experience with cultures. Because NAATs provide highly sensitive detection of organisms and their specificity approaches that of culture, the AAP recommends the use of NAATs when evaluating children and adolescents for genital infections with *C trachomatis* and *N gonorrhoeae*.

All positive test results should be considered presumptive evidence of infection and, if used, should be interpreted with caution. Positive results should be confirmed using additional tests in populations with a low prevalence of the infection or when a false-positive test could have an adverse outcome. When establishing a protocol to evaluate positive NAAT results for *N gonorrhoeae* or *C trachomatis*, experts in laboratory medicine and pediatric infectious diseases should be consulted to determine appropriate secondary tests. All positive specimens in suspected abuse cases should be retained by the laboratory for additional testing.

Recently, various rapid antigen tests, DNA hybridization tests, and NAATs have been developed for *Candida* species, *Gardnerella vaginalis*, and *T vaginalis*.[64] These tests have not been extensively studied in children and should not be used at this time. Bacterial vaginosis (the vaginosis associated with *G vaginalis*) and genital candidiasis are not specific indicators of sexual abuse.

By recommending the use of NAATs for *N gonorrhoeae* and *C trachomatis* in cases of suspected sexual abuse of children, the AAP recognizes that pediatricians' first priority should be protecting the health of children. The pediatrician should be considered primarily a provider of health care for children and should prioritize ensuring the health and well-being of their patients rather than focusing on the legal outcome of criminal cases. In practice, rarely have cases of suspected sexual abuse been adjudicated on the basis of a positive test result for an STI alone in the absence of a history, physical finding, or other confirmatory evidence of abuse. Although properly collected, tested, and confirmed laboratory specimens can aid in the prosecution of sex offenders, the pediatrician's main responsibility lies in protecting the child's health.

The Food and Drug Administration has not approved NAATs for the diagnosis of *C trachomatis* or *N gonorrhoeae* infections of the throat or anus. The Food and Drug Administration does allow laboratories to use NAATs for testing nongenital specimens if the individual laboratory undergoes internal validation of the method used in a method verification study. In verification studies, positive and negative specimens are compared with reference standards or with results from a second laboratory.[65] No studies have been published evaluating the use of nongenital-site NAATs in prepubertal children. However, studies in adults have had promising results when using some NAATs to test for rectal or pharyngeal *N gonorrhoeae* and *Chlamydia* infections in high-risk populations.[66–68] At this point, the use of NAATs in children for rectal or pharyngeal specimens is not warranted until more research is available. If used, they should be interpreted with caution.

If diagnosed with an STI, the child should be treated promptly. When there is a possibility that the child has been exposed to HIV, proper follow-up or prophylaxis is needed. When appropriate, consideration should be given to treating the patient with emergency contraception.

WORKING WITH FAMILIES TO MITIGATE THE ADVERSE EFFECTS OF SEXUAL ABUSE

When children disclose sexual abuse, people close to them are usually deeply affected. Parents often have feelings of guilt for not protecting their children[68,69] and might experience intense anger at the abusers. A child's disclosure can exacerbate a parent's own feelings about his or her adverse childhood experiences. Previous family conflict (eg, marital conflict, substance abuse issues) can be aggravated. Some parents want to sweep the disclosure under the rug to avoid dealing with the painful reality. Family members can feel protective of the accused abuser, especially if that person is another family member. Families should be given the following guidance about how to respond to children who disclose abuse.

1. Parents should understand that medical professionals are required to report suspected abuse to the proper authorities for investigation. It is not an option for the pediatrician to keep the disclosure secret.

2. It is important for families to cooperate with agencies investigating the alleged abuse.

3. Studies have shown that the long-term outcomes of children who have experienced sexual abuse are better if they are believed and supported after a disclosure.[11,70] The parents' initial response to the disclosure is important. If the parents show extreme distress and become nonfunctional, the child will feel less secure and less protected. If the parents are openly emotional and weeping, the child might feel that he or she has to recant or minimize the abuse to decrease the parents' distress.

Parents should respond in a calm and protective manner, assuring the child that the abuse was not his or her fault and that they will do all they can to protect the child and keep him or her safe.

4. Parents should not independently try to question the child or accuse the child of lying. If the child wants to talk about the abuse experience, the parent should listen and be supportive, but it is not helpful to repeatedly question the child or force the child to describe the abuse in detail. This type of questioning can be damaging to the legal adjudication of the case.

5. Pediatricians can provide guidance to families by recognizing the importance of mental health assessment after childhood trauma and by familiarizing themselves with mental health treatments that have been shown to be effective in ameliorating the effects of abuse.[71] Children should be treated by therapists with proper training and experience in dealing with child trauma. Options are available to facilitate the delivery of psychological services to abused children through child advocacy centers, community mental health centers, and victims' compensation programs.

GUIDANCE FOR PEDIATRICIANS

1. Pediatricians should understand the mandatory child abuse reporting laws in their states and should know how to make a report to the responsible agency in their jurisdiction that investigates cases of alleged child sexual abuse.

2. Pediatricians should recognize that sexual abuse of children occurs commonly, and they should be prepared to respond appropriately in their clinical practices.

3. Pediatricians should be aware of normal, developmentally appropriate variations in children's sexual behaviors.[29]

4. Pediatricians should be aware of community resources available to assist in the evaluation of alleged child abuse.

5. Pediatricians should be educated about normal and abnormal genital and anal anatomy in children.

6. Pediatricians should seek a second expert opinion in cases of child sexual abuse when the child's anal or genital examination is thought to be abnormal.

7. Pediatricians should know when and where to refer cases of acute alleged sexual abuse or assault that require forensic testing, prophylaxis for STIs and HIV, and emergency contraception.

8. Pediatricians should know the importance of using nonleading, open-ended questions if they are asking questions about possible abuse.

9. Pediatricians should understand how to support children and families when child sexual abuse is suspected.

10. Pediatricians should be aware of the effects of sexual abuse on children's mental health and be able to refer abused children to mental health professionals who have expertise in treating child trauma.

11. Advice on protection of children from sexual abuse should be part of the anticipatory guidance given to parents in the medical home. The AAP Web site provides guidance for pediatricians (http://www.aap.org/en-us/advocacy-and-policy/aap-health-initiatives/Medical-Home-for-Children-and-Adolescents-Exposed-to-Violence/Pages/Sexual-Abuse.aspx) and for parents (http://www.aap.org/en-us/about-the-aap/aap-press-room/news-features-and-safety-tips/Pages/Parent-Tips-for-Preventing-and-Identifying-Child-Sexual-Abuse.aspx) about preventing child sexual abuse. In addition, the AAP developed an educational toolkit for "Preventing Sexual Violence" (https://www2.aap.org/pubserv/PSVpreview/pages/main.html).

LEAD AUTHORS

Carole Jenny, MD, MBA, FAAP Former Committee Member
James E. Crawford-Jakubiak, MD, FAAP

COMMITTEE ON CHILD ABUSE AND NEGLECT, 2011–2012

Cindy W. Christian, MD, Chairperson, FAAP
James E. Crawford-Jakubiak, MD, FAAP
Emalee G. Flaherty, MD, FAAP
John M. Leventhal, MD, FAAP
James L. Lukefahr, MD, FAAP
Robert D. Sege MD, PhD, FAAP

LIAISONS

Harriet MacMillan, MD, American Academy of Child and Adolescent Psychiatry
Catherine M. Nolan, MSW, ACSW, Administration for Children, Youth, and Families
Janet Saul, PhD, Centers for Disease Control and Prevention

STAFF

Tammy Piazza Hurley

REFERENCES

1. Kellogg N; American Academy of Pediatrics Committee on Child Abuse and Neglect. The evaluation of sexual abuse in children. *Pediatrics*. 2005;116(2):506–512

2. Sedlak AJ, Mettenburg J, Basena M, et al. Fourth National Incidence Study of Child Abuse and Neglect (NIS-4): 2004–2009. Washington, DC: US Department of Health and Human Services, Administration for Children and Families; 2010. Available at: www.acf.hhs.gov/programs/opre/abuse_neglect/natl_incid/index.html. Accessed November 4, 2012

3. Saunders BE, Kilpatrick DG, Hanson RF, Resnick HS, Walker ME. Prevalence, case characteristics, and long-term psychological correlates of child rape among women: a national survey. *Child Maltreat.* 1999;4(3):187–200

4. Tjaden P, Thoennes N. Full Report of the Prevalence, Incidence, and Consequences of Violence Against Women: Findings From the National Violence Against Women Survey. Washington, DC: US Department of Justice, National Institute of Justice; 2000. Available at: https://www.ncjrs.gov/pdffiles1/nij/183781.pdf. Accessed November 4, 2012

5. Finkelhor D. Current information on the scope and nature of child sexual abuse. *Future Child.* 1994;4(2):31–53

6. Finkelhor D, Turner H, Ormrod R, Hamby SL. Violence, abuse, and crime exposure in a national sample of children and youth. *Pediatrics.* 2009;124(5):1411–1423

7. Finkelhor D, Ormrod RK, Turner HA. Lifetime assessment of poly-victimization in a national sample of children and youth. *Child Abuse Negl.* 2009;33(7):403–411

8. Hanson RF, Self-Brown S, Fricker-Elhai AE, Kilpatrick DG, Saunders BE, Resnick HS. The relations between family environment and violence exposure among youth: findings from the national survey of adolescents. *Child Maltreat.* 2006;11(1):3–15

9. Kogan SM. Disclosing unwanted sexual experiences: results from a national sample of adolescent women. *Child Abuse Negl.* 2004;28(2):147–165

10. Smith DW, Letourneau EJ, Saunders BE, Kilpatrick DG, Resnick HS, Best CL. Delay in disclosure of childhood rape: results from a national survey. *Child Abuse Negl.* 2000;24(2):273–287

11. Roesler TA. Reactions to disclosure of childhood sexual abuse. The effect on adult symptoms. *J Nerv Ment Dis.* 1994;182(11):618–624

12. Jonas S, Bebbington P, McManus S, et al. Sexual abuse and psychiatric disorder in England: results from the 2007 Adult Psychiatric Morbidity Survey. *Psychol Med.* 2011;41(4):709–719

13. Deblinger E, Mannarino AP, Cohen JA, Steer RA. A follow-up study of a multisite, randomized, controlled trial for children with sexual abuse–related PTSD symptoms. *J Am Acad Child Adolesc Psychiatry.* 2006;45(12):1474–1484

14. Swanston HY, Plunkett AM, O'Toole BI, Shrimpton S, Parkinson PN, Oates RK. Nine years after child sexual abuse. *Child Abuse Negl.* 2003;27(8):967–984

15. Simon NM, Herlands NN, Marks EH, et al. Childhood maltreatment linked to greater symptom severity and poorer quality of life and function in social anxiety disorder. *Depress Anxiety.* 2009;26(11):1027–1032

16. Boxer P, Terranova AM. Effects of multiple maltreatment experiences among psychiatrically hospitalized youth. *Child Abuse Negl.* 2008;32(6):637–647

17. DiLillo D, Guiffre D, Tremblay GC, Peterson L. A closer look at the nature of intimate partner violence reported by women with a history of child sexual abuse. *J Interpers Violence.* 2001;16(2):116–132

18. Messman-Moore TL, Walsh KL, DiLillo D. Emotion dysregulation and risky sexual behavior in revictimization. *Child Abuse Negl.* 2010;34(12):967–976

19. Midei AJ, Matthews KA. Interpersonal violence in childhood as a risk factor for obesity: a systematic review of the literature and proposed pathways. *Obes Rev.* 2011;12(5):e159–e172

20. Feiring C, Simon VA, Cleland CM. Childhood sexual abuse, stigmatization, internalizing symptoms, and the development of sexual difficulties and dating aggression. *J Consult Clin Psychol.* 2009;77(1):127–137

21. Walker EA, Gelfand AN, Gelfand MD, Katon WJ. Psychiatric diagnoses, sexual and physical victimization, and disability in patients with irritable bowel syndrome or inflammatory bowel disease. *Psychol Med.* 1995;25(6):1259–1267

22. Finestone HM, Stenn P, Davies F, Stalker C, Fry R, Koumanis J. Chronic pain and health care utilization in women with a history of childhood sexual abuse. *Child Abuse Negl.* 2000;24(4):547–556

23. Jones DJ, Runyan DK, Lewis T, et al. Trajectories of childhood sexual abuse and early adolescent HIV/AIDS risk behaviors: the role of other maltreatment, witnessed violence, and child gender. *J Clin Child Adolesc Psychol.* 2010;39(5):667–680

24. Mosack KE, Randolph ME, Dickson-Gomez J, Abbott M, Smith E, Weeks MR. Sexual risk-taking among high-risk urban women with and without histories of childhood sexual abuse: mediating effects of contextual factors. *J Child Sex Abuse.* 2010;19(1):43–61

25. Arnow BA, Hart S, Scott C, Dea R, O'Connell L, Taylor CB. Childhood sexual abuse, psychological distress, and medical use among women. *Psychosom Med.* 1999;61(6):762–770

26. Topitzes J, Mersky JP, Reynolds AJ. Child maltreatment and adult cigarette smoking: a long-term developmental model. *J Pediatr Psychol.* 2010;35(5):484–498

27. Khoury L, Tang YL, Bradley B, Cubells JF, Ressler KJ. Substance use, childhood traumatic experience, and posttraumatic stress disorder in an urban civilian population. *Depress Anxiety.* 2010;27(12):1077–1086

28. Najdowski CJ, Ullman SE. Prospective effects of sexual victimization on PTSD and problem drinking. *Addict Behav.* 2009;34(11):965–968

29. Kellogg ND; Committee on Child Abuse and Neglect, American Academy of Pediatrics. Clinical report: the evaluation of sexual behaviors in children. *Pediatrics.* 2009;124(3):992–998

30. Lowen D, Reece RM. *Visual Diagnosis of Child Abuse on CD-ROM,* 3rd ed. Elk Grove Village, IL: American Academy of Pediatrics; 2008

31. Finkel MA, Giardino AP, eds. *Medical Evaluation of Child Sexual Abuse: A Practical Guide,* 3rd ed. Elk Grove Village, IL: American Academy of Pediatrics; 2009

32. Reece RM, Christian C, eds. *Child Abuse: Medical Diagnosis and Management,* 3rd ed. Elk Grove Village, IL: American Academy of Pediatrics; 2008

33. Flaherty EG, Sege RD, Griffith J, et al; PROS network; NMAPedsNet. From suspicion of physical child abuse to reporting: primary care clinician decision-making. *Pediatrics.* 2008;122(3):611–619

34. Flaherty EG, Jones R, Sege R; Child Abuse Recognition Experience Study Research Group. Telling their stories: primary care practitioners' experience evaluating and reporting injuries caused by child abuse. *Child Abuse Negl.* 2004;28(9):939–945

35. American Academy of Pediatrics Committee on Child Abuse and Neglect. Guidelines for the evaluation of sexual abuse of children: subject review. *Pediatrics.* 1999;103(1):186–191

36. Young KL, Jones JG, Worthington T, Simpson P, Casey PH. Forensic laboratory evidence in sexually abused children and adolescents. *Arch Pediatr Adolesc Med.* 2006;160(6):585–588

37. Christian CW, Lavelle JM, De Jong AR, Loiselle J, Brenner L, Joffe M. Forensic evidence findings in prepubertal victims of sexual assault. *Pediatrics.* 2000;106(1 pt 1):100–104

38. Thackeray JD, Hornor G, Benzinger EA, Scribano PV. Forensic evidence collection and DNA identification in acute child sexual assault. *Pediatrics.* 2011;128(2):227–232

39. Girardet R, Bolton K, Lahoti S, et al. Collection of forensic evidence from pediatric

victims of sexual assault. *Pediatrics.* 2011; 128(2):233–238

40. Fajman N, Wright R. Use of antiretroviral HIV post-exposure prophylaxis in sexually abused children and adolescents treated in an inner-city pediatric emergency department. *Child Abuse Negl.* 2006;30(8): 919–927

41. Workowski KA, Berman S; Centers for Disease Control and Prevention (CDC). Sexually transmitted diseases treatment guidelines, 2010. *MMWR Recomm Rep.* 2010;59(RR-12):1–110

42. Lentsch KA, Johnson CF. Do physicians have adequate knowledge of child sexual abuse? The results of two surveys of practicing physicians, 1986 and 1996. *Child Maltreat.* 2000;5(1):72–78

43. Narayan AP, Socolar RR, St Claire K. Pediatric residency training in child abuse and neglect in the United States. *Pediatrics.* 2006;117(6):2215–2221

44. Starling SP, Heisler KW, Paulson JF, Youmans E. Child abuse training and knowledge: a national survey of emergency medicine, family medicine, and pediatric residents and program directors. *Pediatrics.* 2009;123(4). Available at: www.pediatrics. org/cgi/content/full/123/4/e595

45. Committee on Practice and Ambulatory Medicine. Policy statement: Use of chaperones during the physical examination of the pediatric patient. *Pediatrics.* 2011;127 (5):991–993

46. Braverman PK, Breech L; Committee on Adolescence. American Academy of Pediatrics. Clinical report: gynecologic examination for adolescents in the pediatric office setting. *Pediatrics.* 2010;126(3):583–590

47. Kaufman M; American Academy of Pediatrics Committee on Adolescence. Care of the adolescent sexual assault victim. *Pediatrics.* 2008;122(2):462–470

48. American College of Obstetricians and Gynecologists. ACOG Committee Opinion No. 463: Cervical cancer in adolescents: screening, evaluation, and management. *Obstet Gynecol.* 2010;116(2 pt 1):469–472

49. Adams JA, Kaplan RA, Starling SP, et al. Guidelines for medical care of children who may have been sexually abused. *J Pediatr Adolesc Gynecol.* 2007;20(3):163–172

50. Makoroff KL, Brauley JL, Brandner AM, Myers PA, Shapiro RA. Genital examinations for alleged sexual abuse of prepubertal girls: findings by pediatric emergency medicine physicians compared with child abuse trained physicians. *Child Abuse Negl.* 2002;26(12):1235–1242

51. Adams JA. Guidelines for medical care of children evaluated for suspected sexual abuse: an update for 2008. *Curr Opin Obstet Gynecol.* 2008;20(5):435–441

52. Adams JA, Harper K, Knudson S, Revilla J. Examination findings in legally confirmed child sexual abuse: it's normal to be normal. *Pediatrics.* 1994;94(3):310–317

53. Muram D. Child sexual abuse: relationship between sexual acts and genital findings. *Child Abuse Negl.* 1989;13(2):211–216

54. Kellogg ND, Menard SW, Santos A. Genital anatomy in pregnant adolescents: "normal" does not mean "nothing happened." *Pediatrics.* 2004;113(1 pt 1). Available at: www. pediatrics.org/cgi/content/full/113/1/e67

55. McCann J, Miyamoto S, Boyle C, Rogers K. Healing of nonhymenal genital injuries in prepubertal and adolescent girls: a descriptive study. *Pediatrics.* 2007;120(5): 1000–1011

56. McCann J, Miyamoto S, Boyle C, Rogers K. Healing of hymenal injuries in prepubertal and adolescent girls: a descriptive study. *Pediatrics.* 2007;119(5). Available at: www. pediatrics.org/cgi/content/full/119/5/e1094

57. Girardet RG, Lahoti S, Howard LA, et al. Epidemiology of sexually transmitted infections in suspected child victims of sexual assault. *Pediatrics.* 2009;124(1):79–86.

58. Whaitiri S, Kelly P. Genital gonorrhoea in children: determining the source and mode of infection. *Arch Dis Child.* 2011;96(3):247–251

59. Bell TA, Stamm WE, Wang SP, Kuo CC, Holmes KK, Grayston JT. Chronic *Chlamydia trachomatis* infections in infants. *JAMA.* 1992;267(3):400–402

60. Hammerschlag MR, Alpert S, Rosner I, et al. Microbiology of the vagina in children: normal and potentially pathogenic organisms. *Pediatrics.* 1978;62(1):57–62

61. Hammerschlag MR, Guillén CD. Medical and legal implications of testing for sexually transmitted infections in children. *Clin Microbiol Rev.* 2010;23(3):493–506

62. Lindegren ML, Hanson IC, Hammett TA, Beil J, Fleming PL, Ward JW. Sexual abuse of children: intersection with the HIV epidemic. *Pediatrics.* 1998;102(4). Available at: www.pediatrics.org/cgi/content/full/102/4/E46

63. Black CM, Driebe EM, Howard LA, et al. Multicenter study of nucleic acid amplification tests for detection of *Chlamydia trachomatis* and *Neisseria gonorrhoeae* in children being evaluated for sexual abuse. *Pediatr Infect Dis J.* 2009;28(7): 608–613

64. Brown HL, Fuller DD, Jasper LT, Davis TE, Wright JD. Clinical evaluation of affirm VPIII in the detection and identification of *Trichomonas vaginalis, Gardnerella vaginalis,* and *Candida* species in vaginitis/vaginosis. *Infect Dis Obstet Gynecol.* 2004;12(1):17–21

65. US Food and Drug Administration. *ORA Laboratory Procedure,* vol. II: *Methods. Method Verification and Validation. Version No 1.5.* Silver Spring, MD: US Food and Drug Administration; 2003

66. Bachmann LH, Johnson RE, Cheng H, et al. Nucleic acid amplification tests for diagnosis of *Neisseria gonorrhoeae* and *Chlamydia trachomatis* rectal infections. *J Clin Microbiol.* 2010;48(5):1827–1832

67. Schachter J, Moncada J, Liska S, Shayevich C, Klausner JD. Nucleic acid amplification tests in the diagnosis of chlamydial and gonococcal infections of the oropharynx and rectum in men who have sex with men. *Sex Transm Dis.* 2008;35(7):637–642

68. Giannini CM, Kim HK, Mortensen J, Mortensen J, Marsolo K, Huppert J. Culture of non-genital sites increases the detection of gonorrhea in women. *J Pediatr Adolesc Gynecol.* 2010;23(4): 246–252

69. Leventhal JM, Murphy JL, Asnes AG. Evaluations of child sexual abuse: recognition of overt and latent family concerns. *Child Abuse Negl.* 2010;34(5):289–295

70. Everson MD, Hunter WM, Runyon DK, Edelsohn GA, Coulter ML. Maternal support following disclosure of incest. *Am J Orthopsychiatry.* 1989;59(2):197–207

71. Cohen JA, Mannarino AP, Deblinger EM. *Treating Trauma and Traumatic Grief in Children and Adolescents.* New York, NY: Guilford Press; 2006

Gastroesophageal Reflux: Management Guidance for the Pediatrician

• *Clinical Report*

CLINICAL REPORT

Gastroesophageal Reflux: Management Guidance for the Pediatrician

abstract

Recent comprehensive guidelines developed by the North American Society for Pediatric Gastroenterology, Hepatology, and Nutrition define the common entities of gastroesophageal reflux (GER) as the physiologic passage of gastric contents into the esophagus and gastroesophageal reflux disease (GERD) as reflux associated with troublesome symptoms or complications. The ability to distinguish between GER and GERD is increasingly important to implement best practices in the management of acid reflux in patients across all pediatric age groups, as children with GERD may benefit from further evaluation and treatment, whereas conservative recommendations are the only indicated therapy in those with uncomplicated physiologic reflux. This clinical report endorses the rigorously developed, well-referenced North American Society for Pediatric Gastroenterology, Hepatology, and Nutrition guidelines and likewise emphasizes important concepts for the general pediatrician. A key issue is distinguishing between clinical manifestations of GER and GERD in term infants, children, and adolescents to identify patients who can be managed with conservative treatment by the pediatrician and to refer patients who require consultation with the gastroenterologist. Accordingly, the evidence basis presented by the guidelines for diagnostic approaches as well as treatments is discussed. Lifestyle changes are emphasized as first-line therapy in both GER and GERD, whereas medications are explicitly indicated only for patients with GERD. Surgical therapies are reserved for children with intractable symptoms or who are at risk for life-threatening complications of GERD. Recent black box warnings from the US Food and Drug Administration are discussed, and caution is underlined when using promoters of gastric emptying and motility. Finally, attention is paid to increasing evidence of inappropriate prescriptions for proton pump inhibitors in the pediatric population. *Pediatrics* 2013;131:e1684–e1695

Jenifer R. Lightdale, MD, MPH, David A. Gremse, MD, and SECTION ON GASTROENTEROLOGY, HEPATOLOGY, AND NUTRITION

KEY WORDS
gastroesophageal reflux, gastroesophageal reflux disease, pediatrics, guidelines, review, global consensus, reflux-related disease, vomiting, regurgitation, rumination, extraesophageal symptoms, Barrett esophagus, proton pump inhibitors, diagnostic imaging, impedance monitoring, gastrointestinal endoscopy, lifestyle changes

ABBREVIATIONS
GER—gastroesophageal reflux
GERD—gastroesophageal reflux disease
GI—gastrointestinal
H2RA—histamine-$_2$ receptor antagonist
MII—multiple intraluminal impedance
PPI—proton pump inhibitor

www.pediatrics.org/cgi/doi/10.1542/peds.2013-0421

doi:10.1542/peds.2013-0421

All clinical reports from the American Academy of Pediatrics automatically expire 5 years after publication unless reaffirmed, revised, or retired at or before that time.

PEDIATRICS (ISSN Numbers: Print, 0031-4005; Online, 1098-4275).

INTRODUCTION

Gastroesophageal reflux (GER) occurs in more than two-thirds of otherwise healthy infants and is the topic of discussion with pediatricians at one-quarter of all routine 6-month infant visits.[1,2] In addition to seeking guidance from their pediatricians, parents often request evaluation by pediatric medical subspecialists.[3] It is, therefore, not surprising that strongly evidence-based guidelines incorporating state-of-the-art approaches to the evaluation and management of pediatric GER have been welcomed by both general pediatricians and pediatric medical subspecialists and surgical specialists. GER, defined as the passage of gastric contents into the esophagus, is distinguished from gastroesophageal reflux disease (GERD), which includes troublesome symptoms or complications associated with GER.[4] Differentiating between GER and GERD lies at the crux of the guidelines jointly developed by the North American Society for Pediatric Gastroenterology, Hepatology, and Nutrition and the European Society for Pediatric Gastroenterology, Hepatology, and Nutrition.[4] These definitions have further been recognized as representing a global consensus.[5] Therefore, it is important that all practitioners who treat children with reflux-related disorders are able to identify and distinguish those children with GERD, who may benefit from further evaluation and treatment, from those with simple GER, in whom conservative recommendations are more appropriate.

GER is considered a normal physiologic process that occurs several times a day in healthy infants, children, and adults. GER is generally associated with transient relaxations of the lower esophageal sphincter independent of swallowing, which permits gastric contents to enter the esophagus. Episodes of GER in healthy adults tend to occur after meals, last less than 3 minutes, and cause few or no symptoms.[6] Less is known about the normal physiology of GER in infants and children, but regurgitation or spitting up, as the most visible symptom, is reported to occur daily in 50% of all infants.[7,8]

In both infants and children, reflux can also be associated with vomiting, defined as a forceful expulsion of gastric contents via a coordinated autonomic and voluntary motor response. Regurgitation and vomiting can be further differentiated from rumination, in which recently ingested food is effortlessly regurgitated into the mouth, masticated, and reswallowed. Rumination syndrome has been identified as a relatively rare clinical entity that involves the voluntary contraction of abdominal muscles.[9] In contrast, both regurgitation and vomiting can be considered common and often nonpathologic manifestations of GER.

Symptoms or conditions associated with GERD are classified by the practice guidelines as being either esophageal or extraesophageal.[4] Both classifications can be used to define the disease, which can be further characterized by findings of mucosal injury on upper endoscopy. Esophageal conditions include vomiting, poor weight gain, dysphagia, abdominal or substernal/retrosternal pain, and esophagitis. Extraesophageal conditions have been subclassified according to both established and proposed associations; established extraesophageal manifestations of GERD can include respiratory symptoms, including cough and laryngitis, as well as wheezing in infancy.[10,11] Although older studies from the 1990s suggested that GERD may aggravate asthma, recent publications have suggested that the impact of GERD on asthma control is considerably less than previously thought.[10,12–18] Other extraesophageal manifestations include dental erosions, and proposed associations include pharyngitis, sinusitis, and recurrent otitis media. Patients can be described clinically by their symptoms or by the endoscopic description of their esophageal mucosa. GERD-associated esophageal injuries and complications found on endoscopy include reflux esophagitis, less commonly peptic stricture, and rarely Barrett esophagus and adenocarcinoma.

Although the reported prevalence of GERD in patients of all ages worldwide is increasing,[5] GERD is nevertheless far less common than GER. Population-based studies suggest reflux disorders are not as common in Eastern Asia, where the prevalence is 8.5%,[19] compared with Western Europe and North America, where the current prevalence of GERD is estimated to be 10% to 20%.[20] New epidemiologic and genetic evidence suggests some heritability of GERD and its complications, including erosive esophagitis, Barrett esophagus, and esophageal adenocarcinoma.[21–23] A few pediatric populations at high risk of GERD have also been identified, including children with neurologic impairment, certain genetic disorders, and esophageal atresia[24,25] (Table 1). The prevalence of severe, chronic GERD is much higher in pediatric patients with these "GERD-promoting" conditions. These patients may be more prone to experiencing complications of severe GERD than patients who are otherwise healthy.[26]

Population trends hypothesized to contribute to a general increase in the prevalence of GERD include global epidemics of both obesity and asthma. In some instances, GERD can be implicated as either the underlying etiology (ie, recurrent pneumonia in

TABLE 1 Pediatric Populations at High Risk for GERD and Its Complications

Neurologic impairment
Obese
History of esophageal atresia (repaired)
Hiatal hernia
Achalasia
Chronic respiratory disorders
    Bronchopulmonary dysplasia
    Idiopathic interstitial fibrosis
    Cystic fibrosis
History of lung transplantation
Preterm infants

the premature infant exacerbated by GERD) or a direct repercussion (ie, obesity leading to GERD) of such conditions. In the great majority of cases, however, GERD and comorbidities are known to occur simultaneously in patients without a clear causal relationship.

CLINICAL FEATURES OF GERD

Troublesome symptoms or complications of pediatric GERD are associated with a number of typical clinical presentations in infants and children, depending on patient age[5] (Table 2). Reflux may occur commonly in preterm newborn infants but is generally nonacidic and improves with maturation. A full discussion of reflux in neonates and preterm infants is beyond the scope of this report.

Guidelines have distinguished between manifestations of GERD in full-term infants (younger than 1 year) from those in children older than 1 year and adolescents. Common symptoms of GERD in infants include regurgitation or vomiting associated with irritability, anorexia or feeding refusal, poor weight gain, dysphagia, presumably painful swallowing, and arching of the back during feedings. Relying on a symptom-based diagnosis of GERD can be difficult in the first year of life, especially because symptoms of GERD in infants do not always resolve with acid-suppression therapy.[5,27] GERD in

TABLE 2 Common Presenting Symptoms of GERD in Pediatric Patients

Infant	Older Child/Adolescent
Feeding refusal	Abdominal pain/heartburn
Recurrent vomiting	Recurrent vomiting
Poor weight gain	Dysphagia
Irritability	Asthma
Sleep disturbance	Recurrent pneumonia
Respiratory symptoms	Upper airway symptoms (chronic cough, hoarse voice)

infants can also be associated with extraesophageal symptoms of coughing, choking, wheezing, or upper respiratory symptoms.[7] The incidence of GERD is reportedly lower in breastfed infants than in formula-fed infants.[27] In line with the natural history of regurgitation, GERD in infants is considered to have a peak incidence of approximately 50% at 4 months of age and then to decline to affect only 5% to 10% of infants at 12 months of age.[7,8]

Common symptoms of GERD in children 1 to 5 years of age include regurgitation, vomiting, abdominal pain, anorexia, and feeding refusal.[28] Generally, GERD causes troublesome symptoms without necessarily interfering with growth; however, children with clinically significant GERD or endoscopically diagnosed esophagitis may also develop an aversion to food, presumably because of a stimulus-response association of eating with pain. This aversion, combined with feeding difficulties associated with repeated episodes of regurgitation, as well as potential and substantial nutrient losses resulting from emesis, may lead to poor weight gain or even malnutrition.

Older children and adolescents are most likely to resemble adults in their clinical presentation with GERD and to complain of heartburn, epigastric pain, chest pain, nocturnal pain, dysphagia, and sour burps. When eliciting a history in school-aged children with suspected GERD, it may be important to directly ask patients themselves about their symptoms rather than relying strongly on parent report. In 1 study, adolescents were significantly more likely than their parents to report themselves to be experiencing symptoms of sour burps or nausea.[1] Extraesophageal symptoms in older children and adolescents can include nocturnal cough, wheezing, recurrent

pneumonia, sore throat, hoarseness, chronic sinusitis, laryngitis, or dental erosions. In a pediatric patient with GERD and dental erosions, the progression of tooth structure loss may be indicative that existing therapy for GERD is not effective. Conversely, stability of dental erosions is 1 measure of adequacy of GERD management.

DIAGNOSTIC STUDIES

For most pediatric patients, a history and physical examination in the absence of warning signs are sufficient to reliably diagnose uncomplicated GER and initiate treatment strategies. Generally speaking, diagnostic testing is not necessary. The reliability of symptoms to make the clinical diagnosis of GERD is particularly high in adolescents, who often present with heartburn typical of adults.[29–31] Nevertheless, dedicating at least part of a clinical visit to obtaining a clinical history and performing a physical examination are also essential to exclude more worrisome diagnoses that can present with reflux or vomiting (Table 3).

To date, no single symptom or cluster of symptoms can reliably be used to diagnose esophagitis or other complications of GERD in children or to predict which patients are most likely

TABLE 3 Concerning Symptoms and Signs ("Warning Signs" in Figures) for Primary Etiologies Presenting With Vomiting

Bilious vomiting
GI tract bleeding
  Hematemesis
  Hematochezia
Consistently forceful vomiting
Fever
Lethargy
Hepatosplenomegaly
Bulging fontanelle
Macro/microcephaly
Seizures
Abdominal tenderness or distension
Documented or suspected genetic/metabolic syndrome
Associated chronic disease

to respond to therapy.[21] Nonetheless, a number of GERD symptom questionnaires have been validated and may be useful in the detection and surveillance of GERD in affected children of all ages. Kleinman et al developed a questionnaire for infants that was validated for documentation and monitoring of parent-reported GERD symptoms.[30] Another questionnaire by Størdal et al[32] for pediatric patients 7 to 16 years of age compared favorably with results of pH monitoring. As yet another example, the GERD Symptom Questionnaire developed by Deal et al[33] appears valid for differentiating children with GERD from healthy controls but has not been compared with objective standards, such as pH monitoring or endoscopic findings.

The strategy of using diagnostic testing to diagnose GERD may also be fraught with complexity, because there is no single test that can rule it in or out. Instead, diagnostic tests must be used in a thoughtful and serial manner to document the presence of reflux of gastric contents in the esophagus, to detect complications, to establish a causal relationship between reflux and symptoms, to evaluate the efficacy of therapies, and to exclude other conditions. The diagnostic methods most commonly used to evaluate pediatric patients with GERD symptoms are upper gastrointestinal (GI) tract contrast radiography, esophageal pH and/or impedance monitoring, and upper endoscopy with esophageal biopsy. Upper GI tract series are useful to delineate anatomy and to occasionally document a motility disorder, whereas esophageal pH monitoring and intraluminal esophageal impedance represent tools to quantify GER. Upper endoscopy with esophageal biopsy represents the primary method to investigate the esophageal mucosa to both exclude other conditions that can cause GERD-like symptoms and evaluate for esophageal injury attributable to GERD.[4]

Upper GI Tract Series

Upper GI tract contrast radiography generally involves obtaining a series of fluoroscopic images of swallowed barium until the ligament of Treitz is visualized. According to the new guidelines, the routine performance of upper GI tract radiographic imaging to diagnose GER or GERD is not justified,[4] because upper GI tract series are too brief in duration to adequately rule out the occurrence of pathologic reflux, and the high frequency of nonpathologic reflux during the examination can encourage false-positive diagnoses. Additionally, observation of the reflux of a barium column into the esophagus during GI tract contrast studies may not correlate with the severity of GERD or the degree of esophageal mucosal inflammation in patients with reflux esophagitis. It is recognized that upper GI tract series are useful in the evaluation of vomiting to screen for possible anatomic abnormalities of the upper GI tract.[4] For example, in infants with bilious vomiting, an upper GI tract series may be useful for evaluating for possible malrotation or duodenal web. Persistent, forceful vomiting in the first few months of life should be evaluated with pyloric ultrasonography to evaluate for possible pyloric stenosis. An upper GI tract series should be reserved if the results of the pyloric ultrasound are equivocal.

Esophageal pH Monitoring

Continuous intraluminal esophageal pH monitoring can be used to quantify the frequency and duration of esophageal acid exposure during a study period. The conventional definition of acid exposure in the esophagus is a pH <4.0, the pH most associated with a complaint of heartburn in adults. Esophageal pH metrics generally include an absolute number of reflux episodes detected during monitoring, the duration of reflux episodes detected, and the reflux index, which is calculated as the percentage of a study period during which esophageal pH is <4.0. Although esophageal pH monitoring may be useful for associating a temporal relationship between a symptom and acid reflux and to evaluate the efficacy of pharmacologic therapy on acid suppression, mounting evidence suggests poor reproducibility of pH testing, as well as a clear continuum between pH findings in physiologic GER and pathologic GERD. In turn, esophageal pH monitoring is losing value as a primary modality for diagnosing or managing pediatric GERD.[34]

Multichannel Intraluminal Impedance Monitoring

Multiple intraluminal impedance (MII) is an emerging technology for detecting the movement of both acidic and nonacidic fluids, solids, and air in the esophagus, thereby providing a more detailed picture of esophageal events than pH monitoring.[34] MII can be used to measure volume, speed, and physical length of both anterograde and retrograde esophageal boluses. Combined pH/MII testing is evolving into the test of choice to detect temporal relationships between specific symptoms and the reflux of both acid and nonacid gastric contents. In particular, MII has been used in recent years to investigate how GER and GERD correlate with apnea, cough, and behavioral symptoms.[35] According to the new guidelines, MII and pH electrodes can and should be combined on a single catheter.[4]

Gastroesophageal Scintigraphy

Gastroesophageal scintigraphy scans for reflux of ^{99m}Tc-labeled solids or liquids into the esophagus or lungs after administration of the test material into the stomach. This nuclear scan evaluates postprandial reflux and can also quantitate gastric emptying; however, the lack of standardized techniques and age-specific normal values limits the usefulness of this test. Therefore, gastroesophageal scintigraphy is not recommended in the routine evaluation of pediatric patients with GER.[4]

Endoscopy and Esophageal Biopsy

It is certainly preferable to pursue conservative measures for treating GERD in children before considering the use of more invasive testing. In particular, any diagnostic benefits of pursuing upper endoscopy in pediatric patients suspected of having GERD must also be weighed against minimal, but not entirely negligible, procedural and sedation risks.[36] Nevertheless, the performance of upper endoscopy allows direct visualization of the esophageal mucosa to determine the presence and severity of injury from the reflux of gastric contents into the esophagus.[26] Esophageal biopsies allow evaluation of the microscopic anatomy.[24] Upper endoscopy with esophageal biopsy may be useful to evaluate inflammation in the esophageal mucosa attributable to GERD and to exclude other associated conditions with symptoms that can mimic GERD, such as eosinophilic esophagitis. Recent data confirm that approximately 25% of infants younger than 1 year will have histologic evidence of esophageal inflammation.[37] This test is indicated in patients with GERD who fail to respond to pharmacologic therapy or as part of the initial management if symptoms of poor weight gain, unexplained anemia or fecal occult blood, recurrent pneumonia, or hematemesis exist.

Upper endoscopy may also be helpful in the assessment of other causes of abdominal pain and vomiting in pediatric patients, such as esophageal or antral webs, Crohn esophagitis, peptic ulcer, *Helicobacter pylori* infection, and infectious esophagitis. Erosive esophagitis is reported less often in infants and children with GERD than in adults with GERD; however, a normal endoscopic appearance of the esophageal mucosa in pediatric patients does not exclude histologic evidence of reflux esophagitis.[5,8] Esophageal biopsy is beneficial in evaluating for conditions that may mimic symptoms of GERD, such as eosinophilic esophagitis, infectious esophagitis (*Candida* esophagitis or herpetic esophagitis), Crohn disease, or Barrett esophagus.[24] Because endoscopic findings correlate poorly with histologic testing in infants and children, performing esophageal biopsies during endoscopy is recommended for the evaluation of GERD in children.[4]

MANAGEMENT

The new guidelines describe several treatment options for treating children with GER and GERD. In particular, lifestyle changes are emphasized, because they can effectively minimize symptoms of both in infants and children. For patients who require medication, options include buffering agents, acid secretion suppressants, and promoters of gastric emptying and motility. Finally, surgical approaches are reserved for children who have intractable symptoms unresponsive to medical therapy or who are at risk for life-threatening complications of GERD.

LIFESTYLE CHANGES

Lifestyle Modifications for Infants

Lifestyle changes to treat GERD in infants may involve a combination of feeding changes and positioning therapy. Modifying maternal diet if infants are breastfed, changing formulas, and reducing the feeding volume while increasing the frequency of feedings may be effective strategies to address GERD in many patients. In particular, the guidelines emphasize that milk protein allergy can cause a clinical presentation that mimics GERD in infants. Therefore, a 2- to 4-week trial of a maternal exclusion diet that restricts at least milk and egg is recommended in breastfeeding infants with GERD symptoms, whereas an extensively hydrolyzed protein or amino acid–based formula may be appropriate in formula-fed infants.[4,30] It is important to note that this recommendation applies to the subset of infants with complications of GER, and not "happy spitters."

In 1 study of formula-fed infants, GERD symptoms resolved in 24% of infants after a 2-week trial of changing to a protein hydrolysate formula thickened with 1 tablespoon rice cereal per ounce, avoiding overfeeding, avoiding seated and supine positions, and avoiding environmental tobacco smoke.[3] Feeding changes can also be recommended in breastfed infants, because it is well known that small amounts of cow milk protein ingested by the mother may be expressed in human milk. Indeed, several studies have found that breastfed infants may benefit from a maternal diet that restricts cow milk and eggs.[38,39]

The feeding management strategy that involves the use of thickened feedings, either by adding up to 1 tablespoon of dry rice cereal per 1 oz of formula[30] or changing to commercially thickened (added rice) formulas for full-term infants who are not cow milk protein intolerant, is recognized as a reasonable management strategy for otherwise healthy infants with both GER and GERD.[4] On the other hand, all pediatric clinicians should be aware of a possible association between thickened feedings and necrotizing enterocolitis in preterm infants.[40] The Food and Drug Administration issued a warning regarding a common commercially available thickening agent in 2011, suggesting that "parents, caregivers and health care providers not...feed 'SimplyThick' to infants born before 37 weeks gestation who are currently receiving hospital care or have been discharged from the hospital in the past 30 days."

Thickened feedings appear to decrease observed regurgitation rather than the actual number of reflux episodes. Little is known about the effect of thickening formula on the natural history of infantile reflux or the potential allergenicity of commercial thickening agents. Excessive energy intake may occur with long-term use of feedings thickened with rice cereal or corn. To this point, it is important to realize that thickening a 20-kcal/oz infant formula with 1 tablespoon of rice cereal per ounce increases the energy density to 34 kcal/oz. Commercially available antiregurgitant formulae contain processed rice, corn, or potato starch; guar gum; or locust bean gum and may present an option that does not involve excess energy intake by infants when consumed in normal volumes. To date, there has been little investigation into any relationship between use of added rice cereal or antiregurgitant formulae and childhood obesity.

Lifestyle changes that may also benefit infants with GERD include keeping them in the completely upright position or even placing them prone. Indeed, a number of recent studies that used impedance and pH monitoring have confirmed older studies that used pH monitoring to demonstrate significantly less GER in infants in the flat prone position compared with the flat supine position.[41,42] However, the guidelines are unequivocal that the risk of sudden infant death syndrome in sleeping infants outweighs the benefits of prone positioning in the management of GERD and, therefore,

that prone positioning should be considered acceptable only if the infant is observed and awake.[4] Prone positioning is suggested to be beneficial in children older than 1 year with either GER or GERD, because the risk of sudden infant death syndrome is greatly decreased in older age groups. Perceived and actual benefits of seated or semisupine positioning are also explored in the new guidelines. Semisupine positioning, particularly in an infant carrier or car seat, may exacerbate GER and should be avoided when possible, especially after feeding.[43] More recent data obtained with esophageal impedance–pH monitoring have confirmed that postprandial reflux occurs similarly when infants are in car seats as when they are supine but also suggests that being in a car seat for 2 hours after a feeding reduces reflux-related respiratory events.[44]

Lifestyle Modifications for Children and Adolescents

Lifestyle changes that may benefit GERD in older children and adolescents are more akin to recommendations made for adult patients, including the importance of weight loss in overweight patients, cessation of smoking, and avoiding alcohol use. Recommendations for conservatively managing GERD in older children and adolescents, likewise, may involve dietary modification and positioning changes, although the effectiveness of the latter as a treatment of GERD in older children has not been as well studied as in infants. In terms of dietary changes, older children and adolescents are advised to avoid caffeine, chocolate, alcohol, and spicy foods as potential symptom triggers. The guidelines also point out that 3 independent studies have demonstrated decreased reflux episodes with

postprandial chewing of sugarless gum.[45–47]

PHARMACOTHERAPEUTIC AGENTS FOR PEDIATRIC GERD

Several medications may be used to treat GERD in infants and children. The 2 major classes of pharmacologic agents for treatment of GERD are acid suppressants and prokinetic agents (Table 4). Growing evidence that demonstrates the former to be more effective than the latter has led to an increased use of acid suppressants to manage suspected GERD in pediatric patients[4,39]; however, there is also significant concern for the overprescription of acid suppressants, particularly proton pump inhibitors (PPIs), and it is important to understand the new guidelines for medication indications.

Acid Suppressants

The main classes of acid suppressants are antacids, histamine-$_2$ receptor antagonists (H2RAs), and PPIs. The principles of using these medications in the treatment of pediatric GERD are similar to those in adults, other than the need to prescribe weight-adjusted doses and the need to consider the form of the drug prescribed (ie, for ease of ingestion in infants and children). Dosage ranges for drugs commonly prescribed for pediatric patients with GERD are listed in Table 4.

Antacids

Antacids are a class of medications that can be used to directly buffer gastric acid in the esophagus or stomach to reduce heartburn and ideally allow mucosal healing of esophagitis. There is limited historical evidence that on-demand use of antacids can lead to symptom relief in infants and children.[48] Instead, although antacids are generally seen as a relatively benign approach to treating pediatric

TABLE 4 Pediatric Doses of Medications Prescribed for GERD

Medications	Doses	Formulations	Ages Indicated by the Food and Drug Administration
Cimetidine	30–40 mg/kg/d, divided in 4 doses	Syrup	≥16 y
Ranitidine	5–10 mg/kg/d, divided in 2 to 3 doses	Peppermint-flavored syrup; Effervescent tablet	1 mo–16 y
Famotidine	1 mg/kg/d, divided in 2 doses	Cherry-banana-mint–flavored oral suspension	1–16 y
Nizatidine	10 mg/kg/d, divided in 2 doses	Bubble gum–flavored solution	≥12 y
Omeprazole	0.7–3.3 mg/kg/d	Sprinkle contents of capsule onto soft foods	2–16 y
Lansoprazole	0.7–3 mg/kg/d	Sprinkle contents of capsule onto soft foods or select juices Administer capsule contents in juice through nasogastric tube Strawberry-flavored disintegrating tablet Orally disintegrating tablet via oral syringe or nasogastric tube (≥8 French)	1–17 y
Esomeprazole	0.7–3.3 mg/kg/d	Sprinkle contents of capsule onto soft foods Administer capsule contents in juice through nasogastric tube	1–17 y
Rabeprazole	20 mg daily	Oral tablet	12–17 y
Dexlansoprazole	30–60 mg daily	Oral tablet	No pediatric indication
Pantoprazole	40 mg daily (adult dose)	Oral tablet	No pediatric indication

GERD, it is important to recognize that they are not entirely without risk. Indeed, several studies link aluminum-containing preparations with aluminum toxicity and its complications in children.[49–51] Similarly, milk-alkali syndrome, a triad of hypercalcemia, alkalosis, and renal failure, has been described in children receiving calcium-containing preparations and adds to a note of caution. According to the new guidelines, chronic antacid therapy is generally not recommended in pediatrics for the treatment of GERD.[4] In addition, the safety and efficacy of surface protective agents, such as alginates or sucralfate, an aluminum-containing preparation, have not been adequately studied in the pediatric population. As such, no surface agent is currently recommended as independent treatment of severe symptoms of GERD or erosive esophagitis in children.[4]

H2RAs

H2RAs represent a major class of medications that has completely revolutionized the treatment of GERD in children. H2RAs decrease the secretion of acid by inhibiting the histamine-$_2$ receptor on the gastric parietal cell. Expert opinion suggests little clinical difference between the various formulations of H2RAs. Randomized placebo-controlled pediatric clinical trials have shown that cimetidine and nizatidine are superior to placebo for the treatment of erosive esophagitis in children.[52,53] Pharmacokinetic studies in school-aged children suggest that gastric pH begins to increase within 30 minutes of administration of an H2RA and reaches peak plasma concentrations 2.5 hours after dosing. The acid-inhibiting effects of H2RAs last for approximately 6 hours, so H2RAs are quite effective if administered 2 or 3 times a day.

However, H2RAs inherently have some limitations. In particular, a fairly rapid tachyphylaxis can develop within 6 weeks of initiation of treatment, limiting its potential for long-term use. In addition, H2RAs have been shown to be less effective than PPIs in symptom relief and healing rates of erosive esophagitis. Although most of these downsides have been demonstrated most clearly in adults, they are also believed to affect children. It is also important to recognize that cimetidine has specifically been linked to an increased risk of liver disease and gynecomastia, and that these associations may be generalizable to other H2RAs.

PPIs

Most recently, PPIs have emerged as the most potent class of acid suppressants by repeatedly demonstrating superior efficacy compared with H2RAs. PPIs decrease acid secretion by inhibition of H^+, K^+-ATPase in the gastric parietal cell canaliculus. PPIs are uniquely able to inhibit meal-induced acid secretion and have a capacity to maintain gastric pH >4 for a longer period of time than H2RAs. These properties contribute to higher and faster healing rates for erosive esophagitis with PPI therapy compared with H2RA therapy. Finally, unlike H2RAs, the acid suppression ability of PPIs has not been observed to diminish with chronic use.

The timing of dosing most PPIs is important for maximum efficacy. Both pediatricians and pediatric medical subspecialists must be diligent at educating their patients to administer PPIs, ideally, approximately 30 minutes before meals.[7] All clinicians should also recognize that the metabolism of PPIs is known to differ in children compared with adults, with a trend toward a shorter half-life, necessitating a higher per-kilogram dose to achieve a peak serum concentration and area under the curve similar to those in adults.[45] A fairly wide range of effective doses is evident in children. For example, an open-label study of omeprazole in children revealed an effective dosage range of 0.7 to 3.3 mg/kg daily, on the basis of improvement in clinical symptoms and the results of esophageal pH monitoring.[47] Lansoprazole, 0.7 to 3.0 mg/kg daily, improved GERD symptoms and healed all cases of erosive esophagitis in the treatment of 1- to 12-year-old children with GERD.[48] Other trials of PPI therapy support the efficacy of treatment of severe esophagitis and esophagitis refractory to H2RAs in children.[4,45]

As in adults, PPIs are considered safe and generally well tolerated with relatively few adverse effects. In terms of their long-term use, published studies have reported PPI use for up to 11 years in small numbers of children.[16] The Food and Drug Administration has approved a number of PPIs for use in pediatric patients in recent years, including omeprazole, lansoprazole, and esomeprazole for people 1 year and older and rabeprazole for people 12 years and older. Nonetheless, the new guidelines strike a note of caution when discussing the dramatic increase in past years in the number of PPI prescriptions written for pediatric patients, particularly infants, who may be at increased risk of lower respiratory tract infections.[54–56]

Overuse or misuse of PPIs in infants with reflux is a matter for great concern. Placebo-controlled trials in infants have not demonstrated superiority of PPIs over placebo for reduction in irritability.[57] Headaches, diarrhea, constipation, and nausea have been described as occurring in up to 14% of older children and adults prescribed PPIs.[25,58] Although considered a benign histologic change, enterochromaffin cell hyperplasia has

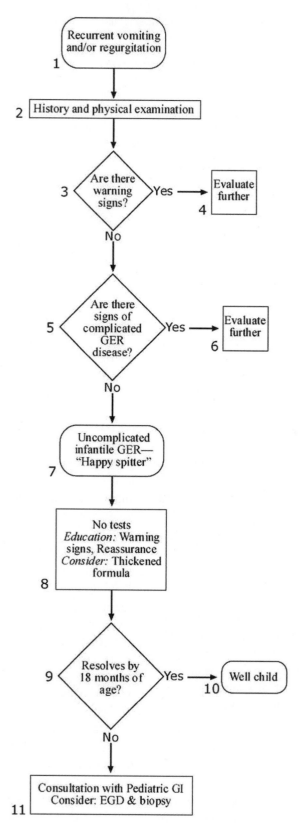

FIGURE 1

Approach to the infant with recurrent regurgitation and vomiting.

recently been demonstrated in up to 50% of children receiving PPIs for more than 2.5 years.[25] Finally, a growing body of evidence suggests that acid suppression, in general, with either H2RAs or PPIs, may be a risk factor for pediatric community-acquired pneumonia, gastroenteritis, candidemia, and necrotizing enterocolitis in preterm infants.[59,60]

Prokinetic Agents

Desired pharmacologic effects of prokinetic agents include improving contractility of the body of the esophagus, increasing lower esophageal sphincter pressure, and increasing the rate of gastric emptying. To date, efforts to design a prokinetic agent with benefits that outweigh adverse effects has proven difficult. Even metoclopramide, the most common prokinetic agent still available, recently received a black box warning regarding its adverse effects. Indeed, adverse effects have been reported in 11% to 34% of patients treated with metoclopramide, including drowsiness, restlessness, and extrapyramidal reactions. Although a meta-analysis of 7 randomized controlled trials of metoclopramide in patients younger than 2 years with GERD confirmed a decrease in GERD symptoms, it was clearly at the cost of such significant adverse effects.[61] Other drugs in this category include bethanechol, cisapride (no longer available commercially in the United States), baclofen, and erythromycin. Each works as a prokinetic by using a different mechanism. Nevertheless, after careful review, guidelines unequivocally state that there is insufficient evidence to support the routine use of any prokinetic agent for the treatment of GERD in infants or older children.[4]

Surgery for Pediatric GERD

Several surgical procedures can be used to decrease GER disorders in children. Fundoplication, whereby the gastric fundus is wrapped around the distal esophagus, is most common and can be performed to prevent reflux by increasing baseline pressure of the lower esophageal sphincter, decreasing the number of transient lower esophageal sphincter relaxations, and increasing the length of the esophagus that is intra-abdominal to accentuate the angle of His and reduce a hiatal hernia, if indicated.[17,56,57] Total esophagogastric dissociation is another operative procedure that is rarely used after failed fundoplication. Both procedures are associated with significant morbidity and do not reduce the risk of direct aspiration of oral contents. Careful patient selection is one of the keys to successful outcome.[17] Children who have failed pharmacologic treatment may be candidates for surgical therapy, as are children at severe risk of aspiration of their gastric contents. In most patients, if acid suppression with PPIs is ineffective, the accuracy of the diagnosis of GERD should be reassessed, because fundoplication may not produce optimum clinical results. Clinical conditions, such as cyclic vomiting, rumination, gastroparesis, and eosinophilic esophagitis, should

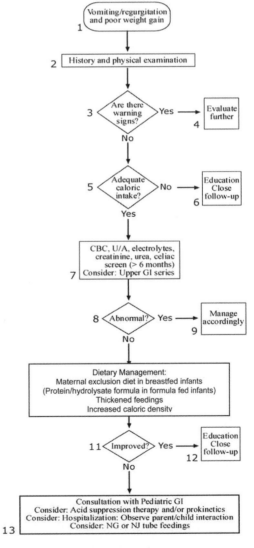

FIGURE 2

Approach to the infant with recurrent regurgitation and weight loss.

be carefully ruled out before surgery, because they are likely to still cause symptoms after surgery. If antireflux surgery is pursued, the new guidelines also stress the importance of providing families with adequate counseling and education before the procedure so that they have a "realistic understanding of the potential complications...including symptom recurrence."[4]

SUMMARY

The updated guidelines published in 2009 are particularly rich with descriptions of typical presentations of GERD across all pediatric age groups.[4] With an emphasis on evidence-based, best practice, they present a number of algorithms that can be of great use to both general pediatricians and pediatric medical subspecialists. The guidelines discuss the evaluation and management of recurrent regurgitation and vomiting in both infants and older children and the importance of distinguishing GERD from numerous other disorders. The figures shown demonstrate the recommended approaches for commonly encountered presentations of GERD in pediatric patients and are summarized here.

In the infant with uncomplicated recurrent regurgitation, it may be important to recognize physiologic GER that is effortless, painless, and not affecting growth (Fig 1). In this situation, pediatricians should focus on minimal testing and conservative management. Overuse of medications in the so-called "happy spitter" should be avoided by all pediatric physicians. Instead, pediatricians are well served to diagnose GER and provide significant parental education, anticipatory guidance, and reassurance. In turn, they will provide high-value, high-quality care without risk to their patients or unnecessary direct and indirect costs.

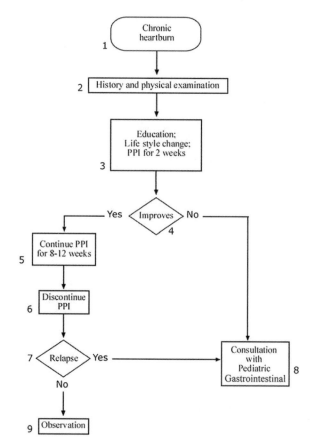

FIGURE 3
Approach to the older child or adolescent with heartburn.

Pediatricians must also be able to recognize infants with recurrent regurgitation and troublesome symptoms of GERD (Fig 2). The new guidelines emphasize weight loss as a crucial warning sign that should alter clinical management. Older children with heartburn may benefit from empirical treatment with PPIs (Fig 3). In general, there is a paucity of studies in pediatrics that demonstrate the effectiveness of this approach. Instead, it is essential to carefully follow all patients empirically treated for GERD to ensure that they are improving, because there are many clinical conditions that may mimic its symptoms. It cannot be overemphasized that pediatric best practice involves both identifying children at risk for complications of GERD and reassuring parents of patients with physiologic GER

who are not at risk for complications to avoid unnecessary diagnostic procedures or pharmacologic therapy.[62–64]

LEAD AUTHORS
Jenifer R. Lightdale, MD, MPH
David A. Gremse, MD

SECTION ON GASTROENTEROLOGY, HEPATOLOGY, AND NUTRITION EXECUTIVE COMMITTEE, 2011–2012
Leo A. Heitlinger, MD, Chairperson
Michael Cabana, MD
Mark A. Gilger, MD
Roberto Gugig, MD
Jenifer R. Lightdale, MD, MPH
Ivor D. Hill, MB, ChB, MD

FORMER EXECUTIVE COMMITTEE MEMBERS
Robert D. Baker, MD, PhD
David A. Gremse, MD
Melvin B. Heyman, MD

STAFF
Debra L. Burrowes, MHA

REFERENCES

1. Nelson SP, Chen EH, Syniar GM, Christoffel KK; Pediatric Practice Research Group. Prevalence of symptoms of gastroesophageal reflux during childhood: a pediatric practice-based survey. *Arch Pediatr Adolesc Med.* 2000;154(2):150–154

2. Campanozzi A, Boccia G, Pensabene L, et al. Prevalence and natural history of gastroesophageal reflux: pediatric prospective survey. *Pediatrics.* 2009;123(3):779–783

3. Shalaby TM, Orenstein SR. Efficacy of telephone teaching of conservative therapy for infants with symptomatic gastroesophageal reflux referred by pediatricians to pediatric gastroenterologists. *J Pediatr.* 2003;142(1):57–61

4. Vandenplas Y, Rudolph CD, Di Lorenzo C, et al; North American Society for Pediatric Gastroenterology Hepatology and Nutrition; European Society for Pediatric Gastroenterology Hepatology and Nutrition. Pediatric gastroesophageal reflux clinical practice guidelines: joint recommendations of the North American Society for Pediatric Gastroenterology, Hepatology, and Nutrition (NASPGHAN) and the European Society for Pediatric Gastroenterology, Hepatology, and Nutrition (ESPGHAN). *J Pediatr Gastroenterol Nutr.* 2009;49(4):498–547

5. Sherman PM, Hassall E, Fagundes-Neto U, et al. A global, evidence-based consensus on the definition of gastroesophageal reflux disease in the pediatric population. *Am J Gastroenterol.* 2009;104(5):1278–1295, quiz 1296

6. Shay S, Tutuian R, Sifrim D, et al. Twenty-four hour ambulatory simultaneous impedance and pH monitoring: a multicenter report of normal values from 60 healthy volunteers. *Am J Gastroenterol.* 2004;99(6):1037–1043

7. Rudolph CD, Mazur LJ, Liptak GS, et al; North American Society for Pediatric Gastroenterology and Nutrition. Guidelines for evaluation and treatment of gastroesophageal reflux in infants and children: recommendations of the North American Society for Pediatric Gastroenterology and Nutrition. *J Pediatr Gastroenterol Nutr.* 2001;32(suppl 2):S1–S31

8. Martin AJ, Pratt N, Kennedy JD, et al. Natural history and familial relationships of infant spilling to 9 years of age. *Pediatrics.* 2002;109(6):1061–1067

9. Fernandez S, Aspirot A, Kerzner B, Friedlander J, Di Lorenzo C. Do some adolescents with rumination syndrome have "supragastric vomiting"? *J Pediatr Gastroenterol Nutr.* 2010;50(1):103–105

10. Sheikh S, Goldsmith LJ, Howell L, Hamlyn J, Eid N. Lung function in infants with wheezing and gastroesophageal reflux. *Pediatr Pulmonol.* 1999;27(4):236–241

11. Sheikh S, Stephen T, Howell L, Eid N. Gastroesophageal reflux in infants with wheezing. *Pediatr Pulmonol.* 1999;28(3):181–186

12. Mastronarde JG, Anthonisen NR, Castro M, et al; American Lung Association Asthma Clinical Research Centers. Efficacy of esomeprazole for treatment of poorly controlled asthma. *N Engl J Med.* 2009;360(15):1487–1499

13. Kiljander TO, Junghard O, Beckman O, Lind T. Effect of esomeprazole 40 mg once or twice daily on asthma: a randomized, placebo-controlled study. *Am J Respir Crit Care Med.* 2010;181(10):1042–1048

14. Littner MR, Leung FW, Ballard ED, II, Huang B, Samra NK Lansoprazole Asthma Study Group. Effects of 24 weeks of lansoprazole therapy on asthma symptoms, exacerbations, quality of life, and pulmonary function in adult asthmatic patients with acid reflux symptoms. *Chest.* 2005;128(3):1128–1135

15. Sopo SM, Radzik D, Calvani M. Does treatment with proton pump inhibitors for gastroesophageal reflux disease (GERD) improve asthma symptoms in children with asthma and GERD? A systematic review. *J Investig Allergol Clin Immunol.* 2009;19(1):1–5

16. Chan WW, Chiou E, Obstein KL, Tignor AS, Whitlock TL. The efficacy of proton pump inhibitors for the treatment of asthma in adults: a meta-analysis. *Arch Intern Med.* 2011;171(7):620–629

17. DiMango E, Holbrook JT, Simpson E, et al; American Lung Association Asthma Clinical Research Centers. Effects of asymptomatic proximal and distal gastroesophageal reflux on asthma severity. *Am J Respir Crit Care Med.* 2009;180(9):809–816

18. Gibson PG, Henry RL, Coughlan JL. Gastro-oesophageal reflux treatment for asthma in adults and children. *Cochrane Database Syst Rev.* 2003;(2):CD001496

19. Jung HK. Epidemiology of gastroesophageal reflux disease in Asia: a systematic review. *J Neurogastroenterol Motil.* 2011;17(1):14–27

20. Dent J, El-Serag HB, Wallander MA, Johansson S. Epidemiology of gastro-oesophageal reflux disease: a systematic review. *Gut.* 2005;54(5):710–717

21. Cameron AJ, Lagergren J, Henriksson C, Nyren O, Locke GR, III, Pedersen NL. Gastroesophageal reflux disease in monozygotic and dizygotic twins. *Gastroenterology.* 2002;122(1):55–59

22. Chak A, Faulx A, Eng C, et al. Gastroesophageal reflux symptoms in patients with adenocarcinoma of the esophagus or cardia. *Cancer.* 2006;107(9):2160–2166

23. Mohammed I, Cherkas LF, Riley SA, Spector TD, Trudgill NJ. Genetic influences in gastro-oesophageal reflux disease: a twin study. *Gut.* 2003;52(8):1085–1089

24. Hassall E. Endoscopy in children with GERD: "the way we were" and the way we should be. *Am J Gastroenterol.* 2002;97(7):1583–1586

25. Hassall E, Kerr W, El-Serag HB. Characteristics of children receiving proton pump inhibitors continuously for up to 11 years duration. *J Pediatr.* 2007;150:262–267, 267.e1

26. Hassall E. Decisions in diagnosing and managing chronic gastroesophageal reflux disease in children. *J Pediatr.* 2005;146 (suppl 3):S3–S12

27. Orenstein SR, McGowan JD. Efficacy of conservative therapy as taught in the primary care setting for symptoms suggesting infant gastroesophageal reflux. *J Pediatr.* 2008;152(3):310–314

28. Gupta SK, Hassall E, Chiu YL, Amer F, Heyman MB. Presenting symptoms of nonerosive and erosive esophagitis in pediatric patients. *Dig Dis Sci.* 2006;51(5):858–863

29. Salvatore S, Hauser B, Vandemaele K, Novario R, Vandenplas Y. Gastroesophageal reflux disease in infants: how much is predictable with questionnaires, pH-metry, endoscopy and histology? *J Pediatr Gastroenterol Nutr.* 2005;40(2):210–215

30. Kleinman L, Revicki DA, Flood E. Validation issues in questionnaires for diagnosis and monitoring of gastroesophageal reflux disease in children. *Curr Gastroenterol Rep.* 2006;8(3):230–236

31. Gold BD, Gunasekaran T, Tolia V, et al. Safety and symptom improvement with esomeprazole in adolescents with gastroesophageal reflux disease. *J Pediatr Gastroenterol Nutr.* 2007;45(5):520–529

32. Størdal K, Johannesdottir GB, Bentsen BS, Sandvik L. Gastroesophageal reflux disease in children: association between symptoms and pH monitoring. *Scand J Gastroenterol.* 2005;40(6):636–640

33. Deal L, Gold BD, Gremse DA, et al. Age-specific questionnaires distinguish GERD symptom frequency and severity in infants and young children: development and initial validation. *J Pediatr Gastroenterol Nutr.* 2005;41(2):178–185

34. Rosen R, Lord C, Nurko S. The sensitivity of multichannel intraluminal impedance and

the pH probe in the evaluation of gastro-esophageal reflux in children. *Clin Gastroenterol Hepatol.* 2006;4(2):167–172

35. Rosen R, Nurko S. The importance of multichannel intraluminal impedance in the evaluation of children with persistent respiratory symptoms. *Am J Gastroenterol.* 2004;99(12):2452–2458

36. Thakkar K, El-Serag HB, Mattek N, Gilger MA. Complications of pediatric EGD: a 4-year experience in PEDS-CORI. *Gastrointest Endosc.* 2007;65(2):213–221

37. Volonaki E, Sebire NJ, Borrelli O, et al. Gastrointestinal endoscopy and mucosal biopsy in the first year of life: indications and outcome. *J Pediatr Gastroenterol Nutr.* 2012;55(1):62–65

38. Isolauri E, Tahvanainen A, Peltola T, Arvola T. Breast-feeding of allergic infants. *J Pediatr.* 1999;134(1):27–32

39. Vance GH, Lewis SA, Grimshaw KE, et al. Exposure of the fetus and infant to hens' egg ovalbumin via the placenta and breast milk in relation to maternal intake of dietary egg. *Clin Exp Allergy.* 2005;35(10):1318–1326

40. Clarke P, Robinson MJ. Thickening milk feeds may cause necrotising enterocolitis. *Arch Dis Child Fetal Neonatal Ed.* 2004;89(3):F280

41. Bhat RY, Rafferty GF, Hannam S, Greenough A. Acid gastroesophageal reflux in convalescent preterm infants: effect of posture and relationship to apnea. *Pediatr Res.* 2007;62(5):620–623

42. Corvaglia L, Rotatori R, Ferlini M, Aceti A, Ancora G, Faldella G. The effect of body positioning on gastroesophageal reflux in premature infants: evaluation by combined impedance and pH monitoring. *J Pediatr.* 2007;151:591–596, 596.e1

43. Orenstein SR, Whitington PF, Orenstein DM. The infant seat as treatment for gastro-esophageal reflux. *N Engl J Med.* 1983;309(13):760–763

44. Jung WJ, Yang HJ, Min TK, et al. The efficacy of the upright position on gastro-esophageal reflux and reflux-related respiratory symptoms in infants with chronic respiratory symptoms. *Allergy Asthma Immunol Res.* 2012;4(1):17–23

45. Avidan B, Sonnenberg A, Schnell TG, Sontag SJ. Walking and chewing reduce postprandial acid reflux. *Aliment Pharmacol Ther.* 2001;15(2):151–155

46. Moazzez R, Bartlett D, Anggiansah A. The effect of chewing sugar-free gum on gastro-esophageal reflux. *J Dent Res.* 2005;84(11):1062–1065

47. Smoak BR, Koufman JA. Effects of gum chewing on pharyngeal and esophageal pH. *Ann Otol Rhinol Laryngol.* 2001;110(12):1117–1119

48. Cucchiara S, Staiano A, Romaniello G, Capobianco S, Auricchio S. Antacids and cimetidine treatment for gastro-oesophageal reflux and peptic oesophagitis. *Arch Dis Child.* 1984;59(9):842–847

49. Sedman A. Aluminum toxicity in childhood. *Pediatr Nephrol.* 1992;6(4):383–393

50. Tsou VM, Young RM, Hart MH, Vanderhoof JA. Elevated plasma aluminum levels in normal infants receiving antacids containing aluminum. *Pediatrics.* 1991;87(2):148–151

51. American Academy of Pediatrics, Committee on Nutrition. Aluminum toxicity in infants and children. *Pediatrics.* 1996;97(3):413–416

52. Gremse DA. GERD in the pediatric patient: management considerations. *MedGenMed.* 2004;6(2):13

53. Simeone D, Caria MC, Miele E, Staiano A. Treatment of childhood peptic esophagitis: a double-blind placebo-controlled trial of nizatidine. *J Pediatr Gastroenterol Nutr.* 1997;25(1):51–55

54. Barron JJ, Tan H, Spalding J, Bakst AW, Singer J. Proton pump inhibitor utilization patterns in infants. *J Pediatr Gastroenterol Nutr.* 2007;45(4):421–427

55. Orenstein SR, Hassall E. Infants and proton pump inhibitors: tribulations, no trials. *J Pediatr Gastroenterol Nutr.* 2007;45(4):395–398

56. Orenstein SR, Hassall E, Furmaga-Jablonska W, Atkinson S, Raanan M. Multicenter, double-blind, randomized, placebo-controlled trial assessing the efficacy and safety of proton pump inhibitor lansoprazole in infants with symptoms of gastroesophageal reflux disease. *J Pediatr.* 2009;154:514–520.e4

57. Moore DJ, Tao BS, Lines DR, Hirte C, Heddle ML, Davidson GP. Double-blind placebo-controlled trial of omeprazole in irritable infants with gastroesophageal reflux. *J Pediatr.* 2003;143(2):219–223

58. Tolia V, Fitzgerald J, Hassall E, Huang B, Pilmer B, Kane R III. Safety of lansoprazole in the treatment of gastroesophageal reflux disease in children. *J Pediatr Gastroenterol Nutr.* 2002;35(suppl 4):S300–S307

59. Canani RB, Cirillo P, Roggero P, et al; Working Group on Intestinal Infections of the Italian Society of Pediatric Gastroenterology, Hepatology and Nutrition (SIGENP). Therapy with gastric acidity inhibitors increases the risk of acute gastroenteritis and community-acquired pneumonia in children. *Pediatrics.* 2006;117(5). Available at: www.pediatrics.org/cgi/content/full/117/5/e817

60. Saiman L, Ludington E, Dawson JD, et al; National Epidemiology of Mycoses Study Group. Risk factors for Candida species colonization of neonatal intensive care unit patients. *Pediatr Infect Dis J.* 2001;20(12):1119–1124

61. Craig WR, Hanlon-Dearman A, Sinclair C, Taback S, Moffatt M. Metoclopramide, thickened feedings, and positioning for gastro-oesophageal reflux in children under two years. *Cochrane Database Syst Rev.* 2004;(4):CD003502

62. Marchant JM, Masters IB, Taylor SM, Cox NC, Seymour GJ, Chang AB. Evaluation and outcome of young children with chronic cough. *Chest.* 2006;129(5):1132–1141

63. Størdal K, Johannesdottir GB, Bentsen BS, et al. Acid suppression does not change respiratory symptoms in children with asthma and gastro-oesophageal reflux disease. *Arch Dis Child.* 2005;90(9):956–960

64. Chang AB, Connor FL, Petsky HL, et al. An objective study of acid reflux and cough in children using an ambulatory pHmetry-cough logger. *Arch Dis Child.* 2011;96(5):468–472

Guidance on Management of Asymptomatic Neonates Born to Women With Active Genital Herpes Lesions

• *Clinical Report*

CLINICAL REPORT

Guidance on Management of Asymptomatic Neonates Born to Women With Active Genital Herpes Lesions

David W. Kimberlin, MD, Jill Baley, MD, COMMITTEE ON INFECTIOUS DISEASES, and COMMITTEE ON FETUS AND NEWBORN

KEY WORDS
newborn, herpes simplex virus, acyclovir, pregnancy

ABBREVIATIONS
CNS—central nervous system
CSF—cerebrospinal fluid
HSV—herpes simplex virus
HSV-1—herpes simplex virus type 1
HSV-2—herpes simplex virus type 2
IgG—immunoglobulin G
PCR—polymerase chain reaction
SEM—skin, eye, mouth

FUNDING: Funded in whole or in part with Federal funds from the National Institute of Allergy and Infectious Diseases, National Institutes of Health, Department of Health and Human Services, under contract (N01-AI-30025, N01-AI-65306, N01-AI-15113, N01-AI-62554), the General Clinical Research Unit (M01-RR00032), and the State of Alabama. Funded by the National Institutes of Health (NIH).

www.pediatrics.org/cgi/doi/10.1542/peds.2012-3216

doi:10.1542/peds.2012-3216

All clinical reports from the American Academy of Pediatrics automatically expire 5 years after publication unless reaffirmed, revised, or retired at or before that time.

PEDIATRICS (ISSN Numbers: Print, 0031-4005; Online, 1098-4275).

abstract

Herpes simplex virus (HSV) infection of the neonate is uncommon, but genital herpes infections in adults are very common. Thus, although treating an infant with neonatal herpes is a relatively rare occurrence, managing infants potentially exposed to HSV at the time of delivery occurs more frequently. The risk of transmitting HSV to an infant during delivery is determined in part by the mother's previous immunity to HSV. Women with primary genital HSV infections who are shedding HSV at delivery are 10 to 30 times more likely to transmit the virus to their newborn infants than are women with recurrent HSV infection who are shedding virus at delivery. With the availability of commercial serological tests that reliably can distinguish type-specific HSV antibodies, it is now possible to determine the type of maternal infection and, thus, further refine management of infants delivered to women who have active genital HSV lesions. The management algorithm presented herein uses both serological and virological studies to determine the risk of HSV transmission to the neonate who is delivered to a mother with active herpetic genital lesions and tailors management accordingly. The algorithm does not address the approach to asymptomatic neonates delivered to women with a history of genital herpes but no active lesions at delivery. *Pediatrics* 2013;131:e635–e646

INTRODUCTION

Herpes simplex virus (HSV) infection of the neonate is an uncommon occurrence, with an estimated 1500 cases diagnosed annually in the United States from a birth cohort of more than 4 000 000. In contrast, genital herpes infections in adults are very common. Between 1 in 4 and 1 in 5 adults in the United States has genital herpes caused by HSV type 2 (HSV-2).[1,2] In addition, HSV type 1 (HSV-1) now accounts for at least 20% and, in some locales, more than 50% of cases of genital herpes in the United States.[3,4] Therefore, managing infants potentially exposed to HSV at the time of delivery is not uncommon, and prevention of the devastating outcomes of neonatal HSV disease is paramount.

Current recommendations for the management of infants after intrapartum exposure are based on expert opinion, because a randomized controlled trial to determine whether an exposed neonate should be treated would be unethical. However, the existing recommendations do not take into account recent information correlating risk of transmission with type of maternal infection (primary versus recurrent) at the time of delivery.[5] The algorithm contained within this American Academy of Pediatrics (AAP) clinical report for the diagnostic and therapeutic approach to the neonate with known potential exposure to HSV during the perinatal period incorporates the most current scientific understanding of the biology, epidemiology, and pathology of HSV infection and disease.

TERMINOLOGY OF HSV INFECTION AND DISEASE

When an individual with no HSV-1 or HSV-2 antibody acquires either virus in the genital tract, a first-episode primary infection results. If a person with pre-existing HSV-1 antibody acquires HSV-2 genital infection (or vice versa), a first-episode nonprimary infection ensues. Viral reactivation from latency and subsequent antegrade translocation of virus back to skin and mucosal surfaces produces a recurrent infection.

Genital HSV infection can be either clinically apparent (eg, genital lesions) or inapparent (asymptomatic, or subclinical). Transmission to the neonate at the time of birth can occur with either presentation.

The distinction between neonatal HSV infection and neonatal HSV disease warrants discussion. Infection occurs when viral replication has been established, but the virus is not causing illness. Disease occurs when viral replication produces clinical signs of illness (eg, skin lesions, encephalitis, hepatitis). Once an infant is infected with HSV, progression to neonatal HSV disease is virtually certain. In an effort to prevent this progression from neonatal infection to neonatal disease, experts have recommended for many years that parenteral acyclovir be administered preemptively to HSV-infected neonates.[6]

RISK OF MATERNAL INFECTION DURING PREGNANCY

Recurrent infections are the most common form of genital HSV during pregnancy.[7] Approximately 10% of HSV-2–seronegative pregnant women have an HSV-2–seropositive sexual partner and, thus, are at risk for contracting a primary HSV-2 infection during the pregnancy[8] and transmitting the virus to their infants during delivery. Approximately one-fifth to one-third of women of childbearing age are seronegative for both HSV-1 and HSV-2,[9,10] and, among discordant couples, the chance that a woman will acquire either virus during pregnancy is estimated to be 3.7%.[11] For women who are already seropositive for HSV-1, the estimated chance of HSV-2 acquisition during the pregnancy is 1.7%.[11] Approximately two-thirds of women who acquire genital herpes during pregnancy remain asymptomatic and have no symptoms to suggest a genital HSV infection.[11] This is consistent with the finding that 60% to 80% of women who deliver an HSV-infected infant have a clinically unapparent genital HSV infection at the time of delivery and have neither a past history of genital herpes nor a sexual partner reporting a history of genital HSV.[12–14]

RISK OF NEONATAL HSV INFECTION

HSV infection of the newborn infant is acquired during 1 of 3 distinct times: intrauterine (in utero), intrapartum (perinatal), and postpartum (postnatal). The time of transmission of HSV-1 or HSV-2 for the overwhelming majority of infected infants (~85%) is in the intrapartum period. An additional 10% of infected neonates acquire HSV-1 postnatally from either a maternal or non-maternal source, and the final 5% are infected with HSV-2 or HSV-1 in utero. Five factors known to influence transmission of HSV from mother to neonate are:

1. Type of maternal infection (primary versus recurrent)[5,15–18];
2. Maternal HSV antibody status[5,14,19,20];
3. Duration of rupture of membranes[18];
4. Integrity of mucocutaneous barriers (eg, use of fetal scalp electrodes)[5,21,22]; and
5. Mode of delivery (cesarean versus vaginal delivery).[5]

Infants born to mothers who have a first episode of genital HSV infection near term and are shedding virus at delivery are at much greater risk of developing neonatal herpes than are infants whose mothers have recurrent genital herpes (Fig 1).[5,15–18]

The largest assessment of the influence of type of maternal infection on likelihood of neonatal transmission is a landmark study involving almost 60 000 women in labor who did not have clinical evidence of genital HSV disease, approximately 40 000 of whom had cultures performed within 48 hours of delivery (Fig 1).[5] Of these, 121 women were identified who were asymptomatically shedding HSV and who had sera available for analysis. In this large trial, 57% of infants delivered to women with first-episode primary HSV infection developed neonatal HSV disease, compared with 25% of infants delivered to women with first-episode nonprimary infection and 2% of infants delivered to women with recurrent HSV disease (Fig 1).[5]

CLINICAL MANIFESTATIONS OF NEONATAL HSV DISEASE

HSV infections acquired either intrapartum or postpartum can be classified as: (1) disease involving multiple visceral organs, including lung, liver, adrenal glands, skin, eye, and/or brain (disseminated disease); (2) central nervous system (CNS) disease, with or without skin lesions (CNS disease); and (3) disease limited to the skin, eyes, and/or mouth (skin, eye, mouth [SEM

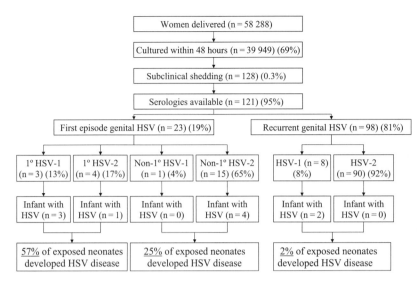

FIGURE 1

Type of maternal infection and risk of HSV transmission to the neonate.[5]

disease). This classification system is predictive of both morbidity and mortality.[23–27] Neonates with disseminated and SEM HSV disease typically present for medical attention at 10 to 12 days of age, whereas infants with CNS disease typically present at 17 to 19 days of age.[24] Overall, approximately half of all infants with neonatal HSV disease will have CNS involvement (CNS disease or disseminated disease with CNS involvement), and approximately 70% will have characteristic vesicular skin lesions (SEM disease, 83%; CNS disease, 63%; disseminated disease, 58%).[24]

DIAGNOSIS OF GENITAL HSV DISEASE

HSV can be detected from genital lesions by polymerase chain reaction (PCR) assay, viral culture, or antigen detection. Of these, PCR assay or viral culture are the testing modalities recommended by the Centers for Disease Control and Prevention for the diagnosis of genital HSV lesions.[28] The sensitivity of viral culture from genital lesions is low, especially for recurrent infection, and declines rapidly as lesions begin to heal. PCR assays for HSV DNA are more sensitive and are increasingly used for the diagnosis of genital HSV.[28,29] A

potential limitation of the PCR assay at the current time relates to its availability in all clinical settings; some smaller or more remote medical facilities have limited or no access to laboratories offering this technology. At many tertiary care centers, PCR assay results may be available within a day, whereas it takes 2 to 5 days for HSV to grow in viral culture. Typing of an HSV culture isolate or PCR assay product to determine if it is HSV-1 or HSV-2 can be accomplished by one of several techniques. The reliability of viral culture depends on the stage of the episode, with higher quantities of virus being present during the prodromal and vesicular stages than during crusting.[30] Antigen detection methods are available commercially but may not distinguish HSV-1 from HSV-2 and are not recommended by the Centers for Disease Control and Prevention for the diagnosis of genital herpes.

Before the year 2000, commercially available serological assays were unable to distinguish between HSV-1 and HSV-2 antibodies, severely limiting their utility. Over the past decade, a number of type-specific serological assays that reliably distinguish between immunoglobulin G (IgG) directed against HSV-1 and HSV-2

have been approved by the US Food and Drug Administration (Table 1). Many of these products are sold in kits that are used by clinical laboratories throughout the United States. Several additional tests that claim to distinguish between HSV-1 and HSV-2 antibody are available commercially, but high cross-reactivity rates attributable to their use of crude antigen preparations limit their utility,[31] and their use is not recommended.

DIAGNOSIS OF NEONATAL HSV DISEASE

Isolation of HSV by culture remains the definitive diagnostic method of establishing neonatal HSV disease. If skin lesions are present, a scraping of the vesicles should be transferred in appropriate viral transport media on ice to a diagnostic virology laboratory.[6] Other sites from which specimens should be obtained for culture of HSV include the conjunctivae, mouth, nasopharynx, and rectum ("surface cultures").[6] Specimens for viral culture from mucosal body sites may be combined before inoculating in cell culture to decrease costs, because the important information gathered from such cultures is the presence or absence of replicating virus rather than its precise body site. The sensitivity of PCR assay on surface specimens has not been studied; if used, surface PCR assay should be performed in addition to (and not instead of) the gold-standard surface culture. Rapid diagnostic techniques also are available, such as direct fluorescent antibody staining of vesicle scrapings or enzyme immunoassay detection of HSV antigens. These techniques are as specific but slightly less sensitive than culture.

The diagnosis of neonatal HSV CNS disease has been greatly enhanced by PCR testing of cerebrospinal fluid (CSF) specimens,[32–38] and PCR assay is now the method of choice for documenting CNS involvement in an infant

TABLE 1 Quick Reference Guide for Blood Tests to Accurately Detect Type-Specific HSV Antibodies

	Biokit HSV-2 Rapid Test (also sold as SureVue HSV-2 Rapid Test by Fisher HealthCare)	BioPlex HSV	Captia ELISA	Euroimmun Anti-HSV-1 and Anti-HSV-2 ELISA	HerpeSelect HSV-1 ELISA and HerpeSelect HSV-2 ELISA	HerpeSelect 1 and 2 Differentiation Immunoblot	Liaison HSV-2	AtheNA MultiLyte
Supplier	Biokit USA	Bio-Rad Laboratories	Trinity Biotech USA	Euroimmun US LLC	Focus Diagnostics	Focus Diagnostics	DiaSorin Inc.	Inverness Medical
FDA approved	1999	2009	2004	2007	2000/2002	2000	2008	2008
Antibodies detected	HSV-2 only	HSV-1 or HSV-2 or both	HSV-1 or HSV-2 or both	HSV-1 or HSV-2	HSV-1 or HSV-2 or both	HSV-1 and/or HSV-2	HSV-1 or HSV-2	HSV-1 and/or HSV-2
Best use of test	POC test to screen or test individuals >3 mo postexposure	Screening or testing (high volume)	Screening or testing pregnant women or STD clinic patients (moderate volume)	Moderate volume	Screening or testing STD patients or pregnant women (moderate volume)	Low volume	High volume	Screening or testing (moderate to high volume)
Collection method	Finger stick, whole blood, or serum in clinic	Blood draw (sent to laboratory)	Blood draw (sent to laboratory)	Blood draw (sent to laboratory)	Blood draw (sent to laboratory)	Blood draw (sent to laboratory)	Blood draw (sent to laboratory)	Blood draw (sent to laboratory)
Test time	10 min	45 min	~2 h	~2 h	~2 h	~2 h	35 min	~2 h
FDA approved for use during pregnancy		Yes	Yes		Yes	Yes		
Test availability	Limited	Limited	Widely available		Widely available			
Web site	www.biokitusa.com	www.bio-rad.com	www.trinitybiotech.com	www.euroimmunus.com	www.herpeselect.com	www.herpeselect.com	www.diasorin.com	www.invernessmedicalpd.com
For more information	800-926-3353	800-224-6723	800-325-3424	800-913-2022			800-328-5669	877-546-8633

FDA, US Food and Drug Administration; POC, point of care; STD, sexually transmitted disease. Adapted from http://www.ashastd.org/ Accessed August 5, 2010.

suspected of having HSV disease. However, PCR assay of CSF should only be performed in conjunction with HSV surface cultures, given that up to 40% of infants with disseminated disease will not have CNS involvement, and, by definition, no infants with SEM disease will have CNS involvement. The sensitivity of CSF PCR testing in neonatal HSV disease ranges from 75% to 100%.[33,36,38] PCR analysis of CSF also should play a role in determining the duration of antiviral therapy, because available data suggest that having HSV DNA detected in CSF at or after completion of intravenous therapy is associated with poor outcomes.[36,37] All infants with a positive CSF PCR assay result for HSV DNA at the beginning of antiviral therapy should have a repeat lumbar puncture near the end of treatment to determine that HSV DNA has been cleared from the CNS.[24] Infants whose PCR assay result remains positive should continue to receive intravenous antiviral therapy until the CSF PCR assay result is negative.[24,36]

Application of PCR testing to blood specimens from infants with suspected HSV disease appears promising,[37–42] and, in the 2012 *Red Book*,[6] PCR assay of blood has been added to the laboratory evaluation for neonatal HSV disease. Data are insufficient at the current time to allow the use of serial PCR assays of blood to establish response to antiviral therapy or to guide decisions about the duration of therapy.

Serological testing is not helpful in the diagnosis of neonatal HSV infection, because transplacentally acquired maternal HSV IgG is present in most infants, given the substantial proportions of the adult American population who are HSV-1 and/or HSV-2 seropositive.

PREVENTION OF NEONATAL HSV DISEASE

Cesarean delivery in a woman with active genital lesions can reduce the infant's risk of acquiring HSV.[5,18] In

1999, the American College of Obstetricians and Gynecologists updated its management guidelines for genital herpes in pregnancy.[43] To reduce the risk of neonatal HSV disease, cesarean delivery should be performed if genital HSV lesions or prodromal symptoms are present at the time of delivery. Neonatal HSV infection has occurred despite cesarean delivery performed before the rupture of membranes.[12,44]

In women with a previous diagnosis of genital herpes, cesarean delivery to prevent neonatal HSV infection is not indicated if there are no genital lesions at the time of labor. In an effort to reduce cesarean deliveries performed for the indication of genital herpes, the use of oral acyclovir or valacyclovir near the end of pregnancy to suppress genital HSV recurrences has become increasingly common in obstetric practice. Several studies with small sample sizes suggest that suppressive acyclovir therapy during the last weeks of pregnancy decreases the occurrence of clinically apparent genital HSV disease at the time of delivery,[45–48] with an associated decrease in cesarean delivery rates for the indication of genital HSV.[45,46,49,50] However, because viral shedding still occurs (albeit with reduced frequency),[47,51] the potential for neonatal infection is not avoided completely, and cases of neonatal HSV disease in newborn infants of women who were receiving antiviral suppression recently have been reported.[52,53]

ALGORITHM FOR MANAGEMENT OF ASYMPTOMATIC NEONATES BORN VAGINALLY OR BY CESAREAN DELIVERY TO WOMEN WITH ACTIVE GENITAL HSV LESIONS (FIGS 2 AND 3)

The risk of transmitting HSV to the newborn infant during delivery is influenced directly by the mother's previous immunity to HSV; women who have primary genital HSV infections who are shedding HSV at delivery are 10 to 30 times more likely to transmit the virus to their newborn infants than women with a recurrent infection.[5] The increased risk is attributable both to lower concentrations of transplacental HSV-specific antibodies (which also are less reactive to expressed polypeptides) in women with primary infection[19] and to the higher quantities of HSV that are shed for a longer period of time in the maternal genital tract in comparison with women who have recurrent genital HSV infection.[54] However, a substantial percentage of women with first clinical episodes of symptomatic genital herpes actually are experiencing reactivation of a previously unrecognized genital herpetic infection.[55] Thus, to tailor management of exposed neonates according to their degree of risk, one must distinguish primary versus recurrent maternal HSV infection in a manner that relies on more than just the history, or lack thereof, of genital herpes in the woman or her partner (s). Ideally, detection of HSV DNA from genital swabs obtained from women in labor would identify both symptomatic and asymptomatic HSV shedding, allowing for focused management of only those infants who are exposed; however, the technology to accomplish this on a broad scale is not readily available commercially at this time.

With the approval of commercially available serological tests that can reliably distinguish type-specific HSV antibodies (Table 1), the means to further refine management of asymptomatic neonates delivered to women with active genital HSV lesions is now possible. The algorithm detailed in Figs 2 and 3 applies only to asymptomatic neonates after vaginal or cesarean (because cesarean delivery reduces but does not eliminate the risk of neonatal HSV disease) delivery to women with active genital HSV lesions. It is intended to outline 1 approach to the management of these infants and may not be feasible in settings with limited access to PCR assays for HSV DNA or to the newer type-specific serological tests. If, at any point during the evaluation outlined in the algorithm, an infant develops symptoms that could possibly indicate neonatal HSV disease (fever, hypothermia, lethargy, irritability, vesicular rash, seizures, etc), a full diagnostic evaluation should be undertaken, and intravenous acyclovir therapy should be initiated. In applying this algorithm, obstetric providers and pediatricians likely will need to work closely with their diagnostic laboratories to ensure that serological and virological testing is available and turnaround times are acceptable. In situations in which this is not possible, the approach detailed in the algorithm will have limited, and perhaps no, applicability.

TESTING OF WOMEN IN LABOR

Women in labor with visible genital lesions that are characteristic of HSV should have the lesions swabbed for HSV PCR and culture (AI). Any positive test result then requires further analysis to determine if the virus is HSV-1 or HSV-2. Correlation of viral type with serological status allows for determination of maternal infection classification (Table 2).

Management of Asymptomatic Neonates After Vaginal or Cesarean Delivery to Women With Lesions at Delivery and History of Genital HSV Preceding Pregnancy

For women with a history of genital herpes preceding the pregnancy, the likelihood that the current outbreak represents reactivation of latent HSV is high, and, therefore, the likelihood of transmission to the infant is low (2%). Skin and mucosal specimens (conjunctivae, mouth, nasopharynx, and rectum, and scalp electrode site, if present) should be obtained from the

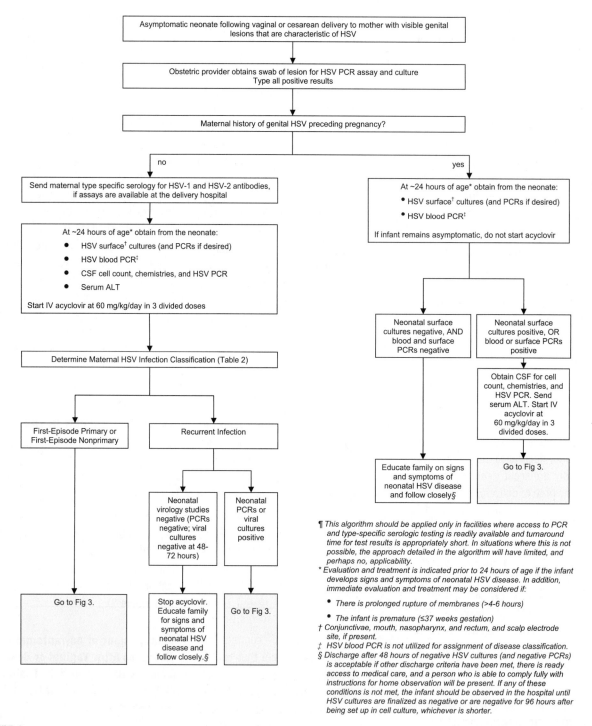

FIGURE 2
Algorithm for the evaluation of asymptomatic neonates after vaginal or cesarean delivery to women with active genital herpes lesions. ALT, alanine aminotransferase; D/C, discontinue.

neonate for culture (and PCR assay, if desired) at approximately 24 hours after delivery (BII), and blood should be sent for HSV DNA PCR assay. Acyclovir need not be started as long as the infant remains asymptomatic (BIII).

The importance of waiting until approximately 24 hours after delivery to obtain virological studies is based on the fact that a positive virological test result at that point represents actively replicating virus on the infant's mucosa,

whereas a positive test result shortly after birth could reflect only transient maternal contamination that may not lead to replication with resulting neonatal HSV disease.[56] It is permissible to discharge an asymptomatic infant after

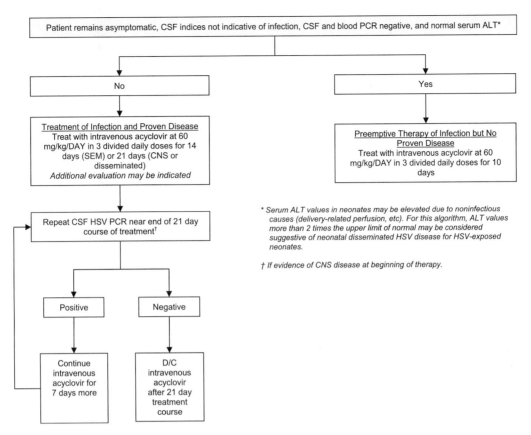

FIGURE 3
Algorithm for the treatment of asymptomatic neonates after vaginal or cesarean delivery to women with active genital herpes lesions. ALT, alanine aminotransferase; D/C, discontinue.

48 hours of negative HSV cultures (and negative PCR assay results) if other discharge criteria have been met, there is ready access to medical care, and a person who is able to comply fully with instructions for home observation will be present (BIII). If any of these conditions is not met, the infant should be observed in the hospital until HSV cultures are finalized as negative or are negative for 96 hours after being set up in cell culture, whichever is shorter.

If the surface and blood virological study results are negative at 5 days, the infant should be evaluated if signs or symptoms of neonatal HSV disease develop during the first 6 weeks of life (AII). Conversely, if the surface and blood virological study results become positive, thus confirming neonatal HSV infection, the infant should undergo a complete evaluation (lumbar puncture with CSF sent for indices and HSV DNA PCR assay, in addition to serum alanine

transaminase) to determine the extent of disease, and intravenous acyclovir should be initiated as soon as possible. If the evaluation findings are normal, indicating that the neonate has HSV infection but that it has not yet progressed to HSV disease, the infant should be treated empirically with intravenous acyclovir for 10 days to prevent progression from infection to disease (preemptive therapy) (BIII). If the evaluation findings are abnormal,

TABLE 2 Maternal Infection Classification by Genital HSV Viral Type and Maternal Serology[a]

Classification of Maternal Infection	PCR/Culture From Genital Lesion	Maternal HSV-1 and HSV-2 IgG Antibody Status
Documented first-episode primary infection	Positive, either virus	Both negative
Documented first-episode nonprimary infection	Positive for HSV-1	Positive for HSV-2 AND negative for HSV-1
	Positive for HSV-2	Positive for HSV-1 AND negative for HSV-2
Assume first-episode (primary or nonprimary) infection	Positive for HSV-1 OR HSV-2	Not available
	Negative OR not available[b]	Negative for HSV-1 and/or HSV-2 OR not available
Recurrent infection	Positive for HSV-1	Positive for HSV-1
	Positive for HSV-2	Positive for HSV-2

[a] To be used for women without a clinical history of genital herpes.
[b] When a genital lesion is strongly suspicious for HSV, clinical judgment should supersede the virological test results for the conservative purposes of this neonatal management algorithm. Conversely, if in retrospect, the genital lesion was not likely to be caused by HSV and the PCR assay result or culture is negative, departure from the evaluation and management in this conservative algorithm may be warranted.

indicating the neonate already has neonatal HSV disease, the infant should be treated for 14 to 21 days with intravenous acyclovir on the basis of the extent of neonatal HSV disease (disseminated, CNS, or SEM) (AII); if the initial CSF PCR assay result is positive for HSV DNA, a repeat lumbar puncture should be obtained near the end of therapy (eg, on day 17 or 18 of an anticipated 21-day course of therapy), and intravenous acyclovir should be discontinued at 21 days if the repeat HSV PCR assay result is negative (AII). If the "end-of-therapy" CSF PCR assay result is positive, intravenous acyclovir should be continued for another 7 days, with another repeat lumbar puncture near the end of therapy, again with decisions regarding cessation of therapy predicated on the repeat HSV CSF PCR assay result (BII). After completion of parenteral acyclovir for treatment of neonatal HSV disease, infants should receive oral acyclovir suppressive therapy for 6 months.[57]

Management of Asymptomatic Neonates After Vaginal or Cesarean Delivery to Women With Lesions at Delivery and No History of Genital HSV Preceding Pregnancy

For women without a history of genital herpes preceding pregnancy, the presence of genital lesions at delivery could represent first-episode primary infection (with a risk of transmission to the newborn infant of 57%), first-episode nonprimary infection (with a risk of transmission to the newborn infant of 25%), or recurrent infection (with a risk of transmission to the newborn infant of 2%). Thus, with the availability of type-specific serological testing, the practitioner can determine which type of infection the outbreak represents, given that the risks to the infant are so disparate. Accordingly, serological testing should be performed to determine the type of HSV infection in the mother to delineate between the 3 (Table 1).

At approximately 24 hours after delivery, neonatal skin and mucosal specimens (conjunctivae, mouth, nasopharynx, and rectum, and scalp electrode site, if present) should be obtained for culture (and PCR assay, if desired), and blood should be sent for HSV DNA PCR assay to evaluate for HSV infection. In addition, the infant should be evaluated for neonatal HSV disease (lumbar puncture with CSF sent for indices and HSV DNA PCR assay, in addition to serum alanine transaminase) at the same time, and intravenous acyclovir should be initiated pending the results of the evaluation, because the possibility is high that this could be a primary maternal infection (BIII). It is acceptable to wait to initiate therapy until approximately 24 hours after delivery in an asymptomatic neonate, because the average age at onset of neonatal HSV disease is between 1.5 and 3 weeks of age. Some practitioners advocate evaluation and treatment immediately after delivery if the infant is preterm or there has been prolonged rupture of membranes (CIII).

Laboratory correlations between virological (PCR/culture) and serological results that define maternal disease classification (first-episode primary, first-episode nonprimary, and recurrent) are presented in Table 2. The table deliberately uses a conservative estimate of first-episode infection, because the likelihood of transmission in such a situation is high. It is intended to be used to determine maternal disease classification in women without a clinical history of genital herpes.

If the mother has a documented or assumed first-episode primary or first-episode nonprimary infection (Table 2) and the neonate's evaluation results are normal, the infant should be treated empirically with intravenous acyclovir for 10 days to prevent progression from neonatal infection to disease (preemptive therapy) (BIII). If

the infant's evaluation results are abnormal, indicating the neonate already has neonatal HSV disease, the infant should be treated for 14 to 21 days with intravenous acyclovir on the basis of the extent of neonatal HSV disease (disseminated, CNS, or SEM) (AII); if the initial CSF PCR assay results are positive for HSV DNA, a repeat lumbar puncture should be obtained near the anticipated end of therapy (eg, on day 17 or 18 of therapy), and intravenous acyclovir should be discontinued at 21 days if the repeat HSV PCR assay result is negative (AII). If the end-of-therapy CSF PCR assay result is positive, the intravenous acyclovir should be continued for another 7 days, with another repeat lumbar puncture near the anticipated new end of therapy, again with decisions regarding cessation of therapy predicated on the HSV CSF PCR assay result (BII). After completion of parenteral acyclovir for treatment of neonatal HSV disease, infants should receive oral acyclovir suppressive therapy for 6 months.[57]

If the mother has recurrent genital HSV infection (that is, she has type-specific antibody to the HSV serotype detected by her genital swab) and the neonatal surface and blood virology study results are negative, acyclovir should be stopped, the parent(s) should receive education regarding signs and symptoms of neonatal HSV, and the infant may be discharged and reevaluated with any signs or symptoms of illness during the first 6 weeks of life (AII). Conversely, if virology study results are positive, confirming neonatal HSV infection, intravenous acyclovir should be continued, with the duration of treatment based on the evaluation for neonatal HSV disease. If the evaluation findings are normal, the infant should be treated empirically with intravenous acyclovir for 10 days to prevent progression from HSV infection to HSV disease (preemptive therapy) (BIII). If the evaluation findings are abnormal, the infant should be treated with intravenous acyclovir for 14 to 21 days on the basis of the extent of neonatal HSV disease (disseminated, CNS, or SEM) (AII); if the initial CSF PCR assay result is positive for HSV DNA, a repeat lumbar puncture should be obtained near the end of therapy (eg, on day 17 or 18 of an anticipated 21-day course of therapy), and intravenous acyclovir should be discontinued at 21 days if the repeat HSV PCR assay result is negative (AII). If the end-of-therapy CSF PCR assay result is positive, intravenous acyclovir should be continued for another 7 days, with another repeat lumbar puncture near the end of therapy, again with decisions regarding cessation of therapy predicated on the basis of HSV CSF PCR assay result (BII). After completion of parenteral acyclovir for treatment of neonatal HSV disease, infants should receive oral acyclovir suppressive therapy for 6 months.[57]

COMMITTEE ON INFECTIOUS DISEASES, 2012–2013

Michael T. Brady, MD, Chairperson
Carrie L. Byington, MD
H. Dele Davies, MD
Kathryn M. Edwards, MD
Mary P. Glode, MD
Mary Anne Jackson, MD
Harry L. Keyserling, MD
Yvonne A. Maldonado, MD
Dennis L. Murray, MD
Walter A. Orenstein, MD
Gordon E. Schutze, MD
Rodney E. Willoughby, MD
Theoklis E. Zaoutis, MD

LIAISONS

Marc A. Fischer, MD – *Centers for Disease Control and Prevention*
Bruce Gellin, MD – *National Vaccine Program Office*
Richard L. Gorman, MD – *National Institutes of Health*
Lucia Lee, MD – *Food and Drug Administration*
R. Douglas Pratt, MD – *Food and Drug Administration*
Jennifer S. Read, MD – *National Vaccine Program Office*
Joan Robinson, MD – *Canadian Pediatric Society*
Marco Aurelio Palazzi Safadi, MD – *Sociedad Latinoamericana de Infectologia Pediatrica (SLIPE)*
Jane Seward, MBBS, MPH – *Centers for Disease Control and Prevention*
Jeffrey R. Starke, MD – *American Thoracic Society*
Geoffrey Simon, MD – *Committee on Practice Ambulatory Medicine*
Tina Q. Tan, MD – *Pediatric Infectious Diseases Society*

EX OFFICIO

Henry H. Bernstein, DO – Red Book Online *Associate Editor*

David W. Kimberlin, MD – Red Book *Editor*
Sarah S. Long, MD – Red Book *Associate Editor*
H. Cody Meissner, MD – Visual Red Book *Associate Editor*

STAFF

Jennifer Frantz, MPH

COMMITTEE ON FETUS AND NEWBORN, 2012–2013

Lu-Ann Papile, MD, Chairperson
Jill E. Baley, MD
William Benitz, MD
Waldemar A. Carlo, MD
James Cummings, MD
Eric Eichenwald, MD
Praveen Kumar, MD
Richard A. Polin, MD
Rosemarie C. Tan, MD, PhD
Kasper S. Wang, MD

FORMER MEMBER

Kristi L. Watterberg, MD

LIAISONS

CAPT Wanda D. Barfield, MD, MPH – *Centers for Disease Control and Prevention*
George Macones, MD – *American College of Obstetricians and Gynecologists*
Ann L. Jefferies, MD – *Canadian Pediatric Society*
Erin L. Keels, APRN, MS, NNP-BC – *National Association of Neonatal Nurses*
Tonse N.K. Raju, MD, DCH – *National Institutes of Health*

STAFF

Jim Couto, MA

REFERENCES

1. Fleming DT, McQuillan GM, Johnson RE, et al. Herpes simplex virus type 2 in the United States, 1976 to 1994. *N Engl J Med.* 1997;337(16):1105–1111

2. Xu F, McQuillan GM, Kottiri BJ, et al. Trends in herpes simplex virus type 2 infection in the United States. In: 42nd Annual Meeting of the Infectious Diseases Society of America; September 30–October 3, 2004; Boston, MA. Abstract 739

3. Lafferty WE, Downey L, Celum C, Wald A. Herpes simplex virus type 1 as a cause of genital herpes: impact on surveillance and prevention. *J Infect Dis.* 2000;181(4):1454–1457

4. Kimberlin DW, Rouse DJ. Clinical practice. Genital herpes. *N Engl J Med.* 2004;350(19):1970–1977

5. Brown ZA, Wald A, Morrow RA, Selke S, Zeh J, Corey L. Effect of serologic status and cesarean delivery on transmission rates of herpes simplex virus from mother to infant. *JAMA.* 2003;289(2):203–209

6. American Academy of Pediatrics. Herpes simplex. In: Pickering LK, Baker CJ, Kimberlin DW, Long SS, eds. *Red Book: 2012 Report of the Committee on Infectious Diseases.* 29th ed. Elk Grove Village, IL: American Academy of Pediatrics; 2012:398–408

7. Whitley RJ. Herpes simplex virus infections. In: Remington JS, Klein JO, eds. *Infectious Diseases of the Fetus and Newborn Infants.* 3rd ed. Philadelphia, PA: WB Saunders Co; 1990:282–305

8. Kulhanjian JA, Soroush V, Au DS, et al. Identification of women at unsuspected risk of primary infection with herpes simplex virus type 2 during pregnancy. *N Engl J Med.* 1992;326(14):916–920

9. Xu F, Schillinger JA, Sternberg MR, et al. Seroprevalence and coinfection with herpes simplex virus type 1 and type 2 in the United States, 1988-1994. *J Infect Dis.* 2002;185(8):1019–1024

10. Xu F, Sternberg MR, Kottiri BJ, et al. Trends in herpes simplex virus type 1 and type 2 seroprevalence in the United States. *JAMA.* 2006;296(8):964–973

11. Brown ZA, Selke S, Zeh J, et al. The acquisition of herpes simplex virus during pregnancy. *N Engl J Med.* 1997;337(8):509–515

12. Whitley RJ, Corey L, Arvin A, et al. Changing presentation of herpes simplex virus

infection in neonates. *J Infect Dis.* 1988; 158(1):109–116

13. Whitley RJ, Nahmias AJ, Visintine AM, Fleming CL, Alford CA. The natural history of herpes simplex virus infection of mother and newborn. *Pediatrics.* 1980;66(4):489–494

14. Yeager AS, Arvin AM. Reasons for the absence of a history of recurrent genital infections in mothers of neonates infected with herpes simplex virus. *Pediatrics.* 1984; 73(2):188–193

15. Brown ZA, Benedetti J, Ashley R, et al. Neonatal herpes simplex virus infection in relation to asymptomatic maternal infection at the time of labor. *N Engl J Med.* 1991;324(18):1247–1252

16. Brown ZA, Vontver LA, Benedetti J, et al. Effects on infants of a first episode of genital herpes during pregnancy. *N Engl J Med.* 1987;317(20):1246–1251

17. Corey L, Wald A. Genital herpes. In: Holmes KK, Sparling PF, Mardh PA, et al, eds. *Sexually Transmitted Diseases.* 3rd ed. New York, NY: McGraw-Hill; 1999:285–312

18. Nahmias AJ, Josey WE, Naib ZM, Freeman MG, Fernandez RJ, Wheeler JH. Perinatal risk associated with maternal genital herpes simplex virus infection. *Am J Obstet Gynecol.* 1971;110(6):825–837

19. Prober CG, Sullender WM, Yasukawa LL, Au DS, Yeager AS, Arvin AM. Low risk of herpes simplex virus infections in neonates exposed to the virus at the time of vaginal delivery to mothers with recurrent genital herpes simplex virus infections. *N Engl J Med.* 1987;316(5):240–244

20. Yeager AS, Arvin AM, Urbani LJ, Kemp JA III. Relationship of antibody to outcome in neonatal herpes simplex virus infections. *Infect Immun.* 1980;29(2):532–538

21. Parvey LS, Ch'ien LT. Neonatal herpes simplex virus infection introduced by fetal-monitor scalp electrodes. *Pediatrics.* 1980; 65(6):1150–1153

22. Kaye EM, Dooling EC. Neonatal herpes simplex meningoencephalitis associated with fetal monitor scalp electrodes. *Neurology.* 1981;31(8):1045–1047

23. Kimberlin DW, Lin CY, Jacobs RF, et al; National Institute of Allergy and Infectious Diseases Collaborative Antiviral Study Group. Safety and efficacy of high-dose intravenous acyclovir in the management of neonatal herpes simplex virus infections. *Pediatrics.* 2001;108(2):230–238

24. Kimberlin DW, Lin CY, Jacobs RF, et al; National Institute of Allergy and Infectious Diseases Collaborative Antiviral Study Group. Natural history of neonatal herpes simplex virus infections in the acyclovir era. *Pediatrics.* 2001;108(2):223–229

25. Whitley R, Arvin A, Prober C, et al; Infectious Diseases Collaborative Antiviral Study Group. A controlled trial comparing vidarabine with acyclovir in neonatal herpes simplex virus infection. *N Engl J Med.* 1991;324(7):444–449

26. Whitley R, Arvin A, Prober C, et al; The National Institute of Allergy and Infectious Diseases Collaborative Antiviral Study Group. Predictors of morbidity and mortality in neonates with herpes simplex virus infections. *N Engl J Med.* 1991;324(7):450–454

27. Whitley RJ, Nahmias AJ, Soong SJ, Galasso GG, Fleming CL, Alford CA. Vidarabine therapy of neonatal herpes simplex virus infection. *Pediatrics.* 1980;66(4):495–501

28. Workowski KA, Berman S; Centers for Disease Control and Prevention (CDC). Sexually transmitted diseases treatment guidelines, 2010 [published correction appears in *MMWR Recomm Rep.* 2011;60(1):18]. *MMWR Recomm Rep.* 2010;59(RR-12):1–110

29. Wald A, Huang ML, Carrell D, Selke S, Corey L. Polymerase chain reaction for detection of herpes simplex virus (HSV) DNA on mucosal surfaces: comparison with HSV isolation in cell culture. *J Infect Dis.* 2003;188 (9):1345–1351

30. Moseley RC, Corey L, Benjamin D, Winter C, Remington ML. Comparison of viral isolation, direct immunofluorescence, and indirect immunoperoxidase techniques for detection of genital herpes simplex virus infection. *J Clin Microbiol.* 1981;13(5):913–918

31. Ashley RL. Sorting out the new HSV type specific antibody tests. *Sex Transm Infect.* 2001;77(4):232–237

32. Rowley AH, Whitley RJ, Lakeman FD, Wolinsky SM. Rapid detection of herpes-simplex-virus DNA in cerebrospinal fluid of patients with herpes simplex encephalitis. *Lancet.* 1990; 335(8687):440–441

33. Troendle-Atkins J, Demmler GJ, Buffone GJ. Rapid diagnosis of herpes simplex virus encephalitis by using the polymerase chain reaction. *J Pediatr.* 1993;123(3):376–380

34. Anderson NE, Powell KF, Croxson MC. A polymerase chain reaction assay of cerebrospinal fluid in patients with suspected herpes simplex encephalitis. *J Neurol Neurosurg Psychiatry.* 1993;56(5):520–525

35. Schlesinger Y, Storch GA. Herpes simplex meningitis in infancy. *Pediatr Infect Dis J.* 1994;13(2):141–144

36. Kimberlin DW, Lakeman FD, Arvin AM, et al; National Institute of Allergy and Infectious Diseases Collaborative Antiviral Study Group. Application of the polymerase chain reaction to the diagnosis and management of neonatal herpes simplex virus disease. *J Infect Dis.* 1996;174(6):1162–1167

37. Malm G, Forsgren M. Neonatal herpes simplex virus infections: HSV DNA in cerebrospinal fluid and serum. *Arch Dis Child Fetal Neonatal Ed.* 1999;81(1):F24–F29

38. Kimura H, Futamura M, Kito H, et al. Detection of viral DNA in neonatal herpes simplex virus infections: frequent and prolonged presence in serum and cerebrospinal fluid. *J Infect Dis.* 1991;164(2): 289–293

39. Barbi M, Binda S, Primache V, Tettamanti A, Negri C, Brambilla C. Use of Guthrie cards for the early diagnosis of neonatal herpes simplex virus disease. *Pediatr Infect Dis J.* 1998;17(3):251–252

40. Diamond C, Mohan K, Hobson A, Frenkel L, Corey L. Viremia in neonatal herpes simplex virus infections. *Pediatr Infect Dis J.* 1999;18(6):487–489

41. Lewensohn-Fuchs I, Osterwall P, Forsgren M, Malm G. Detection of herpes simplex virus DNA in dried blood spots making a retrospective diagnosis possible. *J Clin Virol.* 2003;26(1):39–48

42. Kimura H, Ito Y, Futamura M, et al. Quantitation of viral load in neonatal herpes simplex virus infection and comparison between type 1 and type 2. *J Med Virol.* 2002;67(3):349–353

43. American College of Obstetricians and Gynecologists. ACOG Practice Bulletin. Clinical management guidelines for obstetrician-gynecologists. No 82 June 2007. Management of herpes in pregnancy. *Obstet Gynecol.* 2007;109(6):1489–1498

44. Peng J, Krause PJ, Kresch M. Neonatal herpes simplex virus infection after cesarean section with intact amniotic membranes. *J Perinatol.* 1996;16(5):397–399

45. Braig S, Luton D, Sibony O, et al. Acyclovir prophylaxis in late pregnancy prevents recurrent genital herpes and viral shedding. *Eur J Obstet Gynecol Reprod Biol.* 2001;96 (1):55–58

46. Scott LL, Sanchez PJ, Jackson GL, Zeray F, Wendel GD Jr. Acyclovir suppression to prevent cesarean delivery after first-episode genital herpes. *Obstet Gynecol.* 1996;87(1): 69–73

47. Scott LL, Hollier LM, McIntire D, Sanchez PJ, Jackson GL, Wendel GD Jr. Acyclovir suppression to prevent recurrent genital herpes at delivery. *Infect Dis Obstet Gynecol.* 2002;10(2):71–77

48. Sheffield JS, Hollier LM, Hill JB, Stuart GS, Wendel GD Jr. Acyclovir prophylaxis to prevent herpes simplex virus recurrence at delivery: a systematic review. *Obstet Gynecol.* 2003;102(6):1396–1403

49. Andrews WW, Kimberlin DF, Whitley R, Cliver S, Ramsey PS, Deeter R. Valacyclovir therapy

to reduce recurrent genital herpes in pregnant women. *Am J Obstet Gynecol.* 2006;194 (3):774–781

50. Sheffield JS, Hill JB, Hollier LM, et al. Valacyclovir prophylaxis to prevent recurrent herpes at delivery: a randomized clinical trial. *Obstet Gynecol.* 2006;108(1): 141–147

51. Watts DH, Brown ZA, Money D, et al. A double-blind, randomized, placebo-controlled trial of acyclovir in late pregnancy for the reduction of herpes simplex virus shedding and cesarean delivery. *Am J Obstet Gynecol.* 2003; 188(3):836–843

52. Pinninti SG, Feja KN, Kimberlin DW, et al. Neonatal herpes disease despite maternal antenatal antiviral suppressive therapy: a multicenter case series of the first such infants reported. In: 48th Annual Meeting of the Infectious Diseases Society of America; October 22, 2010; Vancouver, British Columbia. Abstract 1841

53. Pinninti SG, Angara R, Feja KN, et al. Neonatal herpes disease following maternal antenatal antiviral suppressive therapy: a multicenter case series. *J Pediatr.* 2012; 161(1):134–138.e1–e3

54. Whitley RJ. Herpes simplex viruses. In: Fields BN, Knipe DM, Howley PM, et al, eds. *Fields Virology.* 3rd ed. Philadelphia, PA: Lippincott Raven Publishers; 1996:2297–2342

55. Diamond C, Selke S, Ashley R, Benedetti J, Corey L. Clinical course of patients with serologic evidence of recurrent genital herpes presenting with signs and symptoms of first episode disease. *Sex Transm Dis.* 1999;26(4): 221–225

56. Turner R, Shehab Z, Osborne K, Hendley JO. Shedding and survival of herpes simplex virus from 'fever blisters'. *Pediatrics.* 1982; 70(4):547–549

57. Kimberlin DW, Whitley RJ, Wan W, et al; National Institute of Allergy and Infectious Diseases Collaborative Antiviral Study Group. Oral acyclovir suppression and neurodevelopment after neonatal herpes. *N Engl J Med.* 2011;365(14):1284–1292

APPENDIX Evidence-based Rating System Used To Determine Strength Of Recommendations

Category	Definition	Recommendation
Strength of recommendation		
A	Strong evidence for efficacy and substantial clinical benefit	Strongly recommended
B	Strong or moderate evidence for efficacy, but only limited clinical benefit	Generally recommended
C	Insufficient evidence for efficacy, or efficacy does not outweigh possible adverse consequences	Optional
D	Moderate evidence against efficacy or for adverse outcome	Generally not recommended
E	Strong evidence against efficacy or for adverse outcome	Never recommended
Quality of evidence supporting recommendation		
I	Evidence from at least 1 well-executed randomized controlled trial or 1 rigorously designed laboratory-based experimental study that has been replicated by an independent investigator	
II	Evidence from at least 1 well-designed clinical trial without randomization; cohort or case-controlled analytic studies (preferably from >1 center); multiple time-series studies; dramatic results from uncontrolled studies; or some evidence from laboratory experiments	
III	Evidence from opinions of respected authorities based on clinical or laboratory experience, descriptive studies, or reports of expert committees	

Adapted from Centers for Disease Control. 2009 guidelines for the prevention and treatment of opportunistic infections among HIV-exposed and HIV-infected children. *MMWR Recomm Rep.* 2009;58(RR-11):5.

Guiding Principles for Managed Care Arrangements for the Health Care of Newborns, Infants, Children, Adolescents, and Young Adults

- *Policy Statement*

POLICY STATEMENT

Guiding Principles for Managed Care Arrangements for the Health Care of Newborns, Infants, Children, Adolescents, and Young Adults

abstract

By including the precepts of primary care and the medical home in the delivery of services, managed care can be effective in increasing access to a full range of health care services and clinicians. A carefully designed and administered managed care plan can minimize patient under- and overutilization of services, as well as enhance quality of care. Therefore, the American Academy of Pediatrics urges the use of the key principles outlined in this statement in designing and implementing managed care programs for newborns, infants, children, adolescents, and young adults to maximize the positive potential of managed care for pediatrics. These principles include the following: *Pediatrics* 2013;132:e1452–e1462

- Access to primary care pediatricians
- Access to pediatric specialty services
- Appropriate eligibility and treatment authorization
- Effective quality improvement and management
- Adequate financing and payment

COMMITTEE ON CHILD HEALTH FINANCING

KEY WORD
Managed care

ABBREVIATIONS
AAP—American Academy of Pediatrics
ACA—Patient Protection and Affordable Care Act
ACO—accountable care organization
CHIP—Children's Health Insurance Program
CPT—*Current Procedural Terminology*
IDS—integrated delivery system
PCMH—primary care medical home
PCP—primary care pediatrician
RVU—relative value unit

All policy statements from the American Academy of Pediatrics automatically expire 5 years after publication unless reaffirmed, revised, or retired at or before that time.

This policy statement replaces the 2006 policy statement, "Guiding Principles for Managed Care Arrangements for the Health Care of Infants, Children, Adolescents, and Young Adults."

INTRODUCTION

Faced with persistent escalation in health care costs, employers, state Medicaid programs, the State Children's Health Insurance Program (CHIP), and other purchasers of health care continue to study and often reconfigure managed care plans to find the most efficient strategies that provide access to quality health care while controlling costs. As a means of coordinating the delivery and financing of health care services, managed care plans have advanced different configurations that may include selective contracting with clinicians, medical management (ie, utilization management), gatekeeper functions, and different payment methodologies. Newer models and market changes have led to further changes, such as integrated delivery systems (IDSs), accountable care organizations (ACOs), payment incentives based on quality indicators, and clinician and payer consolidations. Additionally, clinicians and payers, including managed

www.pediatrics.org/cgi/doi/10.1542/peds.2013-2655

doi:10.1542/peds.2013-2655

Accepted for publication Aug 19, 2013

PEDIATRICS (ISSN Numbers: Print, 0031-4005; Online, 1098-4275).

Copyright © 2013 by the American Academy of Pediatrics

care plans, are in the midst of adjusting to the mandated components of the Patient Protection and Affordable Care Act (ACA; Pub L No. 111-148, 2010). As the delivery and financing of health care services continues to face profound challenges, diligent and focused efforts are needed to ensure that managed care plans serve the varied health care needs of neonates, infants, children, adolescents, and young adults (hereinafter referred to as children) and their families.

The effects of managed care on children's access to services and actual health outcomes are not yet clear. Some studies report positive effects (lower emergency department use and higher outpatient use; reduced costs, especially for hospitalizations), but also report concerns regarding access to care and satisfaction.[1] Other studies suggest no statistically significant differences in self-reported outcomes for children enrolled in managed care versus traditional health plans.[2]

The effectiveness of managed care in linking more low-income children to a medical home is uncertain. The proportion of Medicaid-enrolled children 0 to 20 years of age registered in managed care plans increased from 52.2% in federal fiscal year 2000 to 69.6% in federal fiscal year 2008.[3] Medicaid program shifts from fee-for-service to managed care plans have had little consistent effect on the health care use pattern by children and satisfaction with care received.[4] States that have expanded Medicaid and CHIP managed care programs for children with special health care needs have reported mixed results in terms of access to care and utilization.[5]

The American Academy of Pediatrics (AAP) urges the use of the following principles outlined in this statement in

designing and implementing managed care for children:

- Access to primary care pediatricians (PCPs)
- Access to pediatric specialty services
- Appropriate eligibility and treatment authorization
- Effective quality improvement and management
- Adequate financing and payment

It is important to monitor the short- and long-term effects of cost-containment measures on the quality and outcome of medical services for children. The financial arrangements inherent in managed care plans often include discounted charges and modified fee schedules, performance incentives, capitation, case rates, and bundled or global fees. Utilization management techniques used by managed care plans include precertification, concurrent review and discharge planning, care coordination, case management, preauthorization, formulary management, and physician practice profiling in comparison with selected benchmarks. Accountability links financial consideration and utilization in addition to quality measures and patient satisfaction. Managed care plans are also incorporating evidence-based review, comparative effectiveness (also known as patient-centered outcomes research), value-based benefits, and tiered-level benefits to manage access to services. These financial and utilization incentives and disincentives should be structured to preserve and, when appropriate, extend access to comprehensive and coordinated preventive, acute, and chronic care for all children. Cost-efficient health care delivery should be driven by performance-incentive programs focused on improved quality of care, actual clinical outcomes, and patient satisfaction, rather than policies that

create barriers to care or discourage a willingness to provide services for children with special health care needs. It is well understood that inadequate physician payment can be a significant barrier to physician service access. Attention should be paid to the relationship of payment on access to care and the quality of care that children and adolescents receive.[6,7] Additionally, market consolidations by managed care plans need to be reviewed in light of the effects on pediatrics and pediatricians, including, but not limited to, coverage benefits and access to pediatricians, pediatric medical subspecialists, and pediatric surgical specialists (unless otherwise indicated, use of the term pediatrician includes PCPs, pediatric medical subspecialists, and pediatric surgical specialists).

By including the precepts of primary care in the delivery of services, managed care can be instrumental in encouraging clinicians to provide access to a full range of evidence-based and evidence-informed pediatric health care services within a medical home. Children who received care in medical homes were less likely to have unmet medical and dental needs and were more likely to receive comprehensive pediatric care.[8] Managed care plans can be instrumental to support the intent and desired outcomes of a medical home. A medical home provides care that is accessible, family centered, continuous, comprehensive, coordinated, compassionate, and culturally effective.[9] The guidelines for care delivered in this environment are well illustrated in *Bright Futures*,[10] as recommended in the ACA.

Medically necessary health interventions that are evidence based or evidence informed are intended to prevent, diagnose, detect, treat, ameliorate, or palliate the effects of a physical, mental, genetic, or congenital condition, injury, or disability that lies outside the range of normal variation. Managed care organizations frequently use medical management guidelines to make coverage determinations. Payers are now looking at value-based benefits, comparative effectiveness, or patient-centered outcomes research to support their medical management and benefits coverage. However, adult-oriented policies frequently cannot be applied to the decision about a child's health care. Many of these "evidence-based" studies are not developed with a pediatric focus, are derived from best-case actuarial data, or are proprietary. The implementation of medical management guidelines that do not address the unique needs of children may adversely affect the health and well-being of pediatric patients, especially those with special health care needs. The development of medical management guidelines and comparative effectiveness studies used to determine benefits coverage should be reviewed regularly to substantiate their validity and reliability in the pediatrics environment. In addition, as part of ACA implementation, each state will establish its own determination of essential health benefits. Therefore, the effect of variability of benefits coverage, which may exist among states because of state determination of essential health benefits, needs to be studied.

Just as fee for service can result in overutilization, payment structures in managed care plans can result in misutilization of appropriate services and reduced quality of care. Underutilization could result from underfunded pediatric services, including inadequately funded primary care capitation or payments and restrictions or limited access to pediatric medical subspecialists, pediatric surgical specialists, and tertiary care centers. Other access restrictions could block the use of

necessary related services that improve outcomes or enhance quality of life, such as behavioral/mental health services, reproductive health services, social work services, developmental evaluation, occupational and physical therapy, vision screening, hearing screening, and speech and language therapies. Many services are, in fact, safety-net services, such as those of school-linked clinics and services of other public entities. To guard against inappropriate utilization and restricted access to necessary services, approaches to managed care must include a definition of medical necessity that addresses the unique needs of children and adolescents, specifically addressing the needs of those who have a functional impairment, chronic condition, or significant and multiple risks.[11] Annual public reporting or monitoring should be considered to inform consumers of the quality of their health care benefits, with specific attention to recognized state or national benchmarks, required medical loss ratios, enrollment retention, and so forth. When a state has mandated participation in Medicaid managed care plans, it must implement rigorous regulatory oversight to ensure that eligible children have access to high-quality health services in a medical home and that pediatricians are adequately paid to provide these services. In addition, in states in which Medicaid enrollees are required to use a Medicaid managed care plan or enroll in state insurance exchanges as proposed by the ACA, beneficiaries should have the freedom to choose among 2 or more managed health care plans.[12] In areas where only 1 managed care plan is available, particularly rural areas, families should be able to choose their individual physicians, and every effort should be made to allow Medicaid patients to remain in the care of

their medical home.[12] Medicaid provisions in the Balanced Budget Act of 1997 (Pub L No. 105-33) require adequate safeguards in every state implementation plan to ensure access to and delivery of quality health care for children.

Despite an exemption for grandfathered plans, the ACA is intended to enhance access and benefits coverage.[13,14] A grandfathered health plan is an existing plan on the market when the ACA was signed into law in March 2010. Grandfathered plans are exempt from several provisions of the ACA as long as the grandfathered plan has not made any significant changes, such as raising premiums or eliminating benefit categories. Insurance plans that undergo such changes forfeit their grandfathered status and are subject to the full scope of ACA provisions. ACA provisions affecting children and adolescents include the following:

- All nongrandfathered health insurance plans are required to cover all well-child visits, including physical examinations; immunizations; screenings for hearing, vision, developmental, and behavioral health; and anticipatory guidance in accordance with *Bright Futures*[10] guidelines.

- Nongrandfathered health insurance plans are required to provide this benefit without copayments or other cost sharing for individual policy years and group plan years, effective September 23, 2010.

- Effective January 1, 2014, new health insurance plans operating under state health insurance exchanges must provide a package of essential benefits, the scope of which must be equal to benefits provided under a "typical" employer-sponsored plan. However, essential health benefits may vary from state to state.

- Preexisting condition exclusions are banned for children up to 19 years of age who are enrolled in nongrandfathered plans (effective September 23, 2010).

- Coverage is extended to young adults under a parent's health insurance plan to 26 years of age if the plan provided dependent coverage (effective September 23, 2010).

- All private insurance plans are barred from rescinding coverage, except in the case of fraud or misrepresentation by the enrollee.

- Private insurance plans are barred from imposing lifetime dollar limits on coverage for "essential health benefits."

- Plan enrollees in all nongrandfathered plans are allowed to choose a participating pediatrician as the child's primary care physician.

Judicial challenges regarding the constitutional nature of the ACA have been resolved. The AAP now seeks to work in partnership with families, other health and health-related professionals, federal and state governments, employers, and the managed care industry to implement the following principles of managed care for children. These principles of access to primary and specialty pediatric services, treatment authorization, coordination of care, and financing and payment are intended to maximize the positive potential of managed care for the benefit of children and guide pediatricians and those providing care to children and adolescents, as well as families, payers, policy makers, and managed care plans.

PRINCIPLES OF MANAGED CARE FOR CHILDREN

1. Access to Appropriate PCPs

a. Choice of primary care physicians for children must include pediatricians.

As the medical specialty concerned with the physical, mental, and social health of children from birth to young adulthood, pediatricians understand the constantly changing functioning status of their patients' growth and development. Numerous studies support the significant relationship between primary care and health outcomes.[15]

b. PCPs should serve as the child's medical home and ensure the delivery of comprehensive preventive, acute, and chronic care services. In areas in which pediatricians are not available, access to pediatric consultation is important. Access to pediatric care/consultation should be available 24 hours a day, 7 days a week, or there should be appropriate coverage arrangements.

c. The primary care medical home (PCMH) implies, first and foremost, care coordination (ie, the PCMH manages all referrals that are medically necessary). The function of the PCP might be transferred to a pediatric medical subspecialist for certain children with complex physical and/or mental health problems (eg, those with special health care needs, including but not limited to cystic fibrosis, juvenile rheumatoid arthritis, renal disease, cancer) if the subspecialist is willing to assume responsibility for care coordination within the context of the patient-/family-centered medical home. Managed care plans should support development of the patient-/family-centered medical home by pediatricians and pediatric medical subspecialists for the pediatric population covered under their plans, particularly children with special health care needs. Children with special health care needs should be defined as those who "have a chronic

physical, developmental, behavioral, or emotional condition and who require coordinated health and related services of a type or amount beyond that required by children generally."[16] For certain physical, developmental, mental health, and social problems, the PCP may seek the assistance of a multidisciplinary team with participation by appropriate public programs (eg, Title V Program for Children with Special Health Care Needs). Managed care plans can assist the PCP in identifying and fostering linkages to available resources.

d. Adolescents, young adults, and other individuals from more vulnerable populations may need multiple sources of care available to ensure that adequate services are provided.

2. Access to Pediatric Specialty Services

a. When children need the services of pediatric medical subspecialists or other health care professionals, managed care plans should use clinicians with appropriate pediatric training and expertise. Pediatric-specialty clinicians include pediatric medical subspecialists, pediatric surgical specialists, and behavioral mental health specialists, who should have completed an appropriate fellowship in their area of expertise and are certified by specialty boards if certification is available. There should be no financial barriers to access to pediatric specialty care above and beyond customary health plan requirements for specialty care.

b. Managed care plans should ensure access within the plan to tertiary-care centers appropriate for children, as well as an appropriate number and mix of geographically accessible pediatric-trained physician specialists.

c. The referral process for pediatric specialty clinicians (pediatric medical subspecialists, pediatric surgical specialists, and pediatric behavioral mental health specialists) should be developed by health plans in collaboration with pediatricians, pediatric specialty clinicians, and families. The criteria for referrals may include age of patient, specific diagnoses, severity of conditions, and logistic considerations (eg, geographic access and cultural competence).

d. Access to specialty services within the managed care organization can be expedited by creating a "presumptive authorization" category (eg, no preauthorization needed for diagnoses including but not limited to hernia, strabismus, appendicitis, and diabetes).

e. Managed care plans must foster and financially support care coordination, such as interdisciplinary communication with the pediatric patient's medical home, including the PCP, pediatric medical subspecialists, pediatric surgical specialists, mental health professionals, and any other professional service providing medical care.

3. Eligibility and Treatment Authorization

a. Managed care plans must provide appropriate written, oral, and Web-based information and counseling to current and potential beneficiaries that allow informed patient choice of a managed care organization, network options for primary care physicians, relevant pediatric medical subspecialists and pediatric surgical specialists, and pediatric hospital and ancillary services.

b. Families should receive education at the time of enrollment to help them understand fully their health plan benefits (including limitations on the amount, duration, and scope of services; cost-sharing requirements; and participating health care professionals). Carriers with multiple managed care plans should provide a clear comparison of pediatric benefits and networks across managed care plans so that families can choose a plan most appropriate for their needs. Materials should be clear, in lay language, and easy for all families to understand.[17] Materials should be available in the patient's/family's primary language.

c. Subsequent to enrollment, health insurance benefits for pediatrics must be clearly defined. Managed care plans must provide details on the scope of pediatric benefits in consumer brochures, Web sites, and, most importantly, in plan evidence of benefit coverage documents and managed care contracts.

d. Families and pediatricians should be fully informed of the plan's participating clinicians. This should include an up-to-date listing of the plan's participating health care professionals whose practices are currently open to patients served by the managed care plan. The roster of the provider network should be continuously updated by the managed care plan to reflect newly participating physicians as well as deletion of nonparticipating providers. The parent's/patient's choice of pediatrician as well as the required copayments should be listed on the patient's insurance card.

e. Managed care plans should provide accurate and current online patient eligibility data, timely authorization review, and real-time claims adjudication with real-time payment information available to clinicians and patients.

f. Managed care plans need to make every effort to provide timely and accurate verification of eligibility to the physician and should not retroactively rescind payments on the basis of the plan's error. Plans must be bound by their confirmation of eligibility, and physicians are to be held harmless and be fully compensated when services are provided after the plan's verification of eligibility.

g. The treatment authorization process for elective services initiated by the PCP should efficiently facilitate timely appropriate referral for specialty consultations, hospital inpatient and outpatient care, and other treatments. Emergency-based services should not require previous authorizations.

h. Plans should provide timely responses to treatment authorization requests (including 24-hour access and approvals in the case of emergencies) on the basis of the nature and urgency of the patient's needs. Managed care plans should allow member access to emergency care consistent with the "prudent layperson" standard.[17] Plans are urged to make transparent their processes for authorizations and are encouraged to evaluate and share studies on the effects of previous authorizations on patient access, costs, and quality of care.

i. Plans should provide a timely appeals process that includes direct discussions between the reviewing panel, the patient's pediatrician, and the relevant specialists and, if appropriate, an external review by an independent third-party reviewer of the same specialty or, if not available, by a physician experienced in the treatment of the pediatric illness.

j. Before making any determination that any item or service furnished to a person younger than 26 years is not medically necessary, the managed care plan should consider whether an item or service (1) is appropriate for the age and health status of the person, and (2) is supported by evidence-based or evidence-informed clinical practice guidelines developed for children's health care services that are endorsed or approved by appropriate medical professional societies or governmental public health agencies. Managed care plans should describe the process by which physicians are to provide justification for medical necessity. Referral to a panel of third-party reviewers with pediatric expertise may be the option of last resort.

k. Pharmacy benefits must be appropriate for children and recognize that off-label use of medications is often a necessity for children, including compounded medications, which are often necessary to meet the unique needs of children. (Off-label use may be defined as using an approved drug to treat a disease that is not indicated on the label or varying from the indicated dosage, regimen, or patient population.)

l. Health plans need to recognize and reward the unique skills of pediatricians in addressing pediatric mental health issues and remove barriers to mental health care, as outlined in the AAP and American Academy of Child and Adolescent Psychiatry joint paper "Improving Mental Health Services in Primary Care: Reducing Administrative and Financial Barriers to Access and Collaboration."[18] Pediatric primary care clinicians have substantial opportunities to affect the mental health of children: preventing mental health problems by guiding parents in behavior management; identifying mental health symptoms as they emerge; intervening early, before symptoms have evolved into disorders; facilitating referral of children and their family members when mental health or substance abuse specialty services are needed; and collaborating with child and adolescent psychiatrists in caring for children with severely impairing mental health and substance abuse disorders. Managed care plans are called on to implement parity in mental health benefits, including diagnostic parity for pediatricians and procedural parity for child and adolescent psychiatrists. By addressing the administrative and financial barriers that primary care clinicians and children's mental health professionals currently encounter in providing behavioral, mental, and brain health services to children and adolescents, managed care plans can improve access, collaboration, and coordination for pediatric mental health care. PCPs should be recognized as often the best equipped to provide initial mental health therapeutic and counseling services for children and their families.

4. Quality Improvement and Management

a. Managed care plans should be transparent and provide written standards that pertain to access to primary care, referrals to specialty physician and other recommended services, the referral process, and protocols for service.

b. Pediatricians, pediatric medical subspecialists, pediatric surgical specialists, and behavioral mental health specialists should have an active role in developing quality improvement mechanisms and patient-centered outcomes research programs. Any cost-containment process, pay-for-performance program, tiered benefits, differential physician payments, or value-based benefit design should be reviewed in light of the effects on pediatric access and quality of care.

c. Managed care plans have developed a broad and diverse clinical database related to utilization of services. As a result, managed care plans should participate in patient registry development and thoughtful quality outcomes research based on the principles articulated in the AAP policy statement "Principles for the Use and Development of Quality Measures."[19] Health care payers are in a unique position to collaborate with the pediatric community to develop and implement changes that systematically advance children's health care. Managed care plans should actively engage pediatricians in both community and hospital settings in outcomes research and quality improvement efforts, such as developing patient registries or working toward a single national pediatric database similar to the Medicare Part B database.[20] Quality management should include appropriate peer review, with pediatric cases reviewed by pediatricians.

d. Use of patient-centered outcomes research studies is increasing as payers look to assess treatments and costs to determine the ideal course of treatment, medication, or medical device for certain conditions. With the establishment of the Council for Comparative Effectiveness Research as part of the American Recovery and Reinvestment Act passed in February 2009,[21] private payers, including managed care payers, have enhanced comparative effectiveness efforts. Also, the Patient-Centered Outcomes Research Institute was established through the 2010 ACA and was created to conduct research to provide information about the best-available evidence to help patients and health care clinicians make more informed decisions.[22] These efforts support incorporation of outcomes-based research to benefit design. Managed care plans are encouraged to share clinical and financial data along the continuum of care to allow for assessment of access, quality, and cost of care. Managed care plans using pediatric comparative effectiveness and patient-centered outcomes research studies for coverage determinations need to make all research public and available for comment by organized medicine and specialty societies. For pediatric comparative effectiveness research, pediatricians, and pediatric specialists must be part of the review.

e. Plans should promote recommended preventive services, early identification, and treatment of health problems in children by providing benefits coverage and appropriate payment to physicians for all recommended screenings and assessments. These measures should be included in incentive programs to physicians as part of pay-for-performance programs.

f. Plans should report a uniform standard set of encounter data in compliance with the Health Insurance Portability and Accountability Act (Pub L No. 104-191 [1996]).

g. States should publish uniform data for health plans that offer consumers and purchasers the opportunity to evaluate and compare performance, including relevant financial information, among competing plans. The measures reported by states on a managed care plan's performance should emphasize quality standards, such as access to care, patient satisfaction, and health outcomes.

h. Managed care contracts shall exclude prohibitions that restrict information and advice that physicians provide about a patient's medical options, including, but not limited to, advice on noncovered treatment options and information about the patient's plan and competing health plans.

i. Managed care plans are encouraged to work collaboratively with pediatricians, pediatric specialists, the AAP, and AAP chapters to develop and/or enhance quality-improvement activities that can benefit all children.

j. Managed care programs should collaborate with their clinicians and community resources to identify appropriate family practice and internal medicine medical homes that provide optimal care for children with special health care needs as they age out of the pediatric medical home and transition to adult care.

5. Financing and Payment

a. Payment methods should be developed that cover all the health care needs of children, as defined by the AAP policy statement "Scope of Health Care Benefits for Newborns, Infants, Children, Adolescents, and Young Adults Through Age 26 Years,"[23] with the periodicity of visits and procedures described in the AAP statement "Recommendations for Preventive Pediatric Health Care"[24] and the current edition of the *Bright Futures*,[10] as well as "The Medical Home for Children: Financing Prin-

ciples."[25] The methods used for pediatric health care payment should consider age, chronicity and severity of underlying health problems (case mix, risk, or severity adjustment), service area market, and geographic considerations. Payments to the PCMH for chronic condition management should support the additional visits and time spent on care plan development and complex disease management, as reflected in *Current Procedural Terminology* (CPT)[26] codes for care plan oversight, non–face-to-face care, complex and transitional care, telephone care,[27] and E-mail consultations, as well as recommended pediatric services provided by nonphysician professionals. The payment structure should encompass recognition of all CPT and Healthcare Common Procedure Coding System codes based on their relative value units (RVUs), the complexity of the physician's patient panel mix, expanded care-management responsibilities, after-hours accessibility, new quality-improvement activities, and up-front investments and support for infrastructure.[25]

b. Managed care plans need to make transparent all policies and procedures regarding coverage and payment determinations, including fee schedules and claims edits. Any changes affecting payment to the pediatrician must be provided in writing and in advance to provide timely notification and allow time for review/appeal/negotiation by the pediatrician. There must be a specified time period for repayment requests applied equally to payers and clinicians, and payment offsets on future claims to adjust contested claims already paid by managed care plans should be prohibited.

c. Appropriate payment for immunizations should be based on the actual cost incurred by the practice and should include a reasonable margin to encourage provision of these services within the medical home. Actual cost calculation should include the purchase price, applicable taxes, shipping/handling charges, and total additional costs associated with vaccine inventory management, including but not limited to finance costs, immunization registry reporting, vaccine administration, personnel costs, and factors for inventory control, loss prevention, inventory shrinkage, and vaccine storage (including specialized refrigerators/freezers, temperature controls, and alarms). Fee schedules and health plan coverage benefits for immunizations must be updated in a timely manner and made effective retroactive to the date new recommendations for new vaccines are published by the AAP or the Advisory Committee on Immunization Practices of the Centers for Disease Control and Prevention.

d. Payment for physician services for newborn care should be separately identified as unique and distinct from maternal services and should ensure adequate and clearly identified payment to attending physicians who provide care for newborn infants to ensure consistent and continuous coverage for the neonatal period and for subsequent pediatric care.

e. All capitated rates should be adjusted for case-mix differences based on age, geographic location, modifiers for children with special health care needs, outlier risk-adjusted methods, more risk-adjusted rating groups, a pediatric diagnostic classification system, or a combination of these. As risk-adjustment techniques are developed by payers, it is necessary to incorporate a pediatric focus and involve PCPs and pediatric specialists experienced in private practice in their design. Contract provisions about carved-out services, outlier payment, stop-loss provisions, reinsurance or shared-risk arrangements for individual children, and aggregate plan loss or profits should be clearly identified. Any additional services (meaningful use reporting, attestations to facilitate data correction, and so forth) to be covered under the capitation rate must be subject to mutual agreement by the health plan and the contracting physician.

f. When primary care is capitated, contracts should include fee-for-service carve-outs for unexpected or high-cost services, including, but not limited to, neonatal and routine newborn hospital care, immunizations, hospitalization, emergency services, transplant services, and, in the case of adolescents, pregnancy and other reproductive health services.[25]

g. All recommended preventive services, including pediatric immunizations, must be covered as first-dollar coverage and not be subject to deductibles and/or copayments or any other cost-sharing mechanism under the health plan. Payment for preventive care services needs to be in full and not be bundled or considered incidental to the office visit. Appropriate payment can be accomplished by paying for each service reported separately at a level that reflects the total RVUs of all the reported services.

h. Health plans paying pediatricians for pediatric care on a fee-for-service schedule should use the most current Resource-Based Relative Value Scale as the basis for their fee schedule. The American Medical Association/Specialty Society Relative Value Scale Update Committee RVU values are appropriate for PCPs, pediatric medical subspecialists, and pediatric surgical specialists. A single multispecialty, regionally adjusted conversion factor applied to the current-year RVUs (ie, at least 100% of the current year Medicare resource-based relative value scale reimbursement rate) should be incorporated. Medicaid fees should be set at a rate that is at least 100% equivalent to those in Medicare.[11,12,28] Health plans should use the most current version of CPT codes and adhere to CPT guidelines regarding the use of codes.

i. In all payment systems and methodologies, pediatric services within the context of the medical home should be appropriately assessed to ensure that pediatric primary and specialty services are not undervalued in terms of practice expense, professional liability, and physician work. Financial incentives to encourage use of the medical home must be paramount, and there should not be financial incentives by the managed care plan to encourage use of nonmedical home service offerings, such as retail-based clinics and/or urgent care centers.

j. In light of evolving payment methodologies, continuation of high-quality services for children must be ensured, and primary care physicians should be protected against undue financial risk as well as arbitrary assignment to tiered or differential payment levels. Risk levels for office-based PCPs should be on an aggregate, not individual, basis and should be adjusted based on case-mix analysis. Any payment incentives, including shifting of risk to the clinician by the managed care plan, need to be fully transparent and supported by data and resources for the clinician to manage the risk and make informed clinical and financial decisions.

k. Mandatory clinician participation in all service offerings by the managed care plan carrier should be prohibited, and physicians need to be allowed to determine their level of participation and acceptable risk, individually or as a physician group, within the health plans.

l. Federal requirements for capitation should apply to all managed care plans. Federal and state governments should preapprove all contracts with managed care plans in which enrollees are primarily beneficiaries of CHIP or Medicaid and require the federal and state governments to guarantee clinician payments if plans become insolvent.

m. Plans should use pediatric quality measures that assess the current status and improvements of care over some relevant time frame. Quality measures on structure, process, health, and functional outcomes need to be based on current acute, chronic, mental, dental, and preventive pediatric care standards, in accordance with the principles promulgated in the AAP policy statement "Principles for the Use and Development of Quality Measures."[19] As physician payment begins to be tied more closely to patient outcomes through pay-for-performance programs, the reporting of CPT category II codes will be necessary

to qualify for supplemental payments.[20]

n. Many of the responsibilities for managing the care of pediatric inpatients are being coordinated between hospitals and physicians as part of IDSs with a variety of payment methodologies: prospective payment, case rate methodologies, or bundled or global fee arrangements. Pediatricians and pediatric medical and surgical specialists are encouraged to work closely with hospitalists, hospital quality assurance managers, case managers, medical directors, and administrators to improve care management and resource utilization continuously and make process changes that are outcome driven. Managed care organizations, ACOs, and health plans could be very influential in enhancing this aspect of health care.

o. To ensure timely and appropriate payment, plans should make available electronically pertinent patient information, including, but not limited to, patient eligibility status and current contact information, benefits, and benefit limitations.

p. Financial incentives are needed to support the medical home infrastructure, including adoption of health information technologies. Despite the benefits to patients and payers attributable to implementation of information technologies, physicians, especially those in private practice, bear the risks and costs of implementation and maintenance as well as associated upgrades but do not see a return on their capital outlay.[29]

q. Managed care plans developing IDSs and ACOs should be aligned with the recommendations by the

AAP.[30,31] The AAP fostered the concept of the medical home and is a staunch advocate for comprehensive essential health care needs of children. The AAP wholeheartedly recommends that managed care plans, ACOs, and IDSs adopt a medical home model for children that adequately addresses the needs of all children, including those with special health care needs.

CONCLUSIONS

Managed care will continue to evolve until the approaches used to finance and deliver health care more consistently meet the needs of patients, clinicians, employers, and society overall. During this evolution in managing health care, specific and consistent attention must be given to the direct relationships between clinician payments, access to care, the quality of care provided, and health outcomes for children as well as patient satisfaction. Primary care physicians, adult and pediatric, are the backbone of managed care systems and key to IDSs. Much of the focus in today's health care reform environment and in managed care has focused, with good reason, on controlling health care costs. In addition to controlling costs, managed care is also in a position to enhance access to and quality of care. To achieve the greatest value in health care for children, payers, employers, and clinicians must all consistently focus on enhancing access to health care, improving outcomes, increasing quality and safety, and achieving greater patient/family participation and satisfaction with their care. Many debilitating adult conditions begin in childhood. Pediatricians need the tools and support of the health care delivery system to ensure the health and readiness of tomorrow's adult population. Comprehensive, coordinated, value-based care with cost control may have great effects and may be best demonstrated in pediatric health care.

LEAD AUTHOR

Thomas Long, MD, FAAP

COMMITTEE ON CHILD HEALTH FINANCING, 2012–2013

Thomas Long, MD, FAAP Chairperson
Molly Droge, MD, FAAP
Norman "Chip" Harbaugh, MD, FAAP
Mark Helm, MD, FAAP
Mark Hudak, MD, FAAP
Andrew Racine, MD, FAAP

Budd Shenkin, MD, FAAP
Iris Snider, MD, FAAP
Patience White, MD, FAAP
Earnestine Willis, MD, FAAP

STAFF

Ed Zimmerman
Lou Terranova

REFERENCES

1. Baker LC, Afendulis C. Medicaid managed care and health care for children. *Health Serv Res.* 2005;40(5 pt 1):1466–1488

2. Newacheck PW, Hung YY, Marchi KS, Hughes DC, Pitter C, Stoddard JJ. The impact of managed care on children's access, satisfaction, use, and quality of care. *Health Serv Res.* 2001;36(2):315–334

3. Federal Fiscal Year 2000 and Federal Fiscal Year 2008 Medicaid State Reports (based on CMS/MSIS2082). Available at: www.aap.org/en-us/professional-resources/Research/research-resources/Pages/Medicaid-State-Reports.aspx. Accessed January 8, 2013

4. Long SK, Coughlin TA. Impacts of Medicaid managed care on children. *Health Serv Res.* 2001;36(1 pt 1):7–23

5. Huffman LC, Brat GA, Chamberlain LJ, Wise PH. Impact of managed care on publicly insured children with special health care needs. *Acad Pediatr.* 2010;10(1):48–55

6. McInerny TK, Cull WL, Yudkowsky BK. Physician reimbursement levels and adherence to American Academy of Pediatrics well-visit and immunization recommendations. *Pediatrics.* 2005;115(4):833–838

7. Yoo BK, Berry A, Kasajima M, Szilagyi PG. Association between Medicaid reimbursement and child influenza vaccination rates. *Pediatrics.* 2010;126(5). Available at: www.pediatrics.org/cgi/content/full/125/5/e998

8. Strickland BB, Jones JR, Ghandour RM, Kogan MD, Newacheck PW. The medical home: health care access and impact for children and youth in the United States. *Pediatrics.* 2011;127(4):604–611

9. American Academy of Pediatrics, Medical Home Initiatives for Children With Special Health Care Needs Project Advisory Committee. The medical home. *Pediatrics.* 2002;110(1):184–186 (Reaffirmed May 2008)

10. Hagan JF, Jr, Shaw JS, Duncan P, eds. *Bright Futures: Guidelines for Health Supervision of Infants, Children, and Adolescents.* 3rd ed. Elk Grove Village, IL: American Academy of Pediatrics; 2008

11. American Academy of Pediatrics Committee on Child Health Financing. Model contractual language for medical necessity for children. *Pediatrics.* 2005;116(1):261–262

12. American Academy of Pediatrics, Committee on Child Health Financing. Medicaid policy statement. *Pediatrics.* 2005;116(1):274-280 (Reaffirmed October 2011)

13. HealthCare.gov The Health Care Law and You. Available at: www.healthcare.gov/law/index.html. Accessed January 8, 2013

14. US Department of Health and Human Services. Patient Protection and Affordable Care Act; requirements for group health plans and health insurance issuers under the Patient Protection and Affordable Care Act relating to preexisting condition exclusions, lifetime and annual limits, rescissions, and patient protections; final rule and proposed rule. *Fed Regist.* 2010;75(123):37187–37241. Available at: http://edocket.access.gpo.gov/2010/2010-15278.htm. Accessed January 8, 2013

15. Starfield B. U.S. child health: what's amiss, and what should be done about it? *Health Aff (Millwood).* 2004;23(5):165–170

16. McPherson M, Arango P, Fox H, et al. A new definition of children with special health care needs. *Pediatrics.* 1998;102(1 pt 1):137–140

17. Balanced Budget Act of 1997. Pub L No. 105-33, Section 4704 (b)(2)(C) (1997)

18. American Academy of Child and Adolescent Psychiatry Committee on Health Care Access and Economics Task Force on Mental Health. Improving mental health services in primary care: reducing administrative and financial barriers to access and collaboration. *Pediatrics.* 2009;123(4):1248–1251

19. Hodgson ES, Simpson L, Lannon CM; American Academy of Pediatrics Steering Committee on Quality Improvement and Management; American Academy of Pediatrics Committee on Practice and Ambulatory Medicine. Principles for use and development of quality measures. *Pediatrics.* 2008;121(2):411–418

20. Committee on Coding and Nomenclature. Application of the resource-based relative value scale system to pediatrics. *Pediatrics.* 2008;122(6):1395–1400

21. US Department of Health and Human Services. Comparative effectiveness research funding. Available at: www.hhs.gov/recovery/programs/cer/index.html. Accessed January 8, 2013

22. Patient Centered Outcomes Research Institute. Available at: www.pcori.org/. Accessed January 8, 2013

23. Committee on Child Health Financing. Scope of health care benefits for children from birth through age 26. *Pediatrics.* 2012;129(1):185–189

24. American Academy of Pediatrics, Committee on Practice and Ambulatory Medicine. Recommendations for preventive pediatric health care. *Pediatrics.* 2007;120(6):1376 (Reaffirmed January 2011)

25. American Academy of Pediatrics, Committee on Child Health Financing. The Medical Home for Children: Financing Principles. Elk Grove Village, IL: American Academy of Pediatrics; 2012. Available at: www.medicalhomeinfo.org/downloads/pdfs/MHfinanceprin.pdf. Accessed January 8, 2013

26. American Medical Association. *Current Procedural Terminology.* Chicago, IL: American Medical Association; 2013

27. Melzer SM, Reuben MS; American Academy of Pediatrics Section on Telephone Care and Committee on Child Health Financing. Payment for telephone care. *Pediatrics.* 2006;118(4):1768–1773

28. Portman RM, Finitzo N, eds. *Model Managed Care Agreement*. Elk Grove Village, IL: American Academy of Pediatrics; 1998

29. Council on Clinical Information Technology. Health information technology and the medical home. *Pediatrics*. 2011;127(5):978–982

30. American Academy of Pediatrics. Accountable care organizations (ACOs) and pediatricians: evaluation and engagement. *AAP News*. 2011;32(1):1

31. American Academy of Family Physicians, American Academy of Pediatrics, American College of Physicians, American Osteopathic Association. Joint principles for accountable care organizations. 2010. Available at: www.acponline.org/advocacy/where_we_stand/other_issues/aco-principles-2010.pdf. Accessed January 8, 2013

Guiding Principles for Pediatric Hospital Medicine Programs

• *Policy Statement*

675

POLICY STATEMENT

Guiding Principles for Pediatric Hospital Medicine Programs

abstract

Pediatric hospital medicine programs have an established place in pediatric medicine. This statement speaks to the expanded roles and responsibilities of pediatric hospitalists and their integrated role among the community of pediatricians who care for children within and outside of the hospital setting. *Pediatrics* 2013;132:782–786

INTRODUCTION

The American Academy of Pediatrics formally recognized pediatric hospital medicine as a discrete area of practice in 1999 when it approved the formation of the Provisional Section on Hospital Care. This entity subsequently became the focal point for general pediatricians with a primary interest in inpatient pediatric medicine and led to the approval of the American Academy of Pediatrics Section on Hospital Medicine. Wachter and Goldman initially coined the term "hospitalist" in 1996,[1] and it is now an easily recognized designation, describing a physician whose primary professional focus is the general medical care of hospitalized patients and whose activities include patient care, teaching, research, and leadership related to hospital medicine.[2] The last policy statement[3] reflected the initiation and introduction of pediatric hospitalists and their expected growth in the form of groups and programs. This statement speaks to the expanded roles and responsibilities of a more defined group of pediatricians and their integrated role among a community of pediatricians within and without the hospital setting. As before, the Section on Hospital Medicine strongly supports a policy of voluntary referrals to pediatric hospital medicine programs and suggests that primary care physicians retain the option to admit and manage their own patients.

DISCUSSION

Construct, Program Setup

Pediatric hospital medicine programs vary considerably in size, scope of practice, and structure. A wide array of programs now exists, ranging from those based in small community hospitals to those found within large academic centers. The range of services provided by a pediatric hospitalist group is dependent on the needs of the institution and the ability of the group to provide these services, which may include the following:

SECTION ON HOSPITAL MEDICINE

KEY WORDS
hospital medicine, hospitalist, inpatient care

This document is copyrighted and is property of the American Academy of Pediatrics and its Board of Directors. All authors have filed conflict of interest statements with the American Academy of Pediatrics. Any conflicts have been resolved through a process approved by the Board of Directors. The American Academy of Pediatrics has neither solicited nor accepted any commercial involvement in the development of the content of this publication.

The recommendations in this statement do not indicate an exclusive course of treatment or serve as a standard of medical care. Variations, taking into account individual circumstances, may be appropriate.

All policy statements from the American Academy of Pediatrics automatically expire 5 years after publication unless reaffirmed, revised, or retired at or before that time.

www.pediatrics.org/cgi/doi/10.1542/peds.2013-2269

doi:10.1542/peds.2013-2269

PEDIATRICS (ISSN Numbers: Print, 0031-4005; Online, 1098-4275).

- General inpatient pediatric care
- Perioperative surgical and medical subspecialty care[4]
- Delivery room services
- Newborn nursery care
- NICU and PICU coverage
- Pediatric emergency department evaluation
- Consultation or short-stay observation unit services
- Sedation services
- Palliative care
- Coordinated, family-centered interdisciplinary admission and discharge planning that includes the essential role of the primary care physician

Pediatric hospital medicine programs may incorporate teaching, mentoring, and other academic responsibilities, especially if programs are affiliated with academic centers. At the community hospital level, programs may be supported by a larger tertiary care center or may be completely independent. Programs may be privately run, supported by hospital-based physician foundations, or funded by other for-profit organizations. Regardless of the many variations in size or scope of these practices, all programs should strive to provide continuity of care with the medical home of primary care physicians, pediatric medical subspecialists, and pediatric surgical specialists for each child.[5]

Transitions of Care

Transitioning patients safely back into the community at the time of discharge is a primary concern of every hospitalist. Admission and discharge planning should emphasize the importance of the medical home, communication with the primary care physician (and vice versa), pediatric medical subspecialists or pediatric surgical specialists, or other service providers involved in the patient's care.[6] The inpatient team should coordinate an interdisciplinary plan of care that includes the patient, family, the primary care provider, and social and other services when necessary. All communication should be timely and complete, including hand-off communication within and between hospitals. Hospitalists should work with their primary care referral centers to establish the preferred means of communication and guidelines for frequency of communication beyond admission and discharge.

Leadership

Developing and maintaining a successful pediatric hospital medicine program requires an understanding of the underlying pediatric vision of the greater institution. It is essential to develop a mission for the program that includes its purpose and scope of services and establishes the basis for organizational support and a long-term viable financial model. This includes understanding the initial goals for the development of the program, the high-priority issues of the program, and its potentials for success and failure. Hospital medicine leaders need to understand the hospital environment in which they work and then define their own program within that environment. This is particularly true in community and non–children's hospitals, where program leaders must be strong advocates for children throughout the hospital. Pediatric hospital medicine leaders should develop a strategic plan for the program that includes stability, expansion of services, and integration into the overall hospital organization and management. In the process of doing this, individual members and program leaders should have a full understanding of the institution's organizational structure and the chain of command. Care needs to be taken to ensure the scope of the program is matched by the abilities of the hospital medicine service, in terms of both clinical skills and manpower. It is important to have well-described agreements for the role of the hospital medicine service that are open to modification with changes in staffing, experience, or other events that affect the scope of practice.

Individual Goals

Physicians serving as pediatric hospitalists should be board certified or board eligible in pediatrics. Ongoing professional practice evaluation should require demonstration of adequate patient volumes, procedural competency, and participation in quality improvement projects. Physicians should participate in continuing medical education and lifelong learning activities with a focus on inpatient pediatrics, systems of care, safety issues, and other topics directly relevant to pediatric hospital medicine.

Pediatric hospital medicine program leadership should identify the skill sets needed for employment and define the roles of its members. These skill sets might include the following:

- Expertise in the care of pediatric inpatients from neonates to adolescents
- Skill in the coordination of medically complex patients
- Understanding of the management of pain, sedation, and palliative care in children
- Ability to provide team leadership and mentoring
- Experience in academic teaching and research
- Participation and leadership in local, state, and national organizations
- Involvement and leadership in hospital committees and initiatives

- Skill in communication practices, both internal and external
- Experience in child health care advocacy and welfare

A full set of knowledge and skills is described in the Pediatric Hospital Medicine Core Competencies.[7]

Leadership should advocate for a stable, defined workforce that promotes healthy work hours, avoids health care worker fatigue,[8] enhances overall career satisfaction, and supports financial viability of the program, including appropriate physician compensation. Program and individual performance target goals and objectives should be consistently and periodically reviewed and monitored for success. Each program, in keeping with its own scope of practice and cognizant of national performance indicators, should set its own practice performance indicators, describe them in a concise and easily understandable format, and review them on a regular basis. Key parameters should focus on both the goals of the pediatric hospital medicine program as part of a larger organization and the goals of its individual members. For example, group program goals could include financial and revenue parameters, recognized safety and clinical quality indicators,[9] and advocacy and leadership roles in the larger organization. Within the group itself, members may have a personal performance review that focuses on individual goals, such as community advocacy, contributions to departmental improvements, academic achievements, research projects, participation in local or national organizations, or other indicators of professional development and excellence.

Advocacy for Patient and Program

Pediatric hospitalists are unequivocal champions for the hospitalized child. Their focus is on the safety of children, and pediatric hospitalists advocate for

services and programs that support the best possible outcomes for children. This is especially true for pediatric programs that exist within a larger, diverse hospital environment in which pediatric patients often represent a small portion of the inpatient population. To do this, pediatric hospitalists should fully participate in hospital committees, policy groups, task forces, and program development initiatives that support these goals. Committees particularly important for pediatric representation include pharmacy and therapeutics, credentials, emergency and transport services, patient safety, quality performance and improvement, and medical executive committees, among others. Pediatric hospitalists are well positioned to take leadership roles in quality improvement, safety, performance improvement, risk management, disaster preparedness, rapid response teams, and medical informatics systems. In addition, hospitalists are ideally suited to develop effective transitions of care, promote patient- and family-centered rounds, coordinate care for medically complex patients, develop efficient and effective methods of communication with primary care and subspecialty physicians, and strengthen the medical home. Hospitalists should play key roles in ensuring compliance with standards of The Joint Commission, National Patient Safety Goals, and other regulatory targets. They should develop evidence-based guidelines for the pediatric service. When pediatric services intersect with other hospital services, benchmarks, outcomes data, and goals should be developed to improve health care outcomes for pediatric inpatients.

Pediatric hospitalists often serve as leaders in patient care: they interface with pediatric medical subspecialists and pediatric surgical specialists, primary care physicians, nurses, and

others in the hospital environment to help provide patients with a consistent message of quality and safety that enables effective medical decision-making.

The hospital setting may serve to magnify health and safety issues in the local environment. Pediatric hospitalists have the opportunity to be advocates in the community by recognizing patterns of illness and injury not easily evident to individual ambulatory physicians and alerting the local medical community to these concerns. It is essential to conclude that the standards set forth in this statement are directed not only at pediatric hospitalists: it is the responsibility of all pediatric physician leaders within hospitals to champion the best and safest medical care for their patients.

GENERALIZABILITY

Hospitalists are not the only providers who work in the hospital setting. Other providers are focused on the care and well-being of their hospitalized patients. Those providers should be equally invested in the care process and can similarly integrate themselves into the hospital environment through interdisciplinary work, care coordination, quality improvement, and leadership activities to produce the best outcomes.

RECOMMENDATIONS

The following basic principles are recommended for pediatric hospital medicine programs:

1. **Each Program Is Unique.** Each pediatric hospital medicine program should be designed to meet the unique needs of the patients, families, and physicians in the community it serves. This may include the option for private pediatricians and other qualified primary (or

subspecialty) care physicians to retain the option to admit and manage their own patients. Regardless of who admits the pediatric patient, attending physicians should strive to meet the unique needs of each patient, maintain continuity with the patient's medical home, and place special emphasis on transitions of care.[10]

2. **Understand the Institution.** Pediatric hospitalists and their leadership should be fully versed in the organizational structure of the institution and seek leadership roles and active participation in the clinical, administrative, and information technology committees of the institution. They should seek strategies for involvement in the hospital systems that ensure quality of care and safety for pediatric patients.

3. **Leadership and Expertise.** Pediatric hospital medicine group members should seek opportunities to develop expertise in areas such as leadership, quality, safety, performance improvement, risk management, disaster relief, rapid response, and other hospital and community health initiatives. These expanded qualifications diversify and strengthen the hospitalist group, provide additional areas of interest, and promote long-term career satisfaction for individual physicians.

4. **Patient- and Family-Centered Care.** Pediatric hospitalists should promote patient- and family-centered care that includes an opportunity for the patient and family to participate in decision-making about treatment plans and effective discharge planning.[11] This should be a part of integrated multidisciplinary care planning that includes other hospital services and the primary care physician.

5. **Coordination of the Care Team.** Pediatric hospitalists should serve as leaders in the coordination of care of the hospitalized patient, champion the medical home, and develop effective admission and discharge planning. They are available to provide the patient and his or her family with a consistent message and optimally communicate with primary care physicians, pediatric medical subspecialists and pediatric surgical specialists, medically complex care teams, nurses, respiratory care therapists, pain management teams, and others. The pediatric hospitalist, as leader of the inpatient team, coordinates interdisciplinary care and promotes an environment for optimal medical decision-making. Primary care physicians are strongly encouraged to participate in the interdisciplinary care of patients and ensure the patients' successful transition back to their medical home.

6. **Outcomes and Data.** Pediatric hospital medicine programs should be supported by data collection and outcome-based assessments to monitor their performance and drive quality improvement for hospitalized children.

7. **Advocacy.** Pediatric hospitalists are in a position to be strong and active champions of pediatric safety and promote the finest pediatric hospital services. They should vigorously advocate for programs that improve the quality and safety of care provided to all children throughout the hospital setting and beyond.

8. **Added Value.** Pediatric hospital medicine and pediatric department leaders should promote recognition of value added by hospitalists to hospital programs[12] and support compensation equity for pediatric hospitalists. Examples of the added value by hospitalists include their support and understanding of hospital systems, their availability for hospital committee participation, their ability to recognize potential areas of quality improvement in patient care, the care of unassigned patients, and the timely management of children with acute changes in medical status.

SUMMARY OF GUIDING PRINCIPLES

The purpose of this statement has been to address the particular roles and responsibilities of pediatric hospitalists, but it is implicit in all the aforementioned recommendations that the overarching goal is always to provide the best possible care for children and protect the safety of children in the hospital setting. This is the responsibility of all physicians who care for children and all leaders in pediatrics and hospital medicine.

LEAD AUTHOR

Laura J. Mirkinson, MD, FAAP,[†] Past Section Executive Committee Chairperson

SECTION ON HOSPITAL MEDICINE EXECUTIVE COMMITTEE, 2011–2012

Jennifer A. Daru, MD, FAAP, Chairperson
Erin R. Stucky Fisher, MD, FAAP
Matthew D. Garber, MD, FAAP
Paul D. Hain, MD, FAAP
A. Steve Narang, MD, FAAP
Ricardo A. Quinonez, MD, FAAP
Daniel A. Rauch, MD, FAAP, Immediate Past Chairperson

LIAISONS

Elena Aragona, MD – *Section on Medical Students, Residents, and Fellowship Trainees*

STAFF

S. Niccole Alexander, MPP
[†]Deceased

REFERENCES

1. Wachter RM, Goldman L. The emerging role of "hospitalists" in the American health care system. *N Engl J Med.* 1996;335(7): 514–517

2. Society of Hospital Medicine. What is a hospitalist? Available at: http://www.hospitalmedicine.org/AM/Template.cfm?Section=FAQs&Template=/FAQ/FAQListAll.cfm. Accessed February 13, 2012

3. Percelay JM, Strong GB; American Academy of Pediatrics Section on Hospital Medicine. Guiding principles for pediatric hospitalist programs. *Pediatrics.* 2005;115(4):1101–1102

4. Rappaport DI, Pressel DM. Pediatric hospitalist comanagement of surgical patients: challenges and opportunities. *Clin Pediatr (Phila).* 2008;47(2):114–121

5. Daru JA. Pediatric hospitalists. *Pediatr Ann.* 2003;32(12):778–780

6. Harlan G, Srivastava R, Harrison L, McBride G, Maloney C. Pediatric hospitalists and primary care providers: a communication needs assessment. *J Hosp Med.* 2009;4(3): 187–193

7. Stucky ER, Maniscalco J, Ottolini MC, et al. The Pediatric Hospital Medicine Core Competencies Supplement: a Framework for Curriculum Development by the Society of Hospital Medicine with acknowledgement to pediatric hospitalists from the American Academy of Pediatrics and the Academic Pediatric Association. *J Hosp Med.* 2010;5(suppl 2):i–xv, 1–114

8. The Joint Commission. Health care worker fatigue and patient safety. *Sentinel Event Alert.* 2011;48(48):1–4. Available at: http://psnet.ahrq.gov/resource.aspx?resourceID=23690. Accessed February 13, 2012

9. Kurtin P, Stucky E. Standardize to excellence: improving the quality and safety of care with clinical pathways. *Pediatr Clin North Am.* 2009;56(4):893–904

10. Lye PS; American Academy of Pediatrics, Committee on Hospital Care and Section on Hospital Medicine. Clinical report—physicians' roles in coordinating care of hospitalized children. *Pediatrics.* 2010;126(4):829–832

11. Committee on Hospital Care. American Academy of Pediatrics. Family-centered care and the pediatrician's role. *Pediatrics.* 2003; 112(3 pt 1):691–697

12. Freed GL, Dunham KM, Switalski KE; Research Advisory Committee of the American Board of Pediatrics. Assessing the value of pediatric hospitalist programs: the perspective of hospital leaders. *Acad Pediatr.* 2009;9(3):192–196

Health and Mental Health Needs of Children in US Military Families

- *Clinical Report*

CLINICAL REPORT

Health and Mental Health Needs of Children in US Military Families

abstract

The wars in Afghanistan and Iraq have been challenging for US uniformed service families and their children. Almost 60% of US service members have family responsibilities. Approximately 2.3 million active duty, National Guard, and Reserve service members have been deployed since the beginning of the wars in Afghanistan and Iraq (2001 and 2003, respectively), and almost half have deployed more than once, some for up to 18 months' duration. Up to 2 million US children have been exposed to a wartime deployment of a loved one in the past 10 years. Many service members have returned from combat deployments with symptoms of posttraumatic stress disorder, depression, anxiety, substance abuse, and traumatic brain injury. The mental health and well-being of spouses, significant others, children (and their friends), and extended family members of deployed service members continues to be significantly challenged by the experiences of wartime deployment as well as by combat mortality and morbidity. The medical system of the Department of Defense provides health and mental health services for active duty service members and their families as well as activated National Guard and Reserve service members and their families. In addition to military pediatricians and civilian pediatricians employed by military treatment facilities, nonmilitary general pediatricians care for >50% of children and family members before, during, and after wartime deployments. This clinical report is for all pediatricians, both active duty and civilian, to aid in caring for children whose loved ones have been, are, or will be deployed. *Pediatrics* 2013;131:e2002–e2015

Benjamin S. Siegel, MD, Beth Ellen Davis, MD, MPH, and THE COMMITTEE ON PSYCHOSOCIAL ASPECTS OF CHILD AND FAMILY HEALTH AND SECTION ON UNIFORMED SERVICES

KEY WORDS
military, families, children, deployment, mental health, health maintenance

This document is copyrighted and is property of the American Academy of Pediatrics and its Board of Directors. All authors have filed conflict of interest statements with the American Academy of Pediatrics. Any conflicts have been resolved through a process approved by the Board of Directors. The American Academy of Pediatrics has neither solicited nor accepted any commercial involvement in the development of the content of this publication.

The guidance in this report does not indicate an exclusive course of treatment or serve as a standard of medical care. Variations, taking into account individual circumstances, may be appropriate.

The views expressed in this article are those of the authors and do not reflect the official policy of the Department of the Army, the Department of Defense, or the US Government.

www.pediatrics.org/cgi/doi/10.1542/peds.2013-0940

doi:10.1542/peds.2013-0940

All clinical reports from the American Academy of Pediatrics automatically expire 5 years after publication unless reaffirmed, revised, or retired at or before that time.

PEDIATRICS (ISSN Numbers: Print, 0031-4005; Online, 1098-4275).

All Americans are challenged in a world changed by terrorism and war. For the past decade, the wars in Iraq (Operation Iraqi Freedom, Operation New Dawn) and Afghanistan (Operation Enduring Freedom) have been especially challenging for US service members and their families. Recent studies describe the physical and mental health issues of US service members involved in wartime deployments, including the toll on American lives.[1,2] Approximately 2.3 million active duty, National Guard, and Reserve service members have deployed since the beginning of the wars (2001, 2003), and over 40% have deployed more than once, some for up to 18 months' duration.[3] Almost 60% of US service members have family responsibilities, resulting in 2 million US children exposed to at least 1 parental wartime deployment in the past 10 years.[4] The US public and its policy makers are increasingly concerned about the health and well-being of the children and families of uniformed service members facing prolonged and multiple wartime deployments. To this end, in January 2011, President and Mrs. Obama announced their commitment to the "care and support of military families as a top national security policy priority."[5]

To a child, wartime deployment means separation from a loved one, usually a parent; an increased sense of danger; and a routine of daily uncertainty. On return of the deployed parent or relative, there are an infinite number of challenges for the child and family members. There are recent and emerging studies specifically describing the effects on children of parental wartime deployments. These studies, outlined in this report, can help inform pediatricians about the needs of military children. Most commonly, children experience separation as loss. Concomitant fear and chronic anxiety have been shown to disrupt the developing architecture of the brain.[6] Children, and even adolescents, watch closely for parental cues to gauge their own degree of distress in a given situation. Maladaptive parental coping or distress may be the single most important predictor of child biopsychosocial symptoms during stressful situations, such as wartime deployment.[7–9] Some military families may be at higher risk of distress, especially if they are young, experiencing a first separation, have recently relocated, include a foreign-born spouse, have young children, are junior enlisted (entry pay level), are single parents, or have children with special needs.[4,9] Service members and families who have not anticipated an extended wartime deployment, such as activated National Guard and Reserve personnel, may be especially challenged.[10]

Pediatricians and other clinicians caring for children are on the front line in the medical home because they identify and assess effects of wartime deployment in children and their family members. More than 50% of military children receive their health and mental health care from nonmilitary providers, outside the gates of military installations, especially children of activated service members in the National Guard and Reserve.[11] One civilian group practice outside a large military treatment facility has 12% of their pediatric patient population enrolled in Tricare Prime, constituting care for more than 22 000 children from military families (Stuart A. Cohen, personal communication, November 21, 2012). Pediatricians need to be aware of common issues during wartime deployments, assess family coping skills, provide anticipatory guidance for the typical cycle of deployment, know where to find appropriate resources, and know when to refer for specialized services or care. For example, during well- or acute-care visits, pediatricians can address family stress and coping in addition to individual child needs related to parental/family military service (see Appendix, General Pediatrician Resources, Home-Base, a toolkit for well-child care of children in military families). This clinical report is intended for all pediatricians, both active duty and civilian, to aid in caring for military children whose loved ones have been, are, or will be deployed.

DEMOGRAPHICS OF MILITARY FAMILIES

US military demographics have changed dramatically since the dissolution of the draft in 1973. As the military became an all-volunteer force with career options, new challenges emerged for the Department of Defense to include housing; family services; over-

seas resources, including education; aging issues; and an increasing retiree population. The addition of more women to the uniformed services (increasing from 1% in 1970 to 15% in 2009) brought with it the need to balance mission and motherhood in a military workplace.[12] Use of the National Guard and Reserve to augment the active duty wartime deployments has resulted in the involvement of even more children and families.

Of the 60% of active duty service members who are married, 93% have female spouses (wives), and 44% have children. On average, military parents marry and have children at a younger age than civilian US parents. Seventy-five percent of all military children are younger than 11 years. The National Guard and Reserve members have similar family demographics as Active Duty service members, except that National Guard and Reserve members and spouses are slightly older, and the greatest proportion of children are schoolage.[12]

Military families have many of the same struggles common to all families, including child care, elder care, parenting concerns, marital issues, education issues, and career choices. However, in the military, families face additional stressors, including frequent relocations, international moves, separations other than war, and wartime deployment and its consequences.

Understanding military structure is important when considering the effects of deployment on children of service members. Each of the active duty services and each of the Selected Reserves have unique qualities that can help pediatricians understand the context of a child's experience with wartime deployment. The Department of Defense has 4 services with an active duty component. The largest is the Army, with 500 000 members, followed by the Navy, Air Force, and Marine Corps. The 5 states with most active duty members are California, Virginia, Texas, North Carolina, and Georgia.[12] As a group, the Reserve and National Guard are often referred to as the Selected Reserve and are made up by the largest group, the Army National Guard, followed by the Army Reserve, the Air National Guard, and the Reserve components from the Navy, Marine Corps, Air Force, and Coast Guard (now under Homeland Security). The 5 states with the largest Selected Reserve members are California, Texas, Pennsylvania, New York, and Florida. In 2005, half of the fighting forces in Iraq and Afghanistan were from the Selected Reserve, and although this has decreased to 15% to 20% of total deployed service members, more than 255 000 National Guard and Reserve service members had deployed by 2008.[13]

Service members are either enlisted or officers. For every officer (average age is 30 years, and >85% have a bachelor's degree), there are approximately 5 enlisted personnel (>50% are younger than 25 years, and 100% have high school diploma or general equivalency diploma). Active duty families often live on or near a military installation, they have neighbors and friends who are also military, and community resources are organized around military activities, including child care, financial and legal supports, and deployments. Typically, new families are "sponsored" or "hosted" by more experienced military families when they move to a new area.

In contrast, the National Guard and Reserve members train and are "activated," as needed. When these members are activated, it means they have been called up for active duty services. Most often, Selected Reserve members are activated for wartime deployment, although recent natural disasters have also resulted in activations of Selected Reserve members

to Southeast Asia and Haiti. The National Guard has state and homeland responsibilities as well. National Guard and Reserve members' families rarely live near a military installation and often seek health care and support from the community in which they live. These service members have primary civilian jobs. Civilian employers are not required to pay National Guard and Reserve members while they are activated and deployed. They are required to vacate or hold a position until return, although sometimes it is for 12 to 15 months.

TRICARE, the health care entitlement program for military families, has eligibility and benefits determined by the US Congress and administered by the Department of Defense via the TRICARE Management Authority.[14] TRICARE unites the direct health care resources (hospitals, clinics, and medical professional services) of the military medical system with networks of civilian professionals, hospitals, and agencies. TRICARE is free to all active duty military service members and their families. When National Guard or Reserve members are activated, they and their families are entitled to the same health coverage as active duty members.[14] This includes medical care and mental health services at any post or base regardless of service type as well as services provided by civilian providers endorsed in the TRICARE network. TRICARE mental health services (whether at a military hospital or clinic or by civilian providers) can be accessed directly by TRICARE beneficiaries without a referral from a primary care provider or previous authorization. Many National Guard and Reserve families switch to the TRICARE health care coverage during deployment because it is basically free, their own company does not cover them during the deployment, or they did not have coverage before

activation. Thus, activation and deployment often mean changing family health care providers temporarily or permanently. There are mechanisms for families who wish to seek care from a non-TRICARE network provider, but this choice requires a deductible and copay. For pediatricians with a number of patients with TRICARE benefits, it may be appropriate to consider TRICARE Preferred Provider status (www.tricare.osd.mil). TRICARE benefits remain up to 180 days after deactivation from duty. Dental coverage for families is also available but is not automatic. Eyeglasses are not covered.

DEPLOYMENT

Deployment is a temporary (3- to 15-month) movement of an individual or military unit away from his or her local work site, resources, and family to accomplish a task or mission. Deployments can occur during peacetime (activated service members during Hurricane Katrina in 2005 or, more recently, 12 000 service members to Haiti in 2010). Peacetime deployments (operations other than war) usually mean travel to safe locations, short duration, and interludes of rest and recovery between absences, and most military families do well. In fact, most military families expect periodic separations from their service member for sea tours or specialized schooling and training. Traditionally, "unaccompanied tours" (1-year remote assignments in which the family stays stateside) have not been described as deployment. Wartime deployments, in contrast, represent hostile, dangerous activity of usually long duration.

This is the first time in our nation's history that families are experiencing war in almost real time, with the use of cell phones, instant computer videos, and media coverage on the battlefield. Media reporters embedded in combat units provide "living room" observation of war activities. Video cameras and web messaging capabilities permit frequent personal contact with deployed services members, which families say is comforting.[15] However, there are also conversations of "near misses," abrupt disruptions in phone calls, and rumors of injury and death (even in the "safe zone") before confirmation, a few examples of a heightened sense of fear experienced by at-home family members not studied in previous wars.

HEALTH AND MENTAL HEALTH OUTCOMES OF RETURNING SERVICE MEMBERS

In the past 5 years, researchers have documented a greater understanding of the effects of war on the psychological well-being of soldiers, many of whom are parents.[1,2,16,17] Complications related to war-combat stress disorder, traumatic brain injury, development of psychiatric illness, and increase in health risk behaviors can complicate family life for a child. After deployment, soldiers' emotional and behavioral responses can range from typical short-term distress, such as change in sleep, decreased sense of safety, or social isolation, to the development of more serious psychiatric conditions, such as posttraumatic stress disorder or depression. It is estimated that more than 30% of returning soldiers have experienced posttraumatic stress disorder, depression, and/or traumatic brain injury.[18] Comorbidities, such as aggression and alcohol misuse, are prevalent in up to half of those with impairment.[1] There has also been an increase in the rates of suicide among military personnel. In 2007–2008, 255 active duty personnel committed suicide (20/100 000), an 80% increase from 2003, the beginning of the major troop deployments in Afghanistan and Iraq. There has also been an increase

in service members seeking mental health support; approximately 280 000 service members sought behavioral treatment in 2011.[19]

Studies of service members and their spouses indicate deployment has an effect on spouses' well-being and on marital relationships. In a 2010 report of more than 250 000 Army wives interviewed between 2003 and 2006, there were 41.3 excess cases of a mental health diagnosis per 1000 wives attributable to 1 to 11 months of wartime deployment. Furthermore, if more than 11 months of deployment occurred in those 3 years, 60.7 excess cases of mental health diagnosis per 1000 wives were identified.[20] It is not surprising that the toll of lengthy and recurrent deployments has been reflected in marital dissolution. The annual divorce rate among active duty soldiers in 2009 was 3.6%, up from 3.3% in 2007.[6] There is a significant body of literature available for informing pediatricians about the effects of parental psychopathology and marital discord on child well-being, distinct

from the stress of wartime deployment. Recognizing the increased vulnerability of children in these circumstances is a role general pediatricians already assume.[21–23]

CYCLE OF DEPLOYMENT

In 2001, Pincus et al reinforced a model describing the typical emotional reactions of family to deployment, called the "emotional cycle of deployment."[24] With onset of longer and repeated exposures, it is unclear whether a cycle is the correct paradigm, but it does provide insight into the diverse and complex nature of deployments, reflecting both the tremendous resilience as well as vulnerability of military families. Table 1 provides guidance for practitioners to assess and intervene with families throughout the cycle of deployment.

Before the wars in Iraq and Afghanistan, deployment was a rare occurrence for the vast majority of military forces. Most families had never experienced a separation to a hostile

TABLE 1 Anticipatory Guidance for Cycle of Deployment to Assess and Intervene in the Family System

Stages of Deployment	Provider Assessment and Anticipatory Guidance
Predicting difficulties with deployment	Assess previous history of family dysfunction, mental health issues in parent, special needs of children, recent family relocation, and previous problems during a deployment.
Predeployment	Discuss responsibilities and expectations of each family member during upcoming deployment. Make plans and goals for family rather than "put lives on hold." Decrease likelihood of misperception and distortion. Prepare for communication strategies and expectations.
Deployment	Initiate plans made during predeployment. Continue family traditions and develop new ones. Facilitate children's understanding of the finite nature of the deployment by developing timelines (as age appropriate).
Sustainment	Establish support systems (extended family, friends, religious group, family support groups, etc). Communicate with deployed service member via e-mail, phone, and letters. Avoid overspending. Spend some time without the children. Ask children how they are doing.
Postdeployment	Take time to communicate and get to know each other. Spend time talking to each other. Take time to make decisions and changes in routine. Lower holiday expectations. Keep plans simple and flexible. Do not try to schedule too many things during the first few weeks. Let absent parent "back into" the family circle.

environment before 2001. Since then, however, families have experienced prolonged and repeated wartime deployments. Deployments have 3 stages, each with typical dynamics: predeployment, deployment (including sustainment), and postdeployment (or redeployment).

1. The predeployment stage begins with the unit sending orders for a service member to deploy. Sometimes there are months of notice and preparation, and sometimes only days. Often, soldiers know their next deployment date when they return from a previous deployment. On 1 survey, spouses indicated that the hardest thing about a deployment was hearing of subsequent deployments.[15] Predeployment can be challenging for both the service member and the at-home parent. Often, the unit requires long hours and lengthy trainings in the months leading up to deployment, resulting in extended absences. Decisions to find alternative or additional child care are often expensive and stressful. For the 40% to 60% of at-home parents who work outside the home, decisions about careers, financial adjustments, or excessive leave to support sick children result in many spouses quitting their jobs. Legal requirements, such as power of attorney and a will, bring up issues of mortality. Unresolved anxieties and expectations from previous deployments interfere with preparation for new deployments.

Although the predeployment stage is stressful for parents, it can be confusing to children, who may not understand why separation is necessary and have no concept of the change about to occur. Children at various developmental ages experience excitement, denial, worry, fear, and anger. Emotional withdrawal is not uncommon immediately before deployment. Last-minute or recurrent goodbyes often increase tension.

2. Deployment typically lasts between 3 and 15 months. The deployment stage usually begins with a tearful ceremony, despite strong feelings of support, patriotism, and duty. This is often followed by a period (usually 1–6 weeks) of emptiness, loss, and abandonment. Spouses report feeling numb, sad, and vulnerable.[15] The intensity leading up to a goodbye can be overwhelming, and the sense of relief that the deployment has actually started can be confusing. After about 6 weeks, most families try to establish a routine. This stage of adjustment may be erratic, with good days and bad days. Finding new resources and new routines and understanding the limits of the family's coping abilities occurs during this time.

Sustainment is the period during the deployment stage (usually between 4 and 13 months) when a new routine without the deployed parent is established. During this time, school-age children and adolescents can develop some positive attributes of a deployment. These difficult life experiences (not dissimilar to family illness, a house fire, etc) can foster maturity, provide opportunities to acquire new skills, encourage independence, build new relationships, and strengthen family cohesion. Deployed service members may come home for 2 weeks for a "midtour" or rest and recuperation leave. Many families have said that rest and recuperation leave is a difficult time for children because it often falls during the school year; children are distracted by anticipation, excitement, and a short period of visitation; and they then have to say goodbye all over again. Despite trying to find resilience and strength, many families describe deployment as a "surviving, not thriving" time. For the month or 2 before homecoming, there may be worry as well as excitement. New independence or self-reliance may have emerged,

and family members are unsure how to reintegrate a deployed parent into a year-older family. This can also be a challenge to the returning service member.

3. At postdeployment (reunion), most families start off with a "honeymoon." The happiness of reuniting is mixed with getting reacquainted and deciding how to share the time lost. There is a sense that problems can be solved, and, to some extent, families can return to "normal." However, the new normal may look different from the roles family members played when a service member left over a year before. The service member is immediately thrust back into a full-time family life, which is desired but often difficult to accommodate while readjusting to daily routines. "Block leave" is 2 to 4 weeks of vacation time given to the postdeployment individual or unit but may not coincide with family member availability from school or work. During this time, at-home parents often want some much-needed respite after a prolonged period of "full-time" parenting.

ASSESSING FAMILY'S RESPONSE TO STRESS

Stress reactions represent an evolutionary advantage in the face of danger, prompting effective adaptations to changing conditions in the environment. Such reactions are often critical and not detrimental. How well or poorly an individual or family responds to a given stressor, such as wartime deployment, is dependent on several factors:

- the individual's previous experiences with stress;

- the meaning of this specific stress;

- the family context where the stress is experienced, including how the parent is coping; and

- the inherent, as well as external, resources available to deal with the stress.

"To assume either widespread pathology or uniform resilience to the stresses of wartime deployments would be superficial and harmful to children and their families."[25] Most families experience substantial stress, and although the risk is present, a minority of families have evidence of being "stressed out," such as maladaptive coping, mental illness, substance use or abuse, or maltreatment.

Resilience appears to play a major factor in all phases of deployment. Overall, studies indicate protective factors, including family readiness, "meaning making" of the situation, receipt of community and social support, acceptance of military lifestyle, ability to develop self-reliant coping skills, and adoption of flexible gender roles. Additionally, at least 5 years of marriage, higher parental education, and civilian spouse working outside the home may contribute to stronger family resilience[9] during deployments.

EFFECT OF WARTIME DEPLOYMENT ON CHILDREN

Previous Research

In the earliest research (1949) on military families coping with postwar settings, Hill studied how the family adjusted to World War II soldiers' return. He proposed that the actual war "time of separation" needed to be considered in the context of family resources. On the basis of family interviews, he noted that the meaning families placed on the war, and the "time of separation" predicted positive versus negative adaptation on return of the soldier.[26] Subsequently, McCubbin and Patterson studied families of Vietnam veterans and concluded that a "pile up" of prewar, during-war, and postwar stressors "added up" to the degree of maladaptation and that a cumulative effect of stress was not purely the result of

wartime deployment.[27] This concept of contextual factors in a family influencing coping and adaptation to stress of war studied during 20th-century US military conflicts may provide important insight into the first war experiences of the 21st century.

In 1978, LaGrone coined the term "military family syndrome" following review of 792 Army charts of children seen in psychology clinics for behavioral problems.[28] He concluded that military families suffer greater psychosocial difficulties than do families in the general population. Later, more methodologically rigorous research, with prospective studies of military versus nonmilitary children, did not find any differences between military versus nonmilitary children. Interestingly, 1 study of Navy families, for whom routine 6-month "sea duty" deployments were a way of life for years, indicated that children demonstrated increased responsibility, independence, and confidence compared with their peers without deployment experiences, suggesting that children develop a different and beneficial parent-child relationship with the at-home parent.[29] In many nonmilitary situations in which parents are absent for periods of time but not in danger, many children demonstrate resilience and strong coping strategies.

Clearly, dangerous combat deployments of parents are significantly more distressing than are peacetime deployments for most children. The first combat deployment studies were conducted during Operation Desert Storm (1990–1991). Children demonstrated moderate degrees of increased internalizing symptoms (such as depression and anxiety)[30,31] and possibly less family cohesion.[32] At-risk groups included those with preexisting psychosocial issues and at-home parents with psychopathologic problems. One study addressing whether gender of

deployed parents affected children found no significant differences in child adaptation between fathers versus mothers who were deployed.[33] An Army family study reported that children who demonstrated strong coping skills during deployment had greater adaptation postdeployment.[34] Additional information about the history of military children and families is available in a recent *Pediatrics* supplement devoted to military pediatrics.[35]

Current Research

Wartime deployment can be stressful for a child, regardless of his or her developmental stage. Changes in behavior, both externalizing and internalizing, and changes in school performance are reported.[7–9,11,36–38] High levels of sadness and worry are reported in most age groups.[7–9,39] Depressive symptoms are reported in approximately 1 in 4 children experiencing deployment of a parent.[39] More than one-third of children report excessive worry about their parent's deployment.[38,39] A parent survey noted 1 in 5 school-age children cope poorly,[9,38,39] and a similar number have academic problems. Length of deployment was associated with significant behavioral health problems.[7] Children and their families were ambivalent about access to a wartime parent, on the one hand comforted by talking to parent on computer[15] and on the other hand identifying media coverage as a source of stress.[39] In addition, a recent population-based study reported increased use of mental-behavioral health services in children whose parents were deployed.[11] Finally, a large population study of 307 520 children of parents in the nonretired active duty military, children 5 to 17 years of age (2003–2006) noted a greater number of mental health diagnoses and more diagnoses correlating with the total time of deployment.[40]

Children of All Ages Are Affected by Wartime Deployments

Infants and Toddlers

In a survey of almost 4000 military spouses with and without deployed partners, researchers investigating depressive symptoms during pregnancy noted that twice as many women with deployed partners reported depressive symptoms before and after delivery compared with those whose partners were at home.[41] In 2008, the first study of preschool-age children affected by current wartime deployments revealed higher emotional reactivity, anxiousness/depression, somatic complaints, and withdrawal than did children whose parents were not deployed.[37] A subsequent study of 57 families with young children found similar findings during deployments.[42]

School Age

The degree of at-home parental stress was the most significant predictor of the child's psychosocial functioning during a wartime deployment. School-age children whose parents were younger, had been married for a shorter period of time, and were junior enlisted rank were at higher risk of having psychosocial problems. Parents who had a college education, a sense of military support, and community support had less parental stress and reported fewer psychosocial problems in their children. Using the Pediatric Symptom Checklist during parental deployment, school-age children scored "high-risk" for emotional and behavioral problems 2.5 times more frequently than national norms. Sleep problems were noted in a majority (56%) of the children.[9] Lester et al found combat deployments had a cumulative negative psychosocial effect on a sample of school-age

children that persisted despite the return of the deployed parent.[7] Mansfield accessed electronic medical records for outpatient care on more than 300 000 school-age children and found a similar "dose-response" pattern between deployment and increased mental health diagnoses.[40]

Adolescents

In a focus group of adolescents whose parents were deployed to Iraq (Operation Iraqi Freedom, Operation New Dawn) and Afghanistan (Operation Enduring Freedom), there were reported changes in relationship with the deployed parent, concern and anxiety about the deployed parent's well-being, and worse performance in school, yet increases in responsibility and maturity in caring for younger siblings.[38] In a telephone survey of 1500 military youth and their at-home parent, Chandra reported increased emotional difficulties associated with longer deployment times and emphasized the importance of positive coping and mental health of the at-home parent.[8] The effects of war can have life-threatening consequences for military children and their families far removed from the battlefields. A study in Texas demonstrated the rate of child maltreatment in the military increased significantly since 2001 and was associated with increased rates of deployment. For military personnel with at least 1 dependent, the rate of child maltreatment increased by approximately 30% for every 1% increase in service members who left for or returned from combat.[43] In another study, from a confidential registry of substantiated cases in the Army, child maltreatment was found to be 42% higher in families of US enlisted soldiers during combat deployment versus nondeployed status and exceeded the comparative civilian rates

of maltreatment, which remained steady during the same time frame. Overall, child maltreatment was 3 times higher during times of deployment, with neglect being 4 times higher and physical abuse being 2 times higher. This study reported the highest increase in maltreatment to be attributed to the at-home caregiver while the service member was deployed.[44]

SUGGESTIONS FOR PEDIATRICIANS

All pediatricians should be prepared to address parental (and other relationships that may be meaningful to the child) wartime deployment issues. This includes recognition of service-specific characteristics of the deployed service member, stage of deployment, and whether there have been previous deployment experiences. The role of the pediatrician is to assess the level of family and child stress that occurs whenever there is a family change, like wartime deployment, and to use the principles of anticipatory guidance, psychoeducation, and continued surveillance and screening as families are seen over time. Asking "How are you doing with this deployment?" may be the single most important family assessment question. Another question is, "Has anyone in your family or close community been involved with wartime experiences?" If yes, the follow-up is "How are your family members coping with this experience?" There are specific situations that warrant additional probing such as, during the postpartum period, when new mothers with a deployed partner may be at heightened risk of depression. Additional guidance during perinatal and postpartum period can be found in this article's Appendix. Another situation to plan for includes speaking confidentially with adolescents, which may help to ensure they are not downplaying their fears and worry. Because of the increased risk of child maltreatment during deployments, child abuse screening and mental health screening of child caregivers are also important elements of the clinical encounter.

Next, the pediatrician should determine the developmental age of the child and assess his or her understanding of deployment (see earlier section, "Cycle of Deployment"). Families need reassurance that children's reactions to a deployed parent are common reactions (see Table 2) and that, for the most part, children adapt to the experience with effective coping skills. Adolescents self-report problems with a similar prevalence as their parents and may have more valid reporting than their parents of their own internalizing symptoms.[38]

Common Child and Adolescent Reactions to Deployment

- Preschool: children at this age have difficulty with change and will not have a full understanding of why a parent is leaving or for how long, compared with the older child and adolescent. Before deployment, they will understand that there has been a change in the family behavior but will not understand the full extent until the parent is absent. Children need reassurance that they will be cared for and kept safe and they did not cause the deployment.

- School-age: children at this age have a greater understanding of why a parent is being deployed, but there still may be confusion. They may hear from other friends and see stories about the war on television and may have heightened worries about the safety of their loved one. It is reasonable for the remaining parent to shelter children from the day-to-day details

TABLE 2 Common Reactions to Deployment[45]

Feelings	Behaviors
Preschool	
Confusion	Clinging, demands for attention
Anger	Problems separating from the remaining parent
Guilt	Irritability and aggression
	Regression (thumb sucking, bedwetting)
	Sleep disturbances
	Feeding issues (more picky)
	Easy frustration and more difficult to comfort
School-age	
Same feelings as preschool plus:	New behavior problems or in intensification of already existing problems
Increased sadness (lack of family normalcy and loss of deployed parent)	Regression
Worry about deployed parent	Rapid mood swings
Fear that remaining parent might leave or die	Changes in eating and sleeping
Anger at parent for missing important events	Anger at both parents for disrupting normalcy
	Changes in behavior at school and with friends (anger, aggression)
	Need to be and do "normal" things (eg, parties)
	Somatic complaints
Adolescent	
Anger	Misdirected or acting-out behavior toward others or themselves
Sadness	School problems
Depression	Apathy, loss of interest, noncommunication, and denial of feelings
Anxiety	Increased importance of friends to the detriment of reasonable family life
Fear	Trying to take charge of the family

of news about the war. Sometimes children feel responsible for the parent being deployed, especially if there has been unresolved tension between the deployed parent and the child. The parent should explain the child's situation to a schoolteacher. It is important to monitor thoughts and feelings about a spouse or partner in front of the child. At this age, children need a trusted adult, either the remaining parent or another adult, with whom they can talk and share their feelings. They need to feel safe and secure.

- Adolescents: teenagers understand the reasons deployment is occurring and the full ramifications of the deployment process. They may feel angry and sad and often get support from their peers outside the family. They may not wish to share their thoughts and feel-

ings with family members. They may not want their parent to inform school of parental deployment. The at-home parent should accept and understand this coping mechanism while monitoring how their teenager is doing in school and with friends.

Helping Children Cope and Foster Resilience During Deployment

Preschool and Elementary School Children (3–9 Years)

To help the child feel connected to the deployed family member, caregivers should do the following:

1. Continue the discussion about the deployed parent on a regular basis.

2. Communicate to the deployed parent frequently and regularly: write letters, draw pictures, put together "goodie" packages.

3. Keep a calendar for each child so he or she can see when the deployed family member is coming home.

4. Have a picture of the deployed parent with the children or with the family. Pictures can be hung up or put in prominent places. This is especially important for the preschool-age child.

5. Protect younger children from seeing or hearing about the war effort or violence on television or in the newspapers.

6. Have deployed parent audio or video record a favorite bedtime story before leaving, especially if reading was a normal routine before leaving.

7. Seek support from extended family or a trusted adult (mentor, for school-age child) who can be available for the children.

8. Ask family and friends not to talk about the painful or scary aspects of deployment.

9. Keep up the family routine.

10. Try to spend extra time with the child or children, if possible and respond empathically to the needs for more attention.

11. Encourage ways for children to express their feelings. For younger children, it may be drawing or playing with dolls, and for older children, it may be telling stories or keeping a journal and possibly sharing the journal, especially at bedtime.

12. Appreciate that young children will act out scary and fearful feelings through play. Support and understand this process and monitor the behaviors and feelings during times of family or school activities.

13. Request the free *Sesame Street* video *Talk, Listen, Connect* (www. militaryonesource.com). Request free Military Child or Youth videos, *Mr. Poe and Friends Discuss Reunion After Deployment* (www. aap.org/sections/uniformedservices/ deployment/videos.html) for younger children.

14. Communicate to teachers about the deployment and continue to check in on their school performance and behaviors.

15. Develop a scrapbook of children's activities and accomplishments to be shared when there is reunion. This will allow the child to "show and tell."

Middle School and Adolescence (10–18 Years)

1. Encourage conversations about deployment and war ("I know this is tough for you and I am here for you. Feel free to talk with me at any time.").

2. Help children maintain regular contact with the deployed parent.

3. Monitor excessive exposure or contact with media coverage of the war.

4. Maintain routines.

5. Do not expect teenagers to act as coparents. They should maintain regular activities and responsibilities.

6. Do not change any of the discipline rules or their consequences.

7. Appreciate the needs of teenagers to be with peers and provide special time with the teenager doing special activities.

8. Be patient and calm in the face of increased anger irritability and withdrawal. Extra support or physical affection can help.

9. Encourage teenagers to get appropriate nutrition, rest, and exercise and monitor for changes in sleep patterns, changes in school, and activities of daily living.

10. Encourage middle-school-age children and teenagers to keep a diary and respect the need for privacy if they wish not to share.

11. Order a free copy of the video *Military Youth Coping With Separation: When Family Members Deploy* (see Appendix for Resources).

12. Encourage children and teenagers to continue extracurricular and community activities.

13. Consider attending "Operation Purple" camp (www.militaryfamily.org) activities or summer camps for students with a deployed parent.

When Should a Primary Care Pediatrician Refer for Additional Help?

If a family is struggling with deployment, the pediatrician can help them contact their "rear detachment chaplain," the "family readiness group," a TRICARE case coordinator, Military One Source, or the local Exceptional Family Member Program; seek deployment-related respite or child care services or offer school-age children "Operation Purple" camp.

The pediatrician may consider a referral to a mental health professional

1. if reassurance and helping the parent cope using a psychoeducational intervention or generally supportive counseling is not working after 2 visits or if there is significant stress at the first visit.

2. if the pediatrician is unsure of his or her counseling and psychoeducational skills and the family is significantly stressed (learn more about motivational interviewing[46]).

3. if the child's behaviors have become more extreme or continue for up to 3 months after the deployed parent has returned home.[47]

4. if there is a significant change in behavior or a drop in grades at school.

5. if there is increased and sustained negativity and reassurance and support does not help.

6. if the teenager is continually away from home and does not check in with the at-home parent.

7. if the at-home parent is not able to cope; is excessively worried, anxious, or simply overwhelmed; and cannot respond to the child's emotional needs.

8. if there is injury of a parent and if other resources provided are not effective (discussed next section).

9. If there is death of a parent and other support programs provided for bereaved families are not effective (see next section).

Injury or Death of a Parent

From October 1, 2001, through February 6, 2012, there were 6351 American casualties in Operation Iraqi Freedom, Operation New Dawn, and Operation Enduring Freedom and 47 545 wounded in action.[48] Although the majority of combat casualties have been active duty soldiers, 11.5% have been service members from the National Guard and 7% have been service members from the Reserve.[47] The combat death or significant injury of a parent is an unexpected and devastating experience for all families.[48,49] The type of injury and degree of disability will determine the way family members cope and adapt. Many families of National Guard and Reserve service members do not have the same community supports as those on active duty. The military medical system and the Office of Veterans Affairs will carry out rehabilitation and medical care of the injured service member. The pediatrician should be available to monitor the social-emotional impact of such an

event on the children and the spouse and refer when appropriate. In this setting, the pediatrician should become familiar with and/or contact the Center for the Study of Traumatic Stress (www.centerforthestudyoftraumaticstress.org), which has expertise and resources specific to combat-injured families.[50]

The death of a parent or significant parenting figure during war is a catastrophically disorganizing event for a child, the surviving parent, and the family. It is one of the unspoken fears that family members endure during wartime deployment. Helping children understand parental death requires a developmentally unique sensitivity, and universal preventive counseling in the face of such a devastating stress should be encouraged.[51,52] The pediatrician should assess the social-emotional reaction of the child in relationship to his or her developmental stage, follow the child over time, and support the remaining parent or life partner. Important policy statements and reports have been provided for pediatricians who desire additional guidance in these skills (see Appendix). When a family is notified of the death of an active duty service member, they are assigned to a Casualty Assistance Representative (CAR), whose sole purpose is to help the family through the military's unique entitlement process and find needed resources. For example, families who reside in government housing (or have a housing allowance) are allowed to remain at their current location (both housing and schooling) for up to 6 months as they determine next steps. Because of the devastating nature of this event, some parents or partners may need referral for social-emotional assessment and therapy, as appropriate. A specific resource for military families is Tragedy Assistance Program for Survivors (www.TAPS.org).[53] The pediatrician can encourage parents

to seek out additional military support through Decedent Affairs, Chaplains' Office, or Commanders of the military unit. This support is usually made available at the time that the spouse or partner is notified of the death of their loved one.

Supporting the Parent

Above all, to have the strength to help children, the nondeployed parent needs to feel in control and have someone to help him or her. The pediatrician can encourage each primary caregiver to stay healthy and connected, including someone with whom to share experiences and opportunities for personal growth, respite, and spiritual wellness. The pediatrician can support and help the parent find a mental health professional so that the parent may be better able to care for his or her children.[54] A resource for all military spouses to access adult mental health services, regardless of location, is www.MilitaryOneSource.com. In the setting of a medical home, pediatricians should be familiar with this Web site to help family caregivers with their own emotional needs. Many deployment-specific resources available to active duty families can be accessed on this Web site for activated National Guard and Reserve families, including military family life consultants, chaplains, legal assistance, social work services, and new parent support programs. Recently the Department of Defense, under the auspices of the United States Bureau of Navy, Medicine and Surgery, initiated a demonstration project titled Family Overcoming Under Stress (FOCUS). This project began in 2008 and as of 2010 included 14 military institutions. The goal of the project was to investigate the impact of a family-centered program on military families, addressing stress and mental health, using a "trauma informed, skill based, family centered prevention intervention designed to mitigate the sequelae of highly stressful deployment-related events on children and parents." The 8-session resiliency psychoeducation program for parents and children used a trained "Resiliency Trainer." Results demonstrated a decrease in parental posttraumatic stress, depression, and anxiety as well as a decrease in childhood conduct problems, emotional symptoms, and total childhood difficulties. In addition, there was significant improvement in "child pro-social functioning and increases in children's use of positive coping strategies."[55–58]

In addition to direct contact with a case manager or mental health locator, at-home parents can request free parenting and support books from the online library and can find local support groups.

The American Academy of Pediatrics Committee on Psychosocial Aspects of Child and Family Health has previously released a report titled "Psychosocial Implications of Disaster or Terrorism on Children: A Guide for the Pediatrician."[47] The report discusses the diagnostic aspects of posttraumatic stress disorder and acute stress disorder, which may be helpful if a child or adolescent is demonstrating excessive or prolonged symptoms associated with parental deployment or reunion, especially in the circumstance of parental injury. Additional military-unique resources for the pediatrician can be found on the Section on Uniformed Services Web site (www.aap.org/sections/unifserv/deployment/index.htm), which includes additional military Web sites, recent research publications, videos for children and adolescents, and information about summer camp experiences, such as Operation Purple camps.

The vast majority of military families can and do cope and adapt to service member deployments. Pediatricians need to recognize when deployment is affecting the emotional and social well-being of children and their parents and relatives and be particularly sensitive to the unique needs of National Guard and Reserve service member families. They need to gather deployment-specific information to assess and monitor the social-emotional reaction of children and family members and refer to mental health professionals or deployment-specific specialists for more extensive diagnostic and therapeutic interventions, as appropriate. By understanding the military family and the experiences of parental wartime deployments, all pediatricians and other health care providers serving children can be the "front line" for the health and well-being of US military children and their family members, especially in time of war.

Appendix

GENERAL INFORMATION RESOURCES FOR PEDIATRICIANS AND PARENTS

General Pediatric Resources

1. The American Academy of Pediatrics, Section on Uniformed Services Web site. Available at: www.aap.org/sections/unifserv/deployment/index.htm. Learn about what primary care providers are doing to take care of military children and teens. Order copies of free military child and youth support videos, including the DVD *Military Youth Coping With Separation*.

2. Ginsburg KR. *Building Resilience in Children and Teens: Giving Kids Roots and Wings*. 2nd ed. Elk Grove Village, IL: American Academy of Pediatrics; 2011.

3. Massachusetts Child Psychiatry Access Project toolkit. Available online for assessing military children at well child visits: www.homebaseprogram.org/community-education/~/media/DDA3707B-C4A648E89F1A7C619C48FC28.pdf.

4. Hooah 4 Health. Available at: www.hooah4health.com. Checklists that pediatricians can help families work through for each stage of deployment, understand reactions postdeployment, and find resources.

5. Center for the Study of Traumatic Stress. Available at: www.centerforthestudyoftraumaticstress.org. Resources and research for health care providers, service members, and their families.

6. American Academy of Pediatrics, Committee on Psychosocial Aspects of Child and Family Health. The pediatrician and childhood bereavement. *Pediatrics.* 2000;105(2):445–447.

7. Bonanno GA, Mancini AD. The human capacity to thrive in the face of potential trauma. *Pediatrics.* 2008;121(2):369–375.

8. Levetown M; American Academy of Pediatrics Committee on Bioethics. Communicating with children and families: from everyday interactions to skill in conveying distressing information. *Pediatrics.* 2008;121(5):e1441–e1460.

9. Madrid PA, Grant R, Reilly MJ, Redlener NB. Challenges in meeting immediate emotional needs: short-term impact of a major disaster on children's mental health: building resiliency in the aftermath of Hurricane Katrina. *Pediatrics.* 2006;117(5 pt 3):S448–S453.

10. Hagan JF Jr; American Academy of Pediatrics Committee on Psychosocial Aspects of Child and Family Health; Task Force on Terrorism. Psychosocial implications of disaster or terrorism on children: a guide for the pediatrician. *Pediatrics.* 2005;116(3):787–795.

11. Earls MF; Committee on Psychosocial Aspects of Child and Family

Health American Academy of Pediatrics. Clinical Report. Incorporating recognition and management of perinatal and postpartum depression into pediatric practice. *Pediatrics.* 2010;126(5):1032–1039. Available at: http://pediatrics. aappublications.org/content/early/ 2010/10/25/peds.2010-2348.full.pdf+ html.

12. Cox JL, Holden JM, Sagovsky R. Detection of postnatal depression. Development of the 10-item Edinburgh Postnatal Depression Scale. *Br J Psychiatry.* 1987;150:782–786

Parent Resources

1. *Sesame Street Talk. Listen, Connect.* Preschool-aged deployment support video program. Learn about the program and order free copies at: www.sesameworkshop.org/tlc.

2. Operation Purple Camps: www.nmfa. org/site/PageServer?pagename= op_default. The goal of these free summer camps is to bring together youth who are experiencing some stage of a deployment and the stress that goes along with it. Operation Purple camps give kids the coping skills and support networks of peers to better handle life's ups and downs.

3. Military One Source. (800) 342-9647 or www.militaryonesource.com. Military support solutions for families. The single best resource for any family in any branch of service.

4. Ginsberg KR. *A Parent's Guide to Building Resilience in Children and Teens: Giving Your Child Roots and Wings*, 2nd ed. Elk Grove Village, IL: American Academy of Pediatrics; 2011.

5. Military Home Front: www.military-homefront.dod.mil.

6. Military Child Education Coalition: www.militarychild.org.7. Military Teens on the Move: www.dod.mil/ mtom/index_t.htm.

7. Tragedy Assistance Program for Survivors: www.taps.org.

8. Zero to Three—Coming Together Around Military Families: www. zerotothree.org/about-us/funded-projects/military-families.

LEAD AUTHORS

Benjamin S. Siegel, MD
COL (ret) Beth Ellen Davis, MD, MPH

COMMITTEE ON PSYCHOSOCIAL ASPECTS OF CHILD AND FAMILY HEALTH, 2011–2012

Benjamin S. Siegel, MD, Chairperson
Mary I. Dobbins, MD
Andrew S. Garner, MD, PhD

Laura J. McGuinn, MD
John M. Pascoe, MD, MPH
David L. Wood, MD, MPH
Michael Yogman, MD

LIAISONS

Ronald T. Brown, PhD — *Society of Pediatric Psychology*
Terry Carmichael, MSW — *National Association of Social Workers*
Mary Jo Kupst, PhD — *Society of Pediatric Psychology*
D. Richard Martini, MD — *American Academy of Child and Adolescent Psychiatry*
Mary Sheppard, MS, RN, PNP, BC — *National Association of Pediatric Nurse Practitioners*

CONSULTANT

George J. Cohen, MD

STAFF

Stephanie Domain

SECTION ON UNIFORMED SERVICES EXECUTIVE COMMITTEE, 2011–2012

LT COL Michael Rajnik, MD, Chairperson
COL (ret) Beth Ellen Davis, MD, MPH, Immediate Past Chairperson
CAPT Wanda Denise Barfield, MD, MPH
CAPT Jerri Curtis, MD
CDR Tony Delgado, MD
LTC Thomas G. Eccles, MD
CDR Christine Leigh Johnson, MD
LTC Catherine Anne Kimball-Eayrs, MD, IBCLC
COL Richard Kynion
LT COL Thomas Charles Newton, MD
COL Laura Place, MD

STAFF

Jackie Burke

REFERENCES

1. Thomas JL, Wilk JE, Riviere LA, McGurk D, Castro CA, Hoge CW. Prevalence of mental health problems and functional impairment among active component and National Guard soldiers 3 and 12 months following combat in Iraq. *Arch Gen Psychiatry.* 2010;67(6):614–623

2. Milliken CS, Auchterlonie JL, Hoge CW. Longitudinal assessment of mental health problems among active and reserve component soldiers returning from the Iraq war. *JAMA.* 2007;298(18):2141–2148

3. Howell A, Wool ZH. *The War Comes Home: The Toll of War and the Shifting Burden of Care.* Providence, RI: Watson Institute for International Studies, Brown University, June 13, 2011. Available at: http://costsofwar. org/article/us-veterans-and-military-families. Accessed January 15, 2013

4. American Psychological Association. *The Psychological Needs of US Military Service Members and Their Families: A Preliminary Report.* Washington, DC: American Psychological Association; 2007. Available at: www. apa.org/about/policy/military-deployment-services.pdf. Accessed July 23, 2012

5. The White House. Presidential initiative supports military families [press release, January 24, 2011]. Available at: www. whitehouse.gov/the-press-office/2011/01/24/ presidential-initiative-supports-military-families. Accessed July 23, 2012

6. National Scientific Council on the Developing Child. *Persistent Fear and Anxiety Can Affect Young Children's Learning and Development: Working Paper No. 9.* Cambridge, MA: National Scientific Council on the Developing Child, Harvard University; 2010. Available at: http://developingchild. harvard.edu/index.php/resources/reports_ and_working_papers/working_papers/wp9/. Accessed July 23, 2012

7. Lester P, Peterson K, Reeves J, et al. The long war and parental combat deployment: effects on military children and at-home

spouses. *J Am Acad Child Adolesc Psychiatry.* 2010;49(4):310–320

8. Chandra A, Lara-Cinisomo S, Jaycox LH, et al. Children on the homefront: the experience of children from military families. *Pediatrics.* 2010;125(1):16–25

9. Flake EM, Davis BE, Johnson PL, Middleton LS. The psychosocial effects of deployment on military children. *J Dev Behav Pediatr.* 2009;30(4):271–278

10. Gorman LA, Blow AJ, Ames BD, Reed PL. National Guard families after combat: mental health, use of mental health services, and perceived treatment barriers. *Psychiatr Serv.* 2011;62(1):28–34

11. Gorman GH, Eide M, Hisle-Gorman E. Wartime military deployment and increased pediatric mental and behavioral health complaints. *Pediatrics.* 2010;126(6):1058–1066

12. Department of Defense. 2009 *Demographics Profile of the Military Community.* Available at: http://www.militaryonesource.mil/12038/MOS/Reports/2009_Demographics_Report.pdf. Accessed July 23, 2012

13. Waterhouse M, O'Bryant J. *National Guard Personnel and Deployments: Fact Sheet.* CRS Report for Congress. Washington, DC: Congressional Research Service, National Library of Medicine; 2008. Available at: www.fas.org/sgp/crs/natsec/RS22451.pdf. Accessed July 23, 2012

14. Tricare Insurance Program Web site. Available at: www.tricare.osd.mil. Accessed July 23, 2012

15. National Military Family Association. *Report on the Cycles of Deployment Survey: An Analysis of Survey Responses From April Through September, 2005.* Available at: www.militaryfamily.org/assets/pdf/NMFACyclesofDeployment9.pdf. Accessed July 23, 2012

16. Hoge CW, Castro CA, Messer SC, McGurk D, Cotting DI, Koffman RL. Combat duty in Iraq and Afghanistan, mental health problems, and barriers to care. *N Engl J Med.* 2004;351(1):13–22

17. Hoge CW, McGurk D, Thomas JL, Cox AL, Engel CC, Castro CA. Mild traumatic brain injury in U.S. Soldiers returning from Iraq. *N Engl J Med.* 2008;358(5):453–463

18. RAND Corporation, Center for Military Health Policy Research. *Invisible Wounds of War. Psychological and Cognitive Injuries, Their Consequences and Services to Assist Recovery.* Santa Monica, CA: RAND Corporation; 2008. Available at: www.oregon.gov/ODVA/TASKFORCE/docs/Resources/InvisibleWoundsOfWar.pdf?ga=t. Accessed July 23, 2012

19. Bachynski KE, Canham-Chervak M, Black SA, Dada EO, Millikan AM, Jones BH. Mental health risk factors for suicides in the US Army, 2007–8. *Inj Prev.* 2012;18(6):405–412

20. Mansfield AJ, Kaufman JS, Marshall SW, Gaynes BN, Morrissey JP, Engel CC. Deployment and the use of mental health services among U.S. Army wives. *N Engl J Med.* 2010;362(2):101–109

21. Woolston JL. A child's reactions to parents' problems. *Pediatr Rev.* 1986;8(6):169–176

22. Committee on Psychosocial Aspects of Child and Family Health and Task Force on Mental Health. Policy Statement—The future of pediatrics: mental health competencies for pediatric primary care. *Pediatrics.* 2009;124(1):410–421

23. Foy JM; American Academy of Pediatrics Task Force on Mental Health. Enhancing pediatric mental health care: algorithms for primary care. *Pediatrics.* 2010;125 (6 suppl 3):S109–S125

24. Pincus SH, House R, Christenson J, Adler LE. Emotional cycle of deployment: a military family perspective. US Army Med Depart J. 2001;Apr/June:15–23. Available at: http://4h.missouri.edu/programs/military/resources/manual/Deployment-Cycles.pdf. Accessed April 9, 2013

25. Cozza SJ, Chun RS, Polo JA. Military families and children during operation Iraqi freedom. *Psychiatr Q.* 2005;76(4):371–378

26. Hill R. *Families Under Stress: Adjustment to the Crisis of War Separation and Reunion.* Westport, CT: Greenwood Press; 1971

27. Patterson J, McCubbin H. Gender role and coping. *J Marriage Fam.* 1984;46(1):95–104

28. Lagrone DM. The military family syndrome. *Am J Psychiatry.* 1978;135(9):1040–1043

29. Drummet AR, Coleman M, Cable S. Military families under stress: implications for family life education. *Fam Relat.* 2003;52(3):279–287

30. Rosen LN, Teitelbaum JM, Westhuis DJ. Children's reactions to the Desert Storm deployment: initial findings from a survey of Army families. *Mil Med.* 1993;158(7):465–469

31. Jensen PS, Martin D, Watanabe HJ. Children's response to parental separation during operation desert storm. *J Am Acad Child Adolesc Psychiatry.* 1996;35(4):433–441

32. Kelley ML. The effects of military-induced separation on family factors and child behavior. *Am J Orthopsychiatry.* 1994;64(1):103–111

33. Applewhite LW, Mays RA. Parent-child separation: a comparison of maternally and paternally separated children in military families. *Child Adolesc Social Work J.* 1986;13(1):23–40

34. Huebner AJ, Mancini JA. *Adjustments Among Adolescents in Military Families When a Parent Is Deployed: Final Report to the Military Family Research Institute and Department of Defense Quality of Life Office.* West Lafayette, IN: Purdue University, Military Family Research Institute; 2005

35. Davis BE, Blaschke GS, Stafford EM. Military children, families, and communities: supporting those who serve. Pediatrics. 2012: 129; S 3–10

36. Chandra A, Burns RM, Tanielain T. RAND Corporation, Center for Military Health Policy Research. Understanding the Impact of Deployment on Children and Families. Findings from a Pilot Study of Operation Purple Camp Participants. Santa Monica, CA: Rand Corporation; April 2008. Available at: www.rand.org/pubs/working_papers/WR566.html. Accessed July 23, 2012

37. Chartrand MM, Frank DA, White LF, Shope TR. Effect of parents' wartime deployment on the behavior of young children in military families. *Arch Pediatr Adolesc Med.* 2008;162(11):1009–1014

38. Aranda MC, Middleton LC, Flake E, Davis BE. Psychosocial screening in children with wartime-deployed parents. *Mil Med.* 2011; 176(4):402–407

39. Orthner D, Den K, Rose R. 2005 SAF V Survey Report: Adjustment of Army Child to Deployment Separation (Survey Report). Chapel Hill, NC: The University of North Carolina at Chapel Hill; 2005. Available at: www.army.mil/cfsc/docs/saf5deployreport15dec05.pdf. Accessed July 23, 2012

40. Mansfield AJ, Kaufman JS, Engel CC, Gaynes BN. Deployment and mental health diagnoses among children of US Army personnel. *Arch Pediatr Adolesc Med.* 2011;165 (11):999–1005

41. Smith DC, Munroe ML, Foglia LM, Nielsen PE, Deering SH. Effects of deployment on depression screening scores in pregnancy at an army military treatment facility. *Obstet Gynecol.* 2010;116(3):679–684

42. Barker LH, Berry KD. Developmental issues impacting military families with young children during single and multiple deployments. *Mil Med.* 2009;174(10):1033–1040

43. Rentz ED, Marshall SW, Loomis D, Casteel C, Martin SL, Gibbs DA. Effect of deployment on the occurrence of child maltreatment in military and nonmilitary families. *Am J Epidemiol.* 2007;165(10):1199–1206

44. Gibbs DA, Martin SL, Kupper LL, Johnson RE. Child maltreatment in enlisted soldiers'

families during combat-related deployments. *JAMA.* 2007;298(5):528–535

45. Strategic Outreach to Families of All Reservists (SOFAR). *The SOFAR Guide for Helping Children and Youth Cope with the Deployment of a Parent in the Military Reserves.* Available at: www.sofarusa.org/ download_brochures_flyers_multimedia_ links.html. Accessed July 23, 2012

46. Lozano P, McPhillips HA, Hartzler B, et al. Randomized trial of teaching brief motivational interviewing to pediatric trainees to promote healthy behaviors in families. *Arch Pediatr Adolesc Med.* 2010;164(6):561–566

47. Hagan JF Jr American Academy of Pediatrics, Committee on Psychosocial Aspects of Child and Family Health, Task Force on Terrorism. Psychosocial implications of disaster or terrorism on children: a guide for the pediatrician. *Pediatrics.* 2005;116 (3):787–795

48. Iraq Coalition Casualty Count. Available at: www.iCasualties.org. Accessed July 23, 2012

49. *Zero to Three. Honoring Our Babies and Toddlers: Supporting Young Children Af-fected by a Military Parent's Deployment, Injury or Death, a Guide for Professionals.* Washington, DC: Zero to Three; 2009. Available at: http://main.zerotothree.org/site/ DocServer/GuideFinalMay27.pdf?docID=9322. Accessed July 23, 2012

50. Cozza SJ, Guimond JM, McKibben JB, et al. Combat-injured service members and their families: the relationship of child distress and spouse-perceived family distress and disruption. *J Trauma Stress.* 2010;23(1): 112–115

51. Levetown M; American Academy of Pediatrics Committee on Bioethics. Communicating with children and families: from everyday interactions to skill in conveying distressing information. *Pediatrics.* 2008; 121(5):e1441–e1460

52. Wessel MA. The primary pediatrician's role when a death occurs in a family in one's practice. *Pediatr Rev.* 2003;24(6):183–185

53. Tragedy Assistance Program for Survivors Web site. Available at: www.TAPS.org. Accessed July 23, 2012

54. American Academy of Pediatrics. Committee on Psychosocial Aspects of Child and Family Health. The pediatrician and childhood bereavement. *Pediatrics.* 2000;105(2): 445–447

55. Beardslee W, Lester P, Klosinski L, et al. Family-centered preventive intervention for military families: implications for implementation science. *Prev Sci.* 2011;12(4): 339–348

56. Saltzman WR, Lester P, Beardslee WR, Layne CM, Woodward K, Nash WP. Mechanisms of risk and resilience in military families: theoretical and empirical basis of a family-focused resilience enhancement program. *Clin Child Fam Psychol Rev.* 2011;14(3):213–230

57. Lester P, Mogil C, Saltzman W, et al. Families overcoming under stress: implementing family-centered prevention for military families facing wartime deployments and combat operational stress. *Mil Med.* 2011; 176(1):19–25

58. Lester P, Saltzman WR, Woodward K, et al. Evaluation of a family-centered prevention intervention for military children and families facing wartime deployments. *Am J Public Health.* 2012;102(S1):S48–S54

Health Supervision for Children With Marfan Syndrome

• *Clinical Report*

CLINICAL REPORT

Health Supervision for Children With Marfan Syndrome

Brad T. Tinkle, MD, PhD, Howard M. Saal, MD, and the COMMITTEE ON GENETICS

KEY WORD
Marfan syndrome

www.pediatrics.org/cgi/doi/10.1542/peds.2013-2063

doi:10.1542/peds.2013-2063

All clinical reports from the American Academy of Pediatrics automatically expire 5 years after publication unless reaffirmed, revised, or retired at or before that time.

PEDIATRICS (ISSN Numbers: Print, 0031-4005; Online, 1098-4275).

abstract

Marfan syndrome is a systemic, heritable connective tissue disorder that affects many different organ systems and is best managed by using a multidisciplinary approach. The guidance in this report is designed to assist the pediatrician in recognizing the features of Marfan syndrome as well as caring for the individual with this disorder. *Pediatrics* 2013;132:e1059–e1072

INTRODUCTION

Marfan syndrome is a heritable, multisystem disorder of connective tissue with extensive clinical variability. It is a relatively common condition, with approximately 1 in 5000 people affected.[1] Cardinal features involve the ocular, musculoskeletal, and cardiovascular systems. Because of the high degree of variability of this disorder, many of these clinical features can be present at birth or can manifest later in childhood or even adulthood.

Marfan syndrome is an autosomal dominant disorder mainly caused by defects in *FBN1*, the gene that codes for the protein fibrillin, although patients with mutations in other genes, including *TGFBR1* and *TGFBR2*, have also been reported, albeit rarely.[2] Mutations in *FBN1* are associated with a wide phenotypic spectrum ranging from classic features of Marfan syndrome presenting in childhood and early adulthood to severe neonatal presentation with rapidly progressive disease. At the other end of the spectrum, isolated phenotypic features, such as ectopia lentis or skeletal manifestations alone, may be the only presenting signs. Mutations in *FBN1* are found in up to 95% of those meeting diagnostic criteria.[3,4] However, the diagnosis of Marfan syndrome is clinically based on well-defined criteria (revised Ghent diagnostic criteria [Tables 1 and 2]) and does not include the whole spectrum of *FBN1*-related disorders, especially the milder, isolated features.[5] Thus, genetic testing of *FBN1* is best reserved for those patients in whom there is a strong clinical suspicion of Marfan syndrome, including those with the "emerging" phenotype, using established guidelines of the interpretation of such results. Because many of the more specific clinical features are age dependent (eg, ectopia lentis, aortic dilation, dural ectasia, protrusio acetabuli), children and adolescents may not fulfill formal diagnostic criteria and are often described as having "potential" Marfan syndrome. Younger patients at risk for Marfan syndrome on the basis of clinical features or a positive family history should be evaluated periodically (eg, at 5, 10, 15, and 18 years of age) in lieu of genetic testing.

TABLE 1 Revised Ghent Diagnostic Criteria for Marfan Syndrome

Diagnosis of definitive Marfan syndrome
(any of the following)
- Aortic root ≥2 z score and ectopia lentis
- Aortic root ≥2 z score and *FBN1* mutation
- Aortic root ≥2 z score and systemic score ≥7
- Ectopia lentis and *FBN1* mutation known to be associated with Marfan syndrome
- Positive family history of Marfan syndrome and ectopia lentis
- Positive family history of Marfan syndrome and systemic score ≥7
- Positive family history of Marfan syndrome and aortic root ≥3 z score in those <20 y of age *or* ≥2 z score in those >20 y of age

Diagnosis of potential Marfan syndrome
- *FBN1* mutation with aortic root with a z score <3 in those <20 y of age

Many features of Marfan syndrome are seen in isolation as well as in other genetic syndromes (Table 3).[6] Diagnosis should be clearly established when possible. For those suspected to have Marfan syndrome based on clinical grounds after physical, cardiac, and ophthalmic evaluation but who may not meet full clinical criteria, one can consider *FBN1* testing.[7]

TABLE 2 Systemic Scoring System for the Revised Ghent Diagnostic Criteria for Marfan Syndrome (Shown in Table 1)

Feature	Value
Wrist *and* thumb sign	3
Wrist *or* thumb sign	1
Pectus carinatum	2
Pectus excavatum or chest asymmetry	1
Hindfoot deformity (eg, valgus)	2
Pes planus	1
Pneumothorax	2
Dural ectasia	2
Protrusio acetabulae	2
Reduced upper-to-lower segment ratio *and* increased arm-span-to-height ratio	1
Scoliosis or thoracolumbar kyphosis	1
Reduced elbow extension	1
Craniofacial features: 3 of the following— dolichocephaly, downward-slanting palpebral fissures, enophthalmos, retrognathia, and malar hypoplasia	1
Skin striae	1
Myopia	1
Mitral valve prolapse	1

Adapted from Loeys et al.[3] Z score calculations are based on Roman et al.[38]

Approximately one-quarter of cases occur as a result of a new mutation, with the remainder inherited from an affected parent. Because of the broad phenotypic variability, some parents will not be readily recognized as having Marfan syndrome.[8] In such cases, both parents and at-risk first-degree relatives should have physical, ophthalmologic, and cardiac evaluation as well, with consideration of genetic testing.

GROWTH AND DEVELOPMENT

Overall growth is characterized by excessive linear growth of the long bones. Typically, most individuals with Marfan syndrome are tall for age (Figs 1 and 2), but it is important to note that not all affected individuals are tall by population standards; they are typically taller than predicted for their family (excluding others with Marfan syndrome).[9] Mean final height was 191.3 ± 9 cm (75 in) for males and 175.4 ± 8.2 cm (69 in) for females.

The growth of the tubular bones is accelerated in Marfan syndrome, resulting in disproportionate features. The extremities are often disproportionately long in comparison with the trunk (dolichostenomelia), altering the upper-to-lower segment and the arm-span-to-height ratios. The arm-span-to-height ratio is relatively fixed during childhood, but the upper-to-lower segment ratio changes during growth (Fig 3). Use of such measurements should take into account racial, gender, and age differences. Similarly, the tubular bones of the hand and fingers are elongated, but the palm is not proportionately wider, resulting in relative arachnodactyly as measured by the thumb and wrist signs (Fig 4).

Excessive growth in Marfan syndrome is attributable, in part, to a peak growth velocity that typically occurs as much as 2 years earlier than the

general population.[9] Hormonal therapy to limit adult height is rarely used in males. Complications can include accelerated growth, early puberty, and the undesirable consequences of associated increased blood pressure, which may increase the progression of the aortic dilation. Prepubertal females have been treated with high-dose estrogen therapy and progesterone to reduce final adult height in the past; however, this treatment remains controversial in both its psychosocial and medical benefits.[10]

Lean muscle mass is also affected. Individuals with Marfan syndrome often show a paucity of muscle mass and fat stores despite adequate caloric intake. Weight is often below the 50th percentile for age.[9]

Cognitive ability in patients with Marfan syndrome is usually within the typical range for the general population. However, poor vision and underlying medical problems may interfere with learning. Q:3 Similarly, many patients report chronic fatigue, which may affect education and can manifest as inattention or poor concentration.[11] The etiology of the fatigue is likely heterogeneous, in part because of the underlying chronic condition, medications such as β-blockers, sleep disturbance (eg, sleep apnea), and/or orthostatic intolerance.[12]

SKELETAL

Skeletal system involvement in Marfan syndrome is characterized by bone overgrowth. Such overgrowth may be noticeable at birth or can develop in young children, with a tendency to progress more rapidly during periods of rapid growth, necessitating close monitoring at such times (Table 4).

Overgrowth of the ribs can push the sternum inward (pectus excavatum) or outward (pectus carinatum). Nearly two-thirds of patients with Marfan

TABLE 3 Differential Diagnoses: Syndromes With Overlapping Features of Marfan Syndrome

Syndrome	Manifestations	Genetic Etiology
Mitral valve prolapse syndrome	Mitral valve prolapse; skeletal manifestations as seen in Marfan syndrome	FBN1(in some)
MASS phenotype	Mitral valve prolapse; myopia; nonprogressive aortic dilation; nonspecific skin and skeletal features	FBN1
Familial ectopia lentis	Eye and skeletal findings of Marfan syndrome	FBN1(in some)
Shprintzen-Goldberg syndrome	Skeletal and cardiac findings of Marfan syndrome; craniosynostosis; hypertelorism; proptosis; abdominal hernias; joint laxity; developmental delay/intellectual disability	FBN1(in some)
Weill-Marchesani syndrome (autosomal dominant form)	Ectopia lentis; short stature; brachydactyly; characteristic facial features	FBN1
Loeys-Dietz syndrome	Skeletal and cardiovascular features of Marfan syndrome; no ectopia lentis; aggressive dilation of large- and medium-sized arteries; most common and unique features include hypertelorism, bifid uvula/cleft palate, blue sclerae, developmental delays, hydrocephalus, translucent skin, arterial tortuosity, and craniosynostosis	TGFBR1 TGFBR2
Congenital contractural arachnodactyly	Marfan-like skeletal features; "crumpled" ears; contractures of the knees, ankles, and digits at birth; progressive kyphoscoliosis; arachnodactyly; cardiac valvular anomalies	FBN2
Familial thoracic aortic aneurysm	Dilation of the aorta and dissections either at the level of the sinuses of Valsalva or the ascending thoracic aorta without the other phenotypic features of Marfan syndrome	Heterogeneous
Ehlers-Danlos syndrome, vascular type	Thin skin with visible veins; easy bruising; small joint laxity; rupture of hollow organs as well as medium- and large-size arteries	COL3A1 COL3A2
Ehlers-Danlos syndrome, kyphoscoliotic form (type VI)	Marfanoid body habitus; kyphoscoliosis; joint laxity; mitral valve prolapse; hypotonia; blue sclerae; ocular fragility; at risk for rupture of medium-sized arteries	PLOD ZNF469
Homocystinuria	Ectopia lentis; skeletal abnormalities such as those seen in Marfan syndrome; variable cognitive impairment; tendency for thrombotic events	CBS
Stickler syndrome	Severe myopia; retinal detachment; hearing loss; midface hypoplasia; cleft palate; spondyloepiphyseal dysplasia	COL2A1 COL11A1 COL11A2 COL9A1
Fragile X syndrome	Often tall; long face; joint laxity; mild dilation of the aorta; mitral valve prolapse; pectus excavatum; variable intellectual disability	FMR1

syndrome will develop pectus excavatum, which is often perceived as a disturbing physical feature by teenagers.[13] The pectus deformity can be severe and, in extreme circumstances, can interfere with pulmonary functioning, warranting surgical intervention.[14] Pectus excavatum may also have a detrimental effect on cardiac function, especially during submaximal exercising[15] and is often repaired before cardiac surgery for aortic root replacement. Pectus deformity is often present before 10 years of age but may worsen during an adolescent growth spurt.

Scoliosis is seen in slightly more than one-half of individuals with Marfan syndrome and can be mild to severe as well as atypically progressive.[16,17] Close monitoring by using the forward-bending test at yearly intervals and management by an orthopedist is preferred because surgical stabilization of the spine may be required.[18] Bracing has a low success rate if the curves are greater than 35° to 40° but may have some preventive value for smaller curves. Those with spinal curvatures less than 30° have an excellent long-term prognosis. Marked progression is often seen by those with spinal curvatures greater than 50°. The progression of scoliosis can occur well into adulthood. Thoracic kyphosis is also common and can be postural or a further complication of bony overgrowth and ligamentous laxity (eg, kyphoscoliosis). Postural education and joint stabilization with core strengthening may be of benefit but are unproven for the treatment of scoliosis in this population. Untreated spinal deformities can lead to chronic back pain and restrictive lung disease. Spinal deformity correction is more prone to complications than in idiopathic deformity and should be performed by those with some experience in treating patients with Marfan syndrome.[19]

The acetabulum of the hip can be abnormally deep (protrusio acetabuli) in some patients with Marfan syndrome and can lead to pelvic or upper leg pain. Protrusio acetabuli is seen commonly in Marfan syndrome[20];

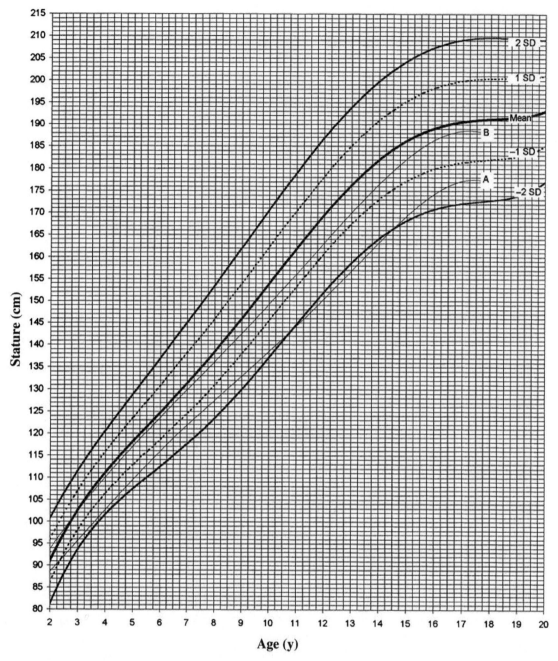

FIGURE 1
Growth curves for males in Marfan syndrome. (A) 50th percentile and (B) 95th percentile for the general population used for comparison. Reprinted with permission from Erkula G, Jones KB, Sponseller PD, Dietz HC, Pyeritz RE. Growth and maturation in Marfan syndrome. *Am J Med Genet.* 2002;109 (2):103.[9]

however, it is not unique to this condition and is seen in a number of infectious, inflammatory, metabolic, genetic, neoplastic, and traumatic conditions.[21] In Marfan syndrome, the protrusio acetabuli is often asymptomatic, and surgical intervention is rarely indicated.[22]

Some people with Marfan syndrome will show reduced mobility of the elbow, but other joints may demonstrate ligamentous laxity. Joint laxity may be more significant in young patients but rarely leads to motor delays. True joint dislocations are rare. Joint laxity can lead to muscle

fatigue and overuse pain/injury.[23] More typically, such individuals demonstrate poor writing skills and complain of hand pain/fatigue with prolonged use. Physical and/or occupational therapy can address these joint laxity issues by using joint stabilization exercises, postural support, education, alternative

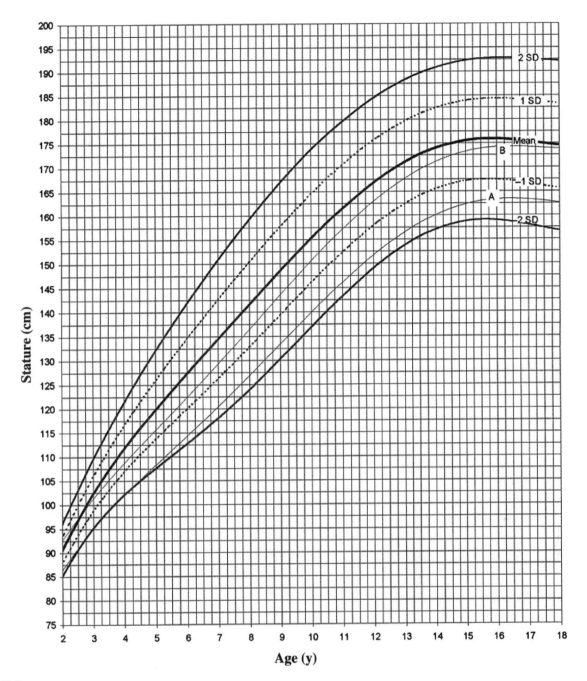

FIGURE 2

Growth curves for females in Marfan syndrome. (A) 50th percentile and (B) 95th percentile for the general population used for comparison. Reprinted with permission from Erkula G, Jones KB, Sponseller PD, Dietz HC, Pyeritz RE. Growth and maturation in Marfan syndrome. *Am J Med Genet*. 2002;109 (2):104.[9]

strategies (eg, use of a laptop for taking notes), and bracing/resting splints if necessary.

Inward rotation of the medial aspect of the ankle can result in pes planus (Fig 5). This condition may lead to foot, ankle, knee, hip, and/or low back pain.[24] Some patients will benefit from the use of shoe orthoses, such as an arch support and more supportive shoes. Surgical intervention is rarely indicated or fully successful. Others will have highly arched feet but have little or no symptoms.

The facial features of Marfan syndrome include a long and narrow face with deeply set eyes (enophthalmos), downward slanting of the eyes, flat cheek bones (malar hypoplasia), and a small chin (micrognathia) (Fig 6). However, facial features are often highly variable and may change with age. In addition, these facial features are not highly sensitive for the

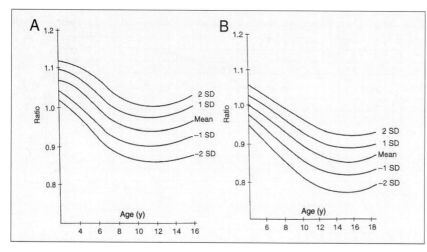

FIGURE 3

Normative upper-to-lower segment ratios for (A) white and (B) African-American subjects. Reprinted with permission from McKusick VA. *Heritable Disorders of Connective Tissue.* Philadelphia, PA: Mosby; 1972.

presence of Marfan syndrome.[25] The palate is often highly arched and narrowed (Fig 7).

Decreased bone density has been documented in the lumbar and hip regions in patients with Marfan syn-

drome.[26,27] The etiology of this bone loss remains speculative, but no significant increase in bone fracture rates has been seen.[28]

OCULAR

Myopia is the most common ocular feature and often progresses rapidly during childhood.[29] Displacement of the lens (ectopia lentis) is a hallmark feature of Marfan syndrome but is only seen in 1 or both eyes in approximately 60% of affected individuals.[30] It is often the presenting feature and occurs much more commonly before 10 years of age. This finding is most reliably diagnosed according to a slit-lamp examination after full pupillary dilation.

The globe is often elongated, and the cornea may be flat or even cone-shaped (keratoconus). People with Marfan syndrome are at increased risk of retinal detachment, glaucoma, and early cataract formation, typically in adulthood. Flashes of light (photopsia) and new floaters are symptoms of posterior vitreous detachment, which may precede retinal detachment.[31,32] Retinal detachment should be considered in any patient with acute onset of visual symptoms, and these patients should be evaluated and treated emergently. Most retinal detachments can be repaired successfully, but the key to optimum visual recovery is prompt diagnosis and treatment.

Affected individuals should be followed up closely by an ophthalmologist familiar with Marfan syndrome at least yearly with slit lamp examinations for lens subluxation and evaluations for glaucoma and cataracts. Most often, eye problems can be controlled adequately with corrective lenses alone. Careful and aggressive refraction and visual correction are mandatory in young children at risk for amblyopia. Lens dislocation can present a clinical

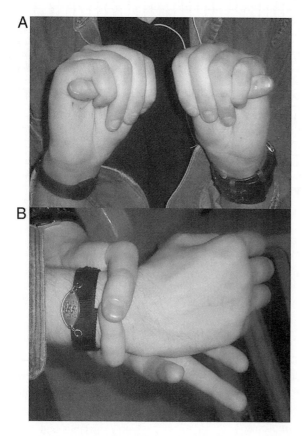

FIGURE 4

(A) Positive thumb sign with the thumbnail extending past the ulnar side of the hand and (B) positive wrist sign with the overlap of the nail beds of the thumb and fifth finger.

TABLE 4 Anticipatory Guidance in Marfan Syndrome

Option	At Diagnosis	0–12 mo	1–5 y	6–12 y[a]	13–18 y[a]	19–22 y
Cardiac examination[b]	√	Each visit	Each visit	Each visit	Yearly	Yearly
Echocardiogram	√	As indicated	Yearly	Yearly	Yearly	Yearly
Ocular (ophthalmology)	√		Yearly	Yearly	Yearly	Yearly
Musculoskeletal[b]						
Scoliosis clinical examination	√	Each visit	Yearly	Every 6 mo	Every 6 mo	Yearly
Joint laxity	√	Each visit	Yearly	Every 6 mo	Every 6 mo	
Pectus deformity	√	Each visit	Yearly	Every 6 mo	Every 6 mo	
Bone age				√[c]		
Review diagnosis	√	PRN	PRN	PRN[d]	PRN[d]	PRN[d]
Examine family members	√	PRN	PRN	PRN	PRN	PRN
Support group information	√	PRN	PRN	PRN	PRN	PRN
Genetic counseling	√				√[e]	√[e]
Lifestyle[f]				√	√	√
Transition					Discuss plans	Begin transition

Many systems should be reviewed regularly at developmentally appropriate stages. PRN, as needed.

[a] Periods of rapid growth require closer supervision.

[b] If abnormal results on examination, refer for further evaluation. Follow-up evaluations as indicated.

[c] Bone age determination in preadolescence. If large discrepancy between bone age and height age, hormonal therapy should be considered.

[d] Review symptoms of potential catastrophic events such as aortic dissection, vision changes, and pneumothorax.

[e] Discuss reproductive and pregnancy risks.

[f] Review physical activity restrictions/lifestyle modifications.

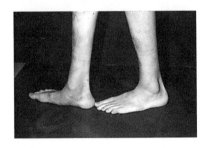

FIGURE 5
Elongated feet with collapse of the medial arch resulting in pes planus.

challenge. Typically, the lens will sublux superiorly with Marfan syndrome. If the lens is subluxed but still within the visual axis, substantial lenticular astigmatism may result, which can require powerful astigmatic spectacle correction. If the lens edge has subluxed at or beyond the center of the visual axis, aphakic spectacle or contact lens correction may improve vision. If there is sufficient optical distortion from lens subluxation, surgical removal of the lens (aphakia) or lens replacement (pseudophakia) may be the treatment of choice.[33] Because of inherently weak zonular support for the Marfan lens, pseudophakia may require supplemental means of attachment to affix the intraocular lens. Although this procedure is currently considered safe when performed in specialized centers, major complications, including retinal detachment, can occur. The long-term stability and safety of sew-in intraocular lenses are unknown. Zonular weakness in Marfan syndrome may also result in complete lens subluxation into the vitreous or result in prolapse of the lens into the anterior chamber of the eye, which may necessitate surgical removal. Corneal refractive surgery for myopia is generally contraindicated in individuals with Marfan syndrome, given the risk of additional eye complications.

CARDIOVASCULAR

The cardiovascular system is the major source of morbidity and mortality in Marfan syndrome. Cardiovascular manifestations include dilation of the aorta, aortic valve insufficiency, a predisposition for aortic tear and rupture, mitral valve prolapse with or without regurgitation, tricuspid valve prolapse, and enlargement of the proximal pulmonary artery.[34]

The aortic dilation in Marfan syndrome tends to progress over time, with the vast majority of cases becoming evident before 18 years of age. The dilation typically is at the level of the sinuses of Valsalva, but dilation of any part of the aorta can be seen in these patients (Fig 8). Histologic examination reveals elastic fiber fragmentation with total loss of elastin content and accumulation of amorphous matrix components in the aortic media. This "cystic medial necrosis" does not distinguish Marfan syndrome from other causes of aortic aneurysm and, therefore, is only a description, not a pathognomonic feature.

The age of onset and rate of progression of aortic dilation are highly variable. As the aneurysm enlarges, the aortic annulus can be overstretched, leading to secondary aortic regurgitation. Valvular dysfunction can lead to volume overload with secondary left ventricular dilation and heart failure. Indeed, mitral valve prolapse with congestive heart failure is the leading cause of cardiovascular morbidity and mortality in young children with Marfan syndrome.[35]

A significant risk of aortic dissection or rupture occurs when the maximal aortic dimension reaches approximately

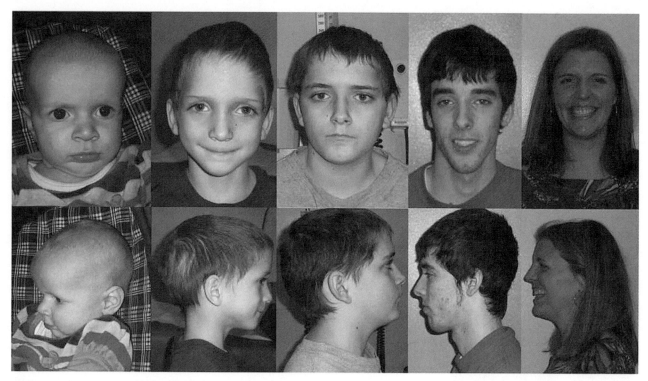

FIGURE 6
Facial features of Marfan syndrome are highly variable, ranging from subtle findings to more "classic" facial features. Photo consents for publication on file.

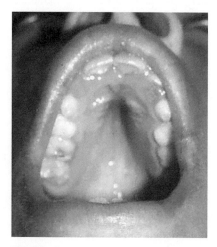

FIGURE 7
High arched ("steepled") palate.

5.0 cm in adults, although rupture at 4.5 cm has been documented among women.[36] Fortunately, aortic dissection is exceedingly rare in early childhood. Acute aortic dissection usually presents as severe chest pain but can also include pallor, pulselessness, paresthesia, and paralysis. Asymmetric blood pressure may also be a sign of dissection.

All individuals with a diagnosis of Marfan syndrome should be followed up by a cardiologist familiar with Marfan syndrome. An echocardiogram should be obtained at diagnosis. A subsequent echocardiogram is often desired in 6 months to assess the rate of progression.[37] Yearly echocardiograms are sufficient when aortic dimensions are small (<4.5 cm in adults) and rates of aortic dilation are low (<0.5 cm per year). Aortic root measurements should be interpreted on the basis of normal values for age and body size.[38] Nomograms are available through the National Marfan Foundation (http://www.marfan.org/marfan/2576/Aortic-Root-Dilatation-Nomogram). More frequent evaluations are indicated when the aortic root diameter exceeds 4.5 cm in adults, when the rate of aortic dilation exceeds 0.5 cm per year, or with the onset of significant valvular or ventricular dysfunction. Aortic root dimensions can also be determined by using computed tomography angiography or magnetic resonance angiography, and they potentially have the benefit of evaluating beyond the aortic root. Because aortic dilation can occur at any age, lifelong monitoring is warranted.

Medications that reduce hemodynamic stress on the aortic wall, such as β-blockers, are often prescribed.[37] Therapy should be considered at the time of diagnosis at any age or on appreciation of progressive aortic root dilation, even in the absence of a definitive diagnosis.[39] The dose needs to be titrated to effect, keeping heart rate after submaximal exercise or agitation less than 110 beats per minute in young children or less than 100 beats per minute in older children or adults. In patients who cannot tolerate β-blockers (eg, individuals with asthma, depression, fatigue), verapamil is commonly used,[40] although recently, concerns have been raised about calcium channel blockers and an increased risk of aortic complications.[41] Currently, randomized controlled trials are underway evaluating the response to the angiotensin receptor blocker losartan, in response to earlier mouse model work[42] and a small cohort study.[43] If congestive heart failure is present as a result of valvular dysfunction, afterload-reducing agents (in combination with a β-blocker)

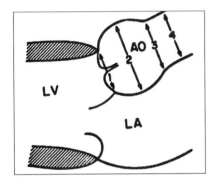

FIGURE 8
Dilation at the level of the aortic root as seen in Marfan syndrome. 1, aortic valve annulus; 2, aortic root (sinuses of Valsalva); 3, sinotubular junction; 4, ascending aorta; AO, aorta; LA, left atrium; LV, left ventricle. Rights to be retained by author (B.T.T.).

can improve cardiovascular function, but surgical intervention may be warranted.

Surgical repair of the aorta is indicated once: (1) the maximal aortic root measurement exceeds 5.0 cm; (2) the rate of increase of the aortic diameter approaches 1.0 cm per year; or (3) there is progressive aortic regurgitation.[44] More aggressive therapy may be indicated in individuals with a family history of early aortic dissection. Many individuals can receive a valve-sparing procedure that precludes the need for chronic anticoagulation therapy.[45,46] Children run the highest risk of requiring repeated cardiac operations, such as valve replacement.[47]

Aortic dilation can also be seen in the descending aorta, although typically at later ages. All people with Marfan syndrome should begin intermittent surveillance of the entire aorta with computed tomography angiography or magnetic resonance angiography scans in young adulthood.[48,49] Such imaging should also be performed at least annually in anyone with a history of aortic root replacement or dissection.

Participation in contact sports, competitive sports, and isometric exercise

should be restricted.[50] However, all people with Marfan syndrome can and should remain active, with aerobic activities performed in moderation.

Agents that stimulate the cardiovascular system, including routine use of decongestants, should be avoided. Caffeine can aggravate a tendency for arrhythmia. The use of psychostimulant medications for chronic fatigue or attention-deficit/hyperactivity disorder should be used with caution and be approved by the cardiologist.

Subacute bacterial endocarditis prophylaxis may be indicated for dental work or other procedures expected to contaminate the bloodstream with bacteria in the presence of significant valvular insufficiency. With proper management, the life expectancy of someone with Marfan syndrome approximates that of the general population.[51,52]

PULMONARY AIRWAY

Pulmonary issues encountered in Marfan syndrome include spontaneous pneumothorax, reduced pulmonary reserve, and sleep apnea. In neonatal Marfan syndrome, an emphysematous lung disease is uniformly present and also occurs in approximately 10% to 15% of those with "classic" Marfan syndrome.

Lung bullae, which develop in 4% to 15% of patients with Marfan syndrome, can develop anywhere on the surface of the lungs but especially in the upper lobes.[53] Such bullae (or blebs) can predispose to spontaneous pneumothorax. Symptoms of pneumothorax include sudden onset of chest pain, dyspnea, and/or cyanosis. Breathing against resistance (eg, playing a brass instrument), scuba diving, or high-altitude sports (eg, skydiving, mountaineering) should be avoided, especially among those with a family history of spontaneous pneumothorax. Those with recurrent pneumothorax

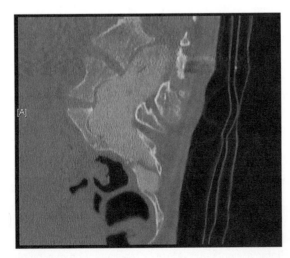

FIGURE 9
Dural ectasia of the lumbar spinal canal. MRI appearance of the dilated dural sac, which can erode the bone and entrap nerves.

may require chemical or surgical pleurodesis or surgical resection of pulmonary blebs.

A restrictive lung disease pattern with increased total and residual lung volume as well as exercise intolerance is typically seen in the majority of those affected.[54] Often, this pattern is related to pectus deformity, chest wall asymmetry, and/or scoliosis. Surgical repair of severe pectus excavatum or scoliosis may improve overall pulmonary lung function. Pulmonary function tests should be performed in any patient with pulmonary complaints or significant pectus deformity and can be monitored after surgical repair.

Obstructive sleep apnea is commonly seen in patients with Marfan syndrome.[55] Increased nasal resistance attributable to craniofacial abnormalities, such as a high arched palate, micrognathia with possible glossoptosis, and laryngotracheomalacia, can cause difficulty with intubation/anesthesia as well as significant upper airway resistance.[56] Sleep apnea is underappreciated among adolescents and young adults with Marfan syndrome. Symptoms commonly seen in Marfan syndrome that may be partially attributable to sleep apnea include fatigue and loss of energy as well as impaired memory and cognition. Symptoms of sleep dysfunction, such as fatigue, decreased sleep duration, nonrestorative sleep, and snoring, should be reviewed at each visit. A formal sleep evaluation should be considered in such cases.

INTEGUMENT

Approximately two-thirds of people with Marfan syndrome develop stretch marks of the skin.[57] Often, these are located across the lower back as well as the inguinal and axillary regions. These stretch marks are signs of rapid growth and are usually perpendicular to the axes of growth.

Because of the defect in connective tissue, individuals with Marfan syndrome are also at risk for hernias. Many will have inguinal herniation that will require surgical repair. However, recurrent hernias or hernias at the site of surgical incisions are a more distinctive hallmark of a connective tissue disorder, such as Marfan syndrome. Primary hernia repair should use a synthetic mesh (or similar artificial construct) in all known or suspected cases of Marfan syndrome to minimize the risk of recurrence.

DURAL ECTASIA

Most individuals with Marfan syndrome often develop stretching of the dural sac in the dependent lumbosacral region, resulting in dural ectasia (Fig 9).[58] This development can lead to bony erosion and nerve entrapment. Symptoms can include pain in the lower back, hip/pelvic region, and proximal leg, as well as weakness/numbness above and below the knees.[59] However, in most patients, the dural ectasia is asymptomatic.[60]

Excessive accumulation or leakage of cerebrospinal fluid from the dural sac can cause postural hypotension and "low-pressure" headaches.[61,62] Damage of the dura from spinal taps or epidurals may not sufficiently heal, causing leakage, which also predisposes the patient to postural headaches. In severe cases of dural ectasia, spinal shunting and/or medication can be used. Complications after surgical repair of the dura include cerebrospinal fluid leakage and recurrence. Detection of dural ectasia can be performed using either MRI or computed tomography scan.

DENTAL

People with Marfan syndrome typically have oromaxillofacial anomalies. Most have an elongated face, malar hypoplasia, high-arched palate, and micrognathia.

Often, these anomalies will cause significant dental crowding and malalignment. Routine dental care is recommended; however, many individuals with Marfan syndrome require orthodontia for proper occlusion as well as appearance. Oral and maxillofacial interventions may also be indicated, such as palatal expansion and/or mandibular distraction.

PHYSICAL ACTIVITY

Although all children are encouraged to participate in physical activity for overall health, skill development, coordination, musculoskeletal health, and socialization, individuals with Marfan syndrome are at significant risk of physical injury and medical complications. Of concern are activities including contact sports and activities involving "burst" exertion (eg, sprinting) and intense static (isometric) exertion, such as weight lifting.[63] In general, patients with Marfan syndrome without aortic dilation or significant mitral valve regurgitation are encouraged to participate in competitive and noncompetitive (recreational) activities, but this action is still limited by the intensity level of the activity and the individual.[50] Sports in which ocular trauma is likely, such as boxing or full-contact karate, should be discouraged. Participation in any activity should be evaluated and discussed before initiation of that activity. Activities of most concern include basketball, body building/weight lifting, hockey, running, skiing, racquetball, surfing, scuba diving, and rock climbing. More acceptable alternatives include modest hiking, stationary cycling, bowling, golf, skating, snorkeling, and brisk walking. Caution is needed for patients with low blood pressure and orthostatic intolerance, including those receiving β-blocker therapy, who may be more susceptible to easy fatigue, near-syncopal/syncopal episodes, and falls.[12]

PSYCHOSOCIAL

Marfan syndrome affects each individual differently. Marfan syndrome has a significant effect on daily activities and perceived quality of life. However, in 2 small series, most affected individuals older than 13 years reported a positive general self-image.[64,65]

Many of those affected by Marfan syndrome benefit from networking and peer relationships. The National Marfan Foundation (www.marfan.org) is an excellent US resource for connections as well as medical advice. Most countries have similar organizations.

TRANSITION/MEDICAL HOME

Because Marfan syndrome can affect the very young and continues throughout a patient's lifetime, it is important that people with Marfan syndrome be recognized and have a medical home. Affected people are often followed up by cardiologists, ophthalmologists, and orthopedists.[66] Care needs to be coordinated among the various specialties, with a special focus on the period of transition from adolescence to adulthood.

PREGNANCY

Pregnancy can lead to significant medical complications for women with Marfan syndrome and should be approached with careful deliberation.[67] If the aortic root is exceeds 4.0 cm, complications can include rapid progression of aortic root enlargement and/or aortic dissection or rupture during pregnancy, delivery, and in the postpartum period. Women whose aorta is greater than 4.5 cm or who previously had an aortic dissection/rupture are at substantially higher risk.[68] Women with aortic dimensions greater than 5.0 cm are at significant risk for aortic rupture, and pregnancy

should be delayed if possible until after definitive treatment of the aorta has been completed. If already pregnant, consideration of immediate aortic replacement, early delivery, or termination of the pregnancy should be considered, given the potentially severe consequences.

A higher-than-expected rate of spontaneous abortion has been reported in women with Marfan syndrome, although the etiology is unknown.[69] In addition, women with Marfan syndrome experience a higher rate of preterm deliveries, premature rupture of membranes, and increased mortality of their offspring.[69,70] Dural ectasia should be considered in any affected individual, and avoidance of spinal anesthesia may be necessary. Epidural anesthesia is safe for most women with Marfan syndrome, although it is not advised for those with moderately severe dural ectasia. General anesthesia has the benefit of avoiding complication of spinal anesthesia with dural ectasia and less stress on the aorta during delivery. Optimally, pregnancy should be considered after appropriate counseling from a geneticist or a cardiologist familiar with Marfan syndrome, a genetic counselor, and a perinatologist.

PRENATAL

The pediatrician is sometimes called on to counsel a family prenatally with regard to Marfan syndrome. The pediatrician may have been previously involved with this family through care of siblings or one of the expectant parents. Families may also seek pediatric advice in the care and management of a fetus at risk. This management may involve a few different scenarios.

1. The pediatrician may be asked about the risk to a child of a parent with Marfan syndrome. The risk of

inheriting the genetic defect in Marfan syndrome is 50%, consistent with autosomal dominant inheritance. Often, expectant parents are concerned about the severity of the disorder in the next generation. Variability of the Marfan phenotype is extensive but is more similar among affected family members, suggesting that the genetic defect is largely responsible for the phenotype. Most people with classic Marfan syndrome do not have children with a much more severe phenotype, such as neonatal Marfan syndrome.[71] One should also be aware of the consequences that may affect the pregnancy outcome for women with Marfan syndrome. As mentioned previously, women with an aortic root greater than 4.5 cm in diameter should avoid pregnancy or undergo elective aortic grafting before becoming pregnant.[72] Aortic dissection or rupture has occurred in women with an aorta less than 5.0 cm, which may result in significant morbidity and mortality of the fetus/infant and the expectant mother.

2. Parents of a child with Marfan syndrome may ask about recurrence risk of Marfan syndrome in subsequent pregnancies. This issue may best be explained by a geneticist. In short, 1 of the parents may either be unrecognized as having Marfan syndrome (therefore, recurrence risk is 50%) or both parents may be unaffected and, therefore, carry only a slight chance of having a low level of germline mosaicism (with anticipated recurrence risk of 2%–3%). Because of a high occurrence of unrecognized Marfan syndrome in parents of a child with Marfan syndrome, it is advisable for both parents to undergo further evaluation to establish their own personal

risk as well as the risk for subsequent pregnancies.

3. An expectant couple may have a fetus with concerning features of neonatal Marfan syndrome discovered through prenatal ultrasonography or even fetal MRI. Ultrasonographic findings may include unusually long limbs and congenital heart disease and are often detected in the third trimester.[73] Genetic testing for *FBN1* mutations by using amniocentesis may be helpful to confirm the diagnosis of Marfan syndrome and to reveal specific mutations in *FBN1* that may be more typically associated with neonatal Marfan syndrome and, therefore, reduced survivability.

NEONATAL MARFAN SYNDROME

Neonatal Marfan syndrome is the most severe disorder attributable to a fibrillinopathy. Features overlap significantly with classic Marfan syndrome but are more severe. Infants with neonatal Marfan syndrome are long with simple/crumpled ears, aged-appearing face, enlarged corneas, ectopia lentis, chest deformity, large feet, arachnodactyly, and contractures.[74] Respiratory insufficiency is common as a result of an abnormally pliant chest wall and emphysematous changes in the lungs.

Cardiac abnormalities are severe and include polyvalvular dysplasia and aortic dilation. Mortality is high within the first year of life because of cardiac failure secondary to severe mitral valve regurgitation.[75] Almost all cases of neonatal Marfan syndrome are sporadic and are associated with mutations clustering within exons 24 through 32 of *FBN1*.

SUPPORT GROUPS

National Marfan Foundation

22 Manhasset Ave,
Port Washington, NY 11050
Phone: 1-800-8-MARFAN ext 10 (1-800-862-7326); 1-516-883-8712
Fax: 1-516-883-8040
E-mail: staff@marfan.org
Web site: www.marfan.org

Canadian Marfan Association

Centre Plaza Postal Outlet
128 Queen St South
PO Box 42257
Mississauga, ONT, L5M4Z0, Canada
Phone: 866-722-1722 (toll-free); 905-826-3223
Fax: 905-826-2125
E-mail: info@marfan.ca
Web site: www.marfan.ca

Marfan Association UK

Rochester House
5 Aldershot Rd
Fleet, Hampshire

GU51 3NG, England
Phone: (0) 1252 810472
E-mail: support@marfan.org.uk
Web site: www.marfan.org.uk

LEAD AUTHORS

Brad T. Tinkle, MD, PhD
Howard M. Saal, MD

COMMITTEE ON GENETICS, 2011–2012

Robert A. Saul, MD, Chairperson
Stephen R. Braddock, MD
Emily Chen, MD, PhD
Debra L. Freedenberg, MD
Marilyn C. Jones, MD
James M. Perrin, MD
Beth Anne Tarini, MD

FORMER COMMITTEE ON GENETICS MEMBERS

Howard M. Saal, MD, Contributor
Brad T. Tinkle, MD, PhD

LIAISONS

Sara Copeland, MD — *Maternal and Child Health Bureau/Health Resources and Services Administration*
Katrina M. Dipple, MD, PhD — *American College of Medical Genetics*
W. Allen Hogge, MD — *American Congress of Obstetricians and Gynecologists*
Melissa A. Parisi, MD, PhD — *Eunice Kennedy Shriver National Institute of Child Health and Human Development*
Stuart K. Shapira, MD, PhD — *Centers for Disease Control and Prevention*

STAFF

Paul Spire

REFERENCES

1. Dietz HC, Loeys B, Carta L, Ramirez F. Recent progress towards a molecular understanding of Marfan syndrome. *Am J Med Genet C Semin Med Genet.* 2005;139C(1):4–9

2. Dean JC. Marfan syndrome: clinical diagnosis and management. *Eur J Hum Genet.* 2007;15(7):724–733

3. Loeys BL, Dietz HC, Braverman AC, et al. The revised Ghent nosology for the Marfan syndrome. *J Med Genet.* 2010;47(7):476–485

4. Attanasio M, Lapini I, Evangelisti L, et al. FBN1 mutation screening of patients with Marfan syndrome and related disorders: detection of 46 novel FBN1 mutations. *Clin Genet.* 2008;74(1):39–46

5. Loeys B, De Backer J, Van Acker P, et al. Comprehensive molecular screening of the FBN1 gene favors locus homogeneity of classical Marfan syndrome. *Hum Mutat.* 2004;24(2):140–146

6. Rybczynski M, Bernhardt AM, Rehder U, et al. The spectrum of syndromes and manifestations in individuals screened for suspected Marfan syndrome. *Am J Med Genet A.* 2008;146A(24):3157–3166

7. Faivre L, Masurel-Paulet A, Collod-Béroud G, et al. Clinical and molecular study of 320 children with Marfan syndrome and related type I fibrillinopathies in a series of 1009 probands with pathogenic FBN1

mutations. *Pediatrics.* 2009;123(1):391–398

8. Summers KM, West JA, Peterson MM, Stark D, McGill JJ, West MJ. Challenges in the diagnosis of Marfan syndrome. *Med J Aust.* 2006;184(12):627–631

9. Erkula G, Jones KB, Sponseller PD, Dietz HC, Pyeritz RE. Growth and maturation in Marfan syndrome. *Am J Med Genet.* 2002; 109(2):100–115

10. Lee JM, Howell JD. Tall girls: the social shaping of a medical therapy. *Arch Pediatr Adolesc Med.* 2006;160(10):1035–1039

11. Rand-Hendriksen S, Sørensen I, Holmström H, Andersson S, Finset A. Fatigue, cognitive

functioning and psychological distress in Marfan syndrome, a pilot study. *Psychol Health Med.* 2007;12(3):305–313

12. van Dijk N, Boer MC, Mulder BJ, van Montfrans GA, Wieling W. Is fatigue in Marfan syndrome related to orthostatic intolerance? *Clin Auton Res.* 2008;18(4): 187–193

13. Scherer LR, Arn PH, Dressel DA, Pyeritz RM, Haller JA Jr. Surgical management of children and young adults with Marfan syndrome and pectus excavatum. *J Pediatr Surg.* 1988;23(12):1169–1172

14. Lawson ML, Mellins RB, Paulson JF, et al. Increasing severity of pectus excavatum is associated with reduced pulmonary function. *J Pediatr.* 2011;159(2):256.e2–261.e2

15. Lesbo M, Tang M, Nielsen HH, et al. Compromised cardiac function in exercising teenagers with pectus excavatum. *Interact Cardiovasc Thorac Surg.* 2011;13(4):377–380

16. Sponseller PD, Hobbs W, Riley LH, III, Pyeritz RE. The thoracolumbar spine in Marfan syndrome. *J Bone Joint Surg Am.* 1995;77 (6):867–876

17. Glard Y, Launay F, Edgard-Rosa G, Collignon P, Jouve JL, Bollini G. Scoliotic curve patterns in patients with Marfan syndrome. *J Child Orthop.* 2008;2(3):211–216

18. Di Silvestre M, Greggi T, Giacomini S, Cioni A, Bakaloudis G, Lolli F, Parisini P. Surgical treatment for scoliosis in Marfan syndrome. *Spine (Phila Pa 1976).* 2005;30(20): E597–E604

19. Shirley ED, Sponseller PD. Marfan syndrome. *J Am Acad Orthop Surg.* 2009;17(9): 572–581

20. Lundby R, Kirkhus E, Rand-Hendriksen S, Hald J, Pripp AH, Smith HJ. CT of the hips in the investigation of protrusio acetabuli in Marfan syndrome. A case control study. *Eur Radiol.* 2011;21(7):1485–1491

21. Dunlop CC, Jones CW, Maffulli N. Protrusio acetabuli. *Bull Hosp Jt Dis.* 2005;62(3–4): 105–114

22. Sponseller PD, Jones KB, Ahn NU, Erkula G, Foran JR, Dietz HC III. Protrusio acetabuli in Marfan syndrome: age-related prevalence and associated hip function. *J Bone Joint Surg Am.* 2006;88(3):486–495

23. Bird HA. Joint hypermobility. *Musculoskelet Care.* 2007;5(1):4–19

24. Dietz HC. Marfan syndrome. In: Pagon RA, Adam MP, Bird TD, et al, eds. *GeneReviews.* Seattle, WA: University of Washington; 1993–2013. Available at: www.ncbi.nlm.nih.gov/books/NBK1335/. Accessed August 18, 2013

25. Ting BL, Mathur D, Loeys BL, Dietz HC, III, Sponseller PD. The diagnostic value of the facial features of Marfan syndrome. *J Child Orthop.* 2010;4(6):545–551

26. Giampietro PF, Peterson M, Schneider R, et al. Assessment of bone mineral density in adults and children with Marfan syndrome. *Osteoporos Int.* 2003;14(7):559–563

27. Moura B, Tubach F, Sulpice M, et al; Multidisciplinary Marfan Syndrome Clinic Group. Bone mineral density in Marfan syndrome. A large case-control study. *Joint Bone Spine.* 2006;73(6):733–735

28. Giampietro PF, Peterson MG, Schneider R, et al. Bone mineral density determinations by dual-energy x-ray absorptiometry in the management of patients with Marfan syndrome—some factors which affect the measurement. *HSS J.* 2007;3(1):89–92

29. Nemet AY, Assia EI, Apple DJ, Barequet IS. Current concepts of ocular manifestations in Marfan syndrome. *Surv Ophthalmol.* 2006;51(6):561–575

30. Maumenee IH. The eye in the Marfan syndrome. *Trans Am Ophthalmol Soc.* 1981;79: 684–733

31. Kang HK, Luff AJ. Management of retinal detachment: a guide for non-ophthalmologists. *BMJ.* 2008;336(7655):1235–1240

32. Hollands H, Johnson D, Brox AC, Almeida D, Simel DL, Sharma S. Acute-onset floaters and flashes: is this patient at risk for retinal detachment? *JAMA.* 2009;302(20):2243–2249

33. Morrison D, Sternberg P, Donahue S. Anterior chamber intraocular lens (ACIOL) placement after pars plana lensectomy in pediatric Marfan syndrome. *J AAPOS.* 2005; 9(3):240–242

34. Stuart AG, Williams A. Marfan's syndrome and the heart. *Arch Dis Child.* 2007;92(4): 351–356

35. Sisk HE, Zahka KG, Pyeritz RE. The Marfan syndrome in early childhood: analysis of 15 patients diagnosed at less than 4 years of age. *Am J Cardiol.* 1983;52(3):353–358

36. Meijboom LJ, Timmermans J, Zwinderman AH, Engelfriet PM, Mulder BJ. Aortic root growth in men and women with the Marfan's syndrome. *Am J Cardiol.* 2005;96 (10):1441–1444

37. Cañadas V, Vilacosta I, Bruna I, Fuster V. Marfan syndrome. Part 2: treatment and management of patients. *Nat Rev Cardiol.* 2010;7(5):266–276

38. Roman MJ, Devereux RB, Kramer-Fox R, O'Loughlin J. Two-dimensional echocardiographic aortic root dimensions in normal children and adults. *Am J Cardiol.* 1989;64 (8):507–512

39. Sharkey AM. Cardiovascular management of Marfan syndrome in the young. *Curr Treat Options Cardiovasc Med.* 2006;8(5): 396–402

40. Rossi-Foulkes R, Roman MJ, Rosen SE, et al. Phenotypic features and impact of beta blocker or calcium antagonist therapy on aortic lumen size in the Marfan syndrome. *Am J Cardiol.* 1999;83(9):1364–1368

41. Kroner BL, Tolunay HE, Basson CT, et al. The National Registry of Genetically Triggered Thoracic Aortic Aneurysms and Cardiovascular Conditions (GenTAC): results from phase I and scientific opportunities in phase II. *Am Heart J.* 2009;162(4):627. e1– 632.e1

42. Habashi JP, Judge DP, Holm TM, et al. Losartan, an AT1 antagonist, prevents aortic aneurysm in a mouse model of Marfan syndrome. *Science.* 2006;312(5770):117–121

43. Brooke BS, Habashi JP, Judge DP, Patel N, Loeys B, Dietz HC III. Angiotensin II blockade and aortic-root dilation in Marfan's syndrome. *N Engl J Med.* 2008;358(26):2787–2795

44. Gott VL, Cameron DE, Alejo DE, et al. Aortic root replacement in 271 Marfan patients: a 24-year experience. *Ann Thorac Surg.* 2002;73(2):438–443

45. Settepani F, Szeto WY, Pacini D, et al. Reimplantation valve-sparing aortic root replacement in Marfan syndrome using the Valsalva conduit: an intercontinental multicenter study. *Ann Thorac Surg.* 2007;83(2): S769–S773, discussion S785–S790

46. Cameron DE, Alejo DE, Patel ND, et al. Aortic root replacement in 372 Marfan patients: evolution of operative repair over 30 years. *Ann Thorac Surg.* 2009;87(5):1344–1349, discussion 1349–1350

47. Gillinov AM, Zehr KJ, Redmond JM, et al. Cardiac operations in children with Marfan's syndrome: indications and results. *Ann Thorac Surg.* 1997;64(4):1140–1144, discussion 1144–1145

48. Finkbohner R, Johnston D, Crawford ES, Coselli J, Milewicz DM. Marfan syndrome. Long-term survival and complications after aortic aneurysm repair. *Circulation.* 1995; 91(3):728–733

49. Yetman AT, Roosevelt GE, Veit N, Everitt MD. Distal aortic and peripheral arterial aneurysms in patients with Marfan syndrome. *J Am Coll Cardiol.* 2011;58(24): 2544–2545

50. Pelliccia A, Zipes DP, Maron BJ. Bethesda Conference #36 and the European Society of Cardiology Consensus Recommendations revisited a comparison of U.S. and European criteria for eligibility and disqualification of competitive athletes with cardiovascular abnormalities. *J Am Coll Cardiol.* 2008;52(24):1990–1996

51. Silverman DI, Burton KJ, Gray J, et al. Life expectancy in the Marfan syndrome. *Am J Cardiol.* 1995;75(2):157–160

52. Gray JR, Bridges AB, West RR, et al. Life expectancy in British Marfan syndrome populations. *Clin Genet.* 1998;54(2):124–128

53. Wood JR, Bellamy D, Child AH, Citron KM. Pulmonary disease in patients with Marfan syndrome. *Thorax.* 1984;39(10):780–784

54. Giske L, Stanghelle JK, Rand-Henriksen S, Strøm V, Wilhelmsen JE, Røe C. Pulmonary function, working capacity and strength in young adults with Marfan syndrome. *J Rehabil Med.* 2003;35(5):221–228

55. Kohler M, Blair E, Risby P, et al. The prevalence of obstructive sleep apnoea and its association with aortic dilatation in Marfan's syndrome. *Thorax.* 2009;64(2):162–166

56. Cistulli PA, Gotsopoulos H, Sullivan CE. Relationship between craniofacial abnormalities and sleep-disordered breathing in Marfan's syndrome. *Chest.* 2001;120(5):1455–1460

57. Cohen PR, Schneiderman P. Clinical manifestations of the Marfan syndrome. *Int J Dermatol.* 1989;28(5):291–299

58. Rand-Henriksen S, Lundby R, Tjeldhorn L, et al. Prevalence data on all Ghent features in a cross-sectional study of 87 adults with proven Marfan syndrome. *Eur J Hum Genet.* 2009;17(10):1222–1230

59. Foran JR, Pyeritz RE, Dietz HC, Sponseller PD. Characterization of the symptoms associated with dural ectasia in the Marfan patient. *Am J Med Genet A.* 2005;134A(1):58–65

60. Nallamshetty L, Ahn NU, Ahn UM, et al. Dural ectasia and back pain: review of the literature and case report. *J Spinal Disord Tech.* 2002;15(4):326–329

61. Milledge JT, Ades LC, Cooper MG, Jaumees A, Onikul E. Severe spontaneous intracranial hypotension and Marfan syndrome in an adolescent. *J Paediatr Child Health.* 2005;41(1–2):68–71

62. Rosser T, Finkel J, Vezina G, Majd M. Postural headache in a child with Marfan syndrome: case report and review of the literature. *J Child Neurol.* 2005;20(2):153–155

63. Maron BJ, Chaitman BR, Ackerman MJ, et al; Working Groups of the American Heart Association Committee on Exercise, Cardiac Rehabilitation, and Prevention; Councils on Clinical Cardiology and Cardiovascular Disease in the Young. Recommendations for physical activity and recreational sports participation for young patients with genetic cardiovascular diseases. *Circulation.* 2004;109(22):2807–2816

64. De Bie S, De Paepe A, Delvaux I, Davies S, Hennekam RC. Marfan syndrome in Europe. *Community Genet.* 2004;7(4):216–225

65. Fusar-Poli P, Klersy C, Stramesi F, Callegari A, Arbustini E, Politi P. Determinants of quality of life in Marfan syndrome. *Psychosomatics.* 2008;49(3):243–248

66. Raanani E, Ghosh P. The multidisciplinary approach to the Marfan patient. *Isr Med Assoc J.* 2008;10(3):171–174

67. Goland S, Barakat M, Khatri N, Elkayam U. Pregnancy in Marfan syndrome: maternal and fetal risk and recommendations for patient assessment and management. *Cardiol Rev.* 2009;17(6):253–262

68. Meijboom LJ, Vos FE, Timmermans J, Boers GH, Zwinderman AH, Mulder BJ. Pregnancy and aortic root growth in the Marfan syndrome: a prospective study. *Eur Heart J.* 2005;26(9):914–920

69. Anum EA, Hill LD, Pandya A, Strauss JF III. Connective tissue and related disorders and preterm birth: clues to genes contributing to prematurity. *Placenta.* 2009;30(3):207–215

70. Meijboom LJ, Drenthen W, Pieper PG, et al; ZAHARA investigators. Obstetric complications in Marfan syndrome. *Int J Cardiol.* 2006;110(1):53–59

71. Tekin M, Cengiz FB, Ayberkin E, et al. Familial neonatal Marfan syndrome due to parental mosaicism of a missense mutation in the FBN1 gene. *Am J Med Genet A.* 2007;143A(8):875–880

72. Volach V, Elami A, Gilon D, Pollak A, Ginosar Y, Ezra Y. Pregnancy in Marfan syndrome after aortic root replacement: a case report and review of the literature. *Congenit Heart Dis.* 2006;1(4):184–188

73. Burke LW, Pyeritz RE. Prenatal diagnosis of connective tissue disorders. In: Milunsky A, ed. *Genetic Disorders and the Fetus: Diagnosis, Prevention and Treatment.* 4th ed. Baltimore, MD: Johns Hopkins University Press; 1998:612–634

74. Sutherell J, Zarate Y, Tinkle BT, et al. Novel fibrillin 1 mutation in a case of neonatal Marfan syndrome: the increasing importance of early recognition. *Congenit Heart Dis.* 2007;2(5):342–346

75. Geva T, Sanders SP, Diogenes MS, Rockenmacher S, Van Praagh R. Two-dimensional and Doppler echocardiographic and pathologic characteristics of the infantile Marfan syndrome. *Am J Cardiol.* 1990;65(18):1230–1237

Infant Feeding and Transmission of Human Immunodeficiency Virus in the United States

- *Policy Statement*

POLICY STATEMENT

Infant Feeding and Transmission of Human Immunodeficiency Virus in the United States

COMMITTEE ON PEDIATRIC AIDS

KEY WORDS

HIV, human milk, mother-to-child transmission

ABBREVIATIONS

AAP—American Academy of Pediatrics
CDC—Centers for Disease Control and Prevention
PEP—postexposure prophylaxis
WHO—World Health Organization

www.pediatrics.org/cgi/doi/10.1542/peds.2012-3543

doi:10.1542/peds.2012-3543

PEDIATRICS (ISSN Numbers: Print, 0031-4005; Online, 1098-4275).

Copyright © 2013 by the American Academy of Pediatrics

abstract

Physicians caring for infants born to women infected with HIV are likely to be involved in providing guidance to HIV-infected mothers on appropriate infant feeding practices. It is critical that physicians are aware of the HIV transmission risk from human milk and the current recommendations for feeding HIV-exposed infants in the United States. Because the only intervention to completely prevent HIV transmission via human milk is not to breastfeed, in the United States, where clean water and affordable replacement feeding are available, the American Academy of Pediatrics recommends that HIV-infected mothers not breastfeed their infants, regardless of maternal viral load and antiretroviral therapy. *Pediatrics* 2013;131:391–396

BACKGROUND

Breastfeeding provides numerous health benefits to infants. In addition to providing optimal infant nutrition, human milk contains immune-modulating factors that protect against morbidity and mortality from infectious diseases, particularly those causing respiratory and gastrointestinal tract illnesses, which is especially important for infants living in resource-limited countries where infectious diseases are a major cause of infant mortality.[1] The American Academy of Pediatrics (AAP) strongly supports exclusive breastfeeding for approximately 6 months, followed by continued breastfeeding as complementary foods are introduced, with continuation of breastfeeding for 1 year or longer as mutually desired by mother and infant.[2]

Given that each year, approximately 8700 HIV-infected women give birth in the United States,[3] it is critical that physicians are aware of the HIV transmission risk from human milk and the current recommendations for feeding HIV-exposed infants in the United States. HIV can be transmitted from mother to child through human milk, with ongoing risk of infection throughout the breastfeeding period.[4] In the absence of antiretroviral prophylaxis, postnatal infection risk appears to be highest in the first 4 to 6 weeks of life, ranging from 0.7% to 1% per week.[5–7] However, risk continues for the duration of breastfeeding; in 2 large studies, late postnatal transmission risk after 4 to 6 weeks of age was 8.9 infections per 100 child-years of breastfeeding (approximately 0.17%/week) and was constant throughout this period.[4,8] Transmission risk is higher for women who acquire HIV infection (acute HIV infection) during lactation than for women with preexisting infection[9]; in 1 study, the cumulative risk of transmission of HIV via human milk was 14% from mothers with chronic HIV infection compared with 25% to 30% among mothers who acquired HIV during late pregnancy or lactation.[8] Other factors associated with increased risk of HIV transmission via human milk include high maternal plasma and human milk viral load, low maternal CD4+ cell count, longer breastfeeding duration, breast abnormalities (eg, mastitis, nipple abnormalities), oral lesions in the infant, mixed breastfeeding and formula feeding in the first few months of life (compared with exclusive breastfeeding), and abrupt weaning.[7]

Recent studies in Africa have revealed that 6 months of antiretroviral prophylaxis, either daily infant nevirapine or a triple-drug antiretroviral regimen administered to the mother, significantly reduced postnatal transmission risk to 1% to 5%.[10] On the basis of these data, the World Health Organization (WHO) published revised feeding guidelines for infants born to HIV-infected mothers living in resource-limited settings where infectious disease and malnutrition are major causes of infant mortality and replacement feeding is not feasible. In such settings, the WHO recommends exclusive breastfeeding for the first 6 months of life, followed by complementary foods and breastfeeding through 12 months of age, accompanied by postnatal infant or maternal antiretroviral prophylaxis to reduce HIV transmission during breastfeeding.[11,12]

However, neither infant nor maternal postpartum antiretroviral prophylaxis completely eliminates the risk of HIV transmission via human milk. In the United States, with current interventions, mother-to-child HIV transmission during pregnancy and labor is very low at under 1%.[13] Breastfeeding transmission rates with antiretroviral prophylaxis administered to either the

infant or the mother, although low, are still 1% to 5%, and transmission can occur despite undetectable maternal plasma RNA concentrations.[14] Maternal prophylaxis with triple-drug regimens may be less effective if first started during the postpartum period or late in pregnancy, because it takes several weeks to months before full viral suppression in human milk is achieved.[15,16] Antiretroviral drugs taken by the mother have differential penetration into human milk, with some drugs achieving concentrations much higher or lower than maternal plasma concentrations.[10,17] Although clinical trials of maternal antiretroviral prophylaxis to prevent postnatal transmission in resource-limited countries have generally shown low infant toxicity, increased rates of severe infant anemia and development of multiclass antiretroviral drug resistance in infants infected despite prophylaxis have been reported.[18,19] Therefore, in the United States, where there is access to clean water and affordable replacement feeding, the AAP continues to recommend complete avoidance of breastfeeding as the best and safest infant feeding option for HIV-infected mothers, regardless of maternal viral load and antiretroviral therapy.

An HIV-infected woman receiving effective antiretroviral therapy with repeatedly undetectable HIV viral loads in rare circumstances may choose to breastfeed despite intensive counseling.[20] This rare circumstance (an HIV-infected mother on effective treatment and fully suppressed who chooses to breastfeed) generally does not constitute grounds for an automatic referral to Child Protective Services agencies. Although this approach is not recommended, a pediatric HIV expert should be consulted on how to minimize transmission risk, including exclusive breastfeeding. Communication with the

mother's HIV specialist is important to ensure careful monitoring of maternal viral load, adherence to maternal therapy, and prompt administration of antimicrobial agents in instances of clinical mastitis. Infant HIV infection status should be monitored by nucleic acid (plasma HIV RNA or DNA) amplification testing throughout lactation and at 4 to 6 weeks and 3 and 6 months after weaning. Breastfeeding by an infected mother with detectable viral load or receiving no antiretroviral therapy despite intensive counseling represents a difficult ethical problem that requires consultation with a team of experts to engage the mother in a culturally effective manner that seeks to address both her health as well as her child's.

The optimal strategy for management of breastfeeding women with suspected acute HIV infection is unknown. In such circumstances, the mother should undergo appropriate evaluation (ie, plasma HIV RNA test as well as an HIV antibody test, because the antibody test result may be negative in acute infection), and breastfeeding should be stopped until HIV infection is confirmed or ruled out. Mothers should be assisted to pump and store expressed milk until a confirmatory test result is available and supported with skin-to-skin care to maintain milk supply; if HIV infection is ruled out, breastfeeding can resume. If the mother is found to be HIV infected, the infant should undergo age-appropriate HIV diagnostic testing evaluation, with follow-up testing at 4 to 6 weeks and 3 and 6 months after breastfeeding cessation if the initial test result is negative.[13]

The use of antiretroviral postexposure prophylaxis (PEP) has not been studied in infants born to mothers with acute HIV infection. Infant PEP may be less effective in this circumstance compared with other nonoccupational exposures, because human milk exposure is likely to have occurred over a prolonged period rather than from a single exposure. A regimen of daily nevirapine given to breastfeeding infants born to women with chronic HIV infection significantly reduces postnatal infection.[10] Whether a combination infant regimen would be more effective is unknown. In a study of infant prophylaxis in Malawi, the combination of daily nevirapine and zidovudine was not more effective in reducing transmission and was associated with more hematologic toxicity.[21] Some experts recommend providing a combination 3-drug regimen to exposed infants that is effective for treatment in HIV-infected infants. The appropriate prophylaxis duration is unknown; 4 weeks is used for nonoccupational exposure PEP. Consultation with a pediatric HIV expert is recommended with regard to decisions about the use of PEP for infants of breastfeeding women diagnosed with acute HIV infection; the National Perinatal HIV Hotline (1-888-448-8765) is a federally funded service providing referrals and free clinical consultation to physicians providing care for HIV-infected women and their infants.

The use of expressed human milk for the nutrition of sick, preterm, and recuperating neonates in ICUs is common practice, and some mothers express milk for feeding their infants in child care settings. The potential for transmission of infectious agents, such as HIV, through donor milk requires appropriate selection and screening of donors and careful collection, processing, and storage of milk. Donor human milk banks that belong to the Human Milk Banking Association of North America (http://www.hmbana.org/) voluntarily follow guidelines of the Centers for Disease Control and Prevention (CDC), which include screening of donors for infectious transmissible agents as well as heat treatment of the milk. Holder pasteurization (ie, heating at 62.5°C for

>30 minutes) is the only method that completely eradicates HIV in all human milk components and is the current standard in human donor milk banks in the United States. Flash-heat pasteurization (heating milk in a water bath to 100°C and removing it when water reaches a rolling boil, then allowing it to cool) has been recommended as a potential method for pasteurizing human milk in developing countries, because it is more feasible for caregivers and preserves more nutritive elements. However, although flash-heat pasteurization destroys cell-free HIV, it does not destroy cell-associated HIV in human milk[22]; therefore, in the United States, where there is access to clean water and affordable replacement feeding, infant feeding of expressed flash-heat–treated human milk from HIV-infected women is not recommended. Informal milk-sharing practices (ie, person-to-person or Internet sharing) are discouraged, because formal procedures for donor laboratory screening and pasteurization of milk cannot be guaranteed through such venues (http://www.fda.gov/downloads/Advisory Committees/CommitteesMeetingMaterials/ PediatricAdvisoryCommittee/UCM238627. pdf).[23] Gloves are not recommended for the routine handling of expressed human milk but should be worn by health care workers in situations in which exposures to human milk might be frequent or prolonged, such as in human milk banking.

Recommendations for management of accidental exposure of an infant to human milk not obtained from his or her mother are available from the CDC (http://www.cdc.gov/breastfeeding). Risk of HIV transmission in the case of an infant consuming human milk from a woman other than the mother in the United States is low, because women with known HIV infection are advised not to breastfeed their infants, HIV

screening of milk donors and heat treatment of human milk is performed by milk banks, and HIV transmission from a single human milk exposure has not been documented.

In 2009, the CDC reported late HIV transmission events in infancy among 3 HIV-infected children suspected to have acquired HIV infection as a result of consuming premasticated (prechewed) food given to them by their HIV-infected caregivers.[24] Phylogenetic comparisons of virus from cases and suspected sources and supporting clinical history and investigations suggest that the feeding of premasticated foods to the infants was the route of transmission. Subsequent investigation has identified additional children with potential HIV acquisition through premastication.[25] In a cross-sectional survey of primary caregivers of HIV-exposed infants 6 months of age or older from 9 pediatric clinics in the United States, 31% reported that the child had received premasticated food from either themselves, someone else, or both. Most primary caregivers were biological mothers and were HIV infected. Physicians should routinely inquire about this feeding practice and should instruct HIV-infected caregivers on potential risks, including premastication, as well as safer feeding options.

CONCLUSIONS

When making infant feeding recommendations, physicians should be aware of the potential for HIV transmission through human milk; knowledge of maternal HIV serostatus is essential to determine whether breastfeeding is appropriate. The WHO has developed recommendations for breastfeeding in resource-limited countries.[11,12] The following recommendations are made by the AAP for the United States, where the risks of infectious diseases and malnutrition for infants who are not breastfed are outweighed by the risks of HIV transmission through human milk and where alternatives to breastfeeding are available. The CDC and the AAP recommend universal opt-out HIV screening of all pregnant women in the United States.[26,27] Because the only intervention to completely prevent HIV transmission via human milk is not to breastfeed, in the United States, where clean water and affordable replacement feeding are available, the AAP recommends that HIV-infected mothers not breastfeed their infants, regardless of maternal viral load and antiretroviral therapy.

RECOMMENDATIONS

1. Women and their physicians need to be aware of the potential risk of HIV transmission to infants during pregnancy, during labor and delivery, and from breastfeeding.

2. Documented routine, opt-out HIV antibody testing should be performed for all women seeking prenatal care in the United States. Knowledge of HIV infection status will facilitate implementation of measures to prevent the acquisition and transmission of HIV and can help to determine whether it is appropriate to breastfeed. Repeat testing may be considered for all HIV-seronegative women in the third trimester and is recommended for women receiving care in jurisdictions with high HIV prevalence (see http://www.cdc.gov/mmwr/preview/mmwrhtml/rr5514a1.htm), for women delivering in health care facilities with an HIV infection prevalence of ≥1 per 1000 pregnant women, for women at increased risk of HIV acquisition, and for women with signs or symptoms of acute HIV infection.

3. For women in labor with undocumented HIV status during the current pregnancy, maternal HIV antibody testing with opt-out consent by using a rapid HIV test is recommended. Rapid antibody testing of the mother, by using either blood or saliva, is preferred over rapid testing of the infant; saliva HIV antibody testing should not be used for infant testing. A positive rapid test result should be confirmed by a standard HIV antibody test. Women with a positive HIV rapid antibody test result should promptly begin receiving antiretroviral prophylaxis to prevent intrapartum transmission (and their infants should receive prophylaxis), without waiting for results of the confirmatory test, and should be advised not to breastfeed. Mothers with a positive HIV rapid test result should be assisted to pump and store expressed human milk until a confirmatory test result is available and supported with skin-to-skin care to maintain milk supply; if HIV infection is ruled out, antiretroviral prophylaxis should be stopped and breastfeeding should be initiated. Women with a negative HIV rapid test result can initiate breastfeeding.

4. In the rare situation in which rapid HIV testing during labor is not immediately available, women with unknown HIV status should be counseled, with documentation in the medical record, regarding the potential high risk of HIV transmission through human milk should she be infected, and that an HIV test would be advised before initiation of breastfeeding.

5. In the United States, HIV-infected women should be counseled not to breastfeed or to provide their milk for the nutrition of their own or other infants, regardless of antiretroviral drug use or viral load; the discussion should be documented in the medical record. If financial resources are identified as a barrier to avoiding breastfeeding, physicians should assist in identifying appropriate financial support to access infant formula (eg, application to the Special Supplemental Nutrition Program for Women, Infants, and Children; http://www.fns.usda.gov/wic).

6. Women who are HIV seronegative should be strongly encouraged to exclusively breastfeed their infants.

7. Women who are HIV seronegative but who are at particularly high risk of seroconversion (eg, injection drug users or sexual partners of known HIV-infected persons or active drug users) should have repeat HIV testing and be provided education about HIV and the risk of transmission through human milk and should be provided an individualized recommendation concerning the appropriateness of breastfeeding.

8. In postpartum lactating women with suspected acute HIV infection, breastfeeding should be stopped until HIV infection is confirmed or ruled out. Pumping and temporarily discarding human milk can be recommended, and if HIV infection is ruled out, breastfeeding can resume. If maternal HIV infection is confirmed, the infant should undergo HIV testing. Consultation with a pediatric HIV expert is recommended regarding decisions about postexposure antiretroviral prophylaxis for the infant.

9. NICUs should develop polices for use of expressed milk for nutrition of neonates. Current standards of the Occupational Safety and Health Administration do not require gloves for routine handling of expressed human milk. However, gloves should be worn by health care workers in situations in which exposure to human

milk might be frequent or pro-longed (eg, human milk banking).

10. Human milk banks should follow guidelines developed by the US Public Health Service, which include donor screening for HIV infection and assessing risk factors that predispose to infection, as well as pasteurization of all human milk specimens.

11. Physicians should routinely inquire about premastication and prewarming feeding practices and instruct HIV-infected care-givers on safer feeding options.

LEAD AUTHOR

Lynne M. Mofenson, MD

COMMITTEE ON PEDIATRIC AIDS, 2011–2012

Patricia M. Flynn, MD, Chairperson
Grace M. Aldrovandi, MD
Ellen Gould Chadwick, MD
Rana Chakraborty, MD
Ellen Rae Cooper, MD

Heidi Schwarzwald, MD
Jaime Martinez, MD
Russell B. Van Dyke, MD

LIAISONS

Kenneth L. Dominguez, MD, MPH – *Centers for Disease Control and Prevention*
Lynne M. Mofenson, MD – *National Institute of Child Health and Human Development*

CONSULTANT

Gordon E. Schutze, MD

STAFF

Anjie Emanuel, MPH

REFERENCES

1. WHO Collaborative Study Team on the Role of Breastfeeding on the Prevention of Infant Mortality. Effect of breastfeeding on infant and child mortality due to infectious diseases in less developed countries: a pooled analysis. *Lancet.* 2000;355(9202): 451–455

2. American Academy of PediatricsSection on Breastfeeding. Breastfeeding and the use of human milk. *Pediatrics.* 2012;129(3). Available at: www.pediatrics.org/cgi/content/full/129/3/e827

3. Whitmore SK, Zhang X, Taylor AW, Blair JM. Estimated number of infants born to HIV-infected women in the United States and five dependent areas, 2006. *J Acquir Immune Defic Syndr.* 2011;57(3):218–222

4. Coutsoudis A, Dabis F, Fawzi W, et al; Breastfeeding and HIV International Transmission Study Group. Late postnatal transmission of HIV-1 in breast-fed children: an individual patient data meta-analysis. *J Infect Dis.* 2004; 189(12):2154–2166

5. Nduati R, John G, Mbori-Ngacha D, et al. Effect of breastfeeding and formula feeding on transmission of HIV-1: a randomized clinical trial. *JAMA.* 2000;283(9):1167–1174

6. Moodley D, Moodley J, Coovadia H, et al; South African Intrapartum Nevirapine Trial (SAINT) Investigators. A multicenter randomized controlled trial of nevirapine versus a combination of zidovudine and lamivudine to reduce intrapartum and early postpartum mother-to-child transmission of human immunodeficiency virus type 1. *J Infect Dis.* 2003;187(5):725–735

7. Bulterys M, Ellington S, Kourtis AP. HIV-1 and breastfeeding: biology of transmission and advances in prevention. *Clin Perinatol.* 2010;37(4):807–824, ix–x

8. Humphrey JH, Marinda E, Mutasa K, et al; ZVITAMBO Study Group. Mother to child transmission of HIV among Zimbabwean women who seroconverted postnatally: prospective cohort study. *BMJ.* 2010;341: c6580

9. Lockman S, Creek T. Acute maternal HIV infection during pregnancy and breast-feeding: substantial risk to infants. *J Infect Dis.* 2009;200(5):667–669

10. Mofenson LM. Antiretroviral drugs to prevent breastfeeding HIV transmission. *Antivir Ther.* 2010;15(4):537–553

11. World Health Organization. *Guidelines on HIV and Infant Feeding 2010: Principles and Recommendations for Infant Feeding in the Context of HIV and a Summary of Evidence.* Geneva, Switzerland: World Health Organization; 2010. Available at: http://whqlibdoc.who.int/publications/2010/9789241599535_eng. pdf. Accessed June 7, 2012

12. World Health Organization. *Antiretroviral Drugs for Treating Pregnant Women and Preventing HIV Infections in Infants: Recommendations for a Public Health Approach, 2010 Version.* Geneva, Switzerland: World Health Organization; 2010. Available at: http://whqlibdoc.who.int/publications/2010/9789241599818_eng.pdf. Accessed June 7, 2012

13. Panel on Treatment of HIV-Infected Pregnant Women and Prevention of Perinatal Transmission. *Recommendations for Use of Antiretroviral Drugs in Pregnant HIV-1-Infected Women for Maternal Health and Interventions to Reduce Perinatal HIV Transmission in the United States.* Washington, DC: Department of Health and Human Services; September 14, 2011. Available at: http://aidsinfo. nih.gov/contentfiles/lvguidelines/perinatalgl. pdf. Accessed June 7, 2012

14. Shapiro RL, Hughes MD, Ogwu A, et al. Antiretroviral regimens in pregnancy and breast-feeding in Botswana. *N Engl J Med.* 2010;362(24):2282–2294

15. Mofenson LM. Protecting the next generation—eliminating perinatal HIV-1 infection. *N Engl J Med.* 2010;362(24):2316–2318

16. Chasela CS, Hudgens MG, Jamieson DJ, et al; BAN Study Group. Maternal or infant antiretroviral drugs to reduce HIV-1 transmission. *N Engl J Med.* 2010;362(24):2271–2281

17. Mirochnick M, Thomas T, Capparelli E, et al. Antiretroviral concentrations in breast-feeding infants of mothers receiving highly active antiretroviral therapy. *Antimicrob Agents Chemother.* 2009;53(3): 1170–1176

18. Dryden-Peterson S, Shapiro RL, Hughes MD, et al. Increased risk of severe infant anemia after exposure to maternal HAART, Botswana. *J Acquir Immune Defic Syndr.* 2011;56(5):428–436

19. Fogel J, Li Q, Taha TE, et al. Initiation of antiretroviral treatment in women after delivery can induce multiclass drug resistance in breastfeeding HIV-infected infants. *Clin Infect Dis.* 2011;52(8):1069–1076

20. Morrison P, Israel-Ballard K, Greiner T. Informed choice in infant feeding decisions can be supported for HIV-infected women even in industrialized countries. *AIDS.* 2011; 25(15):1807–1811

21. Kumwenda NI, Hoover DR, Mofenson LM, et al. Extended antiretroviral prophylaxis to reduce breast-milk HIV-1 transmission. *N Engl J Med.* 2008;359(2):119–129

22. Orloff SL, Wallingford JC, McDougal JS. In-activation of human immunodeficiency virus type I in human milk: effects of intrinsic factors in human milk and of pasteurization. *J Hum Lact.* 1993;9(1):13–17

23. Israel-Ballard K, Donovan R, Chantry C, et al. Flash-heat inactivation of HIV-1 in human milk: a potential method to reduce postnatal transmission in developing countries. *J Acquir Immune Defic Syndr.* 2007;45(3):318–323

24. Gaur AH, Dominguez KL, Kalish ML, et al. Practice of feeding premasticated food to infants: a potential risk factor for HIV transmission. *Pediatrics.* 2009;124(2):658–666

25. Ivy W, III, Dominguez KL, Rakhmanina NY, et al. Premastication as a route of pediatric HIV transmission: case-control and cross-sectional investigations. *J Acquir Immune Defic Syndr.* 2012;59(2):207–212

26. Branson BM, Handsfield HH, Lampe MA, et al; Centers for Disease Control and Prevention (CDC). Revised recommendations for HIV testing of adults, adolescents, and pregnant women in health-care settings. *MMWR Recomm Rep.* 2006;55(RR-14):1–17, quiz CE1–CE4

27. American Academy of Pediatrics Committee on Pediatric AIDS. HIV testing and prophylaxis to prevent mother-to-child transmission in the United States. *Pediatrics.* 2008;122(5):1127–1134

Medicaid Policy Statement

- *Policy Statement*

POLICY STATEMENT

Medicaid Policy Statement

COMMITTEE ON CHILD HEALTH FINANCING

KEY WORDS
Medicaid, Child Health Insurance Program, benefits, coverage, financing, payment, eligibility, outreach, enrollment, managed care, quality improvement

ABBREVIATIONS
AAP—American Academy of Pediatrics
AARA—American Recovery and Reinvestment Act
ACA—Patient Protection and Affordable Care Act
CHIP—Children's Health Insurance Program
CMS—Centers for Medicare and Medicaid Services
CPT—*Current Procedural Terminology*
DHHS—Department of Health and Human Services
EHB—essential health benefits
EPSDT—Early and Periodic Screening, Diagnosis and Treatment
FMAP—federal medical assistance percentage
FPL—federal poverty level
HMO—health maintenance organization
MCO—managed care organization
MOE—maintenance of effort
PCMH—patient-centered medical home

www.pediatrics.org/cgi/doi/10.1542/peds.2013-0419

doi:10.1542/peds.2013-0419

PEDIATRICS (ISSN Numbers: Print, 0031-4005; Online, 1098-4275).

abstract

Medicaid insures 39% of the children in the United States. This revision of the 2005 Medicaid Policy Statement of the American Academy of Pediatrics reflects opportunities for changes in state Medicaid programs resulting from the 2010 Patient Protection and Affordable Care Act as upheld in 2012 by the Supreme Court. Policy recommendations focus on the areas of benefit coverage, financing and payment, eligibility, outreach and enrollment, managed care, and quality improvement. *Pediatrics* 2013;131:e1697–e1706

HISTORY OF MEDICAID PROGRAM

The Medicaid program was enacted in 1965 as Title XIX of the Social Security Act with funding streams derived from both federal and state governments. All states have participated in this voluntary program since Arizona joined in 1982. Federal law designates which groups of people must be eligible for Medicaid enrollment and what core medical benefits must be provided. Each state may then expand eligibility criteria, enhance benefits, contract with managed care organizations (MCOs) to administer the Medicaid program, and apply for waivers to develop specialized programs for particular populations. For instance, states have had the option to enroll children whose families have an income at or below 200% of the federal poverty level (FPL) in Medicaid, although only 6 states had chosen to do so by 1997 when the State Children's Health Insurance Program (CHIP) was enacted by Congress as Title XXI of the Social Security Act.

By 2009, total Medicaid enrollment had grown to include 34.2 million infants, children, and adolescents younger than 21 years. Medicaid provided benefits to 39% of the US pediatric population and covered 48% of all births. In 2009, Medicaid payments to providers for all age groups had expanded to $326.0 billion.* Although children younger than 21 years represented 53% of all Medicaid enrollees, they

---

*These figures differ from the Medicaid data provided by the Centers for Medicare and Medicaid Services (CMS) Office of the Actuary[1] for several reasons. The higher CMS estimate of total Medicaid costs for fiscal year 2009 of $380.6 billion includes nonprovider expenses such as disproportionate share hospital payments, administration costs, the Vaccines for Children Program, and other adjustments. Calculated costs per participant also differ for 3 reasons: (1) CMS uses estimated "person-year equivalents" (50.1 million) for fiscal year 2009 rather than "ever participants" (62.9 million unique participants covered by Medicaid for at least 1 month) as the basis for the calculation; (2) the AAP considers 19- and 20-year-old participants to be children, whereas CMS considers them to be adults; and (3) CMS segregates both children and adults who are blind and/or disabled into a separate "disabled" category.

accounted for only 29% of all Medicaid provider payments. In 2009, Medicaid expenditures averaged $2630 per child younger than 21 years compared with $6459 per adult between the ages of 21 and 64 years and $11 812 per senior citizen 65 years or older.[2]

Except for a few special programs (eg, family planning services, American Indian/Alaskan Native populations, administrative costs), the federal government funds a different proportion of each state's Medicaid budget.[3] This federal medical assistance percentage (FMAP) for each state is based on a formula that relates the 3-year rolling average per capita income in the state to that for the entire United States. By law, the minimum and maximum FMAPs are 50% and 83%, respectively.[3] Before the passage of the 2009 American Recovery and Reinvestment Act (ARRA: Pub L No. 111-5), the FMAP varied across states from 50% to 76%. Under ARRA and other FMAP "extension legislation" (Education, Jobs, and Medicaid Assistance Act of 2010 [Pub L No. 111-226]), FMAPs temporarily increased through June 2011 (eg, to a range of 62%–85% in the second quarter of fiscal year 2010). These enhanced FMAPs transiently decreased state Medicaid expenditures for fiscal year 2009 through fiscal year 2011. However, with the sunset of ARRA FMAP legislation and more Medicaid beneficiaries due to continued poor economic conditions and other factors, state Medicaid costs increased sharply in fiscal year 2012 and are expected to continue to climb through fiscal year 2019.[†]

[†]Beginning in 2020, the federal government will still fund 90% of the additional costs associated with newly eligible participants under the ACA. If the ACA Medicaid expansion were to be adopted by all states, the Congressional Budget Office had estimated that the total increased cost of the Medicaid program attributable to Medicaid expansion from 2014 to 2019 would be $564 billion dollars, of which $500 billion, or 89%, would have been funded by the federal government.[3]

IMPACT OF THE ACA AND THE 2012 SUPREME COURT DECISION ON THE MEDICAID PROGRAM

Passage of the Patient Protection and Affordable Care Act (ACA)[‡] in 2010[4] profoundly changed the Medicaid program through its expansion of Medicaid eligibility to all legal residents younger than 65 years with individual or family incomes at or below 138% of the FPL.[§] Hence, the ACA not only added a large population of adults (ages 19 through 64) who became newly eligible for Medicaid, but in many states, the expansion also increased the number of eligible children (through age 18) by mandating a higher minimum income eligibility.[||] The ACA directed the federal government to fund Medicaid expansion in full through 2016 and then at lower but still significant levels thereafter (tapering to 90% funding by 2020). The landmark Supreme Court decision upheld the constitutionality of the ACA

[‡]Encompassing the Patient Protection and Affordable Care Act and the amendment law associated with that act, the Health Care and Education Reconciliation Act (Pub L No. 111-152).

[§]The ACA established a new national floor of Medicaid coverage at 133% of the FPL with a standard 5% of income disregard that constituted part of a simplified modified adjusted gross income calculation designed to harmonize means-tested eligibility (Medicaid disregards the first 5% of one's income before calculating the proportion to the FPL). The ACA had mandated a minimum income level for Medicaid eligibility at 138% of the FPL beginning in 2014.

[||]The number of children newly eligible for Medicaid in a given state as a result of the change in qualifying FPL will depend on that state's current choice of percentage of FPL as the eligibility criterion for Medicaid for older children as well as that state's implementation of and enrollment within CHIP. There are currently 2.8 million children below 138% of the FPL who are not currently insured by Medicaid or by CHIP. In addition, an unknown number of children with family incomes between 100% and 138% of the FPL who are currently insured by CHIP would rollover to Medicaid coverage and about 4.3 million children with family incomes between 100% and 138% of the FPL who are now covered by private insurance would potentially be eligible for Medicaid.

with respect to the contested "individual mandate" for every American to obtain health insurance by a 5 to 4 margin.[5] However, the Court also struck down as unconstitutional an enforcement provision of the ACA that would have allowed the Department of Health and Human Services (DHHS) to withhold all federal Medicaid funding from states that declined to participate in Medicaid expansion. By a 7 to 2 majority, the Court ruled that this provision constituted undue coercion on states by the federal government; in a remedy, however, the Court upheld the constitutionality of the Medicaid expansion as an individual state option.

Legal scholars generally agree that the narrowly written Court decision did not invalidate other changes made by the ACA to the Medicaid program that pertained to existing populations.[6] The constitutionality of 3 provisions in particular has special importance for the pediatric population. First, Section 2001(b) of the ACA imposes a "maintenance of effort" (MOE) requirement that disallows states from restricting eligibility or reducing benefits for current child Medicaid beneficiaries until 2019. Second, Section 2001(a) (5) (b) expanded Medicaid eligibility for children under 19 by raising the minimum qualifying family income level to 138% of the FPL. Third, the ACA required states to improve outreach to and simplify enrollment of any person currently eligible for Medicaid.[6]

Many children now covered by Medicaid lose health insurance as they become young adults, so that how states choose to respond to the opportunity afforded by the ACA to participate in the adult Medicaid expansion can have a great impact on many pediatric patients. It is likely that additional negotiations will ensue in the future between the secretary of the federal DHHS and state Medicaid agencies that have initially signaled reluctance to pursue full-scale Medicaid expansion.[6]

This revision of the American Academy of Pediatrics (AAP) Medicaid Policy Statement advocates for the provision and funding of children's services in the Medicaid program and highlights changes in or new opportunities for state advocacy efforts as a result of the passage of the ACA and the 2012 Supreme Court decision.

The AAP continues to voice strong support for the Medicaid program and over the years has offered a continuing series of recommendations aimed at enhancing care and improving outcomes for children.[7] In particular, the AAP has long advocated innovative approaches to care (such as pediatric medical homes) that aim to achieve better health outcomes while reducing costs of care. The AAP stands ready to support newer population health-based programs (eg, Medicaid accountable care organizations) that seek to attain those same objectives. AAP members have been integral providers in both regular Medicaid and in state-specific Medicaid waiver programs and consequently have working experience with reform efforts of varying success.

BENEFITS AND MEDICAL HOME

Beyond a core set of mandated benefits, federal guidelines provide states with wide discretion in benefit design. The AAP recommends that all state Medicaid agencies:

1. Provide all children at a minimum the Early and Periodic Screening, Diagnosis, and Treatment (EPSDT) benefit and all other mandatory and optional benefits as outlined in the AAP statement "Scope of Health Care Benefits for Children From Birth Through Age 26."[8] Ensure that the medical necessity definitions used by each state for purposes of justifying medical services covered by Medicaid payment are consistent with the EPSDT policy. Furthermore, each state's process for determining medical necessity should rely on the expertise of pediatricians, pediatric medical subspecialists, and pediatric surgical specialists. Ensure that in the process of making decisions on the basis of medical necessity, the medical, behavioral health, and developmental care needs of the child are fully considered and that appropriate comprehensive benefits are available to address the full range of these needs.[9]

Develop appropriate benefits that address the needs of pregnant women. Pregnant women should be afforded the full range of maternity care (preconception, prenatal, labor, delivery, and postpartum) recommended in the Guidelines for Perinatal Care issued jointly by the American College of Obstetricians and Gynecologists and the American Academy of Pediatrics. Detail the full scope of pediatric Medicaid benefits in consumer brochures, on Web sites, and, most importantly, in state plan documents and managed care contracts. State agencies should provide a clear comparison of pediatric Medicaid benefits and networks among managed care plans so that families can choose a plan that is most appropriate for the needs of their child(ren).

2. Provide pharmacy benefits appropriate for children and broad enough to pay for medicines and specialized nutritional products required for children with special health care needs and for children with rare diseases. State Medicaid Pharmacy and Therapeutics committees should populate and operate a pediatric formulary with the recognition that less expensive (usually generic) drugs may not be as effective as alternative but more costly (usually brand name) drugs of the same class in all patients under all circumstances. Pharmacy benefits should acknowledge that many medications are appropriately prescribed to children in the absence of a pediatric label indication or dosing information. Optimally, states should mandate that all Medicaid MCOs operating in the state adopt the same state pediatric Medicaid formulary to ensure continuous and consistent treatment of patients (especially those with special health care needs or rare diseases) because they often transition between Medicaid insurers.

3. Ensure that all children have timely access to appropriate services from those qualified pediatric medical subspecialists and pediatric surgical specialists who are needed to optimize their health and well-being.

4. Ensure that Medicaid provider networks are sufficient to guarantee that children who transition from pediatric to adult care providers do not experience disruption in services.

5. Adopt periodicity schedules as defined in the AAP guidelines.[10] Immunization schedules should also be consistent with national guidelines as periodically revised by the Advisory Committee on Immunization Practices of the Centers for Disease Control and Prevention, the American Academy of Pediatrics, and the American Academy of Family Physicians.[11]

New or continuing efforts in which the AAP and its members can participate that can result in enhanced benefits for children enrolled in Medicaid programs include the following:

1. Develop and then facilitate the implementation of a working pediatric medical home model that

incorporates Bright Futures guidelines[12] and treatment services as codified in EPSDT.

2. Work with Medicaid and private insurance companies to standardize parameters for the medical home concept.[13,14] The wide variation in both panel size and family demographics encountered across pediatric practices suggests that a variety of models may be needed.

3. Develop and direct a program that educates parents, patients, and physicians about the advantages of a pediatric medical home.[15]

4. Partner with AAP state chapters, other pediatric health care providers, and families with children who are Medicaid beneficiaries to monitor and recommend improvements to state Medicaid programs and to the Centers for Medicare and Medicaid Services (CMS).

5. Assist parents, patients, and physicians to understand the full scope of Medicaid benefits.

FINANCING AND PAYMENT

Medicaid fee schedules and capitated payments to primary care and subspecialty providers are significantly lower than payments for comparable services from Medicare and private insurance companies. Low Medicaid payment is the primary reason that physicians limit participation in the program with resulting barriers to patient access for primary care and subspecialty health care services.[16–22] Even at academic medical centers that serve as "safety nets" for uninsured or underinsured patients, reduced access may be reflected by significantly longer wait times for subspecialty care.[23] Hence, the initial intent of Title XIX to provide truly equal access to quality primary and subspecialty care has not been fulfilled. Other documented reasons why providers decline or

limit participation in Medicaid include delayed or unpredictable payments, confusing or burdensome payment policies and paperwork, and nonadherence to scheduled visits.[17,18,22]

Although the MOE provision in the ACA proscribes states from restricting their current Medicaid eligibility rules until 2019 for children, states may choose instead to reduce their expenses by limiting nonmandatory services for adults, trimming payments for services, revoking any higher payments to specific groups of physicians, and cutting hospital payments. States have voiced alarm that high unemployment rates and increasing numbers of families enrolled in Medicaid will critically affect their budgets. In addition, as the US population ages, the growing number of seniors who become eligible for Medicare will also swell the ranks of seniors dually eligible for Medicaid coverage. The CMS Office of the Actuary has estimated that if each state fully implemented the ACA Medicaid expansion, state Medicaid expenditures would more than double over the decade from 2009 to 2019, from $132.3 billion to $313.3 billion.[24] To the extent that any state chooses to participate in the ACA Medicaid expansion, it will be vital that federal and state governments not compromise necessary coverage for children nor fail to provide adequate payment for pediatric care. In addition, states must be cognizant that ACA discontinued federal disproportionate share hospital payments to all states, anticipating that Medicaid expansion to the adult population would provide replacement revenue for safety net hospitals. Hence, states that choose not to participate in Medicaid expansion may risk the viability of some safety net hospitals.

In 2011, Medicaid payments for evaluation and management services across all states averaged ~64% of the

Medicare rates and lagged even farther behind payments by private insurers.[25] The ACA provides federal funding to Medicaid programs and state-financed Medicaid managed care plans to pay eligible physicians at Medicare rates for certain evaluation and management services, preventive care, and immunization administration during 2013 and 2014 (but not subsequently), including well-child ("checkup") codes (*Current Procedural Terminology* [CPT] codes 99381–99385; 99391–99395). Payment at this level should be sustained beyond 2014 and expanded to include all Medicaid services. This will require intense federal and state-specific advocacy.

The AAP proposes the following recommendations for federal and/or state action:

1. Ensure that Medicaid payments to providers for the goods and services involved in caring for children not only pay for the related work and practice expenses but also provide a sufficient return to make continued operation of a practice or facility economically feasible. In a broader context, payments should be sufficient to enroll enough providers and facilities so that, as required by federal law, Medicaid patients have "equal access" to care and services as do nongovernmentally insured patients in that geographic region. Failure to provide this fair level of payment will lead to continued early attrition of current pediatric providers as well as failure to attract physicians to pursue careers in primary or subspecialty pediatric care. To achieve this aim, the AAP recommends the following:

   a. Increase base Medicaid payment rates for all CPT codes, including pediatric specific CPT codes (eg, well-child checkup, counseling, and developmental assessment), to all providers to the 2012 or 2009 regional Medicare fee schedule rate, whichever is higher, or, in the case of preventive services without a Medicare payment, to a rate calculated by applying Medicare fee schedule methodology to the published values of work, practice expense, and professional liability insurance relative value units adjusted for the geographic region. These payment rate principles should be made permanent (ie, extended beyond the 2014 termination date) with the minimum level of payment per CPT code established as the greater of the 2012 Medicare actual or calculated rate or the current year's rate.

b. Establish a methodology to provide additional fair payment to a practice that recognizes the extra resources that might be invested on behalf of its Medicaid patients to promote wellness (eg, to pay for more vigorous outreach to increase participation rates with well-child checkups) and to provide care coordination of infants and children with complicated physical and/or mental health illnesses (eg, to pay for care coordinators, social workers, extended office hours, home visitations, dental care, durable medical equipment, etc). At present, fee-for-service payments (even if increased to Medicare rates) and current Federally Qualified Health Center payments do not fully pay for these extra resources.

c. Reward practices that meet or exceed AAP-approved predefined quality and performance metrics with incentive payments.[26]

d. Require Medicaid managed care plans to determine payment based on the principles outlined in (a) and (b) so that pediatric providers and patient-centered medical home (PCMH) programs are appropriately compensated. Similarly, require managed care plans to make providers eligible for additional incentive payments, as in (c), if, for instance, providers demonstrate improved outcomes, reduction of total Medicaid costs, and robust efforts to transition children with special health care needs to adult care. Provide input to Medicaid managed care plans about possible designs and implementations of structured incentive programs based on quality and performance parameters advocated by the AAP.

e. Explore the feasibility of adjusting fee-for-service or capitated payments to a provider on the basis of a risk-adjustment mechanism that accounts for the extra costs associated with caring for children with chronic conditions and other key pediatric diagnoses among the children in the provider panel.

f. Establish a mechanism within state Medicaid agencies and Medicaid MCOs for rapid adjustment of fee-for-service or capitated payments to providers for recommended new vaccines and other new technologies that rapidly achieve translation from clinical trials to standard clinical practice.

g. Require that paperwork in support of claims is not unduly burdensome and that clean claims are paid within 30 to 45 days of submission, so that practices can meet their cash flow obligations.

2. Oppose the conversion of Medicaid financing to an annual allotment or block grant programs with a fixed budget. Block grant proposals typically result in cost shifting from federal to state budgets and do not reduce overall health costs or improve quality of care. In fact, institution of block grants in combination with revocation of the MOE provision in ACA would likely restrict eligibility and reduce benefits for children to result in the loss of the individual child's guarantee to access Medicaid services. Recently, the concept of using "per capita caps" to control Medicaid expenditures has resurfaced, but ultimately, this mechanism of funding poses the same risks for children as do block grants.

3. Work with the AAP to study the feasibility of implementing pediatric-specific accountable care organizations through carefully structured demonstration projects.[27,28]

4. Pay primary care physicians for behavioral health services that physicians are qualified and competent to provide. Eliminate carve-outs for behavioral health coverage.

5. Mandate that states perform an in-depth assessment of the fiscal viability of any health plan before contracting with that plan to administer a Medicaid program and conduct annual audits to verify continued fiscal stability of the health plan. Require states that contract with MCOs to publish their physician payment methodologies and rates for each child eligibility group on an annual basis.

6. Advocate for federal and state agencies to partner with organizations, such as the AAP, to educate

physicians about programmatic changes in Medicaid fee-for-service or managed care environments (eg, pay-for-performance and PCMH programs). Physicians should understand the quality and cost control objectives of new initiatives and the linkage between fully documenting achievement of these goals and payments to physician practices.

7. Pay for the administration of immunizations (including multiantigen vaccines) and for counseling using the current CPT code set. Payments for vaccines should be at least 125% of the current Centers for Disease Control and Prevention private sector price list and payment for immunization administration should be, at minimum, 100% of the Medicare rate for each vaccine administration CPT code.

8. Ensure, wherever possible, the availability of at least 2 financially viable Medicaid MCOs in every region to allow for patient choice. Requests for proposals for organizations to serve as Medicaid third-party administrators and the ensuing selection process should be fully transparent.

9. Explore innovative methods to establish trust funds to support graduate medical education specific to the provision of primary and subspecialty care for Medicaid participants that will help maintain a qualified pediatric provider workforce.

10. Require Medicaid to provide full payment for trained interpreter services for patients with limited English proficiency. This will assist in thorough and accurate communication between provider and participant, increased accuracy of diagnosis and more appropriate treatment plan, and increased participant understanding and adherence to treatment, thus avoiding adverse clinical consequences.

11. Pay for observational care, urgent care, day medicine services, and necessary interhospital transport services, including transport of neonates from tertiary or quaternary neonatal or pediatric intensive care units to step-down convalescent units.

12. Implement policies and procedures to ensure equitable and prompt payment to providers and facilities for pediatric services rendered to Medicaid patients out of state. States should work together and with the federal government to achieve uniform and seamless processes to pay for these services.

13. Require all payers to report financial data on an annual basis so that the medical loss ratios (the percentage of total funding that is spent on patient care functions) are clearly delineated and transparent to the public.

14. Require states to develop clear and transparent rules and regulations related to ACA provisions for recovery audit contracting processes. Each state must ensure that physicians who are licensed and have practiced in the state supervise the work of certified professional coders with expertise in pediatric primary and subspecialty care. Key stakeholders, including physicians and the public, must have direct input in the process to avoid flawed statistical analysis. Payment errors due to both undercoding and overcoding should be included in a final reconciliation report. A clear and fair appeals procedure that is accomplished in a timely manner must be part of the formal recovery audit contracting process.

ELIGIBILITY

The AAP endorses the ACA-mandated expansion of Medicaid eligibility to

include all children who live in families with an income below 138% of FPL.¶ The AAP recommends that states implement the following additional measures to facilitate enrollment of children eligible for Medicaid or CHIP benefits:

1. Remove the 5-year waiting period for eligible children and/or pregnant women who are lawfully residing in the United States consistent with the provisions of the CHIP Reauthorization Act (Pub L No. 111-3).

2. Identify uninsured children who are not financially eligible for Medicaid and if possible facilitate enrolling them in CHIP.

3. Ensure that children who are moved by the state into a foster care program are tracked and immediately enrolled in and covered by Medicaid until age 21 using the Chafee option.# In 2014, if chosen by the foster child alumna, Medicaid coverage becomes mandatory under the ACA until age 26.

4. Ensure that newborn infants eligible for Medicaid are assigned to a specific plan immediately after birth so that timely provision of services in the first few months of life is not impeded by anticipated difficulties in payments of claims.

OUTREACH, ENROLLMENT, AND RETENTION

The AAP recommends that states strengthen their outreach, enrollment, and retention efforts to enroll all eligible uninsured children in Medicaid, CHIP, or exchange coverage.

¶For fiscal year 2012, the FPL thresholds are $15 415 for a single adult and $31 809 for a family of 4, with the exception of Alaska and Hawaii, where thresholds are 25% and 15% higher, respectively.

#A Medicaid option, known as the Chafee option, allows states to extend Medicaid to former foster children but only up to age 21. Currently, there are 21 states that use the Chafee option to provide health care coverage to former foster youth (Chafee Foster Care Independence Act of 1999).

1. Use multiple sites and replicate other effective strategies as have been implemented in CHIP to maximize and maintain enrollment of individuals eligible for Medicaid.

2. Optimize coordination of Medicaid, CHIP, and exchange program outreach through the use of streamlined eligibility determination, redetermination and enrollment processes including the use of short and easily understood common application forms, and expanded use of online enrollment. Once a child is enrolled, coverage should continue for 12 months.

3. Consider using the medical home to enroll patients and provide a fair payment for the administrative expense of this procedure.

4. Adopt practices that result in a "no wrong doors" approach to enrollment. All venues for Medicaid, CHIP, and exchange program enrollment should be able to evaluate an applicant's eligibility for any of these programs and to process the appropriate application.

5. Advocate support for federal policies to provide incentives to states to increase enrollment and retention in Medicaid and to continue those incentives for CHIP programs.

MANAGED CARE

In recent years, fiscal and policy considerations have encouraged states to contract with MCOs to administer the Medicaid program. As of fiscal year 2009, an estimated 61% of Medicaid beneficiaries 0 through 20 years of age were enrolled in a Medicaid health maintenance organization (HMO).[2] The AAP recommends that all MCOs should adopt a pediatric medical home model for all children that adequately addresses their needs, including those with special health care needs. Network adequacy should be determined

by periodic evaluation of the number of Medicaid providers whose panels are open to all new Medicaid patients.[29]

The AAP recommends that states adopt the following minimum set of practices and standards in their approach to Medicaid MCOs:

1. Ensure that MCOs (these may be either HMOs or provider-sponsored networks) provide educational materials to families that are culturally effective and written at literacy levels and in languages used by Medicaid recipients. The use of audiovisual aids should be encouraged.

2. Provide appropriate written, oral, and Web-based information and counseling to Medicaid eligible patients that allow informed patient choice of MCO-based network options for primary care physicians, pediatric medical subspecialists and pediatric surgical specialists, and pediatric hospital and ancillary services.

3. Assign Medicaid participants to an MCO that allows retention of the patient's medical home.

4. Recognize that pediatricians are primary care physicians who are eligible for pediatric patient assignment in all default enrollment systems.

5. Ensure that the provider network of all Medicaid MCOs contains the following components:

   a. Sufficient numbers of providers trained in primary care and subspecialty pediatrics, as well as pediatric surgical specialists.

   b. Sufficient numbers of physicians and other licensed providers of oral health, mental health, developmental, behavioral, and substance-abuse services so that medically necessary services are accessible within a reasonable length of time.

   c. When possible, a minimum of 1 hospital that specializes in the care of children.

   d. Vendors of durable medical equipment and home health care agencies that have experience caring for children, especially those with special health care needs.

6. License an MCO as a pediatric Medicaid provider only if its comprehensive pediatric network can provide children with quality care across the full continuum of care and hold that MCO accountable.

7. For Medicaid programs to be responsive to the needs of both patients and providers, it is essential that the programs be subject to either competition among at least 2 and when possible 3 MCOs in a region or to regulation that is regularly updated to reflect continuing input from patients and providers. Provider service networks (not-for-profit organizations created and governed by providers) should be evaluated and approved on a level playing field with HMOs.

8. Require that Medicaid administrative processes such as site visits and audits are simplified to minimize the burden for providers and office staff. Results of these processes should be available as a report card and transparent to prospective Medicaid enrollees.

9. Implement dedicated planning and oversight when MCOs contract for care delivery to children with special health care needs (including children with complex and/or rare diseases, children with behavioral/mental health conditions, and foster care children).

10. Establish an All Payer Claims Database and require MCOs to participate fully in reporting encounter

data. This would allow health policy analysts and researchers in government, academia, and the private sector to examine regional patterns of utilization, access to care, and quality of care and inform efforts to construct "best practice" models of care.

QUALITY IMPROVEMENT AND PROGRAM INTEGRITY

The AAP recommends that, as appropriate, CMS and the AAP, or state Medicaid agencies and state AAP chapters, should work collaboratively to develop and/or enhance quality-improvement activities that can benefit all children.

1. CMS should encourage collaboration among the Agency for Healthcare Research and Quality, the National Committee for Quality Assurance, the National Quality Forum, the AAP, and the CHIP Reauthorization Act Pediatric Healthcare Quality Measures Centers of Excellence. These organizations can evaluate current quality and performance measures with a goal of recommending modifications or achieving consensus around new measures that pertain to pediatric patients, including children with special health care needs. These measures should align with the recommendations outlined in the AAP policy statement "Principles for the Development and Use of Quality Measures."[26]

2. States should require health plans to use the core set of pediatric quality improvement measures that were created as part of the CHIP Reauthorization Act. These measures quantitate access to care, utilization of services, effectiveness of care, patient outcomes, and satisfaction of both patients and providers related to preventive, primary, acute, and chronic care for children. States should develop mechanisms for public reporting of these measures

that allow Medicaid beneficiaries to compare outcomes among MCOs. Consistent with federal statute, states should require that all Medicaid programs provide access to quality primary and subspecialty pediatric care that is equal to that achieved through private payers ("equal access" mandate).

3. At a minimum, states should establish Medicaid Advisory Committees whose membership includes pediatric primary care and subspecialty providers. These committees can advise state Medicaid agencies on issues related to the identification, implementation, and evaluation of quality measures and improvement programs as well as issues related to eligibility, enrollment, formulary, network adequacy, access, and medical necessity. To achieve maximal benefit, each state Medicaid agency should employ a physician with pediatric expertise who can continuously assist the agency with these issues as they relate to pediatrics.

4. Federal and state agencies should work with the AAP to develop tools and measures to monitor potential changes in the quality of pediatric care and the outcomes of the pediatric population. These tools and measures will be helpful in evaluating the effect of PCMHs and the impact of reform on children with special health care needs.

5. States should assume central responsibility for key administrative procedures that pertain to all Medicaid providers. These procedures could include meaningful provider assessment, education (eg, fraud and abuse training), and credentialing activities that would apply for all payers within the Medicaid or CHIP programs.

6. States should report results of peer review and reviews of medical records in a timely manner to

providers, plans, and beneficiaries consistent with applicable federal and state laws related to confidentiality, peer review privilege, and care review privilege.

7. States should monitor enrollment patterns and develop prospective means to assess reasons for changes in enrollment to ensure that MCOs do not encourage children with a high level of need to switch to other plans.

8. States should provide timely, meaningful, linguistically and culturally appropriate summaries of quality and performance measure and programs to beneficiaries to guide their choice of Medicaid plan.

CONCLUSIONS

By 2019, if the ACA Medicaid expansion were to be implemented by all states, 16 million additional individuals would gain insurance coverage through Medicaid and CHIP. Regardless of state variations in participation in the ACA Medicaid expansion, Medicaid will remain as the largest single insurer of children.[30] Additional legal proceedings and federal/state negotiations may clarify how DHHS will implement Medicaid expansion in the new adult population. In the meantime, the AAP supports state chapter advocacy efforts to expand Medicaid to the newly eligible population. Although AAP chapters might not take the lead in advocacy, they can provide pediatric expertise to coalition efforts and highlight the positive effects expansion will have on young adults.

To date, governmental health policy on both state and federal levels has not adequately met the medical, behavioral, and developmental needs of children. The ACA has provided a framework to redress some of these deficiencies. The AAP, through its network of chapters, sections, committees, councils, and staff and in partnership with other allied organizations, can collaborate with both federal and state agencies to monitor implementation of those aspects of the ACA that promise to enhance the care and outcomes of children and young adults and perhaps suggest refinements for future regulations. Success in these endeavors will not only enhance the health and well-being of the children for whom pediatricians care but also will enrich our ability to provide the quality of care to which we aspire.

LEAD AUTHORS
Thomas Chiu, MD, MBA
Mark L. Hudak, MD
Iris Grace Snider, MD

COMMITTEE ON CHILD HEALTH FINANCING, 2012–2013
Thomas F. Long, MD, Chairperson
Norman "Chip" Harbaugh, Jr, MD
Mark Helm, MD, MBA
Mark L. Hudak, MD
Andrew D. Racine, MD, PhD
Budd N. Shenkin, MD
Iris Grace Snider, MD
Patience Haydock White, MD, MA

PAST COMMITTEE MEMBERS
Thomas Chiu, MD, MBA
Russell Clark Libby, MD

STAFF
Edward P. Zimmerman, MS
Dan Walter
Robert Hall, JD, MPAff

REFERENCES

1. 2010 Actuarial Report on the Financial Outlook for Medicaid. Office of the Actuary, Centers for Medicare and Medicaid Services. Available at: https://www.cms.gov/ActuarialStudies/downloads/MedicaidReport2010.pdf

2. Medicaid State Reports FFY2009 [based on Medicaid Statistical Information System (MSIS) published by the Centers for Medicare & Medicaid Services through its State Summary Datamart]. *Elk Grove Village, IL:* American Academy of Pediatrics. Available at: http://www.aap.org/en-us/professional-resources/Research/research-resources/Pages/Medicaid-State-Reports.aspx. Accessed March 20, 2013

3. Peters CP. Medicaid financing: how the FMAP formula works and why it falls short (Issue Brief No. 828). December 11, 2008. Available at: http://nhpf.org/library/details.cfm/2705

4. Patient Protection and Affordable Care Act, Pub L No 111-148.

5. *National Federation of Independent Business et al. v. Sebelius, Secretary of Health and Human Services, et al.* Supreme Court of the United States No. 11-393. Available at: www.supremecourt.gov/opinions/11pdf/11-393c3a2.pdf

6. Rosenbaum S, Westmoreland TM. The Supreme Court's surprising decision on the Medicaid expansion: how will the federal government and states proceed? *Health Aff (Millwood).* 2012;31(8):1663–1672

7. American Academy of Pediatrics Committee on Child Health Financing. Medicaid policy statement. *Pediatrics.* 2005;116(1):274–280

8. Committee On Child Health Financing. Scope of health care benefits for children from birth through age 26. *Pediatrics.* 2012;129(1):185–189

9. Committee on Child Health Financing. Model contractual language for medical necessity for children. *Pediatrics.* 2005;116 (1):261–262

10. American Academy of Pediatrics. Recommendations for Preventive Pediatric Health Care. 2008. Available at: http://www.aap.org/en-us/search/pages/results.aspx?k=recommendations%20for%20preventive%20pediatric%20health%20%202008

11. Kroger AT, Atkinson WL, Marcuse EK, Pickering LK; Advisory Committee on Immunization Practices (ACIP) Centers for Disease Control and Prevention (CDC). General recommendations on immunization: recommendations of the Advisory Committee on Immunization Practices (ACIP). *MMWR Recomm Rep.* 2011;60(2):1–64

12. American Academy of Pediatrics. *Bright Futures: Guidelines for Health Supervision of Infants, Children, and Adolescents.* 3rd ed. 2008. Available at: http://brightfutures.aap.org/

13. American Academy of Pediatrics, Committee on Child Health Financing. Medical Home for Children: Financing Principles. November 11, 2011. Available at: http://www.medicalhomeinfo.org/downloads/pdfs/MHfinanceprin.pdf

14. National Committee for Quality Assurance's Patient-Centered Medical Home (PCMH) 2011. November 11, 2011. Available at: www.ncqa.org/tabid/631/default.aspx

15. Long WE, Bauchner H, Sege RD, Cabral HJ, Garg A. The value of the medical home for children without special health care needs. *Pediatrics.* 2012;129(1):87–98

16. Cohen JW, Cunningham PJ. Medicaid physician fee levels and children's access to care. *Health Aff (Millwood).* 1995;14(1):255–262

17. Coburn AF, Long SH, Marquis MS. Effects of changing Medicaid fees on physician participation and enrollee access. *Inquiry.* 1999;36(3):265–279

18. Berman S, Dolins J, Tang SF, Yudkowsky B. Factors that influence the willingness of private primary care pediatricians to accept more Medicaid patients. *Pediatrics.* 2002;110(2 pt 1):239–248

19. Cunningham PJ, Nichols LM. The effects of medicaid reimbursement on the access to care of medicaid enrollees: a community perspective. *Med Care Res Rev.* 2005;62(6):676–696

20. Decker SL. Medicaid physician fees and the quality of medical care of Medicaid patients in the U.S.A. *Rev Econ Househ.* 2007;5(1):95–112

21. Bisgaier J, Rhodes KV. Auditing access to specialty care for children with public insurance. *N Engl J Med.* 2011;364(24):2324–2333

22. AAP Survey of Pediatrician Participation in Medicaid, *CHIP and VFC.* Elk Grove Village, IL: *American Academy of Pediatrics;* 2012

23. Bisgaier J, Polsky D, Rhodes KV. Academic medical centers and equity in specialty care access for children. *Arch Pediatr Adolesc Med.* 2012;166(4):304–310

24. Office of the Actuary, Centers for Medicare and Medicaid Services. Actuarial Report on the Financial Outlook for Medicaid. 2011. Available at: https://www.cms.gov/ActuarialStudies/downloads/MedicaidReport2011.pdf

25. Methodology and Documentation. Exhibit 1: 2011 Payment Ratio Study. 2011 AAP Pediatric Medical Cost Model. [Actuarial study commissioned by the American Academy of Pediatrics and conducted by OptumInsight, Inc.]. Available at: www.aap.org/en-us/

professional-resources/practice-support/ pediatric-cost-model/Pages/Pediatric-Cost-Model.aspx

26. Hodgson ES, Simpson L, Lannon CM; American Academy of Pediatrics Steering Committee on Quality Improvement and Management; American Academy of Pediatrics Committee on Practice and Ambulatory Medicine. Principles for the development and use of quality measures. *Pediatrics*. 2008;121(2):411–418

27. American Academy of Pediatrics. Accountable Care Organizations (ACOs) and Pediatricians: Evaluation and Engagement. *AAP News*. 2011; 32(1):189–193

28. McClellan M, McKethan AN, Lewis JL, Roski J, Fisher ES. A national strategy to put accountable care into practice. *Health Aff (Millwood)*. 2010;29(5):982–990

29. Henry J. Kaiser Family Foundation, Commission on Medicaid and the Uninsured. Medicaid and Managed Care: Key Data Trends and issues. The Kaiser Commission Policy Brief. February 2010. Available at: http://www.kff.org/medicaid/upload/8046. pdf

30. Congressional Budget Office. Cost Estimate of H.R. 4872, Reconciliation Act of 2010. March 20, 2010. Available at: www.cbo.gov/sites/ default/files/cbofiles/ftpdocs/113xx/doc11379/ amendreconprop.pdf

Motor Delays: Early Identification and Evaluation

• •

• *Clinical Report*

CLINICAL REPORT

Motor Delays: Early Identification and Evaluation

abstract

Pediatricians often encounter children with delays of motor development in their clinical practices. Earlier identification of motor delays allows for timely referral for developmental interventions as well as diagnostic evaluations and treatment planning. A multidisciplinary expert panel developed an algorithm for the surveillance and screening of children for motor delays within the medical home, offering guidance for the initial workup and referral of the child with possible delays in motor development. Highlights of this clinical report include suggestions for formal developmental screening at the 9-, 18-, 30-, and 48-month well-child visits; approaches to the neurologic examination, with emphasis on the assessment of muscle tone; and initial diagnostic approaches for medical home providers. Use of diagnostic tests to evaluate children with motor delays are described, including brain MRI for children with high muscle tone, and measuring serum creatine kinase concentration of those with decreased muscle tone. The importance of pursuing diagnostic tests while concurrently referring patients to early intervention programs is emphasized. *Pediatrics* 2013;131:e2016–e2027

INTRODUCTION

The American Academy of Pediatrics (AAP) recommends developmental surveillance at all preventive care visits and standardized developmental screening of all children at ages 9, 18, and 30 months.[1] Recently, developmental screening instruments and their clinical interpretations have emphasized the early detection of delays in language and social development, responsive to rising prevalence rates of autism spectrum disorders in US children.[2] The most commonly used developmental screening instruments have not been validated on children with motor delays.[3,4] Recognizing the equal importance of surveillance and screening for motor development in the medical home, this clinical report reviews the motor evaluation of children and offers guidelines to the pediatrician regarding an approach to children who demonstrate motor delays and variations in muscle tone. (This report is aimed at all pediatric primary care providers, including pediatricians, family physicians, nurse practitioners, and physician assistants. Generic terms, such as clinician and provider, are intended to encompass all pediatric primary care providers.)

RATIONALE

Gross motor development follows a predictable sequence, reflecting the functional head-to-toe maturation of the central nervous system.

Garey H. Noritz, MD, Nancy A. Murphy, MD, and
NEUROMOTOR SCREENING EXPERT PANEL

KEY WORDS
motor delays, development, screening, neurologic examination, early intervention

ABBREVIATIONS
AAP—American Academy of Pediatrics
CK—creatine phosphokinase
CPT—*Current Procedural Terminology*
DCD—developmental coordination disorder
DMD—Duchenne muscular dystrophy

www.pediatrics.org/cgi/doi/10.1542/peds.2013-1056

doi:10.1542/peds.2013-1056

All clinical reports from the American Academy of Pediatrics automatically expire 5 years after publication unless reaffirmed, revised, or retired at or before that time.

PEDIATRICS (ISSN Numbers: Print, 0031-4005; Online, 1098-4275).

Although parents are reliable in reporting their child's gross motor development,[5,6] it is up to the clinician to use the parent's report and his or her own observations to detect a possible motor delay.[7]

Gross motor delays are common and vary in severity and outcome. Some children with gross motor delays attain typical milestones at a later age. Other children have a permanent motor disability, such as cerebral palsy, which has a prevalence of 3.3 per 1000.[8] Other children have developmental coordination disorder (DCD), which affects up to 6% of the population and generally becomes more evident when children enter kindergarten.[9] When motor delays are pronounced and/or progressive, a specific neuromuscular disorder is more likely to be diagnosed. Motor delays may be the first or most obvious sign of a global developmental disorder. For infants, motor activities are manifestations of early development. It is often the case that children whose developmental trajectories are at risk may experience challenges in meeting early motor milestones. Establishing a specific diagnosis can inform prognostication, service planning, and monitoring for associated developmental and medical disorders. When the underlying etiology of motor delays is genetic, early recognition may assist parents with family planning. A timely diagnosis may reduce family stress related to diagnostic and prognostic uncertainties.[5] For children with the few neuromuscular diseases for which treatments are available, outcomes may be improved when therapy is implemented early.[10]

Focus groups were conducted with 49 pediatricians at the AAP National Conference and Exhibition in 2010, and members of the AAP Quality Improvement Innovation Network were surveyed to ascertain current provider practices and needs regarding neuromotor screening.[11] Pediatricians described widely varying

approaches to motor examinations and identification of delays and expressed uncertainty regarding their ability to detect, diagnose, and manage motor delays in children. Participants requested more education, training, and standardization of the evaluation process, including an algorithm to guide clinical care (Fig 1).

THE ALGORITHM: IDENTIFYING CHILDREN WITH MOTOR DELAYS: AN ALGORITHM FOR SURVEILLANCE AND SCREENING

Step 1. Pediatric Patient at Preventive Care Visit

Each child's motor development should be addressed with other developmental and health topics at every pediatric preventive care visit.

Step 2. Is This a 9-, 18-, 30-, or 48-Month Visit?

All children should receive periodic developmental screening by using a standardized test, as recommended in the 2006 AAP policy statement "Identifying Infants and Children With Developmental Disorders in the Medical Home: An Algorithm for Developmental Surveillance and Screening."[1] Most children will demonstrate typical development without identifiable risks for potential delays. In the absence of established risk factors or parent or provider concerns, completion of a general developmental screening test is recommended at the 9-, 18-, and 30-month visits. These ages were selected, in part, on the basis of critical observations of motor skills development.

At the recommended screening visits, the following motor skills should be observed in the young child. These skills are typically acquired at earlier ages, and their absence at these ages signifies delay:

- 9-month visit: The infant should roll to both sides, sit well without support,

and demonstrate motor symmetry without established handedness. He or she should be grasping and transferring objects hand to hand.

- 18-month visit: The toddler should sit, stand, and walk independently. He or she should grasp and manipulate small objects. Mild motor delays undetected at the 9-month screening visit may be apparent at 18 months.

- 30-month visit: Most motor delays will have already been identified during previous visits. However, more subtle gross motor, fine motor, speech, and oral motor impairments may emerge at this visit. Progressive neuromuscular disorders may begin to emerge at this time and manifest as a loss of previously attained gross or fine motor skills.

An additional general screening test is recommended at the 48-month visit to identify problems in coordination, fine motor, and graphomotor skills before a child enters kindergarten.

- 48-month visit: The preschool-aged child should have early elementary school skills, with emerging fine motor, handwriting, gross motor, communication, and feeding abilities that promote participation with peers in group activities. Preschool or child care staff concerns about motor development should be addressed. Loss of skills should alert the examiner to the possibility of a progressive disorder.

Continuous developmental surveillance should also occur throughout childhood, with additional screenings performed whenever concerns are raised by parents, child health professionals, or others involved in the care of the child.

A summary of screening and surveillance for motor development based on the AAP "Recommendations for Preventive Pediatric Health Care" (also

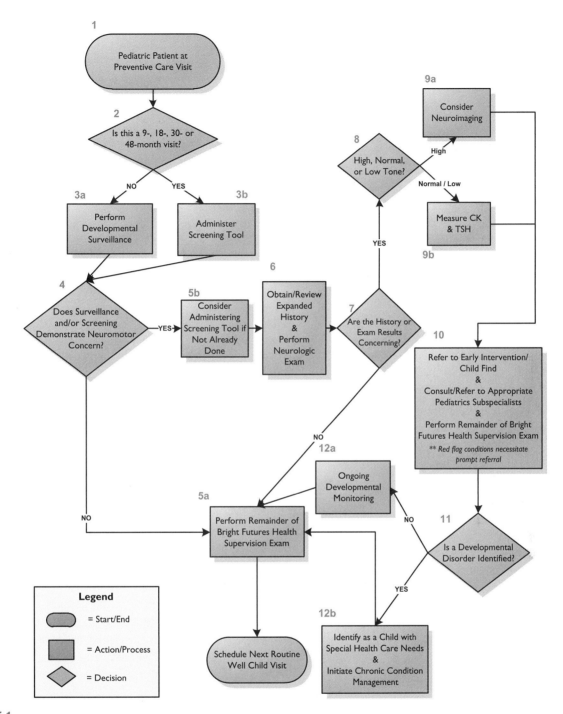

FIGURE 1
Identifying children with motor delays: an algorithm for surveillance and screening.

known as the periodicity schedule) is described in Table 1.[12] Listed are the mean ages at which typically developing children will achieve motor milestones. Marked delay beyond these ages warrants attention but does not necessarily signify a neuromotor disease.

Step 3a. Perform Developmental Surveillance

As the 2006 policy states, "Developmental surveillance is a flexible, longitudinal, continuous and cumulative process whereby knowledgeable health care professionals identify children who may have developmental problems.

Surveillance can be useful for determining appropriate referrals, providing patient education and family-centered care in support of healthy development, and monitoring the effects of developmental health promotion through early intervention and therapy." The 5 components of

TABLE 1 Motor Milestones for Developmental Surveillance at Preventive Care Visits[a]

Age	Gross Motor Milestones	Fine Motor Milestones
2 mo	Lifts head and chest in prone	
4 mo	Rolls over prone to supine; supports on elbows and wrists in prone	Hands unfisted; plays with fingers in midline; grasps object
6 mo	Rolls over supine to prone; sits without support	Reaches for cubes and transfers; rakes small object with 4 fingers
9 mo[b]	Pulls to stand; comes to sit from lying; crawls	Picks up small object with 3 fingers
1 y	Walks independently; stands	Puts 1 block in a cup; bangs 2 objects together; picks up small object with 2-finger pincer grasp
15 mo	Walks backward; runs	Scribbles in imitation; dumps small object from bottle, with demonstration
18 mo[b]	Walks up steps with hand held	Dumps small object from bottle spontaneously; tower of 2 cubes; scribbles spontaneously; puts 10 blocks in a cup
2 y	Rides on toy without pedals; jumps up	Builds tower and horizontal train with 3 blocks
2.5 y[b]	Begins to walk up steps alternating feet	Imitates horizontal and vertical lines; builds a train with a chimney with 4 blocks
3 y	Pedals; climbs on and off furniture	Copies a circle drawing; draws a person with head and one other body part; builds a bridge with 3 blocks
4 y	Climbs stairs without support; skips on 1 foot	Draw a person with 6 parts, simple cross; buttons medium-sized buttons

Adapted from Capute AJ, Shapiro BK, Palmer FB, Ross A, Wachtel RC. Normal gross motor development: the influences of race, sex and socioeconomic status. *Dev Med Child Neurol.* 1985;27 (5):635–643; Accardo PJ, Capute AJ. *The Capute Scales: Cognitive Adaptive Test/Clinical Linguistic and Auditory Milestone Scale (CAT/CLAMS).* Baltimore, MD: Paul H. Brooks; 2005; and Beery KE, Beery NA. *The Beery-Buktenica Developmental Test of Visual-Motor Integration (Beery VMI) Administration, Scoring and Teaching Manual.* Minneapolis, MN: NCS Pearson Inc; 2004.
[a] These milestones generally represent mean age of performance of these skills.
[b] It is recommended that a standardized developmental test be performed at these visits.

developmental surveillance are as follows: eliciting and attending to the parents' concerns about their child's development, documenting and maintaining a developmental history, making accurate observations of the child, identifying risk and protective factors, and maintaining an accurate record of documenting the process and findings.

A great breadth and depth of information is considered in comprehensive developmental surveillance. Much of this information, including prenatal, perinatal, and interval history will accumulate in the child's health record and should be reviewed at each screening visit.

Step 3b. Administer Screening Tool

Developmental screening involves the administration of a brief standardized tool that aids in the identification of children at risk for a developmental disorder. Many screening tools can be completed by parents and scored by nonphysician personnel; pediatric providers interpret the screening results. The aforementioned 2006 policy statement on developmental surveillance and screening provides a list of developmental screening tools and a discussion of how to choose an appropriate screening tool.

Step 4. Do Surveillance and/or Screening Demonstrate Neuromotor Concern?

Step 5a. Perform Remainder of Bright Futures Health Supervision Examination

Step 5b. Consider Administering Screening Tool if Not Already Done

The concerns of both parents and child health professionals should be included in determining whether surveillance suggests that the child may be at risk for developmental problems. If parents or health care providers express concern about the child's development, administration of a developmental screening tool to address the concern may be added.

Step 6. Obtain/Review Expanded History and Perform Neurologic Examination

Pediatricians can elicit key clinical information about a child's motor development from the child, parents, and family. Key elements are listed in Table 2. It is essential to ask parents broad, open-ended questions and listen carefully for any concerns. Some

concerns will be stated explicitly; others may be suggested through statements of perceived differences between a child's abilities and those of their age-matched peers. To broaden historical perspectives, clinicians can ask if extended family members, educators, or others who know the child well express any concerns about motor development. In instances of birth at earlier than 36 weeks' gestation, most experts recommend correcting for prematurity for at least the first 24 months of life.[13] Last, while taking the history, clinicians should carefully watch the child's posture, play, and spontaneous motor function without the stressful demands of performance under deliberate observation. When children are tired or stressed, direct observation of motor skills may not be possible, and full reliance on historical information is needed.

Children with increased tone may attain motor milestones early, asymmetrically, or "out of order." These aberrant milestones may include rolling supine to prone before prone to supine, asymmetric propping with sitting, asymmetric grasp, development of handedness before 18 months,[14] and standing before sitting.[15]

TABLE 2 Key Elements of the Motor History

Key Elements of Motor History	Example
Delayed acquisition of skill	Is there anything your child is <u>not</u> doing that you think he or she should be able to do?
Involuntary movements or coordination impairments	Is there anything your child <u>is</u> doing that you are concerned about?
Regression of skill	Is there anything your child <u>used</u> to be able to do that he or she can <u>no longer</u> do?
Strength, coordination, and endurance issues	Is there anything <u>other children</u> your child's age can do that are difficult for your child?

Physical Examination

The examination maneuvers described here are focused on medical home visits of children in the ambulatory setting. A discussion of newborn examination within the nursery setting is beyond the scope of this report; however, *Guidelines for Perinatal Care*, developed by the AAP Committee on Fetus and Newborn and American College of Obstetrics and Gynecology Committee on Obstetric Practice, provides further information.[16]

General Examination

When there are concerns regarding the quality or progression of a child's motor development, evaluation begins with a complete physical examination, with special attention to the neurologic examination and evaluation of vision and hearing. Children with motor delays related to systemic illness often show alterations in their level of interaction with their environment and general arousal. Careful assessments of head circumference, weight, and length/height with interpretation of percentiles according to Centers for Disease Control and Prevention or World Health Organization growth curves are essential and may facilitate early identification of children with microcephaly, macrocephaly, and growth impairments. Often, poor cooperation by the child may interfere with proper measurements, so any unexpected change in growth pattern should be rechecked by the clinician. Drooling or poor weight gain may suggest facial and oral motor weaknesses, and ptosis should prompt clinicians to consider congenital myopathies or lower motor neuron disorders. Respiratory problems, such as tachypnea, retractions, and ineffective airway clearance, can accompany many neuromotor conditions. Careful palpation of the abdomen may reveal organomegaly suggesting glycogen storage diseases, sphingolipidoses, or mucopolysaccharidoses. The astute clinician can use findings from the general pediatric examination to individualize a diagnostic approach for a child with motor delays.

Neuromotor Examination

Ideally, children should be well rested and comfortable for neuromotor examinations. However, when toddlers and preschoolers are uncooperative, clinicians can still gain important diagnostic information by observing the quality and quantity of movement.

The cranial nerve examination includes eye movements, response to visual confrontation, and pupillary reactivity. Although fundoscopic examination may be difficult, red reflexes should be detectable and symmetric. The quality of eye opening and closure and facial expression, including smile and cry, should be observed. Oromotor movement can be observed and, in the older child formally tested, by observing palate and tongue movement and, if possible, by drinking through a straw or blowing kisses. Observation for tongue fasciculations and quality of shoulder shrug should be assessed.

Strength is most easily assessed by functional observation. Attention to the quality and quantity of body posture and movement includes antigravity movement in the infant and the sequential transition from tripod sitting with symmetrical posture to walking and then running, climbing, hopping, and skipping in the older child. Clinicians should note any use of a Gower maneuver, characterized by an ambulatory child's inability to rise from the floor without pulling or pushing up with his arms. Muscle bulk and texture, joint flexibility, and presence or absence of atrophy should be observed. Quality and intensity of grasp is most easily assessed by observation during play.

For the infant, postural tone is assessed by ventral suspension in the younger infant and truncal positioning when sitting and standing in the older infant.[17] Extremity tone can be monitored during maturation by documenting the scarf sign in infants[18,19] and popliteal angles after the first year (see Fig 2).[20] Persistence of primitive reflexes and asymmetry or absence of protective reflexes suggest neuromotor dysfunction. Unsteady gait or tremor can be a sign of muscle weakness. Diminution or absence of deep tendon reflexes can occur with lower motor neuron disorders, whereas increased reflexes and an abnormal plantar reflex can be signs of upper motor neuron dysfunction. Neuromotor dysfunction can be accompanied by sensory deficits and should be assessed by testing touch and pain sensation.

In older children, difficulties with sequential motor planning, or praxis, should be differentiated from strength and extrapyramidal problems. Dyspraxia refers to the inability to formulate, plan, and execute complex movements. Assessment includes the presence and quality of age-appropriate gross motor skills (stair climb, 1-foot stand, hop, run, skip, and throw) and fine motor skills (button, zip, snap, tie, cut, use objects, and draw). Many of these children also have hypotonia.[21]

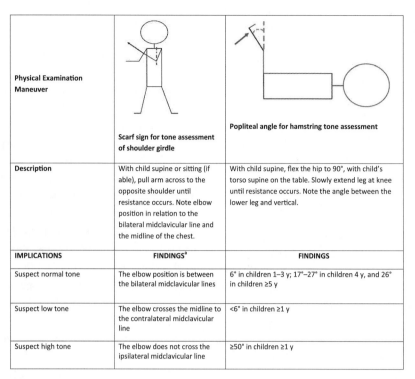

Physical Examination Maneuver	Scarf sign for tone assessment of shoulder girdle	Popliteal angle for hamstring tone assessment
Description	With child supine or sitting (if able), pull arm across to the opposite shoulder until resistance occurs. Note elbow position in relation to the bilateral midclavicular line and the midline of the chest.	With child supine, flex the hip to 90°, with child's torso supine on the table. Slowly extend leg at knee until resistance occurs. Note the angle between the lower leg and vertical.
IMPLICATIONS	FINDINGS[a]	FINDINGS
Suspect normal tone	The elbow position is between the bilateral midclavicular lines	6° in children 1–3 y; 17°–27° in children 4 y, and 26° in children ≥5 y
Suspect low tone	The elbow crosses the midline to the contralateral midclavicular line	<6° in children ≥1 y
Suspect high tone	The elbow does not cross the ipsilateral midclavicular line	≥50° in children ≥1 y

FIGURE 2

Examples of physical examination maneuvers. Adapted from Nercuri E, Haataja L, Dubowitz L. Neurological assessment in normal young infants. In: Cioni C, Mercuri E, eds. *Neurological Assessment in the First Two Years of Life.* London, UK: Mac Keith Press; 2007:30–31. [a] In term infants, these findings do not change significantly after 3 months of age.

Step 7. Are the History or Examination Results Concerning?

After identifying concerns of motor development, primary care clinicians can perform key diagnostic tests. All testing should be performed in the context of the child's past medical history, including prenatal complications and exposures, perinatal problems, feeding, and growth. Family history is also important to identify any other relatives with developmental or motor issues, recurrent pregnancy loss, stillbirth, or infant death, which may lead to identification of an underlying genetic etiology. Findings on physical examination, such as unusual facial features or other known visceral anomalies, may suggest a specific genetic condition. The state-mandated newborn screening laboratory results should be reviewed, because normal results exclude many disorders and avoid unnecessary testing. Although newborn screening is comprehensive, it does not test for all inborn biochemical disorders.

The algorithm (Fig 1) can be used to help guide appropriate initial testing. Table 3 lists "red flags" that should prompt the primary care pediatrician to expedite referral to diagnostic resources.

Step 8. High, Normal, or Low Tone?

Step 9a. Consider Neuroimaging

Increased tone in a child with neuromotor delay suggests an upper motor neuron problem, such as cerebral palsy. The American Academy of Neurology recommends imaging of the brain, preferably by MRI, for patients suspected of having cerebral palsy.[22] This test can be ordered within the medical home at the same time the patient is referred for specialist consultation for diagnosis.

Step 9b. Measure Creatine Phosphokinase and Thyroid-Stimulating Hormone Concentrations

When low to normal tone is identified, especially with concomitant weakness, investigations should target diseases of the lower motor neurons or muscles. Among the most common is Duchenne muscular dystrophy (DMD), characterized by weakness, calf hypertrophy, and sometimes cognitive or social delays. DMD usually presents at 2 to 4 years of age, but signs of weakness may be evident earlier. Becker muscular dystrophy is allelic to DMD but typically presents in older children and with a milder phenotype. Initial testing for all children with motor delay and low tone can be performed within the medical home by measuring the serum creatine phosphokinase (CK) concentration. The CK concentration is significantly elevated in DMD, usually >1000 U/L. As an X-linked disorder, there may be a family history of other affected male family members on the maternal side. However, DMD often presents in the absence of a family history for this disorder, with approximately one-third of cases being new mutations.[23] If the CK concentration is elevated, the diagnosis of DMD can usually be confirmed with molecular sequencing of the DMD gene. Other neuromuscular disorders include diseases of the peripheral motor nerves or muscles, such as myotonic dystrophy, spinal muscular atrophy, mitochondrial disorders, and congenital myasthenia gravis. Testing for these diseases should be performed by subspecialists, because these patients often require electrodiagnostic or specific genetic testing.

Although congenital hypothyroidism will be identified by newborn screening, acquired hypothyroidism and hyperthyroidism can present in later infancy or childhood with motor delay

TABLE 3 "Red Flags" in the Evaluation of a Child With Neuromotor Delay

Red Flags: Indications for Prompt Referral	Implications
Elevated CK to greater than 3× normal values (boys and girls)	Muscle destruction, such as in DMD, Becker muscular dystrophy, other disorders of muscles
Fasciculations (most often but not exclusively seen in the tongue)	Lower motor neuron disorders (spinal muscular atrophy; risk of rapid deterioration in acute illness)
Facial dysmorphism, organomegaly, signs of heart failure, and early joint contractures	Glycogen storage diseases (mucopolysaccharidosis, Pompe disease may improve with early enzyme therapy)
Abnormalities on brain MRI	Neurosurgical consultation if hydrocephalus or another surgical condition is suspected
Respiratory insufficiency with generalized weakness	Neuromuscular disorders with high risk of respiratory failure during acute illness (consider inpatient evaluation)
Loss of motor milestones	Suggestive of neurodegenerative process
Motor delays present during minor acute illness	Mitochondrial myopathies often present during metabolic stress

and low to normal tone. It is reasonable to perform thyroid function studies (thyroxine [T4] and thyroid-stimulating hormone) as part of the general laboratory evaluation for children with low tone or neuromuscular weakness, even without classic signs of thyroid disease.

Cerebral palsy classically presents with spasticity, dystonia, or athetosis, but may also result in hypotonia. Children with cerebral palsy may have a history of perinatal insult with concomitant abnormalities on brain imaging. Other causes of hypotonia should be considered before the diagnosis of hypotonic cerebral palsy is given to a child with an uneventful perinatal history and normal brain imaging.

DCD may be present when a child's motor coordination performance is significantly below norms for age and intellect, unrelated to a definable medical condition that affects neuromotor function (such as cerebral palsy, ataxia, or myopathy). It can affect gait, handwriting, sports and academic participation, and self-help skills. More than half of individuals with DCD remain symptomatic through adolescence and young adulthood. Intervention, especially task-oriented approaches, can improve motor ability.[8]

Children with neuromotor abnormalities, who also have failure to thrive, growth abnormalities, dysmorphic facial features, or other visceral anomalies, may have a chromosome abnormality, either common or rare. The American College of Medical Genetics and Genomics recommends microarray testing as the first-line chromosome study.[24] Because of the difficulty often encountered in interpretation of results, this test is typically ordered by a subspecialist familiar with this testing. Routine chromosome testing may be appropriate for children with weakness suspected as having recognizable disorders, such as Down syndrome (including mosaic Down syndrome), Turner syndrome, and Klinefelter syndrome. Fragile X syndrome is the most common inherited cause of cognitive impairment, and children with fragile X syndrome may have some element of motor delay. Genetic testing for fragile X syndrome should be considered in both boys and girls, whether they have dysmorphic facial features or a family history.

Common genetic conditions may present with early motor delays (Table 4). The 22q11.2 deletion syndrome (velocardiofacial syndrome) may present with hypotonia and feeding disorder in infancy and delayed motor milestones.[25] Noonan syndrome is also a common disorder, and although it is classically associated with short stature, webbed neck, ptosis, and pulmonary stenosis, the phenotype is highly variable, and developmental delays, especially motor delays, are common. Noonan syndrome is genetically heterogeneous and may be caused by mutations in genes in the *ras* pathway.[26] Neurofibromatosis type 1, associated with mutations in the NF1 gene, can lead to developmental delays and hypotonia in infancy and early childhood. This condition should be suspected in children with hypotonia and multiple (greater than 6) café au lait spots.[27] Children with known or suspected genetic disorders may benefit from genetic consultation and genetic counseling for the family.

Step 10. Refer to Early Intervention/Child Find, and Consult/Refer to Appropriate Pediatric Subspecialists, and Perform Remainder of Bright Futures Health Supervision Examination

Observation

Mild abnormalities that are not accompanied by "red flag" findings (red flag conditions necessitate prompt referral) may be closely followed through "observation," but a plan for new or worsening symptoms as well as a time-definite follow-up plan must be developed. Families should understand that clinical changes should prompt urgent reevaluation. This includes regression of motor skills, loss of strength, or any concerns with respiration or swallowing. This ensures that the progressive disorders are brought to medical attention immediately.

TABLE 4 Common Genetic Disorders for Which Neuromotor Delays May Be a Presenting Feature

Condition	Inheritance	Clinical Testing	Clinical Caveats
Angelman syndrome	Sporadic	Methylation testing for Prader-Willi/Angelman syndrome critical region, gene sequencing of UBE3A gene	Infantile hypotonia and delayed motor milestones, usually present with global delays; dysmorphic features are subtle in infancy.
Chromosome disorders	Many sporadic; high recurrence risk for unbalanced translocations if 1 parent has a balanced translocation	Chromosome analysis, single nucleotide polymorphism microarray	Some patients will have multiple anomalies and will have global developmental delays. Some may present in infancy or early childhood with delayed motor and/or speech milestones.
Down syndrome Klinefelter syndrome Rare deletions and duplications			Chromosome mosaicism also seen.
Deletion 22q11 syndrome (velocardiofacial syndrome)	Autosomal dominant (most cases new mutations)	Fluorescence in situ hybridization (FISH) for deletion 22q11.2	90% of cases new mutations. Feeding and speech disorders and cognitive impairment also seen. >50% will have a congenital heart defect.
DMD Becker muscular dystrophy	X-linked recessive	CK, sequencing of dystrophin gene	Becker and Duchenne muscular dystrophies are caused by mutations in different regions of the dystrophin gene. Becker muscular dystrophy has a later onset of symptoms with a less severe course; 67% of cases are inherited, 33% are new mutations.
Fragile X syndrome	X-linked	Gene sequencing and methylation analysis of FMR1 gene	Usually have global delays and cognitive impairment but may present in infancy or early childhood with predominantly motor delays. Males affected primarily, but females with FMR1 expansions may also be affected.
Mitochondrial myopathies	Autosomal recessive; X-linked recessive mitochondrial inheritance	Constitutional and mitochondrial genetic testing, lactate/pyruvate levels and ratio, serum amino acids	Genetic heterogeneity. May not present in infancy. Also at risk for cardiomyopathy, vision loss, hearing loss, cognitive disabilities.
Myotonic muscular dystrophy	Autosomal dominant	Gene sequencing for DMPK gene	May see anticipation with progression of phenotype in subsequent generations.
Neurofibromatosis type 1 (NF1)	Autosomal dominant	Usually a clinical diagnosis, gene sequencing NF1 gene	50% new mutations. Hypotonia most evident in infancy and early childhood. Suspect NF1 if hypotonia seen with multiple café au lait spots.
Noonan syndrome	Autosomal dominant	Gene sequencing for PTPN11 gene, genetically heterogeneous and multiple gene sequencing panels are available	Genetic heterogeneity. Commonly associated with short stature, ptosis, learning and developmental delays, hypotonia, pulmonary stenosis, cryptorchidism, cardiomyopathy.
Prader-Willi syndrome	Sporadic	DNA methylation testing for Prader-Willi/Angelman syndrome critical region	Hypogonadism, especially in boys. Hypotonia most evident in infancy and may be profound.
Spinal muscular atrophy, including congenital axonal neuropathy, Werdnig-Hoffmann disease, Kugelberg-Welander disease	Autosomal recessive	Gene deletion or truncation studies for SMN1 gene (95% to 98% of cases)	Usually presents in early infancy with severe hypotonia. Milder forms identified at later ages.

Depending on the nature of the suspected condition and the age of the child, it may be appropriate to have the child return to his or her medical home for a follow-up visit before the next Bright Futures health supervision visit. This will afford the opportunity for an interval review of noted symptoms, new concerns, and changes in physical examination or other developmental findings.

Education with the family should not be overlooked or delayed, as a suspected condition can cause significant anxiety.[28] Although the discussion may not be as in-depth as a situation in which diagnostic studies or referral is involved, families deserve a cogent and appropriate discussion of the findings that are being evaluated and what developmental trajectory is expected.

This may help assuage fears and increase compliance with follow-up plans.

Resources

All children with suspected neuromotor delay should be referred to early intervention or special education resources. Additionally, concurrent referrals should be made to physical and/or occupational therapists while diagnostic investigations are proceeding.[29] Even when a specific neuromotor diagnosis has not been identified, children with motor delays benefit from educationally and medically based therapies.

Each medical home must develop its own local resources and network of subspecialists for assistance with the diagnosis and management of young children with suspected motor delay. Depending on the setting, such subspecialists may include neurologists, developmental pediatricians, geneticists, physiatrists, or orthopedists. In some areas, availability of these resources may be limited, and waiting times may be long.[30] Direct physician-to-physician communication is recommended when red flags are identified (Table 3). Sharing digital photographs via a secure Internet connection may further expedite evaluations. However, the absence of red flags does not rule out the presence of significant neuromotor disease, and all children with motor delays should be thoroughly and serially evaluated.

Step 11. Is a Developmental Disorder Identified?

If a developmental disorder is identified, the child should be identified as a child with special health care needs, and chronic-condition management should be initiated (see Step 12b).

Step 12a. Ongoing Developmental Monitoring

If a developmental disorder is not identified through medical and developmental evaluation, the child should be scheduled for an early return visit for further surveillance, as mentioned previously. More frequent visits, with particular attention paid to areas of concern, will facilitate prompt referrals for further evaluation when indicated.

Step 12b. Identify as a Child With Special Health Care Needs and Initiate Chronic Condition Management

When a child has delays of motor development, that child is identified as a child with special health care needs even if that child does not have a specific disease etiology. Children with special health care needs are defined by the Department of Health and Human Services, Health Resources and Services Administration, Maternal and Child Health Bureau as "...those who have or are at increased risk for a chronic physical, developmental, behavioral, or emotional condition and who also require health and related services of a type or amount beyond that required by children generally."[31]

Children with special health care needs benefit from chronic-condition management, coordination of care, and regular monitoring in the context of their medical homes. Primary care practices are encouraged to create and maintain a registry for the children in the practice who have special health care needs. The medical home provides a triad of key primary care services, including preventive care, acute illness management, and chronic-condition management. A program of chronic-condition management provides proactive care for children and youth with special health care needs, including condition-related office visits, written care plans, explicit comanagement with specialists, appropriate patient education, and effective information systems for monitoring and tracking. Management plans should be based on a comprehensive needs assessment conducted with the family. Management plans should include relevant, measurable, and valid outcomes. These plans should be reviewed and updated regularly. The clinician should actively participate in all care-coordination activities for children with identified motor disorders. Evidence-based decisions regarding appropriate therapies and their scope and intensity should be determined in consultation with the child's family, therapists, pediatric medical subspecialists, and educators (including early intervention or school-based programs).

Children with established motor disorders often benefit from referral to community-based family-support services, such as respite care, parent-to-parent programs, and advocacy organizations. Some children may qualify for additional benefits, such as supplemental security income, public insurance, waiver programs, and state programs for children and youth with special health care needs (Title V). Parent organizations, such as Family Voices, and condition-specific associations can provide parents with information and support and can also provide an opportunity for advocacy.

RESOURCES

Internet resources are available (www.childmuscleweakness.org) for clinicians to view both typical and atypical motor findings. The identification of motor delays (or any chronic condition) in a child can trigger significant psychosocial stress for families.[32] The effects of repeated medical visits, testing, and modifications to home and school environments can place a significant burden on even well-functioning families.[33] Appropriate psychological support should be implemented early. A consumer health librarian or medical librarian can be used by families to provide specific resources tailored to individual needs (http://www.nlm.nih.gov/medlineplus/libraries.html).

For conditions with genetic basis or implications for family planning, medical genetics consultation and genetic counseling should be recommended. An international directory of genetics and prenatal diagnosis clinics can be found at http://www.ncbi.nlm.nih.gov/sites/ GeneTests/. Additional Web sites, such as www.rarediseases.org, offer information for both physicians and families.

Information on financial assistance programs should also be provided to families of children with established developmental disorders. They may qualify for benefits, such as supplemental security income (http://www.ssa.gov/pgm/ssi.htm), public insurance (http://www.medicaid.gov), and Title V programs for children and youth with special health care needs (http://internet.dscc.uic.edu/dsccroot/titlev.asp). There also may be local community programs that can provide transportation and other assistance.

TABLE 5 CPT Codes for Developmental Screening

Services/Step in Algorithm	Notes	CPT Code	Comments
Pediatric preventive care visit	All preventive care visits should include developmental surveillance; screening is performed as needed or at periodic intervals	99381–99394 (EPSDT)	
Developmental/medical evaluation: Office or Other Outpatient Services Codes; New Patient	If performed by the physician as a new patient outpatient office visit	99201-99205	99204 is used for evaluations performed by the physician that are detailed and moderately complex or take at least 45 min (with more than half spent counseling); 99205 is used for evaluations that are comprehensive and highly complex or take 60 min (with more than half spent counseling)
Developmental/medical evaluation: Office or Other Outpatient Services Codes; Established Patient	If performed by the physician as an outpatient office visit	99210–99215	99214 is used for evaluations performed by the physician that are detailed and moderately complex or take at least 25 min (with more than half spent counseling); 99215 is used for evaluations that are comprehensive and highly complex or take 40 min (with more than half spent counseling)
Developmental/medical evaluation/Office or Other Outpatient Consultations Codes	If performed by the physician as an outpatient office visit	99241–99245	99244 is used for "moderate activities" of up to 60 min (with more than half spent counseling); 99245 is used for "high" activity of up to 80 min (with more than half spent counseling)
Developmental screening	Does not require any physician work; rather, clinical staff can score results and provide to physician for interpretation as part of E/M	96110	Reported in addition to E/M services provided on the same date
Developmental testing	Used for extended developmental testing typically provided by the medical provider (often up to 1 h), including the evaluation interpretation and report	96111	Reported in addition to E/M services provided on the same date
Identify as a child with special health care needs, and initiate chronic condition management	Children with special health care needs are likely to require expanded time and a higher level of medical decision-making found in these "higher-level" outpatient codes; these codes are appropriate for services in the office and for outpatient facility services for established patients; these codes may be reported using time alone as the factor if more than half of the reported time is spent in counseling	99211–99215	As above
Prolonged services	At any point during the algorithm when outpatient office or consultation codes are used, prolonged physician service codes may be reported in addition when visits require considerably more time than typical for the base code alone; both face-to-face and non–face-to-face codes are available in CPT	99354 99355 99358 99359	99354 for first 30–74 min of outpatient face-to-face prolonged services 99355 for each additional 30 min 99358 for first 30–74 min of non–face-to-face prolonged services 99359 for each additional 30 min

E/M, evaluation and management; EPSDT, Early and Periodic Screening, Diagnostic and Treatment program.

DEVELOPMENTAL SCREENING BILLING AND CODING

Separate *Current Procedural Terminology* (CPT) codes exist for developmental screening (96110: developmental screening) and testing (96111: developmental testing) when completing neuromotor screening and assessment. The relative values for these codes are published in the Medicare Resource-Based Relative Value Scale and reflect physician work, practice expenses, and professional liability expenses. Table 5 outlines the appropriate codes to use when billing for the processes described in the algorithm. Billing processes related to developmental screening and surveillance should be carefully reviewed to ensure that appropriate CPT codes are used to document screening procedures and ensure proper payment. CPT code 96110 does not include any payment for medical provider services. The expectation is that a nonphysician will administer the screening tool(s) to the parent and score the responses. The physician reviews and interprets the screening results; the physician's work is included in the evaluation and management code used for the child's visit. The preventive care (or new, consultative, or return visit) code is used with the modifier 25 appended and 96110 listed for each screening tool administered. The CPT code 96111 includes medical provider work. This code would more appropriately be used when the medical provider observes the child performing a neuromotor task and demonstrating a specific developmental skill, using a standardized developmental tool.

CONCLUSIONS

The initial responsibility for identifying a child with motor delay rests with the medical home. By using the algorithm presented here, the medical home provider can begin the diagnostic process and make referrals as appropriate. Both during and after diagnosis, communication between the medical home and subspecialists is important,[34] and the medical home should remain fully engaged with the child's care as an integral part of chronic-condition management.

ACKNOWLEDGMENT

The development of this clinical report was funded by the American Academy of Pediatrics through the Public Health Program to Enhance the Health and Development of Infants and Children through a cooperative agreement (5U58DD000587) with the Centers for Disease Control and Prevention's National Center on Birth Defects and Developmental Disabilities.

NEUROMOTOR SCREENING EXPERT PANEL

Nancy A. Murphy, MD, Chairperson – *Council on Children With Disabilities*

Joseph F. Hagan, Jr, MD – *Bright Futures Initiatives*

Paul H. Lipkin, MD – *Council on Children With Disabilities*

Michelle M. Macias, MD – *Section on Developmental and Behavioral Pediatrics*

Dipesh Navsaria, MD, MPH, MSLIS

Garey H. Noritz, MD – *Council on Children With Disabilities*

Georgina Peacock, MD, MPH – *Centers for Disease Control and Prevention/National Center on Birth Defects*

Peter L. Rosenbaum, MD

Howard M. Saal, MD – *Committee on Genetics*

John F. Sarwark, MD – *Section on Orthopedics*

Mark E. Swanson, MD, MPH – *Centers for Disease Control and Prevention/National Center on Birth Defects*

Max Wiznitzer, MD – *Section on Neurology*

Marshalyn Yeargin-Allsopp, MD – *Centers for Disease Control and Prevention/National Center on Birth Defects*

STAFF

Rachel Daskalov, MHA

Michelle Zajac Esquivel, MPH

Holly Noteboom Griffin

Stephanie Mucha, MPH

PROJECT CONSULTANT

Jane Bernzweig, PhD

REFERENCES

1. Council on Children With Disabilities; Section on Developmental Behavioral Pediatrics; Bright Futures Steering Committee; Medical Home Initiatives for Children With Special Needs Project Advisory Committee. Identifying infants and young children with developmental disorders in the medical home: an algorithm for developmental surveillance and screening. *Pediatrics.* 2006;118(1):405–420

2. Centers for Disease Control and Prevention, Division of News and Electronic Media. CDC estimates 1 in 88 children in United States has been identified as having an autism spectrum disorder [press release]. Available at: www.cdc.gov/media/releases/2012/p0329_autism_disorder.html. Accessed November 14, 2012

3. Squires J, Twombly E, Bricker D, Potter L. *ASQ 3 User's Guide.* Baltimore, MD: Paul H. Brookes Publishing Co; 2009

4. Glascoe FP. *PEDS. Collaborating With Parents.* 2nd ed. Nolensville, TN: PEDSTest.com LLC; 2013

5. Harris SR. Parents' and caregivers' perceptions of their children's development. *Dev Med Child Neurol.* 1994;36(10):918–923

6. Ciafaloni E, Fox DJ, Pandya S, et al. Delayed diagnosis in Duchenne muscular dystrophy: data from the Muscular Dystrophy Surveillance, Tracking, and Research Network (MD STARnet). *J Pediatr.* 2009;155(3):380–385

7. Ehrmann Feldman D, Couture M, Grilli L, Simard MN, Azoulay L, Gosselin J. When and by whom is concern first expressed for children with neuromotor problems? *Arch Pediatr Adolesc Med.* 2005;159(9):882–886

8. Centers for Disease Control and Prevention. Data and statistics for cerebral palsy: prevalence and characteristics. Available at: www.cdc.gov/NCBDDD/cp/data.html. Accessed November 14, 2012

9. Blank R, Smits-Engelsman B, Polatajko H, Wilson P; European Academy for Childhood Disability. European Academy for Childhood

Disability (EACD): recommendations on the definition, diagnosis and intervention of developmental coordination disorder (long version). *Dev Med Child Neurol.* 2012;54(1): 54–93

10. Kishnani PS, Beckemeyer AA, Mendelsohn NJ. The new era of Pompe disease: advances in the detection, understanding of the phenotypic spectrum, pathophysiology, and management. *Am J Med Genet C Semin Med Genet.* 2012;160(1):1–7

11. American Academy of Pediatrics, National Center for Medical Home Implementation/ Centers for Disease Control and Prevention. Neuromotor screening. Available at: www.medicalhomeinfo.org/national/pehdic/neuro-motor_screening.aspx. Accessed November 14, 2012

12. Hagan JF, Shaw JS, Duncan PM, eds. *Bright Futures: Guidelines for Health Supervision of Infants, Children, and Adolescents.* 3rd ed. Elk Grove Village, IL: American Academy of Pediatrics; 2008

13. Aylward GP, Aylward BS. The changing yardstick in measurement of cognitive abilities in infancy. *J Dev Behav Pediatr.* 2011;32(6):465–468

14. Kraus EH. Handedness in children. In: Henderson A, Pehoski C, eds. *Hand Function in the Child: Foundations for Remediation.* St Louis, MO: Mosby/Elsevier; 2010:161–192

15. Capute AJ, Accardo PJ. The infant neuro-developmental assessment: a clinical interpretive manual for CAT-CLAMS in the first two years of life, part 1. *Curr Probl Pediatr.* 1996;26(7):238–257

16. Lemons JA, Lockwood J, Blackmon L, Riley L, eds. American Academy of Pediatrics, Committee on Fetus and Newborn; American College of Obstetrics and Gynecology, Committee on Obstetric Practice. *Guidelines for Perinatal Care.* 6th ed. Elk Grove Village, IL: American Academy of Pediatrics; 2007

17. Heineman KR, Hadders-Algra M. Evaluation of neuromotor function in infancy: a systematic review of available methods. *J Dev Behav Pediatr.* 2008;29(4):315–323

18. Amiel-Tison C, Grenier A. Normal development during the first year of life: identification of anomalies and use of the grid. In: Amiel-Tison C, Grenier A, eds. *Neurological Assessment During the First Year of Life.* New York, NY: Oxford University Press; 1986:46–95

19. Amiel-Tison C, Gosselin J. *Neurological Development from Birth to Six Years: Guide for Examination and Evaluation.* Baltimore, MD: Johns Hopkins University Press; 1998

20. Katz K, Rosenthal A, Yosipovitch Z. Normal ranges of popliteal angle in children. *J Pediatr Orthop.* 1992;12(2):229–231

21. Hadders-Algra M. The neuromotor examination of the preschool child and its prognostic significance. *Ment Retard Dev Disabil Res Rev.* 2005;11(3):180–188

22. Ashwal S, Russman BS, Blasco PA, et al; Quality Standards Subcommittee of the American Academy of Neurology; Practice Committee of the Child Neurology Society. Practice parameter: diagnostic assessment of the child with cerebral palsy: report of the Quality Standards Subcommittee of the American Academy of Neurology and the Practice Committee of the Child Neurology Society. *Neurology.* 2004;62(6):851–863

23. Dent KM, Dunn DM, von Niederhausern AC, et al. Improved molecular diagnosis of dystrophinopathies in an unselected clinical cohort. *Am J Med Genet A.* 2005;134(3): 295–298

24. Manning M, Hudgins L; Professional Practice and Guidelines Committee. Array-based technology and recommendations for utilization in medical genetics practice for detection of chromosomal abnormalities. *Genet Med.* 2010;12(11):742–745

25. Bassett AS, McDonald-McGinn DM, Devriendt K, et al; International 22q11.2 Deletion Syndrome Consortium. Practical guidelines for managing patients with 22q11.2 deletion syndrome. *J Pediatr.* 2011;159(2):332–339, e1

26. Jorge AAL, Malaquias AC, Arnhold IJP, Mendonca BB. Noonan syndrome and related disorders: a review of clinical features and mutations in genes of the RAS/MAPK pathway. *Horm Res.* 2009;71(4):185–193

27. Soucy EA, Gao F, Gutmann DH, Dunn CM. Developmental delays in children with neurofibromatosis type 1. *J Child Neurol.* 2012;27(5):641–644

28. Dodgson JE, Garwick A, Blozis SA, Patterson JM, Bennett FC, Blum RW. Uncertainty in childhood chronic conditions and family distress in families of young children. *J Fam Nurs.* 2000;6(3):252–266

29. Committee on Children With Disabilities. Role of the pediatrician in family-centered early intervention services. *Pediatrics.* 2001;107(5):1155–1157

30. Bale JF, Jr, Currey M, Firth S, Larson R Executive Committee of the Child Neurology Society. The Child Neurology Workforce Study: pediatrician access and satisfaction. *J Pediatr.* 2009;154(4):602–606, e1

31. McPherson M, Arango P, Fox H, et al. A new definition of children with special health care needs. *Pediatrics.* 1998;102(1 pt 1):137–140

32. Eiser C. Psychological effects of chronic disease. *J Child Psychol Psychiatry.* 1990;31 (1):85–98

33. Hamlett KW, Pellegrini DS, Katz KS. Childhood chronic illness as a family stressor. *J Pediatr Psychol.* 1992;17(1):33–47

34. Stille CJ, Primack WA, Savageau JA. Generalist-subspecialist communication for children with chronic conditions: a regional physician survey. *Pediatrics.* 2003;112(6 pt 1):1314–1320

Office-Based Care for Lesbian, Gay, Bisexual, Transgender, and Questioning Youth

• •

- *Policy Statement*

POLICY STATEMENT

Office-Based Care for Lesbian, Gay, Bisexual, Transgender, and Questioning Youth

abstract

The American Academy of Pediatrics issued its last statement on homosexuality and adolescents in 2004. Although most lesbian, gay, bisexual, transgender, and questioning (LGBTQ) youth are quite resilient and emerge from adolescence as healthy adults, the effects of homophobia and heterosexism can contribute to health disparities in mental health with higher rates of depression and suicidal ideation, higher rates of substance abuse, and more sexually transmitted and HIV infections. Pediatricians should have offices that are teen-friendly and welcoming to sexual minority youth. Obtaining a comprehensive, confidential, developmentally appropriate adolescent psychosocial history allows for the discovery of strengths and assets as well as risks. Referrals for mental health or substance abuse may be warranted. Sexually active LGBTQ youth should have sexually transmitted infection/HIV testing according to recommendations of the Sexually Transmitted Diseases Treatment Guidelines of the Centers for Disease Control and Prevention based on sexual behaviors. With appropriate assistance and care, sexual minority youth should live healthy, productive lives while transitioning through adolescence and young adulthood. *Pediatrics* 2013;132:198–203

INTRODUCTION

The American Academy of Pediatrics issued its first statement on sexual minority teenagers in 1983, with revisions in 1993 and 2004. Since the last report, research areas have rapidly expanded and hundreds of new publications have been produced about lesbian, gay, bisexual, transgender, and questioning (LGBTQ) youth, including an Institute of Medicine publication entitled "The Health of Lesbian, Gay, Bisexual, and Transgender People: Building a Foundation for Better Understanding."[1] Being a member of this group of teenagers is not, in itself, a risk behavior and many sexual minority youth are quite resilient; sexual minority youth should not be considered abnormal. However, the presence of stigma from homophobia and heterosexism often leads to psychological distress, which may be accompanied by an increase in risk behaviors. Health disparities exist in mental health, substance abuse, and sexually transmitted infection (STI)/HIV.

LGBTQ will be used whenever discussing studies and recommendations for all self-identified lesbian, gay, bisexual, transgender, or questioning youth. Many adolescents do not define themselves as a member of a sexual minority group but may have had same gender sexual

COMMITTEE ON ADOLESCENCE

KEY WORDS
sexual orientation, sexual identity, sexual behaviors, adolescents, sexual minority, homosexuality, gay, lesbian, bisexual, transgender

ABBREVIATIONS
CDC—Centers for Disease Control and Prevention
HPV—human papillomavirus
LGBTQ—lesbian, gay, bisexual, transgender, and questioning
MSM—men who have sex with men
STI—sexually transmitted infection
WSW—women who have sex with women

This document is copyrighted and is property of the American Academy of Pediatrics and its Board of Directors. All authors have filed conflict of interest statements with the American Academy of Pediatrics. Any conflicts have been resolved through a process approved by the Board of Directors. The American Academy of Pediatrics has neither solicited nor accepted any commercial involvement in the development of the content of this publication.

The recommendations in this statement do not indicate an exclusive course of treatment or serve as a standard of medical care. Variations, taking into account individual circumstances, may be appropriate.

All policy statements from the American Academy of Pediatrics automatically expire 5 years after publication unless reaffirmed, revised, or retired at or before that time.

www.pediatrics.org/cgi/doi/10.1542/peds.2013-1282

doi:10.1542/peds.2013-1282

PEDIATRICS (ISSN Numbers: Print, 0031-4005; Online, 1098-4275).

COMPANION PAPER: A companion to this article can be found on page e297, and online at www.pediatrics.org/cgi/doi/10.1542/peds.2013-1283.

behaviors (men who have sex with men [MSM] and women who have sex with women [WSW]). For this statement, the term "sexual minority" includes LGBTQ and MSM/WSW individuals.

DEFINITIONS

Typically, a young person's sexual orientation emerges before or early in adolescence.[2,3] Sexual orientation is referred to as "an individual's pattern of physical and emotional arousal toward other persons." Individuals who self-identify as heterosexual are attracted to people of the opposite gender; homosexual individuals self-identify as attracted to people of the same gender; bisexual teens report attraction to people of both genders. In common usage, self-identified homosexual people are often referred to as "gay" if male, and "lesbian" if female.[4] Many adolescents struggle with their sexual attractions and identity formation, and some may be referred to as "questioning."[2] For other definitions, please see Table 1 in the accompanying technical report.

Gender identity and gender expression usually conform to anatomic sex for both homosexual and heterosexual teenagers.[5] Gender dysphoria refers to the emotional distress of having a gender identity that is different from natal sex. Many young children with gender dysphoria will resolve their dysphoria by adolescence, but others will maintain it and desire transition to the opposite gender. These teenagers are "transgender."[6,7] Transgender people are often also identified by the natal gender and transition to the desired gender; MTF refers to males transitioning to females and FTM are females transitioning to males.[1,5,7–9]

Many adolescents who self-report as lesbian will still occasionally have sex with males, and many males who self-report as gay may have sex with

females; behaviors do not equal identity.[1,10] This range of sexuality may be reflected in the higher rate of teenage pregnancies experienced by WSW compared with their exclusively heterosexual peers.[11,12]

HOMOPHOBIA, HETEROSEXISM, AND IDENTITY FORMATION

Homophobia and heterosexism may damage the emerging self-image of an LGBTQ adolescent.[13–15] Homophobia perceived by LGBTQ youth may lead to self-destructive behaviors.[16] Societal homophobia is reflected in the higher rates of bullying and violence suffered by sexual minority youth.[17] With proper support and guidance, the majority of LGBTQ youth emerge as adults with sexual identities that are associated with little or no significant increase in risk behaviors compared with other youth. These resilient young adults lead happy, productive lives.[18,19]

HEALTH DISPARITIES FOR SEXUAL MINORITY YOUTH

Stigmatization, ostracism, and parental rejection remain common. Resulting struggles with self-image and self-esteem put sexual minority youth at risk.[11,20,21] Many sexual minority youth become homeless as a consequence of coming out to their families; sexual minority youth who are homeless may engage in riskier behaviors including survival sex.[22]

Significant health disparities exist for sexual minority youth related to depression and suicidality, substance abuse, social anxiety, altered body image, and other mental health issues.[1,13,17,23] Sexual minority youth suffer higher rates of depression and were more than twice as likely to have considered suicide.[1,13,17,24–26] Protective factors against depression, suicidal ideation, and suicide attempts

included family connectedness, caring adults, and school safety.[27]

Referral for "conversion" or "reparative therapy" is never indicated; therapy is not effective and may be harmful to LGBTQ individuals by increasing internalized stigma, distress, and depression.[1]

When sexual minority teenagers "come out" and acknowledge their sexuality as adolescents, there are often significant repercussions, especially victimization.[1,4,17,28] Even if not open about sexuality, 16% of MSM reported experiencing violence. Of adolescents who were open about their LGBTQ sexual orientation, 84% reported verbal harassment; 30% reported being punched, kicked, or injured; and 28% dropped out of school because of harassment.[17,29] Sometimes it is simply the perception that an individual might be LGBTQ that may lead to bullying, harassment, violence, injury, and homicide.[30,31]

Studies on the use of legal and illegal substances revealed significantly higher rates of tobacco, alcohol, marijuana, cocaine, ecstasy, methamphetamine, and heroin in sexual minority youth.[1,17,32,33] Use of club drugs (eg, cocaine, methamphetamine, ecstasy, GHB [γ-hydroxybutyric acid], ketamine, and LSD [lysergic acid diethylamide]) is especially concerning because of the association with unprotected sexual intercourse.[34]

Health disparities exist in sexual health outcomes with respect to HIV/AIDS, other STIs, and teenage pregnancy among LGBTQ youth. Sexual minority youth were more likely than heterosexual youth to report having had intercourse, to have had intercourse before 13 years of age, and to have had intercourse with ≥ 4 people. Gay or lesbian youth were about half as likely as heterosexual youth to have used a condom at the last intercourse.[22] During the past 15 years, reported rates of gonorrhea, chlamydia, and syphilis have trended downward for all adolescents, except for MSM.[35–37] One particular disparity is in HIV infection. Data from the Centers for Disease Control and Prevention (CDC) show that HIV rates continue to increase among young MSM 13 to 24 years of age.[38]

Information on sexual health disparities experienced by WSW is limited. High rates of STIs have been documented in lesbians and bisexual women with recent sexual contact with men, but there were also low but significant rates of STIs in exclusive WSW relationships. Viral infections, such as human papillomavirus (HPV) and herpes simplex virus infection, may be transmitted via exclusive female-to-female sexual contact.[39,40]

LGBTQ youth are less likely to report the use of hormonal or barrier contraceptives at last sexual encounter when having sex with the opposite gender.[22] Due to high rates of earlier sexual initiation, a greater number of partners, and less contraceptive use, WSW are at higher risk of teenage pregnancy than are teenagers who only have sex with the opposite gender.[1]

HEALTH DISPARITIES FOR TRANSGENDER YOUTH

Challenges faced by such youth and the potential of family and societal disapproval increase the risk that transgender adolescents will experience mental health issues, substance abuse, and sexual risk-taking behaviors. Transgender people face alarmingly high rates of verbal harassment and physical violence, including at home and at school.[1] Transgender youth face significant mental health issues as a consequence, including depression and suicidality, anxiety, body image distortion, substance abuse, and post-traumatic stress dis-

order. Supportive families can buffer an adolescent from these negative outcomes and promote positive health and well-being.[8]

MTF transgender youth face even more sexual health disparities than other sexual minority youth, with very high rates of HIV and other STIs.[41] There were higher rates of STIs and HIV in African American and Hispanic, compared with white, transgender individuals.[42,43] Contributing factors included history of incarceration, homelessness, exchanging sex for resources, nonconsensual sex, and difficulty accessing health care. Many had injected liquid silicone in their lifetime, with some sharing needles for hormone or silicone injection. Transgender individuals who purchase or obtain transgenic hormones on the street or from the Internet may cause significant health problems if used improperly, even if they are pure.[23]

PROMOTING SEXUAL HEALTH FOR LGBTQ YOUTH

Pediatricians and their office staff should encourage teenagers to feel comfortable talking with them about their emerging sexual identities and concerns about their sexual activities. Care should be confidential, and it is not the role of the pediatrician to inform parents/guardians about the teenager's sexual identity or behavior; doing so could expose the youth to harm.[44]

Pediatricians' use of gender-neutral terms can encourage teenagers to discuss any questions they have about their sexual behaviors or sexual orientation.[19] Table 2 in the technical report offers suggestions for gender-neutral questions.[45] Confidentiality must be emphasized.[19]

Teenagers who are abstinent should have their abstinence acknowledged and reinforced.[19] If the adolescent notes that they have engaged in sex-

ual activity, 1 classic question is "Are you having sex with males, females, or both?"[46] Table 3 in the technical report offers some additional suggestions for asking about specific sexual behaviors.

STI/HIV TESTING AND PREVENTION

Recent guidelines from the CDC recommend assessing for STI risk including asking about the gender of all partners. Pediatricians should then make decisions about STI testing on the basis of the sexual behaviors identified by the sexual history.[47] Adolescents who have not engaged in high-risk sex should be tested once per year. However, adolescents with multiple or anonymous partners, having unprotected intercourse, or having substance abuse issues should be tested at shorter intervals.[47] Specific STI screening recommendations for MSM are described in Table 4 in the technical report. Because of the increased incidence of anal cancer in HIV-infected MSM, screening for anal cytologic abnormalities has been proposed.[48] Condoms should be encouraged for all insertive/receptive sexual activities.[47] WSW are at risk of acquiring bacterial, viral, and protozoan infections from current and previous partners, both male and female. STD treatment guidelines from the CDC recommend a frank discussion of sexual behavioral risk so that the physician can make decisions about which STI tests to perform. Additionally, because many WSW have also had sex with men, HPV vaccine and routine cervical cancer screening should be offered to women according to recommended guidelines. Condoms for sex toys and dental dam for oral-vaginal contact should be emphasized.[47]

The CDC recommends routine immunization of males and females 11 or 12 years of age with HPV-4; catch-up immunization is recommended for WSW and MSM through 26 years of age.[47,49,50] HPV-2 has been approved for females 8 through 25 years of age.[51]

Because many teenagers who self-identify as LGBTQ may have sexual encounters that may not be predicted by their orientation, conversation about highly effective birth control methods and emergency contraception is important.[11,12]

TREATMENT OF TRANSGENDER YOUTH

See the technical report for additional details on the medical and surgical transition of transgender youth. Supportive counseling is paramount to assist the teenager with any dysphoria and to explore gender roles before altering the body. The therapy consists of potentially delaying puberty with gonadotropin-releasing hormone analogs, then use of hormonal therapy, and finally surgery.[5]

ASSISTING PARENTS

Another critically important role of the pediatrician is to assist parents of sexual minority youth. Pediatricians should acknowledge the parents' feelings but should provide information and support for the adolescent who has disclosed. Parents' reactions and attitudes may adjust over time, and the pediatrician should check in regularly and offer support to the entire family. Please see Table 5 in the technical report for resources to assist sexual minority youth and their parents and families.

RECOMMENDATIONS

- Pediatricians' offices should be teen-friendly and welcoming to all adolescents, regardless of sexual orientation and behavior; this includes training all office staff and ensuring that office forms do not presume heterosexuality of patients (or parents).

- If a pediatrician does not feel competent to provide specialized care for sexual minority teenagers and their families, he or she has the responsibility to evaluate families and then refer for medically appropriate care.

- Pediatricians who provide care to sexual minority youth should follow prevention and screening guidelines as outlined in *Bright Futures.*[19]

- All adolescents should have a confidential adolescent psychosocial history. Verbal histories and/or written questionnaires should use a gender-neutral approach. Screening and referral for depression, suicidality, other mood disorders, substance abuse, and eating disorders should be included.

- LGBTQ adolescents and MSM and WSW should have sexual behaviors and risks assessed and should be provided STI/HIV testing according to recommendations in the most recent sexually transmitted diseases treatment guidelines from the CDC.

- Contraception, including use of emergency contraceptives, should be offered to women regardless of their stated sexual orientation, and the importance of consistent condom/dental dam use should be discussed.

- Strengths, resources, and risks should be assessed, and targeted behavioral interventions should be implemented to allow the adolescent to maximize strengths and acknowledge and minimize risky behaviors.

- Pediatricians should be available to answer questions, to correct misinformation, and to provide the context that being LGBTQ is normal, just different.

- Transgender adolescents need to be supported and affirmed; they need education and referral for the process of transition and about avoiding the pitfalls of using treatments that were not prescribed by a licensed physician.

- Pediatricians should support parents in working through adjustment issues related to having a child who is LGBTQ while continuing to demonstrate love and support for their children.

- Pediatricians should support or create gay-straight alliances at schools and support the development and enforcement of zero-tolerance policies for homophobic teasing, bullying, harassment, and violence.

- Pediatricians should educate themselves about organizations that serve sexual minority youth and families in local communities and national organizations with information, support Web sites, and hotlines.

LEAD AUTHOR

David A. Levine, MD

COMMITTEE ON ADOLESCENCE, 2012–2013

Paula K. Braverman, MD, Chairperson
William P. Adelman, MD
Cora C. Breuner, MD, MPH
David A. Levine, MD
Arik V. Marcell, MD, MPH
Pamela J. Murray, MD, MPH
Rebecca F. O'Brien, MD, MD

LIAISONS

Loretta E. Gavin, PhD, MPH – *Centers for Disease Control and Prevention*
Rachel J. Miller, MD – *American College of Obstetricians and Gynecologists*
Jorge L. Pinzon, MD – *Canadian Pediatric Society*
Benjamin Shain, MD, PhD – *American Academy of Child and Adolescent Psychiatry*

STAFF

Karen S. Smith
James Baumberger

REFERENCES

1. Institute of Medicine, Committee on Lesbian, Gay, Bisexual, and Transgender Health Issues and Research Gaps and Opportunities. *The Health of Lesbian, Gay, Bisexual, and Transgender People: Building a Foundation for Better Understanding.* Washington, DC: National Academies Press; 2011

2. Spigarelli MG. Adolescent sexual orientation. *Adolesc Med State Art Rev.* 2007;18(3): 508–518, vii

3. Glover JA, Galliher RV, Lamere TG. Identity development and exploration among sexual minority adolescents: examination of a multidimensional model. *J Homosex.* 2009;56(1):77–101

4. Frankowski BL; American Academy of Pediatrics Committee on Adolescence. Sexual orientation and adolescents. *Pediatrics.* 2004;113(6):1827–1832

5. World Professional Association for Transgender Health. *Standards of Care for the Health of Transsexual, Transgender, and Gender Nonconforming People.* Minneapolis, MN: World Professional Association for Transgender Health; 2011. Available at: www.wpath.org. Accessed June 11, 2012

6. Wallien MS, Cohen-Kettenis PT. Psychosexual outcome of gender-dysphoric children. *J Am Acad Child Adolesc Psychiatry.* 2008; 47(12):1413–1423

7. Zucker K, Bradley S. Gender identity and psychosexual disorders. *Focus.* 2005;3(4): 598–617

8. Olson J, Forbes C, Belzer M. Management of the transgender adolescent. *Arch Pediatr Adolesc Med.* 2011;165(2):171–176

9. Hembree WC, Cohen-Kettenis P, Delemarre-van de Waal HA, et al; Endocrine Society. Endocrine treatment of transsexual persons: an Endocrine Society clinical practice guideline. *J Clin Endocrinol Metab.* 2009;94 (9):3132–3154

10. Igartua K, Thombs BD, Burgos G, Montoro R. Concordance and discrepancy in sexual identity, attraction, and behavior among adolescents. *J Adolesc Health.* 2009;45(6): 602–608

11. Herrick AL, Matthews AK, Garofalo R. Health risk behaviors in an urban sample of young women who have sex with women. *J Lesbian Stud.* 2010;14(1):80–92

12. Goodenow C, Szalacha LA, Robin LE, Westheimer K. Dimensions of sexual orientation and HIV-related risk among adolescent females: evidence from a statewide survey. *Am J Public Health.* 2008;98(6):1051–1058

13. Almeida J, Johnson RM, Corliss HL, Molnar BE, Azrael D. Emotional distress among LGBT youth: the influence of perceived discrimination based on sexual orientation. *J Youth Adolesc.* 2009;38(7):1001–1014

14. Walls NE. Toward a multidimensional understanding of heterosexism: the changing nature of prejudice. *J Homosex.* 2008;55(1): 20–70

15. Chesir-Teran D, Hughes D. Heterosexism in high school and victimization among lesbian, gay, bisexual, and questioning students. *J Youth Adolesc.* 2009;38(7):963–975

16. McDermott E, Roen K, Scourfield J. Avoiding shame: young LGBT people, homophobia and self-destructive behaviours. *Cult Health Sex.* 2008;10(8):815–829

17. Kann L, Olsen EO, McManus T, et al; Centers for Disease Control and Prevention. Sexual identity, sex of sexual contacts, and health-risk behaviors among students in grades 9-12—youth risk behavior surveillance, selected sites, United States, 2001-2009. *MMWR Surveill Summ.* 2011;60(7):1–133

18. Saewyc EM, Homma Y, Skay CL, Bearinger LH, Resnick MD, Reis E. Protective factors in the lives of bisexual adolescents in North America. *Am J Public Health.* 2009;99(1): 110–117

19. Hagan JF, Shaw JS, Duncan P, eds. *Bright Futures: Guidelines for Health Supervision of Infants, Children, and Adolescents.* 3rd ed. Elk Grove Village, IL: American Academy of Pediatrics; 2008

20. Kipke MD, Kubicek K, Weiss G, et al. The health and health behaviors of young men who have sex with men. *J Adolesc Health.* 2007;40(4):342–350

21. Coker TR, Austin SB, Schuster MA. Health and healthcare for lesbian, gay, bisexual, and transgender youth: reducing disparities through research, education, and practice. *J Adolesc Health.* 2009;45(3):213–215

22. Physicians for Reproductive Choice and Health. *Gay, Lesbian, Bisexual, Transgender, and Questioning Youth.* 4th ed. New York, NY: The Adolescent Reproductive and Sexual Health Education Program; 2011. Available at: www.prch.org/arshep. Accessed June 13, 2012

23. Berg MB, Mimiaga MJ, Safren SA. Mental health concerns of gay and bisexual men seeking mental health services. *J Homosex.* 2008;54(3):293–306

24. Silenzio VM, Pena JB, Duberstein PR, Cerel J, Knox KL. Sexual orientation and risk factors for suicidal ideation and suicide attempts among adolescents and young adults. *Am J Public Health.* 2007;97(11): 2017–2019

25. Walls NE, Freedenthal S, Wisneski H. Suicidal ideation and attempts among sexual minority youths receiving social services. *Soc Work.* 2008;53(1):21–29

26. D'Augelli AR, Grossman AH, Salter NP, Vasey JJ, Starks MT, Sinclair KO. Predicting the suicide attempts of lesbian, gay, and bisexual youth. *Suicide Life Threat Behav.* 2005;35(6):646–660

27. Eisenberg ME, Resnick MD. Suicidality among gay, lesbian and bisexual youth: the role of protective factors. *J Adolesc Health.* 2006;39(5):662–668

28. Kelley TM, Robertson RA. Relational aggression and victimization in gay male relationships: the role of internalized homophobia. *Aggress Behav.* 2008;34(5):475–485

29. Consortium of Higher Education LGBT Resource Professionals. Press release. Syracuse, NY: Consortium of Higher Education LGBT Resource Professionals; October 4, 2004. Available at: www.lgbtcampus.org/about/news-2010-10-04-deaths. Accessed June 13, 2012

30. Lampinen TM, Chan K, Anema A, et al. Incidence of and risk factors for sexual orientation-related physical assault among young men who have sex with men. *Am J Public Health.* 2008;98(6):1028–1035

31. Herek GM, Sims C. Sexual orientation and violence victimization: hate crimes and intimate partner violence among gay and bisexual men in the US. In: Wolitski RJ, Stall R, Valdiserri RO, eds. *Unequal Opportunity: Health Disparities Affecting Gay and Bisexual Men in the US.* New York, NY: Oxford University Press; 2008:35–71

32. D'Augelli AR. High tobacco use among lesbian, gay, and bisexual youth: mounting evidence about a hidden population's health risk behavior. *Arch Pediatr Adolesc Med.* 2004;158(4):309–310

33. Ridner SL, Frost K, Lajoie AS. Health information and risk behaviors among lesbian, gay, and bisexual college students. *J Am Acad Nurse Pract.* 2006;18(8):374–378

34. Parsons JT, Kelly BC, Weiser JD. Initiation into methamphetamine use for young gay and bisexual men. *Drug Alcohol Depend.* 2007;90(2-3):135–144

35. Benson PA, Hergenroeder AC. Bacterial sexually transmitted infections in gay, lesbian, and bisexual adolescents: medical and public health perspectives. *Semin Pediatr Infect Dis.* 2005;16(3):181–191

36. Kipke MD, Weiss G, Wong CF. Residential status as a risk factor for drug use and HIV risk among young men who have sex with men. *AIDS Behav.* 2007;11(suppl 6):56–69

37. Rudy ET, Shoptaw S, Lazzar M, Bolan RK, Tilekar SD, Kerndt PR. Methamphetamine use and other club drug use differ in relation to HIV status and risk behavior among gay and bisexual men. *Sex Transm Dis.* 2009;36(11):693–695

38. Centers for Disease Control and Prevention. Trends in HIV/AIDS diagnoses among men who have sex with men—33 states, 2001-2006. *MMWR Morb Mortal Wkly Rep.* 2008;57(25):681–686

39. Robertson P, Schachter J. Failure to identify venereal disease in a lesbian population. *Sex Transm Dis.* 1981;8(2):75–76

40. Lindley LL, Barnett CL, Brandt HM, Hardin JW, Burcin M. STDs among sexually active female college students: does sexual orientation make a difference? *Perspect Sex Reprod Health.* 2008;40(4):212–217

41. Clements-Nolle K, Marx R, Guzman R, Katz M. HIV prevalence, risk behaviors, health care use, and mental health status of transgender persons: implications for public health intervention. *Am J Public Health.* 2001; 91(6):915–921

42. Nuttbrock L, Hwahng S, Bockting W, et al. Lifetime risk factors for HIV/sexually transmitted infections among male-to-female transgender persons. *J Acquir Immune Defic Syndr.* 2009;52(3):417–421

43. Garofalo R, Deleon J, Osmer E, Doll M, Harper GW. Overlooked, misunderstood and at-risk: exploring the lives and HIV risk of ethnic minority male-to-female transgender youth. *J Adolesc Health.* 2006;38(3): 230–236

44. Perrin E. *Sexual Orientation in Child and Adolescent Health Care.* New York, NY: Kluwer Academic; 2002

45. Goldenring JM, Rosen DS. Getting into adolescent heads: an essential update. *Contemp Pediatr.* 2004;21(1):64–90

46. Kaiser Permanente National Diversity Council. *A Provider's Handbook on Culturally Competent Care.* 2nd ed. Oakland, CA: Kaiser Foundation Health Plan Inc; 2004

47. Workowski KA, Berman SM; Centers for Disease Control and Prevention. Sexually transmitted diseases treatment guidelines, 2010. *MMWR Recomm Rep.* 2010;59(RR-12): 1–110

48. Ho KS, Cranston RD. Anal cytology screening in HIV-positive men who have sex with men: what's new and what's now? *Curr Opin Infect Dis.* 2010;23(1):21–25

49. Centers for Disease Control and Prevention. FDA licensure of quadrivalent human papillomavirus vaccine (HPV4, Gardasil) for use in males and guidance from the Advisory Committee on Immunization Practices (ACIP). *MMWR Morb Mortal Wkly Rep.* 2010; 59(20):630–632

50. Centers for Disease Control and Prevention. Recommendations on the use of quadrivalent human papillomavirus vaccine in males—Advisory Committee on Immunization Practices (ACIP), 2011. *MMWR Morb Mortal Wkly Rep.* 2011;60(50):1705–1708

51. Centers for Disease Control and Prevention. FDA licensure of bivalent human papillomavirus vaccine (HPV2, Cervarix) for use in females and updated HPV vaccination recommendations from the Advisory Committee on Immunization Practices (ACIP). *MMWR Morb Mortal Wkly Rep.* 2010; 59(20):626–629

Office-Based Care for Lesbian, Gay, Bisexual, Transgender, and Questioning Youth

- *Technical Report*

TECHNICAL REPORT

Office-Based Care for Lesbian, Gay, Bisexual, Transgender, and Questioning Youth

David A. Levine, MD, and the COMMITTEE ON ADOLESCENCE

KEY WORDS

sexual orientation, sexual identity, sexual behaviors, adolescents, sexual minority, homosexuality, gay, lesbian, bisexual, transgender

ABBREVIATIONS

CDC—Centers for Disease Control and Prevention
FTM—females transitioning to males
GnRH—gonadotropin-releasing hormone
HPV—human papillomavirus
HSV—herpes simplex virus
IOM—Institute of Medicine
LGBTQ—lesbian, gay, bisexual, transgender, and questioning
MSM—men who have sex with men
MTF—males transitioning to females
STI—sexually transmitted infection
WSW—women who have sex with women
YRBS—Youth Risk Behavior Surveillance

www.pediatrics.org/cgi/doi/10.1542/peds.2013-1283

doi:10.1542/peds.2013-1283

All clinical reports from the American Academy of Pediatrics automatically expire 5 years after publication unless reaffirmed, revised, or retired at or before that time.

(Continued on last page)

abstract

The American Academy of Pediatrics issued its last statement on homosexuality and adolescents in 2004. This technical report reflects the rapidly expanding medical and psychosocial literature about sexual minority youth. Pediatricians should be aware that some youth in their care may have concerns or questions about their sexual orientation or that of siblings, friends, parents, relatives, or others and should provide factual, current, nonjudgmental information in a confidential manner. Although most lesbian, gay, bisexual, transgender, and questioning (LGBTQ) youth are quite resilient and emerge from adolescence as healthy adults, the effects of homophobia and heterosexism can contribute to increased mental health issues for sexual minority youth. LGBTQ and MSM/WSW (men having sex with men and women having sex with women) adolescents, in comparison with heterosexual adolescents, have higher rates of depression and suicidal ideation, higher rates of substance abuse, and more risky sexual behaviors. Obtaining a comprehensive, confidential, developmentally appropriate adolescent psychosocial history allows for the discovery of strengths and assets as well as risks. Pediatricians should have offices that are teen-friendly and welcoming to sexual minority youth. This includes having supportive, engaging office staff members who ensure that there are no barriers to care. For transgender youth, pediatricians should provide the opportunity to acknowledge and affirm their feelings of gender dysphoria and desires to transition to the opposite gender. Referral of transgender youth to a qualified mental health professional is critical to assist with the dysphoria, to educate them, and to assess their readiness for transition. With appropriate assistance and care, sexual minority youth should live healthy, productive lives while transitioning through adolescence and young adulthood. *Pediatrics* 2013;132:e297–e313

INTRODUCTION

The American Academy of Pediatrics issued its first statement on sexual minority teens in 1983, with revisions in 1993 and 2004. Since the last report, research areas have rapidly expanded and hundreds of new publications have been produced about lesbian, gay, bisexual, transgender, and questioning (LGBTQ) youth. In 2011, the Institute of Medicine (IOM) published "The Health of Lesbian, Gay, Bisexual, and Transgender People: Building a Foundation for Better Understanding."[1]

The comprehensive IOM publication includes a section on childhood and adolescence. This updated clinical report provides definitions and the best information available about the demographics of this group of adolescents. Being a member of this group of teens is not, in itself, a risk behavior; nor should sexual minority youth be considered abnormal. However, the presence of stigma reflected in the terms "homophobia" and "heterosexism" often leads to psychological distress, which may be accompanied by an increase in risk behaviors. "Homophobia" refers to an irrational fear and resulting hatred of homosexual individuals. "Heterosexism" is the societal expectation that heterosexuality is the expected norm and that, somehow, LGBTQ individuals are abnormal. Although limited, studies on the resilience of sexual minority youth will be discussed. Studies specifically focused on the disparities in the health of these teens in mental health, substance abuse, and sexuality will be presented, along with new research about emerging effective individual and community health strategies for reducing risks. Finally, issues in providing clinical care and modifying patient care approaches will be discussed.

Although most LGBTQ youth are quite resilient and emerge from adolescence relatively unscathed, the health disparities of this vulnerable population can be significant and often daunting for pediatricians or other health care providers who are assisting youth in their care. For this report, the term LGBTQ will be used whenever discussing studies and recommendations for all lesbian, gay, bisexual, transgender youth. Some of the studies discussed did not include questioning youth – for these, the term LGBT (lesbian, gay, bisexual, and transgender) will be used. Because

many adolescents do not define themselves as a member of a sexual minority group, assisting teens who are men having sex with men (MSM) and women having sex with women (WSW) will also be discussed. Some of the studies in this clinical report reference self-identified LGBTQ individuals, and others reference only sexual behavior (MSM and WSW). For this report, the term "sexual minority" includes LGBTQ and MSM/WSW individuals.

DEFINITIONS

Adolescence is characterized as a time of rapid physical, emotional, and sexual change, during which sexual discovery, exploration, and experimentation are part of the process of incorporating sexuality into one's own identity. Adolescents solidify their gender identification and expression by observing the gender roles of their parents and adults, siblings, peers, and others. Typically, a young person's sexual orientation emerges before or early in adolescence.[2,3] In the previous American Academy of Pediatrics clinical report on sexual minority youth published in June 2004, sexual orientation was referred to as "an individual's pattern of physical and emotional arousal toward other persons." In strict definition, individuals who self-identify as heterosexual are attracted to people of the opposite gender; homosexual individuals self-identify as attracted to people of the same gender; bisexual teens report attraction to people of both genders.[4] As noted in later sections, sexuality is much more complex than these classic definitions. Most self-identified gay and lesbian individuals have had sex with the opposite gender, and some continue to do so. Many heterosexuals have had sex with the same gender, yet self-identify as heterosexual.[1] In common usage, self-identified

homosexual people are often referred to as "gay" if male, and "lesbian" if female.[4] Many adolescents struggle with their sexual attractions and identity formation, and some may be referred to as "questioning."[2] Many individuals also resist definition; when reporting same-gender sexual behavior, these individuals are referred to as MSM or WSW.[1]

Gender identity and gender expression usually conform to anatomic and chromosomal sex or "natal" sex for both homosexual and heterosexual teens. Gender identity is knowledge of one's self as being male or female, whereas gender expression is an outward expression of being male or female. For transgender individuals, their gender or identity does not match their natal sex. Gender nonconforming (or variant) refers to people who do not follow other people's ideas about how they should act according to gender roles. They may or may not be distressed from the nonconformity.[5] Gender dysphoria refers to dislike or distress about one's own gender and about the outward manifestations of gender (eg, hair style, clothing, sports, toys). Children often begin to express this dysphoria in the preschool period. Many young children with gender dysphoria will resolve their dysphoria by adolescence, but others will maintain it. It is difficult to predict, however, whether a young child with gender dysphoria will be transgender as a teenager or adult. Thus, it is best to help families to manage this uncertainty and make it clear in the family that all options remain acceptable and available as the child grows up.[2,6]

Transgender people may be heterosexual, homosexual, or bisexual.[7] Transgender people are often also identified by the natal gender and transition to the desired gender; MTF refers to males transitioning to females and FTM are females transitioning to males. Transgender people may or may not desire to alter their body to match their perceived gender. When people have undergone hormonal and/or surgical alteration, they are often referred to as "transsexual." Gender dysphoria refers to the emotional distress of having a gender identity that is different from natal sex.[1,5,7] In the *Diagnostic and Statistical Manual of Mental Disorders, Fourth Edition, Text Revision*, there was also a set of diagnostic criteria for "gender identity disorder," but critics have noted that this "pathologizes" the issue for the patient. In the forthcoming *Diagnostic and Statistical Manual of Mental Disorders, Fifth Edition*, there will be continued diagnostic criteria for gender dysphoria, but "gender identity disorder" will probably be eliminated.[8,9] "Transition" is defined as the process and time when a person goes from living as one gender to living as the other.[7,10,11]

As a society, our culture assumes that individuals who self-identify a sexual identity will have sexual behaviors that remain consistent with that identity. It is assumed that men or women who self-identify as gay or lesbian will only have attractions to or sexual activity with the same gender. However, the paradigm of sexuality is much more complex, according to qualitative studies in sexual minority youth. Sexual attraction is a term that is easy for all youth to understand. In contrast, for a measure describing sexual orientation using the choices heterosexual, bisexual, gay/lesbian, or unsure, most teens preferred the answers "mostly heterosexual" and "mostly homosexual."[12] This range of sexuality may be reflected in the surprising rate of teen pregnancies experienced by women who report having sex with women. WSW have reported lower rates of

contraceptive use than do women having sex with men.[13,14]

Many adolescents who self-report as lesbian will still occasionally have sex with males, and many males who self-report as gay may have sex with females; thus, behaviors do not always equal identity.[1,15] Some men who have sex with men (MSM) or women who have sex with women (WSW) actively resist being identified as gay or lesbian. And some individuals who are not yet sexually experienced already self-identify as gay, lesbian, or bisexual.[2] Questioning adolescents struggle with sexuality issues more than others, and their sexual behaviors may be diverse. Studies examining how questioning adolescents resolve their inner struggles and reach a stable sexual identity are ongoing.[16] Definitions are summarized in Table 1.

GENDER IDENTITY FORMATION

Awareness of gender identity happens very early in life. Between ages 1 and 2 years, children become conscious of physical differences between the 2 sexes. By age 3, children can identify themselves as a boy or a girl, and, by age 4, gender identity is stable. In middle

childhood, gender identification continues to become more firmly established, reflected in children's interests in playing more exclusively with youngsters of their own gender and also in their interest in acting like, looking like, and having things like their same-sex peers. Occasionally, a child may seem to display gender-role confusion. More than just lacking an interest in what society defines as traditionally masculine activities, some boys actually tend to identify with females and/or feminine traits. Likewise, some girls identify more with males and/or masculine traits. Conflicted about their gender, they may come to dislike that part of themselves that is a boy or a girl.[5,11,17] Many children resolve their dysphoria by the time they complete adolescence. Others will continue to feel dysphoria and may seek treatment to transition to the opposite gender.[1] The etiology of transgender is unknown and likely quite complex.[10]

HETEROSEXISM, HOMOPHOBIA, AND IDENTITY FORMATION

Although overt homophobia may damage the emerging self-image of an LGBTQ adolescent, often, heterosexism

TABLE 1 Definitions

Term	Definition
Homophobia	An irrational fear and resulting hatred of homosexual individuals
Heterosexism	The societal expectation that heterosexuality is the expected normal
MSM	Men having sex with men
WSW	Women having sex with women
Gender identity	Knowledge of one's self as male or female
Gender expression	Outward expression of being male or female
Gender nonconforming	Does not follow society's ideas about how they should act according to gender roles
Natal sex	Chromosomal and anatomic gender
Transition	Process and time when a person goes from living as one gender to living as the other
MTF	Male transitioning to female
FTM	Female transitioning to male
Conversion or reparative therapy	Attempts to "convert" the individual to heterosexual
Survival sex	Engaging in sexual intercourse in exchange for shelter, food, or money; often includes high-risk or unprotected sexuality

is more insidious and damaging. Homophobia refers to an irrational fear and resulting hatred of homosexuality and homosexual individuals. Pervasive in our culture, homophobia is institutionalized in stereotypes promoted in the media and in casual conversation.[18] Heterosexism is the societal expectation that heterosexuality is the expected norm and that somehow LGBTQ teens are "abnormal." Although it is often easy for the majority of sexual minority youth to hide their sexuality from family and friends, nondisclosure may ultimately be damaging to adolescents' developing self-image.[19,20] Homophobia perceived by LGBTQ youth may lead to self-destructive behaviors.[21] Societal homophobia is reflected in the higher rates of bullying and violence suffered by sexual minority youth.[22] Many sexuality education curricula taught in schools limit discussion to "'abstinence-only' until heterosexual marriage." This expected standard may serve to further isolate and alienate many sexual minority youth and contributes to increased risks of personal violence, mental health issues, substance abuse, and risky sexual behaviors.[19,23–25]

With proper support and guidance, the majority of LGBTQ youth emerge as adults with sexual identities that are associated with little or no significant increase in risk behaviors compared with other youth. These resilient young adults lead happy, productive lives.[26] Pediatricians have a role in helping teenagers sort through their feelings and behaviors. Young people need information about healthy, positive expressions of sexuality, and pediatricians should assist adolescents as they develop their identities and to avoid the consequences of unwanted pregnancy and sexually transmitted infections (STIs), regardless of sexual orientation.[27] Research suggests that LGBTQ youth really value these

opportunities for discussions with their pediatricians or primary health care providers.[28] The role of the pediatrician is further described in the section "Making the Office Teen-Friendly for Sexual Minority Youth."

There may be several barriers for pediatricians in working with LGBTQ youth. Until recently, there was not a focus on LGBTQ issues in medical education. The Association of American Medical Colleges has recently begun to develop additional resources for medical educators to use in implementing curricular reform on this topic.[29] The Joint Commission also recently published a comprehensive guidebook for hospital organizations.[30] Although confidentiality is recommended for all adolescents, there may be inadvertent breaches related to electronic health record access and insurers that send explanations of benefit information to parents.

Parental and other adult reactions to "coming out" vary, and often, adolescents and their families will also need support from their pediatrician during this process. Parents play a critical role in support of development for their sexual minority children. The IOM report noted that "parental support either partially or fully mediated associations related to suicidal thoughts, recent drug use, and depressive symptomatology."[1] Negative parental reactions were also associated with higher rates of risk behaviors.[1,31] Parent support organizations, such as Parents, Families and Friends of Lesbians and Gays (www.pflag.org), can provide essential resources for parents.

NATIONAL STATISTICS

There are inherent difficulties in obtaining accurate data about sexual minority youth. Virtually all of the available information is self-report data on survey instruments; sample

bias and general limitations of self-reported data limit accuracy.[32] Although some adolescents are comfortable enough to reveal their sexuality on these instruments, many may not trust that their information will truly be protected. It may take some time for an adolescent to come to an understanding of his/her sexual identity before it is possible to label or describe it or discuss it with others. Some of the best data about the number of gay or lesbian teenagers are state or city specific. Some states and communities have added questions to the Centers for Disease Control and Prevention's (CDC's) Youth Risk Behavior Surveillance (YRBS) System: at the time of this writing, Minnesota,[33] Vermont,[34] Massachusetts,[35] and New York City[36] have added these questions. More nationally representative data are found in the few recent national studies available.

In the 2006–2008 National Survey of Family Growth, 13.4% of females and 4.0% of males 15 to 24 years of age self-reported that they had sex with someone of the same gender.[37] This number is much larger than those who would describe themselves as gay, lesbian, or bisexual. Among participants in the Growing Up Today Study, a US community-based longitudinal cohort study in 9039 female and 7843 male children recruited at 9 to 14 years of age whose mothers were participating in the Nurses' Health Study II, 16.3% of females and 8.7% of males reported a sexual orientation other than heterosexual.[38] In wave 1 of the National Longitudinal Study of Adolescent Health administered to students in grades 7 through 12, same-gender relationships or attractions were reported in 7% of girls and 8.4% of boys.[39] Recently, the CDC combined data from several YRBS survey administrations studying behaviors among 9th through 12th grade sexual minority youth in the states that inquired about sexual identity and the gender of sexual contacts. Seven states (Delaware, Maine, Massachusetts, Rhode Island, Vermont, Connecticut, and Wisconsin) and 6 large urban school districts (Boston, Chicago, Milwaukee, New York, San Diego, and San Francisco) elected to participate and used questions offered by the CDC. Across the 12 sites that assessed gender of sexual contacts, 53.5% reported having had sex with the opposite gender, 2.5% reported having had sex with the same gender, 3.3% reported having had sexual contact with both genders, and 40.5% reported having had no sexual contact.[22]

Estimation of the prevalence of gender identity disorder and transgender youth is more difficult because of the lack of population-based studies. The World Professional Association for Transgender Health published their seventh version of Standards of Care in 2011. Acknowledging the difficulty in obtaining true prevalence data, the World Professional Association for Transgender Health estimated prevalences of 1 in 11 900 to 1 in 45 000 for MTF youth and 1 in 30 400 to 1 in 200 000 for FTM youth.[5] Because most studies have been performed in services providing transition care, population-based studies are needed to capture the hidden populations not accessing such care.[10]

HEALTH DISPARITIES FOR GAY, LESBIAN, AND BISEXUAL YOUTH

Stigmatization, ostracism, and parental rejection remain common. Resulting struggles with self-image and self-esteem often put sexual minority youth at risk. Depression and other mental health issues may be manifest as these teens struggle with developing a stable self-identity and family/community acceptance.[13,40,41] As many as 25% to 40% of homeless youth may be LGBTQ or MSM/WSW, leading to

additional risk-taking behaviors. Many sexual minority youth become homeless as a consequence of coming out to their families. After coming out or being discovered, many LGBTQ youth have been thrown out of their homes or mistreated, leading to runaway status and homelessness. Unfortunately, sexual minority youth who are homeless may engage in survival sex, leading to riskier behaviors and contributing to health disparities.[42]

Mental Health Disparities

Significant health disparities exist for sexual minority youth related to depression and suicidality, substance abuse, social anxiety, altered body image, and other mental health issues.[1,18,22,43] Data from the 2007 Washington, DC, administration of the YRBS survey revealed that 40% of sexual minority youth, compared with 26% of heterosexual youth, reported feeling sad or hopeless in the past 2 weeks. LGBTQ youth were more than twice as likely to have considered suicide in the past year (31% vs 14%).[18] This increased risk has been extensively replicated in other studies and communities.[1,22,44,45] Even for these teens, however, protective factors come into play. Data from the 2004 Minnesota Student Survey of 9th and 12th graders, in which 2255 respondents reported a same-gender romantic or sexual experience, revealed that more than half of LGBTQ students had thought about suicide, and 37.4% had reported a suicide attempt. In this study, the factors that were significantly protective against suicidal ideation and attempts included family connectedness, caring adults, and school safety.[46] Another study found that suicide attempts among sexual minority youth were positively correlated with parental psychological abuse of the child, being considered gender atypical in childhood by parents, and parental efforts to discourage gender atypical

behavior.[47] Sexual minority teens who run away or are put out by their families after acknowledging their sexuality are often victimized, which leads to further mental health issues. Homeless LGBTQ teens are more likely than heterosexual teens to meet criteria for each of 4 mental disorders: major depressive disorder, post-traumatic stress disorder, substance abuse, and conduct disorder.[48]

Social anxiety symptoms are experienced more often by LGBTQ adolescents. In a study in 100 young gay men in a 3-state area of the US East Coast, it was discovered that social anxiety predicted an increased probability of having engaged in unprotected anal intercourse in the previous 6 months.[49] Another study comparing 87 heterosexual and gay male undergraduates at the State University of New York at Stonybrook found that gay men reported greater fear of negative evaluation, greater social interaction anxiety, and lower self-esteem than did heterosexual men.[50]

Unfortunately, an additional barrier to care for LGBTQ (and other) adolescents may be a lack of mental health services in certain communities or mental health services that are not adolescent or sexual minority friendly. Services for adolescents in poverty may be even more limited.[51] In no situation is a referral for conversion or reparative therapy indicated. An American Psychological Association task force to review peer-reviewed studies on efforts to change sexual orientation concluded that conversion therapy is not effective and may be harmful to LGBT individuals by increasing internalized stigma, distress, and depression.[1]

Bullying and Victimization

When sexual minority teens "come out" and acknowledge their sexuality as adolescents, there are often significant repercussions, especially victimization.[1,4,22,23,25] Even if not open about sexuality, 16% of MSM reported experiencing violence. Sometimes it is simply the perception that an individual might be LGBT that may lead to bullying, harassment, and violence.[52] LGBTQ and MSM individuals report that the violence directed toward them is because of perceived sexual orientation or femininity.[53] When sexual minority youth are victimized, the physical assault may lead to death (homicide). Victimized LGBTQ, MSM, and WSW youth may experience increased mental health disorders including depression, sometimes leading to death by suicide. There is a strong association between victimization and suicidality among sexual minority adolescents recruited from gay youth community or university-based organizations.[54]

Bullying at school with resultant adolescent suicide has received increased national attention.[55] Of adolescents who are open about their LGBTQ sexual orientation, 84% reported verbal harassment; 30% reported being punched, kicked, or injured; and 28% dropped out of school because of harassment. The Consortium of Higher Education LGBT Resource Professions published a press release in October 2010 documenting the violence, injuries, and in some cases, deaths of LGBTQ adolescents.[56] The study of pooled CDC data from the 2001–2009 administrations of the YRBS survey to examine risk behaviors faced by sexual minority youth included questions on being victims of threats or violence. In the 9 communities that included relevant questions, sexual minority youth were more likely than heterosexual youth to be in a physical fight, to be injured in a fight, to be threatened on school grounds, and to stay home from school because of perceived risk of violence.[22]

Positive, supportive school environments, those with zero or at least low tolerance for homophobic teasing, bullying, or abuse, were recently shown to be protective, with significantly lower rates of depression and suicidality for sexual minority youth.[25] Supporting the development of policies in school districts that limit teasing and bullying is an important role of the pediatrician. The US Department of Health and Human Services recently has increased antibullying efforts, and among other initiatives, has launched a new Web site, http://www.StopBullying.gov, which includes a specific section for sexual minority youth.[57]

Unfortunately, schools are not the only source of homophobic/heterosexist bullying. Although less research has focused on nonschool settings, LGBT youth experience victimization in their homes, communities, and other institutions.[1] Even after the repeal of the "Don't ask, don't tell" policy, there continues to be victimization in the military.[58] Although many churches are offering education to their members about the issue of bullying in general, some churches continue to bully sexual minority youth.[59] "Cyberbullying," or bullying with electronic means (eg, Internet, texting), is rampant; 32% of all teens say they have been targeted in some form.[60] In 1 study, 52% of LGBT adolescents noted they had been cyberbullied in the past 30 days.[61]

Eating Disorders

Although 10% to 15% of all cases of eating disorders are in men, as many as 42% of young men affected may be gay or bisexual.[62] Male sexual minority youth demonstrated more binge eating and purging than did male heterosexual youth.[63,64] The IOM report acknowledged these findings but noted that they were from small studies and that additional research is necessary.[1] There also may be an association with eating disorders in transgender MTF individuals, but more research is necessary.[65]

Substance Abuse

With the psychosocial and anxiety-provoking stressors of homophobia and heterosexism, the enticement and escape of getting high may be addictive and can lead to increasing use of substances. The pooled YRBS study combining 2001–2009 data revealed significantly higher rates of current alcohol use in the past 30 days in self-identified sexual minority youth (bisexual, 55.6%; gay/lesbian, 47.5%; questioning, 35.1%; and heterosexual, 37.6%).For current use of marijuana, the rates were 36.8% among bisexual youth, 34.5% among gay/lesbian youth, 25.4% among questioning youth, and 21.8% among heterosexual youth. More striking differences were observed among youth for the following: (1) current cocaine use (gay/lesbian, 16.6%; bisexual, 11%; questioning, 11.4%; and heterosexual, 1.8%), (2) ever having used ecstasy (gay/lesbian, 22.9%; bisexual, 20.4%; questioning, 11.4%; and heterosexual, 4.6%), (3) ever having used heroin (gay/lesbian, 17.7%; bisexual, 9.6%; questioning, 13%; and heterosexual, 1.8%), and (4) ever having used methamphetamine (gay/lesbian, 21.5%; bisexual, 14.9%; questioning, 13.2%; and heterosexual, 3.4%).[22] Because this study combined the data for MSM and WSW and included information only from the 7 states and 6 school districts that volunteered to ask more sexuality questions, the data may not be as nationally representative. Tobacco use is also overrepresented among gay and lesbian youth.[1,66–69] Research into best practices to prevent and reduce tobacco use in sexual minority youth is underway.[70–72]

The Young Men's Survey, from 1994 to 1998, was the first study that was considered to have a nationally representative sample of substance-using young MSM. The sample was from 7 major cities, with young men 15 to 22 years of age. The primary objective was to improve access to HIV testing in a high-risk population. In the study, 93% had used alcohol, 71% had used marijuana, 31% had used cocaine, 28% had used methamphetamine, and 27% had used ectasy.[73] A more recent study from 2007 attempted to assess the substance abuse rates for MSM 18 to 22 years of age in Los Angeles. Ninety percent of the sample reported use of alcohol (including 21% who had engaged in binge drinking), 64% reported use of marijuana, 23% reported use of cocaine, 20% reported use of methamphetamine, and 21% reported use of ectasy. The comparison group used was the national sample from the 2006 Monitoring the Future Study (sexual minority and heterosexual youth combined), in which 75% reported alcohol use, 45% reported marijuana use, 8% reported cocaine use, 5% reported methamphetamine use, and 5% reported ecstasy use. Rates of crack cocaine and heroin use were low in both study groups.[74]

Many studies have examined substance use by gay men, but fewer studies have explored WSW or lesbian youth's and young adults' substance use. WSW at a Midwestern university were 4.9 times more likely to smoke, 10.7 times more likely to drink, and 4.9 times as likely to smoke marijuana compared with women having sex with men.[75]

Use of club drugs (eg, cocaine, methamphetamine, and ecstasy, along with GHB [γ-hydroxybutyric acid], ketamine, and LSD [lysergic acid diethylamide] or "acid") is especially a health concern because of the association with other risk behaviors, including unprotected sexual intercourse. Initiation of young MSM into methamphetamine use seems to occur in social, not specifically sexual, settings, with users admitting to limited knowledge of its adverse effects and consequences.[76] Sexual minority youth who "party and play" (PNP) advertise

every day on Web sites that attract LGBTQ youth and young adults. When young men attend gay clubs and other gay-oriented activities, their risk of alcohol and marijuana use increases. Interventions designed to address safety and responsible behaviors in these venues for young MSM need to be developed, implemented, and evaluated.[77]

Sexual and Reproductive Health Disparities

Significant health disparities exist in sexual health outcomes with respect to HIV/AIDS, other STIs, and teen pregnancy among LGBTQ youth. As mentioned previously, sexual minority youth do not necessarily engage in sexual behaviors that are predicted by their orientation. In the CDC's pooled YRBS study, although 1.3% identified themselves as gay or lesbian, 2.5% reported having intercourse with the same gender only and 3.3% reported having sex with both genders.[22]

Regarding sexual behavior, the YRBS pooled data study found that sexual minority youth were more likely than heterosexual youth to report having had intercourse, to have had intercourse before 13 years of age, and to have had intercourse with ≥4 people. Gay or lesbian youth were about half as likely as heterosexual youth (35.8% vs 65.5%) to have used a condom at the last intercourse.[22] In a study in young gay men in college, even after adjusting for age, race, academic classification, and residence, gay men reported higher odds of inconsistent condom use, increased numbers of multiple partners in the past 30 days, and increased risk of illicit drug use than did their heterosexual peers.[78] Between 27% and 48% of young MSM have engaged in unprotected anal intercourse in the previous 6 months.[42] Involvement in these behaviors may explain, in part, why during the past

15 years, reported rates of gonorrhea, chlamydia, and syphilis have trended downward for all adolescents, except for MSM.[79] Substance-abusing gay or lesbian teens may also have more risky sexual behaviors, leading to higher rates of HIV seropositivity.[80,81]

One particular disparity is in HIV infection. The IOM report notes that "the burden of HIV infection among young people falls disproportionally on young men under 25 who have sex with men, particularly those who belong to racial/ethnic minority groups."[1] Data from the CDC reveal that HIV rates continue to increase among young MSM 13 to 24 years of age. For all men, HIV rates between 2001 and 2006 increased by 9%, whereas rates for young MSM (13 to 24 years of age) increased by 12.4% and rates for young black MSM increased by 14.9%. In the age range of 13 to 24 years, MSM of all ethnicities accounted for 60% of the total HIV infections.[82] Despite these alarming data, the IOM report noted that there has been no commensurate response to develop interventions to decrease this risk. The vast majority of published reports on HIV-prevention programs focus on heterosexual adolescents and young adults.[1]

Information on sexual health disparities experienced by WSW is limited; until recently, little research was devoted to lesbian health and many, including physicians, incorrectly assumed that lesbians were at minimal risk of STIs.[83] As noted, many WSW have also had intercourse with men.[1] High rates of STIs have been documented in lesbians and bisexual women with recent sexual contact with men. Viral infections, such as human papillomavirus (HPV) and herpes simplex virus infection (HSV), may be transmitted via exclusive female-to-female sexual contact. In a study in bisexual and lesbian college women, 9% of those who had had sex with both men and women reported that they had had an STI, but 2% of women who exclusively had sex with women also reported that they had had an STI.[84]

LGBTQ youth are less likely to report use of hormonal or barrier contraceptives at last sexual encounter when having sex with the opposite gender. Young women who identified themselves as "unsure" of their sexual orientation were half as likely to report using contraception at last intercourse.[42] Given the high rates of earlier sexual initiation, a greater number of partners, and less contraceptive use, WSW are at higher risk of teen pregnancy than are teens who only have sex with the opposite gender. In the 1999 Minnesota Adolescent Health Survey, lesbian and bisexual women, when compared with heterosexual youth, were found to be about as likely to have had vaginal intercourse (33% vs 29%) but had twice the rate of pregnancy (12% vs 6%) and were more likely to have had ≥2 pregnancies (23.5% vs. 9.8%). In a small study in 137 young women having sex with women (ages 16 to 24 years), 20% reported having had been pregnant.[1]

WSW and MSM report high rates of physical and sexual abuse.[85,86] In 1 study, the rate was 19% to 22%.[87] Consequences for sexual minority youth who have experienced physical or sexual abuse include higher rates of intimate partner violence as adults,[86] frequent drug use and higher-risk sex,[88] and higher rates of HIV.[89] Homeless sexual minority youth are more likely to report histories of physical and sexual abuse and report engaging in risky sexual behaviors as survival strategies.[48] Childhood sexual abuse does not cause children to become LGBTQ.[90]

Health Disparities for Transgender Youth

National data detailing the scope of medical, mental health, and substance abuse issues for transgender youth are lacking. Like other sexual minority youth, self-identifying as transgender does not necessarily indicate the existence of other mental health issues.[91] However, challenges faced by such youth and the potential of family and societal disapproval may increase the risk that transgender adolescents will experience mental health issues, substance abuse, and sexual risk-taking behaviors.[1] Family rejection, peer rejection, harassment, trauma, abuse, legal problems, educational problems, and resulting poverty and homelessness are faced by transgender youth and adults. Transgender people face alarmingly high rates of verbal harassment and physical violence, including at home and at school.[1] Transgender youth face significant mental health issues as a consequence, including depression and suicidality, anxiety, body image distortion, substance abuse, and post-traumatic stress disorder. As with all teens, supportive families can buffer an adolescent from these negative outcomes and promote positive health and well-being.[10]

MTF transgender youth face even more sexual health disparities than other sexual minority youth, with very high rates of HIV and other STIs. One study by the Department of Public Health in San Francisco revealed that HIV prevalence among MTF transgender individuals was 38% (the rate for FTM transgender individuals was much lower, at 2%). Risk factors for HIV infection among MTF transgender individuals in this study included African American race, attaining low education status, having a history of injection drug use, and reporting multiple sexual partners.[92] Another study addressing racial disparity in MTF transgender individuals in New York revealed higher rates of STIs and HIV in African American and Hispanic, compared with white, individuals. The higher STI rates in the study were associated with more lifetime partners, having engaged in commercial sex, unemployment, and injection drug use.[93] An HIV risk study examined 51 transgender MTF ethnic minority adolescents and young adults 16 to 25 years of age in Chicago and found that 22% were HIV-positive. Contributing factors included history of incarceration (37%), homelessness (18%), exchanging sex for resources (59%), nonconsensual sex (52%), and difficulty accessing health care (41%). Among HIV-positive MTF transgender individuals, 98% reported having had sex with men, including unprotected receptive anal intercourse (49%). The study also noted that 53% had had sex while under the influence of drugs or alcohol and 8% had used injection drugs. Twenty-nine percent had injected liquid silicone (as part of their MTF transition) in their lifetime; 8% had shared needles for hormone or silicone injection, increasing HIV transmission risk. For transgender individuals who purchase or obtain transgenic hormones (estrogen or testosterone) on the street or from the Internet, there may be significant health problems if used improperly, even if they are pure.[94]

THE RESILIENCE OF LGBTQ YOUTH

Even with the unique challenges faced by sexual minority youth, the majority grow up healthy and lead happy, productive lives. Research is now beginning to analyze the patterns of resilience in LGBTQ youth. A qualitative study in gay male youth 16 to 22 years of age noted that "general developmental dysfunction is not inevitable for gay adolescents, nor is identifiable personal or family pathology directly related to sexual identity."[95] Similar to other studies in adolescents, another study found that family connectedness, school connectedness, and religious involvement were protective factors, leading to fewer risk behaviors.[26]

Several studies have confirmed that a supportive family network, supportive teachers, and access to gay-straight student alliances at school were all significantly protective.[96,97]

HEALTH CARE FOR SEXUAL MINORITY YOUTH

Pediatricians have the responsibility to provide culturally effective care to help reduce health disparities. Such care should be individualized and meet the needs of the patient regardless of social, educational, or cultural background. This requires an understanding of a patient's ethnic group, neighborhood group, family identification, and religious affiliation.[98] Understanding sexual orientation, behavior, and gender identity is another part of this process.

Being gay, lesbian, bisexual, transgender, or questioning, is not a "problem" or "risk behavior" in itself. These teens, like all teens, should be individually assessed for challenges, vulnerabilities, strengths, and assets. Positive behaviors should be reinforced; teens can be engaged in targeted behavioral interventions to reduce existing risk behaviors. As noted in *Bright Futures*,[27] it is part of the responsibility of the pediatrician to help adolescents identify their strengths and build on their existing talents. Pediatricians and their office staff can encourage teenagers to feel comfortable to talk to them about their emerging sexual identity and concerns about their sexual activities. On the other hand, it is not the role of pediatricians to identify a young person as being gay, or lesbian, unless the teenager has chosen to discuss this. Care should be confidential, and it is not the role of the pediatrician to inform parents/guardians about the teenager's sexual identity or behavior; doing so could expose the youth to harm.[88]

Making the Office Teen-Friendly for Sexual Minority Youth

One of the challenges to health care is removing barriers to care and creating an environment welcoming all teens. Even LGBTQ youth who are open about their sexuality may not feel comfortable disclosing sexuality to their pediatrician. In a study in 131 sexual minority youth attending an empowerment conference, only 35% reported that their physician knew that they were lesbian, gay, or bisexual.[99] LGBTQ adolescents who are hiding their sexuality become quite adept at using gender-neutral terms to describe their relationships and sexual behaviors. Pediatricians' use of gender-neutral terms can encourage teenagers to discuss any questions they have about their sexual behaviors or sexual orientation.[27] Table 2 offers suggestions for gender-neutral questions a pediatrician can use as components of the psychosocial interview.[100] Although pediatricians may use gender-neutral items in obtaining histories, some teens may still choose not to disclose or may delay doing so until a subsequent visit.[101]

It is just as important that the pediatrician's office staff is nonjudgmental and welcoming. Internalized homophobia and heterosexism in the office setting may not be recognized by staff members but will inadvertently interfere with appropriate care. A nurse asking a teenage girl who is in a relationship with another woman about her boyfriend may be interpreted as nonaccepting of her relationship. This negative interaction may then hinder the health care provider's ability to form a trusting relationship.[88,102] Likewise, intake forms and questionnaires should not assume heterosexuality. Another advantage of altering intake forms is to be welcoming to parents who are in same-sex relationships. As for all adolescents, confidentiality

should be ensured. An environment that respects the confidentiality of each client is critical for a facility that provides care for MSM/WSW and LGBTQ youth. Confidentiality must be emphasized at all levels of the clinic staff; many offices and teen clinics have developed a clinic confidentiality policy statement that should be shared with the patient and his or her identified caregiver. Parents should not have access to protected information without the adolescent's consent.[27,28] Current electronic health records may need to be modified to protect adolescents' confidentiality.

The office environment can be made welcoming for all teens by placing in the waiting room items such as brochures on a variety of adolescent topics, including sexual orientation, posters showing both same- and opposite-gender couples, and notices about support groups, if available in the region.[103] Brochures and information left in the privacy of the examination room may be more likely to be picked up by adolescent patients who are not open about their sexuality. If there are no local support groups, Web sites can be suggested so that the sexual minority adolescent does not feel isolated.[42] Even a small "rainbow" button (often a symbol of acceptance of sexual minority individuals) or decal on an office bulletin board or door symbolizes openness and acceptance of diverse sexual orientation and will be appreciated by sexual minority teens and their parents.[88]

Sexuality and Obtaining a Sexual History

For pediatricians to offer optimal clinical care, it is crucial to promote healthy sexuality, even if the teen is not sexually active. Creating an accepting environment will optimize opportunities to learn about a youth's sexual behaviors. Teens who are abstinent should have their abstinence acknowledged and reinforced as a preferred method of prevention for both STIs and unwanted pregnancies.[27] If the adolescent notes that he or she has engaged in sexual activity, 1 classic question is "Are you having sex with males, females, or both?" For adolescents who are not yet sexually active, inquiring "Are you attracted to males, females, or both" will allow for discussions to prevent sexual risk behaviors. If the pediatrician gets an unusual response from the adolescent, a bridging statement such as "Many teenagers your age have sex with members of the opposite or the same sex" can facilitate communication.[101] It may be difficult for some teenagers to answer these questions if they have not yet established trust in the pediatrician. Previous negative experiences in health care or internalized shame as a result of societal homophobia/heterosexism may cause some teenagers to not disclose their sexual orientation or same-gender sexual activity. Sexual minority adolescents also may not trust that their confidential information will truly be kept confidential from their parents/guardians or others. It has been shown that it is easier for some teens to reveal sensitive information (eg, sexual behavior and sexual orientation) before face-to-face visits with the pediatrician.[104] The most comfortable method is on a computer, and the next best is on a paper questionnaire.[105] Once a teen has acknowledged on a previsit form that he or she has a question about sexual activity or sexual identity, it is the responsibility of the pediatrician to introduce a conversation during the subsequent interview. Often, sexuality is disclosed at a future visit after the pediatrician has built a trusting relationship with the patient.

Sexual practices are not dissimilar for heterosexual and lesbian, gay, or bisexual or MSM/WSW teens. Many heterosexual youth engage in oral intercourse, and some engage in anal intercourse.[106] Table 3 offers some suggestions for asking about specific sexual behaviors.

Once sexual history is obtained, in the context of the remainder of the psychosocial history, then specific health-promotion activities can be encouraged. Use of substances, depression, and other mental health disorders place youth at higher sexual risk because of lack of ability to make good decisions regarding use of condoms or contraception, and these issues should be addressed.[107] Using a strength- and asset-based approach and encouraging positive youth development is an effective way to reduce risks in all teenagers, including sexual minority youth.[27,108] Frankowski et al's[109] "Strength-Based Interviewing" is a method that can be applied to all adolescents and young adults.

Pediatricians also may assist sexual minority youth in coming out to their parents/families on the patient's own terms and timetable. This includes offering supportive suggestions and counseling and providing resources to assist the patient and family.[42]

STI/HIV Testing and Prevention Recommendations for Sexual Minority Youth

Recent guidelines from the CDC recommend assessing for STI risk, which includes asking about the gender of all partners. Pediatricians should then make decisions about STI testing on the basis of the sexual behaviors identified by the sexual history.[110] Similar to other populations of adolescents, if adolescents are having protected intercourse (monogamous relationship, using condoms 100% of the time and correctly, and no substance abuse involved), it is reasonable to test them once per year. However, adolescents with multiple or anonymous partners, having unprotected intercourse, or having substance abuse issues or any other risk factors should be tested at shorter intervals.[110] Condoms should be promoted for all sexual activities that involve insertive or receptive intercourse. STI screening recommendations for MSM are described in Table 4.

A growing number of experts recommend testing for HSV (by serology) if infection status is unknown. Because of the increased incidence of anal cancer in HIV-infected MSM, screening

TABLE 2 Using Gender Neutral Terms in the Psychosocial History

Heterosexist Question	Instead Ask
"Do you have a girlfriend?"	"Are you dating anybody?"
	"Are you involved any romantic relationship?"
"What do you and your boyfriend do together?"	"What do the 2 of you do together?"
	"Tell me about your partner."
"Are you and your girlfriend sexually active?"	"Are you having sex?"
	"Are the 2 of you in a sexual relationship?"

TABLE 3 Sexual History Questions About Sexual Behaviors

- Have you ever had sex? What have you done sexually with a partner?
- Have you ever had oral sex? Has a partner ever "gone down" on you or have you ever "gone down" on a partner?
- Have you ever had vaginal sex? Have you ever engaged in penile-vaginal sex?
- Have you ever had anal sex? Did you put your penis in your partner's anus or did your partner put his penis in your anus?
- *If there was any insertive or receptive sex:* Do you use condoms? What percentage of the time? What about last time?
- *If there was any oral-genital contact:* Do you use dental dam or another barrier? What percentage of the time? What about last time?

for anal cytologic abnormalities has been proposed.[110,111] An Atlanta study investigated cytologic screening results from HIV-positive patients, and the authors found highly significant rates of anal dysplasia (47%).[112] However, evidence is limited concerning the natural history of anal intraepithelial neoplasia, the reliability of screening methods, and the safety and response to treatments.[110] WSW are at risk of acquiring bacterial, viral, and protozoan infections from current and previous partners, both male and female. STD treatment guidelines from the CDC recommend a frank discussion of sexual identity and behavioral risk so that the physician can make decisions about which STI tests to perform. Digital-vaginal and digital-anal contact, especially with shared insertive devices, can transmit cervicovaginal secretions. Skin-to-skin or skin-to-mucosa transmission of HPV can occur. Additionally, because many WSW have also had sex with men, HPV vaccine and routine cervical cancer screening should be offered to women according to recommended guidelines. Limited data show inefficient transmission of HSV-2; however, the relatively frequent practice of orogenital sex may increase the risk of HSV-1. Bacterial vaginosis is common among women in general and even more so among WSW. Chlamydia and syphilis transmission may have been more common than previously thought; STD treatment guidelines from the CDC endorse targeted testing on the basis of sexual history. Reports by young women of sex with someone of the same gender should not deter pediatricians from screening them for STIs because of the possibility of a past history of sexual contact with male partners. Condoms should be promoted if using sex toys and dental dam should be promoted for any oral-vaginal or oral-anal contact.[110]

TABLE 4 Summary of Sexually Transmitted Diseases Screening Guidelines for MSM

- HIV serology, if HIV negative or not tested within the previous year
- Syphilis serology
- Test for urethral infection with *Neisseria gonorrheae* and *Chlamydia trachomatis* using NAATs in men who have had insertive anal intercourse during the preceding year
- Test for rectal infection with *N gonorrheae* and *Ctrachomatis* in men who have had receptive anal intercourse during the preceding year, using either preferred NAATs (for laboratories that have met regulatory requirements for an off-label procedure) or culture for *N gonorrheae* and enzyme immunoassay or direct fluorescent antibody assay for *C trachomatis*
- Test for pharyngeal infection with *N gonorrheae* in men who have acknowledged practicing receptive oral intercourse during the preceding year using NAATs (for those laboratories that have met regulatory requirements for an off-label procedure) or culture; testing for *Ctrachomatis* pharyngeal infection is not recommended[98]

NAAT, nucleic acid amplification test.

In 2011, the CDC expanded its recommendations for the quadrivalent HPV vaccine (HPV-4 [Gardasil, Merck Sharp & Dohme Corp, Whitehouse Station, NJ]). The CDC recommends routine immunization of males and females 11 or 12 years of age with HPV-4, administered as a 3-dose series. The immunization series may be started as early as 9 years of age, and if not started at 11 or 12 years of age catch-up immunization is recommended for females 12 through 26 years of age and males at 13 through 21 years of age. HPV-4 is recommended in males for the prevention of genital warts and precancerous/dysplastic lesions of the anus caused by the 4 strains in the vaccine (6, 11, 16, and 18). HPV-4 was noted to be 78% effective at preventing anal intraepithelial neoplasia from strains 16 and 18 in males. Ninety percent of all anal cancer is caused by HPV. For females, HPV-4 is recommended for prevention of genital warts and precancerous/dysplastic lesions of the cervix, vagina, vulva, and anus caused by the 4

strains contained in the vaccine. For MSM, the CDC recommends routine immunization through 26 years of age.[110,113–115] Bivalent HPV vaccine (HPV-2 [Cervarix, GlaxoSmithKline, Middlesex, United Kingdom]) has been approved for the prevention of cervical cancer and precancerous/dysplastic lesions of the cervix caused by HPV types 16 and 18 in females 8 through 25 years of age and may be offered. There are no special recommendations for sexual minority adolescents and young adults.[116]

The 2010 STD treatment guidelines from the CDC also recommend that all MSM should be tested for hepatitis B by testing blood for hepatitis B surface antigen.[110] This test may not need to be performed, however, if the pediatrician has clear evidence that the adolescent has received all doses of the hepatitis B vaccine. If not already immunized against hepatitis B or hepatitis A, all MSM should receive these vaccines. Hepatitis C testing should be conducted if the patient is a current or past drug user or if HIV infected.[117]

Because many teens who self-identify as gay, lesbian, or bisexual may have sexual encounters that may not be predicted by their orientation, conversation about birth control is important.[13,14] Emergency contraception should also be discussed. Emergency contraception is available over-the-counter if the patient is older than 17 years. A prescription may be required for a patient younger than 17 years; additional requirements vary by state.[117]

Treatment of Transgender Youth

In 2009, the Endocrine Society published "Endocrine Treatment of Transsexual Persons: An Endocrine Society Clinical Practice Guideline."[11] This was a refinement of the 2001 publication of The World Professional Association for Transgender Health's Standards of

Care, which was updated in 2011.[5] These documents integrate the best available evidence with clinical experience from experts in the field of assisting transgender patients with transition. The guidelines were further refined by Olson et al[10] in a subsequent publication on the basis of clinical experiences with a large number of transgender patients in Los Angeles. These publications discuss the importance of psychological treatment approaches. The mental health professional is called on to accurately diagnose gender dysphoria and any comorbid conditions, to counsel about the range of treatment options, to ascertain readiness for hormone and surgical therapy, to make formal recommendations to medical and surgical colleagues as part of the team of care, to educate the patient and family, and to provide follow-up. The skilled therapist will use affirming strategies: affirming the adolescent's sense of self, allowing for exploration of gender and self-definition, and conveying the message that it is "entirely acceptable to be whoever you turn out to be." It is recommended that all transgender adolescents be involved in psychological therapy, even those who are functioning well, to ensure that they have the necessary support they need and a safe place to explore identities and consider the transitioning experience.[5,10,11]

Classifications for the process of gender transition include reversible, partially reversible, and irreversible phases. Reversible transition includes the adoption of outward gender expression: wearing preferred clothing, adopting preferred hairstyles, and perhaps acquiring a new name. The use of gonadatropin-releasing hormone (GnRH) analogs is also part of the reversible stage. The Endocrine Society guidelines state, "suppression of pubertal hormones starts when girls and boys first exhibit physical changes of puberty (confirmed by pubertal levels of estradiol and testosterone, respectively) but no earlier than Tanner stages 2-3." Suppression is similar to the treatment of precocious puberty. In general, it is recommended that transgender adolescents be maintained on suppressive GnRH analogs until they are emotionally and cognitively ready for cross-gender sex hormones.[10,11] The rationale for using GnRH analogs early (at sexual maturity rating 2) and then waiting to begin hormonal therapy is so that MTF adolescents experience desired outcomes. However, as noted from 1 large center treating transgender youth, they commonly present at older ages with pubertal development too far advanced for suppressive therapy. The average age of presentation at this center was 14.8 years, with an average sexual maturity rating of 4.1.[118] Waiting too long may result in male voice pitch, laryngeal prominences, and facial hair pattern, which precludes the option of pubertal suppressive therapy.[10,11,118]

The partially reversible treatment phase involves the use of cross-gender hormone therapies. The Endocrine Society guidelines state that "pubertal development of the desired opposite gender be initiated at about the age of 16 years, using a gradually increasing dose schedule of cross-sex steroids."[11] Olson's group follows these guidelines but may choose to provide therapy earlier after careful review of the risks and benefits with the youth and parents.[10] It is recommended that cross-gender hormone therapy begin after assessment of readiness by a medical professional, including a careful review of any hormone contraindications, and by the mental health professional who documents psychological readiness. For FTM patients, testosterone is used. For MTF patients, estrogen is used, sometimes in combination with an androgen inhibitor, such as spironolactone.[10,11,118]

Adolescents undergoing partially reversible cross-gender hormone therapy should be monitored for progress in transition and for any potential medical complications. MTF patients started on estrogen might develop deep venous thrombosis, prolactinomas, hypertension, liver disease, and decreased libido and are at increased risk of breast cancer. Spironolactone can lead to hyperkalemia and decreased blood pressure. FTM patients receiving testosterone may develop hyperlipidemia, polycythemia, male pattern baldness, acne, and other significant side effects.[10,11]

Irreversible therapy occurs during the surgical phase, with many different procedures now available to create a more masculine or feminine appearance. The Endocrine Society guidelines and the World Professional Association for Transgender Health's Standards of Care recommend deferring surgery until an individual is at least 18 years of age.[5,11]

There are many barriers to transgender adolescents receiving desired medical therapies. It is difficult for transgender youth and their families to find comprehensive medical and mental health services. Pediatricians may not feel comfortable or knowledgeable enough to assist transition plans in transgender youth, in which case they should refer to another physician with experience or expertise around gender nonconformity. Most insurance companies do not pay for this care, and the use of GnRH analogs is quite expensive. Medical treatments are neither standardized nor approved by the Food and Drug Administration, although they are increasingly supported by medical literature.[11] Consent is another obstacle, and only Illinois' and West Virginia's state statutes can be interpreted favorably for transgender adolescents to be able to consent for care.[120]

Injectable medical-grade silicone gel and oil have been used by physicians for soft-tissue augmentation.[121] Many transgender adolescents who do not have parental support or who are homeless have injected themselves or others with impure, nonmedical silicone, with significant health consequences. In the Chicago study in ethnic minority transgender youth, the authors found that 29% had injected silicone and 8% had shared needles, half of which were obtained on the street or via the Internet.[94] Injected industrial (nonmedical) silicones or medical silicones used incorrectly have been shown to cause multiorgan dysfunction,[122] silicone pulmonary embolization,[123] and death.[124]

ASSISTING PARENTS OF SEXUAL MINORITY YOUTH

Another critically important role of the pediatrician is to assist parents of sexual minority youth. Some parents have emotional reactions related to societal homophobia and may have extreme difficulty accepting their LGBT teens. Others mourn the loss of the image of the adolescent that they had before the disclosure. Pediatricians should acknowledge the parents' feelings but should provide information and support for the adolescent who has disclosed. Parents' reactions and attitudes may adjust over time and the pediatrician should check in regularly and offer support to the entire family. Organizations like Parents, Families and Friends of Lesbians and Gays (http://www.pflag.org) or Gay Family Support (http://www.gayfamily-support.com) provide valuable resources for discussion. Lead with Love is another excellent resource that includes a film for viewing and discussion (http://leadwithlovefilm.com). For sexual minority youth who have been bullied or victimized, the It Gets Better Project may assist parents and families (http://www.itgetsbetter.org/).

RESOURCES FOR SEXUAL MINORITY YOUTH

Pediatricians' knowledge about national and local resources to assist sexual minority youth is critical to provide LGBTQ patients and their families guidance and support as they progress through adolescence into young adulthood. Nonprofit organizations, such as the United Way in some communities, are a great place to start, as are adult LGBTQ and sexual health advocacy organizations. Table 5 provides selected Web sites of LGBTQ-serving organizations and resources for sexual minority youth, their families, and communities.

SUMMARY

Pediatricians and other health care providers already have many of the skills needed to provide culturally effective, developmentally appropriate care for sexual minority youth. LGBTQ teens/young adults and MSM/WSW are an underserved population, many of whom struggle with acceptance of their sexuality at the same time that they are managing the other rigors of adolescence. The adolescent psychosocial history will allow for discovery of any high-risk behaviors, and targeted behavioral interventions may be developed with the adolescent.

TABLE 5 LGBTQ Support and Advocacy Organizations

- The Gay, Lesbian, and Straight Education Network mission is "Every student deserves a safe space" (http://www.glsen.org).
- Parents, Families, and Friends of Lesbians and Gays (PFLAG) is a long-standing support and advocacy organization (http://community.pflag.org).
- The National Youth Advocacy Coalition (NYAC) is a social justice organization that advocates for and with young people who are lesbian, gay, bisexual, transgender, or questioning in an effort to end discrimination against these youth and to ensure their physical and emotional well-being (http://www.nyacyouth.org).
- The Trevor Project (http://www.thetrevorproject.org) operates the only nationwide, around-the-clock crisis and suicide prevention hotline for sexual minority youth (866-4-U-TREVOR).
- Youth Resource is a Web site created by and for LGBTQ young people. Sponsored by Advocates for Youth, Youth Resource takes a holistic approach to sexual health and exploring issues of concern to LGBTQ youth, by providing information and offering support on sexual and reproductive health issues through education and advocacy (http://www.amplifyyourvoice.org/youthresource).
- For patients, communities, and health care professionals, the Gay and Lesbian Medical Association (http://glma.org) has referral and information resources.
- TransKids Purple Rainbow is a foundation that advocates and organizes events on behalf of transgender children (http://www.transkidspurplerainbow.org).
- The World Professional Association for Transgender Health, Inc (WPATH). Formerly known as the Harry Benjamin International Gender Dysphoria Association, Inc, WPATH is a professional organization devoted to the understanding and treatment of gender identity disorders (http://www.wpath.org).
- Transfamily provides support and education for transgender people, their families, friends, and significant others. The group is associated with PFLAG to bring awareness to school systems, through their principals and counselors, by offering literature, speakers, consultation, and support (http://www.transfamily.org).
- Family Acceptance Project (Marian Wright Education Institute—Resource for LGBTQ youth and families) (http://familyproject.sfsu.edu)
- Other resources are available on the Adolescent Reproductive and Sexual Health Education Project Web site at the end of the presentations, "Gay, Lesbian, Bisexual, Transgender, and Questioning Youth" and "Caring for Transgender Adolescent Patients" found at http://www.prh.org/ARSHEP. These presentations are also outstanding for both self-education and for use in training current and future medical professionals.

Referrals for mental health and substance abuse treatment may be warranted. Pediatricians have an obligation to ensure that sexual minority youth have access to a full range of appropriate health care services. As with all adolescents and young adults, sexual minority youth need honest answers and compassion in dealing with issues and questions around sexual orientation, identity, and sexual behaviors.

LEAD AUTHOR

David A. Levine, MD

COMMITTEE ON ADOLESCENCE, 2012–2013

Paula K. Braverman, MD, Chairperson
William P. Adelman, MD
Cora C. Breuner, MD, MPH
David A. Levine, MD
Arik V. Marcell, MD, MPH
Pamela J. Murray, MD, MPH
Rebecca F. O'Brien, MD, MD

LIAISONS

Loretta E. Gavin, PhD, MPH – *Centers for Disease Control and Prevention*
Rachel J. Miller, MD – *American College of Obstetricians and Gynecologists*
Jorge L. Pinzon, MD – *Canadian Pediatric Society*
Benjamin Shain, MD, PhD – *American Academy of Child and Adolescent Psychiatry*

STAFF

Karen S. Smith
James Baumberger

REFERENCES

1. Institute of Medicine, Committee on Lesbian, Gay, Bisexual, and Transgender Health Issues and Research Gaps and Opportunities. *The Health of Lesbian, Gay, Bisexual, and Transgender People: Building a Foundation for Better Understanding.* Washington, DC: National Academies Press; 2011

2. Spigarelli MG. Adolescent sexual orientation. *Adolesc Med State Art Rev.* 2007;18 (3):508–518, vii

3. Glover JA, Galliher RV, Lamere TG. Identity development and exploration among sexual minority adolescents: examination of a multidimensional model. *J Homosex.* 2009;56(1):77–101

4. Frankowski BL; American Academy of Pediatrics Committee on Adolescence. Sexual orientation and adolescents. *Pediatrics.* 2004;113(6):1827–1832

5. World Professional Association for Transgender Health. Standards of care for the health of transsexual, transgender, and gender nonconforming people. Minneapolis, MN: World Professional Association for Transgender Health; 2011. Available at: www.wpath.org. Accessed June 11, 2012

6. Wallien MS, Cohen-Kettenis PT. Psychosexual outcome of gender-dysphoric children. *J Am Acad Child Adolesc Psychiatry.* 2008;47(12):1413–1423

7. Zucker K, Bradley S. Gender identity and psychosexual disorders. *J Lifelong Learn Psychiatry.* 2005;3(4):598–617

8. American Psychiatric Association. *Diagnostic and Statistical Manual of Mental Disorders.* 4th ed, text revision. Washington, DC: American Psychiatric Association; 2000

9. Sexual and Gender Disorders Work Group for American Psychiatric Association DSM-5 Development. 2011. Available at: www.dsm5.org/ProposedRevision/Pages/ GenderDysphoria.aspx. Accessed June 11, 2012

10. Olson J, Forbes C, Belzer M. Management of the transgender adolescent. *Arch Pediatr Adolesc Med.* 2011;165(2):171–176

11. Hembree WC, Cohen-Kettenis P, Delemarre-van de Waal HA, et al; Endocrine Society. Endocrine treatment of transsexual persons: an Endocrine Society clinical practice guideline. *J Clin Endocrinol Metab.* 2009;94 (9):3132–3154

12. Austin SB, Conron K, Patel A, Freedner N. Making sense of sexual orientation measures: findings from a cognitive processing study with adolescents on health survey questions. *J LGBT Health Res.* 2007;3(1): 55–65

13. Herrick AL, Matthews AK, Garofalo R. Health risk behaviors in an urban sample of young women who have sex with women. *J Lesbian Stud.* 2010;14(1):80–92

14. Goodenow C, Szalacha LA, Robin LE, Westheimer K. Dimensions of sexual orientation and HIV-related risk among adolescent females: evidence from a statewide survey. *Am J Public Health.* 2008;98(6):1051–1058

15. Igartua K, Thombs BD, Burgos G, Montoro R. Concordance and discrepancy in sexual identity, attraction, and behavior among adolescents. *J Adolesc Health.* 2009;45(6): 602–608

16. Wilson BD, Harper GW, Hidalgo MA, Jamil OB, Torres RS, Fernandez MI; Adolescent Medicine Trials Network for HIV/AIDS Interventions. Negotiating dominant masculinity ideology: strategies used by gay, bisexual and questioning male adolescents. *Am J Community Psychol.* 2010;45 (1–2):169–185

17. American Academy of Pediatrics. Gender identity and gender confusion in children. Elk Grove Village, IL: American Academy of Pediatrics; 2010. Available at: www. healthychildren.org/English/ages-stages/ gradeschool/Pages/Gender-Identity-and-Gender-Confusion-In-Children.aspx. Accessed June 11, 2012

18. Almeida J, Johnson RM, Corliss HL, Molnar BE, Azrael D. Emotional distress among LGBT youth: the influence of perceived discrimination based on sexual orientation. *J Youth Adolesc.* 2009;38(7):1001–1014

19. Walls NE. Toward a multidimensional understanding of heterosexism: the changing nature of prejudice. *J Homosex.* 2008; 55(1):20–70

20. Chesir-Teran D, Hughes D. Heterosexism in high school and victimization among lesbian, gay, bisexual, and questioning students. *J Youth Adolesc.* 2009;38(7):963–975

21. McDermott E, Roen K, Scourfield J. Avoiding shame: young LGBT people, homophobia and self-destructive behaviours. *Cult Health Sex.* 2008;10(8):815–829

22. Kann L, Olsen EO, McManus T, et al; Centers for Disease Control and Prevention. Sexual identity, sex of sexual contacts, and health-risk behaviors among students in grades 9-12—youth risk behavior surveillance, selected sites, United States, 2001-2009. *MMWR Surveill Summ.* 2011;60 (7):1–133

23. Kelley TM, Robertson RA. Relational aggression and victimization in gay male relationships: the role of internalized homophobia. *Aggress Behav.* 2008;34(5): 475–485

24. Friedman MS, Marshal MP, Stall R, Cheong J, Wright ER. Gay-related development, early abuse and adult health outcomes among gay males. *AIDS Behav.* 2008;12(6): 891–902

25. Birkett M, Espelage DL, Koenig B. LGB and questioning students in schools: the

moderating effects of homophobic bullying and school climate on negative outcomes. *J Youth Adolesc.* 2009;38(7): 989–1000

26. Saewyc EM, Homma Y, Skay CL, Bearinger LH, Resnick MD, Reis E. Protective factors in the lives of bisexual adolescents in North America. *Am J Public Health.* 2009; 99(1):110–117

27. Hagan JF, Shaw JS, Duncan P, eds. *Bright Futures: Guidelines for Health Supervision of Infants, Children, and Adolescents.* 3rd ed. Elk Grove Village, IL: American Academy of Pediatrics; 2008

28. Hoffman ND, Freeman K, Swann S. Healthcare preferences of lesbian, gay, bisexual, transgender and questioning youth. *J Adolesc Health.* 2009;45(3):222–229

29. American Association of Medical Colleges. Diversity policy and programs: who we are, what we do, where we're going. Washington, DC: American Association of Medical Colleges; 2011. Available at: https://www.aamc.org/download/266998/data/dpp-briefing-book-2011.pdf. Accessed June 11, 2012

30. The Joint Commission. Advancing effective communication, cultural competence, and patient- and family- centered care for the lesbian, gay, bisexual, and transgender (LGBT) community: a field guide. Oakbrook Terrace, IL: 2011. Available at: www.jointcommission.org/assets/1/18/LGBTFieldGuide.pdf. Accessed June 11, 2012

31. Bouris A, Guilamo-Ramos V, Pickard A, et al. A systematic review of parental influences on the health and well-being of lesbian, gay, and bisexual youth: time for a new public health research and practice agenda. *J Prim Prev.* 2010;31(5–6):273–309

32. Bauhoff S. Systematic self-report bias in health data: impact on estimating cross-sectional and treatment effects. *Health Serv Outcomes Res Methodol.* 2011;11(1–2): 44–53

33. Anfinson A, ed. 2007 Minnesota Student Survey statewide tables. Minnesota Student Survey Interagency Team. Roseville, MN: Minnesota Department of Education; 2007. Available at: http://education.state.mn.us/mdeprod/idcplg?IdcService=GET_FILE&RevisionSelectionMethod=latestReleased&Rendition=primary&dDocName=042114. Accessed June 11, 2012

34. Moffat S, Cate R. *The 2007 Vermont Youth Risk Behavior Survey.* Burlington, VT: Vermont Department of Health, Division of Health Surveillance; 2007

35. Massachusetts Department of Elementary and Secondary Education, Massachusetts Department of Public Health. Massachusetts high school students and sexual orientation: results of the 2007 Youth Risk Behavior Survey. Malden, MA: Massachusetts Department of Elementary and Secondary Education; 2008. Available at: www.mass.gov/cgly/yrbs07.pdf. Accessed June 13, 2012

36. Pathela P, Schillinger JA. Sexual behaviors and sexual violence: adolescents with opposite-, same-, or both-sex partners. *Pediatrics.* 2010;126(5):879–886

37. Chandra A, Mosher WD, Copen C, Sionean C. Sexual behavior, sexual attraction, and sexual identity in the United States: data from the 2006-2008 National Survey of Family Growth. *Natl Health Stat Rep.* 2011: Mar 3(36):1–36

38. Corliss HL, Rosario M, Wypij D, Fisher LB, Austin SB. Sexual orientation disparities in longitudinal alcohol use patterns among adolescents: findings from the Growing Up Today Study. *Arch Pediatr Adolesc Med.* 2008;162(11):1071–1078

39. Russell ST, Joyner K. Adolescent sexual orientation and suicide risk: evidence from a national study. *Am J Public Health.* 2001;91(8):1276–1281

40. Kipke MD, Kubicek K, Weiss G, et al. The health and health behaviors of young men who have sex with men. *J Adolesc Health.* 2007;40(4):342–350

41. Coker TR, Austin SB, Schuster MA. Health and healthcare for lesbian, gay, bisexual, and transgender youth: reducing disparities through research, education, and practice. *J Adolesc Health.* 2009;45(3): 213–215

42. Physicians for Reproductive Choice and Health. Gay, lesbian, bisexual, transgender, and questioning youth. 4th ed. New York, NY: The Adolescent Reproductive and Sexual Health Education Program; 2011. Available at: www.prch.org/arshep. Accessed June 13, 2012

43. Berg MB, Mimiaga MJ, Safren SA. Mental health concerns of gay and bisexual men seeking mental health services. *J Homosex.* 2008;54(3):293–306

44. Silenzio VM, Pena JB, Duberstein PR, Cerel J, Knox KL. Sexual orientation and risk factors for suicidal ideation and suicide attempts among adolescents and young adults. *Am J Public Health.* 2007;97(11): 2017–2019

45. Walls NE, Freedenthal S, Wisneski H. Suicidal ideation and attempts among sexual minority youths receiving social services. *Soc Work.* 2008;53(1):21–29

46. Eisenberg ME, Resnick MD. Suicidality among gay, lesbian and bisexual youth: the role of protective factors. *J Adolesc Health.* 2006;39(5):662–668

47. D'Augelli AR, Grossman AH, Salter NP, Vasey JJ, Starks MT, Sinclair KO. Predicting the suicide attempts of lesbian, gay, and bisexual youth. *Suicide Life Threat Behav.* 2005;35(6):646–660

48. Whitbeck LB, Chen X, Hoyt DR, Tyler KA, Johnson KD. Mental disorder, subsistence strategies, and victimization among gay, lesbian, and bisexual homeless and runaway adolescents. *J Sex Res.* 2004;41(4): 329–342

49. Hart TA, Heimberg RG. Social anxiety as a risk factor for unprotected intercourse among gay and bisexual male youth. *AIDS Behav.* 2005;9(4):505–512

50. Pachankis JE, Goldfried MR. Social anxiety in young gay men. *J Anxiety Disord.* 2006; 20(8):996–1015

51. Schwartz SW. Adolescent mental health in the United States. New York, NY: National Center for Children in Poverty, Mailman School of Public Health, Columbia University; 2009. Available at: http://nccp.org/publications/pdf/text_878.pdf. Accessed June 13, 2012

52. Lampinen TM, Chan K, Anema A, et al. Incidence of and risk factors for sexual orientation-related physical assault among young men who have sex with men. *Am J Public Health.* 2008;98(6):1028–1035

53. Herek GM, Sims C. Sexual orientation and violence victimization: hate crimes and intimate partner violence among gay and bisexual men in the US. In: Wolitski RJ, Stall R, Valdiserri RO, eds. *Unequal Opportunity: Health Disparities Affecting Gay and Bisexual Men in the US.* New York, NY: Oxford University Press; 2008:35–71

54. Friedman MS, Koeske GF, Silvestre AJ, Korr WS, Sites EW. The impact of gender-role nonconforming behavior, bullying, and social support on suicidality among gay male youth. *J Adolesc Health.* 2006;38(5): 621–623

55. Cloud J. Bullied to death. Time. 2010;176(16): 60–63

56. Consortium of Higher Education LGBT Resource Professionals. Press release. Syracuse, NY: Consortium of Higher Education LGBT Resource Professionals; October 4, 2004. Available at: www.lgbtcampus.org/about/news-2010-10-04-deaths. Accessed June 13, 2012

57. US Department of Health and Human Services. stopbullying.org Web site. Available at: www.stopbullying.gov. Accessed June 13, 2012

58. Burks DJ. Lesbian, gay, and bisexual victimization in the military: an unintended

consequence of "Don't Ask, Don't Tell"? *Am Psychol.* 2011;66(7):604–613

59. Hand K. United States: Mormon apostle bullies gay youth. *Green Left Weekly.* Octo 10, 2010. Available at: www.greenleft.org.au/node/45676. Accessed June 13, 2012

60. Parents, Families and Friends of Lesbians and Gays. Seven: cyber bullying. Available at: http://community.pflag.org/page.aspx?pid=1025. Accessed June 13, 2012

61. Blumenfeld WJ, Cooper RM. LGBT and allied youth responses to cyberbullying: policy implications. *Int J Crit Pedagogy.* 2010;3(1):114–133

62. Russell CJ, Keel PK. Homosexuality as a specific risk factor for eating disorders in men. *Int J Eat Disord.* 2002;31(3):300–306

63. Austin SB, Ziyadeh NJ, Corliss HL, et al. Sexual orientation disparities in purging and binge eating from early to late adolescence. *J Adolesc Health.* 2009;45(3):238–245

64. Feldman MB, Meyer IH. Childhood abuse and eating disorders in gay and bisexual men. *Int J Eat Disord.* 2007;40(5):418–423

65. Hepp U, Milos G. Gender identity disorder and eating disorders. *Int J Eat Disord.* 2002;32(4):473–478

66. D'Augelli AR. High tobacco use among lesbian, gay, and bisexual youth: mounting evidence about a hidden population's health risk behavior. *Arch Pediatr Adolesc Med.* 2004;158(4):309–310

67. Remafedi G, Jurek AM, Oakes JM. Sexual identity and tobacco use in a venue-based sample of adolescents and young adults. *Am J Prev Med.* 2008;35(6 suppl):S463–S470

68. Lee JG, Griffin GK, Melvin CL. Tobacco use among sexual minorities in the USA, 1987 to May 2007: a systematic review. *Tob Control.* 2009;18(4):275–282

69. Ortiz-Hernández L, Tello BL, Valdés J. The association of sexual orientation with self-rated health, and cigarette and alcohol use in Mexican adolescents and youths. *Soc Sci Med.* 2009;69(1):85–93

70. Remafedi G, Carol H. Preventing tobacco use among lesbian, gay, bisexual, and transgender youths. *Nicotine Tob Res.* 2005;7(2):249–256

71. Remafedi G. Lesbian, gay, bisexual, and transgender youths: who smokes, and why? *Nicotine Tob Res.* 2007;9(suppl 1):S65–S71

72. Schwappach DL. Queer quit: gay smokers' perspectives on a culturally specific smoking cessation service. *Health Expect.* 2009;12(4):383–395

73. Valleroy LA, MacKellar DA, Karon JM, et al; Young Men's Survey Study Group. HIV prevalence and associated risks in young men who have sex with men. *JAMA.* 2000;284(2):198–204

74. Kipke MD, Weiss G, Ramirez M, et al. Club drug use in Los Angeles among young men who have sex with men. *Subst Use Misuse.* 2007;42(11):1723–1743

75. Ridner SL, Frost K, Lajoie AS. Health information and risk behaviors among lesbian, gay, and bisexual college students. *J Am Acad Nurse Pract.* 2006;18(8):374–378

76. Parsons JT, Kelly BC, Weiser JD. Initiation into methamphetamine use for young gay and bisexual men. *Drug Alcohol Depend.* 2007;90(2–3):135–144

77. Rosario M, Schrimshaw EW, Hunter J. Predictors of substance abuse over time among gay, lesbian, and bisexual youths: an examination of three hypotheses. *Addict Behav.* 2004;29(8):1623–1631

78. Rhodes SD, McCoy T, Hergenrather KC, Omli MR, Durant RH. Exploring the health behavior disparities of gay men in the United States: comparing gay male university students to their heterosexual peers. *J LGBT Health Res.* 2007;3(1):15–23

79. Benson PA, Hergenroeder AC. Bacterial sexually transmitted infections in gay, lesbian, and bisexual adolescents: medical and public health perspectives. *Semin Pediatr Infect Dis.* 2005;16(3):181–191

80. Kipke MD, Weiss G, Wong CF. Residential status as a risk factor for drug use and HIV risk among young men who have sex with men. *AIDS Behav.* 2007;11(6 suppl):56–69

81. Rudy ET, Shoptaw S, Lazzar M, Bolan RK, Tilekar SD, Kerndt PR. Methamphetamine use and other club drug use differ in relation to HIV status and risk behavior among gay and bisexual men. *Sex Transm Dis.* 2009;36(11):693–695

82. Centers for Disease Control and Prevention. Trends in HIV/AIDS diagnoses among men who have sex with men—33 states, 2001-2006. *MMWR Morb Mortal Wkly Rep.* 2008;57(25):681–686

83. Robertson P, Schachter J. Failure to identify venereal disease in a lesbian population. *Sex Transm Dis.* 1981;8(2):75–76

84. Lindley LL, Barnett CL, Brandt HM, Hardin JW, Burcin M. STDs among sexually active female college students: does sexual orientation make a difference? *Perspect Sex Reprod Health.* 2008;40(4):212–217

85. Stoddard JP, Dibble SL, Fineman N. Sexual and physical abuse: a comparison between lesbians and their heterosexual sisters. *J Homosex.* 2009;56(4):407–420

86. Welles SL, Corbin TJ, Rich JA, Reed E, Raj A. Intimate partner violence among men having sex with men, women, or both: early-life sexual and physical abuse as antecedents. *J Community Health.* 2011;36(3):477–485

87. Saewyc EM, Bearinger LH, Blum RW, Resnick MD. Sexual intercourse, abuse and pregnancy among adolescent women: does sexual orientation make a difference? *Fam Plann Perspect.* 1999;31(3):127–131

88. Arreola S, Neilands T, Pollack L, Paul J, Catania J. Childhood sexual experiences and adult health sequelae among gay and bisexual men: defining childhood sexual abuse. *J Sex Res.* 2008;45(3):246–252

89. Mimiaga MJ, Noonan E, Donnell D, et al. Childhood sexual abuse is highly associated with HIV risk-taking behavior and infection among MSM in the EXPLORE Study. *J Acquir Immune Defic Syndr.* 2009;51(3):340–348

90. Perrin E. *Sexual Orientation in Child and Adolescent Health Care.* New York, NY: Kluwer Academic; 2002

91. American Psychological Association. *Task Force on Gender Identity and Gender-Variance. Report of the Task Force on Gender Identity and Gender Variance.* Washington, DC: American Psychological Association; 2009

92. Clements-Nolle K, Marx R, Guzman R, Katz M. HIV prevalence, risk behaviors, health care use, and mental health status of transgender persons: implications for public health intervention. *Am J Public Health.* 2001;91(6):915–921

93. Nuttbrock L, Hwahng S, Bockting W, et al. Lifetime risk factors for HIV/sexually transmitted infections among male-to-female transgender persons. *J Acquir Immune Defic Syndr.* 2009;52(3):417–421

94. Garofalo R, Deleon J, Osmer E, Doll M, Harper GW. Overlooked, misunderstood and at-risk: exploring the lives and HIV risk of ethnic minority male-to-female transgender youth. *J Adolesc Health.* 2006;38(3):230–236

95. Eccles TA, Sayegh MA, Fortenberry JD, Zimet GD. More normal than not: a qualitative assessment of the developmental experiences of gay male youth. *J Adolesc Health.* 2004;35(5):425.e11–425.e18

96. Cohn TJ, Hastings SL. Resilience among rural lesbian youth. *J Lesbian Stud.* 2010;14(1):71–79

97. Russell ST, Muraco A, Subramaniam A, Laub C. Youth empowerment and high school gay-straight alliances. *J Youth Adolesc.* 2009;38(7):891–903

98. Satcher D. The Surgeon General's call to action to promote sexual health and

responsible sexual behavior. Washington, DC: US Department of Health and Human Services; 2001. Available at: www.surgeongeneral.gov/library/sexualhealth/index.html. Accessed June 13, 2012

99. Meckler GD, Elliott MN, Kanouse DE, Beals KP, Schuster MA. Nondisclosure of sexual orientation to a physician among a sample of gay, lesbian, and bisexual youth. *Arch Pediatr Adolesc Med.* 2006;160(12): 1248–1254

100. Levine DA. Office-based care for gay, lesbian, bisexual, and questioning youth. *Adolesc Med State Art Rev.* 2009;20(1): 223–242, xi–xii

101. Goldenring JM, Rosen DS. Getting into adolescent heads: an essential update. *Contemp Pediatr.* 2004;21(1):64–90

102. Mayer KH, Bradford JB, Makadon HJ, Stall R, Goldhammer H, Landers S. Sexual minority health: what do we know and where do we need to go? *Am J Public Health.* 2008;98(6):989–995

103. Canadian Paediatric Society, Adolescent Health Committee. Adolescent sexual orientation. *Paediatr Child Health (Oxford).* 2008;13(7):619–623

104. Moyer C. LGBT patients: reluctant and underserved. *Am Med News.* Sept 5 2011. Available at: www.ama-assn.org/amednews/2011/09/05/prsa0905.htm. Accessed June 13, 2012

105. Gutiérrez JP, Torres-Pereda P. Acceptability and reliability of an adolescent risk behavior questionnaire administered with audio and computer support. *Rev Panam Salud Publica.* 2009;25(5):418–422

106. Kaiser Permanente National Diversity Council. *A Provider's Handbook on Culturally Competent Care.* 2nd ed. Oakland, CA: Kaiser Foundation Health Plan Inc; 2004

107. Rosario M, Schrimshaw EW, Hunter J. A model of sexual risk behaviors among young gay and bisexual men: longitudinal associations of mental health, substance abuse, sexual abuse, and the coming-out process. *AIDS Educ Prev.* 2006;18(5):444–460

108. Duncan PM, Garcia AC, Frankowski BL, et al. Inspiring healthy adolescent choices: a rationale for and guide to strength promotion in primary care. *J Adolesc Health.* 2007;41(6):525–535

109. Frankowski BL, Leader IC, Duncan PM. Strength-based interviewing. *Adolesc Med State Art Rev.* 2009;20(1):22–40, vii–viii

110. Workowski KA, Berman SM; Centers for Disease Control and Prevention. Sexually transmitted diseases treatment guidelines, 2010. *MMWR Recomm Rep.* 2010;59 (RR-12):1–110

111. Ho KS, Cranston RD. Anal cytology screening in HIV-positive men who have sex with men: what's new and what's now? *Curr Opin Infect Dis.* 2010;23(1):21–25

112. Bakotic WL, Willis D, Birdsong G, Tadros TS. Anal cytology in an HIV-positive population: a retrospective analysis. *Acta Cytol.* 2005;49(2):163–168

113. US Food and Drug Administration. FDA: Gardasil approved to prevent anal cancer [news release]. Silver Spring, MD: US Food and Drug Administration; December 22, 2010

114. Centers for Disease Control and Prevention. FDA licensure of quadrivalent human papillomavirus vaccine (HPV4, Gardasil) for use in males and guidance from the Advisory Committee on Immunization Practices (ACIP). *MMWR Morb Mortal Wkly Rep.* 2010;59(20):630–632

115. Centers for Disease Control and Prevention. Recommendations on the use of quadrivalent human papillomavirus vaccine in males—Advisory Committee on Immunization Practices (ACIP), 2011. *MMWR Morb Mortal Wkly Rep.* 2011;60 (50):1705–1708

116. Centers for Disease Control and Prevention. FDA licensure of bivalent human papillomavirus vaccine (HPV2, Cervarix) for use in females and updated HPV vaccination recommendations from the Advisory Committee on Immunization Practices (ACIP). *MMWR Morb Mortal Wkly Rep.* 2010; 59(20):626–629

117. Blythe MJ, Diaz A; American Academy of Pediatrics Committee on Adolescence. Contraception and adolescents. *Pediatrics.* 2007;120(5):1135–1148

118. Spack NP, Edwards-Leeper L, Feldman HA, et al. Children and adolescents with gender identity disorder referred to a pediatric medical center. *Pediatrics.* 2012;129(3): 418–425

119. Ashbee O, Goldberg J. Trans care gender transition: hormones: a guide for MTFs. Vancouver, British Columbia, Canada: Vancouver Coastal Health, Transcend Transgender Support & Education Society and Canadian Rainbow Health Coalition; 2006. Available at: http://transhealth.vch.ca/resources/library/tcpdocs/consumer/hormones-MTF.pdf. Accessed June 13, 2012

120. Carroll M. Transgender youth, adolescent decision making, and Roper v. Simmons. *UCLA Law Rev.* 2009;56(3–4):725–753

121. Chasan PE. The history of injectable silicone fluids for soft-tissue augmentation. *Plast Reconstr Surg.* 2007;120(7):2034–2040, discussion 2041–2043

122. Clark RF, Cantrell FL, Pacal A, Chen W, Betten DP. Subcutaneous silicone injection leading to multi-system organ failure. *Clin Toxicol (Phila).* 2008;46(9):834–837

123. Schmid A, Tzur A, Leshko L, Krieger BP. Silicone embolism syndrome: a case report, review of the literature, and comparison with fat embolism syndrome. *Chest.* 2005;127(6):2276–2281

124. Rosioreanu A, Brusca-Augello GT, Ahmed QA, Katz DS. CT visualization of silicone-related pneumonitis in a transsexual man. *AJR Am J Roentgenol.* 2004;183(1): 248–249

Oral Health Care for Children With Developmental Disabilities

- *Clinical Report*

CLINICAL REPORT

Oral Health Care for Children With Developmental Disabilities

abstract

Children with developmental disabilities often have unmet complex health care needs as well as significant physical and cognitive limitations. Children with more severe conditions and from low-income families are particularly at risk with high dental needs and poor access to care. In addition, children with developmental disabilities are living longer, requiring continued oral health care. This clinical report describes the effect that poor oral health has on children with developmental disabilities as well as the importance of partnerships between the pediatric medical and dental homes. Basic knowledge of the oral health risk factors affecting children with developmental disabilities is provided. Pediatricians may use the report to guide their incorporation of oral health assessments and education into their well-child examinations for children with developmental disabilities. This report has medical, legal, educational, and operational implications for practicing pediatricians. *Pediatrics* 2013;131:614–619

Kenneth W. Norwood, Jr, MD, Rebecca L. Slayton, DDS, PhD, COUNCIL ON CHILDREN WITH DISABILITIES, and SECTION ON ORAL HEALTH

KEY WORDS
children, developmental disabilities, oral health, dental care, medical home

The guidance in this report does not indicate an exclusive course of treatment or serve as a standard of medical care. Variations, taking into account individual circumstances, may be appropriate.

www.pediatrics.org/cgi/doi/10.1542/peds.2012-3650

doi:10.1542/peds.2012-3650

All clinical reports from the American Academy of Pediatrics automatically expire 5 years after publication unless reaffirmed, revised, or retired at or before that time.

PEDIATRICS (ISSN Numbers: Print, 0031-4005; Online, 1098-4275).

Good oral health is an important component of overall health and implies that teeth, gums, and oral mucosal tissues are intact and free of disease. Conversely, poor oral health may affect quality of life and a person's ability to eat, sleep, and function without pain. For many children with developmental disabilities, their smile is their most effective way of interacting with the world. Poor oral health may also contribute to systemic illness (aspiration pneumonia, systemic infection, and systemic inflammation).[1] The most common disease of teeth is dental caries (cavities), and the most common diseases of the gingiva and supporting structures of the teeth are gingivitis and periodontal disease, respectively. Dental caries occur when bacteria in the mouth metabolize carbohydrates to produce acid. The regular exposure of tooth surfaces to acid results in loss of mineral from the tooth and subsequent cavities. Gingivitis and periodontal disease are also caused by bacteria and by lack of routine oral hygiene procedures. Bacteria-containing plaque forms on tooth surfaces and causes inflammation of the adjacent gingival tissues. If plaque is permitted to remain on the tooth for a period of time, it becomes mineralized. This tartar or calculus provides a physical irritation to the gingival tissues, eventually resulting in loss of the attachment of gums to teeth and loss of supporting bone.

Children with developmental disabilities, including conditions that affect behavior and cognition, often have limitations in their abilities to perform activities of daily living. They may have special health care needs as well. Examples include children with autism spectrum disorders, intellectual disability, cerebral palsy, craniofacial anomalies, and other health conditions. As a group, children with developmental disabilities are more likely to have unmet dental needs than are typically developing children[2,3] and are considered to be at greater risk of developing dental disease. The reasons include frequent use of medicine high in sugar, dependence on a caregiver for regular oral hygiene, reduced clearance of foods from the oral cavity, impaired salivary function, preference for carbohydrate-rich foods, a liquid or puréed diet, and oral aversions.[4] Medications to manage seizures may cause gingival overgrowth. Other medications, such as glycopyrrolate, trihexyphenidyl, and some attention-deficit/hyperactivity disorder medications (amphetamine, atomoxetine), can result in xerostomia, which increases the risk of dental caries. In addition, recent policies promoting community-based living arrangements and increased independence for people with developmental disabilities may also contribute to the increased risk of dental caries by decreasing direct caregiver supports.[4] The oral health needs of this population have also increased because children with disabilities are much more likely to survive into adulthood than they were in previous decades.[5]

ACCESS TO MEDICAL AND DENTAL CARE

Access to dental care may pose a challenge for children with developmental disabilities because of lack of or inadequate dental insurance or difficulty finding a dentist who is willing and able to care for young children or children and adolescents with complex medical conditions. In some cases, behavioral conditions may make it difficult to provide dental care in the traditional setting. In a survey of families of children with special health care needs, 24% reported that their children needed dental care other than preventive care in the 12 months before the interview and 8.9% of respondents reported that they were unable to obtain the needed care.[1] In the group with unmet dental needs, the more severely affected children were more likely to have unmet dental needs than were children whose medical condition only mildly affected their lives. The access to care for these children was also significantly affected by family income. Medicaid reimbursement rates are often below the usual and customary fees. Low-income families were much less likely to report being able to obtain care than were higher-income families,[2] making it imperative that health care providers advocate for low-income families with children who are at risk of dental problems.

BARRIERS TO ACCESS TO CARE

Barriers to accessing dental care for children with developmental disabilities include transportation difficulties, limited numbers of dentists with the necessary expertise, and overall workforce capacity shortages.[6] Pediatric dentists have the needed training to be able to treat patients with developmental disabilities. However, there are only 5000 practicing pediatric dentists in the United States, and this number as well as their distribution cannot adequately address the treatment needs of these patients. As a result, general dentists often treat children with special health care needs in their practices. It is estimated that there are 11.2 million children with special health care needs in the United States (www.childhealthdata.

org). Not all of these children fit into the category of having a developmental disability. Kerins et al[6] estimated that for general dentists who currently treat children with special health care needs in their practice, one-third of their available visits would need to be for this patient population to meet capacity needs.

Nelson et al[7] divided barriers from the parents' perspective into 2 categories: environmental and nonenvironmental. Significant environmental barriers included the inability to find a dentist who would treat their child and to find a dental office where the staff members were not nervous about caring for a child with special needs. Included are financial barriers resulting from Medicaid reimbursement rates that are below the usual and customary fees. Many children with special health care needs have Medicaid insurance for dental care, but many dentists, including pediatric dentists, do not accept Medicaid insurance. Nonenvironmental barriers included the child's perceived fear of the dentist, the child's inability to cooperate for dental exams, other health care needs that were more urgent, and the child's having an aversion to things in his or her mouth.[7]

ORAL HEALTH CONDITIONS ASSOCIATED WITH DEVELOPMENTAL DISABILITIES

Children Who Do Not Take Food or Fluids Orally

Children who are unable to meet their fluid and nutritional needs orally and who depend on gastrostomy tube feedings are at significantly increased risk of poor oral health, particularly a build-up of tartar and subsequent gingivitis.[4,8,9] The increased calculus formation that is seen in children who are primarily fed via a gastrostomy tube may result from the lack of normal clearance of the oral cavity that takes place when food is chewed and swallowed. Children with quadriplegic cerebral palsy often have increased periodontal disease as a result of poor oral hygiene, in part because of dependence on caregivers.[10] The risk of dental caries is increased by enamel hypoplasia, poor nutritional status, and medicines that reduce saliva or contain sugar. Children with oral dysphagia often pocket food and fluids, further promoting dental decay. Puréed foods may adhere to the teeth longer than regular foods. Gagging, choking, and reflux can expose teeth to acidic gastric contents. The lack of oral experiences and severe motor impairments can result in hyperactive bite and gag reflexes, which can interfere with not only oral hygiene but also with the dentist's access to the child's mouth.

Children With Oral Aversion

Increasing numbers of children with oral aversions are being seen in pediatricians' and dentists' offices. Some children have developed oral aversions as a result of being born preterm and having had prolonged intubation and other noxious experiences to the mouth. Children with autism spectrum disorders often have oral aversions characterized by hypersensitivities to textures, smells, tastes, and colors, thus significantly limiting the foods they will eat. Resultant nutritional deficiencies can affect oral health. Deficiencies of vitamins A and C can result in poor healing and increased gum bleeding. Vitamin D deficiency can result in soft teeth. Malnutrition can affect the immune system and result in increased gingivitis and other oral infections. Preferences for soft foods can lead to increased food adherence to teeth. Oral aversion can interfere with oral hygiene such as brushing or flossing. Poor oral hygiene may be the most influential risk indicator associated with new caries in children with autism.[11] Children with oral aversion may need to be sedated or be provided general anesthesia so that dentists can adequately examine, clean, and restore their teeth.

Children With Functional Limitations in Self-care

Self-care skills in children with intellectual disability and neurodevelopmental disabilities are compromised because of delays in motor and cognitive abilities, which leads to an increased reliance on others for health and oral health care activities.[12] Children with functional limitations in self-care are at increased risk of dental caries and periodontal disease as a result. It is not uncommon for children with intellectual disability to also have oral aversions and to have behavioral problems in the traditional dental office setting. Behavioral problems create an additional barrier to care, because parents are hesitant to bring the child to the dentist and because many dentists are not comfortable managing difficult behavior.

Children with Down syndrome have dental issues similar to those in other children with intellectual disabilities, but in addition, they are more likely to have crowding of teeth, making it more difficult to perform oral hygiene, and are more susceptible to periodontal disease.[13] Because there is a large range in the functional status of children with Down syndrome, generalizations about behavior in the dental office have minimal value. There is the perception that children with Down syndrome are at decreased risk of dental caries, possibly because of factors related to salivary function; however, scientific evidence is lacking.

Children With Craniofacial Anomalies

Orofacial clefts are one of the more common birth defects in the United States, with a prevalence that varies by racial/ethnic background, and are estimated to be present in ~1 in 1000 births.[14] Children with structural anomalies of the face and mouth (eg, cleft lip, cleft palate, Crouzon syndrome, Apert syndrome, and Pierre Robin sequence) frequently require multiple surgeries and experience disturbances in dental and speech development. They may have extra teeth located in or around the cleft, missing teeth, or malformed teeth. The position of the teeth can make it difficult to thoroughly remove plaque and increases the risk of dental caries.[15] In addition, these children often have oral aversions and resist home oral hygiene activities. Orthodontic care is commonly required to correct dental malocclusions in these patients, and orthodontic appliances significantly increase the risk of dental caries. Failure of palate repair and bone grafting is more likely in the presence of unhealthy gingival tissues, making oral hygiene particularly important in these children.

One example of a disorder with craniofacial anomalies is Goldenhar syndrome. Children with Goldenhar syndrome have distinctive clinical features, including mandibular hypoplasia, facial asymmetry, vertebral anomalies, microtia, and central nervous system anomalies.[16] In some cases, cleft lip and palate are present, and the oral manifestations can range from malocclusion to complete lack of the mandibular ramus. Intellectual disability is also a common finding in children with Goldenhar syndrome, and therefore their ability to perform oral hygiene and other self-care activities is compromised. Also, because children with Goldenhar syndrome can have limited oral opening and/or a malocclusion, oral hygiene is more difficult, putting them at increased risk of both dental caries and gingivitis.[17]

Children With Chronic Dental Erosions Secondary to Maladaptive Behaviors

Children with neurodevelopmental disabilities may have increased maladaptive behaviors that can affect oral health, such as bruxism (teeth clenching or grinding) and repetitive biting on nonfood objects. However, there is little information in the literature on these issues, especially biting on nonfood objects. One study showed significantly more physical signs of bruxism in children who had autism spectrum disorders.[18] Bruxism is more common during sleep and is one of the most common sleep disorders. Bruxism can result in occlusal trauma, such as abnormal wear patterns and even teeth fractures. It can result in gum recession and tooth loss. Some risk factors for bruxism are common in individuals with disabilities such as sleep disorders and malocclusion. The usual approaches to bruxism that require the ability to cooperate with and tolerate appliances may not be successful. A systematic review of 11 studies in individuals with developmental disabilities and bruxism suggested that behavior modification and dental treatment may be the best approaches to this problem.[19]

INTERPROFESSIONAL PARTNERSHIPS

Oral Health Education in Medical and Residency Training

Education in oral health during medical and residency training is very limited. In a survey of pediatricians, only 36% said they had received previous training in oral health, with 13% reporting training during medical school.[20] The majority of survey respondents recognized the importance of evaluating their patients for dental caries, but only 41% felt that their ability to identify caries was very good or excellent. This survey focused on healthy young children rather than those with special health care needs, but presumably, their responses would apply to children with special health care needs as well. There are similar findings in family medicine residency programs. In a survey of residency directors, 95% of respondents agreed that oral health knowledge is important for family medicine residents, but the likelihood that residents were taught about oral health screening measures ranged from 9% to 84%. The oral health measure least taught to residents was asking about the mother's oral health.[21]

Identification of Children Who Require Referral for Dental Treatment

The American Academy of Pediatrics recommends the establishment of a dental home by 1 year of age for children at high risk of dental caries.[22] Pediatricians should encourage parents of children with developmental disabilities to seek dental care at their first birthday and to help them identify resources to overcome any barriers such as transportation. The American Academy of Pediatric Dentistry recommends that all children visit a pediatric dentist when the first tooth comes in, usually between 6 and 12 months of age ("first visit by first birthday").[23] In addition to determining caries risk, an early first visit offers opportunities to establish a pediatric dental home and to provide dental-related anticipatory guidance. Currently, 40 states have Medicaid programs that reimburse medical providers for preventive dental care, including fluoride varnish application.[24] Fluoride varnish is a concentrated topical fluoride that is applied to the teeth by using a small brush and sets on contact with saliva. The advantages of this modality are that it is well tolerated by infants and children, has minimal risk for ingestion, has a prolonged therapeutic effect, and can be applied by both dental and nondental health professionals in a variety of settings.[25] The application of fluoride varnish during an oral screening is a great benefit to children at high risk of caries and who may have limited access to dental care. Thus, it should be a high priority for children with developmental disabilities.

Unfortunately, access to pediatric dentists is limited in many areas. General dentists may not begin seeing children until 3 to 5 years of age and often lack the expertise to manage the oral health needs of children with developmental disabilities. Children with disabilities should follow the "first visit by first birthday" recommendation even if it means traveling a long distance to see a pediatric dentist. The importance of the pediatric medical home to coordinate with a pediatric dental home cannot be overstated. Children with certain craniofacial abnormalities and other at-risk conditions should have their initial pediatric dental visit during the first 6 months of life. The early establishment of regular pediatric dental care at the age of 6 to 12 months with 3- to 6-month follow-up visits throughout childhood means that the pediatrician should rarely have to make a decision about when to refer a child with developmental disabilities for dental treatment. The Oral Health Risk Assessment Tool was developed by an expert group of pediatricians and pediatric dentists and is available online (http://www2.aap.org/oralhealth/RiskAssessmentTool.html). This tool can be used to document the caries risk of a child patient and assist with decisions regarding referral to a pediatric or general dentist.

Safe Use of Procedural Sedation and Analgesia/Anesthesia

Many children and adults with developmental disabilities find treatment in the traditional dental setting challenging. Even routine dental procedures involve sounds, tastes, and other stimulation that can be difficult to tolerate. To make preventive and restorative care more comfortable for patients with developmental disabilities, treatment is often provided with the use of either sedation or general anesthesia. Sedation may be provided in the dental office or in an outpatient surgical center following appropriate guidelines to ensure patient safety. General anesthesia is primarily provided in a hospital setting where the necessary precautions can be taken to minimize complications. The pediatrician should be aware that children with disabilities often have exaggerated and unpredictable responses to sedation and conscious anesthesia.

Sedation guidelines were developed collaboratively between the American Academy of Pediatrics and the American Academy of Pediatric Dentistry in 2006.[26,27] These guidelines describe the types of precautions that should be taken for mild and moderate levels of sedation in the dental or pediatric office. Children who are considered candidates for in-office mild or moderate sedation include those that are categorized by the American Society of Anesthesiologists (ASA) Physical Status classification system as ASA I or II. For children with ASA classification III or IV or those with special health care needs or anatomic airway abnormalities, it is recommended that the practitioner take additional precautions and seriously consider consultation with an anesthesiologist.

SUGGESTIONS FOR PEDIATRICIANS

1. Learn how to assess dental and periodontal health in children with special health care needs.

2. Recognize risk factors that contribute to poor oral health with the use of the Oral Health Risk Assessment Tool (http://www2.aap.org/oralhealth/RiskAssessmentTool.html).

3. Identify dental professionals in the community who will provide a dental home for children with developmental disabilities (including providers for children who require sedation/anesthesia).

4. Include anticipatory guidance on appropriate oral hygiene and habits for all children, especially those at high risk because of special health care needs or developmental disabilities.

5. Advocate for oral care for children with developmental disabilities.

6. Develop collaborations with dental partners to coordinate care for children with developmental disabilities.

LEAD AUTHORS

Kenneth W. Norwood, Jr, MD
Rebecca L. Slayton, DDS, PhD

COUNCIL ON CHILDREN WITH DISABILITIES EXECUTIVE COMMITTEE, 2011–2012

Gregory S. Liptak, MD, MPH, Chairperson[†]

Nancy A. Murphy, MD, Interim Chairperson
Richard C. Adams, MD
Robert T. Burke, MD, MPH
Sandra L. Friedman, MD, MPH
Amy J. Houtrow, MD, MPH, PhD
Miriam A. Kalichman, MD
Dennis Z. Kuo, MD, MHS
Susan Ellen Levy, MD
Kenneth W. Norwood, Jr, MD
Renee M. Turchi, MD, MPH
Susan E. Wiley, MD

LIAISONS

Carolyn Bridgemohan, MD – *Section on Developmental and Behavioral Pediatrics*
Georgina Peacock, MD, MPH – *Centers for Disease Control and Prevention*
Bonnie Strickland, PhD – *Maternal and Child Health Bureau*
Nora Wells, MSEd – *Family Voices*
Max Wiznitzer, MD – *Section on Neurology*

STAFF

Stephanie Mucha, MPH

SECTION ON ORAL HEALTH EXECUTIVE COMMITTEE, 2011–2012

Adriana Segura, DDS, MS, Chairperson
Suzanne Boulter, MD
Melinda Clark, MD
Rani Gereige, MD
David Krol, MD, MPH
Wendy Mouradian, MD
Rocio Quinonez, DMD, MPH
Francisco Ramos-Gomez, DDS
Rebecca Slayton, DDS, PhD
Martha Ann Keels, DDS, PhD, Immediate Past Chairperson

LIAISONS

Robert Delarosa, DMD – *American Academy of Pediatric Dentistry*
Sheila Strock, DMD, MPH – *American Dental Association Liaison*

STAFF

Lauren Barone, MPH

REFERENCES

1. Babu NC, Gomes AJ. Systemic manifestations of oral diseases. *J Oral Maxillofac Pathol.* 2011;15(2):144–147

2. Lewis CW. Dental care and children with special health care needs: a population-based perspective. *Acad Pediatr.* 2009;9(6):420–426

3. Kagihara LE, Huebner CE, Mouradian WE, Milgrom P, Anderson BA. Parents' perspectives on a dental home for children with special health care needs. *Spec Care Dentist.* 2011;31(5):170–177

4. Thikkurissy S, Lal S. Oral health burden in children with systemic diseases. *Dent Clin North Am.* 2009;53(2):351–357, xi

5. Seirawan H, Schneiderman J, Greene V, Mulligan R. Interdisciplinary approach to oral health for persons with developmental disabilities. *Spec Care Dentist.* 2008;28(2):43–52

6. Kerins C, Casamassimo PS, Ciesla D, Lee Y, Seale NS. A preliminary analysis of the US dental health care system's capacity to treat children with special health care needs. *Pediatr Dent.* 2011;33(2):107–112

7. Nelson LP, Getzin A, Graham D, et al. Unmet dental needs and barriers to care for

[†]Deceased.

children with significant special health care needs. *Pediatr Dent.* 2011;33(1):29–36

8. Hidas A, Cohen J, Beeri M, Shapira J, Steinberg D, Moskovitz M. Salivary bacteria and oral health status in children with disabilities fed through gastrostomy. *Int J Paediatr Dent.* 2010;20(3):179–185

9. Jawadi AH, Casamassimo PS, Griffen A, Enrile B, Marcone M. Comparison of oral findings in special needs children with and without gastrostomy. *Pediatr Dent.* 2004;26 (3):283–288

10. National Institute of Dental and Craniofacial Research. *Practical Oral Care for People with Cerebral Palsy.* Bethesda, MD: National Institute of Dental and Craniofacial Research; 2009. NIH Publication No. 09-5192

11. Marshall J, Sheller B, Mancl L. Caries-risk assessment and caries status of children with autism. *Pediatr Dent.* 2010;32(1):69–75

12. McIver FT. Access to care: a clinical perspective. In: Mouradian W, ed. *Proceedings: Promoting Oral Health of Children with Neurodevelopmental Disabilities and Other Special Health Care Needs: A Meeting to Develop Training and Research Agendas, Center on Human Development and Disability.* Seattle, WA: University of Washington; 2001: 167–171. Available at: www.healthychild.ucla. edu/nohpc/National%20oral%20Health% 20Policy%20Center/Publications/Promoting %20Oral%20Health.pdf. Accessed July 19, 2012

13. Abanto J, Ciamponi AL, Francischini E, Murakami C, de Rezende NP, Gallottini M. Medical problems and oral care of patients

with Down syndrome: a literature review. *Spec Care Dentist.* 2011;31(6):197–203

14. National Institute of Dental and Craniofacial Research. Prevalence (number) of cases of cleft lip and cleft palate. Available at: www. nidcr.nih.gov/DataStatistics/FindDataByTopic/ CraniofacialBirthDefects/PrevalenceCleft+Lip-CleftPalate.htm. Accessed July 19, 2012

15. Kirchberg A, Treide A, Hemprich A. Investigation of caries prevalence in children with cleft lip, alveolus, and palate. *J Craniomaxillofac Surg.* 2004;32(4):216–219

16. Martelli H, Jr, Miranda RT, Fernandes CM, et al. Goldenhar syndrome: clinical features with orofacial emphasis. *J Appl Oral Sci.* 2010;18(6):646–649

17. OMIM—Online Mendelian Inheritance in Man. Hemifacial microsomia; HFM. Available at: http://omim.org/entry/164210. Accessed July 19, 2012

18. DeMattei R, Cuvo A, Maurizio S. Oral assessment of children with an autism spectrum disorder. *J Dent Hyg.* 2007;81(3):65

19. Lang R, White PJ, Machalicek W, et al. Treatment of bruxism in individuals with developmental disabilities: a systematic review. *Res Dev Disabil.* 2009;30(5):809–818

20. Lewis CW, Boulter S, Keels MA, et al. Oral health and pediatricians: results of a national survey. *Acad Pediatr.* 2009;9(6):457–461

21. Gonsalves WC, Skelton J, Heaton L, Smith T, Feretti G, Hardison JD. Family medicine residency directors' knowledge and attitudes about pediatric oral health education

for residents. *J Dent Educ.* 2005;69(4):446–452

22. Hale KJ; American Academy of Pediatrics Section on Pediatric Dentistry. Oral health risk assessment timing and establishment of the dental home. *Pediatrics.* 2003;111(5 pt 1):1113–1116

23. American Academy of Pediatric Dentistry. *Dental Care for Your Baby* [brochure]. Available at: www.aapd.org/publications/ brochures/. Accessed July 19, 2012

24. The Pew Center on the States. Available at: www.pewcenteronthestates.org/initiatives_ detail.aspx?initiativeID=328928. Accessed July 19, 2012

25. American Dental Association Council on Scientific Affairs. Professionally applied topical fluoride: evidence-based clinical recommendations. *J Am Dent Assoc.* 2006; 137(8):1151–1159

26. American Academy of Pediatric Dentistry. Guideline for monitoring and management of pediatric patients during and after sedation for diagnostic and therapeutic procedures. *American Academy of Pediatric Dentistry Clinical Guidelines Reference Manual.* 2006;33 (6):185–201. Available at: www.aapd.org/media/ policies_guidelines/g_sedation.pdf. Accessed July 19, 2012

27. American Academy of Pediatrics. Guideline for monitoring and management of pediatric patients during and after sedation for diagnostic and therapeutic procedures: an update. *Pediatrics.* 2006;118(6):2587–2602 (Reaffirmed March 2011)

Out-of-School Suspension and Expulsion

- *Policy Statement*

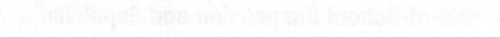

POLICY STATEMENT

Out-of-School Suspension and Expulsion

abstract

The primary mission of any school system is to educate students. To achieve this goal, the school district must maintain a culture and environment where all students feel safe, nurtured, and valued and where order and civility are expected standards of behavior. Schools cannot allow unacceptable behavior to interfere with the school district's primary mission. To this end, school districts adopt codes of conduct for expected behaviors and policies to address unacceptable behavior. In developing these policies, school boards must weigh the severity of the offense and the consequences of the punishment and the balance between individual and institutional rights and responsibilities. Out-of-school suspension and expulsion are the most severe consequences that a school district can impose for unacceptable behavior. Traditionally, these consequences have been reserved for offenses deemed especially severe or dangerous and/or for recalcitrant offenders. However, the implications and consequences of out-of-school suspension and expulsion and "zero-tolerance" are of such severity that their application and appropriateness for a developing child require periodic review. The indications and effectiveness of exclusionary discipline policies that demand automatic or rigorous application are increasingly questionable. The impact of these policies on offenders, other children, school districts, and communities is broad. Periodic scrutiny of policies should be placed not only on the need for a better understanding of the educational, emotional, and social impact of out-of-school suspension and expulsion on the individual student but also on the greater societal costs of such rigid policies. Pediatricians should be prepared to assist students and families affected by out-of-school suspension and expulsion and should be willing to guide school districts in their communities to find more effective and appropriate alternatives to exclusionary discipline policies for the developing child. A discussion of preventive strategies and alternatives to out-of-school suspension and expulsion, as well as recommendations for the role of the physician in matters of out-of-school suspension and expulsion are included. School-wide positive behavior support/positive behavior intervention and support is discussed as an effective alternative. *Pediatrics* 2013;131:e1000–e1007

COUNCIL ON SCHOOL HEALTH

KEY WORDS
suspension, expulsion, school, discipline

ABBREVIATIONS
AAP—American Academy of Pediatrics
IEP—individualized education plan
PBIS—positive behavior intervention and support
SWBS—school-wide positive behavior support

www.pediatrics.org/cgi/doi/10.1542/peds.2012-3932

doi:10.1542/peds.2012-3932

PEDIATRICS (ISSN Numbers: Print, 0031-4005; Online, 1098-4275).

Copyright © 2013 by the American Academy of Pediatrics

RATIONALE FOR OUT-OF-SCHOOL SUSPENSION AND EXPULSION

Perhaps no public institution more closely mirrors the community in which it is found than does the public school system. The school system comprises children from a wide variety of socioeconomic backgrounds and a wide range of academic abilities and challenges. The primary mission of any school system is to educate the students for which it is responsible. To achieve this mission, the school district must maintain a culture and environment in which all students feel safe, nurtured, and valued. Order and civility must be maintained while expecting an appropriate standard of behavior from faculty, staff, and students. Traditionally, the goals for out-of-school suspension and expulsion policies were to promote a safe environment for students and staff by decreasing violent behavior, combating statutorily criminal activities (especially illicit drug usage and trafficking), and discouraging inappropriate behavior and limiting its influence on others. Out-of-school suspension and expulsion ensure that an offending act is punished; thus, in theory, a standard of acceptable behavior is maintained. It has been traditionally held that, in removing the offending student from the school environment, the student's influence on others would be limited, the school environment would thereby be improved, and a message would be sent that certain behaviors will not be tolerated.[1] Research has demonstrated, however, that schools with higher rates of out-of-school suspension and expulsion are not safer for students or faculty.[2]

"ZERO TOLERANCE"

The Gun-Free Schools Act of 1994 (Pub L No. 103-882, §14601) popularized the concept of zero tolerance in the theory and practice of behavior control and discipline in schools and, in many cases, profoundly altered the entire discussion of these topics. As its title implies, that legislation focused specifically on the bringing of weapons to school and mandated a specific response from school districts. The offense for which the Gun-Free Schools Act was intended (that is, bringing

a weapon to school) may account for <2% of the offenses for which students are suspended or expelled.[3] Many school districts, however, quickly seized on zero-tolerance policies as a means of addressing a variety of infractions, including nonviolent offenses, such as drug and alcohol violations, verbal disrespect to teachers, and truancy. The concept of zero tolerance was readily embraced as inherently fair, and its harshness was accepted as a massive deterrent to undesirable behavior. However, problems with zero-tolerance policies began to occur soon thereafter, precisely because of its inflexibility and harshness. It is interesting to note that, although zero-tolerance legislation was prompted by violent acts perpetrated by white students, the vast majority of out-of-school suspension and expulsion occurring with zero-tolerance policy applications involve black or Hispanic students.[2]

One of the first questions to surface was what "zero tolerance" should mean. A zero-tolerance policy that mandates a disciplinary hearing concerning certain unacceptable behaviors allows school boards and administrators flexibility and discretion in dealing with serious infractions. On the other hand, a policy that mandates a particular consequence (for example, that a student be suspended or expelled without consideration being given to the extenuating and mitigating circumstances of the case) allows authorities no such leeway. It should be noted that a school district may not want discretion in its zero-tolerance policy, feeling that such inflexibility sends the clearest message to offenders and best ensures the well-being of the rest of the student body. However, "research indicates a negative relationship between the use of suspension and expulsion and school-wide academic achievement, even when controlling for demographics

such as socioeconomic status."[4] In other words, aggressive out-of-school suspension and expulsion policies may not only hurt those against whom they are applied but may also paradoxically hurt those students the policies were supposedly designed to protect and help. Problems with fairness, impartiality, uniformity, and flexibility have caused the effectiveness, validity, and justification of zero-tolerance policies to be questioned.[2,4] Moreover, a student who has an individualized education plan (IEP) and/or has been identified with a disability may be entitled to a hearing to determine whether the student's alleged misconduct was directly related to his or her disability or a direct consequence of the disability. The Individuals With Disabilities Education Act and relevant state statues should be referenced in this regard. If a student is thought to have a disability and is denied a hearing, the legality of such a denial may be open to question.

DISADVANTAGES OF OUT-OF-SCHOOL SUSPENSION AND EXPULSION TO STUDENT AND FAMILY

The adverse effects of out-of-school suspension and expulsion on the student can be profound. The student is separated from the educational process, and the school district may not be obligated to provide any further educational or counseling services for the student.[5] Data suggest that students who are involved in the juvenile justice system are likely to have been suspended or expelled.[4] Further, students who experience out-of-school suspension and expulsion are as much as 10 times more likely to ultimately drop out of high school than are those who do not.[5,6] The student who does not complete high school can expect to earn considerably less over a working career and to have far fewer educational and employment opportunities from which to choose than a student who has completed high school. If the student's parent(s) work, there may be no one at home during the day to supervise the student's activity, making it more likely that the student (1) will not pursue a home-based education program; (2) will engage in more inappropriate behavior; and (3) will associate with other individuals who will further increase the aforementioned risks.[2]

DISADVANTAGES OF OUT-OF-SCHOOL SUSPENSION AND EXPULSION POLICIES TO A SCHOOL DISTRICT

There are risks and disadvantages associated with the use of any powerful intervention or remedy, and out-of-school suspension and expulsion is no exception. Out-of-school suspension and expulsion are drastic responses to instances of severe misconduct. They can also be very superficial if, in using them, school districts avoid dealing with underlying issues affecting the child or the district, such as drug abuse, racial and ethnic tensions, and cultural anomalies associated with violence and bullying.[7,8] There is also a risk of inconsistent and capricious application. In one 2006 study of statewide school suspension and expulsion rates, it was revealed that 10% of schools were responsible for 50% of suspensions.[3,9] Moreover, "drastic" is not synonymous with "effective." The Zero Tolerance Task Force of the American Psychological Association determined that schools with higher rates of suspension tend to have lower academic quality, pay less attention to school climate (social, cultural, academic, ethical), and receive lower ratings on school governance measures.[4] Ironically, out-of-school suspension and expulsion often place the child back into the very environment that may

have contributed to the antisocial behaviors in the first place, thereby negating the effectiveness of a "lesson-learned" from out-of-school suspension and expulsion. Atkins et al[10] demonstrated that the use of suspension as discipline increased the number of students to whom suspension was applied, whereas when suspension was no longer used as punishment, that number declined.

GREATER FISCAL COSTS

Any discussion of a school district out-of-school suspension and expulsion policy must consider the fiscal implications of such a policy. Besides the loss of capitation funds for student attendance, there are other significant costs to the district associated with the process of suspending or expelling a student, including time spent in meetings, seeking expert testimony, and preparing for the disciplinary hearing itself. Unlike time spent by staff, consultants, and administrators working to educate children, time spent on suspension and expulsion preparation yields no measurable educational benefit, so it is especially costly to the district's primary mission. Moreover, the cost to the district continues to mount after the expulsion hearing. States may require districts to have mechanisms whereby an expelled or suspended student receives services and may become eligible for reinstatement into the district, provided certain conditions are met and maintained.

Recalling that students who experience out-of-school suspension and expulsion are far more likely to ultimately drop out of high school, it is worthwhile to consider critically the potential adverse long-term fiscal consequences to the student and society as a whole. If the student does not graduate from high school, the long-term costs are profound. A high-school dropout will earn $400 000 ($485 000 for males) less over

a lifetime than a high school graduate.[11] The dropout will pay $60 000 less in taxes than the high school graduate. This represents a loss to federal and state governments of billions of dollars per year in income tax revenue. The average high school dropout experiences worse health[12] than the average high school graduate and has a life expectancy that is 6 to 9 years shorter.[13] The implications for the health care system are significant. For economic reasons alone, it is in the best interests of students and society to seek alternatives to out-of-school suspension and expulsion whenever possible.[14]

PREVENTION OF OUT-OF-SCHOOL SUSPENSION AND EXPULSION

As outlined previously, out-of-school suspension and expulsion represent an enormously costly and largely unsatisfactory solution to behavior problems in school, whether from the standpoint of the school district, the student, or the community. Out-of-school suspension and expulsion have short- and long-term consequences that are best avoided if at all possible.

Three strategies schools can use that can lessen the incidence of out-of-school suspension and expulsion are as follows: (1) early intervention programs for preschool children; (2) early identification of children at risk for school difficulties and intensive intervention before problem behaviors occur; and (3) annual implementation of clearly articulated and carefully taught age-appropriate codes of conducts with stated alternatives and supports for students to use before they engage in inappropriate behaviors, such as school-wide positive behavior support (SWBS). These strategies can also instill short- and long-term positive change in individual students and in the school district as a whole. It is important to note that they depend not just on the efforts of the school district, but on the coordinated resources of the entire community for their success.

Early Intervention for Preschool Children[15–17]

The education of a community's children is generally regarded as the responsibility of the local school district. The challenge and glory of the public school district is that it has an obligation to accept any and all children within its geographic boundaries into its programs. The school district does not, however, have much control over how well prepared children are to learn when they enter kindergarten at 4, 5, or 6 years of age. A great deal of neurocognitive development occurs in the first years after birth[18]; moreover, children who do not receive nurturing early in life or who are subject to stressful or toxic stimuli carry the effects of these adverse experiences for years afterward and may never be entirely free of their influence.[19–22] Recent studies in infant and early child brain development have highlighted the critical influence of parenting, attachment, and early childhood education on the emotional, social, and cognitive development of young children and the role of attachment disturbances in many child and adult disorders. On the basis of these new developments, many communities have begun offering services such as nurse visits to at-risk pregnant women and parents, parenting programs, child care consultation, and therapeutic child care settings.[23] Thus, meeting a child's need for care and nurturing early on is critical to normal development and can have a significant effect on the child's ability to adapt socially and succeed academically in school. Families and infants at risk for neglect and domestic violence can be identified by pediatricians and other care providers at prenatal visits and before discharge after delivery. Protocols to screen for

and follow-up on at-risk families ensure fair and equitable treatment; many families in need may not fit a particular socioeconomic stereotype. Identified families should then be referred to public health and other community resources that can provide family support and services. These programs, which have been shown to be effective, at least with low-income families, play an important and, in some instances, essential role in promoting the positive functioning of families and ensuring the well-being of children.[23] The American Academy of Pediatrics (AAP) report, "Preparing the Community for Addressing Mental Health Concerns," provides resources to assist in determining which of these programs targeting young children are most promising.[24] Pediatricians should become familiar with and make appropriate referrals to these programs as well as cooperative educational services and other public school universal pre-K or early education and child care programs that provide early childhood intervention to identified high-risk or at-need children. Early Head Start and Head Start programs are also important resources that pediatricians and other professionals can use for eligible families. Finally, children should be screened for medical and toxicologic etiologies that might result in behavioral problems, consistent with AAP *Bright Futures* guidelines.[25]

Early Identification of School Difficulties and Intensive Intervention

Early identification and intensive intervention is a continuation of the efforts made during birth-to-preschool early intervention efforts. Ideally, this represents a coordinated effort among the primary pediatrician or specialists, the school district, and other community agencies to support families and children at risk. This support can come from many sources, including

public health or social services agencies, service organizations such as Boys' and Girls' Clubs, local health care providers, and specialists at regional medical centers. In its 2004 policy statement, "School-Based Mental Health Services," the AAP supports the development of school-based mental health programs as a means of "improving access to diagnosis and treatment for the mental health problems of children and adolescents."[26] Further research should be performed in this area to explore the question of whether mental health services would be more effective if provided in conjunction with a change in school-wide behavior expectations, as may be achieved through a program such as school-wide positive behavior support.

SWBS/Positive Behavior Intervention and Support

SWBS[27–29] is based on group behavior theory; that is, behavior change occurs when desired behaviors are actively taught, clearly and consistently expected, and positively recognized and acknowledged. When SWBS is practiced, the proportion of students with serious behavior problems decreases, and the school's overall climate improves. SWBS is based on 3 main components: (1) prevention; (2) multitiered support; and (3) data-based decision making. It comprises 3 tiers of intervention.[1] The first focuses on school-wide primary prevention, involving all students, staff, and school settings. The second focuses on groups and students engaging in at-risk behaviors. The third tier focuses individualized intervention on students engaging in at-risk behaviors. The process is developed and driven by a group of 5 to 10 individuals representing administrators, staff, parents, community members, and students. This group learns the key practices of SWBS and develops the behavior goals to be achieved. All school staff members need to reinforce desirable behavior and be consistent in responding to such behavior and respond in a consistent fashion to such behavior.[27]

Prevention involves defining and consistently teaching school behavior expectations and developing a consistent system to acknowledge and reward appropriate behavior.

Multitiered support refers to an equally consistent continuum of interventions for inappropriate behavior and supportive re-education for students who misbehave. Minor violations might entail a reminder to a student; a major violation would entail a specific intervention. These interventions may include (1) problem-solving and negotiation of a behavior contract; (2) in-kind restitution; (3) behavior-focused study courses or self-study modules; (4) parent involvement and "buy-in" in decision-making regarding their child's schooling; (5) psychological evaluation and counseling; (6) community service (apart from restitution); (7) behavior monitoring based on the general tenets of the SWBS plan but tailored to the needs of the individual student; (8) coordinated behavior modification plans based on the general tenets of the SWBS plan but tailored to the needs of the individual student; (9) alternative programming, including curriculum, scheduling, site, and/or program, such as independent study or work-study; and (10) an appropriate in-school suspension program, which may be necessary to provide intensive supervision, academic tutoring, and behavior counseling. The goals of the in-school suspension program should be tailored to the needs of the student.[30] Medical evaluation may also be considered.

Data-based decision-making refers to the practice of gathering aggregate data about student behavior and discipline issues for review by administration and the SWBS team. This analysis allows the development of strategies to reduce the problems identified.[2]

The key to the SWBS approach is that it does not stress fixing the student's past as much as it stresses the gains to be made by improving behavior in the future. In so doing, it does not make demands for counseling and psychological resources that the school district itself may not be able to provide; rather, it creates around each student and all students an environment of support such that even those students being disciplined can feel that it is being done supportively rather than punitively. It is cost-effective, not only in terms of demands on resources, but in terms of success. The effectiveness of SWBS is such that the US Department of Education, through its Office of Special Education Programs, established the Technical Assistance Center on Positive Behavior Interventions and Supports (PBIS) "to give schools capacity-building information and technical assistance for identifying, adapting and sustaining effective school-wide disciplinary practices." Evidence-based analysis of results cited by school districts nationwide indicates that SWBS is effective in achieving these aims.[31–33] More than 16 000 school districts nationwide have already adopted this approach to maintaining school discipline and reducing out-of-school suspension and expulsion, and most states have SWBS/PBIS (www.pbis. org). According to the Association for Positive Behavior Support "over 40 states have a state-level leadership team and action plan for PBIS implementation" (www.apbs.org). Some states have gone so far as to issue official statements citing the inequities and ineffectiveness of zero-tolerance policies and recommending SWBS models instead (Letter to Wisconsin Department of Public Instruction, Letter to Administration, March 2009).

BULLYING

A brief mention of bullying is made here because the problem of bullying among school children is receiving a great deal of well-deserved and overdue attention among various social and governmental institutions, and because SWBS/PBIS has been shown to be effective in addressing the problem of bullying as well. Effective management of bullying via SWBS is specifically addressed by the Technical Assistance Center on Positive Behavior Interventions and Supports.[34]

The recently published AAP policy statement "Role of the Pediatrician in Youth Violence Prevention" addresses bullying defined as "a form of aggression in which 1 or more children repeatedly and intentionally intimidate, harass, or physically harm a victim who is perceived as unable to defend herself or himself."[35–37] The sociologic phenomenon of bullying is complex. Historically, it has been widely practiced and is the most common form of violence. Annually, 3.7 million youth engage in it and more than 3.2 million youth are victims annually.[37] It involves essentially all children, as bullies, victims, or both or as knowledgeable bystanders. Put another way, few if any children are unaware whether bullying is occurring among their peers. Moreover, bullying has historically been ignored, condoned as "normal" or a "rite of passage," and even modeled by adults. It has been suggested that schools themselves may encourage bullying through the widespread practice of labeling and separating students on the basis of physical or academic ability or limitation.[38] Twenty-five percent of teachers in 2003 saw nothing wrong with bullying or harassment and intervened in only 4% of cases of bullying.[38] Bullying among school-aged children, thus, represents an anomalous and distorted social norm, in which attitudes and behavior that would be unacceptable elsewhere in society are condoned or even encouraged.[38]

CONCLUSIONS AND RECOMMENDATIONS

A child's ability to succeed in school depends, to a great extent, on factors affecting the child's life well before the child begins school. Recognizing and addressing the socioeconomic and cultural risk factors affecting a child and the child's family are essential to maximizing a child's chances of success in school and to preventing, insofar as possible, the circumstances that may eventually lead to serious school behavior and discipline problems.

Out-of-school suspension and expulsion can contribute to the risk of a student dropping out of high school. The costs of a person's failure to complete his or her secondary education are significant and are borne by society as a whole. These costs to society should be kept in mind as schools, communities, and states consider how to pay for medical, psychological, counseling, and other needed services for children at risk.

The AAP recognizes the importance of bringing the expertise of various professions to bear in a coordinated way to best help children who are not succeeding in school. More research is indicated to identify the most effective means of eliciting positive behaviors in a child with the greatest benefits to society.

Research continues to demonstrate that so-called zero-tolerance policies and out-of-school suspension and expulsion that are used too readily are ineffective deterrents to inappropriate behavior and are harmful and counterproductive to the student, the family, the school district, and the community as a whole, both short- and long-term.

The AAP does not support the concept of zero tolerance for the developing child. The AAP maintains that out-of-school suspension and expulsion are counterproductive to the intended goals, rarely if ever are necessary, and should not be considered as appropriate discipline in any but the most extreme and dangerous circumstances, as determined on an individual basis rather than as a blanket policy.

The aforementioned AAP policy statement "Role of the Pediatrician in Youth Violence Prevention" provides recommendations that are applicable to the reduction of youth violence and bullying and are consistent with the school-wide behavior modification programs that appear to be effective in reducing behaviors that lead to out-of-school suspension and expulsion.[37] Beyond that, and especially in regard to out-of-school suspension and expulsion specifically, the pediatrician can play a variety of roles within the community and school district with respect to discipline issues:

1. The pediatrician should screen for and recognize early childhood and preschool behavior problems. Once a pediatrician identifies a high-risk child, the pediatrician should refer the child to age-appropriate community resources, such as Birth to 3, Head Start, or other school district and community resources. Early identification of and intervention to address potential mental health concerns are critical.

2. As the primary care physician to a school-aged student who is exhibiting problem behavior, the pediatrician should establish communication with the school nurse and/or counselor to verify how the child's behaviors compare with peer behaviors in the school setting. The pediatrician should work with the school, the child and family, and most effectively, mental health care professionals to facilitate and coordinate care of the student. This should occur as early as possible in the onset of behaviors that fail to respond to standard interventions.

3. The pediatrician should be familiar with safeguards as provided by the Individuals With Disabilities Education Act for those patients who have an IEP or 504 Plan. The pediatrician may act as an advisor, advocate, and mediator in special education IEP or 504 Plan meetings and disciplinary or manifestation hearings. The pediatrician should provide written documentation outlining bona fide need for medical accommodations to assist the school in providing reasonable assistance and therapeutic interventions.

4. Pediatricians should become familiar with local school districts' policies on out-of-school suspension and expulsion and zero tolerance. They should advocate for policy changes that support focus on prevention strategies and alternatives to out-of-school suspension and expulsion, such as positive behavior change programs both individually and school wide.

5. The pediatrician can also serve in a larger capacity as a school district physician, a paid consultant, a medical advisor, or a local school board member to help develop school district policy regarding student behavior and discipline. Any professional services provided by a pediatrician on behalf of a specific student whether through diagnosis, treatment, counseling, or advocacy should be recognized as such and the pediatrician appropriately compensated.

LEAD AUTHOR
Jeffrey H. Lamont, MD

COUNCIL ON SCHOOL HEALTH EXECUTIVE COMMITTEE, 2011–2012
Cynthia D. Devore, MD, Chairperson
Mandy Allison, MD, MSPH

REFERENCES

1. Technical Assistance Center on Positive Behavior Interventions and Supports, Office of Special Education Programs, US Department of Education. School-wide PBIS (positive behavior interventions and supports). Eugene, OR: Technical Assistance Center on Positive Behavior Interventions and Supports, Office of Special Education Programs, US Department of Education; 2009. Available at: www.pbis.org. Accessed October 17, 2012

2. *Opportunities Suspended: The Devastating Consequences of Zero Tolerance and School Discipline Policies.* Cambridge, MA: Civil Rights Project, Harvard University; 2000. Available at: www.eric.ed.gov/ERICWebPortal/contentdelivery/servlet/ERICServlet?accno=ED454314. Accessed October 17, 2012

3. Sundis J, Farneth M. Putting kids out of school: what's causing high suspension rates and why they are detrimental to students, schools and communities. Open Society Institute-Baltimore's Student Attendance Series Policy Paper #2. Baltimore, MD: Open Society Institute; September 2008:2

4. Skiba RJ, Reynolds CR, Graham S, Shera P, Conoley JC, Garcia-Vasquez E; American Psychological Association, Zero Tolerance Task Force. *Are Zero-Tolerance Policies Effective in Schools?* Washington, DC: American Psychological Association; 2006:4–5

5. Wraight S. Services for expelled students: overview of research and policy. Naperville, IL: Regional Educational Laboratory Midwest at Learning Point Associates; 2010. Available at: http://dpi.wi.gov/sspw/doc/services4expelled.doc. Accessed October 17, 2012

6. Colorado Foundation for Families and Children. Youth out of school: linking absence to delinquency. Denver, CO: Colorado Foundation for Families and Children; 2002:2–5.

Available at: www.schoolengagement.org/TruancypreventionRegistry/Admin/Resources/Resources/YouthOutofSchoolLinkingAbsencetoDelinquency.pdf. Accessed October 17, 2012

7. Skiba RJ, Eaton J, Sotoo N. *Factors Associated With State Rates of Out-of-School Suspension and Expulsion.* Bloomington, IN: Indiana University, Center for Evaluation and Education Policy; 2004

8. Skiba RJ, Michael RS, Nardo AC, Peterson R. *The Color of Discipline: Sources of Racial and Gender Disproportionality in School Discipline.* Bloomington, IN: Indiana University, Indiana Education Policy Center; 2000

9. Skiba RJ, Rausch MK. Zero tolerance, suspension and expulsion: questions of equity and effectiveness. In: Evertson CM, Weinstein CS, eds. *Handbook of Classroom Management: Research, Practice and Contemporary Issues.* Mahwah, NJ: Erlbaum; 2006:1063–1089

10. Atkins MS, McKay MM, Frazier SL, et al. Suspensions and detentions in an urban, low-income school: punishment or reward? *J Abnorm Child Psychol.* 2002;30(4):361–371

11. Shore R, Shore B. Kids count indicator brief: reducing the high school dropout rate. Baltimore, MD: The Anna E. Casey Foundation; 2009. Available at: www.aecf.org/~/media/Pubs/Initiatives/KIDS%20COUNT/K/KIDSCOUNTIndicatorBriefReducingtheHighSchoolD/HighSchoolDropouts.pdf. Accessed October 17, 2012

12. National Institutes of Health. Pathways linking education to health. Washington, DC: National Institutes of Health; 2003. Available at: www.federalgrants.com/PATHWAYS-LINKING-EDUCATION-TO-HEALTH-4663.html. Accessed October 17, 2012

13. Wong MD, Shapiro MF, Boscardin WJ, Ettner SL. Contribution of major diseases to dis-

parities in mortality. *N Engl J Med.* 2002;347 (20):1585–1592

14. Meuning P, ed. Issue brief: healthier and wealthier: decreasing healthcare costs by increasing educational attainment. November 1, 2006; Washington, DC: Alliance for Excellent Education; 2006. Available at: www.all4ed.org/files/HandW.pdf. Accessed October 17, 2012

15. Gilliam WS. Implementing policies to reduce the likelihood of preschool expulsion. FCP Policy Brief No 7. New York, NY: Foundation for Child Development; January 2008. Available at: www.fcd-us.org/. Accessed October 17, 2012

16. Gilliam WS, Shahar G. Preschool and child care expulsion and suspension: rates and predictors in one state. *Infants Young Child.* 2006;19(3):228–245

17. Kochhar-Bryant CA, White DL. Issue Brief: Early Care and Education. *Hamilton Fish Institute Reports and Essays Serial.* Washington, DC: Hamilton Fish Institute, The George Washington University; April 2007

18. National Scientific Council on the Developing Child. *The Science of Early Childhood Development: Closing the Gap Between What We Know and What We Do.* Cambridge, MA: Harvard University, National Scientific Council on the Developing Child; 2007

19. Division of Adolescent and School Health, National Center for Chronic Disease Prevention and Health Promotion, Centers for Disease Control and Prevention; Public Health Law Program, Office of Chief of Public Health Practice, Centers for Disease Control and Prevention; the Centers for Law and the Public's Health: A Collaborative at Johns Hopkins and Georgetown Universities. A CDC review of school laws and policies concerning child and adolescent health. *J Sch Health.* 2008;78(2):69–128

20. Zimmerman FJ, Glew GM, Christakis DA, Katon W. Early cognitive stimulation, emotional support, and television watching as predictors of subsequent bullying among grade-school children. *Arch Pediatr Adolesc Med.* 2005;159(4): 384–388

21. Shonkoff JP, Garner AS; Committee on Psychosocial Aspects of Child and Family Health; Committee on Early Childhood, Adoption, and Dependent Care; Section on Developmental and Behavioral Pediatrics. The lifelong effects of early childhood adversity and toxic stress. *Pediatrics.* 2012; 129(1). Available at: www.pediatrics.org/cgi/content/full/129/1/e232

22. American Academy of Pediatrics, Committee on Psychosocial Aspects of Child and Family Health, Committee on Early Childhood, Adoption, and Dependent Care, Section on Developmental and Behavioral Pediatrics. Policy statement: early childhood adversity, toxic stress, and the role of the pediatrician: translating developmental science into lifelong health. *Pediatrics.* 2012;129(1). Available at: www.pediatrics.org/cgi/content/full/129/1/e224

23. Begle AM, Dumas JE. Child and parental outcomes following involvement in a preventive intervention: efficacy of the PACE program. *J Prim Prev.* 2011;32(2):67–81

24. Foy JM, Perrin J; American Academy of Pediatrics Task Force on Mental Health. Enhancing pediatric mental health care:

strategies for preparing a community. *Pediatrics.* 2010;125(suppl 3):S75–S86

25. Hagan JF, Jr, Shaw JS, Duncan P, eds. *Bright Futures: Guidelines for Health Supervision of Infants, Children, and Adolescents*, 3rd ed. Elk Grove Village, IL: American Academy of Pediatrics; 2008

26. Taras HL; American Academy of Pediatrics Committee on School Health. School-based mental health services. *Pediatrics.* 2004;113 (6):1839–1845

27. Skiba RJ, Sprague J. Safety without suspensions. *Educ Leadersh.* 2008;66(1):38–43

28. Horner R, Sugai G. *School-wide Positive Behavior Support: Implementers' Blueprint and Self-Assessment.* Eugene, OR: OSEP Center on Positive Behavioral Interventions and Supports, University of Oregon; 2004

29. Alberto PA, Troutman AC. *Applied Behavioral Analysis for Teachers*, 8th ed. Englewood Cliffs, NJ: Merrill/Prentice-Hall; 2009

30. Peterson RL. Ten alternatives to suspension. In: Gaylord V, Quinn M, McComas J, Lehr C, eds. *Impact: Feature Issue on Fostering Success in School and Beyond for Students With Emotional/Behavioral Disorders.* 2005;18(2). Available at: http://ici.umn.edu/products/impact/182/over5.html. Accessed October 17, 2012

31. Wisconsin Department of Public Instruction, Student Services Prevention and Wellness Team. Alternatives to expulsion: case studies in Wisconsin school districts. Madison, WI: Wisconsin Department of Public Instruction;

March 2009. Available at: http://dpi.wi.gov/sspw/index.html. Accessed October 17, 2012

32. Horner RH, Sugai G, Anderson CM. Examining the evidence base for school-wide positive behavior support. *Focus on Exceptional Children.* 2010;42(8):1–14

33. Bradshaw CP, Waasdorp TE, Leaf PJ. Effects of school-wide positive behavioral interventions and supports on child behavior problems. *Pediatrics.* 2012;130(5). Available at: www.pediatrics.org/cgi/content/full/130/5/e1136

34. US Department of Education, Office of Special Education Programs Technical Assistance Center on Positive Behavior Interventions and Supports. Available at: www.pbis.org. Accessed October 17, 2012

35. Glew GM, Fan MY, Katon W, Rivara FP. Bullying and school safety. *J Pediatr.* 2008;152 (1):123–128, 128, e1

36. Olweus D. What we know about bullying. In: Dunn J, ed. *Bullying at School.* Malden, MA: Blackwell; 1993:9

37. Committee on Injury, Violence, and Poison Prevention. Policy statement—Role of the pediatrician in youth violence prevention. *Pediatrics.* 2009;124(1):393–402

38. Hoover J, Stenhjem P. Bullying and teasing of youth with disabilities: creating positive school environments for effective inclusion. National Center on Secondary Education and Transition Issue Brief. 2003;2(3). Available at: www.ncset.org/publications/issue/ncsetissuebrief_2.3.pdf. Accessed October 17, 2012

Parental Leave for Residents and Pediatric Training Programs

- *Policy Statement*

POLICY STATEMENT

Parental Leave for Residents and Pediatric Training Programs

SECTION ON MEDICAL STUDENTS, RESIDENTS, AND FELLOWSHIP TRAINEES and COMMITTEE ON EARLY CHILDHOOD

KEY WORDS
Family and Medical Leave Act, FMLA, parental leave, residency program

ABBREVIATIONS
AAP—American Academy of Pediatrics
ABP—American Board of Pediatrics
ACGME—Accreditation Council for Graduate Medical Education
FMLA—Family and Medical Leave Act

www.pediatrics.org/cgi/doi/10.1542/peds.2012-3542

doi:10.1542/peds.2012-3542

PEDIATRICS (ISSN Numbers: Print, 0031-4005; Online, 1098-4275).

abstract

The American Academy of Pediatrics (AAP) is committed to the development of rational, equitable, and effective parental leave policies that are sensitive to the needs of pediatric residents, families, and developing infants and that enable parents to spend adequate and good-quality time with their young children. It is important for each residency program to have a policy for parental leave that is written, that is accessible to residents, and that clearly delineates program practices regarding parental leave. At a minimum, a parental leave policy for residents and fellows should conform legally with the Family Medical Leave Act as well as with respective state laws and should meet institutional requirements of the Accreditation Council for Graduate Medical Education for accredited programs. Policies should be well formulated and communicated in a culturally sensitive manner. The AAP advocates for extension of benefits consistent with the Family Medical Leave Act to all residents and interns beginning at the time that pediatric residency training begins. The AAP recommends that regardless of gender, residents who become parents should be guaranteed 6 to 8 weeks, at a minimum, of parental leave with pay after the infant's birth. In addition, in conformance with federal law, the resident should be allowed to extend the leave time when necessary by using paid vacation time or leave without pay. Coparenting, adopting, or fostering of a child should entitle the resident, regardless of gender, to the same amount of paid leave (6–8 weeks) as a person who takes maternity/paternity leave. Flexibility, creativity, and advanced planning are necessary to arrange schedules that optimize resident education and experience, cultivate equity in sharing workloads, and protect pregnant residents from overly strenuous work experiences at critical times of their pregnancies. *Pediatrics* 2013;131:387–390

INTRODUCTION

The Family and Medical Leave Act (FMLA) of 1993 requires employers to grant workers up to 12 weeks of annual unpaid leave for a family member's serious illness. It also specifies that parents be allowed this same amount of leave for the birth or adoption of a child.[1] This federal legislation regarding maternity leave significantly affects residency training programs because approximately one-half of women who enter the field of medicine give birth to their first child during their residency training.[2] This impact is growing, as the percentage of women graduating from medical school has been consistently increasing over the years, from 9.2% in 1970 to 48.8% in 2009.[3] Specific to pediatrics, 53.3% of pediatricians in 2006 were women and that percentage had increased to 69% by 2009.[3,4]

As an advocate for children and their families, the American Academy of Pediatrics (AAP) supported the passage of the FMLA and is concerned with the need to ensure healthy outcomes for pediatricians and their families. The AAP is committed to the development of rational, equitable, and effective parental leave policies that are sensitive to the needs of pediatric residents, families, and developing infants and that enable parents to spend adequate and good-quality time with their young children. Parent–infant attachment is of paramount importance in the first weeks of life, and protected time at home fosters the development of healthy relationships and practices, such as breastfeeding.[5]

A position statement on parental leave for residents by the American College of Physicians in 1989 noted the increasing number of residents having children and raised concerns about both the health outcomes of the children and the emotional outcomes of the parents.[6] The American Medical Association subsequently adopted a policy that supports maternity, paternity, and adoption leave for residents and recommends that programs develop a detailed written policy regarding leave for residents.[7] All accredited residency training programs are required by the Institutional Requirements of the Accreditation Council for Graduate Medical Education (ACGME) to provide written policies on residents' vacations and other leaves of absence (with or without pay), including parental and sick leave, and these policies must comply with applicable laws, such as the FMLA.[8] By 2006, 90% of pediatric

residency program directors surveyed reported that they have a parental leave policy in place for their program. The mean leave time allowed without having to make up the time was 3 weeks, with a range of maternity leave reported from 0 to 12 weeks.[9]

It is important for each residency program to have a policy for parental leave that is written, that is accessible to residents, and that clearly delineates program practices regarding parental leave. Lack of such a policy forces residents to rely on departmental policies, which are often unclear or not as relevant to a resident in training. Lack of clarity regarding leave practices can lead to anxiety for the resident expecting a child, and the resident often faces resentment from colleagues for the extra work they must do in the resident's prolonged absence. Without a clear, written policy outlining expectations for the program and for the resident who is expecting a child, advance planning is not as likely to occur, and unplanned absences can adversely affect the work schedules of peers. Morale problems among residency groups may be exacerbated by surprise or sudden strategies that are used to replace or to cover absent residents, and inconsistencies in departmental policies within and among programs can cause discord. In addition, from a patient-care standpoint, conflicts regarding the balance of work and personal life among residents and faculty members are associated with increased reports of stress and burnout,[10,11] which can be linked to increased rates of medical errors.[12,13]

Although each program must develop its own methods to provide appropriate coverage for anticipated or unanticipated parental leave, certain basic guidelines should apply. At a minimum, a parental leave policy for residents and fellows should conform

legally with the FMLA as well as respective state laws and should meet Institutional Requirements of the ACGME for accredited programs. Policies should be well formulated and communicated in a culturally sensitive manner.

SUMMARY OF RECOMMENDATIONS

FMLA

Federal law requires that employees be eligible for FMLA benefits after they have been employed for 12 months, which means that, during the first year of pediatric residency training, "interns" (eg, postgraduate year 1 trainees) would not be eligible for the FMLA. The AAP advocates for extension of benefits consistent with FMLA to all residents and interns beginning at the time that pediatric residency training begins, which would give a resident or intern 3 months per year of leave without pay and mandates that health insurance benefits be continued by the employer during this time. The AAP advocates for the same coverage for fellows at the beginning of training.

Parental Leave

The duration of maternity leave, both before and after the infant's birth, should be determined in conjunction with the pregnant resident and her physician and should be based on her condition and needs and on the condition of the child. The AAP recommends that regardless of gender, the resident who becomes a parent should be guaranteed 6 to 8 weeks, at a minimum, of parental leave with pay after the infant's birth. In addition, in conformance with federal law, the resident should be allowed to extend the leave time when necessary by using paid vacation time or leave without pay. The resident who is a new parent but not the primary caregiver is also entitled to parental leave. For these residents, program directors may require that parental leave in excess of 2 weeks draw on unused vacation time followed by leave without pay. It is preferable, however, to protect and preserve vacation, sick leave, and time scheduled for elective rotations. Parents in nontraditional families should receive the same leave as parents in traditional families.

Adoption and Foster Care Leave

Adoption or fostering of a child should entitle the resident, regardless of gender, to the same amount of paid leave (6–8 weeks) as a person who takes maternity leave. Extensions should be allowed as leave without pay.

Work Conditions During Pregnancy

Attention should be paid to tailoring resident work schedules during pregnancy to the medical and emotional needs of the pregnant resident while maintaining an emphasis on professional responsibilities. Increases in adverse pregnancy outcomes have been observed with strenuous working conditions.[14] Specifically, increases in pregnancy complications, such as preterm labor, pre-eclampsia, and fetal growth restriction, have been associated with strenuous working conditions during residency training.[15–17] Flexibility, creativity, and advanced planning are necessary to arrange schedules that optimize resident education and experience, cultivate equity in sharing workloads, and protect pregnant residents from overly strenuous work experiences at critical times of their pregnancy.

Training Status and Makeup Time

The duration of training in an accredited program required by the American Board of Pediatrics (ABP) is 36 months, with 33 months of clinical training required (allowing for vacation, illness, and parental leave). Res-

idents who take maternity, paternity, or adoption leave should, therefore, have no loss in training status if their total leave from training has not been more than 3 months. Total absences in excess of 3 months require a written explanation and justification by the program director and would present unique salary complications requiring case-by-case resolution. The program director, therefore, plays an essential role in the certification process, but the Credentials Committee of the ABP must review the circumstances and approve the extended leave. Makeup time for an absence beyond 3 months is indicated to meet the training requirements for board certification. The topic of leave and makeup time for residents in combined training programs (eg, internal medicine and pediatrics) is more complicated and is beyond the scope of this policy statement; the ABP Web site offers more information on this topic (https://www.abp.org/abpwebsite/publicat/certboi.pdf).

Issues Regarding Staffing and Scheduling

Each program should determine the most satisfactory and cost-effective approach to providing appropriate coverage during parental leave. Residency program staffing levels should be flexible enough to allow for coverage without creating an intolerable burden on the other residents. Some programs might rely on physician assistants and/or advanced practice nurses to provide intermittent coverage for residents in these cases. Programs could consider offering incentives or otherwise recognizing those residents who take on additional work for a resident on leave (realizing additional work cannot exceed work-hour limitations). Each residency program should attempt to anticipate the number of residents who will take parental leave to project

staffing needs and to prepare annual program budgets. To accomplish this effectively, residents should be professional and responsible and should notify the program director of anticipated leave far in advance, whenever possible. Such notification should be a requirement written into program policy. Programs should consider incorporating training regarding these professional challenges when planning residency curriculum.

Other Issues

Programs need to develop specific written policies for providing family medical leave for residents to permit them to be at home to care for an ill child, spouse, life partner, or parent.

Flexibility of staffing and scheduling issues are affected by current and future limitations that the ACGME places on the number of hours each resident is allowed to work per day or per week. Work hours are limited for the sake of patient safety; such policies do, however, limit the ability of other residents to take on the workload of residents who are on leave and limit the degree to which program directors can allow flexibility for residents to make up leave time. Decisions regarding leave time and makeup time, therefore, must not negatively affect patient safety and must be in accordance with ACGME work-hour requirements.

LEAD AUTHORS
Jill J. Fussell, MD
Lara W. Johnson, MD

SECTION ON MEDICAL STUDENTS, RESIDENTS, AND FELLOWSHIP TRAINEES, 2011–2012
Sarosh Batlivala, MD, Chairperson
Natalie Riedmann, MD
Gayle Haischer-Rollo, MD
Julia Von Oettingen, MD
Yuen Lie Tjoeng, MD
Erin Kelly, MD
Padma Garg, MD
Sara Slovin, MD, MSPH
David Myles, MD

Lauren Becton, MD
Bijoy Thattaliyath, MD
Matthew Hornik, DO
Kimberly Reynolds, MD
Jessie Marks, MD
Maggie Kuehler, MD
Rupal M. Patel, MD
Ashley Lucke, MD
Neha Patel, MD
Faisal Malik, MD
Elizabeth Van Dyne, MD
Nicole Chao, MD
Oneka Marriott, DO, MPH

Melissa Diamond, MD
Renee Matos, MD

COMMITTEE ON EARLY CHILDHOOD, 2011–2012

Elaine Donoghue, MD, Chairperson
Jill J. Fussell, MD
Mary Margaret Gleason, MD
Veronnie F. Jones, MD
Alan L. Mendelsohn, MD
Elaine E. Schulte, MD, MPH
Patricia Gail Williams, MD

LIAISONS

Barbara U. Hamilton, MA – *Maternal and Child Health Bureau*
Claire Lerner, LCSW – *Zero to Three*
Stephanie Olmore – *National Association for the Education of Young Children*

STAFF

Sonya Clay
Julie Raymond
Charlotte Zia, MPH, CHES

REFERENCES

1. United States Department of Labor. Family Medical Leave Act of 1993. Pub L No. 103-3, 29 USC 2601. Available at: www.dol.gov/whd/fmla/index.htm. Accessed March 12, 2012

2. American Medical Women's Association. Position paper: pregnancy during schooling, training, and early practice years. Available at: www.amwa-doc.org/gallery2-216/PregnancyDuringSchooling. Accessed March 12, 2012

3. Leadley J. Women in U.S. academic medicine: statistics and medical school benchmarking, 2008-2009. Available at: https://www.aamc.org/download/53502/data/wimstatisticsreport2009.pdf. Accessed March 12, 2012

4. American Medical Association. *Physician Characteristics and Distribution in the US, 2008 Edition.* Chicago, IL: American Medical Association; 2008

5. Sattari M, Levine D, Serwint JR. Physician mothers: an unlikely high risk group-call for action. *Breastfeed Med.* 2010;5(1):35–39

6. American College of Physicians. Parental leave for residents. *Ann Intern Med.* 1989;111(12):1035–1038

7. American Medical Association Policy H-420. 987: maternity leave policies. Available at: https://ssl3.ama-assn.org/apps/ecomm/PolicyFinderForm.pl?site=www.ama-assn.org&uri=%2fresources%2fdoc%2fPolicyFinder%2fpolicyfiles%2fHnE%2fH-420.967.HTM. Accessed March 12, 2012

8. Accreditation Council of Graduate Medical Education. Institutional Requirements, Benefits and Conditions of Appointment, Requirement II.C. Available at: www.acgme.org/acWebsite/irc/irc_IRCpr07012007.pdf. Accessed March 12, 2012

9. McPhillips HA, Burke AE, Sheppard K, Pallant A, Stapleton FB, Stanton B. Toward creating family-friendly work environments in pediatrics: baseline data from pediatric department chairs and pediatric program directors. *Pediatrics.* 2007;119(3). Available at: www.pediatrics.org/cgi/content/full/119/3/e596

10. Barton LL, Friedman AD, Locke CJ. Stress in pediatric faculty. Results of a national survey. *Arch Pediatr Adolesc Med.* 1995;149(7):751–757

11. Kahn JA, Parsons SK, Pizzo PA, Newburger JW, Homer CJ. Work-family issues and perceptions of stress among pediatric faculty and house staff. *Ambul Pediatr.* 2001;1(3):141–149

12. Shanafelt TD, Bradley KA, Wipf JE, Back AL. Burnout and self-reported patient care in an internal medicine residency program. *Ann Intern Med.* 2002;136(5):358–367

13. Fahrenkopf AM, Sectish TC, Barger LK, et al. Rates of medication errors among depressed and burnt out residents: prospective cohort study. *BMJ.* 2008;336(7642):488–491

14. Mozurkewich EL, Luke B, Avni M, Wolf FM. Working conditions and adverse pregnancy outcome: a meta-analysis. *Obstet Gynecol.* 2000;95(4):623–635

15. Klebanoff MA, Shiono PH, Rhoads GG. Outcomes of pregnancy in a national sample of resident physicians. *N Engl J Med.* 1990;323(15):1040–1045

16. Gabbe SG, Morgan MA, Power ML, Schulkin J, Williams SB. Duty hours and pregnancy outcome among residents in obstetrics and gynecology. *Obstet Gynecol.* 2003;102(5 pt 1):948–951

17. Finch SJ. Pregnancy during residency: a literature review. *Acad Med.* 2003;78(4):418–428

Pediatric Palliative Care and Hospice Care Commitments, Guidelines, and Recommendations

- *Policy Statement*

POLICY STATEMENT

Pediatric Palliative Care and Hospice Care Commitments, Guidelines, and Recommendations

abstract

Pediatric palliative care and pediatric hospice care (PPC-PHC) are often essential aspects of medical care for patients who have life-threatening conditions or need end-of-life care. PPC-PHC aims to relieve suffering, improve quality of life, facilitate informed decision-making, and assist in care coordination between clinicians and across sites of care. Core commitments of PPC-PHC include being patient centered and family engaged; respecting and partnering with patients and families; pursuing care that is high quality, readily accessible, and equitable; providing care across the age spectrum and life span, integrated into the continuum of care; ensuring that all clinicians can provide basic palliative care and consult PPC-PHC specialists in a timely manner; and improving care through research and quality improvement efforts. PPC-PHC guidelines and recommendations include ensuring that all large health care organizations serving children with life-threatening conditions have dedicated interdisciplinary PPC-PHC teams, which should develop collaborative relationships between hospital- and community-based teams; that PPC-PHC be provided as integrated multimodal care and practiced as a cornerstone of patient safety and quality for patients with life-threatening conditions; that PPC-PHC teams should facilitate clear, compassionate, and forthright discussions about medical issues and the goals of care and support families, siblings, and health care staff; that PPC-PHC be part of all pediatric education and training curricula, be an active area of research and quality improvement, and exemplify the highest ethical standards; and that PPC-PHC services be supported by financial and regulatory arrangements to ensure access to high-quality PPC-PHC by all patients with life-threatening and life-shortening diseases. *Pediatrics* 2013;132:966–972

SECTION ON HOSPICE AND PALLIATIVE MEDICINE AND COMMITTEE ON HOSPITAL CARE

KEY WORDS
pediatric, fetus, newborn, infant, child, adolescent, young adult, palliative care, hospice care

ABBREVIATIONS
AAP—American Academy of Pediatrics
PPC-PHC—pediatric palliative care and pediatric hospice care

www.pediatrics.org/cgi/doi/10.1542/peds.2013-2731

doi:10.1542/peds.2013-2731

PEDIATRICS (ISSN Numbers: Print, 0031-4005; Online, 1098-4275).

INTRODUCTION

Over the past two decades, pediatric palliative care has emerged as an established field of medical expertise and practice.[1–3] Recognized in 2006 by the American Board of Medical Specialties, hospice and palliative medicine is the field of medical expertise that seeks to improve quality of life and reduce various forms of distress for patients and their families in the face of serious life-threatening or inevitably life-shortening conditions or when end-of-life care or bereavement services are needed. Pediatric palliative care addresses the needs of infants, children, adolescents, and young adults (subsequently referred to collectively as "children") with these conditions and the needs of their families, providing treatments that aim to (1) relieve suffering across multiple realms, including the physical (eg, pain or dyspnea), psychological (depression, anxiety, or sense of guilt), social (isolation), practical (home-based services or financial stress), and existential or spiritual (why is this happening?); (2) improve the child's quality and enjoyment of life while helping families adapt and function during the illness and through bereavement; (3) facilitate informed decision-making by patients, families, and health care professionals; and (4) assist with ongoing coordination of care among clinicians and across various sites of care.[4–7]

Hospice care is a particular form of palliative care, delivered in the United States by licensed hospice agencies. As mandated by federal regulation, these agencies provide a bundle of services, including nursing, physician, psychosocial, and spiritual services; medications; durable medical equipment; and a range of diagnostic tests and therapeutic interventions. These services are financed by an all-inclusive per-diem rate and most often are provided in the home setting for pediatric patients. As with adult patients, these services also can be provided in dedicated inpatient hospice beds or units within hospitals, self-standing hospice centers, and long-term care facilities. Also by regulation, hospice care is provided by an interdisciplinary team including physicians, nurses, chaplains, social workers, home health aides, therapists, volunteers, and bereavement counselors. At present, hospice is a widely available palliative care option in the United States for adults but often is not a viable option for pediatric patients, for two principal reasons. First, few hospices currently have the capacity to care for infants,

children, and adolescents, because pediatric treatment plans are sometimes too unfamiliar, complex, and costly for traditional hospice programs. Second, insurance coverage is often restricted or limited. Following the mandates specified in the Medicare hospice benefit, most public and private payers specify that to qualify for hospice services, the patient must have a life expectancy of 6 months or less if the disease follows its expected course, and enrolling in hospice typically entails curtailment of other health care services. However, the Patient Protection and Affordable Care Act (2010 [Pub L No. 111-148]) specifies that children enrolled in Medicaid or the Children's Health Insurance Program can concurrently receive both hospice services and life-extending disease-directed therapy.[8] Although individual physician consultation is a billable service, pediatric palliative care services per se, particularly those performed by nonclinician members of the interdisciplinary team, are typically not covered by either public or private insurance payers except for small pilot programs.[9]

Pediatric palliative care and pediatric hospice care (PPC-PHC) teams collaborate to serve the needs of families and children living with life-threatening conditions. These services are more extensive and of much longer duration than end-of-life services, because PPC-PHC teams are often appropriately used by most patients for months to years.[10]

The American Academy of Pediatrics (AAP) continues to advocate for the development, adoption, and adherence to clinical policies and guidelines that promote the welfare of children living with life-threatening conditions and their families, with goals including the provision of accessible, equitable, and effective support for cure-directed, life-prolonging, and palliative care. While incorporating advances in this field and

acknowledging the need for additional clinical and health service research, this statement reflects current expert consensus as it reaffirms the principles of the original AAP statement published in 2000.[11]

PALLIATIVE CARE AND HOSPICE CARE COMMITMENTS

The following core commitments serve as the foundation for an integrated model of PPC-PHC.

Patient Centered and Family Engaged

PPC-PHC is centered on the child, with a constant commitment to providing the best possible care for that child in a manner that fully engages, respects, and partners with the patient's family.[12]

Respect and Partnering

Respect is manifested by partnering with the child and family, soliciting their understanding of the child's medical condition, eliciting and clarifying their values and preferences, and formulating a plan of care based on those values and preferences in partnership with the patient and family. The child should participate to the fullest extent possible, given his or her preferences, cultural and spiritual tradition, illness experience, developmental capacity, and level of consciousness. Consistent with this principle of respect, information about palliative care should be readily available, and policies should allow patients and parents to initiate referral to a pediatric palliative care program.

Quality, Access, and Equity

PPC-PHC seeks to provide equal access for all patients and families to high-quality and effective interventions to ameliorate pain and other distressing physical and psychological symptoms as well as social, practical, and spiritual sources of distress.[13] PPC-PHC programs should adhere to established

PPC-PHC quality metrics and guidelines.[14]

In contrast to quality metrics being monitored in adult hospice and palliative medicine, the place where death occurs is not an appropriate quality of care indicator for PPC-PHC.[15] The location may depend on such factors as the wishes of the child and family, the physical layout and geographic location of the home, and for children who reside in a facility, the policies of the facility and the desire and ability of staff to provide the necessary care. For these reasons, admission (or readmission) to the hospital of a patient for symptom management or end-of-life care may be warranted.

Care Across Age Spectrum and Life Span

The PPC-PHC team is committed to caring for patients with conditions and illnesses that develop prenatally or during infancy, childhood, or adolescence, even when these patients age into adulthood (which is occurring for an increasing number of patients with a wide range of serious life-threatening conditions). Ideally, this commitment should be honored by promoting timely transitioning of care to comprehensive, high-quality adult-oriented services for people with pediatric-specialty conditions, and these services should be developed and supported so that transitions can occur smoothly and safely.[16] When such transitions cannot be guaranteed, however, the commitment to high-quality care remains for the pediatric providers. Furthermore, when a patient dies, the commitment to the family continues during the period of bereavement.

Integration Into the Continuum of Care

For all patients, high-quality PPC-PHC should routinely prevent and treat distressing symptoms, such as pain, nausea, or anxiety, and seek to maximize quality of life, which may entail various interventions depending on the patient's specific goals. Dedicated specialty PPC-PHC teams should be consulted for advanced clinical treatments and complicated decision-making and for social and spiritual needs beyond what the primary care team can provide. These consultations can occur throughout a child's illness experience, including at initial diagnosis, when the goals of care are focused on cure. PPC-PHC should be integrated throughout the illness course, providing interventions to support the goals of care, which often shift over time. After initiating a PPC-PHC consultation, the patient's medical home and all providers (including primary pediatricians or family medicine physicians, pediatric specialists, and surgeons) should remain fully engaged in the well-coordinated care for the child.

Universal Preparedness and Consultation

All physicians should be trained in basic approaches to prevent, assess, and manage symptoms and to communicate in a clear, caring, and collaborative manner with patients and families. All physicians should also be able to recognize when and how to consult with PPC-PHC specialists and how to inform patients and families of the role PPC-PHC specialists play to ensure that patient care is consistent with best practices.

Research and Continuous Improvement

PPC-PHC should vigorously promote and pursue rigorous research and quality improvement projects in all aspects of interdisciplinary care, including evaluation of specific pharmacologic and nonpharmacologic interventions to alleviate symptoms; medical and psychosocial interventions to improve quality of decision-making and quality of life for patients and family members; various modes of education and training to improve clinicians' knowledge, attitudes, skills, and behaviors; and different program or service delivery models to improve access, outcomes, and cost-effectiveness.[17–21]

GUIDELINES AND RECOMMENDATIONS

The following 12 guidelines and recommendations are based on a combination of published observational studies, expert opinion, and consensus statements.

1. Composition and Capacity of PPC-PHC Specialty Teams

All hospitals and large health care organizations that frequently provide care to children with life-threatening conditions and routinely provide end-of-life care should have dedicated interdisciplinary specialty PPC-PHC teams. These teams should support decision-making, provide timely and effective interventions to minimize suffering while maximizing quality of life, and manage and coordinate the logistics of care to provide seamless transitions between settings and maintain the highest possible quality of care. Teams should have sufficient collective expertise to address the physical, psychosocial, emotional, practical, and spiritual needs of the child and family. Although programs often start with only a few team members, mature teams should include physicians, nurses, social workers, case managers, spiritual care providers, bereavement specialists, and child life specialists. To ensure quality and safety, teams must have an adequate number of dedicated staff, ideally trained in PPC-PHC, be paid specifically to provide pediatric palliative care, and be available for consultation anytime. These consultative activities should bridge the physical locations of patients, from their homes or schools to the hospital and, potentially, to other partnering facilities.

2. Relationships With Hospices and Hospice Pediatric Standards

PPC-PHC teams in geographic regions should proactively develop collaborative relationships.[22,23] Despite steady growth in the hospice industry, recent evidence indicates that hospices willing to care for children are decreasing in number.[24] All hospices are encouraged to provide care to children to maintain a core level of competency; hospices caring for children should adhere to the National Hospice and Palliative Care Organization Standards of Practice for Pediatric Palliative Care and Hospice.[14,25]

3. Collaborative Integrated Multimodal Care

PPC-PHC should be provided as collaborative integrated multimodal care, including cure-seeking, life-prolonging (when in the child's best interest), comfort-enhancing, and quality-of-life enriching modes of care, along with psychological, spiritual, and social support for the family.[26] Collaboration is essential; patient, parents, other involved extended family members and friends, schools, parental employers, and all involved members of the primary and specialty health care team must collaborate to meet the needs of patients most effectively. The medical homes and pediatricians who provide primary and specialty care to children with life-threatening conditions remain invaluable, must advocate for and involve interdisciplinary PPC-PHC in the care of these patients and their families, and, for their patients, may become active members of the interdisciplinary palliative care team.

4. Patient Care Safety and Quality

PPC-PHC is a cornerstone of patient care safety and quality for patients with life-threatening conditions.[15,27] Consultation with PPC-PHC professionals should be considered for complicated pain and other symptom management or when difficult decision-making and communication issues arise. Once consulted, PPC-PHC teams should review all of a child's diagnoses and, if any are uncertain, seek to confirm them. PPC-PHC teams should assist primary and specialty care teams in providing a realistic appraisal of prognosis, including anticipatory guidance about the likelihood of future symptoms, impairments, and mortality, and the timeframe during which these outcomes are likely to occur. Distressing symptoms should be managed promptly and effectively to minimize suffering and avoid unintentional consequences of polypharmacy. Symptom management should be augmented by other services and therapies to maximize the child's quality of life.[28] Bereavement care should be provided for anticipatory grief and continue after the death of a child throughout the bereavement period (which often lasts longer than a year). PPC-PHC teams should conduct ongoing quality improvement reviews and projects aiming to improve patient and family experiences and outcomes.

5. Communication and Decision Support

PPC-PHC clinicians should facilitate clear, compassionate, and forthright discussions with patients and families about therapeutic goals and concerns, the benefits and burdens of specific therapies, and the value of advance care planning. At a minimum, goals of care and treatment choices should be revisited whenever requested by the patient or family, with every hospitalization or with any significant change

in treatment course or prognosis, and at least annually for children with complex chronic conditions. Any changes in goals of care or treatment plan should be communicated to all involved members of the child's care team and medical home. The ability of health care professionals to communicate difficult messages effectively can be learned through directed education and practice.[29–35]

6. Family Support

PPC-PHC clinicians should aim to partner with and support parents throughout the course of the child's illness experience. In addition to addressing issues about the ongoing care of the child, PPC-PHC should aim to facilitate decision-making and help the parents and family cope with the ramifications of living with a serious medical condition. Practical support should include addressing family financial problems or facilitating access to mental health services. Spiritual support should be offered throughout the trajectory of care. Ideally, respite care should be provided. The family should be supported in carrying out important family, religious, or cultural rituals before and after a child dies. Counseling should be provided to the family regarding the potential benefits of additional genetic or metabolic testing of the patient for other family members or future reproductive decision-making. The possibility of organ donation should be addressed by qualified personnel. In addition to providing bereavement services before and after the patient's death, the PPC-PHC team is also encouraged to send a note of sympathy or attend the funeral.[36] Whether an autopsy is performed, provisions should be available to facilitate meetings of clinical staff and families who want to review the course of treatment or causes of the child's death.[37,38]

7. Sibling Support

Siblings of children with life-threatening conditions need attention and support. Health care team members should partner with parents to provide siblings who ask questions with age-appropriate and honest answers and to incorporate siblings in the routine activities of daily living and care of their ill brother or sister. Child life, art, music, and other therapists, as well as psychological and bereavement counselors based in the hospital or community, should be available to help siblings express and process their thoughts and emotions.

8. Health Care Staff Support

Support of all health care professionals, including the PPC-PHC team, is crucial to the well-being and continued ability of staff to meet the needs of families and children who have serious life-threatening or inevitably life-shortening conditions. The psychological, spiritual, and ethical needs of these health care professionals should be proactively addressed by PPC-PHC clinicians via peer-to-peer discussions, group debriefings, psychological and spiritual counseling, and educational programs.

9. Education and Training

All general and subspecialty pediatricians, family physicians, pain specialists, and pediatric surgeons should be able and willing to provide basic pain and symptom management to children and to request timely and appropriate pediatric palliative care consultations. PPC-PHC competencies should be a core part of medical school, residency, fellowship, and continuing education curricula as well as pediatric and subspecialty board certifying examinations. Specifically, these competencies should address interventions to manage pain and symptoms (including pharmacologic and nonpharmacologic methods), specific aspects of end-of-life care, communication skills, decision-making support, ethical issues, and psychological and spiritual dimensions of life and illness, including personal feelings about anxiety and grief. Furthermore, dedicated efforts and initiatives to increase the workforce of PPC-PHC–trained subspecialty clinicians are vital.

10. Research and Quality Improvement

Rigorous observational and experimental research studies using quantitative, qualitative, and mixed methods are needed to improve the effectiveness of PPC-PHC interventions and policies. PPC-PHC teams should support and engage in research endeavors; all programs should have an active quality improvement agenda.

11. Ethical Considerations

The provision of high-quality PPC-PHC can raise a variety of important ethical considerations. The AAP has addressed the ethics of limiting or withdrawing life-sustaining medical treatment, including when anesthesia or a surgical procedure is needed to improve the quality of remaining life or to allow a patient to die at home.[39–43] The AAP has also addressed the special needs of children who have been abused.[44]

On occasion, the relief of severe intractable symptoms, such as pain or dyspnea, may include a rapid escalation in doses of analgesics and sedatives to the point of deep sedation, with the overriding goal of relieving the patient of pain or distress. Whereas palliative sedation for otherwise intractable suffering can be performed in an ethically appropriate manner, requests for euthanasia, assisted suicide, or hastening death cannot be granted but instead should be acknowledged and serve as a starting point of a conversation to elucidate the sources of suffering that often underlie such requests.[45]

PPC-PHC teams should ensure that their organizations have up-to-date institutional policies that address these issues and develop mutually informative relationships with hospital or organizational ethics committees.[46]

12. Financial and Regulatory Issues

PPC-PHC services must be paid equitably in hospital, ambulatory, and home settings by both private and public insurance. Payment systems based on relative value units and other current productivity measures do not compensate adequately for clinician time in providing decision support, complex symptom management, phone conversations, tele–health care, home visits, and care coordination, and therefore staffing of PPC-PHC teams should not be constrained by these metrics. In addition to patient-specific interventions, payment should also be provided for clinical decision-making support activities (eg, meetings with the patient or family, including perinatal meetings), respite for family caregivers, and bereavement interventions for the family even after the patient's death.

Current regulations should be modified by (1) broadening hospice eligibility criteria by expanding life expectancy criteria, (2) specifying that concurrent care includes all routine forms of life-prolonging care (eg, home nursing care) in addition to palliative care, (3) enabling provision of respite care and other therapies that benefit the child by benefiting other members of the child's family, and (4) ensuring that adequate payment accompanies these regulatory changes.

CONCLUSIONS

High-quality PPC-PHC embodies core commitments that represent a fundamental promise to care for all children with serious life-threatening and inevitably life-shortening conditions and their families. Adherence to the guidelines and recommendations affirmed in this policy will advance our ability to keep this promise and ensure that health care teams are appropriately resourced, trained, and positioned to provide excellent care.

LEAD AUTHORS

Chris Feudtner, MD, PhD, MPH, FAAP
Sarah Friebert, MD, FAAP
Jennifer Jewell, MD, FAAP

SECTION ON HOSPICE AND PALLIATIVE MEDICINE EXECUTIVE COMMITTEE, 2012–2013

Brian Carter, MD, FAAP, Chairperson
Sarah Friebert, MD, FAAP, Immediate Past Chairperson
Chris Feudtner, MD, PhD, MPH, FAAP
Jeffrey Klick, MD, FAAP
Kelly Komatz, MD, FAAP

Jennifer Linebarger, MD, MPH, FAAP
Julie Hauer, MD, FAAP

FORMER EXECUTIVE COMMITTEE MEMBERS

Margaret Hood, MD, FAAP
Sonia Imaizumi, MD, FAAP

STAFF

Madra Guinn-Jones, MPH

COMMITTEE ON HOSPITAL CARE, 2012–2013

Jack M. Percelay, MD, MPH, FAAP, Chairperson
James M. Betts, MD, FAAP
Maribeth B. Chitkara, MD, FAAP
Jennifer A. Jewell, MD, FAAP
Claudia K. Preuschoff, MD, FAAP

FORMER COMMITTEE MEMBER

Patricia S. Lye, MD, FAAP

LIAISONS

Richard A. Salerno, MD, MS, FAAP – *Section on Critical Care*
Charles D. Vinocur, MD, FAAP – *Section on Surgery*
Chris Brown, MS, CCLS – *Child Life Council*
Charlotte Ipsan, MSN, NNP – *American Hospital Association*
Lynne Lostocco, RN, MSN – *Children's Hospital Association*

CONSULTANTS

Matthew Scanlon, MD, FAAP – *The Joint Commission Hospital Professional and Technical Advisory Committee*
Martin Wakeham, MD, FAAP – *Alternate Consultant, The Joint Commission Hospital Professional and Technical Advisory Committee*

STAFF

S. Niccole Alexander, MPP

REFERENCES

1. Carter BS, Levetown M, Friebert SE. *Palliative Care for Infants, Children, and Adolescents: A Practical Handbook.* 2nd ed. Baltimore: Johns Hopkins University Press; 2011

2. Goldman A, Hain R, Liben S. *Oxford Textbook of Palliative Care for Children.* Oxford: Oxford University Press; 2006

3. Wolfe J, Hinds PS, Sourkes BM. *Textbook of Interdisciplinary Pediatric Palliative Care.* Philadelphia: Elsevier/Saunders; 2011

4. Himelstein BP, Hilden JM, Boldt AM, Weissman D. Pediatric palliative care. *N Engl J Med.* 2004;350(17):1752–1762

5. Liben S, Papadatou D, Wolfe J. Paediatric palliative care: challenges and emerging ideas. *Lancet.* 2008;371(9615):852–864

6. Hain R, Heckford E, McCulloch R. Paediatric palliative medicine in the UK: past, present, future. *Arch Dis Child.* 2012;97(4):381–384

7. Kang T, Hoehn KS, Licht DJ, et al. Pediatric palliative, end-of-life, and bereavement care. *Pediatr Clin North Am.* 2005;52(4):1029–1046, viii.

8. United States Congress. *Compilation of Patient Protection and Affordable Care Act: As Amended Through November 1, 2010 Including Patient Protection and Affordable Care Act Health-Related Portions of the Health Care and Education Reconciliation Act of 2010.* Washington, DC: U.S. Government Printing Office; 2010

9. The Catalyst Center. Improving Financing of Care for Children and Youth with Special Health Care Needs. Financing Pediatric Palliative and Hospice Care Programs. Available at: http://hdwg.org/catalyst/node/197. Accessed June 25, 2013

10. Feudtner C, Kang TI, Hexem KR, et al. Pediatric palliative care patients: a prospective multicenter cohort study. *Pediatrics.* 2011; 127(6):1094–1101

11. American Academy of Pediatrics. Committee on Bioethics and Committee on Hospital Care. Palliative care for children. *Pediatrics.* 2000;106(2 pt 1):351–357.

12. Committee on Hospital Care and Institute for Patient- and Family-Centered Care. Patient- and family-centered care and the pediatrician's role. *Pediatrics.* 2012;129(2):394–404

13. Council on Community Pediatrics and Committee on Native American Child Health. Policy statement: health equity and children's rights. *Pediatrics.* 2010;125(4):838–849

14. National Hospice and Palliative Care Organization. Standards of Practice for Hospice Programs. Alexandria, VA: National Hospice and Palliative Care Organization; 2010. Available at: http://www.nhpco.org/sites/default/files/public/quality/Standards/NHPCO_STANDARDS_2010CD.pdf. Accessed September 13, 2013

15. Hodgson ES, Simpson L, Lannon CM; American Academy of Pediatrics Steering Committee on Quality Improvement and Management; American Academy of Pediatrics Committee on Practice and Ambulatory Medicine. Principles for the development and use of quality measures. *Pediatrics.* 2008; 121(2):411–418

16. Cooley WC, Sagerman PJ; American Academy of Pediatrics; American Academy of Family Physicians; American College of Physicians; Transitions Clinical Report Authoring Group. Supporting the health care transition from adolescence to adulthood in the medical home. *Pediatrics.* 2011; 128(1):182–200

17. Feudtner C. Perspectives on quality at the end of life. *Arch Pediatr Adolesc Med.* 2004; 158(5):415–418

18. Solomon MZ, Sellers DE, Heller KS, et al. New and lingering controversies in pediatric end-of-life care. *Pediatrics.* 2005;116(4):872–883

19. Browning DM, Solomon MZ. Relational learning in pediatric palliative care: transformative education and the culture of medicine. *Child Adolesc Psychiatr Clin N Am.* 2006;15(3):795–815

20. Ullrich C, Morrison RS. Pediatric palliative care research comes of age: what we stand to learn from children with life-threatening illness. *J Palliat Med.* 2013;16(4):334–336

21. Keele L, Keenan HT, Sheetz J, Bratton SL. Differences in characteristics of dying children who receive and do not receive palliative care. *Pediatrics*. 2013;132(1):72–78

22. Carroll JM, Torkildson C, Winsness JS. Issues related to providing quality pediatric palliative care in the community. *Pediatr Clin North Am*. 2007;54(5):813–827, xiii.

23. Carroll JM, Santucci G, Kang TI, Feudtner C. Partners in Pediatric Palliative Care: a program to enhance collaboration between hospital and community palliative care services. *Am J Hosp Palliat Care*. 2007;24 (3):191–195

24. Lindley LC, Mark BA, Daniel Lee SY, Domino M, Song MK, Jacobson Vann J. Factors associated with the provision of hospice care for children. *J Pain Symptom Manage*. 2013;45(4):701–711

25. National Hospice and Palliative Care Organization. Standards of Practice for Pediatric Palliative Care and Hospice. Alexandria, VA: National Hospice and Palliative Care Organization; 2010. Available at: http://www. nhpco.org/sites/default/files/public/quality/ Ped_Pall_Care%20_Standard.pdf. Accessed September 13, 2013

26. Feudtner C, Mott AR. Expanding the envelope of care. *Arch Pediatr Adolesc Med*. 2012;166(8):772–773

27. Steering Committee on Quality Improvement and Management and Committee on Hospital Care. Policy statement—principles of pediatric patient safety: reducing harm due to medical care. *Pediatrics*. 2011;127(6): 1199–1210

28. Wilson JM; American Academy of Pediatrics Child Life Council and Committee on Hospital Care. Child life services. *Pediatrics*. 2006;118(4):1757–1763

29. Hurwitz CA, Duncan J, Wolfe J. Caring for the child with cancer at the close of life:

"there are people who make it, and I'm hoping I'm one of them." *JAMA*. 2004;292 (17):2141–2149

30. Han PK, Keranen LB, Lescisin DA, Arnold RM. The Palliative Care Clinical Evaluation Exercise (CEX): an experience-based intervention for teaching end-of-life communication skills. *Acad Med*. 2005;80(7):669–676

31. Back AL, Arnold RM, Baile WF, Tulsky JA, Fryer-Edwards K. Approaching difficult communication tasks in oncology. *CA Cancer J Clin*. 2005;55(3):164–177

32. Mack JW, Wolfe J. Early integration of pediatric palliative care: for some children, palliative care starts at diagnosis. *Curr Opin Pediatr*. 2006;18(1):10–14

33. Feudtner C. Collaborative communication in pediatric palliative care: a foundation for problem-solving and decision-making. *Pediatr Clin North Am*. 2007;54(5):583–607, ix.

34. Levetown M; American Academy of Pediatrics Committee on Bioethics. Communicating with children and families: from everyday interactions to skill in conveying distressing information. *Pediatrics*. 2008; 121(5). Available at: www.pediatrics.org/ cgi/content/full/121/5/e1460

35. Harrison ME, Walling A. What do we know about giving bad news? A review. *Clin Pediatr (Phila)*. 2010;49(7):619–626

36. American Academy of Pediatrics. Committee on Psychosocial Aspects of Child and Family Health. The pediatrician and childhood bereavement. *Pediatrics*. 2000;105(2): 445–447

37. Meert KL, Eggly S, Pollack M, et al. Parents' perspectives regarding a physician–parent conference after their child's death in the pediatric intensive care unit. *J Pediatr*. 2007;151(1):50–55, e51–52.

38. Meert KL, Briller SH, Schim SM, Thurston C, Kabel A. Examining the needs of bereaved

parents in the pediatric intensive care unit: a qualitative study. *Death Stud*. 2009;33(8): 712–740

39. Fallat ME, Deshpande JK; American Academy of Pediatrics Section on Surgery, Section on Anesthesia and Pain Medicine, and Committee on Bioethics. Do-not-resuscitate orders for pediatric patients who require anesthesia and surgery. *Pediatrics*. 2004;114(6):1686–1692

40. Bell EF; American Academy of Pediatrics Committee on Fetus and Newborn. Noninitiation or withdrawal of intensive care for high-risk newborns. *Pediatrics*. 2007; 119(2):401–403

41. Murray RD, Antommaria AH; Council on School Health and Committee on Bioethics. Honoring do-not-attempt-resuscitation requests in schools. *Pediatrics*. 2010;125(5): 1073–1077

42. American Academy of Pediatrics. Withdrawal from dialysis. *Pediatrics*. 2011;127 (2):395

43. Diekema DS, Botkin JR; Committee on Bioethics. Clinical report: forgoing medically provided nutrition and hydration in children. *Pediatrics*. 2009;124(2):813–822

44. American Academy of Pediatrics. American Academy of Pediatrics. Committee on Child Abuse and Neglect and Committee on Bioethics. Foregoing life-sustaining medical treatment in abused children. *Pediatrics*. 2000;106(5):1151–1153

45. Dussel V, Joffe S, Hilden JM, Watterson-Schaeffer J, Weeks JC, Wolfe J. Considerations about hastening death among parents of children who die of cancer. *Arch Pediatr Adolesc Med*. 2010;164(3): 231–237

46. Carter BS, Wocial LD. Ethics and palliative care: which consultant and when? *Am J Hosp Palliat Care*. 2012;29(2):146–150

Pediatrician Workforce Policy Statement

- *Policy Statement*

POLICY STATEMENT

Pediatrician Workforce Policy Statement

abstract

This policy statement reviews important trends and other factors that affect the pediatrician workforce and the provision of pediatric health care, including changes in the pediatric patient population, pediatrician workforce, and nature of pediatric practice. The effect of these changes on pediatricians and the demand for pediatric care are discussed. The American Academy of Pediatrics (AAP) concludes that there is currently a shortage of pediatric medical subspecialists in many fields, as well as a shortage of pediatric surgical specialists. In addition, the AAP believes that the current distribution of primary care pediatricians is inadequate to meet the needs of children living in rural and other underserved areas, and more primary care pediatricians will be needed in the future because of the increasing number of children who have significant chronic health problems, changes in physician work hours, and implementation of current health reform efforts that seek to improve access to comprehensive patient- and family-centered care for all children in a medical home. The AAP is committed to being an active participant in physician workforce policy development with both professional organizations and governmental bodies to ensure a pediatric perspective on health care workforce issues. The overall purpose of this statement is to summarize policy recommendations and serve as a resource for the AAP and other stakeholders as they address pediatrician workforce issues that ultimately influence the quality of pediatric health care provided to children in the United States. *Pediatrics* 2013;132:390–397

COMMITTEE ON PEDIATRIC WORKFORCE

KEY WORDS
pediatric medical subspecialists, pediatric surgical specialists, pediatrician workforce, medical home

ABBREVIATIONS
AAP—American Academy of Pediatrics
GME—graduate medical education
IMG—international medical graduates
NP—nurse practitioner
PA—physician assistant

www.pediatrics.org/cgi/doi/10.1542/peds.2013-1517

doi:10.1542/peds.2013-1517

PEDIATRICS (ISSN Numbers: Print, 0031-4005; Online, 1098-4275).

Copyright © 2013 by the American Academy of Pediatrics

INTRODUCTION

To achieve optimal health and well-being for all infants, children, adolescents, and young adults, sufficient numbers of appropriately trained primary care pediatricians, pediatric medical subspecialists, and pediatric surgical specialists (as a group henceforth referred to as "pediatric physicians") must be available to provide care. This statement is meant to be inclusive of all physicians who focus on care for children, including pediatric hospitalists, medicine/pediatrics-trained physicians, and other physicians who limit their practice to the care of children (eg, child and adolescent psychiatrists). There are important trends that affect the pediatrician workforce directly or indirectly. Some of the trends that affect the pediatric workforce are changes in the pediatric patient population, including increases in the number of children with chronic health conditions and complex medical needs and increasing diversity of the US child population. In addition, there are important trends in the pediatrician workforce, including changes in work hours, employment status, and interest in primary care versus subspecialty careers that will affect the supply of pediatricians available to meet the needs of this changing population. Finally, the nature of pediatric practice is evolving as health care systems encourage the formation of accountable care organizations and emphasize implementation of the patient-centered medical home. Other factors significantly affect the pediatrician supply, such as availability of funding for pediatric graduate medical education (GME), pay inequities between those who provide care to children and those who provide similar care to adults, and shortages and maldistribution of the pediatrician workforce, geographically and among medical subspecialties and surgical subspecialties. The overall purpose of this statement is to summarize policy recommendations and resources for the American Academy of Pediatrics (AAP) and other stakeholders as they address the pediatrician workforce issues that ultimately influence the quality of pediatric health care provided to children in the United States.

CHANGES IN THE PEDIATRIC PATIENT POPULATION

The adequacy of the pediatric physician workforce is affected by the health status of the nation's children. Approximately 26.6% of children have a chronic health condition, such as asthma, obesity, diabetes, or mental health disorders.[1] The increased prevalence of chronic diseases in children has expanded the need for pediatric physicians, including primary care pediatricians, pediatric medical subspecialists, and pediatric surgical specialists. Optimal health care for these children requires the availability of a medical home, in which physicians manage all aspects of pediatric primary care, including provision of health maintenance and acute care; advocating for patients with insurers, schools, and other community agencies; and referral to and coordination of care with other physicians. These services should be provided in a longitudinal manner that engenders trust in the relationship and ensures a family-centered format.[2]

Because of the increasing racial and ethnic diversity of the pediatric population, the pediatrician workforce must continually strive to provide culturally effective care.[3] Educational and recruitment strategies to increase culturally effective care and multilingual abilities of the pediatrician workforce should be encouraged. In addition, there is an ongoing need to increase racial and ethnic diversity among the pediatrician workforce, in part because minority pediatricians continue to be more likely to provide care to minority children and their families in a disproportionate manner.[4–6]

CHANGES IN THE PEDIATRICIAN WORKFORCE

Data from the US Residency Match demonstrate a strong interest in pediatric residency positions. National Residency Matching Program data from 2011 reveal that 98% of first-year positions in pediatrics filled, and, from 1997 to 2011, the percentage of first-year positions that filled has exceeded 90%.[7]

However, a simple comparison of the number of pediatric physicians per child population does not provide an accurate picture of the adequacy of the workforce, because many variables incorporated into supply calculations are changing, including the percentage of pediatric physicians who work full-time, average number of work hours per week, complexity of patients, and the percentage of pediatric physicians who leave the workforce for extended periods. For example, the number of pediatric physicians who work part-time continues to increase, from 15% in 2000 to 23% in 2006.[8] Among graduating residents who are applying for nonfellowship positions, as many as 38% are seeking part-time positions.[9] Because part-time physicians work, on average, 14.3 fewer hours per week in direct patient care, the number of pediatricians needed to provide clinical care may be greater than if all pediatricians worked full-time.[10] Although the growth in part-time practice has been attributed largely to the increasing number of women entering pediatrics, a recent AAP member survey revealed that the percentage of men working part-time has significantly increased as well, doubling from 4% in 2000 to 8% in 2006.[8] This survey also revealed that the percentage of pediatricians younger than 40 years who work part-time significantly increased from 18% in 2000 to 29% in 2006. Among pediatricians older than 49 years, the percentage working part-time tripled from 6% in 2000 to 18% in 2006.[8]

In addition to part-time practice, increased numbers of pediatricians are temporarily suspending their clinical practice or assuming nonclinical roles in medicine or other fields, which may affect the availability of pediatric physicians to meet demands for clinical care.[11,12] If pediatric physician work environments do not provide the opportunity for pediatric physicians to adjust their clinical workload so that they have sufficient time to manage other responsibilities (eg, child or elder care) and pursue other interests outside of medicine, more pediatric physicians may abandon clinical practice completely. Therefore, removing barriers to part-time practice and enabling more physicians to reenter clinical practice after periods of inactivity could improve the future supply of pediatric physicians.[13]

Another factor that is increasing the demand for primary care pediatricians is the decreasing role of family physicians in caring for children. From 1996 to 2006, the percentage of visits for children younger than 18 years to nonpediatric generalists declined from 28% to 22%, whereas the percentage of visits for children younger than 18 years to general pediatricians increased from 61% to 71%.[14]

Although nonphysician clinicians, such as nurse practitioners (NPs) and physician assistants (PAs), are not the focus of this policy statement, they are important and valuable participants in the health care team that provides care for children. However, NP and PA training and skills are not interchangeable with those of pediatric primary care physicians; therefore, they cannot be substituted for them as leaders of the pediatric medical home. In addition to differences in training and experience, the numbers of nonphysician clinicians who care for children is insufficient to replace the care provided by pediatric physicians.[15–17] Only a small percentage of PAs and NPs choose pediatric careers. For example, most states have fewer than 50 pediatric PAs, and fewer than 15% of NP students choose pediatric careers.[16,17] Indeed, the number of NP programs offering a pediatric track declined from 1996 to 2008, and only approximately 600 pediatric NPs complete training each year in the United States.[17]

Although family NPs may provide care for children, pediatric patients represent only a small fraction of their patients.[18] Some groups have suggested that NPs can be used to address the shortages of primary care physicians and pediatric specialists, especially in rural areas.[19] However, the percentage of NPs interested in working in areas of physician shortage is small, and few pediatric NPs

choose to practice without a physician.[15] In states where NPs can practice independently, only 11% choose to do so,[15] and fewer than 3% of NPs work in small rural communities.[20] In addition, it is not likely that NPs will provide the full scope of care that pediatric physicians provide. Indeed, a minority of pediatric NPs provide emergency or inpatient care.[15] Because of these issues, it is unlikely that pediatric PAs and NPs can play a significant role in addressing the shortage/maldistribution of primary care pediatricians or pediatric medical subspecialists.

With the increase in the percentage of children who are insured as a result of health care reform, the number of children who will be able to obtain pediatrician services will increase. However, many children will remain uninsured despite health care reform, such as undocumented children, because they are not eligible for enrollment.[21] Poor payment rates for pediatric services adversely affect the pediatrician workforce by threatening the economic viability of pediatric practices, and the combined effect of lack of insurance and poor payment rates have detrimental effects on the health of entire communities.[22,23] When the supply of pediatric primary care physicians in a community is inadequate, children will not have access to a pediatric medical home and may receive care in alternative settings, such as emergency departments and retail-based clinics, where the focus is on acute and episodic treatment rather than health supervision and preventive services.

Other factors that may affect the pediatrician workforce include the supply of international medical graduates (IMGs) entering the US workforce. The current expansion of US medical schools and medical school class sizes may adversely affect the number of

IMGs able to obtain residency training in the United States. In addition, a decrease in the number of J1 visas issued may adversely affect the number of IMGs who choose to practice in rural or other underserved communities. Thus, underserved areas may be faced with increasing shortages of pediatric primary care physicians if the increased output of US medical schools is not accompanied by an increase in the number of those graduates who enter primary care or underserved practice areas.[24]

CHANGES IN THE NATURE OF PEDIATRIC PRACTICE

The primary care pediatrician's role in providing health care for children has been significantly affected by the need to spend increased time coordinating care services; counseling families; and advocating for their patients with insurers, schools, and other community agencies, important functions in a true medical home but not compensated well by current payment mechanisms.[25] Furthermore, the increased complexity of pediatric patients requires greater time and resources of the pediatrician to manage their care. Although primary care pediatricians may have fewer inpatient responsibilities because of the emergence of hospitalists, this decrease in responsibility has been accompanied by an increased need for them to provide coordination of care for children after hospital discharge, care that is often not covered by insurers.[26]

The clinical availability of pediatric physicians has also been adversely affected by the increased amount of time they must spend on practice management because of the ever-increasing amount of paperwork required to obtain payment.[27] Thus, strategies that decrease time spent on these nonclinical responsibilities can effectively increase the clinical availability and effectiveness of all pediatric physicians. Providing medical home–based, comprehensive care also would improve clinical effectiveness by increasing the pediatrician's ability to provide the full range of services needed for optimal child health. However, current payment systems do not adequately provide for the expanded team necessary to provide comprehensive care in a medical home for children that support all of the services needed by the pediatric care team. Payment mechanisms should be developed that support all members of the pediatric care team, including case managers and social workers. Inadequate payment for services provided by pediatricians and other members of their medical home team creates a barrier to providing the full range of pediatric services needed for optimal child health. For example, states with lower payment levels for vaccine administration also have lower rates of age-appropriate vaccination.[28,29]

Children who are uninsured or underinsured are less able to obtain care.[23] In addition, uninsured children create a greater demand on the sector of the pediatrician workforce that provides inpatient and emergency department care, because these children lack access to preventive care services, which can decrease the need for hospitalization and emergency department visits. Thus, decreasing the number of children who are uninsured or underinsured is a critical pediatrician workforce issue. When families lack adequate insurance coverage and cannot afford preventive and acute care services, pediatric physicians may not be able to establish and maintain an economically viable practice, and young physicians may be dissuaded from choosing a career in pediatrics.

PEDIATRIC GME AND ACCESS TO CARE

Because appropriate care for children requires primary care pediatricians, pediatric medical subspecialists, and pediatric surgical specialists, the availability of training positions to meet all of these needs is critical. Limited funding for pediatric GME, including fellowship training, will decrease the availability of training opportunities in pediatrics and lead to a decrease in the number of graduating residents available to meet the demand for care.[30]

To increase the number of pediatric medical subspecialists and maintain the supply of primary care pediatricians, the number of general pediatric residency positions needs to be increased, because most physicians wishing to pursue a career in a pediatric medical subspecialty must first complete a general pediatric residency. Without increases in general pediatric residency positions, there will be insufficient graduates to meet the demands for both pediatric medical subspecialists and primary care pediatricians. Indeed, the percentage of pediatric residency program graduates planning careers in general pediatrics has declined from 68% in 2000 to 61% in 2010, whereas the percentage interested in pursuing a career in a pediatric medical subspecialty has increased from 23% in 2000 to 33% in 2010.[31] Thus, the need to increase entry into pediatric medical subspecialty careers will adversely affect the number of primary care pediatricians, unless the total number of general pediatric residency positions is increased. In contrast, the availability of general pediatric residency positions does not affect pediatric surgical specialists, because they begin their training in surgical residencies.

Many hospital regions in the United States lack pediatric medical subspecialists and surgical specialists, and

primary care pediatricians report difficulty obtaining pediatric medical subspecialty and surgical specialty care for their patients.[32] The shortage of mental health subspecialists (eg, child psychiatrists, developmental/ behavioral pediatric specialists) is especially critical, because it is estimated that approximately 21% of children in the United States meet criteria for a mental health disorder.[33] It is imperative, therefore, that GME funding initiatives designed to increase interest in primary care do not erode entry into pediatric medical subspecialties and surgical specialties. Health policy changes designed to address the shortage of primary care physicians for adults by dissuading entry into adult subspecialties should not be extended to pediatrics. In addition to geographic disparities in the availability of pediatric medical subspecialists, there is wide variation in both the supply and demand among the various pediatric medical subspecialties. For example, the population-weighted average distances to care range from 15 miles for a neonatologist to 78 miles for a pediatric sports medicine specialist.[34] In addition, data from 2003 to 2006 suggest that increases in the number of pediatric medical subspecialists may not address maldistribution, because pediatric medical subspecialists and surgical specialists tend to enter practice where similar physicians already practice, with few entering new markets.[35] Thus, increased GME funding for pediatric medical subspecialty training should be targeted to the subspecialties experiencing the greatest shortages and incentivize subspecialty practices that provide care for children who are currently underserved by subspecialists, including children living in poverty as well as those living in small and rural communities.[34,36] Without increases in GME funding, the current shortage of pediatric medical subspecialists is likely to worsen. Pediatric medical subspecialists also spend less time than generalists in direct patient care, averaging 33.7 hours per week for those working full-time and 21 hours per week for those working part-time, compared with an average of 42 hours per week for full-time generalists and 25.7 hours per week for part-time generalists.[8] Because most pediatric departmental teaching faculty members at academic centers are pediatric medical subspecialists, a shortage of pediatric medical subspecialists not only affects patient care but also adversely affects the ability to train pediatric residents and conduct research. Indeed, a sufficient number of academic pediatric physician faculty members in all medical and surgical disciplines is required to adequately train the future pediatrician workforce, and the demand for academic pediatricians is likely to increase with the increase in primary care training positions and medical school enrollment.

Payment inequities between those who provide care for children and those who provide similar care to adults can provide a significant disincentive for physicians to choose pediatric careers.[37,38] This lack of parity in payment affects all fields of pediatrics, including (but not limited to) primary care, pediatric medical subspecialties, pediatric surgical specialties, and other pediatric physicians, such as pediatric radiologists, pathologists, and others. Even among pediatric medical subspecialties, significant differences in payment and, thus, salary potential exist. These differences lead to greater workforce shortages in some pediatric subspecialties compared with others. The supply of pediatric surgical specialists and many pediatric medical subspecialists is not adequate to meet the needs of children, especially those with complex health problems. If pediatric surgeons and medical subspecialists continue to be paid less to

provide care for children than physicians who provide similar care for adults, there will be a financial disincentive for graduating residents to pursue pediatric surgical or subspecialty careers.[39,40]

WORKFORCE POLICY ISSUES

The pediatrician workforce is influenced by health care policy decisions made at the local, state, and national levels. Thus, the AAP is committed to actively participating in policy development with both professional organizations and governmental bodies to ensure that these deliberations have a pediatric perspective. Pediatrics is unique among the primary care specialties for having strong trainee interest in the field over the past decade, but the nature of pediatric practice is rapidly evolving because of changes in gender mix, patient mix, and work format. Market forces, including changes in health care and medical education financing, affect both the workforce supply and need for health care. The state-to-state variation in payment for pediatric care adversely affects pediatric physicians and makes recruitment of pediatric physicians difficult, especially in underserved communities, where payment is often inadequate.

Additional research is needed to more fully understand the effective supply of all types of pediatric physicians, adjusting for clinical productivity as well as the current and anticipated needs of our communities. The AAP does not believe that simply increasing the number of pediatric physicians or increasing their pay will address all the pediatrician workforce issues discussed in this statement. Indeed, many of the issues that result in workforce shortages and geographic maldistribution must be innovatively addressed, including renewed emphasis on recruitment incentives for

physicians who practice in communities and fields where there is the greatest need, payment parity between physicians who care for adults and those who care for children, loan forgiveness, and stable GME funding for children's hospitals that train most pediatric medical subspecialists and surgical specialists. The current health care reform effort has reinforced Title VII of the Public Health Services Act (health professions education) and the National Health Service Corps, but ongoing support of these programs is essential to improving access to primary care for many underserved populations. Greater attention to pediatrician workforce planning can help reduce geographic disparities and ensure that the proportion of pediatric residents who choose either generalist or subspecialist careers is adequate to meet the demands for clinical care as well as the needs for future academicians and researchers in pediatrics.

SUMMARY

The AAP concludes that there is currently a shortage of pediatric medical subspecialists in many fields, as well as a shortage of pediatric surgical specialists. In addition, the AAP believes that the current supply of primary care pediatricians is inadequate to meet the needs of children living in rural and other underserved areas. In the future, more primary care pediatricians will be needed to care for the increasing number of children who have significant chronic health problems and who will require more medical and surgical care from pediatric physicians throughout their childhood. In addition, there will be an increased demand for general pediatricians because of the decrease in the number of family physicians providing care for children and the limited number of nonphysician clinicians interested in pediatric careers. Other factors that are expected to increase the demand for general pediatricians include changes in physician work hours and implementation of current health reform efforts that seek to improve access to comprehensive patient-centered care for all children in a medical home. Thus, although primary care pediatrics is currently experiencing sustained interest as a career pathway, many factors reviewed in this statement lead to the conclusion that the United States must increase the number of general pediatric residency program graduates to increase the supply of pediatric medical subspecialists and maintain the current supply of primary care pediatricians. Payment structures should be revised to allow pediatric physicians to provide quality care to all children, including the increasing number of children with chronic health conditions. Without adequate payment, general pediatricians are unable to provide the full range of services needed for optimal child health within a patient-centered medical home, and recruiting physicians into medical fields that focus on children will remain challenging because of payment inequities. The AAP maintains that current health care reform efforts that seek to improve access to comprehensive, patient-centered care for all children cannot be successful without an adequate pediatrician workforce to provide such care. All adults once were children, and healthy children who grow to be productive adults are critical to our nation's growth. Therefore, the provision of optimal care to the nation's children is an investment in our nation's future. On the basis of review of these known and evolving factors, the AAP is committed to the following:

STATEMENT OF PRINCIPLES

1. Infants, children, adolescents, and young adults must have access to sufficient numbers of appropriately trained primary care pediatricians, pediatric medical subspecialists, and pediatric surgical specialists to achieve their optimal health and well-being. The AAP believes that the current pediatrician workforce is not meeting the primary care, subspecialty, or surgical needs to provide quality health care for US children and that critical workforce shortages exist in pediatric medical subspecialties and pediatric surgical specialties. The AAP, working collaboratively with other appropriate groups, should advocate for and participate in professional and governmental efforts to achieve a sufficient, balanced pediatrician workforce and encourage members and AAP chapters to do the same.

2. The AAP is committed to participating in national, state, and local efforts to address workforce issues to ensure that the unique needs of the pediatric population and the pediatrician workforce to care for them are addressed in health care policy and legislative efforts.

3. The AAP is committed to promoting pediatrics as a career choice to medical students and residents and to appropriating funding for pediatric GME programs, general pediatric and pediatric subspecialty training positions, academic faculty, and long-term GME funding for children's hospitals.

4. The AAP is committed to advocating for initiatives that support and encourage careers in pediatric medical subspecialties, including funding for the Children's Hospitals GME program and the pediatric subspecialty loan forgiveness program.

5. The AAP is committed to advocating for the needs of children in any initiatives to recruit or train medical students and residents in specific disciplines and/or geographic regions.

6. The AAP is committed to supporting programs that address maldistribution of the pediatrician workforce, such as Title VII health professions education funding, National Health Service Corps, and incentives to enter pediatrics, such as loan forgiveness programs and tax credits.

7. The AAP is committed to promoting flexible practice environments and providing resources for pediatricians interested in part-time practice or desiring to reenter the workforce so that they will have increased opportunities to practice and, thereby, maximize the number of pediatricians in clinical practice.

8. The AAP is committed to supporting and/or coordinating activities to encourage recruitment into pediatric surgical specialties.

9. The AAP is committed to working to achieve parity in payment so that physicians who care for children receive the same payment for similar services as physicians who care for adults.

10. The AAP is committed to working to reduce geographic and socioeconomic barriers that prevent children from obtaining access to appropriate primary care pediatricians, pediatric medical subspecialists, and pediatric surgical specialists. This includes appropriate insurance benefits for patients, adequate payment of physicians, and oversight by governmental agencies of public and private insurers to ensure access to care.

11. The AAP is committed to increasing the diversity, cultural effectiveness, and multilingual skills of the

pediatrician workforce to meet the needs of an increasingly diverse child population.

12. The AAP is committed to promoting research regarding the changing pediatrician workforce. This research should examine the current supply and future needs for pediatric physicians by geographic area. It should also monitor changes in demand for pediatric care as a result of (1) the changing demographics of pediatric patients, (2) the changing demographics of pediatricians, and (3) modifications

in health policy that will influence both patients and physicians.

13. The AAP is committed to promoting comprehensive, high-quality health insurance coverage for all infants, children, adolescents, and young adults, which should be the right of every child.

LEAD AUTHORS

William T. Basco, MD, MS, FAAP
Mary E. Rimsza, MD, FAAP

COMMITTEE ON PEDIATRIC WORKFORCE, 2011-2012

Mary E. Rimsza, MD, FAAP, Chairperson

Andrew J. Hotaling, MD, FAAP
Ted D. Sigrest, MD, FAAP
Frank A. Simon, MD, FAAP

FORMER COMMITTEE MEMBERS

William T. Basco, MD, MS, FAAP
Beth A. Pletcher, MD, FAAP
Luisa I. Alvarado-Domenech, MD, FAAP

LIAISONS

Christopher E. Harris, MD, FAAP – *Section Forum Management Committee*
Gail A. McGuinness, MD, FAAP – *American Board of Pediatrics*

STAFF

Holly J. Mulvey, MA
Carrie L. Radabaugh, MPP

REFERENCES

1. Van Cleave J, Gortmaker SL, Perrin JM. Dynamics of obesity and chronic health conditions among children and youth. *JAMA*. 2010;303(7):623–630

2. Medical Home Initiatives for Children With Special Needs Project Advisory Committee. American Academy of Pediatrics. The medical home. *Pediatrics*. 2002;110(1 pt 1): 184–186

3. Britton CV; American Academy of Pediatrics Committee on Pediatric Workforce. Ensuring culturally effective pediatric care: implications for education and health policy. *Pediatrics*. 2004;114(6):1677–1685

4. Friedman AL; American Academy of Pediatrics Committee on Pediatric Workforce. Enhancing the diversity of the pediatrician workforce. *Pediatrics*. 2007;119(4):833–837

5. Basco WT, Jr, Cull WL, O'Connor KG, Shipman SA. Assessing trends in practice demographics of underrepresented minority pediatricians, 1993-2007. *Pediatrics*. 2010; 125(3):460–467

6. Saha S, Komaromy M, Koepsell TD, Bindman AB. Patient-physician racial concordance and the perceived quality and use of health care. *Arch Intern Med*. 1999;159(9): 997–1004

7. American Academy of Pediatrics, Division of Workforce and Medical Education Policy. Resident match continues to grow. *AAP News*. 2011;32(5):1, 8

8. Cull WL, O'Connor KG, Olson LM. Part-time work among pediatricians expands. *Pediatrics*. 2010;125(1):152–157

9. Cull WL, Caspary GL, Olson LM. Many pediatric residents seek and obtain part-time positions. *Pediatrics*. 2008;121(2):276–281

10. McMurray JE, Heiligers PJ, Shugerman RP, et al; Society of General Internal Medicine Career Satisfaction Study Group (CSSG). Part-time medical practice: where is it headed? *Am J Med*. 2005;118(1):87–92

11. Goodman DC; Committee on Pediatric Workforce. The pediatrician workforce: current status and future prospects. *Pediatrics*. 2005;116(1). Available at: www.pediatrics.org/cgi/content/full/116/1/e156

12. Freed GL, Dunham KM, Switalski KE. Clinical inactivity among pediatricians: prevalence and perspectives. *Pediatrics*. 2009;123(2): 605–610

13. Cull WL, Mulvey HJ, O'Connor KG, Sowell DR, Berkowitz CD, Britton CV. Pediatricians working part-time: past, present, and future. *Pediatrics*. 2002;109(6):1015–1020

14. Freed GL, Dunham KM, Gebremariam A, Wheeler JR. Which pediatricians are providing care to America's children? *J Pediatr*. 2010;157(1):148.e1–152.e1

15. Freed GL, Dunham KM, Lamarand KE, Loveland-Cherry C, Martyn KK; American Board of Pediatrics Research Advisory Committee. Pediatric nurse practitioners: roles and scope of practice. *Pediatrics*. 2010;126(5): 846–850

16. Freed GL, Dunham KM, Moote MJ, Lamarand KE; American Board of Pediatrics Research Advisory Committee. Pediatric physician assistants: distribution and scope of practice. *Pediatrics*. 2010;126(5):851–855

17. Freed GL, Dunham KM, Loveland-Cherry CJ, Martyn KK. Pediatric nurse practitioners in the United States: current distribution and recent trends in training. *J Pediatr*. 2010; 157(4):589.e1–593.e1

18. Freed GL, Dunham KM, Loveland-Cherry CJ, Martyn KK; American Board of Pediatrics Research Advisory Committee. Family nurse practitioners: roles and scope of practice in the care of pediatric patients. *Pediatrics*. 2010;126(5):861–864

19. Institute of Medicine, Committee on the Robert Wood Johnson Foundation Initiative on the Future of Nursing. *The Future of Nursing: Leading Change, Advancing Health*. Washington, DC: The National Academies Press; 2011

20. American Nurses Credentialing Center. *2008 Role Delineation Study: Pediatric Nurse Practitioner—National Results*. Silver Spring, MD: American Nurses Credentialing Center; 2009

21. Passel JF, Taylor P. *Unauthorized Immigrants and Their U.S.-Born Children*. Washington, DC: The Pew Hispanic Center; 2010

22. Institute of Medicine, Committee on the Consequences of Uninsurance. *A Shared Destiny: Effects of Uninsurance on Individuals, Families, and Communities*. Washington, DC: National Academies Press; 2003

23. Olson LM, Tang SF, Newacheck PW. Children in the United States with discontinuous health insurance coverage. *N Engl J Med*. 2005;353(4):382–391

24. American Medical Association, AMA-IMG Section Governing Council. *International Medical Graduates in American Medicine: Contemporary Challenges and Opportunities.* Chicago, IL: American Medical Association; 2010

25. Cooley WC, McAllister JW, Sherrieb K, Kuhlthau K. Improved outcomes associated with medical home implementation in pediatric primary care. *Pediatrics.* 2009;124(1):358–364

26. Percelay JM; Committee on Hospital Care. Physicians' roles in coordinating care of hospitalized children. *Pediatrics.* 2003;111(3):707–709

27. Berman S, Dolins J, Tang SF, Yudkowsky B. Factors that influence the willingness of private primary care pediatricians to accept more Medicaid patients. *Pediatrics.* 2002;110(2 pt 1):239–248

28. McInerny TK, Cull WL, Yudkowsky BK. Physician reimbursement levels and adherence to American Academy of Pediatrics well-visit and immunization recommendations. *Pediatrics.* 2005;115(4):833–838

29. Yoo BK, Berry A, Kasajima M, Szilagyi PG. Association between Medicaid reimbursement and child influenza vaccination rates. *Pediatrics.* 2010;126(5). Available at: www.pediatrics.org/cgi/content/full/126/5/e998 PubMed

30. Shipman SA, Pan RJ; American Academy of Pediatrics Committee on Pediatric Workforce. Financing graduate medical education to meet the needs of children and the future pediatrician workforce. *Pediatrics.* 2008;121(4):855–861

31. American Board of Pediatrics. *Workforce Data 2010–2011.* Chapel Hill, NC: American Board of Pediatrics; 2010

32. Pletcher BA, Rimsza ME, Cull WL, Shipman SA, Shugerman RP, O'Connor KG. Primary care pediatricians' satisfaction with subspecialty care, perceived supply, and barriers to care. *J Pediatr.* 2010;156(6):1011.e1–1015.e1

33. Shaffer D, Fisher P, Dulcan MK, et al. The NIMH Diagnostic Interview Schedule for Children Version 2.3 (DISC-2.3): description, acceptability, prevalence rates, and performance in the MECA Study. Methods for the Epidemiology of Child and Adolescent Mental Disorders Study. *J Am Acad Child Adolesc Psychiatry.* 1996;35(7):865–877

34. Mayer ML. Are we there yet? Distance to care and relative supply among pediatric medical subspecialties. *Pediatrics.* 2006;118(6):2313–2321

35. Mayer ML, Skinner AC. Influence of changes in supply on the distribution of pediatric subspecialty care. *Arch Pediatr Adolesc Med.* 2009;163(12):1087–1091

36. Mayer ML. Disparities in geographic access to pediatric subspecialty care. *Matern Child Health J.* 2008;12(5):624–632

37. DeZee KJ, Maurer D, Colt R, et al. Effect of financial remuneration on specialty choice of fourth-year U.S. medical students. *Acad Med.* 2011;86(2):187–193

38. Ebell MH. Future salary and US residency fill rate revisited. *JAMA.* 2008;300(10):1131–1132

39. Rochlin JM, Simon HK. Does fellowship pay: what is the long-term financial impact of subspecialty training in pediatrics? *Pediatrics.* 2011;127(2):254–260

40. Burton OM. Does fellowship pay? Challenges and opportunities. *Pediatrics.* 2011;127(4):779–780

Planned Home Birth

- *Policy Statement*

POLICY STATEMENT

Planned Home Birth

abstract

The American Academy of Pediatrics concurs with the recent statement of the American College of Obstetricians and Gynecologists affirming that hospitals and birthing centers are the safest settings for birth in the United States while respecting the right of women to make a medically informed decision about delivery. This statement is intended to help pediatricians provide supportive, informed counsel to women considering home birth while retaining their role as child advocates and to summarize the standards of care for newborn infants born at home, which are consistent with standards for infants born in a medical care facility. Regardless of the circumstances of his or her birth, including location, every newborn infant deserves health care that adheres to the standards highlighted in this statement, more completely described in other publications from the American Academy of Pediatrics, including *Guidelines for Perinatal Care*. The goal of providing high-quality care to all newborn infants can best be achieved through continuing efforts by all participating health care providers and institutions to develop and sustain communications and understanding on the basis of professional interaction and mutual respect throughout the health care system. *Pediatrics* 2013;131:1016–1020

COMMITTEE ON FETUS AND NEWBORN

KEY WORDS
birth, delivery, newborn infant, home birth, midwife, obstetrician, pediatrician

ABBREVIATIONS
ACOG—American College of Obstetricians and Gynecologists
AAP—American Academy of Pediatrics

This document is copyrighted and is the property of the American Academy of Pediatrics and its Board of Directors. All authors have filed conflict of interest statements with the American Academy of Pediatrics. Any conflicts have been resolved through a process approved by the Board of Directors. The American Academy of Pediatrics has neither solicited nor accepted any commercial involvement in the development of the content of this publication.

The recommendations in this statement do not indicate an exclusive course of treatment or serve as a standard of medical care. Variations, taking into account individual circumstances, may be appropriate.

All policy statements from the American Academy of Pediatrics automatically expire 5 years after publication unless reaffirmed, revised, or retired at or before that time.

www.pediatrics.org/cgi/doi/10.1542/peds.2013-0575

doi:10.1542/peds.2013-0575

PEDIATRICS (ISSN Numbers: Print, 0031-4005; Online, 1098-4275).

Copyright © 2013 by the American Academy of Pediatrics

INTRODUCTION

Women and their families may desire a home birth for a variety of reasons, including hopes for a more family-friendly setting, increased control of the process, decreased obstetric intervention, and lower cost. Although the incidence of home birth remains below 1% of all births in the United States, the rate of home birth has increased during the past several years for white, non-Hispanic women.[1] However, a woman's choice to plan a home birth is not well supported in the United States. Obstacles are pervasive and systemic and include wide variation in state laws and regulations, lack of appropriately trained and willing providers, and lack of supporting systems to ensure the availability of specialty consultation and timely transport to a hospital. Geography also may adversely affect the safety of planned home birth, because travel times >20 minutes have been associated with increased risk of adverse neonatal outcomes, including mortality.[2] Whether for these reasons or others, planned home birth in the United States appears to be associated with a two- to threefold increase in neonatal mortality or an absolute risk increase of approximately 1 neonatal death per 1000 nonanomalous live births.[3–5] Evidence also suggests that infants born at home in the United States have an increased incidence of low Apgar scores and neonatal seizures.[3,4] In contrast, a smaller study of all planned home births attended by midwives in British Columbia, Canada, from 2000 to 2004 revealed no increase in neonatal mortality over planned hospital births attended by either midwives or physicians.[6] Registered midwives in British Columbia are mandated to offer women the choice to deliver in a hospital or at home if they meet the eligibility criteria for home birth defined by the College of Midwifery of British Columbia (Table 1).

In a recent position statement, the Committee on Obstetric Practice of the American College of Obstetricians and Gynecologists (ACOG) stated, "although the Committee on Obstetric Practice believes that hospitals and birthing centers are the safest setting for birth, it respects the right of a woman to make a medically informed decision about delivery. Women inquiring about planned home birth should be informed of its risks and benefits based on recent evidence."[7] The statement reviewed appropriate candidates for home delivery and outlined the health care system components "critical to reducing perinatal mortality rates and achieving favorable home birth outcomes" (Table 1).

Pediatricians must be prepared to provide supportive, informed counsel to women considering home birth while retaining their role as child advocates in assessing whether the situation is appropriate to support a planned home birth (Table 1). In addition to apprising the expectant mother of the increase in neonatal mortality and other neonatal complications with planned home birth, the pediatrician should advise her that the American Academy of Pediatrics (AAP) and ACOG support provision of care only by midwives who are certified by the American Midwifery Certification Board and should make her aware that some women who plan to deliver at home will need transfer to a hospital before delivery because of unanticipated complications. This percentage varies widely among reports, from approximately 10% to 40%, with a higher transfer rate for primiparous women.[8,9] The mother should be encouraged to see successful transfer not as a failure of the home birth but rather as a success of the system.

Care of the newborn infant born at home is a particularly important topic, because infants born at home are cared for outside the safeguards of the systems-based protocols required of

hospitals and birthing centers. This situation places a larger burden on individual health care providers to remember and carry out all components of assessment and care of the newborn infant. To assist providers, this policy statement addresses 2 specific areas: resuscitation and evaluation of the newborn infant immediately after birth and essential elements of care and follow-up for the healthy term newborn infant.

ASSESSMENT, RESUSCITATION, AND CARE OF THE NEWBORN INFANT IMMEDIATELY AFTER BIRTH

As recommended by the AAP and the American Heart Association, there should be at least 1 person present at every delivery whose primary responsibility is the care of the newborn infant.[10] Situations in which both the mother and the newborn infant simultaneously require urgent attention are infrequent but will nonetheless occur. Thus, each delivery should be attended by 2 individuals, at least 1 of whom has the appropriate training, skills, and equipment to perform a full resuscitation of the infant in accordance of the principles of the Neonatal Resuscitation Program.[10] To facilitate obtaining emergency assistance when needed, the operational integrity of the telephone or other communication system should be tested before the delivery (as should every other piece of medical equipment), and the weather should be monitored. In addition, a previous arrangement with a medical facility needs to be in place to ensure a safe and timely transport in the event of an emergency.

Care of the newborn infant immediately after delivery should adhere to standards of practice as described in *Guidelines for Perinatal Care*[11] and include provision of warmth, initiation of appropriate resuscitation measures,

---

TABLE 1 Recommendations When Considering Planned Home Birth

Candidate for home delivery[a]
- Absence of preexisting maternal disease
- Absence of significant disease occurring during the pregnancy
- A singleton fetus estimated to be appropriate for gestational age
- A cephalic presentation
- A gestation of 37 to <41 completed weeks of pregnancy
- Labor that is spontaneous or induced as an outpatient
- A mother who has not been referred from another hospital

Systems needed to support planned home birth
- The availability of a certified nurse-midwife, certified midwife, or physician practicing within an integrated and regulated health system
- Attendance by at least 1 appropriately trained individual (see text) whose primary responsibility is the care of the newborn infant
- Ready access to consultation
- Assurance of safe and timely transport to a nearby hospital with a preexisting arrangement for such transfers

Data are from refs 6, 7, 10, 11, and 13.
[a] ACOG considers previous cesarean delivery to be an absolute contraindication to planned home birth.[7]

and assignment of Apgar scores. Although skin-to-skin contact with mother is the most effective way to provide warmth, portable warming pads should be available in case a newborn infant requires resuscitation and cannot be placed on the mother's chest. A newborn infant who requires any resuscitation should be monitored frequently during the immediate postnatal period, and infants who receive extensive resuscitation (eg, positive-pressure ventilation for more than 30–60 seconds) should be transferred to a medical facility for close monitoring and evaluation. In addition, any infant who has respiratory distress, continued cyanosis, or other signs of illness should be immediately transferred to a medical facility.

CARE OF THE NEWBORN

Subsequent newborn care should adhere to the AAP standards as described in *Guidelines for Perinatal Care* as well as to the AAP statement regarding care of the well newborn infant.[11–13] Although a detailed review of these standards would be far too lengthy to include in this statement, a few practice points are worthy of specific mention:

- *Transitional care (first 4–8 hours)*: The infant should be kept warm and undergo a detailed physical examination that includes an assessment of gestational age and intrauterine growth status (weight, length, and head circumference), as well as a comprehensive risk assessment for neonatal conditions that require additional monitoring or intervention. Temperature, heart and respiratory rates, skin color, peripheral circulation, respiration, level of consciousness, tone, and activity should be monitored and recorded at least once every 30 minutes until the newborn's condition is considered normal and

has remained stable for 2 hours. An infant who is thought to be <37 weeks' gestational age should be transferred to a medical facility for continuing observation for conditions associated with prematurity, including respiratory distress, poor feeding, hypoglycemia, and hyperbilirubinemia, as well as for a car safety seat study.

- *Monitoring for group B streptococcal disease*: As recommended by the Centers for Disease Control and Prevention and the AAP, all pregnant women should be screened for group B streptococcal colonization at 35 to 37 weeks of gestation.[14] Women who are colonized should receive ≥4 hours of intravenous penicillin, ampicillin, or cefazolin. If the mother has received this intrapartum treatment and both she and her newborn infant remain asymptomatic, they can remain at home if the infant can be observed frequently by an experienced and knowledgeable health care provider. If the mother shows signs of chorioamnionitis or if the infant does not appear completely well, the infant should be transferred rapidly to a medical facility for additional evaluation and treatment.[14]

- *Glucose screening*: Infants who have abnormal fetal growth (estimated to be small or large for gestational age) or whose mothers have diabetes should be delivered in a hospital or birthing center because of the increased risk of hypoglycemia and other neonatal complications. If, after delivery, an infant is discovered to be small or large for gestational age or has required resuscitation, he or she should be screened for hypoglycemia as outlined in the AAP statement.[15] If hypoglycemia is identified and persists after feeding (glucose <45 mg/dL), the infant should be

transferred promptly to a medical facility for continuing evaluation and treatment.

- *Eye prophylaxis*: Every newborn infant should receive prophylaxis against gonococcal ophthalmia neonatorum.

- *Vitamin K*: Every newborn infant should receive a single parenteral dose of natural vitamin K_1 oxide (phytonadione [0.5–1 mg]) to prevent vitamin K–dependent hemorrhagic disease of the newborn. Oral administration of vitamin K has not been shown to be as efficacious as parenteral administration for the prevention of late hemorrhagic disease. This dose should be administered shortly after birth but may be delayed until after the first breastfeeding.

- *Hepatitis B vaccination*: Early hepatitis B immunization is recommended for all medically stable infants with a birth weight >2 kg.

- *Assessment of feeding*: Breastfeeding, including observation of position, latch, and milk transfer, should be evaluated by a trained caregiver. The mother should be encouraged to record the time and duration of each feeding, as well as urine and stool output, during the early days of breastfeeding.

- *Screening for hyperbilirubinemia*: Infants whose mothers are Rh negative should have cord blood sent for a Coombs direct antibody test; if the mother's blood type is O, the cord blood may be tested for the infant's blood type and direct antibody test, but it is not required provided that there is appropriate surveillance, risk assessment, and follow-up.[16] All newborn infants should be assessed for risk of hyperbilirubinemia and undergo bilirubin screening between 24 and 48 hours. The bilirubin value should be plotted on the hour-specific nomogram to determine the risk of severe hyperbilirubinemia and the need for repeat determinations.[13]

- *Universal newborn screening*: Every newborn infant should undergo universal newborn screening in accordance with individual state mandates, with the first blood specimen ideally collected between 24 and 48 hours of age. (A list of conditions for which screening is performed in each state is maintained online by the National Newborn Screening and Genetic Resource Center, available at http://genes-r-us.uthscsa.edu/resources/consumer/statemap.htm.)

- *Hearing screening*: The newborn infant's initial caregiver should ensure that the hearing of any infant born outside the hospital setting is screened by 1 month of age, in accordance with AAP recommendations.

- *Provision of follow-up care*: Comprehensive documentation and communication with the follow-up provider are essential. Written records should describe prenatal care, delivery, and immediate postnatal course, clearly documenting which screenings and medications have been provided by the birth attendant, and which remain to be performed. All newborn infants should be evaluated by a health care professional who is knowledgeable and experienced in pediatrics within 24 hours of birth and subsequently within 48 hours of

that first evaluation. The initial follow-up visit should include infant weight and physical examination, especially for jaundice and hydration. If the mother is breastfeeding, the visit should include evaluation of any maternal history of breast problems (eg, pain or engorgement), infant elimination patterns, and a formal observed evaluation of breastfeeding, including position, latch, and milk transfer. The results of maternal and neonatal laboratory tests should be reviewed; clinically indicated tests, such as serum bilirubin, should be performed; and screening tests should be completed in accordance with state regulations. Screening for congenital heart disease should be performed by using oxygen saturation testing as recommended by the AAP.[17]

CONCLUSIONS

The AAP concurs with the recent position statement of the ACOG, affirming that hospitals and birthing centers are the safest settings for birth in the United States, while respecting the right of women to make a medically informed decision about delivery.[7] In addition, the AAP in concert with the ACOG does not support the provision of care by lay midwives or other midwives who are not certified by the American Midwifery Certification Board.[7]

Regardless of the circumstances of his or her birth, including location, every newborn infant deserves health care

that adheres to the standards highlighted in this statement and more completely described in other AAP publications.[11–16] The goal of providing high-quality care to all newborn infants can best be achieved through continuing efforts by all participating providers and institutions to develop and sustain communications and understanding on the basis of professional interaction and mutual respect throughout the health care system.

LEAD AUTHOR

Kristi L. Watterberg, MD

COMMITTEE ON FETUS AND NEWBORN, 2012–2013

Lu-Ann Papile, MD, Chairperson
Jill E. Baley, MD
William Benitz, MD
James Cummings, MD
Waldemar A. Carlo, MD
Eric Eichenwald, MD
Praveen Kumar, MD
Richard A. Polin, MD
Rosemarie C. Tan, MD, PhD

PAST COMMITTEE MEMBER

Kristi L. Watterberg, MD

LIAISONS

Capt. Wanda Denise Barfield, MD, MPH – *Centers for Disease Control and Prevention*
George Macones, MD – *American College of Obstetricians and Gynecologists*
Ann L. Jefferies, MD – *Canadian Pediatric Society*
Erin L. Keels, APRN, MS, NNP-BC – *National Association of Neonatal Nurses*
Tonse N. K. Raju, MD, DCH – *National Institutes of Health*
Kasper S. Wang, MD – *Section on Surgery*

STAFF

Jim Couto, MA

REFERENCES

1. MacDorman MF, Mathews TJ, Declercq E. Home births in the United States, 1990–2009. *NCHS Data Brief.* 2012;Jan(84):1–8

2. Ravelli AC, Jager KJ, de Groot MH, et al. Travel time from home to hospital and adverse perinatal outcomes in women at term in the Netherlands. *BJOG.* 2011;118(4):457–465

3. Malloy MH. Infant outcomes of certified nurse midwife attended home births: United States 2000 to 2004. *J Perinatol.* 2010;30(9):622–627

4. Chang JJ, Macones GA. Birth outcomes of planned home births in Missouri: a population-based study. *Am J Perinatol.* 2011;28(7):529–536

5. Wax JR, Lucas FL, Lamont M, Pinette MG, Cartin A, Blackstone J. Maternal and newborn

outcomes in planned home birth vs planned hospital births: a meta-analysis [published correction appears in *Am J Obstet Gynecol.* 2011;204(4):e7–e13]. *Am J Obstet Gynecol.* 2010;203(3):243.e1–243.e8

6. Janssen PA, Saxell L, Page LA, Klein MC, Liston RM, Lee SK. Outcomes of planned home birth with registered midwife versus planned hospital birth with midwife or physician [published correction appears in *CMAJ.* 2009;181(9):617]. *CMAJ.* 2009;181(6–7):377–383

7. ACOG Committee on Obstetric Practice. ACOG Committee opinion no. 476: planned home birth [published correction appears in *Obstet Gynecol.* 2011;117(5):1232]. *Obstet Gynecol.* 2011;117(2 pt 1):425–428

8. Lindgren HE, Rådestad IJ, Hildingsson IM. Transfer in planned home births in Sweden—effects on the experience of birth: a nationwide population-based study. *Sex Reprod Healthc.* 2011;2(3):101–105

9. Symon A, Winter C, Inkster M, Donnan PT. Outcomes for births booked under an independent midwife and births in NHS maternity units: matched comparison study. *BMJ.* 2009;Jun 11(338):b2060

10. Kattwinkel J, Perlman JM, Aziz K, et al; American Heart Association. Neonatal resuscitation: 2010 American Heart Association guidelines for cardiopulmonary resuscitation and emergency cardiovascular care. *Pediatrics.* 2010;126(5). Available at: www.pediatrics.org/cgi/content/full/126/5/e1400

11. American Academy of Pediatrics; American College of Obstetricians and Gynecologists. Care of the newborn. In: Riley LE, Stark AR, Kilpatrick SJ, Papile L-A, eds. *Guidelines for Perinatal Care.* 7th ed. Elk Grove Village, IL: American Academy of Pediatrics; 2012:265–320

12. American Academy of Pediatrics Committee on Fetus and Newborn. Hospital stay for healthy term newborns. *Pediatrics.* 2010;125(2):405–409

13. American Academy of Pediatrics; American College of Obstetricians and Gynecologists. Neonatal complications and management of high-risk infants. In: Riley LE, Stark AR, Kilpatrick SJ, Papile L-A, eds. *Guidelines for Perinatal Care.* 7th ed. Elk Grove Village, IL: American Academy of Pediatrics; 2012:321–382

14. Baker CJ, Byington CL, Polin RA; Committee on Infectious Diseases; Committee on Fetus and Newborn. Policy statement—recommendations for the prevention of perinatal group B streptococcal (GBS) disease. *Pediatrics.* 2011;128(3):611–616

15. Adamkin DH; Committee on Fetus and Newborn. Postnatal glucose homeostasis in late-preterm and term infants. *Pediatrics.* 2011;127(3):575–579

16. American Academy of Pediatrics Subcommittee on Hyperbilirubinemia. Management of hyperbilirubinemia in the newborn infant 35 or more weeks of gestation [published correction appears in *Pediatrics.* 2004;114(4):1138]. *Pediatrics.* 2004;114(1):297–316

17. Kemper AR, Mahle WT, Martin GR, et al. Strategies for implementing screening for critical congenital heart disease. *Pediatrics.* 2011;128(5). Available at: www.pediatrics.org/cgi/content/full/128/5/e1259

Prenatal Substance Abuse: Short- and Long-term Effects on the Exposed Fetus

- *Technical Report*

TECHNICAL REPORT

Prenatal Substance Abuse: Short- and Long-term Effects on the Exposed Fetus

Marylou Behnke, MD, Vincent C. Smith, MD, COMMITTEE ON SUBSTANCE ABUSE, and COMMITTEE ON FETUS AND NEWBORN

KEY WORDS

prenatal drug exposure, alcohol, nicotine, marijuana, cocaine, methamphetamine, growth and development

ABBREVIATIONS

AAP—American Academy of Pediatrics
THC—tetrahydrocannabinol

www.pediatrics.org/cgi/doi/10.1542/peds.2012-3931

doi:10.1542/peds.2012-3931

PEDIATRICS (ISSN Numbers: Print, 0031-4005; Online, 1098-4275).

abstract

Prenatal substance abuse continues to be a significant problem in this country and poses important health risks for the developing fetus. The primary care pediatrician's role in addressing prenatal substance exposure includes prevention, identification of exposure, recognition of medical issues for the exposed newborn infant, protection of the infant, and follow-up of the exposed infant. This report will provide information for the most common drugs involved in prenatal exposure: nicotine, alcohol, marijuana, opiates, cocaine, and methamphetamine. *Pediatrics* 2013;131:e1009–e1024

Substance abuse has been a worldwide problem at all levels of society since ancient times. Attention has been directed toward the use of legal and illegal substances by pregnant women over the past several decades. Almost all drugs are known to cross the placenta and have some effect on the fetus. The effects on the human fetus of prenatal cigarette use have been identified and studied since the 1960s,[1] the effects of alcohol and opiate use have been studied since the 1970s,[2–4] and the effects a variety of other illicit drugs have been studied since the 1980s.[5–7] This report reviews data regarding the prevalence of exposure and available technologies for identifying exposure as well as current information regarding short- and long-term outcomes of exposed infants, with the aim of facilitating pediatricians in fulfilling their role in the promotion and maintenance of infant and child health.

PREVALENCE

Prevalence estimates for prenatal substance use vary widely and have been difficult to establish. Differences are likely attributable to such things as the use of different sampling methods and drug-detection methods, screening women in different settings, and obtaining data at different points in time. For example, prevalence will vary depending on whether history or testing of biological specimens is used; whether the biological specimen is hair, urine, or meconium; and whether the specimens are merely screened for drugs or screened and confirmed with additional testing. There also will be differences depending on whether the sample being investigated is a community sample or a targeted sample, such as women who are in drug treatment or are incarcerated. Lastly, prevalence must be interpreted in light of the fact that the use of specific drugs waxes and wanes over time nationwide as the popularity of certain substances changes.

Although a variety of prevalence studies have been conducted over the past 2 decades, there is 1 national survey that regularly provides information on trends in substance abuse among pregnant women. The National Survey on Drug Use and Health (formerly called the National Household Survey on Drug Abuse), sponsored by the Substance Abuse and Mental Health Services Administration (http://www.oas.samhsa.gov/nhsda.htm), is an annual survey providing national and state level information on the use of alcohol, tobacco, and illicit drugs in a sample of more than 67 000 noninstitutionalized people older than 12 years. Data are combined into 2-year epochs and include reported drug use for pregnant women between the ages of 15 and 44 years. Current illegal drug use among pregnant women remained relatively stable from 2007–2008 (5.1%) to 2009–2010 (4.4%). These average prevalence rates are significantly lower than reported current illicit drug use rates for nonpregnant women (10.9%). Importantly, the rate of current drug use among the youngest and possibly the most vulnerable pregnant women was highest (16.2% for 15- to 17-year-olds, compared with 7.4% among 18- to 25-year-olds and 1.9% among 26- to 44-year-olds). Table 1 summarizes these data along with information regarding current alcohol use, binge drinking,

TABLE 1 Comparison of Drug Use Among Women 15 to 44 Years of Age by Pregnancy Status: 2009–2010

	Pregnant Women, %	Nonpregnant Women, %
Illicit drug use	4.4	10.9
Alcohol use	10.8	54.7
Binge drinking	3.7	24.6
Cigarette use	16.3	26.7

and cigarette use by pregnant and nonpregnant women. An additional important finding from this survey was that the rate of cigarette smoking for those 15 to 17 years of age actually was higher for pregnant women than for nonpregnant women (22.7% vs 13.4%, respectively). This report details many sociodemographic variables related to drug use in the American population, and the reader is referred to the Substance Abuse and Mental Health Services Administration Web site for the full report (http://www.oas.samhsa.gov/nhsda.htm).

IDENTIFICATION OF PRENATAL EXPOSURE

Two basic methods are used to identify drug users: self-report or biological specimens. Although no single approach can accurately determine the presence or amount of drug used during pregnancy, it is more likely that fetal exposure will be identified if a biological specimen is collected along with a structured interview.[8]

Self-reported history is an inexpensive and practical method for identifying prenatal drug exposure and is the only method available in which information can be obtained regarding the timing of the drug use during pregnancy and the amount used. Unfortunately, self-report suffers from problems with the veracity of the informant and recall accuracy.[9,10] Histories obtained by trusted, nonjudgmental individuals or via computerized survey forms; questions referring back to the previous trimester or prepregnancy usage, not current use; and pregnancy calendars used to assist recollection each improve the accuracy of the information obtained.[11–13]

Several biological specimens can be used to screen for drug exposure. Each specimen has its own individual variations with regard to the window of detection, the specific drug metabolites

used for identification, methods of adulteration of the sample, and analytical techniques, thus altering the sensitivity and specificity for each drug of interest. The most common analytical method used for screening biological specimens is an immunoassay designed to screen out drug-free samples. Threshold values generally are set high to minimize false-positive test results but may be too high to detect low-dose or remote exposure. Because immunoassay is a relatively nonspecific test, positive results require confirmation by using gas chromatography/mass spectrometry. In addition, confirmation of the presence of a drug is not always associated with drug abuse. Alternative explanations include passive exposure to the drug, ingestion of other products contaminated with the drug, or use of prescription medications that either contain the drug or are metabolized to the drug.[14] Thus, careful patient histories remain essential to the process of identification.

The 3 most commonly used specimens to establish drug exposure during the prenatal and perinatal period are urine, meconium, and hair; however, none is accepted as a "gold standard." Urine has been the most frequently tested biological specimen because of its ease of collection. Urine testing identifies only recent drug use, because threshold levels of drug metabolites generally can be detected in urine only for several days. A notable exception to this is marijuana, the metabolites of which can be excreted for as long as 10 days in the urine of regular users[15] or up to 30 days in chronic, heavy users. Urine is a good medium as well for the detection of nicotine, opiate, cocaine, and amphetamine exposure.[16,17]

Meconium is also easy to collect noninvasively. It is hypothesized that drugs accumulate in meconium throughout pregnancy, and thus, meconium is thought to reflect exposure during the second and third trimester of pregnancy when meconium forms. However, use of meconium to determine the timing or extent of exposure during pregnancy is controversial[18] because of a lack of studies regarding the effects of the timing and quantity of the postpartum specimen collection as well as the effects of urine or transitional stool contamination of the meconium samples.[19] Meconium has been used for the detection of nicotine, alcohol, marijuana, opiate, cocaine, and amphetamine exposure.[16,20]

Hair is easy to collect, although some people decline this sampling method because of cosmetic concerns and societal taboos. Drugs become trapped within the hair and, thus, can reflect drug use over a long period of time. Unfortunately, using hair to determine timing and quantity of exposure also is controversial. In addition, environmental contamination, natural hair colors and textures, cosmetic hair processing, and volume of the hair sample available all affect the rational interpretation of the results.[21–24] Hair is useful for the detection of nicotine, opiate, cocaine, and amphetamine exposure.[16,25]

Other biological specimens have been studied for use in the detection of in utero drug exposure but are not commonly used in the clinical setting. These include such specimens as cord blood, human milk, amniotic fluid, and umbilical cord tissue.[8,19,26] In the case of umbilical cord tissue, drug class-specific immunoassays for amphetamines, opiates, cocaine, and cannabinoids appear to be as reliable as meconium testing, with the additional benefit of availability of the tissue at the time of birth.[27]

Beginning in the early 1980s, states began to enact legislation in response to the increasingly popular use of "crack" cocaine in our society. Such laws required the reporting of women who used drugs during pregnancy to the legal system through states' child abuse statutes. In 2003, the Keeping Children and Families Safe Act (Public Law 108-36) was passed by Congress, requiring physicians to notify their state child protective services agency of any infant identified as affected by illegal substances at birth or experiencing drug withdrawal. Currently, issues of whether to use biological specimens to screen for drug abuse; whether to screen the mother, her infant, or both; and which women and infants to screen are issues complicated by legal, ethical, social, and scientific concerns. Each of these concerns must be taken into account as obstetricians, neonatologists, and pediatricians work to develop protocols for identifying prenatal drug exposure. For example, there is no biological specimen that, when obtained randomly, identifies prenatal drug use with 100% accuracy; hence, a negative drug screening result does not ensure that the pregnancy was drug free. Targeted screening of high-risk women is problematic, because it can be biased toward women of racial or ethnic minorities and those who are economically disadvantaged or socially disenfranchised. Universal screening of pregnant women is impractical and not cost-effective.[28–30] Finally, testing of biological specimens when the maternal history is positive for drug use increases medical costs and does not necessarily provide information that guides the medical care of the infant.[31]

MECHANISMS OF ACTION OF DRUGS ON THE FETUS

Drugs can affect the fetus in multiple ways. Early in gestation, during the embryonic stage, drugs can have significant teratogenic effects. However, during the fetal period, after major structural development is complete, drugs have more subtle effects, including abnormal growth and/or maturation, alterations in neurotransmitters and their receptors, and brain organization. These are considered to be the direct effects of drugs. However, drugs also can exert a pharmacologic effect on the mother and, thus, indirectly affect the fetus. For example, nicotine acts on nicotinic cholinergic receptors within the mesolimbic pathway, and neuropathways activated by alcohol enhance inhibitory γ-aminobutyric acid (GABA) receptors and reduce glutamate receptor activity. Drugs of abuse mimic naturally occurring neurotransmitters, such that marijuana acts as anandamides, opiates act as endorphins, and cocaine and stimulants act within the mesolimbic dopaminergic pathways to increase dopamine and serotonin within the synapses.[32] Other indirect effects of drugs of abuse on the fetus include altered delivery of substrate to the fetus for nutritional purposes, either because of placental insufficiency or altered maternal health behaviors attributable to the mother's addiction. These altered behaviors, which include poor nutrition, decreased access/compliance with health care, increased exposure to violence, and increased risk of mental illness and infection, may place the fetus at risk.[33]

Nicotine concentrations are higher in the fetal compartment (placenta, amniotic fluid, fetal serum) compared with maternal serum concentrations.[34–36] Nicotine is only 1 of more than 4000 compounds to which the fetus is exposed through maternal smoking. Of these, ~30 compounds have been associated with adverse health outcomes. Although the exact mechanisms by which nicotine produces adverse fetal effects are unknown, it is likely that hypoxia, undernourishment of the fetus, and direct vasoconstrictor effects on the placental and umbilical vessels all play a role.[37,38] Nicotine also has been shown to have significant deleterious effects on brain development, including alterations in brain metabolism and neurotransmitter systems and abnormal brain development.[39–43] Additional toxicity from compounds in smoke, such as cyanide and cadmium, contribute to toxicity.[44–48]

Ethanol easily crosses the placenta into the fetus, with a significant concentration of the drug identified in the amniotic fluid as well as in maternal and fetal blood.[49,50] A variety of mechanisms explaining the effects of alcohol on the fetus have been hypothesized. These include direct teratogenic effects during the embryonic and fetal stage of development as well as toxic effects of alcohol on the placenta, altered prostaglandin and protein synthesis, hormonal alterations, nutritional effects, altered neurotransmitter levels in the brain, altered brain morphology and neuronal development, and hypoxia (thought to be attributable to decreased placental blood flow and alterations in vascular tone in the umbilical vessels).[51–69]

Although the main chemical compound in marijuana, δ-9-tetrahydrocannabinol (THC), crosses the placenta rapidly, its major metabolite, 11-nor-9-carboxy-THC, does not.[70] Unlike other drugs, the placenta appears to limit fetal exposure to marijuana, as fetal THC concentrations have been documented to be lower than maternal concentrations in studies of various animal species.[15,70–72] The deleterious effects of marijuana on the fetus are thought to be attributable to complex pharmacologic actions on developing biological systems, altered uterine blood flow, and altered maternal health behaviors.[73–75] Similar to other drugs, marijuana has been shown to alter brain neurotransmitters as well

as brain biochemistry, resulting in decreased protein, nucleic acid, and lipid synthesis.[74,76–79] Marijuana can remain in the body for up to 30 days, thus prolonging fetal exposure. In addition, smoking marijuana produces as much as 5 times the amount of carbon monoxide as does cigarette smoking, perhaps altering fetal oxygenation.[80]

In humans, opiates rapidly cross the placenta, with drug equilibration between the mother and the fetus.[81] Opiates have been shown to decrease brain growth and cell development in animals, but studies of their effects on neurotransmitter levels and opioid receptors have produced mixed results.[82–89]

Pharmacologic studies of cocaine in animal models using a variety of species have demonstrated that cocaine easily crosses both the placenta and the blood-brain barrier and can have significant teratogenic effects on the developing fetus, directly and indirectly.[90] Cocaine's teratogenic effects most likely result from interference with the neurotrophic roles of monoaminergic transmitters during brain development,[91–94] which can significantly affect cortical neuronal development and may lead to morphologic abnormalities in several brain structures, including the frontal cingulate cortex.[94] It also appears that the development of areas of the brain that regulate attention and executive functioning are particularly vulnerable to cocaine. Thus, functions such as arousal, attention, and memory may be adversely affected by prenatal cocaine exposure.[89,91,95–97] Furthermore, insults to the nervous system during neurogenesis, before homeostatic regulatory mechanisms are fully developed, differ from those on mature systems. Thus, cocaine exposure occurring during development of the nervous system might be expected to

result in permanent changes in brain structure and function, which can produce altered responsiveness to environmental or pharmacologic challenges later in life.[98]

Methamphetamine is a member of a group of sympathomimetic drugs that stimulate the central nervous system. It readily passes through the placenta and the blood-brain barrier and can have significant effects on the fetus.[99–101] After a single dose of methamphetamine to pregnant mice, levels of substance in the fetal brain were found to be similar to those found in human infants after prenatal methamphetamine exposure, with accumulation and distribution of the drug most likely dependent on the monoaminergic transport system. It is possible that the mechanism of action of methamphetamine is an interaction with and alteration of these neurotransmitter systems in the developing fetal brain[100] as well as alterations in brain morphogenesis.[102]

MEDICAL ISSUES IN THE NEWBORN PERIOD

Fetal Growth

Fetal tobacco exposure has been a known risk factor for low birth weight and intrauterine growth restriction for more than 50 years,[103] with decreasing birth weight shown to be related to the number of cigarettes smoked.[104–107] Importantly, by 24 months of age, most studies no longer demonstrate an effect of fetal tobacco exposure on somatic growth parameters of prenatally exposed infants.[108–114] Growth restriction is 1 of the hallmarks of prenatal alcohol exposure and must be present to establish a diagnosis of fetal alcohol syndrome.[3,115] However, even moderate amounts of alcohol use during pregnancy is associated with a decrease in size at birth.[116–119] In general, marijuana has not been associated with fetal growth restriction, particularly after controlling for other prenatal drug exposures.[109,120-122] Fetal growth effects are reported in studies of prenatal opiate exposure; however, confounding variables known to be associated with poor growth, such as multiple drug use and low socioeconomic status, were not well controlled in many of the studies.[123] Using data from the Maternal Lifestyle Study, Bada et al[124] reported lower birth weight in opiate-exposed newborn infants born at ≥33 weeks' gestation, independent of use of other drugs, prenatal care, or other medical risk factors. An independent effect of prenatal cocaine exposure on intrauterine growth has been the most consistent finding across studies of prenatally exposed infants.[122,125-130] Early studies on prenatal methamphetamine exposure[131] as well as recent studies[132] reveal independent effects of the drug on fetal growth. However, the literature available is limited at this time. Several reviews on the effects of prenatal drug exposure on growth contain additional details.[133–135]

Congenital Anomalies

Nicotine has been associated with oral facial clefts in exposed newborn infants,[136–140] although the data are relatively weak. There is a vast literature on the teratogenic effects of prenatal alcohol exposure after the first description of fetal alcohol syndrome in 1973.[3] The American Academy of Pediatrics (AAP) policy statement "Fetal Alcohol Syndrome and Alcohol-Related Neurodevelopmental Disorders" contains more information.[141] No clear teratogenic effect of marijuana or opiates is documented in exposed newborn infants.[142] Original reports regarding cocaine teratogenicity have not been further documented.[133,143] Studies of fetal methamphetamine exposure in humans are

limited. However, Little et al[131] reported no increase in the frequency of major anomalies in a small sample of exposed infants when compared with non-exposed infants.

Withdrawal

No convincing studies are available that document a neonatal withdrawal syndrome for prenatal nicotine exposure. Although several authors describe abnormal newborn behavior of exposed infants immediately after delivery, the findings are more consistent with drug toxicity, which steadily improves over time,[144,145] as opposed to an abstinence syndrome, in which clinical signs would escalate over time as the drug is metabolized and eliminated from the body. There is 1 report of withdrawal from prenatal alcohol exposure in infants with fetal alcohol syndrome born to mothers who drank heavily during pregnancy,[146] but withdrawal symptoms have not been reported in longitudinal studies available in the extant literature. Neonatal abstinence symptoms have not been observed in marijuana-exposed infants, although abnormal newborn behavior has been reported with some similarities to that associated with narcotic exposure.[147] An opiate withdrawal syndrome was first described by Finnegan et al[148] in 1975. Neonatal abstinence syndrome includes a combination of physiologic and neurobehavioral signs that include such things as sweating, irritability, increased muscle tone and activity, feeding problems, diarrhea, and seizures. Infants with neonatal abstinence syndrome often require prolonged hospitalization and treatment with medication. Methadone exposure has been associated with more severe withdrawal than has exposure to heroin.[149] Early reports regarding buprenorphine, a more recent alternative to methadone, suggest minimal to mild withdrawal in exposed

neonates. A large multicenter trial evaluating buprenorphine's effect on exposed infants documented decreased morphine dose, hospital length of stay, and length of treatment.[150–152] There has been no substantiation of early reports regarding cocaine withdrawal.[153] Currently, no prospective studies of withdrawal in methamphetamine-exposed infants are available. A retrospective study by Smith et al[154] reported withdrawal symptoms in 49% of their sample of 294 methamphetamine-exposed newborn infants. However, only 4% required pharmacologic intervention. The AAP clinical report on neonatal drug withdrawal contains in-depth information on neonatal drug withdrawal, including treatment options.[155]

Neurobehavior

Abnormalities of newborn neurobehavior, including impaired orientation and autonomic regulation[156] and abnormalities of muscle tone,[144,147,157] have been identified in a number of prenatal nicotine exposure studies. Poor habituation and low levels of arousal along with motor abnormalities have been identified in women who drank alcohol heavily during their pregnancy.[80,158] Prenatal marijuana exposure is associated with increased startles and tremors in the newborn.[120] Abnormal neurobehavior in opiate-exposed newborn infants is related to neonatal abstinence (see earlier section on Withdrawal). Using the Brazelton Newborn Behavioral Assessment Scale,[159] reported effects of prenatal cocaine exposure on infants have included irritability and lability of state, decreased behavioral and autonomic regulation, and poor alertness and orientation.[160] Recent data from the Infant Development, Environment, and Lifestyle multicenter study on the effects of prenatal methamphetamine exposure documented abnormal neurobehavioral patterns in exposed newborn infants consisting of poor movement quality, decreased arousal, and increased stress.[161]

Breastfeeding

Few sources are available documenting the prevalence of drug use during breastfeeding. Lacking recent data, the 1988 National Maternal and Infant Health Survey (http://www.cdc.gov/nchs/about/major/nmihs/abnmihs.htm) revealed that the prevalence of drug use during pregnancy was comparable to the prevalence of use among women who breastfed their infants. Women who used various amounts of alcohol or marijuana and moderate amounts of cocaine during their pregnancy were not deterred from breastfeeding their infants. Thus, the pediatrician is faced with weighing the risks of exposing an infant to drugs during breastfeeding against the many known benefits of breastfeeding.[162] For women who are abstinent at the time of delivery or who are participating in a supervised treatment program and choose to breastfeed, close postpartum follow-up of the mother and infant are essential.

For most street drugs, including marijuana, opiates, cocaine, and methamphetamine, the risks to the infant of ongoing, active use by the mother outweigh the benefits of breastfeeding, because most street drugs have been shown to have some effect on the breastfeeding infant.[163–166] In addition, the dose of drug being used and the contaminants within the drug are unknown for most street drugs. Nicotine is secreted into human milk[167,168] and has been associated with decreased milk production, decreased weight gain of the infant, and exposure of the infant to environmental tobacco smoke.[169–171] Alcohol is concentrated in human milk. Heavy alcohol use has been shown to be associated with decreased milk

supply and neurobehavioral effects on the infant.[172–174] However, for nicotine and alcohol, the benefits of breastfeeding in the face of limited use of these drugs outweigh the potential risks. Marijuana has an affinity for lipids and accumulates in human milk,[175] as can cocaine[26] and amphetamines.[101,165] Although the AAP considers the use of marijuana, opiates, cocaine, and methamphetamine to be a contraindication to breastfeeding, supervised methadone use not only is considered to be compatible with breastfeeding, with no effect on the infant or on lactation, but also is a potential benefit in reducing the symptoms associated with neonatal abstinence syndrome. Several available reviews provide more detailed information with regard to breastfeeding and substance abuse.[162,176] The reader is also referred to the AAP policy statement "Breastfeeding and the Use of Human Milk."[177]

LONG-TERM EFFECTS RELATED TO PRENATAL DRUG EXPOSURE

Growth

The effects of prenatal tobacco exposure on long-term growth are not clear-cut. Reports in the literature of effects on height and weight[178–181] have not been substantiated by research teams able to control for other drug use in the sample.[109,117,182,183] Recent studies, some of which include adolescents, have suggested that the effect on growth might be attributable to a disproportionate weight for height, such that prenatally exposed children were more likely to be obese as evidenced by a higher BMI, increased Ponderal index, and increased skinfold thickness.[113,183,184] A robust and extensive literature is available documenting the effects of prenatal alcohol exposure on long-term growth. Although poor growth is 1 of the hallmarks of fetal alcohol

syndrome, it is the least sensitive of the diagnostic criteria.[185] No independent effect of prenatal marijuana exposure on growth has been documented throughout early childhood and adolescence.[109,182,184] Long-term effects on growth have not been documented in the opiate-exposed child.[186] The available literature on the effect of prenatal cocaine exposure on growth throughout childhood is not conclusive. Although several studies document the negative effects of prenatal cocaine exposure on postnatal growth,[187–189] others do not.[126,190,191] No studies are available linking prenatal methamphetamine exposure to postnatal growth problems. However, 1 study of unspecified amphetamine use suggests that in utero exposure may be associated with poor growth throughout early childhood.[192]

Behavior

After controlling for a variety of potentially confounding socioeconomic, psychosocial, family, and health variables, a number of studies have identified independent effects of prenatal tobacco exposure on long-term behavioral outcomes extending from early childhood into adulthood. For example, impulsivity and attention problems have been identified in children prenatally exposed to nicotine.[193–195] In addition, prenatal tobacco exposure has been associated with hyperactivity[196] and negative[197] and externalizing behaviors in children,[198–200] which appear to continue through adolescence and into adulthood in the form of higher rates of delinquency, criminal behavior, and substance abuse.[201–206] Prenatal alcohol exposure is linked with significant attention problems in offspring[207–210] as well as adaptive behavior problems spanning early childhood to adulthood.[211] Problems identified included disrupted school experiences, delinquent and criminal behavior, and substance abuse. Kelly et al[212] published an in-depth review of the effects of prenatal alcohol exposure on social behavior. Inattention and impulsivity at 10 years of age have been associated with prenatal marijuana exposure.[213] Hyperactivity and short attention span have been noted in toddlers prenatally exposed to opiates,[214] and older exposed children have demonstrated memory and perceptual problems.[215] Caregiver reports of child behavior problems in preschool-aged[216] and elementary school-aged children[217,218] have not been related to cocaine exposure, except in combination with other risk factors.[219–221] However, in longitudinal modeling of caregiver reports at 3, 5, and 7 years of age, the multisite Maternal Lifestyles Study revealed that prenatal cocaine exposure had an independent negative effect on trajectories of behavior problems.[222] There have been teacher reports of behavior problems in prenatally exposed children,[223] although again, findings have not been consistent across studies,[190] and some have been moderated by other risks.[224] There also have been reports in this age group of deficits in attention processing[190] and an increase in symptoms of attention-deficit/hyperactivity disorder and oppositional defiant disorder self-reported by the exposed children.[217,218] To date, no studies are available that link prenatal methamphetamine exposure with long-term behavioral problems. However, 1 study of unspecified amphetamine use during pregnancy suggests a possible association with externalizing behaviors and peer problems.[225,226]

Cognition/Executive Functioning

The link between prenatal nicotine exposure and impaired cognition is not nearly as strong as the link with behavioral problems. However, studies of both young and older children prenatally exposed to nicotine have revealed abnormalities in learning and memory[227,228] and slightly lower IQ scores.[201,229–231] Prenatal alcohol exposure frequently is cited as the most common, preventable cause of nongenetic intellectual disability. Although IQ scores are lower in alcohol-exposed offspring,[207,232] they can be variable. Additionally, prenatal alcohol exposure has been associated with poorer memory and executive functioning skills.[233] Marijuana has not been shown to affect general IQ, but it has been associated with deficits in problem-solving skills that require sustained attention and visual memory, analysis, and integration[230,231,234–236] and with subtle deficits in learning and memory.[237] Longitudinal studies of prenatal opiate exposure have not produced consistent findings with regard to developmental sequelae. Although developmental scores tend to be lower in exposed infants, these differences no longer exist when appropriate medical and environmental controls are included in the analyses.[238–240] With little exception,[241] prenatal cocaine exposure has not predicted overall development, IQ, or school readiness among toddlers, elementary school-aged children, or middle school-aged children.[190,242–250] However, several studies have revealed alterations in various aspects of executive functioning,[221,241] including visual-motor ability,[244] attention,[251–253] and working memory.[254] To date, limited data are available revealing an association between prenatal methamphetamine exposure and IQ.[255]

Language

Poor language development in early childhood after prenatal nicotine exposure has been reported,[227,256,257] as have poor language and reading abilities in 9- to 12-year-olds.[258] Prenatal alcohol exposure has been shown to interfere with the development and use of language,[259] possibly leading to long-term problems in social interaction.[260] No effect of prenatal marijuana exposure on language development has been identified in children through 12 years of age.[227,258] Subtle language delays have been associated with prenatal cocaine exposure.[256,261,262] Currently, no data are available relating the prenatal use of opiates or methamphetamine to language development in exposed offspring.

Achievement

The literature available evaluating academic achievement is limited. In nicotine-exposed children, Batstra et al[200] identified poorer performance on arithmetic and spelling tasks that were part of standardized Dutch achievement tests. Howell et al[232] reported poorer performance in mathematics on achievement tests in adolescents who had been exposed prenatally to alcohol. Streissguth et al[263] describe a variety of significant academic and school problems related to prenatal alcohol exposure, primarily associated with deficits in reading and math skills throughout the school years.[263–266] Prenatal marijuana exposure has been associated with academic underachievement, particularly in the areas of reading and spelling.[267] School achievement is not an area that has been studied adequately with regard to prenatal opiate exposure. Reported effects of cocaine exposure on school achievement are variable. In the longitudinal Maternal Lifestyle Study, 7-year-old children with prenatal cocaine exposure had a 79% increased odds of having an individualized educational plan (adjusted for IQ),[268] and Morrow et al[249] found 2.8 times the risk of learning disabilities among children with prenatal cocaine exposure compared with their peers who were not exposed to drugs prenatally. However, other studies do not support significant cocaine effects on school achievement.[190,269] No data are available for the effects of methamphetamine on school achievement. Cernerud et al[270] reported on 65 children prenatally exposed to amphetamines. At 14 to 15 years of age, the children in their cohort scored significantly lower on mathematics tests than did their classmates who were not exposed to amphetamines prenatally and had a higher rate of grade retention than the Swedish norm.

Predisposed to Own Drug Use

A limited number of studies are available that have investigated the association between prenatal substance exposure and subsequent drug abuse in exposed offspring. These studies did not document cause and effect, and it remains to be determined how much of the association can be linked to prenatal exposure versus socioeconomic, environmental, and genetic influences. Studies available for prenatal nicotine exposure suggest an increased risk of early experimentation[271] and abuse of nicotine in exposed offspring.[272,273] Brennan et al[274] reported an association of prenatal nicotine exposure with higher rates of hospitalization for substance abuse in adult offspring.

Mounting clinical data support an increased risk of ethanol abuse later in life after prenatal exposure.[275,277] Prenatal marijuana exposure has been associated with an increased risk for marijuana and cigarette use in exposed offspring.[273] Insufficient data are available to draw any conclusions relative to the affects of prenatal opiate, cocaine, or methamphetamine exposure on the risk for tobacco, problem alcohol, or illicit drug use later in life.

SUMMARY

Although methodologic differences between studies and limited data in the extant literature make generalization of the results for several of the drugs difficult, some summary statements can be made by using the current knowledge base (Table 2).

The negative effect of prenatal nicotine exposure on fetal growth has been known for decades; however, longitudinal studies do not reveal a consistent effect on long-term growth. Clinical studies have failed to reach a consensus regarding congenital anomalies, and there is no evidence of a withdrawal syndrome in the newborn infant. Recent studies document a negative effect of prenatal exposure on infant neurobehavior as well as on long-term behavior, cognition, language, and achievement.

Alcohol remains the most widely studied prenatal drug of abuse, and the evidence is strong for fetal growth problems, congenital anomalies, and abnormal infant neurobehavior. There has been no convincing evidence of a neonatal withdrawal syndrome. Ongoing longitudinal studies continue to document long-term effects on growth, behavior, cognition, language, and achievement, and alcohol is the most common identifiable teratogen associated with intellectual disability.

Although there have been studies revealing subtle abnormalities in infant neurobehavior related to prenatal marijuana exposure, there have been no significant effects documented for fetal growth, congenital anomalies, or withdrawal. Long-term studies reveal effects of prenatal exposure on behavior, cognition, and achievement but not on language or growth.

The most significant effect of prenatal opiate exposure is neonatal abstinence syndrome. There have been documented effects on fetal growth (but not on long-term growth) and infant neurobehavior as well as long-term effects on behavior. There is not a consensus as to the effects of prenatal opiate exposure on cognition, and few data are available regarding language and achievement.

TABLE 2 Summary of Effects of Prenatal Drug Exposure

	Nicotine	Alcohol	Marijuana	Opiates	Cocaine	Methamphetamine
Short-term effects/birth outcome						
Fetal growth	Effect	Strong effect	No effect	Effect	Effect	Effect
Anomalies	No consensus on effect	Strong effect	No effect	No effect	No effect	No effect
Withdrawal	No effect	No effect	No effect	Strong effect	No effect	*
Neurobehavior	Effect	Effect	Effect	Effect	Effect	Effect
Long-term effects						
Growth	No consensus on effect	Strong effect	No effect	No effect	No consensus on effect	*
Behavior	Effect	Strong effect	Effect	Effect	Effect	*
Cognition	Effect	Strong effect	Effect	No consensus on effect	Effect	*
Language	Effect	Effect	No effect	*	Effect	*
Achievement	Effect	Strong effect	Effect	*	No consensus on effect	*

* Limited or no data available.

Prenatal cocaine exposure has a negative effect on fetal growth and subtle effects on infant neurobehavior. However, there is little evidence to support an association with congenital anomalies or withdrawal. There is not a consensus regarding the effects of prenatal cocaine exposure on either long-term growth or achievement; however, there are documented long-term effects on behavior and subtle effects on language. Although there is little evidence to support an effect on overall cognition, a number of studies have documented effects on specific areas of executive function.

Studies on prenatal methamphetamine exposure are still in their infancy. Early studies have documented an effect of prenatal exposure on fetal growth and infant neurobehavior but no association with congenital anomalies and no data regarding infant withdrawal or any long-term effects.

LEAD AUTHORS

Marylou Behnke, MD
Vincent C. Smith, MD

COMMITTEE ON SUBSTANCE ABUSE, 2012–2013

Sharon Levy, MD, Chairperson
Seth D. Ammerman, MD
Pamela Kathern Gonzalez, MD
Sheryl Ann Ryan, MD
Lorena M. Siqueira, MD, MSPH
Vincent C. Smith, MD

PAST COMMITTEE MEMBERS

Marylou Behnke, MD
Patricia K. Kokotailo, MD, MPH
Janet F. Williams, MD, Immediate Past Chairperson

LIAISON

Vivian B. Faden, PhD – *National Institute on Alcohol Abuse and Alcoholism*
Deborah Simkin, MD – *American Academy of Child and Adolescent Psychiatry*

STAFF

Renee Jarrett
James Baumberger

COMMITTEE ON FETUS AND NEWBORN, 2012–2013

Lu-Ann Papile, MD, Chairperson
Jill E. Baley, MD
William Benitz, MD
Waldemar A. Carlo, MD
James J. Cummings, MD
Eric Eichenwald, MD
Praveen Kumar, MD
Richard A. Polin, MD
Rosemarie C. Tan, MD, PhD
Kasper S. Wang, MD

FORMER COMMITTEE MEMBER

Kristi L. Watterberg, MD

LIAISONS

CAPT Wanda D. Barfield, MD, MPH – *Centers for Disease Control and Prevention*
Ann L. Jefferies, MD – *Canadian Pediatric Society*
George A. Macones, MD – *American College of Obstetricians and Gynecologists*
Erin L. Keels APRN, MS, NNP-BC – *National Association of Neonatal Nurses*
Tonse N. K. Raju, MD, DCH – *National Institutes of Health*

STAFF

Jim Couto, MA

REFERENCES

1. Becker RF, Little CR, King JE. Experimental studies on nicotine absorption in rats during pregnancy. 3. Effect of subcutaneous injection of small chronic doses upon mother, fetus, and neonate. *Am J Obstet Gynecol.* 1968;100(7):957–968

2. Jones KL, Smith DW. Recognition of the fetal alcohol syndrome in early infancy. *Lancet.* 1973;302(7836):999–1001

3. Jones KL, Smith DW, Ulleland CN, Streissguth P. Pattern of malformation in offspring of chronic alcoholic mothers. *Lancet.* 1973;1(7815):1267–1271

4. Finnegan LP. Pathophysiological and behavioural effects of the transplacental transfer of narcotic drugs to the foetuses and neonates of narcotic-dependent mothers. *Bull Narc.* 1979;31(3-4):1–58

5. Chasnoff IJ, Burns WJ, Schnoll SH, Burns KA. Cocaine use in pregnancy. *N Engl J Med.* 1985;313(11):666–669

6. Oro AS, Dixon SD. Perinatal cocaine and methamphetamine exposure: maternal and neonatal correlates. *J Pediatr.* 1987;111(4):571–578

7. Fried PA. Postnatal consequences of maternal marijuana use in humans. *Ann N Y Acad Sci.* 1989;562:123–132

8. Eyler FD, Behnke M, Wobie K, Garvan CW, Tebbett I. Relative ability of biologic specimens and interviews to detect prenatal cocaine use. *Neurotoxicol Teratol.* 2005;27(4):677–687

9. Harrell AV. Validation of self-report: the research record. *NIDA Res Monogr.* 1985;57:12–21

10. Maisto SA, McKay JR, Connors GJ. Self-report issues in substance abuse: state of the art and future directions. *Behav Assess.* 1990;12(1):117–134

11. Day NL, Wagener DK, Taylor PM. Measurement of substance use during pregnancy: methodologic issues. *NIDA Res Monogr.* 1985;59:36–47

12. Magura S, Moses B. *Assessing Risk and Measuring Change in Families: The Family Risk Scales.* Washington, DC: Child Welfare League of America; 1987

13. Jacobson SW, Chiodo LM, Sokol RJ, Jacobson JL. Validity of maternal report of prenatal alcohol, cocaine, and smoking in relation to neurobehavioral outcome. *Pediatrics.* 2002;109(5):815–825

14. Kwong TC, Shearer D. Detection of drug use during pregnancy. *Obstet Gynecol Clin North Am.* 1998;25(1):43–64

15. Lee MJ. Marihuana and tobacco use in pregnancy. *Obstet Gynecol Clin North Am.* 1998;25(1):65–83

16. Lozano J, García-Algar O, Vall O, de la Torre R, Scaravelli G, Pichini S. Biological matrices for the evaluation of in utero exposure to drugs of abuse. *Ther Drug Monit.* 2007;29(6):711–734

17. Chiu HT, Isaac Wu HD, Kuo HW. The relationship between self-reported tobacco exposure and cotinines in urine and blood for pregnant women. *Sci Total Environ.* 2008;406(1-2):331–336

18. Lester BM, ElSohly M, Wright LL, et al. The Maternal Lifestyle Study: drug use by meconium toxicology and maternal self-report. *Pediatrics.* 2001;107(2):309–317

19. Casanova OQ, Lombardero N, Behnke M, Eyler FD, Conlon M, Bertholf RL. Detection of cocaine exposure in the neonate. Analyses of urine, meconium, and

amniotic fluid from mothers and infants exposed to cocaine. *Arch Pathol Lab Med.* 1994;118(10):988–993

20. Köhler E, Avenarius S, Rabsilber A, Gerloff C, Jorch G. Assessment of prenatal tobacco smoke exposure by determining nicotine and its metabolites in meconium. *Hum Exp Toxicol.* 2007;26(6):535–544

21. Bailey DN. Drug screening in an unconventional matrix: hair analysis. [editorial; comment] *JAMA.* 1989;262(23):3331

22. Joseph RE, Jr, Su TP, Cone EJ. In vitro binding studies of drugs to hair: influence of melanin and lipids on cocaine binding to Caucasoid and Africoid hair. *J Anal Toxicol.* 1996;20(6):338–344

23. Jurado C, Kintz P, Menéndez M, Repetto M. Influence of the cosmetic treatment of hair on drug testing. *Int J Legal Med.* 1997;110(3):159–163

24. Henderson GL, Harkey MR, Zhou C, Jones RT, Jacob P III. Incorporation of isotopically labeled cocaine into human hair: race as a factor. *J Anal Toxicol.* 1998;22(2):156–165

25. Jacqz-Aigrain E, Zhang D, Maillard G, Luton D, André J, Oury JF. Maternal smoking during pregnancy and nicotine and cotinine concentrations in maternal and neonatal hair. *BJOG.* 2002;109(8):909–911

26. Winecker RE, Goldberger BA, Tebbett IR, et al. Detection of cocaine and its metabolites in breast milk. *J Forensic Sci.* 2001;46(5):1221–1223

27. Montgomery D, Plate C, Alder SC, Jones M, Jones J, Christensen RD. Testing for fetal exposure to illicit drugs using umbilical cord tissue vs meconium. *J Perinatol.* 2006;26(1):11–14

28. Hansen RL, Evans AT, Gillogley KM, Hughes CS, Krener PG. Perinatal toxicology screening. *J Perinatol.* 1992;12(3):220–224

29. Behnke M, Eyler FD, Conlon M, Woods NS, Casanova OQ. Multiple risk factors do not identify cocaine use in rural obstetrical patients. *Neurotoxicol Teratol.* 1994;16(5):479–484

30. Ellsworth MA, Stevens TP, D'Angio CT. Infant race affects application of clinical guidelines when screening for drugs of abuse in newborns. *Pediatrics.* 2010;125(6). Available at: www.pediatrics.org/cgi/content/full/125/6/e1379

31. Behnke M, Eyler FD, Conlon M, Casanova OQ, Woods NS. How fetal cocaine exposure increases neonatal hospital costs. *Pediatrics.* 1997;99(2):204–208

32. Stahl SM. *Essential Psychopharmacology: Neuroscience Basis and Practical Application,* 2nd ed. New York, NY: Cambridge Press; 2000

33. Bauer CR, Shankaran S, Bada HS, et al. The Maternal Lifestyle Study: drug exposure during pregnancy and short-term maternal outcomes. *Am J Obstet Gynecol.* 2002;186(3):487–495

34. Mosier HD, Jr, Jansons RA. Distribution and fate of nicotine in the rat fetus. *Teratology.* 1972;6(3):303–311

35. Luck W, Nau H, Hansen R, Steldinger R. Extent of nicotine and cotinine transfer to the human fetus, placenta and amniotic fluid of smoking mothers. *Dev Pharmacol Ther.* 1985;8(6):384–395

36. Koren G. Fetal toxicology of environmental tobacco smoke. *Curr Opin Pediatr.* 1995;7(2):128–131

37. Lehtovirta P, Forss M. The acute effect of smoking on intervillous blood flow of the placenta. *Br J Obstet Gynaecol.* 1978;85(10):729–731

38. Ahlsten G, Ewald U, Tuvemo T. Maternal smoking reduces prostacyclin formation in human umbilical arteries. A study on strictly selected pregnancies. *Acta Obstet Gynecol Scand.* 1986;65(6):645–649

39. Joschko MA, Dreosti IE, Tulsi RS. The teratogenic effects of nicotine in vitro in rats: a light and electron microscope study. *Neurotoxicol Teratol.* 1991;13(3):307–316

40. Lichtensteiger W, Schlumpf M. Prenatal nicotine exposure: biochemical and neuroendocrine bases of behavioral dysfunction. *Dev Brain Dysfunc.* 1993;6(4–5):279–304

41. Seidler FJ, Albright ES, Lappi SE, Slotkin TA. In search of a mechanism for receptor-mediated neurobehavioral teratogenesis by nicotine: catecholamine release by nicotine in immature rat brain regions. *Brain Res Dev Brain Res.* 1994;82(1-2):1–8

42. Slotkin TA. Fetal nicotine or cocaine exposure: which one is worse? *J Pharmacol Exp Ther.* 1998;285(3):931–945

43. Hellström-Lindahl E, Seiger A, Kjaeldgaard A, Nordberg A. Nicotine-induced alterations in the expression of nicotinic receptors in primary cultures from human prenatal brain. *Neuroscience.* 2001;105(3):527–534

44. Holsclaw DS, Jr, Topham AL. The effects of smoking on fetal, neonatal, and childhood development. *Pediatr Ann.* 1978;7(3):201–222

45. Abel EL. Smoking and pregnancy. *J Psychoactive Drugs.* 1984;16(4):327–338

46. Hazelhoff Roelfzema W, Roelofsen AM, Copius Peereboom-Stegeman JH. Light microscopic aspects of the rat placenta after chronic cadmium administration. *Sci Total Environ.* 1985;42(1-2):181–184

47. Aaronson LS, Macnee CL. Tobacco, alcohol, and caffeine use during pregnancy. *J Obstet Gynecol Neonatal Nurs.* 1989;18(4):279–287

48. Floyd RL, Zahniser SC, Gunter EP, Kendrick JS. Smoking during pregnancy: prevalence, effects, and intervention strategies. *Birth.* 1991;18(1):48–53

49. Brien JF, Clarke DW, Smith GN, Richardson B, Patrick J. Disposition of acute, multiple-dose ethanol in the near-term pregnant ewe. *Am J Obstet Gynecol.* 1987;157(1):204–211

50. Szeto HH. Kinetics of drug transfer to the fetus. *Clin Obstet Gynecol.* 1993;36(2):246–254

51. Sulik KK, Johnston MC, Webb MA. Fetal alcohol syndrome: embryogenesis in a mouse model. *Science.* 1981;214(4523):936–938

52. West JR, Hodges CA, Black AC Jr. Prenatal exposure to ethanol alters the organization of hippocampal mossy fibers in rats. *Science.* 1981;211(4485):957–959

53. Kennedy LA. The pathogenesis of brain abnormalities in the fetal alcohol syndrome: an integrating hypothesis. *Teratology.* 1984;29(3):363–368

54. Fisher SE. Selective fetal malnutrition: the fetal alcohol syndrome. *J Am Coll Nutr.* 1988;7(2):101–106

55. Hoff SF. Synaptogenesis in the hippocampal dentate gyrus: effects of in utero ethanol exposure. *Brain Res Bull.* 1988;21(1):47–54

56. Clarren SK, Astley SJ, Bowden DM, et al. Neuroanatomic and neurochemical abnormalities in nonhuman primate infants exposed to weekly doses of ethanol during gestation. *Alcohol Clin Exp Res.* 1990;14(5):674–683

57. Druse MJ, Tajuddin N, Kuo A, Connerty M. Effects of in utero ethanol exposure on the developing dopaminergic system in rats. *J Neurosci Res.* 1990;27(2):233–240

58. Jollie WP. Effects of sustained dietary ethanol on the ultrastructure of the visceral yolk-sac placenta of the rat. *Teratology.* 1990;42(5):541–552

59. Michaelis EK. Fetal alcohol exposure: cellular toxicity and molecular events involved in toxicity. *Alcohol Clin Exp Res.* 1990;14(6):819–826

60. Schenker S, Becker HC, Randall CL, Phillips DK, Baskin GS, Henderson GI. Fetal alcohol syndrome: current status of pathogenesis. *Alcohol Clin Exp Res.* 1990;14(5):635–647

61. West JR, Goodlett CR, Bonthius DJ, Hamre KM, Marcussen BL. Cell population depletion associated with fetal alcohol brain

damage: mechanisms of BAC-dependent cell loss. *Alcohol Clin Exp Res.* 1990;14 (6):813–818

62. Wigal SB, Amsel A, Wilcox RE. Fetal ethanol exposure diminishes hippocampal beta-adrenergic receptor density while sparing muscarinic receptors during development. *Brain Res Dev Brain Res.* 1990;55(2):161–169

63. Brien JF, Smith GN. Effects of alcohol (ethanol) on the fetus. *J Dev Physiol.* 1991; 15(1):21–32

64. Ledig M, Megias-Megias L, Tholey G. Maternal alcohol exposure before and during pregnancy: effect on development of neurons and glial cells in culture. *Alcohol Alcohol.* 1991;26(2):169–176

65. Miller MW, Nowakowski RS. Effect of prenatal exposure to ethanol on the cell cycle kinetics and growth fraction in the proliferative zones of fetal rat cerebral cortex. *Alcohol Clin Exp Res.* 1991;15(2): 229–232

66. Smith GN, Patrick J, Sinervo KR, Brien JF. Effects of ethanol exposure on the embryo-fetus: experimental considerations, mechanisms, and the role of prostaglandins. *Can J Physiol Pharmacol.* 1991;69(5):550–569

67. Gressens P, Lammens M, Picard JJ, Evrard P. Ethanol-induced disturbances of gliogenesis and neuronogenesis in the developing murine brain: an in vitro and in vivo immunohistochemical and ultrastructural study. *Alcohol Alcohol.* 1992;27 (3):219–226

68. Kotch LE, Sulik KK. Experimental fetal alcohol syndrome: proposed pathogenic basis for a variety of associated facial and brain anomalies. *Am J Med Genet.* 1992;44 (2):168–176

69. Miller MW, Robertson S. Prenatal exposure to ethanol alters the postnatal development and transformation of radial glia to astrocytes in the cortex. *J Comp Neurol.* 1993;337(2):253–266

70. Bailey JR, Cunny HC, Paule MG, Slikker W Jr. Fetal disposition of delta 9-tetrahydrocannabinol (THC) during late pregnancy in the rhesus monkey. *Toxicol Appl Pharmacol.* 1987;90(2):315–321

71. Abrams RM, Cook CE, Davis KH, Niederreither K, Jaeger MJ, Szeto HH. Plasma delta-9-tetrahydrocannabinol in pregnant sheep and fetus after inhalation of smoke from a marijuana cigarette. *Alcohol Drug Res.* 1985-1986;6(5):361–369

72. Hutchings DE, Martin BR, Gamagaris Z, Miller N, Fico T. Plasma concentrations of delta-9-tetrahydrocannabinol in dams and fetuses following acute or multiple prenatal dosing in rats. *Life Sci.* 1989;44 (11):697–701

73. Murthy NV, Melville GN, Wynter HH. Contractile responses of uterine smooth muscle to acetylcholine and marihuana extract. *Int J Gynaecol Obstet.* 1983;21(3):223–226

74. Dalterio SL. Cannabinoid exposure: effects on development. *Neurobehav Toxicol Teratol.* 1986;8(4):345–352

75. Fisher SE, Atkinson M, Chang B. Effect of delta-9-tetrahydrocannabinol on the in vitro uptake of alpha-amino isobutyric acid by term human placental slices. *Pediatr Res.* 1987;21(1):104–107

76. Walters DE, Carr LA. Changes in brain catecholamine mechanisms following perinatal exposure to marihuana. *Pharmacol Biochem Behav.* 1986;25(4):763–768

77. Morgan B, Brake SC, Hutchings DE, Miller N, Gamagaris Z. Delta-9-tetrahydrocannabinol during pregnancy in the rat: effects on development of RNA, DNA, and protein in offspring brain. *Pharmacol Biochem Behav.* 1988;31(2):365–369

78. Walters DE, Carr LA. Perinatal exposure to cannabinoids alters neurochemical development in rat brain. *Pharmacol Biochem Behav.* 1988;29(1):213–216

79. Rodríguez de Fonseca F, Cebeira M, Fernández-Ruiz JJ, Navarro M, Ramos JA. Effects of pre- and perinatal exposure to hashish extracts on the ontogeny of brain dopaminergic neurons. *Neuroscience.* 1991;43(2-3):713–723

80. Chiriboga CA. Fetal alcohol and drug effects. *Neurologist.* 2003;9(6):267–279

81. Gerdin E, Rane A, Lindberg B. Transplacental transfer of morphine in man. *J Perinat Med.* 1990;18(4):305–312

82. Zagon IS, McLaughlin PJ, Weaver DJ, Zagon E. Opiates, endorphins and the developing organism: a comprehensive bibliography. *Neurosci Biobehav Rev.* 1982;6(4):439–479

83. Lee CC, Chiang CN. Maternal-fetal transfer of abused substances: pharmacokinetic and pharmacodynamic data. *NIDA Res Monogr.* 1985;60:110–147

84. Wang C, Pasulka P, Perry B, Pizzi WJ, Schnoll SH. Effect of perinatal exposure to methadone on brain opioid and alpha 2-adrenergic receptors. *Neurobehav Toxicol Teratol.* 1986;8(4):399–402

85. Hammer RP, Jr, Ricalde AA, Seatriz JV. Effects of opiates on brain development. *Neurotoxicology.* 1989;10(3):475–483

86. Ricalde AA, Hammer RP Jr. Perinatal opiate treatment delays growth of cortical dendrites. *Neurosci Lett.* 1990;115(2-3):137–143

87. Hauser KF, Stiene-Martin A. Characterization of opioid-dependent glial development

in dissociated and organotypic cultures of mouse central nervous system: critical periods and target specificity. *Brain Res Dev Brain Res.* 1991;62(2):245–255

88. Zagon IS, McLaughlin PJ. The perinatal opioid syndrome: laboratory findings and clinical implications. In: Sonderegger TB, ed. *Perinatal Substance Abuse: Research Findings and Clinical Implications.* Baltimore, MD: Johns Hopkins University Press; 1992:207–223

89. Malanga CJ, III, Kosofsky BE. Mechanisms of action of drugs of abuse on the developing fetal brain. *Clin Perinatol.* 1999; 26(1):17–37, v–vi

90. Mayes LC. Neurobiology of prenatal cocaine exposure effect on developing monoamine systems. *Infant Ment Health J.* 1994;15(2):121–133

91. Dow-Edwards DL. Developmental toxicity of cocaine: mechanisms of action. In: Lewis M, Bendersky M, eds. *Mothers, Babies, and Cocaine: The Role of Toxins in Development.* Hillsdale, NJ: Lawrence Erlbaum Associates Inc; 1995:5–17

92. Levitt P, Harvey JA, Friedman E, Simansky K, Murphy EH. New evidence for neurotransmitter influences on brain development. *Trends Neurosci.* 1997;20(6): 269–274

93. Whitaker-Azmitia PM. Role of the neurotrophic properties of serotonin in the delay of brain maturation induced by cocaine. *Ann N Y Acad Sci.* 1998;846:158–164

94. Harvey JA. Cocaine effects on the developing brain: current status. *Neurosci Biobehav Rev.* 2004;27(8):751–764

95. Lauder JM. Discussion: neuroteratology of cocaine relationship to developing monoamine systems. *NIDA Res Monogr.* 1991; 114:233–247

96. Woods JR Jr. Adverse consequences of prenatal illicit drug exposure. *Curr Opin Obstet Gynecol.* 1996;8(6):403–411

97. Mayes LC. Developing brain and in utero cocaine exposure: effects on neural ontogeny. *Dev Psychopathol.* 1999;11(4):685–714

98. Stanwood GD, Levitt P. Drug exposure early in life: functional repercussions of changing neuropharmacology during sensitive periods of brain development. *Curr Opin Pharmacol.* 2004;4(1):65–71

99. Burchfield DJ, Lucas VW, Abrams RM, Miller RL, DeVane CL. Disposition and pharmacodynamics of methamphetamine in pregnant sheep. *JAMA.* 1991;265(15): 1968–1973

100. Won L, Bubula N, McCoy H, Heller A. Methamphetamine concentrations in fetal and maternal brain following prenatal

exposure. *Neurotoxicol Teratol.* 2001;23(4): 349–354

101. Golub M, Costa L, Crofton K, et al. NTP-CERHR Expert Panel Report on the reproductive and developmental toxicity of amphetamine and methamphetamine. *Birth Defects Res B Dev Reprod Toxicol.* 2005;74(6):471–584

102. Cui C, Sakata-Haga H, Ohta K, et al. Histological brain alterations following prenatal methamphetamine exposure in rats. *Congenit Anom (Kyoto).* 2006;46(4):180–187

103. Simpson WJ. A preliminary report on cigarette smoking and the incidence of prematurity. *Am J Obstet Gynecol.* 1957;73(4):807–815

104. Yerushalmy J. The relationship of parents' cigarette smoking to outcome of pregnancy—implications as to the problem of inferring causation from observed associations. *Am J Epidemiol.* 1971;93(6):443–456

105. Persson PH, Grennert L, Gennser G, Kullander S. A study of smoking and pregnancy with special references to fetal growth. *Acta Obstet Gynecol Scand Suppl.* 1978;78(S78):33–39

106. Olsen J. Cigarette smoking in pregnancy and fetal growth. Does the type of tobacco play a role? *Int J Epidemiol.* 1992;21(2):279–284

107. Zarén B, Lindmark G, Gebre-Medhin M. Maternal smoking and body composition of the newborn. *Acta Paediatr.* 1996;85(2):213–219

108. Hoff C, Wertelecki W, Blackburn WR, Mendenhall H, Wiseman H, Stumpe A. Trend associations of smoking with maternal, fetal, and neonatal morbidity. *Obstet Gynecol.* 1986;68(3):317–321

109. Day N, Cornelius M, Goldschmidt L, Richardson G, Robles N, Taylor P. The effects of prenatal tobacco and marijuana use on offspring growth from birth through 3 years of age. *Neurotoxicol Teratol.* 1992;14(6):407–414

110. Barnett E. Race differences in the proportion of low birth weight attributable to maternal cigarette smoking in a low-income population. *Am J Health Promot.* 1995;10(2):105–110

111. Lightwood JM, Phibbs CS, Glantz SA. Short-term health and economic benefits of smoking cessation: low birth weight. *Pediatrics.* 1999;104(6):1312–1320

112. DiFranza JR, Aligne CA, Weitzman M. Prenatal and postnatal environmental tobacco smoke exposure and children's health. *Pediatrics.* 2004;113(suppl 4):1007–1015

113. Fried PA, Watkinson B, Gray R. Growth from birth to early adolescence in offspring prenatally exposed to cigarettes and marijuana. *Neurotoxicol Teratol.* 1999;21(5):513–525

114. Fenercioglu AK, Tamer I, Karatekin G, Nuhoglu A. Impaired postnatal growth of infants prenatally exposed to cigarette smoking. *Tohoku J Exp Med.* 2009;218(3):221–228

115. Mills JL, Graubard BI, Harley EE, Rhoads GG, Berendes HW. Maternal alcohol consumption and birth weight. How much drinking during pregnancy is safe? *JAMA.* 1984;252(14):1875–1879

116. Streissguth AP, Martin DC, Martin JC, Barr HM. The Seattle longitudinal prospective study on alcohol and pregnancy. *Neurobehav Toxicol Teratol.* 1981;3(2):223–233

117. Fried PA, O'Connell CM. A comparison of the effects of prenatal exposure to tobacco, alcohol, cannabis and caffeine on birth size and subsequent growth. *Neurotoxicol Teratol.* 1987;9(2):79–85

118. Greene T, Ernhart CB, Sokol RJ, et al. Prenatal alcohol exposure and preschool physical growth: a longitudinal analysis. *Alcohol Clin Exp Res.* 1991;15(6):905–913

119. Jacobson JL, Jacobson SW, Sokol RJ. Effects of prenatal exposure to alcohol, smoking, and illicit drugs on postpartum somatic growth. *Alcohol Clin Exp Res.* 1994;18(2):317–323

120. Fried PA. Marijuana use during pregnancy: consequences for the offspring. *Semin Perinatol.* 1991;15(4):280–287

121. English DR, Hulse GK, Milne E, Holman CD, Bower CI. Maternal cannabis use and birth weight: a meta-analysis. *Addiction.* 1997;92(11):1553–1560

122. Eyler FD, Behnke M, Conlon M, Woods NS, Wobie K. Birth outcome from a prospective, matched study of prenatal crack/cocaine use: I. Interactive and dose effects on health and growth. *Pediatrics.* 1998;101(2):229–237

123. Hulse GK, Milne E, English DR, Holman CD. The relationship between maternal use of heroin and methadone and infant birth weight. *Addiction.* 1997;92(11):1571–1579

124. Bada HS, Das A, Bauer CR, et al. Gestational cocaine exposure and intrauterine growth: maternal lifestyle study. *Obstet Gynecol.* 2002;100(5 pt 1):916–924

125. Chouteau M, Namerow PB, Leppert P. The effect of cocaine abuse on birth weight and gestational age. *Obstet Gynecol.* 1988;72(3 pt 1):351–354

126. Amaro H, Zuckerman B, Cabral H. Drug use among adolescent mothers: profile of risk. *Pediatrics.* 1989;84(1):144–151

127. Zuckerman B, Frank DA, Hingson R, et al. Effects of maternal marijuana and cocaine use on fetal growth. *N Engl J Med.* 1989;320(12):762–768

128. Zuckerman B, Frank DA. Prenatal cocaine exposure: nine years later. [editorial; comment] *J Pediatr.* 1994;124(5 pt 1):731–733

129. Richardson GA. Prenatal cocaine exposure. A longitudinal study of development. *Ann N Y Acad Sci.* 1998;846:144–152

130. Bauer CR, Langer JC, Shankaran S, et al. Acute neonatal effects of cocaine exposure during pregnancy. *Arch Pediatr Adolesc Med.* 2005;159(9):824–834

131. Little BB, Snell LM, Gilstrap LC III. Methamphetamine abuse during pregnancy: outcome and fetal effects. *Obstet Gynecol.* 1988;72(4):541–544

132. Nguyen D, Smith LM, Lagasse LL, et al. Intrauterine growth of infants exposed to prenatal methamphetamine: results from the infant development, environment, and lifestyle study. *J Pediatr.* 2010;157(2):337–339

133. Bauer CR. Perinatal effects of prenatal drug exposure. Neonatal aspects. *Clin Perinatol.* 1999;26(1):87–106

134. Cornelius MD, Day NL. The effects of tobacco use during and after pregnancy on exposed children. *Alcohol Res Health.* 2000;24(4):242–249

135. Nordstrom-Klee B, Delaney-Black V, Covington C, Ager J, Sokol R. Growth from birth onwards of children prenatally exposed to drugs: a literature review. *Neurotoxicol Teratol.* 2002;24(4):481–488

136. Wyszynski DF, Duffy DL, Beaty TH. Maternal cigarette smoking and oral clefts: a meta-analysis. *Cleft Palate Craniofac J.* 1997;34(3):206–210

137. Wyszynski DF, Wu T. Use of US birth certificate data to estimate the risk of maternal cigarette smoking for oral clefting. *Cleft Palate Craniofac J.* 2002;39(2):188–192

138. Lammer EJ, Shaw GM, Iovannisci DM, Van Waes J, Finnell RH. Maternal smoking and the risk of orofacial clefts: Susceptibility with NAT1 and NAT2 polymorphisms. *Epidemiology.* 2004;15(2):150–156

139. Little J, Cardy A, Arslan MT, Gilmour M, Mossey PA; United Kingdom-based case-control study. Smoking and orofacial clefts: a United Kingdom-based case-control study. *Cleft Palate Craniofac J.* 2004;41(4):381–386

140. Little J, Cardy A, Munger RG. Tobacco smoking and oral clefts: a meta-analysis. *Bull World Health Organ.* 2004;82(3):213–218

141. American Academy of Pediatrics, Committee on Substance Abuse and Committee on Children With Disabilities. Fetal alcohol syndrome and alcohol-related neurodevelopmental disorders. *Pediatrics*. 2000;106(2 pt 1):358–361

142. Astley SJ, Clarren SK, Little RE, Sampson PD, Daling JR. Analysis of facial shape in children gestationally exposed to marijuana, alcohol, and/or cocaine. *Pediatrics*. 1992;89(1):67–77

143. Behnke M, Eyler FD, Garvan CW, Wobie K. The search for congenital malformations in newborns with fetal cocaine exposure. *Pediatrics*. 2001;107(5). Available at: www.pediatrics.org/cgi/content/full/107/5/e74

144. Law KL, Stroud LR, LaGasse LL, Niaura R, Liu J, Lester BM. Smoking during pregnancy and newborn neurobehavior. *Pediatrics*. 2003;111(6 pt 1):1318–1323

145. Godding V, Bonnier C, Fiasse L, et al. Does in utero exposure to heavy maternal smoking induce nicotine withdrawal symptoms in neonates? *Pediatr Res*. 2004; 55(4):645–651

146. Pierog S, Chandavasu O, Wexler I. Withdrawal symptoms in infants with the fetal alcohol syndrome. *J Pediatr*. 1977;90(4): 630–633

147. Fried PA, Makin JE. Neonatal behavioural correlates of prenatal exposure to marihuana, cigarettes and alcohol in a low risk population. *Neurotoxicol Teratol*. 1987;9(1):1–7

148. Finnegan LP, Connaughton JF, Jr, Kron RE, Emich JP. Neonatal abstinence syndrome: assessment and management. *Addict Dis*. 1975;2(1-2):141–158

149. Chasnoff IJ, Hatcher R, Burns WJ. Polydrug- and methadone-addicted newborns: a continuum of impairment? *Pediatrics*. 1982;70(2): 210–213

150. Fischer G, Johnson RE, Eder H, et al. Treatment of opioid-dependent pregnant women with buprenorphine. *Addiction*. 2000;95(2):239–244

151. Johnson RE, Jones HE, Fischer G. Use of buprenorphine in pregnancy: patient management and effects on the neonate. *Drug Alcohol Depend*. 2003;70(suppl 2):S87–S101

152. Jones HE, Kaltenbach K, Heil SH, et al. Neonatal abstinence syndrome after methadone or buprenorphine exposure. *N Engl J Med*. 2010;363(24):2320–2331

153. Eyler FD, Behnke M, Garvan CW, Woods NS, Wobie K, Conlon M. Newborn evaluations of toxicity and withdrawal related to prenatal cocaine exposure. *Neurotoxicol Teratol*. 2001;23(5):399–411

154. Smith L, Yonekura ML, Wallace T, Berman N, Kuo J, Berkowitz C. Effects of prenatal methamphetamine exposure on fetal growth and drug withdrawal symptoms in infants born at term. *J Dev Behav Pediatr*. 2003;24(1):17–23

155. Hudak ML, Tan RC; American Academy of Pediatrics, Committee on Drugs, Committee on Fetus and Newborn. Clinical report: neonatal drug withdrawal. *Pediatrics*. 1998;101(6):1079–1088

156. Picone TA, Allen LH, Olsen PN, Ferris ME. Pregnancy outcome in North American women. II. Effects of diet, cigarette smoking, stress, and weight gain on placentas, and on neonatal physical and behavioral characteristics. *Am J Clin Nutr*. 1982;36(6):1214–1224

157. Dempsey DA, Hajnal BL, Partridge JC, et al. Tone abnormalities are associated with maternal cigarette smoking during pregnancy in in utero cocaine-exposed infants. *Pediatrics*. 2000;106(1 pt 1):79–85

158. Streissguth AP, Barr HM, Martin DC. Maternal alcohol use and neonatal habituation assessed with the Brazelton scale. *Child Dev*. 1983;54(5):1109–1118

159. Brazelton TB. *Neonatal Behavioral Assessment Scale*, 2nd ed. Philadelphia, PA: JB Lippincott Co; 1984

160. Eyler FD, Behnke M. Early development of infants exposed to drugs prenatally. *Clin Perinatol*. 1999;26(1):107–150, vii

161. Smith LM, Lagasse LL, Derauf C, et al. Prenatal methamphetamine use and neonatal neurobehavioral outcome. *Neurotoxicol Teratol*. 2008;30(1):20–28

162. Howard CR, Lawrence RA. Breast-feeding and drug exposure. *Obstet Gynecol Clin North Am*. 1998;25(1):195–217

163. Cobrinik RW, Hood RT, Jr, Chusid E. The effect of maternal narcotic addiction on the newborn infant; review of literature and report of 22 cases. *Pediatrics*. 1959;24(2):288–304

164. Perez-Reyes M, Wall ME. Presence of delta9-tetrahydrocannabinol in human milk. *N Engl J Med*. 1982;307(13):819–820

165. Steiner E, Villén T, Hallberg M, Rane A. Amphetamine secretion in breast milk. *Eur J Clin Pharmacol*. 1984;27(1):123–124

166. Chasnoff IJ, Lewis DE, Squires L. Cocaine intoxication in a breast-fed infant. *Pediatrics*. 1987;80(6):836–838

167. Ferguson BB, Wilson DJ, Schaffner W. Determination of nicotine concentrations in human milk. *Am J Dis Child*. 1976;130(8): 837–839

168. Steldinger R, Luck W, Nau H. Half lives of nicotine in milk of smoking mothers: implications for nursing. *J Perinat Med*. 1988;16(3):261–262

169. Luck W, Nau H. Nicotine and cotinine concentrations in serum and urine of infants exposed via passive smoking or milk from smoking mothers. *J Pediatr*. 1985;107(5):816–820

170. Schwartz-Bickenbach D, Schulte-Hobein B, Abt S, Plum C, Nau H. Smoking and passive smoking during pregnancy and early infancy: effects on birth weight, lactation period, and cotinine concentrations in mother's milk and infant's urine. *Toxicol Lett*. 1987;35(1):73–81

171. Hopkinson JM, Schanler RJ, Fraley JK, Garza C. Milk production by mothers of premature infants: influence of cigarette smoking. *Pediatrics*. 1992;90(6):934–938

172. Cobo E. Effect of different doses of ethanol on the milk-ejecting reflex in lactating women. *Am J Obstet Gynecol*. 1973;115(6): 817–821

173. Little RE, Anderson KW, Ervin CH, Worthington-Roberts B, Clarren SK. Maternal alcohol use during breast-feeding and infant mental and motor development at one year. *N Engl J Med*. 1989;321(7):425–430

174. Anderson PO. Alcohol and breastfeeding. *J Hum Lact*. 1995;11(4):321–323

175. Jakubovic A, Tait RM, McGeer PL. Excretion of THC and its metabolites in ewes' milk. *Toxicol Appl Pharmacol*. 1974;28(1):38–43

176. American Academy of Pediatrics Committee on Drugs. Transfer of drugs and other chemicals into human milk. *Pediatrics*. 2001;108(3):776–789

177. Gartner LM, Morton J, Lawrence RA, et al; American Academy of Pediatrics Section on Breastfeeding. Breastfeeding and the use of human milk. *Pediatrics*. 2005;115 (2):496–506

178. Dunn HG, McBurney AK, Ingram S, Hunter CM. Maternal cigarette smoking during pregnancy and the child's subsequent development: I. Physical growth to the age of 6 1/2 years. *Can J Public Health*. 1976; 67(6):499–505

179. Naeye RL. Influence of maternal cigarette smoking during pregnancy on fetal and childhood growth. *Obstet Gynecol*. 1981;57 (1):18–21

180. Rantakallio P. A follow-up study up to the age of 14 of children whose mothers smoked during pregnancy. *Acta Paediatr Scand*. 1983;72(5):747–753

181. Fogelman KR, Manor O. Smoking in pregnancy and development into early adulthood. *BMJ*. 1988;297(6658):1233–1236

182. Day NL, Richardson GA, Geva D, Robles N. Alcohol, marijuana, and tobacco: effects of prenatal exposure on offspring growth and morphology at age six. *Alcohol Clin Exp Res*. 1994;18(4):786–794

183. Vik T, Jacobsen G, Vatten L, Bakketeig LS. Pre- and post-natal growth in children of

women who smoked in pregnancy. *Early Hum Dev.* 1996;45(3):245–255

184. Fried PA, James DS, Watkinson B. Growth and pubertal milestones during adolescence in offspring prenatally exposed to cigarettes and marihuana. *Neurotoxicol Teratol.* 2001;23(5):431–436

185. Davies JK, Bledsoe JM. Prenatal alcohol and drug exposures in adoption. *Pediatr Clin North Am.* 2005;52(5):1369–1393, vii

186. Shankaran S, Lester BM, Das A, et al. Impact of maternal substance use during pregnancy on childhood outcome. *Semin Fetal Neonatal Med.* 2007;12(2):143–150

187. Hurt H, Brodsky NL, Betancourt L, Braitman LE, Malmud E, Giannetta J. Cocaine-exposed children: follow-up through 30 months. *J Dev Behav Pediatr.* 1995;16(1):29–35

188. Covington CY, Nordstrom-Klee B, Ager J, Sokol R, Delaney-Black V. Birth to age 7 growth of children prenatally exposed to drugs: a prospective cohort study. *Neurotoxicol Teratol.* 2002;24(4):489–496

189. Minnes S, Robin NH, Alt AA, et al. Dysmorphic and anthropometric outcomes in 6-year-old prenatally cocaine-exposed children. *Neurotoxicol Teratol.* 2006;28(1):28–38

190. Richardson GA, Conroy ML, Day NL. Prenatal cocaine exposure: effects on the development of school-age children. *Neurotoxicol Teratol.* 1996;18(6):627–634

191. Kilbride H, Castor C, Hoffman E, Fuger KL. Thirty-six-month outcome of prenatal cocaine exposure for term or near-term infants: impact of early case management. *J Dev Behav Pediatr.* 2000;21(1):19–26

192. Eriksson M, Jonsson B, Steneroth G, Zetterström R. Cross-sectional growth of children whose mothers abused amphetamines during pregnancy. *Acta Paediatr.* 1994;83(6):612–617

193. Kristjansson EA, Fried PA, Watkinson B. Maternal smoking during pregnancy affects children's vigilance performance. *Drug Alcohol Depend.* 1989;24(1):11–19

194. Fried PA, Watkinson B, Gray R. A follow-up study of attentional behavior in 6-year-old children exposed prenatally to marihuana, cigarettes, and alcohol. *Neurotoxicol Teratol.* 1992;14(5):299–311

195. Thapar A, Fowler T, Rice F, et al. Maternal smoking during pregnancy and attention deficit hyperactivity disorder symptoms in offspring. *Am J Psychiatry.* 2003;160(11):1985–1989

196. Kotimaa AJ, Moilanen I, Taanila A, et al. Maternal smoking and hyperactivity in 8-year-old children. *J Am Acad Child Adolesc Psychiatry.* 2003;42(7):826–833

197. Brook JS, Brook DW, Whiteman M. The influence of maternal smoking during pregnancy on the toddler's negativity. *Arch Pediatr Adolesc Med.* 2000;154(4):381–385

198. Day NL, Richardson GA, Goldschmidt L, Cornelius MD. Effects of prenatal tobacco exposure on preschoolers' behavior. *J Dev Behav Pediatr.* 2000;21(3):180–188

199. Wakschlag LS, Hans SL. Maternal smoking during pregnancy and conduct problems in high-risk youth: a developmental framework. *Dev Psychopathol.* 2002;14(2):351–369

200. Batstra L, Hadders-Algra M, Neeleman J. Effect of antenatal exposure to maternal smoking on behavioural problems and academic achievement in childhood: prospective evidence from a Dutch birth cohort. *Early Hum Dev.* 2003;75(1-2):21–33

201. Naeye RL. Cognitive and behavioral abnormalities in children whose mothers smoked cigarettes during pregnancy. *J Dev Behav Pediatr.* 1992;13(6):425–428

202. Fergusson DM, Horwood LJ, Lynskey MT. Maternal smoking before and after pregnancy: effects on behavioral outcomes in middle childhood. *Pediatrics.* 1993;92(6):815–822

203. Fergusson DM, Woodward LJ, Horwood LJ. Maternal smoking during pregnancy and psychiatric adjustment in late adolescence. *Arch Gen Psychiatry.* 1998;55(8):721–727

204. Williams GM, O'Callaghan M, Najman JM, et al. Maternal cigarette smoking and child psychiatric morbidity: a longitudinal study. *Pediatrics.* 1998;102(1). Available at: www.pediatrics.org/cgi/content/full/102/1/e11

205. Räsänen P, Hakko H, Isohanni M, Hodgins S, Järvelin MR, Tiihonen J. Maternal smoking during pregnancy and risk of criminal behavior among adult male offspring in the Northern Finland 1966 Birth Cohort. *Am J Psychiatry.* 1999;156(6):857–862

206. Weissman MM, Warner V, Wickramaratne PJ, Kandel DB. Maternal smoking during pregnancy and psychopathology in offspring followed to adulthood. *J Am Acad Child Adolesc Psychiatry.* 1999;38(7):892–899

207. Nanson JL, Hiscock M. Attention deficits in children exposed to alcohol prenatally. *Alcohol Clin Exp Res.* 1990;14(5):656–661

208. Streissguth AP, Sampson PD, Olson HC, et al. Maternal drinking during pregnancy: attention and short-term memory in 14-year-old offspring—a longitudinal prospective study. *Alcohol Clin Exp Res.* 1994;18(1):202–218

209. Streissguth AP, Bookstein FL, Sampson PD, Barr HM. Attention: prenatal alcohol and continuities of vigilance and attentional problems from 4 through 14 years. *Dev Psychopathol.* 1995;7(3):419–446

210. Coles CD, Platzman KA, Raskind-Hood CL, Brown RT, Falek A, Smith IE. A comparison of children affected by prenatal alcohol exposure and attention deficit, hyperactivity disorder. *Alcohol Clin Exp Res.* 1997;21(1):150–161

211. Streissguth AP, Bookstein FL, Barr HM, Sampson PD, O'Malley K, Young JK. Risk factors for adverse life outcomes in fetal alcohol syndrome and fetal alcohol effects. *J Dev Behav Pediatr.* 2004;25(4):228–238

212. Kelly SJ, Day N, Streissguth AP. Effects of prenatal alcohol exposure on social behavior in humans and other species. *Neurotoxicol Teratol.* 2000;22(2):143–149

213. Goldschmidt L, Day NL, Richardson GA. Effects of prenatal marijuana exposure on child behavior problems at age 10. *Neurotoxicol Teratol.* 2000;22(3):325–336

214. Rosen TS, Johnson HL. Long-term effects of prenatal methadone maintenance. *NIDA Res Monogr.* 1985;59:73–83

215. Lifschltz MH, Wilson GS. Patterns of growth and development in narcotic-exposed children. *NIDA Res Monogr.* 1991;114:323–339

216. Warner TD, Behnke M, Hou W, Garvan CW, Wobie K, Eyler FD. Predicting caregiver-reported behavior problems in cocaine-exposed children at 3 years. *J Dev Behav Pediatr.* 2006;27(2):83–92

217. Accornero VH, Anthony JC, Morrow CE, Xue L, Bandstra ES. Prenatal cocaine exposure: an examination of childhood externalizing and internalizing behavior problems at age 7 years. *Epidemiol Psichiatr Soc.* 2006;15(1):20–29

218. Linares TJ, Singer LT, Kirchner HL, et al. Mental health outcomes of cocaine-exposed children at 6 years of age. *J Pediatr Psychol.* 2006;31(1):85–97

219. Sood BG, Nordstrom Bailey B, Covington C, et al. Gender and alcohol moderate caregiver reported child behavior after prenatal cocaine. *Neurotoxicol Teratol.* 2005;27(2):191–201

220. Bendersky M, Bennett D, Lewis M. Aggression at age 5 as a function of prenatal exposure to cocaine, gender, and environmental risk. *J Pediatr Psychol.* 2006;31(1):71–84

221. Dennis T, Bendersky M, Ramsay D, Lewis M. Reactivity and regulation in children prenatally exposed to cocaine. *Dev Psychol.* 2006;42(4):688–697

222. Bada HS, Das A, Bauer CR, et al. Impact of prenatal cocaine exposure on child behavior problems through school age. Pediatrics. 2007;119(2). Available at: www.pediatrics.org/cgi/content/full/119/2/e348

223. Delaney-Black V, Covington C, Templin T, et al. Teacher-assessed behavior of children prenatally exposed to cocaine. Pediatrics. 2000;106(4):782–791

224. Nordstrom Bailey B, Sood BG, Sokol RJ, et al. Gender and alcohol moderate prenatal cocaine effects on teacher-report of child behavior. Neurotoxicol Teratol. 2005;27(2):181–189

225. Eriksson M, Billing L, Steneroth G, Zetterström R. Health and development of 8-year-old children whose mothers abused amphetamine during pregnancy. Acta Paediatr Scand. 1989;78(6):944–949

226. Billing L, Eriksson M, Jonsson B, Steneroth G, Zetterström R. The influence of environmental factors on behavioural problems in 8-year-old children exposed to amphetamine during fetal life. Child Abuse Negl. 1994;18(1):3–9

227. Fried PA, O'Connell CM, Watkinson B. 60- and 72-month follow-up of children prenatally exposed to marijuana, cigarettes, and alcohol: cognitive and language assessment. J Dev Behav Pediatr. 1992;13(6):383–391

228. Cornelius MD, Ryan CM, Day NL, Goldschmidt L, Willford JA. Prenatal tobacco effects on neuropsychological outcomes among preadolescents. J Dev Behav Pediatr. 2001;22(4):217–225

229. Olds DL, Henderson CR, Jr, Tatelbaum R. Intellectual impairment in children of women who smoke cigarettes during pregnancy. Pediatrics. 1994;93(2):221–227

230. Fried PA. Adolescents prenatally exposed to marijuana: examination of facets of complex behaviors and comparisons with the influence of in utero cigarettes. J Clin Pharmacol. 2002;42(suppl 11):97S–102S

231. Fried PA, Watkinson B, Gray R. Differential effects on cognitive functioning in 13- to 16-year-olds prenatally exposed to cigarettes and marihuana. Neurotoxicol Teratol. 2003;25(4):427–436

232. Howell KK, Lynch ME, Platzman KA, Smith GH, Coles CD. Prenatal alcohol exposure and ability, academic achievement, and school functioning in adolescence: a longitudinal follow-up. J Pediatr Psychol. 2006;31(1):116–126

233. Kodituwakku PW, Kalberg W, May PA. The effects of prenatal alcohol exposure on executive functioning. Alcohol Res Health. 2001;25(3):192–198

234. Fried PA, Watkinson B, Gray R. Differential effects on cognitive functioning in 9- to

12-year olds prenatally exposed to cigarettes and marihuana. Neurotoxicol Teratol. 1998;20(3):293–306

235. Fried PA, Smith AM. A literature review of the consequences of prenatal marihuana exposure. An emerging theme of a deficiency in aspects of executive function. Neurotoxicol Teratol. 2001;23(1):1–11

236. Fried PA, Watkinson B. Differential effects on facets of attention in adolescents prenatally exposed to cigarettes and marihuana. Neurotoxicol Teratol. 2001;23(5):421–430

237. Richardson GA, Ryan C, Willford J, Day NL, Goldschmidt L. Prenatal alcohol and marijuana exposure: effects on neuropsychological outcomes at 10 years. Neurotoxicol Teratol. 2002;24(3):309–320

238. Lifschitz MH, Wilson GS, Smith EO, Desmond MM. Factors affecting head growth and intellectual function in children of drug addicts. Pediatrics. 1985;75(2):269–274

239. Kaltenbach K, Finnegan LP. Children exposed to methadone in utero: assessment of developmental and cognitive ability. Ann N Y Acad Sci. 1989;562:360–362

240. Kaltenbach KA, Finnegan LP. Prenatal narcotic exposure: perinatal and developmental effects. Neurotoxicology. 1989;10(3):597–604

241. Bennett DS, Bendersky M, Lewis M. Children's intellectual and emotional-behavioral adjustment at 4 years as a function of cocaine exposure, maternal characteristics, and environmental risk. Dev Psychol. 2002;38(5):648–658

242. Wasserman GA, Kline JK, Bateman DA, et al. Prenatal cocaine exposure and school-age intelligence. Drug Alcohol Depend. 1998;50(3):203–210

243. Hurt H, Malmud E, Betancourt LM, Brodsky NL, Giannetta JM. A prospective comparison of developmental outcome of children with in utero cocaine exposure and controls using the Battelle Developmental Inventory. J Dev Behav Pediatr. 2001;22(1):27–34

244. Arendt RE, Short EJ, Singer LT, et al. Children prenatally exposed to cocaine: developmental outcomes and environmental risks at seven years of age. J Dev Behav Pediatr. 2004;25(2):83–90

245. Messinger DS, Bauer CR, Das A, et al. The maternal lifestyle study: cognitive, motor, and behavioral outcomes of cocaine-exposed and opiate-exposed infants through three years of age. Pediatrics. 2004;113(6):1677–1685

246. Pulsifer MB, Radonovich K, Belcher HM, Butz AM. Intelligence and school readiness

in preschool children with prenatal drug exposure. Child Neuropsychol. 2004;10(2):89–101

247. Singer LT, Minnes S, Short E, et al. Cognitive outcomes of preschool children with prenatal cocaine exposure. JAMA. 2004;291(20):2448–2456

248. Frank DA, Rose-Jacobs R, Beeghly M, Wilbur M, Bellinger D, Cabral H. Level of prenatal cocaine exposure and 48-month IQ: importance of preschool enrichment. Neurotoxicol Teratol. 2005;27(1):15–28

249. Morrow CE, Culbertson JL, Accornero VH, Xue L, Anthony JC, Bandstra ES. Learning disabilities and intellectual functioning in school-aged children with prenatal cocaine exposure. Dev Neuropsychol. 2006;30(3):905–931

250. Hurt H, Betancourt LM, Malmud EK, et al. Children with and without gestational cocaine exposure: a neurocognitive systems analysis. Neurotoxicol Teratol. 2009;31(6):334–341

251. Leech SL, Richardson GA, Goldschmidt L, Day NL. Prenatal substance exposure: effects on attention and impulsivity of 6-year-olds. Neurotoxicol Teratol. 1999;21(2):109–118

252. Bandstra ES, Morrow CE, Anthony JC, Accornero VH, Fried PA. Longitudinal investigation of task persistence and sustained attention in children with prenatal cocaine exposure. Neurotoxicol Teratol. 2001;23(6):545–559

253. Savage J, Brodsky NL, Malmud E, Giannetta JM, Hurt H. Attentional functioning and impulse control in cocaine-exposed and control children at age ten years. J Dev Behav Pediatr. 2005;26(1):42–47

254. Mayes L, Snyder PJ, Langlois E, Hunter N. Visuospatial working memory in school-aged children exposed in utero to cocaine. Child Neuropsychol. 2007;13(3):205–218

255. Chang L, Smith LM, LoPresti C, et al. Smaller subcortical volumes and cognitive deficits in children with prenatal methamphetamine exposure. Psychiatry Res. 2004;132(2):95–106

256. Delaney-Black V, Covington C, Templin T, et al. Expressive language development of children exposed to cocaine prenatally: literature review and report of a prospective cohort study. J Commun Disord. 2000;33(6):463–480, quiz 480–481

257. Fried PA, Watkinson B. 36- and 48-month neurobehavioral follow-up of children prenatally exposed to marijuana, cigarettes, and alcohol. J Dev Behav Pediatr. 1990;11(2):49–58

258. Fried PA, Watkinson B, Siegel LS. Reading and language in 9- to 12-year olds prenatally

exposed to cigarettes and marijuana. *Neurotoxicol Teratol.* 1997;19(3):171–183

259. Mattson SN, Riley EP. A review of the neurobehavioral deficits in children with fetal alcohol syndrome or prenatal exposure to alcohol. *Alcohol Clin Exp Res.* 1998; 22(2):279–294

260. Coggins TE, Timler GR, Olswang LB. A state of double jeopardy: impact of prenatal alcohol exposure and adverse environments on the social communicative abilities of school-age children with fetal alcohol spectrum disorder. *Lang Speech Hear Serv Sch.* 2007;38(2):117–127

261. Bandstra ES, Morrow CE, Vogel AL, et al. Longitudinal influence of prenatal cocaine exposure on child language functioning. *Neurotoxicol Teratol.* 2002;24(3):297–308

262. Lewis BA, Singer LT, Short EJ, et al. Four-year language outcomes of children exposed to cocaine in utero. *Neurotoxicol Teratol.* 2004;26(5):617–627

263. Streissguth AP, Barr HM, Sampson PD. Moderate prenatal alcohol exposure: effects on child IQ and learning problems at age 7 1/2 years. *Alcohol Clin Exp Res.* 1990;14(5):662–669

264. Coles CD, Brown RT, Smith IE, Platzman KA, Erickson S, Falek A. Effects of prenatal alcohol exposure at school age. I. Physical and cognitive development. *Neurotoxicol Teratol.* 1991;13(4):357–367

265. Goldschmidt L, Richardson GA, Stoffer DS, Geva D, Day NL. Prenatal alcohol exposure and academic achievement at age six: a nonlinear fit. *Alcohol Clin Exp Res.* 1996; 20(4):763–770

266. Olson HC, Streissguth AP, Sampson PD, Barr HM, Bookstein FL, Thiede K. Association of prenatal alcohol exposure with behavioral and learning problems in early adolescence. *J Am Acad Child Adolesc Psychiatry.* 1997;36(9):1187–1194

267. Goldschmidt L, Richardson GA, Cornelius MD, Day NL. Prenatal marijuana and alcohol exposure and academic achievement at age 10. *Neurotoxicol Teratol.* 2004; 26(4):521–532

268. Levine TP, Liu J, Das A, et al. Effects of prenatal cocaine exposure on special education in school-aged children. *Pediatrics.* 2008;122(1). Available at: www.pediatrics.org/cgi/content/full/122/1/e83

269. Hurt H, Brodsky NL, Roth H, Malmud E, Giannetta JM. School performance of children with gestational cocaine exposure. *Neurotoxicol Teratol.* 2005;27(2):203–211

270. Cernerud L, Eriksson M, Jonsson B, Steneroth G, Zetterström R. Amphetamine addiction during pregnancy: 14-year follow-up of growth and school performance. *Acta Paediatr.* 1996;85(2):204–208

271. Cornelius MD, Leech SL, Goldschmidt L, Day NL. Prenatal tobacco exposure: is it a risk factor for early tobacco experimentation? *Nicotine Tob Res.* 2000;2(1):45–52

272. Buka SL, Shenassa ED, Niaura R. Elevated risk of tobacco dependence among offspring of mothers who smoked during pregnancy: a 30-year prospective study. *Am J Psychiatry.* 2003;160(11):1978–1984

273. Porath AJ, Fried PA. Effects of prenatal cigarette and marijuana exposure on drug use among offspring. *Neurotoxicol Teratol.* 2005;27(2):267–277

274. Brennan PA, Grekin ER, Mortensen EL, Mednick SA. Relationship of maternal smoking during pregnancy with criminal arrest and hospitalization for substance abuse in male and female adult offspring. *Am J Psychiatry.* 2002;159(1):48–54

275. Baer JS, Barr HM, Bookstein FL, Sampson PD, Streissguth AP. Prenatal alcohol exposure and family history of alcoholism in the etiology of adolescent alcohol problems. *J Stud Alcohol.* 1998;59(5):533–543

276. Yates WR, Cadoret RJ, Troughton EP, Stewart M, Giunta TS. Effect of fetal alcohol exposure on adult symptoms of nicotine, alcohol, and drug dependence. *Alcohol Clin Exp Res.* 1998;22(4):914–920

277. Alati R, Al Mamun A, Williams GM, O'Callaghan M, Najman JM, Bor W. In utero alcohol exposure and prediction of alcohol disorders in early adulthood: a birth cohort study. *Arch Gen Psychiatry.* 2006;63(9):1009–1016

Principles of Judicious Antibiotic Prescribing for Upper Respiratory Tract Infections in Pediatrics

- *Clinical Report*

CLINICAL REPORT

Principles of Judicious Antibiotic Prescribing for Upper Respiratory Tract Infections in Pediatrics

abstract

Most upper respiratory tract infections are caused by viruses and require no antibiotics. This clinical report focuses on antibiotic prescribing strategies for bacterial upper respiratory tract infections, including acute otitis media, acute bacterial sinusitis, and streptococcal pharyngitis. The principles for judicious antibiotic prescribing that are outlined focus on applying stringent diagnostic criteria, weighing the benefits and harms of antibiotic therapy, and understanding situations when antibiotics may not be indicated. The principles can be used to amplify messages from recent clinical guidelines for local guideline development and for patient communication; they are broadly applicable to antibiotic prescribing in general. *Pediatrics* 2013;132:1146–1154

INTRODUCTION

More than 1 in 5 pediatric ambulatory visits to a physician result in an antibiotic prescription, which accounts for nearly 50 million antibiotic prescriptions annually in the United States.[1] It is widely documented that inappropriate antibiotic prescribing, especially for upper respiratory tract infections (URIs) of viral origin, is common in ambulatory care.[1–3] As many as 10 million antibiotic prescriptions per year are directed toward respiratory conditions for which they are unlikely to provide benefit.[1] Recent evidence shows that broad-spectrum antibiotic prescribing has increased and frequently occurs when either no therapy is necessary or when narrower-spectrum alternatives are appropriate.[1,2] Such overuse of antibiotics causes avoidable drug-related adverse events,[4–6] contributes to antibiotic resistance,[7,8] and adds unnecessary medical costs. This is compounded by the fact that few new antibiotics to treat antibiotic-resistant infections are under development.[9] The growing health and economic threats of antibiotic resistance make promoting judicious antibiotic prescribing, which encompasses both reducing overuse and ensuring that appropriate agents are prescribed, an urgent public health and patient safety priority (http://www.cdc.gov/drugresistance/threat-report-2013).

Clinical decision-making about whether to prescribe antibiotics for a patient with URI symptoms is a daily occurrence for ambulatory-care physicians and other health care professionals who provide care for children. Although antibiotic prescribing is a routine part of clinical

Adam L. Hersh, MD, PhD, Mary Anne Jackson, MD, Lauri A. Hicks, DO, and the COMMITTEE ON INFECTIOUS DISEASES

KEY WORDS
respiratory tract infections, antibacterial agents

ABBREVIATIONS
AAP—American Academy of Pediatrics
AOM—acute otitis media
GAS—group A *Streptococcus*
NNT—number needed to treat
PTA—peritonsillar abscess
TM—tympanic membrane
URI—upper respiratory tract infection

The guidance in this report does not indicate an exclusive course of treatment or serve as a standard of medical care. Variations, taking into account individual circumstances, may be appropriate.

www.pediatrics.org/cgi/doi/10.1542/peds.2013-3260

doi:10.1542/peds.2013-3260

All clinical reports from the American Academy of Pediatrics automatically expire 5 years after publication unless reaffirmed, revised, or retired at or before that time.

PEDIATRICS (ISSN Numbers: Print, 0031-4005; Online, 1098-4275).

care, judicious antibiotic prescribing is challenging because it is difficult to distinguish between viral and bacterial URIs. A major objective of this clinical report is to provide a framework for clinical decision-making regarding antibiotic use for pediatric URIs. A point of emphasis is the importance of using stringent and validated clinical criteria when diagnosing acute otitis media (AOM), acute bacterial sinusitis, and pharyngitis caused by group A *Streptococcus* (GAS), as established through clinical guidelines. Additionally, this document emphasizes situations in which the use of antibiotics is not indicated, in particular for viral respiratory infections. Considering the frequency of URIs and the large proportion of antibiotic prescribing attributable to URI visits, these conditions represent a high-impact target for guidelines and other interventions designed to optimize antibiotic prescribing. The careful application of these criteria has the potential to mitigate overuse of antibiotics for pediatric URIs.

The first "Principles of Judicious Use of Antimicrobial Agents for Pediatric Upper Respiratory Tract Infections" were published in 1998 in response to concerns over the emergence and spread of antibiotic-resistant organisms.[10] The Centers for Disease Control and Prevention, in collaboration with the American Academy of Pediatrics (AAP), sought to update these principles in a current context. Antibiotic resistance remains a major public health concern, and appropriate antibiotic use is an important health care quality goal. Although the introduction of a 7-valent pneumococcal polysaccharide-protein conjugate vaccine (PCV7) in 2000 led to large declines in the incidence of invasive pneumococcal infections,[11] an increase in the prevalence of nonvaccine serotypes, most notably serotype 19A, a commonly antibiotic-resistant serotype,[12,13] prompted the 2010 introduction of

a 13-valent pneumococcal polysaccharide-protein conjugate vaccine (PCV13). Provider concerns about antibiotic resistance may be 1 factor leading to increasing use of broad-spectrum antibiotics. In recent years, several high-quality randomized controlled trials, meta-analyses, and new and updated clinical guidelines have been published that better define the effectiveness of antibiotic use for selected URIs, including AOM and acute bacterial sinusitis.[14–23] At the same time, new evidence highlighting the extent to which antibiotics lead to adverse events requiring medical attention[4–6] or potentially life-threatening events[24,25] has emerged.

This clinical report focuses on antibiotic prescribing for key pediatric URIs that, in certain instances, may benefit from antibiotic therapy: AOM, acute bacterial sinusitis, and pharyngitis. The specific recommendations are applicable to healthy children who do not have underlying medical conditions (eg, immunosuppression) placing them at increased risk of developing serious complications. The purpose of this report is to provide practitioners specific context using the most current recommendations and guidelines while applying 3 principles of judicious antibiotic use: (1) determination of the likelihood of a bacterial infection, (2) weighing the benefits and harms of antibiotics, and (3) implementing judicious prescribing strategies (Table 1).

PRINCIPLE 1: DETERMINE THE LIKELIHOOD OF A BACTERIAL INFECTION

Many aspects of the clinical history, symptoms, and signs of bacterial URIs overlap with or mirror those of viral infections or noninfectious conditions. To make a judicious decision about antibiotic use, it is essential first to determine the likelihood of a bacterial

infection. When a practitioner has made the diagnosis of viral infection and has reasonably excluded the presence of concurrent bacterial infection, antibiotics should not be used because the potential for harm outweighs the potential benefit. In the specific cases of AOM, acute bacterial sinusitis, and pharyngitis, there are well-established stringent criteria that aid in distinguishing bacterial from nonbacterial causes.

AOM

The AAP and American Academy of Family Physicians released updated clinical practice guidelines for the diagnosis and treatment of AOM in 2013.[22] AOM may be defined as "the rapid onset of signs and symptoms of inflammation in the middle ear." The signs include bulging with or without erythema of the tympanic membrane (TM), and the symptoms may include otalgia, irritability, otorrhea, and fever. The diagnosis of AOM always requires a careful otoscopic examination to confirm the presence of inflammatory changes in the TM. The AAP guideline recommends that physicians diagnose AOM definitively under either of 2 conditions: (1) evidence of middle-ear effusion, as demonstrated by moderate to severe bulging of the TM, or (2) new onset of otorrhea that is not attributable to otitis externa. AOM may also be diagnosed when a child presents with only mild bulging of the TM but with additional symptoms of recent onset of ear pain or with intense erythema of the TM. Although clear visualization of the TM at times is difficult and because AOM is typically a self-limiting disease, a high degree of diagnostic certainty is essential to minimize antibiotic overuse. After AOM is diagnosed, judicious antibiotic use can be enhanced by further categorizing patients on the basis of illness severity (severe otalgia, otalgia lasting

TABLE 1 Application of Judicious Antibiotic Principles for Pediatric URIs

Principles	AOM	Acute Bacterial Sinusitis	Acute Pharyngitis
Principle 1: Determine the likelihood of a bacterial infection	Requires middle ear effusion and signs of inflammation:	URI symptoms that are either worsening, severe, or persistent	Diagnosis of GAS pharyngitis requires confirmation by rapid testing or culture
	• moderate or severe bulging of TM; or	• Worsening symptoms: worsening or new onset fever, daytime cough, or nasal discharge after improvement of viral URI	• Only test if 2 of the following are present: fever, tonsillar exudate/swelling, swollen/tender anterior cervical nodes, absence of cough
	• otorrhea not due to otitis externa; or	• Severe symptoms: fever ≥39°C, purulent nasal discharge	• Do not treat empirically
	• mild bulging of TM with ear pain or erythema of TM	• Persistent symptoms without improvement: nasal discharge or daytime cough >10 d No role for routine imaging	
Principle 2: Weigh benefits versus harms of antibiotics	Benefits: for strictly defined AOM, NNT of as few as 4 patients to achieve improvements in symptoms	Benefits: for strictly defined bacterial sinusitis, antibiotics improve symptoms at 3 and 14 d	Benefits: for confirmed GAS, antibiotics shorten symptom duration, prevent rheumatic fever and may limit secondary transmission.
	• no significant benefits in preventing complications such as mastoiditis	• no evidence that antibiotic therapy prevents complications such as brain abscess	• Limited evidence that therapy prevents complications such as PTA
First-line therapy	Amoxicillin with or without clavulanate	Amoxicillin with or without clavulanate	Amoxicillin or penicillin
	Harms: for all conditions, no benefits to therapy when bacterial infection is not likely. Increased risk of adverse events including diarrhea, dermatitis, *C difficile* colitis, antibiotic resistance		
Principle 3: Implement judicious prescribing strategies	• Consider watchful waiting for older patients (>2 y), those with unilateral disease and without severe symptoms • Shorter-duration therapy (7 d)	• Consider watchful waiting for patients with persistent symptoms only	• Once daily dosing of amoxicillin
	Not recommended: azithromycin and oral third-generation cephalosporins are generally not recommended for these conditions attributable to *S pneumoniae* resistance.		

>48 hours, or temperature ≥39°C), laterality of infection (bilateral versus unilateral), and age (≤23 months vs ≥24 months). Patients with more severe symptoms, bilateral involvement, and younger age are more likely to benefit from antibiotics. Watchful waiting is reasonable for patients who are older and have nonsevere, unilateral disease.

Acute Bacterial Sinusitis

The AAP[23] and the Infectious Diseases Society of America[21] recently developed evidence-based clinical guidelines for the diagnosis and treatment of acute bacterial sinusitis. These guidelines support use of strict diagnostic criteria to distinguish bacterial from viral URIs. In particular, acute bacterial sinusitis is diagnosed on the basis of symptoms that are (1) persistent and not improving, (2) worsening, or (3) severe. Persistent symptoms are most common

and include nasal discharge (of any quality) or daytime cough not improving by 10 days. Worsening symptoms include a worsening or new onset of fever, daytime cough, or nasal discharge after improvement of a typical viral URI. Severe symptoms include persistent fever (temperature ≥39°C) and purulent nasal discharge for at least 3 days. These clinical criteria are the basis for the diagnosis of acute bacterial sinusitis. Because many children with viral URI will have radiographic abnormalities, imaging should not be performed routinely.

Acute Pharyngitis

Pharyngitis, or sore throat, may be accompanied by other nonspecific symptoms including cough, congestion, and fever. The most important diagnostic consideration is whether β-hemolytic GAS is the cause. Unlike AOM and acute bacterial sinusitis, the diagnosis of GAS

infection can be confirmed with laboratory testing (either a rapid-antigen detection test or culture).[26,27] Scoring systems (Modified Centor or McIsaac Scores[28]) can assist in identifying candidates for testing. Patients with 2 or more of the following features should undergo testing: (1) absence of cough, (2) presence of tonsillar exudates or swelling, (3) history of fever, (4) presence of swollen and tender anterior cervical lymph nodes, and (5) age younger than 15 years. Children with URI signs and symptoms, including cough, nasal congestion, conjunctivitis, hoarseness, diarrhea, or oropharyngeal lesions (ulcers, vesicles) more likely have viral illnesses and not GAS infection and should not be tested for GAS. Testing should generally not be performed in children younger than 3 years in whom GAS rarely causes pharyngitis and in whom rheumatic fever is uncommon. GAS should not be diagnosed in the absence of testing, even among patients with all of the aforementioned clinical criteria, with rare exceptions (eg, symptomatic and household contact with confirmed GAS pharyngitis). The importance of limiting testing to children with appropriate clinical criteria is further supported by the fact that colonization rates can reach 15% to 20% even among asymptomatic children.

Common Cold, Nonspecific URI, Acute Cough Illness, and Acute Bronchitis

Symptoms of the common cold, nonspecific URI, and bronchitis may overlap with or mirror those of bacterial URIs and can include cough, congestion, and sore throat. Collectively, these viral conditions account for millions of office visits per year. Acute bronchitis, in particular, is a cough illness that is diagnosed during more than 2 million pediatric office visits annually, and antibiotics are prescribed more than 70% of the time.[1] Application of diagnostic clinical criteria for AOM, sinusitis, and pharyngitis should aid clinicians in excluding these conditions. Management of the common cold, nonspecific URI, acute cough illness, and acute bronchitis should focus on symptomatic relief. Antibiotics should not be prescribed for these conditions.

PRINCIPLE 2: WEIGH BENEFITS VERSUS HARMS OF ANTIBIOTICS

If a bacterial infection is determined to be likely, the next step is to compare the evidence about the benefits of antibiotic therapy for each condition to the potential for harms. Relevant outcomes to consider for benefits include the cure rate, symptom reduction, prevention of complications, and secondary cases. Outcomes for harms include antibiotic-related adverse events (eg, abdominal pain, diarrhea, rash), *Clostridium difficile* colitis, development of resistance, and cost.

AOM

Benefits

Several high-quality randomized controlled trials and meta-analyses have been published since the publication of the first principles of judicious use of antibiotics.[18–20,29–33] Collectively, these have emphasized the following: (1) at least half of patients with AOM will recover without antibiotic therapy; (2) recovery is more likely and is hastened for children who receive antibiotic therapy compared with placebo; and (3) recovery without antibiotic therapy is less likely for younger children, those with bilateral versus unilateral disease, and those with more severe signs and symptoms. These observations underlie the rationale for treatment recommendations for AOM.

Multiple meta-analyses indicate that children receiving antibiotic therapy are more likely to achieve clinical success in terms of symptom resolution compared with placebo with a number needed to treat (NNT) of 7 or 8 patients.[18,33] Two recent randomized controlled trials among younger children that used even more stringent diagnostic criteria demonstrated that children who received antibiotics had more favorable symptom scores than those who received placebo, achieved faster symptom recovery, and had significantly lower rates of clinical failure as measured by otoscopic examination and persistence of symptoms, with an NNT closer to 4.[19,20] Nonetheless, it is important to note that in numerous studies of antibiotic efficacy for AOM, the majority of patients have symptoms that ultimately resolve spontaneously regardless of therapy and without complications. The potential for preventing complications, such as mastoiditis, may contribute, in part, to the clinical decision to use antibiotics for AOM. However, across the aforementioned controlled studies and meta-analyses, antibiotics have not demonstrated significant benefit in preventing these rare but serious complications. Observational data from the United Kingdom including more than 1 million AOM episodes indicates that when mastoiditis occurs, it typically is present at time of initial clinical presentation to care.[34] The estimated NNT to prevent 1 episode of mastoiditis is nearly 5000.[34]

The AAP recommends antibiotic therapy for children diagnosed with AOM on the basis of presence of established clinical criteria. Observation can be considered for selected children, particularly children older than 2 years with nonsevere symptoms and unilateral disease.

Acute Bacterial Sinusitis

Benefits

The evidence base evaluating the effectiveness of antibiotics for treatment of acute bacterial sinusitis in children is limited and mixed. Three randomized controlled trials have assessed the effectiveness of antibiotics versus placebo for clinically diagnosed acute bacterial sinusitis in children, 2 of which have been published since the 1998 principles of judicious use of antibiotics.[14,17,35] Two trials concluded that antibiotics significantly improved the likelihood of symptom resolution after both 3 and 14 days,[14,35] but 1 study revealed no benefit of antibiotics over placebo.[17] Key differences in the study design between these studies likely contributed to the differences in outcomes; the trials showing benefit included patients with more severe symptoms and applied more strict diagnostic criteria. This emphasizes the importance of careful attention to clinical diagnosis because antibiotics confer no clinical benefit for patients without diagnostic criteria suggesting acute bacterial sinusitis.

The benefit of antibiotic therapy in preventing suppurative complications, such as orbital cellulitis or intracranial abscess, is unproven. Individual efficacy trials lack the statistical power to demonstrate effectiveness against these rare complications, and a meta-analysis of randomized controlled trials in children and adults found no significant association between antibiotic use and the rate of complications.[36]

The AAP recommends antibiotic therapy for children with clinical features of acute bacterial sinusitis, especially those with symptoms that are worsening or severe. Observation with close follow-up or antibiotic therapy can be considered for those with persistent symptoms (>10 days).

GAS Pharyngitis

Benefits

Antibiotic treatment of acute pharyngitis has been studied with respect to the effects on symptom resolution, transmission, and prevention of complications, including rheumatic fever. Five randomized controlled studies and 1 meta-analysis have examined the effect of immediate antibiotics on resolution of symptoms, 1 of which was completed since publication of the first principles of judicious use of antibiotics.[37–41] These studies provide strong evidence that antibiotic therapy for children with pharyngitis and confirmation of GAS shortens the duration of symptoms, including sore throat and headache, by approximately 1 day. These benefits are apparent within as few as 3 days. However, the benefits of antibiotic therapy on shortening duration of fever are uncertain. Although data are somewhat limited, antibiotic therapy for index cases of GAS may reduce horizontal transmission and thereby prevent secondary cases.[40,42] These benefits are especially relevant in large households, child care settings, schools, and military settings.

Historically, the primary motivation for prescribing antibiotics for GAS pharyngitis was prevention of rheumatic fever. Randomized controlled trials in children before 1975 showed a four-fold benefit in preventing the onset of rheumatic fever, which occurred in approximately 3% of untreated patients.[43] Although localized outbreaks have occurred in recent decades, the incidence of rheumatic fever in most developed countries has declined dramatically.[44] Some of this decline might be attributable to better recognition and antibiotic treatment,[45] but more likely this relates to a decline in the prevalence of rheumatogenic strains of GAS.[46]

Antibiotics may also have a role in preventing suppurative complications associated with GAS pharyngitis, such as peritonsillar abscess (PTA), AOM, and acute sinusitis. One meta-analysis suggested that antibiotic treatment prevents PTA; however, the majority of cases were derived from a single study conducted in 1951.[43] Data from a large observational cohort conducted in the United Kingdom suggest that antibiotic treatment may prevent development of PTA, but with an NNT >4000.[47]

The AAP recommends antibiotic therapy for children with pharyngitis confirmed to be caused by GAS.

Common Cold, Nonspecific URI, Acute Cough Illness, and Acute Bronchitis

Because the predominant etiologies for these conditions are viruses, antibiotic therapy is not indicated. Because of uncertainty about the relevance of the diagnosis of acute bronchitis for children, data are limited. Nonetheless, a large meta-analysis concluded that there was no benefit to antibiotic therapy (including for delayed prescriptions) for patients with nonspecific cough and cold.[48]

Harms of Antibiotic Therapy

It is crucial to account for the potential for antibiotics to cause harm when used for treatment of URIs. The significance of potential harms should be directly balanced against the potential for benefit on a case-by-case basis. The importance of harms associated with antibiotic use is directly related to (1) an assessment of the magnitude of potential benefit (eg, greater benefit achieved for young children with bilateral AOM than unilateral) and (2) the extent to which uncertainty remains in the diagnosis. The preponderance of evidence for benefits of antibiotic therapy in treatment of bacterial URIs relates to attenuation of symptoms. When it is unclear whether the URI represents an acute bacterial infection, in general, the harms of antibiotic use have the potential to outweigh benefits. The importance of applying stringent clinical criteria to establish the diagnosis of a bacterial infection aids in differentiating children with nonspecific URI and common cold. Prescribing antibiotics for nonspecific URI and colds generally does not provide benefit and only exposes these children to potential harm.

Antibiotics are responsible for the largest number of unplanned medical visits for medication-related adverse events among children, which exceeds 150 000 per year and incurs substantial potential morbidity and cost.[4] Antibiotic-associated adverse events can range from mild (diarrhea and rash), to more severe (Stevens-Johnson syndrome), to life-threatening (anaphylaxis or sudden cardiac death) reactions. Most clinical trials conducted to assess the treatment of AOM, sinusitis, and pharyngitis have used amoxicillin or amoxicillin-clavulanate, and these remain the first-line recommended agents for antibiotic therapy for these conditions. Studies comparing antibiotic treatment to placebo for AOM suggest a modestly increased rate of adverse events among treated patients, particularly diarrhea and rash. Two meta-analyses estimated rate differences of approximately 5% for adverse events.[18,32] Not included in these are the results from 2 recent trials using amoxicillin-clavulanate (older studies frequently used amoxicillin), which demonstrated even higher rates of diarrhea and dermatitis among patients receiving antibiotic therapy.[19,20] Among studies of sinusitis, in the most recent trial that demonstrated a benefit of antibiotic therapy, adverse events (defined as rash, diarrhea, vomiting, and abdominal pain) occurred in 44% of patients treated with high-dose amoxicillin-clavulanate compared with 14% in the placebo group.[14]

The adverse events described previously occur relatively frequently, although are relatively mild in most cases. Antibiotics can produce serious allergic reactions such as Stevens-Johnson syndrome.[25] There is rapidly growing evidence that antibiotic exposures early in life may disrupt the microbial balance of the intestines and other parts of the body in such a way as to contribute to long-term adverse health effects, such as inflammatory bowel disease, obesity, eczema, and asthma.[49–51] A recent study highlighted risk of sudden death in adults treated with azithromycin, likely related to drug-associated prolongation of the QT interval.[24] Azithromycin is not a first-line antibiotic for any pediatric URI and is the antibiotic most likely to be used inappropriately (inadequate coverage for the most common pathogens causing AOM and sinusitis).[1] The incidence of *C difficile* colitis in hospitalized children has increased substantially during the past decade.[52] Although

children with comorbid conditions are at greatest risk, community-onset infections occur,[53] with recent antibiotic exposure as an important risk factor.

The relationship between antibiotic exposure and development of antibiotic resistance at the level of the individual patient and at the level of the community is well established.[7,8] Because of limited therapeutic options, antibiotic-resistant infections are difficult to treat and, in some cases, are associated with poor clinical outcomes.[54] Application of stringent diagnostic criteria and use of therapy only when the diagnosis and potential benefits are well established is essential to minimizing the impact of antibiotic overuse on resistance in individuals and within communities.

PRINCIPLE 3: IMPLEMENT JUDICIOUS PRESCRIBING STRATEGIES

When evidence suggests that antibiotics may provide benefit, several aspects of judicious prescribing should be considered. These include selecting an appropriate antibiotic agent that treats the most likely pathogens (including accounting for local resistance patterns), selecting the appropriate dose, and treating for the shortest duration required. Additionally, physicians may consider the role of observation and use of delayed prescribing strategies.

The treatment of AOM and acute bacterial sinusitis illustrates several key aspects of judicious antibiotic use. Amoxicillin has traditionally been the recommended first-line agent for these conditions because *Streptococcus pneumoniae* is the most important cause. However, in some communities, the prevalence of amoxicillin-resistant β-lactamase-producing *Haemophilus influenzae* among bacterial URIs has increased significantly.[55] This underlies (in part) the recommendation to

consider amoxicillin-clavulanate in certain instances (eg, severe symptoms, recent [<6 weeks] antibiotic exposure, known high local prevalence of amoxicillin-resistant *H influenzae*). It is important to note, however, that the benefits of antibiotic therapy appear to be greatest for patients with *S pneumoniae* infection, compared with other bacterial causes of URI, including *H influenzae* and *Moraxella* species, which may have higher rates of spontaneous resolution.[16] In recognition of the possibility of a higher rate of adverse events caused by amoxicillin-clavulanate compared with amoxicillin, some physicians may choose to use amoxicillin as the first-line agent in most instances.

An understanding of local epidemiology and resistance patterns is especially important for understanding appropriate antibiotic selection. The rates of pneumococcal resistance to macrolides[56] and oral third-generation cephalosporins[57,58] make these agents poor choices for treating most children with suspected bacterial URIs. Emergence of macrolide resistance to GAS is also an important problem, although susceptibility testing is not routinely performed.

The role of observation (also termed "wait and see" or "delayed prescribing") instead of immediate antibiotic therapy is an important consideration for children with AOM and acute bacterial sinusitis. Studies among patients with AOM have shown that this approach reduces antibiotic use, is well accepted by families, and, when supported by close follow-up, does not result in worse clinical outcomes.[22] Observation therapy may be considered as an alternative strategy to immediate therapy for AOM and sinusitis for older patients without severe symptoms.[22,23] The use of this approach is an opportunity to engage in shared decision-making with patients and families to include a discussion about the potential benefits and risks associated with immediate antibiotic therapy.

Another important consideration for judicious antibiotic use is overall magnitude of exposure. Relatively short courses of therapy may achieve the same clinical benefits as longer courses while minimizing the risks of adverse events and development of resistance and lead to better compliance. Important examples are the use of once-daily amoxicillin for GAS pharyngitis[26] (vs 2 or 3 times daily dosing but the same daily dose of 50 mg/kg) and short-course therapy (eg, 7 days vs 10 days) for older children with AOM.[22]

CONCLUSIONS

This clinical report discusses principles of judicious antibiotic use for pediatric URIs. There is a strong emphasis on appropriate diagnosis, which is the foundation for making judicious decisions about prescribing antibiotics. Although focused on specific URIs, the main message has broader application for antibiotic use in general. These principles can be used to promote educational efforts for physicians, amplify the messages from recent clinical guidelines, assist with communication about appropriate antibiotic use to patients and families, and support local guideline development for judicious antibiotic use.

COMMITTEE ON INFECTIOUS DISEASES, 2013–2014

Michael T. Brady, MD, Chairperson, *Red Book* Associate Editor
Carrie L. Byington, MD
H. Dele Davies, MD
Kathryn M. Edwards, MD
Mary Anne Jackson, MD, *Red Book* Associate Editor
Yvonne A. Maldonado, MD
Dennis L. Murray, MD
Walter A. Orenstein, MD
Mobeen Rathore, MD
Mark Sawyer, MD
Gordon E. Schutze, MD
Rodney E. Willoughby, MD
Theoklis E. Zaoutis, MD

LIAISONS

Marc A. Fischer, MD – *Centers for Disease Control and Prevention*
Bruce Gellin, MD – *National Vaccine Program Office*
Richard L. Gorman, MD – *National Institutes of Health*
Lucia Lee, MD – *Food and Drug Administration*
R. Douglas Pratt, MD – *Food and Drug Administration*
Jennifer S. Read, MD – *National Vaccine Program Office*

Joan Robinson, MD – *Canadian Pediatric Society*
Marco Aurelio Palazzi Safadi, MD – *Sociedad Latinoamericana de Infectologia Pediatrica (SLIPE)*
Jane Seward, MBBS, MPH – *Centers for Disease Control and Prevention*
Jeffrey R. Starke, MD – *American Thoracic Society*
Geoffrey Simon, MD – *Committee on Practice Ambulatory Medicine*
Tina Q. Tan, MD – *Pediatric Infectious Diseases Society*

EX OFFICIO

Henry H. Bernstein, DO, *Red Book* Online Associate Editor
David W. Kimberlin, MD, *Red Book* Editor
Sarah S. Long, MD, *Red Book* Associate Editor
H. Cody Meissner, MD, *Visual Red Book* Associate Editor

CONSULTANTS

Adam L. Hersh, MD, PhD
Lauri A. Hicks, DO

STAFF

Jennifer Frantz, MPH

ACKNOWLEDGMENTS

The authors acknowledge the contributions of Daniel Shapiro and Jeffrey Gerber for assistance in systematic review and critical review of early versions of this report.

REFERENCES

1. Hersh AL, Shapiro DJ, Pavia AT, Shah SS. Antibiotic prescribing in ambulatory pediatrics in the United States. *Pediatrics.* 2011; 128(6):1053–1061

2. Grijalva CG, Nuorti JP, Griffin MR. Antibiotic prescription rates for acute respiratory tract infections in US ambulatory settings. *JAMA.* 2009;302(7):758–766

3. Nyquist AC, Gonzales R, Steiner JF, Sande MA. Antibiotic prescribing for children with colds, upper respiratory tract infections, and bronchitis. *JAMA.* 1998;279(11):875–877

4. Bourgeois FT, Mandl KD, Valim C, Shannon MW. Pediatric adverse drug events in the outpatient setting: an 11-year national analysis. *Pediatrics.* 2009;124(4). Available at: www.pediatrics.org/cgi/content/full/124/4/e744

5. Shehab N, Patel PR, Srinivasan A, Budnitz DS. Emergency department visits for antibiotic-associated adverse events. *Clin Infect Dis.* 2008;47(6):735–743

6. Cohen AL, Budnitz DS, Weidenbach KN, et al. National surveillance of emergency department visits for outpatient adverse drug events in children and adolescents. *J Pediatr.* 2008;152(3):416–421

7. Hicks LA, Chien YW, Taylor TH, Jr, Haber M, Klugman KP Active Bacterial Core Surveillance (ABCs) Team. Outpatient antibiotic prescribing and nonsusceptible Streptococcus pneumoniae in the United States, 1996–2003. *Clin Infect Dis.* 2011;53(7):631–639

8. Costelloe C, Metcalfe C, Lovering A, Mant D, Hay AD. Effect of antibiotic prescribing in primary care on antimicrobial resistance in individual patients: systematic review and meta-analysis. *BMJ.* 2010;340:c2096

9. Boucher HW, Talbot GH, Bradley JS, et al. Bad bugs, no drugs: no ESKAPE! An update from the Infectious Diseases Society of America. *Clin Infect Dis.* 2009;48(1):1–12

10. Dowell SF, Marcy SM, Philips WR. Principles of judicious use of antimicrobial agents for pediatric upper respiratory tract infections. *Pediatrics.* 1998;101(suppl 1):163–165

11. Pavia M, Bianco A, Nobile CG, Marinelli P, Angelillo IF. Efficacy of pneumococcal vaccination in children younger than 24 months: a meta-analysis. *Pediatrics.* 2009; 123(6). Available at: www.pediatrics.org/cgi/content/full/123/6/e1103

12. Centers for Disease Control and Prevention (CDC). Invasive pneumococcal disease in

children 5 years after conjugate vaccine introduction—eight states, 1998–2005. *MMWR Morb Mortal Wkly Rep.* 2008;57(6):144–148

13. Kyaw MH, Lynfield R, Schaffner W, et al; Active Bacterial Core Surveillance of the Emerging Infections Program Network. Effect of introduction of the pneumococcal conjugate vaccine on drug-resistant Streptococcus pneumoniae. *N Engl J Med.* 2006;354(14):1455–1463

14. Wald ER, Nash D, Eickhoff J. Effectiveness of amoxicillin/clavulanate potassium in the treatment of acute bacterial sinusitis in children. *Pediatrics.* 2009;124(1):9–15

15. American Academy of Pediatrics. Subcommittee on Management of Sinusitis and Committee on Quality Improvement. Clinical practice guideline: management of sinusitis. *Pediatrics.* 2001;108(3):798–808

16. American Academy of Pediatrics Subcommittee on Management of Acute Otitis Media. Diagnosis and management of acute otitis media. *Pediatrics.* 2004;113(5):1451–1465

17. Garbutt JM, Goldstein M, Gellman E, Shannon W, Littenberg B. A randomized, placebo-controlled trial of antimicrobial treatment for children with clinically diagnosed acute sinusitis. *Pediatrics.* 2001;107(4):619–625

18. Coker TR, Chan LS, Newberry SJ, et al. Diagnosis, microbial epidemiology, and antibiotic treatment of acute otitis media in children: a systematic review. *JAMA.* 2010;304(19):2161–2169

19. Hoberman A, Paradise JL, Rockette HE, et al. Treatment of acute otitis media in children under 2 years of age. *N Engl J Med.* 2011;364(2):105–115

20. Tähtinen PA, Laine MK, Huovinen P, Jalava J, Ruuskanen O, Ruohola A. A placebo-controlled trial of antimicrobial treatment for acute otitis media. *N Engl J Med.* 2011;364(2):116–126

21. Chow AW, Benninger MS, Brook I, et al; Infectious Diseases Society of America. IDSA clinical practice guideline for acute bacterial rhinosinusitis in children and adults. *Clin Infect Dis.* 2012;54(8):e72–e112

22. Lieberthal AS, Carroll AE, Chonmaitree T, et al. The diagnosis and management of acute otitis media. *Pediatrics.* 2013;131(3). Available at: www.pediatrics.org/cgi/content/full/131/3/e964

23. Wald ER, Applegate KE, Bordley C, et al; American Academy of Pediatrics. Clinical practice guideline for the diagnosis and management of acute bacterial sinusitis in children aged 1 to 18 years. *Pediatrics.* 2013;132(1). Available at: www.pediatrics.org/cgi/content/full/132/1/e262

24. Ray WA, Murray KT, Hall K, Arbogast PG, Stein CM. Azithromycin and the risk of cardiovascular death. *N Engl J Med.* 2012;366(20):1881–1890

25. Goldman JL, Jackson MA, Herigon JC, Hersh AL, Shapiro DJ, Leeder JS. Trends in adverse reactions to trimethoprim-sulfamethoxazole. *Pediatrics.* 2013;131(1). Available at: www.pediatrics.org/cgi/content/full/131/1/e103

26. American Academy of Pediatrics. In: Pickering LK, Baker CJ, Kimberlin DW, Long SS, eds. *Red Book: 2012 Report of the Committee on Infectious Diseases.* Elk Grove Village, IL: American Academy of Pediatrics; 2012

27. Shulman ST, Bisno AL, Clegg HW, et al. Clinical practice guideline for the diagnosis and management of group A streptococcal pharyngitis: 2012 update by the Infectious Diseases Society of America. *Clin Infect Dis.* 2012;55(10):1279–1282

28. Fine AM, Nizet V, Mandl KD. Large-scale validation of the Centor and McIsaac scores to predict group A streptococcal pharyngitis. *Arch Intern Med.* 2012;172(11):847–852

29. Damoiseaux RA, van Balen FA, Hoes AW, Verheij TJ, de Melker RA. Primary care based randomised, double blind trial of amoxicillin versus placebo for acute otitis media in children aged under 2 years. *BMJ.* 2000;320(7231):350–354

30. Le Saux N, Gaboury I, Baird M, et al. A randomized, double-blind, placebo-controlled noninferiority trial of amoxicillin for clinically diagnosed acute otitis media in children 6 months to 5 years of age. *CMAJ.* 2005;172(3):335–341

31. Vouloumanou EK, Karageorgopoulos DE, Kazantzi MS, Kapaskelis AM, Falagas ME. Antibiotics versus placebo or watchful waiting for acute otitis media: a meta-analysis of randomized controlled trials. *J Antimicrob Chemother.* 2009;64(1):16–24

32. Glasziou PP, Del Mar CB, Sanders SL, Hayem M. Antibiotics for acute otitis media in children. *Cochrane Database Syst Rev.* 2004;(1):CD000219

33. Rovers MM, Glasziou P, Appelman CL, et al. Antibiotics for acute otitis media: a meta-analysis with individual patient data. *Lancet.* 2006;368(9545):1429–1435

34. Thompson PL, Gilbert RE, Long PF, Saxena S, Sharland M, Wong IC. Effect of antibiotics for otitis media on mastoiditis in children: a retrospective cohort study using the United Kingdom general practice research database. *Pediatrics.* 2009;123(2):424–430

35. Wald ER, Chiponis D, Ledesma-Medina J. Comparative effectiveness of amoxicillin and amoxicillin-clavulanate potassium in acute paranasal sinus infections in children: a double-blind, placebo-controlled trial. *Pediatrics.* 1986;77(6):795–800

36. Falagas ME, Giannopoulou KP, Vardakas KZ, Dimopoulos G, Karageorgopoulos DE. Comparison of antibiotics with placebo for treatment of acute sinusitis: a meta-analysis of randomised controlled trials. *Lancet Infect Dis.* 2008;8(9):543–552

37. Zwart S, Rovers MM, de Melker RA, Hoes AW. Penicillin for acute sore throat in children: randomised, double blind trial. *BMJ.* 2003;327(7427):1324

38. el-Daher NT, Hijazi SS, Rawashdeh NM, al-Khalil IA, Abu-Ektaish FM, Abdel-Latif DI. Immediate vs. delayed treatment of group A beta-hemolytic streptococcal pharyngitis with penicillin V. *Pediatr Infect Dis J.* 1991;10(2):126–130

39. Krober MS, Bass JW, Michels GN. Streptococcal pharyngitis. Placebo-controlled double-blind evaluation of clinical response to penicillin therapy. *JAMA.* 1985;253(9):1271–1274

40. Pichichero ME, Disney FA, Talpey WB, et al. Adverse and beneficial effects of immediate treatment of group A beta-hemolytic streptococcal pharyngitis with penicillin. *Pediatr Infect Dis J.* 1987;6(7):635–643

41. Nelson JD. The effect of penicillin therapy on the symptoms and signs of streptococcal pharyngitis. *Pediatr Infect Dis.* 1984;3(1):10–13

42. Kikuta H, Shibata M, Nakata S, et al. Efficacy of antibiotic prophylaxis for intrafamilial transmission of group A beta-hemolytic streptococci. *Pediatr Infect Dis J.* 2007;26(2):139–141

43. Del Mar CB, Glasziou PP, Spinks AB. Antibiotics for sore throat. *Cochrane Database Syst Rev.* 2004;(2):CD000023

44. Robertson KA, Volmink JA, Mayosi BM. Antibiotics for the primary prevention of acute rheumatic fever: a meta-analysis. *BMC Cardiovasc Disord.* 2005;5(1):11

45. Massell BF, Chute CG, Walker AM, Kurland GS. Penicillin and the marked decrease in morbidity and mortality from rheumatic fever in the United States. *N Engl J Med.* 1988;318(5):280–286

46. Shulman ST, Stollerman G, Beall B, Dale JB, Tanz RR. Temporal changes in streptococcal M protein types and the near-disappearance of acute rheumatic fever in the United States. *Clin Infect Dis.* 2006;42(4):441–447

47. Petersen I, Johnson AM, Islam A, Duckworth G, Livermore DM, Hayward AC. Protective effect of antibiotics against serious complications of common respiratory tract infections: retrospective cohort study with

the UK General Practice Research Database. *BMJ.* 2007;335(7627):982

48. Spurling GK, Del Mar CB, Dooley L, Foxlee R, Farley R. Delayed antibiotics for respiratory infections. *Cochrane Database Syst Rev.* 2013;4:CD004417

49. Kronman MP, Zaoutis TE, Haynes K, Feng R, Coffin SE. Antibiotic exposure and IBD development among children: a population-based cohort study. *Pediatrics.* 2012;130 (4). Available at: www.pediatrics.org/cgi/content/full/130/4/e794

50. Tsakok T, McKeever TM, Yeo L, Flohr C. Does early life exposure to antibiotics increase the risk of eczema? A systematic review [published online ahead of print June 21, 2013]. *Br J Dermatol.* doi:doi:10.1111/bjd.12476

51. Jedrychowski W, Perera F, Maugeri U, et al. Wheezing and asthma may be enhanced by broad spectrum antibiotics used in early childhood. Concept and results of a pharmacoepidemiology study. *J Physiol Pharmacol.* 2011;62(2):189–195

52. Lessa FC, Gould CV, McDonald LC. Current status of Clostridium difficile infection epidemiology. *Clin Infect Dis.* 2012;55(suppl 2): S65–S70

53. Khanna S, Baddour LM, Huskins WC, et al. The epidemiology of Clostridium difficile infection in children: a population-based study. *Clin Infect Dis.* 2013;56(10):1401–1406

54. Cosgrove SE. The relationship between antimicrobial resistance and patient outcomes: mortality, length of hospital stay, and health care costs. *Clin Infect Dis.* 2006; 42(suppl 2):S82–S89

55. Pichichero ME, Casey JR. Evolving microbiology and molecular epidemiology of acute otitis media in the pneumococcal conjugate vaccine era. *Pediatr Infect Dis J.* 2007;26(10 suppl):S12–S16

56. Jenkins SG, Farrell DJ. Increase in pneumococcus macrolide resistance, United States. *Emerg Infect Dis.* 2009;15(8):1260–1264

57. Pottumarthy S, Fritsche TR, Jones RN. Comparative activity of oral and parenteral cephalosporins tested against multidrug-resistant Streptococcus pneumoniae: report from the SENTRY Antimicrobial Surveillance Program (1997–2003). *Diagn Microbiol Infect Dis.* 2005;51(2):147–150

58. Fritsche TR, Biedenbach DJ, Jones RN. Update of the activity of cefditoren and comparator oral beta-lactam agents tested against community-acquired Streptococcus pneumoniae isolates (USA, 2004–2006). *J Chemother.* 2008;20(2):170–174

Promoting the Well-Being of Children Whose Parents are Gay or Lesbian

- *Policy Statement*

POLICY STATEMENT

Promoting the Well-Being of Children Whose Parents Are Gay or Lesbian

COMMITTEE ON PSYCHOSOCIAL ASPECTS OF CHILD AND FAMILY HEALTH

KEY WORDS
civil marriage, adoption, foster care, nurturing children, children of gay and lesbian parents, marriage equality

www.pediatrics.org/cgi/doi/10.1542/peds.2013-0376

doi:10.1542/peds.2013-0376

PEDIATRICS (ISSN Numbers: Print, 0031-4005; Online, 1098-4275).

Copyright © 2013 by the American Academy of Pediatrics

abstract

To promote optimal health and well-being of all children, the American Academy of Pediatrics (AAP) supports access for all children to (1) civil marriage rights for their parents and (2) willing and capable foster and adoptive parents, regardless of the parents' sexual orientation. The AAP has always been an advocate for, and has developed policies to support, the optimal physical, mental, and social health and well-being of all infants, children, adolescents, and young adults. In so doing, the AAP has supported families in all their diversity, because the family has always been the basic social unit in which children develop the supporting and nurturing relationships with adults that they need to thrive. Children may be born to, adopted by, or cared for temporarily by married couples, nonmarried couples, single parents, grandparents, or legal guardians, and any of these may be heterosexual, gay or lesbian, or of another orientation. Children need secure and enduring relationships with committed and nurturing adults to enhance their life experiences for optimal social-emotional and cognitive development. Scientific evidence affirms that children have similar developmental and emotional needs and receive similar parenting whether they are raised by parents of the same or different genders. If a child has 2 living and capable parents who choose to create a permanent bond by way of civil marriage, it is in the best interests of their child(ren) that legal and social institutions allow and support them to do so, irrespective of their sexual orientation. If 2 parents are not available to the child, adoption or foster parenting remain acceptable options to provide a loving home for a child and should be available without regard to the sexual orientation of the parent(s). *Pediatrics* 2013;131:827–830

INTRODUCTION

All children need support and nurturing from stable, healthy, and well-functioning adults to become resilient and effective adults. On the basis of a review of extensive scientific literature, the American Academy of Pediatrics (AAP) affirms that "children's well-being is affected much more by their relationships with their parents, their parents' sense of competence and security, and the presence of social and economic support for the family than by the gender or the sexual orientation of their parents."[1]

Families' structural forms are varied. In 2010, married adults were raising 65.3% of all children in this country.[2] The other 34.7% of children (25.9 million of 74.63 million children) were living in a variety of situations. Many were being raised by parents who were single or cohabiting, either by choice or by circumstance. Growing numbers of grandparents are stepping in as parents to 2.5 million children when necessary.[2] When none of a child's biological relatives is available or able to provide necessary nurturing and support, other arrangements exist to nurture children. Foster parenting and adoption are substitute arrangements that can provide financial, emotional, social, and legal support for children. In 2007, >400 000 children were in foster care, and 130 000 children were adopted by unrelated adults.[3,4]

Increasing numbers of same-gender couples are raising children today, and the numbers are likely to increase in the future. The US 2010 Census reported that 646 464 households included 2 adults of the same gender.[5,6] These same-gender couples are raising ~115 000 children aged ≤18 years and are living in essentially all counties of the United States.[5,6] When these children are combined with single gay and lesbian parents who are raising children, almost 2 million children are being raised by gay and lesbian parents in the United States.[7]

Civil marriage is the legal and social institution in modern society that serves as the basic building block for family structure and child-rearing. Marriage is generally considered the optimal relationship between 2 adults who share responsibility for children. Marriage brings 2 extended families together to provide long-term security and social and emotional support to all members of the newly formed family. Marriage offers many legal rights and responsibilities, including the joint responsibility to care for children and to make decisions (including medical decisions) for them. A report from the AAP Task Force on the Family noted that married couples have more financial and social resources to nurture and raise children.[8] Additionally, "married men and women are physically and emotionally healthier and are less likely to engage in health risk behaviors . . . than are unmarried adults."[8] A number of studies have documented "a positive relationship between the quality of marital life and family functioning."[9] The Task Force report emphasized: "As we move forward, the Academy and pediatricians stand ready to serve all children in all families, regardless of the family structure in which they live."[8]

There are few social or legal restrictions limiting the ability of 2 unrelated adults to marry in the United States. These include (1) age: states have different age limits before which parental permission is required for marriage; (2) numerosity: there is a long-standing prohibition on bigamy/polygamy; (3) the existence of blood relationships; and (4) cognitive capacity to consent. The only other exception applies to adults seeking same-gender relationships (in most states).

There is extensive research documenting that there is no causal relationship between parents' sexual orientation and children's emotional, psychosocial, and behavioral development.[1,10–19] Many studies attest to the normal development of children of same-gender couples when the child is wanted, the parents have a commitment to shared parenting, and the parents have strong social and economic supports. Indeed, current research has concluded that "In all, it is now well-established that the adjustment of children and adolescents is best accounted for by variations in the quality of the relationships with their parents, the quality of the relationship between the parents or significant adults in the children's and adolescents' lives, and the availability of economic and socio-economic resources."[19]

Therefore, the AAP has endorsed, for more than a decade, a policy supporting the benefits of both parents in a same-gender couple having legal rights and responsibilities for their child(ren), for example, through second-parent or coparent adoption.[20] A special article in *Pediatrics* in 2006 reviewed the legal issues associated with civil marriage, civil union, and domestic partnership and noted a number of disparities for children growing up in various legal arrangements.[10] The American Medical Association has recently noted the disparities that exist for parents of the same gender who lack marriage equality as well as for their children.[21] Many other professional organizations have adopted policies urging legislative changes and legal mechanisms, including adoption, foster parenting, and civil marriage, for gay and lesbian adults who wish to be parents.* Civil unions and domestic partnerships do not confer the same legal rights, protections, and benefits to children that civil marriage provides.[10]

Public policy related to marriage and family is largely a state function. Consequently, the laws across the country that regulate marriage, adoption, and foster parenting by gay men and lesbians are an inconsistent patchwork. Even civil marriage in a state that

*National organizations that support marriage equality: American Civil Liberties Union (June 1998), National Association of Social Workers (June 2004), American Psychological Association (July 2004), American Psychiatric Association (May 2005), American Psychoanalytic Association (January 2008), American Bar Association (August 2010), American College of Nursing (July 2012), and American Academy of Family Physicians (October 2012). National organizations that support gay and lesbian parenting and the nurturing of children: American Academy of Child and Adolescent Psychiatry, American College of Obstetrics and Gynecology, American Medical Association, Child Welfare League of America, National Adoption Center, National Education Association, North American Council on Adoptable Children, and Voice for Adoption.

permits it does not ensure access to federal benefits. The federal Defense of Marriage Act (1996; Pub. L. No. 104-199) denies members of married same-gender households access and benefits equivalent to those available to households headed by married parents of different genders, such as (1) Social Security and related programs, (2) housing and food stamps, (3) federal civilian and military service benefits, (4) employment benefits, (5) immigration and nationality status, (6) remedies and protections for crimes and family violence, and (7) certain loans and financial guarantees.[10,21] For this reason, the AAP has joined with other national organizations in support of the position that the Defense of Marriage Act is unconstitutional.[†]

A core mission of the AAP is to support the best interests of all children, regardless of their home or family

---

[†]Amici Curiae: Brief of the American Psychological Association, the Massachusetts Psychological Association, the American Psychiatric Association, the National Association of Social Workers and its Massachusetts Chapter, the American Medical Association, and the American Academy of Pediatrics Nos. 10-2204, 10-2207, and 102214 in the United States Court of Appeals for the First Circuit. *The Commonwealth of Massachusetts v the United States Department of Health and Humans Services et al*, November 3, 2011; Brief of the American Psychological Association, the American Academy of Pediatrics, the American Psychiatric Association, the American Psychoanalytic Association, the National Association of Social Workers and its New York City and State Chapters, and the New York State Psychological Association. No. 12-2335(L), 12-2435(Con) in the United States Court of Appeals for the Second Circuit; *Windsor v United States of America and Bipartisan Legal Advisory Group of the US House of Representatives*; Brief of the American Psychological Association, the California Psychological Association, the American Psychiatric Association, the National Association of Social Workers and its California Chapter, the American Medical Association, the American Academy of Pediatrics, and the American Psychoanalytic Association, Nos. 12-15388 and 12-15409 in the United States Court of Appeals for the Ninth Circuit; *Golinski v United States Office of Personnel Management and Berry and Bipartisan Legal Advisory Group of the US House of Representatives*.

structure, on the basis of the common principles of justice. If a child has 2 living and capable parents who choose to create a permanent bond by way of civil marriage, it is in the best interests of their child(ren) that legal and social institutions allow and support them to do so. If 2 parents are not available to the child, adoption or foster parenting remain acceptable options to provide a loving home for a child and should be available without regard to the sexual orientation of the parent(s).

RECOMMENDATIONS

The AAP works to ensure that public policies help all parents, regardless of sexual orientation and other characteristics, to build and maintain strong, stable, and healthy families that are able to meet the needs of their children. In particular, the AAP supports:

1. Marriage equality for all capable and consenting couples, including those who are of the same gender, as a means of guaranteeing all federal and state rights and benefits, and long-term security for their children.

2. Adoption by single parents, coparents adopting together, or a second parent when 1 parent is already a legal parent by birth or adoption, without regard to the sexual orientation of the adoptive parent(s).

3. Foster care placement for eligible children to qualified adults without regard to their sexual orientation.

ACKNOWLEDGMENT

The authors and the committee thank James G. Pawelski, MS, for his valuable contributions to the development of this policy statement.

LEAD AUTHORS

Benjamin S. Siegel, MD
Ellen C. Perrin, MD, MA

COMMITTEE ON PSYCHOSOCIAL ASPECTS OF CHILD AND FAMILY HEALTH, 2012–2013

Benjamin S. Siegel, MD, Chairperson
Mary I. Dobbins, MD
Arthur Lavin, MD
Gerri Mattson, MD
John Pascoe, MD, MPH
Michael Yogman, MD

LIAISONS

Ronald T. Brown, PhD—*Society of Pediatric Psychology*
Mary Jo Kupst, PhD—*Society of Pediatric Psychology*
D. Richard Martini, MD—*American Academy of Child and Adolescent Psychiatry*
Barbara Blue, MSN, RN, CPNP, PMHNP-BC—*National Association of Pediatric Nurse Practitioners*
Terry Carmichael, MSW—*National Association of Social Workers*

CONSULTANT

George J. Cohen, MD

STAFF

Stephanie Domain, MS, CHES

REFERENCES

1. Perrin EC, Siegel BS; American Academy of Pediatrics, Committee on Psychosocial Aspects of Child and Family Health. Technical report: promoting the well-being of children whose parents are gay or lesbian. *Pediatrics*. 2013, In press

2. US Census Bureau. America's Families and Living Arrangements. Available at: www.census.gov/population/www/socdemo/hh-fam/cps2011.html. Accessed November 26, 2012

3. US Department of Health and Human Services. Foster Care Statistics. Child Welfare Information Gateway, 2010. Available at: www.childwelfare.gov/pubs/factsheets/foster.pdf. Accessed July 1, 2012

4. US Department of Health and Human Services, Administration for Children and Families. How Many Children Were Adopted in 2007 and 2008? Child Welfare Information Gateway. Available at: www.childwelfare.gov/pubs/adopted0708.cfm. Accessed November 26, 2012

5. O'Connell M, Feliz S. Same-sex couple household statistics from the 2010 Census.

SEHSD Working Paper Number 2011-26. Washington, DC: Fertility and Family Statistics Branch Social, Economic and Housing Statistics Division, US Census Bureau; 2011. Available at: www.census.gov/hhes/samesex/files/ss-report.doc. Accessed November 26, 2012

6. US Census Bureau. Same sex couple households. *American Community Survey Briefs.* September 2011. Available at: www.census.gov/prod/2011pubs/acsbr10-03.pdf. Accessed November 26, 2012

7. Family Equality Council. All Children Matter. Available at: www.familyequality.org/equal_family_blog/2011/10/25/1066/all_children_matter. Accessed November 26, 2012

8. Schor EL; American Academy of Pediatrics Task Force on the Family. Family pediatrics: report of the task force on the family. *Pediatrics.* 2003;111(6 pt 2):1541–1571

9. American Academy of Pediatrics, Board of Directors. Preface to the report of the task force on the family. *Pediatrics.* 2003;111(6 pt 2):1539–1540

10. Pawelski JG, Perrin EC, Foy JM, et al. The effects of marriage, civil union, and domestic partnership laws on the health and well-being of children. *Pediatrics.* 2006;118(1):349–364

11. Perrin EC, Cohen KM, Gold M, Ryan C, Savin-Williams RC, Schorzman CM. Gay and lesbian issues in pediatric health care. *Curr Probl Pediatr Adolesc Health Care.* 2004;34(10):355–398

12. Goldberg AE. *Lesbian and Gay Parents and Their Children.* Washington, DC: American Psychological Association Press; 2010

13. Biblarz TJ, Stacey J. How does the sexual orientation of parents matter? *Am Sociol Rev.* 2001;66(2):159–183

14. Tasker F. Lesbian mothers, gay fathers, and their children: a review. *J Dev Behav Pediatr.* 2005;26(3):224–240

15. Golombok S, Badger S. Children raised in mother-headed families from infancy: a follow-up of children of lesbian and single heterosexual mothers, at early adulthood. *Hum Reprod.* 2010;25(1):150–157

16. Perrin EC. *Sexual Orientation in Child and Adolescent Health Care.* New York, NY: Kluwer/Plenum Publishers; 2002

17. Wainright JL, Russell ST, Patterson CJ. Psychosocial adjustment, school outcomes, and romantic relationships of adolescents with same-sex parents. *Child Dev.* 2004;75(6):1886–1898

18. Farr RH, Forssell SL, Patterson CJ. Parenting and child development in adoptive families: does sexual orientation matter? *Appl Dev Sci.* 2010;14(3):164–178

19. Lamb ME. Mothers, fathers, families, and circumstances: factors affecting children's adjustment. *Appl Dev Sci.* 2012;16(2):98–111

20. American Academy of Pediatrics, Committee on Psychosocial Aspects of Child and Family Health. Coparent or second-parent adoption by same-sex parents. *Pediatrics.* 2002;109(2):339–340

21. American Medical Association. Policy Statement: Health Disparities Among Gay, Lesbian, Bisexual and Transgender Families. Res. 445, A-05. Chicago, IL: American Medical Association; November 10, 2009. Available at: www.ama-assn.org/resources/doc/glbt/glbt-policy.pdf. Accessed November 26, 2012

Promoting the Well-Being of Children Whose Parents are Gay or Lesbian

- *Technical Report*

TECHNICAL REPORT

Promoting the Well-Being of Children Whose Parents Are Gay or Lesbian

abstract

Extensive data available from more than 30 years of research reveal that children raised by gay and lesbian parents have demonstrated resilience with regard to social, psychological, and sexual health despite economic and legal disparities and social stigma. Many studies have demonstrated that children's well-being is affected much more by their relationships with their parents, their parents' sense of competence and security, and the presence of social and economic support for the family than by the gender or the sexual orientation of their parents. Lack of opportunity for same-gender couples to marry adds to families' stress, which affects the health and welfare of all household members. Because marriage strengthens families and, in so doing, benefits children's development, children should not be deprived of the opportunity for their parents to be married. Paths to parenthood that include assisted reproductive techniques, adoption, and foster parenting should focus on competency of the parents rather than their sexual orientation. *Pediatrics* 2013;131: e1374–e1383

Ellen C. Perrin, MD, MA, Benjamin S. Siegel, MD, and the COMMITTEE ON PSYCHOSOCIAL ASPECTS OF CHILD AND FAMILY HEALTH

KEY WORDS
civil marriage, adoption, foster care, nurturing children, gay parents, lesbian parents, health disparities, legal disparities, same sex, same gender, marriage equality

This document is copyrighted and is property of the American Academy of Pediatrics and its Board of Directors. All authors have filed conflict of interest statements with the American Academy of Pediatrics. Any conflicts have been resolved through a process approved by the Board of Directors. The American Academy of Pediatrics has neither solicited nor accepted any commercial involvement in the development of the content of this publication.

The guidance in this report does not indicate an exclusive course of treatment or serve as a standard of medical care. Variations, taking into account individual circumstances, may be appropriate.

All technical reports from the American Academy of Pediatrics automatically expire 5 years after publication unless reaffirmed, revised, or retired at or before that time.

INTRODUCTION

The mission of the American Academy of Pediatrics (AAP) is to promote optimal physical, mental, and social health and well-being for all infants, children, adolescents, and young adults. Historically, the AAP has worked, through its educational, research, advocacy, and policy efforts, to highlight the powerful connection between children's well-being and the functioning of their most enduring source of support and influence—their parents. It is vital that pediatricians understand the unique and complex characteristics of their patients' families and support them to ensure optimal development of children.

All children have the same needs for, and the right to, nurturing, security, and social stability. Children whose parents are gay and lesbian have historically been subjected to laws, social policies, and disapproving attitudes that create social distance and ostracism and challenge the stability of their families as well as their optimal social and psychological development. This technical report provides the scientific rationale, based on the current available evidence, to support the recommendations outlined in the policy statement "Promoting the Well-Being of Children Whose Parents are Gay or Lesbian"[1]: support for marriage equality, including repeal of the federal Defense of

www.pediatrics.org/cgi/doi/10.1542/peds.2013-0377

doi:10.1542/peds.2013-0377

PEDIATRICS (ISSN Numbers: Print, 0031-4005; Online, 1098-4275).

Marriage Act and similar public policies that limit access to federal benefits associated with civil marriage for gay and lesbian couples, and the right of gay and lesbian adults to adopt and provide foster care for eligible children.

Children depend on their parents for guidance, nurturing, protection, support, and love. Their resiliency derives from their sense of permanence, security, and unconditional attachment. As a consequence of this central value to their children, modern societies have developed the legal and social contract of marriage to ensure the permanent commitment of parents to each other and to their children, and thus to provide an optimal environment for children to thrive. The value of children to society is reflected also in the many public policies and programs that are designed to ensure adequate resources and support to parents who are raising a child alone, by choice or circumstance, and to families that because of physical or mental illness, abuse, neglect, and/or financial difficulty, cannot function successfully in their capacity as parents. Families created by gay and lesbian adults are no exception to these broad social policies.

Because of the value of marriage to the society, there are few legal restrictions on who can marry. The only legal limitations to marriage equality for consenting adults in the United States are for adults who are certified as mentally/emotionally incompetent, for whom marriage would lead to a polygamous relationship, who are of minor age, who are related by blood, or who are the same gender (in a majority of the states). Even a history of child abuse, domestic violence, or other criminal activity does not disqualify adults from civil marriage. Despite conflicts based on individuals' political and religious beliefs, it is important to recognize that laws restricting competent adults of the same gender from codifying their commitment to each other and their children via civil marriage may result not only in pain and hardship for their children but also in legal, economic, psychological, social, and health disparities that can no longer be justified.

DIVERSE FAMILIES

The 2003 report of the AAP Task Force on the Family stated that: "No particular family constellation makes poor or good outcomes for children inevitable."[2] The report continued: "A stable, well-functioning family that consists of 2 parents and children is potentially the most secure, supportive, and nurturing environment in which children may be raised. That children can be successfully brought to adulthood without this basic functioning unit is a tribute to those involved who have developed the skill and resiliency to overcome a difficult and fundamental challenge."[2]

Families are diverse, complex, and changing. Most US public policy is built on the presumption that the majority of families are composed of a married mother and father raising their biological children. In contrast, the 2010 US Census revealed that the proportion of children living with 2 married biological parents had declined to 65.3%, down from 69.2% in 2001.[3] See Table 1 for further elucidation of family types based on the 2010 Census.

Determining the number of children being raised by lesbian and gay parents is challenging, because most surveys do not ask about parents' sexual orientation. Starting with the 2000 Census, gay and lesbian couples have had the option to identify themselves as spouses.[4] The 2010 Census identified 131 729 self-reported married same-gender households and 514 735 same-gender unmarried partner households located in essentially all counties of the United States.[4–6]

Thirty-one percent of same-gender couples who identified as spouses and 14% of those who identified as unmarried partners indicated that they were raising children, more than 111 000 in all.[5] In addition to these parents, many single gay men and lesbians are also raising children. Combined, current estimates suggest that almost 2 million children younger than 18 years are being raised by at least 1 gay or lesbian parent in the United States.[6,7]

Families with a gay or lesbian parent (or parents) are, themselves, a diverse group.[8,9] For example, 55% to 59% of same-gender couples with children identify as white compared with 70% to 73% of married heterosexual couples with children.[7] Same-gender couples, like heterosexual couples, may become parents by having children in previous heterosexual relationships or through fostering, adoption, donor insemination, and/or surrogacy.[10]

LEGAL DISPARITIES CREATED BY STATE LAWS

Regulations and laws about the rights and responsibilities of parenthood are primarily state specific, resulting in

TABLE 1 Children in the United States 2010: Family Status

Family Status	Number of Children (Millions)[a]	Children in the United States, %
Children in 2-parent households	51.456	73.0
Children with married parents living together	48.516	65.3
Children with unmarried parents	2.940	3.9
Children with single/separated parents	20.263	27.1
Children being raised by 1 or more grandparents	2.595	3.5

[a] Total number of children in the United States: 74.630 million.

great variability among the states. Many legal and social disparities exist for same-gender couples and their children.[11]

- A critical disparity for children of unmarried parents is the absence of the protections reflected in divorce law. Thus, in the event of the dissolution of the couple's relationship, these families lack the protections that exist for children whose parents are married, such as:

  1. Access to the courts for a legally structured arrangement for dissolution of the relationship;

  2. A court-approved legal arrangement for visitation rights and/or custody of children; and

  3. Entitlement for children to financial support from and ongoing relationships with both parents.

- The majority of states prohibit, by statute or state constitutional amendment, recognition of same-gender marriage.[12] A few states extend other forms of relationship recognition, such as civil union or domestic partnership.

- A few states, either by statute, regulation, or legal interpretation, restrict or prohibit foster parenting by same-gender couples and/or lesbians and gay men.

- Laws regarding joint adoption by same gender couples, wherein both individuals become the legal parents of a biologically unrelated child, vary from state to state.[13] Joint adoption by lesbian and gay couples is expressly prohibited in a few states, granted by law in fewer than half, and not addressed by statutes in most states.

- Only in states that recognize civil marriage or other forms of domestic relationships can a lesbian or gay spouse or partner be recognized

as a legal parent or step-parent to the child(ren) she or he is helping raise. In the majority of states, this is not a legal option.

- In the United States (but not in much of Europe), sperm and egg donors may choose to remain anonymous and take on no legal responsibility for any children born. In a few states, a donor may be considered a legally recognized parent and have related responsibilities. A few states have laws ensuring that both parents are legally recognized as "presumed parents" of the child.

- Most states lack a formal mechanism to ensure basic rights and responsibilities to nonbiological, nonadoptive coparents. Such laws are important to children when adult couple relationships are in dissolution and appropriate custody is under consideration.

- Legal arrangements with a surrogate carrier are available in only a few states to gay men who wish to have a biologically related child.

- In the event of death of a spouse, partner, or parent, state laws do not provide for Social Security or veteran's survivor benefits for the surviving spouse/partner and children.

LEGAL DISPARITIES CREATED BY FEDERAL LAWS AND REGULATIONS

Restrictions against civil marriage for same-gender couples, such as the federal Defense of Marriage Act (Pub L No. 104-199 [1996]) and replications of it in state statutes and constitutions, deny these couples and their children numerous other protections and benefits deemed valuable by society and government to which heterosexual married couples and their children have access. Under the Defense of Marriage Act, these benefits are not

available to couples of the same gender even if they are legally married in a state that recognizes same-gender marriage. The US Government Accountability Office has identified a total of 1138 federal statutory provisions in which marital status was a factor in determining or receiving rights, benefits, and protections. These have been outlined elsewhere in detail[14]; a few examples are presented here:

- Legal recognition of a couple's commitment to and responsibility for one another and legal recognition of a child's relationship to both parents and joint parenting rights;

- Tax-exempt employer-sponsored health and other insurance benefits for spouse/partner and nonbiological/not jointly adopted children;

- Ability to consent to medical care or authorize emergency medical treatment of nonbiological/not jointly adopted children;

- The ability to travel with a child if it will require proof of being a legal parent;

- The ability to file joint income tax returns and take advantage of family-related deductions, including the ability to use the child tax credit, child and dependent care tax credit, dependency exemption, earned income tax credit, and gift and estate tax exemption; and

- A surviving parent's right to the custody of and care for, and children's right to maintain a relationship with, a nonbiological or not legally recognized parent in the event of the death of the other parent.

HEALTH DISPARITIES

- Because children cannot legally consent to medical treatment, the lack of uniform legal recognition of lesbian and gay parents results in parents being prohibited from accompanying their child(ren) and making medical decisions for them in routine and even emergency situations. Parents may even be barred from visiting their child in the hospital if their parental status is ambiguous.

- Another challenge for same-gender couples and their families is obtaining health insurance. As a result of the federal Defense of Marriage Act, employers are not required to, although some choose to, offer health benefits to same-gender spouses or partners or children of lesbian and gay employees, even if those workers are legally married in their state. As a result, same-gender couples are 2 to 3 times less likely to have health insurance than are heterosexual couples.[7,15] This disparity affects children directly, because the vast majority of children (more than 84%) have the same health insurance status as their parents (public or private insurance or uninsured[16]). Evidence that health insurance coverage is directly associated with health status is undeniable.[17]

- Even when employers do make health insurance benefits available to same-gender spouses, partners, and related children, these families are faced with an economic disadvantage compared with their heterosexual counterparts. Such benefits are considered by the Internal Revenue Code to be taxable or "imputed" income to the employee unless the spouse or partner or child qualifies as a legal dependent. In addition, employers must also pay taxes on this imputed income for their share of the employee's payroll tax.

- Lesbian- and gay-headed families are at greater peril than heterosexual-headed families when a parent loses a job or takes a cut in pay. The Consolidated Omnibus Budget Reconciliation Act of 1995 (COBRA [Pub L No. 99-272]) provides workers and their families who lose their health benefits the capacity to continue group health benefits provided by their employer group health plan for limited periods of time. However, the COBRA, as federal legislation, does not require employers, even those who provide benefits for same-gender spouses/partners and their dependents, to offer lesbian and gay employees the opportunity to enroll their spouses, partners, or children.

- Additional challenges exist in the provision of health care. Physicians, hospitals, and other health care professionals and environments may not offer a welcoming environment for same-gender parents and their children. The reaction a family may encounter ranges from acceptance to disdain: sometimes pediatricians and others encountered in health care settings or institutions may express stigmatizing attitudes or refuse to recognize an unmarried parent, especially when that parent is part of a gay or lesbian couple. Among respondents in a survey of gay and lesbian parents in New York, 42% reported that dislike of lesbian and gay people was a barrier to accessing health care and reported a lack of appropriately trained, competent professionals to deliver health care to lesbian and gay people.[18] According to the October 2011 report, *All Children Matter: How Legal and Social Inequalities Hurt LGBT Children*, "a family may shy away from scheduling a child's

doctor's visit in an effort to shield him or her from hostile questions or misunderstandings. For parents who must rely on medical professionals with unknown attitudes toward lesbian and gay patients, concerns linger about treatment of them and their children, which can make care more difficult to obtain."[7] Some parents report worries about being blamed for their child's physical or emotional disorders because of their sexual orientation or family constellation.[19]

CHILDREN'S DEVELOPMENTAL TRAJECTORY AND PSYCHOLOGICAL OUTCOMES

Many factors confer risk to children's healthy development and adult outcomes, such as poverty, parental depression, parental substance abuse, divorce, and domestic violence, but the sexual orientation of their parents is not among them. Many studies have assessed the developmental and psychosocial outcomes of children whose parents are gay or lesbian and note that a family's social and economic resources and the strength of the relationships among members of the family are far more important variables than parental gender or sexual orientation in affecting children's development and well-being.[20] A large body of scientific literature demonstrates that children and adolescents who grow up with gay and/or lesbian parents fare as well in emotional, cognitive, social, and sexual functioning as do children whose parents are heterosexual.[21–37] Although the methodologic challenges are daunting in addressing phenomena as complex and multifactorial as children's long-term developmental and psychosocial outcomes, the literature accumulated over more than 30 years, taken together, provides robust, reliable, and valid assurance about the well-being of children raised by parents of the same gender.[28,29]

The first review of available data regarding the well-being of children living with lesbian or gay parents concluded that "While research on these topics is relatively new....there is no evidence that the development of children with lesbian and gay parents is compromised in any significant respect relative to that among children of heterosexual parents in otherwise comparable circumstances."[30]

Another early review summarized 23 articles published before 2000 that, together, described 615 offspring of lesbian mothers and gay fathers and 387 controls by using a variety of psychological tests and interviews. The conclusion drawn from these studies was that children raised by gay and lesbian parents did not systematically differ from other children in emotional/behavioral functioning, sexual orientation, experiences of stigmatization, gender role behavior, or cognitive functioning.[31]

A more recent comprehensive review of the experiences of gay and lesbian parents and their children reaffirmed that most children raised by lesbian and gay parents are developmentally and socially well-adjusted and that the societal presence of stigma, heterosexism, family circumstance, structure, and process are more important influences on children's developmental trajectory than is the gender or sexual orientation of their parents.[32]

Much of this early research about children with gay and lesbian parents was, by necessity, based on relatively small convenience samples. Nevertheless, more than 100 scientific publications over 30 years, taken together, have demonstrated that children's well-being is affected much more by their relationships with their parents, their parents' sense of competence and security, and the presence of social and economic support for the family than by the gender or the sexual orientation of their parents.[20,33,34]

Increasing recognition and acceptance of lesbian and gay parents has allowed for larger, community-based and national studies in the United States and Europe. Three studies are of particular note. Using data obtained in a large US population-based survey, the National Longitudinal Study of Adolescent Health, the 44 adolescents who reported being raised by 2 women in a "marriage-like" family arrangement were compared with a random sample of 44 adolescents raised by heterosexual parents.[35,36] There were no differences noted in measures of self-esteem, depression, anxiety, school connectedness, and school success. The authors concluded that "adolescents were functioning well and their adjustment was not associated with family type." In both groups of adolescents, those who described a "closer relationship with their parents" reported less delinquent behavior and substance abuse; that is, the quality of parent-adolescent relationships better predicted adolescent outcomes than did family type.

Another community-wide study was based on data from a cohort of 14 000 mothers of children born within a particular county in England during 1 year.[37] The study examined the quality of parent-child relationships and socioemotional and gender development in a community sample of 5- to 7-year-old children with lesbian mothers. Thirty-nine lesbian mother families were compared with 74 two-parent heterosexual families and 60 families headed by single heterosexual mothers. No differences were found in maternal warmth, emotional involvement, enjoyment of motherhood, frequency of conflicts, supervision of the child, abnormal behaviors reported by parents or teachers in the child, children's self-esteem, or psychiatric disorders. Both mothers and teachers reported more behavioral problems among children in single-parent families than among children who had 2 parents in the home, irrespective of their sexual orientation.

A recent publication was based on a large national sample of US adults who were asked whether their parents had ever had a relationship with a person of the same gender while they were growing up and whether they had ever lived with that parent while the parent was involved in such a relationship.[38] Parents who were said to have had a same-gender relationship were categorized as lesbian or gay parents, although their sexual orientation was not directly determined. In comparison with those who did not report that a parent had had a same-gender relationship, a number of adverse outcomes were identified, including being on public assistance, being unemployed, and having poorer educational attainment. Extensive critique of this study[39–44] has pointed out that:

- It is well known that family instability, and in particular divorce, is a risk factor for children,[45,46] and almost all of the respondents whose parent had had a same-gender relationship had also experienced the divorce of their parents.

- These data reflect an era when stigmatization and discrimination toward same-gender couples and their children were strong and were likely to have contributed to less-than-optimal child-rearing environments.[40]

- Respondents were certainly not children "raised by" lesbian or gay parents, because only half were living with these parents, and the sexual orientation of the parents was not determined.[41,42]

- The great variability in the form and characteristics of both same-gender and heterosexual relationships, combined with the small number of those relationships, even in a large data set like this one, makes it impossible to sort out true evidence of causality.[43]

A longstanding longitudinal study of children born to lesbian parents in the United States provides further insight into the well-being of children raised from birth by lesbian parents. The National Longitudinal Lesbian Family Study began in 1986, enrolling 154 lesbian mothers who became pregnant through donor insemination (70 birth mothers, 70 comothers, and 14 single mothers). These mothers have been enrolled in the study for more than 17 years, maintaining a retention rate of 92%. Recent publications describe the outcome of 78 adolescent offspring at age 17 (39 girls and 39 boys) on the basis of mothers' and adolescents' reports and comparing them with national standardization samples. The mothers' reports about their 17-year-old sons and daughters indicated that they had high levels of social, school/academic, and total competence and fewer social problems, rule breaking, and aggressive and externalizing behavior compared with their age-matched counterparts in the Achenbach Child Behavior Checklist's standardization sample. There were no differences between offspring who were conceived by known or anonymous donors or between offspring whose parents were still together and those whose mothers had separated.[47] An accompanying editorial noted, "Can these data reassure those who fear that homosexual relationships with or without children will herald the end of the family as we know it? Our experience

tells us of the resilience of children who are loved and know that love. ... And when we see these moms or dads with their kids in our practice, we call them families."[48]

The self-reported quality of life of the adolescents in this sample was similar to that reported by a comparable sample of adolescents with heterosexual parents.[49] Lesbian parents reported that they planned to expose their children to male role models as an important child-rearing strategy. Half of both the girls and the boys had identified a male role model in their lives. There were no significant associations between gender role traits, adolescent psychological adjustment, gender of the adolescent, and the presence or absence of male role models.[50]

More data are available to document the well-being of children whose parents are lesbian than of those whose parents are gay men, because the numbers of gay men parenting have, until recently, been small. Recent studies affirm that families created by gay men resemble closely those created by lesbians.[51] For example, a recent study assessed child development and parenting among 27 lesbian, 29 gay, and 50 heterosexual couples who had adopted a child.[52] Lesbian and gay parents were similar in a variety of parenting characteristics to their heterosexual counterparts. Children in all family types were functioning similarly and had few behavior problems. Average scores for internalizing, externalizing, and total behavior problems reported by parents and teachers were similar to population averages for the child development instruments. In particular, there were no differences among the family types in children's adjustment, parenting stress, parent discipline techniques, and couple adjustment. As in previous studies, teachers' ratings

of behavior noted that behavior problems were more likely in children with single parents than with 2 parents, irrespective of their sexual orientation. Instead, "parents who reported less parenting stress, use of more effective disciplinary techniques and who had greater happiness in their couple relationships had children who were described as well off."[51]

Some authors have investigated children's academic performance as an indicator of their well-being. Two articles compared the academic achievement of children whose parents were gay or lesbian with children whose parents were heterosexual. Although the studies were performed with different methodologies and in different population groups, both revealed similar academic achievement in the 2 groups. Using an analysis of US Census data to perform the first large-sample, nationally representative analysis of educational outcomes, the author concluded that "children of same-sex couples are as likely to make normal progress through school as the children of most other family structures."[53] Another study demonstrated that lower academic achievement was related more to the number of family transitions experienced by children than to the sexual orientation of their parents.[54]

A few publications have suggested less positive outcomes for children raised by same-gender parents. For example, a small study from Australia[55] has sometimes been cited in support of the proposition that children raised by lesbians and gay men are less well-adjusted than those raised by heterosexual couples. The study was based on a comparison of teachers' reports about 58 children in each of 3 groups of parents: married, heterosexual cohabiting, and gay or lesbian cohabiting. A primary goal of the study was to understand possible disadvantages to children's school and social performance on the basis of the marriage versus cohabitation of their parents. It is critical to note that:

- At the time of the research, marriage was available only to heterosexual parents, and therefore, all gay or lesbian couples were, by definition, cohabiting.

- There is strong evidence provided in the article that the children with gay or lesbian parents were severely stigmatized in their schools and communities.

- Most of the children with gay or lesbian parents had experienced the divorce of their heterosexual birth parents, in many cases shortly before the time of study, thus potentially adding to the children's stress.[45,46]

The study's findings included considerable variation in the ratings given by teachers with regard to the children's school behavior and performance. For example, children with gay or lesbian parents were rated as performing less well in language and math but better in social studies and as having a better attitude toward learning, compared with the children being raised by cohabiting or married heterosexual parents. The deleterious effects of divorce and of stigmatization on children's development are described by the author as likely contributors to the areas of poorer performance of the children with gay or lesbian parents. Overall, the author's conclusions emphasized the benefits of marriage: "married couples seem to offer the best environment for a child's social and educational development."[55] In another article, the same author reported a comparison of cohabiting adults of the same and of different genders and concluded that, in substantial

ways, the relationships of cohabiting adults are similar, whether the partners are of the same or different genders.[56]

A 2012 commentary has described various shortcomings of the aforementioned research in support of adoption rights and marriage equality for same-gender couples.[57] In general, this critique pointed out that most studies have included small and selective samples; have rarely reported longitudinal data and, therefore, have reported only short-term outcomes; and often have not included a comparison group. While agreeing with the imperfections of past research in this area, others have pointed out the intrinsic complexities of this research agenda[40] and commented that, despite these imperfections, it is likely that the extensive research efforts that have been carried out would have documented serious and significant damages if they existed. In addition, it is important to note that all past research about children growing up with gay or lesbian parents has taken place in the context of pervasive social stigma and includes a majority of children whose parents were either single or divorced, each of which can be expected to contribute to poor outcomes for children.[39]

Although studies of uncommon and varied phenomena are difficult to perform and yield incomplete and imperfect results, there is an emerging consensus, based on an extensive review of the scientific literature, that children growing up in households headed by gay men or lesbians are not disadvantaged in any significant respect relative to children of heterosexual parents. Indeed, the fact that most data suggest that children grow up successfully in families created by gay and lesbian parents despite the almost-universal family disruption and social stigma they have experienced

attests to the resilience of these families. Greater acceptance and support of these families will provide an environment even more conducive to successful social and emotional development.

Over the past decade, 11 countries have recognized marriage equality and, thus, allow marriage between 2 partners of the same gender: Argentina, Belgium, Canada, Denmark, Iceland, Netherlands, Norway, Portugal, Spain, South Africa, and Sweden. There has been no evidence that children in these countries have experienced difficulties as a result of these social changes.

WHEN MARRIAGE IS NOT AN OPTION

The AAP recognizes that some children are members of families headed by a single parent or by 2 parents who do not choose to be legally married and that it is possible for these parents to overcome the challenges involved in raising children in these circumstances. The AAP also acknowledges that some children have been removed from severely challenged families and are in temporary custody of a state agency or a related adult. There is no evidence that restricting these children's access to loving and nurturing adoptive or foster care homes on the basis of gender or sexual orientation of the parents is in their best interests.[52,58]

MARRIAGE MATTERS

The AAP Task Force on the Family reported that "married men and women are physically and emotionally healthier and are less likely to engage in health risk behaviors, such as alcohol or drug abuse, than are unmarried adults."[2] Both men and women live longer when married, presumably in part because they have healthier lifestyles, eat better, and monitor each other's health.[2] They tend to have relationships with more people and social institutions, which increases their level of social support. It has been well established that permanently married parents can create the best environment for children's development.[2,59]

Marriage supports permanence and security (the basic ingredients for the healthy development of children). Marriage is also the official societal mechanism for conferring rights, benefits, and protections that support couples as spouses and parents and their children financially and legally. In a survey of married same-gender couples in Massachusetts, the first state to allow civil marriage for same-gender couples, 24% of the respondents noted that their children had previously been explicitly teased or taunted about having a gay or lesbian parent, but 93% of respondents stated that marriage has made their children happier and better off.[60] Eighty-four percent of parents stated that their being married made them feel more comfortable working with their child (ren)'s teachers at school.

CONCLUSIONS

On the basis of this comprehensive review of the literature regarding the development and adjustment of children whose parents are the same gender, as well as the existing evidence for the legal, social, and health benefits of marriage to children, the AAP concludes that it is in the best interests of children that they be able to partake in the security of permanent nurturing and care that comes with the civil marriage of their parents, without regard to their parents' gender or sexual orientation.

Marriage equality can help reduce social stigma faced by lesbian and gay parents and their children, thereby enhancing social stability, acceptance, and support. Children who are raised by married parents benefit from the social and legal status that civil marriage conveys to their parents.

When marriage of their parents is not a viable option, children should not be deprived of the opportunity for temporary foster care or adoption by single parents or couples, irrespective of their sexual orientation. Public policy and community support are vital to the success of children in these circumstances.

Pediatricians working to eliminate disparities and establish support, stability, and security of all families through marriage equality and legal parental recognition honor the AAP mission to promote the optimal physical, mental, and social health and well-being of all infants, children, adolescents, and young adults.

ACKNOWLEDGMENT

The authors and the committee thank James G. Pawelski, MS, for his valuable contributions to the development of this technical report.

LEAD AUTHORS
Ellen C. Perrin, MD, MA
Benjamin S. Siegel, MD

COMMITTEE ON PSYCHOSOCIAL ASPECTS OF CHILD AND FAMILY HEALTH, 2012–2013
Benjamin S. Siegel, MD, Chairperson
Mary I. Dobbins, MD
Arthur Lavin, MD
Gerri Mattson, MD
John Pascoe, MD, MPH
Michael Yogman, MD

LIAISONS
Ronald T. Brown, PhD – *Society of Pediatric Psychology*
Mary Jo Kupst, PhD – *Society of Pediatric Psychology*
D. Richard Martini, MD – *American Academy of Child and Adolescent Psychiatry*
Barbara Blue, MSN, RN, CPNP, PMHNP-BC – *National Association of Pediatric Nurse Practitioners*
Terry Carmichael, MSW – *National Association of Social Workers*

CONSULTANT
George J. Cohen, MD

STAFF
Stephanie Domain, MS, CHES

REFERENCES

1. American Academy of Pediatrics, Committee on the Psychosocial Aspects of Child and Family Health. Promoting the well-being of children whose parents are gay or lesbian. *Pediatrics*. 2013; in press

2. American Academy of Pediatrics, Task Force on the Family. Family pediatrics. *Pediatrics*. 2003;111(6 suppl 2):1541–1571

3. United States Census Bureau. America's families and living arrangements: 2011. Table C3. Living arrangements of children under 18 years/1 and marital status of parents, by age, sex, race, and Hispanic origin/2 and selected characteristics of the child for all children. Available at: www.census.gov/population/www/socdemo/hh-fam/cps2011.html. Accessed November 28, 2012

4. US Census Bureau. Same-sex couple household statistics from the 2010 census. September 27, 2011. Washington, DC: US Census Bureau, Social, Economic and Housing Statistics Division; 2011. Working paper 2011-26. Available at: www.census.gov/hhes/samesex/files/ss-report.doc. Accessed November 28, 2012

5. US Census Bureau and American Community Survey. Same-sex unmarried partner or spouse households by sex of householder by presence of own children. Washington, DC: US Census Bureau; 2010. Available at: www.census.gov/hhes/samesex/files/supp-table-AFF.xls. Accessed November 28, 2012

6. The Williams Institute. Census snapshot 2010. Available at: http://williamsinstitute.

law.ucla.edu/wp-content/uploads/Census2010 Snapshot-US-v2.pdf. Accessed November 28, 2012

7. Movement Advancement Project, Family Equality Council, and Center for American Progress. *All Children Matter: How Legal and Social Inequalities Hurt LGBT Families*. Boston, MA: Family Equality Council; October 2011. Available at: http://www.lgbtmap.org/file/all-children-matter-full-report.pdf. Accessed February 22, 2013

8. Cianciotto J. Hispanic and Latino same-sex couple households in the United States: a report from the 2000 census. Washington, DC: National Gay and Lesbian Task Force Policy Institute and National Latino/a Coalition for Justice; 2005. Available at: www.thetaskforce.org/downloads/reports/reports/HispanicLatinoHouseholdsUS.pdf. Accessed November 28, 2012

9. Dang A, Frazer S. Black same-sex households in the United States: a report from the 2000 census. 2nd ed. Washington, DC: National Gay and Lesbian Task Force Policy Institute; 2005. Available at: www.thetaskforce.org/reports_and_research/blackcouples_census. Accessed November 28, 2012

10. Sears RB, Gates GJ, Rubenstein WB. *Same-Sex Couples and Same-Sex Couples Raising Children in the United States: Data From Census 2000*. Los Angeles, CA: The Williams Institute; 2005

11. American Academy of Pediatrics, Division of State Government Affairs. Available at: www.aap.org/en-us/advocacy-and-policy/state-advocacy/Pages/Division-of-State-Government-Affair.aspx. Accessed November 28, 2012

12. National Conference of State Legislatures. Defining marriage: defense of marriage acts and same-sex marriage laws. Available at: www.ncsl.org/issues-research/human-services/same-sex-marriage-overview.aspx. Accessed November 28, 2012

13. Adoption and Foster Care Analysis and Reporting System. Preliminary FY 2010 estimates. Available at: www.acf.hhs.gov/programs/cb/resource/afcars-report-18. Accessed November 28, 2012

14. Shah DK, Associate General Counsel. Letter to Honorable Bill Frist, Majority Leader, United State Senate, January 23, 2004. Defense of Marriage Act: update to prior report. Available at: www.gao.gov/new.items/d04353r.pdf. Accessed November 28, 2012

15. Kaiser Family Foundation. Health coverage of children: the role of Medicaid and CHIP. Washington, DC: Kaiser Family Foundation; 2010. Available at: www.kff.org/uninsured/upload/7698-04.pdf. Accessed November 28, 2012

16. Ash MA, Badgett MV. Separate and unequal: the effect of unequal access to employment-based health insurance on same-sex and unmarried different-sex couples. *Contemp Econ Policy*. 2006:24(4):582–599

17. US Government Accountability Office. Report to Congressional Committees. Medicaid and CHIP: given the association between parent and child insurance status, new expansions may benefit families. February 2011. Available at: www.gao.gov/new.items/d11264.pdf. Accessed November 28, 2012

18. Frazer MS. LGBT health and human services needs in New York State. Albany, NY: Empire State Pride Agenda Foundation; 2009. Available at: www.prideagenda.org/Portals/0/pdfs/LGBT%20Health%20and%20Human%20Services%20Needs%20in%20New%20York%20State.pdf. Accessed November 28, 2012

19. Perrin EC, Kulkin H. Pediatric care for children whose parents are gay or lesbian. *Pediatrics*. 1996;97(5):629–635

20. Lamb ME. Mothers, fathers, families, and circumstances: factors affecting children's adjustment. *Appl Dev Sci*. 2012;16(2):98–111

21. Stacey J, Biblarz TJ. How does the sexual orientation of parents matter? *Am Sociol Rev*. 2001;66(2):159–183

22. Golombok S, Badger S. Children raised in mother-headed families from infancy: a follow-up of children of lesbian and single heterosexual mothers in early adulthood. *Hum Reprod*. 2010;25(1):150–157

23. Bos HM, Sandfort TG, de Bruyn EH, et al. Same-sex attraction, social relationships, psychosocial functioning, and school performance in early adolescence. *Dev Psychol*. 2008;44(1):59–68

24. MacCallum F, Golombok S. Children raised in fatherless families from infancy: a follow-up of children of lesbian and single heterosexual mothers at early adolescence. *J Child Psychol Psychiatry*. 2004;45(8):1407–1419

25. Vanfraussen K, Ponjaert-Kristofferson I, Brewaeys A. What does it mean for youngsters to grow up in a lesbian family created by means of donor insemination? *J Reprod Infant Psychol*. 2002;20(4):237–252

26. Patterson CJ. Children of lesbian and gay parents. *Curr Dir Psychol Sci*. 2006;15(5):241–244

27. Wainright L, Russell ST, Patterson CJ. Psychosocial adjustment, school outcomes, and romantic relationships of adolescents with same sex parents. *Child Dev*. 2004;75(6):1886–1898

28. Tasker F. Lesbian mothers, gay fathers, and their children: a review. *J Dev Behav Pediatr*. 2005; 26(3):224–240

29. Perrin EC. *Sexual Orientation in Child and Adolescent Health Care*. New York, NY: Wolters Kluwer; 2002

30. Patterson CJ. Children of lesbian and gay parents. *Child Dev*. 1992;63(5):1025–1042

31. Anderssen N, Amlie C, Ytterøy EA. Outcomes for children with lesbian and gay parents. A review of the studies from 1978 to 2000. *Scand J Psychol*. 2002;43(4):335–351

32. Goldberg AE. *Lesbian and Gay Parents and Their Children: Research on the Family Life Cycle*. Washington, DC: American Psychological Association; 2010

33. Perrin EC; American Academy of Pediatrics, Committee on Psychosocial Aspects of Child and Family Health. Technical report: coparent or second-parent adoption by same-sex parents. *Pediatrics*. 2002;109(2):341–344

34. Pawelski JG, Perrin EC, Foy JM, et al. The effects of marriage, civil union, and domestic partnership laws on the health and well-being of children. *Pediatrics*. 2006;118(1):349–364

35. Wainwright JL, Patterson CJ. Delinquency, victimization, and substance abuse among adolescents with female same-sex parents. *J Family Psychol*. 2006;20(3):526–530

36. Wainwright JL, Patterson CJ. Peer relations among adolescents with female same-sex parents. *Dev Psychol*. 2008;44(1):117–126

37. Golombok S, Perry B, Burston A, et al. Children with lesbian parents: a community study. *Dev Psychol*. 2003;39(1):20–33

38. Regnerus M. How different are the adult children of parents who have same-sex relationships? Findings from the New Family Structures Study. *Soc Sci Res*. 2012;41(4):752–770

39. Eggebeen DJ. What can we learn from studies of children raised by gay or lesbian parents? *Soc Sci Res*. 2012;41(4):775–778

40. Amato PR. The well-being of children with gay and lesbian parents. *Soc Sci Res*. 2012;41(4):771–774

41. Gates G. Letter to the editors. *Soc Sci Res*. 2012:41(6):1350–1351

42. Barrett D. Presentation, politics, and editing: the Marks/Regnerus articles. *Soc Sci Res*. 2012;41(6):1354–1356

43. Osborne C. Further comments on the papers by Marks and Regnerus. *Soc Sci Res*. 2012;41(4):779–783

44. Perrin AJ, Cohen P, Caren N. Are children of parents who had same-sex relationships disadvantaged? A scientific evaluation of the no-difference hypothesis. *J Gay Lesbian Mental Health*. 2013;17(3). In press

45. Cherlin AJ, Chase-Lansdale PL, McRae C. Effects of parental divorce on mental

health throughout the life course. *Am Sociol Rev.* 1998;63(2):239–249

46. Cherlin AJ, Kiernan KE, Chase-Lansdale PL. Parental divorce in childhood and demographic outcomes in young adulthood. *Demography.* 1995;32(3):299–318

47. Gartrell N, Bos HN. US national longitudinal lesbian family study: psychological adjustment of 17-year-old adolescents. *Pediatrics.* 2010;126(1):28–36

48. Hagan J. What shall we call them? *Pediatrics.* 2010;126(1):175–176

49. Van Gelderen L, Bos HN, Gartrell N, et al Quality of life of adolescents raised from birth by lesbian mothers: the national longitudinal study. *J Dev Behav Pediatr.* 2012;33(1):17–23

50. Bos H, Goldberg N, Van Gelderen L, Gartrell N. Adolescents of the U.S. national longitudinal lesbian family study: male role models, gender role traits, and psychological adjustment. *Gender Soc.* 2012;26(4):603–638

51. Goldberg A. *Gay Dads: Transitions to Adoptive Fatherhood.* New York, NY: New York University Press; 2012

52. Farr RH, Forssell SL, Patterson CJ. Parenting and child development in adoptive families: does sexual orientation matter? *Appl Dev Sci.* 2010;14(3):164–178

53. Rosenfeld MJ. Nontraditional families and childhood progress through school. *Demography.* 2010;47(3):755–775

54. Potter D. Same-sex parent families and children's academic achievement. *J Marriage Fam.* 2012;74(3):556–571

55. Sarantakos S. Children in three contexts: family, education and social development. *Children Austr.* 1996;21(3):23–30

56. Sarantakos S. Same-sex couples: problems and prospects. *J Fam Studies.* 1996;2(2):147–163

57. Marks L. Same-sex parenting and children's outcomes: a closer examination of the American psychological association's brief on lesbian and gay parenting. *Soc Sci Res.* 2012;41(4):735–751

58. Lavner JA, Waterman J, Peplau LA. Can gay and lesbian parents promote healthy development in high risk children adopted from foster care? *Am J Orthopsychiatry.* 2012;82(4):465–472

59. Brown S. Marriage and child well-being: research and policy perspectives. *J Marriage Fam.* 2010;72(5):1059–1077

60. Ramos C, Goldberg NG, Lee Badgett MV. The effects of marriage equality in Massachusetts: a survey of the experiences and impact of marriage on same sex couples. Los Angeles, CA: The Williams Institute; May 2009. Available at: www.policyarchive.org/handle/10207/bitstreams/18503.pdf. Accessed November 28, 2012

Providing Care for Children and Adolescents Facing Homelessness and Housing Insecurity

- *Policy Statement*

POLICY STATEMENT

Providing Care for Children and Adolescents Facing Homelessness and Housing Insecurity

abstract

Child health and housing security are closely intertwined, and children without homes are more likely to suffer from chronic disease, hunger, and malnutrition than are children with homes. Homeless children and youth often have significant psychosocial development issues, and their education is frequently interrupted. Given the overall effects that homelessness can have on a child's health and potential, it is important for pediatricians to recognize the factors that lead to homelessness, understand the ways that homelessness and its causes can lead to poor health outcomes, and when possible, help children and families mitigate some of the effects of homelessness. Through practice change, partnership with community resources, awareness, and advocacy, pediatricians can help optimize the health and well-being of children affected by homelessness. *Pediatrics* 2013;131:1206–1210

COUNCIL ON COMMUNITY PEDIATRICS

KEY WORDS

homelessness, housing insecurity, children, adolescents, pediatrician, health, poverty, toxic stress

This article was written by members of the American Academy of Pediatrics. It does not represent the views of the US government or any US government agency.

INTRODUCTION

An estimated 1.6 million children, or nearly 1 in 45 American children, experienced homelessness in 2010.[1] Although a national economic downturn and an increase in housing foreclosures contribute to family homelessness, additional adversity and risk factors often contribute to this complex problem. Children affected by homelessness may experience a variety of challenges to their health because of difficulty accessing health care, inadequate nutrition, education interruptions, trauma, and family dynamics. By recognizing these challenges, pediatricians can help improve the care of these children in practices and communities.

DEFINING AND MEASURING HOMELESSNESS

The US Department of Education defines a homeless individual as "(A) an individual who lacks a fixed, regular, and adequate nighttime residence . . . and (B) includes (i) children and youths who are sharing the housing of other persons due to loss of housing, economic hardship, or a similar reason; are living in motels, hotels, trailer parks, or camping grounds due to the lack of alternative accommodations; are living in emergency or transitional shelters; are abandoned in hospitals; or are awaiting foster care placement; (ii) children and youths who have a primary nighttime residence that is a public or private place not designed for or ordinarily used as

www.pediatrics.org/cgi/doi/10.1542/peds.2013-0645

doi:10.1542/peds.2013-0645

PEDIATRICS (ISSN Numbers: Print, 0031-4005; Online, 1098-4275).

a regular sleeping accommodation for human beings ...; (iii) children and youths who are living in cars, parks, public spaces, abandoned buildings, substandard housing, bus or train stations, or similar settings; and (iv) migratory children who qualify as homeless for the purposes of this subtitle because the children are living in circumstances described in clauses (i) through (iii)."[2]

Measuring the homeless population is difficult, and there are no definitive counts of homeless persons in the United States. The US Census Bureau does not currently attempt to estimate the total homeless population; however, the US Department of Housing and Urban Development collects data on shelter usage and makes point-in-time estimates of homelessness. The 2011 Annual Homeless Assessment Report to Congress estimates that approximately 1.5 million homeless people used an emergency shelter or transitional housing during 2010–2011, and on a single night in January 2011, 636 017 people were homeless. From 2007 to 2011, the number of children in shelters increased by 1.9% and families with children comprised 35.8% of the total sheltered population in 2011. In addition, from 2007 to 2011, the number of families that moved from stable housing arrangements to the shelter system increased by 38.5%.[3] These estimates did not include homeless persons who were unsheltered or living temporarily with other families. The incidence of homelessness in the United States in a given year is thought to be much higher.

RISK FACTORS

Although all populations experience homelessness, some populations are disproportionately affected. Major risk factors for homelessness among parents include unemployment, substance abuse, mental illness, previous military service, and a previous history of domestic violence or physical or sexual abuse.[4] An analysis of homelessness in a national cohort of US adolescents revealed that poor family relationship quality, school adjustment problems, and victimization during adolescence were each independent predictors of homelessness in adulthood.[5] Among homeless youth, a sexual orientation other than heterosexual and a history of foster care placement and school expulsion are all potential predictors of homelessness as well.[6,7] Racial and ethnic minorities are significantly overrepresented in the sheltered homeless population. In 2011, 71.9% of sheltered families were racial minorities.[3] Recognition of these risk factors is an important part of understanding and supporting homeless children and families.

Homeless children and families often experience a number of negative exposures and life events that create a cumulative risk for poor health outcomes. For example, children who live in poverty, are exposed to violence, or experience food insecurity also have poor health care service attainment, increased emergency department utilization, and overall poor health outcomes, independent of housing status.[8,9] However, these risks can be additionally compounded by homelessness. A series of studies on adverse childhood experiences has shown that multiple toxic stressors that begin in childhood can have long-term adverse effects on a child's neurobiological make-up, cognitive ability, mental health, and ability to manage stressors as an adult.[10,11] It is therefore important to understand and address these stressors both separately and in totality.

HEALTH EFFECTS OF HOMELESSNESS

Homelessness and housing insecurity negatively impact child health and development in many ways. Homeless children have shown higher rates of acute and chronic health problems than low-income children with homes. Cross-sectional surveys conducted in the 1990s reveal increased rates of multiple infectious, respiratory, gastrointestinal, and dermatologic diseases and otitis media, diarrhea, bronchitis, scabies, lice, and dental caries.[12,13] Both the prevalence and severity of asthma are markedly increased among homeless children, and homeless children suffer from higher rates of accidents and injuries than low-income children with homes.[12,14] In an evaluation completed in a school-based health center, homeless children were 2.5 times more likely to have health problems and 3 times more likely to have severe health problems than children with homes.[15] Children without a stable home are more likely to skip meals, worry about the availability of food, and consume foods with low nutritional quality and high fat content.[16,17] As a result, they suffer from high rates of malnutrition, stunting, and obesity.[8,18] Homeless children are at an increased risk of abuse, exposure to violence, and psychological trauma. Emotional distress, developmental delays, and decreased academic achievement are all more common in this population.[19–21] Speech and language deficits lead to significantly decreased literacy rates in school-aged children.[19,21] Homeless children may experience frequent moves that interrupt their education and impact school performance. In a study in elementary school students, homeless children scored lower on math and reading achievement tests than low-income students living in homes.[21] A study in homeless adolescents who received crisis services at a homeless shelter revealed just 34% of those students attained a high school diploma or general equivalency diploma (GED) by 18 years of age.[22]

Unaccompanied homeless and runaway youth differ from homeless children in families. They are more often separated from their families and more frequently exposed to violence and exploitation. Unaccompanied homeless youth are more likely to engage in high-risk sexual behaviors, have teenage pregnancies, engage in drug use, experience mood and anxiety disorders, and face violence than youth with homes.[23,24]

ACCESS TO HOUSING

Homeless families face many barriers to accessing appropriate housing. In the 2012 Hunger and Homelessness Survey conducted by the US Conference of Mayors, 64% of the surveyed cities reported that shelters turn away families with children experiencing homelessness because of lack of available beds.[25] Access to shelters is challenging in urban settings and rural communities. Although homeless families are more likely to be sheltered than individuals, age and gender restrictions in many shelters often lead to family separations. Homeless mothers are also more likely than housed mothers to have their children separated from them by the child welfare system.[26]

ACCESS TO HEALTH CARE

Children and families in unstable housing often receive fragmented health care and rely on the emergency department as a primary source of care.[27] Some of the barriers that prevent homeless children and families from accessing optimal care include the following:

- difficulty obtaining affordable, accessible, and coordinated health care services;
- frequent and unpredictable changes in living circumstances that prevent timely presentation for care, follow-up,

and communications with health care providers;

- inadequate access to storage places for medication and medical supplies; and
- potential exposure to violence or fear of violence that limits freedom.

Despite these barriers, pediatricians can support homeless children. By partnering with community resources and making changes in practice, pediatricians have the opportunity to help families establish a stable source of quality health care, improve family dynamics, and obtain housing and needed services. Addressing these barriers has been shown to have a positive effect on the health outcomes of those who have experienced homelessness.[21,22,28,29]

RECOMMENDATIONS

The following recommendations address how pediatricians can help improve the health of homeless children through practice strategies.

1. Pediatricians should help homeless children increase access to health care services by promoting and, when possible, facilitating Medicaid enrollment to eligible children and families.

2. Pediatricians should familiarize themselves with best practices for care of homeless populations and the management of chronic diseases in homeless populations.

3. Pediatricians should optimize acute care visits to best resolve patient concerns and provide comprehensive care when possible. For example, pediatricians can update immunizations if a patient is significantly behind rather than having him or her schedule a separate appointment.

4. Pediatricians should seek to identify the issues of homelessness and housing insecurity in their patient

populations. Pediatricians can use methods such as routine screening on intake and making note of frequent address changes or a history of scattered care provision.

5. Pediatricians should seek to identify underlying causes of homelessness in specific families and help facilitate connection to appropriate resources. This may include asking sensitive questions about unemployment, intimate partner violence, substance abuse, and sexual and gender identity issues. Supporting families to address these difficult issues in addition to their housing needs is critical to improving child health and development.

6. Pediatricians should partner with families to develop care plans that acknowledge barriers posed by homelessness. This can involve a variety of innovations, such as making a communications plan that takes into consideration patient access to telephone and mail services, assisting with transportation through vouchers, offering more flexible office visit scheduling, and prescribing the most affordable treatments available. Pediatricians can also learn about the availability of mobile health services in communities to facilitate care that is convenient for homeless children and families.

7. Pediatricians should become familiar with government and community-based services that assist families with unmet social and economic needs. These include such programs as Temporary Assistance for Needy Families (TANF), Special Nutrition Assistance for Nutrition (SNAP), and the Special Supplemental Nutrition Program for Women, Infants, and Children (WIC). Medical-legal partnerships and local departments of health

and human services are also helpful resources.

8. Pediatricians should support and assist in the development of shelter-based care, including partnering with mental health, dental, and other health programs when possible.

9. Pediatricians can learn about the causes and prevalence of homelessness in their communities. The State Report Card on Child Homelessness (www.homelesschildrenameric.org) issued by the National Coalition on Family Homelessness (www.familyhomelessness.org) is one of many good resources.

Pediatricians and the American Academy of Pediatrics can advocate for the needs of homeless children and families in the following ways:

1. Support local, state, and federal policies that lead to increased availability of low-income, transitional, and permanent housing.

2. Support policies and programs, such as the "Homelessness Prevention and Rapid Re-Housing Program," that aim to quickly place families in stable, permanent housing rather than a continuum of emergency and temporary housing. Permanent housing has been demonstrated to be more cost-effective and more stabilizing for families, who can be exposed to significant trauma while experiencing homelessness.

3. Support violence protection policies such as the Family Violence Prevention and Services Act and Child Abuse Prevention and Treatment Act, which provide substantial funding for shelter in addition to social services and legal aid for victims of family violence.

4. Support creative approaches to providing stable health insurance to homeless and unemployed populations, and promote strategies that enable homeless families to enroll and maintain health coverage without requiring a permanent address.

5. Support policies to eliminate any barriers for children without addresses to enroll in school.

6. Support local, state, and federal policies that provide child care vouchers for homeless families.

7. Support reformation of the foster care system to allow longer time in foster care, increased resources for maintaining families when children are aging out of foster care, and greater resources toward training/supporting foster children as they transition into independent adulthood.

Homelessness is a complex issue that presents a number of challenges for children and families. Pediatricians can support all children who are impacted, by implementing practice-level strategies and engaging in advocacy to promote their health and well-being.

LEAD AUTHOR

Melissa A. Briggs, MD, MPH

COUNCIL ON COMMUNITY PEDIATRICS, 2011–2012

Deise C. Granado-Villar, MD, MPH, Chairperson
Benjamin A. Gitterman, MD, Vice Chairperson
Jeffrey M. Brown, MD, MPH
Lance A. Chilton, MD
William H. Cotton, MD
Thresia B. Gambon, MD
Peter A. Gorski, MD, MPA
Colleen A. Kraft, MD
Alice A. Kuo, MD, PhD
Gonzalo J. Paz-Soldan, MD
Barbara Zind, MD

LIAISONS

Benjamin Hoffman, MD – Chairperson, *Indian Health Special Interest Group*
Melissa A. Briggs, MD – *Section on Medical Students, Residents, and Fellowship Trainees*
Frances J. Dunston, MD, MPH
Charles R. Feild, MD, MPH – Chairperson, *Prevention and Public Health Special Interest Group*
M. Edward Ivancic, MD – Chairperson, *Rural Health Special Interest Group*
David M. Keller, MD – Chairperson, *Community Pediatrics Education and Training Special Interest Group*

STAFF

Camille Watson, MS

REFERENCES

1. The National Center on Family Homelessness. America's youngest outcasts 2010: state report card on child homelessness. Available at: www.FamilyHomelessness.org. Accessed January 30, 2013

2. McKinney-Vento Act §725(2), 42USC 11435 (2) (2002)

3. US Department of Housing and Urban Development. The 2011 annual homeless assessment report to Congress. Washington, DC: US Department of Housing and Urban Development, Office of Community Planning and Development; 2011. Available at: https://www.onecpd.info/resources/documents/2011AHAR_FinalReport.pdf. Accessed January 30, 2013

4. US Department of Housing and Urban Development. The 2010 annual homeless assessment report to Congress. Washington, DC: US Department of Housing and Urban Development, Office of Community Planning and Development; 2010. Available at: www.hurhre.info/documents/2010HomelessAssessmentReport.pdf. Accessed January 30, 2013

5. van den Bree MB, Shelton K, Bonner A, Moss S, Thomas H, Taylor PJ. A longitudinal population-based study of factors in adolescence predicting homelessness in young adulthood. *J Adolesc Health*. 2009;45(6):571–578

6. US Interagency Council on Homelessness. Opening doors: federal strategic plan to

prevent and end homelessness. Washington, DC: US Interagency Council on Homelessness; 2010. Available at: www.ich.gov/PDF/Opening-Doors_2010_FSPPreventEndHomeless.pdf. Accessed January 30, 2013

7. Cook R. *A National Evaluation of Title IV-E Foster Care Independent Living Programs for Youth, Phase 2*. Rockville, MD: Westat Inc; 1991

8. Ma CT, Gee L, Kushel MB. Associations between housing instability and food insecurity with health care access in low-income children. *Ambul Pediatr.* 2008;8(1):50–57

9. Park JM, Fertig AR, Allison PD. Physical and mental health, cognitive development, and health care use by housing status of low-income young children in 20 American cities: a prospective cohort study. *Am J Public Health.* 2011;101(suppl 1):S255–S261

10. Anda RF, Felitti VJ, Bremner JD, et al. The enduring effects of abuse and related adverse experiences in childhood: a convergence of evidence from neurobiology and epidemiology. *Eur Arch Psychiatry Clin Neurosci.* 2006;256(3):174–186

11. Shonkoff JP, Garner AS; Committee on Psychosocial Aspects of Child and Family Health; Committee on Early Childhood, Adoption, and Dependent Care; Section on Developmental and Behavioral Pediatrics. The lifelong effects of early childhood adversity and toxic stress. *Pediatrics.* 2012;129(1). Available at: www.pediarics.org/cgi/content/full/129/1/e232

12. Weinreb L, Goldberg R, Bassuk E, Perloff J. Determinants of health and service use patterns in homeless and low-income housed children. *Pediatrics.* 1998;102(3 pt 1):554–562

13. Karr C, Kline S. Homeless children: what every clinician should know. *Pediatr Rev.* 2004;25(7):235–241

14. McLean DE, Bowen S, Drezner K, et al. Asthma among homeless children: undercounting and undertreating the underserved. *Arch Pediatr Adolesc Med.* 2004;158(3):244–249

15. Berti LC, Zylbert S, Rolnitzky L. Comparison of health status of children using a school-based health center for comprehensive care. *J Pediatr Health Care.* 2001;15(5):244–250

16. Wood DL, Valdez RB, Hayashi T, Shen A. Health of homeless children and housed, poor children. *Pediatrics.* 1990;86(6):858–866

17. Smith C, Richards R. Dietary intake, overweight status, and perceptions of food insecurity among homeless Minnesotan youth. *Am J Hum Biol.* 2008;20(5):550–563

18. Wiecha JL, Dwyer JT, Dunn-Strohecker M. Nutrition and health services needs among the homeless. *Public Health Rep.* 1991;106(4):364–374

19. Rubin DH, Erickson CJ, San Agustin M, Cleary SD, Allen JK, Cohen P. Cognitive and academic functioning of homeless children compared with housed children. *Pediatrics.* 1996;97(3):289–294

20. Zima BT, Wells KB, Freeman HE. Emotional and behavioral problems and severe academic delays among sheltered homeless children in Los Angeles County. *Am J Public Health.* 1994;84(2):260–264

21. Obradović J, Long JD, Cutuli JJ, et al. Academic achievement of homeless and highly mobile children in an urban school district: longitudinal evidence on risk, growth, and resilience. *Dev Psychopathol.* 2009;21(2):493–518

22. Barber CC, Fonagy P, Fultz J, Simulinas M, Yates M. Homeless near a thousand homes: outcomes of homeless youth in a crisis shelter. *Am J Orthopsychiatry.* 2005;75(3):347–355

23. Edidin JP, Ganim Z, Hunter SJ, Karnik NS. The mental and physical health of homeless youth: a literature review. *Child Psychiatry Hum Dev.* 2012;43(3):354–375

24. Thompson SJ, Bender KA, Lewis CM, Watkins R. Runaway and pregnant: risk factors associated with pregnancy in a national sample of runaway/homeless female adolescents. *J Adolesc Health.* 2008;43(2):125–132

25. US Conference of Mayors. *Hunger and Homelessness Survey: A Status Report on Hunger and Homelessness in America's Cities. A 25-City Survey.* Washington, DC: US Conference of Mayors; 2012

26. Cowal K, Shinn M, Weitzman BC, Stojanovic D, Labay L. Mother-child separations among homeless and housed families receiving public assistance in New York City. *Am J Community Psychol.* 2002;30(5):711–730

27. Morris DM, Gordon JA. The role of the emergency department in the care of homeless and disadvantaged populations. *Emerg Med Clin North Am.* 2006;24(4):839–848

28. Martinez TE, Burt MR. Impact of permanent supportive housing on the use of acute care health services by homeless adults. *Psychiatr Serv.* 2006;57(7):992–999

29. Sadowski LS, Kee RA, VanderWeele TJ, Buchanan D. Effect of a housing and case management program on emergency department visits and hospitalizations among chronically ill homeless adults: a randomized trial. *JAMA.* 2009;301(17):1771–1778

Providing Care for Immigrant, Migrant, and Border Children

- *Policy Statement*

POLICY STATEMENT

Providing Care for Immigrant, Migrant, and Border Children

abstract

This policy statement, which recognizes the large changes in immigrant status since publication of the 2005 statement "Providing Care for Immigrant, Homeless, and Migrant Children," focuses on strategies to support the health of immigrant children, infants, adolescents, and young adults. Homeless children will be addressed in a forthcoming separate statement ("Providing Care for Children and Adolescents Facing Homelessness and Housing Insecurity"). While recognizing the diversity across and within immigrant, migrant, and border populations, this statement provides a basic framework for serving and advocating for all immigrant children, with a particular focus on low-income and vulnerable populations. Recommendations include actions needed within and outside the health care system, including expansion of access to high-quality medical homes with culturally and linguistically effective care as well as education and literacy programs. The statement recognizes the unique and special role that pediatricians can play in the lives of immigrant children and families. Recommendations for policies that support immigrant child health are included. *Pediatrics* 2013;131:e2028–e2034

COUNCIL ON COMMUNITY PEDIATRICS

KEY WORDS
immigrant, migrant, border, underserved communities

ABBREVIATIONS
CHIP—Children's Health Insurance Program

www.pediatrics.org/cgi/doi/10.1542/peds.2013-1099

doi:10.1542/peds.2013-1099

PEDIATRICS (ISSN Numbers: Print, 0031-4005; Online, 1098-4275).

INTRODUCTION

Many children in immigrant communities face multiple barriers to accessing comprehensive, affordable, and culturally and linguistically effective health care services. Some of these barriers include poverty, fear and stigma, high mobility, limited English proficiency, little information or misunderstandings about how the US health care system works, and lack of insurance and/or access to care. Many children of immigrant families belong to racial and ethnic minority groups that face health status disparities resulting from complex determinants that are exacerbated by children's living circumstances. Inadequate availability of basic necessities, such as housing, and lack of information regarding previous medical care are among the persistent challenges faced by these vulnerable families. For some, the fear of violence or harassment because of their immigrant status compounds their already fragile living conditions. For many within this population, care can be episodic, fragmented, and oriented to care of acute conditions.[1] Although many children in these circumstances face similar challenges, there are some differences of experiences among migrant and border immigrant subgroups (see Fig 1).

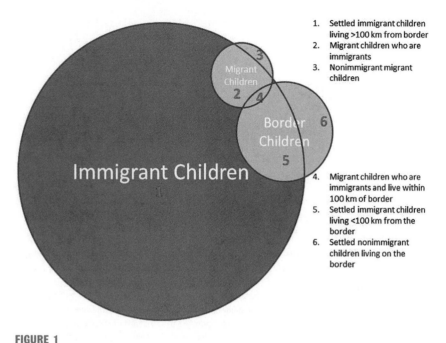

1. Settled immigrant children living >100 km from border
2. Migrant children who are immigrants
3. Nonimmigrant migrant children
4. Migrant children who are immigrants and live within 100 km of border
5. Settled immigrant children living <100 km from the border
6. Settled nonimmigrant children living on the border

FIGURE 1

Representation of the populations of immigrant, border, and migrant children: separate and overlapping groups.

DEFINITIONS

"Immigrant children" are defined as children who are foreign-born or children born in the United States who live with at least 1 parent who is foreign-born.[2]

Many immigrant children are in migrant families that move across the country seeking seasonal or temporary employment in a variety of industries. "Migrant children" may work in the industries in which their family members are employed and move frequently because of changes in their parents' employment. Migrant families are often located in areas that have many agricultural workers and/or where rapid growth is occurring.

"Border children" are those who live within 100 km of the US-Mexico border.[3] Immigrant children have a significant presence in the border states of Arizona, California, New Mexico, and Texas. Many border children are of Mexican origin, and a significant number are US citizens whose ancestors have been US citizens for generations. For the purposes of this discussion, only children living north of the Mexican border are described, although many children south of the border share similar characteristics. Children living along the Canadian border are not discussed in this statement, because there is far less immigration across that border and discrete immigrant communities there have been rare.

DEMOGRAPHICS

Immigrant children represent the fastest growing segment of the US population. One in every 4 children in the United States, approximately 18.4 million children, live in an immigrant family. Eighty-nine percent of these children are born in the United States and are US citizens.[4] Immigrant children accounted for most of the US child population growth over the past decade. Although 64% of all children of immigrants live in 6 states (California, Texas, New York, Florida, Illinois, and New Jersey), immigrant children are dispersed throughout the country. Since 1990, the largest growth in percentage of immigrant children has occurred in North Carolina, Nevada, Georgia, and Arkansas.[5] Families immigrate for a variety of reasons that may include seeking opportunity, fleeing war/chaos, or escaping persecution.

Pediatricians may be surprised by the high degree of diversity of the immigrant population and by the variety of immigrant communities within their midst, such as Haitians in Florida and eastern Virginia or Somali families in Seattle and Minneapolis. Hmong families are present in the Central Valley of California.[6] In response to the growth of these immigrant communities, some health care and social/community service providers have begun providing culturally appropriate care and services.

Approximately 43% of immigrant children have parents of Mexican origin, and 20% are of Central American descent. An estimated 22% of immigrant children have parents of Asian or Middle Eastern origin. Fifteen percent of children have parents with origins in Africa, Central and Eastern Europe, Western Europe, Canada, and Australia.[7] Given this rapid demographic growth, most pediatricians will provide care for immigrant children in their practices.

COMMON CHALLENGES FOR IMMIGRANT, MIGRANT, AND BORDER CHILDREN

All 3 groups of children face a variety of challenges to their health and well-being, including poverty, lack of health insurance, low educational attainment, substandard housing, and language barriers.

Poverty is a strong determinant of child well-being and is very common among immigrant children. Poverty is closely linked to negative physical, developmental, and mental health–related outcomes.[8] A family's socioeconomic status has a direct effect on its ability to access high-quality health care services and to achieve good health, social, and emotional outcomes. In 2010, 30% of children in immigrant families lived below the federal poverty level, compared with 19% of children with US-born parents.[4] This is despite the fact that immigrant children are more likely to live in 2-parent families and have parents who work and work more hours compared with parents of US-born children.[9] Immigrant children tend to live in larger families, with 19% having 4 or more siblings, compared with 14% of US-born families.[10] Housing is often substandard and/or overcrowded for these families.

Lack of health care coverage is more common among children in each of these groups than for nonimmigrant children. Children of immigrants are nearly twice as likely to be uninsured (15%) as are children of nonimmigrant families (8%).[4] Many of the immigrant children who are uninsured are eligible for Medicaid or the Children's Health Insurance Program (CHIP) but are not enrolled. Many immigrant parents fear that accessing services for their eligible children will lead them to be considered a "public charge" (a person dependent on the government for the expenses of living[11]) and worry about how that may negatively affect their immigration status and prospects. They may also fear that agencies offering assistance will share information with immigration enforcement agencies. Other families may not be aware of their children's eligibility for coverage. These same reasons may affect parents' ability and willingness to access other programs and benefits that their children may be eligible for, such as the Special Supplemental Nutrition Program for Women, Infants, and Children; Supplemental Nutrition Assistance Program; the Temporary Assistance for Needy Families program; and Supplemental Security Income.

Current federal law allows states to apply waiting periods for up to 5 years for legal permanent residents to become eligible for Medicaid coverage. Medicaid also excludes undocumented children from all but emergency health care. Although states may choose to cover children sooner, waiting periods can exacerbate the lack of health insurance coverage for immigrant children. The Affordable Care Act of 2010 (Pub L No. 111-148) also restricts the access to health insurance exchanges of children and adults who are undocumented immigrants.[12]

Language and communication barriers may impede medical care for many children in each of these 3 groups. Although many immigrant children speak English, their parents may not, creating a barrier that can prevent families from accessing health services and/or causing inadequate communication with health care providers. Without access to qualified medical interpreters in health care settings, language barriers can place English-speaking children in the difficult position of interpreting between health care providers and their family members. Use of children and other family members as untrained interpreters should be avoided. These challenges can result in major barriers to accessing health care and decreased satisfaction with services received. Providing care to families with limited English proficiency without appropriate medical interpretation services can ultimately lead to a higher incidence of medical errors when delivering care.[13]

Educational levels and health literacy are often lower among parents of immigrant, border, and migrant families than among native-born US families. Thirty-one percent of immigrant children have a mother without a high school education; the proportion of fathers without a high school education is similar.[4] It is important to note

that the level of maternal education is an important determinant of child health. Lower education levels are associated with lower health literacy. Low health literacy creates a barrier for patients in understanding medical information and is associated with poor health outcomes.

Health Status and Health Disparities

Although immigrant children may be vulnerable to many risk factors for poorer health outcomes, some groups of immigrant children enjoy a healthier infancy than expected. For example, Latino families have a relatively low incidence of low birth weight, preterm birth, and infant mortality compared with children of US-born parents.[4] This phenomenon has been called the "healthy immigrant phenomenon."[9] Immigrant mothers are more likely to breastfeed their infants than mothers born in the United States.[14] Immigrant children also seem to benefit from some additional protective factors, such as growing up in 2-parent or extended families,[9] as well as close identification with the cultural and spiritual practices of their family and community. In addition, as they grow up, immigrant children may also display relatively better adjustment and behavior in school compared with nonimmigrant peers. This phenomenon has been shown to fade with increased length of stay in the United States and is, therefore, an infrequent protective factor for health outcomes.

On the other hand, the health of immigrant children as a group is, in some respects, worse than US-born children. For example, they are less likely to be perceived by their parents to be in excellent/good health and are less likely to have a usual source of medical care and to obtain specialty care when needed.[15] They also have less access to dental care, despite the fact that they have a higher prevalence of dental caries.[16] The Affordable Care Act excluded undocumented immigrants from health care coverage made available through the Act, leaving that group of adults and children as the largest group who still will not have health insurance after the changes of 2014.[12]

Immigrant children who are foreign-born may not have been screened at birth for congenital syphilis, hemoglobinopathies, hearing deficits, and inborn errors of metabolism. In comparison with US-born children, they also have lower immunization rates, especially for vaccines that are not routinely administered in their countries of origin. Some children may lack immunization records. Foreign-born immigrant children have a higher incidence or prevalence of some infectious diseases, such as tuberculosis, hepatitis A, amebiasis, and parasitosis.[17] Immigrant children with asthma are less likely to be prescribed the recommended preventive medications.[18] Immigrant families may be uniquely vulnerable to mental health problems and experience high levels of stress, depression, grief, and traumatic events compared with nonimmigrant families.[19] Additionally, many experience the stress of family separation, in which some of the siblings or, in some cases, 1 or both of the parents do not reside in this country with them.

Development, Early Education, and School Success

Many immigrant, migrant, and border children also experience educational disparities compared with US-born children. As noted, immigrant children may enjoy a healthy start as infants but may experience developmental stagnation as toddlers compared with nonimmigrant children.[20]

In general, children who grow up in bilingual homes should attain major language developmental milestones at the normally expected times. At the same time, children raised in homes with impoverished language have a greater chance of being delayed in language acquisition, whether their families are monolingual or bilingual. When language delays are suspected in children growing up in limited English proficiency households, they present complex evaluation and intervention issues. When in doubt about a suspected language delay in a bilingual child, timely referral to a knowledgeable, bilingual speech and language pathologist is ideal.

Many immigrant children have less access to quality early education programs and are less likely to be enrolled in preschool programs, such as Head Start.[4] Once enrolled in school, cultural and linguistic barriers between parents and schools can lead to decreased family interaction and involvement. As they advance in their schooling, children in immigrant families are less likely to graduate from high school than are their nonimmigrant peers.[4]

Fear and Discrimination

Immigrant children and families may face discrimination and be fearful of attitudes and behaviors of the people they interact with outside their communities, including health care providers, which can reduce access to health care and lead to negative child health outcomes. Families may face anti-immigrant sentiment. Fear and discrimination can exacerbate a feeling of isolation and contribute to mental health problems, such as child and family depression, leaving these populations vulnerable.

Family Separation

Immigrant children may have 1 or more undocumented family members. An undocumented immigrant lacks the proper records and identification to live in the United States.[21] Immigration enforcement and related policies can lead to the sudden removal of an undocumented parent or other key family member without notice or preparation. Children whose parents are taken into custody and/or deported have been shown to experience mental and emotional health problems, including sleeping and eating disturbances, anxiety, depression, poor school performance, and other types of distress. Forced separations because of immigration enforcement can also result in the loss of family income and have been shown to result in family housing and food instability.[22] This can negatively affect a child's safety, health, and development.

FACTORS SPECIFIC TO MIGRANT CHILDREN

A large number of migrant children are also immigrants. For that reason, virtually all of the points made earlier about immigrant children may also apply to those who are migrants. Because of their migration patterns, migrant children are even more likely to lack medical coverage and a medical home than other immigrant children. They are also more likely to be socially, culturally, and linguistically isolated because of their mobile lifestyle.

Many migrant children face a panoply of health problems related to their living and working conditions, including workplace injuries, substandard housing, and unreliable transportation.[23] These factors can contribute to higher rates of respiratory tract and ear infections, bacterial and viral gastroenteritis, tuberculosis, nutritional deficiencies, intestinal parasites, skin infections, dental problems, lead and pesticide exposure, and undiagnosed congenital anomalies.[24] Additionally, at times, migrant adolescents travel on their own from 1 job site to another, putting them at increased risk of many health-related problems.

FACTORS SPECIFIC TO BORDER CHILDREN

Immigrant children living at the US-Mexico border share almost all of the characteristics of other immigrant children but may experience additional challenges. Children who have crossed the border to enter the United States may have experienced trauma in the form of threat of death, abuse, and exploitation that leave serious psychological scars. Once in the United States, these children may experience an enhanced fear of a family member's deportation, imprisonment, or abuse because of documentation status. Children and families who have recently crossed the border can also experience difficulty adapting to the new cultural environment of the United States and experience stress from the absence of an extended family (including a parent or head of household) that is located in another country. Border children may be even more stigmatized or mistreated by the nonimmigrant populations living nearby, as their families are falsely presumed to take advantage of scarce resources and not pay taxes.

Many border communities are poor and lacking in resources, including medical care. In general, border communities lack sufficient numbers of primary care pediatricians, and those present may lack appropriate cultural and linguistic capacity to serve minority border children. In addition, primary care providers bear an especially high proportion of Medicaid, CHIP, and self-pay patients, with few privately insured patients to whom costs may be shifted. As a consequence of these deficiencies and because of high costs of medical care in the United States, families living close

to the border may use medical care and pharmaceutical resources south of the border.

RECOMMENDATIONS

Immigrant children represent a considerable part of the economic and social future of the nation. It is in the national interest that we work to ensure that all children within the United States, including immigrant, border, and migrant children, grow up physically and developmentally healthy. The future prosperity and well-being of the United States depends on the health and vitality of all of its children, without exception. The following recommendations address how pediatricians can help support immigrant child health in practice.

1. Pediatricians and the American Academy of Pediatrics should advocate for health insurance coverage for every child and every individual living in the United States, as lack of coverage for any family member affects the health of the entire family.[25] This advocacy should focus on expanding access to quality health care within a medical home. Barriers to enrollment must be addressed, including the removal of any waiting periods for documented immigrant children to enroll into coverage. Efforts must also address barriers to enrollment for children who are potentially eligible for Medicaid and CHIP but not enrolled. Simplified enrollment for both programs and federal or state funding for those who are not currently eligible for Medicaid or CHIP is also essential.

2. The provision of comprehensive, coordinated, culturally and linguistically effective care, and continuous health services provided in a quality medical home should be integral to all efforts on behalf

of immigrant children.[26] This is especially critical for children with chronic health care needs and emotional or behavioral health problems. Private and public insurance payers should pay for qualified medical interpretation services.

3. Pediatricians caring for immigrant children should evaluate immunization adequacy and should conduct careful developmental surveillance and screening at regular intervals as recommended by the American Academy of Pediatrics.[27] Appropriate referral for early intervention services or psychoeducational evaluation should be initiated as soon as a concern is identified.

4. Pediatricians should recognize the barriers to health that are faced by immigrant children and take these barriers into account while providing care. They should inquire about beliefs and practices related to health, illness, and disability, as well as traditional healing practices and medication use while obtaining a patient's medical history. Knowledge, attitude, and skill development in culturally and linguistically effective practices and cross-cultural communication should be part of every pediatrician's professional agenda.

5. Pediatricians should be knowledgeable about the unique emotional, behavioral, mental, and physical health advantages and problems that may be faced by immigrant children, including those related to family separation. Appropriate screening to identify family, environmental, and social circumstances, as well as biological factors, should be incorporated into routine pediatric assessments, such as in Bright Futures history forms.

6. Pediatricians should have access to information regarding federal, state, and community programs that can serve as resources to at-risk children and families. Culturally relevant programs that address social and economic challenges, such as food and housing security, English literacy, and legal services, are particularly important. Medical-legal partnerships should be supported to help immigrant families with these issues.

7. Pediatricians should play a key role in helping immigrant parents assess and review the educational progress of the child and encouraging parents to become involved in and interact with teachers and the school community. If a child exhibits difficulty or academic underachievement, pediatricians are in a unique position to advocate for the child and encourage and help parents to obtain appropriate evaluation and intervention from the school system.

8. Pediatricians should routinely use available screening and diagnostic protocols for evaluating foreign-born children for infectious diseases and other medical conditions when providing care for newly arrived immigrant children.[28] Additional screenings, including lead, vision, and hearing screenings, should be considered whether required for school entry or not.

9. Pediatricians should advocate for an array of culturally effective early intervention services, including the establishment of evidence-based early literacy promotion programs, such as Reach Out and Read, in immigrant, border, and migrant communities. Because reading is such an important skill, these programs are important tools for improving the school readiness of all children, just as fostering health literacy in parents is important to the well-being of their children.

10. Pediatricians should use their positions of respect in communities to promote the value of diversity and inclusion and to advocate for children and families of all backgrounds.

Given the challenging circumstances many immigrant children face because of their family's immigration status, the following recommendations address how immigration policies can support child health and well-being.

11. The health, well-being, and safety of children should be prioritized in all immigration proceedings. Whenever possible, the separation of a child from his or her family and home environment should be prevented, and family reunions should be expedited.

12. In no circumstances should a child have to represent himself or herself in an immigration proceeding.

13. Health care facilities should be safe settings for immigrant children and families to access health care. Medical records and health care facilities should not be used in any immigration enforcement action.

LEAD AUTHORS
Lance A. Chilton, MD
Gilbert A. Handal, MD
Gonzalo J. Paz-Soldan, MD

COUNCIL ON COMMUNITY PEDIATRICS EXECUTIVE COMMITTEE, 2011–2012
Deise C. Granado-Villar, MD, MPH, Chairperson
Benjamin A. Gitterman, MD, Vice Chairperson
Jeffrey M. Brown, MD, MPH
Lance A. Chilton, MD
William H. Cotton, MD
Thresia B. Gambon, MD
Peter A. Gorski, MD, MPA
Colleen A. Kraft, MD
Alice A. Kuo, MD, PhD
Gonzalo J. Paz-Soldan, MD
Barbara Zind, MD

CONTRIBUTOR
Ricky Choi, MD, MPH – *Chairperson, Special Interest Group on Immigrant Health*

LIAISONS
Benjamin Hoffman, MD – *Chairperson, Indian Health Special Interest Group*
Melissa A. Briggs, MD – *Section on Medical Students, Residents, and Fellowship Trainees*
Frances J. Dunston, MD, MPH – *Commission to End Health Care Disparities*
Charles R. Feild, MD, MPH – *Chairperson, Prevention and Public Health Special Interest Group*
M. Edward Ivancic, MD – *Chairperson, Rural Health Special Interest Group*
David M. Keller, MD – *Chairperson, Community Pediatrics Education and Training Special Interest Group*

STAFF
Camille Watson, MS

REFERENCES

1. Okie S. Immigrants and health care—at the intersection of two broken systems. *N Engl J Med.* 2007;357(6):525–529

2. Child Trends. Immigrant children. Available at: www.childtrendsdatabank.org/?q=node/333. Accessed July 19, 2012

3. United States-Mexico Border Health Commission. What is defined as the border region? Available at: www.borderhealth.org/show_faq.php?id=16. Accessed July 19, 2012

4. Foundation for Child Development. Children in immigrant families: essential to America's future. Available at: http://fcd-us.org/node/1232. Accessed July 19, 2012

5. Fortuny K, Ajay C. *Children of Immigrants: Growing National and State Diversity. Brief 5.* Washington, DC: The Urban Institute; 2011

6. Fadiman A. *The Spirit Catches You and You Fall Down: A Hmong Child, Her American Doctors, and the Collision of Two Cultures.* New York, NY: Noonday Press; 1998

7. Fortuny K, Hernandez DJ, Ajay C. *Young Children of Immigrants: The Leading Edge of America's Future. Brief 3.* Washington, DC: The Urban Institute; 2010

8. Conroy K, Sandel M, Zuckerman B. Poverty grown up: how childhood socioeconomic status impacts adult health. *J Dev Behav Pediatr.* 2010;31(2):154–160

9. Mendoza FS. Health disparities and children in immigrant families: a research agenda. *Pediatrics.* 2009;124(suppl 3): S187–S195

10. Lansford JE, Deater-Deckard K, Bornstein MH, eds. *Immigrant Families in Contemporary Society.* New York, NY: Guilford Press; 2007

11. US Citizenship and Immigration Services. Public Charge Fact Sheet, April 2011. Available at: www.uscis.gov/portal/site/uscis/menuitem.5af9bb95919f35e66f614176543f6d1a/?vgnextoid=775d23cbea6bf210VgnVCM100000082ca60aRCRD&vgnextchannel=8a2f6d26d17df110VgnVCM1000004718190aRCRD. Accessed July 19, 2012

12. National Immigration Law Center. How are immigrants included in health care reform? Washington, DC: National Immigration Law Center; April 2010. Available at: www.nilc.org/contact_us.html. Accessed July 19, 2012

13. Flores G, Laws MB, Mayo SJ, et al. Errors in medical interpretation and their potential clinical consequences in pediatric encounters. *Pediatrics.* 2003;111(1):6–14

14. Singh GK, Kogan MD, Dee DL. Nativity/immigrant status, race/ethnicity, and socioeconomic determinants of breastfeeding initiation and duration in the United States, 2003. *Pediatrics.* 2007;119(1 suppl 1):S38–S46

15. Capps R, Fix M, Ost J, Reardon-Anderson J, Passel JS. *The Health and Well-Being of Young Children of Immigrants.* Washington, DC: The Urban Institute; 2004

16. Liu J, Probst JC, Martin AB, Wang JY, Salinas CF. Disparities in dental insurance coverage and dental care among US children: the National Survey of Children's Health. *Pediatrics.* 2007;119(suppl 1):S12–S21

17. Strine TW, Barker LE, Mokdad AH, Luman ET, Sutter RW, Chu SY. Vaccination coverage of foreign-born children 19 to 35 months of age: findings from the National Immunization Survey, 1999-2000. *Pediatrics.* 2002;110 (2 pt 1):e15

18. Tienda M, Haskin R. Immigrant children: introducing the issue. *Immigrant Children.* 2011;21(1):3–18

19. Kupersmidt JB, Martin SL. Mental health problems of children of migrant and seasonal farm workers: a pilot study. *J Am Acad Child Adolesc Psychiatry.* 1997;36(2):1–9

20. Fuller B, Bridges M, Bein E, et al. The health and cognitive growth of Latino toddlers: at risk or immigrant paradox? *Matern Child Health J.* 2009;13(6):755–768

21. Legal Information Institute. Immigration law: an overview. Available at: www.law.cornell.edu/wex/Immigration. Accessed July 19, 2012

22. Chaudry A, Capps R, Pedroza JM, Castenada RM, Santos R, Scott MM. *Facing Our Future: Children in the Aftermath of Immigration Enforcement.* Washington, DC: The Urban Institute; 2010

23. McLaurin J, ed; American Academy of Pediatrics. *Guidelines for the Care of Migrant Farmworker's Children.* Elk Grove Village, IL: American Academy of Pediatrics; 2000

24. Migrant Clinician's Network. Children's health. Available at: www.migrantclinician.org/issues/childrens-health.html. Accessed July 19, 2012

25. Ku L, Broaddus M. *Coverage for Parents Helps Children, Too.* Washington, DC: Center on Budget and Policy Priorities; 2006

26. American Academy of Pediatrics Committee on Pediatric Workforce. Culturally effective pediatric care: education and training issues. *Pediatrics.* 1999;103(1):167–170

27. Hagan JF, Jr, Shaw JS, Duncan P, eds. *Bright Futures: Guidelines for Health Supervision of Infants, Children, and Adolescents.* 3rd ed. Elk Grove Village, IL: American Academy of Pediatrics; 2008

28. Pickering LK, Baker CJ, Kimberlin DW, Long SS, eds; American Academy of Pediatrics. *Red Book: 2012 Report of the Committee on Infectious Diseases.* 29th ed. Elk Grove Village, IL: American Academy of Pediatrics; 2012

Recognition and Management of Iatrogenically Induced Opioid Dependence and Withdrawal in Children

• •

- *Clinical Report*

CLINICAL REPORT

Recognition and Management of Iatrogenically Induced Opioid Dependence and Withdrawal in Children

abstract

Opioids are often prescribed to children for pain relief related to procedures, acute injuries, and chronic conditions. Round-the-clock dosing of opioids can produce opioid dependence within 5 days. According to a 2001 Consensus Paper from the American Academy of Pain Medicine, American Pain Society, and American Society of Addiction Medicine, dependence is defined as "a state of adaptation that is manifested by a drug class specific withdrawal syndrome that can be produced by abrupt cessation, rapid dose reduction, decreasing blood level of the drug, and/or administration of an antagonist." Although the experience of many children undergoing iatrogenically induced withdrawal may be mild or goes unreported, there is currently no guidance for recognition or management of withdrawal for this population. Guidance on this subject is available only for adults and primarily for adults with substance use disorders. The guideline will summarize existing literature and provide readers with information currently not available in any single source specific for this vulnerable pediatric population. *Pediatrics* 2014;133:152–155

Jeffrey Galinkin, MD, FAAP, Jeffrey Lee Koh, MD, FAAP, COMMITTEE ON DRUGS, and SECTION ON ANESTHESIOLOGY AND PAIN MEDICINE

KEY WORDS
opioids, dependence, withdrawal, sedation, analgesia

This document is copyrighted and is property of the American Academy of Pediatrics and its Board of Directors. All authors have filed conflict of interest statements with the American Academy of Pediatrics. Any conflicts have been resolved through a process approved by the Board of Directors. The American Academy of Pediatrics has neither solicited nor accepted any commercial involvement in the development of the content of this publication.

The guidance in this report does not indicate an exclusive course of treatment or serve as a standard of medical care. Variations, taking into account individual circumstances, may be appropriate.

www.pediatrics.org/cgi/doi/10.1542/peds.2013-3398

doi:10.1542/peds.2013-3398

All clinical reports from the American Academy of Pediatrics automatically expire 5 years after publication unless reaffirmed, revised, or retired at or before that time.

PEDIATRICS (ISSN Numbers: Print, 0031-4005; Online, 1098-4275).

INTRODUCTION

Opioids are commonly prescribed to children of all ages.[1] Primarily, they are used in short duration for pain related to either a procedure or an acute injury. Utilization of opioids in these circumstances is widely accepted and generally considered low risk. Even in this circumstance, it is important to realize that children prescribed opioids for as little as 7 days can develop opioid dependence and exhibit drug-specific withdrawal symptoms on abrupt discontinuation of medications. Children in ICU settings are especially prone to these issues, because they are often exposed to opioids for longer periods of time when they have ongoing pain or require long-term sedation/analgesia as part of their care.

To understand the consequences of opioid use, it is important that one understands some basic definitions related to opioid use and adaptation to this use. The most commonly accepted definitions for these behaviors are based on a 2001 Consensus Paper from the American Academy of Pain Medicine, American Pain Society, and American Society of Addiction Medicine.[2] The definitions are as follows:

- Addiction is a primary, chronic, neurobiological disease with genetic, psychosocial, and environmental factors influencing its development and manifestations. It is characterized by behaviors that include one or more of the following: impaired control over drug use, compulsive use, continued use despite harm, and craving.

- Physical dependence is a state of adaptation that is manifested by a drug class—specific withdrawal syndrome that can be produced by abrupt cessation, rapid dose reduction, decreasing blood level of the drug, and/or administration of an antagonist.

- Tolerance is a state of adaptation in which exposure to a drug induces changes that result in a diminution of one or more of the drug's effects over time.

The consensus paper also noted, "most specialists in pain medicine and addiction agree that patients treated with prolonged opioid therapy do develop physical dependence and sometimes tolerance, but do not usually develop addictive disorders."

Although the experience of many children undergoing iatrogenically induced withdrawal may be mild or go unreported, there is currently no guidance for recognition or management of withdrawal for this population. (Guidance for newborn infants is available from the American Academy of Pediatrics.[3]) Guidance available on this subject is mostly from adults and primarily from literature on adults with substance use disorders. This clinical report summarizes existing literature on this subject and provides readers with information currently not available in any single source specific for this vulnerable pediatric population. The scope of this document is limited to children who received opioid medications outside the neonatal and infant period.

EPIDEMIOLOGY OF OPIOID USE IN THE PEDIATRIC POPULATION

In 2009, approximately 7.2 million outpatient opioid prescriptions were dispensed for children in the United States.[1] The frequency of opioid prescriptions to children has doubled in the past decade.[4] The vast majority of these prescriptions were written for children between the ages of 10 and 17 years, with many of these prescriptions for postprocedural and postoperative use.

BEHAVIORAL AND PHYSIOLOGIC CHARACTERISTICS OF OPIOID DEPENDENCE AND WITHDRAWAL

In most clinical situations, opioid dependence does not manifest any symptoms until opioid administration is abruptly decreased or discontinued (sometimes in favor of nonopioid analgesics), resulting in symptoms of withdrawal. Withdrawal also occurs when an alteration in gastrointestinal absorption leads to decreased absorption of oral opioid and a subsequent decrease in opioid blood concentration. Finally, transition from intravenous to oral administration is not always a predictable conversion, and withdrawal symptoms can occur when oral dosing results in a significantly lower blood concentration of opioid than the previous intravenous dosing. The signs and symptoms associated with withdrawal in the pediatric population can vary somewhat by age but are relatively consistent overall.[5,6]

Behavioral changes are often the primary manifestation of withdrawal and include anxiety, agitation, insomnia, and tremors. In addition to behavioral symptoms, physiologic changes commonly seen in withdrawal include increased muscle tone, nausea, vomiting, diarrhea, decreased appetite, tachypnea, tachycardia, fever, sweating, and hypertension. Care must be taken to

rule out other causes of these symptoms, such as infection and sepsis.

Many of these symptoms are assessed in tools used to monitor children undergoing potential opioid withdrawal.[5] Specific scales for children include the Modified Narcotic Abstinence Scale, the Sedation Withdrawal Score, the Sophia Observation Withdrawal Symptoms Scale, and the Opioid Benzodiazepine Withdrawal Scale. Of these pediatric-specific scales, only the Sophia Observation Withdrawal Symptoms Scale has been validated.[7] The only validated scales to measure withdrawal in adults are the Clinical Opiate Withdrawal Scale (an 11-item clinician-administered scale assessing opioid withdrawal) and the Clinical Institute Narcotic Assessment scale, but these are not specific for children.[8] Consistently using and becoming familiar with any of these scales (adult or pediatric) will allow a clinician a means of detecting early signs of withdrawal so a treatment strategy can be implemented. Clinicians should also interpret results from the use of these scales within the clinical context of each individual patient, because there may be reasons other than opioid withdrawal that could explain certain behaviors being scored.

MANAGEMENT STRATEGIES FOR APPROPRIATE WEANING OF OPIOIDS AND TREATMENT OF WITHDRAWAL SYMPTOMS

Prevention is the preferred approach to management of opioid withdrawal symptoms and is achieved by decreasing the dose of opioid over time rather than abruptly discontinuing the medication, commonly referred to as "weaning." When discontinuing an opioid, the first step is to decide whether a patient is at risk for opioid withdrawal. Opioid withdrawal symptoms have been reported in as little as 5 days,[6] but there seems to be considerable interpatient variability. Most patients who have received an opioid for less than 7 days do not suffer from withdrawal and can have their medication discontinued quickly. Patients who have been exposed to an opioid for longer than 14 days will usually need to follow a weaning protocol to prevent withdrawal symptoms. Those patients with opioid exposure lasting between 7 and 14 days may need to be weaned off their opioid but usually can be weaned more quickly than those with exposure longer than 14 days. It is critical to assess a patient's pain status at the time of anticipated weaning. A patient should not have ongoing painful stimuli or a condition that requires continuation or escalation of opioid dose to adequately manage pain before weaning.

After it is determined that a patient should be weaned from an opioid, a weaning protocol is developed taking into account the length of opioid exposure and total daily opioid dose. Unfortunately, there is no clear outcome-based evidence to support an ideal weaning protocol, but it does seem logical that individual patient response to weaning is more important than following a rigid schedule. It is beyond the scope of this article to prescribe specific guidelines; the generally accepted approach involves transition to a longer-acting opioid formulation, such as methadone, extended-release morphine, or extended-release oxycodone (this is an off-label use for these drugs). Once the patient is stabilized on the long-acting opioid, weaning is usually accomplished by steps of a 10% to 20% decrease in the original dose every 24 to 48 hours.[6] During opioid weaning, parents and care providers should carefully monitor for signs of withdrawal. If withdrawal symptoms are observed, the planned dose of opioid, from the weaning schedule, should be administered, and administration of additional rescue opioid should be considered if withdrawal symptoms are severe. A shorter-acting opioid should be available for signs of withdrawal, painful procedures, or for breakthrough pain. Adjunctive medications, such as clonidine, gabapentin, and dexmedetomidine, have been used[6] to decrease withdrawal symptoms and to help in the opioid-weaning process. These drugs are not labeled for this indication, and there is little information, other than the articles referenced in this clinical report, to provide guidance on their use.

Another common clinical scenario in patients with opioid dependence is concomitant long-term benzodiazepine exposure. Again, there are no clear guidelines for the concurrent weaning of benzodiazepines and opioids. It would seem prudent to have patients wean from 1 medication at a time rather than attempt to wean from both at the same time. This way, any signs of withdrawal can be more clearly attributed to 1 medication.

There is little in the literature describing the use of behavioral strategies for management of iatrogenic opioid withdrawal symptoms in children and adolescents. However, there are reports of the successful use of these interventions for the management of benzodiazepine withdrawal in adult patients with insomnia.[9,10] Behavioral intervention has also been used as part of treatment programs in adolescents who are dependent on either prescription opioids or heroin.[11] Given the success of multidisciplinary pain management interventions that include some form of behavioral therapy, it would seem logical that behavioral intervention would be a useful part of any weaning program to help with sleep hygiene, anxiety/mood symptoms, and pain-related symptoms that may occur during the weaning period.

Overall, the management of opioid dependence and tolerance can be managed safely and comfortably for most patients. The most common difficulties in the process are using a weaning schedule that is too rapid or not understanding that the patient's weaning protocol may not provide adequate analgesia if there are ongoing (or new) painful stimuli.

CONCLUSIONS

There is a high prevalence in the use of prescription opioids in the pediatric population (see the earlier section "Epidemiology of Opioid Use in the Pediatric Population") for durations exceeding 1 week. It is essential to realize that abrupt discontinuation of opioids can lead to drug-specific withdrawal symptoms. For patients receiving prolonged opioid therapy, it is best to develop strategies in conjunction with the patient's care team and family to minimize withdrawal symptoms while following a set opioid-weaning strategy. Understanding opioid withdrawal is key to its prevention. Research in this field is just beginning and should be looked at as a priority, because the frequency of prescribed opioid use in children has doubled in the past decade.[4]

LEAD AUTHORS
Jeffrey L. Galinkin, MD, FAAP
Jeffrey Lee Koh, MD, FAAP

COMMITTEE ON DRUGS, 2012–2013
Daniel A. C. Frattarelli, MD, FAAP, Chairperson
Jeffrey L. Galinkin, MD, FAAP
Thomas P. Green, MD, FAAP
Timothy D. Johnson, DO, MMM, FAAP
Kathleen A. Neville, MD, FAAP
Ian M. Paul, MD, MSc, FAAP
John N. Van Den Anker, MD, PhD, FAAP

LIAISONS
John J. Alexander, MD, FAAP — *Food and Drug Administration*
James D. Goldberg, MD — *American College of Obstetricians and Gynecologists*
Janet D. Cragan, MD, MPH, FAAP — *Centers for Disease Control and Prevention*

REFERENCES

1. Volkow ND, McLellan TA, Cotto JH, Karithanom M, Weiss SR. Characteristics of opioid prescriptions in 2009. *JAMA*. 2011;305(13):1299–1301

2. American Academy of Pain Medicine; American Pain Society; American Society of Addiction Medicine. *Definitions Related to the Use of Opioids for the Treatment of Pain*. Glenview, IL, and Chevy Chase, MD: American Academy of Pain Medicine, American Pain Society, American Society of Addiction Medicine; 2001

3. Hudak ML, Tan RC; American Academy of Pediatrics Committee on Drugs; Committee on Fetus and Newborn. Neonatal drug withdrawal. *Pediatrics*. 2012;129(2). Available at: www.pediatrics.org/cgi/content/full/129/2/e540

4. Fortuna RJ, Robbins BW, Caiola E, Joynt M, Halterman JS. Prescribing of controlled medications to adolescents and young adults in the United States. *Pediatrics*. 2010;126(6):1108–1116

5. Ista E, van Dijk M, Gamel C, Tibboel D, de Hoog M. Withdrawal symptoms in critically ill children after long-term administration of sedatives and/or analgesics: a first evaluation. *Crit Care Med*. 2008;36(8):2427–2432

6. Anand KJ, Willson DF, Berger J, et al; Eunice Kennedy Shriver National Institute of Child Health and Human Development Collaborative Pediatric Critical Care Research Network. Tolerance and withdrawal from prolonged opioid use in critically ill children. *Pediatrics*. 2010;125(5). Available at: www.pediatrics.org/cgi/content/full/125/5/e1208

7. Ista E, de Hoog M, Tibboel D, Duivenvoorden HJ, van Dijk M. Psychometric evaluation of the Sophia observation withdrawal symptoms scale in critically ill children. *Pediatr Crit Care Med*. 2013;14(8):761–769

8. Tompkins DA, Bigelow GE, Harrison JA, Johnson RE, Fudala PJ, Strain EC. Concurrent validation of the Clinical Opiate Withdrawal Scale (COWS) and single-item indices against the Clinical Institute Narcotic Assessment (CINA) opioid withdrawal instrument. *Drug Alcohol Depend*. 2009;105(1–2):154–159

9. Morin CM, Bastien C, Guay B, Radouco-Thomas M, Leblanc J, Vallières A. Randomized clinical trial of supervised tapering and cognitive behavior therapy to facilitate benzodiazepine discontinuation in older adults with chronic insomnia. *Am J Psychiatry*. 2004;161(2):332–342

10. Baillargeon L, Landreville P, Verreault R, Beauchemin JP, Grégoire JP, Morin CM. Discontinuation of benzodiazepines among older insomniac adults treated with cognitive-behavioural therapy combined with gradual tapering: a randomized trial. *CMAJ*. 2003;169(10):1015–1020

11. Motamed M, Marsch LA, Solhkhah R, Bickel WK, Badger GJ. Differences in treatment outcomes between prescription opioid-dependent and heroin-dependent adolescents. *J Addict Med*. 2008;2(3):158–164

Recommendations for Prevention and Control of Influenza in Children, 2013–2014

- *Policy Statement*

  - *PPI: AAP Partnership for Policy Implementation See Appendix 2 for more information.*

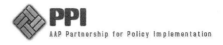

POLICY STATEMENT

Recommendations for Prevention and Control of Influenza in Children, 2013–2014

COMMITTEE ON INFECTIOUS DISEASES

KEY WORDS
influenza, immunization, live-attenuated influenza vaccine, inactivated influenza vaccine, vaccine, children, pediatrics

ABBREVIATIONS
AAP—American Academy of Pediatrics
ccIIV3—trivalent cell culture-based inactivated influenza vaccine
CDC—Centers for Disease Control and Prevention
FDA—US Food and Drug Administration
ID—intradermal
IIV—inactivated influenza vaccine
IIV3—trivalent inactivated influenza vaccine
IIV4—quadrivalent inactivated influenza vaccine
IM—intramuscular
HCP—health care personnel
LAIV—live-attenuated influenza vaccine
LAIV3—trivalent live-attenuated influenza vaccine
LAIV4—quadrivalent live-attenuated influenza vaccine
PCV13—13-valent pneumococcal conjugate vaccine
pH1N1—influenza A (H1N1) pdm09 pandemic virus
RIV3—trivalent recombinant influenza vaccine

(Continued on last page)

abstract

The purpose of this statement is to update recommendations for routine use of seasonal influenza vaccine and antiviral medications for the prevention and treatment of influenza in children. Highlights for the upcoming 2013–2014 season include (1) this year's trivalent influenza vaccine contains an A/California/7/2009 (H1N1) pdm09-like virus (same as 2012–2013); an A/Texas/50/2012 (H3N2) virus (antigenically like the 2012–2013 strain); and a B/Massachusetts/2/2012-like virus (a B/Yamagata lineage like 2012–2013 but a different virus); (2) new quadrivalent influenza vaccines with an additional B virus (B/Brisbane/60/2008-like virus [B/Victoria lineage]) have been licensed by the US Food and Drug Administration; (3) annual universal influenza immunization is indicated with either a trivalent or quadrivalent vaccine (no preference); and (4) the dosing algorithm for administration of influenza vaccine to children 6 months through 8 years of age is unchanged from 2012–2013. As always, pediatricians, nurses, and all health care personnel should promote influenza vaccine use and infection control measures. In addition, pediatricians should promptly identify influenza infections to enable rapid antiviral treatment, when indicated, to reduce morbidity and mortality. *Pediatrics* 2013;132:e1089–e1104

INTRODUCTION

The American Academy of Pediatrics (AAP) recommends annual seasonal influenza immunization for all people, including *all* children and adolescents, 6 months of age and older during the 2013–2014 influenza season. In addition, special effort should be made to vaccinate people in the following groups:

- All children, including infants born preterm, who are 6 months of age and older with conditions that increase the risk of complications from influenza (eg, children with chronic medical conditions, such as asthma, diabetes mellitus, hemodynamically significant cardiac disease, immunosuppression, or neurologic and neurodevelopmental disorders)

- Children of American Indian/Alaskan Native heritage

- All household contacts and out-of-home care providers of
  - children with high-risk conditions; and
  - children younger than 5 years, especially infants younger than 6 months

- All health care personnel (HCP)
- All women who are pregnant, are considering pregnancy, have recently delivered, or are breastfeeding during the influenza season

KEY POINTS RELEVANT FOR THE 2013–2014 INFLUENZA SEASON

1. **Annual seasonal influenza vaccine is recommended for *all* people, including all children and adolescents, 6 months of age and older during the 2013–2014 influenza season.** It is important that household contacts and out-of-home care providers of children younger than 5 years, especially infants younger than 6 months and children of any age at high risk of complications of influenza (eg, children with chronic medical conditions, such as asthma, diabetes mellitus, hemodynamically significant cardiac disease, immunosuppression, or neurologic and neurodevelopmental disorders) receive annual influenza vaccine. In the United States, more than two-thirds of children younger than 6 years and almost all children 6 years and older spend significant time in child care and school settings outside the home. Exposure to groups of children increases the risk of contracting infectious diseases. Children younger than 2 years are at an increased risk of hospitalization and complications attributable to influenza. School-age children bear a large influenza disease burden and have a significantly higher chance of seeking influenza-related medical care compared with healthy adults. Therefore, reducing influenza virus transmission among children who attend child care or school has been shown to decrease the burden of childhood influenza and transmission of influenza virus to household contacts and community members of all ages.

2. The 2012–2013 influenza season was moderately severe, with a higher percentage of outpatient visits for influenza-like illness, higher rates of hospitalization, and more deaths attributed to pneumonia and influenza compared with the 2011–2012 influenza season. As of August 10, 2013, 158 laboratory-confirmed influenza-associated pediatric deaths were reported to the Centers for Disease Control and Prevention (CDC) during the 2012–2013 influenza season. Influenza A (H3N2) viruses predominated overall, but influenza B viruses and, to a lesser extent, A (H1N1) pdm09 (pH1N1) viruses also were reported in the United States. Eighty-two of the 158 deaths were associated with influenza B viruses, 32 deaths were associated with influenza A (H3) viruses, and 4 deaths were associated with pH1N1 viruses. Thirty-seven deaths were associated with an influenza A virus for which the subtype was not determined, 1 death was associated with an undetermined type of influenza virus, and 2 deaths were associated with both influenza A and B viruses. The majority of pediatric deaths were among children who had not been immunized against influenza. Among children hospitalized with influenza and for whom medical chart data were available, approximately 44% did not have any recorded underlying condition, whereas 23% had underlying asthma or reactive airway disease (Fig 1). Although children with certain conditions are at higher risk of complications, substantial proportions of seasonal influenza morbidity and mortality occur among healthy children.

3. Both trivalent and quadrivalent influenza vaccines are licensed and available in the United States for the 2013–2014 season. Neither vaccine formulation is preferred over the other. The trivalent vaccine contains an A/California/7/2009 (H1N1) pdm09-like virus (same as 2012–2013), an A/Texas/50/2012 (H3N2) virus (antigenically like the 2012–2013 strain), and a B/Massachusetts/2/2012-like virus (a B/Yamagata lineage like 2012-2013 but a different virus). The new quadrivalent influenza vaccines include an additional B virus (B/Brisbane/60/2008-like virus [B/Victoria lineage]). In addition, 2 trivalent influenza vaccines manufactured using new technologies that do not use eggs will also be available during the 2013–2014 season: cell culture-based inactivated influenza vaccine (ccIIV3) and recombinant influenza vaccine (RIV3).

4. The number of seasonal influenza vaccine doses to be administered in the 2013–2014 influenza season depends on the child's age at the time of the first administered dose and his or her vaccine history (Fig 2):

- Influenza vaccines are not licensed for administration to infants younger than 6 months of age.
- Children 9 years and older need only 1 dose.
- Children 6 months through 8 years of age receiving the seasonal influenza vaccine for the first time should receive a second dose this season at least 4 weeks after the first dose.
- Children 6 months through 8 years of age who received seasonal influenza vaccine before the 2013–2014 influenza season
  - need only 1 dose of vaccine, if they previously received 2 or more doses of seasonal vaccine since July 1, 2010.
  - need 2 doses of vaccine, if they have not previously received 2 or more doses of seasonal vaccine since July 1, 2010.

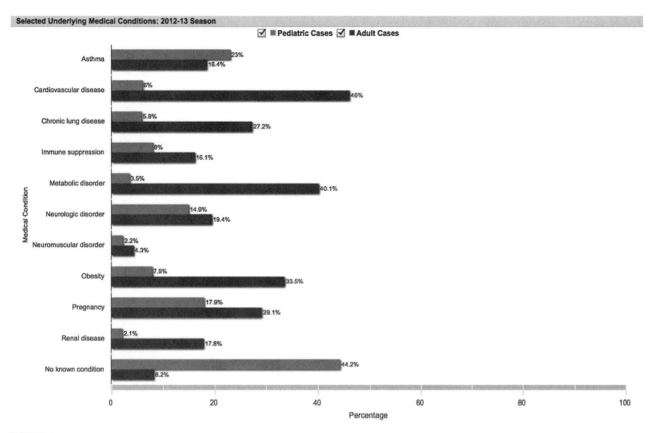

FIGURE 1

Selected underlying medical conditions in patients hospitalized with influenza, FluSurv-NET 2012–2013. Source: Centers for Disease Control and Prevention. FluView 2012–2013 Preliminary Data as of August 10, 2013. Available at: http://gis.cdc.gov/grasp/fluview/FluHospChars.html. FluSurv-NET data are preliminary and displayed as they become available. Therefore, figures are based on varying denominators because some variables represent information that may require more time to be collected. Data are refreshed and updated weekly. Asthma includes a medical diagnosis of asthma or reactive airway disease. Cardiovascular disease includes include conditions such as coronary heart disease, cardiac valve disorders, congestive heart failure, pulmonary hypertension, and aortic stenosis. It does not include hypertension disease only. Chronic lung disease includes conditions such as bronchitis obliterans, chronic aspiration pneumonia, and interstitial lung disease. Immune suppression includes conditions such as immunoglobulin deficiency, leukemia, lymphoma, HIV/AIDS, and individuals taking immunosuppression medications. Metabolic disorder includes conditions such as diabetes mellitus, thyroid dysfunction, adrenal insufficiency, and liver disease. Neurologic disorder includes conditions such as seizure disorders, cerebral palsy, and cognitive dysfunction. Neuromuscular disorder includes conditions such as multiple sclerosis and muscular dystrophy. Obesity was assigned if indicated in patients' medical chart or if BMI was >30. Pregnancy percentage was calculated using number of female cases aged between 15 and 44 years as the denominator. Renal disease includes conditions such as acute or chronic renal failure, nephrotic syndrome, glomerulonephritis, and impaired creatinine clearance. No known condition indicates that the case did not have any known underlying medical condition indicated in the medical chart at the time of hospitalization.

- need only 1 dose of influenza vaccine if there is clear documentation of having received at least 2 seasonal influenza vaccines from any previous season and at least 1 dose of a pH1N1-containing vaccine, which could have been in 1 of the seasonal vaccines (2010–2011, 2011–2012, or 2012–2013) or as the monovalent pH1N1 vaccine from 2009–2010.

Vaccination should not be delayed to obtain a specific product for either dose. Any available, age-appropriate trivalent or quadrivalent vaccine can be used. A child who receives only 1 of the 2 doses as a quadrivalent formulation is likely to be less primed against the additional B virus.

5. Pediatric offices should consider serving as alternate venues for providing influenza immunization to parents and other adults who care for children, if this approach is acceptable to both the pediatrician and the adult to be immunized.[1] There are important medical liability issues and medical record documentation requirements that need to be addressed before a pediatrician begins immunizing adults (see details at www.aapredbook.org/implementation). Pediatricians are reminded to document the recommendation for adult immunization in the vulnerable child's medical record. In addition, adults should still be encouraged to have a medical home and communicate their immunization status to their primary care provider. Immunization of close contacts of children at high risk of influenza-related complications is

Number of Seasonal Influenza Doses for Children 6 months through 8 years of age

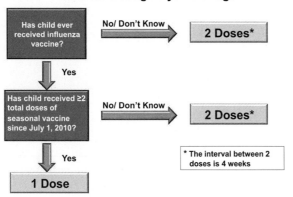

FIGURE 2

Number of 2013–2014 seasonal influenza vaccine doses for children 6 months through 8 years of age.

intended to reduce their risk of contagion (ie, "cocooning"). The concept of cocooning is particularly important to help protect infants younger than 6 months, because they are too young to be immunized with influenza vaccine. Infants younger than 6 months of age can also be protected through vaccination of their mothers during pregnancy with transplacental transfer of antibodies. The risk of influenza-associated hospitalization in healthy children aged younger than 24 months has been shown to be greater than the risk of hospitalization in previously recognized high-risk groups, such as the elderly, during influenza season. Children 24 through 59 months of age have shown increased rates of outpatient visits and antimicrobial use associated with influenza-like illnesses.

6. As soon as the seasonal influenza vaccine is available locally, HCP should be immunized, parents and caregivers should be notified about vaccine availability, and immunization of all children 6 months and older, especially children at high risk of complications from influenza, should begin. HCP endorsement plays a major role in vaccine uptake.

A strong correlation exists between HCP endorsement of influenza vaccine and patient acceptance.[2] Prompt initiation of influenza immunization and continuance of immunization throughout the influenza season, whether or not influenza is circulating (or has circulated) in the community, are critical components of an effective immunization strategy. Giving the vaccine promptly and early during the influenza season is not felt to pose a significant risk that immunity might wane before the end of the season. The seasonal vaccine is not perfect, but it still is the best strategy available for preventing illness from influenza. It is moderately effective in reducing the risk for outpatient medical visits caused by circulating influenza viruses by approximately one-half to two-thirds in most people. Even a moderately effective influenza vaccine has been shown to reduce illness, antibiotic use, doctor visits, time lost from work, hospitalizations, and deaths.

7. Providers should continue to offer vaccine until the vaccine expiration date because influenza is unpredictable. Protective immune responses persist throughout the influenza season, which can have >1 disease peak and often extends into March or later. Although most influenza activity in the United States tends to occur in January through March, influenza activity can occur in early fall (ie, October and November) or late spring (eg, influenza circulated through the third week in May during the 2012–2013 season). This approach also provides ample opportunity to administer a second dose of vaccine because children aged <9 years may require 2 doses to confer optimal protection. In addition, with international travel so common, there is potential exposure to influenza at virtually all times of the year.

8. HCP, influenza campaign organizers, and public health agencies should collaborate to develop improved strategies for planning, communication, and administration of vaccines.

● Plan to make seasonal influenza vaccine easily accessible for all children. Examples include creating walk-in influenza clinics; extending hours beyond routine times during peak vaccination periods; administering influenza vaccine during both well and sick visits; considering how to immunize parents, adult caregivers, and siblings at the same time in the same office setting as children[1]; and working with other institutions (eg, schools, child-care centers, and religious organizations) or alternative care sites, such as emergency departments, to expand venues for administering vaccine. If a child or adult receives influenza vaccine outside of his or her medical home, such as at a pharmacy or other retail-based clinic, appropriate documentation of immunization must be provided to the medical home.

- Concerted efforts among the aforementioned groups, plus vaccine manufacturers, distributors, and payers, also are necessary to prioritize distribution appropriately to the primary care office setting and patient-centered medical home before other venues, especially when vaccine supplies are delayed or limited.

- Vaccine safety, effectiveness, and indications must be properly communicated to the public. HCP should act as role models by receiving influenza immunization annually as well as recommending annual immunizations to both colleagues and patients. Influenza immunization programs for HCP benefit the health of employees, their patients, and members of the community.[2] Beginning in 2012, as an immunization core measure, the Centers for Medicare and Medicaid Services, the US federal agency that administers Medicare, Medicaid, and the State Children's Health Insurance Program, began requiring hospitals and certain other inpatient facilities to screen for a history of influenza vaccination and to administer influence vaccine to all unimmunized hospitalized patients 6 months and older between October and March unless contraindicated or the patient or family refuses.

9. Antiviral medications also are important in the control of influenza but are not a substitute for influenza immunization. The neuraminidase inhibitors oral oseltamivir (Tamiflu; Roche Laboratories, Nutley, NJ) and inhaled zanamivir (Relenza; GlaxoSmithKline, Research Triangle Park, NC) are the only antiviral medications routinely recommended for chemoprophylaxis or treatment of influenza during the 2013–2014 season. Intravenous preparations of oseltamivir, zanamivir, and peramivir are not currently approved by the US Food and Drug Administration (FDA) and are not routinely available. However, with consultation with infectious diseases specialists, experimental intravenous antiviral medications could be considered for some critically ill children, especially those who are immunocompromised. Recent viral surveillance and resistance data indicate that the majority of currently circulating influenza viruses likely to cause 2013–2014 seasonal influenza in North America continue to be sensitive to oseltamivir and zanamivir. In contrast, amantadine and rimantadine should not be used because circulating influenza A viruses have sustained high levels of resistance to these drugs, and they are not effective against influenza B viruses. Resistance characteristics may change rapidly; pediatricians should verify susceptibility data at the start of the influenza season and monitor it during the season. Up-to-date information can be found on the AAP Web site (www.aap.org or www.aapredbook.org/flu), through state-specific AAP chapter Web sites, or on the CDC Web site (www.cdc.gov/flu/index.htm).

SEASONAL INFLUENZA VACCINES

During previous influenza seasons, only trivalent influenza vaccines that included antigen from 1 influenza B virus were available. However, since 1985, 2 antigenically distinct lineages (ie, Victoria or Yamagata) of influenza B viruses have circulated globally. In most years, vaccination against a B virus of 1 lineage confers little cross-protection against a B virus strain from the other lineage. Thus, trivalent vaccines offer limited immunity against circulating influenza B strains of the lineage not present in the vaccine. Furthermore, in recent years, it has proven difficult to consistently predict which B lineage will predominate during a given influenza season. Therefore, a quadrivalent influenza vaccine with influenza B strains of both lineages may offer improved protection. Post-marketing safety and vaccine effectiveness data are not yet available, prohibiting a full risk-benefit analysis of newer versus previously available products.

For the 2013–2014 season, the inactivated influenza vaccines (IIVs) will be available for intramuscular (IM) injection in both trivalent (IIV3) and quadrivalent (IIV4) formulations. Note that the abbreviation IIV has replaced TIV (trivalent inactivated influenza vaccine) because inactivated influenza vaccines now contain either 3 or 4 virus strains. The intranasally administered live-attenuated influenza vaccine (LAIV) will be available only in a quadrivalent formulation (LAIV4). IIV4 and LAIV4 will contain the identical influenza strains anticipated to circulate during the 2013–2014 influenza season.

IIVs contain no live virus. IIV3 formulations are now available for IM and intradermal (ID) use. The IM formulation of IIV3 is licensed and recommended for children 6 months of age and older and adults, including people with and without chronic medical conditions. The most common adverse events after IIV administration are local injection site pain and tenderness. Fever may occur within 24 hours after immunization in approximately 10% to 35% of children younger than 2 years but rarely in older children and adults. Mild systemic symptoms, such as nausea, lethargy, headache, muscle aches, and chills, may occur after administration of IIV3.

An ID formulation of IIV3 is licensed for use in people 18 through 64 years of age. ID vaccine administration involves a microinjection with a shorter needle than needles used for IM administration. The most common adverse events are redness, induration, swelling, pain, and itching, which occur at the site of administration; although all adverse events occur at a slightly higher rate with the IM formulation of IIV3, the rate of pain was similar between ID and IM. Headache, myalgia, and malaise may occur and tend to occur at the same rate as that with the IM formulation of IIV3. There is no preference for IM or ID immunization with IIV3 in people 18 years or older. Therefore, pediatricians may choose to use either the IM or ID product in their late adolescent and young adult patients as well as for any adults they may be vaccinating (ie, as part of a cocooning strategy).

IIV4 is available in IM but not ID formulations. One formulation is licensed for use in children as young as 6 months of age. In children, the most common injection site adverse reactions were pain, redness, and swelling. The most common systemic adverse events were drowsiness, irritability, loss of appetite, fatigue, muscle aches, headache, arthralgia, and gastrointestinal tract symptoms. These events were reported with comparable frequency among participants receiving the licensed comparator trivalent vaccines. IIV4 is an acceptable alternative to other approved vaccines indicated for persons 6 months or older when otherwise appropriate and may offer greater protection than IIV3. The relative quantity of doses of IIV4 that will be available is not certain and likely to be limited.

During the 2010–2011 and 2011–2012 influenza seasons, increased reports of febrile seizures in the United States were noted by the Vaccine Adverse Event Reporting System and were associated with IIV3 manufactured by Sanofi Pasteur (Fluzone), mainly in children in the 12- through 23-month age group (the peak age for febrile seizures). The most common vaccine administered concomitantly with IIV3 when a febrile seizure was reported was the 13-valent pneumococcal conjugate vaccine (PCV13). This disproportionate reporting of febrile seizures did not persist through the most recent 2012–2013 influenza season. On the basis of these data, simultaneous administration of IIV and PCV13 for the 2013–2014 influenza season continues to be recommended when both vaccines are indicated.

LAIV4 is a quadrivalent live-attenuated influenza vaccine that is administered intranasally and replaces the previous trivalent formulation of LAIV (LAIV3). It is licensed by the FDA for previously healthy people aged 2 through 49 years. It is not recommended for people with a history of asthma, diabetes mellitus, or other high-risk medical conditions associated with an increased risk of complications from influenza (see Contraindications and Precautions). LAIV4 has a similar safety profile to that of LAIV3. The most commonly reported reactions in children were runny nose/nasal congestion, headache, decreased activity/lethargy, and sore throat. LAIV should not be administered to people with notable nasal congestion that would impede vaccine delivery.

Two trivalent influenza vaccines manufactured using new technologies that do not use eggs will also be available for people 18 years or older during the 2013–2014 season: ccIIV3 and recombinant influenza vaccine (RIV3). These manufacturing methods are beneficial because they would be expected to permit a more rapid scale up of vaccine production when needed, such as during a pandemic.

ccIIV3 is a trivalent cell culture–based inactivated influenza vaccine indicated for people 18 years or older, administered as an IM injection. ccIIV3 has comparable immunogenicity to US-licensed comparator vaccines. Although ccIIV3 is manufactured from virus propagated in Madin Darby Canine Kidney cells rather than embryonated eggs, before production, seed virus is created using the World Health Organization reference virus strains that have been passaged in eggs. However, egg protein is not detectable in the final vaccine, and egg allergy is not mentioned in the package insert. Contraindications are similar to those for other IIVs. The most common solicited adverse reactions included injection site pain, erythema at the injection site, headache, fatigue, myalgia, and malaise.

RIV3 is a recombinant hemagglutinin vaccine. It is indicated for people 18 through 49 years of age and is administered via IM injection. The most frequently reported adverse events were pain, headache, myalgia, and fatigue.

Tables 1 and 2 summarize information on the types of 2013–2014 seasonal influenza vaccines licensed for immunization of children and adults. With the addition of 5 newly licensed vaccines, it is likely that more than 1 type or brand of vaccine may be appropriate for vaccine recipients. However, no preferential recommendation is made for use of any influenza vaccine product over another. Vaccination should not be delayed to obtain a specific product.

A large body of scientific evidence demonstrates that thimerosal-containing vaccines are not associated with increased risk of autism spectrum disorders in children. As such, the AAP extends its strongest support to the recent World Health Organization recommendations to retain the use of thimerosal in the global vaccine supply.

Some people may still raise concerns about the minute amounts of thimerosal in IIV vaccines, and in some states, there is a legislated restriction on the use of thimerosal-containing vaccines. The benefits of protecting children against the known risks of influenza are clear. Therefore, children should receive any available formulation of IIV rather than delaying immunization while waiting for vaccines with reduced-thimerosal content or thimerosal-free vaccine. Although some formulations of IIV contain only a trace amount of thimerosal, certain types can be obtained thimerosal free. LAIV does not contain thimerosal. Vaccine manufacturers are delivering increasing amounts of thimerosal-free influenza vaccine each year.

INFLUENZA VACCINES AND EGG ALLERGY

Almost all IIV and LAIV are produced in eggs and contain measurable amounts of egg protein, expressed as the concentration of ovalbumin per dose. However, recent data have shown that IIV administered in a single, age-appropriate dose is well tolerated by virtually all recipients who have egg allergy. More conservative approaches, such as skin testing or a 2-step graded challenge, are no longer recommended. No data exist on the safety of administering LAIV to egg-allergic recipients.

As a precaution, pediatricians should continue to determine whether the presumed egg allergy is based on a mild (ie, hives alone) or severe (ie, anaphy-

laxis involving cardiovascular changes, respiratory and/or gastrointestinal tract symptoms, or reactions that required the use of epinephrine) reaction. Pediatricians should consult with an allergist for children with a history of severe reaction. Most vaccine administration to individuals with egg allergy can happen without the need for referral. Data indicate that approximately 1% of children have immunoglobulin E-mediated sensitivity to egg, and of those, a rare minority has a severe allergy.

Standard immunization practice should include the ability to respond to acute hypersensitivity reactions. Therefore, influenza vaccine should be given to people with egg allergy with the following preconditions (Fig 3):

TABLE 1 Recommended Seasonal Influenza Vaccines for Different Age Groups: United States, 2013–2014 Influenza Season

Vaccine	Trade Name	Manufacturer	Presentation	Thimerosal Mercury Content[a]	Age Group
Inactivated					
IIV3	Fluzone	Sanofi Pasteur	0.25-mL prefilled syringe	0	6–35 mo
			0.5-mL prefilled syringe	0	≥36 mo
			0.5-mL vial	0	≥36 mo
			5.0-mL multidose vial	25	≥6 mo
IIV3	Fluzone Intradermal	Sanofi Pasteur	0.1-mL prefilled microinjection	0	18–64 y
IIV3	Fluzone HD	Sanofi Pasteur	0.5-mL prefilled syringe	0	≥65 y
IIV3	Fluvirin	Novartis	0.5-mL prefilled syringe	≤1.0	≥4 y
			5.0-mL multidose vial	25	≥4 y
IIV3	Agriflu	Novartis	0.5-mL prefilled syringe	0	≥18 y
IIV3	Fluarix	GlaxoSmithKline	0.5-mL prefilled syringe	0	≥36 mo
IIV3	FluLaval	ID Biomedical Corporation of Quebec (distributed by GlaxoSmithKline)	5.0-mL multidose vial	25	≥3 y
IIV3	Afluria	CSL Biotherapies (distributed by Merck)	0.5-mL prefilled syringe	0	≥9 y[b]
			5-mL multidose vial	24.5	≥9 y[b]
ccIIV3	Flucelvax	Novartis Vaccines	0.5-mL prefilled syringe	0	≥18 y
IIV4	Fluzone Quadrivalent	Sanofi Pasteur	0.25-mL prefilled syringe	0	6-35 mo
			0.5-mL prefilled syringe	0	≥36 mo
			0.5-mL vial	0	≥36 mo
IIV4	Fluarix Quadrivalent	GlaxoSmithKline	0.5-mL prefilled syringe	0	≥36 mo
IIV4	FluLaval Quadrivalent	ID Biomedical Corporation of Quebec (distributed by GlaxoSmithKline)	5.0-mL multidose vial	25	≥3 y
Recombinant					
RIV3	FluBlok	Protein Sciences	0.5-mL vial	0	18–49 y
Live-attenuated					
LAIV4	FluMist Quadrivalent	MedImmune	0.2-mL sprayer	0	2–49 y

Data sources: American Academy of Pediatrics, Committee on Infectious Diseases. Recommendations for prevention and control of influenza in children, 2012–2013. *Pediatrics.* 2012;130 (4):780–792; Centers for Disease Control and Prevention. Prevention and control of influenza with vaccines: recommendations of the Advisory Committee on Immunization Practices (ACIP)—United States, 2012–13 influenza season. *MMWR Morb Mortal Wkly Rep.* 2012;61(32):613–618; and Centers for Disease Control and Prevention. Prevention and control of influenza with vaccines: interim recommendations of the Advisory Committee on Immunization Practices (ACIP), 2013. *MMWR Morb Mortal Wkly Rep.* 2013;62(18):356.

[a] Microgram of Hg/0.5-mL dose.

[b] Age indication per package insert is ≥5 y; however, the Advisory Committee on Immunization Practices recommends Afluria not be used in children 6 months through 8 years of age because of increased reports of febrile reactions noted in this age group. If no other age-appropriate, licensed, inactivated seasonal influenza vaccine is available for a child 5 through 8 years of age who has a medical condition that increases the child's risk of influenza complications, Afluria can be used; however, pediatricians should discuss with the parents or caregivers the benefits and risks of influenza vaccination with Afluria before administering this vaccine.

TABLE 2 LAIV4 Compared With IIV3 and IIV4

Vaccine Characteristic	LAIV4	IIV3	IIV4
Route of administration	Intranasal spray	IM or ID injection[a]	IM injection[a]
Type of vaccine	Live virus	Killed virus	Killed virus
Product	Attenuated, cold-adapted	Inactivated subvirion or surface antigen	Inactivated subvirion or surface antigen
No. of included virus strains	4 (2 influenza A, 2 influenza B)	3 (2 influenza A, 1 influenza B)	4 (2 influenza A, 2 influenza B)
Vaccine virus strains updated	Annually	Annually	Annually
Frequency of administration[b]	Annually	Annually	Annually
Approved age groups	All healthy people aged 2–49 y	All people aged ≥6 mo (ID 18–64 y)	All people aged ≥6 mo
Interval between 2 doses in children	4 wk	4 wk	4 wk
Can be given to people with medical risk factors for influenza-related complications?	No	Yes	Yes
Can be given to children with asthma or children aged 2–4 y with wheezing in the previous year?	No[c]	Yes	Yes
Can be simultaneously administered with other vaccines?	Yes[d]	Yes[d]	Yes[d]
If not simultaneously administered, can be administered within 4 wk of another live vaccine?	No, prudent to space 4 wk apart	Yes	Yes
Can be administered within 4 wk of an inactivated vaccine?	Yes	Yes	Yes

Data sources: American Academy of Pediatrics, Committee on Infectious Diseases. Recommendations for prevention and control of influenza in children, 2012–2013. *Pediatrics.* 2012;130 (4):780–792; Centers for Disease Control and Prevention. Prevention and control of influenza with vaccines: recommendations of the Advisory Committee on Immunization Practices (ACIP)—United States, 2012–13 influenza season. *MMWR Morb Mortal Wkly Rep.* 2012;61(32):613–618; and Centers for Disease Control and Prevention. Prevention and control of influenza with vaccines: interim recommendations of the Advisory Committee on Immunization Practices (ACIP), 2013. *MMWR Morb Mortal Wkly Rep.* 2013;62(18):356.

[a] The preferred site of IIV intramuscular injection for infants and young children is the anterolateral aspect of the thigh.

[b] See Fig 2 for decision algorithm to determine number of doses of seasonal influenza vaccine recommended for children during the 2013–2014 influenza season.

[c] LAIV4 is not recommended for children with a history of asthma. In the 2- through 4-year age group, there are children who have a history of wheezing with respiratory illnesses in whom reactive airways disease is diagnosed and in whom asthma may later be diagnosed. Therefore, because of the potential for increased wheezing after immunization, children 2 through 4 years of age with recurrent wheezing or a wheezing episode in the previous 12 months should not receive LAIV4. When offering LAIV4 to children in this age group, a pediatrician should screen those who might be at higher risk of asthma by asking the parents/guardians of 2-, 3-, and 4-year-olds (24- through 59-month-olds) the question: "In the previous 12 months, has a health care professional ever told you that your child had wheezing?" If the parents answer yes to this question, LAIV4 is not recommended for these children.

[d] LAIV4 coadministration has been evaluated systematically only among children 12 to 15 months of age with measles-mumps-rubella and varicella vaccines. IIV coadministration has been evaluated systematically only among adults with pneumococcal polysaccharide and zoster vaccines.

- Appropriate resuscitative equipment must be readily available.[3]
- The vaccine recipient should be observed in the office for 30 minutes after immunization, the standard observation time for receiving immunotherapy.

Providers may consider use of ccIIV3 or RIV3 vaccines produced via non-egg-based technologies for adults with egg allergy in settings in which these vaccines are available and otherwise age appropriate. Because there is no known safe threshold for ovalbumin content in vaccines, ccIIV3, which does contain trace amounts of ovalbumin, should be administered according to the guidance for other IIVs (Fig 3). In contrast, RIV3, which contains no ovalbumin, may be administered to people with egg allergy of any severity who are 18 through 49 years of age and do not have other contraindications.

However, vaccination of individuals with mild egg allergy should not be delayed if RIV3 or ccIIV3 are not available. Instead, any licensed, age-appropriate IIV should be used.

VACCINE STORAGE AND ADMINISTRATION

The AAP Storage and Handling Tip Sheet provides resources for practices to develop comprehensive vaccine management protocols to keep their vaccine supply safe during a power failure or other disaster (www2. aap.org/immunization/pediatricians/ pdf/DisasterPlanning.pdf). Any of the influenza vaccines can be administered at the same visit with all other recommended routine vaccines.

IM Vaccine

The IM formulation of IIV is shipped and stored at 2°C to 8°C (35°F–46°F). It is

administered intramuscularly into the anterolateral thigh of infants and young children and into the deltoid muscle of older children and adults. The volume of vaccine is age dependent; infants and toddlers 6 months through 35 months of age should receive a dose of 0.25 mL, and all people 3 years (36 months) and older should receive 0.5 mL/dose.

ID Vaccine

The ID formulation of IIV is also shipped and stored at 2°C to 8°C (35°F–46°F). It is administered intradermally only to people 18 through 64 years of age, preferably over the deltoid muscle, and only using the device included in the vaccine package. Vaccine is supplied in a single-dose, prefilled microinjection system (0.1 mL) for adults. The package insert should be reviewed for full administration details of this product.

Approach to Children With Presumed Egg Allergy

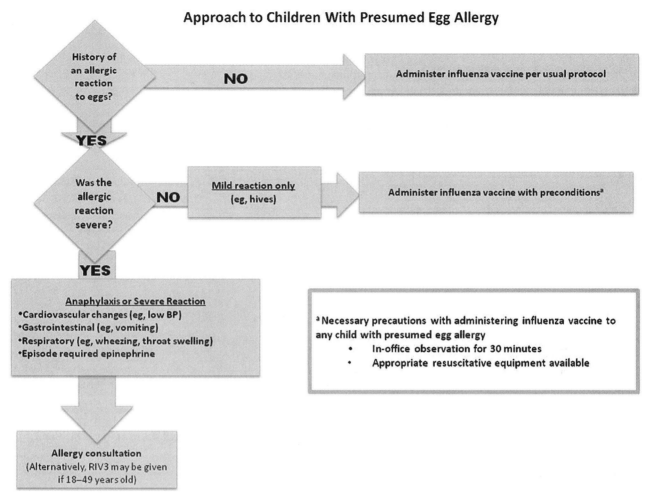

FIGURE 3
Precautions for administering IIV to presumed egg-allergic individuals. BP, blood pressure.

Live-Attenuated (Intranasal) Vaccine

The cold-adapted, temperature sensitive LAIV formulation currently licensed in the United States must be shipped and stored at 2°C to 8°C (35°F–46°F) and administered intranasally in a prefilled, single-use sprayer containing 0.2 mL of vaccine. A removable dose-divider clip is attached to the sprayer to administer 0.1 mL separately into each nostril. After administration of any live-virus vaccine, at least 4 weeks should pass before another live-virus vaccine is administered.

CURRENT RECOMMENDATIONS

Seasonal influenza immunization is recommended for all children 6 months and older. Healthy children 2 years and older can receive either IIV or LAIV. Particular focus should be on the administration of IIV for all children and adolescents with underlying medical conditions associated with an increased risk of complications from influenza, including the following:

- Asthma or other chronic pulmonary diseases, including cystic fibrosis.
- Hemodynamically significant cardiac disease.
- Immunosuppressive disorders or therapy.
- HIV infection.
- Sickle cell anemia and other hemoglobinopathies.

- Diseases that require long-term aspirin therapy, including juvenile idiopathic arthritis or Kawasaki disease.
- Chronic renal dysfunction.
- Chronic metabolic disease, including diabetes mellitus
- Any condition that can compromise respiratory function or handling of secretions or can increase the risk of aspiration, such as neurodevelopmental disorders, spinal cord injuries, seizure disorders, or neuromuscular abnormalities.

Although universal immunization for all people 6 months and older is recommended for the 2013–2014 influenza season, particular immunization

efforts with either IIV or LAIV should be made for the following groups to prevent transmission of influenza to those at risk, unless contraindicated:

- Household contacts and out-of-home care providers of children younger than 5 years of age and at-risk children of all ages (healthy contacts 2 through 49 years of age can receive either IIV or LAIV).

- Any woman who is pregnant, is considering pregnancy, has recently delivered, or is breastfeeding during the influenza season (IIV only). Studies have shown that infants born to immunized women have better influenza-related health outcomes. However, according to Internet panel surveys conducted by the CDC, only 47% of pregnant women reported receiving an influenza vaccine during the 2011–2012 season, even though both pregnant women and their infants are at higher risk of complications. In addition, data from some studies suggest that influenza vaccination in pregnancy may decrease the risk of preterm birth as well as giving birth to infants who are small for gestational age. Pregnant women can safely receive the influenza vaccine during any trimester.

- Children and adolescents of American Indian/Alaskan Native heritage.

- HCP or health care volunteers. Despite the recent AAP recommendation for mandatory influenza immunization for all HCP,[2] many HCP remain unvaccinated. As of November 2012, the CDC estimated that only 62.9% of HCP received the seasonal influenza vaccine. The AAP recommends mandatory vaccination of HCP, because they frequently come into contact with patients at high risk of influenza illness in their clinical settings.

- Close contacts of immunosuppressed people.

CONTRAINDICATIONS AND PRECAUTIONS

Minor illnesses, with or without fever, are not contraindications to the use of influenza vaccines, particularly among children with mild upper respiratory infection symptoms or allergic rhinitis.

Children Who Should Not Be Vaccinated With IIV

- Infants younger than 6 months.

- Children who have a moderate-to-severe febrile illness on the basis of clinical judgment of the clinician.

Children Who Should Not Be Vaccinated With LAIV

- Children younger than 2 years.

- Children who have a moderate-to-severe febrile illness.

- Children with an amount of nasal congestion that would notably impede vaccine delivery.

- Children with chronic underlying medical conditions, including metabolic disease, diabetes mellitus, asthma, other chronic disorders of the pulmonary or cardiovascular systems, renal dysfunction, or hemoglobinopathies.

- Children 2 through 4 years of age with a history of recurrent wheezing or a medically attended wheezing episode in the previous 12 months because of the potential for increased wheezing after immunization. In this age range, many children have a history of wheezing with respiratory tract illnesses and are eventually diagnosed with asthma. Therefore, when offering LAIV to children 24 through 59 months of age, the pediatrician should screen them by asking the parent/guardian the question, "In the previous 12 months, has a health care professional ever told you that your child had wheezing?" If a parent

answers yes to this question, LAIV is not recommended for the child. IIV would be recommended for the child to whom LAIV is not given.

- Children who have received other live-virus vaccines within the past 4 weeks; however, other live-virus vaccines can be given on the same day as LAIV.

- Children who have known or suspected immunodeficiency disease or who are receiving immunosuppressive or immunomodulatory therapies.

- Children who are receiving aspirin or other salicylates.

- Any woman who is pregnant or considering pregnancy.

- Children with any condition that can compromise respiratory function or handling of secretions or can increase the risk for aspiration, such as neurodevelopmental disorders, spinal cord injuries, seizure disorders, or neuromuscular abnormalities.

- Children taking an influenza antiviral medication should not receive LAIV until 48 hours after stopping the influenza antiviral therapy. If a child recently received LAIV but has an influenza illness for which antiviral agents are appropriate, the antiviral agents should be given. Reimmunization may be indicated because of the potential effects of antiviral medications on LAIV replication and immunogenicity.

IIV is the vaccine of choice for anyone in close contact with a subset of severely immunocompromised people (ie, individuals in a protected environment). IIV is preferred over LAIV for contacts of severely immunocompromised people (ie, in a protected environment) because of the theoretical risk of infection in an immunocompromised contact of a LAIV-immunized person. Available data indicate a low risk of transmission of the virus in both children and adults vaccinated with LAIV. HCP immunized with LAIV may continue to work in most units of a hospital, including the NICU and general oncology wards, using standard infection-control techniques. As a precautionary measure, people recently vaccinated with LAIV should restrict contact with severely immunocompromised patients (eg, hematopoietic stem cell transplant recipients during periods that require a protected environment) for 7 days after immunization, although there have been no reports of LAIV transmission from a vaccinated person to an immunocompromised person. In the theoretical scenario in which symptomatic LAIV infection develops in an immunocompromised host, oseltamivir or zanamivir could be prescribed because LAIV strains are susceptible to these antiviral medications.

SURVEILLANCE

Information about influenza surveillance is available through the CDC Voice Information System (influenza update, 888-232-3228) or at www.cdc.gov/flu/index.htm. Although current influenza season data on circulating strains do not necessarily predict which and in what proportion strains will circulate in the subsequent season, it is instructive to be aware of 2012–2013 influenza surveillance data and use them as a guide to empirical therapy until current seasonal data are available from the CDC. Information is posted weekly on the CDC Web site (www.cdc.gov/flu/weekly/fluactivity.htm).

VACCINE IMPLEMENTATION

These updated recommendations for prevention and control of influenza in children will have considerable operational and fiscal effects on pediatric practice. Therefore, the AAP has developed implementation guidance on supply, payment, coding, and liability issues; these documents can be found at www.aapredbook.org/implementation.

In addition, the AAP's Partnership for Policy Implementation has developed a series of definitions using accepted health information technology standards to assist in the implementation of this guideline in computer systems and quality measurement efforts. This document is available at www2.aap.org/informatics/PPI.html.

USE OF ANTIVIRAL MEDICATIONS

Oseltamivir remains the antiviral drug of choice for the management of influenza infections. Zanamivir is an acceptable alternative but is more difficult to administer. Antiviral resistance can emerge quickly from one season to the next. If local or national influenza surveillance data indicate a predominance of a particular influenza strain with known antiviral susceptibility profile, then empirical treatment can be directed toward that strain. For example, among 2123 influenza A (H3N2) viruses tested, 1 (0.05%) was found to be resistant to oseltamivir alone and 1 (0.05%) to both oseltamivir and zanamivir. Among the 542 pH1N1 viruses tested for resistance to oseltamivir, 2 (0.4%) were resistant, and all of the 258 viruses tested for resistance to zanamivir were sensitive. In contrast, high levels of resistance to amantadine and rimantadine exist, so these drugs should not be used in the upcoming season unless resistance patterns change significantly.

- Current treatment guidelines for antiviral medications (Table 3) are applicable to both infants and children with suspected influenza when known virus strains are circulating in the community or when infants or children are confirmed to have seasonal influenza.
- Oseltamivir is available in capsule and oral-suspension formulations. The commercially manufactured liquid formulation has a concentration of 6 mg/mL. If the commercially manufactured oral suspension is

not available, the capsule may be opened and the contents mixed with simple syrup or Oral-Sweet SF (sugar-free) by retail pharmacies to a final concentration of 6 mg/mL (Table 3, footnote a).
- Continuous monitoring of the epidemiology, change in severity, and resistance patterns of influenza strains may lead to new guidance.

Treatment should be offered for the following:

- Any child hospitalized with presumed influenza or with severe, complicated, or progressive illness attributable to influenza, regardless of influenza immunization status.
- Influenza infection of any severity in children at high risk of complications of influenza infection (Table 4).

Treatment should be considered for the following:

- Any otherwise healthy child with influenza infection for whom a decrease in duration of clinical symptoms is felt to be warranted by his or her pediatrician; the greatest impact on outcome will occur if treatment can be initiated within 48 hours of illness onset.

Reviews of available studies by the CDC, the World Health Organization, and independent investigators have consistently found that timely oseltamivir treatment can reduce the risks of complications, including those resulting in hospitalization and death. Although a 2012 Cochrane review suggested that oseltamivir may not be effective in preventing complications or hospitalizations from influenza, its authors correctly pointed out that the data reviewed were not always complete, were analyzed in a variety of treated populations, and used a number of clinical trial designs. Regardless, treatment with oseltamivir for children with presumed serious, complicated, or progressive disease, irrespective of influenza immunization status and/or even if illness began > 48 hours before admission, continues to be recommended. Earlier treatment provides optimal clinical responses. However, treatment after 48 hours of symptoms in adults and children with moderate-to-severe disease or with progressive disease has been shown to provide some benefit and should be strongly considered.

Dosages for antiviral agents for both treatment and chemoprophylaxis in children can be found in Table 3 and on the CDC Web site (http://www.cdc.gov/flu/professionals/antivirals/index.htm). Children younger than 2 years are at an increased risk of hospitalization and complications attributable to influenza. The FDA recently licensed

oseltamivir down to 2 weeks of age. Given its known safety profile, oseltamivir can be used to treat influenza in both term and preterm infants from birth.

Clinical judgment (on the basis of underlying conditions, disease severity, time since symptom onset, and local influenza activity) is an important factor in treatment decisions for pediatric patients who present with influenza-like illness. Antiviral treatment should be started as soon as possible after illness onset and should not be delayed while waiting for a definitive influenza test result. Currently available rapid antigen tests have low sensitivity, particularly for the pH1N1 virus strain, and should not be used to exclude influenza infection. Although negative results from

rapid antigen tests should not be used to make treatment or infection-control decisions, positive results are helpful because they may reduce additional testing to identify the cause of the child's influenza-like illness. Nucleic-acid-based molecular diagnostic techniques (eg, polymerase chain reaction–based) are more widely available and have greater sensitivity than antigen tests for influenza infection.

People with suspected influenza who present with an uncomplicated febrile illness typically do not require treatment with antiviral medications unless they are at higher risk of influenza complications (eg, children with chronic medical conditions such as asthma, diabetes mellitus, hemodynamically significant

TABLE 3 Recommended Dosage and Schedule of Influenza Antiviral Medications for Treatment and Chemoprophylaxis for the 2013–2014 Influenza Season: United States

Medication	Treatment (5 d)	Chemoprophylaxis (10 d)
Oseltamivir[a]		
Adults	75 mg twice daily	75 mg once daily
Children ≥12 mo		
≤15 kg (≤33 lb)	30 mg twice daily	30 mg once daily
>15–23 kg (33–51 lb)	45 mg twice daily	45 mg once daily
>23–40 kg (>51–88 lb)	60 mg twice daily	60 mg once daily
>40 kg (>88 lb)	75 mg twice daily	75 mg once daily
Infants 9 through 11 mo[b]	3.5 mg/kg/dose twice daily	3.5 mg/kg/dose once per day
Term Infants 0 through 8 mo[b]	3 mg/kg/dose twice daily[c]	3 mg/kg/dose once daily for infants 3 through 8 mo; not recommended for infants younger than 3 mo, unless situation judged critical, because of limited safety and efficacy data in this age group
Zanamivir[d]		
Adults	10 mg (two 5-mg inhalations) twice daily	10 mg (two 5-mg inhalations) once daily
Children (≥7 y for treatment, ≥5 y for chemoprophylaxis)	10 mg (two 5-mg inhalations) twice daily	10 mg (two 5-mg inhalations) once daily

Sources: Centers for Disease Control and Prevention. Antiviral agents for the treatment and chemoprophylaxis of influenza: recommendations of the Advisory Committee on Immunization Practices (ACIP). *MMWR Recomm Rep.* 2011;60(RR-1):1–24; Kimberlin DW, Acosta EP, Prichard MN, et al. National Institute of Allergy and Infectious Diseases Collaborative Antiviral Study Group. Oseltamivir pharmacokinetics, dosing, and resistance among children aged <2 y with influenza. *J Infect Dis.* 2013;207(5):709–720.

[a] Oseltamivir is administered orally without regard to meals, although administration with meals may improve gastrointestinal tolerability. Oseltamivir is available as Tamiflu in 30-mg, 45-mg, and 75-mg capsules and as a powder for oral suspension that is reconstituted to provide a final concentration of 6 mg/mL. For the 6-mg/mL suspension, a 30-mg dose is given with 5 mL of oral suspension, a 45-mg dose is given with 7.5 mL oral suspension; a 60-mg dose is given with 10 mL oral suspension, and a 75-mg dose is given with 12.5 mL oral suspension. If the commercially manufactured oral suspension is not available, a suspension can be compounded by retail pharmacies (final concentration also 6 mg/mL), based on instructions on the package label. In patients with renal insufficiency, the dose should be adjusted on the basis of creatinine clearance. For treatment of patients with creatinine clearance 10 to 30 mL/min: 75 mg once daily for 5 days. For chemoprophylaxis of patients with creatinine clearance 10 to 30 mL/min: 30 mg, once daily, for 10 days after exposure or 75 mg, once every other day, for 10 days after exposure (5 doses). See http://www.cdc.gov/flu/professionals/antivirals/antiviral-drug-resistance.htm.

[b] Approved by the FDA down to 2 weeks of age. Given its known safety profile, oseltamivir can be used to treat influenza in both term and preterm infants from birth.

[c] Oseltamivir dosing for preterm infants. The weight-based dosing recommendation for preterm infants is lower than for term infants. Preterm infants may have lower clearance of oseltamivir because of immature renal function, and doses recommended for full-term infants may lead to high drug concentrations in this age group. Limited data from the National Institute of Allergy and Infectious Diseases Collaborative Antiviral Study Group provide the basis for dosing preterm infants using their postmenstrual age (gestational age + chronological age): 1.0 mg/kg/dose, orally, twice daily, for those <38 weeks' postmenstrual age; 1.5 mg/kg/dose, orally, twice daily, for those 38 through 40 weeks' postmenstrual age; 3.0 mg/kg/dose, orally, twice daily, for those >40 weeks' postmenstrual age.

[d] Zanamivir is administered by inhalation using a proprietary "Diskhaler" device distributed together with the medication. Zanamivir is a dry powder, not an aerosol, and should not be administered using nebulizers, ventilators, or other devices typically used for administering medications in aerosolized solutions. Zanamivir is not recommended for people with chronic respiratory diseases, such as asthma or chronic obstructive pulmonary disease, which increase the risk of bronchospasm.

TABLE 4 People at Higher Risk of Influenza Complications Recommended for Antiviral Treatment of Suspected or Confirmed Influenza

Children <2 y

Adults ≥65 y

People with chronic pulmonary (including asthma), cardiovascular (except hypertension alone), renal, hepatic, hematologic (including sickle cell disease), or metabolic disorders (including diabetes mellitus) or neurologic and neurodevelopment conditions (including disorders of the brain, spinal cord, peripheral nerve, and muscle such as cerebral palsy, epilepsy [seizure disorders], stroke, intellectual disability [mental retardation], moderate to severe developmental delay, muscular dystrophy, or spinal cord injury)

People with immunosuppression, including that caused by medications or by HIV infection

Women who are pregnant or postpartum (within 2 wk after delivery)

People <19 y who are receiving long-term aspirin therapy

American Indian/Alaska Native people

People who are morbidly obese (ie, BMI ≥40)

Residents of nursing homes and other chronic-care facilities

Source: Centers for Disease Control and Prevention. Antiviral agents for the treatment and chemoprophylaxis of influenza: recommendations of the Advisory Committee on Immunization Practices (ACIP). *MMWR Recomm Rep.* 2011;60(RR-1):1–24

cardiac disease, immunosuppression, or neurologic and neurodevelopmental disorders), especially in situations with limited antiviral medication availability. Should there be a shortage of antiviral medications, local public health authorities will provide additional guidance about testing and treatment.

Randomized placebo-controlled studies showed that oseltamivir and zanamivir were efficacious when administered as chemoprophylaxis to household contacts after a family member had laboratory confirmed influenza. During the 2009 pandemic, the emergence of oseltamivir resistance was observed among people receiving postexposure prophylaxis. Decisions on whether to administer antiviral agents for chemoprophylaxis should take into account the exposed person's risk of influenza complications, vaccination status, the type and duration of contact, recommendations from local or public health authorities, and clinical judgment. Optimally, postexposure chemoprophylaxis should only be used when antiviral agents can be started within 48 hours of exposure. Early treatment of high-risk patients without waiting for laboratory confirmation is an alternative strategy.

Although immunization is the preferred approach to prevention of infection, chemoprophylaxis during an influenza outbreak, as defined by the CDC, is recommended:

● For children at high risk of complications from influenza for whom influenza vaccine is contraindicated.

● For children at high risk during the 2 weeks after influenza immunization.

● For family members or HCP who are unimmunized and are likely to have ongoing, close exposure to

  ● unimmunized children at high risk; or

  ● unimmunized infants and toddlers who are younger than 24 months.

● For control of influenza outbreaks for unimmunized staff and children in a closed institutional setting with children at high risk (eg, extended-care facilities).

● As a supplement to immunization among children at high risk, including children who are immunocompromised and may not respond to vaccine.

● As postexposure prophylaxis for family members and close contacts of an infected person if those people are at high risk of complications from influenza.

● For children at high risk and their family members and close contacts, as well as HCP, when circulating strains of influenza virus in the community are not matched with seasonal influenza vaccine strains, on the basis of current data from the CDC and local health departments.

These recommendations apply to routine circumstances, but it should be noted that guidance may change on the basis of updated recommendations from the CDC in concert with antiviral availability, local resources, clinical judgment, recommendations from local or public health authorities, risk of influenza complications, type and duration of exposure contact, and change in epidemiology or severity of influenza. Chemoprophylaxis is not recommended for infants younger than 3 months, unless the situation is judged critical, because of limited safety and efficacy data in this age group.

Chemoprophylaxis should not be considered a substitute for immunization.

Influenza vaccine should always be offered when not contraindicated, even when influenza virus is circulating in the community. Antiviral medications currently licensed are important adjuncts to influenza immunization for control and prevention of influenza disease, but there are toxicities associated with antiviral agents, and indiscriminate use might limit availability. Pediatricians should inform recipients of antiviral chemoprophylaxis that risk of influenza is lowered but remains while taking the medication, and susceptibility to influenza returns when medication is discontinued. For recommendations about treatment and chemoprophylaxis against influenza, see Table 3. Updates will be available at www.aapredbook.org/flu and http://www.cdc.gov/flu/professionals/antivirals/index.htm.

FUTURE NEEDS

Currently, within the approved indications and recommendations, no preferential recommendation is made for any type or brand of influenza vaccine over another. This is partly because the supply of newer vaccines may be limited during the 2013–2014 season. Moreover, postmarketing safety and vaccine effectiveness data are not yet available, prohibiting a full risk-benefit analysis of newer versus previously available products. However, such analyses will be performed as the data become available and, in the future, specific vaccines may be preferentially recommended for particular groups.

A large body of evidence indicates that even children with severe (anaphylactic) allergic reactions to the ingestion of eggs tolerate IIV in a single, age-appropriate dose. Examination of Vaccine Adverse Event Reporting System data after new Advisory Committee on Immunization Practices guidelines recommending influenza vaccine for egg-allergic recipients indicated no disproportionate reporting of allergy or anaphylaxis. Studies are also underway examining the safety of LAIV in egg-allergic recipients. If, as expected, additional safety monitoring continues to show no increased risk for anaphylactic reactions in egg-allergic recipients of influenza vaccine, special precautions regarding allergy referral and waiting periods after administration to egg-allergic recipients beyond those recommended for any vaccine may no longer be recommended.

Efforts should be made to create adequate outreach and infrastructure to ensure an optimal distribution of vaccine so that more people are immunized. Pediatricians should also become more involved in pandemic preparedness or disaster planning efforts. A bidirectional partner dialogue between pediatricians and public health decision makers ensures that children's issues are addressed during the initial state, regional, and local plan development stages. Further information concerning disaster preparedness can be found at www.aap.org/en-us/advocacy-and-policy/aap-health-initiatives/children-and-disasters/Pages/Pediatric-Preparedness-Resource-Kit.aspx.

Health care for children should be provided in the child's medical home. However, medical homes may have limited capacity to accommodate all patients (and their families) seeking influenza immunization. Because of the increased demand for immunization during each influenza season, the AAP and the CDC recommend vaccine administration at any visit to the medical home during influenza season when it is not contraindicated, at specially arranged "vaccine-only" sessions, and through cooperation with community sites, schools, and child care centers to provide influenza vaccine. If alternate venues are used, including pharmacies and other retail-based clinics, a system of patient record transfer is beneficial to ensuring maintenance of accurate immunization records. Immunization information systems should be used whenever available. The use of 2-dimensional barcodes may help facilitate more efficient and accurate documentation of vaccine administration. Multiple barriers appear to have an impact on influenza vaccination coverage for children in foster care, refugee and immigrant children, and homeless children. Access to care issues, lack of immunization records, and questions regarding who can provide consent may be addressed by linking children with a medical home, using all health care encounters as vaccination opportunities, and more consistently using immunization registry data.

Cost-effectiveness and logistic feasibility of vaccinating everyone continue to be concerns. With universal immunization, particular attention is being paid to vaccine supply, distribution, implementation, and financing. Potential benefits of more widespread childhood immunization among recipients, their contacts, and the community include fewer influenza cases, fewer outpatient visits and hospitalizations for influenza infection, and a decrease in the use of antimicrobial agents, absenteeism from school, and lost parent work time. To optimally administer antiviral therapy in hospitalized patients with influenza who cannot tolerate oral or inhaled antiviral agents, FDA-approved intravenous neuraminidase inhibitors for children also are needed.

Continued evaluation of the safety, immunogenicity, and effectiveness of influenza vaccine, especially for children younger than 2 years, is important. The potential role of previous influenza vaccination on overall vaccine effectiveness by virus strain and subject age in preventing outpatient medical visits, hospitalizations, and deaths continues to be explored. There is also a need for more systematic health services research on influenza vaccine uptake and refusal as well as identification of methods to enhance uptake. In addition, development of a safe, immunogenic vaccine for infants younger than 6 months is essential. Until such a vaccine is available for infants younger than 6 months, vaccination of their mothers while pregnant is the best way to protect them. Breastfeeding is also recommended to protect against influenza viruses by activating innate antiviral mechanisms, specifically type 1 interferons, in the host. Mandatory annual influenza immunization of all HCP has been implemented successfully at an increasing number of pediatric institutions. Future efforts should include broader implementation of mandatory immunization programs. Optimal prevention of influenza in the health care setting depends on the vaccination of at least 90% of HCP.

Additional studies are needed to investigate the extent of offering to immunize parents and adult child care providers in the pediatric office setting; the level of family contact satisfaction with this practice; how practices handle the logistic, liability, legal, and financial barriers that limit or complicate this service; and, most important, how this practice will affect disease rates in children and adults. In addition, adjuvants have been shown to enhance immune responses to influenza vaccines, but certain adjuvants have been associated with the development of narcolepsy in some studies. Additional studies on the effectiveness and safety of influenza vaccines containing adjuvants are needed. Finally, as mentioned earlier, efforts to improve the vaccine-development process to allow for a shorter interval between identification of vaccine strains and vaccine production continue.

COMMITTEE ON INFECTIOUS DISEASES, 2013–2014

Michael T. Brady, MD, Chairperson, *Red Book* Associate Editor
Carrie L. Byington, MD
H. Dele Davies, MD

Kathryn M. Edwards, MD
Mary Anne Jackson, MD, *Red Book* Associate Editor
Yvonne A. Maldonado, MD
Dennis L. Murray, MD
Walter A. Orenstein, MD
Mobeen Rathore, MD
Mark Sawyer, MD
Gordon E. Schutze, MD
Rodney E. Willoughby, MD
Theoklis E. Zaoutis, MD

FORMER COMMITTEE MEMBERS

John Bradley, MD
Mary P. Glode, MD
Harry L. Keyserling, MD

LIAISONS

Marc A. Fischer, MD – *Centers for Disease Control and Prevention*
Bruce Gellin, MD – *National Vaccine Program Office*
Richard L. Gorman, MD – *National Institutes of Health*
Lucia Lee, MD – *Food and Drug Administration*
R. Douglas Pratt, MD – *Food and Drug Administration*
Jennifer S. Read, MD – *Food and Drug Administration*
Joan Robinson, MD – *Canadian Pediatric Society*
Marco Aurelio Palazzi Safadi, MD – *Sociedad Latinoamericana de Infectologia Pediatrica*
Jane Seward, MBBS, MPH – *Centers for Disease Control and Prevention*
Jeffrey R. Starke, MD – *American Thoracic Society*

Geoffrey Simon, MD – *Committee on Practice Ambulatory Medicine*
Tina Q. Tan, MD – *Pediatric Infectious Diseases Society*

EX OFFICIO

Henry H. Bernstein, DO, *Red Book Online* Associate Editor
David W. Kimberlin, MD, *Red Book* Editor
Sarah S. Long, MD, *Red Book* Associate Editor
H. Cody Meissner, MD, *Visual Red Book* Associate Editor

CONTRIBUTORS

Stuart T. Weinberg, MD – *Partnership for Policy Implementation*
Jenna A. Katz, BA, and Rebecca J. Schneyer, BA – *Research Assistants, Cohen Children's Medical Center of NY*
John M. Kelso, MD

STAFF

Jennifer Frantz, MPH

ACKNOWLEDGMENTS

This AAP policy statement was prepared in parallel with CDC recommendations and reports. Much of this statement is based on literature reviews, analyses of unpublished data, and deliberations of CDC staff in collaborations with the Advisory Committee on Immunization Practices (ACIP) Influenza Working Group, with liaison from the AAP.

REFERENCES

1. Lessin HR, Edwards KM; Committee On Practice And Ambulatory Medicine; Committee on Infectious Diseases. Immunizing parents and other close family contacts in the pediatric office setting. *Pediatrics*. 2012;129(1). Available at: www.pediatrics.org/cgi/content/full/129/1/e247

2. Bernstein HH, Starke JR; American Academy of Pediatrics. Committee on Infectious Diseases. Policy statement—recommendation for mandatory influenza immunization of all health care personnel. *Pediatrics*. 2010;126 (4):809–815

3. Frush K; American Academy of Pediatrics Committee on Pediatric Emergency Medicine. Preparation for emergencies in the offices of pediatricians and pediatric primary care providers. *Pediatrics*. 2007;120 (1):200–212

ADDITIONAL RESOURCES

Committee on Infectious Diseases, American Academy of Pediatrics. Recommendations for prevention and control of influenza in children, 2012–2013. *Pediatrics*. 2012;130(4):780–792
American Academy of Pediatrics. Influenza. In: Pickering LK, Baker CJ, Long SS, Kimberlin DW, eds. *Red Book: 2012 Report of the Committee on Infectious Diseases*. 29th ed. Elk Grove Village, IL: American Academy of Pediatrics; 2012:439–453.

Available at: http://aapredbook.aappublications.org/flu
Bradley JS, Bernstein HH, Kimberlin DW, Brady MT. Antiviral therapy options critical for high-risk patients with influenza. *AAP News*. 2012;33(12):12
Fiore AE, Fry A, Shay D, Gubareva L, Bresee JS, Uyeki TM; Centers for Disease Control and Prevention. Antiviral agents for the treatment and chemoprophylaxis of influenza—recommendations

of the Advisory Committee on Immunization Practices (ACIP). *MMWR Recomm Rep*. 2011;60 (1 RR-1):1–24
Centers for Disease Control and Prevention. Prevention and control of seasonal influenza with vaccines: recommendations of the Advisory Committee on Immunization Practices (ACIP)—United States, 2013–2014 influenza season. *MMWR Recomm Rep*. 2013, in press

Englund JA, Walter EB, Fairchok MP, Monto AS, Neuzil KM. A comparison of 2 influenza vaccine schedules in 6- to 23-month-old children. *Pediatrics*. 2005;115(4):1039–1047

Harper SA, Bradley JS, Englund JA, et al; Expert Panel of the Infectious Diseases Society of America. Seasonal influenza in adults and children—diagnosis, treatment, chemoprophylaxis, and institutional outbreak management: clinical practice guidelines of the Infectious Diseases Society of America. *Clin Infect Dis*. 2009;48(8):1003–1032

Kelso JM, Greenhawt MJ, Li JT, et al. Adverse reactions to vaccines practice parameter 2012 update. *J Allergy Clin Immunol*. 2012;130(1):25–43

Kimberlin DW, Acosta EP, Prichard MN, et al; National Institute of Allergy and Infectious Diseases Collaborative Antiviral Study Group. Oseltamivir pharmacokinetics, dosing, and resistance among children aged <2 years with influenza. *J Infect Dis*. 2013;207(5):709–720

Pickering LK, Baker CJ, Freed GL, et al; Infectious Diseases Society of America. Immunization programs for infants, children, adolescents, and adults: clinical practice guidelines by the Infectious Diseases Society of America. *Clin Infect Dis*. 2009;49(6):817–840

Recommended Childhood and Adolescent Immunization Schedule—United States, 2014

• •

- *Policy Statement*

POLICY STATEMENT

Recommended Childhood and Adolescent Immunization Schedule—United States, 2014

COMMITTEE ON INFECTIOUS DISEASES

www.pediatrics.org/cgi/doi/10.1542/peds.2013-3965

doi:10.1542/peds.2013-3965

Accepted for publication Dec 4, 2013

PEDIATRICS (ISSN Numbers: Print, 0031-4005; Online, 1098-4275).

The 2014 recommended childhood and adolescent immunization schedules have been approved by the American Academy of Pediatrics, the Advisory Committee on Immunization Practices of the Centers for Disease Control and Prevention, the American Academy of Family Physicians, and the American College of Obstetricians and Gynecologists. The 2014 format is similar to last year and includes a single schedule for persons 0 through 18 years of age (Fig 1). The yellow bars indicate the recommended age range for all children and contain a notation indicating the recommended dose number by age. The green bars indicate the recommended catch-up age. The purple bars designate the range for immunization for certain groups at high risk. The combined green and purple bar indicates the recommended age when hepatitis A vaccine catch-up is recommended. The white boxes show the ages when a vaccine is not recommended routinely. The catch-up schedule offers recommendations for children and adolescents who start late or are >1 month behind (Fig 2).

Footnotes contain recommendations for routine vaccination, for catch-up vaccination, and for vaccination of children and adolescents with high-risk conditions or in special circumstances. Numerous changes have been made to improve the clarity and readability of the footnotes. A parent-friendly vaccine schedule for children and adolescents is available at http://www.cdc.gov/vaccines/schedules/index.html. An adult immunization schedule also is published in February of each year and is available at www.cdc.gov/vaccines. These schedules are revised annually to reflect current recommendations for the use of vaccines licensed by the US Food and Drug Administration and include the following specific changes from last year:

- Both generic names and trade names are referenced in the title of each vaccine footnote; thereafter, only the trade name is used, as in the rotavirus footnote.

- The Tdap footnote includes information on vaccination of persons 7 years and older with a single lifetime dose of Tdap, except for pregnant adolescents, who should be vaccinated with each pregnancy. For pregnant adolescents, administration is preferred during week 27 through week 36 of gestation, regardless of time since previous Td or Tdap.

- The *Haemophilus influenzae* type b footnote clarifies vaccination of children 12 through 59 months of age who are at increased risk because of incomplete vaccination, asplenia, HIV infection, receipt of hematopoietic stem cell transplant, or receipt of chemotherapy or radiation treatment.

- The pneumococcal vaccine footnote itemizes recommendations for PCV13 and PPSV23 use in children and adolescents at increased risk on the basis of age and degree of risk.

- The influenza vaccine footnote describes vaccine dosing for children 6 months through 8 years of age and for those 9 years of age and older for the 2013–2014 season.

- The hepatitis A vaccine footnote includes the list of persons at increased risk of hepatitis A disease.

- The HPV footnote clarifies the intervals between vaccine doses.

- The meningococcal footnote includes guidance for use of Menveo (Novartis, Cambridge, MA) starting at 2 months of age for certain persons at increased risk. Clarification is added regarding immunization of children with sickle cell disease or persistent complement component deficiency, travelers to areas where meningococcal disease is hyperendemic/epidemic, and children at risk during a community outbreak. Catch-up recommendations for persons at high risk are addressed.

Clinically significant adverse events that follow immunization should be reported to the Vaccine Adverse Event Reporting System (VAERS). Guidance about how to obtain and complete a VAERS form can be obtained at www.vaers.hhs.gov or by calling 800-822-7967. Additional information can be found in the *Red Book* and at *Red Book* Online (http://aapredbook.aappublications.org/). Statements from the Advisory Committee on Immunization Practices of the Centers for Disease Control and Prevention that contain details of recommendations for individual vaccines, including recommendations for children with high-risk conditions, are available at www.cdc.gov/vaccines/pubs/ACIP-list.htm. Information on new vaccine releases, vaccine supplies, and interim recommendations resulting from vaccine shortages and statements on specific vaccines can be found at www.aapredbook.org/news/vaccstatus.shtml and www.cdc.gov/vaccines/pubs/ACIP-list.htm.

COMMITTEE ON INFECTIOUS DISEASES, 2013–2014

Michael T. Brady, MD, Chairperson, *Red Book* Associate Editor
Carrie L. Byington, MD
H. Dele Davies, MD
Kathryn M. Edwards, MD
Mary Anne Jackson, MD, *Red Book* Associate Editor
Yvonne A. Maldonado, MD
Dennis L. Murray, MD
Walter A. Orenstein, MD
Mobeen Rathore, MD
Mark Sawyer, MD
Gordon E. Schutze, MD
Rodney E. Willoughby, MD
Theoklis E. Zaoutis, MD

LIAISONS

Marc A. Fischer, MD – *Centers for Disease Control and Prevention*
Bruce Gellin, MD – *National Vaccine Program Office*
Richard L. Gorman, MD – *National Institutes of Health*
Lucia Lee, MD – *Food and Drug Administration*
R. Douglas Pratt, MD – *Food and Drug Administration*
Jennifer S. Read, MD – *National Vaccine Program Office*
Joan Robinson, MD – *Canadian Pediatric Society*
Marco Aurelio Palazzi Safadi, MD – *Sociedad Latinoamericana de Infectologia Pediatrica (SLIPE)*
Jane Seward, MBBS, MPH – *Centers for Disease Control and Prevention*
Jeffrey R. Starke, MD – *American Thoracic Society*
Geoffrey Simon, MD – *Committee on Practice Ambulatory Medicine*
Tina Q. Tan, MD – *Pediatric Infectious Diseases Society*

EX OFFICIO

Henry H. Bernstein, DO, *Red Book* Online Associate Editor
David W. Kimberlin, MD, *Red Book* Editor
Sarah S. Long, MD, *Red Book* Associate Editor
H. Cody Meissner, MD, *Visual Red Book* Associate Editor

STAFF

Jennifer Frantz, MPH

FIGURE 1

Recommended immunization schedule for persons aged 0 through 18 years—2014. (For those who fall behind or start late, see the catch-up schedule [Fig 2].)

These recommendations must be read with the footnotes that follow. For those who fall behind or start late, provide catch-up vaccination at the earliest opportunity as indicated by the green bars in Figure 1. To determine minimum intervals between doses, see the catch-up schedule (Figure 2). School entry and adolescent vaccine age groups are in bold.

Vaccines	Birth	1 mo	2 mos	4 mos	6 mos	9 mos	12 mos	15 mos	18 mos	19–23 mos	2–3 yrs	4–6 yrs	7–10 yrs	11–12 yrs	13–15 yrs	16–18 yrs
Hepatitis B[1] (HepB)	1st dose	←—— 2nd dose ——→			←————————— 3rd dose —————————→											
Rotavirus[2] (RV) RV1 (2-dose series); RV5 (3-dose series)			1st dose	2nd dose	See footnote 2											
Diphtheria, tetanus, & acellular pertussis[3] (DTaP: <7 yrs)			1st dose	2nd dose	3rd dose			←—— 4th dose ——→				5th dose				
Tetanus, diphtheria, & acellular pertussis[4] (Tdap: ≥7 yrs)														(Tdap)		
Haemophilus influenzae type b[5] (Hib)			1st dose	2nd dose	See footnote 5		←— 3rd or 4th dose, See footnote 5 —→									
Pneumococcal conjugate[6] (PCV13)			1st dose	2nd dose	3rd dose		←—— 4th dose ——→									
Pneumococcal polysaccharide[6] (PPSV23)																
Inactivated Poliovirus[7] (IPV) (<18 yrs)			1st dose	2nd dose	←————————— 3rd dose —————————→							4th dose				
Influenza[8] (IIV; LAIV) 2 doses for some: See footnote 8					Annual vaccination (IIV only)							Annual vaccination (IIV or LAIV)				
Measles, mumps, rubella[9] (MMR)							←— 1st dose —→					2nd dose				
Varicella[10] (VAR)							←— 1st dose —→					2nd dose				
Hepatitis A[11] (HepA)							←——— 2-dose series, See footnote 11 ———→									
Human papillomavirus[12] (HPV2: females only; HPV4: males and females)														(3-dose series)		
Meningococcal[13] (Hib-MenCY ≥ 6 weeks; MenACWY-D ≥9 mos; MenACWY-CRM ≥ 2 mos)			←————————————————— See footnote 13 —————————————————→											1st dose		Booster

Legend:

- Range of recommended ages for all children
- Range of recommended ages for catch-up immunization
- Range of recommended ages for certain high-risk groups
- Range of recommended ages during which catch-up is encouraged and for certain high-risk groups
- Not routinely recommended

This schedule includes recommendations in effect as of January 1, 2014. Any dose not administered at the recommended age should be administered at a subsequent visit, when indicated and feasible. The use of a combination vaccine generally is preferred over separate injections of its equivalent component vaccines. Vaccination providers should consult the relevant Advisory Committee on Immunization Practices (ACIP) statement for detailed recommendations, available online at http://www.cdc.gov/vaccines/hcp/acip-recs/index.html. Clinically significant adverse events that follow vaccination should be reported to the Vaccine Adverse Event Reporting System (VAERS) online (http://www.vaers.hhs.gov) or by telephone (800-822-7967).Suspected cases of vaccine-preventable diseases should be reported to the state or local health department. Additional information, including precautions and contraindications for vaccination, is available from CDC online (http://www.cdc.gov/vaccines/acip) or by telephone (800-CDC-INFO [800-232-4636]).

This schedule is approved by the Advisory Committee on Immunization Practices (http://www.cdc.gov/vaccines/acip), the American Academy of Pediatrics (http://www.aap.org), the American Academy of Family Physicians (http://www.aafp.org), and the American College of Obstetricians and Gynecologists (http://www.acog.org).

NOTE: The above recommendations must be read along with the footnotes of this schedule.

FIGURE 2

Catch-up immunization schedule for persons aged 4 months through 18 years who start late or who are >1 month behind—United States, 2014.

The figure below provides catch-up schedules and minimum intervals between doses for children whose vaccinations have been delayed. A vaccine series does not need to be restarted, regardless of the time that has elapsed between doses. Use the section appropriate for the child's age. Always use this table in conjunction with Figure 1 and the footnotes that follow.

Vaccine	Minimum Age for Dose 1	Minimum Interval Between Doses			
		Dose 1 to dose 2	Dose 2 to dose 3	Dose 3 to dose 4	Dose 4 to dose 5
Persons aged 4 months through 6 years					
Hepatitis B[1]	Birth	4 weeks	8 weeks and at least 16 weeks after first dose; minimum age for the final dose is 24 weeks		
Rotavirus[2]	6 weeks	4 weeks	4 weeks		
Diphtheria, tetanus, & acellular pertussis[3]	6 weeks	4 weeks	4 weeks	6 months	6 months[3]
Haemophilus influenzae type b[5]	6 weeks	4 weeks if first dose administered at younger than age 12 months / 8 weeks (as final dose) if first dose administered at age 12 through 14 months / No further doses needed if first dose administered at age 15 months or older	4 weeks[5] if current age is younger than 12 months and first dose administered at < 7 months old / 8 weeks (as final dose)[5] if current age is younger than 12 months and first dose administered between 7 through 11 months (regardless of Hib vaccine [PRP-T or PRP-OMP] used for first dose); OR if current age is 12 through 59 months and first dose administered at younger than age 12 months; OR first 2 doses were PRP-OMP and administered at younger than 12 months. / No further doses needed if previous dose administered at age 15 months or older	8 weeks (as final dose) This dose only necessary for children aged 12 through 59 months who received 3 (PRP-T) doses before age 12 months and started the primary series before age 7 months	
Pneumococcal[6]	6 weeks	4 weeks if first dose administered at younger than age 12 months / 8 weeks (as final dose for healthy children) if first dose administered at age 12 months or older / No further doses needed for healthy children if first dose administered at age 24 months or older	4 weeks if current age is younger than 12 months / 8 weeks (as final dose for healthy children) if current age is 12 months or older / No further doses needed for healthy children if previous dose administered at age 24 months or older	8 weeks (as final dose) This dose only necessary for children aged 12 through 59 months who received 3 doses before age 12 months or for children at high risk who received 3 doses at any age	
Inactivated poliovirus[7]	6 weeks	4 weeks[7]	4 weeks[7]	6 months[7] minimum age 4 years for final dose	
Meningococcal[13]	6 weeks	8 weeks[13]	See footnote 13	See footnote 13	
Measles, mumps, rubella[9]	12 months	4 weeks			
Varicella[10]	12 months	3 months			
Hepatitis A[11]	12 months	6 months			
Persons aged 7 through 18 years					
Tetanus, diphtheria; tetanus, diphtheria, & acellular pertussis[4]	7 years[4]	4 weeks	4 weeks if first dose of DTaP/DT administered at younger than age 12 months / 6 months if first dose of DTaP/DT administered at age 12 months or older and then no further doses needed for catch-up	6 months if first dose of DTaP/DT administered at younger than age 12 months	
Human papillomavirus[12]	9 years	Routine dosing intervals are recommended[12]			
Hepatitis A[11]	12 months	6 months			
Hepatitis B[1]	Birth	4 weeks	8 weeks (and at least 16 weeks after first dose)		
Inactivated poliovirus[7]	6 weeks	4 weeks[7]	4 weeks[7]	6 months[7]	
Meningococcal[13]	6 weeks	8 weeks[13]	See footnote 13		
Measles, mumps, rubella[9]	12 months	4 weeks			
Varicella[10]	12 months	3 months if person is younger than age 13 years / 4 weeks if person is aged 13 years or older			

NOTE: The above recommendations must be read along with the footnotes of this schedule.

Footnotes — Recommended immunization schedule for persons aged 0 through 18 years—United States, 2014

For further guidance on the use of the vaccines mentioned below, see: http://www.cdc.gov/vaccines/hcp/acip-recs/index.html.
For vaccine recommendations for persons 19 years of age and older, see the adult immunization schedule.

Additional information

- For contraindications and precautions to use of a vaccine and for additional information regarding that vaccine, vaccination providers should consult the relevant ACIP statement available online at http://www.cdc.gov/vaccines/hcp/acip-recs/index.html.
- For purposes of calculating intervals between doses, 4 weeks = 28 days. Intervals of 4 months or greater are determined by calendar months.
- Vaccine doses administered 4 days or less before the minimum interval are considered valid. Doses of any vaccine administered ≥5 days earlier than the minimum interval or minimum age should not be counted as valid doses and should be repeated as age-appropriate. The repeat dose should be spaced after the invalid dose by the recommended minimum interval. For further details, see MMWR, General Recommendations on Immunization and Reports / Vol. 60 / No. 2; Table 2. Recommended and minimum ages and intervals between vaccine doses available online at http://www.cdc.gov/mmwr/pdf/rr/rr6002.pdf.
- Information on travel vaccine requirements and recommendations is available at http://wwwnc.cdc.gov/travel/page/vaccinations.htm.
- For vaccination of persons with primary and secondary immunodeficiencies, see Table 13, "Vaccination of persons with primary and secondary immunodeficiencies," in General Recommendations on Immunization (ACIP), available at http://www.cdc.gov/mmwr/pdf/rr/rr6002.pdf; and American Academy of Pediatrics. Immunization in Special Clinical Circumstances, in Pickering LK, Baker CJ, Kimberlin DW, Long SS eds. Red Book: 2012 report of the Committee on Infectious Diseases. 29th ed. Elk Grove Village, IL: American Academy of Pediatrics.

1. Hepatitis B (HepB) vaccine. (Minimum age: birth)

Routine vaccination:

At birth
- Administer monovalent HepB vaccine to all newborns before hospital discharge.
- For infants born to hepatitis B surface antigen (HBsAg)-positive mothers, administer HepB vaccine and 0.5 mL of hepatitis B immune globulin (HBIG) within 12 hours of birth. These infants should be tested for HBsAg and antibody to HBsAg (anti-HBs) 1 to 2 months after completion of the HepB series, at age 9 through 18 months (preferably at the next well-child visit).
- If mother's HBsAg status is unknown, within 12 hours of birth administer HepB vaccine regardless of birth weight. For infants weighing less than 2,000 grams, administer HBIG in addition to HepB vaccine within 12 hours of birth. Determine mother's HBsAg status as soon as possible and, if mother is HBsAg-positive, also administer HBIG for infants weighing 2,000 grams or more as soon as possible, but no later than age 7 days.

Doses following the birth dose
- The second dose should be administered at age 1 or 2 months. Monovalent HepB vaccine should be used for doses administered before age 6 weeks.
- Infants who did not receive a birth dose should receive 3 doses of a HepB-containing vaccine on a schedule of 0, 1 to 2 months, and 6 months starting as soon as feasible. See Figure 2.
- Administer the second dose 1 to 2 months after the first dose (minimum interval of 4 weeks).
- Administer the third dose at least 8 weeks after the second dose AND at least 16 weeks after the **first** dose. The final (third or fourth) dose in the HepB vaccine series should be administered **no earlier than** age 24 weeks.
- Administration of a total of 4 doses of HepB vaccine is permitted when a combination vaccine containing HepB is administered after the birth dose.

Catch-up vaccination:
- Unvaccinated persons should complete a 3-dose series.
- A 2-dose series (doses separated by at least 4 months) of adult formulation Recombivax HB is licensed for use in children aged 11 through 15 years.
- For other catch-up guidance, see Figure 2.

2. Rotavirus (RV) vaccines. (Minimum age: 6 weeks for both RV1 [Rotarix] and RV5 [RotaTeq])

Routine vaccination:
Administer a series of RV vaccine to all infants as follows:
1. If Rotarix is used, administer a 2-dose series at 2 and 4 months of age.
2. If RotaTeq is used, administer a 3-dose series at ages 2, 4, and 6 months.
3. If any dose in the series was RotaTeq or vaccine product is unknown for any dose in the series, a total of 3 doses of RV vaccine should be administered.

Catch-up vaccination:
- The maximum age for the first dose in the series is 14 weeks, 6 days; vaccination should not be initiated for infants aged 15 weeks, 0 days or older.
- The maximum age for the final dose in the series is 8 months, 0 days.
- For other catch-up guidance, see Figure 2.

3. Diphtheria and tetanus toxoids and acellular pertussis (DTaP) vaccine. (Minimum age: 6 weeks. Exception: DTaP-IPV [Kinrix]: 4 years)

Routine vaccination:
- Administer a 5-dose series of DTaP vaccine at ages 2, 4, 6, 15 through 18 months, and 4 through 6 years. The fourth dose may be administered as early as age 12 months, provided at least 6 months have elapsed since the third dose.

Catch-up vaccination:
- The fifth dose of DTaP vaccine is not necessary if the fourth dose was administered at age 4 years or older.
- For other catch-up guidance, see Figure 2.

4. Tetanus and diphtheria toxoids and acellular pertussis (Tdap) vaccine. (Minimum age: 10 years for Boostrix, 11 years for Adacel)

Routine vaccination:
- Administer 1 dose of Tdap vaccine to all adolescents aged 11 through 12 years.
- Tdap may be administered regardless of the interval since the last tetanus and diphtheria toxoid-containing vaccine.
- Administer 1 dose of Tdap vaccine to pregnant adolescents during each pregnancy (preferred during 27 through 36 weeks gestation) regardless of time since prior Td or Tdap vaccination.

Catch-up vaccination:
- Persons aged 7 years and older who are not fully immunized with DTaP vaccine should receive Tdap vaccine as 1 (preferably the first) dose in the catch-up series; if additional doses are needed, use Td vaccine. For children 7 through 10 years who receive a dose of Tdap as part of the catch-up series, an adolescent Tdap vaccine dose at age 11 through 12 years should NOT be administered. Td should be administered instead 10 years after the Tdap dose.
- Persons aged 11 through 18 years who have not received Tdap vaccine should receive a dose followed by tetanus and diphtheria toxoids (Td) booster doses every 10 years thereafter.
- Inadvertent doses of DTaP vaccine:
  - If administered inadvertently to a child aged 7 through 10 years may count as part of the catch-up series. This dose may count as the adolescent Tdap dose, or the child can later receive a Tdap booster dose at age 11 through 12 years.
  - If administered inadvertently to an adolescent aged 11 through 18 years, the dose should be counted as the adolescent Tdap booster.
- For other catch-up guidance, see Figure 2.

5. Haemophilus influenzae type b (Hib) conjugate vaccine. (Minimum age: 6 weeks for PRP-T [ACTHIB, DTaP-IPV/Hib (Pentacel) and Hib-MenCY (MenHibrix)], PRP-OMP [PedvaxHIB or COMVAX], 12 months for PRP-T [Hiberix])

Routine vaccination:
- Administer a 2- or 3-dose Hib vaccine primary series and a booster dose (dose 3 or 4 depending on vaccine used in primary series) at age 12 through 15 months to complete a full Hib vaccine series.
- The primary series with ActHIB, MenHibrix, or Pentacel consists of 3 doses and should be administered at 2, 4, and 6 months of age. The primary series with PedvaxHIB or COMVAX consists of 2 doses and should be administered at 2 and 4 months of age; a dose at age 6 months is not indicated.
- One booster dose (dose 3 or 4 depending on vaccine used in primary series) of any Hib vaccine should be administered at age 12 through 15 months. An exception is Hiberix vaccine. Hiberix should only be used for the booster (final) dose in children aged 12 months through 4 years who have received at least 1 prior dose of Hib-containing vaccine.

For further guidance on the use of the vaccines mentioned below, see: http://www.cdc.gov/vaccines/hcp/acip-recs/index.html.

5. **Haemophilus influenzae type b (Hib) conjugate vaccine (cont'd)**
- For recommendations on the use of MenHibrix in patients at increased risk for meningococcal disease, please refer to the meningococcal vaccine footnotes and also to *MMWR* March 22, 2013 / 62(RR02); 1-22, available at http://www.cdc.gov/mmwr/pdf/rr/rr6202.pdf.

Catch-up vaccination:
- If dose 1 was administered at ages 12 through 14 months, administer a second (final) dose at least 8 weeks after dose 1, regardless of Hib vaccine used in the primary series.
- If the first 2 doses were PRP-OMP (PedvaxHIB or COMVAX), and were administered at age 11 months or younger, the third (and final) dose should be administered at age 12 through 15 months and at least 8 weeks after the second dose.
- If the first dose was administered at age 7 through 11 months, administer the second dose at least 4 weeks later and a third (and final) dose at age 12 through 15 months or 8 weeks after second dose, whichever is later, regardless of Hib vaccine used for first dose.
- If first dose is administered at younger than 12 months of age and second dose is given between 12 through 14 months of age, a third (and final) dose should be given 8 weeks later.
- For unvaccinated children aged 15 months or older, administer only 1 dose.
- For other catch-up guidance, see Figure 2. For catch-up guidance related to MenHibrix, please see the meningococcal vaccine footnotes and also *MMWR* March 22, 2013 / 62(RR02); 1-22, available at http://www.cdc.gov/mmwr/pdf/rr/rr6202.pdf.

Vaccination of persons with high-risk conditions:
- Children aged 12 through 59 months who are at increased risk for Hib disease, including chemotherapy recipients and those with anatomic or functional asplenia (including sickle cell disease), human immunodeficiency virus (HIV) infection, immunoglobulin deficiency, or early component complement deficiency, who have received either no doses or only 1 dose of Hib vaccine before 12 months of age, should receive 2 additional doses of Hib vaccine 8 weeks apart; children who received 2 or more doses of Hib vaccine before 12 months of age should receive 1 additional dose.
- For patients younger than 5 years of age undergoing chemotherapy or radiation treatment who received a Hib vaccine dose(s) within 14 days of starting therapy or during therapy, repeat the dose(s) at least 3 months following therapy completion.
- Recipients of hematopoietic stem cell transplant (HSCT) should be revaccinated with a 3-dose regimen of Hib vaccine starting 6 to 12 months after successful transplant, regardless of vaccination history; doses should be administered at least 4 weeks apart.
- A single dose of any Hib-containing vaccine should be administered to unimmunized* children and adolescents 15 months of age and older undergoing an elective splenectomy; if possible, vaccine should be administered at least 14 days before procedure.
- Hib vaccine is not routinely recommended for patients 5 years or older. However, 1 dose of Hib vaccine should be administered to unimmunized* persons aged 5 years or older who have anatomic or functional asplenia (including sickle cell disease) and unvaccinated persons 5 through 18 years of age with human immunodeficiency virus (HIV) infection.
  * Patients who have not received a primary series and booster dose or at least 1 dose of Hib vaccine after 14 months of age are considered unimmunized.

6. **Pneumococcal vaccines. (Minimum age: 6 weeks for PCV13, 2 years for PPSV23)**
Routine vaccination with PCV13:
- Administer a 4-dose series of PCV13 vaccine at ages 2, 4, and 6 months and at age 12 through 15 months.
- For children aged 14 through 59 months who have received an age-appropriate series of 7-valent PCV (PCV7), administer a single supplemental dose of 13-valent PCV (PCV13).

Catch-up vaccination with PCV13:
- Administer 1 dose of PCV13 to all healthy children aged 24 through 59 months who are not completely vaccinated for their age.
- For other catch-up guidance, see Figure 2.

Vaccination of persons with high-risk conditions with PCV13 and PPSV23:
- All recommended PCV13 doses should be administered prior to PPSV23 vaccination if possible.
- For children 2 through 5 years of age with any of the following conditions: chronic heart disease (particularly cyanotic congenital heart disease and cardiac failure); chronic lung disease (including asthma if treated with high-dose oral corticosteroid therapy); diabetes mellitus; cerebrospinal fluid leak; cochlear implant; sickle cell disease and other hemoglobinopathies; anatomic or functional asplenia; HIV infection; chronic renal failure; nephrotic syndrome; diseases associated with treatment with immunosuppressive drugs or radiation therapy, including malignant neoplasms, leukemias, lymphomas, and Hodgkin disease; solid organ transplantation; or congenital immunodeficiency:
  1. Administer 1 dose of PCV13 if 3 doses of PCV (PCV7 and/or PCV13) were received previously.
  2. Administer 2 doses of PCV13 at least 8 weeks apart if fewer than 3 doses of PCV (PCV7 and/or PCV13) were received previously.

6. Pneumococcal vaccines (cont'd)
  3. Administer 1 supplemental dose of PCV13 if 4 doses of PCV7 or other age-appropriate complete PCV7 series was received previously.
  4. The minimum interval between doses of PCV (PCV7 or PCV13) is 8 weeks.
  5. For children with no history of PPSV23 vaccination, administer PPSV23 at least 8 weeks after the most recent dose of PCV13.
- For children aged 6 through 18 years who have cerebrospinal fluid leak; cochlear implant; sickle cell disease and other hemoglobinopathies; anatomic or functional asplenia; congenital or acquired immunodeficiencies; HIV infection; chronic renal failure; nephrotic syndrome; diseases associated with treatment with immunosuppressive drugs or radiation therapy, including malignant neoplasms, leukemias, lymphomas, and Hodgkin disease; generalized malignancy; solid organ transplantation; or multiple myeloma:
  1. If neither PCV13 nor PPSV23 has been received previously, administer 1 dose of PCV13 now and 1 dose of PPSV23 at least 8 weeks later.
  2. If PCV13 has been received previously but PPSV23 has not, administer 1 dose of PPSV23 at least 8 weeks after the most recent dose of PCV13.
  3. If PPSV23 has been received but PCV13 has not, administer 1 dose of PCV13 at least 8 weeks after the most recent dose of PPSV23.
- For children aged 6 through 18 years with chronic heart disease (particularly cyanotic congenital heart disease and cardiac failure), chronic lung disease (including asthma if treated with high-dose oral corticosteroid therapy), diabetes mellitus, alcoholism, or chronic liver disease, who have not received previously, then PPSV23 should be administered at least 8 weeks after any prior PCV13 dose.
- A single revaccination with PPSV23 should be administered 5 years after the first dose to children with sickle cell disease or other hemoglobinopathies; anatomic or functional asplenia; congenital or acquired immunodeficiencies; HIV infection; chronic renal failure; nephrotic syndrome; diseases associated with treatment with immunosuppressive drugs or radiation therapy, including malignant neoplasms, leukemias, lymphomas, and Hodgkin disease; generalized malignancy; solid organ transplantation; or multiple myeloma.

7. **Inactivated poliovirus vaccine (IPV). (Minimum age: 6 weeks)**
Routine vaccination:
- Administer a 4-dose series of IPV at ages 2, 4, 6 through 18 months, and 4 through 6 years. The final dose in the series should be administered on or after the fourth birthday and at least 6 months after the previous dose.

Catch-up vaccination:
- In the first 6 months of life, minimum age and minimum intervals are only recommended if the person is at risk for imminent exposure to circulating poliovirus (i.e., travel to a polio-endemic region or during an outbreak).
- If 4 or more doses are administered before age 4 years, an additional dose should be administered at age 4 through 6 years and at least 6 months after the previous dose.
- A fourth dose is not necessary if the third dose was administered at age 4 years or older and at least 6 months after the previous dose.
- If both OPV and IPV were administered as part of a series, a total of 4 doses should be administered, regardless of the child's current age. IPV is not routinely recommended for U.S. residents aged 18 years or older.
- For other catch-up guidance, see Figure 2.

8. **Influenza vaccines. (Minimum age: 6 months for inactivated influenza vaccine [IIV], 2 years for live, attenuated influenza vaccine [LAIV])**
Routine vaccination:
- Administer influenza vaccine annually to all children beginning at age 6 months. For most healthy, nonpregnant persons aged 2 through 49 years, either LAIV or IIV may be used. However, LAIV should NOT be administered to some persons, including 1) those with asthma, 2) children 2 through 4 years who had wheezing in the past 12 months, or 3) those who have any other underlying medical conditions that predispose them to influenza complications. For all other contraindications to use of LAIV, see *MMWR* 2013; 62 (No. RR-7):1-43, available at http://www.cdc.gov/mmwr/pdf/rr/rr6207.pdf.

For children aged 6 months through 8 years:
- For the 2013-14 season, administer 2 doses (separated by at least 4 weeks) to children who are receiving influenza vaccine for the first time. Some children in this age group who have been vaccinated previously will also need 2 doses. For additional guidance, follow dosing guidelines in the 2013-14 ACIP influenza vaccine recommendations, *MMWR* 2013; 62 (No. RR-7):1-43, available at http://www.cdc.gov/mmwr/pdf/rr/rr6207.pdf.
- For the 2014-15 season, follow dosing guidelines in the 2014 ACIP influenza vaccine recommendations.

For persons aged 9 years and older:
- Administer 1 dose.

For further guidance on the use of the vaccines mentioned below, see: http://www.cdc.gov/vaccines/hcp/acip-recs/index.html.

9. **Measles, mumps, and rubella (MMR) vaccine. (Minimum age: 12 months for routine vaccination)**

Routine vaccination:
- Administer a 2-dose series of MMR vaccine at ages 12 through 15 months and 4 through 6 years. The second dose may be administered before age 4 years, provided at least 4 weeks have elapsed since the first dose.
- Administer 1 dose of MMR vaccine to infants aged 6 through 11 months before departure from the United States for international travel. These children should be revaccinated with 2 doses of MMR vaccine, the first at age 12 through 15 months (12 months if the child remains in an area where disease risk is high), and the second dose at least 4 weeks later.
- Administer 2 doses of MMR vaccine to children aged 12 months and older before departure from the United States for international travel. The first dose should be administered on or after age 12 months and the second dose at least 4 weeks later.

Catch-up vaccination:
- Ensure that all school-aged children and adolescents have had 2 doses of MMR vaccine; the minimum interval between the 2 doses is 4 weeks.

10. **Varicella (VAR) vaccine. (Minimum age: 12 months)**

Routine vaccination:
- Administer a 2-dose series of VAR vaccine at ages 12 through 15 months and 4 through 6 years. The second dose may be administered before age 4 years, provided at least 3 months have elapsed since the first dose. If the second dose was administered at least 4 weeks after the first dose, it can be accepted as valid.

Catch-up vaccination:
- Ensure that all persons aged 7 through 18 years without evidence of immunity (see *MMWR* 2007; 56 [No. RR-4], available at http://www.cdc.gov/mmwr/pdf/rr/rr5604.pdf) have 2 doses of varicella vaccine. For children aged 7 through 12 years, the recommended minimum interval between doses is 3 months (if the second dose was administered at least 4 weeks after the first dose, it can be accepted as valid); for persons aged 13 years and older, the minimum interval between doses is 4 weeks.

11. **Hepatitis A (HepA) vaccine. (Minimum age: 12 months)**

Routine vaccination:
- Initiate the 2-dose HepA vaccine series at 12 through 23 months; separate the 2 doses by 6 to 18 months.
- Children who have received 1 dose of HepA vaccine before age 24 months should receive a second dose 6 to 18 months after the first dose.
- For any person aged 2 years and older who has not already received the HepA vaccine series, 2 doses of HepA vaccine separated by 6 to 18 months may be administered if immunity against hepatitis A virus infection is desired.

Catch-up vaccination:
- The minimum interval between the two doses is 6 months.

Special populations:
- Administer 2 doses of HepA vaccine at least 6 months apart to previously unvaccinated persons who live in areas where vaccination programs target older children, or who are at increased risk for infection. This includes persons traveling to or working in countries that have high or intermediate endemicity of infection; men having sex with men; users of injection and non-injection illicit drugs; persons who work with HAV-infected primates or with HAV in a research laboratory; persons with clotting-factor disorders; persons with chronic liver disease; and persons who anticipate close, personal contact (e.g., household or regular babysitting) with an international adoptee during the first 60 days after arrival in the United States from a country with high or intermediate endemicity. The first dose should be administered as soon as the adoption is planned, ideally 2 or more weeks before the arrival of the adoptee.

12. **Human papillomavirus (HPV) vaccines. (Minimum age: 9 years for HPV2 [Cervarix] and HPV4 [Gardasil])**

Routine vaccination:
- Administer a 3-dose series of HPV vaccine on a schedule of 0, 1-2, and 6 months to all adolescents aged 11 through 12 years. Either HPV4 or HPV2 may be used for females, and only HPV4 may be used for males.
- The vaccine series may be started at age 9 years.
- Administer the second dose 1 to 2 months after the first dose (minimum interval of 4 weeks), administer the third dose 24 weeks after the first dose and 16 weeks after the second dose (minimum interval of 12 weeks).

Catch-up vaccination:
- Administer the vaccine series to females (either HPV2 or HPV4) and males (HPV4) at age 13 through 18 years if not previously vaccinated.
- Use recommended routine dosing intervals (see above) for vaccine series catch-up.

13. **Meningococcal conjugate vaccines. (Minimum age: 6 weeks for Hib-MenCY [MenHibrix], 9 months for MenACWY-D [Menactra], 2 months for MenACWY-CRM [Menveo])**

Routine vaccination:
- Administer a single dose of Menactra or Menveo vaccine at age 11 through 12 years, with a booster dose at age 16 years.
- Adolescents aged 11 through 18 years with human immunodeficiency virus (HIV) infection should receive a 2-dose primary series of Menactra or Menveo with at least 8 weeks between doses.
- For children aged 2 months through 18 years with high-risk conditions, see below.

Catch-up vaccination:
- Administer Menactra or Menveo vaccine at age 13 through 18 years if not previously vaccinated.
- If the first dose is administered at age 13 through 15 years, a booster dose should be administered at age 16 through 18 years with a minimum interval of at least 8 weeks between doses.
- If the first dose is administered at age 16 years or older, a booster dose is not needed.
- For other catch-up guidance, see Figure 2.

Vaccination of persons with high-risk conditions and other persons at increased risk of disease:
- Children with anatomic or functional asplenia (including sickle cell disease):
  1. For children younger than 19 months of age, administer a 4-dose infant series of MenHibrix or Menveo at 2, 4, 6, and 12 through 15 months of age.
  2. For children aged 19 through 23 months who have not completed a series of MenHibrix or Menveo, administer 2 primary doses of Menveo at least 3 months apart.
  3. For children aged 24 months and older who have not received a complete series of MenHibrix or Menveo or Menactra, administer 2 primary doses of either Menactra or Menveo at least 2 months apart. If Menactra is administered to a child with asplenia (including sickle cell disease), do not administer Menactra until 2 years of age and at least 4 weeks after the completion of all PCV13 doses.
- Children with persistent complement component deficiency:
  1. For children younger than 19 months of age, administer a 4-dose infant series of either MenHibrix or Menveo at 2, 4, 6, and 12 through 15 months of age.
  2. For children 7 through 23 months who have not initiated vaccination, two options exist depending on age and vaccine brand:
     a. For children who initiate vaccination with Menveo at 7 months through 23 months of age, a 2-dose series should be administered with the second dose after 12 months of age and at least 3 months after the first dose.
     b. For children who initiate vaccination with Menactra at 9 months through 23 months of age, a 2-dose series of Menactra should be administered at least 3 months apart.
     c. For children aged 24 months and older who have not received a complete series of MenHibrix, Menveo, or Menactra, administer 2 primary doses of either Menactra or Menveo at least 2 months apart.
- For children who travel to or reside in countries in which meningococcal disease is hyperendemic or epidemic, including countries in the African meningitis belt or the Hajj, administer an age-appropriate formulation and series of Menactra or Menveo for protection against serogroups A and W meningococcal disease. Prior receipt of MenHibrix is not sufficient for children traveling to the meningitis belt or the Hajj because it does not contain serogroups A or W.
- For children at risk during a community outbreak attributable to a vaccine serogroup, administer or complete an age- and formulation-appropriate series of MenHibrix, Menactra, or Menveo.
- For booster doses among persons with high-risk conditions, refer to *MMWR* 2013 62(RR02); 1-22, available at http://www.cdc.gov/mmwr/preview/mmwrhtml/rr6202a1.htm.

Catch-up recommendations for persons with high-risk conditions:
  1. If MenHibrix is administered to achieve protection against meningococcal disease, a complete age-appropriate series of MenHibrix should be administered.
  2. If the first dose of MenHibrix is given at or after 12 months of age, a total of 2 doses should be given at least 8 weeks apart to ensure protection against serogroups C and Y meningococcal disease.
  3. For children who initiate vaccination with Menveo at 7 months through 9 months of age, a 2-dose series should be administered with the second dose after 12 months of age and at least 3 months after the first dose.
  4. For other catch-up recommendations for these persons, refer to *MMWR* 2013 62(RR02); 1-22, available at http://www.cdc.gov/mmwr/preview/mmwrhtml/rr6202a1.htm.

For complete information on use of meningococcal vaccines, including guidance related to vaccination of persons at increased risk of infection, see *MMWR* March 22, 2013 / 62(RR02);1-22, available at http://www.cdc.gov/mmwr/pdf/rr/rr6202.pdf.

Respiratory Support in Preterm Infants at Birth

- *Policy Statement*

POLICY STATEMENT

Respiratory Support in Preterm Infants at Birth

COMMITTEE ON FETUS AND NEWBORN

KEY WORDS

respiratory distress syndrome, preterm infant, neonate, surfactant, continuous positive airway pressure, bronchopulmonary dysplasia

ABBREVIATIONS

BPD—bronchopulmonary dysplasia
CI—confidence interval
CPAP—continuous positive airway pressure
INSURE—intubation, surfactant, and extubation
RDS—respiratory distress syndrome
RR—relative risk

www.pediatrics.org/cgi/doi/10.1542/peds.2013-3442

doi:10.1542/peds.2013-3442

PEDIATRICS (ISSN Numbers: Print, 0031-4005; Online, 1098-4275).

abstract

Current practice guidelines recommend administration of surfactant at or soon after birth in preterm infants with respiratory distress syndrome. However, recent multicenter randomized controlled trials indicate that early use of continuous positive airway pressure with subsequent selective surfactant administration in extremely preterm infants results in lower rates of bronchopulmonary dysplasia/death when compared with treatment with prophylactic or early surfactant therapy. Continuous positive airway pressure started at or soon after birth with subsequent selective surfactant administration may be considered as an alternative to routine intubation with prophylactic or early surfactant administration in preterm infants. *Pediatrics* 2014;133:171–174

BACKGROUND

Current practice guidelines in neonatology recommend administration of surfactant at or soon after birth in preterm infants with respiratory distress syndrome (RDS).[1] However, recent multicenter randomized controlled trials indicate that nasal continuous positive airway pressure (CPAP) may be an effective alternative to prophylactic or early surfactant administration.[2–8] Respiratory support is being achieved more frequently with CPAP and other less invasive approaches, such as the technique of intubation, surfactant, and extubation (INSURE).[9]

Experimental evidence documents that mechanical ventilation, particularly in the presence of surfactant deficiency, results in lung injury. Early randomized clinical trials demonstrated that surfactant administration in infants with established RDS decreased mortality, bronchopulmonary dysplasia (BPD), and pneumothorax.[10] Subsequent trials indicated that early selective administration of surfactant results in fewer pneumothoraces, less pulmonary interstitial emphysema, less BPD, and lower mortality compared with delayed selective surfactant therapy.[11] Trials of prophylactic administration of surfactant demonstrated decreased air leaks and mortality compared with selective surfactant therapy.[12] However, infants enrolled in these trials did not consistently receive early CPAP, an alternative therapy for the maintenance of functional residual capacity. Furthermore, control infants were intubated and mechanically ventilated without exogenous surfactant.

The INSURE strategy also resulted in fewer air leaks and shorter duration of ventilation when compared with later selective surfactant administration with continued ventilation. However, oxygen need and survival at 36 weeks' postmenstrual age or longer-term outcomes were not assessed in these trials.[13] It is also worth noting that the INSURE studies did not consistently use early CPAP in the control group. In fact, a recent large trial not included in this meta-analysis did not show a benefit of the INSURE strategy when compared with early CPAP.[7] The INSURE strategy may be more efficacious if an infant can be rapidly extubated. Studies in baboons have demonstrated an increase in the severity of pulmonary injury when extubation to CPAP is delayed, thus reducing the benefits of surfactant administration.[14] Decisions on extubation may have to be individualized, because some critically ill infants may not benefit from rapid extubation. Further research is needed to test the potential benefits of the INSURE strategy on important long-term outcomes. However, rapid extubation after surfactant administration may not be achievable or desirable in the most immature infants, and decisions to extubate should be individualized.

CPAP can be delivered by several noninvasive techniques such as nasal prongs, nasopharyngeal tube, or mask by using a water-bubbling system (bubble CPAP) or a ventilator. Although physician preference for bubble or ventilator CPAP is common, physiologic and clinical studies have been inconclusive. It is feasible to provide noninvasive nasal CPAP starting in the delivery room, even in extremely preterm infants (24–27 weeks' gestation), but the most immature infants had the highest risk of failure.[6] Noninvasive modes of ventilation, such as nasal intermittent ventilation, do not appear to provide further benefits compared with CPAP.[15]

RANDOMIZED CONTROLLED TRIALS OF NASAL CPAP STARTING AT BIRTH

Recently published large, multicenter randomized controlled trials of prophylactic or early CPAP have enrolled very immature infants, a group that, in previous trials, benefited from surfactant treatment. The COIN (CPAP or INtubation) Trial of the Australasian Trial Network compared the effectiveness of nasal CPAP (8 cm of water pressure) to intubation and mechanical ventilation in preterm infants who were breathing spontaneously at 5 minutes after birth.[4] There was a trend for a lower rate of death or BPD in infants who received CPAP and used fewer corticosteroids postnatally. The mean duration of ventilation was shorter in the CPAP group (3 days in the CPAP group and 4 days in the ventilator group). However, the CPAP group had a higher rate of pneumothorax than the ventilator group (9% vs 3%; $P < .001$). Although surfactant therapy was not required for intubated infants, three-quarters of the intubation cohort received surfactant. Similarly, 46% of infants in the CPAP group required ventilator support, and 50% received surfactant. Therefore, the comparison was between early CPAP (with 50% of infants ultimately receiving surfactant) and intubation and ventilation, mostly but not always with surfactant administration.

The largest CPAP trial ($N = 1310$), the Surfactant Positive Pressure and Pulse Oximetry Randomized Trial (SUPPORT) conducted by the *Eunice Kennedy Shriver* National Institutes of Health and Human Development Neonatal Research Network investigators, was designed to evaluate nasal CPAP started immediately after birth by using a limited-ventilation strategy compared with prophylactic surfactant therapy and ventilator support started within 60 minutes after birth by using a limited ventilation strategy in infants born at 24 to 27 weeks' gestation.[5] This trial used prospectively defined criteria for intubation and extubation. The rate of death or BPD in the CPAP group was 48% compared with 51% in the surfactant group (relative risk [RR]: 0.91; 95% confidence interval [CI]: 0.83–1.01; $P = .07$). Among infants born at 24 and 25 weeks' gestation, the death rate was lower in the CPAP group than in the surfactant group (20% vs 29%; RR: 0.68; 95% CI: 0.5–0.92; $P = .01$). Two-thirds of the infants in the CPAP group ultimately received surfactant. In addition, duration of mechanical ventilation was shorter (25 vs 28 days), and use of postnatal corticosteroid therapy was reduced in the CPAP group (7% vs 13%). The rate of air leaks did not differ between the groups, and there were no adverse effects of the CPAP strategy despite a reduction in the use of surfactant. This trial demonstrated that nasal CPAP started immediately after birth is an effective and safe alternative to prophylactic or early surfactant administration and may be superior. A follow-up study at 18 to 22 months' corrected age showed that death or neurodevelopmental impairment occurred in 28% of the infants in the CPAP group compared with 30% of those in the surfactant/ventilation group (RR: 0.93; 95% CI: 0.78–1.10; $P = .38$).[16] CPAP and the limited-ventilation strategy, rather than intubation and surfactant, resulted in less respiratory morbidity by 18 to 22 months' corrected age.[17]

The Vermont Oxford Network Delivery Room Management Trial randomly assigned infants born at 26 to 29 weeks' gestation to 1 of 3 treatment groups: prophylactic surfactant and continued ventilation, prophylactic surfactant and extubation to CPAP, or CPAP (without surfactant).[7] There were no statistically significant differences between the 3 groups, but when compared with the prophylactic surfactant group, the RR of BPD or death was 0.83 (95% CI: 0.64–1.09) for the CPAP group and 0.78 (95% CI: 0.59–1.03) for the INSURE group.

Other trials have compared early CPAP with prophylactic or early surfactant administration. The CURPAP[2] and Colombian Network[3] trials did not demonstrate a difference in the rate of BPD between the 2 treatment strategies. Moreover, in the Columbian Network trial,[3] infants randomly assigned to prophylactic CPAP had a higher risk of pneumothorax (9%) than infants randomly assigned to INSURE (2%). Infants in the South American Neocosur Network trial were randomly assigned to early CPAP (with rescue using an INSURE strategy) or oxygen hood (with rescue using mechanical ventilation).[8] The early CPAP strategy (and selective of INSURE, if needed) reduced the need for mechanical ventilation and surfactant.

Standard but diverse CPAP systems have been used in these and other large randomized controlled trials reviewed, including bubble CPAP and ventilator CPAP. A detailed description of the practical aspects of using CPAP systems are beyond the scope of this statement but are available in the published literature.[18,19]

Preterm infants are frequently born precipitously in hospitals without the capability of CPAP. CPAP can be provided with a bag and mask or other comparable devices in these circumstances. However, special expertise is necessary because CPAP may not be easy to use without specific training. Safe transport before delivery may be preferable depending on clinical circumstances.

Thus, care should be individualized on the basis of the capabilities of health workers in addition to the patient's condition.

A meta-analysis of prophylactic surfactant versus prophylactic stabilization with CPAP and subsequent selective surfactant administration in preterm infants showed that prophylactic administration of surfactant compared with stabilization with CPAP and selective surfactant administration was associated with a higher risk of death or BPD (RR: 1.12; 95% CI: 1.02–1.24; $P <$ .05).[11] The previously reported benefits of prophylactic surfactant could no longer be demonstrated.

It is notable that infants as immature as 24 weeks' gestational age were enrolled in many of the trials. In a subgroup analysis in the SUPPORT trial, the most immature infants (born at 24 and 25 weeks' gestation) benefited the most from the CPAP strategy. Many extremely preterm infants can be managed with CPAP only; early application of nasal CPAP (without surfactant administration) was successful in 50% of infants weighing ≤750 g at birth in 1 retrospective review.[20]

Surfactant administration can be expensive, particularly in low-resource settings. Additionally, intubation and mechanical ventilation may not be possible or desirable in institutions with limited resources. CPAP provides an alternative for early respiratory support in resource-limited settings. Emerging evidence indicates that early CPAP is an effective strategy for respiratory support in extremely preterm infants, including very immature infants. CPAP appears to be at least as safe and effective as early surfactant therapy with mechanical ventilation.[9]

CONCLUSIONS

1. Based on a meta-analysis of prophylactic surfactant versus CPAP

as well as on other trials of more selective early use of surfactant versus CPAP not included in the meta-analysis, the early use of CPAP with subsequent selective surfactant administration in extremely preterm infants results in lower rates of BPD/death when compared with treatment with prophylactic or early surfactant therapy (Level of Evidence: 1).

2. Preterm infants treated with early CPAP alone are not at increased risk of adverse outcomes if treatment with surfactant is delayed or not given (Level of Evidence: 1).

3. Early initiation of CPAP may lead to a reduction in duration of mechanical ventilation and postnatal corticosteroid therapy (Level of Evidence: 1).

4. Infants with RDS may vary markedly in the severity of the respiratory disease, maturity, and presence of other complications, and thus it is necessary to individualize patient care. Care for these infants is provided in a variety of care settings, and thus the capabilities of the health care team need to be considered.

RECOMMENDATION

1. Using CPAP immediately after birth with subsequent selective surfactant administration may be considered as an alternative to routine intubation with prophylactic or early surfactant administration in preterm infants (Level of Evidence: 1, Strong Recommendation).[21] If it is likely that respiratory support with a ventilator will be needed, early administration of surfactant followed by rapid extubation is preferable to prolonged ventilation (Level of Evidence: 1, Strong Recommendation).[21]

LEAD AUTHORS

Waldemar A. Carlo, MD, FAAP
Richard A. Polin, MD, FAAP

**COMMITTEE ON FETUS AND
NEWBORN, 2012–2013**

Lu-Ann Papile, MD, FAAP, Chairperson
Richard A. Polin, MD, FAAP
Waldemar A. Carlo, MD, FAAP
Rosemarie Tan, MD, FAAP

Praveen Kumar, MD, FAAP
William Benitz, MD, FAAP
Eric Eichenwald, MD, FAAP
James Cummings, MD, FAAP
Jill Baley, MD, FAAP

LIAISONS

Tonse N. K. Raju, MD, FAAP — *National Institutes
of Health*
CAPT Wanda Denise Barfield, MD, FAAP — *Centers
for Disease Control and Prevention*

Erin Keels, MSN — *National Association of
Neonatal Nurses*
Anne Jefferies, MD — *Canadian Pediatric Society*
Kasper S. Wang, MD, FAAP — *AAP Section on
Surgery*
George Macones, MD — *American College of
Obstetricians and Gynecologists*

STAFF

Jim Couto, MA

REFERENCES

1. Engle WA; American Academy of Pediatrics Committee on Fetus and Newborn. Surfactant-replacement therapy for respiratory distress in the preterm and term neonate. *Pediatrics.* 2008;121(2):419–432

2. Sandri F, Ancora G, Lanzoni A, et al. Prophylactic nasal continuous positive airways pressure in newborns of 28-31 weeks gestation: multicentre randomised controlled clinical trial. *Arch Dis Child Fetal Neonatal Ed.* 2004;89(5):F394–F398

3. Rojas MA, Lozano JM, Rojas MX, et al; Colombian Neonatal Research Network. Very early surfactant without mandatory ventilation in premature infants treated with early continuous positive airway pressure: a randomized, controlled trial. *Pediatrics.* 2009;123(1):137–142

4. Morley CJ, Davis PG, Doyle LW, Brion LP, Hascoet JM, Carlin JB; COIN Trial Investigators. Nasal CPAP or intubation at birth for very preterm infants. *N Engl J Med.* 2008;358(7):700–708

5. Finer NN, Carlo WA, Walsh MC, et al; SUPPORT Study Group of the Eunice Kennedy Shriver NICHD Neonatal Research Network. Early CPAP versus surfactant in extremely preterm infants. *N Engl J Med.* 2010;362 (21):1970–1979

6. Finer NN, Carlo WA, Duara S, et al; National Institute of Child Health and Human Development Neonatal Research Network. Delivery room continuous positive airway pressure/positive end-expiratory pressure in extremely low birth weight infants: a feasibility trial. *Pediatrics.* 2004;114(3):651–657

7. Dunn MS, Kaempf J, de Klerk A, et al; Vermont Oxford Network DRM Study Group. Randomized trial comparing 3 approaches

to the initial respiratory management of preterm neonates. *Pediatrics.* 2011;128(5). Available at: www.pediatrics.org/cgi/content/full/128/5/e1069

8. Tapia JL, Urzua S, Bancalari A, et al; South American Neocosur Network. Randomized trial of early bubble continuous positive airway pressure for very low birth weight infants. *J Pediatr.* 2012;161(1):75–80, e1

9. Pfister RH, Soll RF. Initial respiratory support of preterm infants: the role of CPAP, the INSURE method, and noninvasive ventilation. *Clin Perinatol.* 2012;39(3):459–481

10. Soll RF, McQueen MC. Respiratory distress syndrome. In: Sinclair JC, Bracken B, eds. *Effective Care of the Newborn Infant.* Oxford, United Kingdom: Oxford University Press; 1992:325–358

11. Bahadue FL, Soll R. Early versus delayed selective surfactant treatment for neonatal respiratory distress syndrome. *Cochrane Database Syst Rev.* 2012;11(11): CD001456

12. Rojas-Reyes MX, Morley CJ, Soll R. Prophylactic versus selective use of surfactant in preventing morbidity and mortality in preterm infants. *Cochrane Database Syst Rev.* 2012;3(3):CD000510

13. Stevens TP, Harrington EW, Blennow M, Soll RF. Early surfactant administration with brief ventilation vs. selective surfactant and continued mechanical ventilation for preterm infants with or at risk for respiratory distress syndrome. *Cochrane Database Syst Rev.* 2007;(4):CD003063

14. Thomson MA, Yoder BA, Winter VT, Giavedoni L, Chang LY, Coalson JJ. Delayed extubation to nasal continuous positive airway pressure in the immature baboon model of

bronchopulmonary dysplasia: lung clinical and pathological findings. *Pediatrics.* 2006; 118(5):2038–2050

15. Kirpalani H, Millar D, Lemyre B, Yoder B, Chiu A, Roberts R. Nasal intermittent positive pressure (NIPPV) does not confer benefit above nasal CPAP (nCPAP) in extremely low birth weight (ELBW) infants <1000 g BW—the NIPPV International Randomized Controlled Trial [abstract]. E-PAS2012:1675.1.Available at: www.abstracts2-view.com/pas/view.php?nu=PAS12L1_511. Accessed February 7, 2013

16. Vaucher YE, Peralta-Carcelen M, Finer NN, et al; SUPPORT Study Group of the Eunice Kennedy Shriver NICHD Neonatal Research Network. Neurodevelopmental outcomes in the early CPAP and pulse oximetry trial. *N Engl J Med.* 2012;367(26):2495–2504

17. Stevens TP, Finer NN, Carlo WA, et al. Respiratory outcomes of the early CPAP and pulse oximetry trial. In: Pediatric Academic Societies Annual Meeting; May 4–7, 2013; Washington, DC. Abstract

18. Polin RA, Sahni R. Continuous positive airway pressure: old questions and new controversies. *J Neo Peri Med.* 2008;1(1):1–10

19. Sahni R, Wung JT. Continuous positive airway pressure (CPAP). *Indian J Pediatr.* 1998;65(2):265–271

20. Ammari A, Suri M, Milisavljevic V, et al. Variables associated with the early failure of nasal CPAP in very low birth weight infants. *J Pediatr.* 2005;147(3):341–347

21. American Academy of Pediatrics Steering Committee on Quality Improvement and Management. Classifying recommendations for clinical practice guidelines. *Pediatrics.* 2004;114(3):874–877

Returning to Learning Following a Concussion

- *Clinical Report*

CLINICAL REPORT

Returning to Learning Following a Concussion

abstract

Following a concussion, it is common for children and adolescents to experience difficulties in the school setting. Cognitive difficulties, such as learning new tasks or remembering previously learned material, may pose challenges in the classroom. The school environment may also increase symptoms with exposure to bright lights and screens or noisy cafeterias and hallways. Unfortunately, because most children and adolescents look physically normal after a concussion, school officials often fail to recognize the need for academic or environmental adjustments. Appropriate guidance and recommendations from the pediatrician may ease the transition back to the school environment and facilitate the recovery of the child or adolescent. This report serves to provide a better understanding of possible factors that may contribute to difficulties in a school environment after a concussion and serves as a framework for the medical home, the educational home, and the family home to guide the student to a successful and safe return to learning. *Pediatrics* 2013;132:948–957

Mark E. Halstead, MD, FAAP, Karen McAvoy, PsyD, Cynthia D. Devore, MD, FAAP, Rebecca Carl, MD, FAAP, Michael Lee, MD, FAAP, Kelsey Logan, MD, FAAP, Council on Sports Medicine and Fitness, and Council on School Health

KEY WORDS
head injury, mild traumatic brain injury, pediatrics, return to school, academics, return to learn, cognitive deficits

ABBREVIATIONS
AT—certified athletic trainer
FERPA—Family Educational Rights and Privacy Act
HIPAA—Health Insurance Portability and Accountability Act
IEP—individualized education plan
IDEA—Individuals with Disabilities Education Act
RTL—return to learn

This document is copyrighted and is property of the American Academy of Pediatrics and its Board of Directors. All authors have filed conflict of interest statements with the American Academy of Pediatrics. Any conflicts have been resolved through a process approved by the Board of Directors. The American Academy of Pediatrics has neither solicited nor accepted any commercial involvement in the development of the content of this publication.

The guidance in this report does not indicate an exclusive course of treatment or serve as a standard of medical care. Variations, taking into account individual circumstances, may be appropriate.

DEFINITIONS

- Individualized education plan (IEP): a formalized educational plan protected under the Individuals with Disabilities Education Act (IDEA; Pub L No. 101-476, 1990), known commonly as special education, that provides for classification or coding of a student under 1 of 13 federally designated categories and allowances for modification of regular education without penalty to the student.

- 504 plan: under Section 504 of the Rehabilitation Act (Pub L No. 93-112, 1973) and the Americans with Disabilities Act (Pub L No. 101-336, 1990), provides for a student who is not eligible for special education under an IEP but who requires accommodations in regular education on the basis of bona fide medical need, as documented by a physician and validation by the educational home.

- Individualized health care plan: a written document created by a school nurse on the basis of information provided by the student's pediatrician to document specific health care needs in the school setting with a plan for addressing each documented need.

- Family Educational Rights and Privacy Act (FERPA): a federal law established in 1974 (Pub L No. 93-380) that protects the privacy of students' "education records," including school health records, and applies to educational agencies and institutions that receive funds under any program administered by the US Department of

www.pediatrics.org/cgi/doi/10.1542/peds.2013-2867

doi:10.1542/peds.2013-2867

All clinical reports from the American Academy of Pediatrics automatically expire 5 years after publication unless reaffirmed, revised, or retired at or before that time.

PEDIATRICS (ISSN Numbers: Print, 0031-4005; Online, 1098-4275).

Education. Schools require FERPA permission from parents to release any information to any entity, including physicians. FERPA does not cover requirements of the Health Insurance Portability and Accountability Act (HIPAA). Other details can be found at: http://www.ed.gov/policy/gen/guid/fpco/index.html.

- Health Insurance Portability and Accountability Act (HIPAA): the Privacy Rule of HIPAA (Pub L No. 104-191, 1996) requires "covered entities," including physicians, to protect individuals' health records and other identifiable health information with appropriate safeguards to protect privacy and sets limits and conditions on the uses and disclosures that may be made of such information without patient authorization. HIPAA covers FERPA requirements. More information is available at http://www.hhs.gov/ocr/privacy.

- Child Find: Child Find is a continuous process of public awareness activities, screening, and evaluation designed to locate, identify, and refer as early as possible all young children with disabilities and their families who are in need of Early Intervention Program (Part C) or Preschool Special Education (Part B/619) services of the IDEA.

INTRODUCTION

Much attention has been paid to concussions in children and adolescents, particularly concussions resulting from sports. The majority of the focus on concussions has been centered on diagnosis, education of key stakeholders regarding the problem, and the timing of safe return to play (that is, to sports and other physical activity). Unfortunately, little attention has been given to academics and learning and how a concussion may affect the young student learner. Developing appropriate guidance and evidence-based recommendations

for a "return to learn" (RTL) for a student following a concussion is a challenge, given the limited research that exists in this area of concussion and its management. Because of this shortage of research, the guidance provided in this clinical report is based primarily on expert opinion and adapted from a program developed in Colorado to address the issue of RTL.[1] Data are currently insufficient to advocate the ideal way to manage the RTL in the pediatric population.

Pediatricians report that inadequate training on concussion management is among the most significant barriers to effectively counseling patients on returning to school following a concussion.[2] There are many published statements that discuss the importance of "cognitive rest" following a concussion.[3–5] Cognitive rest refers to avoiding potential cognitive stressors, such as texting, video games, TV exposure, and schoolwork, as examples. However, to date, there is no research documenting the benefits or harm of these methods in either the prolongation of symptoms or the ultimate outcome for the student following a concussion. Given the disruptive nature that concussion symptoms may pose for the student and his or her family, adding additional restrictions that may not be needed has the potential to create further emotional stress during the recovery. This calls for an individualized approach for the student when a pediatrician is making recommendations for cognitive rest and the student's RTL in the school setting.

BACKGROUND

With an estimated 1.7 million traumatic brain injuries occurring annually, many of them concussions, the need for specific recommendations for returning a student to learning after concussion is necessary.[6] Given that students typically appear well physically after

a concussion, it may be difficult for educators, school administrators, and peers of the student to fully understand the extent of deficits experienced by a student with a concussion. This lack of outward physical appearance of illness may also make it difficult for school officials to accept the need for adjustments for a student with a concussion.

Cognitive difficulties following a concussion have long been recognized and can clearly affect a student's learning capabilities. With recent increased attention to concussions, more focus has been placed on appropriate management for this specific injury. Neurocognitive testing, particularly the commercially available computerized versions, and its use after concussion has become more widespread, but the focus has been primarily on sports-related concussions. Although these neurocognitive tests may be helpful as a tool in assessing a student after a concussion, they have not been applied systematically to determine when and how a student is ready to take on the typical cognitive demands in a school setting.

Although a concussion can have obvious direct effects on learning, there is also increasing evidence that using a concussed brain to learn may worsen concussion symptoms and perhaps even prolong recovery.[7,8] Increasing cognitive activities are hypothesized to add additional stress to an energy-deprived brain, which may worsen symptoms. The goal during concussion recovery is to avoid overexerting the brain to the level of worsening or reproducing symptoms. Determining the appropriate balance between how much cognitive exertion and rest is needed is the hallmark of the management plan during cognitive recovery.

There is insufficient research on the role of cognitive rest, although recent research suggests benefit to the concept of cognitive rest both early and late in the recovery of the student.[9]

SIGNS AND SYMPTOMS OF CONCUSSION AFFECTING STUDENTS

Many aspects of a concussion can affect the student in the classroom. The common signs and symptoms the student may experience can be physical, cognitive, emotional, or related to sleep. Fortunately, research has demonstrated that recovery for the school-age student occurs usually within 3 weeks from the injury, but school adjustments during this recovery period may be necessary.[10]

When evaluating the student, recognizing the common signs and symptoms of a concussion and how they may affect the student in the school setting is important (Table 1). A thorough understanding of potential problems the student can encounter will help the pediatrician make appropriate recommendations to the school, the student, and the student's family. Allowing adequate cognitive rest may help minimize a worsening of symptoms and potentially facilitate a quicker recovery without significant disruption to the student's life.

Use of symptom checklists may help not only in evaluating what symptoms the student may be experiencing but also in rating them in severity (Figs 1 and 2). These checklists can also be used serially to follow the student through his or her recovery and identify areas that may need more targeted interventions.[11] Because the diagnosis of concussion is largely symptom driven, it is important not only to recognize but also to inquire further about the specific nature of the symptoms reported by the student or observed by the parent because many of the symptoms reported after a concussion may not be unique to a concussion. For example, some students may have preexisting depression, chronic daily or intermittent headaches, learning disabilities, or attention-deficit/hyperactivity disorder, which can affect reporting on a symptom checklist.

TABLE 1 Signs and Symptoms of a Concussion and the Potential Problems They May Pose to the Student

Sign/Symptom	Potential Implications in School
Headache	Most common symptom reported in concussions
	Can distract the student from concentration
	Can vary throughout the day and may be triggered by various exposures, such as fluorescent lighting, loud noises, and focusing on tasks
Dizziness/lightheadedness	May be an indication of injury to vestibular system
	May make standing quickly or walking in crowded environment challenging
	Often provoked by visual stimulus (rapid movements, videos, etc)
Visual symptoms: light sensitivity, double vision, blurry vision	Troubles with various aspects of the school building
	Slide presentations
	Movies
	Smart boards
	Computers
	Handheld computers (tablets)
	Artificial lighting
	Difficulty reading and copying
	Difficulty paying attention to visual tasks
Noise sensitivity	Troubles with various aspects of the school building
	Lunchroom
	Shop classes
	Music classes (band/choir)
	Physical education classes
	Hallways
	Organized sports practices
Difficulty concentrating or remembering	Challenges learning new tasks and comprehending new materials
	Difficulty with recalling and applying previously learned material
	Lack of focus in the classroom
	Troubles with test taking
	Troubles with standardized testing
	Reduced ability to take drivers education classes safely
Sleep disturbances	Excessive fatigue can hamper memory for new or past learning or ability to attend and focus
	Insufficient sleep can lead to tardiness or excessive absences
	Difficulty getting to sleep or frequent waking at night may lead to sleeping in class
	Excessive napping due to fatigue may lead to further disruptions of the sleep cycle

Careful history taking to account for any possible preinjury conditions is useful in assessing the student with concussion, especially one with protracted postconcussive symptoms. The pediatrician should account for these preexisting conditions and continue to manage the concussion and as well as the preexisting problems concurrently. It is also worthwhile to discuss other potential stressors that may affect symptom reporting, such as family or relationship problems, pressures from coaches and teammates if the child is involved in organized sports, and the restriction from participation in important upcoming life events. Symptom checklists and their scores may help in determining what symptoms may need to be addressed when returning to the school environment but should not be the sole determining factor in deciding when to return a child to school after a concussion.

THE RETURN TO LEARNING TEAM

A student returning to school after a concussion may benefit from a multi-disciplinary team to maximize his or her recovery (Table 2).[1] Because state laws differ, the accessibility for some

CIRCLE ONE FOR EACH LISTED	NONE	MILD		MODERATE		SEVERE	
Headache	0	1	2	3	4	5	6
"Pressure in head"	0	1	2	3	4	5	6
Neck pain	0	1	2	3	4	5	6
Nausea or vomiting	0	1	2	3	4	5	6
Dizziness	0	1	2	3	4	5	6
Blurred or double vision	0	1	2	3	4	5	6
Balance problems	0	1	2	3	4	5	6
Sensitive to light	0	1	2	3	4	5	6
Sensitive to noise	0	1	2	3	4	5	6
Feeling slowed down	0	1	2	3	4	5	6
Feeling "in a fog"	0	1	2	3	4	5	6
"Don't feel right"	0	1	2	3	4	5	6
Difficulty concentrating	0	1	2	3	4	5	6
Difficulty remembering	0	1	2	3	4	5	6
Fatigue or low energy	0	1	2	3	4	5	6
Confusion	0	1	2	3	4	5	6
Drowsiness	0	1	2	3	4	5	6
Trouble falling asleep	0	1	2	3	4	5	6
More emotional	0	1	2	3	4	5	6
Irritability	0	1	2	3	4	5	6
Sadness	0	1	2	3	4	5	6
Nervous or anxious	0	1	2	3	4	5	6

FIGURE 1

Example postconcussion symptom score checklist (recommended for seventh grade and up).[5] Use of the postconcussion symptom scale: the student should complete the form, on his or her own, by circling a subjective value for each symptom. This form can be used with each encounter to track progress toward symptom resolution. Many students may have some of these reported symptoms at a baseline, such as concentration difficulties in the patient with attention-deficit disorder or sadness in a student with underlying depression. This must be taken into consideration when interpreting the score. Students do not need a total score of 0 to return to play if they had symptoms before their concussion. This scale has not been validated to determine concussion severity.

CIRCLE ONE FOR EACH LISTED	NONE	RARELY	SOMETIMES	OFTEN
I have trouble paying attention	0	1	2	3
I get distracted easily	0	1	2	3
I have a hard time concentrating	0	1	2	3
I have problems remembering what people tell me	0	1	2	3
I have problems following directions	0	1	2	3
I daydream too much	0	1	2	3
I get confused	0	1	2	3
I forget things	0	1	2	3
I have problems finishing things	0	1	2	3
I have trouble figuring things out	0	1	2	3
It's hard for me to learn new things	0	1	2	3
I have headaches	0	1	2	3
I feel dizzy	0	1	2	3
I feel like the room is spinning	0	1	2	3
I feel like I'm going to faint	0	1	2	3
Things are blurry when I look at them	0	1	2	3
I see double/two of things	0	1	2	3
I feel sick to my stomach	0	1	2	3
I get tired a lot	0	1	2	3
I get tired easily	0	1	2	3

FIGURE 2

Example of postconcussion symptom score checklist (recommended for kindergarten to sixth grade).[5]

students to a school physician or a school nurse may be less likely in some communities. It remains essential that all schools recognize the importance of team management for a student after concussion and ensure that all students recovering from concussion have assigned staff who will be responsible for smooth reentry to school. Yet in the ideal situation, there is a school physician in every district and a school nurse in every school, so that a medical team in the educational home can readily work with the student's medical home toward a child or adolescent's optimal benefit and outcome.[12,13]

Even though a student may be having symptoms, ultimately, the goal is to keep disruptions to the student's life to a minimum and to return the recovering student to school as soon as possible. The challenge of the multidisciplinary team is to balance the need for the student to be at school with the appropriate adjustments for the cognitive demands at school that have the potential for increasing symptoms. To reach the right balance at home and school, the multidisciplinary teams should be well versed in their roles and responsibilities in concussion management and keep communication open among all parties regarding decisions to progress, regress, or hold steady during the RTL process.

After a concussion, the student already has individuals in place for each of the teams described (Table 2). Ideally, at least 1 person from each team is involved in the concussion management and communicating with each other to help facilitate the recovery. The pediatrician does not need to create the teams or roles, but it will help to understand what roles and responsibilities each team has in the recovery of the student.

The role and responsibility of the family team is to enforce rest and to reduce stimulation to the student during recovery. In the early phases of a concussion,

TABLE 2 Multidisciplinary Team to Facilitate "Return to Learning"[1]

Team	Members of the Team
Family team	Student, parents, guardians, grandparents, peers, teammates, and family friends
Medical team	Emergency department, primary care provider, concussion specialist (primary care sports medicine physicians, neurologists, neurosurgeons, as examples), clinical psychologist, neuropsychologist, team and/or school physician
School academic team	Teacher, school counselor, school psychologist, social worker, school nurse, school administrator, school physician
School physical activity team	School nurse, athletic trainer, coach, physical education teacher, playground supervisor, school physician

All members listed for a team do not need to be involved for successful concussion management. An individual, such as an emergency department physician, may only be involved in the initial assessment and suggestion for initiating academic adjustments. Some members may serve roles on various teams. Some schools may have access to only certain individuals suggested for a team. This list is meant to serve as a framework to help pediatricians and others involved with concussion management, possible roles they can serve for a student with a concussion.

TABLE 3 Sample Approach for Determining a Students' Readiness to Return to Learning Following a Concussion[17]

If a student/athlete experiences symptoms enough to affect his or her ability to concentrate or tolerate stimulation for even up to 30 minutes, the student should likely remain at home. The student may consider light mental activities, such as watching TV, light reading, and interaction with the family, until they provoke symptoms. Computer use, texting, and video games should remain at a minimum.

When the student/athlete is able to tolerate symptoms comfortably for up to 30 to 45 minutes, the parent may consider returning him or her back to learning, either through home tutoring or in-school instruction with programming adjustment as needed. However, it is the parent who should communicate with the school about the concussion and sign a release of information for school personnel to coordinate adjustments that may be needed as recommended by the primary care provider. The level of adjustments are decided collectively by the parent, school, and primary care provider based on severity, type, and duration of symptoms present.

symptoms may be so severe that they may prevent the student from attending school or even accepting home tutoring. However, as symptoms become tolerable, short-lived, and/or amenable to rest and intervention, the student may return to school, often with the use of supplemental academic adjustments. Therefore, it is the parent who will ultimately make the decision when the student should return to school. It is not unusual for a student to be extremely symptomatic in the doctor's office initially but minimally symptomatic at home within several days. Some guidance to help decision making for return to school can be found in Table 3.

The role and responsibility of the medical team is to evaluate the concussion, assess for a more serious structural or neurologic injury, and prescribe physical and cognitive rest, as appropriate, until symptoms improve. As recovery continues, the medical team should gather data from the family and from the school teams to aid in the decision of when to start to allow safe progression back to increasing physical activity.

Two school teams are involved in the recovery process for the student with a concussion, the school physical activity team and the school academic team. The roles and responsibilities of the 2 school teams are extensive and varied. In the early stages of the

concussion, the primary goal of the school physical activity team is to safeguard the student from any further potential injury to the brain. If a concussion has been suspected, it is recommended that the student be removed from physical activity and be evaluated by his or her pediatrician or other appropriate health care professionals for further diagnosis and management before returning to physical activity. Pediatricians should counsel patients on the current recommended return to activity progressions, as outlined in the clinical report from the American Academy of Pediatrics titled "Sport-Related Concussion in Children and Adolescents," which may be applied to both athletes and nonathletes.[3]

Similarly, in the early phases of a concussion, the school academic team must coordinate the return of the student to cognitive exertion and help to facilitate the appropriate level of academic adjustments necessary to reduce or eliminate symptoms. Whether communication occurs directly with a single teacher or is coordinated across all teachers via the designated case manager, such as the school nurse, counselor, or school psychologist, it is essential for all adults working with the student to understand the effects of a concussion on learning and how best to reduce cognitive demands during this

period of recovery. The parent is encouraged to return the student to school, even if the day is shortened, when the student can tolerate cognitive activity or stimulation for approximately 30 to 45 minutes. This arbitrary cutoff is based on the observation that a good amount of learning takes place in 30- to 45-minute increments. High schools with 7 to 8 consecutive classes often schedule periods at 30- to 45-minute intervals. A student with a concussion can benefit from 30 minutes of instruction and a 15-minute "rest period" before changing classes. High schools on a "block schedule" usually run 90-minute blocks (two 45-minute periods), which may require allowances for a planned rest midway through the block. The concussed student may maximize learning in 30- to 45-minute increments before needing to take a rest (Table 3). Missing instruction, however, may necessitate the need for the provision of class notes, supplemental tutoring, or an easing of assignments or course expectations.

When the student returns to school, observing which classes exacerbate symptoms will allow for further adjustments to be made to help reduce symptom provocation. Students may be able to tolerate some classes better than others, and consideration should be given for reduced exposure for those classes that the student cannot tolerate as well by substituting a study hall period, allowing for rest periods, or making adjustments to class schedules.

As the concussion symptoms improve, the school academic team and the family team should feel comfortable increasing mental and social activities, as tolerated by the student, and involving the medical team only as needed, apart from preplanned follow-up visits. This may translate into parents allowing their child to attend a social gathering, watch a game, or return to driving. At school, this should translate into a teacher requiring more work from a student who is obviously feeling better and able to tolerate longer periods of time of mental exertion without provoking symptoms.

Pediatricians should encourage teachers to pick and choose the academic adjustments most amenable to their class teaching style and content and most appropriate for the phase of recovery of the concussion on the basis of a child's tolerance. Teachers and those on the school academic team should reassess progress at weekly intervals to determine the effectiveness and continued need of adjustments. Direct communication and attention to symptoms with the student is helpful, because the student may not be willing to mention problems specifically to the teacher. Communication with a student should be conducted in a private setting, because many students prefer not to be singled out or draw additional attention to themselves following the injury. Younger students may be apprehensive or not know how to effectively express their academic struggles. High-achieving students may also be unwilling to "give in" to adjustments that are offered.

STRATEGIES TO RETURN TO LEARN IN THE CLASSROOM

Returning a student to the classroom while symptomatic from a concussion requires an individualized approach. Most students will likely return to the classroom while symptomatic from their concussion. Each concussion is unique and may encompass a different constellation and severity of symptoms. Concussion symptoms may vary from student to student and even from concussion to concussion in the same individual who may sustain more than one concussion. Therefore, a "cookie-cutter" approach to managing a concussion and a return to the classroom cannot be applied. However, most of the difficulties that arise in students can be handled with similar adjustments, depending on the signs or symptoms they are experiencing.

In the first few weeks after a concussion, most interventions can be made in the general education classroom, by the general education teacher, with minimal support and check-ins with the school physician, school nurse, school counselor, school psychologist, school social worker, or certified athletic trainer (AT).[14,15] Parents should be encouraged to follow up with the school and student to assess whether academic adjustments are occurring to minimize worsening of students' symptoms during their early recovery.

Physicians should learn educational terminology to assist them in being precise in what they are requesting of schools. The term "academic adjustment" is used intentionally to refer to nonformalized adjustments made to the student's environment during the typical 1- to 3-week recovery period that do not jeopardize the curriculum or require alterations in standardized testing. The term "academic accommodations" is used to address longer-term needs, beyond 3 weeks, which may include standardized testing arrangement,

extra time on work, changes in class schedule, for example, and access to the grade-level curriculum but still within the context of regular education and may be formalized in a 504 plan. The term "academic modification" is used when considering more prolonged and more permanent changes to an educational plan, necessitating special education with needs specified in an IEP. Teachers' understanding and putting a few reasonable adjustments in place in the early stages of the concussion will often help bring the student through recovery in the typical, expected timeframe of 1 to 3 weeks. The type of academic adjustments put in place should depend on the severity of the symptoms, the type of symptom, specific teaching styles used by a teacher in the classroom, and pattern of the symptoms (Table 4).

Concussion education can be conducted by the pediatrician via direct communication with school personnel on a case-by-case basis to facilitate better understanding among appropriate school personnel during the RTL process; restrictions and adjustments should be specifically listed on a school note at each visit and during the interim, if needed. Unfortunately, simply requesting this in written form does not guarantee the school can or will comply. It would be helpful for the pediatrician if the school could identify a "point person" or case manager to contact at the school and likewise for the school to be given a "point person" in the pediatrician's office who will communicate with each other during the RTL process. FERPA permission is needed by educational agencies, and HIPAA permission is required by medical personnel; therefore, a signed parent permission on a document that satisfies both is required for communication among team members. The school point person is often a member of the school academic team. The medical home point person is someone with enough knowledge of the situation and of the child to communicate concerns back to the pediatrician. Parents should also be involved with this communication.

The team approach between the medical home and a school staff member is helpful in assisting the school with problems it encounters in the process and identifying solutions to these problems. A team approach also can reduce the likelihood of a pediatrician's office from receiving frequent phone calls from many individuals about the same situation. For many schools, the point person would be a guidance counselor, school psychologist, school physician, or school nurse. In schools in which a AT is present, the AT can help reinforce communication of any school or sports restrictions to safeguard

against the student-athlete beginning a return to play protocol but still having academic adjustments.[15] For this reason, communication with the AT by the treating physician or a representative of the school who has been communicating with the physician is also encouraged.[16] In some circumstances, the AT may be limited to support only the students in organized sports for the school rather than the student body as a whole. It would be helpful to the pediatrician to understand how ATs can assist the pediatrician with the management of their patients.

Encouraging parents to communicate with the school, especially the designated case manager, about how recommended adjustments are being applied can be helpful. Pediatricians should also encourage parents to communicate with their child to make sure any adjust-

ments that are being offered are also being used, as needed, and are helping.

PROLONGED SYMPTOMS

Fortunately, most students with a concussion will recover within the first 3 weeks from their injury.[10] For students with symptoms lasting longer than 3 weeks, further medical management considerations and accommodations, rather than academic adjustments, may be needed. Schools currently have in place a system for accommodations (504 plan) for students expected to have temporary interference with learning or modifications (IEP) for students with a classifiable chronic condition. However, applying these systems to concussions, in some schools, may be a newer concept. Although healing may be considered "protracted" with some concussions, the expectation is still for a full recovery that no longer would require academic adjustments, accommodations, or modifications. Referral to a concussion specialist (licensed physician, such as a pediatrician, neurologist, primary care sports medicine specialist, or neurosurgeon with expanded knowledge and experience in pediatric concussion management) should also be considered, if not already initiated, for the student with prolonged symptoms.

Because laws, regulations, policies, and practices vary among states, districts, and schools, it is important that the pediatrician be familiar with the level of flexibility and creativity that a particular school will provide or permit. Differences also exist among long-term modifications, midterm accommodations, and short-term adjustments. Pediatricians should understand that the IDEA provides for longer-term accommodations. For example, there are provisions for school-based problem-solving teams to determine the appropriateness of an IEP for a child in need of long-term modifications through special education on the basis of a given classification.

TABLE 4 Signs and Symptoms of a Concussion and the Strategies to Help in the School Setting

Sign/Symptom	Potential Adjustments in School Setting
Headache	Frequent breaks
	Identifying aggravators and reducing exposure to them
	Rests, planned or as needed, in nurses office or quiet area
Dizziness	Allow student to put head down if symptoms worsen
	Give student early dismissal from class and extra time to get from class to class to avoid crowded hallways
Visual symptoms: light sensitivity, double vision, blurry vision	Reduce exposure to computers, smart boards, videos
	Reduce brightness on the screens
	Allow the student to wear a hat or sunglasses in school
	Consider use of audiotapes of books
	Turn off fluorescent lights as needed
	Seat student closer to the center of classroom activities (blurry vision)
	Cover 1 eye with patch/tape 1 lens if glasses are worn (double vision)
Noise sensitivity	Allow the student to have lunch in quiet area with a classmate
	Limit or avoid band, choir, or shop classes
	Avoid noisy gyms and organized sports practices/games
	Consideration of the use of earplugs
	Give student early dismissal from class and extra time to get from class to class to avoid crowded hallways during pass time
Difficulty concentrating or remembering	Avoid testing or completion of major projects during recovery when possible
	Provide extra time to complete nonstandardized tests
	Postpone standardized testing (may require that 504 plan is in place)
	Consider 1 test per day during exam periods
	Consider the use of preprinted notes, notetaker, scribe, or reader for oral test taking
Sleep disturbances	Allow for late start or shortened school day to catch up on sleep
	Allow rest breaks

In addition, a 504 plan is available through the Rehabilitation Act of 1973 and Americans with Disabilities Act of 1990 for a child who needs longer-term academic accommodations in regular education but does not qualify for special education through 1 of the 13 classifications available via an IEP. Most adjustments can and should be short term and through the child's educational team, with guidance from the medical home and approval by the principal and family team. The key to this process is that the pediatrician provides the school with medical documentation based on persisting signs and symptoms that might significantly limit a child's ability to access full instruction. It is also helpful for the pediatrician to realize that, often, schools will not allow a child to participate in extracurricular activities until he or she is fully participating in curricular activities.

Early in the recovery, a student may need simple academic adjustments in the classroom. Students who do not respond in the first few months may need a more targeted level of intervention. At this level, school teams may need to brainstorm and problem solve what other interventions may be helpful and decide whether more formalized assessments need to occur. Often, the family team is a critical part of the problem-solving process, as is the medical team. All 3 teams must be actively involved in managing the concussion on behalf of the recovering student. At this level, some of the interventions can no longer be easily applied in the general education classroom without formal intervention. For example, students may require some amount of pullout from the regular classroom for a small-group intervention, tutoring, or 1-on-1 instruction. Customized plans at this point may be more formalized into an Individualized Health Plan, a learning plan, or a 504 plan. Interventions at this level are usually accommodations to the environment (ie, large-print books, extra set of books at home, audio books, extended time on tests, note takers).

If symptoms remain severe or prolonged, typically longer than 5 to 6 months, more intensive intervention may be needed. In these cases, a potentially more permanent disability is considered, necessitating most school districts to trigger their Child Find (a component of IDEA) obligations, provide appropriate testing, and develop an IEP. The family team and medical team should continue to be involved and consulted during the development of the IEP. Interventions at this level are often considered modifications of the curriculum, implying that the student may not be held responsible for the regular education curriculum required of all other same-age peers. Instead, the student may be taught without penalty on a level appropriate for him or her, often at a level lower than peers, and will only be held accountable for his or her own personal academic growth rather than being compared with typical grade-level peers.[17,18] In addition, the concussion would be so severe at this level as to potentially necessitate specialized instruction and/or specialized programming. It is uncommon, however, for the student with a concussion to need an IEP.

When considering the implementation of a 504 plan or IEP, involving the school academic teams or special education teams is beneficial and necessary. The school academic team, including the school psychologist, can provide formal recommendations to the school to make the creation of the 504 plan or IEP that is most relevant to the particular student's greatest needs in the academic setting. Regardless of the problems, it is essential the medical team, the school team, and the family team work together, if further testing seems indicated to help in the development of an educational program through an IEP or 504 plan. In the majority of these assessments, the recommendations and development of an IEP or 504 plan will be developed by the schools. A medical diagnosis of concussion can prompt the school academic team to collect other sources of information and consider developing a 504 plan or IEP. Importantly, 504 plans and IEPs are governed by different laws. A 504 plan can be provided when a school determines the concussion to substantially limit one or more major life activities, such as learning. On the other hand, an IEP can be provided if it is determined that the concussion results in total or partial impairment that adversely affects educational performance such that a student cannot benefit from regular education alone and requires modification of curriculum, specialized instruction, programming, and/or placement.

Although not expected or common after a concussion, a student with prolonged symptoms who does not seem to be responding to various interventions should also be evaluated for issues related to anxiety about school or school avoidance. This may be more likely in the child who sustained a concussion from an incidence of bullying or assault. Keeping a child out of school and away from friends for extended periods also may risk development of fear and isolation in a child or adolescent on attempting to return to school and might require the assistance of a mental health specialist in extreme cases.

EDUCATION

Given the large number of concussions occurring each year, both in and out of formal sport activities, most schools will encounter a child who is dealing with symptoms from a concussion. Education of all individuals involved is paramount to helping students who may need assistance in the school setting.

Education regarding concussion, generally, and the role of cognitive and physical rest and return to school, specifically, is essential for the teams of individuals helping a student with concussion during assessment, management, and recovery. This education should extend to both school personnel (eg, administrators, athletic directors, teachers, guidance counselors, school psychologists, coaches, school physicians, school nurses, ATs) and individuals likely not employed by the school (eg, primary physicians, sports/team physicians, emergency department physicians, parents, and other caregivers). Even in states with legislation for concussion education and management, nonathletic personnel in schools are often left out of concussion education efforts. However, a comprehensive team approach to care may help reduce mistakes in management, which could potentially risk reinjury during the healing phase, lengthen recovery, or result in untoward long-term outcomes.

Education, on a larger scale, should be conducted to instruct school groups on the concepts of concussion management, particularly when introducing models of cognitive rest. Education can be tailored to various school personnel as needed. Education sessions are especially helpful as sport seasons begin in the fall, winter, and spring. Several groups have developed educational materials, such as online tutorials, relevant to this topic and provide excellent resources for schools, parents, students, and health care providers (see Resources).

FUTURE DIRECTIONS

Given the paucity of studies that have been conducted thus far regarding the effects and role of cognitive rest after concussion, further research is needed. Future research is also needed to clarify best practices for RTL. Developing a better understanding of the best methods to assist a student in the school environment, determining whether cognitive rest can assist in speed

of recovery, and evaluating written and educational resources on this topic are all areas that require additional research and review. Studies comparing outcomes in school settings that have concussion management teams with case management versus those that do not would also be of value.

Continued education of all individuals involved with a student with a concussion should help facilitate better outcomes and less resistance to developing appropriate concussion management guidelines and programs.

CONCLUSIONS AND GUIDANCE FOR PHYSICIANS

1. Students with a concussion may need academic adjustments in school to help minimize a worsening of symptoms.

2. Given that most concussions resolve within 3 weeks of the injury, adjustments may often be made in the individual classroom setting without formal written plans, such as a 504 plan or IEP.

3. Students with symptoms lasting longer than 3 to 4 weeks may benefit from a more detailed assessment by a concussion specialist (licensed physician, such as a pediatrician, neurologist, primary care sports medicine specialist, or neurosurgeon with expanded knowledge and experience in pediatric concussion management) and recommendations specific to the educational environment. Considerations should be given to developing a 504 plan or, subsequently, but unlikely, an IEP, in the student with a lengthy recovery.

4. A team approach consisting of the medical team, the school team, and the family team to assist the student in his or her return to learning is ideal.

5. Students should be performing at their academic "baseline" before returning to sports, full physical activity, or other extracurricular activities following a concussion.

6. Education of all individuals involved with students who sustain a concussion is necessary to provide adequate adjustments, accommodations, and long-term program modifications for the students.

7. Additional research is necessary to strengthen and provide more evidence-based recommendations for appropriate adjustments for students following a concussion.

RESOURCES

- Brain 101: Concussion Handbook: http://brain101.orcasinc.com/1000

- REAP (Reduce/Educate/Accommodate/Pace) Program: a community-based concussion management program: http://www.rockymountainhospital-forchildren.com/sports-medicine/concussion-management/reap-guidelines.htm

- CDC Foundation Online Training for Clinicians: http://preventingconcussions.org/

- Centers for Disease Control and Prevention: Fact Sheet for School Professionals on Returning to School after a Concussion: http://www.cdc.gov/concussion/pdf/TBI_Returning_to_School-a.pdf

- Centers for Disease Control and Prevention: Heads Up for Schools: http://www.cdc.gov/concussion/HeadsUp/schools.html

- Centers for Disease Control and Prevention: Online Coaches Training: http://www.cdc.gov/concussion/HeadsUp/online_training.html

- Dr. Mike Evans Concussions 101 Video: http://www.myfavouritemedicine.com/concussions-101/

- Frequently Asked Questions about 504 Plans: http://www2.ed.gov/about/offices/list/ocr/504faq.html

- Sample Return to Learning Note for Physicians: http://www.aap.org/en-us/

about-the-aap/Committees-Councils-Sections/Council-on-sports-medicine-and-fitness/Documents/returntoschool.pdf and http://www2.aap.org/sections/schoolhealth/returntoschool.pdf

LEAD AUTHORS
Mark E. Halstead, MD, FAAP
Karen McAvoy, PsyD
Cynthia D. Devore, MD, FAAP

CONTRIBUTING AUTHORS
Rebecca Carl, MD, FAAP
Michael Lee, MD, FAAP
Kelsey Logan, MD, FAAP

COUNCIL ON SPORTS MEDICINE AND FITNESS EXECUTIVE COMMITTEE, 2012–2013
Joel S. Brenner, MD, MPH, FAAP, Chairperson
Rebecca A. Demorest, MD, FAAP
Mark E. Halstead, MD, FAAP
Amanda K. Weiss Kelly, MD, FAAP
Chris G. Koutures, MD, FAAP
Cynthia R. LaBella, MD, FAAP
Michele LaBotz, MD, FAAP
Keith J. Loud, MDCM, MSc, FAAP

Kody A. Moffatt, MD, FAAP
M. Alison Brooks, MD, FAAP
Stephanie S. Martin, MD, FAAP

LIAISONS
Andrew Gregory, MD, FAAP – *American Medical Society for Sports Medicine*
Lisa K. Kluchurosky, MEd, ATC – *National Athletic Trainers Association*
John F. Philpott, MD, FAAP – *Canadian Paediatric Society*

STAFF
Anjie Emanuel, MPH

COUNCIL ON SCHOOL HEALTH EXECUTIVE COMMITTEE, 2012–2013
Cynthia D. Devore, MD, FAAP, Chairperson
Mandy A. Allison, MD, MSPH, FAAP
Richard Ancona, MD, FAAP
Elliott Attisha, DO, FAAP
Stephen Barnett, MD, FAAP
Breena Welch Holmes, MD, FAAP
Chris Kjolhede, MD, MPH, FAAP
Marc Lerner, MD, FAAP
Mark Minier, MD, FAAP
Jeffrey Okamoto MD, FAAP
Thomas Young, MD, FAAP

LIAISONS
Carolyn Duff, RN, MS – *National Association of School Nurses*
Linda M. Grant, MD, MPH, FAAP – *American School Health Association*
Veda Johnson, MD, FAAP – *School-Based Health Alliance*
Mary Vernon-Smiley, MD, MPH, MDiv – *Centers for Disease Control Division of Adolescents and School Health (DASH)*

CONSULTANTS
Gerry Giola, PhD
K. Brooke Pengel, MD, FAAP
Keith Yeates, PhD

STAFF
Madra Guinn-Jones, MPH

ORGANIZATIONS THAT HAVE ENDORSED THIS REPORT
American Medical Society for Sports Medicine
Brain Injury Association of America
Canadian Paediatric Society
National Association of School Nurses
National Association of School Psychologists
National Federation of State High School Associations

REFERENCES

1. Rocky Mountain Youth Sports Medicine Institute, Center for Concussion. REAP Guidelines. Available at: http://www.rockymountainhospitalforchildren.com/sports-medicine/concussion-management/reap-guidelines.htm. Accessed June 18, 2013

2. Zonfrillo MR, Master CL, Grady MF, Winston FK, Callahan JM, Arbogast KB. Pediatric providers' self-reported knowledge, practices, and attitudes about concussion. *Pediatrics*. 2012;130(6):1120–1125

3. Halstead ME, Walter KD; Council on Sports Medicine and Fitness. American Academy of Pediatrics. Clinical report—sport-related concussion in children and adolescents. *Pediatrics*. 2010;126(3):597–615

4. Harmon KG, Drezner JA, Gammons M, et al; American Medical Society for Sports Medicine. American Medical Society for Sports Medicine position statement: concussion in sport. *Clin J Sport Med*. 2013;23(1):1–18

5. McCrory P, Meeuwisse W, Aubry M, et al; Kathryn Schneider, PT, PhD, Charles H. Tator, MD, PHD. Consensus statement on concussion in sport—the 4th International Conference on Concussion in Sport held in Zurich, November 2012. *Clin J Sport Med*. 2013;23(2):89–117

6. Faul M, Xu L, Wald M, Coronado V. *Traumatic Brain Injury in the United States: Emergency Department Visits, Hospitalizations, and Death*. Atlanta, GA: Centers for Disease Control and Prevention, National Center for Injury Prevention; 2010

7. Sady MD, Vaughan CG, Gioia GA. School and the concussed youth: recommendations for concussion education and management. *Phys Med Rehabil Clin N Am*. 2011;22(4):701–719, ix

8. Howell D, Osternig L, Van Donkelaar P, Mayr U, Chou LS. Effects of concussion on attention and executive function in adolescents. *Med Sci Sports Exerc*. 2013;45(6):1030–1037

9. Moser RS, Glatts C, Schatz P. Efficacy of immediate and delayed cognitive and physical rest for treatment of sports-related concussion. *J Pediatr*. 2012;161(5):922–926

10. Collins M, Lovell MR, Iverson GL, Ide T, Maroon J. Examining concussion rates and return to play in high school football players wearing newer helmet technology: a three-year prospective cohort study. *Neurosurgery*. 2006;58(2):275–286, discussion 275–286

11. Master C, Giola G, Leddy J, Grady M. The importance of "return-to-learn" in pediatric and adolescent concussion. *Pediatr Ann*. 2012;41(9):1–6

12. Magalnick H, Mazyck D; American Academy of Pediatrics Council on School Health. Role of the school nurse in providing school health services. *Pediatrics*. 2008;121(5):1052–1056

13. Devore CD, Wheeler LS; American Academy of Pediatrics, Council on School Health. Role of the school physician. *Pediatrics*. 2013;131(1):178–182

14. Piebes SK, Gourley M, Valovich McLeod TC. Caring for student-athletes following a concussion. *J Sch Nurs*. 2009;25(4):270–281

15. McGrath N. Supporting the student-athlete's return to the classroom after a sport-related concussion. *J Athl Train*. 2010;45(5):492–498

16. Valovich-McLeod T, Giola G. Cognitive rest: the often neglected aspect of concussion management. *Athl Ther Today*. 2010;15(2):1–3

17. McAvoy K. Return to learning: going back to school following a concussion. *Communique*. 2012;40(6):23–25

18. McAvoy K. Providing a continuum of care for concussion using existing educational frameworks. *Brain Inj Professional*. 2012;9(1):26–27

Scope of Practice Issues in the Delivery of Pediatric Health Care

- *Policy Statement*

POLICY STATEMENT

Scope of Practice Issues in the Delivery of Pediatric Health Care

COMMITTEE ON PEDIATRIC WORKFORCE

KEY WORDS
delegate, family physician, independent practice, medical home, pediatric nurse practitioner, pediatrician, physician assistant, nonphysician clinician, team-based care

ABBREVIATIONS
AAP—American Academy of Pediatrics
NP—nurse practitioner
PA—physician assistant

This document is copyrighted and is property of the American Academy of Pediatrics and its Board of Directors. All authors have filed conflict of interest statements with the American Academy of Pediatrics. Any conflicts have been resolved through a process approved by the Board of Directors. The American Academy of Pediatrics has neither solicited nor accepted any commercial involvement in the development of the content of this publication.

The recommendations in this statement do not indicate an exclusive course of treatment or serve as a standard of medical care. Variations, taking into account individual circumstances, may be appropriate.

All policy statements from the American Academy of Pediatrics automatically expire 5 years after publication unless reaffirmed, revised, or retired at or before that time.

www.pediatrics.org/cgi/doi/10.1542/peds.2013-0943

doi:10.1542/peds.2013-0943

PEDIATRICS (ISSN Numbers: Print, 0031-4005; Online, 1098-4275).

Copyright © 2013 by the American Academy of Pediatrics

abstract

The American Academy of Pediatrics (AAP) believes that optimal pediatric health care depends on a team-based approach with supervision by a physician leader, preferably a pediatrician. The pediatrician, here defined to include not only pediatric generalists but all pediatric medical subspecialists, all surgical specialists, and internal medicine/pediatric physicians, is uniquely qualified to manage, coordinate, and supervise the entire spectrum of pediatric care, from diagnosis through all stages of treatment, in all practice settings. The AAP recognizes the valuable contributions of nonphysician clinicians, including nurse practitioners and physician assistants, in delivering optimal pediatric care. However, the expansion of the scope of practice of nonphysician pediatric clinicians raises critical public policy and child health advocacy concerns. Pediatricians should serve as advocates for optimal pediatric care in state legislatures, public policy forums, and the media and should pursue opportunities to resolve scope of practice conflicts outside state legislatures. The AAP affirms the importance of appropriate documentation and standards in pediatric education, training, skills, clinical competencies, examination, regulation, and patient care to ensure safety and quality health care for all infants, children, adolescents, and young adults. *Pediatrics* 2013;131:1211–1216

INTRODUCTION

The American Academy of Pediatrics (AAP) advocates that every child receive high-quality, accessible, family-centered, continuous, coordinated, comprehensive care in a medical home. To this end, optimal pediatric care is best delivered in a team-based approach that is led by a primary physician, ideally a pediatrician, who assumes responsibility for managing the patient's care. All professionals who provide pediatric care must hold to the highest standards of education and training and continually demonstrate their skills and competencies.

COMPREHENSIVE TEAM-BASED CARE WITH PHYSICIAN LEADERSHIP

The provision of optimal pediatric care depends on a team-based approach to health care that is ideally led by a pediatrician. In this team-based model of pediatric care, the physician assumes overall responsibility for the care of the patient. As leader of the pediatric health care team, the physician oversees the delivery of care and, when appropriate, delegates patient care responsibilities to nurse practitioners (NPs), physician assistants (PAs), and other valued members of the heath care team. The pediatrician who leads the health care team also determines when referral to other physicians is warranted. When patient care responsibilities must be shared by multiple providers, the pediatrician should assume primary responsibility for managing the full range of health care services to ensure continuity of care within the child's medical home.[1] For some children, a general pediatrician and a pediatric medical subspecialist or surgical specialist may decide to comanage care. The medical home's team-based model of pediatric care provides high-quality, cost-effective care by minimizing duplication of clinical effort, promoting the appropriate and timely use of all health care providers on the team, and ensuring that the care provided is accessible, continuous, comprehensive, family-centered, coordinated, compassionate, and culturally effective.[2]

UNIQUE QUALIFICATIONS OF PEDIATRICIANS

As a direct result of their extensive training and experience, pediatricians possess the broad range of competencies required to best assess and manage health issues in children. Pediatric illness runs the gamut from basic to complex, from common behavioral disorders to rare metabolic and genetic diseases. In addition, diseases that present initially as a common condition such as a cold may sometimes progress to a severe and complex illness such as pneumonia or respiratory failure. The pediatrician is the clinician most extensively educated in pediatric health care and has the depth and breadth of knowledge, skills,

and experience to deliver optimal care to children.

PROFESSIONAL STANDARDS TO ENSURE SAFETY AND QUALITY CARE

The AAP supports safe, quality care for all children and their families and believes that any health care professional who wishes to actively participate in the care of children must demonstrate appropriate education, training, skills, and ongoing competencies in pediatric health within his or her scope of practice to ensure the highest standards of care. All members of the health care team should provide care consistent with their education, training, and licensure.

In recent years, the health care market has seen a significant increase in the number of nonphysician clinicians who seek to care for children. Professional associations for psychologists, pharmacists, massage therapists, physical therapists, occupational therapists, optometrists, acupuncturists, naturopaths, homeopaths, and chiropractors have actively sought expanded scopes of practice in the care of children. In an evergrowing and more complicated health care delivery system, patients and families need to know what services these clinicians are licensed and trained to provide and understand the differences in education and skills among them.

Support for such transparency is increasing and resulting in requirements that medical and health professionals be required to display or advertise their degrees, credential(s), or licenses according to a standard that is easier for consumers to understand. In addition, truth-in-advertising laws help patients distinguish between medical doctors and other health professions with doctoral degrees who are licensed to provide care.

KEY MEMBERS OF THE PEDIATRIC HEALTH CARE TEAM

For many years, pediatricians have worked closely with physicians in disciplines across the field of medicine to optimize the care of children. The AAP specifically acknowledges the key role that family physicians have played in providing care to children and the importance of their continuing collaboration with pediatricians. Pediatricians need to collaborate closely with family physicians in practice to provide pediatric support and consultation.

Nonphysician clinicians play an invaluable role in the provision of health care to infants, children, adolescents, and young adults as part of the physician-led team that provides pediatric health care. Learning to work in teams should begin in pediatric residency training, where collaborative learning with nonphysician clinicians can expose future pediatricians to the benefits of team-based care. In particular, the AAP also affirms that these nonphysician clinicians have been important participants in the care of children in the United States for many years.

PAs are educated in the medical model to provide medical care specifically under the direction and supervision of a physician. PAs must graduate from an accredited master's-level educational program that includes didactic education and clinical rotations in pediatrics and must also pass the national certifying examination administered by the National Commission on Certification of Physician Assistants. The AAP is involved in the development of educational standards and national certification for PAs through appointed representatives on the boards of the Accreditation Review Commission on Education for the Physician Assistant and the National Commission on Certification of Physician Assistants. PAs support the concept of physician-directed, team-based care.

NPs are educated in graduate-level training programs, and the majority of NPs are certified by either the American Nurses Credentialing Center or the American Academy of Nurse Practitioners. In 7 states, national board certification is not required for licensing. The care provided by NPs can vary considerably on the basis of the laws in the state in which they practice. States may limit or deny NPs the authority to prescribe medications, to admit patients to the hospital, or to practice independently. As of 2012, more than half of the states required physician involvement (eg, collaborative practice agreement, physician delegation and supervision) for NPs to practice diagnosis and treatment and for prescriptive authority (for information on current state laws, please contact the AAP Division of State Government Affairs at stgov@aap. org).[3] Full admitting privileges for NPs would allow them to admit, provide care for, and discharge patients without physician supervision. Although NPs are rarely granted full admitting privileges, it is not uncommon for them to obtain associate privileges that permit them to admit a patient to a supervising physician. NPs can play an important role in the inpatient setting, but the AAP believes that a pediatrician should lead the health care team that is providing pediatric inpatient care.

In states that do not allow independent practice, a structured agreement with a physician is required. Recent studies have shown that even in states which allow independent practice for NPs, fewer than 15% of pediatric NPs actually choose to practice independently.[4] Regardless of the state in which they practice, the vast majority of pediatric NPs choose to practice under the supervision of general pediatricians, pediatric medical subspecialists, or pediatric surgical specialists. The AAP endorses this collaborative and structured relationship and believes this choice reflects both a shared commitment to patient safety and the positive nature of current pediatrician–NP relationships in US health care.

Of note, some reports have called for changes in the education of NPs so that they might spend additional time in clinical training and increase their likelihood of independent practice. These reports have also called for changes in the scope of practice for NPs in efforts to meet a workforce demand in areas with physician shortages.[5–7]

Considering the educational aspect, NPs generally receive a master's degree or postmaster's certificate. These NP training programs provide 500 to 720 hours of clinical training.[8] However, in 2004, the American Association of Colleges of Nursing endorsed a position statement calling for NP training programs to move the current level of preparation necessary for advanced nursing practice from a master's-level to a doctorate-level degree (eg, Doctor of Nursing Practice [DNP] or Doctor of Philosophy [PhD] in Nursing) by 2015.[9] The American Association of Colleges of Nursing's *The Essentials of Doctoral Education for Advanced Nursing Practice* (2006) recommends that programs—designed for individuals who have already acquired the competencies in *The Essentials of Baccalaureate Education for Professional Nursing Practice* (1998)—be "three calendar years, or 36 months of full-time study (including summers) or four years on a traditional academic calendar."[10] This requirement is equivalent to the currently required 3 years of graduate training for the master's degree program. Subsequently, the number of doctorate-level nursing programs in the United States has grown from 20 in 2006 to 182 in 2011.[9]

Increases in the duration of education or the final degree (eg, a DNP or PhD in Nursing) will not achieve educational parity with physicians. In comparison, with 4 years of medical school and 3 years of pediatric residency at a minimum, the pediatrician has invested between 12 000 and 14 000 clinical hours at the completion of basic pediatric training alone. Therefore, the AAP believes that pediatricians and NPs are not interchangeable in the delivery of pediatric health care.

A recent study of the geographic distribution of pediatric NPs found that the majority of states have fewer than 25 pediatric NPs per 100 000 children and that a state's independent practice laws are not related to its density of pediatric NPs.[11] In 2010, almost 85% of all NPs reported practicing in urban areas.[12] Furthermore, a recent study from the University of Washington Rural Health Research Center found no statistically significant link between states that allow NPs greater practice autonomy and higher rates of NP practice in rural areas.

Because a greater supply of NPs in a state does not necessarily lead to an equitable distribution to areas that are underserved, the AAP does not support changes in scope of practice for NPs in these areas and believes it is ill-advised to create a system of care based on independent practice without any supervision or oversight by a physician. Rather, the AAP recommends incentives for physician relocation, including loan forgiveness, payment reform, and expanded health insurance coverage for children.[13]

Some have called for an expansion of retail-based clinics as a means to increase the provision of care for children in underserved areas. However, retail-based clinics are not staffed by physicians, and the nonphysician clinicians that are staffing these clinics often work without supervision or oversight by a physician (ie, independent practice). Also, a recent study of more than 900 retail clinics throughout the United States found that "retail clinics are currently located in more advantaged neighborhoods, which may make them less accessible for those most in need."[14] In light of its commitment to comprehensive team-based care, the AAP does not support the use of retail-based clinics for the medical care of infants, children, and adolescents.[15] Because retail-based clinics are not founded on a medical home model, use of these clinics as a source of care for children poses a significant risk for fragmentation of care, limited follow-up, missed diagnoses, and decreased quality of care overall.

SCOPE OF PRACTICE LEGISLATION

Scope of practice legislation falls under the jurisdiction of individual states. State legislatures are therefore the loci of deliberations on these issues. The competing political agendas and perspectives expressed during these deliberations often generate highly charged debates. To bring a uniformity of approach and an essential level of civility to this discourse, the AAP endorses the 2005 recommendations of the Federation of State Medical Boards regarding the approach to scope of practice legislation.[16] A portion of the Federation of State Medical Boards statement follows:

> "Changing or creating a new scope of practice for a health profession necessitates establishment of a legitimate need for the change, along with a systematic review of the impact of the proposed change on public health, safety, and welfare. Patient safety and public protection must be the primary objectives in making decisions on scope of practice. It is important for boards and legislatures to recognize that there

are often significant differences in the prerequisites, the scope, and the duration of education provided to other health care practitioners when compared with that provided to physicians. Policy makers must ensure that all practitioners are prepared, by virtue of education and training, to provide the services authorized in their scope of practice in a safe, effective, and economical manner."

LIABILITY

The expansion of the scope of practice of NPs, PAs, and other nonphysician clinicians has created new challenges for physicians in all specialties in addressing professional and medical liability issues. Specific areas of risk for physicians when supervising nonphysician clinicians include improper delegation of authority, vicarious liability for medical care provided by nonphysician clinicians, and liability for nonmedical acts committed by nonphysician clinicians in which the physician is responsible for the negligent hiring, training, supervising, or retaining of the nonphysician clinicians. When delegating authority to nonphysician clinicians, physicians should consider the proper method of delegation and their oversight responsibilities for the delegated duties.

It is important that lawmakers and regulators remain attentive to the fact that a physician's ability to delegate authority is often governed by contractual limitations as well as by statutes that govern health care facilities. Moreover, health care entities, such as hospitals or managed care organizations, may not authorize the delegation of more authority than is permitted by state statutes or regulations, but they may impose limitations on the delegation of authority that are more restrictive than state laws. These policies may also be admissible in a medical liability lawsuit as evidence of the standard of care. Physicians violating such policies may

risk loss of employment or revocation of privileges. Physicians and health care entities must therefore be knowledgeable about the terms of these state statutes and regulations, as well as health care entity policies, and should seek advice from a qualified attorney.

For nonphysician clinicians who practice independently of a physician, public policy should require both exclusive professional responsibility for the care they provide and adequate liability insurance to allow for appropriate financial remedy for adverse settlements or decisions. States that license nonphysician clinicians should therefore require that these nonphysician clinicians abide by the same rules regarding liability insurance as do physicians. Because physicians can be held accountable for clinicians acting under their supervision, a pediatrician should consider potential professional or medical liability issues before establishing a supervisory relationship.

CONCLUSIONS

The AAP believes that optimal pediatric care is best rendered by using a team-based approach led by a pediatrician. As the clinician most extensively educated in pediatric health care, the pediatrician has the depth and breadth of knowledge, skills, and experience to assume this role and should be held to the highest standards. Collaboration with family physicians is an important component of pediatric health care delivery, as are partnerships with nonphysician clinicians in an effort to provide safe and effective quality health care for all infants, children, adolescents, and young adults in the United States. The AAP recognizes the importance of team-based education and training. Furthermore, the AAP maintains that to ensure safe and effective care, all members of the health care team must be required to demonstrate adequate education, training, skills, and competencies in pediatric health within their scope of practice, and all members of the health care team must provide care that is consistent with their education, training, and licensure. Patient safety and public protection must be the primary benchmarks in making any decision on changes involving the scope of practice of those who care for children.

The AAP affirms the following policy recommendations:

1. A pediatrician should serve as the leader of the pediatric health care team. This leadership role is based on the pediatrician's ability to manage, coordinate, and supervise the entire spectrum of pediatric care, from diagnosis through all stages of treatment and in all practice settings.

2. Pediatricians must assume responsibility for educating patients, families, health care purchasers, policy makers, the media, and the public about scope of practice issues.

3. Pediatricians should participate in the training and educational experiences of nonphysician pediatric clinicians, using evidenced-based and best-practice sources whenever possible. Similarly, training of pediatricians should include collaborative learning experiences in team care.

4. The AAP supports limitations on the scope of practice of nonphysician clinicians and opposes legislation that expands their scope of practice, including independent practice, hospital admitting privileges, and independent prescriptive authority.

5. Although the AAP opposes independent practice for nonphysician clinicians, in states that do allow independent practice, nonphysician clinicians acting independently of physicians should be held to the equivalent degree of professional and medical liability and abide by the same rules regarding liability insurance as would physicians.

6. To promote the highest standards of care in each state, scope of practice issues should be resolved according to the current guidelines developed by the Federation of State Medical Boards. These guidelines were designed to assist policy makers in ensuring that all practitioners are prepared, by virtue of education, training, and ongoing evaluation of competency, to provide services authorized in their scopes of practice in a safe, effective, and cost-efficient manner.

7. AAP chapters should encourage, recruit, and train their members to serve as advocates of optimal pediatric health care in state-level policy initiatives concerning nonphysician scope of practice. Such activities depend on physicians who are knowledgeable about lawmaking and policy-making processes and who have the skills necessary to be effective advocates in legislative deliberations.

8. AAP chapters and state medical and specialty societies, as well as national medical and specialty societies, should be proactive in scope of practice advocacy and should partner in informing policy makers, health care purchasers, the media, and the public about the differences in the education, skills, and knowledge of various health care professionals.

LEAD AUTHORS
Richard P. Shugerman, MD
Mary E. Rimsza, MD, Chairperson

COMMITTEE ON PEDIATRIC WORKFORCE, 2011–2012
William T. Basco, MD, MS
Andrew J. Hotaling, MD
Ted D. Sigrest, MD
Frank A. Simon, MD

FORMER COMMITTEE MEMBERS
Beth A. Pletcher, MD
Luisa I. Alvarado-Domenech, MD

LIAISONS
Christopher E. Harris, MD – *Section Forum Management Committee*
Gail A. McGuinness, MD – *American Board of Pediatrics*

STAFF
Holly J. Mulvey, MA
Carrie L. Radabaugh, MPP

ACKNOWLEDGMENT
The Committee acknowledges the contributions of Ethan Alexander Jewett, MA, a former member of the AAP Division of Workforce & Medical Education Policy, to the development of this policy statement.

REFERENCES

1. American Academy of Pediatrics, Ad Hoc Task Force on Definition of the Medical Home. The medical home. *Pediatrics*. 1992; 90(5):774

2. Grumbach K, Grundy P. Patient-Centered Primary Care Collaborative. Outcomes of implementing patient centered medical home interventions: a review of the evidence from prospective evaluation studies in the United States. Available at: http://www.pcpcc.net/content/results-evidence. Accessed September 14, 2012

3. American Medical Association, Advocacy Resource Center. 50-State Survey: Nurse Practitioner Prescriptive Authority. Chicago, IL: American Medical Association; 2012

4. Freed GL, Dunham KM, Lamarand KE, Loveland-Cherry C, Martyn KK; American Board of Pediatrics Research Advisory Committee. Pediatric nurse practitioners: roles and scope of practice. *Pediatrics*. 2010;126(5):846–850

5. Pearson LJ. The Pearson report. *Am J Nurse Pract*. 2009;13(2):8–82

6. Institute of Medicine, Committee on the Robert Wood Johnson Foundation Initiative on the Future of Nursing. *The Future of Nursing: Leading Change, Advancing Health*. Washington, DC: The National Academies Press; 2011

7. Cronenwett L, Dzau V. In: Culliton B, Russell S, eds. *Who Will Provide Primary Care and How Will They Be Trained? Proceedings of a Conference Sponsored by the Josiah Macy, Jr. Foundation*. Durham, NC: Josiah Macy Jr. Foundation; 2010

8. American Medical Association. AMA scope of practice data series: nurse practitioners. Available at: www.tnaonline.org/Media/pdf/apn-ama-sop-1109.pdf. Accessed September 19, 2012

9. American Association of Colleges of Nursing. DNP fact sheet: the doctor of nursing practice (DNP). Available at: www.aacn.nche.edu/media-relations/fact-sheets/dnp. Accessed September 19, 2012

10. American Association of Colleges of Nursing. The essentials of doctoral education for advanced nursing practice. Available at: www.aacn.nche.edu/publications/position/DNPEssentials.pdf. Accessed September 19, 2012

11. Freed GL, Dunham KM, Loveland-Cherry CJ, Martyn KK; Research Advisory Committee of the American Board of Pediatrics. Pediatric nurse practitioners in the United States: current distribution and recent trends in training. *J Pediatr*. 2010;157(4):589–593, 593.e1

12. Skillman SM, Kaplan L, Fordyce MA, McMenamin PD, Doescher MP. *Understanding Advanced Practice Registered Nurse Distribution in Urban and Rural Areas of the United States Using National Provider Identifier Data*. Seattle, WA: WWAMI Rural Health Research Center, University of Washington; 2012

13. American Academy of Pediatrics Committee on Pediatric Workforce. Pediatrician workforce statement. *Pediatrics*. 2005;116(1):263–269

14. Pollack CE, Armstrong K. The geographic accessibility of retail clinics for underserved populations. *Arch Intern Med*. 2009;169(10):945–949, discussion 950–953

15. Retail-Based Clinic Policy Work Group, AAP. AAP principles concerning retail-based clinics. *Pediatrics*. 2006;118(6):2561–2562

16. Federation of State Medical Boards. Assessing scope of practice in health care delivery: critical questions in assuring public access and safety. Available at: www.fsmb.org/pdf/2005_grpol_scope_of_practice.pdf. Accessed September 14, 2011

Surfactant Replacement Therapy for Preterm and Term Neonates With Respiratory Distress

- *Clinical Report*

CLINICAL REPORT

Surfactant Replacement Therapy for Preterm and Term Neonates With Respiratory Distress

abstract

Respiratory failure secondary to surfactant deficiency is a major cause of morbidity and mortality in preterm infants. Surfactant therapy substantially reduces mortality and respiratory morbidity for this population. Secondary surfactant deficiency also contributes to acute respiratory morbidity in late-preterm and term neonates with meconium aspiration syndrome, pneumonia/sepsis, and perhaps pulmonary hemorrhage; surfactant replacement may be beneficial for these infants. This statement summarizes the evidence regarding indications, administration, formulations, and outcomes for surfactant-replacement therapy. The clinical strategy of intubation, surfactant administration, and extubation to continuous positive airway pressure and the effect of continuous positive airway pressure on outcomes and surfactant use in preterm infants are also reviewed. *Pediatrics* 2014;133:156–163

Richard A. Polin, MD, FAAP, Waldemar A. Carlo, MD, FAAP, and COMMITTEE ON FETUS AND NEWBORN

KEY WORDS
surfactant, antenatal steroids, respiratory distress syndrome, meconium aspiration syndrome, neonatal pneumonia, neonatal sepsis, congenital diaphragmatic hernia, pulmonary hemorrhage, persistent pulmonary hypertension, preterm, term

ABBREVIATIONS
BPD—bronchopulmonary dysplasia
CI—confidence interval
CPAP—continuous positive airway pressure
ECMO—extracorporeal membrane oxygenation
INSURE—intubation, surfactant administration, and extubation
LOE—level of evidence
NNTB—number needed to benefit
RDS—respiratory distress syndrome
RR—relative risk
SP-B—surfactant protein B

INTRODUCTION

Surfactant replacement was established as an effective and safe therapy for immaturity-related surfactant deficiency by the early 1990s.[1] Systematic reviews of randomized, controlled trials confirmed that surfactant administration in preterm infants with established respiratory distress syndrome (RDS) reduces mortality, decreases the incidence of pulmonary air leak (pneumothoraces and pulmonary interstitial emphysema), and lowers the risk of chronic lung disease or death at 28 days of age (Table 1).[2–11] Subsequent trials indicated that prophylactic or early administration of surfactant resulted in fewer pneumothoraces, less pulmonary interstitial emphysema, and improved survival without bronchopulmonary dysplasia (BPD). However, recent randomized clinical trials indicate that the benefits of prophylactic surfactant are no longer evident in groups of infants when continuous positive airway pressure (CPAP) is used routinely.[5]

This clinical report updates a 2008 report from the American Academy of Pediatrics.[1] As in the previous report, a number of clinically important topics are reviewed surrounding use of surfactant, including prophylactic versus rescue replacement, preparations and administration techniques, the synergistic effects of surfactant and antenatal steroids, and surfactant therapy for respiratory disorders other than RDS. In addition, the effect of CPAP on RDS and surfactant replacement and the

www.pediatrics.org/cgi/doi/10.1542/peds.2013-3443

doi:10.1542/peds.2013-3443

All clinical reports from the American Academy of Pediatrics automatically expire 5 years after publication unless reaffirmed, revised, or retired at or before that time.

PEDIATRICS (ISSN Numbers: Print, 0031-4005; Online, 1098-4275).

TABLE 1 Meta-analyses of Surfactant Replacement: Prophylaxis and Rescue Treatment With Animal-Derived and Synthetic Surfactant[2,3,8,11]

Outcome	Prophylactic Surfactant		Rescue Surfactant	
	Animal Derived	Synthetic	Animal Derived	Synthetic
	N RR (95% CI)	N RR (95% CI)	N RR (95% CI)	N RR (95% CI)
Neonatal mortality	8 0.60 (0.47–0.77)	7 0.70 (0.58–0.85)	10 0.68 (0.57–0.82)	6 0.73 (0.61–0.88)
Pneumothorax	9 0.40 (0.29–0.54)	6 0.67 (0.50–0.90)	12 0.42 (0.34–0.52)	5 0.64 (0.55–0.76)
PIE	6 0.46 (0.36–0.59)	2 0.68 (0.50–0.93)	8 0.45 (0.37–0.55)	4 0.62 (0.54–0.71)
BPD[a]	8 0.91 (0.79–1.05)	4 1.06 (0.83–1.36)	12 0.95 (0.84–1.08)	5 0.75 (0.61–0.92)
BPD/death[a]	8 0.80 (0.72–0.88)	4 0.89 (0.77–1.03)	12 0.83 (0.77–0.90)	4 0.73 (0.65–0.83)

N, number; PIE, pulmonary interstitial emphysema.

[a] Defined at 28 d.

efficacy of the INSURE approach (intubation, surfactant administration, and extubation to CPAP) are reviewed.

PRETERM INFANTS AND SURFACTANT EFFECTIVENESS IN CLINICAL TRIALS

Surfactant trials have included infants born between 23 and 34 weeks' gestation and/or with birth weight between 500 and 2000 g.[1–12] The results of subgroup analyses from such studies indicated that surfactant therapy decreased mortality rates most effectively in infants born at less than 30 weeks' gestation or with birth weight <1250 g.[12] In addition, surfactant replacement reduced the incidence of pneumothorax, pulmonary interstitial emphysema, and the combined outcome of death or BPD, compared with no surfactant replacement[12]; these findings suggest that lung injury is mitigated after surfactant replacement. The incidence of other medical morbidities, such as BPD, intraventricular hemorrhage, necrotizing enterocolitis, health care–associated infections, retinopathy of prematurity, and patent ductus arteriosus, has not changed with surfactant replacement, but this may be attributable, in part, to the large reduction in mortality with surfactant replacement therapy.[13] The onset of clinical signs of patent ductus arteriosus may occur earlier, and the incidence of pulmonary hemorrhage, especially in infants born at less than 27 weeks' gestation, may be increased with surfactant therapy. Surfactant replacement is effective for larger and more mature preterm infants with established RDS.

PROPHYLACTIC VERSUS RESCUE SURFACTANT

A prophylactic, or preventive, surfactant strategy is defined as intubation and surfactant administration to infants at high risk of developing RDS for the primary purpose of preventing worsening RDS rather than treatment of established RDS; this has been operationalized in clinical studies as surfactant administration in the delivery room before initial resuscitation efforts or the onset of respiratory distress or, most commonly, after initial resuscitation but within 10 to 30 minutes after birth. This contrasts with a rescue or treatment surfactant strategy, in which surfactant is given only to preterm infants with established RDS. Rescue surfactant is most often administered within the first 12 hours after birth, when specified threshold criteria of severity of RDS are met.

The meta-analysis of studies conducted before routine application of CPAP demonstrated a lower mortality rate (relative risk [RR] 0.69; 95% confidence interval [CI] 0.56–0.85; number needed to benefit [NNTB] 20) and a decrease in the risk of air leak (RR 0.79; 95% CI 0.63–0.98) in preterm infants receiving prophylactic surfactant versus rescue surfactant.[14] However, when the studies that allowed for routine application of CPAP were included in the meta-analysis (National Institute of Child Health and Human Development SUPPORT Trial and Vermont Oxford Network Delivery Room Management Trial), the benefits of prophylactic surfactant on mortality (RR 0.89; 95% CI 0.76–1.04) and air leak (RR 0.86; 95% CI 0.71–1.04) could no longer be demonstrated.[5] Furthermore, infants receiving prophylactic surfactant had a higher incidence of BPD or death than did infants stabilized on CPAP (RR 1.12; 95% CI 1.02–1.24). Secondary analyses of studies that did or did not use CPAP to stabilize infants demonstrated a trend to a lower risk of intraventricular hemorrhage (RR 0.91; 95% CI 0.82–1.00) and severe intraventricular hemorrhage (RR 0.87; 95% CI 0.70–1.04) with prophylactic surfactant. That finding cannot be explained; however, there was considerable heterogeneity in the trials included in the meta-analysis. The risks of developing other complications of prematurity, such as retinopathy of prematurity, patent ductus arteriosus, and periventricular leukomalacia, were not significantly different.

When studies investigating infants born at <30 weeks' gestation were analyzed separately,[5] similar findings were noted. However, there was a trend for an increased risk of chronic lung disease in infants born at <30 weeks' gestation who received prophylactic surfactant (RR 1.13; 95% CI 1.00–1.28) and a significant increase in death or chronic lung disease (RR 1.13; 95% CI 1.02–1.25) with use of prophylactic surfactant.

EARLY VERSUS DELAYED SELECTIVE SURFACTANT TREATMENT OF RDS

Although there are no statistically significant benefits to prophylactic use of surfactant when compared with prophylactic CPAP, several studies have investigated whether administration of surfactant early in the course of respiratory insufficiency improves clinical outcomes. Early rescue is defined as surfactant treatment within 1 to 2 hours of birth, and late rescue is defined as surfactant treatment 2 or more hours after birth. A recent meta-analysis of early (within 2 hours) versus delayed surfactant treatment concluded that the risks of mortality (RR 0.84; 95% CI 0.74–0.95), air leak (RR 0.61; 95% CI 0.48–0.78), chronic lung disease (RR 0.69; 95% CI 0.55–0.86), and chronic lung disease or death (RR 0.83; 95% CI 0.75–0.91) were significantly decreased. There were no differences in other complications of prematurity.[7]

EARLY ADMINISTRATION OF SURFACTANT FOLLOWED BY BRIEF VENTILATION AND EXTUBATION TO CPAP (INSURE STRATEGY)

The INSURE strategy is widely used throughout the world. In randomized clinical trials performed before 2008, the INSURE approach, compared with rescue surfactant administration in infants with RDS, was associated with a significantly reduced need for mechanical ventilation (RR 0.67; 95% CI 0.57–0.79) and a reduced need for oxygen at 28 days.[6] In an analysis stratified by fraction of inspired oxygen requirement at study entry, a significantly higher frequency of patent ductus arteriosus was observed among infants in the rescue surfactant group, who required a fraction of inspired oxygen greater than 0.45 (RR 2.15; 95% CI 1.09–4.23). The Vermont Oxford Network Delivery Room Management Trial (n = 648) randomly assigned infants born at 26 to 29 weeks' gestation to 1 of 3 treatment groups: prophylactic surfactant and continued ventilation, prophylactic surfactant and rapid extubation to CPAP (INSURE), or nasal

CPAP without surfactant.[15] When compared with the group of infants receiving prophylactic surfactant and continued ventilation, the RR of death or BPD was 0.78 (95% CI 0.59–1.03) for the INSURE group and 0.83 (95% CI 0.64–1.09) for the CPAP group. However, in the nasal CPAP group, 48% were managed without intubation and 54% without surfactant treatment. A recent meta-analysis demonstrated that prophylactic surfactant (with rapid extubation to CPAP) was associated with a higher risk of death or BPD (RR 1.12; 95% CI 1.02–1.24; number needed to harm of 17) when compared with early stabilization with CPAP and selective surfactant administration.[5] In infants with birth weight ≥1250 g and mild to moderate RDS, elective intubation and administration of surfactant decreased the need for mechanical ventilation but had no effect on the duration of oxygen therapy, ventilator therapy, or hospital stay.[16]

ANIMAL-DERIVED VERSUS SYNTHETIC SURFACTANT

A wide variety of animal-derived and synthetic surfactants are available commercially (Table 2); both are beneficial as therapy for RDS in preterm infants. Animal-derived surfactants are modified or purified from bovine or porcine lungs. Treatment with animal-derived surfactants (beractant [Survanta; Abbvie Inc, North Chicago, IL], calfactant [Infasurf; ONY Inc, Amherst, NY], and poractant [Curosurf; Chiesi Farmaceutici, Parma, Italy]) has several advantages over first-generation, protein-free synthetic surfactants (eg, colfosceril palmitate [Exosurf; GlaxoSmithKline, Middlesex, UK]).[3] These include lower mortality rates (RR 0.86; 95% CI 0.76–0.98; number needed to harm of 40) and fewer pneumothoraces (RR 0.63; 95% CI 0.53–0.75; NNTB 22).[4] Animal-derived surfactants contain variable amounts

of surfactant protein B (SP-B). SP-B enhances the rate of adsorption of phospholipids at the air-water interface, is involved in the formation of tubular myelin, and has antiinflammatory properties. However, it is unclear whether significant differences in clinical outcomes exist among the available animal-derived products.

A synthetic surfactant (lucinactant) that contains a 21-amino acid peptide that mimics SP-B activity has recently been approved for the prevention and treatment of RDS in preterm infants.[18,19] When compared with animal-derived surfactant (beractant or poractant), lucinactant was shown to be equivalent.[18,19] Neonatal morbidities (intraventricular hemorrhage, periventricular leukomalacia, pulmonary hemorrhage, sepsis, patent ductus arteriosus, retinopathy of prematurity, necrotizing enterocolitis, and BPD) were not significantly different between preterm infants treated with animal-derived surfactants and those treated with synthetic surfactants.

SURFACTANT ADMINISTRATION

Surfactant administration strategies have been based on manufacturer guidelines for individual surfactants.[1] The dose of surfactant, frequency of administration, and treatment procedures have been modeled after research protocols. Furthermore, repeated doses of surfactants given at intervals for predetermined indications have decreased mortality and morbidity compared with placebo or single surfactant doses.[10] However, given the long half-life for surfactant in preterm infants with RDS,[20] redosing should not be needed more often than every 12 hours, unless surfactant is being inactivated by an infectious process, meconium, or blood. Dosing intervals shorter than 12 hours recommended by some manufacturers are not based on human pharmacokinetic data.

TABLE 2 Composition and Dosage of Surfactants[17]

Surfactant	Main Phospholipids	Proteins	Phospholipid Concentration	Suggested Dose	Phospholipid per Dose
Animal-derived					
Beractant (Survanta[a]) minced bovine lung extract	DPPC and PG	(<0.1%) SP-B and (1%) SP-C	25 mg/mL	4 mL/kg	100 mg/kg
Calfactant (Infasurf[b]) bovine calf lung lavage	DPPC and PG	(0.7%) SP-B and (1%) SP-C	35 mg/mL	3 mL/kg	105 mg/kg
Poractant (Curosurf[c]) minced porcine lung extract	DPPC and PG	(0.6%)SP-B and (1%) SP-C	80 mg/mL	2.5 mL/kg and	100-200 mg/kg
				1.25 mL/kg	100 mg/kg
Synthetic					
Colfosceril (Exosurf[d])	DPPC (100%)	None	13.5 mg/mL	5 mL/kg	67.5 mg/kg
Synthetic, protein analog					
Lucinactant (Surfaxin[e])	DPPC and POPG	KL4 peptide as SP-B	30 mg/mL	5.8 mL/kg	175 mg/kg

DPPC, dipalmitoyl phosphatidylcholine; PG, phosphatidylglycerol; POPG, palmitoyloleyl phosphatidylglycerol; SP-C, surfactant protein C.
[a] Abbvie Inc, North Chicago, IL.
[b] ONY Inc, Amherst, NY.
[c] Chiesi Farmaceutici, Parma, Italy.
[d] GlaxoSmithKline, Middlesex, UK.
[e] Discovery Laboratories, Warrington, PA.

Surfactant administration procedures may be complicated by transient airway obstruction, oxygen desaturation, bradycardia, and alterations in cerebral blood flow and brain electrical activity. The delivery of surfactant can also result in rapid improvement in lung volume, functional residual capacity, and compliance. Thus, expeditious changes in mechanical ventilator settings may be necessary to minimize the risks of lung injury and air leak. Clinicians with expertise in these procedures should be responsible for surfactant administration whenever surfactant is given.

Surfactant has traditionally been administered through an endotracheal tube either as bolus, in smaller aliquots,[21] or by infusion through an adaptor port on the proximal end of the endotracheal tube.[19] In an animal model, administration of surfactant as an intratracheal bolus while disconnected from the mechanical ventilator resulted in more uniform distribution than an infusion administered over 30 minutes through a side-hole adapter.[22] However, a small clinical trial of human preterm infants showed no significant differences in clinical outcomes between methods.[23] During surfactant administration, reflux into the endotracheal tube occurred more often when the infusion technique was used. Similar clinical outcomes were also found when surfactant was administered as a bolus or as a 1-minute infusion through a side-hole adapter.[24] Because data are conflicting and limited, the optimal method of surfactant administration in preterm infants has yet to be clearly proven. Additionally, there is insufficient evidence to recommend the optimal number of fractional doses of surfactant or what body position is best when surfactant is administered.

A number of alternatives to intratracheal administration of surfactant have been evaluated in clinical trials.[25-32] These include use of aerosolized surfactant preparations, laryngeal mask airway-aided delivery of surfactant, instillation of pharyngeal surfactant, and administration of surfactant using thin intratracheal catheters. Theoretically, each of these methods could allow administration of surfactant without intubation in spontaneously breathing infants. In a recent study, Göpel et al[25] randomized 220 preterm infants born at 26 to 28 weeks' gestation to receive either surfactant administered via a thin plastic catheter (using laryngoscopy) or surfactant administered as a rescue therapy. All infants were maintained on CPAP. The administration of surfactant through a thin plastic catheter significantly reduced the need for mechanical ventilation and decreased the need for oxygen therapy at 28 days. More data are needed to recommend any of the alternative techniques for surfactant administration.

SURFACTANT REPLACEMENT THERAPY FOR RESPIRATORY DISORDERS OTHER THAN RDS

Surfactant inactivation and secondary dysfunction may occur with conditions such as meconium aspiration syndrome, persistent pulmonary hypertension of the newborn, neonatal pneumonia, and pulmonary hemorrhage.[33,34] Surfactant administration techniques, surfactant dosage, patient populations, entry criteria, and study outcomes in the small randomized trials and case series of surfactant replacement in neonates with secondary surfactant deficiency vary considerably.[35-42]

Meconium aspiration syndrome with severe respiratory failure and persistent pulmonary hypertension may be complicated by surfactant inactivation. Surfactant replacement by bolus or slow infusion in infants with severe meconium aspiration syndrome improved oxygenation and reduced the need for extracorporeal membrane oxygenation (ECMO) (RR 0.64; 95% CI 0.46–0.91; NNTB 6).[35] Surfactant did not reduce mortality or decrease the frequency of air leaks (pneumothoraces or pulmonary interstitial emphysema). In a blinded randomized clinical trial of infants receiving ECMO, administration of surfactant shortened the duration of the ECMO. Notably, there were no infants with congenital diaphragmatic hernia in that study.[36]

Surfactant inactivation may be associated with pneumonia.[37,38] In a small randomized trial of surfactant rescue therapy, the subgroup of infants with sepsis showed improved oxygenation and a reduced need for ECMO compared with a similar group of control infants.[37] Newborn infants with pneumonia or sepsis receiving rescue surfactant also demonstrated improved gas exchange compared with infants without surfactant treatment. The number of neonates who received surfactant for sepsis and pneumonia in these clinical reports is small, and no recommendation can be made.

Surfactant treatment of pulmonary hemorrhage is plausible, because blood inhibits surfactant function. However, only a few retrospective and observational reports have documented the benefits of such therapy, and the magnitude of benefit remains to be established.[39]

Congenital diaphragmatic hernia may be associated with surfactant insufficiency.[40] Although measurements of disaturated phosphatidylcholine from lungs of infants with congenital diaphragmatic hernia show synthetic rates similar to those from infants without diaphragmatic hernia, pool sizes and kinetics are altered.[40] However, surfactant treatment of a large series of infants with congenital diaphragmatic hernia did not improve

outcomes. In fact, the need for ECMO, the incidence of chronic lung disease, and mortality rate were increased with surfactant administration.[41,42]

ANTENATAL STEROIDS AND SURFACTANT REPLACEMENT

Surfactant trials that proved efficacy were performed at a time when antenatal steroid therapy was given infrequently.[43] By the late 1990s, most mothers of preterm infants born at less than 30 weeks' gestation had received antenatal steroids (58% to 92%).[44–46] Antenatal steroids significantly reduce mortality (RR 0.62; 95% CI 0.51–0.77; NNTB 23), RDS (RR 0.65; 95% CI 0.47–0.75; NNTB 12), and surfactant use in preterm infants (RR 0.45; 95% CI 0.22–0.93; NNTB 9),[47] most consistently in those born between 28 and 34 weeks' gestation.

Results of observational studies and clinical trials have inferred that antenatal steroids may reduce the need for prophylactic and early rescue surfactant replacement in infants born after 27 to 28 weeks' gestation,[16,48] but no randomized, controlled trials have addressed this issue. In infants born at or earlier than 27 weeks' gestation, the incidence of RDS is not reduced after exposure to antenatal steroids; however, in a recently published study, death or neurodevelopment impairment at 18 to 22 months was significantly lower for infants who had been

exposed to antenatal steroids at 23 to 25 weeks' gestation.[49] Infants born before 32 weeks' gestation who received both antenatal steroids and postnatal surfactant were found on subgroup analyses to have significant reductions in mortality, severity of respiratory distress, and air leaks when compared with subgroups that received neither steroids nor surfactant, antenatal steroids only, or surfactant only.[50–52] This finding corroborates evidence from animal models of RDS that the combination of antenatal steroids and postnatal surfactant improves lung function more than either treatment alone.[53–55]

An important additional benefit of antenatal steroids is a reduction in risk of intraventricular hemorrhage, an advantage not found with surfactant replacement alone.[56] The effects of antenatal steroids on other neonatal morbidities, such as necrotizing enterocolitis and patent ductus arteriosus, have been inconsistent. However, antenatal steroids have not significantly decreased the incidence of BPD.[50,51]

CPAP AND SURFACTANT

Randomized clinical trials suggest that nasal CPAP is acceptable as an alternative to surfactant administration in preterm infants with RDS. A clinical report from the American Academy of Pediatrics, "Respiratory Support of the Preterm Infant," is forthcoming.[57]

TABLE 3 Levels of Evidence[59]

Recommendation LOE	LOE	Grade of Recommendation
Preterm infants born at <30 wk of gestation who need mechanical ventilation because of severe RDS should be given surfactant after initial stabilization.	1	Strong Recommendation
Using CPAP immediately after birth with subsequent selective surfactant administration should be considered as an alternative to routine intubation with prophylactic or early surfactant administration in preterm infants.	1	Strong Recommendation
Rescue surfactant may be considered for infants with hypoxic respiratory failure attributable to secondary surfactant deficiency (eg, meconium aspiration syndrome or sepsis/pneumonia).	2	Recommendation

SUMMARY OF SCIENCE

1. Surfactant replacement, given as prophylaxis or rescue treatment, reduces the incidence of RDS, air leaks, and mortality in preterm infants with RDS (level of evidence [LOE] 1).

2. Both animal-derived and newer synthetic surfactants with SP-B–like activity decrease acute respiratory morbidity and mortality in preterm infants with RDS (LOE 1).

3. Early rescue surfactant treatment (<2 hours of age) in infants with RDS decreases the risk of mortality, air leak, and chronic lung disease in preterm infants (LOE 1).

4. Early initiation of CPAP with subsequent selective surfactant administration in extremely preterm infants results in lower rates of BPD/death when compared with treatment with prophylactic surfactant therapy (LOE 1).

5. Surfactant replacement has not been shown to affect the incidence of neurologic, developmental, behavioral, medical, or educational outcomes in preterm infants (LOE 2).

6. Surfactant treatment improves oxygenation and reduces the need for ECMO without an increase in morbidity in neonates with meconium aspiration syndrome (LOE 2).

7. Surfactant treatment of infants with congenital diaphragmatic hernia does not improve clinical outcomes (LOE 2).

8. Antenatal steroids and postnatal surfactant replacement independently and additively reduce mortality, the severity of RDS, and air leaks in preterm infants (LOE 2).

CLINICAL IMPLICATIONS (TABLE 3)

1. Preterm infants born at <30 weeks' gestation who need mechanical ventilation because of severe RDS should be given surfactant after initial stabilization (Strong Recommendation).

2. Using CPAP immediately after birth with subsequent selective surfactant administration should be considered as an alternative to routine intubation with prophylactic or early surfactant administration in preterm infants (Strong Recommendation).

3. Rescue surfactant may be considered for infants with hypoxic respiratory failure attributable to secondary surfactant deficiency (eg, pulmonary hemorrhage, meconium aspiration syndrome, or sepsis/pneumonia) (Recommendation).

4. Preterm and term neonates who are receiving surfactant should be managed by nursery and transport personnel with the technical and clinical expertise to administer surfactant safely and deal with multisystem illness. Therefore, pediatric providers who are without expertise, or who are inexperienced or uncomfortable with surfactant administration or managing an infant who has received surfactant should wait for the transport team to arrive.

LEAD AUTHORS

Richard A. Polin, MD, FAAP
Waldemar A. Carlo, MD, FAAP

COMMITTEE ON FETUS AND NEWBORN, 2012–2013

Lu-Ann Papile, MD, FAAP, Chairperson
Richard A. Polin, MD, FAAP
Waldemar A. Carlo, MD, FAAP
Rosemarie Tan, MD, FAAP
Praveen Kumar, MD, FAAP
William Benitz, MD, FAAP
Eric Eichenwald, MD, FAAP
James Cummings, MD, FAAP
Jill Baley, MD, FAAP

CONSULTANT

Roger F. Soll, MD, FAAP

LIAISONS

Tonse N. K. Raju, MD, FAAP – *National Institutes of Health*
CAPT Wanda Denise Barfield, MD, FAAP – *Centers for Disease Control and Prevention*
Erin Keels, MSN – *National Association of Neonatal Nurses*
Anne Jefferies, MD – *Canadian Pediatric Society*
Kasper S. Wang, MD, FAAP – *AAP Section on Surgery*
George Macones, MD – *American College of Obstetricians and Gynecologists*

STAFF

Jim Couto, MA

DISCLOSURES

Dr Carlo is on the Mednax Board of Directors. Dr Polin is a consultant for Discovery Laboratories.

REFERENCES

1. Engle WA; American Academy of Pediatrics Committee on Fetus and Newborn. Surfactant-replacement therapy for respiratory distress in the preterm and term neonate. *Pediatrics.* 2008;121(2):419–432

2. Soll RF. Synthetic surfactant for respiratory distress syndrome in preterm infants. *Cochrane Database Syst Rev.* 2000;(2):CD001149

3. Seger N, Soll R. Animal derived surfactant extract for treatment of respiratory distress syndrome. *Cochrane Database Syst Rev.* 2009; (2):CD007836

4. Soll RF, Blanco F. Natural surfactant extract versus synthetic surfactant for neonatal respiratory distress syndrome. *Cochrane Database Syst Rev.* 2001;(2):CD000144

5. Rojas-Reyes MX, Morley CJ, Soll R. Prophylactic versus selective use of surfactant in preventing morbidity and mortality in preterm infants. *Cochrane Database Syst Rev.* 2012;3(3):CD000510

6. Stevens TP, Harrington EW, Blennow M, Soll RF. Early surfactant administration with brief ventilation vs. selective surfactant

and continued mechanical ventilation for preterm infants with or at risk for respiratory distress syndrome. *Cochrane Database Syst Rev.* 2007;(4):CD003063

7. Bahadue FL, Soll R. Early versus delayed selective surfactant treatment for neonatal respiratory distress syndrome. *Cochrane Database Syst Rev.* 2012;11(11):CD001456

8. Soll R, Ozek E. Prophylactic protein free synthetic surfactant for preventing morbidity and mortality in preterm infants. *Cochrane Database Syst Rev.* 2010;(1):CD001079

9. Pfister RH, Soll R, Wiswell TE. Protein-containing synthetic surfactant versus protein-free synthetic surfactant for the prevention and treatment of respiratory distress syndrome. *Cochrane Database Syst Rev.* 2009;(4):CD006180

10. Soll R, Ozek E. Multiple versus single doses of exogenous surfactant for the prevention or treatment of neonatal respiratory distress syndrome. *Cochrane Database Syst Rev.* 2009;(1):CD000141

11. Soll RF. Prophylactic natural surfactant extract for preventing morbidity and mortality in preterm infants. *Cochrane Database Syst Rev.* 2000;(2):CD000511

12. Suresh GK, Soll RF. Overview of surfactant replacement trials. *J Perinatol.* 2005;25 (suppl 2):S40–S44

13. Philip AG. Neonatal mortality rate: is further improvement possible? *J Pediatr.* 1995;126(3):427–433

14. Soll RF, Morley CJ. Prophylactic versus selective use of surfactant in preventing morbidity and mortality in preterm infants. *Cochrane Database Syst Rev.* 2001;(2):CD000510

15. Dunn MS, Kaempf J, de Klerk A, et al; Vermont Oxford Network DRM Study Group. Randomized trial comparing 3 approaches to the initial respiratory management of preterm neonates. *Pediatrics.* 2011;128(5). Available at: www.pediatrics.org/cgi/content/full/128/5/e1069

16. Escobedo MB, Gunkel JH, Kennedy KA, et al; Texas Neonatal Research Group. Early surfactant for neonates with mild to moderate respiratory distress syndrome: a multicenter, randomized trial. *J Pediatr.* 2004;144(6):804–808

17. Moya F, Javier MC. Myth: all surfactants are alike. *Semin Fetal Neonatal Med.* 2011;16 (5):269–274

18. Sinha SK, Lacaze-Masmonteil T, Valls i Soler A, et al; Surfaxin Therapy Against Respiratory Distress Syndrome Collaborative Group. A multicenter, randomized, controlled trial of lucinactant versus poractant alfa among very premature infants at high

risk for respiratory distress syndrome. *Pediatrics.* 2005;115(4):1030–1038

19. Moya F, Sinha S, Gadzinowski J, et al; SELECT and STAR Study Investigators. One-year follow-up of very preterm infants who received lucinactant for prevention of respiratory distress syndrome: results from 2 multicenter randomized, controlled trials. *Pediatrics.* 2007;119(6). Available at: www.pediatrics.org/cgi/content/full/119/6/e1361

20. Cogo PE, Facco M, Simonato M, et al. Pharmacokinetics and clinical predictors of surfactant redosing in respiratory distress syndrome. *Intensive Care Med.* 2011;37(3):510–517

21. Kendig JW, Ryan RM, Sinkin RA, et al. Comparison of two strategies for surfactant prophylaxis in very premature infants: a multicenter randomized trial. *Pediatrics.* 1998;101(6):1006–1012

22. Ueda T, Ikegami M, Rider ED, Jobe AH. Distribution of surfactant and ventilation in surfactant-treated preterm lambs. *J Appl Physiol (1985).* 1994;76(1):45–55

23. Zola EM, Gunkel JH, Chan RK, et al. Comparison of three dosing procedures for administration of bovine surfactant to neonates with respiratory distress syndrome. *J Pediatr.* 1993;122(3):453–459

24. Valls-i-Soler A, López-Heredia J, Fernández-Ruanova MB, Gastiasoro E; Spanish Surfactant Collaborative Group. A simplified surfactant dosing procedure in respiratory distress syndrome: the "side-hole" randomized study. *Acta Paediatr.* 1997;86(7):747–751

25. Göpel W, Kribs A, Ziegler A, et al; German Neonatal Network. Avoidance of mechanical ventilation by surfactant treatment of spontaneously breathing preterm infants (AMV): an open-label, randomised, controlled trial. *Lancet.* 2011;378(9803):1627–1634

26. Schmölzer GM, Agarwal M, Kamlin CO, Davis PG. Supraglottic airway devices during neonatal resuscitation: an historical perspective, systematic review and meta-analysis of available clinical trials. *Resuscitation.* 2013;84(6):722–730

27. Kribs A. How best to administer surfactant to VLBW infants? *Arch Dis Child Fetal Neonatal Ed.* 2011;96(4):F238–F240

28. Mehler K, Grimme J, Abele J, Huenseler C, Roth B, Kribs A. Outcome of extremely low gestational age newborns after introduction of a revised protocol to assist preterm infants in their transition to extrauterine life. *Acta Paediatr.* 2012;101(12):1232–1239

29. Abdel-Latif ME, Osborn DA. Laryngeal mask airway surfactant administration for pre-

vention of morbidity and mortality in preterm infants with or at risk of respiratory distress syndrome. *Cochrane Database Syst Rev.* 2011;(7):CD008309

30. Abdel-Latif ME, Osborn DA. Nebulised surfactant in preterm infants with or at risk of respiratory distress syndrome. *Cochrane Database Syst Rev.* 2012;(10):CD008310

31. Abdel-Latif ME, Osborn DA. Pharyngeal instillation of surfactant before the first breath for prevention of morbidity and mortality in preterm infants at risk of respiratory distress syndrome. *Cochrane Database Syst Rev.* 2011;(3):CD008311

32. Abdel-Latif ME, Osborn DA, Challis D. Intra-amniotic surfactant for women at risk of preterm birth for preventing respiratory distress in newborns. *Cochrane Database Syst Rev.* 2010;(1):CD007916

33. Finer NN. Surfactant use for neonatal lung injury: beyond respiratory distress syndrome. *Paediatr Respir Rev.* 2004;5(suppl A):S289–S297

34. Donn SM, Dalton J. Surfactant replacement therapy in the neonate: beyond respiratory distress syndrome. *Respir Care.* 2009;54(9):1203–1208

35. El Shahed AI, Dargaville P, Ohlsson A, Soll RF. Surfactant for meconium aspiration syndrome in full term/near term infants. *Cochrane Database Syst Rev.* 2007;(3):CD002054

36. Lotze A, Knight GR, Martin GR, et al. Improved pulmonary outcome after exogenous surfactant therapy for respiratory failure in term infants requiring extracorporeal membrane oxygenation. *J Pediatr.* 1993;122(2):261–268

37. Tan K, Lai NM, Sharma A. Surfactant for bacterial pneumonia in late preterm and term infants. *Cochrane Database Syst Rev.* 2012;(2):CD008155

38. Vento GM, Tana M, Tirone C, et al. Effectiveness of treatment with surfactant in premature infants with respiratory failure and pulmonary infection. *Acta Biomed.* 2012;83(suppl 1):33–36

39. Aziz A, Ohlsson A. Surfactant for pulmonary haemorrhage in neonates. *Cochrane Database Syst Rev.* 2012;(7):CD005254

40. Cogo PE, Zimmermann LJ, Meneghini L, et al. Pulmonary surfactant disaturated-phosphatidylcholine (DSPC) turnover and pool size in newborn infants with congenital diaphragmatic hernia (CDH). *Pediatr Res.* 2003;54(5):653–658

41. Van Meurs K; Congenital Diaphragmatic Hernia Study Group. Is surfactant therapy beneficial in the treatment of the term newborn infant with congenital diaphragmatic hernia? *J Pediatr.* 2004;145(3):312–316

42. Lally KP, Lally PA, Langham MR, et al; Congenital Diaphragmatic Hernia Study Group. Surfactant does not improve survival rate in preterm infants with congenital diaphragmatic hernia. *J Pediatr Surg.* 2004; 39(6):829–833

43. Wright LL, Horbar JD, Gunkel H, et al. Evidence from multicenter networks on the current use and effectiveness of antenatal corticosteroids in low birth weight infants. *Am J Obstet Gynecol.* 1995;173(1):263–269

44. Chien LY, Ohlsson A, Seshia MM, Boulton J, Sankaran K, Lee SK; Canadian Neonatal Network. Variations in antenatal corticosteroid therapy: a persistent problem despite 30 years of evidence. *Obstet Gynecol.* 2002;99(3):401–408

45. Horbar JD, Badger GJ, Carpenter JH, et al; Members of the Vermont Oxford Network. Trends in mortality and morbidity for very low birth weight infants, 1991-1999. *Pediatrics.* 2002;110(1 pt 1):143–151

46. St John EB, Carlo WA. Respiratory distress syndrome in VLBW infants: changes in management and outcomes observed by the NICHD Neonatal Research Network. *Semin Perinatol.* 2003;27(4):288–292

47. Roberts D, Dalziel S. Antenatal corticosteroids for accelerating fetal lung maturation for women at risk of preterm birth. *Cochrane Database Syst Rev.* 2006;(3): CD004454

48. Gortner L, Wauer RR, Hammer H, et al. Early versus late surfactant treatment in preterm infants of 27 to 32 weeks' gestational age: a multicenter controlled clinical trial. *Pediatrics.* 1998;102(5):1153–1160

49. Carlo WA, McDonald SA, Fanaroff AA, et al; Eunice Kennedy Shriver National Institute of Child Health and Human Development Neonatal Research Network. Association of antenatal corticosteroids with mortality and neurodevelopmental outcomes among infants born at 22 to 25 weeks' gestation. *JAMA.* 2011;306(21):2348–2358

50. Jobe AH, Mitchell BR, Gunkel JH. Beneficial effects of the combined use of prenatal corticosteroids and postnatal surfactant on preterm infants. *Am J Obstet Gynecol.* 1993;168(2):508–513

51. Kari MA, Hallman M, Eronen M, et al. Prenatal dexamethasone treatment in conjunction with rescue therapy of human surfactant: a randomized placebo-controlled multicenter study. *Pediatrics.* 1994;93(5):730–736

52. White A, Marcucci G, Andrews E, Edwards K, Long W; The American Exosurf Neonatal Study Group I and The Canadian Exosurf Neonatal Study Group. Antenatal steroids and neonatal outcomes in controlled clinical trials of surfactant replacement. *Am J Obstet Gynecol.* 1995;173(1):286–290

53. Seidner S, Pettenazzo A, Ikegami M, Jobe A. Corticosteroid potentiation of surfactant dose response in preterm rabbits. *J Appl Physiol (1985).* 1988;64(6):2366–2371

54. Ikegami M, Jobe AH, Seidner S, Yamada T. Gestational effects of corticosteroids and surfactant in ventilated rabbits. *Pediatr Res.* 1989;25(1):32–37

55. Gladstone IM, Mercurio MR, Devenny SG, Jacobs HC. Antenatal steroids, postnatal surfactant, and pulmonary function in premature rabbits. *J Appl Physiol (1985).* 1989;67(4):1377–1382

56. National Institutes of Health. Effect of corticosteroids for fetal maturation on perinatal outcomes. *NIH Consens Statement.* 1994;12(2):1–24

57. Carlo W, Polin RA; American Academy of Pediatrics, Committee on Fetus and Newborn. Respiratory support in preterm infants at birth. *Pediatrics.* In press

58. US Preventive Services Task Force. Grade definition recommendations after 2007. Available at: www.uspreventiveservicestaskforce.org/uspstf/grades.htm. Accessed June 7, 2013

The Transfer of Drugs and Therapeutics Into Human Breast Milk: An Update on Selected Topics

- *Clinical Report*

CLINICAL REPORT

The Transfer of Drugs and Therapeutics Into Human Breast Milk: An Update on Selected Topics

abstract

Many mothers are inappropriately advised to discontinue breastfeeding or avoid taking essential medications because of fears of adverse effects on their infants. This cautious approach may be unnecessary in many cases, because only a small proportion of medications are contraindicated in breastfeeding mothers or associated with adverse effects on their infants. Information to inform physicians about the extent of excretion for a particular drug into human milk is needed but may not be available. Previous statements on this topic from the American Academy of Pediatrics provided physicians with data concerning the known excretion of specific medications into breast milk. More current and comprehensive information is now available on the Internet, as well as an application for mobile devices, at LactMed (http://toxnet.nlm.nih.gov). Therefore, with the exception of radioactive compounds requiring temporary cessation of breastfeeding, the reader will be referred to LactMed to obtain the most current data on an individual medication. This report discusses several topics of interest surrounding lactation, such as the use of psychotropic therapies, drugs to treat substance abuse, narcotics, galactagogues, and herbal products, as well as immunization of breastfeeding women. A discussion regarding the global implications of maternal medications and lactation in the developing world is beyond the scope of this report. The World Health Organization offers several programs and resources that address the importance of breastfeeding (see http://www.who.int/topics/breastfeeding/en/). *Pediatrics* 2013;132:e796–e809

Hari Cheryl Sachs, MD, FAAP* and COMMITTEE ON DRUGS

KEY WORD
human milk

ABBREVIATIONS
AAP—American Academy of Pediatrics
FDA—Food and Drug Administration
HBV—hepatitis B vaccine
HPV—human papillomavirus vaccine
NSAID—nonsteroidal antiinflammatory drug

www.pediatrics.org/cgi/doi/10.1542/peds.2013-1985

doi:10.1542/peds.2013-1985

All clinical reports from the American Academy of Pediatrics automatically expire 5 years after publication unless reaffirmed, revised, or retired at or before that time.

PEDIATRICS (ISSN Numbers: Print, 0031-4005; Online, 1098-4275).

INTRODUCTION

Lactating women can be exposed to medications or other therapeutics, either on a limited or long-term basis, depending on the need to treat acute or chronic conditions. Many women are advised to discontinue nursing or avoid taking necessary medications because of concerns about possible adverse effects in their infants.[1] Such advice is often not based on evidence, because information about the extent of drug excretion into human milk may be unavailable, and for many drugs, information is limited to data from animal studies, which may not correlate with human experience. In addition, not all drugs are excreted in clinically significant amounts into human milk, and the presence of a drug in human milk may not pose a risk for the infant. To weigh the risks and benefits of breastfeeding, physicians need to consider multiple factors. These factors include the need for the drug by the mother, the potential effects of the drug on milk production, the amount of the drug excreted into human milk, the extent of oral absorption by the breastfeeding infant, and potential adverse effects on the breastfeeding infant. The age of the infant is also an important factor in the decision-making process, because adverse events associated with drug exposure via lactation occur most often in neonates younger than 2 months and rarely in infants older than 6 months.[2] In the near future, pharmacogenetics may also provide important guidance for individualized decisions.

In large part because of efforts by Cheston Berlin, Jr, MD, a statement by the American Academy of Pediatrics (AAP) on the transfer of drugs and chemicals into human milk was first published in 1983[3] and underwent several subsequent revisions,[4,5] the most recent of which was published in 2001.[6] Previous editions were intended to list drugs potentially used during lactation and to describe possible effects on the infant and/or on lactation. Revisions for the statement can no longer keep pace with the rapidly changing information available via the Internet, published studies, and new drug approvals. A more comprehensive and current database is available at LactMed (http://toxnet. nlm.nih.gov). LactMed includes up-to-date information on drug levels in human milk and infant serum, possible adverse effects on breastfeeding infants, potential effects on lactation, and recommendations for possible alternative drugs to consider. Common herbal products are also included. For this reason, with the exception of radioactive compounds that require temporary or permanent cessation of breastfeeding, the reader will be referred to LactMed to obtain the most current data on an individual medication.

This statement reviews proposed changes in US Food and Drug Administration (FDA) labeling that are designed to provide useful information to the physician and to outline general

---

LactMed is part of the National Library of Medicine's Toxicology Data Network (TOXNET)

Each record includes the following information:

- Generic name: refers to US-adopted name of active portion of the drug
- Scientific name: genus and species of botanical products (when applicable)
- Summary of use during lactation (includes discussion of conflicting recommendations and citations)
- Drug levels
  - Maternal levels: based on studies that measure concentration in breast milk; includes relative infant dose (weight-adjusted percentage of maternal dose) when possible
  - Infant levels: serum or urine concentrations from the literature
- Effects in breastfed infants: adverse events with Naranjo* assessment of causality (definite, probably, possibly, unlikely)
- Possible effects on lactation: if known, including effects on infants that may interfere with nursing (eg, sedation)
- Alternative drugs to consider: may not be comprehensive
- References
- Chemical Abstracts Service Registry Number
- Drug class
- LactMed record number
- Last revision date

Primary Author: Philip O. Anderson, PharmD

Contributor: Jason Sauberan, PharmD

Peer Review Panel:

  Cheston M. Berlin, Jr, MD
  Shinya Ito, MD
  Kathleen Uhl, MD
  Sonia Neubauer, MD

* The Naranjo probability scale is a method used to estimate the probability that an adverse event is caused by a drug.[7]

considerations for individual risk/benefit counseling. An update regarding the use of antidepressants, anxiolytics, and antipsychotics in the lactating woman is also provided, because the use of psychotropic agents during lactation is still debated. Since publication of the last statement, numerous questions have been raised regarding the use of methadone in the lactating woman. For this reason, therapies for substance abuse and smoking cessation are discussed. Given the finding that codeine use may be associated with toxicity in patients, including neonates with ultrarapid metabolism, a brief review of alternative agents to treat pain in the lactating woman is provided. The use of galactagogues is also reviewed because more women now endeavor to breastfeed adopted infants or preterm neonates. The increasing use of herbal products has invited a discussion of the merits of these alternative therapies in the nursing woman. Finally, immunization of breastfeeding women and their infants will be reviewed to assist pediatricians in encouraging immunization when needed in lactating women and addressing parental reluctance to immunize breastfed infants.

GENERAL CONSIDERATIONS

Several factors should be considered when advising a woman regarding a decision to breastfeed her infant while she is on drug therapy. The benefits of breastfeeding for both the infant and mother need to be weighed against the risks of drug exposure to the infant (or to the mother, in the case of agents intended to induce lactation). Many factors affect the individual risk/benefit decision, including specific information about chemical and pharmacologic properties of the drug, which may be available from resources such as LactMed and in product labeling. In general, chemical properties of a drug, such as lack of ionization, small molecular weight, low volume of distribution, low maternal serum protein binding, and high lipid solubility, facilitate drug excretion into human milk. Drugs with long half-lives are more likely to accumulate in human milk, and drugs with high oral bioavailability are more easily absorbed by the infant.[8] The adverse event profile of the drug is another property that affects the individual risk/benefit ratio. Use of a drug with a significant adverse effect in a lactating woman (such as an arrhythmia) may be acceptable to treat a serious illness in the mother; however, use of the same drug to increase milk production would not be acceptable. For drugs with an adverse event profile that correlates with increasing dosage, higher maternal doses may be associated with greater neonatal toxicity. In addition, the timing of exposure and the duration of therapy are other important considerations. A decision to breastfeed when continuing treatment with an agent for which in utero exposure also has occurred differs from a decision to initiate a novel therapy in the early postpartum period. Similarly, the risks of a single-dose therapy or short-term treatment may differ from those of a chronic therapy.

In addition to pharmacokinetic or chemical properties of the drug, the infant's expected drug exposure is influenced by infant and maternal factors beyond basic known pharmacokinetic and chemical properties of the drug itself. For example, the risk of adverse reactions in a preterm infant or an infant with underlying chronic medical conditions may be higher than that for a more mature or healthier infant. Certain drugs may accumulate in the breastfed infant because of reduced clearance or immaturity of metabolic pathways. However, for other drugs (eg, acetaminophen), the immaturity of these same pathways may protect an infant from toxic drug metabolites. Similarly, patients with specific genotypes may experience drug toxicity, as evidenced by fatalities observed in individuals who demonstrate ultrarapid metabolism of codeine.[9] Finally, certain infant conditions, such as metabolic diseases, and maternal health conditions may preclude nursing (eg, HIV) or require multiple therapies that are particularly toxic (eg, cancer treatment).

CHANGES IN DRUG LABELING

In the past, the lactation section in FDA-approved labeling was often limited to statements that advise caution or contain an admonition to discontinue breastfeeding or discontinue therapy, depending on the importance to the mother. In 2008, the FDA published a proposed revision to the regulations, which affects the pregnancy and lactation sections of labeling. The agency is currently working on the final rule, which is intended to provide a clinically oriented framework for placement of pregnancy and lactation information into drug labeling and to permit the patient and physician to explore the risk/benefit on the basis of the best available data. Under the proposed rule, the current Nursing Mothers section is replaced by a section called Lactation. The Lactation section of labeling will contain 3 subsections: Risk Summary, Clinical Considerations, and Data. The Risk Summary section will include a summary of what is known about the excretion of the drug into human milk and potential effects on the breastfed infant, as well as maternal milk production. The Clinical Considerations section will include methods to minimize exposure of the breastfed infant to the drug when applicable, as well as information about monitoring for expected adverse drug effects on the infant. The Data component will provide a detailed overview of the existing data that forms the evidence base for the other 2 sections.

In addition to the proposed rule, the FDA published "Guidance for Industry: Clinical Lactation Studies: Study Design, Data Analysis, and Recommendations for Labeling."[10]

Along with outlining recommendations regarding lactation study design as well as the timing and indications for these studies, this draft guidance includes advice on parameters (several of which are used in LactMed) that can be used to inform physicians about the extent of drug exposure. Using these parameters, drug exposure to the infant may be measured directly in infant serum or estimated on the basis of pharmacokinetic parameters. These estimates of infant exposure (for example, relative infant dose) can be expressed as a percent of weight-adjusted maternal or, when known, weight-adjusted pediatric dose.

ESTIMATES OF DRUG EXPOSURE

Daily Infant Dosage (mg/day) =

$\sum$(drug concentration in each milk collection × expressed volume in each milk collection)

OR

C_{milk}[average drug concentration in milk(mg/mL)] × V_{milk}(volume in mL of milk ingested in 24 hours)

Note: V_{milk} is typically estimated to be 150 mL/kg/day

Relative Infant Dose

% Maternal Dose = [Daily Infant Dosage (mg/kg/day) ÷ Maternal Dose (mg/kg/day)] × 100

% Infant or Pediatric Dose = [Daily Infant Dosage (mg/kg/day) ÷ Infant or Pediatric dose(mg/kg/day)] × 100

ANTIDEPRESSANTS, ANXIOLYTICS, AND ANTIPSYCHOTICS

Previous statements from the AAP categorized the effect of psychoactive drugs on the nursing infant as "unknown but may be of concern." Although new data have been published since 2001, information on the long-term effects of these compounds is still limited. Most publications regarding psychoactive drugs describe the pharmacokinetics in small numbers of lactating women with short-term observational studies of their infants. In addition, interpretation of the effects on the infant from the small number of longer-term studies is confounded by prenatal treatment or exposure to multiple therapies. For these reasons, the long-term effect on the developing infant is still largely unknown.[11,12]

Many antianxiety drugs, antidepressants, and mood stabilizers appear in low concentrations in human milk, with estimated relative infant doses less than 2% of weight-adjusted maternal dose and/or milk-plasma ratios less than 1.[13] However, the percentage of maternal doses that approach clinically significant levels (10% or more) have been reported for bupropion,[14] diazepam,[13] fluoxetine,[15] citalopram,[16] lithium,[17] lamotrigine,[18] and venlafaxine.[19] Data on drug excretion in human milk are not available for up to one-third of psychoactive therapies.[13]

Because of the long half-life of some of these compounds and/or their metabolites, coupled with an infant's immature hepatic and renal function, nursing infants may have measurable amounts of the drug or its metabolites in plasma and potentially in neural tissue. Infant plasma concentrations that exceed 10% of therapeutic maternal plasma concentrations have been reported for a number of selective serotonin reuptake inhibitors,

---

TABLE 1 Psychoactive Drugs With Infant Serum Concentrations Exceeding 10% of Maternal Plasma Concentrations[a]

Agent	Reference
Citalopram	Weissman 2004[20]
Clomipramine	Schimmell 1991[21]
Diazepam	Wesson 1985[22]
Doxepin	Moretti 2009[16]
Fluoxetine	Weissman 2004,[20] product labeling
Fluvoxamine	Weissman 2004[20]
Lamotrigine	Newport 2008,[18] Fotopoulou 2009[23]
Lithium	Viguerra 2007,[24] Grandjean 2009,[25] Bogen 2012[26]
Mirtazapine	Tonn 2009[27]
Nortriptyline	Weissman 2004[20]
Olanzapine	Whitworth 2008[28]
Sertraline	Hendrick 2001,[29] Stowe 2003[30]
Venlafaxine	Newport 2009[19]

[a] Based on individual maternal-infant pair(s); may include active metabolites.

---

antipsychotics, anxiolytics, and mood stabilizers (see Table 1).

Mothers who desire to breastfeed their infant(s) while taking these agents should be counseled about the benefits of breastfeeding as well as the potential risk that the infant may be exposed to clinically significant levels and that the long-term effects of this exposure are unknown. Consideration should be given to monitoring growth and neurodevelopment of the infant.

DRUGS FOR SMOKING CESSATION OR TO TREAT SUBSTANCE ABUSE/ ALCOHOL DEPENDENCE

Although many women are appropriately advised to refrain from smoking, drinking, and using recreational drugs during and after pregnancy, in part because of adverse effects on their infants (see Table 2), some are unable to do so and may seek assistance after delivery. Maternal smoking is not an absolute contraindication to breastfeeding.[31] Nonetheless, for multiple reasons, including the association of sudden infant death syndrome with

TABLE 2 Drugs of Abuse for Which Adverse Effects on the Breastfeeding Infant Have Been Reported[a]

Drug	Reported Effect or Reason for Concern	Reference
Alcohol	Impaired motor development or postnatal growth, decreased milk consumption, sleep disturbances.	Koren 2002,[34] Backstrand 2004,[35] Mennella 2007[36]
	Note: Although binge drinking should be avoided, occasional, limited ingestion (0.5 g of alcohol/kg/d; equivalent to 8 oz wine or 2 cans of beer per day) may be acceptable.	National Academy of Sciences 1991[37]
Amphetamines	Hypertension, tachycardia, and seizures.	Product labeling
	In animal studies of postnatal exposure, long-term behavioral effects, including learning and memory deficits and altered locomotor activity, were observed.	
Benzodiazepines	Accumulation of metabolite, prolonged half-life in neonate or preterm infant is noted; chronic use not recommended.	Jain 2005,[38] Malone 2004[39]
	Apnea, cyanosis, withdrawal, sedation, cyanosis, and seizures.	
Cocaine	Intoxication, seizures, irritability, vomiting, diarrhea, tremulousness.	Chasnoff 1987,[40] Winecker 2001[41]
Heroin	Withdrawal symptoms, tremors, restlessness, vomiting, poor feeding.	vandeVelde 2007[42]
LSD	Potent hallucinogen.	
Methamphetamine	Fatality, persists in breast milk for 48 h.	Ariagno 1995,[43] Bartu 2009[44]
Methylene dioxy-methamphetamine (ecstasy)	Closely related products (amphetamines) are concentrated in human milk.	
Marijuana (cannabis)	Neurodevelopmental effects, delayed motor development at 1 y, lethargy, less frequent and shorter feedings, high milk-plasma ratios in heavy users.	Djulus 2005,[45] Campolongo 2009,[46] Garry 2010[47]
Phencyclidine	Potent hallucinogen, infant intoxication.	AAP 2001,[6] Academy of Breastfeeding Medicine[48]

[a] Effect on maternal judgment or mood may affect ability to care for infant.

tobacco exposure,[32,33] lactating women should be strongly encouraged to stop smoking and to minimize secondhand exposure. Exposure to alcohol or recreational drugs may impair a mother's judgment and interfere with her care of the infant and can cause toxicity to the breastfeeding infant (see Table 2).

Limited information is available regarding the use of medications in lactating women to treat substance abuse or alcohol dependence or for smoking cessation. However, the presence of behaviors, such as continued ingestion of illicit drugs or alcohol, and underlying conditions, such as HIV infection, are not compatible with breastfeeding.[49,50] Patients also require ongoing psychosocial support to maintain abstinence.[48]

Methadone, buprenorphine, and naltrexone are 3 agents approved by the FDA for use in the treatment of opioid dependence. Continued breastfeeding by women undergoing such treatment presumes that the patient remains abstinent, is HIV negative, and is en-

rolled in and closely monitored by an appropriate drug treatment program with significant social support.[48,51]

Potential adverse effects on breastfeeding infants from methadone (according to product labeling) and buprenorphine include lethargy, respiratory difficulty, and poor weight gain.[52] The long-term effects of methadone in humans are unknown. Nonetheless, methadone levels in human milk are low, with calculated infant exposures less than 3% of the maternal weight-adjusted dose.[53,54] Plasma concentrations in infants are also low (less than 3% of maternal trough concentrations) during the neonatal period and up to 6 months postpartum.[55,56] For these reasons, guidelines from the Academy of Breastfeeding Medicine encourage breastfeeding for women treated with methadone who are enrolled in methadone-maintenance programs.[48]

Buprenorphine is excreted into human milk and achieves a level similar to that in maternal plasma.[57] Infant exposure

appears to be up to 2.4% of the maternal weight-adjusted dose.[55,56,58] However, buprenorphine can be abused, and although the significance in humans is unknown, labeling for buprenorphine and buprenorphine/naloxone combinations states that use is not advised by lactating women, because animal lactation studies have shown decreased milk production and viability of the offspring. FDA labeling also advises caution for use of naltrexone in nursing infants of opioid-dependent women. Of note, published information on naltrexone is limited to 1 case report that estimates infant exposure to be low (7 µg/kg/d, or 0.86% of the maternal weight-adjusted dose).[59]

Transferred amounts of methadone or buprenorphine are insufficient to prevent symptoms of neonatal abstinence syndrome.[49,60] Neonatal abstinence syndrome can occur after abrupt discontinuation of methadone.[51,61] Thus, breastfeeding should not be stopped abruptly, and gradual weaning is advised if a decision is made to discontinue breastfeeding.

Limited information is available for disulfiram and naltrexone, agents that are used to treat alcohol dependence. As noted previously, a low relative infant dose (<1%) was observed in a single case report of naltrexone exposure in a 6-week-old breastfed infant.[59] FDA labeling discourages use of disulfiram and both the injectable and oral form of naltrexone in lactating women.

Only one-third of women successfully discontinue smoking without pharmacologic aids.[62] Nicotine replacement therapy, bupropion, and varenicline are agents indicated for use as aids to smoking cessation treatment. Nicotine replacement therapy is compatible with breastfeeding as long as the dose (assuming a cigarette delivers ~1 mg of nicotine) is less than the number of cigarettes typically smoked, because nicotine passes freely into human milk and is orally absorbed as nicotine. Cotinine concentrations are lower than those related to tobacco use. Short-acting products (eg, gum or lozenges) are recommended.[62] Infant exposure decreases proportionally with maternal patch doses.[63]

In contrast, bupropion is excreted into human milk with exposures that may exceed 10% (range, 1.4%–10.6%) of the maternal dose.[14] Although infant levels were not measured, there is a case report of a seizure in a 6-month-old breastfed infant potentially related to bupropion.[64] Limited published information is available for varenicline, but the varenicline label includes a boxed warning for serious neuropsychiatric adverse events, including suicidal ideation or behavior. FDA labeling discourages use of both these agents in lactating women.

PAIN MEDICATIONS

Rarely, normal doses of codeine given to lactating women may result in dangerously high levels of its active metabolite morphine in breastfeeding infants. A fatality has been noted in an infant of a mother with ultrarapid metabolism.[65] In this infant, the postmortem level of morphine (87 ng/mL) greatly exceeded a typical level in a breastfeeding infant (2.2 ng/mL), as well as the therapeutic range for neonates (10–12 ng/mL). In addition, unexplained apnea, bradycardia, cyanosis, and sedation have been reported in nursing infants of mothers receiving codeine.[2,66] Hydrocodone is also metabolized via the CYP2D6 pathway. On the basis of pharmacokinetic data, infants exposed to hydrocodone through human milk may receive up to 9% of the relative maternal dose.[67] Given the reduced clearance of hydrocodone in neonates and the adverse events observed in ultrarapid metabolizers of codeine, caution is advised for use of codeine and hydrocodone in both the mother and nursing infant. Close monitoring for signs and symptoms of neonatal as well as maternal toxicity is recommended. A commercial test to identify ultrarapid metabolizers is not yet widely available. The incidence of this specific CYP2D6 genotype varies with racial and ethnic group as follows: Chinese, Japanese, or Hispanic, 0.5% to 1.0%; Caucasian, 1.0% to 10.0%; African American, 3.0%; and North African, Ethiopian, and Saudi Arabian, 16.0% to 28.0%.[68]

For these reasons, when narcotic agents are needed to treat pain in the breastfeeding woman, agents other than codeine (eg, butorphanol, morphine, or hydromorphone) are preferred. Clinically insignificant levels of butorphanol are excreted into human milk. Morphine appears to be tolerated by the breastfeeding infant, although there is 1 case report of an infant with plasma concentrations within the therapeutic range.[69] Clear-ance of morphine is decreased in infants younger than 1 month and approaches 80% of adult values by 6 months of age.[70] Limited data suggest that use of hydromorphone for brief periods may be compatible with breastfeeding[71,72]; however, FDA labeling discourages use. Regardless of the choice of therapy, to minimize adverse events for both the mother and her nursing infant, the lowest dose and shortest duration of therapy should be prescribed. Drug delivery via patient-controlled anesthesia or administration by the epidural route may also minimize infant exposure.

Other narcotic agents, such as oxycodone, pentazocine, propoxyphene, and meperidine, are not recommended in the lactating mother. Relatively high amounts of oxycodone are excreted into human milk, and therapeutic concentrations have been detected in the plasma of a nursing infant.[73] Central nervous system depression was noted in 20% of infants exposed to oxycodone during breastfeeding.[74] Thus, use of oxycodone should be discouraged. Limited published data are available about pentazocine. However, respiratory depression and apnea occur frequently in infants, particularly in neonates or in preterm infants, who are treated with pentazocine. Propoxyphene has been associated with unexplained apnea, bradycardia, and cyanosis, as well as hypotonia in nursing infants.[75,76] Moreover, propoxyphene was withdrawn from the market because significant QT prolongation occurred at therapeutic doses.[77] Meperidine use is associated with decreased alertness of the infant and is likely to interfere with breastfeeding.[71] Although estimates of meperidine exposure are low (approximately 2% to 3% of the maternal weight-adjusted dose), the half-life of the active metabolite for meperidine is prolonged, and it may accumulate in infant blood or tissue.[71,72]

When narcotics are not required to relieve mild to moderate pain, other analgesic agents can be used. Presuming that pain relief is adequate, short-acting agents, such as ibuprofen and acetaminophen, are acceptable.[78] Although the half-life of ibuprofen may be prolonged in neonates, particularly in preterm infants (according to product labeling), minimal amounts of ibuprofen are excreted into human milk.[72] Despite reduced clearance of acetaminophen,[79] hepatotoxicity is less common in neonates than in older infants, in part because of low levels of certain cytochrome P-450 enzymes, which convert acetaminophen into toxic metabolites.[80] Acetaminophen is available for both oral and intravenous administration.

Although all nonsteroidal antiinflammatory drugs (NSAIDs) carry a boxed warning regarding gastrointestinal bleeding and potential long-term cardiac toxicity, according to their product labeling and Gardiner et al,[81] celecoxib, flurbiprofen, and naproxen are considered to be compatible with breastfeeding, because less than 1% is excreted into human milk. In addition, a breastfeeding infant would receive less than 1% of the relative pediatric dose of celecoxib prescribed for a 2-year-old (according to product labeling). However, long-term use of naproxen is not recommended because of the drug's long half-life and case reports of gastrointestinal tract bleeding and emesis. Avoiding NSAIDs in breastfeeding infants with ductal-dependent cardiac lesions may be prudent.

Limited published data on other NSAIDs (etodolac, fenoprofen, meloxicam, oxaprozin, piroxicam, sulindac, and tolmetin) are available, and FDA labeling discourages their use for a variety of reasons. Although the implications for humans are unknown, meloxicam concentrations in milk of lactating animals exceed plasma concentrations. Diflunisal has a long half-life and is not recommended because of potential adverse events, including cataracts and fatality, in neonatal animals. Similarly, mefenamic acid has a prolonged half-life in preterm infants. Injectable and oral forms of ketorolac are contraindicated in nursing women, according to product labeling, because of potential adverse effects related to closure of the ductus arteriosus in neonates. Less than 1% of ketorolac nasal spray is excreted into human milk, and unlike the oral and intravenous forms of ketorolac, use is not contraindicated (product labeling).

Carisoprodol and its active metabolite, meprobamate, are concentrated in human milk (2–4 times maternal plasma concentrations). Impaired milk production has been observed, and animal studies suggest maternal use may lead to less effective infant feeding (because of sedation) and/or decreased milk production (according to product labeling).

Low doses (75–162 mg/d) of aspirin may be acceptable[82]; however, use of high-dose aspirin therapy during breastfeeding is not advised, because the serum concentration of salicylate in breastfeeding infants has been reported to reach approximately 40% of therapeutic concentrations. Adverse events, such as rash, platelet abnormalities, bleeding, and metabolic acidosis have also been reported.[71]

GALACTAGOGUES

Galactagogues, or agents to stimulate lactation, are often used to facilitate lactation, particularly for mothers of preterm infants. They also may be used to induce lactation in an adoptive mother. However, evidence to support these agents, including use of dopamine antagonists, such as domperidone and metoclopramide; herbal treatments; and hormonal manipulation, is lacking.[83]

Although a placebo-controlled study (*n* = 42) suggested that domperidone may increase milk volume in mothers of preterm infants,[84] maternal safety has not been established. The FDA issued a warning in June 2004 regarding use of domperidone in breastfeeding women because of safety concerns based on published reports of arrhythmia, cardiac arrest, and sudden death associated with intravenous therapy. Furthermore, treatment with oral domperidone is associated with QT prolongation in children and infants.[85,86] Domperidone is not an approved product in the United States, and labeling for oral formulations marketed outside the United States do not recommend use during lactation.

Several small trials (each with fewer than 25 subjects) published before 1990 suggested that metoclopramide increases prolactin concentrations and/or milk production in mothers of both term and preterm infants.[87] However, more recent controlled studies do not replicate this finding.[88,89] Human milk concentrations of metoclopramide are similar to therapeutic concentrations in adult plasma,[88] and measurable amounts can be detected in breastfeeding infants.[90] Clearance of metoclopramide in neonates is prolonged, which may result in excessive serum concentrations and the risk of conditions associated with overdose, such as methemoglobinemia. Of concern, prolactin concentrations were increased in 4 of 7 infants exposed to metoclopramide via human milk.[90] The safety profile for metoclopramide includes adverse reactions, such as dystonia, depression, suicidal ideation, and gastrointestinal tract disturbances, as well as a boxed warning about the risk of tardive dyskinesia. These risks to the mother limit the usefulness of this therapy.

Although a pilot study in 8 lactating women performed decades ago suggested that oxytocin nasal spray increased human milk production, a larger placebo-controlled trial in 51 women has not confirmed that observation.[91] Oxytocin nasal spray is no longer marketed in the United States. Similarly, anecdotal reports supporting the use of the herb fenugreek to facilitate lactation have not been confirmed by controlled studies.[92,93] Fenugreek contains coumarin, which may interact with NSAIDs.[94] Use of fenugreek in lactating women also is associated with maple-syrup odor in infants.[95] Available data do not support the routine use of other herbal products, such as fennel, to facilitate lactation.[96]

In summary, galactagogues have a limited role in facilitating lactation and have not been subject to full assessments of safety for the nursing infant. Nursing mothers should seek consultation with a lactation specialist and use non-pharmacologic measures to increase milk supply, such as ensuring proper technique, using massage therapy, increasing the frequency of milk expression, prolonging the duration of pumping, and maximizing emotional support.

COMMONLY USED HERBAL PRODUCTS

Despite the frequent use of herbal products in breastfeeding women (up to 43% of lactating mothers in a 2004 survey),[97] reliable information on the safety of many herbal products is lacking. Herbal products are not subject to the same standards for manufacturing and proven effectiveness and safety as are drug products before they are marketed.[98] In fact, the use of several herbal products may be harmful, including kava and yohimbe. For example, the FDA has issued a warning that links kava supplementation to severe liver damage.[99] Breastfeeding mothers should not use yohimbe because of reports of associated fatalities in children.[100] In addition, from 2008 through 2010, the FDA recalled 10 or more dietary supplements each year because of the presence of potentially toxic undeclared ingredients in the supplement.[101] Similarly, the US Government Accountability Office found that 16 of 40 common herbal dietary supplements obtained from retail stores contained pesticide residues.[102]

Safety data are lacking for many herbs commonly used during breastfeeding, such as chamomile,[103] black cohosh,[104] blue cohosh,[105] chastetree,[106] echinacea,[107] ginseng,[108] gingko,[109] Hypericum (St John's wort),[110,111] and valerian.[112] Adverse events have been reported in both breastfeeding infants and mothers. For example, St John's wort may cause colic, drowsiness, or lethargy in the breastfed infant even though milk production and infant weight do not appear to be adversely affected[110] and relative maternal dose and infant plasma concentrations are low.[113] Prolonged use of fenugreek may require monitoring of coagulation status and serum glucose concentrations.[114] For these reasons, these aforementioned herbal products are not recommended for use by nursing women.

Although supplementation of nursing mothers with iron and vitamins is safe as long as recommended daily allowances are not exceeded, the use of other nutritional supplements may not be. For instance, L-tryptophan has been associated with eosinophilic myositis.[115] Therefore, physicians should inquire about the use of herbal products and dietary supplements in lactating women and discuss the need for caution because of the paucity of data available.

DIAGNOSTIC IMAGING

When feasible, elective imaging procedures should be delayed until a woman is no longer breastfeeding. For most radiopharmaceuticals, breastfeeding should be interrupted for a time period based on the rate of decline of the agent and dosimetry to avoid infant exposures greater than 1 mSv (100 mrem). For agents that may be concentrated in breast tissue, close contact of the mother with the infant and, consequently, nursing may need to be avoided for a period of time, although expressed milk that has been refrigerated until the radioactivity has decayed may be safe. General guidelines based on Nuclear Regulatory Commission regulations and International Commission on Radiologic Protection guidelines[116] are cited in Tables 3 and 4. However, because there is considerable variability in milk radioactivity, and close contact with an infant may result in additional exposure, consultation with a radiologist should be sought. If deemed necessary, individualized testing of expressed milk may be performed to ensure that radioactivity has reached background levels before breastfeeding is resumed.[117]

Notably, because radiolabeled iodinated products are concentrated in the developing thyroid and radioactivity persists after imaging with most ^{131}I and ^{125}I radiopharmaceuticals (with the exception of ^{125}I- hippurate), breastfeeding should be interrupted for a minimum of 3 weeks. Similarly, ^{22}Na and ^{67}Ga (gallium) administration also require a prolonged (3-week) interruption in breastfeeding. Because the lactating breast has a greater ^{131}I affinity than does the nonlactating breast, women should cease breastfeeding at least 4 weeks before whole-body procedures with ^{131}I and should discontinue breastfeeding thereafter. Doing so will reduce the radiation dose and potential cancer risk to maternal breast tissue.

Traditionally, lactating women receiving intravascular gadolinium or iodinated contrast (as opposed to radiolabeled iodine) are advised to discontinue nursing for 24 hours. However, a minimal amount (0.04%) of the intravenous dose reaches human milk, and, of that, less than 1% to

TABLE 3 Radioactive Compounds That May Require Temporary Cessation of Breastfeeding: Recommendations of the International Commission on Radiologic Protection

Compound	Examples	Example of Procedures	Recommended Time for Cessation of Breastfeeding	Comments
[14]C-labeled	Triolein, glycocholic acid, urea	*Helicobacter pylori* breath test	None	No approved US products
[99m]Tc-labeled	DMSA, DTPA, phosphonates (MDP), PYP, tetrofosmin	Multiple: imaging of kidney, bone, lung, heart, tumors	0 to 4 h, as long as no free pertechnetate	Consider discarding at least 1 meal after procedure
	Microspheres, pertechnetate, WBC		12–24 h	Range depends on dose
	Sulfur-colloids, RBC in vivo		6 h	
I-labeled	[123]I, ^{125}I or ^{131}I-iodo hippurate	Thyroid imaging	12 h	Note: whole-body irradiation with ^{131}I requires prolonged cessation
Others	[11]C- [11]N or [11]O-labeled	PET scans	None	Short physical half-life
	[57]Co-labeled vitamin B$_{12}$	Schilling test	24 h	Pomeroy 2005[119]
	^{18}F-FDG	PET scans	None, first feeding should be expressed breast milk to avoid direct contact[120]	Use alternatives for 10 half-lives (10×109 min= 18 h)[a]
	^{51}Cr-EDTA	Renal imaging	None	
	[81m]Kr-gas	Pulmonary imaging	None	No approved US products
	[82]Rb chloride	PET scan of myocardium	May resume 1 h after last infusion	Half-life 75 s[a]
	^{111}In-octreotide	SPECT, neuroendocrine tumors	None	
	[111]In -WBC		1 wk	Depends on dose
	[133]Xe	Cardiac, pulmonary, and cerebral imaging	None	Half-life 5 d[a]

DMSA, dimercaptosuccinic acid; DTPA, diethylenetriaminepentaacetate; EDTA, ethylenediaminetetraacetic acid; FDG, fludeoxyglucose; PET, positron emission tomography; PYP, pyrophosphate; RBC, red blood cell; SPECT, single-photon emission computed tomography; WBC, white blood cell.
[a] FDA-approved drug labeling.

TABLE 4 Radioactive Compounds Requiring Prolonged Cessation of Breastfeeding

Compound	Examples	Example of Procedures	Recommended Time for Cessation of Breastfeeding	Comments
I-labled	[123]I- BMIPP, -HSA, -IPPA, -MIBG, -NaI, or -HSA	Imaging of tumors	Greater than 3 wk	Essentially need to stop breastfeeding
	^{131}I-MIBG or -NaI			
Others	^{201}Tl-chloride	Cardiac imaging	48 h to 2 wk	Half-life 73 h[a]
	^{67}Ga-citrate	Imaging of tumors	1 wk to 1 mo	Depends on dose
	[22]Na, [75]Se		Greater than 3 wk	Essentially need to stop breastfeeding

Use of expressed human milk recommended because of exposure via direct contact.[120] BMIPP, β-methyl-p-iodophenyl-pentadecanoic acid; HSA, human serum albumin; IPPA, iodophe-nylpentadecanoic; MIBG, metaiodobenzylguanidine; NaI, sodium iodide.
[a] FDA-approved drug labeling.

2% is absorbed by the infant. Therefore, breastfeeding can be continued without interruption after the use of iodinated contrast or gadolinium.[118]

BREASTFEEDING AND VACCINES

With rare exceptions, maternal immunization does not create any problems for breastfeeding infants, although questions concerning 2 topics often arise regarding lactation and immunization: the effect of lactation on the infant's immune response to a vaccine and a potential adverse effect on the infant from maternal immunization. Breastfeeding does not interfere with the infant's immune response to most routine immunizations (eg, diphtheria and tetanus toxoids and acellular pertussis vaccine, inactivated poliovirus vaccine, and hepatitis B vaccine [HBV]),[121] despite the presence of maternal antibodies in human milk. Seroconversion rates are also similar between breastfed and formula-fed infants receiving rotavirus vaccine; however, vaccine efficacy for severe rotavirus gastroenteritis appears to be higher in formula-fed infants compared with exclusively breastfed infants, particularly during the second season (98% vs 88%) when breastfeeding has been discontinued.[122] Nonetheless, protection during the first year is similar. Moreover, breastfeeding enhances the antibody response to pneumococcal and *Haemophilus influenzae* type b vaccines.[123] Breastfeeding may also decrease the incidence of fever after infant immunization.[124] Therefore, the timing of infant feeding (including human milk) relative to immunization is not restricted, even for live vaccines, such as rotavirus.

Lactating women may need to be immunized. Inactivated vaccines (such as tetanus toxoid, reduced diphtheria toxoid, and acellular pertussis vaccine; inactivated poliovirus vaccine; influenza; hepatitis A vaccine; HBV; or human papillomavirus vaccine [HPV]) given to a nursing mother do not pose a risk to the breastfeeding infant. Several vaccines, such as tetanus toxoid, reduced diphtheria toxoid, and acellular pertussis vaccine and influenza vaccine, are recommended for the mother during the postpartum period to protect the infant as well as the mother. Other routine or catch-up vaccines, such as HPV, hepatitis A vaccine, and HBV, can be given to the lactating mother. HPV immunization is recommended for women younger than 27 years. The incidence of adverse reactions in nursing infants within 30 days of maternal immunization with HPV was similar to nursing infants of women receiving the control except for acute respiratory illness (according to Gardasil labeling). Hence, caution is warranted when immunizing mothers of infants who are vulnerable to respiratory illnesses (eg, preterm infants, infants with congenital heart disease or chronic respiratory problems).

Most live vaccines are not associated with virus secretion in human milk. For example, despite maternal seroconversion, neither the varicella virus nor antibody to varicella DNA has been detected in breastfeeding infants.[125] Although attenuated rubella can be secreted into human milk and transmitted to breastfed infants, infections are usually asymptomatic or mild. Consequently, postpartum immunization with measles-mumps-rubella vaccine is recommended for women who lack immunity, especially to rubella.[126] In contrast, infants are considered to be at high risk of developing vaccinia

after exposure to smallpox vaccine or encephalitis after yellow fever vaccine. Two cases of meningoencephalitis in nursing infants whose mothers had been immunized against yellow fever are documented in the literature.[127,128] Therefore, most vaccines, with the exception of smallpox or yellow-fever vaccine, which are contraindicated in nonemergency situations, may be administered during lactation.

SUMMARY

The benefits of breastfeeding outweigh the risk of exposure to most therapeutic agents via human milk. Although most drugs and therapeutic agents do not pose a risk to the mother or nursing infant, careful consideration of the individual risk/benefit ratio is necessary for certain agents, particularly those that are concentrated in human milk or result in exposures in the infant that may be clinically significant on the basis of relative infant dose or detectable serum concentrations. Caution is also advised for drugs and agents with unproven benefits, with long half-lives that may lead to drug accumulation, or with known toxicity to the mother or infant. In addition, specific infants may be more vulnerable to adverse events because of immature organ function (eg, preterm infants or neonates) or underlying medical conditions. Several excellent resources are available for the pediatrician, including product labeling and the peer-reviewed database, LactMed. Consultation with a specialist may be indicated, particularly when the

use of radiopharmaceuticals, oncologic drugs, or other therapies not addressed by LactMed is contemplated. Additional information about topics outside the scope of this report, such as environmental agents, can be obtained from the third edition of the AAP textbook *Pediatric Environmental Health*.[129]

LEAD AUTHOR

Hari Cheryl Sachs, MD, FAAP

COMMITTEE ON DRUGS, 2012–2013

Daniel A. C. Frattarelli, MD, FAAP, Chairperson
Jeffrey L. Galinkin, MD, FAAP
Thomas P. Green, MD, FAAP
Timothy Johnson, DO, FAAP
Kathleen Neville, MD, FAAP
Ian M. Paul, MD, MSc, FAAP
John Van den Anker, MD, PhD, FAAP

FORMER COMMITTEE MEMBERS

Mark L. Hudak, MD, FAAP
Matthew E. Knight, MD, FAAP

LIAISONS

John J. Alexander, MD, FAAP – *Food and Drug Administration*
Sarah J. Kilpatrick, MD, PhD – *American College of Obstetricians and Gynecologists*
Janet D. Cragan, MD, MPH, FAAP – *Centers for Disease Control and Prevention*
Michael J. Rieder, MD, FAAP – *Canadian Pediatric Society*
Adelaide Robb, MD – *American Academy of Child and Adolescent Psychiatry*
Hari Cheryl Sachs, MD, FAAP – *Food and Drug Administration*
Anne Zajicek, MD, PharmD, FAAP – *National Institutes of Health*

CONTRIBUTOR

Ashley Moss, MD, FAAP

STAFF

Tamar Haro, JD
Raymond J. Koteras, MHA

REFERENCES

1. Berlin CM, Briggs GG. Drugs and chemicals in human milk. *Semin Fetal Neonatal Med*. 2005;10(2):149–159
2. Anderson PO, Pochop SL, Manoguerra AS. Adverse drug reactions in breastfed infants: less than imagined. *Clin Pediatr (Phila)*. 2003;42(4):325–340
3. American Academy of Pediatrics, Committee on Drugs. The transfer of drugs and other chemicals into human breast milk. *Pediatrics*. 1983;72(3):375–383
4. American Academy of Pediatrics, Committee on Drugs. The transfer of drugs and other chemicals into human breast milk. *Pediatrics*. 1989;84(5):924–936
5. American Academy of Pediatrics, Committee on Drugs. The transfer of drugs and other chemicals into human breast milk. *Pediatrics*. 1994;93(1):137–150

6. American Academy of Pediatrics Committee on Drugs. Transfer of drugs and other chemicals into human milk. *Pediatrics.* 2001;108(3):776–789

7. Naranjo CA, Busto U, Sellers EM, et al. A method for estimating the probability of adverse drug reactions. *Clin Pharmacol Ther.* 1981;30(2):239–245

8. Hale TW. Maternal medications during breastfeeding. *Clin Obstet Gynecol.* 2004; 47(3):696–711

9. Berlin CM, Jr, Paul IM, Vesell ES. Safety issues of maternal drug therapy during breastfeeding. *Clin Pharmacol Ther.* 2009; 85(1):20–22

10. Food and Drug Administration. Draft guidance for industry: clinical lactation studies —study design, data analysis, and recommendations for labeling. February 2005. Available at: www.fda.gov/downloads/RegulatoryInformation/Guidances/ucm127505. pdf. Accessed November 26, 2012

11. Gentile S. SSRIs in pregnancy and lactation: emphasis on neurodevelopmental outcome. *CNS Drugs.* 2005;19(7):623–633

12. Gentile S. The safety of newer antidepressants in pregnancy and breastfeeding. *Drug Saf.* 2005;28(2):137–152

13. Fortinguerra F, Clavenna A, Bonati M. Psychotropic drug use during breastfeeding: a review of the evidence. *Pediatrics.* 2009;124(4). Available at: www.pediatrics.org/cgi/content/full/124/4/e547

14. Davis MF, Miller HS, Nolan PE Jr. Bupropion levels in breast milk for 4 mother-infant pairs: more answers to lingering questions. *J Clin Psychiatry.* 2009;70(2):297–298

15. Kristensen JH, Ilett KF, Hackett LP, Yapp P, Paech M, Begg EJ. Distribution and excretion of fluoxetine and norfluoxetine in human milk. *Br J Clin Pharmacol.* 1999;48 (4):521–527

16. Moretti ME. Psychotropic drugs in lactation— Motherisk Update 2008. *Can J Clin Pharmacol.* 2009;16(1):e49–e57

17. Ostrea EM, Jr, Mantaring JB, III, Silvestre MA. Drugs that affect the fetus and newborn infant via the placenta or breast milk. *Pediatr Clin North Am.* 2004;51(3): 539–579, vii

18. Newport DJ, Pennell PB, Calamaras MR, et al. Lamotrigine in breast milk and nursing infants: determination of exposure. *Pediatrics.* 2008;122(1). Available at: www.pediatrics.org/cgi/content/full/122/1/e223

19. Newport DJ, Ritchie JC, Knight BT, Glover BA, Zach EB, Stowe ZN. Venlafaxine in human breast milk and nursing infant

plasma: determination of exposure. *J Clin Psychiatry.* 2009;70(9):1304–1310

20. Weissman AM, Levy BT, Hartz AJ, et al. Pooled analysis of antidepressant levels in lactating mothers, breast milk, and nursing infants. *Am J Psychiatry.* 2004;161 (6):1066–1078

21. Schimmell MS, Katz EZ, Shaag Y, Pastuszak A, Koren G. Toxic neonatal effects following maternal clomipramine therapy. *J Toxicol Clin Toxicol.* 1991;29(4):479–484

22. Wesson DR, Camber S, Harkey M, Smith DE. Diazepam and desmethyldiazepam in breast milk. *J Psychoactive Drugs.* 1985; 17(1):55–56

23. Fotopoulou C, Kretz R, Bauer S, et al. Prospectively assessed changes in lamotrigine-concentration in women with epilepsy during pregnancy, lactation and the neonatal period. *Epilepsy Res.* 2009;85 (1):60–64

24. Viguera AC, Newport DJ, Ritchie J, et al. Lithium in breast milk and nursing infants: clinical implications. *Am J Psychiatry.* 2007;164(2):342–345

25. Grandjean EM, Aubry JM. Lithium: updated human knowledge using an evidence-based approach: part III: clinical safety. *CNS Drugs.* 2009;23(5):397–418

26. Bogen DL, Sit D, Genovese A, Wisner KL. Three cases of lithium exposure and exclusive breastfeeding. *Arch Women Ment Health.* 2012;15(1):69–72

27. Tonn P, Reuter SC, Hiemke C, Dahmen N. High mirtazapine plasma levels in infant after breast feeding: case report and review of the literature. *J Clin Psychopharmacol.* 2009;29(2):191–192

28. Whitworth A, Stuppaeck C, Yazdi K, et al. Olanzapine and breast-feeding: changes of plasma concentrations of olanzapine in a breast-fed infant over a period of 5 months. *J Psychopharmacol.* 2010;24(1): 121–123

29. Hendrick V, Fukuchi A, Altshuler L, Widawski M, Wertheimer A, Brunhuber MV. Use of sertraline, paroxetine and fluvoxamine by nursing women. *Br J Psychiatry.* 2001;179:163–166

30. Stowe ZN, Hostetter AL, Owens MJ, et al. The pharmacokinetics of sertraline excretion into human breast milk: determinants of infant serum concentrations. *J Clin Psychiatry.* 2003;64(1):73–80

31. Section on Breastfeeding. Breastfeeding and the use of human milk. *Pediatrics.* 2012;129(3). Available at: www.pediatrics. org/cgi/content/full/129/3/e827

32. Liebrechts-Akkerman G, Lao O, Liu F, et al. Postnatal parental smoking: an important

risk factor for SIDS. *Eur J Pediatr.* 2011; 170(10):1281–1291

33. Moon RY; Task Force on Sudden Infant Death Syndrome. SIDS and other sleep-related infant deaths: expansion of recommendations for a safe infant sleeping environment. *Pediatrics.* 2011;128(5): 1030–1039

34. Koren G. MotherRisk update: drinking alcohol while breastfeeding. *Can Fam Physician.* 2002;48:29–41

35. Backstrand JR, Goodman AH, Allen LH, Pelto GH. Pulque intake during pregnancy and lactation in rural Mexico: alcohol and child growth from 1 to 57 months. *Eur J Clin Nutr.* 2004;58(12):1626–1634

36. Mennella JA, Yourshaw LM, Morgan LK. Breastfeeding and smoking: short-term effects on infant feeding and sleep. *Pediatrics.* 2007;120(3):497–502

37. Institute of Medicine, Subcommittee on Nutrition During Lactation. *Nutrition During Lactation.* Washington, DC: National Academies Press; 1991

38. Jain AE, Lacy T. Psychotropic drugs in pregnancy and lactation. *J Psychiatr Pract.* 2005;11(3):177–191

39. Malone K, Papagni K, Ramini S, Keltner NL. Antidepressants, antipsychotics, benzodiazepines, and the breastfeeding dyad. *Perspect Psychiatr Care.* 2004;40 (2):73–85

40. Chasnoff IJ, Lewis DE, Squires L. Cocaine intoxication in a breast-fed infant. *Pediatrics.* 1987;80(6):836–838

41. Winecker RE, Goldberger BA, Tebbett IR, et al. Detection of cocaine and its metabolites in breast milk. *J Forensic Sci.* 2001;46(5):1221–1223

42. vande Velde S, Verloo P, Van Biervliet S, et al. Heroin withdrawal leads to metabolic alkalosis in an infant with cystic fibrosis. *Eur J Pediatr.* 2007;166(1):75–76

43. Ariagno R, Karch SB, Middleberg R, Stephens BG, Valdès-Dapena M. Methamphetamine ingestion by a breast-feeding mother and her infant's death: People v Henderson. *JAMA.* 1995;274(3):215

44. Bartu A, Dusci LJ, Ilett KF. Transfer of methylamphetamine and amphetamine into breast milk following recreational use of methylamphetamine. *Br J Clin Pharmacol.* 2009;67(4):455–459

45. Djulus J, Moretti M, Koren G. Marijuana use and breastfeeding. *Can Fam Physician.* 2005;51:349–350

46. Campolongo P, Trezza V, Palmery M, Trabace L, Cuomo V. Developmental exposure to cannabinoids causes subtle and enduring neurofunctional alterations. *Int Rev Neurobiol.* 2009;85:117–133

47. Garry A, Rigourd V, Amirouche A, et al. Cannabis and breastfeeding. *J Toxicol.* 2009;2009:596149

48. Jansson LM; Academy of Breastfeeding Medicine Protocol Committee. ABM clinical protocol #21: guidelines for breastfeeding and the drug-dependent woman. *Breastfeed Med.* 2009;4(4):225–228

49. Jones HE, Martin PR, Heil SH, et al. Treatment of opioid-dependent pregnant women: clinical and research issues. *J Subst Abuse Treat.* 2008;35(3):245–259

50. Centers for Disease Control and Prevention. Human immunodeficiency virus (HIV), and acquired immunodeficiency syndrome (AIDS). Available at: www.cdc.gov/breastfeeding/disease/hiv.htm. Accessed November 3, 2012

51. Jansson LM, Velez M, Harrow C. Methadone maintenance and lactation: a review of the literature and current management guidelines. *J Hum Lact.* 2004;20(1):62–71

52. Hirose M, Hosokawa T, Tanaka Y. Extradural buprenorphine suppresses breast feeding after caesarean section. *Br J Anaesth.* 1997;79(1):120–121

53. Glatstein MM, Garcia-Bournissen F, Finkelstein Y, Koren G. Methadone exposure during lactation. *Can Fam Physician.* 2008;54(12):1689–1690

54. Farid WO, Dunlop SA, Tait RJ, Hulse GK. The effects of maternally administered methadone, buprenorphine and naltrexone on offspring: review of human and animal data. *Curr Neuropharmacol.* 2008;6(2):125–150

55. Jansson LM, Choo R, Velez ML, Lowe R, Huestis MA. Methadone maintenance and long-term lactation. *Breastfeed Med.* 2008;3(1):34–37

56. Jansson LM, Choo R, Velez ML, et al. Methadone maintenance and breastfeeding in the neonatal period. *Pediatrics.* 2008;121(1):106–114

57. Johnson RE, Jones HE, Jasinski DR, et al. Buprenorphine treatment of pregnant opioid-dependent women: maternal and neonatal outcomes. *Drug Alcohol Depend.* 2001;63(1):97–103

58. Lindemalm S, Nydert P, Svensson JO, Stahle L, Sarman I. Transfer of buprenorphine into breast milk and calculation of infant drug dose. *J Hum Lact.* 2009;25(2):199–205

59. Chan CF, Page-Sharp M, Kristensen JH, O'Neil G, Ilett KF. Transfer of naltrexone and its metabolite 6,beta-naltrexol into human milk. *J Hum Lact.* 2004;20(3):322–326

60. Abdel-Latif ME, Pinner J, Clews S, Cooke F, Lui K, Oei J. Effects of breast milk on the severity and outcome of neonatal abstinence syndrome among infants of drug-dependent mothers. *Pediatrics.* 2006;117(6). Available at: www.pediatrics.org/cgi/content/full/117/6/e1163

61. Malpas TJ, Darlow BA. Neonatal abstinence syndrome following abrupt cessation of breastfeeding. *N Z Med J.* 1999;112(1080):12–13

62. Molyneux A. Nicotine replacement therapy. *BMJ.* 2004;328(7437):454–456

63. Ilett KF, Hale TW, Page-Sharp M, Kristensen JH, Kohan R, Hackett LP. Use of nicotine patches in breast-feeding mothers: transfer of nicotine and cotinine into human milk. *Clin Pharmacol Ther.* 2003;74(6):516–524

64. Chaudron LH, Schoenecker CJ. Bupropion and breastfeeding: a case of a possible infant seizure. *J Clin Psychiatry.* 2004;65(6):881–882

65. Madadi P, Shirazi F, Walter FG, Koren G. Establishing causality of CNS depression in breastfed infants following maternal codeine use. *Paediatr Drugs.* 2008;10(6):399–404

66. Madadi P, Koren G, Cairns JU, et al. Safety of codeine during breastfeeding: fatal morphine poisoning in the breastfed neonate of a mother prescribed codeine. *Can Fam Physician.* 2007;53(1):33–35

67. Sauberan JB, Anderson PO, Lane JR, et al. Breast milk hydrocodone and hydromorphone levels in mothers using hydrocodone for postpartum pain. *Obstet Gynecol.* 2011;117(3):611–617

68. Food and Drug Administration. FDA Alert. Information for healthcare professionals: use of codeine products in nursing mothers. August 17, 2007. Available at: www.fda.gov/drugs/drugsafety/postmarketdrugsafetyinformationforpatientsandproviders/ucm124889.htm. Accessed November 26, 2012

69. Robieux I, Koren G, Vandenbergh H, Schneiderman J. Morphine excretion in breast milk and resultant exposure of a nursing infant. *J Toxicol Clin Toxicol.* 1990;28(3):365–370

70. Bouwmeester NJ, Anderson BJ, Tibboel D, Holford NH. Developmental pharmacokinetics of morphine and its metabolites in neonates, infants and young children. *Br J Anaesth.* 2004;92(2):208–217

71. Bar-Oz B, Bulkowstein M, Benyamini L, et al. Use of antibiotic and analgesic drugs during lactation. *Drug Saf.* 2003;26(13):925–935

72. Spigset O, Hägg S. Analgesics and breastfeeding: safety considerations. *Paediatr Drugs.* 2000;2(3):223–238

73. Seaton S, Reeves M, McLean S. Oxycodone as a component of multimodal analgesia for lactating mothers after Caesarean section: relationships between maternal plasma, breast milk and neonatal plasma levels. *Aust N Z J Obstet Gynaecol.* 2007;47(3):181–185

74. Lam J, Kelly L, Ciszkowski C, et al. Central nervous system depression of neonates breastfed by mothers receiving oxycodone for postpartum analgesia. *J Pediatr.* 2011;160(1):33.e2–37.e2

75. Rigourd V, Amirouche A, Tasseau A, Kintz P, Serreau R. Retrospective diagnosis of an adverse drug reaction in a breastfed neonate: liquid chromatography-tandem mass spectrometry quantification of dextropropoxyphene and norpropoxyphene in newborn and maternal hair. *J Anal Toxicol.* 2008;32(9):787–789

76. Naumburg EG, Meny RG. Breast milk opioids and neonatal apnea. *Am J Dis Child.* 1988;142(1):11–12

77. Food and Drug Administration. Medwatch Safety Information. Propoxyphene: withdrawal – risk of cardiac toxicity. November 19, 2010. Available at: www.fda.gov/Safety/MedWatch/SafetyInformation/SafetyAlertsforHumanMedicalProducts/ucm234389.htm. Accessed November 26, 2012

78. Spencer J, Gonzalez L, Barnhart D. Medications in the breastfeeding mother. *Am Fam Physician.* 2001;64(1):119–126

79. Jacqz-Aigrain E, Serreau R, Boissinot C, et al. Excretion of ketoprofen and nalbuphine in human milk during treatment of maternal pain after delivery. *Ther Drug Monit.* 2007;29(6):815–818

80. van der Marel CD, Anderson BJ, van Lingen RA, et al. Paracetamol and metabolite pharmacokinetics in infants. *Eur J Clin Pharmacol.* 2003;59(3):243–251

81. Gardiner SJ, Doogue MP, Zhang M, Begg EJ. Quantification of infant exposure to celecoxib through breast milk. *Br J Clin Pharmacol.* 2006;61(1):101–104

82. Bell AD, Roussin A, Cartier R, et al; Canadian Cardiovascular Society. The use of antiplatelet therapy in the outpatient setting: Canadian Cardiovascular Society guidelines. *Can J Cardiol.* 2011;27(suppl A):S1–S59

83. Academy of Breastfeeding Medicine Protocol Committee. ABM Clinical Protocol #9: use of galactogogues in initiating or augmenting the rate of maternal secretion. *Breastfeed Med.* 2011;6(1):41–49

84. Campbell-Yeo ML, Allen AC, Joseph KS, et al. Effect of domperidone on the composition of preterm human breast milk. *Pediatrics.* 2010;125(1). Available at: www.pediatrics.org/cgi/content/full/125/1/e107

85. Collins KK, Sondheimer JM. Domperidone-induced QT prolongation: add another drug to the list. *J Pediatr.* 2008;153(5):596–598

86. Djeddi D, Kongolo G, Lefaix C, Mounard J, Léké A. Effect of domperidone on QT interval in neonates. *J Pediatr.* 2008;153(5):663–666

87. Zuppa AA, Sindico P, Orchi C, Carducci C, Cardiello V, Romagnoli C. Safety and efficacy of galactogogues: substances that induce, maintain and increase breast milk production. *J Pharm Pharm Sci.* 2010;13(2):162–174

88. Hansen WF, McAndrew S, Harris K, Zimmerman MB. Metoclopramide effect on breastfeeding the preterm infant: a randomized trial. *Obstet Gynecol.* 2005;105(2):383–389

89. Fife S, Gill P, Hopkins M, Angello C, Boswell S, Nelson KM. Metoclopramide to augment lactation, does it work? A randomized trial. *J Matern Fetal Neonatal Med.* 2011;24(11):1317–1320

90. Kauppila A, Arvela P, Koivisto M, Kivinen S, Ylikorkala O, Pelkonen O. Metoclopramide and breast feeding: transfer into milk and the newborn. *Eur J Clin Pharmacol.* 1983;25(6):819–823

91. Fewtrell MS, Loh KL, Blake A, Ridout DA, Hawdon J. Randomised, double blind trial of oxytocin nasal spray in mothers expressing breast milk for preterm infants. *Arch Dis Child Fetal Neonatal Ed.* 2006;91(3):F169–F174

92. Betzold CM. Galactagogues. *J Midwifery Womens Health.* 2004;49(2):151–154

93. Ulbricht C, Basch E, Burke D, et al. Fenugreek (*Trigonella foenum-graecum* L. Leguminosae): an evidence-based systematic review by the natural standard research collaboration. *J Herb Pharmacother.* 2007;7(3-4):143–177

94. Abebe W. Herbal medication: potential for adverse interactions with analgesic drugs. *J Clin Pharm Ther.* 2002;27(6):391–401

95. Korman SH, Cohen E, Preminger A. Pseudo-maple syrup urine disease due to maternal prenatal ingestion of fenugreek. *J Paediatr Child Health.* 2001;37(4):403–404

96. Jackson PC. Complementary and alternative methods of increasing breast milk supply for lactating mothers of infants in the NICU. *Neonatal Netw.* 2010;29(4):225–230

97. Nordeng H, Havnen GC. Use of herbal drugs in pregnancy: a survey among 400 Norwegian women. *Pharmacoepidemiol Drug Saf.* 2004;13(6):371–380

98. Denham BE. Dietary supplements—regulatory issues and implications for public health. *JAMA.* 2011;306(4):428–429

99. Food and Drug Administration. Consumer advisory: kava-containing dietary supplements may be associated with severe liver injury. March 25, 2002. Available at: www.fda.gov/Food/ResourcesForYou/Consumers/ucm085482.htm. Accessed November 26, 2012

100. Medline Plus. Yohimbe. Available at: www.nlm.nih.gov/medlineplus/druginfo/natural/759.html. Accessed November 26, 2012

101. Food and Drug Administration. Safety alerts for human medical products 2008-2010. Available at: www.fda.gov/Safety/MedWatch/SafetyInformation/default.htm. Accessed November 26, 2012

102. US Government Accountability Office. Herbal dietary supplements: examples of deceptive or questionable marketing practices and potentially dangerous advice. May 26, 2010. Available at: www.gao.gov/products/GAO-10-662T. Accessed November 26, 2012

103. Gardiner P. Complementary, holistic, and integrative medicine: chamomile. *Pediatr Rev.* 2007;28(4):e16–e18

104. Dugoua JJ, Seely D, Perri D, Koren G, Mills E. Safety and efficacy of black cohosh (*Cimicifuga racemosa*) during pregnancy and lactation. *Can J Clin Pharmacol.* 2006;13(3):e257–e261

105. Dugoua JJ, Perri D, Seely D, Mills E, Koren G. Safety and efficacy of blue cohosh (*Caulophyllum thalictroides*) during pregnancy and lactation. *Can J Clin Pharmacol.* 2008;15(1):e66–e73

106. Dugoua JJ, Seely D, Perri D, Koren G, Mills E. Safety and efficacy of chastetree (*Vitex agnus-castus*) during pregnancy and lactation. *Can J Clin Pharmacol.* 2008;15(1):e74–e79

107. Perri D, Dugoua JJ, Mills E, Koren G. Safety and efficacy of echinacea (*Echinacea angustafolia*, *E. purpurea* and *E. pallida*) during pregnancy and lactation. *Can J Clin Pharmacol.* 2006;13(3):e262–e267

108. Seely D, Dugoua JJ, Perri D, Mills E, Koren G. Safety and efficacy of panax ginseng during pregnancy and lactation. *Can J Clin Pharmacol.* 2008;15(1):e87–e94

109. Dugoua JJ, Mills E, Perri D, Koren G. Safety and efficacy of ginkgo (*Ginkgo biloba*) during pregnancy and lactation. *Can J Clin Pharmacol.* 2006;13(3):e277–e284

110. Dugoua JJ, Mills E, Perri D, Koren G. Safety and efficacy of St. John's wort (hypericum) during pregnancy and lactation. *Can J Clin Pharmacol.* 2006;13(3):e268–e276

111. Budzynska K, Gardner ZE, Dugoua JJ, Low Dog T, Gardiner P. Systematic review of breastfeeding and herbs. *Breastfeed Med.* 2012;7(6):489–503

112. Drugs and Lactation Database (LactMed). Available at: http://toxnet.nlm.nih.gov/cgi-bin/sis/htmlgen?LACT. Accessed May 8, 2013

113. Klier CM, Schmid-Siegel B, Schäfer MR, et al. St. John's wort (*Hypericum perforatum*) and breastfeeding: plasma and breast milk concentrations of hyperforin for 5 mothers and 2 infants. *J Clin Psychiatry.* 2006;67(2):305–309

114. Tiran D. The use of fenugreek for breast feeding women. *Complement Ther Nurs Midwifery.* 2003;9(3):155–156

115. Dourmishev LA, Dourmishev AL. Activity of certain drugs in inducing of inflammatory myopathies with cutaneous manifestations. *Expert Opin Drug Saf.* 2008;7(4):421–433

116. ICRP . Radiation dose to patients from radiopharmaceuticals. Addendum 3 to ICRP Publication 53. ICRP Publication 106. Approved by the Commission in October 2007. *Ann ICRP.* 2008;38(1-2):1–197

117. Stabin MG, Breitz HB. Breast milk excretion of radiopharmaceuticals: mechanisms, findings, and radiation dosimetry. *J Nucl Med.* 2000;41(5):863–873

118. Chen MM, Coakley FV, Kaimal A, Laros RK Jr. Guidelines for computed tomography and magnetic resonance imaging use during pregnancy and lactation. *Obstet Gynecol.* 2008;112(2 pt 1):333–340

119. Pomeroy KM, Sawyer LJ, Evans MJ. Estimated radiation dose to breast feeding infant following maternal administration of 57Co labelled to vitamin B12. *Nucl Med Commun.* 2005;26(9):839–841

120. Devine CE, Mawlawi O. Radiation safety with positron emission tomography and computed tomography. *Semin Ultrasound CT MR.* 2010;31(1):39–45

121. Atkinson WL, Pickering LK, Schwartz B, Weniger BG, Iskander JK, Watson JC; Centers for Disease Control and Prevention. General recommendations on immunization. Recommendations of the Advisory Committee on Immunization Practices (ACIP) and the American Academy of Family Physicians (AAFP). *MMWR Recomm Rep.* 2002;51(RR-2):1–35

122. Vesikari T, Prymula R, Schuster V, et al. Efficacy and immunogenicity of live-attenuated human rotavirus vaccine in breast-fed and formula-fed European infants. *Pediatr Infect Dis J.* 2012;31(5):509–513

123. Silfverdal SA, Ekholm L, Bodin L. Breastfeeding enhances the antibody response

to Hib and Pneumococcal serotype 6B and 14 after vaccination with conjugate vaccines. *Vaccine.* 2007;25(8):1497–1502

124. Pisacane A, Continisio P, Palma O, Cataldo S, De Michele F, Vairo U. Breastfeeding and risk for fever after immunization. *Pediatrics.* 2010;125(6). Available at: www.pediatrics.org/cgi/content/full/125/6/e1448

125. Bohlke K, Galil K, Jackson LA, et al. Postpartum varicella vaccination: is the vaccine virus excreted in breast milk? *Obstet Gynecol.* 2003;102(5 pt 1):970–977

126. Kroger AT, Atkinson WL, Marcuse EK, Pickering LK; Advisory Committee on Immunization Practices (ACIP) Centers for Disease Control and Prevention (CDC). General recommendations on immunization: recommendations of the Advisory Committee on Immunization Practices (ACIP). *MMWR Recomm Rep.* 2006;55(RR-15):1–48

127. Centers for Disease Control and Prevention (CDC). Transmission of yellow fever vaccine virus through breast-feeding - Brazil, 2009. *MMWR Morb Mortal Wkly Rep.* 2010;59(5):130–132

128. Traiber C, Coelho-Amaral P, Ritter VR, Winge A. Infant meningoencephalitis caused by yellow fever vaccine virus transmitted via breastmilk. *J Pediatr (Rio J).* 2011;87(3): 269–272

129. American Academy of Pediatrics, Council on Environmental Health. In: Etzel RA, Balk SJ, eds. *Pediatric Environmental Health.* 3rd ed. Elk Grove Village, IL: American Academy of Pediatrics; 2012

Transitioning HIV-Infected Youth Into Adult Health Care

- *Policy Statement*

POLICY STATEMENT

Transitioning HIV-Infected Youth Into Adult Health Care

abstract

With advances in antiretroviral therapy, most HIV-infected children survive into adulthood. Optimal health care for these youth includes a formal plan for the transition of care from primary and/or subspecialty pediatric/adolescent/family medicine health care providers (medical home) to adult health care provider(s). Successful transition involves the early engagement and participation of the youth and his or her family with the pediatric medical home and adult health care teams in developing a formal plan. Referring providers should have a written policy for the transfer of HIV-infected youth to adult care, which will guide in the development of an individualized plan for each youth. The plan should be introduced to the youth in early adolescence and modified as the youth approaches transition. Assessment of developmental milestones is important to define the readiness of the youth in assuming responsibility for his or her own care before initiating the transfer. Communication among all providers is essential and should include both personal contact and a written medical summary. Progress toward the transition should be tracked and, once completed, should be documented and assessed. *Pediatrics* 2013;132:192–197

COMMITTEE ON PEDIATRIC AIDS

KEY WORDS
adolescents, adults, HIV, transition, young adults

ABBREVIATIONS
AAP—American Academy of Pediatrics
ART—antiretroviral treatment
EHR—electronic health record
MSM—males who have sex with men

INTRODUCTION

In the United States, the prevalence of HIV infection in adolescents and young adults continues to increase as a result of the improved survival of perinatally infected youth as well as those horizontally infected through adult risk behaviors.[1] The Centers for Disease Control and Prevention estimated that in 2009, there were approximately 77 000 HIV-infected youth between 13 and 24 years of age in the United States. Currently, HIV infection is the seventh leading cause of death in this age group. Youths accounted for 12 200 (25.7%) of all new HIV infections in 2010. More than one-half (59.5%) were unaware of their infection, the highest for any age group.[2]

The rate of new HIV infections is highest in African-American youth, including males who have sex with men (MSM) and females with heterosexual contact. HIV infection rates are sevenfold higher among non-Hispanic African Americans and 2.5-fold higher among Hispanic Americans than among non-Hispanic white Americans.[3] AIDS rates nearly doubled from 1997 to 2006 in male subjects between 15 and 19 years of age, largely because of the dramatic increase in HIV infection among MSM from lower socioeconomic classes.[4] In addition, female subjects between 10 and 14 years of age are at a higher risk of

www.pediatrics.org/cgi/doi/10.1542/peds.2013-1073

doi:10.1542/peds.2013-1073

PEDIATRICS (ISSN Numbers: Print, 0031-4005; Online, 1098-4275).

Copyright © 2013 by the American Academy of Pediatrics

infection than similarly aged male subjects.[2] The disease disproportionately affects minorities and individuals residing in the South and the Northeast regions of the United States. Risk factors include sex with older men, lack of access to HIV prevention services, and lack of perceived personal risk despite frequent anonymous sexual encounters and unprotected anal intercourse. The HIV incidence rate for African-American women is nearly 15 times that of white women and nearly 4 times that of Hispanic/Latina women.[5] Risk factors among these groups include poverty, stigma, limited access to health care, higher rates of concurrent sexually transmitted infections, and drug use.[2]

Adolescence is a developmental stage characterized by immature concrete reasoning often manifested by denial of illness, a sense of invulnerability reflected by risk taking, and behaviors that are strongly influenced by peer norms. These characteristics all have a direct negative effect on the ability to adhere to complex medical regimens. With the dramatic improvement in HIV care over the past 3 decades, the infected adolescent and his or her caregivers are now faced with managing a chronic illness. In addition to caring for the physical needs of the HIV-infected adolescent, it is important to recognize and address the psychosocial barriers to optimal health and enable delivery of uninterrupted, high-quality medically and developmentally appropriate health care as the individual transitions from adolescence to adulthood.[6]

The increasing incidence and prevalence of HIV infection affect the nation's youth at an age when individual psychosocial and physical developmental processes are evolving and maturing. Physically, the pubertal growth spurt is associated with hormonal and bodily changes reflected in secondary sexual characteristics that influence adolescents' long-term self-image and self-esteem. Furthermore, the social environment and responses of peers and significant others have to be constantly integrated into an evolving identity. Among HIV-infected adolescents and young adults, these changes often occur on a background of denial, depression, marginalization and stigmatization, and medical comorbidities associated with HIV infection.[6] Accompanying psychosocial stressors include parental loss, placement in foster care, poverty, homelessness, unemployment, discrimination, and abuse. HIV-infected youth may have less social support because of stigmatization associated with their infection and/or their sexual orientation. Planning for the transition to adult health care should consider potential cultural differences in different populations of infected youth.

HIV-infected youth consist of 2 distinct populations: those who acquired HIV infection perinatally and those infected horizontally through risk behaviors including consensual or nonconsensual sex. Although the course of the infections in these populations may differ, the challenges faced can be similar, including the stigma of HIV infection and the resulting need for confidentiality, which conflicts with the need for disclosure of their infection status to sexual partners.[7] Youth with horizontal acquisition of HIV may be reluctant to disclose an abusive relationship or sexual exploitation to parents and authorities. Differences between the clinical and psychosocial presentations of youth with perinatally and horizontally acquired HIV infection influence the acceptance of illness, self-efficacy, and antiretroviral treatment (ART) adherence. Among young MSM, unique stressors include homophobia and discrimination, which can lead to a cascade of adverse outcomes, including homelessness and unemployment,

and directly affect clinical follow-up and adherence to life-saving medications. Adolescents with newly diagnosed infection may present with an opportunistic and/or sexually transmitted infection associated with advanced immunosuppression. The development of individual disease management skills may be essential for adherence to ART and treatment of associated comorbidities. However, these expectations may be incongruous with the developmental stage of the individual newly diagnosed with HIV along with the complex social situations in which these teenagers may find themselves. Many perinatally infected children have survived into adolescence with multiple courses of combination ART not infrequently associated with periods of poor adherence, often reflecting treatment fatigue, leading to viral resistance.[8] With HIV resistance, therapeutic options become limited, necessitating increasingly more complex treatment regimens. Such regimens can be particularly difficult to implement in treatment-weary adolescents with challenges such as stunted growth, delayed puberty, and physical disabilities arising from earlier complications of perinatal HIV infection or from long-term ART.

Adolescents who have chronic health conditions are often followed up in pediatric or adolescent clinics through adolescence or into young adulthood, although the upper age limit varies. Seamless and successful transition from pediatric- to adult-oriented health care is dependent on these youth acquiring skills to allow them to be responsible for the management of their own health care.[9–12] In situations in which youth have both a primary care provider (medical home) and a subspecialty HIV care provider, both primary care and HIV care will need to be transitioned to adult providers. This situation could allow for the transition of primary care and subspecialty care at different times. With good communication and careful planning, this strategy could help smooth the transition and improve retention in care.

HIV-infected youth face many of the same challenges in transitioning to adult health care as do individuals with other chronic health conditions.[10] These include the loss of close and supportive relationships with their individual pediatric/adolescent/family medicine providers. The neurocognitive delay and behavioral problems commonly experienced by HIV-infected youth may pose additional challenges for the adult health care provider.[6,13,14] The adult care site may not provide the level of support and encouragement to which the youth is accustomed in his or her pediatric medical home. At 1 site, HIV-infected youth aged 17 to 24 years who received care in an adult health clinic had poorer outcomes than did older adults in the same clinic, with lower rates of viral suppression and nearly 4 times the rate of loss to follow-up.[15] However, increases in CD4+ T-lymphocyte counts were similar in the 2 groups. High rates of substance use and mental health problems, difficulties in adjustment, and reduced emotional support may lead to loss to follow-up and disease progression.[15,16] In addition, in many states, youth who have received public health insurance coverage become ineligible at 18 to 21 years of age, limiting their access to care and medications. Among HIV-infected youth older than 18 years who transitioned from National Institutes of Health clinical research protocols to adult care, 15% reported not having health insurance.[16] Protocols and linkages to care in anticipation of the transition can help avert such consequences.

Several models of transition to adult health care have been proposed, with considerable variability among institutions and individual providers. This variability is reflected in differences in addressing comprehensive care needs as part of the transition, including medical, psychosocial, and financial aspects of transitioning.[17–21] In a survey of providers of pediatric HIV care in the United States, 81% had designated a transition coordinator, but few had established policies to define the details of the transition.[22] One university-based program elected to begin the process at 23 years of age because of a high failure rate when initiated at 21 years of age.[20] Results of this strategy are not yet available. Most models are characterized by flexibility, allowing youth to move back and forth between stages of the transition with the anticipation of completing the process by 25 years of age.

Data are limited regarding the outcomes of HIV-infected youth after transition to adult health care.[23,24] Fewer than one-half of children with congenital heart disease at 1 large pediatric center successfully transitioned to adult health care.[25] Qualitative studies emphasize the importance of an adult-based case manager and mental health providers to assist in the transition as well as an individualized approach to the transition process, including addressing health insurance, alcohol and drug treatment, housing, transportation, education, training, and employment needs.[16,26] Predictors of a successful transition included good adherence to care[24] and effective management of psychiatric comorbidities[6,27] before transition. Further studies to define the outcome of transition and identify the determinants of a successful transfer of care are urgently needed.

RECOMMENDATIONS

Guidelines for transitioning youth with chronic diseases to adult health care have been published by the Society for Adolescent Health and Medicine (formerly known as the Society for Adolescent Medicine)[28] and the American Academy of Pediatrics (AAP [with endorsement by the American Academy of Family Physicians and the American College of Physicians]).[10,29] Broad recommendations include the development of a formal, multidisciplinary, transitional program that involves individual youths and their families and the identification of an adult health care provider before the transition. These guidelines provide guidance on care planning and the transfer of medical information. Their conclusions remain widely accepted as a gold standard that can serve as a framework for the transition of HIV-infected youth. However, a national survey of AAP members revealed that pediatricians remain poorly informed about the conclusions of the AAP consensus statement and that most pediatric practices neither initiate transition planning early in adolescence nor offer transition support services.[30] Identified gaps included limited personnel and training of staff, limited time and workforce shortages, inadequate reimbursement, and anxiety on the part of treating clinicians, adolescents, and their parents about planning for future health care. Guidelines specific to transitioning HIV-infected youth are also available.[20,21]

There are 4 major steps in the transition process:

1. The primary and/or subspecialty pediatric, adolescent, or family medicine HIV care team, in collaboration with adult HIV care providers, develops a formal written policy for transition of youth to adult health care. Written supporting documents, such as brochures and Web-based information, can be helpful in implementing the policy. The transition policy should describe the goals and timeline of transition and explain how the practice evaluates this process.

The policy should be shared with all members of the health care team and implemented with appropriate staff training. An important component of the plan is to establish a system, such as a registry, to identify and track youth as they approach and progress through the transition process because these youth may frequently change where they are living.

2. The patient and his or her family should be introduced to the concept of transition to adult health care early in adolescence, well in anticipation of the actual transfer of care. Although opinions differ regarding the appropriate age to first introduce the transition process, early adolescence is generally regarded as the most appropriate time. Many recommend beginning the discussion of transition by 12 years of age or at an appropriate time after the initial diagnosis, if it occurs at an older age.[10] HIV infection status must be fully disclosed to the patient and explained before introducing the plan. Factors to consider in choosing the age to introduce the plan include individual developmental stage and neurocognitive abilities. Providers may use a readiness assessment tool to reveal areas of strength and weakness to which patient education can be focused to achieve self-management. Specific tools are available for downloading from the Internet, such as the New York State guidelines.[21] It is important to encourage independence through personal ownership and management of health care. Particular attention should be paid to identifying and addressing behavioral, emotional, and mental health problems. In conjunction with the patient and family, the referring provider develops an individualized written transition plan with realistic goals to delineate the process of transition to adult health care. The plan should emphasize education of all involved parties and empowerment of the HIV-infected youth to assume responsibility for his or her own health care. The plan should anticipate and address challenges that patients, parents, and caregivers encounter during transition, including the loss of an established provider. Patient education during office visits and peer group sessions can reinforce the value of independence and decision-making as part of the transition. The creation of a portable medical summary and an emergency care plan is an important component of the plan.

Ongoing discussions of the transition plan should occur at least annually at subsequent visits, with modification of the plan as appropriate. The health care coverage of the youth should be evaluated regularly to ensure that health care coverage and access to medications remains uninterrupted during the transition. The 2010 Patient Protection and Affordable Care Act health care reform legislation includes provision for children to remain on their parents' insurance until 26 years of age and eliminates insurers' ability to exclude coverage on the basis of preexisting conditions.

3. The actual transition to adult health care is initiated. The age at which this transition is initiated is generally between 18 and 25 years and can be influenced by the upper age at which health care is provided by the referring team and the comfort of the adult health care provider in caring for younger adults. Once a suitable adult HIV medicine provider is identified, a pretransfer visit to meet the adult health care provider can help to establish a successful long-term relationship. The pediatric, adolescent, or family medicine provider should communicate directly with the adult health care provider and supply appropriate documentation, including a transfer letter, the portable medical summary, and/or electronic health record (EHR), before the initial encounter between the adult health care provider and the patient. The portable medical summary and/or EHR should address all medical and psychosocial needs, including advance directives. Ideally, the youth would be introduced to the adult health care provider personally by the pediatric, adolescent, or family medicine provider, either in the referring or adult clinic. It is likely that most youth will need ongoing support from the pediatric adolescent or family medicine health care team during the process for transition to be successful. This support could consist of periodic contact by a member of the referring health care team, such as a nurse or social worker. A peer support group may assist youth with dealing with anxiety resulting from the transition process.

4. The final step in the transition process is to document the completion of the transition and evaluate the outcome of the process. The referring health care provider should document that the young adult has established his or her care in the adult clinic and should be available to provide ongoing encouragement to maintain the youth in adult health care. The referring team should be available to the adult health care provider to serve as a resource during the immediate posttransfer period. However, once the youth has established ongoing care with the adult health care provider, it is appropriate for the

pediatric, adolescent, or family medicine provider to withdraw from providing care to prevent confusion in the patient and to reinforce the role of the adult health care provider.

CONCLUSIONS

A well-planned transition of HIV-infected youth from pediatric, adolescent, or family medicine clinics, often from a medical home to adult health care, enables them to optimize their ability to assume adult roles and activities. Transition planning should be a standard part of providing health care for all HIV-infected youth. Pediatricians and adolescent and family medicine providers have a pivotal role in facilitating seamless and effective transition at a very vulnerable and anxious time of life for both HIV-infected youth and their families. These essential transitional activities can improve health outcomes for HIV-infected adolescents.

Specific Recommendations

1. Pediatric, adolescent, and family medicine HIV care providers, in collaboration with suitable adult HIV care providers, should develop a formal process for transition of youth to adult health care.

2. The patient and his or her family should be introduced to the concept of transition to adult health care early in adolescence well in anticipation of the actual transfer of care. The youth should be informed of his or her HIV status before initiating the process.

3. There are 4 key steps in the transition process:

a. The referring provider should develop written policies to define the process of transition of HIV-infected youth to adult health care. The plan should be shared with all pediatric/adolescent or family medicine providers, staff, and patients and their families with appropriate staff training. Written documents, such as brochures and Web-based information, can be helpful in implementing the policy. Providers should establish a system to identify and track youth as they progress through the transition process.

b. The provider, the youth, and the family should jointly create an individualized transition plan well in anticipation of transition, which should include creation of a portable medical summary and/or EHR and an emergency care plan. Providers may use a readiness assessment tool, and the transition plan should be revised on the basis of these assessments.

c. Transition to the adult HIV care provider should be initiated with appropriate communication, including a transfer letter and portable medical summary. A pretransfer visit by the patient to meet the adult health care provider can assist in establishing a successful long-term relationship.

d. Completion of the transition should be documented, and the outcome of the process should be evaluated. The referring health care team should be available to the adult health care provider to serve as a resource during the immediate posttransfer period.

4. The health care coverage of the youth should be evaluated regularly to ensure that health care coverage and access to medications remains uninterrupted during transition.

5. The transition process should ensure that the youth's health care, educational, vocational, and social service needs are discussed and addressed.

LEAD AUTHORS

Rana Chakraborty, MD
Russell B. Van Dyke, MD

COMMITTEE ON PEDIATRIC AIDS, 2011–2012

Patricia M. Flynn, MD, Chairperson
Grace M. Aldrovandi, MD
Ellen Gould Chadwick, MD
Rana Chakraborty, MD
Ellen Rae Cooper, MD
Heidi Schwarzwald, MD
Jaime Martinez, MD

FORMER COMMITTEE MEMBER

Russell B. Van Dyke, MD

LIAISONS

Kenneth L. Dominguez MD, MPH – *Centers for Disease Control and Prevention*
Lynne M. Mofenson MD – *Eunice Kennedy Shriver National Institute of Child Health and Human Development*

CONSULTANT

Gordon E. Schutze, MD

STAFF

Anjie Emanuel, MPH

REFERENCES

1. Brady MT, Oleske JM, Williams PL, et al. Declines in mortality rates and changes in causes of death in HIV-1-infected children during the HAART era. *J Acquir Immune Defic Syndr.* 2010;53(1):86–94

2. Centers for Disease Control and Prevention. Vital signs: HIV infection, testing, and risk behaviors among youths—United States. *MMWR Morb Mortal Wkly Rep.* 2012; 61(47):971–976

3. Hall HI, Song R, Rhodes P, et al. Estimation of HIV incidence in the United States. *JAMA.* 2008;300(5):520–529

4. Gavin L, MacKay AP, Brown K, et al. Sexual and reproductive health of persons aged

10-24 years—United States, 2002-2007. *MMWR Surveill Summ.* 2009;58(6):1–58

5. Centers for Disease Control and Prevention. Subpopulation estimates from the HIV incidence surveillance system—United States, 2006. *MMWR Morb Mortal Wkly Rep.* 2008;57(36):985–989

6. Mellins CA, Tassiopoulos K, Malee K, et al. Behavioral health risks in perinatally HIV-exposed youth: co-occurrence of sexual and drug use behavior, mental health problems, and nonadherence to antiretroviral treatment. *AIDS Patient Care STDS.* 2011;25(7):413–422

7. Vijayan T, Benin AL, Wagner K, Romano S, Andiman WA. We never thought this would happen: transitioning care of adolescents with perinatally acquired HIV infection from pediatrics to internal medicine. *AIDS Care.* 2009;21(10):1222–1229

8. Van Dyke RB, Patel K, Siberry GK, et al. Antiretroviral treatment of U.S. children with perinatally-acquired HIV infection: temporal changes in therapy between 1991 and 2009 and predictors of immunologic and virologic outcomes. *J Acquir Immune Defic Syndr.* 2011;57(2):165–173

9. Spiegel HM, Futterman DC. Adolescents and HIV: prevention and clinical care. *Curr HIV/AIDS Rep.* 2009;6(2):100–107

10. Cooley WC, Sagerman PJ. Supporting the health care transition from adolescence to adulthood in the medical home. *Pediatrics.* 2011;128(1):182–200

11. Crowley R, Wolfe I, Lock K, McKee M. Improving the transition between paediatric and adult healthcare: a systematic review. *Arch Dis Child.* 2011;96(6):548–553

12. van Staa A, van der Stege HA, Jedeloo S, Moll HA, Hilberink SR. Readiness to transfer to adult care of adolescents with chronic conditions: exploration of associated factors. *J Adolesc Health.* 2011;48(3):295–302

13. Malee KM, Tassiopoulos K, Huo Y, et al. Mental health functioning among children and adolescents with perinatal HIV infection and perinatal HIV exposure. *AIDS Care.* 2011;23(12):1533–1544

14. Nozyce ML, Lee SS, Wiznia A, et al. A behavioral and cognitive profile of clinically stable HIV-infected children. *Pediatrics.* 2006;117(3):763–770

15. Ryscavage P, Anderson EJ, Sutton SH, Reddy S, Taiwo B. Clinical outcomes of adolescents and young adults in adult HIV care. *J Acquir Immune Defic Syndr.* 2011;58(2):193–197

16. Wiener LS, Kohrt BA, Battles HB, Pao M. The HIV experience: youth identified barriers for transitioning from pediatric to adult care. *J Pediatr Psychol.* 2011;36(2):141–154

17. Gilliam PP, Ellen JM, Leonard L, Kinsman S, Jevitt CM, Straub DM. Transition of adolescents with HIV to adult care: characteristics and current practices of the Adolescent Trials Network for HIV/AIDS Interventions. *J Assoc Nurses AIDS Care.* 2011;22(4):283–294

18. Wiener LS, Zobel M, Battles H, Ryder C. Transition from a pediatric HIV intramural clinical research program to adolescent and adult community-based care services: assessing transition readiness. *Soc Work Health Care.* 2007;46(1):1–19

19. Machado DM, Succi RC, Turato ER. Transitioning adolescents living with HIV/AIDS to adult-oriented health care: an emerging challenge. *J Pediatr (Rio J).* 2010;86(6):465–472

20. Maturo D, Powell A, Major-Wilson H, Sanchez K, De Santis JP, Friedman LB. Development of a protocol for transitioning adolescents with HIV infection to adult care. *J Pediatr Health Care.* 2011;25(1):16–23

21. New York State Department of Health. Transitioning HIV-infected adolescents into adult care. Available at: www.hivguidelines.org/clinical-guidelines/adolescents/transitioning-hiv-infected-adolescents-into-adult-care/. Accessed March 11, 2013

22. Andiman WA. Transition from pediatric to adult healthcare services for young adults with chronic illnesses: the special case of human immunodeficiency virus infection. *J Pediatr.* 2011;159(5):714–719

23. Dowshen N, D'Angelo L. Health care transition for youth living with HIV/AIDS. *Pediatrics.* 2011;128(4):762–771

24. Arazi-Caillaud S, Mecikovsky D, Miranda C, et al. Transition of HIV-infected adolescents to adult HIV care: a pilot study in Buenos Aires, Argentina. Presented at: 5th IAS Conference on HIV Pathogenesis and Treatment; July 17–20, 2011; Capetown, South Africa

25. Reid GJ, Irvine MJ, McCrindle BW, et al. Prevalence and correlates of successful transfer from pediatric to adult health care among a cohort of young adults with complex congenital heart defects. *Pediatrics.* 2004;113(3 pt 1). Available at: www.pediatrics.org/cgi/content/full/113/3/e197

26. Valenzuela JM, Buchanan CL, Radcliffe J, et al. Transition to adult services among behaviorally infected adolescents with HIV—a qualitative study. *J Pediatr Psychol.* 2011;36(2):134–140

27. Kapetanovic S, Wiegand RE, Dominguez K, et al. Associations of medically documented psychiatric diagnoses and risky health behaviors in highly active antiretroviral therapy-experienced perinatally HIV-infected youth. *AIDS Patient Care STDS.* 2011;25(8):493–501

28. Rosen DS, Blum RW, Britto M, Sawyer SM, Siegel DM; Society for Adolescent Medicine. Transition to adult health care for adolescents and young adults with chronic conditions: position paper of the Society for Adolescent Medicine. *J Adolesc Health.* 2003;33(4):309–311

29. American Academy of Pediatrics, American Academy of Family Physicians, American College of Physicians-American Society of Internal Medicine. A consensus statement on health care transitions for young adults with special health care needs. *Pediatrics.* 2002;110(6 pt 2):1304–1306

30. American Academy of Pediatrics, Department of Research. Survey: transition services lacking for teens with special needs. *AAP News.* 2009;30:12

Use of Inhaled Nitric Oxide in Preterm Infants

• *Clinical Report*

CLINICAL REPORT

Use of Inhaled Nitric Oxide in Preterm Infants

abstract

Nitric oxide, an important signaling molecule with multiple regulatory effects throughout the body, is an important tool for the treatment of full-term and late-preterm infants with persistent pulmonary hypertension of the newborn and hypoxemic respiratory failure. Several randomized controlled trials have evaluated its role in the management of preterm infants ≤34 weeks' gestational age with varying results. The purpose of this clinical report is to summarize the existing evidence for the use of inhaled nitric oxide in preterm infants and provide guidance regarding its use in this population. *Pediatrics* 2014;133:164–170

INTRODUCTION

Nitric oxide (NO) is an important signaling molecule with multiple regulatory effects throughout the body. In perinatal medicine, inhaled nitric oxide (iNO) was initially studied for its pulmonary vasodilating effects in infants with pulmonary hypertension and has since become an important tool for the treatment of full-term and late-preterm infants with persistent pulmonary hypertension of the newborn and hypoxemic respiratory failure.[1] Inhaled NO also has multiple and complex systemic and pulmonary effects. In animal models of neonatal chronic lung disease, iNO stimulates angiogenesis, augments alveolarization, improves surfactant function, and inhibits proliferation of smooth muscle cells and abnormal elastin deposition.[2–6] Although the evidence for similar benefits in preterm infants is lacking, the off-label use of iNO in this population has escalated.[7] A study published in 2010 reported a sixfold increase (from 0.3% to 1.8%) in the use of iNO among infants born at less than 34 weeks' gestation between 2000 and 2008.[7] The greatest increase occurred among infants who were born at 23 to 26 weeks' gestation (0.8% to 6.6%). The National Institutes of Health convened a consensus panel in October 2010 to evaluate the evidence for safety and efficacy of iNO therapy in preterm infants. After reviewing the published evidence, the panel concluded that the available evidence does not support the use of iNO in early routine, early rescue, or later rescue regimens in the care of infants born at less than 34 weeks' gestation and that hospitals, clinicians, and the pharmaceutical industry should avoid marketing iNO for this group of infants.[8] An individual-patient data meta-analysis of 14 randomized controlled trials reached similar conclusions.[9] The purpose of this clinical report is to summarize the

Praveen Kumar MD, FAAP, and COMMITTEE ON FETUS AND NEWBORN

KEY WORDS
inhaled nitric oxide, preterm infants, hypoxic respiratory failure, bronchopulmonary dysplasia

ABBREVIATIONS
BPD—bronchopulmonary dysplasia
iNO—inhaled nitric oxide
NO—nitric oxide
NOCLD—Nitric Oxide Chronic Lung Disease study group

The guidance in this report does not indicate an exclusive course of treatment or serve as a standard of medical care. Variations, taking into account individual circumstances, may be appropriate.

www.pediatrics.org/cgi/doi/10.1542/peds.2013-3444

doi:10.1542/peds.2013-3444

All clinical reports from the American Academy of Pediatrics automatically expire 5 years after publication unless reaffirmed, revised, or retired at or before that time.

PEDIATRICS (ISSN Numbers: Print, 0031-4005; Online, 1098-4275).

existing evidence for the use of iNO in preterm infants and provide guidance regarding its use in this population.

LITERATURE REVIEW

Use of iNO in Preterm Infants With Respiratory Failure

The benefits associated with iNO therapy in full-term and late-preterm infants with persistent pulmonary hypertension of the newborn and hypoxemic respiratory failure initiated interest in exploring whether iNO could reduce the rates of death and neonatal morbidities in more immature infants. Pilot studies reported short-term improvement in oxygenation with iNO, but no significant benefit was observed in mortality or other morbidities.[10–15] Subsequently, several randomized clinical trials were undertaken.[16–23] Table 1 outlines the study population, entry criteria, and dose and duration of iNO treatment and summarizes the outcomes for all published randomized controlled trials. Only 1 small trial of 40 patients reported a beneficial effect on survival (Table 1). Subgroup analyses of secondary outcomes have provided conflicting results. Post hoc analysis of the Neonatal Research Network study suggested that iNO therapy was associated with reduced rates of death and bronchopulmonary dysplasia (BPD) in infants with a birth weight greater than 1000 g, but higher mortality and increased risk of severe intracranial hemorrhage in infants weighing 1000 g or less at birth.[17] In contrast, another large multicenter US trial reported no significant difference in the primary outcome of death or BPD between treated and control groups; however, infants treated with iNO had fewer brain lesions (eg, grade 3 or 4 intracranial hemorrhage, periventricular leukomalacia, and/or ventriculomegaly) noted on cranial ultrasonography.[20] A European multicenter study reported that

infants randomized to iNO treatment had longer duration of ventilation, time on oxygen therapy, and length of hospital stay compared with the placebo group, although none of these results were statistically significant.[19]

Use of iNO in Preterm Infants to Improve the Rate of Survival Without BPD

Lung pathology in preterm infants with BPD is characterized by reduced numbers of large alveoli and abnormal pulmonary vasculature development. Surfactant deficiency, ventilator-induced lung injury, oxygen toxicity, and inflammation appear to play important roles in its pathogenesis.[26,27] In animal models of neonatal lung injury, iNO promotes angiogenesis, decreases apoptosis, and reduces lung inflammation and oxidant injury.[28–30] In an early study of iNO use in preterm infants, the incidence of BPD was reduced in treated infants who required ventilator support.[16] Of 3 subsequent large randomized trials designed to evaluate the effect of iNO therapy on survival without BPD,[20,24,25] 2 found no significant benefit[20,25] (Table 1). A third trial, which featured late treatment (7–21 days of age), a longer duration of drug exposure (25 days), and a higher cumulative dose, demonstrated a modest but statistically significant beneficial effect (44% iNO vs 37% placebo; $P = .042$).[24] A subgroup analysis showed that the beneficial effect was seen in infants enrolled between 7 and 14 days of age but not those enrolled between the ages of 15 and 21 days.[24]

EFFECTS OF iNO THERAPY ON NEURODEVELOPMENTAL OUTCOME

Studies in animal models suggest that iNO may have direct beneficial effects on the brain through mechanisms involving the cerebral vasculature and/or neuronal maturation.[31,32] Other investigators have described a possible role

for intravascular NO-derived molecules in conserving and stabilizing NO bioactivity that may contribute to the regulation of regional blood flow and oxygen delivery.[33,34] Neurodevelopmental outcome has been reported for 6 clinical trials,[35–40] and of these, 1 noted a more favorable neurodevelopmental outcome at 1 year of age among the preterm cohort treated with iNO but no difference in the rate of cerebral palsy.[36]

EFFECTS OF iNO THERAPY ON LONG-TERM PULMONARY OUTCOME OF SURVIVORS

In animal models, iNO decreases baseline airway resistance and may increase the rate of alveolarization.[2–6] To date, only 2 studies have reported respiratory outcomes of preterm infants treated with iNO.[41,42] In a telephone survey that included 456 infants in the Nitric Oxide Chronic Lung Disease (NOCLD) study group, the use of bronchodilators, inhaled steroids, systemic steroids, diuretics, and supplemental oxygen during the first year of life was less in the iNO-treated group, but there were no significant differences in the frequency of wheezing or the rate of rehospitalization. In the Inhaled Nitric Oxide Versus Ventilatory Support Without Inhaled Nitric Oxide multicenter trial, follow-up at 1 year of age showed no difference in maximal expiratory flow at functional residual capacity, wheezing, readmission rate, or use of respiratory medications.[42]

RESULTS OF META-ANALYSES OF STUDIES EVALUATING THE USE OF iNO IN PRETERM INFANTS

Two published meta-analyses found no overall significant effect of iNO on the rate of mortality, BPD, intraventricular hemorrhage, or neurodevelopmental impairment.[43,44] In view of the limitations

TABLE 1 Randomized Controlled Trials of iNO in Preterm Infants

Author, Year	n	Gestational Age, wk	Birth Weight, g	Age at Enrollment	Entry Criteria	iNO Protocol	Primary Outcome	Study Results
Subhedar, 1997[11]	42	<32	—	96 h	Need for mechanical ventilation and high risk of developing CLD	20 ppm for at least first 2 h and then 5 ppm for 3–4 d	Death and/or CLD before discharge	No difference in primary outcome
Kinsella, 1999[12]	80	≤34	—	≤7 d	aAO$_2$ ratio <0.1 on 2 consecutive blood gases in first 7 d of life	5 ppm for 7–14 d	Survival	No difference in primary outcome; no difference in rate of IVH or CLD
The French-Belgian iNO Trial, 1999[13]	85	<33	—	<7 d	OI between 12.5 and 30.0 on 2 consecutive blood gases at least 1 h apart	10–20 ppm for a minimum of 2 h	OI reduction of ≥33% or at least 10 points	More treated infants achieved primary outcome; no difference in median OI at 2 h; no difference in survival or other outcomes
Srisuparp, 2002[15]	34	—	<2000	<72 h	OI ranging from >4 to >12 based on birth wt	20 ppm for 24–48 h and then 5 ppm for maximum of 7 d	Change in oxygenation	Improved oxygenation with treatment but no difference in survival or IVH
Schreiber, 2003[16]	207	<34	<2000	<72 h	Need for mechanical ventilation	10 ppm for first day then 5 ppm for 6 d	Death and survival without BPD at 36 wk postmenstrual age	Treatment associated with a decrease in the combined incidence of BPD and death; no difference in mortality alone
Van Meurs, 2005[17]	420	<34	401–1500	4–120 h; mean 26–28 h	OI ≥10 on 2 consecutive blood gases between 30 min and 12 h apart	5–10 ppm for maximum of 14 d	Incidence of death or BPD	No difference in primary outcome; no difference in rate of BPD, severe IVH, or PVL. Post hoc analyses: Decrease in primary outcome in cohort with birth weight >1000 g; higher rate of mortality and severe IVH in cohort with birth wt <1000 g
Hascoet, 2005[18]	145	<32	—	6–48 h	aAO$_2$ ratio <0.22	5 ppm for first h of treatment and further dosage were adjusted based on response; total duration of treatment not clearly defined but varied from 4 h in nonresponders to few days in responders	Intact survival at 28 d	No difference in primary outcome; iNO was an independent risk factor for the combined risk of death or brain lesion
Field, 2005[19]	108	<34	—	<28 d; median 1 d	Severe respiratory failure requiring assisted ventilation	5–40 ppm depending on patient response; total duration of treatment not clearly defined	Death or severe disability at 1 y corrected age; death or CLD	No difference in primary outcome
Kinsella, 2006[20]	793	≤34	500–1250	<48 h	Need for mechanical ventilation	5 ppm for maximum of 21 d	Death or BPD at 36 wk postmenstrual age	No difference in primary outcome but had a decreased risk of brain injury; decreased incidence of BPD in cohort with birth weight ≤1000 g
Dani, 2006[21]	40	<30	—	≤7 d	aAO$_2$ ratio <0.15	10 ppm for 4 h then 6 ppm until extubation	Death and BPD	Primary outcome less with iNO treatment

TABLE 1 Continued

Author, Year	n	Gestational Age, wk	Birth Weight, g	Age at Enrollment	Entry Criteria	iNO Protocol	Primary Outcome	Study Results
Ballard, 2006[24]	582	≤32	500–1250	7–21 d	Need for mechanical ventilation for lung disease between 7 and 21 d; infants with birth weight 500–799 g were eligible if requiring nasal CPAP	20 ppm for 48–96 h followed by 10, 5, and 2 ppm at weekly intervals, with a minimum treatment duration of 24 d	Survival without BPD at 36 wk of postmenstrual age	Improved survival without BPD at 36 wk postmenstrual age; post hoc analysis showed most benefit when iNO treatment was started between 7–14 d of age
Van Meurs, 2007[23]	29	<34	>1500	4–120 h; mean 24–25 h	OI ≥15 on 2 consecutive blood gases between 30 min and 12 h apart	5–10 ppm for maximum of 14 d	Incidence of death or BPD	No difference in primary outcome
Su and Chen, 2008[22]	65	<32	≤1500	Mean 2.5 d	OI ≥25	5–20 ppm based on patient response; treatment duration at physician discretion (mean duration 4.9 ± 2.3 d)	OI at 24 h after randomization	Improved oxygenation with iNO treatment; no difference in survival, CLD, IVH, PDA, ROP, or duration of intubation
Mercier, 2010[25]	800	<29	>500	First day of life	Need for surfactant or CPAP within 24 h of birth	5 ppm for minimum of 7 d and maximum of 21 d	Survival without BPD at 36 wk postmenstrual age	No difference in primary outcome; no difference in survival alone; no difference in BPD; no difference in brain injury

Dash indicates not part of enrollment criteria.

aAO₂, arterial-alveolar oxygen ratio; CLD, chronic lung disease; CPAP, continuous positive airway pressure; IVH, intraventricular hemorrhage; OI, oxygenation index; PDA, patent ductus arteriosus; PVL, periventricular leukomalacia; ROP, retinopathy of prematurity.

of meta-analysis using aggregate data from different trials and to identify any patient or treatment characteristics that might predict benefit, Askie et al[9] conducted an individual-patient data meta-analysis. Data from 3298 infants in 11 trials that included 96% of published data showed no statistically significant effect of iNO on the rate of death or chronic lung disease (relative risk 0.96; 95% confidence interval 0.92–1.01) or severe brain lesions on cranial imaging (relative risk 1.12; 95% confidence interval 0.98–1.28). There were no statistically significant differences in iNO effect according to any of the patient-level characteristics tested; however, the authors cautioned that they could not exclude the possibility of a small reduction in the combined outcome of death or chronic lung disease if a higher dose of iNO (20 ppm) was used after >7 days of age, as observed in the NOCLD study.[9,24]

COST-BENEFIT ANALYSES OF ROUTINE USE OF INO IN PRETERM INFANTS

Treatment with iNO is expensive and can add significantly to health care costs.[8] A retrospective economic evaluation using patient-level data from the NOCLD trial (the only trial showing clinical benefit) reported that the overall mean cost per infant for the initial hospitalization was similar in the treated and placebo groups; however, when iNO therapy was initiated between 7 and 14 days of age, there was a 71% probability that the treatment decreased costs and improved outcomes.[45] Cost-benefit analysis from 2 other studies failed to show any cost-benefit.[37,39] Among preterm infants in the Inhaled Nitric Oxide Versus Ventilatory Support Without Inhaled Nitric Oxide trial, there was no difference in resource use and cost of care through the 4-year assessment.[37] Using more robust research methodology, including data on postdischarge resource utilization and health-related quality of life evaluations, Watson et al[39] found that costs of care did not vary significantly by treatment arm through 1 year of age. Although quality-adjusted survival was slightly better with iNO therapy, the estimated incremental cost-effectiveness ratio was $2.25 million per quality-adjusted life year, with only a 12.9% probability that the incremental cost-effectiveness ratio would be less than $500 000 per quality-adjusted life year. Additionally, in subgroup analysis, total costs were significantly higher for the iNO-treated group in the smallest birth weight stratum (500–749 g).

SAFETY OF INO USE IN PRETERM INFANTS

The only information regarding the safety of iNO use in preterm infants is derived from the NOCLD trial.[46–49] The limited data suggest that iNO is safe and does not increase lung inflammation or oxidative stress.[46,48]

SUMMARY

1. The results of randomized controlled trials, traditional meta-analyses, and an individualized patient data meta-analysis study indicate that neither rescue nor routine use of iNO improves survival in preterm infants with respiratory failure (Evidence quality, A; Grade of recommendation, strong).[50]

2. The preponderance of evidence does not support treating preterm infants who have respiratory failure with iNO for the purpose of preventing/ameliorating BPD, severe intraventricular hemorrhage, or other neonatal morbidities (Evidence quality, A; Grade of recommendation, strong).

3. The incidence of cerebral palsy, neurodevelopmental impairment, or cognitive impairment in preterm infants treated with iNO is similar to that of control infants (Evidence quality, A).

4. The results of 1 multicenter, randomized controlled trial suggest that treatment with a high dose of iNO (20 ppm) beginning in the second postnatal week may provide a small reduction in the rate of BPD. However, these results need to be confirmed by other trials.

5. An individual-patient data meta-analysis that included 96% of preterm infants enrolled in all published iNO trials found no statistically significant differences in iNO effect according to any of the patient-level characteristics, including gestational age, race, oxygenation index, postnatal age at enrollment, evidence of pulmonary hypertension, and mode of ventilation.

6. There are limited data and inconsistent results regarding the effects of iNO treatment on pulmonary outcomes of preterm infants in early childhood.

LEAD AUTHOR
Praveen Kumar, MD, FAAP

COMMITTEE ON FETUS AND NEWBORN, 2012–2013
Lu-Ann Papile, MD, FAAP, Chairperson
Richard A. Polin, MD, FAAP
Waldemar A. Carlo, MD, FAAP
Rosemarie Tan, MD, FAAP
Praveen Kumar, MD, FAAP
William Benitz, MD, FAAP
Eric Eichenwald, MD, FAAP
James Cummings, MD, FAAP
Jill Baley, MD, FAAP

LIAISONS
Tonse N. K. Raju, MD, FAAP – *National Institutes of Health*
CAPT Wanda Denise Barfield, MD, FAAP – *Centers for Disease Control and Prevention*
Erin Keels, MSN – *National Association of Neonatal Nurses*
Anne Jefferies, MD – *Canadian Pediatric Society*
Kasper S. Wang, MD, FAAP – *AAP Section on Surgery*
George Macones, MD – *American College of Obstetricians and Gynecologists*

STAFF
Jim Couto, MA

REFERENCES

1. American Academy of Pediatrics, Committee on Fetus and Newborn. American Academy of Pediatrics. Committee on Fetus and Newborn. Use of inhaled nitric oxide. *Pediatrics.* 2000;106(2 pt 1):344–345

2. Lin YJ, Markham NE, Balasubramaniam V, et al. Inhaled nitric oxide enhances distal lung growth after exposure to hyperoxia in neonatal rats. *Pediatr Res.* 2005;58(1):22–29

3. McCurnin DC, Pierce RA, Chang LY, et al. Inhaled NO improves early pulmonary function and modifies lung growth and elastin deposition in a baboon model of neonatal chronic lung disease. *Am J Physiol Lung Cell Mol Physiol.* 2005;288(3):L450–L459

4. Ballard PL, Gonzales LW, Godinez RI, et al. Surfactant composition and function in a primate model of infant chronic lung disease: effects of inhaled nitric oxide. *Pediatr Res.* 2006;59(1):157–162

5. Bland RD, Albertine KH, Carlton DP, MacRitchie AJ. Inhaled nitric oxide effects on lung structure and function in chronically ventilated preterm lambs. *Am J Respir Crit Care Med.* 2005;172(7):899–906

6. Tang JR, Markham NE, Lin YJ, et al. Inhaled nitric oxide attenuates pulmonary hypertension and improves lung growth in infant rats after neonatal treatment with a VEGF receptor inhibitor. *Am J Physiol Lung Cell Mol Physiol.* 2004;287(2):L344–L351

7. Clark RH, Ursprung RL, Walker MW, Ellsbury DL, Spitzer AR. The changing pattern of inhaled nitric oxide use in the neonatal

intensive care unit. *J Perinatol.* 2010;30 (12):800–804

8. Cole FS, Alleyne C, Barks JD, et al. NIH Consensus Development Conference statement: inhaled nitric-oxide therapy for premature infants. *Pediatrics.* 2011;127(2): 363–369

9. Askie LM, Ballard RA, Cutter GR, et al; Meta-analysis of Preterm Patients on Inhaled Nitric Oxide Collaboration. Inhaled nitric oxide in preterm infants: an individual-patient data meta-analysis of randomized trials. *Pediatrics.* 2011;128(4):729–739

10. Skimming JW, Bender KA, Hutchison AA, Drummond WH. Nitric oxide inhalation in infants with respiratory distress syndrome. *J Pediatr.* 1997;130(2):225–230

11. Subhedar NV, Ryan SW, Shaw NJ. Open randomised controlled trial of inhaled nitric oxide and early dexamethasone in high risk preterm infants. *Arch Dis Child Fetal Neonatal Ed.* 1997;77(3):F185–F190

12. Kinsella JP, Walsh WF, Bose CL, et al. Inhaled nitric oxide in premature neonates with severe hypoxaemic respiratory failure: a randomised controlled trial. *Lancet.* 1999; 354(9184):1061–1065

13. The Franco-Belgium Collaborative NO Trial Group. Early compared with delayed inhaled nitric oxide in moderately hypoxaemic neonates with respiratory failure: a randomised controlled trial. *Lancet.* 1999; 354(9184):1066–1071

14. Truffert P, Llado-Paris J, Mercier JC, Dehan M, Bréart G; Franco-Belgian iNO Study Group. Early inhaled nitric oxide in moderately hypoxemic preterm and term newborns with RDS: the RDS subgroup analysis of the Franco-Belgian iNO Randomized Trial. *Eur J Pediatr.* 2003;162(9):646–647

15. Srisuparp P, Heitschmidt M, Schreiber MD. Inhaled nitric oxide therapy in premature infants with mild to moderate respiratory distress syndrome. *J Med Assoc Thai.* 2002; 85(suppl 2):S469–S478

16. Schreiber MD, Gin-Mestan K, Marks JD, Huo D, Lee G, Srisuparp P. Inhaled nitric oxide in premature infants with the respiratory distress syndrome. *N Engl J Med.* 2003;349 (22):2099–2107

17. Van Meurs KP, Wright LL, Ehrenkranz RA, et al; Preemie Inhaled Nitric Oxide Study. Inhaled nitric oxide for premature infants with severe respiratory failure. *N Engl J Med.* 2005;353(1):13–22

18. Hascoet JM, Fresson J, Claris O, et al. The safety and efficacy of nitric oxide therapy in premature infants. *J Pediatr.* 2005;146(3): 318–323

19. Field D, Elbourne D, Truesdale A, et al; INNOVO Trial Collaborating Group. Neonatal ventilation with inhaled nitric oxide versus ventilatory support without inhaled nitric oxide for preterm infants with severe respiratory failure: the INNOVO multicentre randomised controlled trial (ISRCTN 17821339). *Pediatrics.* 2005;115(4):926–936

20. Kinsella JP, Cutter GR, Walsh WF, et al. Early inhaled nitric oxide therapy in premature newborns with respiratory failure. *N Engl J Med.* 2006;355(4):354–364

21. Dani C, Bertini G, Pezzati M, Filippi L, Cecchi A, Rubaltelli FF. Inhaled nitric oxide in very preterm infants with severe respiratory distress syndrome. *Acta Paediatr.* 2006;95 (9):1116–1123

22. Su PH, Chen JY. Inhaled nitric oxide in the management of preterm infants with severe respiratory failure. *J Perinatol.* 2008; 28(2):112–116

23. Van Meurs KP, Hintz SR, Ehrenkranz RA, et al. Inhaled nitric oxide in infants >1500 g and <34 weeks gestation with severe respiratory failure. *J Perinatol.* 2007;27(6): 347–352

24. Ballard RA, Truog WE, Cnaan A, et al; NO CLD Study Group. Inhaled nitric oxide in preterm infants undergoing mechanical ventilation. *N Engl J Med.* 2006;355(4):343–353

25. Mercier JC, Hummler H, Durrmeyer X, et al; EUNO Study Group. Inhaled nitric oxide for prevention of bronchopulmonary dysplasia in premature babies (EUNO): a randomised controlled trial. *Lancet.* 2010;376(9738):346–354

26. Jobe AH, Bancalari E. Bronchopulmonary dysplasia. *Am J Respir Crit Care Med.* 2001; 163(7):1723–1729

27. Stenmark KR, Abman SH. Lung vascular development: implications for the pathogenesis of bronchopulmonary dysplasia. *Annu Rev Physiol.* 2005;67:623–661

28. Balasubramaniam V, Maxey AM, Morgan DB, Markham NE, Abman SH. Inhaled NO restores lung structure in eNOS-deficient mice recovering from neonatal hypoxia. *Am J Physiol Lung Cell Mol Physiol.* 2006; 291(1):L119–L127

29. Tang JR, Seedorf G, Balasubramaniam V, Maxey A, Markham N, Abman SH. Early inhaled nitric oxide treatment decreases apoptosis of endothelial cells in neonatal rat lungs after vascular endothelial growth factor inhibition. *Am J Physiol Lung Cell Mol Physiol.* 2007;293(5):L1271–L1280

30. Gutierrez HH, Nieves B, Chumley P, Rivera A, Freeman BA. Nitric oxide regulation of superoxide-dependent lung injury: oxidant-protective actions of endogenously produced and exogenously administered nitric oxide. *Free Radic Biol Med.* 1996;21(1):43–52

31. Zhang YT, Zhang DL, Cao YL, Zhao BL. Developmental expression and activity varia-tion of nitric oxide synthase in the brain of golden hamster. *Brain Res Bull.* 2002;58(4): 385–389

32. Soygüder Z, Karadağ H, Nazli M. Neuronal nitric oxide synthase immunoreactivity in ependymal cells during early postnatal development. *J Chem Neuroanat.* 2004;27(1):3–6

33. Cannon RO, III, Schechter AN, Panza JA, et al. Effects of inhaled nitric oxide on regional blood flow are consistent with intravascular nitric oxide delivery. *J Clin Invest.* 2001;108(2):279–287

34. McMahon TJ, Moon RE, Luschinger BP, et al. Nitric oxide in the human respiratory cycle. *Nat Med.* 2002;8(7):711–717

35. Bennett AJ, Shaw NJ, Gregg JE, Subhedar NV. Neurodevelopmental outcome in high-risk preterm infants treated with inhaled nitric oxide. *Acta Paediatr.* 2001;90(5):573–576

36. Mestan KK, Marks JD, Hecox K, Huo D, Schreiber MD. Neurodevelopmental outcomes of premature infants treated with inhaled nitric oxide. *N Engl J Med.* 2005;353(1):23–32

37. Huddy CL, Bennett CC, Hardy P, et al; INNOVO Trial Collaborating Group. The INNOVO multicentre randomised controlled trial: neonatal ventilation with inhaled nitric oxide versus ventilatory support without nitric oxide for severe respiratory failure in preterm infants: follow up at 4–5 years. *Arch Dis Child Fetal Neonatal Ed.* 2008;93(6):F430–F435

38. Hintz SR, Van Meurs KP, Perritt R, et al; NICHD Neonatal Research Network. Neurodevelopmental outcomes of premature infants with severe respiratory failure enrolled in a randomized controlled trial of inhaled nitric oxide. *J Pediatr.* 2007;151(1): 16–22, 22.e1–e3

39. Watson RS, Clermont G, Kinsella JP, et al; Prolonged Outcomes After Nitric Oxide Investigators. Clinical and economic effects of iNO in premature newborns with respiratory failure at 1 year. *Pediatrics.* 2009; 124(5):1333–1343

40. Walsh MC, Hibbs AM, Martin CR, et al; NO CLD Study Group. Two-year neurodevelopmental outcomes of ventilated preterm infants treated with inhaled nitric oxide. *J Pediatr.* 2010;156(4):556–561.e1

41. Hibbs AM, Walsh MC, Martin RJ, et al. One-year respiratory outcomes of preterm infants enrolled in the Nitric Oxide (to prevent) Chronic Lung Disease trial. *J Pediatr.* 2008;153(4):525–529

42. Hoo AF, Beardsmore CS, Castle RA, et al; INNOVO Trial Collaborating Group. Respiratory function during infancy in survivors of the INNOVO trial. *Pediatr Pulmonol.* 2009;44(2):155–161

43. Barrington KJ, Finer N. Inhaled nitric oxide for respiratory failure in preterm infants.

Cochrane Database Syst Rev. 2010;(12): CD000509

44. Donohue PK, Gilmore MM, Cristofalo E, et al. Inhaled nitric oxide in preterm infants: a systematic review. *Pediatrics.* 2011;127(2). Available at: www.pediatrics.org/cgi/content/full/127/2/e414

45. Zupancic JA, Hibbs AM, Palermo L, et al; NO CLD Trial Group. Economic evaluation of inhaled nitric oxide in preterm infants undergoing mechanical ventilation. *Pediatrics.* 2009;124(5):1325–1332

46. Truog WE, Ballard PL, Norberg M, et al; Nitric Oxide (to Prevent) Chronic Lung Disease Study Investigators. Inflammatory markers and mediators in tracheal fluid of premature infants treated with inhaled nitric oxide. *Pediatrics.* 2007;119(4):670–678

47. Ballard PL, Merrill JD, Truog WE, et al. Surfactant function and composition in premature infants treated with inhaled nitric oxide. *Pediatrics.* 2007;120(2):346–353

48. Ballard PL, Truog WE, Merrill JD, et al. Plasma biomarkers of oxidative stress: relationship to lung disease and inhaled nitric oxide therapy in premature infants. *Pediatrics.* 2008;121(3):555–561

49. Posencheg MA, Gow AJ, Truog WE, et al; NO CLD Investigators. Inhaled nitric oxide in premature infants: effect on tracheal aspirate and plasma nitric oxide metabolites. *J Perinatol.* 2010;30(4):275–280

50. American Academy of Pediatrics Steering Committee on Quality Improvement and Management. Classifying recommendations for clinical practice guidelines. *Pediatrics.* 2004;114(3):874–877

Section 5

Current Policies

From the American Academy of Pediatrics

• •

(Through January 1, 2014)

- *Policy Statements*
  ORGANIZATIONAL PRINCIPLES TO GUIDE AND DEFINE THE CHILD HEALTH CARE SYSTEM
  AND TO IMPROVE THE HEALTH OF ALL CHILDREN

- *Clinical Reports*
  GUIDANCE FOR THE CLINICIAN IN RENDERING PEDIATRIC CARE

- *Technical Reports*
  BACKGROUND INFORMATION TO SUPPORT AMERICAN ACADEMY OF PEDIATRICS POLICY

AMERICAN ACADEMY OF PEDIATRICS

Policy Statements, Clinical Reports, Technical Reports

Current through January 1, 2014

Full text of all titles listed below is available on the *Pediatric Clinical Practice Guidelines & Policies* CD-ROM included with this manual.

AAP PRINCIPLES CONCERNING RETAIL-BASED CLINICS
Retail-Based Clinic Policy Work Group (12/06, reaffirmed 1/11)

ABUSIVE HEAD TRAUMA IN INFANTS AND CHILDREN
Cindy W. Christian, MD; Robert Block, MD; and Committee on Child Abuse and Neglect
ABSTRACT. Shaken baby syndrome is a term often used by physicians and the public to describe abusive head trauma inflicted on infants and young children. Although the term is well known and has been used for a number of decades, advances in the understanding of the mechanisms and clinical spectrum of injury associated with abusive head trauma compel us to modify our terminology to keep pace with our understanding of pathologic mechanisms. Although shaking an infant has the potential to cause neurologic injury, blunt impact or a combination of shaking and blunt impact cause injury as well. Spinal cord injury and secondary hypoxic ischemic injury can contribute to poor outcomes of victims. The use of broad medical terminology that is inclusive of all mechanisms of injury, including shaking, is required. The American Academy of Pediatrics recommends that pediatricians develop skills in the recognition of signs and symptoms of abusive head injury, including those caused by both shaking and blunt impact, consult with pediatric subspecialists when necessary, and embrace a less mechanistic term, abusive head trauma, when describing an inflicted injury to the head and its contents. (4/09, reaffirmed 3/13)

ACCESS TO OPTIMAL EMERGENCY CARE FOR CHILDREN
Committee on Pediatric Emergency Medicine
ABSTRACT. Millions of pediatric patients require some level of emergency care annually, and significant barriers limit access to appropriate services for large numbers of children. The American Academy of Pediatrics has a strong commitment to identifying barriers to access to emergency care, working to surmount these obstacles, and encouraging, through education and system changes, improved levels of emergency care available to all children. (1/07, reaffirmed 8/10)

ACCF/AHA/AAP RECOMMENDATIONS FOR TRAINING IN PEDIATRIC CARDIOLOGY
American College of Cardiology Foundation, American Heart Association, and American Academy of Pediatrics (12/05, reaffirmed 1/09)

ACHIEVING QUALITY HEALTH SERVICES FOR ADOLESCENTS
Committee on Adolescence
ABSTRACT. In recent years, there has been an increased national focus on assessing and improving the quality of health care. This statement provides recommendations and criteria for assessment of the quality of primary care delivered to adolescents in the United States. Consistent implementation of American Academy of Pediatrics recommendations (periodicity of visits and confidentiality issues), renewed attention to professional quality-improvement activities (access and immunizations) and public education, and modification of existing quality-measurement activities to ensure that quality is delivered are proposed as strategies that would lead to improved care for youth. (6/08, reaffirmed 3/13)

ACTIVE HEALTHY LIVING: PREVENTION OF CHILDHOOD OBESITY THROUGH INCREASED PHYSICAL ACTIVITY
Council on Sports Medicine and Fitness and Council on School Health
ABSTRACT. The current epidemic of inactivity and the associated epidemic of obesity are being driven by multiple factors (societal, technologic, industrial, commercial, financial) and must be addressed likewise on several fronts. Foremost among these are the expansion of school physical education, dissuading children from pursuing sedentary activities, providing suitable role models for physical activity, and making activity-promoting changes in the environment. This statement outlines ways that pediatric health care providers and public health officials can encourage, monitor, and advocate for increased physical activity for children and teenagers. (5/06, reaffirmed 5/09, 8/12)

ADDITIONAL RECOMMENDATIONS FOR USE OF TETANUS TOXOID, REDUCED-CONTENT DIPHTHERIA TOXOID, AND ACELLULAR PERTUSSIS VACCINE (TDAP)
Committee on Infectious Diseases
ABSTRACT. The American Academy of Pediatrics and the Centers for Disease Control and Prevention are amending previous recommendations and making additional recommendations for the use of tetanus toxoid, reduced-content diphtheria toxoid, and acellular pertussis vaccine (Tdap). Review of the results from clinical trials and other studies has revealed no excess reactogenicity when Tdap is given within a short interval after other tetanus- or diphtheria-containing toxoid products, and accrual of postmarketing adverse-events reports reveals an excellent safety record for Tdap. Thus, the recommendation for caution regarding Tdap use within any interval after a tetanus- or

diphtheria-containing toxoid product is removed. Tdap should be given when it is indicated and when no contraindication exists. In further efforts to protect people who are susceptible to pertussis, the American Academy of Pediatrics and Centers for Disease Control and Prevention recommend a single dose of Tdap for children 7 through 10 years of age who were underimmunized with diphtheria-tetanus-acellular pertussis (DTaP). Also, the age for recommendation for Tdap is extended to those aged 65 years and older who have or are likely to have contact with an infant younger than 12 months (eg, health care personnel, grandparents, and other caregivers). (9/11)

ADMISSION AND DISCHARGE GUIDELINES FOR THE PEDIATRIC PATIENT REQUIRING INTERMEDIATE CARE (CLINICAL REPORT)

Committee on Hospital Care and Section on Critical Care
  (joint with Society of Critical Care Medicine)

ABSTRACT. During the past 3 decades, the specialty of pediatric critical care medicine has grown rapidly, leading to a number of pediatric intensive care units opening across the country. Many patients who are admitted to the hospital require a higher level of care than routine inpatient general pediatric care, yet not to the degree of intensity of pediatric critical care; therefore, an intermediate care level has been developed in institutions providing multidisciplinary subspecialty pediatric care. These patients may require frequent monitoring of vital signs and nursing interventions, but usually they do not require invasive monitoring. The admission of the pediatric intermediate care patient is guided by physiologic parameters depending on the respective organ system involved relative to an institution's resources and capacity to care for a patient in a general care environment. This report provides admission and discharge guidelines for intermediate pediatric care. Intermediate care promotes greater flexibility in patient triage and provides a cost-effective alternative to admission to a pediatric intensive care unit. This level of care may enhance the efficiency of care and make health care more affordable for patients receiving intermediate care. (5/04, reaffirmed 2/08, 1/13)

ADOLESCENT PREGNANCY: CURRENT TRENDS AND ISSUES (CLINICAL REPORT)

Jonathan D. Klein, MD, MPH, and Committee on Adolescence

ABSTRACT. The prevention of unintended adolescent pregnancy is an important goal of the American Academy of Pediatrics and our society. Although adolescent pregnancy and birth rates have been steadily decreasing, many adolescents still become pregnant. Since the last statement on adolescent pregnancy was issued by the Academy in 1998, efforts to prevent adolescent pregnancy have increased, and new observations, technologies, and prevention effectiveness data have emerged. The purpose of this clinical report is to review current trends and issues related to adolescent pregnancy, update practitioners on this topic, and review legal and policy implications of concern to pediatricians. (7/05)

ADOLESCENTS AND HIV INFECTION: THE PEDIATRICIAN'S ROLE IN PROMOTING ROUTINE TESTING

Committee on Pediatric AIDS

ABSTRACT. Pediatricians can play a key role in preventing and controlling HIV infection by promoting risk-reduction counseling and offering routine HIV testing to adolescent and young adult patients. Most sexually active youth do not feel that they are at risk of contracting HIV and have never been tested. Obtaining a sexual history and creating an atmosphere that promotes nonjudgmental risk counseling is a key component of the adolescent visit. In light of increasing numbers of people with HIV/AIDS and missed opportunities for HIV testing, the Centers for Disease Control and Prevention recommends universal and routine HIV testing for all patients seen in health care settings who are 13 to 64 years of age. There are advances in diagnostics and treatment that help support this recommendation. This policy statement reviews the epidemiologic data and recommends that routine screening be offered to all adolescents at least once by 16 to 18 years of age in health care settings when the prevalence of HIV in the patient population is more than 0.1%. In areas of lower community HIV prevalence, routine HIV testing is encouraged for all sexually active adolescents and those with other risk factors for HIV. This statement addresses many of the real and perceived barriers that pediatricians face in promoting routine HIV testing for their patients. (10/11)

ADOLESCENTS AND HUMAN IMMUNODEFICIENCY VIRUS INFECTION: THE ROLE OF THE PEDIATRICIAN IN PREVENTION AND INTERVENTION

Committee on Pediatric AIDS and Committee on Adolescence

ABSTRACT. Half of all new human immunodeficiency virus (HIV) infections in the United States occur among young people between the ages of 13 and 24. Sexual transmission accounts for most cases of HIV during adolescence. Pediatricians can play an important role in educating adolescents about HIV prevention, transmission, and testing, with an emphasis on risk reduction, and in advocating for the special needs of adolescents for access to information about HIV. (1/01, reaffirmed 10/03, 1/05)

THE ADOLESCENT'S RIGHT TO CONFIDENTIAL CARE WHEN CONSIDERING ABORTION

Committee on Adolescence

ABSTRACT. In this statement, the American Academy of Pediatrics (AAP) reaffirms its position that the rights of adolescents to confidential care when considering abortion should be protected. The AAP supports the recommendations presented in the report on mandatory parental consent to abortion by the Council on Ethical and Judicial Affairs of the American Medical Association. Adolescents should be strongly encouraged to involve their parents and other trusted adults in decisions regarding pregnancy termination, and the majority of them voluntarily do so. Legislation mandating parental involvement does not achieve the intended benefit of promoting family communication, but it does increase the risk of harm to the adolescent by delaying access to appropriate medical care.

The statement presents a summary of pertinent current information related to the benefits and risks of legislation requiring mandatory parental involvement in an adolescent's decision to obtain an abortion. The AAP acknowledges and respects the diversity of beliefs about abortion and affirms the value of voluntary parental involvement in decision making by adolescents. (5/96, reaffirmed 5/99, 11/02)

ADVANCED PRACTICE IN NEONATAL NURSING
Committee on Fetus and Newborn
ABSTRACT. The participation of advanced practice registered nurses in neonatal care continues to be accepted and supported by the American Academy of Pediatrics. Recognized categories of advanced practice neonatal nursing are the neonatal clinical nurse specialist and the neonatal nurse practitioner. (5/09)

AGE LIMITS OF PEDIATRICS
Child and Adolescent Health Action Group (5/88, reaffirmed 9/92, 1/97, 3/02, 1/06, 10/11)

AGE TERMINOLOGY DURING THE PERINATAL PERIOD
Committee on Fetus and Newborn
ABSTRACT. Consistent definitions to describe the length of gestation and age in neonates are needed to compare neurodevelopmental, medical, and growth outcomes. The purposes of this policy statement are to review conventional definitions of age during the perinatal period and to recommend use of standard terminology including gestational age, postmenstrual age, chronological age, corrected age, adjusted age, and estimated date of delivery. (11/04, reaffirmed 10/07, 11/08, 1/09)

ALCOHOL USE BY YOUTH AND ADOLESCENTS: A PEDIATRIC CONCERN
Committee on Substance Abuse
ABSTRACT. Alcohol use continues to be a major problem from preadolescence through young adulthood in the United States. Results of recent neuroscience research have substantiated the deleterious effects of alcohol on adolescent brain development and added even more evidence to support the call to prevent and reduce underaged drinking. Pediatricians should be knowledgeable about substance abuse to be able to recognize risk factors for alcohol and other substance abuse among youth, screen for use, provide appropriate brief interventions, and refer to treatment. The integration of alcohol use prevention programs in the community and our educational system from elementary school through college should be promoted by pediatricians and the health care community. Promotion of media responsibility to connect alcohol consumption with realistic consequences should be supported by pediatricians. Additional research into the prevention, screening and identification, brief intervention, and management and treatment of alcohol and other substance use by adolescents continues to be needed to improve evidence-based practices. (4/10)

ALLERGY TESTING IN CHILDHOOD: USING ALLERGEN-SPECIFIC IGE TESTS (CLINICAL REPORT)
Scott H. Sicherer, MD; Robert A. Wood, MD; and Section on Allergy and Immunology
ABSTRACT. A variety of triggers can induce common pediatric allergic diseases which include asthma, allergic rhinitis, atopic dermatitis, food allergy, and anaphylaxis. Allergy testing serves to confirm an allergic trigger suspected on the basis of history. Tests for allergen-specific immunoglobulin E (IgE) are performed by in vitro assays or skin tests. The tests are excellent for identifying a sensitized state in which allergen-specific IgE is present, and may identify triggers to be eliminated and help guide immunotherapy treatment. However, a positive test result does not always equate with clinical allergy. Newer enzymatic assays based on anti-IgE antibodies have supplanted the radioallergosorbent test (RAST). This clinical report focuses on allergen-specific IgE testing, emphasizing that the medical history and knowledge of disease characteristics are crucial for rational test selection and interpretation. (12/11)

ALL-TERRAIN VEHICLE INJURY PREVENTION: TWO-, THREE-, AND FOUR-WHEELED UNLICENSED MOTOR VEHICLES
Committee on Injury and Poison Prevention
ABSTRACT. Since 1987, the American Academy of Pediatrics (AAP) has had a policy about the use of motorized cycles and all-terrain vehicles (ATVs) by children. The purpose of this policy statement is to update and strengthen previous policy. This statement describes the various kinds of motorized cycles and ATVs and outlines the epidemiologic characteristics of deaths and injuries related to their use by children in light of the 1987 consent decrees entered into by the US Consumer Product Safety Commission and the manufacturers of ATVs. Recommendations are made for public, patient, and parent education by pediatricians; equipment modifications; the use of safety equipment; and the development and improvement of safer off-road trails and responsive emergency medical systems. In addition, the AAP strengthens its recommendation for passage of legislation in all states prohibiting the use of 2- and 4-wheeled off-road vehicles by children younger than 16 years, as well as a ban on the sale of new and used 3-wheeled ATVs, with a recall of all used 3-wheeled ATVs. (6/00, reaffirmed 5/04, 1/07)

AMBIENT AIR POLLUTION: HEALTH HAZARDS TO CHILDREN
Committee on Environmental Health
ABSTRACT. Ambient (outdoor) air pollution is now recognized as an important problem, both nationally and worldwide. Our scientific understanding of the spectrum of health effects of air pollution has increased, and numerous studies are finding important health effects from air pollution at levels once considered safe. Children and infants are among the most susceptible to many of the air pollutants. In addition to associations between air pollution and respiratory symptoms, asthma exacerbations, and asthma hospitalizations, recent studies have found links between air pollution and preterm birth, infant mortality, deficits in lung growth, and possibly, develop-

ment of asthma. This policy statement summarizes the recent literature linking ambient air pollution to adverse health outcomes in children and includes a perspective on the current regulatory process. The statement provides advice to pediatricians on how to integrate issues regarding air quality and health into patient education and children's environmental health advocacy and concludes with recommendations to the government on promotion of effective air-pollution policies to ensure protection of children's health. (12/04, reaffirmed 4/09)

ANTENATAL COUNSELING REGARDING RESUSCITATION AT AN EXTREMELY LOW GESTATIONAL AGE (CLINICAL REPORT)

Daniel G. Batton, MD, and Committee on Fetus and Newborn
ABSTRACT. The anticipated delivery of an extremely low gestational age infant raises difficult questions for all involved, including whether to initiate resuscitation after delivery. Each institution caring for women at risk of delivering extremely preterm infants should provide comprehensive and consistent guidelines for antenatal counseling. Parents should be provided the most accurate prognosis possible on the basis of all the factors known to affect outcome for a particular case. Although it is not feasible to have specific criteria for when the initiation of resuscitation should or should not be offered, the following general guidelines are suggested. If the physicians involved believe there is no chance for survival, resuscitation is not indicated and should not be initiated. When a good outcome is considered very unlikely, the parents should be given the choice of whether resuscitation should be initiated, and clinicians should respect their preference. Finally, if a good outcome is considered reasonably likely, clinicians should initiate resuscitation and, together with the parents, continually reevaluate whether intensive care should be continued. Whenever resuscitation is considered an option, a qualified individual, preferably a neonatologist, should be involved and should be present in the delivery room to manage this complex situation. Comfort care should be provided for all infants for whom resuscitation is not initiated or is not successful. (6/09)

ANTIVIRAL THERAPY AND PROPHYLAXIS FOR INFLUENZA IN CHILDREN (CLINICAL REPORT)

Committee on Infectious Diseases
ABSTRACT. Antiviral agents are available that are safe and effective for the treatment and prophylaxis of influenza virus infections in children. The neuraminidase inhibitors (oseltamivir [Tamiflu] and zanamivir [Relenza]) are preferred agents because of current widespread resistance to the adamantanes (amantadine [Symmetrel] and rimantadine [Flumadine]). Therapy should be provided to children with influenza infection who are at high risk of severe infection and to children with moderate-to-severe influenza infection who may benefit from a decrease in the duration of symptoms. Prophylaxis should be provided (1) to high-risk children who have not yet received immunization and during the 2 weeks after immunization, (2) to unimmunized family members and health care professionals with close contact with high-risk unimmunized children or infants who are younger than 6 months, and (3) for control of influenza outbreaks in unimmunized

staff and children in an institutional setting. Testing of current H5N1 avian influenza virus isolates, the potential agents of pandemic influenza, suggests susceptibility to oseltamivir and zanamivir. Because no prospective data exist on the efficacy of these agents in humans for H5N1 strains, the dosage and duration of therapy in adults and children may differ from those documented to be effective for epidemic influenza strains. (4/07, reaffirmed 7/10)

THE APGAR SCORE

Committee on Fetus and Newborn (joint with American College of Obstetricians and Gynecologists)
ABSTRACT. The Apgar score provides a convenient shorthand for reporting the status of the newborn infant and the response to resuscitation. The Apgar score has been used inappropriately to predict specific neurologic outcome in the term infant. There are no consistent data on the significance of the Apgar score in preterm infants. The Apgar score has limitations, and it is inappropriate to use it alone to establish the diagnosis of asphyxia. An Apgar score assigned during resuscitation is not equivalent to a score assigned to a spontaneously breathing infant. An expanded Apgar score reporting form will account for concurrent resuscitative interventions and provide information to improve systems of perinatal and neonatal care. (4/06, reaffirmed 1/09)

APPLICATION OF THE RESOURCE-BASED RELATIVE VALUE SCALE SYSTEM TO PEDIATRICS

Committee on Coding and Nomenclature
ABSTRACT. With an increased focus on payment and productivity measurement in health care, it is essential to understand the genesis and principles behind the Medicare Resource-Based Relative Value Scale (RBRVS) physician fee schedule. The majority of third-party payers, including a growing number of Medicaid programs and commercial payers, use variations of the Medicare RBRVS as their basis for physician payment. Many group practices have also adopted this system to benchmark physician productivity and determine variable compensation and bonus payments. Because pediatric care is underrepresented in any Medicare-based payment system analysis, unique aspects of physician work and practice expense may not be accurately reflected in the total relative value units (RVUs) for certain pediatric services. Despite this potential limitation, the American Academy of Pediatrics supports the use of *Current Procedural Terminology* (CPT) codes to report unique physician work and the RBRVS physician fee schedule as a uniform payment system. The American Academy of Pediatrics will continue to work to rectify perceived inequities of the RBRVS system as they pertain to pediatrics. (12/08)

ASSESSMENT AND MANAGEMENT OF INGUINAL HERNIA IN INFANTS (CLINICAL REPORT)

Kasper S. Wang, MD; Committee on Fetus and Newborn; and Section on Surgery
ABSTRACT. Inguinal hernia repair in infants is a routine surgical procedure. However, numerous issues, including timing of the repair, the need to explore the contralateral groin, use of laparoscopy, and anesthetic approach, remain unsettled. Given the lack of compelling data, con-

sideration should be given to large, prospective, randomized controlled trials to determine best practices for the management of inguinal hernias in infants. (9/12)

ATHLETIC PARTICIPATION BY CHILDREN AND ADOLESCENTS WHO HAVE SYSTEMIC HYPERTENSION

Rebecca A. Demorest, MD; Reginald L. Washington, MD; and Council on Sports Medicine and Fitness

ABSTRACT. Children and adolescents who have hypertension may be at risk for complications when exercise causes their blood pressure to rise even higher. The purpose of this statement is to update recommendations concerning the athletic participation of individuals with hypertension, including special populations such as those with spinal cord injuries or obesity, by using the guidelines from "The 36th Bethesda Conference: Eligibility Recommendations for Competitive Athletes with Cardiovascular Abnormalities"; "The Fourth Report on the Diagnosis, Evaluation, and Treatment of High Blood Pressure in Children and Adolescents"; and "The Seventh Report of the Joint National Committee on Prevention, Detection, Evaluation, and Treatment of High Blood Pressure." (5/10, reaffirmed 5/13)

AUDITORY INTEGRATION TRAINING AND FACILITATED COMMUNICATION FOR AUTISM

Committee on Children With Disabilities

ABSTRACT. This statement reviews the basis for two new therapies for autism—auditory integration training and facilitative communication. Both therapies seek to improve communication skills. Currently available information does not support the claims of proponents that these treatments are efficacious. Their use does not appear warranted at this time, except within research protocols. (8/98, reaffirmed 5/02, 1/06, 12/09)

BASEBALL AND SOFTBALL

Council on Sports Medicine and Fitness

ABSTRACT. Baseball and softball are among the most popular and safest sports in which children and adolescents participate. Nevertheless, traumatic and overuse injuries occur regularly, including occasional catastrophic injury and even death. Safety of the athlete is a constant focus of attention among those responsible for modifying rules. Understanding the stresses placed on the arm, especially while pitching, led to the institution of rules controlling the quantity of pitches thrown in youth baseball and established rest periods between pitching assignments. Similarly, field maintenance and awareness of environmental conditions as well as equipment maintenance and creative prevention strategies are critically important in minimizing the risk of injury. This statement serves as a basis for encouraging safe participation in baseball and softball. This statement has been endorsed by the Canadian Paediatric Society. (2/12)

BICYCLE HELMETS

Committee on Injury and Poison Prevention

ABSTRACT. Bicycling remains one of the most popular recreational sports among children in America and is the leading cause of recreational sports injuries treated in emergency departments. An estimated 23 000 children younger than 21 years sustained head injuries (excluding the face) while bicycling in 1998. The bicycle helmet is a very effective device that can prevent the occurrence of up to 88% of serious brain injuries. Despite this, most children do not wear a helmet each time they ride a bicycle, and adolescents are particularly resistant to helmet use. Recently, a group of national experts and government agencies renewed the call for all bicyclists to wear helmets. This policy statement describes the role of the pediatrician in helping attain universal helmet use among children and teens for each bicycle ride. (10/01, reaffirmed 1/05, 2/08, 11/11)

BONE DENSITOMETRY IN CHILDREN AND ADOLESCENTS (CLINICAL REPORT)

Laura K. Bachrach, MD; Irene N. Sills, MD; and Section on Endocrinology

ABSTRACT. Concern for bone fragility in children and adolescents has led to increased interest in bone densitometry. Pediatric patients with genetic and acquired chronic diseases, immobility, and inadequate nutrition may fail to achieve the expected gains in bone size, mass, and strength, which leaves them vulnerable to fracture. In older adults, bone densitometry has been shown to predict fracture risk and reflect response to therapy. The role of densitometry in the management of children at risk of bone fragility is less certain. This clinical report summarizes the current knowledge about bone densitometry in the pediatric population, including indications for its use, interpretation of results, and its risks and costs. This report emphasizes consensus statements generated at the 2007 Pediatric Position Development Conference of the International Society of Clinical Densitometry by an international panel of bone experts. Some of these recommendations are evidence-based, and others reflect expert opinion, because the available data are inadequate. The statements from this and other expert panels have provided general guidance to the pediatrician, but decisions about ordering and interpreting bone densitometry still require clinical judgment. Ongoing studies will help to better define the indications and best methods for assessing bone strength in children and the clinical factors that contribute to fracture risk. (12/10)

BOXING PARTICIPATION BY CHILDREN AND ADOLESCENTS

Council on Sports Medicine and Fitness (joint with Canadian Paediatric Society Healthy Active Living and Sports Medicine Committee)

ABSTRACT. Thousands of boys and girls younger than 19 years participate in boxing in North America. Although boxing provides benefits for participants, including exercise, self-discipline, and self-confidence, the sport of boxing encourages and rewards deliberate blows to the head and face. Participants in boxing are at risk of head, face, and neck injuries, including chronic and even fatal neurologic injuries. Concussions are one of the most common injuries that occur with boxing. Because of the risk of head and facial injuries, the American Academy of Pediatrics and the Canadian Paediatric Society oppose boxing as a sport for children and adolescents. These organizations recommend that physicians vigorously oppose boxing in youth and encourage patients to participate in alternative sports in which intentional head blows are not central to the sport. (8/11)

BREASTFEEDING AND THE USE OF HUMAN MILK
Section on Breastfeeding
ABSTRACT. Breastfeeding and human milk are the normative standards for infant feeding and nutrition. Given the documented short- and long-term medical and neurodevelopmental advantages of breastfeeding, infant nutrition should be considered a public health issue and not only a lifestyle choice. The American Academy of Pediatrics reaffirms its recommendation of exclusive breastfeeding for about 6 months, followed by continued breastfeeding as complementary foods are introduced, with continuation of breastfeeding for 1 year or longer as mutually desired by mother and infant. Medical contraindications to breastfeeding are rare. Infant growth should be monitored with the World Health Organization (WHO) Growth Curve Standards to avoid mislabeling infants as underweight or failing to thrive. Hospital routines to encourage and support the initiation and sustaining of exclusive breastfeeding should be based on the American Academy of Pediatrics-endorsed WHO/UNICEF "Ten Steps to Successful Breastfeeding." National strategies supported by the US Surgeon General's Call to Action, the Centers for Disease Control and Prevention, and The Joint Commission are involved to facilitate breastfeeding practices in US hospitals and communities. Pediatricians play a critical role in their practices and communities as advocates of breastfeeding and thus should be knowledgeable about the health risks of not breastfeeding, the economic benefits to society of breastfeeding, and the techniques for managing and supporting the breastfeeding dyad. The "Business Case for Breastfeeding" details how mothers can maintain lactation in the workplace and the benefits to employers who facilitate this practice. (2/12)

THE BUILT ENVIRONMENT: DESIGNING COMMUNITIES TO PROMOTE PHYSICAL ACTIVITY IN CHILDREN
Committee on Environmental Health
ABSTRACT. An estimated 32% of American children are overweight, and physical inactivity contributes to this high prevalence of overweight. This policy statement highlights how the built environment of a community affects children's opportunities for physical activity. Neighborhoods and communities can provide opportunities for recreational physical activity with parks and open spaces, and policies must support this capacity. Children can engage in physical activity as a part of their daily lives, such as on their travel to school. Factors such as school location have played a significant role in the decreased rates of walking to school, and changes in policy may help to increase the number of children who are able to walk to school. Environment modification that addresses risks associated with automobile traffic is likely to be conducive to more walking and biking among children. Actions that reduce parental perception and fear of crime may promote outdoor physical activity. Policies that promote more active lifestyles among children and adolescents will enable them to achieve the recommended 60 minutes of daily physical activity. By working with community partners, pediatricians can participate in establishing communities designed for activity and health. (5/09, reaffirmed 1/13)

CALCIUM AND VITAMIN D REQUIREMENTS OF ENTERALLY FED PRETERM INFANTS (CLINICAL REPORT)
Steven A. Abrams, MD, and Committee on Nutrition
ABSTRACT. Bone health is a critical concern in managing preterm infants. Key nutrients of importance are calcium, vitamin D, and phosphorus. Although human milk is critical for the health of preterm infants, it is low in these nutrients relative to the needs of the infants during growth. Strategies should be in place to fortify human milk for preterm infants with birth weight <1800 to 2000 g and to ensure adequate mineral intake during hospitalization and after hospital discharge. Biochemical monitoring of very low birth weight infants should be performed during their hospitalization. Vitamin D should be provided at 200 to 400 IU/day both during hospitalization and after discharge from the hospital. Infants with radiologic evidence of rickets should have efforts made to maximize calcium and phosphorus intake by using available commercial products and, if needed, direct supplementation with these minerals. (4/13)
See full text on page 461.

CARDIOVASCULAR HEALTH SUPERVISION FOR INDIVIDUALS AFFECTED BY DUCHENNE OR BECKER MUSCULAR DYSTROPHY (CLINICAL REPORT)
Section on Cardiology and Cardiac Surgery
ABSTRACT. Duchenne muscular dystrophy is the most common and severe form of the childhood muscular dystrophies. The disease is typically diagnosed between 3 and 7 years of age and follows a predictable clinical course marked by progressive skeletal muscle weakness with loss of ambulation by 12 years of age. Death occurs in early adulthood secondary to respiratory or cardiac failure. Becker muscular dystrophy is less common and has a milder clinical course but also results in respiratory and cardiac failure. The natural history of the cardiomyopathy in these diseases has not been well established. As a result, patients traditionally present for cardiac evaluation only after clinical symptoms become evident. The purpose of this policy statement is to provide recommendations for optimal cardiovascular evaluation to health care specialists caring for individuals in whom the diagnosis of Duchenne or Becker muscular dystrophy has been confirmed. (12/05, reaffirmed 1/09)

CARDIOVASCULAR MONITORING AND STIMULANT DRUGS FOR ATTENTION-DEFICIT/HYPERACTIVITY DISORDER
James M. Perrin, MD; Richard A. Friedman, MD; Timothy K. Knilans, MD; Black Box Working Group; and Section on Cardiology and Cardiac Surgery
ABSTRACT. A recent American Heart Association (AHA) statement recommended electrocardiograms (ECGs) routinely for children before they start medications to treat attention-deficit/hyperactivity disorder (ADHD). The AHA statement reflected the thoughtful work of a group committed to improving the health of children with heart disease. However, the recommendation to obtain

an ECG before starting medications for treating ADHD contradicts the carefully considered and evidence-based recommendations of the American Academy of Child and Adolescent Psychiatry and the American Academy of Pediatrics (AAP). These organizations have concluded that sudden cardiac death (SCD) in persons taking medications for ADHD is a very rare event, occurring at rates no higher than those in the general population of children and adolescents. Both of these groups also noted the lack of any evidence that the routine use of ECG screening before beginning medication for ADHD treatment would prevent sudden death. The AHA statement pointed out the importance of detecting silent but clinically important cardiac conditions in children and adolescents, which is a goal that the AAP shares. The primary purpose of the AHA statement is to prevent cases of SCD that may be related to stimulant medications. The recommendations of the AAP and the rationale for these recommendations are the subject of this statement. (8/08)

CARE OF ADOLESCENT PARENTS AND THEIR CHILDREN (CLINICAL REPORT)

Jorge L. Pinzon, MD; Veronnie F. Jones, MD; Committee on Adolescence; and Committee on Early Childhood
ABSTRACT. Teen pregnancy and parenting remain an important public health issue in the United States and the world, and many children live with their adolescent parents alone or as part of an extended family. A significant proportion of teen parents reside with their family of origin, significantly affecting the multigenerational family structure. Repeated births to teen parents are also common. This clinical report updates a previous policy statement on care of the adolescent parent and their children and addresses medical and psychosocial risks specific to this population. Challenges unique to teen parents and their children are reviewed, along with suggestions for the pediatrician on models for intervention and care. (11/12)

CARE OF THE ADOLESCENT SEXUAL ASSAULT VICTIM (CLINICAL REPORT)

Miriam Kaufman, MD, and Committee on Adolescence
ABSTRACT. Sexual assault is a broad-based term that encompasses a wide range of sexual victimizations including rape. Since the American Academy of Pediatrics published its last policy statement on sexual assault in 2001, additional information and data have emerged about sexual assault and rape in adolescents and the treatment and management of the adolescent who has been a victim of sexual assault. This report provides new information to update physicians and focuses on assessment and care of sexual assault victims in the adolescent population. (8/08)

CARE COORDINATION IN THE MEDICAL HOME: INTEGRATING HEALTH AND RELATED SYSTEMS OF CARE FOR CHILDREN WITH SPECIAL HEALTH CARE NEEDS

Council on Children With Disabilities
ABSTRACT. Care coordination is a process that facilitates the linkage of children and their families with appropriate services and resources in a coordinated effort to achieve good health. Care coordination for children with special health care needs often is complicated because there is no single point of entry into the multiple systems of care, and complex criteria frequently determine the availability of funding and services among public and private payers. Economic and sociocultural barriers to coordination of care exist and affect families and health care professionals. In their important role of providing a medical home for all children, primary care physicians have a vital role in the process of care coordination, in concert with the family. (11/05)

CAREGIVER-FABRICATED ILLNESS IN A CHILD: A MANIFESTATION OF CHILD MALTREATMENT (CLINICAL REPORT)

Emalee G. Flaherty, MD; Harriet L. MacMillan, MD; and Committee on Child Abuse and Neglect
ABSTRACT. Caregiver-fabricated illness in a child is a form of child maltreatment caused by a caregiver who falsifies and/or induces a child's illness, leading to unnecessary and potentially harmful medical investigations and/or treatment. This condition can result in significant morbidity and mortality. Although caregiver-fabricated illness in a child has been widely known as Munchausen syndrome by proxy, there is ongoing discussion about alternative names, including pediatric condition falsification, factitious disorder (illness) by proxy, child abuse in the medical setting, and medical child abuse. Because it is a relatively uncommon form of maltreatment, pediatricians need to have a high index of suspicion when faced with a persistent or recurrent illness that cannot be explained and that results in multiple medical procedures or when there are discrepancies between the history, physical examination, and health of a child. This report updates the previous clinical report "Beyond Munchausen Syndrome by Proxy: Identification and Treatment of Child Abuse in the Medical Setting." The authors discuss the need to agree on appropriate terminology, provide an update on published reports of new manifestations of fabricated medical conditions, and discuss approaches to assessment, diagnosis, and management, including how best to protect the child from further harm. (8/13)
See full text on page 471.

THE CHANGING CONCEPT OF SUDDEN INFANT DEATH SYNDROME: DIAGNOSTIC CODING SHIFTS, CONTROVERSIES REGARDING THE SLEEPING ENVIRONMENT, AND NEW VARIABLES TO CONSIDER IN REDUCING RISK

Task Force on Sudden Infant Death Syndrome
ABSTRACT. There has been a major decrease in the incidence of sudden infant death syndrome (SIDS) since the American Academy of Pediatrics (AAP) released its recommendation in 1992 that infants be placed down for sleep in a nonprone position. Although the SIDS rate continues to fall, some of the recent decrease of the last several years may be a result of coding shifts to other causes of unexpected infant deaths. Since the AAP published its last statement on SIDS in 2000, several issues have become relevant, including the significant risk of side sleeping position; the AAP no longer recognizes side sleeping as a reasonable alternative to fully supine sleeping. The AAP also stresses the need to avoid redundant soft bedding and soft objects in the infant's sleeping environment, the hazards of adults sleeping with an infant in the same bed, the SIDS risk reduction associated with having infants sleep

in the same room as adults and with using pacifiers at the time of sleep, the importance of educating secondary caregivers and neonatology practitioners on the importance of "back to sleep," and strategies to reduce the incidence of positional plagiocephaly associated with supine positioning. This statement reviews the evidence associated with these and other SIDS-related issues and proposes new recommendations for further reducing SIDS risk. (11/05, reaffirmed 5/08)

CHEERLEADING INJURIES: EPIDEMIOLOGY AND RECOMMENDATIONS FOR PREVENTION
Council on Sports Medicine and Fitness

ABSTRACT. Over the last 30 years, cheerleading has increased dramatically in popularity and has evolved from leading the crowd in cheers at sporting events into a competitive, year-round sport involving complex acrobatic stunts and tumbling. Consequently, cheerleading injuries have steadily increased over the years in both number and severity. Sprains and strains to the lower extremities are the most common injuries. Although the overall injury rate remains relatively low, cheerleading has accounted for approximately 66% of all catastrophic injuries in high school girl athletes over the past 25 years. Risk factors for injuries in cheerleading include higher BMI, previous injury, cheering on harder surfaces, performing stunts, and supervision by a coach with low level of training and experience. This policy statement describes the epidemiology of cheerleading injuries and provides recommendations for injury prevention. (10/12)

CHEMICAL-BIOLOGICAL TERRORISM AND ITS IMPACT ON CHILDREN
Committee on Environmental Health and Committee on Infectious Diseases

ABSTRACT. Children remain potential victims of chemical or biological terrorism. In recent years, children have even been specific targets of terrorist acts. Consequently, it is necessary to address the needs that children would face after a terrorist incident. A broad range of public health initiatives have occurred since September 11, 2001. Although the needs of children have been addressed in many of them, in many cases, these initiatives have been inadequate in ensuring the protection of children. In addition, public health and health care system preparedness for terrorism has been broadened to the so-called all-hazards approach, in which response plans for terrorism are blended with plans for a public health or health care system response to unintentional disasters (eg, natural events such as earthquakes or pandemic flu or manmade catastrophes such as a hazardous-materials spill). In response to new principles and programs that have appeared over the last 5 years, this policy statement provides an update of the 2000 policy statement. The roles of both the pediatrician and public health agencies continue to be emphasized; only a coordinated effort by pediatricians and public health can ensure that the needs of children, including emergency protocols in schools or child care centers, decontamination protocols, and mental health interventions, will be successful. (9/06, reaffirmed 1/11)

CHEMICAL-MANAGEMENT POLICY: PRIORITIZING CHILDREN'S HEALTH
Council on Environmental Health

ABSTRACT. The American Academy of Pediatrics recommends that chemical-management policy in the United States be revised to protect children and pregnant women and to better protect other populations. The Toxic Substance Control Act (TSCA) was passed in 1976. It is widely recognized to have been ineffective in protecting children, pregnant women, and the general population from hazardous chemicals in the marketplace. It does not take into account the special vulnerabilities of children in attempting to protect the population from chemical hazards. Its processes are so cumbersome that in its more than 30 years of existence, the TSCA has been used to regulate only 5 chemicals or chemical classes of the tens of thousands of chemicals that are in commerce. Under the TSCA, chemical companies have no responsibility to perform premarket testing or postmarket follow-up of the products that they produce; in fact, the TSCA contains disincentives for the companies to produce such data. Voluntary programs have been inadequate in resolving problems. Therefore, chemical-management policy needs to be rewritten in the United States. Manufacturers must be responsible for developing information about chemicals before marketing. The US Environmental Protection Agency must have the authority to demand additional safety data about a chemical and to limit or stop the marketing of a chemical when there is a high degree of suspicion that the chemical might be harmful to children, pregnant women, or other populations. (4/11)

CHILD ABUSE, CONFIDENTIALITY, AND THE HEALTH INSURANCE PORTABILITY AND ACCOUNTABILITY ACT
Committee on Child Abuse and Neglect

ABSTRACT. The federal Health Insurance Portability and Accountability Act (HIPAA) of 1996 has significantly affected clinical practice, particularly with regard to how patient information is shared. HIPAA addresses the security and privacy of patient health data, ensuring that information is released appropriately with patient or guardian consent and knowledge. However, when child abuse or neglect is suspected in a clinical setting, the physician may determine that release of information without consent is necessary to ensure the health and safety of the child. This policy statement provides an overview of HIPAA regulations with regard to the role of the pediatrician in releasing or reviewing patient health information when the patient is a child who is a suspected victim of abuse or neglect. This statement is based on the most current regulations provided by the US Department of Health and Human Services and is subject to future changes and clarifications as updates are provided. (12/09)

THE CHILD IN COURT: A SUBJECT REVIEW (CLINICAL REPORT)
Committee on Psychosocial Aspects of Child and Family Health

ABSTRACT. When children come to court as witnesses, or when their needs are decided in a courtroom, they face unique stressors from the legal proceeding and from the social predicament that resulted in court action. Effective pediatric support and intervention requires an understanding of the situations that bring children to court and the issues that will confront children and child advocates in different court settings. (11/99, reaffirmed 11/02)

CHILD FATALITY REVIEW

Cindy W. Christian, MD; Robert D. Sege, MD, PhD;
Committee on Child Abuse and Neglect; Committee on
Injury, Violence, and Poison Prevention; and Council on
Community Pediatrics

ABSTRACT. Injury remains the leading cause of pediatric mortality and requires public health approaches to reduce preventable deaths. Child fatality review teams, first established to review suspicious child deaths involving abuse or neglect, have expanded toward a public health model of prevention of child fatality through systematic review of child deaths from birth through adolescence. Approximately half of all states report reviewing child deaths from all causes, and the process of fatality review has identified effective local and state prevention strategies for reducing child deaths. This expanded approach can be a powerful tool in understanding the epidemiology and preventability of child death locally, regionally, and nationally; improving accuracy of vital statistics data; and identifying public health and legislative strategies for reducing preventable child fatalities. The American Academy of Pediatrics supports the development of federal and state legislation to enhance the child fatality review process and recommends that pediatricians become involved in local and state child death reviews. (8/10)

CHILD LIFE SERVICES

Committee on Hospital Care and Child Life Council

ABSTRACT. Child life programs have become standard in most large pediatric centers and even on some smaller pediatric inpatient units to address the psychosocial concerns that accompany hospitalization and other health care experiences. The child life specialist focuses on the strengths and sense of well-being of children while promoting their optimal development and minimizing the adverse effects of children's experiences in health care or other potentially stressful settings. Using play and psychological preparation as primary tools, child life interventions facilitate coping and adjustment at times and under circumstances that might prove overwhelming otherwise. Play and age-appropriate communication may be used to (1) promote optimal development, (2) present information, (3) plan and rehearse useful coping strategies for medical events or procedures, (4) work through feelings about past or impending experiences, and (5) establish therapeutic relationships with children and parents to support family involvement in each child's care, with continuity across the care continuum. The benefits of this collaborative work with the family and health care team are not limited to the health care setting; it may also optimize reintegration into schools and the community. (10/06, reaffirmed 2/12)

CHILD PASSENGER SAFETY

Committee on Injury, Violence,
and Poison Prevention

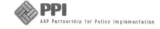

ABSTRACT. Child passenger safety has dramatically evolved over the past decade; however, motor vehicle crashes continue to be the leading cause of death of children 4 years and older. This policy statement provides 4 evidence-based recommendations for best practices in the choice of a child restraint system to optimize safety in passenger vehicles for children from birth through adolescence: (1) rear-facing car safety seats for most infants up to 2 years of age; (2) forward-facing car safety seats for most children through 4 years of age; (3) belt-positioning booster seats for most children through 8 years of age; and (4) lap-and-shoulder seat belts for all who have outgrown booster seats. In addition, a fifth evidence-based recommendation is for all children younger than 13 years to ride in the rear seats of vehicles. It is important to note that every transition is associated with some decrease in protection; therefore, parents should be encouraged to delay these transitions for as long as possible. These recommendations are presented in the form of an algorithm that is intended to facilitate implementation of the recommendations by pediatricians to their patients and families and should cover most situations that pediatricians will encounter in practice. The American Academy of Pediatrics urges all pediatricians to know and promote these recommendations as part of child passenger safety anticipatory guidance at every health-supervision visit. (3/11)

CHILD PASSENGER SAFETY (TECHNICAL REPORT)

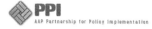

Dennis R. Durbin, MD, MSCE,
and Committee on Injury, Violence, and Poison Prevention

ABSTRACT. Despite significant reductions in the number of children killed in motor vehicle crashes over the past decade, crashes continue to be the leading cause of death for children 4 years and older. Therefore, the American Academy of Pediatrics continues to recommend inclusion of child passenger safety anticipatory guidance at every health-supervision visit. This technical report provides a summary of the evidence in support of 5 recommendations for best practices to optimize safety in passenger vehicles for children from birth through adolescence that all pediatricians should know and promote in their routine practice. These recommendations are presented in the revised policy statement on child passenger safety in the form of an algorithm that is intended to facilitate their implementation by pediatricians with their patients and families. The algorithm is designed to cover the majority of situations that pediatricians will encounter in practice. In addition, a summary of evidence on a number of additional issues that affect the safety of children in motor vehicles, including the proper use and installation of child restraints, exposure to air bags, travel in pickup trucks, children left in or around vehicles, and the importance of restraint laws, is provided. Finally, this technical report provides pediatricians with a number of resources for additional information to use when providing anticipatory guidance to families. (3/11)

CHILDREN, ADOLESCENTS, AND ADVERTISING
Committee on Communications

ABSTRACT. Advertising is a pervasive influence on children and adolescents. Young people view more than 40 000 ads per year on television alone and increasingly are being exposed to advertising on the Internet, in magazines, and in schools. This exposure may contribute significantly to childhood and adolescent obesity, poor nutrition, and cigarette and alcohol use. Media education has been shown to be effective in mitigating some of the negative effects of advertising on children and adolescents. (12/06, reaffirmed 3/10)

CHILDREN, ADOLESCENTS, AND THE MEDIA
Council on Communications and Media

ABSTRACT. Media, from television to the "new media" (including cell phones, iPads, and social media), are a dominant force in children's lives. Although television is still the predominant medium for children and adolescents, new technologies are increasingly popular. The American Academy of Pediatrics continues to be concerned by evidence about the potential harmful effects of media messages and images; however, important positive and prosocial effects of media use should also be recognized. Pediatricians are encouraged to take a media history and ask 2 media questions at every well-child visit: How much recreational screen time does your child or teenager consume daily? Is there a television set or Internet-connected device in the child's bedroom? Parents are encouraged to establish a family home use plan for all media. Media influences on children and teenagers should be recognized by schools, policymakers, product advertisers, and entertainment producers. (10/13)

See full text on page 481.

CHILDREN, ADOLESCENTS, OBESITY, AND THE MEDIA
Council on Communications and Media

ABSTRACT. Obesity has become a worldwide public health problem. Considerable research has shown that the media contribute to the development of child and adolescent obesity, although the exact mechanism remains unclear. Screen time may displace more active pursuits, advertising of junk food and fast food increases children's requests for those particular foods and products, snacking increases while watching TV or movies, and late-night screen time may interfere with getting adequate amounts of sleep, which is a known risk factor for obesity. Sufficient evidence exists to warrant a ban on junk-food or fast-food advertising in children's TV programming. Pediatricians need to ask 2 questions about media use at every well-child or well-adolescent visit: (1) How much screen time is being spent per day? and (2) Is there a TV set or Internet connection in the child's bedroom? (7/11)

CHILDREN, ADOLESCENTS, SUBSTANCE ABUSE, AND THE MEDIA
Victor C. Strasburger, MD, and Council on Communications and Media

ABSTRACT. The causes of adolescent substance use are multifactorial, but the media can play a key role. Tobacco and alcohol represent the 2 most significant drug threats to adolescents. More than $25 billion per year is spent on advertising for tobacco, alcohol, and prescription drugs, and such advertising has been shown to be effective. Digital media are increasingly being used to advertise drugs. In addition, exposure to PG-13– and R-rated movies at an early age may be a major factor in the onset of adolescent tobacco and alcohol use. The American Academy of Pediatrics recommends a ban on all tobacco advertising in all media, limitations on alcohol advertising, avoiding exposure of young children to substance-related (tobacco, alcohol, prescription drugs, illegal drugs) content on television and in PG-13– and R-rated movies, incorporating the topic of advertising and media into all substance abuse–prevention programs, and implementing media education programs in the classroom. (9/10)

CHILDREN, ADOLESCENTS, AND TELEVISION
Committee on Public Education

ABSTRACT. This statement describes the possible negative health effects of television viewing on children and adolescents, such as violent or aggressive behavior, substance use, sexual activity, obesity, poor body image, and decreased school performance. In addition to the television ratings system and the v-chip (electronic device to block programming), media education is an effective approach to mitigating these potential problems. The American Academy of Pediatrics offers a list of recommendations on this issue for pediatricians and for parents, the federal government, and the entertainment industry. (2/01)

CHILDREN AS HEMATOPOIETIC STEM CELL DONORS
Committee on Bioethics

ABSTRACT. In the past half-century, hematopoietic stem cell transplantation has become standard treatment for a variety of diseases in children and adults, including selected hematologic malignancies, immunodeficiencies, hemoglobinopathies, bone marrow failure syndromes, and congenital metabolic disorders. There are 3 sources of allogeneic hematopoietic stem cells: bone marrow, peripheral blood, and umbilical cord blood; each has its own benefits and risks. Children often serve as hematopoietic stem cell donors, most commonly for their siblings. HLA-matched biological siblings are generally preferred as donors because of reduced risks of transplant-related complications as compared with unrelated donors. This statement includes a discussion of the ethical considerations regarding minors serving as stem cell donors, using the traditional benefit/burden calculation from the perspectives of both the donor and the recipient. The statement also includes an examination of the circumstances under which a minor may ethically participate as a hematopoietic stem cell donor, how the risks can be minimized, what the informed-consent process should entail, the role for a donor advocate (or some similar mechanism), and other ethical concerns. The American Academy of Pediatrics holds that minors can ethically serve as stem cell donors when specific criteria are fulfilled. (1/10)

CHILDREN IN PICKUP TRUCKS

Committee on Injury and Poison Prevention

ABSTRACT. Pickup trucks have become increasingly popular in the United States. A recent study found that in crashes involving fatalities, cargo area passengers were 3 times more likely to die than were occupants in the cab. Compared with restrained cab occupants, the risk of death for those in the cargo area was 8 times higher. Furthermore, the increased use of extended-cab pickup trucks and air bag-equipped front passenger compartments creates concerns about the safe transport of children. The most effective preventive strategies are the legislative prohibition of travel in the cargo area and requirements for age-appropriate restraint use and seat selection in the cab. Parents should select vehicles that are appropriate for the safe transportation needs of the family. Physicians have an important role in counseling families and advocating public policy measures to reduce the number of deaths and injuries to occupants of pickup trucks. (10/00, reaffirmed 5/04, 1/07)

CHRONIC ABDOMINAL PAIN IN CHILDREN (CLINICAL REPORT)

Subcommittee on Chronic Abdominal Pain (joint
   with North American Society for Pediatric
   Gastroenterology, Hepatology, and Nutrition)

ABSTRACT. Children and adolescents with chronic abdominal pain pose unique challenges to their caregivers. Affected children and their families experience distress and anxiety that can interfere with their ability to perform regular daily activities. Although chronic abdominal pain in children is usually attributable to a functional disorder rather than organic disease, numerous misconceptions, insufficient knowledge among health care professionals, and inadequate application of knowledge may contribute to a lack of effective management. This clinical report accompanies a technical report (see page e370 in this issue) on childhood chronic abdominal pain and provides guidance for the clinician in the evaluation and treatment of children with chronic abdominal pain. The recommendations are based on the evidence reviewed in the technical report and on consensus achieved among subcommittee members. (3/05)

CHRONIC ABDOMINAL PAIN IN CHILDREN (TECHNICAL REPORT)

Subcommittee on Chronic Abdominal Pain (joint
   with North American Society for Pediatric
   Gastroenterology, Hepatology, and Nutrition)

ABSTRACT. Chronic abdominal pain, defined as long-lasting intermittent or constant abdominal pain, is a common pediatric problem encountered by primary care physicians, medical subspecialists, and surgical specialists. Chronic abdominal pain in children is usually functional, that is, without objective evidence of an underlying organic disorder. The Subcommittee on Chronic Abdominal Pain of the American Academy of Pediatrics and the North American Society for Pediatric Gastroenterology, Hepatology, and Nutrition has prepared this report based on a comprehensive, systematic review and rating of the medical literature. This report accompanies a clinical report based on the literature review and expert opinion.

The subcommittee examined the diagnostic and therapeutic value of a medical and psychological history, diagnostic tests, and pharmacologic and behavioral therapy. The presence of alarm symptoms or signs (such as weight loss, gastrointestinal bleeding, persistent fever, chronic severe diarrhea, and significant vomiting) is associated with a higher prevalence of organic disease. There was insufficient evidence to state that the nature of the abdominal pain or the presence of associated symptoms (such as anorexia, nausea, headache, and joint pain) can discriminate between functional and organic disorders. Although children with chronic abdominal pain and their parents are more often anxious or depressed, the presence of anxiety, depression, behavior problems, or recent negative life events does not distinguish between functional and organic abdominal pain. Most children who are brought to the primary care physician's office for chronic abdominal pain are unlikely to require diagnostic testing. Pediatric studies of therapeutic interventions were examined and found to be limited or inconclusive. (3/05)

CIRCUMCISION POLICY STATEMENT

Task Force on Circumcision

ABSTRACT. Male circumcision is a common procedure, generally performed during the newborn period in the United States. In 2007, the American Academy of Pediatrics (AAP) formed a multidisciplinary task force of AAP members and other stakeholders to evaluate the recent evidence on male circumcision and update the Academy's 1999 recommendations in this area. Evaluation of current evidence indicates that the health benefits of newborn male circumcision outweigh the risks and that the procedure's benefits justify access to this procedure for families who choose it. Specific benefits identified included prevention of urinary tract infections, penile cancer, and transmission of some sexually transmitted infections, including HIV. The American College of Obstetricians and Gynecologists has endorsed this statement. (8/12)

CLASSIFYING RECOMMENDATIONS FOR CLINICAL PRACTICE GUIDELINES

*Steering Committee on Quality Improvement and
   Management*

ABSTRACT. Clinical practice guidelines are intended to improve the quality of clinical care by reducing inappropriate variations, producing optimal outcomes for patients, minimizing harm, and promoting cost-effective practices. This statement proposes an explicit classification of recommendations for clinical practice guidelines of the American Academy of Pediatrics (AAP) to promote communication among guideline developers, implementers, and other users of guideline knowledge, to improve consistency, and to facilitate user understanding. The statement describes 3 sequential activities in developing evidence-based clinical practice guidelines and related policies: 1) determination of the aggregate evidence quality in support of a proposed recommendation; 2) evaluation of the anticipated balance between benefits and harms when the recommendation is carried out; and

3) designation of recommendation strength. An individual policy can be reported as a "strong recommendation," "recommendation," "option," or "no recommendation." Use of this classification is intended to improve consistency and increase the transparency of the guideline-development process, facilitate understanding of AAP clinical practice guidelines, and enhance both the utility and credibility of AAP clinical practice guidelines. (9/04)

CLIMATIC HEAT STRESS AND EXERCISING CHILDREN AND ADOLESCENTS

Council on Sports Medicine and Fitness and Council on School Health

ABSTRACT. Results of new research indicate that, contrary to previous thinking, youth do not have less effective thermoregulatory ability, insufficient cardiovascular capacity, or lower physical exertion tolerance compared with adults during exercise in the heat when adequate hydration is maintained. Accordingly, besides poor hydration status, the primary determinants of reduced performance and exertional heat-illness risk in youth during sports and other physical activities in a hot environment include undue physical exertion, insufficient recovery between repeated exercise bouts or closely scheduled same-day training sessions or rounds of sports competition, and inappropriately wearing clothing, uniforms, and protective equipment that play a role in excessive heat retention. Because these known contributing risk factors are modifiable, exertional heat illness is usually preventable. With appropriate preparation, modifications, and monitoring, most healthy children and adolescents can safely participate in outdoor sports and other physical activities through a wide range of challenging warm to hot climatic conditions. (8/11)

CLINICAL GENETIC EVALUATION OF THE CHILD WITH MENTAL RETARDATION OR DEVELOPMENTAL DELAYS (CLINICAL REPORT)

John B. Moeschler, MD; Michael Shevell, MD; and Committee on Genetics

ABSTRACT. This clinical report describes the clinical genetic evaluation of the child with developmental delays or mental retardation. The purpose of this report is to describe the optimal clinical genetics diagnostic evaluation to assist pediatricians in providing a medical home for children with developmental delays or mental retardation and their families. The literature supports the benefit of expert clinical judgment by a consulting clinical geneticist in the diagnostic evaluation. However, it is recognized that local factors may preclude this particular option. No single approach to the diagnostic process is supported by the literature. This report addresses the diagnostic importance of clinical history, 3-generation family history, dysmorphologic examination, neurologic examination, chromosome analysis (≥650 bands), fragile X molecular genetic testing, fluorescence in situ hybridization studies for subtelomere chromosome rearrangements, molecular genetic testing for typical and atypical presentations of known syndromes, computed tomography and/or magnetic resonance brain imaging, and targeted studies for metabolic disorders. (6/06, reaffirmed 5/12)

CLOSTRIDIUM DIFFICILE INFECTION IN INFANTS AND CHILDREN

Committee on Infectious Diseases

ABSTRACT. Infections caused by *Clostridium difficile* in hospitalized children are increasing. The recent publication of clinical practice guidelines for *C difficile* infection in adults did not address issues that are specific to children. The purpose of this policy statement is to provide the pediatrician with updated information and recommendations about *C difficile* infections affecting pediatric patients. (12/12)

COCHLEAR IMPLANTS IN CHILDREN: SURGICAL SITE INFECTIONS AND PREVENTION AND TREATMENT OF ACUTE OTITIS MEDIA AND MENINGITIS

Lorry G. Rubin, MD; Blake Papsin, MD; Committee on Infectious Diseases; and Section on Otolaryngology–Head and Neck Surgery

ABSTRACT. The use of cochlear implants is increasingly common, particularly in children younger than 3 years. Bacterial meningitis, often with associated acute otitis media, is more common in children with cochlear implants than in groups of control children. Children with profound deafness who are candidates for cochlear implants should receive all age-appropriate doses of pneumococcal conjugate and *Haemophilus influenzae* type b conjugate vaccines and appropriate annual immunization against influenza. In addition, starting at 24 months of age, a single dose of 23-valent pneumococcal polysaccharide vaccine should be administered. Before implant surgery, primary care providers and cochlear implant teams should ensure that immunizations are up-to-date, preferably with completion of indicated vaccines at least 2 weeks before implant surgery. Imaging of the temporal bone/inner ear should be performed before cochlear implantation in all children with congenital deafness and all patients with profound hearing impairment and a history of bacterial meningitis to identify those with inner-ear malformations/cerebrospinal fluid fistulas or ossification of the cochlea. During the initial months after cochlear implantation, the risk of complications of acute otitis media may be higher than during subsequent time periods. Therefore, it is recommended that acute otitis media diagnosed during the first 2 months after implantation be initially treated with a parenteral antibiotic (eg, ceftriaxone or cefotaxime). Episodes occurring 2 months or longer after implantation can be treated with a trial of an oral antimicrobial agent (eg, amoxicillin or amoxicillin/clavulanate at a dose of approximately 90 mg/kg per day of amoxicillin component), provided the child does not appear toxic and the implant does not have a spacer/positioner, a wedge that rests in the cochlea next to the electrodes present in certain implant models available between 1999 and 2002. "Watchful waiting" without antimicrobial therapy is inappropriate for children with implants with acute otitis media. If feasible, tympanocentesis should be performed for acute otitis media, and the material should be sent for culture, but performance of this procedure should not result in an undue delay in initiating antimicrobial therapy. For patients with suspected meningitis, cerebrospinal fluid as well as middle-ear fluid, if present, should be sent for culture. Empiric antimicrobial therapy for meningitis occurring within 2 months of implantation should include an agent with broad activity against Gram-negative bacilli (eg, meropenem) plus vancomycin. For meningitis occurring 2 months or longer after implantation, standard empiric antimicrobial therapy for meningitis (eg, ceftriaxone plus vancomycin) is indicated. For patients with meningitis, urgent evaluation by an otolaryngologist is indicated for consideration of imaging and surgical exploration. (7/10)

COLLABORATIVE ROLE OF THE PEDIATRICIAN IN THE DIAGNOSIS AND MANAGEMENT OF BIPOLAR DISORDER IN ADOLESCENTS (CLINICAL REPORT)

Benjamin N. Shain, MD, PhD, and Committee on Adolescence
ABSTRACT. Despite the complexity of diagnosis and management, pediatricians have an important collaborative role in referring and partnering in the management of adolescents with bipolar disorder. This report presents the classification of bipolar disorder as well as interviewing and diagnostic guidelines. Treatment options are described, particularly focusing on medication management and rationale for the common practice of multiple, simultaneous medications. Medication adverse effects may be problematic and better managed with collaboration between mental health professionals and pediatricians. Case examples illustrate a number of common diagnostic and management issues. (11/12)

COMMUNICATING WITH CHILDREN AND FAMILIES: FROM EVERYDAY INTERACTIONS TO SKILL IN CONVEYING DISTRESSING INFORMATION (TECHNICAL REPORT)

Marcia Levetown, MD, and Committee on Bioethics
ABSTRACT. Health care communication is a skill that is critical to safe and effective medical practice; it can and must be taught. Communication skill influences patient disclosure, treatment adherence and outcome, adaptation to illness, and bereavement. This article provides a review of the evidence regarding clinical communication in the pediatric setting, covering the spectrum from outpatient primary care consultation to death notification, and provides practical suggestions to improve communication with patients and families, enabling more effective, efficient, and empathic pediatric health care. (5/08, reaffirmed 5/11)

COMMUNITY PEDIATRICS: NAVIGATING THE INTERSECTION OF MEDICINE, PUBLIC HEALTH, AND SOCIAL DETERMINANTS OF CHILDREN'S HEALTH

Council on Community Pediatrics
ABSTRACT. This policy statement provides a framework for the pediatrician's role in promoting the health and well-being of all children in the context of their families and communities. It offers pediatricians a definition of community pediatrics, emphasizes the importance of recognizing social determinants of health, and delineates the need to partner with public health to address population-based child health issues. It also recognizes the importance of pediatric involvement in child advocacy at local, state, and federal levels to ensure all children have access to a high-quality medical home and to eliminate child health disparities. This statement provides a set of specific recommendations that underscore the critical nature of this dimension of pediatric practice, teaching, and research. (2/13)
See full text on page 487.

COMPREHENSIVE HEALTH EVALUATION OF THE NEWLY ADOPTED CHILD (CLINICAL REPORT)

Veronnie F. Jones, MD, PhD, MSPH, and Committee on Early Childhood, Adoption, and Dependent Care
ABSTRACT. Children who join families through the process of adoption often have multiple health care needs. After placement in an adoptive home, it is essential that these children have a timely comprehensive health evaluation. This evaluation should include a review of all available medical records and a complete physical examination. Evaluation should also include diagnostic testing based on the findings from the history and physical examination as well as the risks presented by the child's previous living conditions. Age-appropriate screens should be performed, including, for example, newborn screening panels, hearing, vision, dental, and formal behavioral/developmental screens. The comprehensive assessment can occur at the time of the initial visit to the physician after adoptive placement or can take place over several visits. Adopted children should be referred to other medical specialists as deemed appropriate. The Section on Adoption and Foster Care is a resource within the American Academy of Pediatrics for physicians providing care for children who are being adopted. (12/11)

CONDOM USE BY ADOLESCENTS

Committee on Adolescence
ABSTRACT. Rates of sexual activity, pregnancies, and births among adolescents have continued to decline during the past decade to historic lows. Despite these positive trends, many adolescents remain at risk for unintended pregnancy and sexually transmitted infections (STIs). This policy statement has been developed to assist the pediatrician in understanding and supporting the use of condoms by their patients to prevent unintended pregnancies and STIs and address barriers to their use. When used consistently and correctly, male latex condoms reduce the risk of pregnancy and many STIs, including HIV. Since the last policy statement published 12 years ago, there is an increased evidence base supporting the protection provided by condoms against STIs. Rates of acquisition of STIs/HIV among adolescents remain unacceptably high. Interventions that increase availability or accessibility to condoms are most efficacious when combined with additional individual, small-group, or community-level activities that include messages about safer sex. Continued research is needed to inform public health interventions for adolescents that increase the consistent and correct use of condoms and promote dual protection of condoms for STI prevention with other effective methods of contraception. (10/13)
See full text on page 495.

CONFIDENTIALITY IN ADOLESCENT HEALTH CARE
Committee on Adolescence (4/89, reaffirmed 1/93, 11/97, 5/00, 5/04)

CONFLICTS BETWEEN RELIGIOUS OR SPIRITUAL BELIEFS AND PEDIATRIC CARE: INFORMED REFUSAL, EXEMPTIONS, AND PUBLIC FUNDING
Committee on Bioethics

ABSTRACT. Although respect for parents' decision-making authority is an important principle, pediatricians should report suspected cases of medical neglect, and the state should, at times, intervene to require medical treatment of children. Some parents' reasons for refusing medical treatment are based on their religious or spiritual beliefs. In cases in which treatment is likely to prevent death or serious disability or relieve severe pain, children's health and future autonomy should be protected. Because religious exemptions to child abuse and neglect laws do not equally protect all children and may harm some children by causing confusion about the duty to provide medical treatment, these exemptions should be repealed. Furthermore, public health care funds should not cover alternative unproven religious or spiritual healing practices. Such payments may inappropriately legitimize these practices as appropriate medical treatment. (10/13)

See full text on page 507.

CONGENITAL ADRENAL HYPERPLASIA (TECHNICAL REPORT)
Section on Endocrinology and Committee on Genetics

ABSTRACT. The Section on Endocrinology and the Committee on Genetics of the American Academy of Pediatrics, in collaboration with experts from the field of pediatric endocrinology and genetics, developed this policy statement as a means of providing up-to-date information for the practicing pediatrician about current practice and controversial issues in congenital adrenal hyperplasia (CAH), including the current status of prenatal diagnosis and treatment, the benefits and problem areas of neonatal screening programs, and the management of children with nonclassic CAH. The reference list is designed to allow physicians who wish more information to research the topic more thoroughly. (12/00, reaffirmed 10/04)

A CONSENSUS STATEMENT ON HEALTH CARE TRANSITIONS FOR YOUNG ADULTS WITH SPECIAL HEALTH CARE NEEDS
American Academy of Pediatrics, American Academy of Family Physicians, and American College of Physicians-American Society of Internal Medicine

ABSTRACT. This policy statement represents a consensus on the critical first steps that the medical profession needs to take to realize the vision of a family-centered, continuous, comprehensive, coordinated, compassionate, and culturally competent health care system that is as developmentally appropriate as it is technically sophisticated. The goal of transition in health care for young adults with special health care needs is to maximize lifelong functioning and potential through the provision of high-quality, developmentally appropriate health care services that continue uninterrupted as the individual moves from adolescence to adulthood. This consensus document has now been approved as policy by the boards of the American Academy of Pediatrics, the American Academy of Family Physicians, and the American College of Physicians-American Society of Internal Medicine. (12/02)

CONSENT FOR EMERGENCY MEDICAL SERVICES FOR CHILDREN AND ADOLESCENTS
Committee on Pediatric Emergency Medicine and Committee on Bioethics

ABSTRACT. Parental consent generally is required for the medical evaluation and treatment of minor children. However, children and adolescents might require evaluation of and treatment for emergency medical conditions in situations in which a parent or legal guardian is not available to provide consent or conditions under which an adolescent patient might possess the legal authority to provide consent. In general, a medical screening examination and any medical care necessary and likely to prevent imminent and significant harm to the pediatric patient with an emergency medical condition should not be withheld or delayed because of problems obtaining consent. The purpose of this policy statement is to provide guidance in those situations in which parental consent is not readily available, in which parental consent is not necessary, or in which parental refusal of consent places a child at risk of significant harm. (7/11)

CONSENT BY PROXY FOR NONURGENT PEDIATRIC CARE (CLINICAL REPORT)
Gary N. McAbee, DO, JD, and Committee on Medical Liability and Risk Management

ABSTRACT. Minor-aged patients are often brought to the pediatrician for nonurgent acute medical care, physical examinations, or health supervision visits by someone other than their legally authorized representative, which, in most situations, is a parent. These surrogates or proxies can be members of the child's extended family, such as a grandparent, adult sibling, or aunt/uncle; a noncustodial parent or stepparent in cases of divorce and remarriage; an adult who lives in the home but is not biologically or legally related to the child; or even a child care professional (eg, au pair, nanny). This report identifies common situations in which pediatricians may encounter "consent by proxy" for nonurgent medical care for minors, including physical examinations, and explains the potential for liability exposure associated with these circumstances. The report suggests practical steps that balance the need to minimize the physician's liability exposure with the patient's access to health care. Key issues to be considered when creating or updating office policies for obtaining and documenting consent by proxy are offered. (10/10)

CONSUMPTION OF RAW OR UNPASTEURIZED MILK AND MILK PRODUCTS BY PREGNANT WOMEN AND CHILDREN
Committee on Infectious Diseases and Committee on Nutrition

ABSTRACT. Sales of raw or unpasteurized milk and milk products are still legal in at least 30 states in the United States. Raw milk and milk products from cows, goats, and sheep continue to be a source of bacterial infections attributable to a number of virulent pathogens, including *Listeria monocytogenes, Campylobacter jejuni, Salmonella* species, *Brucella* species, and *Escherichia coli* O157. These infections can occur in both healthy and immunocompromised individuals, including older adults, infants, young children, and pregnant women and their unborn fetuses, in whom life-threatening infections and fetal miscarriage can occur. Efforts to limit the sale of raw milk products have met with opposition from those who are proponents of the purported health benefits of consuming raw milk products, which contain natural or unprocessed factors not inactivated by pasteurization. However, the benefits of these natural factors have not been clearly demonstrated in evidence-based studies and, therefore, do not outweigh the risks of raw milk consumption. Substantial data suggest that pasteurized milk confers equivalent health benefits compared with raw milk, without the additional risk of bacterial infections. The purpose of this policy statement was to review the risks of raw milk consumption in the United States and to provide evidence of the risks of infectious complications associated with consumption of unpasteurized milk and milk products, especially among pregnant women, infants, and children. (12/13)

See full text on page 513.

CONTRACEPTION AND ADOLESCENTS
Committee on Adolescence
ABSTRACT. Although adolescent pregnancy rates in the United States have decreased significantly over the past decade, births to adolescents remain both an individual and public health issue. As advocates for the health and well-being of all young people, the American Academy of Pediatrics strongly supports the recommendation that adolescents postpone consensual sexual activity until they are fully ready for the emotional, physical, and financial consequences of sex. The academy recognizes, however, that some young people will choose not to postpone sexual activity, and as health care providers, the responsibility of pediatricians includes helping teens reduce risks and negative health consequences associated with adolescent sexual behaviors, including unintended pregnancies and sexually transmitted infections. This policy statement provides the pediatrician with updated information on contraception methods and guidelines for counseling adolescents. (11/07)

CONTROVERSIES CONCERNING VITAMIN K AND THE NEWBORN
Committee on Fetus and Newborn
ABSTRACT. Prevention of early vitamin K deficiency bleeding (VKDB) of the newborn, with onset at birth to 2 weeks of age (formerly known as classic hemorrhagic disease of the newborn), by oral or parenteral administration of vitamin K is accepted practice. In contrast, late VKDB, with onset from 2 to 12 weeks of age, is most effectively prevented by parenteral administration of vitamin K. Earlier concern regarding a possible causal association between parenteral vitamin K and childhood cancer has not been substantiated. This revised statement presents updated recommendations for the use of vitamin K in the prevention of early and late VKDB. (7/03, reaffirmed 5/06, 5/09)

COPARENT OR SECOND-PARENT ADOPTION BY SAME-SEX PARENTS
Committee on Psychosocial Aspects of Child and Family Health
ABSTRACT. Children who are born to or adopted by 1 member of a same-sex couple deserve the security of 2 legally recognized parents. Therefore, the American Academy of Pediatrics supports legislative and legal efforts to provide the possibility of adoption of the child by the second parent or coparent in these families. (2/02, reaffirmed 5/09)

COPARENT OR SECOND-PARENT ADOPTION BY SAME-SEX PARENTS (TECHNICAL REPORT)
Committee on Psychosocial Aspects of Child and Family Health
ABSTRACT. A growing body of scientific literature demonstrates that children who grow up with 1 or 2 gay and/or lesbian parents fare as well in emotional, cognitive, social, and sexual functioning as do children whose parents are heterosexual. Children's optimal development seems to be influenced more by the nature of the relationships and interactions within the family unit than by the particular structural form it takes. (2/02, reaffirmed 5/09)

CORPORAL PUNISHMENT IN SCHOOLS
Committee on School Health
ABSTRACT. The American Academy of Pediatrics recommends that corporal punishment in schools be abolished in all states by law and that alternative forms of student behavior management be used. (8/00, reaffirmed 6/03, 5/06, 2/12)

COUNSELING THE ADOLESCENT ABOUT PREGNANCY OPTIONS
Committee on Adolescence
ABSTRACT. When consulted by a pregnant adolescent, pediatricians should be able to make a timely diagnosis and to help the adolescent understand her options and act on her decision to continue or terminate her pregnancy. Pediatricians may not impose their values on the decision-making process and should be prepared to support the adolescent in her decision or refer her to a physician who can. (5/98, reaffirmed 1/01, 1/06)

COUNSELING FAMILIES WHO CHOOSE COMPLEMENTARY AND ALTERNATIVE MEDICINE FOR THEIR CHILD WITH CHRONIC ILLNESS OR DISABILITY
Committee on Children With Disabilities
ABSTRACT. The use of complementary and alternative medicine (CAM) to treat chronic illness or disability is increasing in the United States. This is especially evident among children with autism and related disorders. It may be challenging to the practicing pediatrician to distinguish among accepted biomedical treatments, unproven therapies, and alternative therapies. Moreover, there are no published guidelines regarding the use of CAM in the care of children with chronic illness or disability. To best serve the interests of children, it is important to maintain a scientific perspective, to provide balanced advice about therapeutic options, to guard against bias, and to establish and maintain a trusting relationship with families. This

statement provides information and guidance for pediatricians when counseling families about CAM. (3/01, reaffirmed 1/05, 5/10)

CREATING HEALTHY CAMP EXPERIENCES
Council on School Health
ABSTRACT. The American Academy of Pediatrics has created recommendations for health appraisal and preparation of young people before participation in day or resident camps and to guide health and safety practices for children at camp. These recommendations are intended for parents, primary health care providers, and camp administration and health center staff. Although camps have diverse environments, there are general guidelines that apply to all situations and specific recommendations that are appropriate under special conditions. This policy statement has been reviewed and is supported by the American Camp Association. (3/11)

THE CRUCIAL ROLE OF RECESS IN SCHOOL
Council on School Health
ABSTRACT. Recess is at the heart of a vigorous debate over the role of schools in promoting the optimal development of the whole child. A growing trend toward reallocating time in school to accentuate the more academic subjects has put this important facet of a child's school day at risk. Recess serves as a necessary break from the rigors of concentrated, academic challenges in the classroom. But equally important is the fact that safe and well-supervised recess offers cognitive, social, emotional, and physical benefits that may not be fully appreciated when a decision is made to diminish it. Recess is unique from, and a complement to, physical education—not a substitute for it. The American Academy of Pediatrics believes that recess is a crucial and necessary component of a child's development and, as such, it should not be withheld for punitive or academic reasons. (12/12)

DEALING WITH THE PARENT WHOSE JUDGMENT IS IMPAIRED BY ALCOHOL OR DRUGS: LEGAL AND ETHICAL CONSIDERATIONS (CLINICAL REPORT)
Committee on Medical Liability
ABSTRACT. An estimated 11 to 17.5 million children are being raised by a substance-abusing parent or guardian. The importance of this statistic is undeniable, particularly when a patient is brought to a pediatric office by a parent or guardian exhibiting symptoms of judgment impairment. Although the physician-patient relationship exists between the pediatrician and the minor patient, other obligations (some perceived and some real) should be considered as well. In managing encounters with impaired parents who may become disruptive or dangerous, pediatricians should be aware of their responsibilities before acting. In addition to fulfilling the duty involved with an established physician-patient relationship, the pediatrician should take reasonable care to safeguard patient confidentiality; protect the safety of the patient and other patients, visitors, and employees; and comply with reporting mandates. This clinical report identifies and discusses the legal and ethical concepts related to these circumstances. The report offers implementation suggestions when establishing anticipatory office procedures and training programs for staff on what to do (and not do) in such situations to maximize the patient's well-being and safety and minimize the liability of the pediatrician. (9/04, reaffirmed 9/10)

DEATH OF A CHILD IN THE EMERGENCY DEPARTMENT (TECHNICAL REPORT)
Jane Knapp, MD; Deborah Mulligan-Smith, MD; and Committee on Pediatric Emergency Medicine
ABSTRACT. Of the estimated 40000 American children ≤14 years old who die each year, approximately 20% die or are pronounced dead in outpatient sites, primarily the emergency department (ED). The ED is distinguishable from other sites at which children die, because the death is often sudden, unexpected, and without a previously established physician-patient care relationship. Despite these difficult circumstances and potentially limited professional experience with the death of a child, the emergency physician must be prepared to respond to the emotional, cultural, procedural, and legal issues that are an inevitable part of caring for ill and injured children who die. All of this must be accomplished while supporting a grieving family. There is also a responsibility to inform the child's pediatrician of the death, who in turn also must be prepared to counsel and support bereaved families. The American Academy of Pediatrics and American College of Emergency Physicians collaborated on the joint policy statement, "Death of a Child in the Emergency Department," agreeing on recommendations on the principles of care after the death of a child in the ED. This technical report provides the background information, consensus opinion, and evidence, where available, used to support the recommendations found in the policy statement. Important among these are the pediatrician's role as an advocate to advise in the formulation of ED policy and procedure that facilitate identification and management of medical examiners' cases, identification and reporting of child maltreatment, requests for postmortem examinations, and procurement of organ donations. (5/05, reaffirmed 8/13)

DEATH OF A CHILD IN THE EMERGENCY DEPARTMENT: JOINT STATEMENT OF THE AMERICAN ACADEMY OF PEDIATRICS AND THE AMERICAN COLLEGE OF EMERGENCY PHYSICIANS
Committee on Pediatric Emergency Medicine (joint with American College of Emergency Physicians) (10/02, reaffirmed 1/06, 1/09, 8/13)

DEVELOPMENTAL DYSPLASIA OF THE HIP PRACTICE GUIDELINE (TECHNICAL REPORT)
Harold P. Lehmann, MD, PhD; Richard Hinton, MD, MPH; Paola Morello, MD; Jeanne Santoli, MD; in conjunction with Committee on Quality Improvement and Subcommittee on Developmental Dysplasia of the Hip
ABSTRACT. *Objective.* To create a recommendation for pediatricians and other primary care providers about their role as screeners for detecting developmental dysplasia of the hip (DDH) in children.
Patients. Theoretical cohorts of newborns.

Method. Model-based approach using decision analysis as the foundation. Components of the approach include the following:

Perspective: Primary care provider.

Outcomes: DDH, avascular necrosis of the hip (AVN).

Options: Newborn screening by pediatric examination; orthopaedic examination; ultrasonographic examination; orthopaedic or ultrasonographic examination by risk factors. Intercurrent health supervision-based screening.

Preferences: 0 for bad outcomes, 1 for best outcomes.

Model: Influence diagram assessed by the Subcommittee and by the methodology team, with critical feedback from the Subcommittee.

Evidence Sources: Medline and EMBASE search of the research literature through June 1996. Hand search of sentinel journals from June 1996 through March 1997. Ancestor search of accepted articles.

Evidence Quality: Assessed on a custom subjective scale, based primarily on the fit of the evidence to the decision model.

Results. After discussion, explicit modeling, and critique, an influence diagram of 31 nodes was created. The computer-based and the hand literature searches found 534 articles, 101 of which were reviewed by 2 or more readers. Ancestor searches of these yielded a further 17 articles for evidence abstraction. Articles came from around the globe, although primarily Europe, British Isles, Scandinavia, and their descendants. There were 5 controlled trials, each with a sample size less than 40. The remainder were case series. Evidence was available for 17 of the desired 30 probabilities. Evidence quality ranged primarily between one third and two thirds of the maximum attainable score (median: 10–21; interquartile range: 8–14).Based on the raw evidence and Bayesian hierarchical meta-analyses, our estimate for the incidence of DDH revealed by physical examination performed by pediatricians is 8.6 per 1000; for orthopaedic screening, 11.5; for ultrasonography, 25. The odds ratio for DDH, given breech delivery, is 5.5; for female sex, 4.1; for positive family history, 1.7, although this last factor is not statistically significant. Postneonatal cases of DDH were divided into mid-term (younger than 6 months of age) and late-term (older than 6 months of age). Our estimates for the mid-term rate for screening by pediatricians is 0.34/1000 children screened; for orthopaedists, 0.1; and for ultrasonography, 0.28. Our estimates for late-term DDH rates are 0.21/1000 newborns screened by pediatricians; 0.08, by orthopaedists; and 0.2 for ultrasonography. The rates of AVN for children referred before 6 months of age is estimated at 2.5/1000 infants referred. For those referred after 6 months of age, our estimate is 109/1000 referred infants. The decision model (reduced, based on available evidence) suggests that orthopaedic screening is optimal, but because orthopaedists in the published studies and in practice would differ, the supply of orthopaedists is relatively limited, and the difference between orthopaedists and pediatricians is statistically insignificant, we conclude that pediatric screening is to be recommended. The place of ultrasonography in the screening process remains to be defined because there are too few data about postneonatal diagnosis by ultrasonographic screening to permit definitive recommendations. These data could be used by others to refine the conclusions based on costs, parental preferences, or physician style. Areas for research are well defined by our model-based approach. (4/00)

DIAGNOSIS OF HIV-1 INFECTION IN CHILDREN YOUNGER THAN 18 MONTHS IN THE UNITED STATES (TECHNICAL REPORT)

Jennifer S. Read, MD, MS, MPH, DTM&H, and Committee on Pediatric AIDS

ABSTRACT. The objectives of this technical report are to describe methods of diagnosis of HIV-1 infection in children younger than 18 months in the United States and to review important issues that must be considered by clinicians who care for infants and young children born to HIV-1–infected women. Appropriate HIV-1 diagnostic testing for infants and children younger than 18 months differs from that for older children, adolescents, and adults because of passively transferred maternal HIV-1 antibodies, which may be detectable in the child's bloodstream until 18 months of age. Therefore, routine serologic testing of these infants and young children is generally only informative before the age of 18 months if the test result is negative. Virologic assays, including HIV-1 DNA or RNA assays, represent the gold standard for diagnostic testing of infants and children younger than 18 months. With such testing, the diagnosis of HIV-1 infection (as well as the presumptive exclusion of HIV-1 infection) can be established within the first several weeks of life among nonbreastfed infants. Important factors that must be considered when selecting HIV-1 diagnostic assays for pediatric patients and when choosing the timing of such assays include the age of the child, potential timing of infection of the child, whether the infection status of the child's mother is known or unknown, the antiretroviral exposure history of the mother and of the child, and characteristics of the virus. If the mother's HIV-1 serostatus is unknown, rapid HIV-1 antibody testing of the newborn infant to identify HIV-1 exposure is essential so that antiretroviral prophylaxis can be initiated within the first 12 hours of life if test results are positive. For HIV-1–exposed infants (identified by positive maternal test results or positive antibody results for the infant shortly after birth), it has been recommended that diagnostic testing with HIV-1 DNA or RNA assays be performed within the first 14 days of life, at 1 to 2 months of age, and at 3 to 6 months of age. If any of these test results are positive, repeat testing is recommended to confirm the diagnosis of HIV-1 infection. A diagnosis of HIV-1 infection can be made on the basis of 2 positive HIV-1 DNA or RNA assay results. In nonbreastfeeding children younger than 18 months with no positive HIV-1 virologic test results, presumptive exclusion of HIV-1 infection can be based on 2 negative virologic test results (1 obtained at ≥2 weeks and 1 obtained at ≥4 weeks of age); 1 negative virologic test result obtained at ≥8 weeks of age; or 1 negative HIV-1 antibody test result obtained at ≥6 months of age. Alternatively, presumptive exclusion of HIV-1 infection can be based on 1 positive HIV-1 virologic test with at least 2 subsequent negative virologic test results (at least 1 of which is performed at ≥8 weeks of age) or negative HIV-1 antibody test results (at least 1 of which is performed at ≥6 months of age). Definitive exclusion of HIV-1 infection is based on 2 negative virologic test results, 1 obtained at ≥1 month of age and 1 obtained at ≥4 months of age, or 2 negative HIV-1 antibody test results from separate specimens obtained at ≥6 months of age. For both presumptive and definitive exclusion of infection, the child should have no other laboratory (eg, no positive virologic test results) or clinical (eg, no AIDS-defining conditions) evidence of HIV-1 infection. Many clinicians confirm the absence of HIV-1 infection with a negative HIV-1 antibody assay result at 12 to 18 months of age. For breastfeeding infants, a similar testing algorithm can be followed, with timing of testing starting from the date of complete cessation of breastfeeding instead of the date of birth. (12/07, reaffirmed 4/10)

DIAGNOSIS AND MANAGEMENT OF CHILDHOOD OBSTRUCTIVE SLEEP APNEA SYNDROME (TECHNICAL REPORT)

Carole L. Marcus, MBBCh; Lee J. Brooks, MD; Sally Davidson Ward, MD; Kari A. Draper, MD; David Gozal, MD; Ann C. Halbower, MD; Jacqueline Jones, MD; Christopher Lehmann, MD; Michael S. Schechter, MD, MPH; Stephen Sheldon, MD; Richard N. Shiffman, MD, MCIS; and Karen Spruyt, PhD

ABSTRACT. *Objective.* This technical report describes the procedures involved in developing recommendations on the management of childhood obstructive sleep apnea syndrome (OSAS).

Methods. The literature from 1999 through 2011 was evaluated.

Results and Conclusions. A total of 3166 titles were reviewed, of which 350 provided relevant data. Most articles were level II through IV. The prevalence of OSAS ranged from 0% to 5.7%, with obesity being an independent risk factor. OSAS was associated with cardiovascular, growth, and neurobehavioral abnormalities and possibly inflammation. Most diagnostic screening tests had low sensitivity and specificity. Treatment of OSAS resulted in improvements in behavior and attention and likely improvement in cognitive abilities. Primary treatment is adenotonsillectomy (AT). Data were insufficient to recommend specific surgical techniques; however, children undergoing partial tonsillectomy should be monitored for possible recurrence of OSAS. Although OSAS improved postoperatively, the proportion of patients who had residual OSAS ranged from 13% to 29% in low-risk populations to 73% when obese children were included and stricter polysomnographic criteria were used. Nevertheless, OSAS may improve after AT even in obese children, thus supporting surgery as a reasonable initial treatment. A significant number of obese patients required intubation or continuous positive airway pressure (CPAP) postoperatively, which reinforces the need for inpatient observation. CPAP was effective in the treatment of OSAS, but adherence is a major barrier. For this reason, CPAP is not recommended as first-line therapy for OSAS when AT is an option. Intranasal steroids may ameliorate mild OSAS, but follow-up is needed. Data were insufficient to recommend rapid maxillary expansion. (8/12)

DIAGNOSIS AND MANAGEMEN OF AN INITIAL UTI IN FEBRILE INFANTS AND YOUNG CHILDREN (TECHNICAL REPORT)

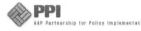

S. Maria E. Finnell, MD, MS; Aaron E. Carroll, MD, MS; Stephen M. Downs, MD, MS; and Subcommittee on Urinary Tract Infection

ABSTRACT. *Objectives.* The diagnosis and management of urinary tract infections (UTIs) in young children are clinically challenging. This report was developed to inform the revised, evidence-based, clinical guideline regarding the diagnosis and management of initial UTIs in febrile infants and young children, 2 to 24 months of age, from the American Academy of Pediatrics Subcommittee on Urinary Tract Infection.

Methods. The conceptual model presented in the 1999 technical report was updated after a comprehensive review of published literature. Studies with potentially new information or with evidence that reinforced the 1999 technical report were retained. Meta-analyses on the effectiveness of antimicrobial prophylaxis to prevent recurrent UTI were performed.

Results. Review of recent literature revealed new evidence in the following areas. Certain clinical findings and new urinalysis methods can help clinicians identify febrile children at very low risk of UTI. Oral antimicrobial therapy is as effective as parenteral therapy in treating UTI. Data from published, randomized controlled trials do not support antimicrobial prophylaxis to prevent febrile UTI when vesicoureteral reflux is found through voiding cystourethrography. Ultrasonography of the urinary tract after the first UTI has poor sensitivity. Early antimicrobial treatment may decrease the risk of renal damage from UTI.

Conclusions. Recent literature agrees with most of the evidence presented in the 1999 technical report, but meta-analyses of data from recent, randomized controlled trials do not support antimicrobial prophylaxis to prevent febrile UTI. This finding argues against voiding cystourethrography after the first UTI. (8/11)

DIAGNOSIS AND PREVENTION OF IRON DEFICIENCY AND IRON-DEFICIENCY ANEMIA IN INFANTS AND YOUNG CHILDREN (0–3 YEARS OF AGE) (CLINICAL REPORT)

Robert D. Baker, MD, PhD; Frank R. Greer, MD; and Committee on Nutrition

ABSTRACT. This clinical report covers diagnosis and prevention of iron deficiency and iron-deficiency anemia in infants (both breastfed and formula fed) and toddlers from birth through 3 years of age. Results of recent basic research support the concerns that iron-deficiency anemia and iron deficiency without anemia during infancy and childhood can have long-lasting detrimental effects on neurodevelopment. Therefore, pediatricians and other health care providers should strive to eliminate iron deficiency and iron-deficiency anemia. Appropriate iron intakes for infants and toddlers as well as methods for screening for iron deficiency and iron-deficiency anemia are presented. (10/10)

DIAGNOSTIC IMAGING OF CHILD ABUSE
Section on Radiology

ABSTRACT. The role of imaging in cases of child abuse is to identify the extent of physical injury when abuse is present and to elucidate all imaging findings that point to alternative diagnoses. Effective diagnostic imaging of child abuse rests on high-quality technology as well as a full appreciation of the clinical and pathologic alterations occurring in abused children. This statement is a revision of the previous policy published in 2000. (4/09)

DISASTER PLANNING FOR SCHOOLS
Council on School Health

ABSTRACT. Community awareness of the school district's disaster plan will optimize a community's capacity to maintain the safety of its school-aged population in the event of a school-based or greater community crisis. This statement is intended to stimulate awareness of the disaster-preparedness process in schools as a part of a global, community-wide preparedness plan. Pediatricians, other health care professionals, first responders, public health officials, the media, school nurses, school staff, and parents all need to be unified in their efforts to support schools in the prevention of, preparedness for, response to, and recovery from a disaster. (10/08, reaffirmed 9/11)

DISCLOSURE OF ILLNESS STATUS TO CHILDREN AND ADOLESCENTS WITH HIV INFECTION
Committee on Pediatric AIDS

ABSTRACT. Many children with human immunodeficiency virus (HIV) infection and acquired immunodeficiency syndrome are surviving to middle childhood and adolescence. Studies suggest that children who know their HIV status have higher self-esteem than children who are unaware of their status. Parents who have disclosed the status to their children experience less depression than those who do not. This statement addresses our current knowledge and recommendations for disclosure of HIV infection status to children and adolescents. (1/99, reaffirmed 2/02, 5/05, 1/09, 1/12)

DISPENSING MEDICATIONS AT THE HOSPITAL UPON DISCHARGE FROM AN EMERGENCY DEPARTMENT (TECHNICAL REPORT)
Loren G. Yamamoto, MD, MPH, MBA; Shannon Manzi, PharmD; and Committee on Pediatric Emergency Medicine

ABSTRACT. Although most health care services can and should be provided by their medical home, children will be referred or require visits to the emergency department (ED) for emergent clinical conditions or injuries. Continuation of medical care after discharge from an ED is dependent on parents or caregivers' understanding of and compliance with follow-up instructions and on adherence to medication recommendations. ED visits often occur at times when the majority of pharmacies are not open and caregivers are concerned with getting their ill or injured child directly home. Approximately one-third of patients fail to obtain priority medications from a pharmacy after discharge from an ED. The option of judiciously dispensing ED discharge medications from the ED's outpatient pharmacy within the facility is a major convenience that overcomes this obstacle, improving the likelihood of medication adherence. Emergency care encounters should be routinely followed up with primary care provider medical homes to ensure complete and comprehensive care. (1/12)

DISTINGUISHING SUDDEN INFANT DEATH SYNDROME FROM CHILD ABUSE FATALITIES (CLINICAL REPORT)
Kent P. Hymel, MD, and Committee on Child Abuse and Neglect (joint with National Association of Medical Examiners)

ABSTRACT. Fatal child abuse has been mistaken for sudden infant death syndrome. When a healthy infant younger than 1 year dies suddenly and unexpectedly, the cause of death may be certified as sudden infant death syndrome. Sudden infant death syndrome is more common than infanticide. Parents of sudden infant death syndrome victims typically are anxious to provide unlimited information to professionals involved in death investigation or research. They also want and deserve to be approached in a nonaccusatory manner. This clinical report provides professionals with information and suggestions for procedures to help avoid stigmatizing families of sudden infant death syndrome victims while allowing accumulation of appropriate evidence in potential cases of infanticide. This clinical report addresses deficiencies and updates recommendations in the 2001 American Academy of Pediatrics policy statement of the same name. (7/06, reaffirmed 4/09, 3/13)

DO-NOT-RESUSCITATE ORDERS FOR PEDIATRIC PATIENTS WHO REQUIRE ANESTHESIA AND SURGERY (CLINICAL REPORT)
Section on Surgery, Section on Anesthesia and Pain Medicine, and Committee on Bioethics

ABSTRACT. This clinical report addresses the topic of preexisting do-not-resuscitate (DNR) orders for children undergoing anesthesia and surgery. Pertinent issues addressed include the rights of children, surrogate decision-making, the process of informed consent, and the roles of surgeons and anesthesiologists. The reevaluation process of DNR orders called "required reconsideration" can be incorporated into the process of informed consent for surgery and anesthesia. Care should be taken to distinguish between goal-directed and procedure-directed approaches to DNR orders. By giving parents or other surrogates and clinicians the option of deciding from among full resuscitation, limitations based on procedures, or limitations based on goals, the child's needs are individualized and better served. (12/04, reaffirmed 1/09, 10/12)

DRINKING WATER FROM PRIVATE WELLS AND RISKS TO CHILDREN
Committee on Environmental Health and Committee on Infectious Diseases

ABSTRACT. Drinking water for approximately one sixth of US households is obtained from private wells. These wells can become contaminated by pollutant chemicals or pathogenic organisms and cause illness. Although the US Environmental Protection Agency and all states offer guidance for construction, maintenance, and testing of private wells, there is little regulation. With few exceptions, well owners are responsible for their own wells. Children may also drink well water at child care or when traveling. Illness resulting from children's ingestion of contaminated water can be severe. This policy statement provides recommendations for inspection, testing, and remediation for wells providing drinking water for children. (5/09, reaffirmed 1/13)

DRINKING WATER FROM PRIVATE WELLS AND RISKS TO CHILDREN (TECHNICAL REPORT)

Walter J. Rogan, MD; Michael T. Brady, MD;
   Committee on Environmental Health; and Committee
   on Infectious Diseases

ABSTRACT. Drinking water for approximately one sixth of US households is obtained from private wells. These wells can become contaminated by pollutant chemicals or pathogenic organisms, leading to significant illness. Although the US Environmental Protection Agency and all states offer guidance for construction, maintenance, and testing of private wells, there is little regulation, and with few exceptions, well owners are responsible for their own wells. Children may also drink well water at child care or when traveling. Illness resulting from children's ingestion of contaminated water can be severe. This report reviews relevant aspects of groundwater and wells; describes the common chemical and microbiologic contaminants; gives an algorithm with recommendations for inspection, testing, and remediation for wells providing drinking water for children; reviews the definitions and uses of various bottled waters; provides current estimates of costs for well testing; and provides federal, national, state, and, where appropriate, tribal contacts for more information. (5/09, reaffirmed 1/13)

EARLY CHILDHOOD ADVERSITY, TOXIC STRESS, AND THE ROLE OF THE PEDIATRICIAN: TRANSLATING DEVELOPMENTAL SCIENCE INTO LIFELONG HEALTH

Committee on Psychosocial Aspects of Child and Family
   Health; Committee on Early Childhood, Adoption, and
   Dependent Care; and Section on Developmental and
   Behavioral Pediatrics

ABSTRACT. Advances in a wide range of biological, behavioral, and social sciences are expanding our understanding of how early environmental influences (the ecology) and genetic predispositions (the biologic program) affect learning capacities, adaptive behaviors, lifelong physical and mental health, and adult productivity. A supporting technical report from the American Academy of Pediatrics (AAP) presents an integrated ecobiodevelopmental framework to assist in translating these dramatic advances in developmental science into improved health across the life span. Pediatricians are now armed with new information about the adverse effects of toxic stress on brain development, as well as a deeper understanding of the early life origins of many adult diseases. As trusted authorities in child health and development, pediatric providers must now complement the early identification of developmental concerns with a greater focus on those interventions and community investments that reduce external threats to healthy brain growth. To this end, AAP endorses a developing leadership role for the entire pediatric community—one that mobilizes the scientific expertise of both basic and clinical researchers, the family-centered care of the pediatric medical home, and the public influence of AAP and its state chapters—to catalyze fundamental change in early childhood policy and services. AAP is committed to leveraging science to inform the development of innovative strategies to reduce the precipitants of toxic stress in young children and to mitigate their negative effects on the course of development and health across the life span. (12/11)

EARLY CHILDHOOD CARIES IN INDIGENOUS COMMUNITIES

Committee on Native American Child Health (joint with
   Canadian Paediatric Society First Nations, Inuit, and
   Métis Committee)

ABSTRACT. The oral health of Indigenous children of Canada (First Nations, Inuit, and Métis) and the United States (American Indian, Alaska Native) is a major child health issue: there is a high prevalence of early childhood caries (ECC) and resulting adverse health effects in this community, as well as high rates and costs of restorative and surgical treatments under general anesthesia. ECC is an infectious disease that is influenced by multiple factors, including socioeconomic determinants, and requires a combination of approaches for improvement. This statement includes recommendations for preventive oral health and clinical care for young infants and pregnant women by primary health care providers, community-based health-promotion initiatives, oral health workforce and access issues, and advocacy for community water fluoridation and fluoride-varnish program access. Further community-based research on the epidemiology, prevention, management, and microbiology of ECC in Indigenous communities would be beneficial. (5/11)

EARLY INTERVENTION, IDEA PART C SERVICES, AND THE MEDICAL HOME: COLLABORATION FOR BEST PRACTICE AND BEST OUTCOMES (CLINICAL REPORT)

Richard C. Adams, MD; Carl Tapia, MD; and Council on
   Children With Disabilities

ABSTRACT. The medical home and the Individuals With Disabilities Education Act Part C Early Intervention Program share many common purposes for infants and children ages 0 to 3 years, not the least of which is a family-centered focus. Professionals in pediatric medical home practices see substantial numbers of infants and toddlers with developmental delays and/or complex chronic conditions. Economic, health, and family-focused data each underscore the critical role of timely referral for relationship-based, individualized, accessible early intervention services and the need for collaborative partnerships in care. The medical home process and Individuals With Disabilities Education Act Part C policy both support nurturing relationships and family-centered care; both offer clear value in terms of economic and health outcomes. Best practice models for early intervention services incorporate learning in the natural environment and coaching models. Proactive medical homes provide strategies for effective developmental surveillance, family-centered resources, and tools to support high-risk groups, and comanagement of infants with special health care needs, including the monitoring of services provided and outcomes achieved. (9/13)

See full text on page 521.

ECHOCARDIOGRAPHY IN INFANTS AND CHILDREN
Section on Cardiology

ABSTRACT. It is the intent of this statement to inform pediatric providers on the appropriate use of echocardiography. Although on-site consultation may be impossible, methods should be established to ensure timely review of echocardiograms by a pediatric cardiologist. With advances in data transmission, echocardiography information can be exchanged, in some cases eliminating the need for a costly patient transfer. By cooperating through training, education, and referral, complete and cost-effective echocardiographic services can be provided to all children. (6/97, reaffirmed 3/03, 3/07)

EDUCATION OF CHILDREN WITH HUMAN IMMUNODEFICIENCY VIRUS INFECTION
Committee on Pediatric AIDS

ABSTRACT. Treatment for human immunodeficiency virus (HIV) infection has enabled more children and youths to attend school and participate in school activities. Children and youths with HIV infection should receive the same education as those with other chronic illnesses. They may require special services, including home instruction, to provide continuity of education. Confidentiality about HIV infection status should be maintained with parental consent required for disclosure. Youths also should assent or consent as is appropriate for disclosure of their diagnosis. (6/00, reaffirmed 3/03, 10/06, 4/10, 3/13)

EFFECTS OF EARLY NUTRITIONAL INTERVENTIONS ON THE DEVELOPMENT OF ATOPIC DISEASE IN INFANTS AND CHILDREN: THE ROLE OF MATERNAL DIETARY RESTRICTION, BREASTFEEDING, TIMING OF INTRODUCTION OF COMPLEMENTARY FOODS, AND HYDROLYZED FORMULAS (CLINICAL REPORT)
Frank R. Greer, MD; Scott H. Sicherer, MD; A. Wesley Burks, MD; Committee on Nutrition; and Section on Allergy and Immunology

ABSTRACT. This clinical report reviews the nutritional options during pregnancy, lactation, and the first year of life that may affect the development of atopic disease (atopic dermatitis, asthma, food allergy) in early life. It replaces an earlier policy statement from the American Academy of Pediatrics that addressed the use of hypoallergenic infant formulas and included provisional recommendations for dietary management for the prevention of atopic disease. The documented benefits of nutritional intervention that may prevent or delay the onset of atopic disease are largely limited to infants at high risk of developing allergy (ie, infants with at least 1 first-degree relative [parent or sibling] with allergic disease). Current evidence does not support a major role for maternal dietary restrictions during pregnancy or lactation. There is evidence that breastfeeding for at least 4 months, compared with feeding formula made with intact cow milk protein, prevents or delays the occurrence of atopic dermatitis, cow milk allergy, and wheezing in early childhood. In studies of infants at high risk of atopy and who are not exclusively breastfed for 4 to 6 months, there is modest evidence that the onset of atopic disease may be delayed or prevented by the use of hydrolyzed formulas compared with formula made with intact cow milk protein, particularly for atopic dermatitis. Comparative studies of the various hydrolyzed formulas also indicate that not all formulas have the same protective benefit. There is also little evidence that delaying the timing of the introduction of complementary foods beyond 4 to 6 months of age prevents the occurrence of atopic disease. At present, there are insufficient data to document a protective effect of any dietary intervention beyond 4 to 6 months of age for the development of atopic disease. (1/08)

ELECTRONIC PRESCRIBING IN PEDIATRICS: TOWARD SAFER AND MORE EFFECTIVE MEDICATION MANAGEMENT
Council on Clinical Information Technology

ABSTRACT. This policy statement identifies the potential value of electronic prescribing (e-prescribing) systems in improving quality and reducing harm in pediatric health care. On the basis of limited but positive pediatric data and on the basis of federal statutes that provide incentives for the use of e-prescribing systems, the American Academy of Pediatrics recommends the adoption of e-prescribing systems with pediatric functionality. The American Academy of Pediatrics also recommends a set of functions that technology vendors should provide when e-prescribing systems are used in environments in which children receive care. (3/13)
See full text on page 537.

ELECTRONIC PRESCRIBING IN PEDIATRICS: TOWARD SAFER AND MORE EFFECTIVE MEDICATION MANAGEMENT (TECHNICAL REPORT)
Kevin B. Johnson, MD, MS; Christoph U. Lehmann, MD; and Council on Clinical Information Technology

ABSRACT. This technical report discusses recent advances in electronic prescribing (e-prescribing) systems, including the evidence base supporting their limitations and potential benefits. Specifically, this report acknowledges that there are limited but positive pediatric data supporting the role of e-prescribing in mitigating medication errors, improving communication with dispensing pharmacists, and improving medication adherence. On the basis of these data and on the basis of federal statutes that provide incentives for the use of e-prescribing systems, the American Academy of Pediatrics recommends the adoption of e-prescribing systems with pediatric functionality. This report supports the accompanying policy statement from the American Academy of Pediatrics recommending the adoption of e-prescribing by pediatric health care providers. (3/13)
See full text on page 537.

ELECTRONIC PRESCRIBING SYSTEMS IN PEDIATRICS: THE RATIONALE AND FUNCTIONALITY REQUIREMENTS
Council on Clinical Information Technology

ABSTRACT. The use of electronic prescribing applications in pediatric practice, as recommended by the federal government and other national health care improvement organizations, should be encouraged. Legislation and policies that foster adoption of electronic prescribing systems by pediatricians should recognize both specific pediatric requirements and general economic incentives required to speed the adoption of these systems. Continued research into improving the effectiveness of these systems, recognizing the unique challenges of providing care to the pediatric population, should be promoted. (6/07)

ELECTRONIC PRESCRIBING SYSTEMS IN PEDIATRICS: THE RATIONALE AND FUNCTIONALITY REQUIREMENTS (TECHNICAL REPORT)

*Robert S. Gerstle, MD; Christoph U. Lehmann, MD; and
    Council on Clinical Information Technology*

ABSTRACT. This technical report discusses electronic prescribing systems and their limitations and potential benefits, particularly to the pediatrician in the ambulatory setting. In the report we acknowledge the benefits of integrating these systems with electronic health records and practice-management systems and recommend that the adoption of electronic prescribing systems be done in the context of ultimately moving toward an electronic health record. This technical report supports the accompanying American Academy of Pediatrics policy-statement recommendations on the adoption of electronic prescribing systems by pediatricians. (6/07)

E-MAIL COMMUNICATION BETWEEN PEDIATRICIANS AND THEIR PATIENTS (CLINICAL REPORT)

Steering Committee on Clinical Information Technology

ABSTRACT. This report addresses specific e-mail patient communication issues relevant to pediatricians and their appropriate use of e-mail in the office setting. The report briefly reviews: 1) e-mail privacy and security concerns; 2) e-mail in the office environment; 3) the legal status of e-mail; and 4) available e-mail technologic solutions. (7/04, reaffirmed 2/08)

EMERGENCY CONTRACEPTION

Committee on Adolescence

ABSTRACT. Despite significant declines over the past 2 decades, the United States continues to have teen birth rates that are significantly higher than other industrialized nations. Use of emergency contraception can reduce the risk of pregnancy if used up to 120 hours after unprotected intercourse or contraceptive failure and is most effective if used in the first 24 hours. Indications for the use of emergency contraception include sexual assault, unprotected intercourse, condom breakage or slippage, and missed or late doses of hormonal contraceptives, including the oral contraceptive pill, contraceptive patch, contraceptive ring (ie, improper placement or loss/expulsion), and injectable contraception. Adolescents younger than 17 years must obtain a prescription from a physician to access emergency contraception in most states. In all states, both males and females 17 years or older can obtain emergency contraception without a prescription. Adolescents are more likely to use emergency contraception if it has been prescribed in advance of need. The aim of this updated policy statement is to (1) educate pediatricians and other physicians on available emergency contraceptive methods; (2) provide current data on safety, efficacy, and use of emergency contraception in teenagers; and (3) encourage routine counseling and advance emergency-contraception prescription as 1 part of a public health strategy to reduce teen pregnancy. This policy focuses on pharmacologic methods of emergency contraception used within 120 hours of unprotected or underprotected coitus for the pre-vention of unintended pregnancy. Emergency contraceptive medications include products labeled and dedicated for use as emergency contraception by the US Food and Drug Administration (levonorgestrel and ulipristal) and the "off-label" use of combination oral contraceptives. (11/12)

EMERGENCY INFORMATION FORMS AND EMERGENCY PREPAREDNESS FOR CHILDREN WITH SPECIAL HEALTH CARE NEEDS

*Committee on Pediatric Emergency Medicine and Council on
    Clinical Information Technology (joint with American
    College of Emergency Physicians Pediatric Emergency
    Medicine Committee)*

ABSTRACT. Children with chronic medical conditions rely on complex management plans for problems that cause them to be at increased risk for suboptimal outcomes in emergency situations. The emergency information form (EIF) is a medical summary that describes medical condition(s), medications, and special health care needs to inform health care providers of a child's special health conditions and needs so that optimal emergency medical care can be provided. This statement describes updates to EIFs, including computerization of the EIF, expanding the potential benefits of the EIF, quality-improvement programs using the EIF, the EIF as a central repository, and facilitating emergency preparedness in disaster management and drills by using the EIF. (3/10)

ENDORSEMENT OF HEALTH AND HUMAN SERVICES RECOMMENDATION FOR PULSE OXIMETRY SCREENING FOR CRITICAL CONGENITAL HEART DISEASE

*Section on Cardiology and Cardiac Surgery Executive
    Committee*

ABSTRACT. Incorporation of pulse oximetry to the assessment of the newborn infant can enhance detection of critical congenital heart disease (CCHD). Recently, the Secretary of Health and Human Services (HHS) recommended that screening for CCHD be added to the uniform screening panel. The American Academy of Pediatrics (AAP) has been a strong advocate of early detection of CCHD and fully supports the decision of the Secretary of HHS.

The AAP has published strategies for the implementation of pulse oximetry screening, which addressed critical issues such as necessary equipment, personnel, and training, and also provided specific recommendations for assessment of saturation by using pulse oximetry as well as appropriate management of a positive screening result. The AAP is committed to the safe and effective implementation of pulse oximetry screening and is working with other advocacy groups and governmental agencies to promote pulse oximetry and to support widespread surveillance for CCHD.

Going forward, AAP chapters will partner with state health departments to implement the new screening strategy for CCHD and will work to ensure that there is an adequate system for referral for echocardiographic/pediatric cardiac evaluation after a positive screening result. It is imperative that AAP members engage their respective policy makers in adopting and funding the recommendations made by the Secretary of HHS. (12/11)

ENHANCING PEDIATRIC WORKFORCE DIVERSITY AND PROVIDING CULTURALLY EFFECTIVE PEDIATRIC CARE: IMPLICATIONS FOR PRACTICE, EDUCATION, AND POLICY MAKING

Committee on Pediatric Workforce

ABSTRACT. This policy statement serves to combine and update 2 previously independent but overlapping statements from the American Academy of Pediatrics (AAP) on culturally effective health care (CEHC) and workforce diversity. The AAP has long recognized that with the ever-increasing diversity of the pediatric population in the United States, the health of all children depends on the ability of all pediatricians to practice culturally effective care. CEHC can be defined as the delivery of care within the context of appropriate physician knowledge, understanding, and appreciation of all cultural distinctions, leading to optimal health outcomes. The AAP believes that CEHC is a critical social value and that the knowledge and skills necessary for providing CEHC can be taught and acquired through focused curricula across the spectrum of lifelong learning.

This statement also addresses workforce diversity, health disparities, and affirmative action. The discussion of diversity is broadened to include not only race, ethnicity, and language but also cultural attributes such as gender, religious beliefs, sexual orientation, and disability, which may affect the quality of health care. The AAP believes that efforts must be supported through health policy and advocacy initiatives to promote the delivery of CEHC and to overcome educational, organizational, and other barriers to improving workforce diversity. (9/13)

See full text on page 553.

EPIDEMIOLOGY AND DIAGNOSIS OF HEALTH CARE–ASSOCIATED INFECTIONS IN THE NICU (TECHNICAL REPORT)

Committee on Fetus and Newborn and Committee on Infectious Diseases

ABSTRACT. Health care–associated infections in the NICU are a major clinical problem resulting in increased morbidity and mortality, prolonged length of hospital stays, and increased medical costs. Neonates are at high risk for health care–associated infections because of impaired host defense mechanisms, limited amounts of protective endogenous flora on skin and mucosal surfaces at time of birth, reduced barrier function of neonatal skin, the use of invasive procedures and devices, and frequent exposure to broad-spectrum antibiotics. This statement will review the epidemiology and diagnosis of health care–associated infections in newborn infants. (3/12)

EQUIPMENT FOR AMBULANCES

American College of Surgeons Committee on Trauma, American College of Emergency Physicians, National Association of EMS Physicians, Pediatric Equipment Guidelines Committee—Emergency Medical Services for Children (EMSC) Partnership for Children Stakeholder Group, and American Academy of Pediatrics

INTRODUCTION (EXCERPT). Almost 4 decades ago, the Committee on Trauma of the American College of Surgeons (ACS) developed a list of standardized equipment for ambulances. Beginning in 1988, the American College of Emergency Physicians (ACEP) published a similar list. The 2 organizations collaborated on a joint document published in 2000, and the National Association of EMS Physicians (NAEMSP) participated in the 2005 revision. The 2005 revision included resources needed on ambulances for appropriate homeland security. All 3 organizations adhere to the principle that emergency medical services (EMS) providers at all levels must have the appropriate equipment and supplies to optimize prehospital delivery of care. The document was written to serve as a standard for the equipment needs of emergency ambulance services in both the United States and Canada.

EMS providers care for patients of all ages, who have a wide variety of medical and traumatic conditions. With permission from the ACS Committee on Trauma, ACEP, and NAEMSP, the current revision includes updated pediatric recommendations developed by members of the federal Emergency Medical Services for Children (EMSC) Stakeholder Group. The EMSC Program has developed several performance measures for the program's state partnership grantees. One of the performance measures evaluates the availability of essential pediatric equipment and supplies for basic life support (BLS) and advanced life support (ALS) patient care units. This document will be used as the standard for this performance measure. The American Academy of Pediatrics (AAP) has also officially endorsed this list. (6/09)

ESSENTIAL CONTRACTUAL LANGUAGE FOR MEDICAL NECESSITY IN CHILDREN

Committee on Child Health Financing

ABSTRACT. The previous policy statement from the American Academy of Pediatrics, "Model Language for Medical Necessity in Children," was published in July 2005. Since that time, there have been new and emerging delivery and payment models. The relationship established between health care providers and health plans should promote arrangements that are beneficial to all who are affected by these contractual arrangements. Pediatricians play an important role in ensuring that the needs of children are addressed in these emerging systems. It is important to recognize that health care plans designed for adults may not meet the needs of children. Language in health care contracts should reflect the health care needs of children and families. Informed pediatricians can make a difference in the care of children and influence the role of primary care physicians in the new paradigms. This policy highlights many of the important elements pediatricians should assess as providers develop a role in emerging care models. (7/13)

See full text on page 567.

ETHICAL CONSIDERATIONS IN RESEARCH WITH SOCIALLY IDENTIFIABLE POPULATIONS

Committee on Native American Child Health and Committee on Community Health Services

ABSTRACT. Community-based research raises ethical issues not normally encountered in research conducted in academic settings. In particular, conventional risk-benefits assessments frequently fail to recognize harms that can occur in socially identifiable populations as a result of research participation. Furthermore, many such communities require more stringent measures of beneficence that must be applied directly to the participating communities. In this statement, the American Academy of Pediatrics sets forth recommendations for minimizing harms that may result from community-based research by emphasizing community involvement in the research process. (1/04, reaffirmed 10/07, 1/13)

ETHICAL CONTROVERSIES IN ORGAN DONATION AFTER CIRCULATORY DEATH

Committee on Bioethics

ABSTRACT. The persistent mismatch between the supply of and need for transplantable organs has led to efforts to increase the supply, including controlled donation after circulatory death (DCD). Controlled DCD involves organ recovery after the planned withdrawal of life-sustaining treatment and the declaration of death according to the cardiorespiratory criteria. Two central ethical issues in DCD are when organ recovery can begin and how to manage conflicts of interests. The "dead donor rule" should be maintained, and donors in cases of DCD should only be declared dead after the permanent cessation of circulatory function. Permanence is generally established by a 2- to 5-minute waiting period. Given ongoing controversy over whether the cessation must also be irreversible, physicians should not be required to participate in DCD. Because the preparation for organ recovery in DCD begins before the declaration of death, there are potential conflicts between the donor's and recipient's interests. These conflicts can be managed in a variety of ways, including informed consent and separating the various participants' roles. For example, informed consent should be sought for premortem interventions to improve organ viability, and organ procurement organization personnel and members of the transplant team should not be involved in the discontinuation of life-sustaining treatment or the declaration of death. It is also important to emphasize that potential donors in cases of DCD should receive integrated interdisciplinary palliative care, including sedation and analgesia. (4/13)

See full text on page 573.

ETHICAL ISSUES WITH GENETIC TESTING IN PEDIATRICS

Committee on Bioethics

ABSTRACT. Advances in genetic research promise great strides in the diagnosis and treatment of many childhood diseases. However, emerging genetic technology often enables testing and screening before the development of definitive treatment or preventive measures. In these circumstances, careful consideration must be given to testing and screening of children to ensure that use of this technology promotes the best interest of the child. This statement reviews considerations for the use of genetic technology for newborn screening, carrier testing, and testing for susceptibility to late-onset conditions. Recommendations are made promoting informed participation by parents for newborn screening and limited use of carrier testing and testing for late-onset conditions in the pediatric population. Additional research and education in this developing area of medicine are encouraged. (6/01, reaffirmed 1/05, 1/09)

ETHICAL AND POLICY ISSUES IN GENETIC TESTING AND SCREENING OF CHILDREN

Committee on Bioethics and Committee on Genetics (joint with American College of Medical Genetics and Genomics)

ABSTRACT. The genetic testing and genetic screening of children are commonplace. Decisions about whether to offer genetic testing and screening should be driven by the best interest of the child. The growing literature on the psychosocial and clinical effects of such testing and screening can help inform best practices. This policy statement represents recommendations developed collaboratively by the American Academy of Pediatrics and the American College of Medical Genetics and Genomics with respect to many of the scenarios in which genetic testing and screening can occur. (2/13)

See full text on page 581.

ETHICS AND THE CARE OF CRITICALLY ILL INFANTS AND CHILDREN

Committee on Bioethics

ABSTRACT. The ability to provide life support to ill children who, not long ago, would have died despite medicine's best efforts challenges pediatricians and families to address profound moral questions. Our society has been divided about extending the life of some patients, especially newborns and older infants with severe disabilities. The American Academy of Pediatrics (AAP) supports individualized decision making about life-sustaining medical treatment for all children, regardless of age. These decisions should be jointly made by physicians and parents, unless good reasons require invoking established child protective services to contravene parental authority. At this time, resource allocation (rationing) decisions about which children should receive intensive care resources should be made clear and explicit in public policy, rather than be made at the bedside. (7/96, reaffirmed 10/99, 6/03)

EVALUATING INFANTS AND YOUNG CHILDREN WITH MULTIPLE FRACTURES (CLINICAL REPORT)

Carole Jenny, MD, MBA, FAAP, for Committee on Child Abuse and Neglect

ABSTRACT. Infants and toddlers with multiple unexplained fractures are often victims of inflicted injury. However, several medical conditions can also cause multiple fractures in children in this age group. In this report, the differential diagnosis of multiple fractures is presented, and diagnostic testing available to the clinician is discussed. The hypothetical entity "temporary brittle-bone disease" is examined also. Although frequently offered in court cases as a cause of multiple infant fractures, there is no evidence that this condition actually exists. (9/06)

EVALUATING FOR SUSPECTED CHILD ABUSE: CONDITIONS THAT PREDISPOSE TO BLEEDING (TECHNICAL REPORT)

Shannon L. Carpenter, MD, MS; Thomas C. Abshire, MD;
James D. Anderst, MD, MS; Section on Hematology/
Oncology; and Committee on Child Abuse and Neglect

ABSTRACT. Child abuse might be suspected when children present with cutaneous bruising, intracranial hemorrhage, or other manifestations of bleeding. In these cases, it is necessary to consider medical conditions that predispose to easy bleeding/bruising. When evaluating for the possibility of bleeding disorders and other conditions that predispose to hemorrhage, the pediatrician must consider the child's presenting history, medical history, and physical examination findings before initiating a laboratory investigation. Many medical conditions can predispose to easy bleeding. Before ordering laboratory tests for a disease, it is useful to understand the biochemical basis and clinical presentation of the disorder, condition prevalence, and test characteristics. This technical report reviews the major medical conditions that predispose to bruising/bleeding and should be considered when evaluating for abusive injury. (3/13)
See full text on page 587.

EVALUATION FOR BLEEDING DISORDERS IN SUSPECTED CHILD ABUSE (CLINICAL REPORT)

James D. Anderst, MD, MS; Shannon L. Carpenter, MD, MS;
Thomas C. Abshire, MD; Section on Hematology/Oncology;
and Committee on Child Abuse and Neglect

ABSTRACT. Bruising or bleeding in a child can raise the concern for child abuse. Assessing whether the findings are the result of trauma and/or whether the child has a bleeding disorder is critical. Many bleeding disorders are rare, and not every child with bruising/bleeding concerning for abuse requires an evaluation for bleeding disorders. In some instances, however, bleeding disorders can present in a manner similar to child abuse. The history and clinical evaluation can be used to determine the necessity of an evaluation for a possible bleeding disorder, and prevalence and known clinical presentations of individual bleeding disorders can be used to guide the extent of the laboratory testing. This clinical report provides guidance to pediatricians and other clinicians regarding the evaluation for bleeding disorders when child abuse is suspected. (3/13)
See full text on page 607.

THE EVALUATION OF CHILDREN IN THE PRIMARY CARE SETTING WHEN SEXUAL ABUSE IS SUSPECTED (CLINICAL REPORT)

Carole Jenny, MD, MBA; James E. Crawford-Jakubiak, MD;
and Committee on Child Abuse and Neglect

ABSTRACT. This clinical report updates a 2005 report from the American Academy of Pediatrics on the evaluation of sexual abuse in children. The medical assessment of suspected child sexual abuse should include obtaining a history, performing a physical examination, and obtaining appropriate laboratory tests. The role of the physician includes determining the need to report suspected sexual abuse; assessing the physical, emotional, and behavioral consequences of sexual abuse; providing information to parents about how to support their child; and coordinating with other professionals to provide comprehensive treatment and follow-up of children exposed to child sexual abuse. (7/13)
See full text on page 619.

EVALUATION AND MANAGEMENT OF THE INFANT EXPOSED TO HIV-1 IN THE UNITED STATES (CLINICAL REPORT)

Peter L. Havens, MD; Lynne M. Mofenson, MD; and
Committee on Pediatric AIDS

ABSTRACT. The pediatrician plays a key role in the prevention of mother-to-child transmission of HIV-1 infection. For infants born to women with HIV-1 infection identified during pregnancy, the pediatrician ensures that antiretroviral prophylaxis is provided to the infant to decrease the risk of acquiring HIV-1 infection and promotes avoidance of postnatal HIV-1 transmission by advising HIV-1–infected women not to breastfeed. The pediatrician should perform HIV-1 antibody testing for infants born to women whose HIV-1 infection status was not determined during pregnancy or labor. For HIV-1–exposed infants, the pediatrician monitors the infant for early determination of HIV-1 infection status and for possible short- and long-term toxicity from antiretroviral exposures. Provision of chemoprophylaxis for *Pneumocystis jiroveci* pneumonia and support of families living with HIV-1 by providing counseling to parents or caregivers are also important components of care. (12/08)

THE EVALUATION OF SEXUAL BEHAVIORS IN CHILDREN (CLINICAL REPORT)

Nancy D. Kellogg, MD, and Committee on Child Abuse
and Neglect

ABSTRACT. Most children will engage in sexual behaviors at some time during childhood. These behaviors may be normal but can be confusing and concerning to parents or disruptive or intrusive to others. Knowledge of age-appropriate sexual behaviors that vary with situational and environmental factors can assist the clinician in differentiating normal sexual behaviors from sexual behavior problems. Most situations that involve sexual behaviors in young children do not require child protective services intervention; for behaviors that are age-appropriate and transient, the pediatrician may provide guidance in supervision and monitoring of the behavior. If the behavior is intrusive, hurtful, and/or age-inappropriate, a more comprehensive assessment is warranted. Some children with sexual behavior problems may reside or have resided in homes characterized by inconsistent parenting, violence, abuse, or neglect and may require more immediate intervention and referrals. (8/09, reaffirmed 3/13)

EVALUATION OF SUSPECTED CHILD PHYSICAL ABUSE (CLINICAL REPORT)

Nancy D. Kellogg, MD, and Committee on Child Abuse
and Neglect

ABSTRACT. This report provides guidance in the clinical approach to the evaluation of suspected physical abuse in children. The medical assessment is outlined with respect to obtaining a history, physical examination, and appropriate ancillary testing. The role of the physician may encompass reporting suspected abuse; assessing the consistency of the explanation, the child's developmental capabilities, and the characteristics of the injury or injuries; and coordination with other professionals to provide immediate and long-term treatment and follow-up for victims. Accurate and timely diagnosis of children who are suspected victims of abuse can ensure appropriate evaluation, investigation, and outcomes for these children and their families. (6/07, reaffirmed 5/12)

EVIDENCE FOR THE DIAGNOSIS AND TREATMENT OF ACUTE UNCOMPLICATED SINUSITIS IN CHILDREN: A SYSTEMATIC REVIEW (TECHNICAL REPORT)

Michael J. Smith, MD, MSCE
In 2001, the American Academy of Pediatrics published clinical practice guidelines for the management of acute bacterial sinusitis (ABS) in children. The technical report accompanying those guidelines included 21 studies that assessed the diagnosis and management of ABS in children. This update to that report incorporates studies of pediatric ABS that have been performed since 2001. Overall, 17 randomized controlled trials of the treatment of sinusitis in children were identified and analyzed. Four randomized, double-blind, placebo-controlled trials of antimicrobial therapy have been published. The results of these studies varied, likely due to differences in inclusion and exclusion criteria. Because of this heterogeneity, formal meta-analyses were not performed. However, qualitative analysis of these studies suggests that children with greater severity of illness at presentation are more likely to benefit from antimicrobial therapy. An additional 5 trials compared different antimicrobial therapies but did not include placebo groups. Six trials assessed a variety of ancillary treatments for ABS in children, and 3 focused on subacute sinusitis. Although the number of pediatric trials has increased since 2001, there are still limited data to guide the diagnosis and management of ABS in children. Diagnostic and treatment guidelines focusing on severity of illness at the time of presentation have the potential to identify those children most likely to benefit from antimicrobial therapy and at the same time minimize unnecessary use of antibiotics. (6/13)
See full text on page 317.

AN EVIDENCE-BASED REVIEW OF IMPORTANT ISSUES CONCERNING NEONATAL HYPERBILIRUBINEMIA (TECHNICAL REPORT)

Stanley Ip, MD; Mei Chung, MPH; John Kulig, MD, MPH; Rebecca O'Brien, MD; Robert Sege, MD, PhD; Stephan Glicken, MD; M. Jeffrey Maisels, MB, BCh; Joseph Lau, MD; and Subcommittee on Hyperbilirubinemia
ABSTRACT. This article is adapted from a published evidence report concerning neonatal hyperbilirubinemia with an added section on the risk of blood exchange transfusion (BET). Based on a summary of multiple case reports that spanned more than 30 years, we conclude that kernicterus, although infrequent, has at least 10% mortality and at least 70% long-term morbidity. It is evident that the preponderance of kernicterus cases occurred in infants with a bilirubin level higher than 20 mg/dL. Given the diversity of conclusions on the relationship between peak bilirubin levels and behavioral and neurodevelopmental outcomes, it is apparent that the use of a single total serum bilirubin level to predict long-term outcomes is inadequate and will lead to conflicting results. Evidence for efficacy of treatments for neonatal hyperbilirubinemia was limited. Overall, the 4 qualifying studies showed that phototherapy had an absolute risk-reduction rate of 10% to 17% for prevention of serum bilirubin levels higher than 20 mg/dL in healthy infants with jaundice. There is no evidence to suggest that phototherapy for neonatal hyperbilirubinemia has any long-term adverse neurodevelopmental effects. Transcutaneous measurements of bilirubin have a linear correlation to total serum bilirubin and may be useful as screening devices to detect clinically significant jaundice and decrease the need for serum bilirubin determinations. Based on our review of the risks associated with BETs from 15 studies consisting mainly of infants born before 1970, we conclude that the mortality within 6 hours of BET ranged from 3 per 1000 to 4 per 1000 exchanged infants who were term and without serious hemolytic diseases. Regardless of the definitions and rates of BET-associated morbidity and the various pre-exchange clinical states of the exchanged infants, in many cases the morbidity was minor (eg, postexchange anemia). Based on the results from the most recent study to report BET morbidity, the overall risk of permanent sequelae in 25 sick infants who survived BET was from 5% to 10%. (7/04)

EXCESSIVE SLEEPINESS IN ADOLESCENTS AND YOUNG ADULTS: CAUSES, CONSEQUENCES, AND TREATMENT STRATEGIES (TECHNICAL REPORT)

Richard P. Millman, MD; Working Group on Sleepiness in Adolescents/Young Adults; and Committee on Adolescence
ABSTRACT. Adolescents and young adults are often excessively sleepy. This excessive sleepiness can have a profound negative effect on school performance, cognitive function, and mood and has been associated with other serious consequences such as increased incidence of automobile crashes. In this article we review available scientific knowledge about normal sleep changes in adolescents (13–22 years of age), the factors associated with chronic insufficient sleep, the effect of insufficient sleep on a variety of systems and functions, and the primary sleep disorders or organic dysfunctions that, if untreated, can cause excessive daytime sleepiness in this population. (6/05)

EXPERT WITNESS PARTICIPATION IN CIVIL AND CRIMINAL PROCEEDINGS

Committee on Medical Liability and Risk Management
ABSTRACT. The interests of the public and both the medical and legal professions are best served when scientifically sound and unbiased expert witness testimony is readily available in civil and criminal proceedings. As members of the medical community, patient advocates, and private citizens, pediatricians have ethical and professional obligations to assist in the administration of justice. The American Academy of Pediatrics believes that the adoption of the recommendations outlined in this statement will improve the quality of medical expert witness testimony in legal proceedings and, thereby, increase

the probability of achieving outcomes that are fair, honest, and equitable. Strategies for enforcing guidance and promoting oversight of expert witnesses are proposed. (6/09)

EXPOSURE TO NONTRADITIONAL PETS AT HOME AND TO ANIMALS IN PUBLIC SETTINGS: RISKS TO CHILDREN (CLINICAL REPORT)

Larry K. Pickering, MD; Nina Marano, DVM, MPH; Joseph A. Bocchini, MD; Frederick J. Angulo, DVM, PhD; and Committee on Infectious Diseases

ABSTRACT. Exposure to animals can provide many benefits during the growth and development of children. However, there are potential risks associated with animal exposures, including exposure to nontraditional pets in the home and animals in public settings. Educational materials, regulations, and guidelines have been developed to minimize these risks. Pediatricians, veterinarians, and other health care professionals can provide advice on selection of appropriate pets as well as prevention of disease transmission from nontraditional pets and when children contact animals in public settings. (10/08, reaffirmed 12/11)

THE EYE EXAMINATION IN THE EVALUATION OF CHILD ABUSE (CLINICAL REPORT)

Alex V. Levin, MD, MHSc; Cindy W. Christian, MD; Committee on Child Abuse and Neglect; and Section on Ophthalmology

ABSTRACT. Retinal hemorrhage is an important indicator of possible abusive head trauma, but it is also found in a number of other conditions. Distinguishing the type, number, and pattern of retinal hemorrhages may be helpful in establishing a differential diagnosis. Identification of ocular abnormalities requires a full retinal examination by an ophthalmologist using indirect ophthalmoscopy through a pupil that has been pharmacologically dilated. At autopsy, removal of the eyes and orbital tissues may also reveal abnormalities not discovered before death. In previously well young children who experience unexpected apparent life-threatening events with no obvious cause, children with head trauma that results in significant intracranial hemorrhage and brain injury, victims of abusive head trauma, and children with unexplained death, premortem clinical eye examination and postmortem examination of the eyes and orbits may be helpful in detecting abnormalities that can help establish the underlying etiology. (7/10)

EYE EXAMINATION IN INFANTS, CHILDREN, AND YOUNG ADULTS BY PEDIATRICIANS

Committee on Practice and Ambulatory Medicine and Section on Ophthalmology (joint with American Association of Certified Orthoptists, American Association for Pediatric Ophthalmology and Strabismus, and American Academy of Ophthalmology)

ABSTRACT. Early detection and prompt treatment of ocular disorders in children is important to avoid lifelong visual impairment. Examination of the eyes should be performed beginning in the newborn period and at all well-child visits. Newborns should be examined for ocular structural abnormalities, such as cataract, corneal opacity, and ptosis, which are known to result in visual problems. Vision assessment beginning at birth has been endorsed by the American Academy of Pediatrics, the American Association for Pediatric Ophthalmology and Strabismus, and the American Academy of Ophthalmology. All children who are found to have an ocular abnormality or who fail vision assessment should be referred to a pediatric ophthalmologist or an eye care specialist appropriately trained to treat pediatric patients. (4/03, reaffirmed 5/07)

FACILITIES AND EQUIPMENT FOR THE CARE OF PEDIATRIC PATIENTS IN A COMMUNITY HOSPITAL (CLINICAL REPORT)

Committee on Hospital Care

ABSTRACT. Many children who require hospitalization are admitted to community hospitals that are more accessible for families and their primary care physicians but vary substantially in their pediatric resources. The intent of this clinical report is to provide basic guidelines for furnishing and equipping a pediatric area in a community hospital. (5/03, reaffirmed 5/07, reaffirmed 8/13)

FAILURE TO THRIVE AS A MANIFESTATION OF CHILD NEGLECT (CLINICAL REPORT)

Robert W. Block, MD; Nancy F. Krebs, MD; Committee on Child Abuse and Neglect; and Committee on Nutrition

ABSTRACT. Failure to thrive is a common problem in infancy and childhood. It is most often multifactorial in origin. Inadequate nutrition and disturbed social interactions contribute to poor weight gain, delayed development, and abnormal behavior. The syndrome develops in a significant number of children as a consequence of child neglect. This clinical report is intended to focus the pediatrician on the consideration, evaluation, and management of failure to thrive when child neglect may be present. Child protective services agencies should be notified when the evaluation leads to a suspicion of abuse or neglect. (11/05, reaffirmed 1/09)

FALLS FROM HEIGHTS: WINDOWS, ROOFS, AND BALCONIES

Committee on Injury and Poison Prevention

ABSTRACT. Falls of all kinds represent an important cause of child injury and death. In the United States, approximately 140 deaths from falls occur annually in children younger than 15 years. Three million children require emergency department care for fall-related injuries. This policy statement examines the epidemiology of falls from heights and recommends preventive strategies for pediatricians and other child health care professionals. Such strategies involve parent counseling, community programs, building code changes, legislation, and environmental modification, such as the installation of window guards and balcony railings. (5/01, reaffirmed 10/04, 5/07, 6/10)

FAMILIES AND ADOPTION: THE PEDIATRICIAN'S ROLE IN SUPPORTING COMMUNICATION (CLINICAL REPORT)

Committee on Early Childhood, Adoption, and Dependent Care

ABSTRACT. Each year, more children join families through adoption. Pediatricians have an important role in assisting adoptive families in the various challenges they may face with respect to adoption. The acceptance of the differences between families formed through birth and those formed through adoption is essential in promoting positive emotional growth within the family. It is important for pediatricians to be informed about adoption and to share this knowledge with adoptive families. Parents need ongoing advice with respect to adoption issues and need to be supported in their communication with their adopted children. (12/03)

FATHERS AND PEDIATRICIANS: ENHANCING MEN'S ROLES IN THE CARE AND DEVELOPMENT OF THEIR CHILDREN (CLINICAL REPORT)

Committee on Psychosocial Aspects of Child and Family Health

ABSTRACT. Research substantiates that fathers' interactions with their children can exert a positive influence on their children's development. This report suggests ways pediatricians can enhance fathers' caregiving involvement by offering specific, culturally sensitive advice and how pediatricians might change their office practices to support and increase fathers' active involvement in their children's care and development. (5/04, reaffirmed 8/13)

FEVER AND ANTIPYRETIC USE IN CHILDREN (CLINICAL REPORT)

Janice E. Sullivan, MD; Henry C. Farrar, MD; Section on Clinical Pharmacology and Therapeutics; and Committee on Drugs

ABSTRACT. Fever in a child is one of the most common clinical symptoms managed by pediatricians and other health care providers and a frequent cause of parental concern. Many parents administer antipyretics even when there is minimal or no fever, because they are concerned that the child must maintain a "normal" temperature. Fever, however, is not the primary illness but is a physiologic mechanism that has beneficial effects in fighting infection. There is no evidence that fever itself worsens the course of an illness or that it causes long-term neurologic complications. Thus, the primary goal of treating the febrile child should be to improve the child's overall comfort rather than focus on the normalization of body temperature. When counseling the parents or caregivers of a febrile child, the general well-being of the child, the importance of monitoring activity, observing for signs of serious illness, encouraging appropriate fluid intake, and the safe storage of antipyretics should be emphasized. Current evidence suggests that there is no substantial difference in the safety and effectiveness of acetaminophen and ibuprofen in the care of a generally healthy child with fever. There is evidence that combining these 2 products is more effective than the use of a single agent alone; however, there are concerns that combined treatment may be more complicated and contribute to the unsafe use of these drugs. Pediatricians should also promote patient safety by advocating for simplified formulations, dosing instructions, and dosing devices. (2/11)

FINANCING GRADUATE MEDICAL EDUCATION TO MEET THE NEEDS OF CHILDREN AND THE FUTURE PEDIATRICIAN WORKFORCE

Committee on Pediatric Workforce

ABSTRACT. This policy statement articulates the positions of the American Academy of Pediatrics on graduate medical education and the associated costs and funding mechanisms. It reaffirms the policy of the American Academy of Pediatrics that graduate medical education is a public good and is an essential part of maintaining a high-quality physician workforce. The American Academy of Pediatrics advocates for lifelong learning across the continuum of medical education. This policy statement focuses on the financing of one component of this continuum, namely residency education. The statement calls on federal and state governments to continue their support of residency education and advocates for stable means of funding such as the establishment of an all-payer graduate medical education trust fund. It further proposes a portable authorization system that would allocate graduate medical education funds for direct medical education costs to accredited residency programs on the basis of the selection of the program by qualified student or residents. This system allows the funding to follow the residents to their program. Recognizing the critical workforce needs of many pediatric medical subspecialties, pediatric surgical specialties, and other pediatric specialty disciplines, this statement maintains that subspecialty fellowship training and general pediatrics research fellowship training should receive adequate support from the graduate medical education financing system, including funding from the National Institutes of Health and other federal agencies, as appropriate. Furthermore, residency education that is provided in freestanding children's hospitals should receive a level of support equivalent to that of other teaching hospitals. The financing of graduate medical education is an important and effective tool to ensure that the future pediatrician workforce can provide optimal heath care for infants, children, adolescents, and young adults. (4/08, reaffirmed 1/12)

FINANCING OF PEDIATRIC HOME HEALTH CARE

Committee on Child Health Financing and Section on Home Care

ABSTRACT. In certain situations, home health care has been shown to be a cost-effective alternative to inpatient hospital care. National health expenditures reveal that pediatric home health costs totaled $5.3 billion in 2000. Medicaid is the major payer for pediatric home health care (77%), followed by other public sources (22%). Private health insurance and families each paid less than 1% of pediatric home health expenses. The most important factors affecting access to home health care are the inadequate supply of clinicians and ancillary personnel, shortages of home health nurses with pediatric expertise, inadequate payment, and restrictive insurance and managed care policies. Many children must stay in the NICU, PICU, and other pediatric wards and intermediate care areas at a much higher cost because of inadequate pediatric home health care services. The main financing problem pertaining to Medicaid is low payment to home health agencies at rates that are insufficient to provide beneficiaries access to home health services. Although home care services may be a covered benefit under private health plans, most do not cover private-duty nursing (83%), home health aides (45%), or home physical, occupational, or speech therapy (33%) and/or impose visit or monetary limits or caps. To advocate for improvements in financing of pediatric home health care, the American Academy of Pediatrics has developed several recommendations for public policy makers, federal and state Medicaid offices, private insurers, managed care plans, Title V officials, and home health care professionals. These recommendations will improve licensing, payment, coverage, and research related to pediatric home health services. (8/06)

FIREARM-RELATED INJURIES AFFECTING THE PEDIATRIC POPULATION
Council on Injury, Violence, and Poison Prevention Executive Committee
ABSTRACT. The absence of guns from children's homes and communities is the most reliable and effective measure to prevent firearm-related injuries in children and adolescents. Adolescent suicide risk is strongly associated with firearm availability. Safe gun storage (guns unloaded and locked, ammunition locked separately) reduces children's risk of injury. Physician counseling of parents about firearm safety appears to be effective, but firearm safety education programs directed at children are ineffective. The American Academy of Pediatrics continues to support a number of specific measures to reduce the destructive effects of guns in the lives of children and adolescents, including the regulation of the manufacture, sale, purchase, ownership, and use of firearms; a ban on semiautomatic assault weapons; and the strongest possible regulations of handguns for civilian use. (10/12)

FIREWORKS-RELATED INJURIES TO CHILDREN
Committee on Injury and Poison Prevention
ABSTRACT. An estimated 8500 individuals, approximately 45% of them children younger than 15 years, were treated in US hospital emergency departments during 1999 for fireworks-related injuries. The hands (40%), eyes (20%), and head and face (20%) are the body areas most often involved. Approximately one third of eye injuries from fireworks result in permanent blindness. During 1999, 16 people died as a result of injuries associated with fireworks. Every type of legally available consumer (so-called "safe and sane") firework has been associated with serious injury or death. In 1997, 20 100 fires were caused by fireworks, resulting in $22.7 million in direct property damage. Fireworks typically cause more fires in the United States on the Fourth of July than all other causes of fire combined on that day. Pediatricians should educate parents, children, community leaders, and others about the dangers of fireworks. Fireworks for individual private use should be banned. Children and their families should be encouraged to enjoy fireworks at public fireworks displays conducted by professionals rather than purchase fireworks for home or private use. (7/01, reaffirmed 1/05, 2/08, 10/11)

FOLIC ACID FOR THE PREVENTION OF NEURAL TUBE DEFECTS
Committee on Genetics
ABSTRACT. The American Academy of Pediatrics endorses the US Public Health Service (USPHS) recommendation that all women capable of becoming pregnant consume 400 µg of folic acid daily to prevent neural tube defects (NTDs). Studies have demonstrated that periconceptional folic acid supplementation can prevent 50% or more of NTDs such as spina bifida and anencephaly. For women who have previously had an NTD-affected pregnancy, the Centers for Disease Control and Prevention (CDC) recommends increasing the intake of folic acid to 4000 µg per day beginning at least 1 month before conception and continuing through the first trimester. Implementation of these recommendations is essential for the primary prevention of these serious and disabling birth defects. Because fewer than 1 in 3 women consume the amount of folic acid recommended by the USPHS, the Academy notes that the prevention of NTDs depends on an urgent and effective campaign to close this prevention gap. (8/99, reaffirmed 11/02, 1/07, 5/12)

FOLLOW-UP MANAGEMENT OF CHILDREN WITH TYMPANOSTOMY TUBES
Section on Otolaryngology and Bronchoesophagology
ABSTRACT. The follow-up care of children in whom tympanostomy tubes have been placed is shared by the pediatrician and the otolaryngologist. Guidelines are provided for routine follow-up evaluation, perioperative hearing assessment, and the identification of specific conditions and complications that warrant urgent otolaryngologic consultation. These guidelines have been developed by a consensus of expert opinions. (2/02)

FORGOING LIFE-SUSTAINING MEDICAL TREATMENT IN ABUSED CHILDREN
Committee on Child Abuse and Neglect and Committee on Bioethics
ABSTRACT. A decision to forgo life-sustaining medical treatment (LSMT) for a critically ill child injured as the result of abuse should be made using the same criteria as those used for any critically ill child. The parent or guardian of an abused child may have a conflict of interest when a decision to forgo LSMT risks changing the legal charge faced by a parent, guardian, relative, or acquaintance from assault to manslaughter or homicide. If a physician suspects that a parent or guardian is not acting in a child's best interest, further review and consultation should be sought in hopes of resolving the conflict. A guardian ad litem who will represent the child's interests regarding LSMT should be appointed in all cases in which a parent or guardian may have a conflict of interest. (11/00, reaffirmed 6/03, 10/06, 4/09)

FORGOING MEDICALLY PROVIDED NUTRITION AND HYDRATION IN CHILDREN (CLINICAL REPORT)
Douglas S. Diekema, MD, MPH; Jeffrey R. Botkin, MD, MPH; and Committee on Bioethics
ABSTRACT. There is broad consensus that withholding or withdrawing medical interventions is morally permissible when requested by competent patients or, in the case of patients without decision-making capacity, when the interventions no longer confer a benefit to the patient or when the burdens associated with the interventions outweigh the benefits received. The withdrawal or withholding of measures such as attempted resuscitation, ventilators, and critical care medications is common in the terminal care of adults and children. In the case of adults, a consensus has emerged in law and ethics that the medical administration of fluid and nutrition is not fundamentally different from other medical interventions such

as use of ventilators; therefore, it can be forgone or withdrawn when a competent adult or legally authorized surrogate requests withdrawal or when the intervention no longer provides a net benefit to the patient. In pediatrics, forgoing or withdrawing medically administered fluids and nutrition has been more controversial because of the inability of children to make autonomous decisions and the emotional power of feeding as a basic element of the care of children. This statement reviews the medical, ethical, and legal issues relevant to the withholding or withdrawing of medically provided fluids and nutrition in children. The American Academy of Pediatrics concludes that the withdrawal of medically administered fluids and nutrition for pediatric patients is ethically acceptable in limited circumstances. Ethics consultation is strongly recommended when particularly difficult or controversial decisions are being considered. (7/09)

THE FUTURE OF PEDIATRICS: MENTAL HEALTH COMPETENCIES FOR PEDIATRIC PRIMARY CARE

Committee on Psychosocial Aspects of Child and Family Health and Task Force on Mental Health

ABSTRACT. Pediatric primary care clinicians have unique opportunities and a growing sense of responsibility to prevent and address mental health and substance abuse problems in the medical home. In this report, the American Academy of Pediatrics proposes competencies requisite for providing mental health and substance abuse services in pediatric primary care settings and recommends steps toward achieving them. Achievement of the competencies proposed in this statement is a goal, not a current expectation. It will require innovations in residency training and continuing medical education, as well as a commitment by the individual clinician to pursue, over time, educational strategies suited to his or her learning style and skill level. System enhancements, such as collaborative relationships with mental health specialists and changes in the financing of mental health care, must precede enhancements in clinical practice. For this reason, the proposed competencies begin with knowledge and skills for systems-based practice. The proposed competencies overlap those of mental health specialists in some areas; for example, they include the knowledge and skills to care for children with attention-deficit/hyperactivity disorder, anxiety, depression, and substance abuse and to recognize psychiatric and social emergencies. In other areas, the competencies reflect the uniqueness of the primary care clinician's role: building resilience in all children; promoting healthy lifestyles; preventing or mitigating mental health and substance abuse problems; identifying risk factors and emerging mental health problems in children and their families; and partnering with families, schools, agencies, and mental health specialists to plan assessment and care. Proposed interpersonal and communication skills reflect the primary care clinician's critical role in overcoming barriers (perceived and/or experienced by children and families) to seeking help for mental health and substance abuse concerns. (6/09, reaffirmed 8/13)

GASTROESOPHAGEAL REFLUX: MANAGEMENT GUIDANCE FOR THE PEDIATRICIAN (CLINICAL REPORT)

Jenifer R. Lightdale, MD, MPH; David A. Gremse, MD; and Section on Gastroenterology, Hepatology, and Nutrition

ABSTRACT. Recent comprehensive guidelines developed by the North American Society for Pediatric Gastroenterology, Hepatology, and Nutrition define the common entities of gastroesophageal reflux (GER) as the physiologic passage of gastric contents into the esophagus and gastroesophageal reflux disease (GERD) as reflux associated with troublesome symptoms or complications. The ability to distinguish between GER and GERD is increasingly important to implement best practices in the management of acid reflux in patients across all pediatric age groups, as children with GERD may benefit from further evaluation and treatment, whereas conservative recommendations are the only indicated therapy in those with uncomplicated physiologic reflux. This clinical report endorses the rigorously developed, well-referenced North American Society for Pediatric Gastroenterology, Hepatology, and Nutrition guidelines and likewise emphasizes important concepts for the general pediatrician. A key issue is distinguishing between clinical manifestations of GER and GERD in term infants, children, and adolescents to identify patients who can be managed with conservative treatment by the pediatrician and to refer patients who require consultation with the gastroenterologist. Accordingly, the evidence basis presented by the guidelines for diagnostic approaches as well as treatments is discussed. Lifestyle changes are emphasized as first-line therapy in both GER and GERD, whereas medications are explicitly indicated only for patients with GERD. Surgical therapies are reserved for children with intractable symptoms or who are at risk for life-threatening complications of GERD. Recent black box warnings from the US Food and Drug Administration are discussed, and caution is underlined when using promoters of gastric emptying and motility. Finally, attention is paid to increasing evidence of inappropriate prescriptions for proton pump inhibitors in the pediatric population. (4/13)

See full text on page 631.

GENERIC PRESCRIBING, GENERIC SUBSTITUTION, AND THERAPEUTIC SUBSTITUTION

Committee on Drugs (5/87, reaffirmed 6/93, 5/96, 6/99, 5/01, 5/05, 10/08, 10/12)

GLOBAL CLIMATE CHANGE AND CHILDREN'S HEALTH

Committee on Environmental Health

ABSTRACT. There is broad scientific consensus that Earth's climate is warming rapidly and at an accelerating rate. Human activities, primarily the burning of fossil fuels, are very likely (>90% probability) to be the main cause of this warming. Climate-sensitive changes in ecosystems are already being observed, and fundamental, potentially irreversible, ecological changes may occur in the coming decades. Conservative environmental estimates of the impact of climate changes that are already in process indicate that they will result in numerous health effects to children. The nature and extent of these changes will be greatly affected by actions taken or not taken now at the global level.

Physicians have written on the projected effects of climate change on public health, but little has been written specifically on anticipated effects of climate change on children's health. Children represent a particularly vulnerable group that is likely to suffer disproportionately from both direct and indirect adverse health effects of climate change. Pediatric health care professionals should understand these threats, anticipate their effects on children's health, and participate as children's advocates for strong mitigation and adaptation strategies now. Any solutions that address climate change must be developed within the context of overall sustainability (the use of resources by the current generation to meet current needs while ensuring that future generations will be able to meet their needs). Pediatric health care professionals can be leaders in a move away from a traditional focus on disease prevention to a broad, integrated focus on sustainability as synonymous with health.

This policy statement is supported by a technical report that examines in some depth the nature of the problem of climate change, likely effects on children's health as a result of climate change, and the critical importance of responding promptly and aggressively to reduce activities that are contributing to this change. (11/07, reaffirmed 5/12)

GLOBAL CLIMATE CHANGE AND CHILDREN'S HEALTH (TECHNICAL REPORT)

Katherine M. Shea, MD, MPH, and Committee on Environmental Health

ABSTRACT. There is a broad scientific consensus that the global climate is warming, the process is accelerating, and that human activities are very likely (>90% probability) the main cause. This warming will have effects on ecosystems and human health, many of them adverse. Children will experience both the direct and indirect effects of climate change. Actions taken by individuals, communities, businesses, and governments will affect the magnitude and rate of global climate change and resultant health impacts. This technical report reviews the nature of the global problem and anticipated health effects on children and supports the recommendations in the accompanying policy statement on climate change and children's health. (11/07, reaffirmed 5/12)

GRADUATE MEDICAL EDUCATION AND PEDIATRIC WORKFORCE ISSUES AND PRINCIPLES

Task Force on Graduate Medical Education Reform (6/94)

GUIDANCE FOR THE ADMINISTRATION OF MEDICATION IN SCHOOL

Council on School Health

ABSTRACT. Many children who take medications require them during the school day. This policy statement is designed to guide prescribing health care professionals, school physicians, and school health councils on the administration of medications to children at school. All districts and schools need to have policies and plans in place for safe, effective, and efficient administration of medications at school. Having full-time licensed registered nurses administering all routine and emergency medications in schools is the best situation. When a licensed registered nurse is not available, a licensed practical nurse may administer medications. When a nurse cannot administer medication in school, the American Academy of Pediatrics supports appropriate delegation of nursing services in the school setting. Delegation is a tool that may be used by the licensed registered school nurse to allow unlicensed assistive personnel to provide standardized, routine health services under the supervision of the nurse and on the basis of physician guidance and school nursing assessment of the unique needs of the individual child and the suitability of delegation of specific nursing tasks. Any delegation of nursing duties must be consistent with the requirements of state nurse practice acts, state regulations, and guidelines provided by professional nursing organizations. Long-term, emergency, and short-term medications; over-the-counter medications; alternative medications; and experimental drugs that are administered as part of a clinical trial are discussed in this statement. This statement has been endorsed by the American School Health Association. (9/09, reaffirmed 2/13)

GUIDANCE FOR EFFECTIVE DISCIPLINE

Committee on Psychosocial Aspects of Child and Family Health

ABSTRACT. When advising families about discipline strategies, pediatricians should use a comprehensive approach that includes consideration of the parent-child relationship, reinforcement of desired behaviors, and consequences for negative behaviors. Corporal punishment is of limited effectiveness and has potentially deleterious side effects. The American Academy of Pediatrics recommends that parents be encouraged and assisted in the development of methods other than spanking for managing undesired behavior. (4/98, reaffirmed 3/01, 1/05, 5/12)

GUIDANCE ON MANAGEMENT OF ASYMPTOMATIC NEONATES BORN TO WOMEN WITH ACTIVE GENITAL HERPES LESIONS (CLINICAL REPORT)

Committee on Infectious Diseases and Committee on Fetus and Newborn

ABSTRACT. Herpes simplex virus (HSV) infection of the neonate is uncommon, but genital herpes infections in adults are very common. Thus, although treating an infant with neonatal herpes is a relatively rare occurrence, managing infants potentially exposed to HSV at the time of delivery occurs more frequently. The risk of transmitting HSV to an infant during delivery is determined in part by the mother's previous immunity to HSV. Women with primary genital HSV infections who are shedding HSV at delivery are 10 to 30 times more likely to transmit the virus to their newborn infants than are women with recurrent HSV infection who are shedding virus at delivery. With the availability of commercial serological tests that reliably can distinguish type-specific HSV antibodies, it is now possible to determine the type of maternal infection and, thus, further refine management of infants delivered to women who have active genital HSV lesions. The management algorithm presented herein uses both serological and virological studies to determine the risk of HSV transmission to the neonate who is delivered to a mother with active herpetic genital lesions and tailors management accordingly. The algorithm does not address the approach to asymptomatic neonates delivered to women with a history of genital herpes but no active lesions at delivery. (1/13)

See full text on page 645.

GUIDELINES FOR CARE OF CHILDREN IN THE EMERGENCY DEPARTMENT

Committee on Pediatric Emergency Medicine (joint with American College of Emergency Physicians Pediatric Committee and Emergency Nurses Association Pediatric Committee)

ABSTRACT. Children who require emergency care have unique needs, especially when emergencies are serious or life-threatening. The majority of ill and injured children are brought to community hospital emergency departments (EDs) by virtue of their geography within communities. Similarly, emergency medical services (EMS) agencies provide the bulk of out-of-hospital emergency care to children. It is imperative, therefore, that all hospital EDs have the appropriate resources (medications, equipment, policies, and education) and staff to provide effective emergency care for children. This statement outlines resources necessary to ensure that hospital EDs stand ready to care for children of all ages, from neonates to adolescents. These guidelines are consistent with the recommendations of the Institute of Medicine's report on the future of emergency care in the United States health system. Although resources within emergency and trauma care systems vary locally, regionally, and nationally, it is essential that hospital ED staff and administrators and EMS systems' administrators and medical directors seek to meet or exceed these guidelines in efforts to optimize the emergency care of children they serve. This statement has been endorsed by the Academic Pediatric Association, American Academy of Family Physicians, American Academy of Physician Assistants, American College of Osteopathic Emergency Physicians, American College of Surgeons, American Heart Association, American Medical Association, American Pediatric Surgical Association, Brain Injury Association of America, Child Health Corporation of America, Children's National Medical Center, Family Voices, National Association of Children's Hospitals and Related Institutions, National Association of EMS Physicians, National Association of Emergency Medical Technicians, National Association of State EMS Officials, National Committee for Quality Assurance, National PTA, Safe Kids USA, Society of Trauma Nurses, Society for Academic Emergency Medicine, and The Joint Commission. (9/09, reaffirmed 4/13)

GUIDELINES FOR THE DETERMINATION OF BRAIN DEATH IN INFANTS AND CHILDREN: AN UPDATE OF THE 1987 TASK FORCE RECOMMENDATIONS (CLINICAL REPORT)

Thomas A. Nakagawa, MD; Stephen Ashwal, MD; Mudit Mathur, MD; and Mohan Mysore, MD (joint with Society of Critical Care Medicine Section on Critical Care and Section on Neurology and Child Neurology Society)

ABSTRACT. *Objective.* To review and revise the 1987 pediatric brain death guidelines.

Methods. Relevant literature was reviewed. Recommendations were developed using the GRADE system.

Conclusions and Recommendations.

(1) Determination of brain death in term newborns, infants and children is a clinical diagnosis based on the absence of neurologic function with a known irreversible cause of coma. Because of insufficient data in the literature, recommendations for preterm infants less than 37 weeks gestational age are not included in this guideline.

(2) Hypotension, hypothermia, and metabolic disturbances should be treated and corrected and medications that can interfere with the neurologic examination and apnea testing should be discontinued allowing for adequate clearance before proceeding with these evaluations.

(3) Two examinations including apnea testing with each examination separated by an observation period are required. Examinations should be performed by different attending physicians. Apnea testing may be performed by the same physician. An observation period of 24 hours for term newborns (37 weeks gestational age) to 30 days of age, and 12 hours for infants and chi (> 30 days to 18 years) is recommended. The first examination determines the child has met the accepted neurologic examination criteria for brain death. The second examination confirms brain death based on an unchanged and irreversible condition. Assessment of neurologic function following cardiopulmonary resuscitation or other severe acute brain injuries should be deferred for 24 hours or longer if there are concerns or inconsistencies in the examination.

(4) Apnea testing to support the diagnosis of brain death must be performed safely and requires documentation of an arterial PaCO2 20 mm Hg above the baseline and 60 mm Hg with no respiratory effort during the testing period. If the apnea test cannot be safely completed, an ancillary study should be performed.

(5) Ancillary studies (electroencephalogram and radionuclide cerebral blood flow) are not required to establish brain death and are not a substitute for the neurologic examination. Ancillary studies may be us d to assist the clinician in making the diagnosis of brain death (i) when components of the examination or apnea testing cannot be completed safely due to the underlying medical condition of the patient; (ii) if there is uncertainty about the results of the neurologic examination; (iii) if a medication effect may be present; or (iv) to reduce the inter-examination observation period. When ancillary studies are used, a second clinical examination and apnea test should be performed and components that can be completed must remain consistent with brain death. In this instance the observation interval may be shortened and the second

neurologic examination and apnea test (or all components that are able to be completed safely) can be performed at any time thereafter.

(6) Death is declared when the above criteria are fulfilled. (8/11)

GUIDELINES FOR DEVELOPING ADMISSION AND DISCHARGE POLICIES FOR THE PEDIATRIC INTENSIVE CARE UNIT (CLINICAL REPORT)

Committee on Hospital Care and Section on Critical Care
  (joint with Society of Critical Care Medicine Pediatric
  Section Admission Criteria Task Force)

ABSTRACT. These guidelines were developed to provide a reference for preparing policies on admission to and discharge from pediatric intensive care units. They represent a consensus opinion of physicians, nurses, and allied health care professionals. By using this document as a framework for developing multidisciplinary admission and discharge policies, use of pediatric intensive care units can be optimized and patients can receive the level of care appropriate for their condition. (4/99, reaffirmed 5/05, 2/08, 1/13)

GUIDELINES FOR THE ETHICAL CONDUCT OF STUDIES TO EVALUATE DRUGS IN PEDIATRIC POPULATIONS (CLINICAL REPORT)

*Robert E. Shaddy, MD; Scott C. Denne, MD; Committee on
  Drugs; and Committee on Pediatric Research*

ABSTRACT. The proper ethical conduct of studies to evaluate drugs in children is of paramount importance to all those involved in these types of studies. This report is an updated revision to the previously published guidelines from the American Academy of Pediatrics in 1995. Since the previous publication, there have been great strides made in the science and ethics of studying drugs in children. There have also been numerous legislative and regulatory advancements that have promoted the study of drugs in children while simultaneously allowing for the protection of this particularly vulnerable group. This report summarizes these changes and advances and provides a framework from which to guide and monitor the ethical conduct of studies to evaluate drugs in children. (3/10)

GUIDELINES ON FORGOING LIFE-SUSTAINING MEDICAL TREATMENT

Committee on Bioethics (3/94, reaffirmed 11/97, 10/00, 1/04, 1/09, 10/12)

GUIDELINES FOR HOME CARE OF INFANTS, CHILDREN, AND ADOLESCENTS WITH CHRONIC DISEASE

Committee on Children With Disabilities (7/95, reaffirmed 4/00, 1/06)

GUIDELINES FOR MONITORING AND MANAGEMENT OF PEDIATRIC PATIENTS DURING AND AFTER SEDATION FOR DIAGNOSTIC AND THERAPEUTIC PROCEDURES: AN UPDATE (CLINICAL REPORT)

*American Academy of Pediatrics; American Academy of
  Pediatric Dentistry; Charles J. Coté, MD; Stephen Wilson,
  DMD, MA, PhD; and Work Group on Sedation*

ABSTRACT. The safe sedation of children for procedures requires a systematic approach that includes the following: no administration of sedating medication without the safety net of medical supervision; careful presedation evaluation for underlying medical or surgical conditions that would place the child at increased risk from sedating medications; appropriate fasting for elective procedures and a balance between depth of sedation and risk for those who are unable to fast because of the urgent nature of the procedure; a focused airway examination for large tonsils or anatomic airway abnormalities that might increase the potential for airway obstruction; a clear understanding of the pharmacokinetic and pharmacodynamic effects of the medications used for sedation, as well as an appreciation for drug interactions; appropriate training and skills in airway management to allow rescue of the patient; age- and size-appropriate equipment for airway management and venous access; appropriate medications and reversal agents; sufficient numbers of people to carry out the procedure and monitor the patient; appropriate physiologic monitoring during and after the procedure; a properly equipped and staffed recovery area; recovery to presedation level of consciousness before discharge from medical supervision; and appropriate discharge instructions. This report was developed through a collaborative effort of the American Academy of Pediatrics and the American Academy of Pediatric Dentistry to offer pediatric providers updated information and guidance in delivering safe sedation to children. (12/06, reaffirmed 3/11)

GUIDELINES FOR PEDIATRIC CANCER CENTERS

Section on Hematology/Oncology

ABSTRACT. Since the American Academy of Pediatrics published guidelines for pediatric cancer centers in 1986 and 1997, significant changes in the delivery of health care have prompted a review of the role of tertiary medical centers in the care of pediatric patients. The potential effect of these changes on the treatment and survival rates of children with cancer led to this revision. The intent of this statement is to delineate personnel and facilities that are essential to provide state-of-the-art care for children and adolescents with cancer. This statement emphasizes the importance of board-certified pediatric hematologists/oncologists, pediatric subspecialty consultants, and appropriately qualified pediatric medical subspecialists and pediatric surgical specialists overseeing the care of all pediatric and adolescent cancer patients and the need for facilities available only at a tertiary center as essential for the initial management and much of the follow-up for pediatric and adolescent cancer patients. (6/04, reaffirmed 10/08)

GUIDELINES FOR PEDIATRIC CARDIOVASCULAR CENTERS

Section on Cardiology and Cardiac Surgery

ABSTRACT. Pediatric cardiovascular centers should aim to provide high-quality therapeutic outcomes for infants and children with congenital and acquired heart diseases. This policy statement describes critical elements and organizational features of centers in which high-quality outcomes have the greatest likelihood of occurring. Center elements include noninvasive diagnostic modalities, cardiac catheterization, cardiovascular surgery, and cardiovascular intensive care. These elements should be organizationally united in centers in which pediatric cardiac physician specialists and specialized pediatric staff work together to achieve and surpass existing quality-of-care benchmarks. (3/02, reaffirmed 10/07)

GUIDELINES FOR REFERRAL TO PEDIATRIC SURGICAL SPECIALISTS
Surgical Advisory Panel (7/02, reaffirmed 1/07)

GUIDING PRINCIPLES FOR MANAGED CARE ARRANGEMENTS FOR THE HEALTH CARE OF NEWBORNS, INFANTS, CHILDREN, ADOLESCENTS, AND YOUNG ADULTS
Committee on Child Health Financing

ABSTRACT. By including the precepts of primary care and the medical home in the delivery of services, managed care can be effective in increasing access to a full range of health care services and clinicians. A carefully designed and administered managed care plan can minimize patient under- and overutilization of services, as well as enhance quality of care. Therefore, the American Academy of Pediatrics urges the use of the key principles outlined in this statement in designing and implementing managed care programs for newborns, infants, children, adolescents, and young adults to maximize the positive potential of managed care for pediatrics. (10/13)
See full text on page 659.

GUIDING PRINCIPLES FOR PEDIATRIC HOSPITAL MEDICINE PROGRAMS
Section on Hospital Medicine

ABSTRACT. Pediatric hospital medicine programs have an established place in pediatric medicine. This statement speaks to the expanded roles and responsibilities of pediatric hospitalists and their integrated role among the community of pediatricians who care for children within and outside of the hospital setting. (9/13)
See full text on page 673.

GYNECOLOGIC EXAMINATION FOR ADOLESCENTS IN THE PEDIATRIC OFFICE SETTING (CLINICAL REPORT)
Paula K. Braverman, MD; Lesley Breech, MD; and Committee on Adolescence

ABSTRACT. The American Academy of Pediatrics promotes the inclusion of the gynecologic examination in the primary care setting within the medical home. Gynecologic issues are commonly seen by clinicians who provide primary care to adolescents. Some of the most common concerns include questions related to pubertal development; menstrual disorders such as dysmenorrhea, amenorrhea, oligomenorrhea, and abnormal uterine bleeding; contraception; and sexually transmitted and non–sexually transmitted infections. The gynecologic examination is a key element in assessing pubertal status and documenting physical findings. Most adolescents do not need an internal examination involving a speculum or bimanual examination. However, for cases in which more extensive examination is needed, the primary care office with the primary care clinician who has established rapport and trust with the patient is often the best setting for pelvic examination. This report reviews the gynecologic examination, including indications for the pelvic examination in adolescents and the approach to this examination in the office setting. Indications for referral to a gynecologist are included. The pelvic examination may be successfully completed when conducted without pressure and approached as a normal part of routine young women's health care. (8/10, reaffirmed 5/13)

HEAD LICE (CLINICAL REPORT)
Barbara L. Frankowski, MD, MPH; Joseph A. Bocchini, Jr, MD; Council on School Health; and Committee on Infectious Diseases

ABSTRACT. Head lice infestation is associated with limited morbidity but causes a high level of anxiety among parents of school-aged children. Since the 2002 clinical report on head lice was published by the American Academy of Pediatrics, patterns of resistance to products available over-the-counter and by prescription have changed, and additional mechanical means of removing head lice have been explored. This revised clinical report clarifies current diagnosis and treatment protocols and provides guidance for the management of children with head lice in the school setting. (7/10)

HEALTH CARE SUPERVISION FOR CHILDREN WITH WILLIAMS SYNDROME
Committee on Genetics

ABSTRACT. This set of guidelines is designed to assist the pediatrician to care for children with Williams syndrome diagnosed by clinical features and with regional chromosomal microdeletion confirmed by fluorescence in situ hybridization. (5/01, reaffirmed 5/05, 1/09)

HEALTH CARE OF YOUTH AGING OUT OF FOSTER CARE
Council on Foster Care, Adoption, and Kinship Care and Committee on Early Childhood

ABSTRACT. Youth transitioning out of foster care face significant medical and mental health care needs. Unfortunately, these youth rarely receive the services they need because of lack of health insurance. Through many policies and programs, the federal government has taken steps to support older youth in foster care and those aging out. The Fostering Connections to Success and Increasing Adoptions Act of 2008 (Pub L No. 110-354) requires states to work with youth to develop a transition plan that addresses issues such as health insurance. In addition, beginning in 2014, the Patient Protection and Affordable Care Act of 2010 (Pub L No. 111-148) makes youth aging out of foster care eligible for Medicaid coverage until age 26 years, regardless of income. Pediatricians can support youth aging out of foster care by working collaboratively with the child welfare agency in their state to ensure that the ongoing health needs of transitioning youth are met. (11/12)

HEALTH CARE FOR YOUTH IN THE JUVENILE JUSTICE SYSTEM
Committee on Adolescence

ABSTRACT. Youth in the juvenile correctional system are a high-risk population who, in many cases, have unmet physical, developmental, and mental health needs. Multiple studies have found that some of these health issues occur at higher rates than in the general adolescent population. Although some youth in the juvenile justice system have interfaced with health care providers in their community on a regular basis, others have had inconsistent or nonexistent care. The health needs of these youth are commonly identified when they are admitted to a juvenile custodial facility. Pediatricians and other health care providers play an important role in the care of these youth, and continuity between the community and the correctional facility is crucial. This policy statement provides an overview of the health needs of youth in the juvenile correctional system, including existing resources and standards for care, financing of health care within correctional facilities, and evidence-based interventions. Recommendations are provided for the provision of health care services to youth in the juvenile correctional system as well as specific areas for advocacy efforts. (11/11)

HEALTH EQUITY AND CHILDREN'S RIGHTS

Council on Community Pediatrics and Committee on Native American Child Health

ABSTRACT. Many children in the United States fail to reach their full health and developmental potential. Disparities in their health and well-being result from the complex interplay of multiple social and environmental determinants that are not adequately addressed by current standards of pediatric practice or public policy. Integrating the principles and practice of child health equity—children's rights, social justice, human capital investment, and health equity ethics—into pediatrics will address the root causes of child health disparities.

Promoting the principles and practice of equity-based clinical care, child advocacy, and child- and family-centered public policy will help to ensure that social and environmental determinants contribute positively to the health and well-being of children. The American Academy of Pediatrics and pediatricians can move the national focus from documenting child health disparities to advancing the principles and practice of child health equity and, in so doing, influence the worldwide practice of pediatrics and child health. All pediatricians, including primary care practitioners and medical and surgical subspecialists, can incorporate these principles into their practice of pediatrics and child health. Integration of these principles into competency-based training and board certification will secure their assimilation into all levels of pediatric practice. (3/10, reaffirmed 10/13)

HEALTH INFORMATION TECHNOLOGY AND THE MEDICAL HOME

Council on Clinical Information Technology

ABSTRACT. The American Academy of Pediatrics (AAP) supports development and universal implementation of a comprehensive electronic infrastructure to support pediatric information functions of the medical home. These functions include (1) timely and continuous management and tracking of health data and services over a patient's lifetime for all providers, patients, families, and guardians, (2) comprehensive organization and secure transfer of health data during patient-care transitions between providers, institutions, and practices, (3) establishment and maintenance of central coordination of a patient's health information among multiple repositories (including personal health records and information exchanges), (4) translation of evidence into actionable clinical decision support, and (5) reuse of archived clinical data for continuous quality improvement. The AAP supports universal, secure, and vendor-neutral portability of health information for all patients contained within the medical home across all care settings (ambulatory practices, inpatient settings, emergency departments, pharmacies, consultants, support service providers, and therapists) for multiple purposes including direct care, personal health records, public health, and registries. The AAP also supports financial incentives that promote the development of information tools that meet the needs of pediatric workflows and that appropriately recognize the added value of medical homes to pediatric care. (4/11)

HEALTH AND MENTAL HEALTH NEEDS OF CHILDREN IN US MILITARY FAMILIES (CLINICAL REPORT)

Benjamin S. Siegel, MD; Beth Ellen Davis, MD, MPH; Committee on Psychosocial Aspects of Child and Family Health; and Section on Uniformed Services

ABSTRACT. The wars in Afghanistan and Iraq have been challenging for US uniformed service families and their children. Almost 60% of US service members have family responsibilities. Approximately 2.3 million active duty, National Guard, and Reserve service members have been deployed since the beginning of the wars in Afghanistan and Iraq (2001 and 2003, respectively), and almost half have deployed more than once, some for up to 18 months' duration. Up to 2 million US children have been exposed to a wartime deployment of a loved one in the past 10 years. Many service members have returned from combat deployments with symptoms of posttraumatic stress disorder, depression, anxiety, substance abuse, and traumatic brain injury. The mental health and well-being of spouses, significant others, children (and their friends), and extended family members of deployed service members continues to be significantly challenged by the experiences of wartime deployment as well as by combat mortality and morbidity. The medical system of the Department of Defense provides health and mental health services for active duty service members and their families as well as activated National Guard and Reserve service members and their families. In addition to military pediatricians and civilian pediatricians employed by military treatment facilities, nonmilitary general pediatricians care for >50% of children and family members before, during, and after wartime deployments. This clinical report is for all pediatricians, both active duty and civilian, to aid in caring for children whose loved ones have been, are, or will be deployed. (5/13)

See full text on page 681.

HEALTH SUPERVISION FOR CHILDREN WITH ACHONDROPLASIA (CLINICAL REPORT)

Tracy L. Trotter, MD; Judith G. Hall, OC, MD; and Committee on Genetics

ABSTRACT. Achondroplasia is the most common condition associated with disproportionate short stature. Substantial information is available concerning the natural history and anticipatory health supervision needs in children with this dwarfing disorder. Most children with achondroplasia have delayed motor milestones, problems with persistent or recurrent middle-ear dysfunction, and bowing of the lower legs. Less often, infants and children may have serious health consequences related to hydrocephalus, craniocervical junction compression, upper-airway obstruction, or thoracolumbar kyphosis. Anticipatory care should be directed at identifying children who are at high risk and intervening to prevent serious sequelae. This report is designed to help the pediatrician care for children with achondroplasia and their families. (9/05, reaffirmed 5/12)

HEALTH SUPERVISION FOR CHILDREN WITH DOWN SYNDROME (CLINICAL REPORT)

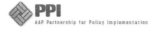

Marilyn J. Bull, MD, and Committee on Genetics

ABSTRACT. These guidelines are designed to assist the pediatrician in caring for the child in whom a diagnosis of Down syndrome has been confirmed by chromosome analysis. Although a pediatrician's initial contact with the child is usually during infancy, occasionally the pregnant woman who has been given a prenatal diagnosis of Down syndrome will be referred for review of the condition and the genetic counseling provided. Therefore, this report offers guidance for this situation as well. (7/11)

HEALTH SUPERVISION FOR CHILDREN WITH FRAGILE X SYNDROME (CLINICAL REPORT)

Joseph H. Hersh, MD; Robert A. Saul, MD; and Committee on Genetics

ABSTRACT. Fragile X syndrome (an FMR1–related disorder) is the most commonly inherited form of mental retardation. Early physical recognition is difficult, so boys with developmental delay should be strongly considered for molecular testing. The characteristic adult phenotype usually does not develop until the second decade of life. Girls can also be affected with developmental delay. Because multiple family members can be affected with mental retardation and other conditions (premature ovarian failure and tremor/ataxia), family history information is of critical importance for the diagnosis and management of affected patients and their families. This report summarizes issues for fragile X syndrome regarding clinical diagnosis, laboratory diagnosis, genetic counseling, related health problems, behavior management, and age-related health supervision guidelines. The diagnosis of fragile X syndrome not only involves the affected children but also potentially has significant health consequences for multiple generations in each family. (4/11)

HEALTH SUPERVISION FOR CHILDREN WITH MARFAN SYNDROME (CLINICAL REPORT)

Brad T. Tinkle, MD, PhD; Howard M. Saal, MD; and Committee on Genetics

ABSTRACT. Marfan syndrome is a systemic, heritable connective tissue disorder that affects many different organ systems and is best managed by using a multidisciplinary approach. The guidance in this report is designed to assist the pediatrician in recognizing the features of Marfan syndrome as well as caring for the individual with this disorder. (9/13)

See full text on page 697.

HEALTH SUPERVISION FOR CHILDREN WITH NEUROFIBROMATOSIS (CLINICAL REPORT)

Joseph H. Hersh, MD, and Committee on Genetics

ABSTRACT. Neurofibromatosis 1 is a multisystem disorder that primarily involves the skin and nervous system. Its population prevalence is 1 in 3500. The condition usually is recognized in early childhood, when cutaneous manifestations are apparent. Although neurofibromatosis 1 is associated with marked clinical variability, most affected children do well from the standpoint of their growth and development. Some features of neurofibromatosis 1 are present at birth, and others are age-related abnormalities of tissue proliferation, which necessitate periodic monitoring to address ongoing health and developmental needs and to minimize the risk of serious medical complications. This clinical report provides a review of the clinical criteria needed to establish a diagnosis, the inheritance pattern of neurofibromatosis 1, its major clinical and developmental manifestations, and guidelines for monitoring and providing intervention to maximize the growth, development, and health of an affected child. (3/08)

HEALTH SUPERVISION FOR CHILDREN WITH PRADER-WILLI SYNDROME (CLINICAL REPORT)

Shawn E. McCandless, MD, and Committee on Genetics

ABSTRACT. This set of guidelines was designed to assist the pediatrician in caring for children with Prader-Willi syndrome diagnosed by clinical features and confirmed by molecular testing. Prader-Willi syndrome provides an excellent example of how early diagnosis and management can improve the long-term outcome for some genetic disorders. (12/10)

HEALTH SUPERVISION FOR CHILDREN WITH SICKLE CELL DISEASE

Section on Hematology/Oncology and Committee on Genetics

ABSTRACT. Sickle cell disease (SCD) is a group of complex genetic disorders with multisystem manifestations. This statement provides pediatricians in primary care and subspecialty practice with an overview of the genetics, diagnosis, clinical manifestations, and treatment of SCD. Specialized comprehensive medical care decreases morbidity and mortality during childhood. The provision of comprehensive care is a time-intensive endeavor that includes ongoing patient and family education, periodic comprehensive evaluations and other disease-specific health maintenance services, psychosocial care, and genetic counseling. Timely and appropriate treatment of acute illness is critical, because life-threatening complications develop rapidly. It is essential that every child with SCD receive comprehensive care that is coordinated through a medical home with appropriate expertise. (3/02, reaffirmed 1/06, 1/11)

HEARING ASSESSMENT IN INFANTS AND CHILDREN: RECOMMENDATIONS BEYOND NEONATAL SCREENING (CLINICAL REPORT)

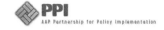

Allen D. "Buz" Harlor Jr, MD; Charles Bower, MD;
Committee on Practice and Ambulatory Medicine; and
Section on Otolaryngology–Head and Neck Surgery

ABSTRACT. Congenital or acquired hearing loss in infants and children has been linked with lifelong deficits in speech and language acquisition, poor academic performance, personal-social maladjustments, and emotional difficulties. Identification of hearing loss through neonatal hearing screening, regular surveillance of developmental milestones, auditory skills, parental concerns, and middle-ear status and objective hearing screening of all infants and children at critical developmental stages can prevent or reduce many of these adverse consequences. This report promotes a proactive, consistent, and explicit process for the early identification of children with hearing loss in the medical home. An algorithm of the recommended approach has been developed to assist in the detection and documentation of, and intervention for, hearing loss. (9/09)

HELPING CHILDREN AND FAMILIES DEAL WITH DIVORCE AND SEPARATION (CLINICAL REPORT)

Committee on Psychosocial Aspects of Child and Family Health

ABSTRACT. More than 1 million children each year experience their parents' divorce. For these children and their parents, this process can be emotionally traumatic from the beginning of parental disagreement and rancor, through the divorce, and often for many years thereafter. Pediatricians are encouraged to be aware of behavioral changes in their patients that might be signals of family dysfunction so they can help parents and children understand and deal more positively with the issue. Age-appropriate explanation and counseling is important so children realize that they are not the cause of, and cannot be the cure for, the divorce. Pediatricians can offer families guidance in dealing with their children through the troubled time as well as appropriate lists of reading material and, if indicated, can refer them to professionals with expertise in the emotional, social, and legal aspects of divorce and its aftermath. (11/02, reaffirmed 1/06)

HIGH-DEDUCTIBLE HEALTH PLANS AND THE NEW RISKS OF CONSUMER-DRIVEN HEALTH INSURANCE PRODUCTS

Committee on Child Health Financing

ABSTRACT. Consumer-driven health care is the most noteworthy development in health insurance since the widespread adoption of health maintenance organizations and preferred provider organizations in the 1980s. The most common consumer-driven health plan is the high-deductible health plan, which is essentially a catastrophic health insurance plan, often linked with tax-advantaged spending accounts, with very high deductibles, fewer benefits, and higher cost-sharing than conventional health maintenance organization or preferred provider organization plans. The financial risks are significant under high-deductible health plans, especially for low- to moderate-income families and for families whose children have special health care needs. Of concern for pediatricians are the potential quality risks that are predictable in high-deductible health plans, in which families are likely to delay or avoid seeking care, especially preventive care (if it is not exempted from the deductible), when they are faced with paying for care before the deductible is met. This policy statement provides background information on the most common consumer-driven health plan model, discusses the implications for pediatricians and families, and offers recommendations pertaining to health plan product design, education, practice administration, and research. (3/07)

HIV TESTING AND PROPHYLAXIS TO PREVENT MOTHER-TO-CHILD TRANSMISSION IN THE UNITED STATES

Committee on Pediatric AIDS

ABSTRACT. Universal HIV testing of pregnant women in the United States is the key to prevention of mother-to-child transmission of HIV. Repeat testing in the third trimester and rapid HIV testing at labor and delivery are additional strategies to further reduce the rate of perinatal HIV transmission. Prevention of mother-to-child transmission of HIV is most effective when antiretroviral drugs are received by the mother during her pregnancy and continued through delivery and then administered to the infant after birth. Antiretroviral drugs are effective in reducing the risk of mother-to-child transmission of HIV even when prophylaxis is started for the infant soon after birth. New rapid testing methods allow identification of HIV-infected women or HIV-exposed infants in 20 to 60 minutes. The American Academy of Pediatrics recommends documented, routine HIV testing for all pregnant women in the United States after notifying the patient that testing will be performed, unless the patient declines HIV testing ("opt-out" consent or "right of refusal"). For women in labor with undocumented HIV-infection status during the current pregnancy, immediate maternal HIV testing with opt-out consent, using a rapid HIV antibody test, is recommended. Positive HIV antibody screening test results should be confirmed with immunofluorescent antibody or Western blot assay. For women with a positive rapid HIV antibody test result, antiretroviral prophylaxis should be administered promptly to the mother and newborn infant on the basis of the positive result of the rapid antibody test without waiting for results of confirmatory HIV testing. If the confirmatory test result is negative, then prophylaxis should be discontinued. For a newborn infant whose mother's HIV serostatus is unknown, the health care professional should perform rapid HIV antibody testing on the mother or on the newborn infant, with results reported to the health care professional no later than 12 hours after the infant's birth. If the rapid HIV antibody test result is positive, antiretroviral prophylaxis should be instituted as soon as possible after birth but certainly by 12 hours after delivery, pending completion of confirmatory HIV testing. The mother should be counseled not to breastfeed the infant. Assistance with immediate initiation of hand and pump expression to stimulate milk production should be offered to the mother, given the possibility that the confirmatory test result may be negative. If the confirmatory test result is negative, then prophylaxis should be stopped and breastfeeding may be initiated. If the confirmatory test result is positive, infants should receive antiretroviral prophylaxis for 6 weeks after birth, and the mother should not breastfeed the infant. (11/08, reaffirmed 6/11)

HOME CARE OF CHILDREN AND YOUTH WITH COMPLEX HEALTH CARE NEEDS AND TECHNOLOGY DEPENDENCIES (CLINICAL REPORT)
Ellen Roy Elias, MD; Nancy A. Murphy, MD; and Council on Children With Disabilities

ABSTRACT. Children and youth with complex medical issues, especially those with technology dependencies, experience frequent and often lengthy hospitalizations. Hospital discharges for these children can be a complicated process that requires a deliberate, multistep approach. In addition to successful discharges to home, it is essential that pediatric providers develop and implement an interdisciplinary and coordinated plan of care that addresses the child's ongoing health care needs. The goal is to ensure that each child remains healthy, thrives, and obtains optimal medical home and developmental supports that promote ongoing care at home and minimize recurrent hospitalizations. This clinical report presents an approach to discharging the child with complex medical needs with technology dependencies from hospital to home and then continually addressing the needs of the child and family in the home environment. (4/12)

HOME, HOSPITAL, AND OTHER NON–SCHOOL-BASED INSTRUCTION FOR CHILDREN AND ADOLESCENTS WHO ARE MEDICALLY UNABLE TO ATTEND SCHOOL
Committee on School Health

ABSTRACT. The American Academy of Pediatrics recommends that school-aged children and adolescents obtain their education in school in the least restrictive setting, that is, the setting most conducive to learning for the particular student. However, at times, acute illness or injury and chronic medical conditions preclude school attendance. This statement is meant to assist evaluation and planning for children to receive non–school-based instruction and to return to school at the earliest possible date. (11/00, reaffirmed 6/03, 5/06)

HONORING DO-NOT-ATTEMPT-RESUSCITATION REQUESTS IN SCHOOLS
Council on School Health and Committee on Bioethics

ABSTRACT. Increasingly, children and adolescents with complex chronic conditions are living in the community. Federal legislation and regulations facilitate their participation in school. Some of these children and adolescents and their families may wish to forego life-sustaining medical treatment, including cardiopulmonary resuscitation, because they would be ineffective or because the risks outweigh the benefits. Honoring these requests in the school environment is complex because of the limited availability of school nurses and the frequent lack of supporting state legislation and regulations. Understanding and collaboration on the part of all parties is essential. Pediatricians have an important role in helping school nurses incorporate a specific action plan into the student's individualized health care plan. The action plan should include both communication and comfort-care plans. Pediatricians who work directly with schools can also help implement policies, and professional organizations can advocate for regulations and legislation that enable students and their families to effectuate their preferences. (4/10, reaffirmed 7/13)

HOSPITAL DISCHARGE OF THE HIGH-RISK NEONATE
Committee on Fetus and Newborn

ABSTRACT. This policy statement updates the guidelines on discharge of the high-risk neonate first published by the American Academy of Pediatrics in 1998. As with the earlier document, this statement is based, insofar as possible, on published, scientifically derived information. This updated statement incorporates new knowledge about risks and medical care of the high-risk neonate, the timing of discharge, and planning for care after discharge. It also refers to other American Academy of Pediatrics publications that are relevant to these issues. This statement draws on the previous classification of high-risk infants into 4 categories: (1) the preterm infant; (2) the infant with special health care needs or dependence on technology; (3) the infant at risk because of family issues; and (4) the infant with anticipated early death. The issues of deciding when discharge is appropriate, defining the specific needs for follow-up care, and the process of detailed discharge planning are addressed as they apply in general to all 4 categories; in addition, special attention is directed to the particular issues presented by the 4 individual categories. Recommendations are given to aid in deciding when discharge is appropriate and to ensure that all necessary care will be available and well coordinated after discharge. The need for individualized planning and physician judgment is emphasized. (11/08, reaffirmed 5/11)

THE HOSPITAL RECORD OF THE INJURED CHILD AND THE NEED FOR EXTERNAL CAUSE-OF-INJURY CODES
Committee on Injury and Poison Prevention

ABSTRACT. Proper record-keeping of emergency department visits and hospitalizations of injured children is vital for appropriate patient management. Determination and documentation of the circumstances surrounding the injury event are essential. This information not only is the basis for preventive counseling, but also provides clues about how similar injuries in other youth can be avoided. The hospital records have an important secondary purpose; namely, if sufficient information about the cause and mechanism of injury is documented, it can be subsequently coded, electronically compiled, and retrieved later to provide an epidemiologic profile of the injury, the first step in prevention at the population level. To be of greatest use, hospital records should indicate the "who, what, when, where, why, and how" of the injury occurrence and whether protective equipment (eg, a seat belt) was used. The pediatrician has two important roles in this area: to document fully the injury event and to advocate the use of standardized external cause-of-injury codes, which allow such data to be compiled and analyzed. (2/99, reaffirmed 5/02, 5/05, 10/08)

HOSPITAL STAY FOR HEALTHY TERM NEWBORNS
Committee on Fetus and Newborn

ABSTRACT. The hospital stay of the mother and her healthy term newborn infant should be long enough to allow identification of early problems and to ensure that the family is able and prepared to care for the infant at home. The length of stay should also accommodate the unique characteristics of each mother-infant dyad, including the health of the mother, the health and stability of the infant, the ability and confidence of the mother to care for her infant, the adequacy of support systems at home, and access to appropriate follow-up care. Input from the mother and her obstetrician should be considered before a decision to discharge a newborn is made, and all efforts should be made to keep mothers and infants together to promote simultaneous discharge. (1/10)

HPV VACCINE RECOMMENDATIONS
Committee on Infectious Diseases
ABSTRACT. On October 25, 2011, the Advisory Committee on Immunization Practices of the Centers for Disease Control and Prevention recommended that the quadrivalent human papillomavirus vaccine (Gardasil; Merck & Co, Inc, Whitehouse Station, NJ) be used routinely in males. The American Academy of Pediatrics has reviewed updated data provided by the Advisory Committee on Immunization Practices on vaccine efficacy, safety, and cost-effectiveness as well as programmatic considerations and supports this recommendation. This revised statement updates recommendations for human papillomavirus immunization of both males and females. (2/12)

HUMAN EMBRYONIC STEM CELL (HESC) AND HUMAN EMBRYO RESEARCH
Committee on Pediatric Research and Committee on Bioethics
ABSTRACT. Human embryonic stem cell research has emerged as an important platform for the understanding and treatment of pediatric diseases. From its inception, however, it has raised ethical concerns based not on the use of stem cells themselves but on objections to the source of the cells—specifically, the destruction of preimplantation human embryos. Despite differences in public opinion on this issue, a large majority of the public supports continued research using embryonic stem cells. Given the possible substantial benefit of stem cell research on child health and development, the American Academy of Pediatrics believes that funding and oversight for human embryo and embryonic stem cell research should continue. (10/12)

HUMAN IMMUNODEFICIENCY VIRUS AND OTHER BLOOD-BORNE VIRAL PATHOGENS IN THE ATHLETIC SETTING
Committee on Sports Medicine and Fitness
ABSTRACT. Because athletes and the staff of athletic programs can be exposed to blood during athletic activity, they have a very small risk of becoming infected with human immunodeficiency virus, hepatitis B virus, or hepatitis C virus. This statement, which updates a previous position statement of the American Academy of Pediatrics, discusses sports participation for athletes infected with these pathogens and the precautions needed to reduce the risk of infection to others in the athletic setting. Each of the recommendations in this statement is dependent upon and intended to be considered with reference to the other recommendations in this statement and not in isolation. (12/99, reaffirmed 1/05, 1/09, 11/11)

HUMAN IMMUNODEFICIENCY VIRUS SCREENING
Committee on Fetus and Newborn and Committee on Pediatric AIDS (joint with American College of Obstetricians and Gynecologists) (7/99, reaffirmed 6/02, 5/05, 10/08, 5/12)

HUMAN MILK, BREASTFEEDING, AND TRANSMISSION OF HUMAN IMMUNODEFICIENCY VIRUS IN THE UNITED STATES
Committee on Pediatric AIDS (11/95, reaffirmed 11/99, 11/03, 2/08)

HUMAN MILK, BREASTFEEDING, AND TRANSMISSION OF HUMAN IMMUNODEFICIENCY VIRUS TYPE 1 IN THE UNITED STATES (TECHNICAL REPORT)
Committee on Pediatric AIDS
ABSTRACT. Transmission of human immunodeficiency virus type 1 (HIV-1) through breastfeeding has been conclusively demonstrated. The risk of such transmission has been quantified, the timing has been clarified, and certain risk factors for breastfeeding transmission have been identified. In areas where infant formula is accessible, affordable, safe, and sustainable, avoidance of breastfeeding has represented one of the main components of mother-to-child HIV-1 transmission prevention efforts for many years. In areas where affordable and safe alternatives to breastfeeding may not be available, interventions to prevent breastfeeding transmission are being investigated. Complete avoidance of breastfeeding by HIV-1-infected women has been recommended by the American Academy of Pediatrics and the Centers for Disease Control and Prevention and remains the only means by which prevention of breastfeeding transmission of HIV-1 can be absolutely ensured. This technical report summarizes the information available regarding breastfeeding transmission of HIV-1. (11/03, reaffirmed 1/07)

IDENTIFICATION AND CARE OF HIV-EXPOSED AND HIV-INFECTED INFANTS, CHILDREN, AND ADOLESCENTS IN FOSTER CARE
Committee on Pediatric AIDS
ABSTRACT. As a consequence of the expanding human immunodeficiency virus (HIV) epidemic and major advances in medical management of HIV-exposed and HIV-infected persons, revised recommendations are provided for HIV testing of infants, children, and adolescents in foster care. Updated recommendations also are provided for the care of HIV-exposed and HIV-infected persons who are in foster care. (7/00, reaffirmed 3/03, 2/08, 6/11)

IDENTIFICATION AND EVALUATION OF CHILDREN WITH AUTISM SPECTRUM DISORDERS (CLINICAL REPORT)

PPI
AAP Partnership for Policy Implementation

Chris Plauché Johnson, MD, MEd; Scott M. Myers, MD; and Council on Children With Disabilities
ABSTRACT. Autism spectrum disorders are not rare; many primary care pediatricians care for several children with autism spectrum disorders. Pediatricians play an important role in early recognition of autism spectrum disorders, because they usually are the first point of contact for parents. Parents are now much more aware of

the early signs of autism spectrum disorders because of frequent coverage in the media; if their child demonstrates any of the published signs, they will most likely raise their concerns to their child's pediatrician. It is important that pediatricians be able to recognize the signs and symptoms of autism spectrum disorders and have a strategy for assessing them systematically. Pediatricians also must be aware of local resources that can assist in making a definitive diagnosis of, and in managing, autism spectrum disorders. The pediatrician must be familiar with developmental, educational, and community resources as well as medical subspecialty clinics. This clinical report is 1 of 2 documents that replace the original American Academy of Pediatrics policy statement and technical report published in 2001. This report addresses background information, including definition, history, epidemiology, diagnostic criteria, early signs, neuropathologic aspects, and etiologic possibilities in autism spectrum disorders. In addition, this report provides an algorithm to help the pediatrician develop a strategy for early identification of children with autism spectrum disorders. The accompanying clinical report addresses the management of children with autism spectrum disorders and follows this report on page 1162 [available at www.pediatrics. org/cgi/content/full/120/5/1162]. Both clinical reports are complemented by the toolkit titled *Autism: Caring for Children With Autism Spectrum Disorders: A Resource Toolkit for Clinicians,* which contains screening and surveillance tools, practical forms, tables, and parent handouts to assist the pediatrician in the identification, evaluation, and management of autism spectrum disorders in children. (11/07, reaffirmed 9/10)

IDENTIFICATION AND MANAGEMENT OF EATING DISORDERS IN CHILDREN AND ADOLESCENTS (CLINICAL REPORT)

David S. Rosen, MD, MPH, and Committee on Adolescence

ABSTRACT. The incidence and prevalence of eating disorders in children and adolescents has increased significantly in recent decades, making it essential for pediatricians to consider these disorders in appropriate clinical settings, to evaluate patients suspected of having these disorders, and to manage (or refer) patients in whom eating disorders are diagnosed. This clinical report includes a discussion of diagnostic criteria and outlines the initial evaluation of the patient with disordered eating. Medical complications of eating disorders may affect any organ system, and careful monitoring for these complications is required. The range of treatment options, including pharmacotherapy, is described in this report. Pediatricians are encouraged to advocate for legislation and policies that ensure appropriate services for patients with eating disorders, including medical care, nutritional intervention, mental health treatment, and care coordination. (11/10)

IDENTIFYING INFANTS AND YOUNG CHILDREN WITH DEVELOPMENTAL DISORDERS IN THE MEDICAL HOME: AN ALGORITHM FOR DEVELOPMENTAL SURVEILLANCE AND SCREENING

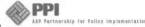

Council on Children With Disabilities, Section on Developmental and Behavioral Pediatrics, Bright Futures Steering Committee, and Medical Home Initiatives for Children With Special Needs Project Advisory Committee

ABSTRACT. Early identification of developmental disorders is critical to the well-being of children and their families. It is an integral function of the primary care medical home and an appropriate responsibility of all pediatric health care professionals. This statement provides an algorithm as a strategy to support health care professionals in developing a pattern and practice for addressing developmental concerns in children from birth through 3 years of age. The authors recommend that developmental surveillance be incorporated at every well-child preventive care visit. Any concerns raised during surveillance should be promptly addressed with standardized developmental screening tests. In addition, screening tests should be administered regularly at the 9-, 18-, and 30-month visits. (Because the 30-month visit is not yet a part of the preventive care system and is often not reimbursable by third-party payers at this time, developmental screening can be performed at 24 months of age. In addition, because the frequency of regular pediatric visits decreases after 24 months of age, a pediatrician who expects that his or her patients will have difficulty attending a 30-month visit should conduct screening during the 24-month visit.) The early identification of developmental problems should lead to further developmental and medical evaluation, diagnosis, and treatment, including early developmental intervention. Children diagnosed with developmental disorders should be identified as children with special health care needs, and chronic-condition management should be initiated. Identification of a developmental disorder and its underlying etiology may also drive a range of treatment planning, from medical treatment of the child to family planning for his or her parents. (7/06, reaffirmed 12/09)

IMMUNIZATION INFORMATION SYSTEMS

Committee on Practice and Ambulatory Medicine

ABSTRACT. The American Academy of Pediatrics continues to support the development and implementation of immunization information systems, previously referred to as immunization registries, and other systems for the benefit of children, pediatricians, and their communities. Pediatricians and others must be aware of the value that immunization information systems have for society, the potential fiscal influences on their practice, the costs and benefits, and areas for future improvement. (9/06, reaffirmed 10/11)

IMMUNIZING PARENTS AND OTHER CLOSE FAMILY CONTACTS IN THE PEDIATRIC OFFICE SETTING (TECHNICAL REPORT)

Herschel R. Lessin, MD; Kathryn M. Edwards, MD;
Committee on Practice and Ambulatory Medicine; and
Committee on Infectious Diseases

ABSTRACT. Additional strategies are needed to protect children from vaccine-preventable diseases. In particular, very young infants, as well as children who are immuno-compromised, are at especially high risk for developing the serious consequences of vaccine-preventable diseases and cannot be immunized completely. There is some evidence that children who become infected with these diseases are exposed to pathogens through household contacts, particularly from parents or other close family contacts. Such infections likely are attributable to adults who are not fully protected from these diseases, either because their immunity to vaccine-preventable diseases has waned over time or because they have not received a vaccine. There are many challenges that have added to low adult immunization rates in the United States. One option to increase immunization coverage for parents and close family contacts of infants and vulnerable children is to provide alternative locations for these adults to be immunized, such as the pediatric office setting. Ideally, adults should receive immunizations in their medical homes; however, to provide greater protection to these adults and reduce the exposure of children to pathogens, immunizing parents or other adult family contacts in the pediatric office setting could increase immunization coverage for this population to protect themselves as well as children to whom they provide care. (12/11)

IMPACT OF MUSIC, MUSIC LYRICS, AND MUSIC VIDEOS ON CHILDREN AND YOUTH

Council on Communications and Media

ABSTRACT. Music plays an important role in the socialization of children and adolescents. Popular music is present almost everywhere, and it is easily available through the radio, various recordings, the Internet, and new technologies, allowing adolescents to hear it in diverse settings and situations, alone or shared with friends. Parents often are unaware of the lyrics to which their children are listening because of the increasing use of downloaded music and headphones. Research on popular music has explored its effects on schoolwork, social interactions, mood and affect, and particularly behavior. The effect that popular music has on children's and adolescents' behavior and emotions is of paramount concern. Lyrics have become more explicit in their references to drugs, sex, and violence over the years, particularly in certain genres. A teenager's preference for certain types of music could be correlated or associated with certain behaviors. As with popular music, the perception and the effect of music-video messages are important, because research has reported that exposure to violence, sexual messages, sexual stereotypes, and use of substances of abuse in music videos might produce significant changes in behaviors and attitudes of young viewers. Pediatricians and parents should be aware of this information. Furthermore, with the evidence portrayed in these studies, it is essential for pediatricians and parents to take a stand regarding music lyrics. (10/09)

THE IMPACT OF SOCIAL MEDIA ON CHILDREN, ADOLESCENTS, AND FAMILIES (CLINICAL REPORT)

Gwenn Schurgin O'Keeffe, MD; Kathleen Clarke-Pearson,
MD; and Council on Communications and Media

ABSTRACT. Using social media Web sites is among the most common activity of today's children and adolescents. Any Web site that allows social interaction is considered a social media site, including social networking sites such as Facebook, MySpace, and Twitter; gaming sites and virtual worlds such as Club Penguin, Second Life, and the Sims; video sites such as YouTube; and blogs. Such sites offer today's youth a portal for entertainment and communication and have grown exponentially in recent years. For this reason, it is important that parents become aware of the nature of social media sites, given that not all of them are healthy environments for children and adolescents. Pediatricians are in a unique position to help families understand these sites and to encourage healthy use and urge parents to monitor for potential problems with cyberbullying, "Facebook depression," sexting, and exposure to inappropriate content. (3/11)

IMPLEMENTATION PRINCIPLES AND STRATEGIES FOR THE STATE CHILDREN'S HEALTH INSURANCE PROGRAM

Committee on Child Health Financing

ABSTRACT. This policy statement presents principles and implementation and evaluation strategies recommended for the State Children's Health Insurance Program (SCHIP). The statement summarizes the current status of SCHIP, the needs of uninsured children, and the potential benefits of SCHIP programs. Principles and recommended strategies include expanding eligibility, maximizing funding, providing comprehensive benefits, including pediatricians in program design and evaluation, providing adequate reimbursement and access to pediatricians, ensuring choices for families and pediatricians, and establishing simple administrative procedures. (5/01)

THE IMPORTANCE OF PLAY IN PROMOTING HEALTHY CHILD DEVELOPMENT AND MAINTAINING STRONG PARENT-CHILD BONDS (CLINICAL REPORT)

Kenneth R. Ginsburg, MD, MSEd; Committee on
Communications; and Committee on Psychosocial Aspects
of Child and Family Health

ABSTRACT. Play is essential to development because it contributes to the cognitive, physical, social, and emotional well-being of children and youth. Play also offers an ideal opportunity for parents to engage fully with their children. Despite the benefits derived from play for both children and parents, time for free play has been markedly reduced for some children. This report addresses a variety of factors that have reduced play, including a hurried lifestyle, changes in family structure, and increased attention to academics and enrichment activities at the expense of recess or free child-centered play. This report offers guidelines on how pediatricians can advocate for children by helping families, school systems, and communities consider how best to ensure that play is protected as they seek the balance in children's lives to create the optimal developmental milieu. (1/07)

THE IMPORTANCE OF PLAY IN PROMOTING HEALTHY CHILD DEVELOPMENT AND MAINTAINING STRONG PARENT-CHILD BOND: FOCUS ON CHILDREN IN POVERTY (CLINICAL REPORT)

Regina M. Milteer, MD; Kenneth R. Ginsburg, MD, MSEd; Council on Communications and Media; and Committee on Psychosocial Aspects of Child and Family Health

ABSTRACT. Play is essential to the social, emotional, cognitive, and physical well-being of children beginning in early childhood. It is a natural tool for children to develop resiliency as they learn to cooperate, overcome challenges, and negotiate with others. Play also allows children to be creative. It provides time for parents to be fully engaged with their children, to bond with their children, and to see the world from the perspective of their child. However, children who live in poverty often face socioeconomic obstacles that impede their rights to have playtime, thus affecting their healthy social-emotional development. For children who are underresourced to reach their highest potential, it is essential that parents, educators, and pediatricians recognize the importance of lifelong benefits that children gain from play. (12/11)

IMPROVING SUBSTANCE ABUSE PREVENTION, ASSESSMENT, AND TREATMENT FINANCING FOR CHILDREN AND ADOLESCENTS

Committee on Child Health Financing and Committee on Substance Abuse

ABSTRACT. The numbers of children, adolescents, and families affected by substance abuse have sharply increased since the early 1990s. The American Academy of Pediatrics recognizes the scope and urgency of this problem and has developed this policy statement for consideration by Congress, federal and state agencies, employers, national organizations, health care professionals, health insurers, managed care organizations, advocacy groups, and families. (10/01)

THE INAPPROPRIATE USE OF SCHOOL "READINESS" TESTS

Committee on Early Childhood, Adoption, and Dependent Care and Committee on School Health (3/95, reaffirmed 4/98, 1/04, 4/10)

INCORPORATING RECOGNITION AND MANAGEMENT OF PERINATAL AND POSTPARTUM DEPRESSION INTO PEDIATRIC PRACTICE (CLINICAL REPORT)

Marian F. Earls, MD, and Committee on Psychosocial Aspects of Child and Family Health

ABSTRACT. Every year, more than 400 000 infants are born to mothers who are depressed, which makes perinatal depression the most underdiagnosed obstetric complication in America. Postpartum depression leads to increased costs of medical care, inappropriate medical care, child abuse and neglect, discontinuation of breastfeeding, and family dysfunction and adversely affects early brain development. Pediatric practices, as medical homes, can establish a system to implement postpartum depression screening and to identify and use community resources for the treatment and referral of the depressed mother and support for the mother-child (dyad) relationship. This system would have a positive effect on the health and well-being of the infant and family. State chapters of the American Academy of Pediatrics, working with state Early Periodic Screening, Diagnosis, and Treatment (EPSDT) and maternal and child health programs, can increase awareness of the need for perinatal depression screening in the obstetric and pediatric periodicity of care schedules and ensure payment. Pediatricians must advocate for workforce development for professionals who care for very young children and for promotion of evidence-based interventions focused on healthy attachment and parent-child relationships. (10/10)

INCREASING ANTIRETROVIRAL DRUG ACCESS FOR CHILDREN WITH HIV INFECTION

Committee on Pediatric AIDS and Section on International Child Health

ABSTRACT. Although there have been great gains in the prevention of pediatric HIV infection and provision of antiretroviral therapy for children with HIV infection in resource-rich countries, many barriers remain to scaling up HIV prevention and treatment for children in resource-limited areas of the world. Appropriate testing technologies need to be made more widely available to identify HIV infection in infants. Training of practitioners in the skills required to care for children with HIV infection is required to increase the number of children receiving antiretroviral therapy. Lack of availability of appropriate antiretroviral drug formulations that are easily usable and inexpensive is a major impediment to optimal care for children with HIV. The time and energy spent trying to develop liquid antiretroviral formulations might be better used in the manufacture of smaller pill sizes or crushable tablets, which are easier to dispense, transport, store, and administer to children. (4/07, reaffirmed 4/10)

INCREASING IMMUNIZATION COVERAGE

Committee on Practice and Ambulatory Medicine and Council on Community Pediatrics

ABSTRACT. In 1977, the American Academy of Pediatrics issued a statement calling for universal immunization of all children for whom vaccines are not contraindicated. In 1995, the policy statement "Implementation of the Immunization Policy" was published by the American Academy of Pediatrics, followed in 2003 with publication of the first version of this statement, "Increasing Immunization Coverage." Since 2003, there have continued to be improvements in immunization coverage, with progress toward meeting the goals set forth in *Healthy People 2010*. Data from the 2007 National Immunization Survey showed that 90% of children 19 to 35 months of age have received recommended doses of each of the following vaccines: inactivated poliovirus (IPV), measles-mumps-rubella (MMR), varicella-zoster virus (VZB), hepatitis B virus (HBV), and *Haemophilus influenzae* type b (Hib). For diphtheria and tetanus and acellular pertussis (DTaP) vaccine, 84.5% have received the recommended 4 doses by 35 months of age. Nevertheless, the *Healthy People 2010* goal of at least 80% coverage for the full series (at least 4 doses of DTaP, 3 doses of IPV, 1 dose of MMR, 3 doses of Hib, 3 doses of HBV, and 1 dose of varicella-zoster virus vaccine) has not yet been met, and immunization coverage of adolescents continues to lag behind the goals set forth in *Healthy People 2010*. Despite these encouraging data, a vast number of new challenges that threaten continued success toward the goal of universal immunization coverage have emerged. These challenges include an increase in new vaccines and new vaccine combinations as well as a significant number of vaccines currently under development; a dramatic increase in the acquisition cost of vaccines, coupled with a lack of adequate payment to practitioners to buy and administer vaccines; unanticipated manufacturing and delivery problems that have caused significant shortages of various vaccine products; and the rise of a public antivaccination movement that uses the Internet as well as standard media outlets to advance a position, wholly unsupported by any scientific evidence, linking vaccines with various childhood conditions, particularly autism. Much remains to be accomplished by physician organizations; vaccine manufacturers; third-party payers; the media; and local, state, and federal governments to ensure dependable vaccine supply and payments that are sufficient to continue to provide immunizations in public and private settings and to promote effective strategies to combat unjustified misstatements by the antivaccination movement.

Pediatricians should work individually and collectively at the local, state, and national levels to ensure that all children without a valid contraindication receive all childhood immunizations on time. Pediatricians and pediatric organizations, in conjunction with government agencies such as the Centers for Disease Control and Prevention, must communicate effectively with parents to maximize their understanding of the overall safety and efficacy of vaccines. Most parents and children have not experienced many of the vaccine-preventable diseases, and the general public is not well informed about the risks and sequelae of these conditions. A number of recommendations are included for pediatricians, individually and collectively, to support further progress toward the goal of universal immunization coverage of all children for whom vaccines are not contraindicated. (5/10)

INDICATIONS FOR MANAGEMENT AND REFERRAL OF PATIENTS INVOLVED IN SUBSTANCE ABUSE
Committee on Substance Abuse
ABSTRACT. This statement addresses the challenge of evaluating and managing the various stages of substance use by children and adolescents in the context of pediatric practice. Approaches are suggested that would assist the pediatrician in differentiating highly prevalent experimental and occasional use from more severe use with adverse consequences that affect emotional, behavioral, educational, or physical health. Comorbid psychiatric conditions are common and should be evaluated and treated simultaneously by child and adolescent mental health specialists. Guidelines for referral based on severity of involvement using established patient treatment-matching criteria are outlined. Pediatricians need to become familiar with treatment professionals and facilities in their communities and to ensure that treatment for adolescent patients is appropriate based on their developmental, psychosocial, medical, and mental health needs. The family should be encouraged to participate actively in the treatment process. (7/00)

INFANT FEEDING AND TRANSMISSION OF HUMAN IMMUNODEFICIENCY VIRUS IN THE UNITED STATES
Committee on Pediatric AIDS
ABSTRACT. Physicians caring for infants born to women infected with HIV are likely to be involved in providing guidance to HIV-infected mothers on appropriate infant feeding practices. It is critical that physicians are aware of the HIV transmission risk from human milk and the current recommendations for feeding HIV-exposed infants in the United States. Because the only intervention to completely prevent HIV transmission via human milk is not to breastfeed, in the United States, where clean water and affordable replacement feeding are available, the American Academy of Pediatrics recommends that HIV-infected mothers not breastfeed their infants, regardless of maternal viral load and antiretroviral therapy. (1/13)
See full text on page 713.

INFANT METHEMOGLOBINEMIA: THE ROLE OF DIETARY NITRATE IN FOOD AND WATER (CLINICAL REPORT)
Frank R. Greer, MD; Michael Shannon, MD; Committee on Nutrition; and Committee on Environmental Health
ABSTRACT. Infants for whom formula may be prepared with well water remain a high-risk group for nitrate poisoning. This clinical report reinforces the need for testing of well water for nitrate content. There seems to be little or no risk of nitrate poisoning from commercially prepared infant foods in the United States. However, reports of nitrate poisoning from home-prepared vegetable foods for infants continue to occur. Breastfeeding infants are not at risk of methemoglobinemia even when mothers ingest water with very high concentrations of nitrate nitrogen (100 ppm). (9/05, reaffirmed 4/09)

INFECTION PREVENTION AND CONTROL IN PEDIATRIC AMBULATORY SETTINGS
Committee on Infectious Diseases
ABSTRACT. Since the American Academy of Pediatrics published a statement titled "Infection Control in Physicians' Offices" (*Pediatrics.* 2000;105[6]:1361–1369), there have been significant changes that prompted this updated statement. Infection prevention and control is an integral part of pediatric practice in ambulatory medical settings as well as in hospitals. Infection prevention and control practices should begin at the time the ambulatory visit is scheduled. All health care personnel should be educated regarding the routes of transmission and techniques used to prevent transmission of infectious agents. Policies for infection prevention and control should be written, readily available, updated annually, and enforced. The standard precautions for hospitalized patients from the Centers for Disease Control and Prevention, with a modification from the American Academy of Pediatrics exempting the use of gloves for routine diaper changes and wiping a well child's nose or tears, are appropriate for most patient encounters. As employers, pediatricians are required by the Occupational Safety and Health Administration to take precautions to identify and protect employees who are likely to be exposed to blood or other potentially infectious materials while on the job. Key principles of standard precautions include hand hygiene

(ie, use of alcohol-based hand rub or hand-washing with soap [plain or antimicrobial] and water) before and after every patient contact; implementation of respiratory hygiene and cough-etiquette strategies for patients with suspected influenza or infection with another respiratory tract pathogen to the extent feasible; separation of infected, contagious children from uninfected children when feasible; safe handling and disposal of needles and other sharp medical devices and evaluation and implementation of needle-safety devices; appropriate use of personal protective equipment such as gloves, gowns, masks, and eye protection; and appropriate sterilization, disinfection, and antisepsis. (9/07, reaffirmed 8/10)

INFORMED CONSENT, PARENTAL PERMISSION, AND ASSENT IN PEDIATRIC PRACTICE
Committee on Bioethics (2/95, reaffirmed 11/98, 11/02, 10/06, 5/11)

INHALANT ABUSE (CLINICAL REPORT)
Janet F. Williams, MD; Michael Storck, MD; Committee on Substance Abuse; and Committee on Native American Child Health
ABSTRACT. Inhalant abuse is the intentional inhalation of a volatile substance for the purpose of achieving an altered mental state. As an important, yet-underrecognized form of substance abuse, inhalant abuse crosses all demographic, ethnic, and socioeconomic boundaries, causing significant morbidity and mortality in school-aged and older children. This clinical report reviews key aspects of inhalant abuse, emphasizes the need for greater awareness, and offers advice regarding the pediatrician's role in the prevention and management of this substance abuse problem. (5/07)

INJURIES ASSOCIATED WITH INFANT WALKERS
Committee on Injury and Poison Prevention
ABSTRACT. In 1999, an estimated 8800 children younger than 15 months were treated in hospital emergency departments in the United States for injuries associated with infant walkers. Thirty-four infant walker-related deaths were reported from 1973 through 1998. The vast majority of injuries occur from falls down stairs, and head injuries are common. Walkers do not help a child learn to walk; indeed, they can delay normal motor and mental development. The use of warning labels, public education, adult supervision during walker use, and stair gates have all been demonstrated to be insufficient strategies to prevent injuries associated with infant walkers. To comply with the revised voluntary standard (ASTM F977-96), walkers manufactured after June 30, 1997, must be wider than a 36-in doorway or must have a braking mechanism designed to stop the walker if 1 or more wheels drop off the riding surface, such as at the top of a stairway. Because data indicate a considerable risk of major and minor injury and even death from the use of infant walkers, and because there is no clear benefit from their use, the American Academy of Pediatrics recommends a ban on the manufacture and sale of mobile infant walkers. If a parent insists on using a mobile infant walker, it is vital that they choose a walker that meets the performance standards of ASTM F977-96 to prevent falls down stairs.

Stationary activity centers should be promoted as a safer alternative to mobile infant walkers. (9/01, reaffirmed 1/05, 2/08, 10/11)

INJURIES IN YOUTH SOCCER (CLINICAL REPORT)
Chris G. Koutures, MD; Andrew J. M. Gregory, MD; and Council on Sports Medicine and Fitness
ABSTRACT. Injury rates in youth soccer, known as football outside the United States, are higher than in many other contact/collision sports and have greater relative numbers in younger, preadolescent players. With regard to musculoskeletal injuries, young females tend to suffer more knee injuries, and young males suffer more ankle injuries. Concussions are fairly prevalent in soccer as a result of contact/collision rather than purposeful attempts at heading the ball. Appropriate rule enforcement and emphasis on safe play can reduce the risk of soccer-related injuries. This report serves as a basis for encouraging safe participation in soccer for children and adolescents. (1/10, reaffirmed 5/13)

INJURY RISK OF NONPOWDER GUNS (TECHNICAL REPORT)
Committee on Injury, Violence, and Poison Prevention
ABSTRACT. Nonpowder guns (ball-bearing [BB] guns, pellet guns, air rifles, paintball guns) continue to cause serious injuries to children and adolescents. The muzzle velocity of these guns can range from approximately 150 ft/second to 1200 ft/second (the muzzle velocities of traditional firearm pistols are 750 ft/second to 1450 ft/second). Both low- and high-velocity nonpowder guns are associated with serious injuries, and fatalities can result from high-velocity guns. A persisting problem is the lack of medical recognition of the severity of injuries that can result from these guns, including penetration of the eye, skin, internal organs, and bone. Nationally, in 2000, there were an estimated 21840 (coefficient of variation: 0.0821) injuries related to nonpowder guns, with approximately 4% resulting in hospitalization. Between 1990 and 2000, the US Consumer Product Safety Commission reported 39 nonpowder gun–related deaths, of which 32 were children younger than 15 years. The introduction of high-powered air rifles in the 1970s has been associated with approximately 4 deaths per year. The advent of war games and the use of paintball guns have resulted in a number of reports of injuries, especially to the eye. Injuries associated with nonpowder guns should receive prompt medical management similar to the management of firearm-related injuries, and nonpowder guns should never be characterized as toys. (11/04, reaffirmed 2/08, 10/11)

IN-LINE SKATING INJURIES IN CHILDREN AND ADOLESCENTS
Committee on Injury and Poison Prevention and Committee on Sports Medicine and Fitness
ABSTRACT. In-line skating has become one of the fastest-growing recreational sports in the United States. Recent studies emphasize the value of protective gear in reducing the incidence of injuries. Recommendations are provided for parents and pediatricians, with special emphasis on the novice or inexperienced skater. (4/98, reaffirmed 1/02, 1/06, 1/09, 11/11)

INSTITUTIONAL ETHICS COMMITTEES
Committee on Bioethics
ABSTRACT. In hospitals throughout the United States, institutional ethics committees (IECs) have become a standard vehicle for the education of health professionals about biomedical ethics, for the drafting and review of hospital policy, and for clinical ethics case consultation. In addition, there is increasing interest in a role for the IEC in organizational ethics. Recommendations are made about the membership and structure of an IEC, and guidelines are provided for those serving on an ethics committee. (1/01, reaffirmed 1/04, 1/09, 10/12)

INSTRUMENT-BASED PEDIATRIC VISION SCREENING POLICY STATEMENT
Section on Ophthalmology and Committee on Practice and Ambulatory Medicine (joint with American Academy of Ophthalmology, American Association for Pediatric Ophthalmology and Strabismus, and American Association of Certified Orthoptists)
ABSTRACT. A policy statement describing the use of automated vision screening technology (instrument-based vision screening) is presented. Screening for amblyogenic refractive error with instrument-based screening is not dependent on behavioral responses of children, as when visual acuity is measured. Instrument-based screening is quick, requires minimal cooperation of the child, and is especially useful in the preverbal, preliterate, or developmentally delayed child. Children younger than 4 years can benefit from instrument-based screening, and visual acuity testing can be used reliably in older children. Adoption of this new technology is highly dependent on third-party payment policies, which could present a significant barrier to adoption. (10/12)

INSURANCE COVERAGE OF MENTAL HEALTH AND SUBSTANCE ABUSE SERVICES FOR CHILDREN AND ADOLESCENTS: A CONSENSUS STATEMENT
Joint Statement (10/00)

INTENSIVE TRAINING AND SPORTS SPECIALIZATION IN YOUNG ATHLETES
Committee on Sports Medicine and Fitness
ABSTRACT. Children involved in sports should be encouraged to participate in a variety of different activities and develop a wide range of skills. Young athletes who specialize in just one sport may be denied the benefits of varied activity while facing additional physical, physiologic, and psychologic demands from intense training and competition.

This statement reviews the potential risks of high-intensity training and sports specialization in young athletes. Pediatricians who recognize these risks can have a key role in monitoring the health of these young athletes and helping reduce risks associated with high-level sports participation. (7/00, reaffirmed 11/04, 1/06, 5/09)

INTIMATE PARTNER VIOLENCE: THE ROLE OF THE PEDIATRICIAN (CLINICAL REPORT)
Jonathan D. Thackeray, MD; Roberta Hibbard, MD; M. Denise Dowd, MD, MPH; Committee on Child Abuse and Neglect; and Committee on Injury, Violence, and Poison Prevention
ABSTRACT. The American Academy of Pediatrics and its members recognize the importance of improving the physician's ability to recognize intimate partner violence (IPV) and understand its effects on child health and development and its role in the continuum of family violence. Pediatricians are in a unique position to identify abused caregivers in pediatric settings and to evaluate and treat children raised in homes in which IPV may occur. Children exposed to IPV are at increased risk of being abused and neglected and are more likely to develop adverse health, behavioral, psychological, and social disorders later in life. Identifying IPV, therefore, may be one of the most effective means of preventing child abuse and identifying caregivers and children who may be in need of treatment and/or therapy. Pediatricians should be aware of the profound effects of exposure to IPV on children. (4/10)

KNEE BRACE USE IN THE YOUNG ATHLETE (TECHNICAL REPORT)
Committee on Sports Medicine and Fitness
ABSTRACT. This statement is a revision of a previous statement on prophylactic knee bracing and provides information for pediatricians regarding the use of various types of knee braces, indications for the use of knee braces, and the background knowledge necessary to prescribe the use of knee braces for children. (8/01, reaffirmed 1/07, 4/10, 5/13)

LACTOSE INTOLERANCE IN INFANTS, CHILDREN, AND ADOLESCENTS (CLINICAL REPORT)
Melvin B. Heyman, MD, MPH, for Committee on Nutrition
ABSTRACT. The American Academy of Pediatrics Committee on Nutrition presents an updated review of lactose intolerance in infants, children, and adolescents. Differences between primary, secondary, congenital, and developmental lactase deficiency that may result in lactose intolerance are discussed. Children with suspected lactose intolerance can be assessed clinically by dietary lactose elimination or by tests including noninvasive hydrogen breath testing or invasive intestinal biopsy determination of lactase (and other disaccharidase) concentrations. Treatment consists of use of lactase-treated dairy products or oral lactase supplementation, limitation of lactose-containing foods, or dairy elimination. The American Academy of Pediatrics supports use of dairy foods as an important source of calcium for bone mineral health and of other nutrients that facilitate growth in children and adolescents. If dairy products are eliminated, other dietary sources of calcium or calcium supplements need to be provided. (9/06, reaffirmed 8/12)

"LATE-PRETERM" INFANTS: A POPULATION AT RISK (CLINICAL REPORT)

William A. Engle, MD; Kay M. Tomashek, MD; Carol
*   Wallman, MSN; and Committee on Fetus and Newborn*

ABSTRACT. Late-preterm infants, defined by birth at 34%₇ through 36%₇ weeks' gestation, are less physiologically and metabolically mature than term infants. Thus, they are at higher risk of morbidity and mortality than term infants. The purpose of this report is to define "late preterm," recommend a change in terminology from "near term" to "late preterm," present the characteristics of late-preterm infants that predispose them to a higher risk of morbidity and mortality than term infants, and propose guidelines for the evaluation and management of these infants after birth. (12/07, reaffirmed 5/10)

LAWN MOWER-RELATED INJURIES TO CHILDREN

Committee on Injury and Poison Prevention

ABSTRACT. Lawn mower-related injuries to children are relatively common and can result in severe injury or death. Many amputations during childhood are caused by power mowers. Pediatricians have an important role as advocates and educators to promote the prevention of these injuries. (6/01, reaffirmed 10/04, 5/07, 6/10)

LAWN MOWER-RELATED INJURIES TO CHILDREN (TECHNICAL REPORT)

Committee on Injury and Poison Prevention

ABSTRACT. In the United States, approximately 9400 children younger than 18 years receive emergency treatment annually for lawn mower-related injuries. More than 7% of these children require hospitalization, and power mowers cause a large proportion of the amputations during childhood. Prevention of lawn mower-related injuries can be achieved by design changes of lawn mowers, guidelines for mower operation, and education of parents, child caregivers, and children. Pediatricians have an important role as advocates and educators to promote the prevention of these injuries. (6/01, reaffirmed 10/04, 5/07, 6/10)

LEARNING DISABILITIES, DYSLEXIA, AND VISION

Section on Ophthalmology and Council on Children
*   With Disabilities* (joint with American Academy of
*   Ophthalmology, American Association for Pediatric*
*   Ophthalmology and Strabismus, and American*
*   Association of Certified Orthoptists)*

ABSTRACT. Learning disabilities, including reading disabilities, are commonly diagnosed in children. Their etiologies are multifactorial, reflecting genetic influences and dysfunction of brain systems. Learning disabilities are complex problems that require complex solutions. Early recognition and referral to qualified educational professionals for evidence-based evaluations and treatments seem necessary to achieve the best possible outcome. Most experts believe that dyslexia is a language-based disorder. Vision problems can interfere with the process of learning; however, vision problems are not the cause of primary dyslexia or learning disabilities. Scientific evidence does not support the efficacy of eye exercises, behavioral vision therapy, or special tinted filters or lenses for improving the long-term educational performance in these complex pediatric neurocognitive conditions. Diagnostic and treatment approaches that lack scientific evidence of efficacy, including eye exercises, behavioral vision therapy, or special tinted filters or lenses, are not endorsed and should not be recommended. (7/09)

LEARNING DISABILITIES, DYSLEXIA, AND VISION (TECHNICAL REPORT)

Sheryl M. Handler, MD; Walter M. Fierson, MD; and
*   Section on Ophthalmology and Council on Children*
*   With Disabilities* (joint with American Academy of
*   Ophthalmology, American Association for Pediatric*
*   Ophthalmology and Strabismus, and American*
*   Association of Certified Orthoptists)*

ABSTRACT. Learning disabilities constitute a diverse group of disorders in which children who generally possess at least average intelligence have problems processing information or generating output. Their etiologies are multifactorial and reflect genetic influences and dysfunction of brain systems. Reading disability, or dyslexia, is the most common learning disability. It is a receptive language-based learning disability that is characterized by difficulties with decoding, fluent word recognition, rapid automatic naming, and/or reading-comprehension skills. These difficulties typically result from a deficit in the phonologic component of language that makes it difficult to use the alphabetic code to decode the written word. Early recognition and referral to qualified professionals for evidence-based evaluations and treatments are necessary to achieve the best possible outcome. Because dyslexia is a language-based disorder, treatment should be directed at this etiology. Remedial programs should include specific instruction in decoding, fluency training, vocabulary, and comprehension. Most programs include daily intensive individualized instruction that explicitly teaches phonemic awareness and the application of phonics. Vision problems can interfere with the process of reading, but children with dyslexia or related learning disabilities have the same visual function and ocular health as children without such conditions. Currently, there is inadequate scientific evidence to support the view that subtle eye or visual problems cause or increase the severity of learning disabilities. Because they are difficult for the public to understand and for educators to treat, learning disabilities have spawned a wide variety of scientifically unsupported vision-based diagnostic and treatment procedures. Scientific evidence does not support the claims that visual training, muscle exercises, ocular pursuit-and-tracking exercises, behavioral/perceptual vision therapy, "training" glasses, prisms, and colored lenses and filters are effective direct or indirect treatments for learning disabilities. There is no valid evidence that children who participate in vision therapy are more responsive to educational instruction than children who do not participate. (3/11)

LEGALIZATION OF MARIJUANA: POTENTIAL IMPACT ON YOUTH

Committee on Substance Abuse and Committee on Adolescence

ABSTRACT. As experts in the health care of children and adolescents, pediatricians may be called on to advise legislators concerning the potential impact of changes in the legal status of marijuana on adolescents. Parents, too, may look to pediatricians for advice as they consider whether to support state-level initiatives that propose to legalize the use of marijuana for medical purposes or to decriminalize possession of small amounts of marijuana. This policy statement provides the position of the American Academy of Pediatrics on the issue of marijuana legalization, and the accompanying technical report (available online) reviews what is currently known about the relationship between adolescents' use of marijuana and its legal status to better understand how change might influence the degree of marijuana use by adolescents in the future. (6/04)

LEGALIZATION OF MARIJUANA: POTENTIAL IMPACT ON YOUTH (TECHNICAL REPORT)

Committee on Substance Abuse and Committee on Adolescence
ABSTRACT. This technical report provides historical perspectives and comparisons of various approaches to the legal status of marijuana to aid in forming public policy. Information on the impact that decriminalization and legalization of marijuana could have on adolescents, in addition to concerns surrounding medicinal use of marijuana, are also addressed in this report. Recommendations are included in the accompanying policy statement. (6/04)

LEVELS OF NEONATAL CARE

Committee on Fetus and Newborn
ABSTRACT. Provision of risk-appropriate care for newborn infants and mothers was first proposed in 1976. This updated policy statement provides a review of data supporting evidence for a tiered provision of care and reaffirms the need for uniform, nationally applicable definitions and consistent standards of service for public health to improve neonatal outcomes. Facilities that provide hospital care for newborn infants should be classified on the basis of functional capabilities, and these facilities should be organized within a regionalized system of perinatal care. (8/12)

THE LIFELONG EFFECTS OF EARLY CHILDHOOD ADVERSITY AND TOXIC STRESS (TECHNICAL REPORT)

Jack P. Shonkoff, MD; Andrew S. Garner, MD, PhD; Committee on Psychosocial Aspects of Child and Family Health; Committee on Early Childhood, Adoption, and Dependent Care; and Section on Developmental and Behavioral Pediatrics
ABSTRACT. Advances in fields of inquiry as diverse as neuroscience, molecular biology, genomics, developmental psychology, epidemiology, sociology, and economics are catalyzing an important paradigm shift in our understanding of health and disease across the lifespan. This converging, multidisciplinary science of human development has profound implications for our ability to enhance the life prospects of children and to strengthen the social and economic fabric of society. Drawing on these multiple streams of investigation, this report presents an eco-biodevelopmental framework that illustrates how early experiences and environmental influences can leave a lasting signature on the genetic predispositions that affect emerging brain architecture and long-term health. The report also examines extensive evidence of the disruptive impacts of toxic stress, offering intriguing insights into causal mechanisms that link early adversity to later

impairments in learning, behavior, and both physical and mental well-being. The implications of this framework for the practice of medicine, in general, and pediatrics, specifically, are potentially transformational. They suggest that many adult diseases should be viewed as developmental disorders that begin early in life and that persistent health disparities associated with poverty, discrimination, or maltreatment could be reduced by the alleviation of toxic stress in childhood. An ecobiodevelopmental framework also underscores the need for new thinking about the focus and boundaries of pediatric practice. It calls for pediatricians to serve as both front-line guardians of healthy child development and strategically positioned, community leaders to inform new science-based strategies that build strong foundations for educational achievement, economic productivity, responsible citizenship, and lifelong health. (12/11)

LONG-TERM FOLLOW-UP CARE FOR PEDIATRIC CANCER SURVIVORS (CLINICAL REPORT)

Section on Hematology/Oncology (joint with Children's Oncology Group)
ABSTRACT. Progress in therapy has made survival into adulthood a reality for most children, adolescents, and young adults diagnosed with cancer today. Notably, this growing population remains vulnerable to a variety of long-term therapy-related sequelae. Systematic ongoing follow-up of these patients, therefore, is important for providing for early detection of and intervention for potentially serious late-onset complications. In addition, health counseling and promotion of healthy lifestyles are important aspects of long-term follow-up care to promote risk reduction for health problems that commonly present during adulthood. Both general and subspecialty pediatric health care providers are playing an increasingly important role in the ongoing care of childhood cancer survivors, beyond the routine preventive care, health supervision, and anticipatory guidance provided to all patients. This report is based on the guidelines that have been developed by the Children's Oncology Group to facilitate comprehensive long-term follow-up of childhood cancer survivors (www.survivorshipguidelines.org). (3/09, reaffirmed 4/13)

MALE ADOLESCENT SEXUAL AND REPRODUCTIVE HEALTH CARE (CLINICAL REPORT)

Arik V. Marcell, MD, MPH; Charles Wibbelsman, MD; Warren M. Seigel, MD; and Committee on Adolescence
ABSTRACT. Male adolescents' sexual and reproductive health needs often go unmet in the primary care setting. This report discusses specific issues related to male adolescents' sexual and reproductive health care in the context of primary care, including pubertal and sexual development, sexual behavior, consequences of sexual behavior, and methods of preventing sexually transmitted infections (including HIV) and pregnancy. Pediatricians are encouraged to address male adolescent sexual and reproductive health on a regular basis, including taking a sexual history, performing an appropriate examination, providing patient-centered and age-appropriate anticipatory guidance, and delivering appropriate vaccinations. Pediatricians should provide these services to male ado-

lescent patients in a confidential and culturally appropriate manner, promote healthy sexual relationships and responsibility, and involve parents in age-appropriate discussions about sexual health with their sons. (11/11)

MALE CIRCUMCISION (TECHNICAL REPORT)
Task Force on Circumcision

ABSTRACT. Male circumcision consists of the surgical removal of some, or all, of the foreskin (or prepuce) from the penis. It is one of the most common procedures in the world. In the United States, the procedure is commonly performed during the newborn period. In 2007, the American Academy of Pediatrics (AAP) convened a multidisciplinary workgroup of AAP members and other stakeholders to evaluate the evidence regarding male circumcision and update the AAP's 1999 recommendations in this area. The Task Force included AAP representatives from specialty areas as well as members of the AAP Board of Directors and liaisons representing the American Academy of Family Physicians, the American College of Obstetricians and Gynecologists, and the Centers for Disease Control and Prevention. The Task Force members identified selected topics relevant to male circumcision and conducted a critical review of peer-reviewed literature by using the American Heart Association's template for evidence evaluation.

Evaluation of current evidence indicates that the health benefits of newborn male circumcision outweigh the risks; furthermore, the benefits of newborn male circumcision justify access to this procedure for families who choose it. Specific benefits from male circumcision were identified for the prevention of urinary tract infections, acquisition of HIV, transmission of some sexually transmitted infections, and penile cancer. Male circumcision does not appear to adversely affect penile sexual function/sensitivity or sexual satisfaction. It is imperative that those providing circumcision are adequately trained and that both sterile techniques and effective pain management are used. Significant acute complications are rare. In general, untrained providers who perform circumcisions have more complications than well-trained providers who perform the procedure, regardless of whether the former are physicians, nurses, or traditional religious providers.

Parents are entitled to factually correct, nonbiased information about circumcision and should receive this information from clinicians before conception or early in pregnancy, which is when parents typically make circumcision decisions. Parents should determine what is in the best interest of their child. Physicians who counsel families about this decision should provide assistance by explaining the potential benefits and risks and ensuring that parents understand that circumcision is an elective procedure. The Task Force strongly recommends the creation, revision, and enhancement of educational materials to assist parents of male infants with the care of circumcised and uncircumcised penises. The Task Force also strongly recommends the development of educational materials for providers to enhance practitioners' competency in discussing circumcision's benefits and risks with parents.

The Task Force made the following recommendations:

- Evaluation of current evidence indicates that the health benefits of newborn male circumcision outweigh the risks, and the benefits of newborn male circumcision justify access to this procedure for those families who choose it.
- Parents are entitled to factually correct, nonbiased information about circumcision that should be provided before conception and early in pregnancy, when parents are most likely to be weighing the option of circumcision of a male child.
- Physicians counseling families about elective male circumcision should assist parents by explaining, in a nonbiased manner, the potential benefits and risks and by ensuring that they understand the elective nature of the procedure.
- Parents should weigh the health benefits and risks in light of their own religious, cultural, and personal preferences, as the medical benefits alone may not outweigh these other considerations for individual families.
- Parents of newborn boys should be instructed in the care of the penis, regardless of whether the newborn has been circumcised or not.
- Elective circumcision should be performed only if the infant's condition is stable and healthy.
- Male circumcision should be performed by trained and competent practitioners, by using sterile techniques and effective pain management.
- Analgesia is safe and effective in reducing the procedural pain associated with newborn circumcision; thus, adequate analgesia should be provided whenever newborn circumcision is performed.
  — Nonpharmacologic techniques (eg, positioning, sucrose pacifiers) alone are insufficient to prevent procedural and postprocedural pain and are not recommended as the sole method of analgesia. They should be used only as analgesic adjuncts to improve infant comfort during circumcision.
  — If used, topical creams may cause a higher incidence of skin irritation in low birth weight infants, compared with infants of normal weight; penile nerve block techniques should therefore be chosen for this group of newborns.
- Key professional organizations (AAP, the American Academy of Family Physicians, the American College of Obstetricians and Gynecologists, the American Society of Anesthesiologists, the American College of Nurse Midwives, and other midlevel clinicians such as nurse practitioners) should work collaboratively to:
  — Develop standards of trainee proficiency in the performance of anesthetic and procedure techniques, including suturing;
  — Teach the procedure and analgesic techniques during postgraduate training programs;
  — Develop educational materials for clinicians to enhance their own competency in discussing the benefits and risks of circumcision with parents;
  — Offer educational materials to assist parents of male infants with the care of both circumcised and uncircumcised penises.

- The preventive and public health benefits associated with newborn male circumcision warrant third-party reimbursement of the procedure.

The American College of Obstetricians and Gynecologists has endorsed this technical report. (8/12)

MALTREATMENT OF CHILDREN WITH DISABILITIES (CLINICAL REPORT)

Roberta A. Hibbard, MD; Larry W. Desch, MD; Committee on Child Abuse and Neglect; and Council on Children With Disabilities

ABSTRACT. Widespread efforts are being made to increase awareness and provide education to pediatricians regarding risk factors of child abuse and neglect. The purpose of this clinical report is to ensure that children with disabilities are recognized as a population that is also at risk of maltreatment. Some conditions related to a disability can be confused with maltreatment. The need for early recognition and intervention of child abuse and neglect in this population, as well as the ways that a medical home can facilitate the prevention and early detection of child maltreatment, are the subject of this report. (5/07, reaffirmed 1/11)

MANAGEMENT OF CHILDREN WITH AUTISM SPECTRUM DISORDERS (CLINICAL REPORT)

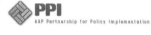

Scott M. Myers, MD; Chris Plauché Johnson, MD, MEd; and Council on Children With Disabilities

ABSTRACT. Pediatricians have an important role not only in early recognition and evaluation of autism spectrum disorders but also in chronic management of these disorders. The primary goals of treatment are to maximize the child's ultimate functional independence and quality of life by minimizing the core autism spectrum disorder features, facilitating development and learning, promoting socialization, reducing maladaptive behaviors, and educating and supporting families. To assist pediatricians in educating families and guiding them toward empirically supported interventions for their children, this report reviews the educational strategies and associated therapies that are the primary treatments for children with autism spectrum disorders. Optimization of health care is likely to have a positive effect on habilitative progress, functional outcome, and quality of life; therefore, important issues, such as management of associated medical problems, pharmacologic and nonpharmacologic intervention for challenging behaviors or coexisting mental health conditions, and use of complementary and alternative medical treatments, are also addressed. (11/07, reaffirmed 9/10)

MANAGEMENT OF FOOD ALLERGY IN THE SCHOOL SETTING (CLINICAL REPORT)

Scott H. Sicherer, MD; Todd Mahr, MD; and Section on Allergy and Immunology

ABSTRACT. Food allergy is estimated to affect approximately 1 in 25 school-aged children and is the most common trigger of anaphylaxis in this age group. School food-allergy management requires strategies to reduce the risk of ingestion of the allergen as well as procedures to recognize and treat allergic reactions and anaphylaxis. The role of the pediatrician or pediatric health care provider may include diagnosing and documenting a potentially life-threatening food allergy, prescribing self-injectable epinephrine, helping the child learn how to store and use the medication in a responsible manner, educating the parents of their responsibility to implement prevention strategies within and outside the home environment, and working with families, schools, and students in developing written plans to reduce the risk of anaphylaxis and to implement emergency treatment in the event of a reaction. This clinical report highlights the role of the pediatrician and pediatric health care provider in managing students with food allergies. (11/10)

MANAGEMENT OF NEONATES WITH SUSPECTED OR PROVEN EARLY-ONSET BACTERIAL SEPSIS (CLINICAL REPORT)

Richard A. Polin, MD, and Committee on Fetus and Newborn

ABSTRACT. With improved obstetrical management and evidence-based use of intrapartum antimicrobial therapy, early-onset neonatal sepsis is becoming less frequent. However, early-onset sepsis remains one of the most common causes of neonatal morbidity and mortality in the preterm population. The identification of neonates at risk for early-onset sepsis is frequently based on a constellation of perinatal risk factors that are neither sensitive nor specific. Furthermore, diagnostic tests for neonatal sepsis have a poor positive predictive accuracy. As a result, clinicians often treat well-appearing infants for extended periods of time, even when bacterial cultures are negative. The optimal treatment of infants with suspected early-onset sepsis is broad-spectrum antimicrobial agents (ampicillin and an aminoglycoside). Once a pathogen is identified, antimicrobial therapy should be narrowed (unless synergism is needed). Recent data suggest an association between prolonged empirical treatment of preterm infants (≥5 days) with broad-spectrum antibiotics and higher risks of late onset sepsis, necrotizing enterocolitis, and mortality. To reduce these risks, antimicrobial therapy should be discontinued at 48 hours in clinical situations in which the probability of sepsis is low. The purpose of this clinical report is to provide a practical and, when possible, evidence-based approach to the management of infants with suspected or proven early-onset sepsis. (4/12)

MANAGEMENT OF PEDIATRIC TRAUMA

Section on Orthopaedics, Committee on Pediatric Emergency Medicine, Section on Critical Care, Section on Surgery, and Section on Transport Medicine (joint with Pediatric Orthopaedic Society of North America)

ABSTRACT. Injury is the number 1 killer of children in the United States. In 2004, injury accounted for 59.5% of all deaths in children younger than 18 years. The financial burden to society of children who survive childhood injury with disability continues to be enormous. The entire process of managing childhood injury is complex and varies by region. Only the comprehensive cooperation of a broadly diverse group of people will have a significant effect on improving the care and outcome of injured children. (4/08, reaffirmed 4/13)

MANAGEMENT OF TYPE 2 DIABETES MELLITUS IN CHILDREN AND ADOLESCENTS (TECHNICAL REPORT)

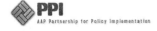

Shelley C. Springer, MD, MBA, MSc, JD; Janet Silverstein, MD; Kenneth Copeland, MD; Kelly R. Moore, MD; Greg E. Prazar, MD; Terry Raymer, MD, CDE; Richard N. Shiffman, MD; Vidhu V. Thaker, MD; Meaghan Anderson, MS, RD, LD, CDE; Stephen J. Spann, MD, MBA; and Susan K. Flinn, MA

ABSTRACT. *Objective.* Over the last 3 decades, the prevalence of childhood obesity has increased dramatically in North America, ushering in a variety of health problems, including type 2 diabetes mellitus (T2DM), which previously was not typically seen until much later in life. This technical report describes, in detail, the procedures undertaken to develop the recommendations given in the accompanying clinical practice guideline, "Management of Type 2 Diabetes Mellitus in Children and Adolescents," and provides in-depth information about the rationale for the recommendations and the studies used to make the clinical practice guideline's recommendations.

Methods. A primary literature search was conducted relating to the treatment of T2DM in children and adolescents, and a secondary literature search was conducted relating to the screening and treatment of T2DM's comorbidities in children and adolescents. Inclusion criteria were prospectively and unanimously agreed on by members of the committee. An article was eligible for inclusion if it addressed treatment (primary search) or 1 of 4 comorbidities (secondary search) of T2DM, was published in 1990 or later, was written in English, and included an abstract. Only primary research inquiries were considered; review articles were considered if they included primary data or opinion. The research population had to constitute children and/or adolescents with an existing diagnosis of T2DM; studies of adult patients were considered if at least 10% of the study population was younger than 35 years. All retrieved titles, abstracts, and articles were reviewed by the consulting epidemiologist.

Results. Thousands of articles were retrieved and considered in both searches on the basis of the aforementioned criteria. From those, in the primary search, 199 abstracts were identified for possible inclusion, 58 of which were retained for systematic review. Five of these studies were classified as grade A studies, 1 as grade B, 20 as grade C, and 32 as grade D. Articles regarding treatment of T2DM selected for inclusion were divided into 4 major subcategories on the basis of type of treatment being discussed: (1) medical treatments (32 studies); (2) nonmedical treatments (9 studies); (3) provider behaviors (8 studies); and (4) social issues (9 studies). From the secondary search, an additional 336 abstracts relating to comorbidities were identified for possible inclusion, of which 26 were retained for systematic review. These articles included the following: 1 systematic review of literature regarding comorbidities of T2DM in adolescents; 5 expert opinions presenting global recommendations not based on evidence; 5 cohort studies reporting natural history of disease and comorbidities; 3 with specific attention to comorbidity patterns in specific ethnic groups (case-control, cohort, and clinical report using adult literature); 3 reporting an association between microalbuminuria and retinopathy (2 case-control, 1 cohort); 3 reporting the prevalence of nephropathy (cohort); 1 reporting peripheral vascular disease (case series); 2 discussing retinopathy (1 case-control, 1 position statement); and 3 addressing hyperlipidemia (American Heart Association position statement on cardiovascular risks; American Diabetes Association consensus statement; case series). A breakdown of grade of recommendation shows no grade A studies, 10 grade B studies, 6 grade C studies, and 10 grade D studies. With regard to screening and treatment recommendations for comorbidities, data in children are scarce, and the available literature is conflicting. Therapeutic recommendations for hypertension, dyslipidemia, retinopathy, microalbuminuria, and depression were summarized from expert guideline documents and are presented in detail in the guideline. The references are provided, but the committee did not independently assess the supporting evidence. Screening tools are provided in the Supplemental Information. (1/13)

See full text on page 97.

MARIJUANA: A CONTINUING CONCERN FOR PEDIATRICIANS

Committee on Substance Abuse

ABSTRACT. Marijuana, the common name for products derived from the plant *Cannabis sativa,* is the most common illicit drug used by children and adolescents in the United States. Despite growing concerns by the medical profession about the physical and psychological effects of its active ingredient, Æ-9-tetrahydrocannabinol, survey data continue to show that increasing numbers of young people are using the drug as they become less concerned about its dangers. (10/99, reaffirmed 4/03)

MATERNAL-FETAL INTERVENTION AND FETAL CARE CENTERS (CLINICAL REPORT)

Committee on Bioethics (joint with American College of Obstetricians and Gynecologists Committee on Ethics)

ABSTRACT. The past 2 decades have yielded profound advances in the fields of prenatal diagnosis and fetal intervention. Although fetal interventions are driven by a beneficence-based motivation to improve fetal and neonatal outcomes, advancement in fetal therapies raises ethical issues surrounding maternal autonomy and decision-making, concepts of innovation versus research, and organizational aspects within institutions in the development of fetal care centers. To safeguard the interests of both the pregnant woman and the fetus, the American College of Obstetricians and Gynecologists and the American Academy of Pediatrics make recommendations regarding informed consent, the role of research subject advocates and other independent advocates, the availability of support services, the multidisciplinary nature of fetal intervention teams, the oversight of centers, and the need to accumulate maternal and fetal outcome data. (7/11)

MATERNAL PHENYLKETONURIA

Committee on Genetics

ABSTRACT. Elevated maternal phenylalanine concentrations during pregnancy are teratogenic and may result in growth retardation, microcephaly, significant developmental delays, and birth defects in the offspring of women with poorly controlled phenylketonuria during pregnancy. Women of childbearing age with all forms of phenylketonuria, including mild variants such as mild hyperphenylalaninemia, should receive counseling concerning their risks for adverse fetal effects, optimally before conceiving. The best outcomes occur when strict control of maternal phenylalanine concentration is achieved before conception and continued throughout pregnancy. Included are brief descriptions of novel treatments for phenylketonuria. (8/08, reaffirmed 1/13)

MEDIA EDUCATION
Committee on Communications and Media
ABSTRACT. The American Academy of Pediatrics recognizes that exposure to mass media (eg, television, movies, video and computer games, the Internet, music lyrics and videos, newspapers, magazines, books, advertising) presents health risks for children and adolescents but can provide benefits as well. Media education has the potential to reduce the harmful effects of media and accentuate the positive effects. By understanding and supporting media education, pediatricians can play an important role in reducing harmful effects of media on children and adolescents. (9/10)

MEDIA USE BY CHILDREN YOUNGER THAN 2 YEARS
Council on Communications and Media
ABSTRACT. In 1999, the American Academy of Pediatrics (AAP) issued a policy statement addressing media use in children. The purpose of that statement was to educate parents about the effects that media—both the amount and the content—may have on children. In one part of that statement, the AAP recommended that "pediatricians should urge parents to avoid television viewing for children under the age of two years." The wording of the policy specifically discouraged media use in this age group, although it is frequently misquoted by media outlets as no media exposure in this age group. The AAP believed that there were significantly more potential negative effects of media than positive ones for this age group and, thus, advised families to thoughtfully consider media use for infants. This policy statement reaffirms the 1999 statement with respect to media use in infants and children younger than 2 years and provides updated research findings to support it. This statement addresses (1) the lack of evidence supporting educational or developmental benefits for media use by children younger than 2 years, (2) the potential adverse health and developmental effects of media use by children younger than 2 years, and (3) adverse effects of parental media use (background media) on children younger than 2 years. (10/11)

MEDIA VIOLENCE
Council on Communications and Media
ABSTRACT. Exposure to violence in media, including television, movies, music, and video games, represents a significant risk to the health of children and adolescents. Extensive research evidence indicates that media violence can contribute to aggressive behavior, desensitization to violence, nightmares, and fear of being harmed. Pediatricians should assess their patients' level of media exposure and intervene on media-related health risks.

Pediatricians and other child health care providers can advocate for a safer media environment for children by encouraging media literacy, more thoughtful and proactive use of media by children and their parents, more responsible portrayal of violence by media producers, and more useful and effective media ratings. Office counseling has been shown to be effective. (10/09)

MEDICAID POLICY STATEMENT
Committee on Child Health Financing
ABSTRACT. Medicaid insures 39% of the children in the United States. This revision of the 2005 Medicaid Policy Statement of the American Academy of Pediatrics reflects opportunities for changes in state Medicaid programs resulting from the 2010 Patient Protection and Affordable Care Act as upheld in 2012 by the Supreme Court. Policy recommendations focus on the areas of benefit coverage, financing and payment, eligibility, outreach and enrollment, managed care, and quality improvement. (4/13)
See full text on page 721.

MEDICAL CONCERNS IN THE FEMALE ATHLETE
Committee on Sports Medicine and Fitness
ABSTRACT. Female children and adolescents who participate regularly in sports may develop certain medical conditions, including disordered eating, menstrual dysfunction, and decreased bone mineral density. The pediatrician can play an important role in monitoring the health of young female athletes. This revised policy statement provides updated and expanded information for pediatricians on these health concerns as well as recommendations for evaluation, treatment, and ongoing assessments of female athletes. (9/00, reaffirmed 5/05, 5/08)

MEDICAL CONDITIONS AFFECTING SPORTS PARTICIPATION (CLINICAL REPORT)
Stephen G. Rice, MD, PhD, MPH, and Council on Sports Medicine and Fitness
ABSTRACT. Children and adolescents with medical conditions present special issues with respect to participation in athletic activities. The pediatrician can play an important role in determining whether a child with a health condition should participate in certain sports by assessing the child's health status, suggesting appropriate equipment or modifications of sports to decrease the risk of injury, and educating the athlete, parent(s) or guardian, and coach regarding the risks of injury as they relate to the child's condition. This report updates a previous policy statement and provides information for pediatricians on sports participation for children and adolescents with medical conditions. (4/08, reaffirmed 5/11)

MEDICAL EMERGENCIES OCCURRING AT SCHOOL
Council on School Health
ABSTRACT. Children and adults might experience medical emergency situations because of injuries, complications of chronic health conditions, or unexpected major illnesses that occur in schools. In February 2001, the American Academy of Pediatrics issued a policy statement titled "Guidelines for Emergency Medical Care in Schools" (available at: http://aappolicy.aappublications.org/cgi/content/full/pediatrics;107/2/435). Since the

release of that statement, the spectrum of potential individual student emergencies has changed significantly. The increase in the number of children with special health care needs and chronic medical conditions attending schools and the challenges associated with ensuring that schools have access to on-site licensed health care professionals on an ongoing basis have added to increasing the risks of medical emergencies in schools. The goal of this statement is to increase pediatricians' awareness of schools' roles in preparing for individual student emergencies and to provide recommendations for primary care and school physicians on how to assist and support school personnel. (10/08, reaffirmed 9/11)

THE MEDICAL HOME
Medical Home Initiatives for Children With Special Needs Project Advisory Committee (7/02, reaffirmed 5/08)

MEDICAL STAFF APPOINTMENT AND DELINEATION OF PEDIATRIC PRIVILEGES IN HOSPITALS (CLINICAL REPORT)
Daniel A. Rauch, MD; Committee on Hospital Care; and Section on Hospital Medicine

ABSTRACT. The review and verification of credentials and the granting of clinical privileges are required of every hospital to ensure that members of the medical staff are competent and qualified to provide specified levels of patient care. The credentialing process involves the following: (1) assessment of the professional and personal background of each practitioner seeking privileges; (2) assignment of privileges appropriate for the clinician's training and experience; (3) ongoing monitoring of the professional activities of each staff member; and (4) periodic reappointment to the medical staff on the basis of objectively measured performance. We examine the essential elements of a credentials review for initial and renewed medical staff appointments along with suggested criteria for the delineation of clinical privileges. Sample forms for the delineation of privileges can be found on the American Academy of Pediatrics Committee on Hospital Care Web site (http://www.aap.org/visit/cmte19.htm). Because of differences among individual hospitals, no 1 method for credentialing is universally applicable. The medical staff of each hospital must, therefore, establish its own process based on the general principles reviewed in this report. The issues of medical staff membership and credentialing have become very complex, and institutions and medical staffs are vulnerable to legal action. Consequently, it is advisable for hospitals and medical staffs to obtain expert legal advice when medical staff bylaws are constructed or revised. (3/12)

MENINGOCOCCAL CONJUGATE VACCINES POLICY UPDATE: BOOSTER DOSE RECOMMENDATIONS
Committee on Infectious Diseases

ABSTRACT. The Advisory Committee on Immunization Practices of the Centers for Disease Control and Prevention and the American Academy of Pediatrics approved updated recommendations for the use of quadravalent (serogroups A, C, W-135, and Y) meningococcal conjugate vaccines (Menactra [Sanofi Pasteur, Swiftwater, PA] and Menveo [Novartis, Basel, Switzerland]) in adolescents and in people at persistent high risk of meningococcal disease. The recommendations supplement previous Advisory Committee on Immunization Practices and American Academy of Pediatrics recommendations for meningococcal vaccinations. Data were reviewed pertaining to immunogenicity in high-risk groups, bactericidal antibody persistence after immunization, current epidemiology of meningococcal disease, meningococcal conjugate vaccine effectiveness, and cost-effectiveness of different strategies for vaccination of adolescents. This review prompted the following recommendations: (1) adolescents should be routinely immunized at 11 through 12 years of age and given a booster dose at 16 years of age; (2) adolescents who received their first dose at age 13 through 15 years should receive a booster at age 16 through 18 years or up to 5 years after their first dose; (3) adolescents who receive their first dose of meningococcal conjugate vaccine at or after 16 years of age do not need a booster dose; (4) a 2-dose primary series should be administered 2 months apart for those who are at increased risk of invasive meningococcal disease because of persistent complement component (eg, C5–C9, properdin, factor H, or factor D) deficiency (9 months through 54 years of age) or functional or anatomic asplenia (2–54 years of age) and for adolescents with HIV infection; and (5) a booster dose should be given 3 years after the primary series if the primary 2-dose series was given from 2 through 6 years of age and every 5 years for persons whose 2-dose primary series or booster dose was given at 7 years of age or older who are at risk of invasive meningococcal disease because of persistent component (eg, C5–C9, properdin, factor H, or factor D) deficiency or functional or anatomic asplenia. (11/11)

MENSTRUATION IN GIRLS AND ADOLESCENTS: USING THE MENSTRUAL CYCLE AS A VITAL SIGN (CLINICAL REPORT)
Committee on Adolescence (joint with American College of Obstetricians and Gynecologists Committee on Adolescent Health Care)

ABSTRACT. Young patients and their parents often are unsure about what represents normal menstrual patterns, and clinicians also may be unsure about normal ranges for menstrual cycle length and amount and duration of flow through adolescence. It is important to be able to educate young patients and their parents regarding what to expect of a first period and about the range for normal cycle length of subsequent menses. It is equally important for clinicians to have an understanding of bleeding patterns in girls and adolescents, the ability to differentiate between normal and abnormal menstruation, and the skill to know how to evaluate young patients' conditions appropriately. Using the menstrual cycle as an additional vital sign adds a powerful tool to the assessment of normal development and the exclusion of pathological conditions. (11/06)

MINORS AS LIVING SOLID-ORGAN DONORS (CLINICAL REPORT)
Lainie Friedman Ross, MD, PhD; J. Richard Thistlethwaite Jr, MD, PhD; and Committee on Bioethics

ABSTRACT. In the past half-century, solid-organ transplantation has become standard treatment for a variety of diseases in children and adults. The major limitation for all transplantation is the availability of donors, and the gap between demand and supply continues to grow despite the increase in living donors. Although rare, children do serve as living donors, and these donations raise serious ethical issues. This clinical report includes a discussion of the ethical considerations regarding minors serving as living donors, using the traditional benefit/burden calculus from the perspectives of both the donor and the recipient. The report also includes an examination of the circumstances under which a minor may morally participate as a living donor, how to minimize risks, and what the informed-consent process should entail. The American Academy of Pediatrics holds that minors can morally serve as living organ donors but only in exceptional circumstances when specific criteria are fulfilled. (8/08, reaffirmed 5/11)

MODEL CONTRACTUAL LANGUAGE FOR MEDICAL NECESSITY FOR CHILDREN
Committee on Child Health Financing
ABSTRACT. The term "medical necessity" is used by Medicare and Medicaid and in insurance contracts to refer to medical services that are generally recognized as appropriate for the diagnosis, prevention, or treatment of disease and injury. There is no consensus on how to define and apply the term and the accompanying rules and regulations, and as a result there has been substantial variation in medical-necessity definitions and interpretations. With this policy statement, the American Academy of Pediatrics hopes to encourage insurers to adopt more consistent medical-necessity definitions that take into account the needs of children. (7/05, reaffirmed 10/11)

MOLECULAR GENETIC TESTING IN PEDIATRIC PRACTICE: A SUBJECT REVIEW (CLINICAL REPORT)
Committee on Genetics
ABSTRACT. Although many types of diagnostic and carrier testing for genetic disorders have been available for decades, the use of molecular methods is a relatively recent phenomenon. Such testing has expanded the range of disorders that can be diagnosed and has enhanced the ability of clinicians to provide accurate prognostic information and institute appropriate health supervision measures. However, the proper application of these tests may be difficult because of their scientific complexity and the potential for negative, sometimes unexpected, consequences for many patients. The purposes of this subject review are to provide background information on molecular genetic tests, to describe specific testing modalities, and to discuss some of the benefits and risks specific to the pediatric population. It is likely that pediatricians will use these testing methods increasingly for their patients and will need to evaluate critically their diagnostic and prognostic implications. (12/00, reaffirmed 5/07)

MOTOR DELAYS: EARLY IDENTIFICATION AND EVALUATION (CLINICAL REPORT)
Garey H. Noritz, MD; Nancy A. Murphy, MD; and Neuromotor Screening Expert Panel
ABSTRACT. Pediatricians often encounter children with delays of motor development in their clinical practices. Earlier identification of motor delays allows for timely referral for developmental interventions as well as diagnostic evaluations and treatment planning. A multidisciplinary expert panel developed an algorithm for the surveillance and screening of children for motor delays within the medical home, offering guidance for the initial workup and referral of the child with possible delays in motor development. Highlights of this clinical report include suggestions for formal developmental screening at the 9-, 18-, 30-, and 48-month well-child visits; approaches to the neurologic examination, with emphasis on the assessment of muscle tone; and initial diagnostic approaches for medical home providers. Use of diagnostic tests to evaluate children with motor delays are described, including brain MRI for children with high muscle tone, and measuring serum creatine kinase concentration of those with decreased muscle tone. The importance of pursuing diagnostic tests while concurrently referring patients to early intervention programs is emphasized. (5/13)
See full text on page 733.

NEONATAL DRUG WITHDRAWAL (CLINICAL REPORT)
Mark L. Hudak, MD; Rosemarie C. Tan, MD, PhD; Committee on Drugs; and Committee on Fetus and Newborn
ABSTRACT. Maternal use of certain drugs during pregnancy can result in transient neonatal signs consistent with withdrawal or acute toxicity or cause sustained signs consistent with a lasting drug effect. In addition, hospitalized infants who are treated with opioids or benzodiazepines to provide analgesia or sedation may be at risk for manifesting signs of withdrawal. This statement updates information about the clinical presentation of infants exposed to intrauterine drugs and the therapeutic options for treatment of withdrawal and is expanded to include evidence-based approaches to the management of the hospitalized infant who requires weaning from analgesics or sedatives. (1/12)

THE NEW MORBIDITY REVISITED: A RENEWED COMMITMENT TO THE PSYCHOSOCIAL ASPECTS OF PEDIATRIC CARE
Committee on Psychosocial Aspects of Child and Family Health
ABSTRACT. In 1993, the American Academy of Pediatrics adopted the policy statement "The Pediatrician and the 'New Morbidity.'" Since then, social difficulties, behavioral problems, and developmental difficulties have become a main part of the scope of pediatric practice, and recognition of the importance of these areas has increased. This statement reaffirms the Academy's commitment to prevention, early detection, and management of behavioral, developmental, and social problems as a focus in pediatric practice. (11/01)

NEWBORN SCREENING EXPANDS: RECOMMENDATIONS FOR PEDIATRICIANS AND MEDICAL HOMES—IMPLICATIONS FOR THE SYSTEM (CLINICAL REPORT)

Newborn Screening Authoring Committee

ABSTRACT. Advances in newborn screening technology, coupled with recent advances in the diagnosis and treatment of rare but serious congenital conditions that affect newborn infants, provide increased opportunities for positively affecting the lives of children and their families. These advantages also pose new challenges to primary care pediatricians, both educationally and in response to the management of affected infants. Primary care pediatricians require immediate access to clinical and diagnostic information and guidance and have a proactive role to play in supporting the performance of the newborn screening system. Primary care pediatricians must develop office policies and procedures to ensure that newborn screening is conducted and that results are transmitted to them in a timely fashion; they must also develop strategies to use should these systems fail. In addition, collaboration with local, state, and national partners is essential for promoting actions and policies that will optimize the function of the newborn screening systems and ensure that families receive the full benefit of them. (1/08)

NEWBORN SCREENING FACT SHEETS, INTRODUCTION TO THE (TECHNICAL REPORT)

Celia I. Kaye, MD, PhD, and Committee on Genetics

ABSTRACT. Newborn screening fact sheets were last revised in 1996 by the Committee on Genetics of the American Academy of Pediatrics. These fact sheets have been revised again because of advances in the field, including technologic innovations such as tandem mass spectrometry, as well as greater appreciation of ethical issues such as informed consent. The fact sheets provide information to assist pediatricians and other professionals who care for children in performing their essential role within the newborn screening public health system. The newborn screening system consists of 5 parts: (1) newborn testing; (2) follow-up of abnormal screening results to facilitate timely diagnostic testing and management; (3) diagnostic testing; (4) disease management, which requires coordination with the medical home and genetic counseling; and (5) continuous evaluation and improvement of the newborn screening system. The following disorders are reviewed in the newborn screening fact sheets (which are available at www.pediatrics.org/cgi/content/full/118/3/e934): biotinidase deficiency, congenital adrenal hyperplasia, congenital hearing loss, congenital hypothyroidism, cystic fibrosis, galactosemia, homocystinuria, maple syrup urine disease, medium-chain acyl-coenzyme A dehydrogenase deficiency, phenylketonuria, sickle cell disease and other hemoglobinopathies, and tyrosinemia. (9/06, reaffirmed 1/11)

NEWBORN SCREENING FACT SHEETS (TECHNICAL REPORT)

Celia I. Kaye, MD, PhD, and Committee on Genetics

ABSTRACT. Newborn screening fact sheets were last revised in 1996 by the American Academy of Pediatrics Committee on Genetics. This revision was prompted by advances in the field since 1996, including technologic innovations, as well as greater appreciation of ethical issues such as those surrounding informed consent. The following disorders are discussed in this revision of the newborn screening fact sheets: biotinidase deficiency, congenital adrenal hyperplasia, congenital hearing loss, congenital hypothyroidism, cystic fibrosis, galactosemia, homocystinuria, maple syrup urine disease, medium-chain acyl-coenzyme A dehydrogenase deficiency, phenylketonuria, sickle cell disease and other hemoglobinopathies, and tyrosinemia. A series of topics related to newborn screening is discussed in a companion publication to this electronic publication of the fact sheets (available at: www.pediatrics.org/cgi/content/full/118/3/1304). These topics are newborn screening as a public health system; factors contributing to the need for review of the newborn screening system; informed consent; tandem mass spectrometry; DNA analysis in newborn screening; status of newborn screening in the United States; and the effect of sample timing, preterm birth, diet, transfusion, and total parenteral nutrition on newborn screening results. (9/06, reaffirmed 1/11)

NONDISCRIMINATION IN PEDIATRIC HEALTH CARE

Committee on Pediatric Workforce

ABSTRACT. This policy statement is a revision of a 2001 statement and articulates the positions of the American Academy of Pediatrics on nondiscrimination in pediatric health care. It addresses both pediatricians who provide health care and the infants, children, adolescents, and young adults whom they serve. (10/07, reaffirmed 6/11)

NONINITIATION OR WITHDRAWAL OF INTENSIVE CARE FOR HIGH-RISK NEWBORNS

Committee on Fetus and Newborn

ABSTRACT. Advances in medical technology have led to dilemmas in initiation and withdrawal of intensive care of newborn infants with a very poor prognosis. Physicians and parents together must make difficult decisions guided by their understanding of the child's best interest. The foundation for these decisions consists of several key elements: (1) direct and open communication between the health care team and the parents of the child with regard to the medical status, prognosis, and treatment options; (2) inclusion of the parents as active participants in the decision process; (3) continuation of comfort care even when intensive care is not being provided; and (4) treatment decisions that are guided primarily by the best interest of the child. (2/07, reaffirmed 5/10)

NONTHERAPEUTIC USE OF ANTIMICROBIAL AGENTS IN ANIMAL AGRICULTURE: IMPLICATIONS FOR PEDIATRICS (TECHNICAL REPORT)

Committee on Environmental Health and Committee on Infectious Diseases

ABSTRACT. Antimicrobial resistance is widespread. Overuse or misuse of antimicrobial agents in veterinary and human medicine is responsible for increasing the crisis of resistance to antimicrobial agents. The American Academy of Pediatrics, in conjunction with the US Public Health Service, has begun to address this problem by disseminating policies on the judicious use of antimicrobial agents in humans. Between 40% and 80% of the antimicrobial agents used in the United States each year are used in food animals; many are identical or very similar to drugs used in humans. Most of this use involves the addition of low doses of antimicrobial agents to the feed of healthy animals over prolonged periods to promote growth and increase feed efficiency or at a range of doses to prevent disease. These nontherapeutic uses contribute to resistance and create health dangers for humans. This report will describe how antimicrobial agents are used in animal agriculture and review the mechanisms by which such uses contribute to resistance in human pathogens. Although therapeutic use of antimicrobial agents in agriculture clearly contributes to the development of resistance, this report will concentrate on nontherapeutic uses in healthy animals. (9/04, reaffirmed 10/08, 4/13)

OFFICE-BASED CARE FOR LESBIAN, GAY, BISEXUAL, TRANSGENDER, AND QUESTIONING YOUTH
Committee on Adolescence
ABSTRACT. The American Academy of Pediatrics issued its last statement on homosexuality and adolescents in 2004. Although most lesbian, gay, bisexual, transgender, and questioning (LGBTQ) youth are quite resilient and emerge from adolescence as healthy adults, the effects of homophobia and heterosexism can contribute to health disparities in mental health with higher rates of depression and suicidal ideation, higher rates of substance abuse, and more sexually transmitted and HIV infections. Pediatricians should have offices that are teen-friendly and welcoming to sexual minority youth. Obtaining a comprehensive, confidential, developmentally appropriate adolescent psychosocial history allows for the discovery of strengths and assets as well as risks. Referrals for mental health or substance abuse may be warranted. Sexually active LGBTQ youth should have sexually transmitted infection/HIV testing according to recommendations of the Sexually Transmitted Diseases Treatment Guidelines of the Centers for Disease Control and Prevention based on sexual behaviors. With appropriate assistance and care, sexual minority youth should live healthy, productive lives while transitioning through adolescence and young adulthood. (6/13)
See full text on page 747.

OFFICE-BASED CARE FOR LESBIAN, GAY, BISEXUAL, TRANSGENDER, AND QUESTIONING YOUTH (TECHNICAL REPORT)
David A. Levine, MD, and Committee on Adolescence
ABSTRACT. The American Academy of Pediatrics issued its last statement on homosexuality and adolescents in 2004.This technical report reflects the rapidly expanding medical and psychosocial literature about sexual minority youth. Pediatricians should be aware that some youth in their care may have concerns or questions about their sexual orientation or that of siblings, friends, parents, relatives, or others and should provide factual, current, nonjudgmental information in a confidential manner. Although most lesbian, gay, bisexual, transgender, and questioning (LGBTQ) youth are quite resilient and emerge from adolescence as healthy adults, the effects of homophobia and heterosexism can contribute to increased

mental health issues for sexual minority youth. LGBTQ and MSM/WSW (men having sex with men and women having sex with women) adolescents, in comparison with heterosexual adolescents, have higher rates of depression and suicidal ideation, higher rates of substance abuse, and more risky sexual behaviors. Obtaining a comprehensive, confidential, developmentally appropriate adolescent psychosocial history allows for the discovery of strengths and assets as well as risks. Pediatricians should have offices that are teen-friendly and welcoming to sexual minority youth. This includes having supportive, engaging office staff members who ensure that there are no barriers to care. For transgender youth, pediatricians should provide the opportunity to acknowledge and affirm their feelings of gender dysphoria and desires to transition to the opposite gender. Referral of transgender youth to a qualified mental health professional is critical to assist with the dysphoria, to educate them, and to assess their readiness for transition. With appropriate assistance and care, sexual minority youth should live healthy, productive lives while transitioning through adolescence and young adulthood. (6/13)
See full text on page 755.

OFFICE-BASED COUNSELING FOR UNINTENTIONAL INJURY PREVENTION (CLINICAL REPORT)
H. Garry Gardner, MD, and Committee on Injury, Violence, and Poison Prevention
ABSTRACT. Unintentional injuries are the leading cause of death for children older than 1 year. Pediatricians should include unintentional injury prevention as a major component of anticipatory guidance for infants, children, and adolescents. The content of injury-prevention counseling varies for infants, preschool-aged children, school-aged children, and adolescents. This report provides guidance on the content of unintentional injury-prevention counseling for each of those age groups. (1/07)

OPHTHALMOLOGIC EXAMINATIONS IN CHILDREN WITH JUVENILE RHEUMATOID ARTHRITIS (CLINICAL REPORT)
James Cassidy, MD; Jane Kivlin, MD; Carol Lindsley, MD; James Nocton, MD; Section on Rheumatology; and Section on Ophthalmology
ABSTRACT. Unlike the joints, ocular involvement with juvenile rheumatoid arthritis is most often asymptomatic; yet, the inflammation can cause serious morbidity with loss of vision. Scheduled slit-lamp examinations by an ophthalmologist at specific intervals can detect ocular disease early, and prompt treatment can prevent vision loss. (5/06)

ORAL AND DENTAL ASPECTS OF CHILD ABUSE AND NEGLECT (CLINICAL REPORT)
Nancy Kellogg, MD, and Committee on Child Abuse and Neglect (joint with American Academy of Pediatric Dentistry)
ABSTRACT. In all 50 states, physicians and dentists are required to report suspected cases of abuse and neglect to social service or law enforcement agencies. The purpose of this report is to review the oral and dental aspects of physical and sexual abuse and dental neglect and the role of physicians and dentists in evaluating such condi-

tions. This report addresses the evaluation of bite marks as well as perioral and intraoral injuries, infections, and diseases that may cause suspicion for child abuse or neglect. Physicians receive minimal training in oral health and dental injury and disease and, thus, may not detect dental aspects of abuse or neglect as readily as they do child abuse and neglect involving other areas of the body. Therefore, physicians and dentists are encouraged to collaborate to increase the prevention, detection, and treatment of these conditions. (12/05, reaffirmed 1/09)

ORAL HEALTH CARE FOR CHILDREN WITH DEVELOPMENTAL DISABILITIES (CLINICAL REPORT)
Kenneth W. Norwood Jr, MD; Rebecca L. Slayton, DDS, PhD; Council on Children With Disabilities; and Section on Oral Health

ABSTRACT. Children with developmental disabilities often have unmet complex health care needs as well as significant physical and cognitive limitations. Children with more severe conditions and from low-income families are particularly at risk with high dental needs and poor access to care. In addition, children with developmental disabilities are living longer, requiring continued oral health care. This clinical report describes the effect that poor oral health has on children with developmental disabilities as well as the importance of partnerships between the pediatric medical and dental homes. Basic knowledge of the oral health risk factors affecting children with developmental disabilities is provided. Pediatricians may use the report to guide their incorporation of oral health assessments and education into their well-child examinations for children with developmental disabilities. This report has medical, legal, educational, and operational implications for practicing pediatricians. (2/13)

See full text on page 775.

ORAL HEALTH RISK ASSESSMENT TIMING AND ESTABLISHMENT OF THE DENTAL HOME
Section on Pediatric Dentistry

ABSTRACT. Early childhood dental caries has been reported by the Centers for Disease Control and Prevention to be perhaps the most prevalent infectious disease of our nation's children. Early childhood dental caries occurs in all racial and socioeconomic groups; however, it tends to be more prevalent in low-income children, in whom it occurs in epidemic proportions. Dental caries results from an overgrowth of specific organisms that are a part of normally occurring human flora. Human dental flora is site specific, and an infant is not colonized until the eruption of the primary dentition at approximately 6 to 30 months of age. The most likely source of inoculation of an infant's dental flora is the mother or another intimate care provider, through shared utensils, etc. Decreasing the level of cariogenic organisms in the mother's dental flora at the time of colonization can significantly impact the child's predisposition to caries. To prevent caries in children, high-risk individuals must be identified at an early age (preferably high-risk mothers during prenatal care), and aggressive strategies should be adopted, including anticipatory guidance, behavior modifications (oral hygiene and feeding practices), and establishment of a dental home by 1 year of age for children deemed at risk. (5/03, reaffirmed 5/09)

ORGANIC FOODS: HEALTH AND ENVIRONMENTAL ADVANTAGES AND DISADVANTAGES (CLINICAL REPORT)
Joel Forman, MD; Janet Silverstein, MD; Committee on Nutrition; and Council on Environmental Health

ABSTRACT. The US market for organic foods has grown from $3.5 billion in 1996 to $28.6 billion in 2010, according to the Organic Trade Association. Organic products are now sold in specialty stores and conventional supermarkets. Organic products contain numerous marketing claims and terms, only some of which are standardized and regulated.

In terms of health advantages, organic diets have been convincingly demonstrated to expose consumers to fewer pesticides associated with human disease. Organic farming has been demonstrated to have less environmental impact than conventional approaches. However, current evidence does not support any meaningful nutritional benefits or deficits from eating organic compared with conventionally grown foods, and there are no well-powered human studies that directly demonstrate health benefits or disease protection as a result of consuming an organic diet. Studies also have not demonstrated any detrimental or disease-promoting effects from an organic diet. Although organic foods regularly command a significant price premium, well-designed farming studies demonstrate that costs can be competitive and yields comparable to those of conventional farming techniques. Pediatricians should incorporate this evidence when discussing the health and environmental impact of organic foods and organic farming while continuing to encourage all patients and their families to attain optimal nutrition and dietary variety consistent with the US Department of Agriculture's MyPlate recommendations.

This clinical report reviews the health and environmental issues related to organic food production and consumption. It defines the term "organic," reviews organic food-labeling standards, describes organic and conventional farming practices, and explores the cost and environmental implications of organic production techniques. It examines the evidence available on nutritional quality and production contaminants in conventionally produced and organic foods. Finally, this report provides guidance for pediatricians to assist them in advising their patients regarding organic and conventionally produced food choices. (10/12)

ORGANIZED SPORTS FOR CHILDREN AND PREADOLESCENTS
Committee on Sports Medicine and Fitness and Committee on School Health

ABSTRACT. Participation in organized sports provides an opportunity for young people to increase their physical activity and develop physical and social skills. However, when the demands and expectations of organized sports exceed the maturation and readiness of the participant, the positive aspects of participation can be negated. The nature of parental or adult involvement can also influence the degree to which participation in organized sports is a positive experience for preadolescents. This updates a previous policy statement on athletics for preadolescents and incorporates guidelines for sports participation for preschool children. Recommendations are offered on how pediatricians can help determine a child's readiness to participate, how risks can be minimized, and how child-oriented goals can be maximized. (6/01, reaffirmed 1/05, 6/11)

OUT-OF-SCHOOL SUSPENSION AND EXPULSION
Council on School Health

ABSTRACT. The primary mission of any school system is to educate students. To achieve this goal, the school district must maintain a culture and environment where all students feel safe, nurtured, and valued and where order and civility are expected standards of behavior. Schools cannot allow unacceptable behavior to interfere with the school district's primary mission. To this end, school districts adopt codes of conduct for expected behaviors and policies to address unacceptable behavior. In developing these policies, school boards must weigh the severity of the offense and the consequences of the punishment and the balance between individual and institutional rights and responsibilities. Out-of-school suspension and expulsion are the most severe consequences that a school district can impose for unacceptable behavior. Traditionally, these consequences have been reserved for offenses deemed especially severe or dangerous and/ or for recalcitrant offenders. However, the implications and consequences of out-of-school suspension and expulsion and "zero-tolerance" are of such severity that their application and appropriateness for a developing child require periodic review. The indications and effectiveness of exclusionary discipline policies that demand automatic or rigorous application are increasingly questionable. The impact of these policies on offenders, other children, school districts, and communities is broad. Periodic scrutiny of policies should be placed not only on the need for a better understanding of the educational, emotional, and social impact of out-of-school suspension and expulsion on the individual student but also on the greater societal costs of such rigid policies. Pediatricians should be prepared to assist students and families affected by out-of-school suspension and expulsion and should be willing to guide school districts in their communities to find more effective and appropriate alternatives to exclusionary discipline policies for the developing child. A discussion of preventive strategies and alternatives to out-of-school suspension and expulsion, as well as recommendations for the role of the physician in matters of out-of-school suspension and expulsion are included. School-wide positive behavior support/positive behavior intervention and support is discussed as an effective alternative. (2/13)
See full text on page 783.

OVERCROWDING CRISIS IN OUR NATION'S EMERGENCY DEPARTMENTS: IS OUR SAFETY NET UNRAVELING?
Committee on Pediatric Emergency Medicine

ABSTRACT. Emergency departments (EDs) are a vital component in our health care safety net, available 24 hours a day, 7 days a week, for all who require care. There has been a steady increase in the volume and acuity of patient visits to EDs, now with well over 100 million Americans (30 million children) receiving emergency care annually. This rise in ED utilization has effectively saturated the capacity of EDs and emergency medical services in many communities. The resulting phenomenon, commonly referred to as ED overcrowding, now threatens access to emergency services for those who need them the most. As managers of the pediatric medical home and advocates for children and optimal pediatric health care, there is a very important role for pediatricians and the American Academy of Pediatrics in guiding health policy decision-makers toward effective solutions that promote the medical home and timely access to emergency care. (9/04, reaffirmed 5/07, 6/11)

OVERUSE INJURIES, OVERTRAINING, AND BURNOUT IN CHILD AND ADOLESCENT ATHLETES (CLINICAL REPORT)
Joel S. Brenner, MD, MPH, and Council on Sports Medicine and Fitness

ABSTRACT. Overuse is one of the most common etiologic factors that lead to injuries in the pediatric and adolescent athlete. As more children are becoming involved in organized and recreational athletics, the incidence of overuse injuries is increasing. Many children are participating in sports year-round and sometimes on multiple teams simultaneously. This overtraining can lead to burnout, which may have a detrimental effect on the child participating in sports as a lifelong healthy activity. One contributing factor to overtraining may be parental pressure to compete and succeed. The purpose of this clinical report is to assist pediatricians in identifying and counseling at-risk children and their families. This report supports the American Academy of Pediatrics policy statement on intensive training and sport specialization. (6/07, reaffirmed 3/11)

PALLIATIVE CARE FOR CHILDREN
Committee on Bioethics and Committee on Hospital Care

ABSTRACT. This statement presents an integrated model for providing palliative care for children living with a life-threatening or terminal condition. Advice on the development of a palliative care plan and on working with parents and children is also provided. Barriers to the provision of effective pediatric palliative care and potential solutions are identified. The American Academy of Pediatrics recommends the development and broad availability of pediatric palliative care services based on child-specific guidelines and standards. Such services will require widely distributed and effective palliative care education of pediatric health care professionals. The Academy offers guidance on responding to requests for hastening death, but does not support the practice of physician-assisted suicide or euthanasia for children. (8/00, reaffirmed 6/03, 10/06, 2/12)

PARENT-PROVIDER-COMMUNITY PARTNERSHIPS: OPTIMIZING OUTCOMES FOR CHILDREN WITH DISABILITIES (CLINICAL REPORT)

Nancy A. Murphy, MD; Paul S. Carbone, MD; and Council on Children With Disabilities

ABSTRACT. Children with disabilities and their families have multifaceted medical, developmental, educational, and habilitative needs that are best addressed through strong partnerships among parents, providers, and communities. However, traditional health care systems are designed to address acute rather than chronic conditions. Children with disabilities require high-quality medical homes that provide care coordination and transitional care, and their families require social and financial supports. Integrated community systems of care that promote participation of all children are needed. The purpose of this clinical report is to explore the challenges of developing effective community-based systems of care and to offer suggestions to pediatricians and policy-makers regarding the development of partnerships among children with disabilities, their families, and health care and other providers to maximize health and well-being of these children and their families. (9/11)

PARENTAL LEAVE FOR RESIDENTS AND PEDIATRIC TRAINING PROGRAMS

Section on Medical Students, Residents, and Fellowship Trainees and Committee on Early Childhood

ABSTRACT. The American Academy of Pediatrics (AAP) is committed to the development of rational, equitable, and effective parental leave policies that are sensitive to the needs of pediatric residents, families, and developing infants and that enable parents to spend adequate and good-quality time with their young children. It is important for each residency program to have a policy for parental leave that is written, that is accessible to residents, and that clearly delineates program practices regarding parental leave. At a minimum, a parental leave policy for residents and fellows should conform legally with the Family Medical Leave Act as well as with respective state laws and should meet institutional requirements of the Accreditation Council for Graduate Medical Education for accredited programs. Policies should be well formulated and communicated in a culturally sensitive manner. The AAP advocates for extension of benefits consistent with the Family Medical Leave Act to all residents and interns beginning at the time that pediatric residency training begins. The AAP recommends that regardless of gender, residents who become parents should be guaranteed 6 to 8 weeks, at a minimum, of parental leave with pay after the infant's birth. In addition, in conformance with federal law, the resident should be allowed to extend the leave time when necessary by using paid vacation time or leave without pay. Coparenting, adopting, or fostering of a child should entitle the resident, regardless of gender, to the same amount of paid leave (6–8 weeks) as a person who takes maternity/paternity leave. Flexibility, creativity, and advanced planning are necessary to arrange schedules that optimize resident education and experience, cultivate equity in sharing workloads, and protect pregnant residents from overly strenuous work experiences at critical times of their pregnancies. (1/13)
See full text on page 793.

PATIENT- AND FAMILY-CENTERED CARE OF CHILDREN IN THE EMERGENCY DEPARTMENT (TECHNICAL REPORT)

Patricia J. O'Malley, MD; Kathleen Brown, MD; Steven E. Krug, MD; and Committee on Pediatric Emergency Medicine

ABSTRACT. Patient- and family-centered care is an innovative approach to the planning, delivery, and evaluation of health care that is grounded in a mutually beneficial partnership among patients, families, and health care professionals. Providing patient- and family-centered care to children in the emergency department setting presents many opportunities and challenges. This technical report draws on previously published policy statements and reports, reviews the current literature, and describes the present state of practice and research regarding patient- and family-centered care for children in the emergency department setting as well as some of the complexities of providing such care. This technical report has been endorsed by the Academic Pediatric Association (formerly the Ambulatory Pediatric Association), the American College of Osteopathic Emergency Physicians, the National Association of Emergency Medical Technicians, the Institute for Family-Centered Care, and the American College of Emergency Physicians. This report is also supported by the Emergency Nurses Association. (8/08)

PATIENT- AND FAMILY-CENTERED CARE AND THE PEDIATRICIAN'S ROLE

Committee on Hospital Care and Institute for Patient- and Family-Centered Care

ABSTRACT. Drawing on several decades of work with families, pediatricians, other health care professionals, and policy makers, the American Academy of Pediatrics provides a definition of patient- and family-centered care. In pediatrics, patient- and family-centered care is based on the understanding that the family is the child's primary source of strength and support. Further, this approach to care recognizes that the perspectives and information provided by families, children, and young adults are essential components of high-quality clinical decision-making, and that patients and family are integral partners with the health care team. This policy statement outlines the core principles of patient- and family-centered care, summarizes some of the recent literature linking patient- and family-centered care to improved health outcomes, and lists various other benefits to be expected when engaging in patient- and family-centered pediatric practice. The statement concludes with specific recommendations for how pediatricians can integrate patient- and family-centered care in hospitals, clinics, and community settings, and in broader systems of care, as well. (1/12)

PATIENT- AND FAMILY-CENTERED CARE AND THE ROLE OF THE EMERGENCY PHYSICIAN PROVIDING CARE TO A CHILD IN THE EMERGENCY DEPARTMENT

Committee on Pediatric Emergency Medicine (joint with American College of Emergency Physicians)

ABSTRACT. Patient- and family-centered care is an approach to health care that recognizes the role of the family in providing medical care; encourages collaboration between the patient, family, and health care professionals; and honors individual and family strengths, cultures, traditions, and expertise. Although there are many opportunities for providing patient- and family-centered care in the emergency department, there are also challenges to doing so. The American Academy of Pediatrics and the American College of Emergency Physicians support promoting patient dignity, comfort, and autonomy; recognizing the patient and family as key decision-makers in the patient's medical care; recognizing the patient's experience and perspective in a culturally sensitive manner; acknowledging the interdependence of child and parent as well as the pediatric patient's evolving independence; encouraging family-member presence; providing information to the family during interventions; encouraging collaboration with other health care professionals; acknowledging the importance of the patient's medical home; and encouraging institutional policies for patient- and family-centered care. (11/06, reaffirmed 6/09, 10/11)

PATIENT SAFETY IN THE PEDIATRIC EMERGENCY CARE SETTING

Committee on Pediatric Emergency Medicine

ABSTRACT. Patient safety is a priority for all health care professionals, including those who work in emergency care. Unique aspects of pediatric care may increase the risk of medical error and harm to patients, especially in the emergency care setting. Although errors can happen despite the best human efforts, given the right set of circumstances, health care professionals must work proactively to improve safety in the pediatric emergency care system. Specific recommendations to improve pediatric patient safety in the emergency department are provided in this policy statement. (12/07, reaffirmed 6/11)

PAYMENT FOR TELEPHONE CARE

Section on Telephone Care and Committee on Child Health Financing

ABSTRACT. Telephone care in pediatrics requires medical judgment, is associated with practice expense and medical liability risk, and can often substitute for more costly face-to-face care. Despite this, physicians are infrequently paid by patients or third-party payors for medical services provided by telephone. As the costs of maintaining a practice continue to increase, pediatricians are increasingly seeking payment for the time and work involved in telephone care. This statement reviews the role of telephone care in pediatric practice, the current state of payment for telephone care, and the practical issues associated with charging for telephone care services, a service traditionally provided gratis to patients and families. Specific recommendations are presented for appropriate documenting, reporting, and billing for telephone care services. (10/06)

PEDESTRIAN SAFETY

Committee on Injury, Violence, and Poison Prevention

ABSTRACT. Each year, approximately 900 pediatric pedestrians younger than 19 years are killed. In addition, 51000 children are injured as pedestrians, and 5300 of them are hospitalized because of their injuries. Parents should be warned that young children often do not have the cognitive, perceptual, and behavioral abilities to negotiate traffic independently. Parents should also be informed about the danger of vehicle back-over injuries to toddlers playing in driveways. Because posttraumatic stress syndrome commonly follows even minor pedestrian injury, pediatricians should screen and refer for this condition as necessary. The American Academy of Pediatrics supports community- and school-based strategies that minimize a child's exposure to traffic, especially to high-speed, high-volume traffic. Furthermore, the American Academy of Pediatrics supports governmental and industry action that would lead to improvements in vehicle design, driver manuals, driver education, and data collection for the purpose of reducing pediatric pedestrian injury. (7/09, reaffirmed 8/13)

PEDIATRIC AND ADOLESCENT MENTAL HEALTH EMERGENCIES IN THE EMERGENCY MEDICAL SERVICES SYSTEM (TECHNICAL REPORT)

Margaret A. Dolan, MD; Joel A. Fein, MD, MPH; and Committee on Pediatric Emergency Medicine

ABSTRACT. Emergency department (ED) health care professionals often care for patients with previously diagnosed psychiatric illnesses who are ill, injured, or having a behavioral crisis. In addition, ED personnel encounter children with psychiatric illnesses who may not present to the ED with overt mental health symptoms. Staff education and training regarding identification and management of pediatric mental health illness can help EDs overcome the perceived limitations of the setting that influence timely and comprehensive evaluation. In addition, ED physicians can inform and advocate for policy changes at local, state, and national levels that are needed to ensure comprehensive care of children with mental health illnesses. This report addresses the roles that the ED and ED health care professionals play in emergency mental health care of children and adolescents in the United States, which includes the stabilization and management of patients in mental health crisis, the discovery of mental illnesses and suicidal ideation in ED patients, and approaches to advocating for improved recognition and treatment of mental illnesses in children. The report also addresses special issues related to mental illness in the ED, such as minority populations, children with special health care needs, and children's mental health during and after disasters and trauma. (4/11)

PEDIATRIC ASPECTS OF INPATIENT HEALTH INFORMATION TECHNOLOGY SYSTEMS (TECHNICAL REPORT)

George R. Kim; Christoph U. Lehmann, MD; and Council on Clinical Information Technology

ABSTRACT. US adoption of health information technology as a path to improved quality of patient care (effectiveness, safety, timeliness, patient-centeredness, efficiency, and equity) has been promoted by the medical community. Children and infants (especially those with special health care needs) are at higher risk than are adults for medical errors and their consequences (particularly in environments in which children are not the primary patient population). However, development and adoption of health information technology tools and practices that promote pediatric quality and patient safety are lagging. Two inpatient clinical processes—medication delivery and patient care transitions—are discussed in terms of health information technology applications that support them and functions that are important to pediatric quality and safety. Pediatricians and their partners (pediatric nurses, pharmacists, etc) must develop awareness of technical and adaptive issues in adopting these tools and collaborate with organizational leaders and developers as advocates for the best interests and safety of pediatric patients. Pediatric health information technology adoption cannot be considered in terms of applications (such as electronic health records or computerized physician order entry) alone but must be considered globally in terms of technical (health information technology applications), organizational (structures and workflows of care), and cultural (stakeholders) aspects of what is best. (12/08)

PEDIATRIC CARE RECOMMENDATIONS FOR FREESTANDING URGENT CARE FACILITIES
Committee on Pediatric Emergency Medicine
ABSTRACT. Freestanding urgent care centers are not emergency departments or medical homes, yet they are sometimes used as a source of pediatric care. The purpose of this policy statement is to provide updated and expanded recommendations for ensuring appropriate stabilization in pediatric emergency situations and timely and appropriate transfer to a hospital for definitive care when necessary. (7/05, reaffirmed 1/09, 6/11)

PEDIATRIC FELLOWSHIP TRAINING
Federation of Pediatric Organizations (7/04)

PEDIATRIC MENTAL HEALTH EMERGENCIES IN THE EMERGENCY MEDICAL SERVICES SYSTEM
Committee on Pediatric Emergency Medicine (joint with American College of Emergency Physicians)
ABSTRACT. Emergency departments are vital in the management of pediatric patients with mental health emergencies. Pediatric mental health emergencies are an increasing part of emergency medical practice because emergency departments have become the safety net for a fragmented mental health infrastructure that is experiencing critical shortages in services in all sectors. Emergency departments must safely, humanely, and in a culturally and developmentally appropriate manner manage pediatric patients with undiagnosed and known mental illnesses, including those with mental retardation, autistic spectrum disorders, and attention-deficit/hyperactivity disorder and those experiencing a behavioral crisis. Emergency departments also manage patients with suicidal ideation, depression, escalating aggression, substance abuse, post-traumatic stress disorder, and maltreatment and those exposed to violence and unexpected deaths. Emergency departments must address not only the physical but also the mental health needs of patients during and after mass-casualty incidents and disasters. The American Academy of Pediatrics and the American College of Emergency Physicians support advocacy for increased mental health resources, including improved pediatric mental health tools for the emergency department, increased mental health insurance coverage, and adequate reimbursement at all levels; acknowledgment of the importance of the child's medical home; and promotion of education and research for mental health emergencies. (10/06, reaffirmed 6/09, 4/13)

PEDIATRIC OBSERVATION UNITS (CLINICAL REPORT)
Gregory P. Conners, MD, MPH, MBA; Sanford M. Melzer, MD, MBA; Committee on Hospital Care; and Committee on Pediatric Emergency Medicine
ABSTRACT. Pediatric observation units (OUs) are hospital areas used to provide medical evaluation and/or management for health-related conditions in children, typically for a well-defined, brief period. Pediatric OUs represent an emerging alternative site of care for selected groups of children who historically may have received their treatment in an ambulatory setting, emergency department, or hospital-based inpatient unit. This clinical report provides an overview of pediatric OUs, including the definitions and operating characteristics of different types of OUs, quality considerations and coding for observation services, and the effect of OUs on inpatient hospital utilization. (6/12)

PEDIATRIC ORGAN DONATION AND TRANSPLANTATION
Committee on Hospital Care, Section on Surgery, and Section on Critical Care
ABSTRACT. Pediatric organ donation and organ transplantation can have a significant life-extending benefit to the young recipients of these organs and a high emotional impact on donor and recipient families. Pediatricians, pediatric medical specialists, and pediatric transplant surgeons need to be better acquainted with evolving national strategies that involve organ procurement and organ transplantation to help acquaint families with the benefits and risks of organ donation and transplantation. Efforts of pediatric professionals are needed to shape public policies to provide a system in which procurement, distribution, and cost are fair and equitable to children and adults. Major issues of concern are availability of and access to donor organs; oversight and control of the process; pediatric medical and surgical consultation and continued care throughout the organ-donation and transplantation process; ethical, social, financial, and follow-up issues; insurance-coverage issues; and public awareness of the need for organ donors of all ages. (3/10)

PEDIATRIC PALLIATIVE CARE AND HOSPICE CARE COMMITMENTS, GUIDELINES, AND RECOMMENDATIONS
Section on Hospice and Palliative Medicine and Committee on Hospital Care
ABSTRACT. Pediatric palliative care and pediatric hospice care (PPC-PHC) are often essential aspects of medical care for patients who have life-threatening conditions or

need end-of-life care. PPC-PHC aims to relieve suffering, improve quality of life, facilitate informed decision-making, and assist in care coordination between clinicians and across sites of care. Core commitments of PPC-PHC include being patient centered and family engaged; respecting and partnering with patients and families; pursuing care that is high quality, readily accessible, and equitable; providing care across the age spectrum and life span, integrated into the continuum of care; ensuring that all clinicians can provide basic palliative care and consult PPC-PHC specialists in a timely manner; and improving care through research and quality improvement efforts. PPC-PHC guidelines and recommendations include ensuring that all large health care organizations serving children with life-threatening conditions have dedicated interdisciplinary PPC-PHC teams, which should develop collaborative relationships between hospital- and community-based teams; that PPC-PHC be provided as integrated multimodal care and practiced as a cornerstone of patient safety and quality for patients with life-threatening conditions; that PPC-PHC teams should facilitate clear, compassionate, and forthright discussions about medical issues and the goals of care and support families, siblings, and health care staff; that PPC-PHC be part of all pediatric education and training curricula, be an active area of research and quality improvement, and exemplify the highest ethical standards; and that PPC-PHC services be supported by financial and regulatory arrangements to ensure access to high-quality PPC-PHC by all patients with life-threatening and life-shortening diseases. (10/13)

See full text on page 799.

PEDIATRIC PRIMARY HEALTH CARE
Committee on Pediatric Workforce (11/93, reaffirmed 6/01
   AAP News, 1/05, 10/07, 9/10)

PEDIATRIC SUDDEN CARDIAC ARREST
Section on Cardiology and Cardiac Surgery
ABSTRACT. Pediatric sudden cardiac arrest (SCA), which can cause sudden cardiac death if not treated within minutes, has a profound effect on everyone: children, parents, family members, communities, and health care providers. Preventing the tragedy of pediatric SCA, defined as the abrupt and unexpected loss of heart function, remains a concern to all. The goal of this statement is to increase the knowledge of pediatricians (including primary care providers and specialists) of the incidence of pediatric SCA, the spectrum of causes of pediatric SCA, disease-specific presentations, the role of patient and family screening, the rapidly evolving role of genetic testing, and finally, important aspects of secondary SCA prevention. This statement is not intended to address sudden infant death syndrome or sudden unexplained death syndrome, nor will specific treatment of individual cardiac conditions be discussed. This statement has been endorsed by the American College of Cardiology, the American Heart Association, and the Heart Rhythm Society. (3/12)

THE PEDIATRICIAN AND CHILDHOOD BEREAVEMENT
*Committee on Psychosocial Aspects of Child and
   Family Health*
ABSTRACT. Pediatricians should understand and evaluate children's reactions to the death of a person important to them by using age-appropriate and culturally sensitive guidance while being alert for normal and complicated grief responses. Pediatricians also should advise and assist families in responding to the child's needs. Sharing, family support, and communication have been associated with positive long-term bereavement adjustment. (2/00, reaffirmed 1/04, 3/13)

THE PEDIATRICIAN AND DISASTER PREPAREDNESS
*Committee on Pediatric Emergency Medicine, Committee on
   Medical Liability, and Task Force on Terrorism*
ABSTRACT. Recent natural disasters and events of terrorism and war have heightened society's recognition of the need for emergency preparedness. In addition to the unique pediatric issues involved in general emergency preparedness, several additional issues related to terrorism preparedness must be considered, including the unique vulnerabilities of children to various agents as well as the limited availability of age- and weight-appropriate antidotes and treatments. Although children may respond more rapidly to therapeutic intervention, they are at the same time more susceptible to various agents and conditions and more likely to deteriorate if not monitored carefully.

The challenge of dealing with the threat of terrorism, natural disasters, and public health emergencies in the United States is daunting not only for disaster planners but also for our medical system and health professionals of all types, including pediatricians. As part of the network of health responders, pediatricians need to be able to answer concerns of patients and families, recognize signs of possible exposure to a weapon of terror, understand first-line response to such attacks, and sufficiently participate in disaster planning to ensure that the unique needs of children are addressed satisfactorily in the overall process. Pediatricians play a central role in disaster and terrorism preparedness with families, children, and their communities. This applies not only to the general pediatrician but also to the pediatric medical subspecialist and pediatric surgical specialist. Families view pediatricians as their expert resource, and most of them expect the pediatrician to be knowledgeable in areas of concern. Providing expert guidance entails educating families in anticipation of events and responding to questions during and after actual events. It is essential that pediatricians educate themselves regarding these issues of emergency preparedness.

For pediatricians, some information is currently available on virtually all of these issues in recently produced printed materials, at special conferences, in broadcasts of various types, and on the Internet. However, selecting appropriate, accurate sources of information and determining how much information is sufficient remain difficult challenges. Similarly, guidance is needed with respect to developing relevant curricula for medical students and postdoctoral clinical trainees. (2/06, reaffirmed 6/09, 9/13)

PEDIATRICIAN-FAMILY-PATIENT RELATIONSHIPS: MANAGING THE BOUNDARIES
Committee on Bioethics

ABSTRACT. All professionals are concerned about maintaining the appropriate limits in their relationships with those they serve. Pediatricians should be aware that, under normal circumstances, caring for one's own children presents significant ethical issues. Pediatricians also must strive to maintain appropriate professional boundaries in their relationships with the family members of their patients. Pediatricians should avoid behavior that patients and parents might misunderstand as having sexual or inappropriate social meaning. Romantic and sexual involvement between physicians and patients is unacceptable. The acceptance of gifts or nonmonetary compensation for medical services has the potential to affect the professional relationship adversely. (11/09)

THE PEDIATRICIAN WORKFORCE: CURRENT STATUS AND FUTURE PROSPECTS (TECHNICAL REPORT)
David C. Goodman, MD, MS, and Committee on Pediatric Workforce

ABSTRACT. The effective and efficient delivery of children's health care depends on the pediatrician workforce. The number, composition, and distribution of pediatricians necessary to deliver this care have been the subject of long-standing policy and professional debate. This technical report reviews current characteristics and recent trends in the pediatric workforce and couples the workforce to a conceptual model of improvement in children's health and well-being. Important recent changes in the workforce include (1) the growth in the number of pediatricians in relation to the child population, (2) increased numbers of female pediatricians and their attainment of majority gender status in the specialty, (3) the persistence of a large number of international medical graduates entering training programs, (4) a lack of ethnic and racial diversity in pediatricians compared with children, and (5) the persistence of marked regional variation in pediatrician supply. Supply models projecting the pediatric workforce are reviewed and generally indicate that the number of pediatricians per child will increase by 50% over the next 20 years. The differing methods of assessing workforce requirements are presented and critiqued. The report finds that the pediatric workforce is undergoing fundamental changes that will have important effects on the professional lives of pediatricians and children's health care delivery. (7/05)

PEDIATRICIAN WORKFORCE POLICY STATEMENT
Committee on Pediatric Workforce

ABSTRACT. This policy statement reviews important trends and other factors that affect the pediatrician workforce and the provision of pediatric health care, including changes in the pediatric patient population, pediatrician workforce, and nature of pediatric practice. The effect of these changes on pediatricians and the demand for pediatric care are discussed. The American Academy of Pediatrics (AAP) concludes that there is currently a shortage of pediatric medical subspecialists in many fields, as well as a shortage of pediatric surgical specialists. In addition, the AAP believes that the current distribution of primary care pediatricians is inadequate to meet the needs of children living in rural and other underserved areas, and more primary care pediatricians will be needed in the future because of the increasing number of children who have significant chronic health problems, changes in physician work hours, and implementation of current health reform efforts that seek to improve access to comprehensive patient- and family-centered care for all children in a medical home. The AAP is committed to being an active participant in physician workforce policy development with both professional organizations and governmental bodies to ensure a pediatric perspective on health care workforce issues. The overall purpose of this statement is to summarize policy recommendations and serve as a resource for the AAP and other stakeholders as they address pediatrician workforce issues that ultimately influence the quality of pediatric health care provided to children in the United States. (7/13)
See full text on page 809.

THE PEDIATRICIAN'S ROLE IN CHILD MALTREATMENT PREVENTION (CLINICAL REPORT)
Emalee G. Flaherty, MD; John Stirling Jr, MD; and Committee on Child Abuse and Neglect

ABSTRACT. It is the pediatrician's role to promote the child's well-being and to help parents raise healthy, well-adjusted children. Pediatricians, therefore, can play an important role in the prevention of child maltreatment. Previous clinical reports and policy statements from the American Academy of Pediatrics have focused on improving the identification and management of child maltreatment. This clinical report outlines how the pediatrician can help to strengthen families and promote safe, stable, nurturing relationships with the aim of preventing maltreatment. After describing some of the triggers and factors that place children at risk for maltreatment, the report describes how pediatricians can identify family strengths, recognize risk factors, provide helpful guidance, and refer families to programs and other resources with the goal of strengthening families, preventing child maltreatment, and enhancing child development. (9/10)

THE PEDIATRICIAN'S ROLE IN COMMUNITY PEDIATRICS
Committee on Community Health Services

ABSTRACT. This policy statement reaffirms the pediatrician's role in community pediatrics. It offers pediatricians a definition of community pediatrics and provides a set of specific recommendations that underscore the critical nature of this important dimension of the profession. (4/05, reaffirmed 1/10)

THE PEDIATRICIAN'S ROLE IN DEVELOPMENT AND IMPLEMENTATION OF AN INDIVIDUAL EDUCATION PLAN (IEP) AND/OR AN INDIVIDUAL FAMILY SERVICE PLAN (IFSP)
Committee on Children With Disabilities

ABSTRACT. The Individual Education Plan and Individual Family Service Plan are legally mandated documents developed by a multidisciplinary team assessment that specifies goals and services for each child eligible for special educational services or early intervention services.

Pediatricians need to be knowledgeable of federal, state, and local requirements; establish linkages with early intervention, educational professionals, and parent support groups; and collaborate with the team working with individual children. (7/99, reaffirmed 11/02, 1/06)

THE PEDIATRICIAN'S ROLE IN FAMILY SUPPORT AND FAMILY SUPPORT PROGRAMS
Committee on Early Childhood, Adoption, and Dependent Care
ABSTRACT. Children's social, emotional, and physical health; their developmental trajectory; and the neurocircuits that are being created and reinforced in their developing brains are all directly influenced by their relationships during early childhood. The stresses associated with contemporary American life can challenge families' abilities to promote successful developmental outcomes and emotional health for their children. Pediatricians are positioned to serve as partners with families and other community providers in supporting the well-being of children and their families. The structure and support of families involve forces that are often outside the agenda of the usual pediatric health supervision visits. Pediatricians must ensure that their medical home efforts promote a holistically healthy family environment for all children. This statement recommends opportunities for pediatricians to develop their expertise in assessing the strengths and stresses in families, in counseling families about strategies and resources, and in collaborating with others in their communities to support family relationships. (11/11)

THE PEDIATRICIAN'S ROLE IN THE PREVENTION OF MISSING CHILDREN (CLINICAL REPORT)
Committee on Psychosocial Aspects of Child and Family Health
ABSTRACT. In 2002, the *Second National Incidence Studies of Missing, Abducted, Runaway, and Thrownaway Children* report was released by the US Department of Justice, providing new data on a problem that our nation continues to face. This clinical report describes the categories of missing children, the prevalence of each, and prevention strategies that primary care pediatricians can share with parents to increase awareness and education about the safety of their children. (10/04)

THE PEDIATRICIAN'S ROLE IN SUPPORTING ADOPTIVE FAMILIES (CLINICAL REPORT)
Veronnie F. Jones, MD, PhD; Elaine E. Schulte, MD, MPH; Committee on Early Childhood; and Council on Foster Care, Adoption, and Kinship Care
ABSTRACT. Each year, more children join families through adoption. Pediatricians have an important role in assisting adoptive families in the various challenges they may face with respect to adoption. The acceptance of the differences between families formed through birth and those formed through adoption is essential in promoting positive emotional growth within the family. It is important for pediatricians to be aware of the adoptive parents' need to be supported in their communication with their adopted children. (9/12)

PERSONAL WATERCRAFT USE BY CHILDREN AND ADOLESCENTS
Committee on Injury and Poison Prevention
ABSTRACT. The use of personal watercraft (PWC) has increased dramatically during the past decade as have the speed and mobility of the watercraft. A similar dramatic increase in PWC-related injury and death has occurred simultaneously. No one younger than 16 years should operate a PWC. The operator and all passengers must wear US Coast Guard-approved personal flotation devices. Other safety recommendations are suggested for parents and pediatricians. (2/00, reaffirmed 5/04, 1/07, 6/10)

PESTICIDE EXPOSURE IN CHILDREN
Council on Environmental Health
ABSTRACT. This statement presents the position of the American Academy of Pediatrics on pesticides. Pesticides are a collective term for chemicals intended to kill unwanted insects, plants, molds, and rodents. Children encounter pesticides daily and have unique susceptibilities to their potential toxicity. Acute poisoning risks are clear, and understanding of chronic health implications from both acute and chronic exposure are emerging. Epidemiologic evidence demonstrates associations between early life exposure to pesticides and pediatric cancers, decreased cognitive function, and behavioral problems. Related animal toxicology studies provide supportive biological plausibility for these findings. Recognizing and reducing problematic exposures will require attention to current inadequacies in medical training, public health tracking, and regulatory action on pesticides. Ongoing research describing toxicologic vulnerabilities and exposure factors across the life span are needed to inform regulatory needs and appropriate interventions. Policies that promote integrated pest management, comprehensive pesticide labeling, and marketing practices that incorporate child health considerations will enhance safe use. (11/12)

PESTICIDE EXPOSURE IN CHILDREN (TECHNICAL REPORT)
James R. Roberts, MD, MPH; Catherine J. Karr, MD, PhD; and Council on Environmental Health
ABSTRACT. Pesticides are a collective term for a wide array of chemicals intended to kill unwanted insects, plants, molds, and rodents. Food, water, and treatment in the home, yard, and school are all potential sources of children's exposure. Exposures to pesticides may be overt or subacute, and effects range from acute to chronic toxicity. In 2008, pesticides were the ninth most common substance reported to poison control centers, and approximately 45% of all reports of pesticide poisoning were for children. Organophosphate and carbamate poisoning are perhaps the most widely known acute poisoning syndromes, can be diagnosed by depressed red blood cell cholinesterase levels, and have available antidotal therapy. However, numerous other pesticides that may cause acute toxicity, such as pyrethroid and neonicotinoid insecticides, herbicides, fungicides, and rodenticides, also have specific toxic effects; recognition of these effects may help identify acute exposures. Evidence is increasingly

emerging about chronic health implications from both acute and chronic exposure. A growing body of epidemiological evidence demonstrates associations between parental use of pesticides, particularly insecticides, with acute lymphocytic leukemia and brain tumors. Prenatal, household, and occupational exposures (maternal and paternal) appear to be the largest risks. Prospective cohort studies link early-life exposure to organophosphates and organochlorine pesticides (primarily DDT) with adverse effects on neurodevelopment and behavior. Among the findings associated with increased pesticide levels are poorer mental development by using the Bayley index and increased scores on measures assessing pervasive developmental disorder, inattention, and attention-deficit/hyperactivity disorder. Related animal toxicology studies provide supportive biological plausibility for these findings. Additional data suggest that there may also be an association between parental pesticide use and adverse birth outcomes including physical birth defects, low birth weight, and fetal death, although the data are less robust than for cancer and neurodevelopmental effects. Children's exposures to pesticides should be limited as much as possible. (11/12)

PHOTOTHERAPY TO PREVENT SEVERE NEONATAL HYPERBILIRUBINEMIA IN THE NEWBORN INFANT 35 OR MORE WEEKS OF GESTATION (TECHNICAL REPORT)

Vinod K. Bhutani, MD, and Committee on Fetus and Newborn

ABSTRACT. *Objective.* To standardize the use of phototherapy consistent with the American Academy of Pediatrics clinical practice guideline for the management of hyperbilirubinemia in the newborn infant 35 or more weeks of gestation.

Methods. Relevant literature was reviewed. Phototherapy devices currently marketed in the United States that incorporate fluorescent, halogen, fiber-optic, or blue light-emitting diode light sources were assessed in the laboratory.

Results. The efficacy of phototherapy units varies widely because of differences in light source and configuration. The following characteristics of a device contribute to its effectiveness: (1) emission of light in the blue-to-green range that overlaps the in vivo plasma bilirubin absorption spectrum (~460–490 nm); (2) irradiance of at least 30 μW·cm^{-2}·nm^{-1} (confirmed with an appropriate irradiance meter calibrated over the appropriate wavelength range); (3) illumination of maximal body surface; and (4) demonstration of a decrease in total bilirubin concentrations during the first 4 to 6 hours of exposure.

Recommendations. The intensity and spectral output of phototherapy devices is useful in predicting potential effectiveness in treating hyperbilirubinemia (group B recommendation). Clinical effectiveness should be evaluated before and monitored during use (group B recommendation). Blocking the light source or reducing exposed body surface should be avoided (group B recommendation). Standardization of irradiance meters, improvements in device design, and lower-upper limits of light intensity for phototherapy units merit further study. Comparing the in vivo performance of devices is not practical, in general, and alternative procedures need to be explored. (9/11)

PHYSICIAN REFUSAL TO PROVIDE INFORMATION OR TREATMENT ON THE BASIS OF CLAIMS OF CONSCIENCE

Committee on Bioethics

ABSTRACT. Health care professionals may have moral objections to particular medical interventions. They may refuse to provide or cooperate in the provision of these interventions. Such objections are referred to as conscientious objections. Although it may be difficult to characterize or validate claims of conscience, respecting the individual physician's moral integrity is important. Conflicts arise when claims of conscience impede a patient's access to medical information or care. A physician's conscientious objection to certain interventions or treatments may be constrained in some situations. Physicians have a duty to disclose to prospective patients treatments they refuse to perform. As part of informed consent, physicians also have a duty to inform their patients of all relevant and legally available treatment options, including options to which they object. They have a moral obligation to refer patients to other health care professionals who are willing to provide those services when failing to do so would cause harm to the patient, and they have a duty to treat patients in emergencies when referral would significantly increase the probability of mortality or serious morbidity. Conversely, the health care system should make reasonable accommodations for physicians with conscientious objections. (11/09)

PHYSICIANS' ROLES IN COORDINATING CARE OF HOSPITALIZED CHILDREN (CLINICAL REPORT)

Patricia S. Lye, MD; Committee on Hospital Care; and Section on Hospital Medicine

ABSTRACT. The care of hospitalized children and adolescents has become increasingly complex and often involves multiple physicians beyond the traditional primary care pediatrician. Hospitalists, medical subspecialists, surgical specialists, and hospital attending physicians may all participate in the care of hospitalized children and youth. This report summarizes the responsibilities of the pediatrician and other involved physicians in ensuring that children receive coordinated and comprehensive medical care delivered within the context of their medical homes as inpatients, and that care is appropriately continued on an outpatient basis. (9/10)

PLANNED HOME BIRTH

Committee on Fetus and Newborn

ABSTRACT. The American Academy of Pediatrics concurs with the recent statement of the American College of Obstetricians and Gynecologists affirming that hospitals and birthing centers are the safest settings for birth in the United States while respecting the right of women to make a medically informed decision about delivery. This statement is intended to help pediatricians provide supportive, informed counsel to women considering home birth while retaining their role as child advocates and to summarize the standards of care for newborn infants born at home, which are consistent with standards for infants born in a medical care facility. Regardless of the circumstances of his or her birth, including location, every newborn infant deserves health care that adheres to the standards highlighted in this statement, more completely described in other publications from the American Academy of Pediatrics, including *Guidelines for Perinatal Care*. The goal of providing high-quality care to all newborn infants can best be achieved through continuing efforts by all participating health care providers and institutions to develop and sustain communications and understanding on the basis of professional interaction and mutual respect throughout the health care system. (4/13)

See full text on page 819.

POLIOVIRUS
Committee on Infectious Diseases

ABSTRACT. Despite marked progress in global polio eradication, the threat of polio importation into the United States remains; therefore, all children should be protected against the disease. The standard schedule for poliovirus immunization remains 4 doses of inactivated poliovirus vaccine at 2, 4, and 6 through 18 months and 4 through 6 years of age. The minimum interval between doses 1 and 2 and between doses 2 and 3 is 4 weeks, and the minimum interval between doses 3 and 4 is 6 months. The minimum age for dose 1 is 6 weeks. Minimal age and intervals should be used when there is imminent threat of exposure, such as travel to an area in which polio is endemic or epidemic. The final dose in the inactivated poliovirus vaccine series should be administered at 4 through 6 years of age, regardless of the previous number of doses administered before the fourth birthday, and at least 6 months since the last dose was received. (9/11)

POSTDISCHARGE FOLLOW-UP OF INFANTS WITH CONGENITAL DIAPHRAGMATIC HERNIA (CLINICAL REPORT)
Section on Surgery and Committee on Fetus and Newborn

ABSTRACT. Infants with congenital diaphragmatic hernia often require intensive treatment after birth, have prolonged hospitalizations, and have other congenital anomalies. After discharge from the hospital, they may have long-term sequelae such as respiratory insufficiency, gastroesophageal reflux, poor growth, neurodevelopmental delay, behavior problems, hearing loss, hernia recurrence, and orthopedic deformities. Structured follow-up for these patients facilitates early recognition and treatment of these complications. In this report, follow-up of infants with congenital diaphragmatic hernia is outlined. (3/08, reaffirmed 5/11)

POSTEXPOSURE PROPHYLAXIS IN CHILDREN AND ADOLESCENTS FOR NONOCCUPATIONAL EXPOSURE TO HUMAN IMMUNODEFICIENCY VIRUS (CLINICAL REPORT)
Committee on Pediatric AIDS

ABSTRACT. Exposure to human immunodeficiency virus (HIV) can occur in a number of situations unique to, or more common among, children and adolescents. Guidelines for postexposure prophylaxis (PEP) for occupational and nonoccupational (eg, sexual, needle-sharing) exposures to HIV have been published by the US Public Health Service, but they do not directly address nonoccupational HIV exposures unique to children (such as accidental exposure to human milk from a woman infected with HIV or a puncture wound from a discarded needle on a playground), and they do not provide antiretroviral drug information relevant to PEP in children.

This clinical report reviews issues of potential exposure of children and adolescents to HIV and gives recommendations for PEP in those situations. The risk of HIV transmission from nonoccupational, nonperinatal exposure is generally low. Transmission risk is modified by factors related to the source and extent of exposure. Determination of the HIV infection status of the exposure source may not be possible, and data on transmission risk by exposure type may not exist. Except in the setting of perinatal transmission, no studies have demonstrated the safety and efficacy of postexposure use of antiretroviral drugs for the prevention of HIV transmission in nonoccupational settings. Antiretroviral therapy used for PEP is associated with significant toxicity. The decision to initiate prophylaxis needs to be made in consultation with the patient, the family, and a clinician with experience in treatment of persons with HIV infection. If instituted, therapy should be started as soon as possible after an exposure—no later than 72 hours—and continued for 28 days. Many clinicians would use 3 drugs for PEP regimens, although 2 drugs may be considered in certain circumstances. Instruction for avoiding secondary transmission should be given. Careful follow-up is needed for psychologic support, encouragement of medication adherence, toxicity monitoring, and serial HIV antibody testing. (6/03, reaffirmed 1/07, 10/08)

POSTNATAL CORTICOSTEROIDS TO PREVENT OR TREAT BRONCHOPULMONARY DYSPLASIA
Kristi L. Watterberg, MD, and Committee on Fetus and Newborn

ABSTRACT. The purpose of this revised statement is to review current information on the use of postnatal glucocorticoids to prevent or treat bronchopulmonary dysplasia in the preterm infant and to make updated recommendations regarding their use. High-dose dexamethasone (0.5 mg/kg per day) does not seem to confer additional therapeutic benefit over lower doses and is not recommended. Evidence is insufficient to make a recommendation regarding other glucocorticoid doses and preparations. The clinician must use clinical judgment when attempting to balance the potential adverse effects of glucocorticoid treatment with those of bronchopulmonary dysplasia. (9/10)

POSTNATAL GLUCOSE HOMEOSTASIS IN LATE-PRETERM AND TERM INFANTS (CLINICAL REPORT)
David H. Adamkin, MD, and Committee on Fetus and Newborn

ABSTRACT. This report provides a practical guide and algorithm for the screening and subsequent management of neonatal hypoglycemia. Current evidence does not support a specific concentration of glucose that can discriminate normal from abnormal or can potentially result in acute or chronic irreversible neurologic damage. Early identification of the at-risk infant and institution of prophylactic measures to prevent neonatal hypoglycemia are recommended as a pragmatic approach despite the absence of a consistent definition of hypoglycemia in the literature. (3/11)

PRECERTIFICATION PROCESS

Committee on Hospital Care

ABSTRACT. Precertification is a process still used by health insurance companies to control health care costs. Although we believe precertification is unnecessary and not cost-effective, in those instances where precertification is still being utilized, we suggest that the following procedures be adopted. This statement suggests guidelines that should help achieve this goal while allowing optimal access to care for children. (8/00, reaffirmed 5/05, 11/08)

PREMEDICATION FOR NONEMERGENCY ENDOTRACHEAL INTUBATION IN THE NEONATE (CLINICAL REPORT)

Praveen Kumar, MD; Susan E. Denson, MD; Thomas J. Mancuso, MD; Committee on Fetus and Newborn; and Section on Anesthesiology and Pain Medicine

ABSTRACT. Endotracheal intubation is a common procedure in newborn care. The purpose of this clinical report is to review currently available evidence on use of premedication for intubation, identify gaps in knowledge, and provide guidance for making decisions about the use of premedication. (2/10, reaffirmed 8/13)

PRENATAL SUBSTANCE ABUSE: SHORT- AND LONG-TERM EFFECTS ON THE EXPOSED FETUS (TECHNICAL REPORT)

Marylou Behnke, MD; Vincent C. Smith, MD; Committee on Substance Abuse; and Committee on Fetus and Newborn

ABSTRACT. Prenatal substance abuse continues to be a significant problem in this country and poses important health risks for the developing fetus. The primary care pediatrician's role in addressing prenatal substance exposure includes prevention, identification of exposure, recognition of medical issues for the exposed newborn infant, protection of the infant, and follow-up of the exposed infant. This report will provide information for the most common drugs involved in prenatal exposure: nicotine, alcohol, marijuana, opiates, cocaine, and methamphetamine. (2/13)

See full text on page 827.

THE PRENATAL VISIT (CLINICAL REPORT)

George J. Cohen, MD, and Committee on Psychosocial Aspects of Child and Family Health

ABSTRACT. As advocates for children and their families, pediatricians can support and guide expectant parents in the prenatal period. Prenatal visits allow the pediatrician to gather basic information from expectant parents, offer them information and advice, and identify high-risk conditions that may require special care. In addition, a prenatal visit is the first step in establishing a relationship between the family and the pediatrician (the infant's medical home) and in helping the parents develop parenting skills and confidence. There are several possible formats for this first visit. The one used depends on the experience and preference of the parents, the style of the pediatrician's practice, and pragmatic issues of reimbursement. (9/09)

PREPARATION FOR EMERGENCIES IN THE OFFICES OF PEDIATRICIANS AND PEDIATRIC PRIMARY CARE PROVIDERS

Committee on Pediatric Emergency Medicine

ABSTRACT. High-quality pediatric emergency care can be provided only through the collaborative efforts of many health care professionals and child advocates working together throughout a continuum of care that extends from prevention and the medical home to prehospital care, to emergency department stabilization, to critical care and rehabilitation, and finally to a return to care in the medical home. At times, the office of the pediatric primary care provider will serve as the entry site into the emergency care system, which comprises out-of-hospital emergency medical services personnel, emergency department nurses and physicians, and other emergency and critical care providers. Recognizing the important role of pediatric primary care providers in the emergency care system for children and understanding the capabilities and limitations of that system are essential if pediatric primary care providers are to offer the best chance at intact survival for every child who is brought to the office with an emergency. Optimizing pediatric primary care provider office readiness for emergencies requires consideration of the unique aspects of each office practice, the types of patients and emergencies that might be seen, the resources on site, and the resources of the larger emergency care system of which the pediatric primary care provider's office is a part. Parent education regarding prevention, recognition, and response to emergencies, patient triage, early recognition and stabilization of pediatric emergencies in the office, and timely transfer to an appropriate facility for definitive care are important responsibilities of every pediatric primary care provider. In addition, pediatric primary care providers can collaborate with out-of-hospital and hospital-based providers and advocate for the best-quality emergency care for their patients. (7/07, reaffirmed 6/11)

PREPARING FOR PEDIATRIC EMERGENCIES: DRUGS TO CONSIDER (CLINICAL REPORT)

Mary A. Hegenbarth, MD, and Committee on Drugs

ABSTRACT. This clinical report provides current recommendations regarding the selection and use of drugs in preparation for pediatric emergencies. It is not intended to be a comprehensive list of all medications that may be used in all emergencies. When possible, dosage recommendations are consistent with those used in current emergency references such as the *Advanced Pediatric Life Support and Pediatric Advanced Life Support* textbooks and the recently revised American Heart Association resuscitation guidelines. (2/08, reaffirmed 10/11)

PRESCRIBING ASSISTIVE-TECHNOLOGY SYSTEMS: FOCUS ON CHILDREN WITH IMPAIRED COMMUNICATION (CLINICAL REPORT)

Larry W. Desch, MD; Deborah Gaebler-Spira, MD; and Council on Children With Disabilities

ABSTRACT. This clinical report defines common terms of use and provides information on current practice, research, and limitations of assistive technology that can be used in systems for communication. The assessment process to determine the best devices for use with a particular child (ie, the best fit of a device) is also reviewed. The primary care pediatrician, as part of the medical home, plays an important role in the interdisciplinary effort to provide appropriate assistive technology and may be asked to make a referral for assessment or prescribe a particular device. This report provides resources to assist pediatricians in this role and reviews the interdisciplinary team functional evaluation using standardized assessments; the multiple funding opportunities available for obtaining devices and ways in which pediatricians can assist families with obtaining them; the training necessary to use these systems once the devices are procured; the follow-up evaluation to ensure that the systems are meeting their goals; and the leadership skills needed to advocate for this technology. The American Academy of Pediatrics acknowledges the need for key resources to be identified in the community and recognizes that these resources are a shared medical, educational, therapeutic, and family responsibility. Although this report primarily deals with assistive technology specific for communication impairments, many of the details in this report also can aid in the acquisition and use of other types of assistive technology. (6/08, reaffirmed 1/12)

PRESCRIBING THERAPY SERVICES FOR CHILDREN WITH MOTOR DISABILITIES (CLINICAL REPORT)
Committee on Children With Disabilities
ABSTRACT. Pediatricians often are called on to prescribe physical, occupational, and speech-language therapy services for children with motor disabilities. This report defines the context in which rehabilitation therapies should be prescribed, emphasizing the evaluation and enhancement of the child's function and abilities and participation in age-appropriate life roles. The report encourages pediatricians to work with teams including the parents, child, teachers, therapists, and other physicians to ensure that their patients receive appropriate therapy services. (6/04, reaffirmed 5/07, 5/11)

PRESERVATION OF FERTILITY IN PEDIATRIC AND ADOLESCENT PATIENTS WITH CANCER (TECHNICAL REPORT)
Mary E. Fallat, MD; John Hutter, MD; Committee on Bioethics; Section on Hematology/Oncology; and Section on Surgery
ABSTRACT. Many cancers that present in children and adolescents are curable with surgery, chemotherapy, and/or radiation therapy. Potential adverse consequences of treatment include sterility, infertility, or subfertility as a result of either gonad removal or damage to germ cells from adjuvant therapy. In recent years, treatment of solid tumors and hematologic malignancies has been modified in an attempt to reduce damage to the gonads. Simultaneously, advances in assisted reproductive techniques have led to new possibilities for the prevention and treatment of infertility. This technical report reviews the topic of fertility preservation in pediatric and adolescent patients with cancer, including ethical considerations. (5/08, reaffirmed 2/12)

PREVENTING AND TREATING HOMESICKNESS (CLINICAL REPORT)
Christopher A. Thurber, PhD; Edward Walton, MD; and Council on School Health
ABSTRACT. Homesickness is the distress and functional impairment caused by an actual or anticipated separation from home and attachment objects such as parents. It is characterized by acute longing and preoccupying thoughts of home. Almost all children, adolescents, and adults experience some degree of homesickness when they are apart from familiar people and environments. Pediatricians and other health care professionals are in a unique position to assist families in understanding the etiology, prevention, and treatment of homesickness. In the case of planned separations, such as summer camp, techniques are provided that may aid in prevention. In the case of unanticipated or traumatic separations, such as hospitalization, effective treatment strategies are available. (1/07, reaffirmed 5/12)

PREVENTION OF AGRICULTURAL INJURIES AMONG CHILDREN AND ADOLESCENTS
Committee on Injury and Poison Prevention and Committee on Community Health Services
ABSTRACT. Although the annual number of farm deaths to children and adolescents has decreased since publication of the 1988 American Academy of Pediatrics statement, "Rural Injuries," the rate of nonfatal farm injuries has increased. Approximately 100 unintentional injury deaths occur annually to children and adolescents on US farms, and an additional 22 000 injuries to children younger than 20 years occur on farms. Relatively few adolescents are employed on farms compared with other types of industry, yet the proportion of fatalities in agriculture is higher than that for any other type of adolescent employment. The high mortality and severe morbidity associated with farm injuries require continuing and improved injury-control strategies. This statement provides recommendations for pediatricians regarding patient and community education as well as public advocacy related to agricultural injury prevention in childhood and adolescence. (10/01, reaffirmed 1/07, 11/11)

PREVENTION OF CHOKING AMONG CHILDREN
Committee on Injury, Violence, and Poison Prevention
ABSTRACT. Choking is a leading cause of morbidity and mortality among children, especially those aged 3 years or younger. Food, coins, and toys are the primary causes of choking-related injury and death. Certain characteristics, including shape, size, and consistency, of certain toys and foods increase their potential to cause choking among children. Childhood choking hazards should be addressed through comprehensive and coordinated prevention activities. The US Consumer Product Safety Commission (CPSC) should increase efforts to ensure that toys that are sold in retail store bins, vending machines, or on the Internet have appropriate choking-hazard warnings; work with manufacturers to improve the effectiveness of recalls of products that pose a choking risk to children; and increase efforts to prevent the resale of these recalled products via online auction sites. Current gaps in choking-prevention standards for children's toys should

be reevaluated and addressed, as appropriate, via revisions to the standards established under the Child Safety Protection Act, the Consumer Product Safety Improvement Act, or regulation by the CPSC. Prevention of food-related choking among children in the United States has been inadequately addressed at the federal level. The US Food and Drug Administration should establish a systematic, institutionalized process for examining and addressing the hazards of food-related choking. This process should include the establishment of the necessary surveillance, hazard evaluation, enforcement, and public education activities to prevent food-related choking among children. While maintaining its highly cooperative arrangements with the CPSC and the US Department of Agriculture, the Food and Drug Administration should have the authority to address choking-related risks of all food products, including meat products that fall under the jurisdiction of the US Department of Agriculture. The existing National Electronic Injury Surveillance System–All Injury Program of the CPSC should be modified to conduct more-detailed surveillance of choking on food among children. Food manufacturers should design new foods and redesign existing foods to avoid shapes, sizes, textures, and other characteristics that increase choking risk to children, to the extent possible. Pediatricians, dentists, and other infant and child health care providers should provide choking-prevention counseling to parents as an integral part of anticipatory guidance activities. (2/10)

PREVENTION OF DROWNING
Committee on Injury, Violence, and Poison Prevention
ABSTRACT. Drowning is a leading cause of injury-related death in children. In 2006, fatal drowning claimed the lives of approximately 1100 US children younger than 20 years. A number of strategies are available to prevent these tragedies. As educators and advocates, pediatricians can play an important role in the prevention of drowning. (5/10)

PREVENTION OF DROWNING (TECHNICAL REPORT)
Committee on Injury, Violence, and Poison Prevention and Jeffrey Weiss, MD
ABSTRACT. Drowning is a leading cause of injury-related death in children. In 2006, approximately 1100 US children younger than 20 years died from drowning. A number of strategies are available to prevent these tragedies. As educators and advocates, pediatricians can play an important role in the prevention of drowning. (5/10)

PREVENTION AND MANAGEMENT OF PAIN IN THE NEONATE: AN UPDATE
Committee on Fetus and Newborn and Section on Surgery
  (joint with Canadian Paediatric Society)
ABSTRACT. The prevention of pain in neonates should be the goal of all caregivers, because repeated painful exposures have the potential for deleterious consequences. Neonates at greatest risk of neurodevelopmental impairment as a result of preterm birth (ie, the smallest and sickest) are also those most likely to be exposed to the greatest number of painful stimuli in the NICU. Although there are major gaps in our knowledge regarding the most effective way to prevent and relieve pain in neonates, proven and safe therapies are currently underused for routine minor yet painful procedures. Every health care facility caring for neonates should implement an effective pain-prevention program, which includes strategies for routinely assessing pain, minimizing the number of painful procedures performed, effectively using pharmacologic and nonpharmacologic therapies for the prevention of pain associated with routine minor procedures, and eliminating pain associated with surgery and other major procedures. (11/06, reaffirmed 5/10)

PREVENTION AND MANAGEMENT OF POSITIONAL SKULL DEFORMITIES IN INFANTS (CLINICAL REPORT)
James Laughlin, MD; Thomas G. Luerssen, MD; Mark S. Dias, MD; Committee on Practice and Ambulatory Medicine; and Section on Neurological Surgery
ABSTRACT. Positional skull deformities may be present at birth or may develop during the first few months of life. Since the early 1990s, US pediatricians have seen an increase in the number of children with cranial asymmetry, particularly unilateral flattening of the occiput, likely attributable to parents following the American Academy of Pediatrics "Back to Sleep" positioning recommendations aimed at decreasing the risk of sudden infant death syndrome. Positional skull deformities are generally benign, reversible head-shape anomalies that do not require surgical intervention, as opposed to craniosynostosis, which can result in neurologic damage and progressive craniofacial distortion. Although associated with some risk of positional skull deformity, healthy young infants should be placed down for sleep on their backs. The practice of putting infants to sleep on their backs has been associated with a drastic decrease in the incidence of sudden infant death syndrome. Pediatricians need to be able to properly differentiate infants with benign skull deformities from those with craniosynostosis, educate parents on methods of proactively decreasing the likelihood of the development of occipital flattening, initiate appropriate management, and make referrals when necessary. This report provides guidance for the prevention, diagnosis, and management of positional skull deformity in an otherwise normal infant without evidence of associated anomalies, syndromes, or spinal disease. (11/11)

PREVENTION OF PEDIATRIC OVERWEIGHT AND OBESITY
Committee on Nutrition
ABSTRACT. The dramatic increase in the prevalence of childhood overweight and its resultant comorbidities are associated with significant health and financial burdens, warranting strong and comprehensive prevention efforts. This statement proposes strategies for early identification of excessive weight gain by using body mass index, for dietary and physical activity interventions during health supervision encounters, and for advocacy and research. (8/03, reaffirmed 10/06)

PREVENTION OF ROTAVIRUS DISEASE: UPDATED GUIDELINES FOR USE OF ROTAVIRUS VACCINE
Committee on Infectious Diseases

ABSTRACT. This statement updates and replaces the 2007 American Academy of Pediatrics statement for prevention of rotavirus gastroenteritis. In February 2006, a live oral human-bovine reassortant rotavirus vaccine (RV5 [RotaTeq]) was licensed as a 3-dose series for use in infants in the United States. The American Academy of Pediatrics recommended routine use of RV5 in infants in the United States. In April 2008, a live, oral, human attenuated rotavirus vaccine (RV1 [Rotarix]) was licensed as a 2-dose series for use in infants in the United States. The American Academy of Pediatrics recommends routine immunization of infants in the United States with rotavirus vaccine. The American Academy of Pediatrics does not express a preference for either RV5 or RV1. RV5 is to be administered orally in a 3-dose series with doses administered at 2, 4, and 6 months of age; RV1 is to be administered orally in a 2-dose series with doses administered at 2 and 4 months of age. The first dose of rotavirus vaccine should be administered from 6 weeks through 14 weeks, 6 days of age. The minimum interval between doses of rotavirus vaccine is 4 weeks. All doses should be administered by 8 months, 0 days of age. Recommendations in this statement also address the maximum ages for doses, contraindications, precautions, and special situations for administration of rotavirus vaccine. (3/09)

PREVENTION OF SEXUAL HARASSMENT IN THE WORKPLACE AND EDUCATIONAL SETTINGS
Committee on Pediatric Workforce

ABSTRACT. The American Academy of Pediatrics is committed to working to ensure that workplaces and educational settings in which pediatricians spend time are free of sexual harassment. The purpose of this statement is to heighten awareness and sensitivity to this important issue, recognizing that institutions, clinics, and office-based practices may have existing policies. (10/06, reaffirmed 5/09, 1/12)

PREVENTION AND TREATMENT OF TYPE 2 DIABETES MELLITUS IN CHILDREN, WITH SPECIAL EMPHASIS ON AMERICAN INDIAN AND ALASKA NATIVE CHILDREN (CLINICAL REPORT)
Committee on Native American Child Health and Section on Endocrinology

ABSTRACT. The emergence of type 2 diabetes mellitus in the American Indian/Alaska Native pediatric population presents a new challenge for pediatricians and other health care professionals. This chronic disease requires preventive efforts, early diagnosis, and collaborative care of the patient and family within the context of a medical home. (10/03, reaffirmed 10/08)

THE PREVENTION OF UNINTENTIONAL INJURY AMONG AMERICAN INDIAN AND ALASKA NATIVE CHILDREN: A SUBJECT REVIEW (CLINICAL REPORT)
Committee on Native American Child Health and Committee on Injury and Poison Prevention

ABSTRACT. Among ethnic groups in the United States, American Indian and Alaska Native (AI/AN) children experience the highest rates of injury mortality and morbidity. Injury mortality rates for AI/AN children have decreased during the past quarter century, but remain almost double the rate for all children in the United States. The Indian Health Service (IHS), the federal agency with the primary responsibility for the health care of AI/AN people, has sponsored an internationally recognized injury prevention program designed to reduce the risk of injury death by addressing community-specific risk factors. Model programs developed by the IHS and tribal governments have led to successful outcomes in motor vehicle occupant safety, drowning prevention, and fire safety. Injury prevention programs in tribal communities require special attention to the sovereignty of tribal governments and the unique cultural aspects of health care and communication. Pediatricians working with AI/AN children on reservations or in urban environments are strongly urged to collaborate with tribes and the IHS to create community-based coalitions and develop programs to address highly preventable injury-related mortality and morbidity. Strong advocacy also is needed to promote childhood injury prevention as an important priority for federal agencies and tribes. (12/99, reaffirmed 12/02 COIVPP, 5/03 CONACH, 1/06, 1/09)

PREVENTION OF VARICELLA: UPDATE OF RECOMMENDATIONS FOR USE OF QUADRIVALENT AND MONOVALENT VARICELLA VACCINES IN CHILDREN
Committee on Infectious Diseases

ABSTRACT. Two varicella-containing vaccines are licensed for use in the United States: monovalent varicella vaccine (Varivax [Merck & Co, Inc, West Point, PA]) and quadrivalent measles-mumps-rubella-varicella vaccine (MMRV) (ProQuad [Merck & Co, Inc]). It is estimated from postlicensure data that after vaccination at 12 through 23 months of age, 7 to 9 febrile seizures occur per 10 000 children who receive the MMRV, and 3 to 4 febrile seizures occur per 10 000 children who receive the measles-mumps-rubella (MMR) and varicella vaccines administered concurrently but at separate sites. Thus, 1 additional febrile seizure is expected to occur per approximately 2300 to 2600 children 12 to 23 months old vaccinated with the MMRV, when compared with separate MMR and varicella vaccine administration. The period of risk for febrile seizures is from 5 through 12 days after receipt of the vaccine(s). No increased risk of febrile seizures is seen among patients 4 to 6 years of age receiving MMRV. Febrile seizures do not predispose to epilepsy or neurodevelopmental delays later in life and are not associated with long-term health impairment. The American Academy of Pediatrics recommends that either MMR and varicella vaccines separately or the MMRV be used for the first dose of measles, mumps, rubella, and varicella vaccines administered at 12 through 47 months of age. For the first dose of measles, mumps, rubella, and varicella vaccines administered at ages 48 months and older, and for dose 2 at any age (15 months to 12 years), use of MMRV generally is preferred over separate injections of MMR and varicella vaccines. (8/11)

PREVENTIVE ORAL HEALTH INTERVENTION FOR PEDIATRICIANS
Section on Pediatric Dentistry and Oral Health

ABSTRACT. This policy is a compilation of current concepts and scientific evidence required to understand and implement practice-based preventive oral health programs designed to improve oral health outcomes for all children and especially children at significant risk of dental decay. In addition, it reviews cariology and caries risk assessment and defines, through available evidence, appropriate recommendations for preventive oral health intervention by primary care pediatric practitioners. (12/08)

PRINCIPLES FOR THE DEVELOPMENT AND USE OF QUALITY MEASURES
Steering Committee on Quality Improvement and Management and Committee on Practice and Ambulatory Medicine

ABSTRACT. The American Academy of Pediatrics and its members are committed to improving the health care system to provide the highest-quality and safest health care for infants, children, adolescents, and young adults. This statement is intended as a guide for pediatricians and pediatric leadership on the appropriate uses of quality measures and the criteria on which they should be based. The statement summarizes the current national efforts on quality measurement and provides a set of principles for the development, use, and evaluation of quality measures for improving children's health and health care. The American Academy of Pediatrics recommends that these measures address important issues for children; be appropriate for children's health and health care, scientifically valid, and feasible; and focus on what can be improved. In addition, the American Academy of Pediatrics supports reasonable principles for the oversight and implementation of pay-for-performance programs. (2/08)

PRINCIPLES OF HEALTH CARE FINANCING
Committee on Child Health Financing

ABSTRACT. The American Academy of Pediatrics advocates that all children must have health insurance coverage that ensures them access to affordable and comprehensive quality care. Access to care depends on the design and implementation of payment systems that ensure the economic viability of the medical home; support and grow the professional pediatric workforce; promote the adoption and implementation of health information technology; enhance medical education, training, and research; and encourage and reward quality-improvement programs that advance and strengthen the medical home. Health insurance plans must be portable from state to state, with administrative procedures to eliminate breaks and gaps in coverage to ensure continuous coverage from year to year. Plans should ensure free choice of clinicians and foster coordination with public and private community-based programs for infants, children, and adolescents through the age of 26. The scope of services provided by all health plans must include preventive, acute and chronic illness, behavioral, inpatient, emergency, and home health care. These plans must be affordable and have cost-sharing policies that protect patients and families from financial strain and are without risk of loss of benefits because of plan design, current illness, or preexisting condition. (10/10, reaffirmed 4/13)

PRINCIPLES OF JUDICIOUS ANTIBIOTIC PRESCRIBING FOR UPPER RESPIRATORY TRACT INFECTIONS IN PEDIATRICS (CLINICAL REPORT)
Committee on Infectious Diseases

ABSTRACT. Most upper respiratory tract infections are caused by viruses and require no antibiotics. This clinical report focuses on antibiotic prescribing strategies for bacterial upper respiratory tract infections, including acute otitis media, acute bacterial sinusitis, and streptococcal pharyngitis. The principles for judicious antibiotic prescribing that are outlined focus on applying stringent diagnostic criteria, weighing the benefits and harms of antibiotic therapy, and understanding situations when antibiotics may not be indicated. The principles can be used to amplify messages from recent clinical guidelines for local guideline development and for patient communication; they are broadly applicable to antibiotic prescribing in general. (11/13)

See full text on page 845.

PRINCIPLES OF PEDIATRIC PATIENT SAFETY: REDUCING HARM DUE TO MEDICAL CARE
Steering Committee on Quality Improvement and Management and Committee on Hospital Care

ABSTRACT. Pediatricians are rendering care in an environment that is increasingly complex, which results in multiple opportunities to cause unintended harm. National awareness of patient safety risks has grown in the 10 years since the Institute of Medicine published its report *To Err Is Human,* and patients and society as a whole continue to challenge health care providers to examine their practices and implement safety solutions. The depth and breadth of harm incurred by the practice of medicine is still being defined as reports continue to uncover a variety of avoidable errors, from those that involve specific high-risk medications to those that are more generalizable, such as patient misidentification. Pediatricians in all venues must have a working knowledge of patient-safety language, advocate for best practices that attend to risks that are unique to children, identify and support a culture of safety, and lead efforts to eliminate avoidable harm in any setting in which medical care is rendered to children. (5/11)

PROBIOTICS AND PREBIOTICS IN PEDIATRICS (CLINICAL REPORT)

Dan W. Thomas, MD; Frank R. Greer, MD; Committee on Nutrition; and Section on Gastroenterology, Hepatology, and Nutrition

ABSTRACT. This clinical report reviews the currently known health benefits of probiotic and prebiotic products, including those added to commercially available infant formula and other food products for use in children. Probiotics are supplements or foods that contain viable microorganisms that cause alterations of the microflora of the host. Use of probiotics has been shown to be modestly effective in randomized clinical trials (RCTs) in (1) treating acute viral gastroenteritis in healthy children; and (2) preventing antibiotic-associated diarrhea in healthy children. There is some evidence that probiotics prevent necrotizing enterocolitis in very low birth weight infants (birth weight between 1000 and 1500 g), but more studies are needed. The results of RCTs in which probiotics were used to treat childhood *Helicobacter pylori* gastritis, irritable bowel syndrome, chronic ulcerative colitis, and infantile colic, as well as in preventing childhood atopy, although encouraging, are preliminary and require further confirmation. Probiotics have not been proven to be beneficial in treating or preventing human cancers or in treating children with Crohn disease. There are also safety concerns with the use of probiotics in infants and children who are immunocompromised, chronically debilitated, or seriously ill with indwelling medical devices.

Prebiotics are supplements or foods that contain a nondigestible food ingredient that selectively stimulates the favorable growth and/or activity of indigenous probiotic bacteria. Human milk contains substantial quantities of prebiotics. There is a paucity of RCTs examining prebiotics in children, although there may be some long-term benefit of prebiotics for the prevention of atopic eczema and common infections in healthy infants. Confirmatory well-designed clinical research studies are necessary. (11/10)

PROFESSIONAL LIABILITY INSURANCE AND MEDICOLEGAL EDUCATION FOR PEDIATRIC RESIDENTS AND FELLOWS

Committee on Medical Liability and Risk Management

ABSTRACT. The American Academy of Pediatrics believes that pediatric residents and fellows should be fully informed of the scope and limitations of their professional liability insurance coverage while in training. The academy states that residents and fellows should be educated by their training institutions on matters relating to medical liability and the importance of maintaining adequate and continuous professional liability insurance coverage throughout their careers in medicine. (8/11)

PROFESSIONALISM IN PEDIATRICS: STATEMENT OF PRINCIPLES

Committee on Bioethics

ABSTRACT. The purpose of this statement is to delineate the concept of professionalism within the context of pediatrics and to provide a brief statement of principles to guide the behavior and professional practice of pediatricians. (10/07, reaffirmed 5/11)

PROFESSIONALISM IN PEDIATRICS (TECHNICAL REPORT)

Mary E. Fallat, MD; Jacqueline Glover, PhD; and Committee on Bioethics

ABSTRACT. The purpose of this report is to provide a concrete overview of the ideal standards of behavior and professional practice to which pediatricians should aspire and by which students and residents can be evaluated. Recognizing that the ideal is not always achievable in the practical sense, this document details the key components of professionalism in pediatric practice with an emphasis on core professional values for which pediatricians should strive and that will serve as a moral compass needed to provide quality care for children and their families. (10/07, reaffirmed 5/11)

PROMOTING EDUCATION, MENTORSHIP, AND SUPPORT FOR PEDIATRIC RESEARCH

Committee on Pediatric Research

ABSTRACT. Pediatricians have an important role to play in the advancement of child health research and should be encouraged and supported to pursue research activities. Education and training in child health research should be part of every level of pediatric training. Continuing education and access to research advisors should be available to practitioners and academic faculty. Recommendations to promote additional research education and support at all levels of pediatric training, from premedical to continuing medical education, as well as suggestions for means to increase support and mentorship for research activities, are outlined in this statement. (6/01, reaffirmed 1/05, 5/08, 10/11)

PROMOTING THE PARTICIPATION OF CHILDREN WITH DISABILITIES IN SPORTS, RECREATION, AND PHYSICAL ACTIVITIES (CLINICAL REPORT)

Nancy A. Murphy, MD; Paul S. Carbone, MD; and Council on Children With Disabilities

ABSTRACT. The benefits of physical activity are universal for all children, including those with disabilities. The participation of children with disabilities in sports and recreational activities promotes inclusion, minimizes deconditioning, optimizes physical functioning, and enhances overall well-being. Despite these benefits, children with disabilities are more restricted in their participation, have lower levels of fitness, and have higher levels of obesity than their peers without disabilities. Pediatricians and parents may overestimate the risks or overlook the benefits of physical activity in children with disabilities. Well-informed decisions regarding each child's participation must consider overall health status, individual activity preferences, safety precautions, and availability of appropriate programs and equipment. Health supervision visits afford pediatricians, children with disabilities, and parents opportunities to collaboratively generate goal-directed activity "prescriptions." Child, family, financial, and societal barriers to participation need to be directly identified and addressed in the context of local, state, and federal laws. The goal is inclusion for all children with disabilities in appropriate activities. This clinical report discusses the importance of physical activity, recreation, and sports participation for children with disabilities and offers practical suggestions to pediatric health care professionals for the promotion of participation. (5/08, reaffirmed 1/12)

PROMOTING THE WELL-BEING OF CHILDREN WHOSE PARENTS ARE GAY OR LESBIAN
Committee on Psychosocial Aspects of Child and Family Health
ABSTRACT. To promote optimal health and well-being of all children, the American Academy of Pediatrics (AAP) supports access for all children to (1) civil marriage rights for their parents and (2) willing and capable foster and adoptive parents, regardless of the parents' sexual orientation. The AAP has always been an advocate for, and has developed policies to support, the optimal physical, mental, and social health and well-being of all infants, children, adolescents, and young adults. In so doing, the AAP has supported families in all their diversity, because the family has always been the basic social unit in which children develop the supporting and nurturing relationships with adults that they need to thrive. Children may be born to, adopted by, or cared for temporarily by married couples, nonmarried couples, single parents, grandparents, or legal guardians, and any of these may be heterosexual, gay or lesbian, or of another orientation. Children need secure and enduring relationships with committed and nurturing adults to enhance their life experiences for optimal social-emotional and cognitive development. Scientific evidence affirms that children have similar developmental and emotional needs and receive similar parenting whether they are raised by parents of the same or different genders. If a child has 2 living and capable parents who choose to create a permanent bond by way of civil marriage, it is in the best interests of their child(ren) that legal and social institutions allow and support them to do so, irrespective of their sexual orientation. If 2 parents are not available to the child, adoption or foster parenting remain acceptable options to provide a loving home for a child and should be available without regard to the sexual orientation of the parent(s). (3/13)
See full text on page 857.

PROMOTING THE WELL-BEING OF CHILDREN WHOSE PARENTS ARE GAY OR LESBIAN (TECHNICAL REPORT)
Ellen C. Perrin, MD, MA; Benjamin S. Siegel, MD;
    and Committee on Psychosocial Aspects of Child and
    Family Health
ABSTRACT. Extensive data available from more than 30 years of research reveal that children raised by gay and lesbian parents have demonstrated resilience with regard to social, psychological, and sexual health despite economic and legal disparities and social stigma. Many studies have demonstrated that children's well-being is affected much more by their relationships with their parents, their parents' sense of competence and security, and the presence of social and economic support for the family than by the gender or the sexual orientation of their parents. Lack of opportunity for same-gender couples to marry adds to families' stress, which affects the health and welfare of all household members. Because marriage strengthens families and, in so doing, benefits children's development, children should not be deprived of the opportunity for their parents to be married. Paths to parenthood that include assisted reproductive techniques, adoption, and foster parenting should focus on competency of the parents rather than their sexual orientation. (3/13)
See full text on page 863.

PROMOTION OF HEALTHY WEIGHT-CONTROL PRACTICES IN YOUNG ATHLETES
Committee on Sports Medicine and Fitness
ABSTRACT. Children and adolescents are often involved in sports in which weight loss or weight gain is perceived as an advantage. This policy statement describes unhealthy weight-control practices that may be harmful to the health and/or performance of athletes. Healthy methods of weight loss and weight gain are discussed, and physicians are given resources and recommendations that can be used to counsel athletes, parents, coaches, and school administrators in discouraging inappropriate weight-control behaviors and encouraging healthy methods of weight gain or loss, when needed. (12/05)

PROTECTING CHILDREN FROM SEXUAL ABUSE BY HEALTH CARE PROVIDERS
Committee on Child Abuse and Neglect
ABSTRACT. Sexual abuse or exploitation of children is never acceptable. Such behavior by health care providers is particularly concerning because of the trust that children and their families place on adults in the health care profession. The American Academy of Pediatrics strongly endorses the social and moral prohibition against sexual abuse or exploitation of children by health care providers. The academy opposes any such sexual abuse or exploitation by providers, particularly by the academy's members. Health care providers should be trained to recognize and abide by appropriate provider-patient boundaries. Medical institutions should screen staff members for a history of child abuse issues, train them to respect and maintain appropriate boundaries, and establish policies and procedures to receive and investigate concerns about patient abuse. Each person has a responsibility to ensure the safety of children in health care settings and to scrupulously follow appropriate legal and ethical reporting and investigation procedures. (6/11)

PROTECTIVE EYEWEAR FOR YOUNG ATHLETES
Committee on Sports Medicine and Fitness (joint with
    American Academy of Ophthalmology)
ABSTRACT. The American Academy of Pediatrics and American Academy of Ophthalmology strongly recommend protective eyewear for all participants in sports in which there is risk of eye injury. Protective eyewear should be mandatory for athletes who are functionally 1-eyed and for athletes whose ophthalmologists recommend eye protection after eye surgery or trauma. (3/04, reaffirmed 2/08, 6/11)

PROVIDING CARE FOR CHILDREN AND ADOLESCENTS FACING HOMELESSNESS AND HOUSING INSECURITY
Council on Community Pediatrics
ABSTRACT. Child health and housing security are closely intertwined, and children without homes are more likely to suffer from chronic disease, hunger, and malnutrition than are children with homes. Homeless children and

youth often have significant psychosocial development issues, and their education is frequently interrupted. Given the overall effects that homelessness can have on a child's health and potential, it is important for pediatricians to recognize the factors that lead to homelessness, understand the ways that homelessness and its causes can lead to poor health outcomes, and when possible, help children and families mitigate some of the effects of homelessness. Through practice change, partnership with community resources, awareness, and advocacy, pediatricians can help optimize the health and well-being of children affected by homelessness. (5/13)

See full text on page 875.

PROVIDING CARE FOR IMMIGRANT, MIGRANT, AND BORDER CHILDREN

Council on Community Pediatrics

ABSTRACT. This policy statement, which recognizes the large changes in immigrant status since publication of the 2005 statement "Providing Care for Immigrant, Homeless, and Migrant Children," focuses on strategies to support the health of immigrant children, infants, adolescents, and young adults. Homeless children will be addressed in a forthcoming separate statement ("Providing Care for Children and Adolescents Facing Homelessness and Housing Insecurity"). While recognizing the diversity across and within immigrant, migrant, and border populations, this statement provides a basic framework for serving and advocating for all immigrant children, with a particular focus on low-income and vulnerable populations. Recommendations include actions needed within and outside the health care system, including expansion of access to high-quality medical homes with culturally and linguistically effective care as well as education and literacy programs. The statement recognizes the unique and special role that pediatricians can play in the lives of immigrant children and families. Recommendations for policies that support immigrant child health are included. (5/13)

See full text on page 883.

PROVIDING A PRIMARY CARE MEDICAL HOME FOR CHILDREN AND YOUTH WITH CEREBRAL PALSY (CLINICAL REPORT)

Gregory S. Liptak, MD, MPH; Nancy A. Murphy, MD; and Council on Children With Disabilities

ABSTRACT. All primary care providers will care for children with cerebral palsy in their practice. In addition to well-child and acute illness care, the role of the medical home in the management of these children includes diagnosis, planning for interventions, authorizing treatments, and follow-up. Optimizing health and well-being for children with cerebral palsy and their families entails family-centered care provided in the medical home; comanagement is the most common model. This report reviews the aspects of care specific to cerebral palsy that a medical home should provide beyond the routine health care needed by all children. (10/11)

PROVIDING A PRIMARY CARE MEDICAL HOME FOR CHILDREN AND YOUTH WITH SPINA BIFIDA (CLINICAL REPORT)

Robert Burke, MD, MPH; Gregory S. Liptak, MD, MPH; and Council on Children With Disabilities

ABSTRACT. The pediatric primary care provider in the medical home has a central and unique role in the care of children with spina bifida. The primary care provider addresses not only the typical issues of preventive and acute health care but also the needs specific to these children. Optimal care requires communication and comanagement with pediatric medical and developmental subspecialists, surgical specialists, therapists, and community providers. The medical home provider is essential in supporting the family and advocating for the child from the time of entry into the practice through adolescence, which includes transition and transfer to adult health care. This report reviews aspects of care specific to the infant with spina bifida (particularly myelomeningocele) that will facilitate optimal medical, functional, and developmental outcomes. (11/11)

PROVISION OF EDUCATIONALLY RELATED SERVICES FOR CHILDREN AND ADOLESCENTS WITH CHRONIC DISEASES AND DISABLING CONDITIONS

Council on Children With Disabilities

ABSTRACT. Children and adolescents with chronic diseases and disabling conditions often need educationally related services. As medical home providers, physicians and other health care professionals can assist children, adolescents, and their families with the complex federal, state, and local laws, regulations, and systems associated with these services. Expanded roles for physicians and other health care professionals in individualized family service plan, individualized education plan, and Section 504 plan development and implementation are recommended. Recent updates to the Individuals With Disabilities Education Act will also affect these services. Funding for these services by private and nonprivate sources also continue to affect the availability of these educationally related services.

The complex range of federal, state, and local laws, regulations, and systems for special education and related services for children and adolescents in public schools is beyond the scope of this statement. Readers are referred to the American Academy of Pediatrics policy statement "The Pediatrician's Role in Development and Implementation of an Individual Education Plan (IEP) and/or an Individual Family Service Plan (IFSP)" for additional background materials. The focus of this statement is the role that health care professionals have in determining and managing educationally related services in the school setting.

This policy statement is a revision of a previous statement, "Provision of Educationally Related Services for Children and Adolescents With Chronic Diseases and Disabling Conditions," published in February 2000 by the Committee on Children With Disabilities (http://aappolicy.aappublications.org/cgi/content/full/pediatrics;105/2/448). (6/07)

PSYCHOLOGICAL MALTREATMENT (CLINICAL REPORT)

Roberta Hibbard, MD; Jane Barlow, Dphil; Harriet MacMillan, MD; Committee on Child Abuse and Neglect (joint with American Academy of Child and Adolescent Psychiatry Child Maltreatment and Violence Committee)

ABSTRACT. Psychological or emotional maltreatment of children may be the most challenging and prevalent form of child abuse and neglect. Caregiver behaviors include acts of omission (ignoring need for social interactions) or commission (spurning, terrorizing); may be verbal or nonverbal, active or passive, and with or without intent to harm; and negatively affect the child's cognitive, social, emotional, and/or physical development. Psychological maltreatment has been linked with disorders of attachment, developmental and educational problems, socialization problems, disruptive behavior, and later psychopathology. Although no evidence-based interventions that can prevent psychological maltreatment have been identified to date, it is possible that interventions shown to be effective in reducing overall types of child maltreatment, such as the Nurse Family Partnership, may have a role to play. Furthermore, prevention before occurrence will require both the use of universal interventions aimed at promoting the type of parenting that is now recognized to be necessary for optimal child development, alongside the use of targeted interventions directed at improving parental sensitivity to a child's cues during infancy and later parent-child interactions. Intervention should, first and foremost, focus on a thorough assessment and ensuring the child's safety. Potentially effective treatments include cognitive behavioral parenting programs and other psychotherapeutic interventions. The high prevalence of psychological abuse in advanced Western societies, along with the serious consequences, point to the importance of effective management. Pediatricians should be alert to the occurrence of psychological maltreatment and identify ways to support families who have risk indicators for, or evidence of, this problem. (7/12)

PSYCHOSOCIAL IMPLICATIONS OF DISASTER OR TERRORISM ON CHILDREN: A GUIDE FOR THE PEDIATRICIAN (CLINICAL REPORT)

Joseph F. Hagan Jr, MD; Committee on Psychosocial Aspects of Child and Family Health; and Task Force on Terrorism

ABSTRACT. During and after disasters, pediatricians can assist parents and community leaders not only by accommodating the unique needs of children but also by being cognizant of the psychological responses of children to reduce the possibility of long-term psychological morbidity. The effects of disaster on children are mediated by many factors including personal experience, parental reaction, developmental competency, gender, and the stage of disaster response. Pediatricians can be effective advocates for the child and family and at the community level and can affect national policy in support of families. In this report, specific children's responses are delineated, risk factors for adverse reactions are discussed, and advice is given for pediatricians to ameliorate the effects of disaster on children. (9/05)

PSYCHOSOCIAL RISKS OF CHRONIC HEALTH CONDITIONS IN CHILDHOOD AND ADOLESCENCE

Committee on Children With Disabilities and Committee on Psychosocial Aspects of Child and Family Health (12/93, reaffirmed 10/96)

QUALITY EARLY EDUCATION AND CHILD CARE FROM BIRTH TO KINDERGARTEN

Committee on Early Childhood, Adoption, and Dependent Care

ABSTRACT. High-quality early education and child care for young children improves their health and promotes their development and learning. Early education includes all of a child's experiences at home, in child care, and in other preschool settings. Pediatricians have a role in promoting access to quality early education and child care beginning at birth for all children. The American Academy of Pediatrics affords pediatricians the opportunity to promote the educational and socioemotional needs of young children with other advocacy groups. (1/05, reaffirmed 12/09)

RABIES-PREVENTION POLICY UPDATE: NEW REDUCED-DOSE SCHEDULE

Committee on Infectious Diseases

ABSTRACT. The Advisory Committee on Immunization Practices of the Centers for Disease Control and Prevention recommends reducing the number of doses from 5 to 4 of human diploid cell vaccine or purified chick embryo cell vaccine required for postexposure prophylaxis to prevent rabies in humans. The vaccine doses should be given on day 0 (first day of prophylaxis) and days 3, 7, and 14 after the first dose. For persons with immune suppression, the 5-dose regimen should continue to be used. Recommendations for the use of human rabies immunoglobulin remain unchanged. The American Academy of Pediatrics endorses these recommendations. (3/11)

RACE/ETHNICITY, GENDER, SOCIOECONOMIC STATUS—RESEARCH EXPLORING THEIR EFFECTS ON CHILD HEALTH: A SUBJECT REVIEW (CLINICAL REPORT)

Committee on Pediatric Research

ABSTRACT. Data on research participants and populations frequently include race, ethnicity, and gender as categorical variables, with the assumption that these variables exert their effects through innate or genetically determined biologic mechanisms. There is a growing body of research that suggests, however, that these variables have strong social dimensions that influence health. Socioeconomic status, a complicated construct in its own right, interacts with and confounds analyses of race/ethnicity and gender. The Academy recommends that research studies include race/ethnicity, gender, and socioeconomic status as explanatory variables only when data relevant to the underlying social mechanisms have been collected and included in the analyses. (6/00, reaffirmed 10/05, 1/09)

RACIAL AND ETHNIC DISPARITIES IN THE HEALTH AND HEALTH CARE OF CHILDREN (TECHNICAL REPORT)

Glenn Flores, MD, and Committee on Pediatric Research

ABSTRACT. *Objective.* This technical report reviews and synthesizes the published literature on racial/ethnic disparities in children's health and health care.

Methods. A systematic review of the literature was conducted for articles published between 1950 and March 2007. Inclusion criteria were peer-reviewed, original research articles in English on racial/ethnic disparities in the health and health care of US children. Search terms used included "child," "disparities," and the Index Medicus terms for each racial/ethnic minority group.

Results. Of 781 articles initially reviewed, 111 met inclusion criteria and constituted the final database. Review of the literature revealed that racial/ethnic disparities in children's health and health care are quite extensive, pervasive, and persistent. Disparities were noted across the spectrum of health and health care, including in mortality rates, access to care and use of services, prevention and population health, health status, adolescent health, chronic diseases, special health care needs, quality of care, and organ transplantation. Mortality-rate disparities were noted for children in all 4 major US racial/ethnic minority groups, including substantially greater risks than white children of all-cause mortality; death from drowning, from acute lymphoblastic leukemia, and after congenital heart defect surgery; and an earlier median age at death for those with Down syndrome and congenital heart defects. Certain methodologic flaws were commonly observed among excluded studies, including failure to evaluate children separately from adults (22%), combining all nonwhite children into 1 group (9%), and failure to provide a white comparison group (8%). Among studies in the final database, 22% did not perform multivariable or stratified analyses to ensure that disparities persisted after adjustment for potential confounders.

Conclusions. Racial/ethnic disparities in children's healthand health care are extensive, pervasive, and persistent, and occur across the spectrum of health and health care. Methodologic flaws were identified in how such disparities are sometimes documented and analyzed. Optimal health and health care for all children will require recognition of disparities as pervasive problems, methodologically sound disparities studies, and rigorous evaluation of disparities interventions. (3/10, reaffirmed 5/13)

RADIATION DISASTERS AND CHILDREN

Committee on Environmental Health

ABSTRACT. The special medical needs of children make it essential that pediatricians be prepared for radiation disasters, including 1) the detonation of a nuclear weapon; 2) a nuclear power plant event that unleashes a radioactive cloud; and 3) the dispersal of radionuclides by conventional explosive or the crash of a transport vehicle. Any of these events could occur unintentionally or as an act of terrorism. Nuclear facilities (eg, power plants, fuel processing centers, and food irradiation facilities) are often located in highly populated areas, and as they age, the risk of mechanical failure increases. The short- and long-term consequences of a radiation disaster are significantly greater in children for several reasons. First, children have a disproportionately higher minute ventilation, leading to greater internal exposure to radioactive gases. Children have a significantly greater risk of developing cancer even when they are exposed to radiation in utero. Finally, children and the parents of young children are more likely than are adults to develop enduring psychologic injury after a radiation disaster. The pediatrician has a critical role in planning for radiation disasters. For example, potassium iodide is of proven value for thyroid protection but must be given before or soon after exposure to radioiodines, requiring its placement in homes, schools, and child care centers. Pediatricians should work with public health authorities to ensure that children receive full consideration in local planning for a radiation disaster. (6/03, reaffirmed 1/07)

RADIATION RISK TO CHILDREN FROM COMPUTED TOMOGRAPHY (CLINICAL REPORT)

Alan S. Brody, MD; Donald P. Frush, MD; Walter Huda, PhD; Robert L. Brent, MD, PhD; and Section on Radiology

ABSTRACT. Imaging studies that use ionizing radiation are an essential tool for the evaluation of many disorders of childhood. Ionizing radiation is used in radiography, fluoroscopy, angiography, and computed tomography scanning. Computed tomography is of particular interest because of its relatively high radiation dose and wide use. Consensus statements on radiation risk suggest that it is reasonable to act on the assumption that low-level radiation may have a small risk of causing cancer. The medical community should seek ways to decrease radiation exposure by using radiation doses as low as reasonably achievable and by performing these studies only when necessary. There is wide agreement that the benefits of an indicated computed tomography scan far outweigh the risks. Pediatric health care professionals' roles in the use of computed tomography on children include deciding when a computed tomography scan is necessary and discussing the risk with patients and families. Radiologists should be a source of consultation when forming imaging strategies and should create specific protocols with scanning techniques optimized for pediatric patients. Families and patients should be encouraged to ask questions about the risks and benefits of computed tomography scanning. The information in this report is provided to aid in decision-making and discussions with the health care team, patients, and families. (9/07)

RECOGNITION AND MANAGEMENT OF IATROGENICALLY INDUCED OPIOID DEPENDENCE AND WITHDRAWAL IN CHILDREN (CLINICAL REPORT)

Jeffrey Galinkin, MD, FAAP; Jeffrey Lee Koh, MD, FAAP; Committee on Drugs; and Section on Anesthesiology and Pain Medicine

ABSTRACT. Opioids are often prescribed to children for pain relief related to procedures, acute injuries, and chronic conditions. Round-the-clock dosing of opioids can produce opioid dependence within 5 days. According to a 2001 consensus paper from the American Academy of Pain Medicine, American Pain Society, and American Society of Addiction Medicine, dependence is defined as "a state of adaptation that is manifested by a drug class specific withdrawal syndrome that can be produced by abrupt cessation, rapid dose reduction, decreasing blood level of the drug, and/or administration of an antagonist." Although the experience of many children undergoing iatrogenically induced withdrawal may be mild or goes unreported, there is currently no guidance for recognition or management of withdrawal for this population. Guidance on this subject is available only for adults and primarily for adults with substance use disorders. The guideline will summarize existing literature and provide readers with information currently not available in any single source specific for this vulnerable pediatric population. (12/13)

See full text on page 893.

RECOGNIZING AND RESPONDING TO MEDICAL NEGLECT (CLINICAL REPORT)

Carole Jenny, MD, MBA, and Committee on Child Abuse and Neglect

ABSTRACT. A caregiver may fail to recognize or respond to a child's medical needs for a variety of reasons. An effective response by a health care professional to medical neglect requires a comprehensive assessment of the child's needs, the parents' resources, the parents' efforts to provide for the needs of the child, and options for ensuring optimal health for the child. Such an assessment requires clear, 2-way communication between the family and the health care professional. Physicians should consider the least intrusive options for managing cases of medical neglect that ensure the health and safety of the child. (12/07, reaffirmed 1/11)

RECOMMENDATION FOR MANDATORY INFLUENZA IMMUNIZATION OF ALL HEALTH CARE PERSONNEL

Henry H. Bernstein, DO; Jeffrey R. Starke, MD; and Committee on Infectious Diseases

ABSTRACT. The purpose of this statement is to recommend implementation of a mandatory influenza immunization policy for all health care personnel. Immunization of health care personnel is a critically important step to substantially reduce health care–associated influenza infections. Despite the efforts of many organizations to improve influenza immunization rates with the use of voluntary campaigns, influenza coverage among health care personnel remains unacceptably low. Mandatory influenza immunization for all health care personnel is ethically justified, necessary, and long overdue to ensure patient safety. (9/10)

RECOMMENDATIONS FOR ADMINISTERING HEPATITIS A VACCINE TO CONTACTS OF INTERNATIONAL ADOPTEES

Committee on Infectious Diseases

ABSTRACT. The Advisory Committee on Immunization Practices of the Centers for Disease Control and Prevention and the American Academy of Pediatrics (AAP) recommend routine administration of hepatitis A vaccine for household members and close contacts, including baby-sitters, when children are adopted from countries with high or intermediate rates of hepatitis A infection. This policy expands previous AAP recommendations to immunize travelers to countries who are seeking to adopt a child in countries with high or medium hepatitis A endemicity. All previously nonimmune unvaccinated people who anticipate close exposure to international adoptees during the 60 days after their arrival should receive hepatitis A immunization, ideally 2 or more weeks before the arrival of the adopted child. (9/11)

RECOMMENDATIONS FOR PREVENTION AND CONTROL OF INFLUENZA IN CHILDREN, 2013–2014

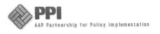

Committee on Infectious Diseases

ABSTRACT. The purpose of this statement is to update recommendations for routine use of seasonal influenza vaccine and antiviral medications for the prevention and treatment of influenza in children. Highlights for the upcoming 2013–2014 season include (1) this year's trivalent influenza vaccine contains an A/California/7/2009 (H1N1) pdm09-like virus (same as 2012–2013); an A/Texas/50/2012 (H3N2) virus (antigenically like the 2012–2013 strain); and a B/Massachusetts/2/2012-like virus (a B/Yamagata lineage like 2012–2013 but a different virus); (2) new quadrivalent influenza vaccines with an additional B virus (B/Brisbane/60/2008-like virus [B/Victoria lineage]) have been licensed by the US Food and Drug Administration; (3) annual universal influenza immunization is indicated with either a trivalent or quadrivalent vaccine (no preference); and (4) the dosing algorithm for administration of influenza vaccine to children 6 months through 8 years of age is unchanged from 2012–2013. As always, pediatricians, nurses, and all health care personnel should promote influenza vaccine use and infection control measures. In addition, pediatricians should promptly identify influenza infections to enable rapid antiviral treatment, when indicated, to reduce morbidity and mortality. (9/13)

See full text on page 899.

RECOMMENDATIONS FOR THE PREVENTION OF PERINATAL GROUP B STREPTOCOCCAL (GBS) DISEASE

Committee on Infectious Diseases and Committee on Fetus and Newborn

ABSTRACT. The Centers for Disease Control and Prevention (CDC) guidelines for the prevention of perinatal group B streptococcal (GBS) disease were initially published in 1996. The American Academy of Pediatrics (AAP) also published a policy statement on this topic in 1997. In 2002, the CDC published revised guidelines that recommended universal antenatal GBS screening; the AAP endorsed these guidelines and published recommendations based on them in the 2003 *Red Book*. Since then, the incidence of early-onset GBS disease in neonates has decreased by an estimated 80%. However, in 2010, GBS disease remained the leading cause of early-onset neonatal sepsis. The CDC issued revised guidelines in 2010 based on evaluation of data generated after 2002. These revised and comprehensive guidelines, which have been endorsed by the AAP, reaffirm the major prevention strategy—universal antenatal GBS screening and intrapartum antibiotic prophylaxis for culture-positive and high-risk women—and include new recommendations for laboratory methods for identification of GBS colonization during pregnancy, algorithms for screening and intrapartum prophylaxis for women with preterm labor and premature rupture of membranes, updated prophylaxis recommendations for women with a penicillin allergy, and a revised algorithm for the care of newborn infants. The purpose of this policy statement is to review and discuss the differences between the 2002 and 2010 CDC guidelines that are most relevant for the practice of pediatrics. (8/11)

RECOMMENDATIONS FOR THE PREVENTION OF *STREPTOCOCCUS PNEUMONIAE* INFECTIONS IN INFANTS AND CHILDREN: USE OF 13-VALENT PNEUMOCOCCAL CONJUGATE VACCINE (PCV13) AND PNEUMOCOCCAL POLYSACCHARIDE VACCINE (PPSV23)

Committee on Infectious Diseases

ABSTRACT. Routine use of the 7-valent pneumococcal conjugate vaccine (PCV7), available since 2000, has resulted in a dramatic reduction in the incidence of invasive pneumococcal disease (IPD) attributable to serotypes of Streptococcus pneumoniae contained in the vaccine. However, IPD caused by nonvaccine pneumococcal serotypes has increased, and nonvaccine serotypes are now responsible for the majority of the remaining cases of IPD occurring in children. A 13-valent pneumococcal conjugate vaccine has been licensed by the US Food and Drug Administration, which, in addition to the 7 serotypes included in the original PCV7, contains the 6 pneumococcal serotypes responsible for 63% of IPD cases now occurring in children younger than 5 years. Because of the expanded coverage provided by PCV13, it will replace PCV7. This statement provides recommendations for (1) the transition from PCV7 to PCV13; (2) the routine use of PCV13 for healthy children and children with an underlying medical condition that increases the risk of IPD; (3) a supplemental dose of PCV13 for (a) healthy children 14 through 59 months of age who have completed the PCV7 series and (b) children 14 through 71 months of age with an underlying medical condition that increases the risk of IPD who have completed the PCV7 series; (4) "catch-up" immunization for children behind schedule; and (5) PCV13 for certain children at high risk from 6 through 18 years of age. In addition, recommendations for the use of pneumococcal polysaccharide vaccine for children at high risk of IPD are also updated. (5/10)

RECOMMENDATIONS FOR PREVENTIVE PEDIATRIC HEALTH CARE

Committee on Practice and Ambulatory Medicine and Bright Futures Steering Committee

ABSTRACT. Each child and family is unique; therefore, these Recommendations for Preventive Pediatric Health Care are designed for the care of children who are receiving competent parenting, have no manifestations of any important health problems, and are growing and developing in satisfactory fashion. Additional visits may become necessary if circumstances suggest variations from normal.

Developmental, psychosocial, and chronic disease issues for children and adolescents may require frequent counseling and treatment visits separate from preventive care visits.

These guidelines represent a consensus by the American Academy of Pediatrics (AAP) and Bright Futures. The AAP continues to emphasize the great importance of continuity of care in comprehensive health supervision and the need to avoid fragmentation of care. (12/07, reaffirmed 1/11)

RECOMMENDED CHILDHOOD AND ADOLESCENT IMMUNIZATION SCHEDULE—UNITED STATES, 2014

Committee on Infectious Diseases (1/14)
See full text on page 917.

RED REFLEX EXAMINATION IN NEONATES, INFANTS, AND CHILDREN

*Section on Ophthalmology (*joint with American Association for Pediatric Ophthalmology and Strabismus, American Academy of Ophthalmology, and American Association of Certified Orthoptists)

ABSTRACT. Red reflex testing is an essential component of the neonatal, infant, and child physical examination. This statement, which is a revision of the previous policy statement published in 2002, describes the rationale for testing, the technique used to perform this examination, and the indications for referral to an ophthalmologist experienced in the examination of children. (12/08)

REDUCING THE NUMBER OF DEATHS AND INJURIES FROM RESIDENTIAL FIRES

Committee on Injury and Poison Prevention

ABSTRACT. Smoke inhalation, severe burns, and death from residential fires are devastating events, most of which are preventable. In 1998, approximately 381 500 residential structure fires resulted in 3250 non-firefighter deaths, 17 175 injuries, and approximately $4.4 billion in property loss. This statement reviews important prevention messages and intervention strategies related to residential fires. It also includes recommendations for pediatricians regarding office anticipatory guidance, work in the community, and support of regulation and legislation that could result in a decrease in the number of fire-related injuries and deaths to children. (6/00)

REDUCING THE RISK OF HIV INFECTION ASSOCIATED WITH ILLICIT DRUG USE

Committee on Pediatric AIDS

ABSTRACT. Substance abuse, specifically the use of illicit drugs that are administered intravenously, continues to play a role in the transmission of human immunodeficiency virus type 1 (HIV-1) among adolescents and young adults (youth). Risks of HIV-1 infection may result from direct exposure to contaminated blood through sharing of injection drug equipment and from unsafe sexual practices (while under the influence of drugs and/or in exchange for drugs). Reducing the risk of HIV-1 infection that is associated with illicit drug use requires prevention education and prompt engagement in treatment. Providing patients with education, instruction on decontamination of used injection drug equipment, improved access to sterile syringes and needles, and postexposure prophylaxis may decrease their risk of acquiring HIV-1 infection. Pediatricians should assess risk behaviors as part of every health care encounter, including queries about tobacco, alcohol, and marijuana use. The risks and benefits of postexposure prophylaxis with antiretroviral drugs should be considered for youth with a single recent (within 72 hours) high-risk exposure to HIV-1 through sharing needles/syringes with an HIV-1–infected individual or having unprotected intercourse with an individual who engages in injection drug use. Such prophylaxis must be accompanied by risk-reduction counseling, appropriate referrals for treatment, and evaluation for pregnancy and associated sexually transmitted infections. There is an urgent need for more substance-abuse prevention and treatment programs, legislation that facilitates unencumbered access to sterile syringes, and expedient availability of reproductive health care services for sexually active youth, including voluntary HIV-1 counseling and testing. (2/06, reaffirmed 5/09, 5/12)

REIMBURSEMENT FOR FOODS FOR SPECIAL DIETARY USE
Committee on Nutrition
ABSTRACT. Foods for special dietary use are recommended by physicians for chronic diseases or conditions of childhood, including inherited metabolic diseases. Although many states have created legislation requiring reimbursement for foods for special dietary use, legislation is now needed to mandate consistent coverage and reimbursement for foods for special dietary use and related support services with accepted medical benefit for children with designated medical conditions. (5/03, reaffirmed 1/06)

RELIEF OF PAIN AND ANXIETY IN PEDIATRIC PATIENTS IN EMERGENCY MEDICAL SYSTEMS (CLINICAL REPORT)
Joel A. Fein, MD, MPH; William T. Zempsky, MD, MPH;
*   Joseph P. Cravero, MD; Committee on Pediatric*
*   Emergency Medicine; and Section on Anesthesiology*
*   and Pain Medicine*
ABSTRACT. Control of pain and stress for children is a vital component of emergency medical care. Timely administration of analgesia affects the entire emergency medical experience and can have a lasting effect on a child's and family's reaction to current and future medical care. A systematic approach to pain management and anxiolysis, including staff education and protocol development, can provide comfort to children in the emergency setting and improve staff and family satisfaction. (10/12)

RELIGIOUS OBJECTIONS TO MEDICAL CARE
Committee on Bioethics
ABSTRACT. Parents sometimes deny their children the benefits of medical care because of religious beliefs. In some jurisdictions, exemptions to child abuse and neglect laws restrict government action to protect children or seek legal redress when the alleged abuse or neglect has occurred in the name of religion. The American Academy of Pediatrics (AAP) believes that all children deserve effective medical treatment that is likely to prevent substantial harm or suffering or death. In addition, the AAP advocates that all legal interventions apply equally whenever children are endangered or harmed, without exemptions based on parental religious beliefs. To these ends, the AAP calls for the repeal of religious exemption laws and supports additional efforts to educate the public about the medical needs of children. (2/97, reaffirmed 10/00, 6/03, 10/06, 5/09)

RESPIRATORY SUPPORT IN PRETERM INFANTS AT BIRTH
Committee on Fetus and Newborn
ABSTRACT. Current practice guidelines recommend administration of surfactant at or soon after birth in preterm infants with respiratory distress syndrome. However, recent multicenter randomized controlled trials indicate that early use of continuous positive airway pressure with subsequent selective surfactant administration in extremely preterm infants results in lower rates of bronchopulmonary dysplasia/death when compared with treatment with prophylactic or early surfactant therapy. Continuous positive airway pressure started at or soon after birth with subsequent selective surfactant administration may be considered as an alternative to routine intubation with prophylactic or early surfactant administration in preterm infants. (12/13)
See full text on page 927.

RESPONDING TO PARENTAL REFUSALS OF IMMUNIZATION OF CHILDREN (CLINICAL REPORT)
Douglas S. Diekema, MD, MPH, and Committee on Bioethics
ABSTRACT. The American Academy of Pediatrics strongly endorses universal immunization. However, for childhood immunization programs to be successful, parents must comply with immunization recommendations. The problem of parental refusal of immunization for children is an important one for pediatricians. The goal of this report is to assist pediatricians in understanding the reasons parents may have for refusing to immunize their children, review the limited circumstances under which parental refusals should be referred to child protective services agencies or public health authorities, and provide practical guidance to assist the pediatrician faced with a parent who is reluctant to allow immunization of his or her child. (5/05, reaffirmed 1/09, 11/12)

RESTRAINT USE ON AIRCRAFT
Committee on Injury and Poison Prevention
ABSTRACT. Occupant protection policies for children younger than 2 years on aircraft are inconsistent with all other national policies on safe transportation. Children younger than 2 years are not required to be restrained or secured on aircraft during takeoff, landing, and conditions of turbulence. They are permitted to be held on the lap of an adult. Preventable injuries and deaths have occurred in children younger than 2 years who were unrestrained in aircraft during survivable crashes and conditions of turbulence. The American Academy of Pediatrics recommends a mandatory federal requirement for restraint use for children on aircraft. The Academy further recommends that parents ensure that a seat is available for all children during aircraft transport and follow current recommendations for restraint use for all children. Physicians play a significant role in counseling families, advocating for public policy mandates, and encouraging technologic research that will improve protection of children in aircraft. (11/01, reaffirmed 5/05, 10/08)

RETURNING TO LEARNING FOLLOWING A CONCUSSION (CLINICAL REPORT)

Mark E. Halstead, MD, FAAP; Karen McAvoy, PsyD; Cynthia D. Devore, MD, FAAP; Rebecca Carl, MD, FAAP; Michael Lee, MD, FAAP; Kelsey Logan, MD, FAAP; Council on Sports Medicine and Fitness; and Council on School Health

ABSTRACT. Following a concussion, it is common for children and adolescents to experience difficulties in the school setting. Cognitive difficulties, such as learning new tasks or remembering previously learned material, may pose challenges in the classroom. The school environment may also increase symptoms with exposure to bright lights and screens or noisy cafeterias and hallways. Unfortunately, because most children and adolescents look physically normal after a concussion, school officials often fail to recognize the need for academic or environmental adjustments. Appropriate guidance and recommendations from the pediatrician may ease the transition back to the school environment and facilitate the recovery of the child or adolescent. This report serves to provide a better understanding of possible factors that may contribute to difficulties in a school environment after a concussion and serves as a framework for the medical home, the educational home, and the family home to guide the student to a successful and safe return to learning. (10/13)

See full text on page 933.

RITUAL GENITAL CUTTING OF FEMALE MINORS

Board of Directors (6/10)

THE ROLE OF HOME-VISITATION PROGRAMS IN IMPROVING HEALTH OUTCOMES FOR CHILDREN AND FAMILIES

Council on Child and Adolescent Health

ABSTRACT. Traditional pediatric care is often based on the assumption that parents have the basic knowledge and resources to provide a nurturing, safe environment and to provide for the emotional, physical, developmental, and health care needs of their infants and young children. Unfortunately, many families have insufficient knowledge of parenting skills and an inadequate support system of friends, extended family, or professionals to help with these vital tasks. Home-visitation programs offer an effective mechanism to ensure ongoing parental education, social support, and linkage with public and private community services. This statement reviews the history and current research on home-visitation programs and provides recommendations about the pediatrician's role in supporting and using home visitation. (3/98, reaffirmed 5/01)

ROLE OF THE MEDICAL HOME IN FAMILY-CENTERED EARLY INTERVENTION SERVICES

Council on Children With Disabilities

ABSTRACT. There is growing evidence that early intervention services have a positive influence on the developmental outcome of children with established disabilities as well as those who are considered to be "at risk" of disabilities. Various federal and state laws now mandate the establishment of community-based, coordinated, multidisciplinary, family-centered programs that are accessible to children and families. The medical home, in close collaboration with the family and the early intervention team, can play a critical role in ensuring that at-risk children receive appropriate clinical and developmental early intervention services. The purpose of this statement is to assist the pediatric health care professional in assuming a proactive role with the interdisciplinary team that provides early intervention services. (11/07)

THE ROLE OF THE PEDIATRICIAN IN RURAL EMERGENCY MEDICAL SERVICES FOR CHILDREN

Committee on Pediatric Emergency Medicine

ABSTRACT. In rural America, pediatricians can play a key role in the development, implementation, and ongoing supervision of emergency medical services for children (EMSC). Pediatricians may represent the only source of pediatric expertise for a large region and are a vital resource for rural physicians (eg, general and family practice, emergency medicine) and other rural health care professionals (physician assistants, nurse practitioners, and emergency medical technicians), providing education about management and prevention of pediatric illness and injury; appropriate equipment for the acutely ill or injured child; and acute, chronic, and rehabilitative care. In addition to providing clinical expertise, the pediatrician may be involved in quality assurance, clinical protocol development, and advocacy, and may serve as a liaison between emergency medical services and other entities working with children (eg, school nurses, child care centers, athletic programs, and programs for children with special health care needs). (10/12)

ROLE OF THE PEDIATRICIAN IN YOUTH VIOLENCE PREVENTION

Committee on Injury, Violence, and Poison Prevention

ABSTRACT. Youth violence continues to be a serious threat to the health of children and adolescents in the United States. It is crucial that pediatricians clearly define their role and develop the appropriate skills to address this threat effectively. From a clinical perspective, pediatricians should become familiar with *Connected Kids: Safe, Strong, Secure,* the American Academy of Pediatrics' primary care violence prevention protocol. Using this material, practices can incorporate preventive education, screening for risk, and linkages to community-based counseling and treatment resources. As advocates, pediatricians may bring newly developed information regarding key risk factors such as exposure to firearms, teen dating violence, and bullying to the attention of local and national policy makers. This policy statement refines the developing role of pediatricians in youth violence prevention and emphasizes the importance of this issue in the strategic agenda of the American Academy of Pediatrics. (6/09)

ROLE OF PEDIATRICIANS IN ADVOCATING LIFE SUPPORT TRAINING COURSES FOR PARENTS AND THE PUBLIC

Committee on Pediatric Emergency Medicine

ABSTRACT. Available literature suggests a need for both initial cardiopulmonary resuscitation basic life support training and refresher courses for parents and the public as well as health care professionals. The promotion of basic life support training courses that establish a pediatric chain of survival spanning from prevention of cardiac arrest and trauma to rehabilitative and follow-up care for victims of cardiopulmonary arrest is advocated in this policy statement and is the focus of an accompanying technical report. Immediate bystander cardiopulmonary resuscitation for victims of cardiac arrest improves survival for out-of-hospital cardiac arrest. Pediatricians will improve the chance of survival of children and adults who experience cardiac arrest by advocating for cardiopulmonary resuscitation training and participating in basic life support training courses as participants and instructors. (12/04, reaffirmed 5/07, 8/10, 8/13)

ROLE OF PEDIATRICIANS IN ADVOCATING LIFE SUPPORT TRAINING COURSES FOR PARENTS AND THE PUBLIC (TECHNICAL REPORT)

Lee A. Pyles, MD; Jane Knapp, MD; and Committee on Pediatric Emergency Medicine

ABSTRACT. Available literature suggests a need for both initial cardiopulmonary resuscitation training and refresher courses. The establishment of a pediatric chain of survival for victims of cardiopulmonary arrest is the focus of this technical report and is advocated in the accompanying policy statement. Immediate bystander cardiopulmonary resuscitation for victims of cardiac arrest improves survival for out-of-hospital cardiac arrest. Pediatricians will improve the chance of survival of children and adults who experience cardiac arrest by advocating for basic life support training and participating in basic life support courses as participants and teachers. (12/04, reaffirmed 5/07, 8/10)

THE ROLE OF PRESCHOOL HOME-VISITING PROGRAMS IN IMPROVING CHILDREN'S DEVELOPMENTAL AND HEALTH OUTCOMES

Council on Community Pediatrics

ABSTRACT. Child health and developmental outcomes depend to a large extent on the capabilities of families to provide a nurturing, safe environment for their infants and young children. Unfortunately, many families have insufficient knowledge about parenting skills and an inadequate support system of friends, extended family, or professionals to help with or advise them regarding child rearing. Home-visiting programs offer a mechanism for ensuring that at-risk families have social support, linkage with public and private community services, and ongoing health, developmental, and safety education. When these services are part of a system of high-quality well-child care linked or integrated with the pediatric medical home, they have the potential to mitigate health and developmental outcome disparities. This statement reviews the history of home visiting in the United States and reaffirms the support of the American Academy of Pediatrics for home-based parenting education and support. (1/09)

ROLE OF PULSE OXIMETRY IN EXAMINING NEWBORNS FOR CONGENITAL HEART DISEASE: A SCIENTIFIC STATEMENT FROM THE AHA AND AAP

William T. Mahle, MD; Jane W. Newburger, MD, MPH; G. Paul Matherne, MD; Frank C. Smith, MD; Tracey R. Hoke, MD; Robert Koppel, MD; Samuel S. Gidding, MD; Robert H. Beekman, III, MD; Scott D. Grosse, PhD; on behalf of American Heart Association Congenital Heart Defects Committee of the Council on Cardiovascular Disease in the Young, Council on Cardiovascular Nursing, and Interdisciplinary Council on Quality of Care and Outcomes Research; and American Academy of Pediatrics Section on Cardiology and Cardiac Surgery and Committee on Fetus and Newborn

ABSTRACT. *Background.* The purpose of this statement is to address the state of evidence on the routine use of pulse oximetry in newborns to detect critical congenital heart disease (CCHD).

Methods and Results. A writing group appointed by the American Heart Association and the American Academy of Pediatrics reviewed the available literature addressing current detection methods for CCHD, burden of missed and/or delayed diagnosis of CCHD, rationale of oximetry screening, and clinical studies of oximetry in otherwise asymptomatic newborns. MEDLINE database searches from 1966 to 2008 were done for English-language papers using the following search terms: congenital heart disease, pulse oximetry, physical examination, murmur, echocardiography, fetal echocardiography, and newborn screening. The reference lists of identified papers were also searched. Published abstracts from major pediatric scientific meetings in 2006 to 2008 were also reviewed. The American Heart Association classification of recommendations and levels of evidence for practice guidelines were used. In an analysis of pooled studies of oximetry assessment performed after 24 hours of life, the estimated sensitivity for detecting CCHD was 69.6%, and the positive predictive value was 47.0%; however, sensitivity varied dramatically among studies from 0% to 100%. False-positive screens that required further evaluation occurred in only 0.035% of infants screened after 24 hours.

Conclusions. Currently, CCHD is not detected in some newborns until after their hospital discharge, which results in significant morbidity and occasional mortality. Furthermore, routine pulse oximetry performed on asymptomatic newborns after 24 hours of life, but before hospital discharge, may detect CCHD. Routine pulse oximetry performed after 24 hours in hospitals that have on-site pediatric cardiovascular services incurs very low cost and risk of harm. Future studies in larger populations and across a broad range of newborn delivery systems are needed to determine whether this practice should become standard of care in the routine assessment of the neonate. (8/09)

ROLE OF THE SCHOOL NURSE IN PROVIDING SCHOOL HEALTH SERVICES

Council on School Health

ABSTRACT. The school nurse has a crucial role in the seamless provision of comprehensive health services to children and youth. Increasing numbers of students enter schools with chronic health conditions that require management during the school day. This policy statement describes for pediatricians the role of the school nurse in serving as a team member in providing preventive services, early identification of problems, interventions, and referrals to foster health and educational success. To optimally care for children, preparation, ongoing education, and appropriate staffing levels of school nurses are important factors for success. Recommendations are offered to facilitate the working relationship between the school nurse and the child's medical home. This statement has been endorsed by the National Association of School Nurses. (5/08)

ROLE OF THE SCHOOL PHYSICIAN
Council on School Health
ABSTRACT. The American Academy of Pediatrics recognizes the important role physicians play in promoting the optimal biopsychosocial well-being of children in the school setting. Although the concept of a school physician has existed for more than a century, uniformity among states and school districts regarding physicians in schools and the laws governing it are lacking. By understanding the roles and contributions physicians can make to schools, pediatricians can support and promote school physicians in their communities and improve health and safety for children. (12/12)

THE ROLE OF SCHOOLS IN COMBATING ILLICIT SUBSTANCE ABUSE
Council on School Health and Committee on Substance Abuse
ABSTRACT. Disturbingly high levels of illicit drug use remain a problem among American teenagers. As the physical, social, and psychological "home away from home" for most youth, schools naturally assume a primary role in substance abuse education, prevention, and early identification. However, the use of random drug testing on students as a component of drug prevention programs requires additional, more rigorous scientific evaluation. Widespread implementation should await the result of ongoing studies to address the effectiveness of testing and evaluate possible inadvertent harm. If drug testing on students is conducted, it should never be implemented in isolation. A comprehensive assessment and therapeutic management program for the student who tests positive should be in place before any testing is performed. Schools have the opportunity to work with parents, health care professionals, and community officials to use programs with proven effectiveness, to identify students who show behavioral risks for drug-related problems, and to make referrals to a student's medical home. When use of an illicit substance is detected, schools can foster relationships with established health care experts to assist them. A student undergoing individualized intervention for using illicit substances merits privacy. This requires that awareness of the student's situation be limited to parents, the student's physician, and only those designated school health officials with a need to know. For the purposes of this statement, alcohol, tobacco, and inhalants are not addressed. (12/07)

SAFE TRANSPORTATION OF NEWBORNS AT HOSPITAL DISCHARGE
Committee on Injury and Poison Prevention
ABSTRACT. All hospitals should set policies that require the discharge of every newborn in a car safety seat that is appropriate for the infant's maturity and medical condition. Discharge policies for newborns should include a parent education component, regular review of educational materials, and periodic in-service education for responsible staff. Appropriate child restraint systems

should become a benefit of coverage by Medicaid, managed care organizations, and other third-party insurers. (10/99, reaffirmed 1/03, 1/06, 10/08)

SAFE TRANSPORTATION OF PRETERM AND LOW BIRTH WEIGHT INFANTS AT HOSPITAL DISCHARGE (CLINICAL REPORT)
Marilyn J. Bull, MD; William A. Engle, MD; Committee on Injury, Violence, and Poison Prevention; and Committee on Fetus and Newborn
ABSTRACT. Safe transportation of preterm and low birth weight infants requires special considerations. Both physiologic immaturity and low birth weight must be taken into account to properly position such infants. This clinical report provides guidelines for pediatricians and other caregivers who counsel parents of preterm and low birth weight infants about car safety seats. (4/09, reaffirmed 8/13)

SAFETY IN YOUTH ICE HOCKEY: THE EFFECTS OF BODY CHECKING
Committee on Sports Medicine and Fitness
ABSTRACT. Ice hockey is a sport enjoyed by many young people. The occurrence of injury can offset what may otherwise be a positive experience. A high proportion of injuries in hockey appear to result from intentional body contact or the practice of checking. The American Academy of Pediatrics recommends limiting checking in hockey players 15 years of age and younger as a means to reduce injuries. Strategies such as the fair play concept can also help decrease injuries that result from penalties or unnecessary contact. (3/00, reaffirmed 1/06, 5/09)

SCHOOL BUS TRANSPORTATION OF CHILDREN WITH SPECIAL HEALTH CARE NEEDS
Committee on Injury and Poison Prevention (8/01, reaffirmed 1/05, 2/08)

SCHOOL HEALTH ASSESSMENTS
Committee on School Health
ABSTRACT. Comprehensive health assessments often are performed in school-based clinics or public health clinics by health professionals other than pediatricians. Pediatricians or other physicians skilled in child health care should participate in such evaluations. This statement provides guidance on the scope of in-school health assessments and the roles of the pediatrician, school nurse, school, and community. (4/00, reaffirmed 6/03, 5/06, 10/11)

SCHOOL HEALTH CENTERS AND OTHER INTEGRATED SCHOOL HEALTH SERVICES
Committee on School Health
ABSTRACT. This statement offers guidelines on the integration of expanded school health services, including school-based and school-linked health centers, into community-based health care systems. Expanded school health services should be integrated so that they enhance accessibility, provide high-quality health care, link children to a medical home, are financially sustainable, and address both long- and short-term needs of children and adolescents. (1/01)

SCHOOL READINESS (TECHNICAL REPORT)
Pamela C. High, MD; Committee on Early Childhood,
*   Adoption, and Dependent Care; and Council on*
*   School Health*

ABSTRACT. School readiness includes the readiness of the individual child, the school's readiness for children, and the ability of the family and community to support optimal early child development. It is the responsibility of schools to be ready for all children at all levels of readiness. Children's readiness for kindergarten should become an outcome measure for community-based programs, rather than an exclusion criterion at the beginning of the formal educational experience. Our new knowledge of early brain and child development has revealed that modifiable factors in a child's early experience can greatly affect that child's learning trajectory. Many US children enter kindergarten with limitations in their social, emotional, cognitive, and physical development that might have been significantly diminished or eliminated through early identification of and attention to child and family needs. Pediatricians have a role in promoting school readiness for all children, beginning at birth, through their practices and advocacy. The American Academy of Pediatrics affords pediatricians many opportunities to promote the physical, social-emotional, and educational health of young children, with other advocacy groups. This technical report supports American Academy of Pediatrics policy statements "Quality Early Education and Child Care From Birth to Kindergarten" and "The Inappropriate Use of School 'Readiness' Tests." (4/08, reaffirmed 9/13)

SCHOOL TRANSPORTATION SAFETY
Committee on Injury, Violence, and Poison Prevention and
*   Council on School Health*

ABSTRACT. This policy statement replaces the previous version published in 1996. It provides new information, studies, regulations, and recommendations related to the safe transportation of children to and from school and school-related activities. Pediatricians can play an important role at the patient/family, community, state, and national levels as child advocates and consultants to schools and early education programs about transportation safety. (7/07, reaffirmed 10/11)

SCHOOL-BASED HEALTH CENTERS AND PEDIATRIC PRACTICE
Council on School Health

ABSTRACT. School-based health centers (SBHCs) have become an important method of health care delivery for the youth of our nation. Although they only represent 1 aspect of a coordinated school health program approach, SBHCs have provided access to health care services for youth confronted with age, financial, cultural, and geographic barriers. A fundamental principle of SBHCs is to create an environment of service coordination and collaboration that addresses the health needs and well-being of youth with health disparities or poor access to health care services. Some pediatricians have concerns that these centers are in conflict with the primary care provider's medical home. This policy provides an overview of SBHCs and some of their documented benefits, addresses the issue of potential conflict with the medical home, and provides recommendations that support the integration and coordination of SBHCs and the pediatric medical home practice. (1/12)

SCHOOL-BASED MENTAL HEALTH SERVICES
Committee on School Health

ABSTRACT. More than 20% of children and adolescents have mental health problems. Health care professionals for children and adolescents must educate key stakeholders about the extent of these problems and work together with them to increase access to mental health resources. School-based programs offer the promise of improving access to diagnosis of and treatment for the mental health problems of children and adolescents. Pediatric health care professionals, educators, and mental health specialists should work in collaboration to develop and implement effective school-based mental health services. (6/04, reaffirmed 5/09)

SCOPE OF HEALTH CARE BENEFITS FOR CHILDREN FROM BIRTH THROUGH AGE 26
Committee on Child Health Financing

ABSTRACT. The optimal health of all children is best achieved with access to appropriate and comprehensive health care benefits. This policy statement outlines and defines the recommended set of health insurance benefits for children through age 26. The American Academy of Pediatrics developed a set of recommendations concerning preventive care services for children, adolescents, and young adults. These recommendations are compiled in the publication *Bright Futures: Guidelines for Health Supervision of Infants, Children, and Adolescents,* third edition. The Bright Futures recommendations were referenced as a standard for access and design of age-appropriate health insurance benefits for infants, children, adolescents, and young adults in the Patient Protection and Affordable Care Act of 2010 (Pub L No. 114–148). (11/11)

SCOPE OF PRACTICE ISSUES IN THE DELIVERY OF PEDIATRIC HEALTH CARE
Committee on Pediatric Workforce

ABSTRACT. The American Academy of Pediatrics (AAP) believes that optimal pediatric health care depends on a team-based approach with supervision by a physician leader, preferably a pediatrician. The pediatrician, here defined to include not only pediatric generalists but all pediatric medical subspecialists, all surgical specialists, and internal medicine/pediatric physicians, is uniquely qualified to manage, coordinate, and supervise the entire spectrum of pediatric care, from diagnosis through all stages of treatment, in all practice settings. The AAP recognizes the valuable contributions of nonphysician clinicians, including nurse practitioners and physician assistants, in delivering optimal pediatric care. However, the expansion of the scope of practice of nonphysician pediatric clinicians raises critical public policy and child health advocacy concerns. Pediatricians should serve as advocates for optimal pediatric care in state legislatures, public policy forums, and the media and should pursue opportunities to resolve scope of practice conflicts outside state legislatures. The AAP affirms the importance of appropriate documentation and standards in pediatric education, training, skills, clinical competencies, examination, regulation, and patient care to ensure safety and quality health care for all infants, children, adolescents, and young adults. (5/13)

See full text on page 945.

SCREENING EXAMINATION OF PREMATURE INFANTS FOR RETINOPATHY OF PREMATURITY

Section on Ophthalmology (joint with American Academy of Ophthalmology, American Association for Pediatric Ophthalmology and Strabismus, and American Association of Certified Orthoptists)

ABSTRACT. This statement revises a previous statement on screening of preterm infants for retinopathy of prematurity (ROP) that was published in 2006. ROP is a pathologic process that occurs only in immature retinal tissue and can progress to a tractional retinal detachment, which can result in functional or complete blindness. Use of peripheral retinal ablative therapy by using laser photocoagulation for nearly 2 decades has resulted in a high probability of markedly decreasing the incidence of this poor visual outcome, but the sequential nature of ROP creates a requirement that at-risk preterm infants be examined at proper times and intervals to detect the changes of ROP before they become permanently destructive. This statement presents the attributes on which an effective program for detecting and treating ROP could be based, including the timing of initial examination and subsequent reexamination intervals. (12/12)

SCREENING FOR RETINOPATHY IN THE PEDIATRIC PATIENT WITH TYPE 1 DIABETES MELLITUS (CLINICAL REPORT)

Gregg T. Lueder, MD; Janet Silverstein, MD; Section on Ophthalmology; and Section on Endocrinology (joint with American Association for Pediatric Ophthalmology and Strabismus)

ABSTRACT. Diabetic retinopathy (DR) is the leading cause of blindness in young adults in the United States. Early identification and treatment of DR can decrease the risk of vision loss in affected patients. This clinical report reviews the risk factors for the development of DR and screening guidance for pediatric patients with type 1 diabetes mellitus. (7/05, reaffirmed 1/09)

SECONDHAND AND PRENATAL TOBACCO SMOKE EXPOSURE (TECHNICAL REPORT)

Dana Best, MD, MPH; Committee on Environmental Health; Committee on Native American Child Health; and Committee on Adolescence

ABSTRACT. Secondhand tobacco smoke (SHS) exposure of children and their families causes significant morbidity and mortality. In their personal and professional roles, pediatricians have many opportunities to advocate for elimination of SHS exposure of children, to counsel tobacco users to quit, and to counsel children never to start. This report discusses the harms of tobacco use and SHS exposure, the extent and costs of tobacco use and SHS exposure, and the evidence that supports counseling and other clinical interventions in the cycle of tobacco use. Recommendations for future research, policy, and clinical practice change are discussed. To improve understanding and provide support for these activities, the harms of SHS exposure are discussed, effective ways to eliminate or reduce SHS exposure are presented, and policies that support a smoke-free environment are outlined. (10/09)

SELECTING APPROPRIATE TOYS FOR YOUNG CHILDREN: THE PEDIATRICIAN'S ROLE (CLINICAL REPORT)

Committee on Early Childhood, Adoption, and Dependent Care

ABSTRACT. Play is essential for learning in children. Toys are the tools of play. Which play materials are provided and how they are used are equally important. Adults caring for children can be reminded that toys facilitate but do not substitute for the most important aspect of nurture—warm, loving, dependable relationships. Toys should be safe, affordable, and developmentally appropriate. Children do not need expensive toys. Toys should be appealing to engage the child over a period of time. Information and resources are provided in this report so pediatricians can give parents advice about selecting toys. (4/03, reaffirmed 10/06, 5/11)

SELF-INJECTABLE EPINEPHRINE FOR FIRST-AID MANAGEMENT OF ANAPHYLAXIS (CLINICAL REPORT)

Scott H. Sicherer, MD; F. Estelle R. Simons, MD; and Section on Allergy and Immunology

ABSTRACT. Anaphylaxis is a severe, potentially fatal systemic allergic reaction that is rapid in onset and may cause death. Epinephrine is the primary medical therapy, and it must be administered promptly. This clinical report focuses on practical issues concerning the administration of self-injectable epinephrine for first-aid treatment of anaphylaxis in the community. The recommended epinephrine dose for anaphylaxis in children, based primarily on anecdotal evidence, is 0.01 mg/kg, up to 0.30 mg. Intramuscular injection of epinephrine into the lateral thigh (vastus lateralis) is the preferred route for therapy in first-aid treatment. Epinephrine autoinjectors are currently available in only 2 fixed doses: 0.15 and 0.30 mg. On the basis of current, albeit limited, data, it seems reasonable to recommend autoinjectors with 0.15 mg of epinephrine for otherwise healthy young children who weigh 10 to 25 kg (22–55 lb) and autoinjectors with 0.30 mg of epinephrine for those who weigh approximately 25 kg (55 lb) or more; however, specific clinical circumstances must be considered in these decisions. This report also describes several quandaries in regard to management, including the selection of dose, indications for prescribing an autoinjector, and decisions regarding when to inject epinephrine. Effective care for individuals at risk of anaphylaxis requires a comprehensive management approach involving families, allergic children, schools, camps, and other youth organizations. Risk reduction entails confirmation of the trigger, discussion of avoidance of the relevant allergen, a written individualized emergency anaphylaxis action plan, and education of supervising adults with regard to recognition and treatment of anaphylaxis. (3/07)

SENSORY INTEGRATION THERAPIES FOR CHILDREN WITH DEVELOPMENTAL AND BEHAVIORAL DISORDERS

Section on Complementary and Integrative Medicine and Council on Children With Disabilities

ABSTRACT. Sensory-based therapies are increasingly used by occupational therapists and sometimes by other types of therapists in treatment of children with developmental and behavioral disorders. Sensory-based therapies involve activities that are believed to organize the sensory system by providing vestibular, proprioceptive, auditory, and tactile inputs. Brushes, swings, balls, and other specially designed therapeutic or recreational equipment are used to provide these inputs. However, it is unclear whether children who present with sensory-based problems have an actual "disorder" of the sensory pathways of the brain or whether these deficits are characteristics associated with other developmental and behavioral disorders. Because there is no universally accepted framework for diagnosis, sensory processing disorder generally should not be diagnosed. Other developmental and behavioral disorders must always be considered, and a thorough evaluation should be completed. Difficulty tolerating or processing sensory information is a characteristic that may be seen in many developmental behavioral disorders, including autism spectrum disorders, attention-deficit/hyperactivity disorder, developmental coordination disorders, and childhood anxiety disorders.

Occupational therapy with the use of sensory-based therapies may be acceptable as one of the components of a comprehensive treatment plan. However, parents should be informed that the amount of research regarding the effectiveness of sensory integration therapy is limited and inconclusive. Important roles for pediatricians and other clinicians may include discussing these limitations with parents, talking with families about a trial period of sensory integration therapy, and teaching families how to evaluate the effectiveness of a therapy. (5/12)

SEXUAL ORIENTATION AND ADOLESCENTS (CLINICAL REPORT)

Committee on Adolescence

ABSTRACT. The American Academy of Pediatrics issued its first statement on homosexuality and adolescents in 1983, with a revision in 1993. This report reflects the growing understanding of youth of differing sexual orientations. Young people are recognizing their sexual orientation earlier than in the past, making this a topic of importance to pediatricians. Pediatricians should be aware that some youths in their care may have concerns about their sexual orientation or that of siblings, friends, parents, relatives, or others. Health care professionals should provide factual, current, nonjudgmental information in a confidential manner. All youths, including those who know or wonder whether they are not heterosexual, may seek information from physicians about sexual orientation, sexually transmitted diseases, substance abuse, or various psychosocial difficulties. The pediatrician should be attentive to various potential psychosocial difficulties, offer counseling or refer for counseling when necessary and ensure that every sexually active youth receives a thorough medical history, physical examination, immunizations, appropriate laboratory tests, and counseling about sexually transmitted diseases (including human immunodeficiency virus infection) and appropriate treatment if necessary.

Not all pediatricians may feel able to provide the type of care described in this report. Any pediatrician who is unable to care for and counsel nonheterosexual youth should refer these patients to an appropriate colleague. (6/04)

SEXUALITY OF CHILDREN AND ADOLESCENTS WITH DEVELOPMENTAL DISABILITIES (CLINICAL REPORT)

Nancy A. Murphy, MD; Ellen Roy Elias, MD; for Council on Children With Disabilities

ABSTRACT. Children and adolescents with developmental disabilities, like all children, are sexual persons. However, attention to their complex medical and functional issues often consumes time that might otherwise be invested in addressing the anatomic, physiologic, emotional, and social aspects of their developing sexuality. This report discusses issues of puberty, contraception, psychosexual development, sexual abuse, and sexuality education specific to children and adolescents with disabilities and their families. Pediatricians, in the context of the medical home, are encouraged to discuss issues of sexuality on a regular basis, ensure the privacy of each child and adolescent, promote self-care and social independence among persons with disabilities, advocate for appropriate sexuality education, and provide ongoing education for children and adolescents with developmental disabilities and their families. (7/06, reaffirmed 12/09, 7/13)

SEXUALITY, CONTRACEPTION, AND THE MEDIA

Victor C. Strasburger, MD, and Council on Communications and Media

ABSTRACT. From a health viewpoint, early sexual activity among US adolescents is a potential problem because of the risk of pregnancy and sexually transmitted infections. New evidence points to the media adolescents use frequently (television, music, movies, magazines, and the Internet) as important factors in the initiation of sexual intercourse. There is a major disconnect between what mainstream media portray—casual sex and sexuality with no consequences—and what children and teenagers need—straightforward information about human sexuality and the need for contraception when having sex. Television, film, music, and the Internet are all becoming increasingly sexually explicit, yet information on abstinence, sexual responsibility, and birth control remains rare. It is unwise to promote "abstinence-only" sex education when it has been shown to be ineffective and when the media have become such an important source of information about "nonabstinence." Recommendations are presented to help pediatricians address this important issue. (8/10)

SEXUALITY EDUCATION FOR CHILDREN AND ADOLESCENTS

Committee on Psychosocial Aspects of Child and Family Health and Committee on Adolescence

ABSTRACT. Children and adolescents need accurate and comprehensive education about sexuality to practice healthy sexual behavior as adults. Early, exploitative, or risky sexual activity may lead to health and social problems, such as unintended pregnancy and sexually transmitted diseases, including human immunodeficiency virus infection and acquired immunodeficiency syndrome. This statement reviews the role of the pediatrician in providing sexuality education to children, adolescents, and their families. Pediatricians should integrate sexuality education into the confidential and longitudinal relationship they develop with children, adolescents, and families to complement the education children obtain at school and at home. Pediatricians must be aware of their own attitudes, beliefs, and values so their effectiveness in discussing sexuality in the clinical setting is not limited. (8/01, reaffirmed 10/04)

SHOPPING CART–RELATED INJURIES TO CHILDREN

Committee on Injury, Violence, and Poison Prevention

ABSTRACT. Shopping cart–related injuries to children are common and can result in severe injury or even death. Most injuries result from falls from carts or cart tip-overs, and injuries to the head and neck represent three fourths of cases. The current US standard for shopping carts should be revised to include clear and effective performance criteria to prevent falls from carts and cart tipovers. Pediatricians have an important role as educators, researchers, and advocates to promote the prevention of these injuries. (8/06, reaffirmed 4/09, 8/13)

SHOPPING CART–RELATED INJURIES TO CHILDREN (TECHNICAL REPORT)

Gary A. Smith, MD, DrPH, for Committee on Injury, Violence, and Poison Prevention

ABSTRACT. An estimated 24 200 children younger than 15 years, 20 700 (85%) of whom were younger than 5 years, were treated in US hospital emergency departments in 2005 for shopping cart–related injuries. Approximately 4% of shopping cart–related injuries to children younger than 15 years require admission to the hospital. Injuries to the head and neck represent three fourths of all injuries. Fractures account for 45% of all hospitalizations. Deaths have occurred from falls from shopping carts and cart tip-overs. Falls are the most common mechanism of injury and account for more than half of injuries associated with shopping carts. Cart tip-overs are the second most common mechanism, responsible for up to one fourth of injuries and almost 40% of shopping cart–related injuries among children younger than 2 years. Public-awareness initiatives, education programs, and parental supervision, although important, are not enough to prevent these injuries effectively. European Standard EN 1929-1:1998 and joint Australian/New Zealand Standard AS/NZS 3847.1:1999 specify requirements for the construction, performance, testing, and safety of shopping carts and have been implemented as national standards in 21 countries. A US performance standard for shopping carts (ASTM [American Society for Testing and Materials] F2372-04) was established in July 2004; however, it does not adequately address falls and cart tip-overs, which are the leading mechanisms of shopping cart–related injuries to children. The current US standard for shopping carts should be revised to include clear and effective performance criteria for shopping cart child-restraint systems and cart stability to prevent falls from carts and cart tip-overs. This is imperative to decrease the number and severity of shopping cart–related injuries to children. Recommendations from the American Academy of Pediatrics regarding prevention of shopping cart–related injuries are included in the accompanying policy statement. (8/06, reaffirmed 4/09, 8/13)

SIDS AND OTHER SLEEP-RELATED INFANT DEATHS: EXPANSION OF RECOMMENDATIONS FOR A SAFE INFANT SLEEPING ENVIRONMENT

Task Force on Sudden Infant Death Syndrome

ABSTRACT. Despite a major decrease in the incidence of sudden infant death syndrome (SIDS) since the American Academy of Pediatrics (AAP) released its recommendation in 1992 that infants be placed for sleep in a nonprone position, this decline has plateaued in recent years. Concurrently, other causes of sudden unexpected infant death that occur during sleep (sleep-related deaths), including suffocation, asphyxia, and entrapment, and ill-defined or unspecified causes of death have increased in incidence, particularly since the AAP published its last statement on SIDS in 2005. It has become increasingly important to address these other causes of sleep-related infant death. Many of the modifiable and nonmodifiable risk factors for SIDS and suffocation are strikingly similar. The AAP, therefore, is expanding its recommendations from focusing only on SIDS to focusing on a safe sleep environment that can reduce the risk of all sleep-related infant deaths, including SIDS. The recommendations described in this policy statement include supine positioning, use of a firm sleep surface, breastfeeding, room-sharing without bed-sharing, routine immunizations, consideration of using a pacifier, and avoidance of soft bedding, overheating, and exposure to tobacco smoke, alcohol, and illicit drugs. The rationale for these recommendations is discussed in detail in the accompanying "Technical Report—SIDS and Other Sleep-Related Infant Deaths: Expansion of Recommendations for a Safe Infant Sleeping Environment." (10/11)

SIDS AND OTHER SLEEP-RELATED INFANT DEATHS: EXPANSION OF RECOMMENDATIONS FOR A SAFE INFANT SLEEPING ENVIRONMENT (TECHNICAL REPORT)

Task Force on Sudden Infant Death Syndrome

ABSTRACT. Despite a major decrease in the incidence of sudden infant death syndrome (SIDS) since the American Academy of Pediatrics (AAP) released its recommendation in 1992 that infants be placed for sleep in a nonprone position, this decline has plateaued in recent years. Concurrently, other causes of sudden unexpected infant death occurring during sleep (sleep-related deaths), including suffocation, asphyxia, and entrapment, and ill-defined or unspecified causes of death have increased in incidence, particularly since the AAP published its last statement on SIDS in 2005. It has become increasingly important to address these other causes of sleep-related infant death. Many of the modifiable and nonmodifiable risk factors for SIDS and suffocation are strikingly similar. The AAP, therefore, is expanding its recommendations from being only SIDS-focused to focusing on a safe sleep environment that can reduce the risk of all sleep-related infant deaths including SIDS. The recommendations described in this report include supine positioning, use of a firm sleep surface, breastfeeding, room-sharing without bed-sharing, routine immunization, consideration of a pacifier, and avoidance of soft bedding, overheating, and exposure to tobacco smoke, alcohol, and illicit drugs. The rationale for these recommendations is discussed in detail in this technical report. The recommendations are published in the accompanying "Policy Statement—Sudden Infant Death Syndrome and Other Sleep-Related Infant Deaths: Expansion of Recommendations for a Safe Infant Sleeping Environment." (10/11)

SKATEBOARD AND SCOOTER INJURIES
Committee on Injury, Violence, and Poison Prevention
ABSTRACT. Skateboard-related injuries account for an estimated 50 000 emergency department visits and 1500 hospitalizations among children and adolescents in the United States each year. Nonpowered scooter-related injuries accounted for an estimated 9400 emergency department visits between January and August 2000, and 90% of these patients were children younger than 15 years. Many such injuries can be avoided if children and youth do not ride in traffic, if proper protective gear is worn, and if, in the absence of close adult supervision, skateboards and scooters are not used by children younger than 10 and 8 years, respectively. (3/02, reaffirmed 5/05, 10/08)

SNOWMOBILING HAZARDS
Committee on Injury and Poison Prevention
ABSTRACT. Snowmobiles continue to pose a significant risk to children younger than 15 years and adolescents and young adults 15 through 24 years of age. Head injuries remain the leading cause of mortality and serious morbidity, arising largely from snowmobilers colliding, falling, or overturning during operation. Children also were injured while being towed in a variety of conveyances by snowmobiles. No uniform code of state laws governs the use of snowmobiles by children and youth. Because evidence is lacking to support the effectiveness of operator safety certification and because many children and adolescents do not have the required strength and skills to operate a snowmobile safely, the recreational operation of snowmobiles by persons younger than 16 years is not recommended. Snowmobiles should not be used to tow persons on a tube, tire, sled, or saucer. Furthermore, a graduated licensing program is advised for snowmobilers 16 years and older. Both active and passive snowmobile injury prevention strategies are suggested, as well as recommendations for manufacturers to make safer equipment for snowmobilers of all ages. (11/00, reaffirmed 5/04, 1/07, 6/10)

SOFT DRINKS IN SCHOOLS
Committee on School Health
ABSTRACT. This statement is intended to inform pediatricians and other health care professionals, parents, superintendents, and school board members about nutritional concerns regarding soft drink consumption in schools. Potential health problems associated with high intake of sweetened drinks are 1) overweight or obesity attributable to additional calories in the diet; 2) displacement of milk consumption, resulting in calcium deficiency with an attendant risk of osteoporosis and fractures; and 3) dental caries and potential enamel erosion. Contracts with school districts for exclusive soft drink rights encourage consumption directly and indirectly. School officials and parents need to become well informed about the health implications of vended drinks in school before making a decision about student access to them. A clearly defined, district-wide policy that restricts the sale of soft drinks will safeguard against health problems as a result of overconsumption. (1/04, reaffirmed 1/09)

SPECIAL REQUIREMENTS OF ELECTRONIC HEALTH RECORD SYSTEMS IN PEDIATRICS (CLINICAL REPORT)
S. Andrew Spooner, MD, MS, and Council on Clinical Information Technology
ABSTRACT. Some functions of an electronic health record system are much more important in providing pediatric care than in adult care. Pediatricians commonly complain about the absence of these "pediatric functions" when they are not available in electronic health record systems. To stimulate electronic health record system vendors to recognize and incorporate pediatric functionality into pediatric electronic health record systems, this clinical report reviews the major functions of importance to child health care providers. Also reviewed are important but less critical functions, any of which might be of major importance in a particular clinical context. The major areas described here are immunization management, growth tracking, medication dosing, data norms, and privacy in special pediatric populations. The American Academy of Pediatrics believes that if the functions described in this document are supported in all electronic health record systems, these systems will be more useful for patients of all ages. (3/07, reaffirmed 5/12)

SPECTRUM OF NONINFECTIOUS HEALTH EFFECTS FROM MOLDS
Committee on Environmental Health
ABSTRACT. Molds are eukaryotic (possessing a true nucleus) nonphotosynthetic organisms that flourish both indoors and outdoors. For humans, the link between mold exposure and asthma exacerbations, allergic rhinitis, infections, and toxicities from ingestion of mycotoxin-contaminated foods are well known. However, the cause-and-effect relationship between inhalational exposure to mold and other untoward health effects (eg, acute idiopathic pulmonary hemorrhage in infants and other illnesses and health complaints) requires additional investigation. Pediatricians play an important role in the education of families about mold, its adverse health effects, exposure prevention, and remediation procedures. (12/06, reaffirmed 1/11)

SPECTRUM OF NONINFECTIOUS HEALTH EFFECTS FROM MOLDS (TECHNICAL REPORT)

Lynnette J. Mazur, MD, MPH; Janice Kim, MD, PhD, MPH; and Committee on Environmental Health

ABSTRACT. Molds are multicellular fungi that are ubiquitous in outdoor and indoor environments. For humans, they are both beneficial (for the production of antimicrobial agents, chemotherapeutic agents, and vitamins) and detrimental. Exposure to mold can occur through inhalation, ingestion, and touching moldy surfaces. Adverse health effects may occur through allergic, infectious, irritant, or toxic processes. The cause-and-effect relationship between mold exposure and allergic and infectious illnesses is well known. Exposures to toxins via the gastrointestinal tract also are well described. However, the cause-and-effect relationship between inhalational exposure to mold toxins and other untoward health effects (eg, acute idiopathic pulmonary hemorrhage in infants and other illnesses and health complaints) is controversial and requires additional investigation. In this report we examine evidence of fungal-related illnesses and the unique aspects of mold exposure to children. Mold-remediation procedures are also discussed. (12/06, reaffirmed 1/11)

SPORT-RELATED CONCUSSION IN CHILDREN AND ADOLESCENTS (CLINICAL REPORT)

Mark E. Halstead, MD; Kevin D. Walter, MD; and Council on Sports Medicine and Fitness

ABSTRACT. Sport-related concussion is a "hot topic" in the media and in medicine. It is a common injury that is likely underreported by pediatric and adolescent athletes. Football has the highest incidence of concussion, but girls have higher concussion rates than boys do in similar sports. A clear understanding of the definition, signs, and symptoms of concussion is necessary to recognize it and rule out more severe intracranial injury. Concussion can cause symptoms that interfere with school, social and family relationships, and participation in sports. Recognition and education are paramount, because although proper equipment, sport technique, and adherence to rules of the sport may decrease the incidence or severity of concussions, nothing has been shown to prevent them. Appropriate management is essential for reducing the risk of long-term symptoms and complications. Cognitive and physical rest is the mainstay of management after diagnosis, and neuropsychological testing is a helpful tool in the management of concussion. Return to sport should be accomplished by using a progressive exercise program while evaluating for any return of signs or symptoms. This report serves as a basis for understanding the diagnosis and management of concussion in children and adolescent athletes. (8/10)

SPORTS DRINKS AND ENERGY DRINKS FOR CHILDREN AND ADOLESCENTS: ARE THEY APPROPRIATE? (CLINICAL REPORT)

Committee on Nutrition and Council on Sports Medicine and Fitness

ABSTRACT. Sports and energy drinks are being marketed to children and adolescents for a wide variety of inappropriate uses. Sports drinks and energy drinks are significantly different products, and the terms should not be used interchangeably. The primary objectives of this clinical report are to define the ingredients of sports and energy drinks, categorize the similarities and differences between the products, and discuss misuses and abuses. Secondary objectives are to encourage screening during annual physical examinations for sports and energy drink use, to understand the reasons why youth consumption is widespread, and to improve education aimed at decreasing or eliminating the inappropriate use of these beverages by children and adolescents. Rigorous review and analysis of the literature reveal that caffeine and other stimulant substances contained in energy drinks have no place in the diet of children and adolescents. Furthermore, frequent or excessive intake of caloric sports drinks can substantially increase the risk for overweight or obesity in children and adolescents. Discussion regarding the appropriate use of sports drinks in the youth athlete who participates regularly in endurance or high-intensity sports and vigorous physical activity is beyond the scope of this report. (5/11)

STANDARD TERMINOLOGY FOR FETAL, INFANT, AND PERINATAL DEATHS (CLINICAL REPORT)

CAPT Wanda Denise Barfield, MD, MPH, and Committee on Fetus and Newborn

ABSTRACT. Accurately defining and reporting perinatal deaths (ie, fetal and infant deaths) is a critical first step in understanding the magnitude and causes of these important events. In addition to obstetric health care providers, neonatologists and pediatricians should know the current US definitions and reporting requirements for live births, fetal deaths, and infant deaths. Correct identification of these vital events will improve our local, state, and national data so that these deaths can be better addressed and reduced. (6/11)

STANDARDS FOR HEALTH INFORMATION TECHNOLOGY TO ENSURE ADOLESCENT PRIVACY

Committee on Adolescence and Council on Clinical Information Technology

ABSTRACT. Privacy and security of health information is a basic expectation of patients. Despite the existence of federal and state laws safeguarding the privacy of health information, health information systems currently lack the capability to allow for protection of this information for minors. This policy statement reviews the challenges to privacy for adolescents posed by commercial health information technology systems and recommends basic principles for ideal electronic health record systems. This policy statement has been endorsed by the Society for Adolescent Health and Medicine. (10/12)

STATE CHILDREN'S HEALTH INSURANCE PROGRAM ACHIEVEMENTS, CHALLENGES, AND POLICY RECOMMENDATIONS

Committee on Child Health Financing

ABSTRACT. This policy statement reviews the impressive progress of the State Children's Health Insurance Program since its enactment in 1997 and identifies outstanding challenges and state and federal policy recommendations. The American Academy of Pediatrics urges Congress to reauthorize SCHIP to strengthen its historic gains. The following set of recommended strategies for reauthorization pertain to funding, eligibility and enrollment, coverage, cost sharing, payment and provider-network capacity, and quality performance. (6/07)

STRATEGIES FOR PREVENTION OF HEALTH CARE–ASSOCIATED INFECTIONS IN THE NICU (CLINICAL REPORT)

Richard A. Polin, MD; Susan Denson, MD; Michael T. Brady, MD; Committee on Fetus and Newborn; and Committee on Infectious Diseases

ABSTRACT. Health care–associated infections in the NICU result in increased morbidity and mortality, prolonged lengths of stay, and increased medical costs. Neonates are at high risk of acquiring health care–associated infections because of impaired host-defense mechanisms, limited amounts of protective endogenous flora on skin and mucosal surfaces at time of birth, reduced barrier function of their skin, use of invasive procedures and devices, and frequent exposure to broad-spectrum antibiotic agents. This clinical report reviews management and prevention of health care–associated infections in newborn infants. (3/12)

STRENGTH TRAINING BY CHILDREN AND ADOLESCENTS

Council on Sports Medicine and Fitness

ABSTRACT. Pediatricians are often asked to give advice on the safety and efficacy of strength-training programs for children and adolescents. This statement, which is a revision of a previous American Academy of Pediatrics policy statement, defines relevant terminology and provides current information on risks and benefits of strength training for children and adolescents. (4/08, reaffirmed 6/11)

SUBSTANCE USE SCREENING, BRIEF INTERVENTION, AND REFERRAL TO TREATMENT FOR PEDIATRICIANS

Committee on Substance Abuse

ABSTRACT. As a component of comprehensive pediatric care, adolescents should receive appropriate guidance regarding substance use during routine clinical care. This statement addresses practitioner challenges posed by the spectrum of pediatric substance use and presents an algorithm-based approach to augment the pediatrician's confidence and abilities related to substance use screening, brief intervention, and referral to treatment in the primary care setting. Adolescents with addictions should be managed collaboratively (or comanaged) with child and adolescent mental health or addiction specialists. This statement reviews recommended referral guidelines that are based on established patient-treatment–matching criteria and the risk level for substance abuse. (10/11)

SUICIDE AND SUICIDE ATTEMPTS IN ADOLESCENTS (CLINICAL REPORT)

Benjamin N. Shain, MD, PhD, and Committee on Adolescence

ABSTRACT. Suicide is the third-leading cause of death for adolescents 15 to 19 years old. Pediatricians can take steps to help reduce the incidence of adolescent suicide by screening for depression and suicidal ideation and behavior. This report updates the previous statement of the American Academy of Pediatrics and is intended to assist the pediatrician in the identification and management of the adolescent at risk of suicide. The extent to which pediatricians provide appropriate care for suicidal adolescents depends on their knowledge, skill, comfort with the topic, and ready access to appropriate community resources. All teenagers with suicidal thoughts or behaviors should know that their pleas for assistance are heard and that pediatricians are willing to serve as advocates to help resolve the crisis. (9/07)

SUPPLEMENTAL SECURITY INCOME (SSI) FOR CHILDREN AND YOUTH WITH DISABILITIES

Council on Children With Disabilities

ABSTRACT. The Supplemental Security Income (SSI) program remains an important source of financial support for low-income families of children with special health care needs and disabling conditions. In most states, SSI eligibility also qualifies children for the state Medicaid program, providing access to health care services. The Social Security Administration (SSA), which administers the SSI program, considers a child disabled under SSI if there is a medically determinable physical or mental impairment or combination of impairments that results in marked and severe functional limitations. The impairment(s) must be expected to result in death or have lasted or be expected to last for a continuous period of at least 12 months. The income and assets of families of children with disabilities are also considered when determining financial eligibility. When an individual with a disability becomes an adult at 18 years of age, the SSA considers only the individual's income and assets. The SSA considers an adult to be disabled if there is a medically determinable impairment (or combination of impairments) that prevents substantial gainful activity for at least 12 continuous months. SSI benefits are important for youth with chronic conditions who are transitioning to adulthood. The purpose of this statement is to provide updated information about the SSI medical and financial eligibility criteria and the disability-determination process. This statement also discusses how pediatricians can help children and youth when they apply for SSI benefits. (11/09)

SUPPORTING THE FAMILY AFTER THE DEATH OF A CHILD (CLINICAL REPORT)

Esther Wender, MD, and Committee on Psychosocial Aspects of Child and Family Health

ABSTRACT. The death of a child can have a devastating effect on the family. The pediatrician has an important role to play in supporting the parents and any siblings still in his or her practice after such a death. Pediatricians may be poorly prepared to provide this support. Also, because of the pain of confronting the grief of family members, they may be reluctant to become involved. This statement gives guidelines to help the pediatrician provide such support. It describes the grief reactions that can be expected in family members after the death of a child. Ways of supporting family members are suggested, and other helpful resources in the community are described. The goal of this guidance is to prevent outcomes that may impair the health and development of affected parents and children. (11/12)

SUPPORTING THE HEALTH CARE TRANSITION FROM ADOLESCENCE TO ADULTHOOD IN THE MEDICAL HOME (CLINICAL REPORT)

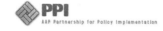

American Academy of Pediatrics, American Academy of Family Physicians, and American College of Physicians Transitions Clinical Report Authoring Group

ABSTRACT. Optimal health care is achieved when each person, at every age, receives medically and developmentally appropriate care. The goal of a planned health care transition is to maximize lifelong functioning and well-being for all youth, including those who have special health care needs and those who do not. This process includes ensuring that high-quality, developmentally appropriate health care services are available in an uninterrupted manner as the person moves from adolescence to adulthood. A well-timed transition from child- to adult-oriented health care is specific to each person and ideally occurs between the ages of 18 and 21 years. Coordination of patient, family, and provider responsibilities enables youth to optimize their ability to assume adult roles and activities. This clinical report represents expert opinion and consensus on the practice-based implementation of transition for all youth beginning in early adolescence. It provides a structure for training and continuing education to further understanding of the nature of adolescent transition and how best to support it. Primary care physicians, nurse practitioners, and physician assistants, as well as medical subspecialists, are encouraged to adopt these materials and make this process specific to their settings and populations. (7/11)

SURFACTANT REPLACEMENT THERAPY FOR PRETERM AND TERM NEONATES WITH RESPIRATORY DISTRESS (CLINICAL REPORT)

Richard A. Polin, MD, FAAP; Waldemar A. Carlo, MD, FAAP; and Committee on Fetus and Newborn

ABSTRACT. Respiratory failure secondary to surfactant deficiency is a major cause of morbidity and mortality in preterm infants. Surfactant therapy substantially reduces mortality and respiratory morbidity for this population. Secondary surfactant deficiency also contributes to acute respiratory morbidity in late-preterm and term neonates with meconium aspiration syndrome, pneumonia/sepsis, and perhaps pulmonary hemorrhage; surfactant replacement may be beneficial for these infants. This statement summarizes the evidence regarding indications, administration, formulations, and outcomes for surfactant-replacement therapy. The clinical strategy of intubation, surfactant administration, and extubation to continuous positive airway pressure and the effect of continuous positive airway pressure on outcomes and surfactant use in preterm infants are also reviewed. (12/13)
    See full text on page 953.

SURVEILLANCE OF PEDIATRIC HIV INFECTION

Committee on Pediatric AIDS

ABSTRACT. Pediatric human immunodeficiency virus (HIV)/acquired immunodeficiency syndrome (AIDS) surveillance should expand to include perinatal HIV exposure and HIV infection as well as AIDS to delineate completely the extent and impact of HIV infection on children and families, accurately assess the resources necessary to provide services to this population, evaluate the efficacy of public health recommendations, and determine any potential long-term consequences of interventions to prevent perinatal transmission to children ultimately determined to be uninfected as well as for those who become infected. Ensuring the confidentiality of information collected in the process of surveillance is critical. In addition, expansion of surveillance must not compromise the established, ongoing surveillance system for pediatric AIDS. An expanded pediatric HIV surveillance program provides an important counterpart to existing American Academy of Pediatrics and American College of Obstetricians and Gynecologists recommendations for HIV counseling and testing in the prenatal setting. (2/98, reaffirmed 2/02, 1/06, 1/11)

SWIMMING PROGRAMS FOR INFANTS AND TODDLERS

Committee on Sports Medicine and Fitness and Committee on Injury and Poison Prevention

ABSTRACT. Infant and toddler aquatic programs provide an opportunity to introduce young children to the joy and risks of being in or around water. Generally, children are not developmentally ready for swimming lessons until after their fourth birthday. Aquatic programs for infants and toddlers have not been shown to decrease the risk of drowning, and parents should not feel secure that their child is safe in water or safe from drowning after participating in such programs. Young children should receive constant, close supervision by an adult while in and around water. (4/00, reaffirmed 5/04)

THE TEEN DRIVER

Committee on Injury, Violence, and Poison Prevention and Committee on Adolescence

ABSTRACT. Motor vehicle–related injuries to adolescents continue to be of paramount importance to society. Since the original policy statement on the teenaged driver was published in 1996, there have been substantial changes in many state laws and much new research on this topic. There is a need to provide pediatricians with up-to-date information and materials to facilitate appropriate counseling and anticipatory guidance. This statement describes why teenagers are at greater risk of motor vehicle–related injuries, suggests topics suitable for office-based counseling, describes innovative programs, and proposes preventive interventions for pediatricians, parents, legislators, educators, and other child advocates. (12/06, reaffirmed 6/10)

TESTING FOR DRUGS OF ABUSE IN CHILDREN AND ADOLESCENTS

Committee on Substance Abuse

ABSTRACT. The American Academy of Pediatrics (AAP) recognizes the abuse of psychoactive drugs as one of the greatest problems facing children and adolescents and condemns all such use. Diagnostic testing for drugs of abuse is frequently an integral part of the pediatrician's evaluation and management of those suspected of such use. "Voluntary screening" is the term applied to many mass non–suspicion-based screening programs, yet such programs may not be truly voluntary as there are often negative consequences for those who choose not to take part. Participation in such programs should not be a prerequisite to participation in school activities. Involuntary testing is not appropriate in adolescents with decisional capacity—even with parental consent—and should be performed only if there are strong medical or legal reasons to do so. The AAP reaffirms its position that the appropriate response to the suspicion of drug abuse in a young person is the referral to a qualified health care professional for comprehensive evaluation. (8/96, reaffirmed 5/99, 5/06)

TESTING FOR DRUGS OF ABUSE IN CHILDREN AND ADOLESCENTS: ADDENDUM—TESTING IN SCHOOLS AND AT HOME

Committee on Substance Abuse and Council on School Health

ABSTRACT. The American Academy of Pediatrics continues to believe that adolescents should not be drug tested without their knowledge and consent. Recent US Supreme Court decisions and market forces have resulted in recommendations for drug testing of adolescents at school and products for parents to use to test adolescents at home. The American Academy of Pediatrics has strong reservations about testing adolescents at school or at home and believes that more research is needed on both safety and efficacy before school-based testing programs are implemented. The American Academy of Pediatrics also believes that more adolescent-specific substance abuse treatment resources are needed to ensure that testing leads to early rehabilitation rather than to punitive measures only. (3/07)

TOBACCO, ALCOHOL, AND OTHER DRUGS: THE ROLE OF THE PEDIATRICIAN IN PREVENTION, IDENTIFICATION, AND MANAGEMENT OF SUBSTANCE ABUSE (CLINICAL REPORT)

John W. Kulig, MD, MPH, and Committee on Substance Abuse

ABSTRACT. Substance abuse remains a major public health concern, and pediatricians are uniquely positioned to assist their patients and families with its prevention, detection, and treatment. The American Academy of Pediatrics has highlighted the importance of such issues in a variety of ways, including its guidelines for preventive services. The harmful consequences of tobacco, alcohol, and other drug use are a concern of medical professionals who care for infants, children, adolescents, and young adults. Thus, pediatricians should include discussion of substance abuse as a part of routine health care, starting with the prenatal visit, and as part of ongoing anticipatory guidance. Knowledge of the nature and extent of the consequences of tobacco, alcohol, and other drug use as well as the physical, psychological, and social consequences is essential for pediatricians. Pediatricians should incorporate substance-abuse prevention into daily practice, acquire the skills necessary to identify young people at risk of substance abuse, and provide or facilitate assessment, intervention, and treatment as necessary. (3/05, reaffirmed 3/13)

TOBACCO AS A SUBSTANCE OF ABUSE (TECHNICAL REPORT)

Tammy H. Sims, MD, MS, and Committee on Substance Abuse

ABSTRACT. Tobacco use is the leading preventable cause of morbidity and death in the United States. Because 80% to 90% of adult smokers began during adolescence, and two thirds became regular, daily smokers before they reached 19 years of age, tobacco use may be viewed as a pediatric disease. Every year in the United States, approximately 1.4 million children younger than 18 years start smoking, and many of them will die prematurely from a smoking-related disease. Moreover, there is recent evidence that adolescents report symptoms of tobacco dependence early in the smoking process, even before becoming daily smokers. The prevalence of tobacco use is higher among teenagers and young adults than among older adult populations. The critical role of pediatricians in helping to reduce tobacco use and addiction and secondhand tobacco-smoke exposure in the pediatric population includes education and prevention, screening and detection, and treatment and referral. (10/09)

TOBACCO USE: A PEDIATRIC DISEASE

Committee on Environmental Health, Committee on Substance Abuse, Committee on Adolescence, and Committee on Native American Child Health

ABSTRACT. Tobacco use and secondhand tobacco-smoke (SHS) exposure are major national and international health concerns. Pediatricians and other clinicians who care for children are uniquely positioned to assist patients and families with tobacco-use prevention and treatment. Understanding the nature and extent of tobacco use and SHS exposure is an essential first step toward the goal of eliminating tobacco use and its consequences in the pediatric population. The next steps include counseling patients and family members to avoid SHS exposures or cease tobacco use; advocacy for policies that protect children from SHS exposure; and elimination of tobacco use in the media, public places, and homes. Three overarching principles of this policy can be identified: (1) there is no safe way to use tobacco; (2) there is no safe level or duration of exposure to SHS; and (3) the financial and political power of individuals, organizations, and government should be used to support tobacco control. Pediatricians are advised not to smoke or use tobacco; to make their homes, cars, and workplaces tobacco free; to consider tobacco control when making personal and professional decisions; to support and advocate for comprehensive tobacco control; and to advise parents and patients not to start using tobacco or to quit if they are already using tobacco. Prohibiting both tobacco advertising and the use of tobacco products in the media is recommended. Recommendations for eliminating SHS exposure and reducing tobacco use include attaining universal (1) smoke-free home, car, school, work, and play environments, both inside and outside, (2) treatment of tobacco use and dependence through employer, insurance, state, and federal supports, (3) implementation and enforcement of evidence-based tobacco-control measures in local, state, national, and international jurisdictions, and (4) financial and systems support for training in and research of effective ways to prevent and treat tobacco use and SHS exposure. Pediatricians, their staff and colleagues, and the American Academy of Pediatrics have key responsibilities in tobacco control to promote the health of children, adolescents, and young adults. (10/09)

TOWARD TRANSPARENT CLINICAL POLICIES
Steering Committee on Quality Improvement and Management
ABSTRACT. Clinical policies of professional societies such as the American Academy of Pediatrics are valued highly, not only by clinicians who provide direct health care to children but also by many others who rely on the professional expertise of these organizations, including parents, employers, insurers, and legislators. The utility of a policy depends, in large part, on the degree to which its purpose and basis are clear to policy users, an attribute known as the policy's transparency. This statement describes the critical importance and special value of transparency in clinical policies, guidelines, and recommendations; helps identify obstacles to achieving transparency; and suggests several approaches to overcome these obstacles. (3/08)

TRAMPOLINE SAFETY IN CHILDHOOD AND ADOLESCENCE
Council on Sports Medicine and Fitness
ABSTRACT. Despite previous recommendations from the American Academy of Pediatrics discouraging home use of trampolines, recreational use of trampolines in the home setting continues to be a popular activity among children and adolescents. This policy statement is an update to previous statements, reflecting the current literature on prevalence, patterns, and mechanisms of trampoline-related injuries. Most trampoline injuries occur with multiple simultaneous users on the mat. Cervical spine injuries often occur with falls off the trampoline or with attempts at somersaults or flips. Studies on the efficacy of trampoline safety measures are reviewed, and although there is a paucity of data, current implementation of safety measures have not appeared to mitigate risk substantially. Therefore, the home use of trampolines is strongly discouraged. The role of trampoline as a competitive sport and in structured training settings is reviewed, and recommendations for enhancing safety in these environments are made. (9/12)

THE TRANSFER OF DRUGS AND THERAPEUTICS INTO HUMAN BREAST MILK: AN UPDATE ON SELECTED TOPICS (CLINICAL REPORT)
Hari Cheryl Sachs, MD, FAAP, and Committee on Drugs
ABSTRACT. Many mothers are inappropriately advised to discontinue breastfeeding or avoid taking essential medications because of fears of adverse effects on their infants. This cautious approach may be unnecessary in many cases, because only a small proportion of medications are contraindicated in breastfeeding mothers or associated with adverse effects on their infants. Information to inform physicians about the extent of excretion for a particular drug into human milk is needed but may not be available. Previous statements on this topic from the American Academy of Pediatrics provided physicians with data concerning the known excretion of specific medications into breast milk. More current and comprehensive information is now available on the Internet, as well as an application for mobile devices, at LactMed (http://toxnet.nlm.nih.gov). Therefore, with the exception of radioactive compounds requiring temporary cessation of breastfeeding, the reader will be referred to LactMed to obtain the most current data on an individual medication. This report discusses several topics of interest surrounding lactation, such as the use of psychotropic therapies, drugs to treat substance abuse, narcotics, galactagogues, and herbal products, as well as immunization of breastfeeding women. A discussion regarding the global implications of maternal medications and lactation in the developing world is beyond the scope of this report. The World Health Organization offers several programs and resources that address the importance of breastfeeding (see http://www.who.int/topics/breastfeeding/en/). (8/13)
See full text on page 963.

TRANSITIONING HIV-INFECTED YOUTH INTO ADULT HEALTH CARE
Committee on Pediatric AIDS
ABSTRACT. With advances in antiretroviral therapy, most HIV-infected children survive into adulthood. Optimal health care for these youth includes a formal plan for the transition of care from primary and/or subspecialty pediatric/adolescent/family medicine health care providers (medical home) to adult health care provider(s). Successful transition involves the early engagement and participation of the youth and his or her family with the pediatric medical home and adult health care teams in developing a formal plan. Referring providers should have a written policy for the transfer of HIV-infected youth to adult care, which will guide in the development of an individualized plan for each youth. The plan should be introduced to the youth in early adolescence and modified as the youth approaches transition. Assessment of developmental milestones is important to define the readiness of the youth in assuming responsibility for his or her own care before initiating the transfer. Communication among all providers is essential and should include both personal contact and a written medical summary. Progress toward the transition should be tracked and, once completed, should be documented and assessed. (6/13)
See full text on page 979.

TRANSPORTING CHILDREN WITH SPECIAL HEALTH CARE NEEDS
Committee on Injury and Poison Prevention
ABSTRACT. Children with special health care needs should have access to proper resources for safe transportation. This statement reviews important considerations for transporting children with special health care needs and provides current guidelines for the protection of children with specific health care needs, including those with a tracheostomy, a spica cast, challenging behaviors, or muscle tone abnormalities as well as those transported in wheelchairs. (10/99, reaffirmed 1/03, 1/06, 3/13)

THE TREATMENT OF NEUROLOGICALLY IMPAIRED CHILDREN USING PATTERNING

Committee on Children With Disabilities

ABSTRACT. This statement reviews patterning as a treatment for children with neurologic impairments. This treatment is based on an outmoded and oversimplified theory of brain development. Current information does not support the claims of proponents that this treatment is efficacious, and its use continues to be unwarranted. (11/99, reaffirmed 11/02, 1/06, 8/10)

ULTRAVIOLET RADIATION: A HAZARD TO CHILDREN AND ADOLESCENTS

Council on Environmental Health and Section on Dermatology

ABSTRACT. Ultraviolet radiation (UVR) causes the 3 major forms of skin cancer: basal cell carcinoma; squamous cell carcinoma; and cutaneous malignant melanoma. Public awareness of the risk is not optimal, overall compliance with sun protection is inconsistent, and melanoma rates continue to rise. The risk of skin cancer increases when people overexpose themselves to sun and intentionally expose themselves to artificial sources of UVR. Yet, people continue to sunburn, and teenagers and adults alike remain frequent visitors to tanning parlors. Pediatricians should provide advice about UVR exposure during health-supervision visits and at other relevant times. Advice includes avoiding sunburning, wearing clothing and hats, timing activities (when possible) before or after periods of peak sun exposure, wearing protective sunglasses, and applying and reapplying sunscreen. Advice should be framed in the context of promoting outdoor physical activity. Adolescents should be strongly discouraged from visiting tanning parlors. Sun exposure and vitamin D status are intertwined. Cutaneous vitamin D production requires sunlight exposure, and many factors, such as skin pigmentation, season, and time of day, complicate efficiency of cutaneous vitamin D production that results from sun exposure. Adequate vitamin D is needed for bone health. Accumulating information suggests a beneficial influence of vitamin D on many health conditions. Although vitamin D is available through the diet, supplements, and incidental sun exposure, many children have low vitamin D concentrations. Ensuring vitamin D adequacy while promoting sun-protection strategies will require renewed attention to children's use of dietary and supplemental vitamin D. (2/11)

ULTRAVIOLET RADIATION: A HAZARD TO CHILDREN AND ADOLESCENTS (TECHNICAL REPORT)

Sophie J. Balk, MD; Council on Environmental Health; and Section on Dermatology

ABSTRACT. Sunlight sustains life on earth. Sunlight is essential for vitamin D synthesis in the skin. The sun's ultraviolet rays can be hazardous, however, because excessive exposure causes skin cancer and other adverse health effects. Skin cancer is a major public health problem; more than 2 million new cases are diagnosed in the United States each year. Ultraviolet radiation (UVR) causes the 3 major forms of skin cancer: basal cell carcinoma; squamous cell carcinoma; and cutaneous malignant melanoma. Exposure to UVR from sunlight and artificial sources early in life elevates the risk of developing skin cancer. Approximately 25% of sun exposure occurs before 18 years of age. The risk of skin cancer is increased when people overexpose themselves to sun and intentionally expose themselves to artificial sources of UVR. Public awareness of the risk is not optimal, compliance with sun protection is inconsistent, and skin-cancer rates continue to rise in all age groups including the younger population. People continue to sunburn, and teenagers and adults are frequent visitors to tanning parlors. Sun exposure and vitamin D status are intertwined. Adequate vitamin D is needed for bone health in children and adults. In addition, there is accumulating information suggesting a beneficial influence of vitamin D on various health conditions. Cutaneous vitamin D production requires sunlight, and many factors complicate the efficiency of vitamin D production that results from sunlight exposure. Ensuring vitamin D adequacy while promoting sun-protection strategies, therefore, requires renewed attention to evaluating the adequacy of dietary and supplemental vitamin D. Daily intake of 400 IU of vitamin D will prevent vitamin D deficiency rickets in infants. The vitamin D supplementation amounts necessary to support optimal health in older children and adolescents are less clear. This report updates information on the relationship of sun exposure to skin cancer and other adverse health effects, the relationship of exposure to artificial sources of UVR and skin cancer, sun-protection methods, vitamin D, community skin-cancer–prevention efforts, and the pediatrician's role in preventing skin cancer. In addition to pediatricians' efforts, a sustained public health effort is needed to change attitudes and behaviors regarding UVR exposure. (3/11)

UNDERINSURANCE OF ADOLESCENTS: RECOMMENDATIONS FOR IMPROVED COVERAGE OF PREVENTIVE, REPRODUCTIVE, AND BEHAVIORAL HEALTH CARE SERVICES

Committee on Adolescence and Committee on Child Health Financing

ABSTRACT. The purpose of this policy statement is to address the serious underinsurance (ie, insurance that exists but is inadequate) problems affecting insured adolescents' access to needed preventive, reproductive, and behavioral health care. In addition, the statement addresses provider payment problems that disproportionately affect clinicians who care for adolescents.

Among adolescents with insurance, particularly private health insurance, coverage of needed services is often inadequate. Benefits are typically limited in scope and amount; certain diagnoses are often excluded; and cost-sharing requirements are often too high. As a result, underinsurance represents a substantial problem among adolescents and adversely affects their health and well-being.

In addition to underinsurance problems, payment problems in the form of inadequate payment, uncompensated care for confidential reproductive services, and the failure of insurers to recognize and pay for certain billing and diagnostic codes are widespread among both private and public insurers. Payment problems negatively affect clinicians' ability to offer needed services to adolescents, especially publicly insured adolescents. (12/08)

UNDERSTANDING THE BEHAVIORAL AND EMOTIONAL CONSEQUENCES OF CHILD ABUSE (CLINICAL REPORT)

John Stirling Jr, MD; Committee on Child Abuse and Neglect; and Section on Adoption and Foster Care (joint with Lisa Amaya-Jackson, MD, MPH; American Academy of Child and Adolescent Psychiatry; and National Center for Child Traumatic Stress)

ABSTRACT. Children who have suffered early abuse or neglect may later present with significant behavior problems including emotional instability, depression, and a tendency to be aggressive or violent with others. Troublesome behaviors may persist long after the abusive or neglectful environment has changed or the child has been in foster care placement. Neurobiological research has shown that early abuse results in an altered physiological response to stressful stimuli, a response that deleteriously affects the child's subsequent socialization. Pediatricians can assist caregivers by helping them recognize the abused or neglected child's altered responses, formulate more effective coping strategies, and mobilize available community resources. (9/08)

UPDATE OF NEWBORN SCREENING AND THERAPY FOR CONGENITAL HYPOTHYROIDISM (CLINICAL REPORT)

Susan R. Rose, MD; Section on Endocrinology; and Committee on Genetics (joint with American Thyroid Association; Rosalind S. Brown, MD; and Lawson Wilkins Pediatric Endocrine Society)

ABSTRACT. Unrecognized congenital hypothyroidism leads to mental retardation. Newborn screening and thyroid therapy started within 2 weeks of age can normalize cognitive development. The primary thyroid-stimulating hormone screening has become standard in many parts of the world. However, newborn thyroid screening is not yet universal in some countries. Initial dosage of 10 to 15 μg/kg levothyroxine is recommended. The goals of thyroid hormone therapy should be to maintain frequent evaluations of total thyroxine or free thyroxine in the upper half of the reference range during the first 3 years of life and to normalize the serum thyroid-stimulating hormone concentration to ensure optimal thyroid hormone dosage and compliance.

Improvements in screening and therapy have led to improved developmental outcomes in adults with congenital hypothyroidism who are now in their 20s and 30s. Thyroid hormone regimens used today are more aggressive in targeting early correction of thyroid-stimulating hormone than were those used 20 or even 10 years ago. Thus, newborn infants with congenital hypothyroidism today may have an even better intellectual and neurologic prognosis. Efforts are ongoing to establish the optimal therapy that leads to maximum potential for normal development for infants with congenital hypothyroidism.

Remaining controversy centers on infants whose abnormality in neonatal thyroid function is transient or mild and on optimal care of very low birth weight or preterm infants. Of note, thyroid-stimulating hormone is not elevated in central hypothyroidism. An algorithm is proposed for diagnosis and management.

Physicians must not relinquish their clinical judgment and experience in the face of normal newborn thyroid test results. Hypothyroidism can be acquired after the newborn screening. When clinical symptoms and signs suggest hypothyroidism, regardless of newborn screening results, serum free thyroxine and thyroid-stimulating hormone determinations should be performed. (6/06, reaffirmed 12/11)

USE OF CHAPERONES DURING THE PHYSICAL EXAMINATION OF THE PEDIATRIC PATIENT

Committee on Practice and Ambulatory Medicine

ABSTRACT. Physicians should always communicate the scope and nature of the physical examination to be performed to the pediatric patient and his or her parent. This statement addresses the use of chaperones and issues of patient comfort, confidentiality, and privacy. The use of a chaperone should be a shared decision between the patient and physician. In some states, the use of a chaperone is mandated by state regulations. (4/11)

USE OF CODEINE- AND DEXTROMETHORPHAN-CONTAINING COUGH REMEDIES IN CHILDREN

Committee on Drugs

ABSTRACT. Numerous prescription and nonprescription medications are currently available for suppression of cough, a common symptom in children. Because adverse effects and overdosage associated with the administration of cough and cold preparations in children have been reported, education of patients and parents about the lack of proven antitussive effects and the potential risks of these products is needed. (6/97, reaffirmed 5/00, 6/03, 10/06)

THE USE OF COMPLEMENTARY AND ALTERNATIVE MEDICINE IN PEDIATRICS (CLINICAL REPORT)

Kathi J. Kemper, MD, MPH; Sunita Vohra, MD; Richard Walls, MD, PhD; Task Force on Complementary and Alternative Medicine; and Provisional Section on Complementary, Holistic, and Integrative Medicine

ABSTRACT. The American Academy of Pediatrics is dedicated to optimizing the well-being of children and advancing family-centered health care. Related to these goals, the American Academy of Pediatrics recognizes the increasing use of complementary and alternative medicine in children and, as a result, the need to provide information and support for pediatricians. From 2000 to 2002, the American Academy of Pediatrics convened and charged the Task Force on Complementary and Alternative Medicine to address issues related to the use of complementary and alternative medicine in children and to develop resources to educate physicians, patients, and families. One of these resources is this report describing complementary and alternative medicine services, current levels of utilization and financial expenditures, and associated legal and ethical considerations. The subject of complementary and alternative medicine is large and diverse, and consequently, an in-depth discussion of each method of complementary and alternative medicine is beyond the scope of this report. Instead, this report will define terms; describe epidemiology; outline common types of complementary and alternative medicine therapies; review medicolegal, ethical, and research implications; review education and training for complementary and alternative medicine providers; provide resources for learning more about complementary and alternative medicine; and suggest communication strategies to use when discussing complementary and alternative medicine with patients and families. (12/08, reaffirmed 10/12, 1/13)

USE OF INHALED NITRIC OXIDE
Committee on Fetus and Newborn
ABSTRACT. Approval of inhaled nitric oxide by the US Food and Drug Administration for hypoxic respiratory failure of the term and near-term newborn provides an important new therapy for this serious condition. This statement addresses the conditions under which inhaled nitric oxide should be administered to the neonate with hypoxic respiratory failure. (8/00, reaffirmed 4/03, 12/09)

USE OF INHALED NITRIC OXIDE IN PRETERM INFANTS (CLINICAL REPORT)
Praveen Kumar, MD, FAAP, and Committee on Fetus and Newborn
ABSTRACT. Nitric oxide, an important signaling molecule with multiple regulatory effects throughout the body, is an important tool for the treatment of full-term and late-preterm infants with persistent pulmonary hypertension of the newborn and hypoxemic respiratory failure. Several randomized controlled trials have evaluated its role in the management of preterm infants ≤34 weeks' gestational age with varying results. The purpose of this clinical report is to summarize the existing evidence for the use of inhaled nitric oxide in preterm infants and provide guidance regarding its use in this population. (12/13)
See full text on page 987.

THE USE AND MISUSE OF FRUIT JUICE IN PEDIATRICS
Committee on Nutrition
ABSTRACT. Historically, fruit juice was recommended by pediatricians as a source of vitamin C and an extra source of water for healthy infants and young children as their diets expanded to include solid foods with higher renal solute. Fruit juice is marketed as a healthy, natural source of vitamins and, in some instances, calcium. Because juice tastes good, children readily accept it. Although juice consumption has some benefits, it also has potential detrimental effects. Pediatricians need to be knowledgeable about juice to inform parents and patients on its appropriate uses. (5/01, reaffirmed 10/06, 8/13)

USE OF PERFORMANCE-ENHANCING SUBSTANCES
Committee on Sports Medicine and Fitness
ABSTRACT. Performance-enhancing substances include dietary supplements, prescription medications, and illicit drugs. Virtually no data are available on the efficacy and safety in children and adolescents of widely used performance-enhancing substances. This statement is intended to provide a generalized but functional definition of performance-enhancing substances. The American Academy of Pediatrics strongly condemns the use of performance-enhancing substances and vigorously endorses efforts to eliminate their use among children and adolescents. (4/05, reaffirmed 5/08)

USE OF SOY PROTEIN-BASED FORMULAS IN INFANT FEEDING (CLINICAL REPORT)
Jatinder Bhatia, MD; Frank Greer, MD; and Committee on Nutrition
ABSTRACT. Soy protein-based formulas have been available for almost 100 years. Since the first use of soy formula as a milk substitute for an infant unable to tolerate a cow milk protein-based formula, the formulation has changed to the current soy protein isolate. Despite very limited indications for its use, soy protein-based formulas in the United States may account for nearly 25% of the formula market. This report reviews the limited indications and contraindications of soy formulas. It will also review the potential harmful effects of soy protein-based formulas and the phytoestrogens contained in these formulas. (5/08)

THE USE OF SYSTEMIC AND TOPICAL FLUOROQUINOLONES (CLINICAL REPORT)
John S. Bradley, MD; Mary Anne Jackson, MD; and Committee on Infectious Diseases
ABSTRACT. Appropriate prescribing practices for fluoroquinolones are essential as evolving resistance patterns are considered, additional treatment indications are identified, and the toxicity profile of fluoroquinolones in children becomes better defined. Earlier recommendations for systemic therapy remain; expanded uses of fluoroquinolones for the treatment of certain infections are outlined in this report. Although fluoroquinolones are reasonably safe in children, clinicians should be aware of the specific adverse reactions. Use of fluoroquinolones in children should continue to be limited to treatment of infections for which no safe and effective alternative exists. (9/11)

USES OF DRUGS NOT DESCRIBED IN THE PACKAGE INSERT (OFF-LABEL USES)
Committee on Drugs
ABSTRACT. New regulatory initiatives have been designed to ensure that new drugs and biologicals include adequate pediatric labeling for the claimed indications at the time of, or soon after, approval. However, because such labeling may not immediately be available, off-label use (or use that is not included in the approved label) of therapeutic agents is likely to remain common in the practice of pediatrics. This policy statement was written to address questions practitioners have regarding off-label use. The purpose of off-label use is to benefit the individual patient. Practitioners may use their professional judgment to determine these uses. Practitioners should understand that the Food and Drug Administration does not regulate off-label use. (7/02, reaffirmed 10/05)

USING PERSONAL HEALTH RECORDS TO IMPROVE THE QUALITY OF HEALTH CARE FOR CHILDREN
Council on Clinical Information Technology
ABSTRACT. A personal health record (PHR) is a repository of information from multiple contributors (eg, patient, family, guardians, physicians, and other health care professionals) regarding the health of an individual. The development of electronic PHRs presents new opportunities and challenges to the practice of pediatrics. This policy statement provides recommendations for actions

that pediatricians can take to support the development and use of PHRs for children.

Pediatric health care professionals must become actively involved in developing and adopting PHRs and PHR systems. The American Academy of Pediatrics supports development of:

- educational programs for families and clinicians on effective and efficient use of PHRs;
- incentives to facilitate PHR use and maintenance; and
- child- and adolescent-friendly standards for PHR content, portability, security, and privacy.

Properly designed PHR systems for pediatric care can empower patients. PHRs can improve access to health information, improve coordination of preventive health and health maintenance activities, and support emergency and disaster management activities. PHRs provide support for the medical home for all children, including those with special health care needs and those in foster care. PHRs can also provide information to serve as the basis for pediatric quality improvement efforts.

For PHRs to be adopted sufficiently to realize these benefits, we must determine how best to support their development and adoption. Privacy and security issues, especially with regard to children and adolescents, must be addressed. (6/09)

VENTRICULAR FIBRILLATION AND THE USE OF AUTOMATED EXTERNAL DEFIBRILLATORS ON CHILDREN

Committee on Pediatric Emergency Medicine and Section on Cardiology and Cardiac Surgery

ABSTRACT. The use of automated external defibrillators (AEDs) has been advocated in recent years as one part of the chain of survival to improve outcomes for adult cardiac arrest victims. When AEDs first entered the market, they had not been tested for pediatric usage and rhythm interpretation. In addition, the presumption was that children do not experience ventricular fibrillation, so they would not benefit from the use of AEDs. Recent literature has shown that children do experience ventricular fibrillation, which has a better outcome than do other cardiac arrest rhythms. At the same time, the arrhythmia software on AEDs has become more extensive and validated for children, and attenuation devices have become available to downregulate the energy delivered by AEDs to allow their use on children. Pediatricians are now being asked whether AED programs should be implemented, and where they are being implemented, pediatricians are being asked to provide guidance on the use of them on children. As AED programs expand, pediatricians must advocate on behalf of children so that their needs are accounted for. For pediatricians to be able to provide guidance and ensure that children are included in AED programs, it is important for pediatricians to know how AEDs work, be up-to-date on the literature regarding pediatric fibrillation and energy delivery, and understand the role of AEDs as life-saving interventions for children. (11/07, reaffirmed 6/11)

WHEN IS LACK OF SUPERVISION NEGLECT? (CLINICAL REPORT)

Kent P. Hymel, MD, and Committee on Child Abuse and Neglect

ABSTRACT. Occasionally, pediatricians become aware of children who are inadequately supervised. More frequently, pediatricians treat children for traumatic injuries or ingestions that they suspect could have been prevented with better supervision. This clinical report contains guidance for pediatricians considering a referral to a child protective services agency on the basis of suspicion of supervisory neglect. (9/06)

WIC PROGRAM

Provisional Section on Breastfeeding

ABSTRACT. This policy statement highlights the important collaboration between pediatricians and local Special Supplemental Nutrition Program for Women, Infants, and Children (WIC) programs to ensure that infants and children receive high-quality, cost-effective health care and nutrition services. Specific recommendations are provided for pediatricians and WIC personnel to help children and their families receive optimum services through a medical home. (11/01)

YEAR 2007 POSITION STATEMENT: PRINCIPLES AND GUIDELINES FOR EARLY HEARING DETECTION AND INTERVENTION PROGRAMS

Joint Committee on Infant Hearing

ABSTRACT. The Joint Committee on Infant Hearing (JCIH) endorses early detection of and intervention for infants with hearing loss. The goal of early hearing detection and intervention (EHDI) is to maximize linguistic competence and literacy development for children who are deaf or hard of hearing. Without appropriate opportunities to learn language, these children will fall behind their hearing peers in communication, cognition, reading, and social-emotional development. Such delays may result in lower educational and employment levels in adulthood. To maximize the outcome for infants who are deaf or hard of hearing, the hearing of all infants should be screened at no later than 1 month of age. Those who do not pass screening should have a comprehensive audiological evaluation at no later than 3 months of age. Infants with confirmed hearing loss should receive appropriate intervention at no later than 6 months of age from health care and education professionals with expertise in hearing loss and deafness in infants and young children. Regardless of previous hearing-screening outcomes, all infants with or without risk factors should receive ongoing surveillance of communicative development beginning at 2 months of age during well-child visits in the medical home. EHDI systems should guarantee seamless transitions for infants and their families through this process. (10/07)

Section 6

Endorsed Policies

· · · · · · · · · · · · · · · · · · ·

The American Academy of Pediatrics endorses
and accepts as its policy the following
documents from other organizations.

AMERICAN ACADEMY OF PEDIATRICS

Endorsed Policies

APPROPRIATE MEDICAL CARE FOR THE SECONDARY SCHOOL-AGE ATHLETE COMMUNICATION
National Athletic Trainers' Association (2004)

BEST PRACTICE FOR INFANT SURGERY: A POSITION STATEMENT FROM THE AMERICAN PEDIATRIC SURGICAL ASSOCIATION
American Pediatric Surgical Association (9/08)

CARDIOVASCULAR RISK REDUCTION IN HIGH-RISK PEDIATRIC POPULATIONS
American Heart Association
ABSTRACT. Although for most children the process of atherosclerosis is subclinical, dramatically accelerated atherosclerosis occurs in some pediatric disease states, with clinical coronary events occurring in childhood and very early adult life. As with most scientific statements about children and the future risk for cardiovascular disease, there are no randomized trials documenting the effects of risk reduction on hard clinical outcomes. A growing body of literature, however, identifies the importance of premature cardiovascular disease in the course of certain pediatric diagnoses and addresses the response to risk factor reduction. For this scientific statement, a panel of experts reviewed what is known about very premature cardiovascular disease in 8 high-risk pediatric diagnoses and, from the science base, developed practical recommendations for management of cardiovascular risk. (*Circulation.* 2006;114:000-000.) (12/06)

A COMPREHENSIVE IMMUNIZATION STRATEGY TO ELIMINATE TRANSMISSION OF HEPATITIS B VIRUS INFECTION IN THE UNITED STATES
Advisory Committee on Immunization Practices and Centers for Disease Control and Prevention
SUMMARY. This report is the first of a two-part statement from the Advisory Committee on Immunization Practices (ACIP) that updates the strategy to eliminate hepatitis B virus (HBV) transmission in the United States. The report provides updated recommendations to improve prevention of perinatal and early childhood HBV transmission, including implementation of universal infant vaccination beginning at birth, and to increase vaccine coverage among previously unvaccinated children and adolescents. Strategies to enhance implementation of the recommendations include 1) establishing standing orders for administration of hepatitis B vaccination beginning at birth; 2) instituting delivery hospital policies and procedures and case management programs to improve identification of and administration of immunoprophylaxis to infants born to mothers who are hepatitis B surface antigen (HBsAg) positive and to mothers with unknown HBsAg status at the time of delivery; and 3) implementing vaccination record reviews for all children aged 11–12 years and children and adolescents aged <19 years who were born in countries with intermediate and high levels of HBV endemicity, adopting hepatitis B vaccine requirements for school entry, and integrating hepatitis B vaccination services into settings that serve adolescents. The second part of the ACIP statement, which will include updated recommendations and strategies to increase hepatitis B vaccination of adults, will be published separately. (7/06)

CONSENSUS STATEMENT: DEFINITIONS FOR CONSISTENT EMERGENCY DEPARTMENT METRICS
American Academy of Emergency Medicine, American Association of Critical Care Nurses, American College of Emergency Physicians, Association of periOperative Registered Nurses, Emergency Department Practice Management Association, Emergency Nurses Association, and National Association of EMS Physicians (2/10)

CONSENSUS STATEMENT ON MANAGEMENT OF INTERSEX DISORDERS
International Consensus Conference on Intersex (Lawson Wilkins Pediatric Endocrine Society and European Society for Paediatric Endocrinology)
INTRODUCTION. The birth of an intersex child prompts a long-term management strategy that involves myriad professionals working with the family. There has been progress in diagnosis, surgical techniques, understanding psychosocial issues, and recognizing and accepting the place of patient advocacy. The Lawson Wilkins Pediatric Endocrine Society and the European Society for Paediatric Endocrinology considered it timely to review the management of intersex disorders from a broad perspective, review data on longer-term outcome, and formulate proposals for future studies. The methodology comprised establishing a number of working groups, the membership of which was drawn from 50 international experts in the field. The groups prepared previous written responses to a defined set of questions resulting from evidence-based review of the literature. At a subsequent gathering of participants, a framework for a consensus document was agreed. This article constitutes its final form. (8/06)

DEFINING PEDIATRIC MALNUTRITION: A PARADIGM SHIFT TOWARD ETIOLOGY-RELATED DEFINITIONS
American Society for Parenteral and Enteral Nutrition
ABSTRACT. Lack of a uniform definition is responsible for underrecognition of the prevalence of malnutrition and its impact on outcomes in children. A pediatric malnutrition definitions workgroup reviewed existing pediatric age group English-language literature from 1955 to 2011, for relevant references related to 5 domains of the definition of *malnutrition* that were a *priori* identified: anthropometric parameters, growth, chronicity of malnutrition, etiology and pathogenesis, and developmental/functional outcomes. Based on available evidence and an iterative process to arrive at multidisciplinary consensus in the group, these domains were included in the overall construct of a new definition. Pediatric malnutrition

(undernutrition) is defined as an imbalance between nutrient requirements and intake that results in cumulative deficits of energy, protein, or micronutrients that may negatively affect growth, development, and other relevant outcomes. A summary of the literature is presented and a new classification scheme is proposed that incorporates chronicity, etiology, mechanisms of nutrient imbalance, severity of malnutrition, and its impact on outcomes. Based on its etiology, malnutrition is either *illness related* (secondary to 1 or more diseases/injury) or *non–illness related*, (caused by environmental/behavioral factors), or both. Future research must focus on the relationship between inflammation and illness-related malnutrition. We anticipate that the definition of malnutrition will continue to evolve with improved understanding of the processes that lead to and complicate the treatment of this condition. A uniform definition should permit future research to focus on the impact of pediatric malnutrition on functional outcomes and help solidify the scientific basis for evidence-based nutrition practices. (3/13)

DIABETES CARE FOR EMERGING ADULTS: RECOMMENDATIONS FOR TRANSITION FROM PEDIATRIC TO ADULT DIABETES CARE SYSTEMS
American Diabetes Association (11/11)

DIAGNOSIS, TREATMENT, AND LONG-TERM MANAGEMENT OF KAWASAKI DISEASE: A STATEMENT FOR HEALTH PROFESSIONALS
American Heart Association (12/04)

DIETARY RECOMMENDATIONS FOR CHILDREN AND ADOLESCENTS: A GUIDE FOR PRACTITIONERS
American Heart Association (9/05)

DIETARY REFERENCE INTAKES FOR CALCIUM AND VITAMIN D
Institute of Medicine (2011)

EMERGENCY EQUIPMENT AND SUPPLIES IN THE SCHOOL SETTING
National Association of School Nurses (1/12)

EVIDENCE REPORT: GENETIC AND METABOLIC TESTING ON CHILDREN WITH GLOBAL DEVELOPMENTAL DELAY
American Academy of Neurology and Child Neurology Society
ABSTRACT. *Objective.* To systematically review the evidence concerning the diagnostic yield of genetic and metabolic evaluation of children with global developmental delay or intellectual disability (GDD/ID).

Methods. Relevant literature was reviewed, abstracted, and classified according to the 4-tiered American Academy of Neurology classification of evidence scheme.

Results and Conclusions. In patients with GDD/ID, microarray testing is diagnostic on average in 7.8% (Class III), G-banded karyotyping is abnormal in at least 4% (Class II and III), and subtelomeric fluorescence in situ hybridization is positive in 3.5% (Class I, II, and III). Testing for X-linked ID genes has a yield of up to 42% in males with an appropriate family history (Class III). *FMR1* testing shows full expansion in at least 2% of patients with mild to moderate GDD/ID (Class II and III), and *MeCP2* testing is diagnostic in 1.5% of females with moderate to severe GDD/ID (Class III). Tests for metabolic disorders have a yield of up to 5%, and tests for congenital disorders of glycosylation and cerebral creatine disorders have yields of up to 2.8% (Class III). Several genetic and metabolic screening tests have been shown to have a better than 1% diagnostic yield in selected populations of children with GDD/ID. These values should be among the many factors considered in planning the laboratory evaluation of such children. (9/11)

EVIDENCE-BASED GUIDELINE UPDATE: MEDICAL TREATMENT OF INFANTILE SPASMS
American Academy of Neurology and Child Neurology Society
ABSTRACT. *Objective.* To update the 2004 American Academy of Neurology/Child Neurology Society practice parameter on treatment of infantile spasms in children.

Methods. MEDLINE and EMBASE were searched from 2002 to 2011 and searches of reference lists of retrieved articles were performed. Sixty-eight articles were selected for detailed review; 26 were included in the analysis. Recommendations were based on a 4-tiered classification scheme combining pre-2002 evidence and more recent evidence.

Results. There is insufficient evidence to determine whether other forms of corticosteroids are as effective as adrenocorticotropic hormone (ACTH) for short-term treatment of infantile spasms. However, low-dose ACTH is probably as effective as high-dose ACTH. ACTH is more effective than vigabatrin (VGB) for short-term treatment of children with infantile spasms (excluding those with tuberous sclerosis complex). There is insufficient evidence to show that other agents and combination therapy are effective for short-term treatment of infantile spasms. Short lag time to treatment leads to better long-term developmental outcome. Successful short-term treatment of cryptogenic infantile spasms with ACTH or prednisolone leads to better long-term developmental outcome than treatment with VGB.

Recommendations. Low-dose ACTH should be considered for treatment of infantile spasms. ACTH or VGB may be useful for short-term treatment of infantile spasms, with ACTH considered preferentially over VGB. Hormonal therapy (ACTH or prednisolone) may be considered for use in preference to VGB in infants with cryptogenic infantile spasms, to possibly improve developmental outcome. A shorter lag time to treatment of infantile spasms with either hormonal therapy or VGB possibly improves long-term developmental outcomes. (6/12)

EXECUTING JUVENILE OFFENDERS: A FUNDAMENTAL FAILURE OF SOCIETY
Society for Adolescent Medicine (10/04)

EXPEDITED PARTNER THERAPY FOR ADOLESCENTS DIAGNOSED WITH CHLAMYDIA OR GONORRHEA: A POSITION PAPER OF THE SOCIETY FOR ADOLESCENT MEDICINE

Society for Adolescent Medicine

ABSTRACT. Chlamydia and gonorrhea, the most frequently reported sexually transmitted infections (STIs), present substantial public health challenges among adolescents. Although these infections are easily treated with antibiotics, many adolescents are reinfected within 3–6 months, usually because their partners remain untreated. The standard approaches to notifying and treating a partner of an STI-infected patient are patient referral, whereby the patient notifies his/her partners to seek care, and provider referral, whereby the provider or public health disease intervention specialist notifies the partner and directs him/her toward treatment. These methods rely on the accuracy of the disclosed partner information as well as other limitations, such as compliance and staffing resources. Another approach to partner notification is expedited partner therapy (EPT), treating sex partners without requiring a prior clinical evaluation. In randomized trials, EPT has reduced the rates of persistent or recurrent gonorrhea and chlamydia infection; however, its routine use is limited by concerns related to liability, cost, compliance, and missed opportunities for prevention counseling. The Society for Adolescent Medicine (SAM) recommends that providers who care for adolescents should do the following: use EPT as an option for STI care among chlamydia- or gonorrhea-infected heterosexual males and females who are unlikely or unable to otherwise receive treatment; through SAM and AAP chapters, collaborate with policy makers to remove EPT legal barriers and facilitate reimbursement; and collaborate with health departments for implementation assistance. (9/09)

EXPERT PANEL ON INTEGRATED GUIDELINES FOR CARDIOVASCULAR HEALTH AND RISK REDUCTION IN CHILDREN AND ADOLESCENTS: SUMMARY REPORT

National Heart, Lung and Blood Institute

INTRODUCTION (EXCERPT). Atherosclerotic cardiovascular disease (CVD) remains the leading cause of death in North Americans, but manifest disease in childhood and adolescence is rare. By contrast, risk factors and risk behaviors that accelerate the development of atherosclerosis begin in childhood, and there is increasing evidence that risk reduction delays progression toward clinical disease. In response, the former director of the National Heart, Lung, and Blood Institute (NHLBI), Dr Elizabeth Nabel, initiated development of cardiovascular health guidelines for pediatric care providers based on a formal evidence review of the science with an integrated format addressing all the major cardiovascular risk factors simultaneously. An expert panel was appointed to develop the guidelines in the fall of 2006. (3/12)

FOSTER CARE MENTAL HEALTH VALUES

American Academy of Child and Adolescent Psychiatry and Child Welfare League of America (2002)

GENERAL RECOMMENDATIONS ON IMMUNIZATION: RECOMMENDATIONS OF THE ADVISORY COMMITTEE ON IMMUNIZATION PRACTICES (ACIP)

Advisory Committee on Immunization Practices

SUMMARY. This report is a revision of General Recommendations on Immunization and updates the 2002 statement by the Advisory Committee on Immunization Practices (ACIP) (CDC. General recommendations on immunization: recommendations of the Advisory Committee on Immunization Practices and the American Academy of Family Physicians. MMWR 2002;51[No. RR-2]). This report is intended to serve as a general reference on vaccines and immunization. The principal changes include 1) expansion of the discussion of vaccination spacing and timing; 2) an increased emphasis on the importance of injection technique/age/body mass in determining appropriate needle length; 3) expansion of the discussion of storage and handling of vaccines, with a table defining the appropriate storage temperature range for inactivated and live vaccines; 4) expansion of the discussion of altered immunocompetence, including new recommendations about use of live-attenuated vaccines with therapeutic monoclonal antibodies; and 5) minor changes to the recommendations about vaccination during pregnancy and vaccination of internationally adopted children, in accordance with new ACIP vaccine-specific recommendations for use of inactivated influenza vaccine and hepatitis B vaccine. The most recent ACIP recommendations for each specific vaccine should be consulted for comprehensive discussion. This report, ACIP recommendations for each vaccine, and other information about vaccination can be accessed at CDC's National Center for Immunization and Respiratory Diseases (proposed) (formerly known as the National Immunization Program) website at http//:www.cdc.gov/nip. (12/06)

GENETIC BASIS FOR CONGENITAL HEART DEFECTS: CURRENT KNOWLEDGE

American Heart Association

ABSTRACT. The intent of this review is to provide the clinician with a summary of what is currently known about the contribution of genetics to the origin of congenital heart disease. Techniques are discussed to evaluate children with heart disease for genetic alterations. Many of these techniques are now available on a clinical basis. Information on the genetic and clinical evaluation of children with cardiac disease is presented, and several tables have been constructed to aid the clinician in the assessment of children with different types of heart disease. Genetic algorithms for cardiac defects have been constructed and are available in an appendix. It is anticipated that this summary will update a wide range of medical personnel, including pediatric cardiologists and pediatricians, adult cardiologists, internists, obstetricians, nurses, and thoracic surgeons, about the genetic aspects of congenital heart disease and will encourage an interdisciplinary approach to the child and adult with congenital heart disease. (*Circulation.* 2007;115:3015-3038.) (6/07)

GIFTS TO PHYSICIANS FROM INDUSTRY

American Medical Association (8/01)

GUIDELINES FOR FIELD TRIAGE OF INJURED PATIENTS
Centers for Disease Control and Prevention (1/12)

GUIDELINES FOR THE PREVENTION AND TREATMENT OF OPPORTUNISTIC INFECTIONS IN HIV-EXPOSED AND HIV-INFECTED CHILDREN
National Institutes of Health, Centers for Disease Control and Prevention, HIV Medicine Association of Infectious Diseases Society of America, and Pediatric Infectious Diseases Society (11/13)

GUIDELINES FOR REFERRAL OF CHILDREN AND ADOLESCENTS TO PEDIATRIC RHEUMATOLOGISTS
American College of Rheumatology (6/02, reaffirmed 5/07)

HELPING THE STUDENT WITH DIABETES SUCCEED: A GUIDE FOR SCHOOL PERSONNEL
National Diabetes Education Program (6/03)

IDENTIFYING AND RESPONDING TO DOMESTIC VIOLENCE: CONSENSUS RECOMMENDATIONS FOR CHILD AND ADOLESCENT HEALTH
Family Violence Prevention Fund (9/02)

IMPORTANCE AND IMPLEMENTATION OF TRAINING IN CARDIOPULMONARY RESUSCITATION AND AUTOMATED EXTERNAL DEFIBRILLATION IN SCHOOLS
American Heart Association Emergency Cardiovascular Care Committee, Council on Cardiopulmonary, Critical Care, Perioperative and Resuscitation, Council on Cardiovascular Diseases in the Young, Council on Cardiovascular Nursing, Council on Clinical Cardiology, and Advocacy Coordinating Committee
ABSTRACT. In 2003, the International Liaison Committee on Resuscitation published a consensus document on education in resuscitation that strongly recommended that "...instruction in CPR [cardiopulmonary resuscitation] be incorporated as a standard part of the school curriculum."[1] The next year the American Heart Association (AHA) recommended that schools "...establish a goal to train every teacher in CPR and first aid and train all students in CPR" as part of their preparation for a response to medical emergencies on campus.[2]

Since that time, there has been an increased interest in legislation that would mandate that school curricula include training in CPR or CPR and automated external defibrillation. Laws or curriculum content standards in 36 states (as of the 2009–2010 school year) now encourage the inclusion of CPR training programs in school curricula. The language in those laws and standards varies greatly, ranging from a suggestion that students "recognize" the steps of CPR to a requirement for certification in CPR. Not surprisingly, then, implementation is not uniform among states, even those whose laws or standards encourage CPR training in schools in the strongest language. This statement recommends that training in CPR and familiarization with automated external defibrillators (AEDs) should be required elements of secondary school curricula and provides the rationale for implementation of CPR training, as well as guidance in overcoming barriers to implementation. (2/11)

INTER-ASSOCIATION CONSENSUS STATEMENT ON BEST PRACTICES FOR SPORTS MEDICINE MANAGEMENT FOR SECONDARY SCHOOLS AND COLLEGES
National Athletic Trainers Association, National Interscholastic Athletic Administrators Association, College Athletic Trainers' Society, National Federation of State High School Associations, American College Health Association, American Orthopaedic Society for Sports Medicine, National Collegiate Athletic Association, American Medical Society for Sports Medicine, National Association of Collegiate Directors of Athletics, and National Association of Intercollegiate Athletics (7/13)

LIGHTNING SAFETY FOR ATHLETICS AND RECREATION
National Athletic Trainers' Association
Abstract. *Objective.* To educate athletic trainers and others about the dangers of lightning, provide lightning-safety guidelines, define safe structures and locations, and advocate prehospital care for lightning-strike victims.
Background. Lightning may be the most frequently encountered severe-storm hazard endangering physically active people each year. Millions of lightning flashes strike the ground annually in the United States, causing nearly 100 deaths and 400 injuries. Three quarters of all lightning casualties occur between May and September, and nearly four fifths occur between 10:00 AM and 7:00 PM, which coincides with the hours for most athletic or recreational activities. Additionally, lightning casualties from sports and recreational activities have risen alarmingly in recent decades.
Recommendations. The National Athletic Trainers' Association recommends a proactive approach to lightning safety, including the implementation of a lightning-safety policy that identifies safe locations for shelter from the lightning hazard. Further components of this policy are monitoring local weather forecasts, designating a weather watcher, and establishing a chain of command. Additionally, a flash-to-bang count of 30 seconds or more should be used as a minimal determinant of when to suspend activities. Waiting 30 minutes or longer after the last flash of lightning or sound of thunder is recommended before athletic or recreational activities are resumed. Lightning safety strategies include avoiding shelter under trees, avoiding open fields and spaces, and suspending the use of land-line telephones during thunderstorms. Also outlined in this document are the prehospital care guidelines for triaging and treating lightning-strike victims. It is important to evaluate victims quickly for apnea, asystole, hypothermia, shock, fractures, and burns. Cardiopulmonary resuscitation is effective in resuscitating pulseless victims of lightning strike. Maintenance of cardiopulmonary resuscitation and first-aid certification should be required of all persons involved in sports and recreational activities. (12/00)

LONG-TERM CARDIOVASCULAR TOXICITY IN CHILDREN, ADOLESCENTS, AND YOUNG ADULTS WHO RECEIVE CANCER THERAPY: PATHOPHYSIOLOGY, COURSE, MONITORING, MANAGEMENT, PREVENTION, AND RESEARCH DIRECTIONS: A SCIENTIFIC STATEMENT FROM THE AMERICAN HEART ASSOCIATION

American Heart Association (9/13)

THE MANAGEMENT OF HYPOTENSION IN THE VERY-LOW-BIRTH-WEIGHT INFANT: GUIDELINE FOR PRACTICE

National Association of Neonatal Nurses

ABSTRACT. This guideline, released in 2011, focuses on the clinical management of systemic hypotension in the very-low-birth-weight (VLBW) infant during the first 3 days of postnatal life. (2011)

MEETING OF THE STRATEGIC ADVISORY GROUP OF EXPERTS ON IMMUNIZATION, APRIL 2012– CONCLUSIONS AND RECOMMENDATIONS

World Health Organization (5/12) (The AAP endorses the recommendation pertaining to the use of thimerosal in vaccines.)

MENTAL HEALTH AND SUBSTANCE USE SCREENING AND ASSESSMENT OF CHILDREN IN FOSTER CARE

American Academy of Child and Adolescent Psychiatry and Child Welfare League of America (2003)

NEURODEVELOPMENTAL OUTCOMES IN CHILDREN WITH CONGENITAL HEART DISEASE: EVALUATION AND MANAGEMENT: A SCIENTIFIC STATEMENT FROM THE AMERICAN HEART ASSOCIATION

American Heart Association (7/12)

NONINHERITED RISK FACTORS AND CONGENITAL CARDIOVASCULAR DEFECTS: CURRENT KNOWLEDGE

American Heart Association

ABSTRACT. Prevention of congenital cardiovascular defects has been hampered by a lack of information about modifiable risk factors for abnormalities in cardiac development. Over the past decade, there have been major breakthroughs in the understanding of inherited causes of congenital heart disease, including the identification of specific genetic abnormalities for some types of malformations. Although relatively less information has been available on noninherited modifiable factors that may have an adverse effect on the fetal heart, there is a growing body of epidemiological literature on this topic. This statement summarizes the currently available literature on potential fetal exposures that might alter risk for cardiovascular defects. Information is summarized for periconceptional multivitamin or folic acid intake, which may reduce the risk of cardiac disease in the fetus, and for additional types of potential exposures that may increase the risk, including maternal illnesses, maternal therapeutic and nontherapeutic drug exposures, environmental exposures, and paternal exposures. Information is highlighted regarding definitive risk factors such as maternal rubella; phenylketonuria; pregestational diabetes; exposure to thalidomide, vitamin A cogeners, or retinoids; and indomethacin tocolysis. Caveats regarding interpretation of possible exposure-outcome relationships from case-control studies are given because this type of study has provided most of the available information. Guidelines for prospective parents that could reduce the likelihood that their child will have a major cardiac malformation are given. Issues related to pregnancy monitoring are discussed. Knowledge gaps and future sources of new information on risk factors are described. (*Circulation.* 2007;115:2995-3014.) (6/07)

PEDIATRIC CARE IN THE EMERGENCY DEPARTMENT

Society for Academic Emergency Medicine

ABSTRACT. Physicians who have successfully completed an accredited Emergency Medicine residency and are certified in emergency medicine by the American Board of Emergency Medicine (ABEM) or the American Osteopathic Board of Emergency Medicine (AOBEM) ABEM/AOBEM or those who are certified in pediatric emergency medicine by ABEM or the American Board of Pediatrics (ABP) possess the knowledge and skills required to provide quality emergency medical care to children of all ages for a wide variety of illnesses, injuries or poisonings. To provide quality care, the emergency physician must have all necessary and age-appropriate medical equipment readily available. The emergency physician must also have access via consultation, admission, or transfer, to appropriate specialty and sub-specialty physicians, to who will provide any needed patient care after emergency department treatment. Physically separated care areas for children are not mandatory in order to provide high-quality care to patients of all ages. Although physically separate care areas for children are ideal, they are not mandatory to provide high-quality care. (11/03)

PREVENTION AND CONTROL OF MENINGOCOCCAL DISEASE: RECOMMENDATIONS OF THE ADVISORY COMMITTEE ON IMMUNIZATION PRACTICES (ACIP)

Centers for Disease Control and Prevention

SUMMARY. Meningococcal disease describes the spectrum of infections caused by Neisseria meningiditis, including meningitdis, bacteremia, and bacteremic pneumonia. Two quadrivalent meningococcal polysaccharide-protein conjugate vaccines that provide protection against meningococcal serogroups A, C, W, and Y (MenACWY-D [Menactra, manufactured by Sanofi Pasteur, Inc., Swiftwater, Pennsylvania] and MenACWY-CRM [Menveo, manufactured by Novartis Vaccines, Cambridge, Massachusetts]) are licensed in the United States for use among persons aged 2 through 55 years. MenACWY-D also is licensed for use among infants and toddlers aged 9 through 23 months. Quadrivalent meningococcal polysaccharide vaccine (MPSV4 [Menommune, manufactured by sanofi pasteur, Inc., Swiftwater, Pennsylvania]) is the only vaccine licensed for use among persons aged ≥56 years. A bivalent meningococcal polysaccharide protein conjugate vaccine that provides protection against meningococcal serogroups C and Y along with Haemophilus influenzae type b (Hib) (Hib-MenCY-TT [MenHibrix, manufactured by GlaxoSmithKline Biologicals, Rixensart, Belgium]) is licensed for use in children aged 6 weeks through 18 months.

This report compiles and summarizes all recommendations from CDC's Advisory Committee on Immunization

Practices (ACIP) regarding prevention and control of meningococcal disease in the United States, specifically the changes in the recommendations published since 2005 (CDC. Prevention and control of meningococcal disease: recommendations of the Advisory Committee on Immunization Practices [ACIP]. MMWR 2005;54 Adobe PDF file [No. RR-7]). As a comprehensive summary of previously published recommendations, this report does not contain any new recommendations; it is intended for use by clinicians as a resource. ACIP recommends routine vaccination with a quadrivalent meningococcal conjugate vaccine (MenACWY) for adolescents aged 11 or 12 years, with a booster dose at age 16 years. ACIP also recommends routine vaccination for persons at increased risk for meningococcal disease (i.e., persons who have persistent complement component deficiencies, persons who have anatomic or functional asplenia, microbiologists who routinely are exposed to isolates of N. meningitidis, military recruits, and persons who travel to or reside in areas in which meningococcal disease is hyperendemic or epidemic). Guidelines for antimicrobial chemoprophylaxis and for evaluation and management of suspected outbreaks of meningococcal disease also are provided. (3/13)

PREVENTION OF RHEUMATIC FEVER AND DIAGNOSIS AND TREATMENT OF ACUTE STREPTOCOCCAL PHARYNGITIS

American Heart Association Rheumatic Fever, Endocarditis, and Kawasaki Disease Committee of the Council on Cardiovascular Disease in the Young, Interdisciplinary Council on Functional Genomics and Translational Biology, and Interdisciplinary Council on Quality of Care and Outcomes Research

ABSTRACT. Primary prevention of acute rheumatic fever is accomplished by proper identification and adequate antibiotic treatment of group A â-hemolytic streptococcal (GAS) tonsillopharyngitis. Diagnosis of GAS pharyngitis is best accomplished by combining clinical judgment with diagnostic test results, the criterion standard of which is the throat culture. Penicillin (either oral penicillin V or injectable benzathine penicillin) is the treatment of choice, because it is cost-effective, has a narrow spectrum of activity, and has long-standing proven efficacy, and GAS resistant to penicillin have not been documented. For penicillin-allergic individuals, acceptable alternatives include a narrow-spectrum oral cephalosporin, oral clindamycin, or various oral macrolides or azalides. The individual who has had an attack of rheumatic fever is at very high risk of developing recurrences after subsequent GAS pharyngitis and needs continuous antimicrobial prophylaxis to prevent such recurrences (secondary prevention). The recommended duration of prophylaxis depends on the number of previous attacks, the time elapsed since the last attack, the risk of exposure to GAS infections, the age of the patient, and the presence or absence of cardiac involvement. Penicillin is again the agent of choice for secondary prophylaxis, but sulfadiazine or a macrolide or azalide are acceptable alternatives in penicillin-allergic individuals. This report updates the 1995 statement by the American Heart Association Rheumatic Fever, Endocarditis, and Kawasaki Disease Committee. It includes new recommendations for the diagnosis and treatment of GAS pharyngi-

tis, as well as for the secondary prevention of rheumatic fever, and classifies the strength of the recommendations and level of evidence supporting them. (2/09)

PROTECTING ADOLESCENTS: ENSURING ACCESS TO CARE AND REPORTING SEXUAL ACTIVITY AND ABUSE
Society for Adolescent Medicine (11/04)

RECOMMENDATION OF WHO STRATEGIC ADVISORY GROUP OF EXPERTS (SAGE) ON IMMUNIZATION
World Health Organization's Strategic Advisory Group of Experts (SAGE) on Immunization (5/12)

REPORT OF THE NATIONAL CONSENSUS CONFERENCE ON FAMILY PRESENCE DURING PEDIATRIC CARDIOPULMONARY RESUSCITATION AND PROCEDURES
Ambulatory Pediatric Association

INTRODUCTION. The National Consensus Conference on Family Presence during Pediatric Cardiopulmonary Resuscitation and Procedures was held in Washington, DC, on September 7–8, 2003. The concept, funding, planning and organization for the conference were the Ambulatory Pediatric Association (APA) Presidential Project of James Seidel, M.D., Ph.D. Dr. Seidel was in the final stages of preparation for chairing the conference when he died on July 25, 2003. In Dr. Seidel's absence, the conference was chaired by Deborah Parkman Henderson R.N., PhD, his co-investigator, and Jane F. Knapp, M.D, a colleague.

The National Consensus Conference on Family Presence during Pediatric Procedures and Cardiopulmonary Resuscitation was funded by a grant to the APA from the Maternal Child Health Bureau (MCHB) Partnership for Children. This meeting brought together a panel of over 20 appointed representatives from a multidisciplinary, diverse group of national organizations interested in the emergency care of children. The conference was part of a multiphase process designed with the goal of publishing consensus guidelines useful for defining policy regarding family presence (FP) during pediatric procedures and CPR in the Emergency Department (ED). It is also possible that the consensus panel recommendations could be applied to other settings.

Panel members completed a review of the literature prior to attending the conference. This review, along with results of a pre-conference questionnaire, formed the basis of the discussion during the conference. During the two day conference the participants completed the outline of the guidelines presented here. We believe these recommendations are a powerful testimony to Dr. Seidel's vision for promoting FP through multidisciplinary consensus building. Beyond that vision, however, we hope that the guidelines will make a difference in improving the quality of children's health care. (9/03)

RESPONSE TO CARDIAC ARREST AND SELECTED LIFE-THREATENING MEDICAL EMERGENCIES: THE MEDICAL EMERGENCY RESPONSE PLAN FOR SCHOOLS. A STATEMENT FOR HEALTHCARE PROVIDERS, POLICYMAKERS, SCHOOL ADMINISTRATORS, AND COMMUNITY LEADERS
American Heart Association (1/04)

SAFE AT SCHOOL CAMPAIGN STATEMENT OF PRINCIPLES
American Diabetes Association (endorsed 2/06)

SCREENING FOR IDIOPATHIC SCOLIOSIS IN ADOLESCENTS
Pediatric Orthopaedic Society of North America, American Academy of Orthopaedic Surgeons, and Scoliosis Research Society

EXECUTIVE SUMMARY. Many states mandate school screening to identify children at risk for scoliosis, though recent studies have cast some controversy on the effectiveness of routine scoliosis screening. Previous studies have both supported and discouraged routine screening.

Prevention of severe scoliosis is a major commitment of physicians caring for children with spinal deformities. For this reason, the American Academy of Orthopaedic Surgeons (AAOS), the Scoliosis Research Society (SRS), the Pediatric Orthopaedic Society of North America (POSNA), and the American Academy of Pediatrics (AAP) convened a task force to examine issues related to scoliosis screening and to put forth the present information statement. The societies acknowledge the important role of a systematic review of the literature as well as the role of consensus expert opinion in the common situation where the available evidence does not yet exist to speak definitely for, or against, an evaluation or intervention.

Costs involved with scoliosis screening are relatively low on a societal level and may justify the possibility of preventing surgery in adolescents with scoliosis. Adolescents without significant spinal deformity who are referred to a specialist for evaluation often do not require radiographs. For those who do need radiographic evaluation, it is important to know that the radiation exposure using current-day radiographic techniques, including digital radiography, is significantly smaller than in the past.

Opponents to scoliosis screening have focused on concerns about a low predictive value of screening and the cost-effectiveness of referral. There have also been concerns about the possibility of unnecessary treatment, including brace use, and the effect of exposure to radiation when radiographs are obtained.

With regard to early treatment in those adolescents detected with moderate scoliosis, the available data neither definitively support nor refute the efficacy of bracing. To most effectively answer this, a well-organized level I study is needed. Such a study, a five-year multicenter randomized controlled trial of bracing sponsored by the National Institutes of Health/National Institute of Arthritis and Musculoskeletal and Skin Diseases (NIH/NIAMS), is currently under way.

In 1996, the United States Preventive Services Task Force (USPSTF) concluded that there was insufficient evidence to make a recommendation for, or against, screening. However, in 2004, the USPSTF changed their position and recommended against the routine screening of asymptomatic adolescents for idiopathic scoliosis. The AAOS, SRS, POSNA, and AAP have concerns that this change in position by the USPSTF came in the absence of any significant change in the available literature, in the absence of any change in position statements by the AAOS, SRS, POSNA, and AAP, and in the absence of any significant input from specialists who commonly care for children with scoliosis.

As the primary care providers for adolescents with idiopathic scoliosis, the AAOS, SRS, POSNA, and AAP do not support any recommendation against scoliosis screening, given the available literature. (1/08)

SELECTED ISSUES FOR THE ADOLESCENT ATHLETE AND THE TEAM PHYSICIAN: A CONSENSUS STATEMENT
American Academy of Family Physicians, American Academy of Orthopaedic Surgeons, American College of Sports Medicine, American Medical Society for Sports Medicine, American Orthopaedic Society for Sports Medicine, and American Osteopathic Academy of Sports Medicine

GOAL. The goal of this document is to help the team physician improve the care of the adolescent athlete by understanding the medical, musculoskeletal and psychological factors common in this age group. To accomplish this goal, the team physician should have knowledge of and be involved with:
- Musculoskeletal injuries of the adolescent athlete, specifically those to the shoulder, knee, elbow and spine
- Medical conditions of the adolescent athlete, especially those pertaining to infectious diseases, concussion, and nutrition and supplementation
- Psychological issues related to sports specialization and overtraining. (11/08)

SKIING AND SNOWBOARDING INJURY PREVENTION
Canadian Paediatric Society

ABSTRACT. Skiing and snowboarding are popular recreational and competitive sport activities for children and youth. Injuries associated with both activities are frequent and can be serious. There is new evidence documenting the benefit of wearing helmets while skiing and snowboarding, as well as data refuting suggestions that helmet use may increase the risk of neck injury. There is also evidence to support using wrist guards while snowboarding. There is poor uptake of effective preventive measures such as protective equipment use and related policy. Physicians should have the information required to counsel children, youth and families regarding safer snow sport participation, including helmet use, wearing wrist guards for snowboarding, training and supervision, the importance of proper equipment fitting and binding adjustment, sun safety and avoiding substance use while on the slopes. (1/12)

SUPPLEMENT TO THE JCIH 2007 POSITION STATEMENT: PRINCIPLES AND GUIDELINES FOR EARLY INTERVENTION AFTER CONFIRMATION THAT A CHILD IS DEAF OR HARD OF HEARING
Joint Committee on Infant Hearing

PREFACE. This document is a supplement to the recommendations in the year 2007 position statement of the Joint Committee on Infant Hearing (JCIH) and provides comprehensive guidelines for early hearing detection and intervention (EHDI) programs on establishing strong early intervention (EI) systems with appropriate expertise to meet the needs of children who are deaf or hard of hearing (D/HH).

EI services represent the purpose and goal of the entire EHDI process. Screening and confirmation that a child is D/HH are largely meaningless without appropriate, individualized, targeted and high-quality intervention. For the infant or young child who is D/HH to reach his or her full potential, carefully designed individualized intervention must be implemented promptly, utilizing service providers with optimal knowledge and skill levels and providing services on the basis of research, best practices, and proven models.

The delivery of EI services is complex and requires individualization to meet the identified needs of the child and family. Because of the diverse needs of the population of children who are D/HH and their families, well-controlled intervention studies are challenging. At this time, few comparative effectiveness studies have been conducted. Randomized controlled trials are particularly difficult for ethical reasons, making it challenging to establish causal links between interventions and outcomes. EI systems must partner with colleagues in research to document what works for children and families and to strengthen the evidence base supporting practices.

Despite limitations and gaps in the evidence, the literature does contain research studies in which all children who were D/HH had access to the same well-defined EI service. These studies indicate that positive outcomes are possible, and they provide guidance about key program components that appear to promote these outcomes. This EI services document, drafted by teams of professionals with extensive expertise in EI programs for children who are D/HH and their families, relied on literature searches, existing systematic reviews, and recent professional consensus statements in developing this set of guidelines.

Terminology presented a challenge throughout document development. The committee noted that many of the frequently occurring terms necessary within the supplement may not reflect the most contemporary understanding and/or could convey inaccurate meaning. Rather than add to the lack of clarity or consensus and to avoid introducing new terminology to stakeholders, the committee opted to use currently recognized terms consistently herein and will monitor the emergence and/or development of new descriptors before the next JCIH consensus statement.

For purposes of this supplement:

- Language refers to all spoken and signed languages.
- Early intervention (EI), according to part C of the Individuals with Disabilities Education Improvement Act (IDEA) of 2004, is the process of providing services, education, and support to young children who are deemed to have an established condition, those who are evaluated and deemed to have a diagnosed physical or mental condition (with a high probability of resulting in a developmental delay), those who have an existing delay, or those who are at risk of developing a delay or special need that may affect their development or impede their education.
- Communication is used in lieu of terms such as communication options, methods, opportunities, approaches, etc.

- Deaf or hard of hearing (D/HH) is intended to be inclusive of all children with congenital and acquired hearing loss, unilateral and bilateral hearing loss, all degrees of hearing loss from minimal to profound, and all types of hearing loss (sensorineural, auditory neuropathy spectrum disorder, permanent conductive, and mixed).
- Core knowledge and skills is used to describe the expertise needed to provide appropriate EI that will optimize the development and well-being of infants/children and their families. Core knowledge and skills will differ according to the roles of individuals within the EI system (eg, service coordinator or EI provider).

This supplement to JCIH 2007 focuses on the practices of EI providers outside of the primary medical care and specialty medical care realms, rather than including the full spectrum of necessary medical, audiologic, and educational interventions. For more information about the recommendations for medical follow-up, primary care surveillance for related medical conditions, and specialty medical care and monitoring, the reader is encouraged to reference the year 2007 position statement of the JCIH as well as any subsequent revision. When an infant is confirmed to be D/HH, the importance of ongoing medical and audiologic management and surveillance both in the medical home and with the hearing health professionals, the otolaryngologist and the audiologist, cannot be overstated. A comprehensive discussion of those services is beyond the scope of this document. (3/13)

TARGETED TUBERCULIN TESTING AND TREATMENT OF LATENT TUBERCULOSIS INFECTION
American Thoracic Society and Centers for Disease Control and Prevention (4/00) (The AAP endorses and accepts as its policy the sections of this statement as they relate to infants and children.)

TIMING OF UMBILICAL CORD CLAMPING AFTER BIRTH
American College of Obstetricians and Gynecologists Committee on Obstetric Practice (12/12)

TYPE 2 DIABETES IN CHILDREN AND ADOLESCENTS
American Diabetes Association (3/00)

UPDATE ON JAPANESE ENCEPHALITIS VACCINE FOR CHILDREN—UNITED STATES, MAY 2011
Centers for Disease Control and Prevention
Inactivated mouse brain-derived Japanese encephalitis (JE) vaccine (JE-MB [manufactured as JE-Vax]), the only JE vaccine that is licensed for use in children in the United States, is no longer available. This notice provides updated information regarding options for obtaining JE vaccine for U.S. children. (8/11)

WEIGHING PEDIATRIC PATIENTS IN KILOGRAMS
Emergency Nurses Association (3/12)

APPENDIX 1

Policies by Committee

· ·

AMERICAN ACADEMY OF PEDIATRICS
Policies by Committee

BLACK BOX WORKING GROUP

Cardiovascular Monitoring and Stimulant Drugs for Attention-Deficit/Hyperactivity Disorder (joint with Section on Cardiology and Cardiac Surgery), 8/08

BOARD OF DIRECTORS

Ritual Genital Cutting of Female Minors, 6/10

BRIGHT FUTURES STEERING COMMITTEE

Identifying Infants and Young Children With Developmental Disorders in the Medical Home: An Algorithm for Developmental Surveillance and Screening (joint with Council on Children With Disabilities, Section on Developmental and Behavioral Pediatrics, and Medical Home Initiatives for Children With Special Needs Project Advisory Committee), 7/06, reaffirmed 12/09

Recommendations for Preventive Pediatric Health Care (joint with Committee on Practice and Ambulatory Medicine), 12/07, reaffirmed 1/11

CHILD AND ADOLESCENT HEALTH ACTION GROUP (FORMERLY COUNCIL ON CHILD AND ADOLESCENT HEALTH)

Age Limits of Pediatrics, 5/88, reaffirmed 9/92, 1/97, 3/02, 1/06, 10/11

The Role of Home-Visitation Programs in Improving Health Outcomes for Children and Families, 3/98, reaffirmed 5/01

COMMITTEE ON ADOLESCENCE

Achieving Quality Health Services for Adolescents, 6/08, reaffirmed 3/13

Adolescent Pregnancy: Current Trends and Issues (Clinical Report), 7/05

Adolescents and Human Immunodeficiency Virus Infection: The Role of the Pediatrician in Prevention and Intervention (joint with Committee on Pediatric AIDS), 1/01, reaffirmed 10/03, 1/05

The Adolescent's Right to Confidential Care When Considering Abortion, 5/96, reaffirmed 5/99, 11/02

Care of Adolescent Parents and Their Children (Clinical Report) (joint with Committee on Early Childhood), 11/12

Care of the Adolescent Sexual Assault Victim (Clinical Report), 8/08

Collaborative Role of the Pediatrician in the Diagnosis and Management of Bipolar Disorder in Adolescents (Clinical Report), 11/12

Condom Use by Adolescents, 10/13

Confidentiality in Adolescent Health Care, 4/89, reaffirmed 1/93, 11/97, 5/00, 5/04

Contraception and Adolescents, 11/07

Counseling the Adolescent About Pregnancy Options, 5/98, reaffirmed 1/01, 1/06

Emergency Contraception, 11/12

Excessive Sleepiness in Adolescents and Young Adults: Causes, Consequences, and Treatment Strategies (Technical Report) (joint with Working Group on Sleepiness in Adolescents/Young Adults), 6/05

Gynecologic Examination for Adolescents in the Pediatric Office Setting (Clinical Report), 8/10, reaffirmed 5/13

Health Care for Youth in the Juvenile Justice System, 11/11

Identification and Management of Eating Disorders in Children and Adolescents (Clinical Report), 11/10

Legalization of Marijuana: Potential Impact on Youth (joint with Committee on Substance Abuse), 6/04

Legalization of Marijuana: Potential Impact on Youth (Technical Report) (joint with Committee on Substance Abuse), 6/04

Male Adolescent Sexual and Reproductive Health Care (Clinical Report), 11/11

Menstruation in Girls and Adolescents: Using the Menstrual Cycle as a Vital Sign (Clinical Report) (joint with American College of Obstetricians and Gynecologists), 11/06

Office-Based Care for Lesbian, Gay, Bisexual, Transgender, and Questioning Youth, 6/13

Office-Based Care for Lesbian, Gay, Bisexual, Transgender, and Questioning Youth (Technical Report), 6/13

Secondhand and Prenatal Tobacco Smoke Exposure (Technical Report) (joint with Committee on Environmental Health and Committee on Native American Child Health), 10/09

Sexual Orientation and Adolescents (Clinical Report), 6/04

Sexuality Education for Children and Adolescents (joint with Committee on Psychosocial Aspects of Child and Family Health), 8/01, reaffirmed 10/04

Standards for Health Information Technology to Ensure Adolescent Privacy (joint with Council on Clinical Information Technology), 10/12

Suicide and Suicide Attempts in Adolescents (Clinical Report), 9/07

The Teen Driver (joint with Committee on Injury, Violence, and Poison Prevention), 12/06, reaffirmed 6/10

Tobacco Use: A Pediatric Disease (joint with Committee on Environmental Health, Committee on Substance Abuse, and Committee on Native American Child Health), 10/09

Underinsurance of Adolescents: Recommendations for Improved Coverage of Preventive, Reproductive, and Behavioral Health Care Services (joint with Committee on Child Health Financing), 12/08

COMMITTEE ON BIOETHICS

Children as Hematopoietic Stem Cell Donors, 1/10

Communicating With Children and Families: From Everyday Interactions to Skill in Conveying Distressing Information (Technical Report), 5/08, reaffirmed 5/11

Conflicts Between Religious or Spiritual Beliefs and Pediatric Care: Informed Refusal, Exemptions, and Public Funding, 10/13

Consent for Emergency Medical Services for Children and Adolescents (joint with Committee on Pediatric Emergency Medicine), 7/11

Do-Not-Resuscitate Orders for Pediatric Patients Who Require Anesthesia and Surgery (Clinical Report) (joint with Section on Surgery and Section on Anesthesia and Pain Medicine), 12/04, reaffirmed 1/09, 10/12

Ethical Controversies in Organ Donation After Circulatory Death, 4/13

Ethical Issues With Genetic Testing in Pediatrics, 6/01, reaffirmed 1/05, 1/09

Ethical and Policy Issues in Genetic Testing and Screening of Children (joint with Committee on Genetics and American College of Medical Genetics and Genomics), 2/13

Ethics and the Care of Critically Ill Infants and Children, 7/96, reaffirmed 10/99, 6/03

Forgoing Life-Sustaining Medical Treatment in Abused Children (joint with Committee on Child Abuse and Neglect), 11/00, reaffirmed 6/03, 10/06, 4/09

Forgoing Medically Provided Nutrition and Hydration in Children (Clinical Report), 7/09

Guidelines on Forgoing Life-Sustaining Medical Treatment, 3/94, reaffirmed 11/97, 10/00, 1/04, 1/09, 10/12

Honoring Do-Not-Attempt-Resuscitation Requests in Schools (joint with Council on School Health), 4/10, reaffirmed 7/13

Human Embryonic Stem Cell (hESC) and Human Embryo Research (joint with Committee on Pediatric Research), 10/12

Informed Consent, Parental Permission, and Assent in Pediatric Practice, 2/95, reaffirmed 11/98, 11/02, 10/06, 5/11

Institutional Ethics Committees, 1/01, reaffirmed 1/04, 1/09, 10/12

Maternal-Fetal Intervention and Fetal Care Centers (Clinical Report) (joint with American College of Obstetricians and Gynecologists), 7/11

Minors as Living Solid-Organ Donors (Clinical Report), 8/08, reaffirmed 5/11

Palliative Care for Children (joint with Committee on Hospital Care), 8/00, reaffirmed 6/03, 10/06, 2/12

Pediatrician-Family-Patient Relationships: Managing the Boundaries, 11/09

Physician Refusal to Provide Information or Treatment on the Basis of Claims of Conscience, 11/09

Preservation of Fertility in Pediatric and Adolescent Patients With Cancer (Technical Report) (joint with Section on Hematology/Oncology and Section on Surgery), 5/08, reaffirmed 2/12

Professionalism in Pediatrics: Statement of Principles, 10/07, reaffirmed 5/11

Professionalism in Pediatrics (Technical Report), 10/07, reaffirmed 5/11

Religious Objections to Medical Care, 2/97, reaffirmed 10/00, 6/03, 10/06, 5/09

Responding to Parental Refusals of Immunization of Children (Clinical Report), 5/05, reaffirmed 1/09

COMMITTEE ON CHILD ABUSE AND NEGLECT

Abusive Head Trauma in Infants and Children, 4/09, reaffirmed 3/13

Caregiver-Fabricated Illness in a Child: A Manifestation of Child Maltreatment (Clinical Report), 8/13

Child Abuse, Confidentiality, and the Health Insurance Portability and Accountability Act, 12/09

Child Fatality Review (joint with Committee on Injury, Violence, and Poison Prevention and Council on Community Pediatrics), 8/10

Distinguishing Sudden Infant Death Syndrome From Child Abuse Fatalities (Clinical Report) (joint with National Association of Medical Examiners), 7/06, reaffirmed 4/09, 3/13

Evaluating Infants and Young Children With Multiple Fractures (Clinical Report), 9/06

Evaluating for Suspected Child Abuse: Conditions That Predispose to Bleeding (Technical Report) (joint with Section on Hematology/Oncology), 3/13

Evaluation for Bleeding Disorders in Suspected Child Abuse (Clinical Report) (joint with Section on Hematology/Oncology), 3/13

The Evaluation of Children in the Primary Care Setting When Sexual Abuse Is Suspected (Clinical Report), 7/13

The Evaluation of Sexual Behaviors in Children (Clinical Report), 8/09, reaffirmed 3/13

Evaluation of Suspected Child Physical Abuse (Clinical Report), 6/07, reaffirmed 5/12

The Eye Examination in the Evaluation of Child Abuse (Clinical Report) (joint with Section on Ophthalmology), 7/10

Failure to Thrive as a Manifestation of Child Neglect (Clinical Report) (joint with Committee on Nutrition), 11/05, reaffirmed 1/09

Forgoing Life-Sustaining Medical Treatment in Abused Children (joint with Committee on Bioethics), 11/00, reaffirmed 6/03, 10/06, 4/09

Intimate Partner Violence: The Role of the Pediatrician (Clinical Report) (joint with Committee on Injury, Violence, and Poison Prevention), 4/10

Maltreatment of Children With Disabilities (Clinical Report) (joint with Council on Children With Disabilities), 5/07, reaffirmed 1/11

Oral and Dental Aspects of Child Abuse and Neglect (Clinical Report) (joint with American Academy of Pediatric Dentistry), 12/05, reaffirmed 1/09

The Pediatrician's Role in Child Maltreatment Prevention (Clinical Report), 9/10

Protecting Children From Sexual Abuse by Health Care Providers, 6/11

Psychological Maltreatment (Clinical Report) (joint with American Academy of Child and Adolescent Psychiatry), 7/12

Recognizing and Responding to Medical Neglect (Clinical Report), 12/07, reaffirmed 1/11

Understanding the Behavioral and Emotional Consequences of Child Abuse (Clinical Report) (joint with Section on Adoption and Foster Care, American Academy of Child and Adolescent Psychiatry, and National Center for Child Traumatic Stress), 9/08

When Is Lack of Supervision Neglect? (Clinical Report), 9/06

COMMITTEE ON CHILD HEALTH FINANCING

Essential Contractual Language for Medical Necessity in Children, 7/13

Financing of Pediatric Home Health Care (joint with Section on Home Care), 8/06

Guiding Principles for Managed Care Arrangements for the Health Care of Newborns, Infants, Children, Adolescents, and Young Adults, 10/13

High-Deductible Health Plans and the New Risks of Consumer-Driven Health Insurance Products, 3/07

Implementation Principles and Strategies for the State Children's Health Insurance Program, 5/01

Improving Substance Abuse Prevention, Assessment, and Treatment Financing for Children and Adolescents (joint with Committee on Substance Abuse), 10/01

Medicaid Policy Statement, 4/13

Model Contractual Language for Medical Necessity for Children, 7/05, reaffirmed 10/11

Payment for Telephone Care (joint with Section on Telephone Care), 10/06

Principles of Health Care Financing, 10/10, reaffirmed 4/13

Scope of Health Care Benefits for Children From Birth Through Age 26, 11/11

State Children's Health Insurance Program Achievements, Challenges, and Policy Recommendations, 6/07

Underinsurance of Adolescents: Recommendations for Improved Coverage of Preventive, Reproductive, and Behavioral Health Care Services (joint with Committee on Adolescence), 12/08

COMMITTEE ON CODING AND NOMENCLATURE

Application of the Resource-Based Relative Value Scale System to Pediatrics, 12/08

COMMITTEE ON DRUGS

Fever and Antipyretic Use in Children (Clinical Report) (joint with Section on Clinical Pharmacology and Therapeutics), 2/11

Generic Prescribing, Generic Substitution, and Therapeutic Substitution, 5/87, reaffirmed 6/93, 5/96, 6/99, 5/01, 5/05, 10/08, 10/12

Guidelines for the Ethical Conduct of Studies to Evaluate Drugs in Pediatric Populations (Clinical Report) (joint with Committee on Pediatric Research), 3/10

Neonatal Drug Withdrawal (Clinical Report) (joint with Committee on Fetus and Newborn), 1/12

Preparing for Pediatric Emergencies: Drugs to Consider (Clinical Report), 2/08, reaffirmed 10/11

Recognition and Management of Iatrogenically Induced Opioid Dependence and Withdrawal in Children (Clinical Report) (joint with Section on Anesthesiology and Pain Medicine), 12/13

The Transfer of Drugs and Therapeutics Into Human Breast Milk: An Update on Selected Topics (Clinical Report), 8/13

Use of Codeine- and Dextromethorphan-Containing Cough Remedies in Children, 6/97, reaffirmed 5/00, 6/03, 10/06

Uses of Drugs Not Described in the Package Insert (Off-Label Uses), 7/02, reaffirmed 10/05

COMMITTEE ON FETUS AND NEWBORN

Advanced Practice in Neonatal Nursing, 5/09

Age Terminology During the Perinatal Period, 11/04, reaffirmed 10/07, 11/08, 1/09

Antenatal Counseling Regarding Resuscitation at an Extremely Low Gestational Age (Clinical Report), 6/09

The Apgar Score (joint with American College of Obstetricians and Gynecologists), 4/06, reaffirmed 1/09

Assessment and Management of Inguinal Hernia in Infants (Clinical Report) (joint with Section on Surgery), 9/12

Controversies Concerning Vitamin K and the Newborn, 7/03, reaffirmed 5/06, 5/09

Epidemiology and Diagnosis of Health Care–Associated Infections in the NICU (Technical Report) (joint with Committee on Infectious Diseases), 3/12

Guidance on Management of Asymptomatic Neonates Born to Women With Active Genital Herpes Lesions (Clinical Report) (joint with Committee on Infectious Diseases), 1/13

Hospital Discharge of the High-Risk Neonate, 11/08, reaffirmed 5/11

Hospital Stay for Healthy Term Newborns, 1/10

Human Immunodeficiency Virus Screening (joint with Committee on Pediatric AIDS and American College of Obstetricians and Gynecologists), 7/99, reaffirmed 6/02, 5/05, 10/08, 5/12

"Late-Preterm" Infants: A Population at Risk (Clinical Report), 12/07, reaffirmed 5/10

Levels of Neonatal Care, 8/12

Management of Neonates With Suspected or Proven Early-Onset Bacterial Sepsis (Clinical Report), 4/12

Neonatal Drug Withdrawal (Clinical Report) (joint with Committee on Drugs), 1/12

Noninitiation or Withdrawal of Intensive Care for High-Risk Newborns, 2/07, reaffirmed 5/10

Phototherapy to Prevent Severe Neonatal Hyperbilirubinemia in the Neonate Infant 35 or More Weeks of Gestation (Technical Report), 9/11

Planned Home Birth, 4/13

Postdischarge Follow-up of Infants With Congenital Diaphragmatic Hernia (Clinical Report) (joint with Section on Surgery), 3/08, reaffirmed 5/11

Postnatal Corticosteroids to Prevent or Treat Bronchopulmonary Dysplasia, 9/10

Postnatal Glucose Homeostasis in Late-Preterm and Term Infants (Clinical Report), 3/11

Premedication for Nonemergency Endotracheal Intubation in the Neonate (Clinical Report) (joint with Section on Anesthesiology and Pain Medicine), 2/10, reaffirmed 8/13

Prenatal Substance Abuse: Short- and Long-term Effects on the Exposed Fetus (Technical Report) (joint with Committee on Substance Abuse), 2/13

Prevention and Management of Pain in the Neonate: An Update (joint with Section on Surgery and Canadian Paediatric Society), 11/06, reaffirmed 5/10

Recommendations for the Prevention of Perinatal Group B Streptococcal (GBS) Disease (joint with Committee on Infectious Diseases), 8/11

Respiratory Support in Preterm Infants at Birth, 12/13

Role of Pulse Oximetry in Examining Newborns for Congenital Heart Disease: A Scientific Statement from the AHA and AAP (joint with Section on Cardiology and Cardiac Surgery and American Heart Association Congenital Heart Defects Committee of the Council on Cardiovascular Disease in the Young, Council on Cardiovascular Nursing, and Interdisciplinary Council on Quality of Care and Outcomes Research), 8/09

Safe Transportation of Preterm and Low Birth Weight Infants at Hospital Discharge (Clinical Report) (joint with Committee on Injury, Violence, and Poison Prevention), 4/09, reaffirmed 8/13

Standard Terminology for Fetal, Infant, and Perinatal Deaths (Clinical Report), 6/11

Strategies for Prevention of Health Care–Associated Infections in the NICU (Clinical Report) (joint with Committee on Infectious Diseases), 3/12

Surfactant Replacement Therapy for Preterm and Term Neonates With Respiratory Distress (Clinical Report), 12/13

Use of Inhaled Nitric Oxide, 8/00, reaffirmed 4/03, 12/09

Use of Inhaled Nitric Oxide in Preterm Infants (Clinical Report), 12/13

COMMITTEE ON GENETICS

Clinical Genetic Evaluation of the Child With Mental Retardation or Developmental Delays (Clinical Report), 6/06, reaffirmed 5/12

Congenital Adrenal Hyperplasia (Technical Report) (joint with Section on Endocrinology), 12/00, reaffirmed 10/04

Ethical and Policy Issues in Genetic Testing and Screening of Children (joint with Committee on Bioethics and American College of Medical Genetics and Genomics), 2/13

Folic Acid for the Prevention of Neural Tube Defects, 8/99, reaffirmed 11/02, 1/07, 5/12

Health Care Supervision for Children With Williams Syndrome, 5/01, reaffirmed 5/05, 1/09

Health Supervision for Children With Achondroplasia (Clinical Report), 9/05, reaffirmed 5/12

Health Supervision for Children With Down Syndrome (Clinical Report), 7/11

Health Supervision for Children With Fragile X Syndrome (Clinical Report), 4/11

Health Supervision for Children With Marfan Syndrome (Clinical Report), 9/13

Health Supervision for Children With Neurofibromatosis (Clinical Report), 3/08

Health Supervision for Children With Prader-Willi Syndrome (Clinical Report), 12/10

Health Supervision for Children With Sickle Cell Disease (joint with Section on Hematology/Oncology), 3/02, reaffirmed 1/06, 1/11

Maternal Phenylketonuria, 8/08, reaffirmed 1/13

Molecular Genetic Testing in Pediatric Practice: A Subject Review (Clinical Report), 12/00, reaffirmed 5/07

Newborn Screening Fact Sheets, Introduction to the (Technical Report), 9/06, reaffirmed 1/11

Newborn Screening Fact Sheets (Technical Report), 9/06, reaffirmed 1/11

Update of Newborn Screening and Therapy for Congenital Hypothyroidism (Clinical Report) (joint with Section on Endocrinology, American Thyroid Association, and Lawson Wilkins Pediatric Endocrine Society), 6/06, reaffirmed 12/11

COMMITTEE ON HOSPITAL CARE

Admission and Discharge Guidelines for the Pediatric Patient Requiring Intermediate Care (Clinical Report) (joint with Section on Critical Care and Society of Critical Care Medicine), 5/04, reaffirmed 2/08, 1/13

Child Life Services (joint with Child Life Council), 10/06, reaffirmed 2/12

Facilities and Equipment for the Care of Pediatric Patients in a Community Hospital (Clinical Report), 5/03, reaffirmed 5/07, 8/13

Guidelines for Developing Admission and Discharge Policies for the Pediatric Intensive Care Unit (Clinical Report) (joint with Section on Critical Care and Society of Critical Care Medicine), 4/99, reaffirmed 5/05, 2/08, 1/13

Medical Staff Appointment and Delineation of Pediatric Privileges in Hospitals (Clinical Report) (joint with Section on Hospital Medicine), 3/12

Palliative Care for Children (joint with Committee on Bioethics), 8/00, reaffirmed 6/03, 10/06, 2/12

Patient- and Family-Centered Care and the Pediatrician's Role (joint with Institute for Patient- and Family-Centered Care), 1/12

Pediatric Observation Units (Clinical Report) (joint with Committee on Pediatric Emergency Medicine), 6/12

Pediatric Organ Donation and Transplantation (joint with Section on Surgery and Section on Critical Care), 3/10

Pediatric Palliative Care and Hospice Care Commitments, Guidelines, and Recommendations (joint with Section on Hospice and Palliative Medicine), 10/13

Physicians' Roles in Coordinating Care of Hospitalized Children (Clinical Report) (joint with Section on Hospital Medicine), 9/10

Precertification Process, 8/00, reaffirmed 5/05, 11/08

Principles of Pediatric Patient Safety: Reducing Harm Due to Medical Care (joint with Steering Committee on Quality Improvement and Management), 5/11

COMMITTEE ON INFECTIOUS DISEASES

Additional Recommendations for Use of Tetanus Toxoid, Reduced Content Diphtheria Toxoid, and Acellular Pertussis Vaccine (Tdap), 9/11

Antiviral Therapy and Prophylaxis for Influenza in Children (Clinical Report), 4/07, reaffirmed 7/10

Chemical-Biological Terrorism and Its Impact on Children (joint with Committee on Environmental Health), 9/06, reaffirmed 1/11

Clostridium difficile Infection in Infants and Children, 12/12

Cochlear Implants in Children: Surgical Site Infections and Prevention and Treatment of Acute Otitis Media and Meningitis (joint with Section on Otolaryngology–Head and Neck Surgery), 7/10

Consumption of Raw or Unpasteurized Milk and Milk Products by Pregnant Women and Children (joint with Committee on Nutrition), 12/13

Drinking Water From Private Wells and Risks to Children (joint with Committee on Environmental Health), 5/09, reaffirmed 1/13

Drinking Water From Private Wells and Risks to Children (Technical Report) (joint with Committee on Environmental Health), 5/09, reaffirmed 1/13

Epidemiology and Diagnosis of Health Care–Associated Infections in the NICU (Technical Report) (joint with Committee on Fetus and Newborn), 3/12

Exposure to Nontraditional Pets at Home and to Animals in Public Settings: Risks to Children (Clinical Report), 10/08, reaffirmed 12/11

Guidance on Management of Asymptomatic Neonates Born to Women With Active Genital Herpes Lesions (Clinical Report) (joint with Committee on Fetus and Newborn), 1/13

Head Lice (Clinical Report) (joint with Council on School Health), 7/10

HPV Vaccine Recommendations, 2/12

Immunizing Parents and Other Close Family Contacts in the Pediatric Office Setting (Technical Report) (joint with Committee on Practice and Ambulatory Medicine), 12/11

Infection Prevention and Control in Pediatric Ambulatory Settings, 9/07, reaffirmed 8/10

Meningococcal Conjugate Vaccines Policy Update: Booster Dose Recommendations, 11/11

Nontherapeutic Use of Antimicrobial Agents in Animal Agriculture: Implications for Pediatrics (Technical Report) (joint with Committee on Environmental Health), 9/04, reaffirmed 10/08, 4/13

Poliovirus, 9/11

Prevention of Rotavirus Disease: Updated Guidelines for Use of Rotavirus Vaccine, 3/09

Prevention of Varicella: Update of Recommendations for Use of Quadrivalent and Monovalent Varicella Vaccines in Children, 8/11

Principles of Judicious Antibiotic Prescribing for Upper Respiratory Tract Infections in Pediatrics (Clinical Report), 11/13

Rabies-Prevention Policy Update: New Reduced-Dose Schedule, 3/11

Recommendation for Mandatory Influenza Immunization of All Health Care Personnel, 9/10

Recommendations for Administering Hepatitis A Vaccine to Contacts of International Adoptees, 9/11

Recommendations for Prevention and Control of Influenza in Children, 2013–2014, 9/13

Recommendations for the Prevention of Perinatal Group B Streptococcal (GBS) Disease (joint with Committee on Fetus and Newborn), 8/11

Recommendations for the Prevention of *Streptococcus pneumoniae* Infections in Infants and Children: Use of 13-Valent Pneumococcal Conjugate Vaccine (PCV13) and Pneumococcal Polysaccharide Vaccine (PPSV23), 5/10

Recommended Childhood and Adolescent Immunization Schedule—United States, 2014, 1/14

Strategies for Prevention of Health Care–Associated Infections in the NICU (Clinical Report) (joint with Committee on Fetus and Newborn), 3/12

The Use of Systemic and Topical Fluoroquinolones (Clinical Report), 9/11

COMMITTEE ON MEDICAL LIABILITY AND RISK MANAGEMENT

Consent by Proxy for Nonurgent Pediatric Care (Clinical Report), 10/10

Dealing With the Parent Whose Judgment Is Impaired by Alcohol or Drugs: Legal and Ethical Considerations (Clinical Report), 9/04, reaffirmed 9/10

Expert Witness Participation in Civil and Criminal Proceedings, 6/09

The Pediatrician and Disaster Preparedness (joint with Committee on Pediatric Emergency Medicine and Task Force on Terrorism), 2/06, reaffirmed 6/09, 9/13

Professional Liability Insurance and Medicolegal Education for Pediatric Residents and Fellows, 8/11

COMMITTEE ON NATIVE AMERICAN CHILD HEALTH

Early Childhood Caries in Indigenous Communities (joint with Canadian Paediatric Society), 5/11

Ethical Considerations in Research With Socially Identifiable Populations (joint with Committee on Community Health Services), 1/04, reaffirmed 10/07, 1/13

Health Equity and Children's Rights (joint with Council on Community Pediatrics), 3/10, reaffirmed 10/13

Inhalant Abuse (Clinical Report) (joint with Committee on Substance Abuse), 5/07

Prevention and Treatment of Type 2 Diabetes Mellitus in Children, With Special Emphasis on American Indian and Alaska Native Children (Clinical Report) (joint with Section on Endocrinology), 10/03, reaffirmed 10/08

The Prevention of Unintentional Injury Among American Indian and Alaska Native Children: A Subject Review (Clinical Report) (joint with Committee on Injury and Poison Prevention), 12/99, reaffirmed 5/03, 1/06, 1/09

Secondhand and Prenatal Tobacco Smoke Exposure (Technical Report) (joint with Committee on Environmental Health and Committee on Adolescence), 10/09

Tobacco Use: A Pediatric Disease (joint with Committee on Environmental Health, Committee on Substance Abuse, and Committee on Adolescence), 10/09

COMMITTEE ON NUTRITION

Calcium and Vitamin D Requirements of Enterally Fed Preterm Infants (Clinical Report), 4/13

Consumption of Raw or Unpasteurized Milk and Milk Products by Pregnant Women and Children (joint with Committee on Infectious Diseases), 12/13

Diagnosis and Prevention of Iron Deficiency and Iron-Deficiency Anemia in Infants and Young Children (0–3 Years of Age) (Clinical Report), 10/10

Effects of Early Nutritional Interventions on the Development of Atopic Disease in Infants and Children: The Role of Maternal Dietary Restriction, Breastfeeding, Timing of Introduction of Complementary Foods, and Hydrolyzed Formulas (Clinical Report) (joint with Section on Allergy and Immunology), 1/08

Failure to Thrive as a Manifestation of Child Neglect (Clinical Report) (joint with Committee on Child Abuse and Neglect), 11/05, reaffirmed 1/09

Infant Methemoglobinemia: The Role of Dietary Nitrate in Food and Water (Clinical Report) (joint with Committee on Environmental Health), 9/05, reaffirmed 4/09

Lactose Intolerance in Infants, Children, and Adolescents (Clinical Report), 9/06, reaffirmed 8/12

Organic Foods: Health and Environmental Advantages and Disadvantages (Clinical Report) (joint with Council on Environmental Health), 10/12

Prevention of Pediatric Overweight and Obesity, 8/03, reaffirmed 10/06

Probiotics and Prebiotics in Pediatrics (Clinical Report) (joint with Section on Gastroenterology, Hepatology, and Nutrition), 11/10

Reimbursement for Foods for Special Dietary Use, 5/03, reaffirmed 1/06

Sports Drinks and Energy Drinks for Children and Adolescents: Are They Appropriate? (Clinical Report) (joint with Council on Sports Medicine and Fitness), 5/11

The Use and Misuse of Fruit Juice in Pediatrics, 5/01, reaffirmed 10/06, 8/13

Use of Soy Protein-Based Formulas in Infant Feeding (Clinical Report), 5/08

COMMITTEE ON PEDIATRIC AIDS

Adolescents and HIV Infection: The Pediatrician's Role in Promoting Routine Testing, 10/11

Adolescents and Human Immunodeficiency Virus Infection: The Role of the Pediatrician in Prevention and Intervention (joint with Committee on Adolescence), 1/01, reaffirmed 10/03, 1/05

Diagnosis of HIV-1 Infection in Children Younger Than 18 Months in the United States (Technical Report), 12/07, reaffirmed 4/10

Disclosure of Illness Status to Children and Adolescents With HIV Infection, 1/99, reaffirmed 2/02, 5/05, 1/09, 1/12

Education of Children With Human Immunodeficiency Virus Infection, 6/00, reaffirmed 3/03, 10/06, 4/10, 3/13

Evaluation and Management of the Infant Exposed to HIV-1 in the United States (Clinical Report), 12/08

HIV Testing and Prophylaxis to Prevent Mother-to-Child Transmission in the United States, 11/08, reaffirmed 6/11

Human Immunodeficiency Virus Screening (joint with Committee on Fetus and Newborn and American College of Obstetricians and Gynecologists), 7/99, reaffirmed 6/02, 5/05, 10/08, 5/12

Human Milk, Breastfeeding, and Transmission of Human Immunodeficiency Virus in the United States, 11/95, reaffirmed 11/99, 11/03, 2/08

Human Milk, Breastfeeding, and Transmission of Human Immunodeficiency Virus Type 1 in the United States (Technical Report), 11/03, reaffirmed 1/07

Identification and Care of HIV-Exposed and HIV-Infected Infants, Children, and Adolescents in Foster Care, 7/00, reaffirmed 3/03, 2/08, 6/11

Increasing Antiretroviral Drug Access for Children With HIV Infection (joint with Section on International Child Health), 4/07, reaffirmed 4/10

Infant Feeding and Transmission of Human Immunodeficiency Virus in the United States, 1/13

Postexposure Prophylaxis in Children and Adolescents for Nonoccupational Exposure to Human Immunodeficiency Virus (Clinical Report), 6/03, reaffirmed 1/07, 10/08

Reducing the Risk of HIV Infection Associated With Illicit Drug Use, 2/06, reaffirmed 5/09, 5/12

Surveillance of Pediatric HIV Infection, 2/98, reaffirmed 2/02, 1/06, 1/11

Transitioning HIV-Infected Youth Into Adult Health Care, 6/13

COMMITTEE ON PEDIATRIC EMERGENCY MEDICINE

Access to Optimal Emergency Care for Children, 1/07, reaffirmed 8/10

Consent for Emergency Medical Services for Children and Adolescents (joint with Committee on Bioethics), 7/11

Death of a Child in the Emergency Department (Technical Report), 5/05, reaffirmed 8/13

Death of a Child in the Emergency Department: Joint Statement of the American Academy of Pediatrics and the American College of Emergency Physicians (joint with American College of Emergency Physicians), 10/02, reaffirmed 1/06, 1/09, 8/13

Dispensing Medications at the Hospital Upon Discharge From an Emergency Department (Technical Report), 1/12

Emergency Information Forms and Emergency Preparedness for Children With Special Health Care Needs (joint with Council on Clinical Information Technology and American College of Emergency Physicians Pediatric Emergency Medicine Committee), 3/10

Guidelines for Care of Children in the Emergency Department (joint with American College of Emergency Physicians and Emergency Nurses Association), 9/09, reaffirmed 4/13

Management of Pediatric Trauma (joint with Section on Orthopaedics, Section on Critical Care, Section on Surgery, Section on Transport Medicine, and Pediatric Orthopaedic Society of North America), 4/08, reaffirmed 4/13

Overcrowding Crisis in Our Nation's Emergency Departments: Is Our Safety Net Unraveling?, 9/04, reaffirmed 5/07, 6/11

Patient- and Family-Centered Care of Children in the Emergency Department (Technical Report), 8/08

Patient- and Family-Centered Care and the Role of the Emergency Physician Providing Care to a Child in the Emergency Department (joint with American College of Emergency Physicians), 11/06, reaffirmed 6/09, 10/11

Patient Safety in the Pediatric Emergency Care Setting, 12/07, reaffirmed 6/11

Pediatric and Adolescent Mental Health Emergencies in the Emergency Medical Services System (Technical Report), 4/11

Pediatric Care Recommendations for Freestanding Urgent Care Facilities, 7/05, reaffirmed 1/09, 6/11

Pediatric Mental Health Emergencies in the Emergency Medical Services System (joint with American College of Emergency Physicians), 10/06, reaffirmed 6/09, 4/13

Pediatric Observation Units (Clinical Report) (joint with Committee on Hospital Care), 6/12

The Pediatrician and Disaster Preparedness (joint with Committee on Medical Liability and Task Force on Terrorism), 2/06, reaffirmed 6/09, 9/13

Preparation for Emergencies in the Offices of Pediatricians and Pediatric Primary Care Providers, 7/07, reaffirmed 6/11

Relief of Pain and Anxiety in Pediatric Patients in Emergency Medical Systems (Clinical Report) (joint with Section on Anesthesiology and Pain Medicine), 10/12

The Role of the Pediatrician in Rural Emergency Medical Services for Children, 10/12

Role of Pediatricians in Advocating Life Support Training Courses for Parents and the Public, 12/04, reaffirmed 5/07, 8/10, 8/13

Role of Pediatricians in Advocating Life Support Training Courses for Parents and the Public (Technical Report), 12/04, reaffirmed 5/07, 8/10

Ventricular Fibrillation and the Use of Automated External Defibrillators on Children (joint with Section on Cardiology and Cardiac Surgery), 11/07, reaffirmed 6/11

COMMITTEE ON PEDIATRIC RESEARCH

Guidelines for the Ethical Conduct of Studies to Evaluate Drugs in Pediatric Populations (Clinical Report) (joint with Committee on Drugs), 3/10

Human Embryonic Stem Cell (hESC) and Human Embryo Research (joint with Committee on Bioethics), 10/12

Promoting Education, Mentorship, and Support for Pediatric Research, 6/01, reaffirmed 1/05, 5/08, 10/11

Race/Ethnicity, Gender, Socioeconomic Status—Research Exploring Their Effects on Child Health: A Subject Review (Clinical Report), 6/00, reaffirmed 10/05, 1/09

Racial and Ethnic Disparities in the Health and Health Care of Children (Technical Report), 3/10, reaffirmed 5/13

COMMITTEE ON PEDIATRIC WORKFORCE

Enhancing Pediatric Workforce Diversity and Providing Culturally Effective Pediatric Care: Implications for Practice, Education, and Policy Making, 9/13

Financing Graduate Medical Education to Meet the Needs of Children and the Future Pediatrician Workforce, 4/08, reaffirmed 1/12

Nondiscrimination in Pediatric Health Care, 10/07, reaffirmed 6/11

Pediatric Primary Health Care, 11/93, reaffirmed 6/01, 1/05, 10/07, 9/10

The Pediatrician Workforce: Current Status and Future Prospects (Technical Report), 7/05

Pediatrician Workforce Policy Statement, 7/13

Prevention of Sexual Harassment in the Workplace and Educational Settings, 10/06, reaffirmed 5/09, 1/12

Scope of Practice Issues in the Delivery of Pediatric Health Care, 5/13

COMMITTEE ON PRACTICE AND AMBULATORY MEDICINE

Eye Examination in Infants, Children, and Young Adults by Pediatricians (joint with Section on Ophthalmology, American Association of Certified Orthoptists, American Association for Pediatric Ophthalmology and Strabismus, and American Academy of Ophthalmology), 4/03, reaffirmed 5/07

Hearing Assessment in Infants and Children: Recommendations Beyond Neonatal Screening (Clinical Report) (joint with Section on Otolaryngology–Head and Neck Surgery), 9/09

Immunization Information Systems, 9/06, reaffirmed 10/11

Immunizing Parents and Other Close Family Contacts in the Pediatric Office Setting (Technical Report) (joint with Committee on Infectious Diseases), 12/11

Increasing Immunization Coverage (joint with Council on Community Pediatrics), 5/10

Instrument-Based Pediatric Vision Screening Policy Statement (joint with Section on Ophthalmology, American Academy of Ophthalmology, American Association for Pediatric Ophthalmology and Strabismus, and American Association of Certified Orthoptists), 10/12

Prevention and Management of Positional Skull Deformities in Infants (Clinical Report) (joint with Section on Neurological Surgery), 11/11

Principles for the Development and Use of Quality Measures (joint with Steering Committee on Quality Improvement and Management), 2/08

Recommendations for Preventive Pediatric Health Care (joint with Bright Futures Steering Committee), 12/07, reaffirmed 1/11

Use of Chaperones During the Physical Examination of the Pediatric Patient, 4/11

COMMITTEE ON PSYCHOSOCIAL ASPECTS OF CHILD AND FAMILY HEALTH

The Child in Court: A Subject Review (Clinical Report), 11/99, reaffirmed 11/02

Coparent or Second-Parent Adoption by Same-Sex Parents, 2/02, reaffirmed 5/09

Coparent or Second-Parent Adoption by Same-Sex Parents (Technical Report), 2/02, reaffirmed 5/09

Early Childhood Adversity, Toxic Stress, and the Role of the Pediatrician: Translating Developmental Science Into Lifelong Health (joint with Committee on Early Childhood, Adoption, and Dependent Care and Section on Developmental and Behavioral Pediatrics), 12/11

Fathers and Pediatricians: Enhancing Men's Roles in the Care and Development of Their Children (Clinical Report), 5/04, reaffirmed 8/13

The Future of Pediatrics: Mental Health Competencies for Pediatric Primary Care (joint with Task Force on Mental Health), 6/09, reaffirmed 8/13

Guidance for Effective Discipline, 4/98, reaffirmed 3/01, 1/05, 5/12

Health and Mental Health Needs of Children in US Military Families (Clinical Report) (joint with Section on Uniformed Services), 5/13

Helping Children and Families Deal With Divorce and Separation (Clinical Report), 11/02, reaffirmed 1/06

The Importance of Play in Promoting Healthy Child Development and Maintaining Strong Parent-Child Bonds (Clinical Report) (joint with Committee on Communications), 1/07

The Importance of Play in Promoting Healthy Child Development and Maintaining Strong Parent-Child Bond: Focus on Children in Poverty (Clinical Report) (joint with Council on Communications and Media), 12/11

Incorporating Recognition and Management of Perinatal and Postpartum Depression Into Pediatric Practice (Clinical Report), 10/10

The Lifelong Effects of Early Childhood Adversity and Toxic Stress (Technical Report) (joint with Committee on Early Childhood, Adoption, and Dependent Care and Section on Developmental and Behavioral Pediatrics), 12/11

The New Morbidity Revisited: A Renewed Commitment to the Psychosocial Aspects of Pediatric Care, 11/01

The Pediatrician and Childhood Bereavement, 2/00, reaffirmed 1/04, 3/13

The Pediatrician's Role in the Prevention of Missing Children (Clinical Report), 10/04

The Prenatal Visit (Clinical Report), 9/09

Promoting the Well-Being of Children Whose Parents Are Gay or Lesbian, 3/13

Promoting the Well-Being of Children Whose Parents Are Gay or Lesbian (Technical Report), 3/13

Psychosocial Implications of Disaster or Terrorism on Children: A Guide for the Pediatrician (Clinical Report) (joint with Task Force on Terrorism), 9/05

Psychosocial Risks of Chronic Health Conditions in Childhood and Adolescence (joint with Committee on Children With Disabilities), 12/93, reaffirmed 10/96

Sexuality Education for Children and Adolescents (joint with Committee on Adolescence), 8/01, reaffirmed 10/04

Supporting the Family After the Death of a Child (Clinical Report), 11/12

COMMITTEE ON SUBSTANCE ABUSE

Alcohol Use by Youth and Adolescents: A Pediatric Concern, 4/10

Improving Substance Abuse Prevention, Assessment, and Treatment Financing for Children and Adolescents (joint with Committee on Child Health Financing), 10/01

Indications for Management and Referral of Patients Involved in Substance Abuse, 7/00

Inhalant Abuse (Clinical Report) (joint with Committee on Native American Child Health), 5/07

Legalization of Marijuana: Potential Impact on Youth (joint with Committee on Adolescence), 6/04

Legalization of Marijuana: Potential Impact on Youth (Technical Report) (joint with Committee on Adolescence), 6/04

Marijuana: A Continuing Concern for Pediatricians, 10/99, reaffirmed 4/03

Prenatal Substance Abuse: Short- and Long-term Effects on the Exposed Fetus (Technical Report) (joint with Committee on Fetus and Newborn), 2/13

The Role of Schools in Combating Illicit Substance Abuse (joint with Council on School Health), 12/07

Substance Use Screening, Brief Intervention, and Referral to Treatment for Pediatricians, 10/11

Testing for Drugs of Abuse in Children and Adolescents, 8/96, reaffirmed 5/99, 5/06

Testing for Drugs of Abuse in Children and Adolescents: Addendum—Testing in Schools and at Home (joint with Council on School Health), 3/07

Tobacco, Alcohol, and Other Drugs: The Role of the Pediatrician in Prevention, Identification, and Management of Substance Abuse (Clinical Report), 3/05, reaffirmed 3/13

Tobacco as a Substance of Abuse (Technical Report), 10/09

Tobacco Use: A Pediatric Disease (joint with Committee on Environmental Health, Committee on Adolescence, and Committee on Native American Child Health), 10/09

COUNCIL ON CHILDREN WITH DISABILITIES (FORMERLY COMMITTEE ON CHILDREN WITH DISABILITIES AND SECTION ON CHILDREN WITH DISABILITIES)

Auditory Integration Training and Facilitated Communication for Autism, 8/98, reaffirmed 5/02, 1/06, 12/09

Care Coordination in the Medical Home: Integrating Health and Related Systems of Care for Children With Special Health Care Needs, 11/05

Counseling Families Who Choose Complementary and Alternative Medicine for Their Child With Chronic Illness or Disability, 3/01, reaffirmed 1/05, 5/10

Early Intervention, IDEA Part C Services, and the Medical Home: Collaboration for Best Practice and Best Outcomes (Clinical Report), 9/13

Guidelines for Home Care of Infants, Children, and Adolescents With Chronic Disease, 7/95, reaffirmed 4/00, 1/06

Home Care of Children and Youth With Complex Health Care Needs and Technology Dependencies (Clinical Report), 4/12

Identification and Evaluation of Children With Autism Spectrum Disorders (Clinical Report), 11/07, reaffirmed 9/10

Identifying Infants and Young Children With Developmental Disorders in the Medical Home: An Algorithm for Developmental Surveillance and Screening (joint with Section on Developmental and Behavioral Pediatrics, Bright Futures Steering Committee, and Medical Home Initiatives for Children With Special Needs Project Advisory Committee), 7/06, reaffirmed 12/09

Learning Disabilities, Dyslexia, and Vision (joint with Section on Ophthalmology, American Academy of Ophthalmology, American Association for Pediatric Ophthalmology and Strabismus, and American Association of Certified Orthoptists), 7/09

Learning Disabilities, Dyslexia, and Vision (Technical Report) (joint with Section on Ophthalmology, American Academy of Ophthalmology, American Association for Pediatric Ophthalmology and Strabismus, and American Association of Certified Orthoptists), 3/11

Maltreatment of Children With Disabilities (Clinical Report) (joint with Committee on Child Abuse and Neglect), 5/07, reaffirmed 1/11

Management of Children With Autism Spectrum Disorders (Clinical Report), 11/07, reaffirmed 9/10

Oral Health Care for Children With Developmental Disabilities (Clinical Report) (joint with Section on Oral Health), 2/13

Parent-Provider-Community Partnerships: Optimizing Outcomes for Children With Disabilities (Clinical Report), 9/11

The Pediatrician's Role in Development and Implementation of an Individual Education Plan (IEP) and/or an Individual Family Service Plan (IFSP), 7/99, reaffirmed 11/02, 1/06

Prescribing Assistive-Technology Systems: Focus on Children With Impaired Communication (Clinical Report), 6/08, reaffirmed 1/12

Prescribing Therapy Services for Children With Motor Disabilities (Clinical Report), 6/04, reaffirmed 5/07, 5/11

Promoting the Participation of Children With Disabilities in Sports, Recreation, and Physical Activities (Clinical Report), 5/08, reaffirmed 1/12

Providing a Primary Care Medical Home for Children and Youth With Cerebral Palsy (Clinical Report), 10/11

Providing a Primary Care Medical Home for Children and Youth With Spina Bifida (Clinical Report), 11/11

Provision of Educationally Related Services for Children and Adolescents With Chronic Diseases and Disabling Conditions, 6/07

Psychosocial Risks of Chronic Health Conditions in Childhood and Adolescence (joint with Committee on Psychosocial Aspects of Child and Family Health), 12/93, reaffirmed 10/96

Role of the Medical Home in Family-Centered Early Intervention Services, 11/07

Sensory Integration Therapies for Children With Developmental and Behavioral Disorders (joint with Section on Complementary and Integrative Medicine), 5/12

Sexuality of Children and Adolescents With Developmental Disabilities (Clinical Report), 7/06, reaffirmed 12/09, 7/13

Supplemental Security Income (SSI) for Children and Youth With Disabilities, 11/09

The Treatment of Neurologically Impaired Children Using Patterning, 11/99, reaffirmed 11/02, 1/06, 8/10

COUNCIL ON CLINICAL INFORMATION TECHNOLOGY (FORMERLY STEERING COMMITTEE ON CLINICAL INFORMATION TECHNOLOGY, SECTION ON COMPUTERS AND OTHER TECHNOLOGIES, AND TASK FORCE ON MEDICAL INFORMATICS)

Electronic Prescribing in Pediatrics: Toward Safer and More Effective Medication Management, 3/13

Electronic Prescribing in Pediatrics: Toward Safer and More Effective Medication Management (Technical Report), 3/13

Electronic Prescribing Systems in Pediatrics: The Rationale and Functionality Requirements, 6/07

Electronic Prescribing Systems in Pediatrics: The Rationale and Functionality Requirements (Technical Report), 6/07

E-mail Communication Between Pediatricians and Their Patients (Clinical Report), 7/04, reaffirmed 2/08

Emergency Information Forms and Emergency Preparedness for Children With Special Health Care Needs (joint with Committee on Pediatric Emergency Medicine and American College of Emergency Physicians Pediatric Emergency Medicine Committee), 3/10

Health Information Technology and the Medical Home, 4/11

Pediatric Aspects of Inpatient Health Information Technology Systems (Technical Report), 12/08

Special Requirements of Electronic Health Record Systems in Pediatrics (Clinical Report), 3/07, reaffirmed 5/12

Standards for Health Information Technology to Ensure Adolescent Privacy (joint with Committee on Adolescence), 10/12

Using Personal Health Records to Improve the Quality of Health Care for Children, 6/09

COUNCIL ON COMMUNICATIONS AND MEDIA (FORMERLY COMMITTEE ON COMMUNICATIONS AND COMMITTEE ON PUBLIC EDUCATION)

Children, Adolescents, and Advertising, 12/06, reaffirmed 3/10

Children, Adolescents, and the Media, 10/13

Children, Adolescents, Obesity, and the Media, 7/11

Children, Adolescents, Substance Abuse, and the Media, 9/10

Children, Adolescents, and Television, 2/01

Impact of Music, Music Lyrics, and Music Videos on Children and Youth, 10/09

The Impact of Social Media on Children, Adolescents, and Families (Clinical Report), 3/11

The Importance of Play in Promoting Healthy Child Development and Maintaining Strong Parent-Child Bonds (Clinical Report) (joint with Committee on Psychosocial Aspects of Child and Family Health), 1/07

The Importance of Play in Promoting Healthy Child Development and Maintaining Strong Parent-Child Bond: Focus on Children in Poverty (Clinical Report) (joint with Committee on Psychosocial Aspects of Child and Family Health), 12/11

Media Education, 9/10

Media Use by Children Younger Than 2 Years, 10/11

Media Violence, 10/09

Sexuality, Contraception, and the Media, 8/10

COUNCIL ON COMMUNITY PEDIATRICS (FORMERLY COMMITTEE ON COMMUNITY HEALTH SERVICES)

Child Fatality Review (joint with Committee on Child Abuse and Neglect and Committee on Injury, Violence, and Poison Prevention), 8/10

Community Pediatrics: Navigating the Intersection of Medicine, Public Health, and Social Determinants of Children's Health, 2/13

Ethical Considerations in Research With Socially Identifiable Populations (joint with Committee on Native American Child Health), 1/04, reaffirmed 10/07, 1/13

Health Equity and Children's Rights (joint with Committee on Native American Child Health), 3/10, reaffirmed 10/13

Increasing Immunization Coverage (joint with Committee on Practice and Ambulatory Medicine), 5/10

The Pediatrician's Role in Community Pediatrics, 4/05, reaffirmed 1/10

Prevention of Agricultural Injuries Among Children and Adolescents (joint with Committee on Injury and Poison Prevention), 10/01, reaffirmed 1/07, 11/11

Providing Care for Children and Adolescents Facing Homelessness and Housing Insecurity, 5/13

Providing Care for Immigrant, Migrant, and Border Children, 5/13

The Role of Preschool Home-Visiting Programs in Improving Children's Developmental and Health Outcomes, 1/09

COUNCIL ON EARLY CHILDHOOD (FORMERLY COMMITTEE ON EARLY CHILDHOOD, ADOPTION, AND DEPENDENT CARE AND COMMITTEE ON EARLY CHILDHOOD)

Care of Adolescent Parents and Their Children (Clinical Report) (joint with Committee on Adolescence), 11/12

Comprehensive Health Evaluation of the Newly Adopted Child (Clinical Report), 12/11

Early Childhood Adversity, Toxic Stress, and the Role of the Pediatrician: Translating Developmental Science Into Lifelong Health (joint with Committee on Psychosocial Aspects of Child and Family Health and Section on Developmental and Behavioral Pediatrics), 12/11

Families and Adoption: The Pediatrician's Role in Supporting Communication (Clinical Report), 12/03

Health Care of Youth Aging Out of Foster Care (joint with Council on Foster Care, Adoption, and Kinship Care), 11/12

The Inappropriate Use of School "Readiness" Tests (joint with Committee on School Health), 3/95, reaffirmed 4/98, 1/04, 4/10

The Lifelong Effects of Early Childhood Adversity and Toxic Stress (Technical Report) (joint with Committee on Psychosocial Aspects of Child and Family Health and Section on Developmental and Behavioral Pediatrics), 12/11

Parental Leave for Residents and Pediatric Training Programs (joint with Section on Medical Students, Residents, and Fellowship Trainees), 1/13

The Pediatrician's Role in Family Support and Family Support Programs, 11/11

The Pediatrician's Role in Supporting Adoptive Families (Clinical Report) (joint with Council on Foster Care, Adoption, and Kinship Care), 9/12

Quality Early Education and Child Care From Birth to Kindergarten, 1/05, reaffirmed 12/09

School Readiness (Technical Report) (joint with Council on School Health), 4/08, reaffirmed 9/13

Selecting Appropriate Toys for Young Children: The Pediatrician's Role (Clinical Report), 4/03, reaffirmed 10/06, 5/11

COUNCIL ON ENVIRONMENTAL HEALTH (FORMERLY COMMITTEE ON ENVIRONMENTAL HEALTH)

Ambient Air Pollution: Health Hazards to Children, 12/04, reaffirmed 4/09

The Built Environment: Designing Communities to Promote Physical Activity in Children, 5/09, reaffirmed 1/13

Chemical-Biological Terrorism and Its Impact on Children (joint with Committee on Infectious Diseases), 9/06, reaffirmed 1/11

Chemical-Management Policy: Prioritizing Children's Health, 4/11

Drinking Water From Private Wells and Risks to Children (joint with Committee on Infectious Diseases), 5/09, reaffirmed 1/13

Drinking Water From Private Wells and Risks to Children (Technical Report) (joint with Committee on Infectious Diseases), 5/09, reaffirmed 1/13

Global Climate Change and Children's Health, 11/07, reaffirmed 5/12

Global Climate Change and Children's Health (Technical Report), 11/07, reaffirmed 5/12

Infant Methemoglobinemia: The Role of Dietary Nitrate in Food and Water (Clinical Report) (joint with Committee on Nutrition), 9/05, reaffirmed 4/09

Nontherapeutic Use of Antimicrobial Agents in Animal Agriculture: Implications for Pediatrics (Technical Report) (joint with Committee on Infectious Diseases), 9/04, reaffirmed 10/08, 4/13

Organic Foods: Health and Environmental Advantages and Disadvantages (Clinical Report) (joint with Committee on Nutrition), 10/12

Pesticide Exposure in Children, 11/12

Pesticide Exposure in Children (Technical Report), 11/12

Radiation Disasters and Children, 6/03, reaffirmed 1/07

Secondhand and Prenatal Tobacco Smoke Exposure (Technical Report) (joint with Committee on Native American Child Health and Committee on Adolescence), 10/09

Spectrum of Noninfectious Health Effects From Molds, 12/06, reaffirmed 1/11

Spectrum of Noninfectious Health Effects From Molds (Technical Report), 12/06, reaffirmed 1/11

Tobacco Use: A Pediatric Disease (joint with Committee on Substance Abuse, Committee on Adolescence, and Committee on Native American Child Health), 10/09

Ultraviolet Radiation: A Hazard to Children and Adolescents (joint with Section on Dermatology), 2/11

Ultraviolet Radiation: A Hazard to Children and Adolescents (Technical Report) (joint with Section on Dermatology), 3/11

COUNCIL ON FOSTER CARE, ADOPTION, AND KIN-SHIP CARE (FORMALLY SECTION ON ADOPTION AND FOSTER CARE, TASK FORCE ON FOSTER CARE, AND COMMITTEE ON EARLY CHILDHOOD, ADOPTION, AND DEPENDENT CARE)

Families and Adoption: The Pediatrician's Role in Supporting Communication (Clinical Report), 12/03

Health Care of Youth Aging Out of Foster Care (joint with Committee on Early Childhood), 11/12

The Inappropriate Use of School "Readiness" Tests (joint with Committee on School Health), 3/95, reaffirmed 4/98, 1/04, 4/10

The Pediatrician's Role in Family Support and Family Support Programs, 11/11

The Pediatrician's Role in Supporting Adoptive Families (Clinical Report) (joint with Committee on Early Childhood), 9/12

Quality Early Education and Child Care From Birth to Kindergarten, 1/05, reaffirmed 12/09

School Readiness (Technical Report) (joint with Council on School Health), 4/08, reaffirmed 9/13

Selecting Appropriate Toys for Young Children: The Pediatrician's Role (Clinical Report), 4/03, reaffirmed 10/06, 5/11

Understanding the Behavioral and Emotional Consequences of Child Abuse (Clinical Report) (joint with Committee on Child Abuse and Neglect, American Academy of Child and Adolescent Psychiatry, and National Center for Child Traumatic Stress), 9/08

COUNCIL ON INJURY, VIOLENCE, AND POISON PREVENTION (FORMALLY COMMITTEE ON INJURY, VIOLENCE, AND POISON PREVENTION)

All-Terrain Vehicle Injury Prevention: Two-, Three-, and Four-Wheeled Unlicensed Motor Vehicles, 6/00, reaffirmed 5/04, 1/07

Bicycle Helmets, 10/01, reaffirmed 1/05, 2/08, 11/11

Child Fatality Review (joint with Committee on Child Abuse and Neglect and Council on Community Pediatrics), 8/10

Child Passenger Safety, 3/11

Child Passenger Safety (Technical Report), 3/11

Children in Pickup Trucks, 10/00, reaffirmed 5/04, 1/07

Falls From Heights: Windows, Roofs, and Balconies, 5/01, reaffirmed 10/04, 5/07, 6/10

Firearm-Related Injuries Affecting the Pediatric Population, 10/12

Fireworks-Related Injuries to Children, 7/01, reaffirmed 1/05, 2/08, 10/11

The Hospital Record of the Injured Child and the Need for External Cause-of-Injury Codes, 2/99, reaffirmed 5/02, 5/05, 10/08

Injuries Associated With Infant Walkers, 9/01, reaffirmed 1/05, 2/08, 10/11

Injury Risk of Nonpowder Guns (Technical Report), 11/04, reaffirmed 2/08, 10/11

In-line Skating Injuries in Children and Adolescents (joint with Committee on Sports Medicine and Fitness), 4/98, reaffirmed 1/02, 1/06, 1/09, 11/11

Intimate Partner Violence: The Role of the Pediatrician (Clinical Report) (joint with Committee on Child Abuse and Neglect), 4/10

Lawn Mower–Related Injuries to Children, 6/01, reaffirmed 10/04, 5/07, 6/10

Lawn Mower–Related Injuries to Children (Technical Report), 6/01, reaffirmed 10/04, 5/07, 6/10

Office-Based Counseling for Unintentional Injury Prevention (Clinical Report), 1/07

Pedestrian Safety, 7/09, reaffirmed 8/13

Personal Watercraft Use by Children and Adolescents, 2/00, reaffirmed 5/04, 1/07, 6/10

Prevention of Agricultural Injuries Among Children and Adolescents (joint with Committee on Community Health Services), 10/01, reaffirmed 1/07, 11/11

Prevention of Choking Among Children, 2/10

Prevention of Drowning, 5/10

Prevention of Drowning (Technical Report), 5/10

The Prevention of Unintentional Injury Among American Indian and Alaska Native Children: A Subject Review (Clinical Report) (joint with Committee on Native American Child Health), 12/99, reaffirmed 12/02, 1/06, 1/09

Reducing the Number of Deaths and Injuries From Residential Fires, 6/00

Restraint Use on Aircraft, 11/01, reaffirmed 5/05, 10/08

Role of the Pediatrician in Youth Violence Prevention, 6/09

Safe Transportation of Newborns at Hospital Discharge, 10/99, reaffirmed 1/03, 1/06, 10/08

Safe Transportation of Preterm and Low Birth Weight Infants at Hospital Discharge (Clinical Report) (joint with Committee on Fetus and Newborn), 4/09, reaffirmed 8/13

School Bus Transportation of Children With Special Health Care Needs, 8/01, reaffirmed 1/05, 2/08

School Transportation Safety (joint with Council on School Health), 7/07, reaffirmed 10/11

Shopping Cart–Related Injuries to Children, 8/06, reaffirmed 4/09, 8/13

Shopping Cart–Related Injuries to Children (Technical Report), 8/06, reaffirmed 4/09, 8/13

Skateboard and Scooter Injuries, 3/02, reaffirmed 5/05, 10/08

Snowmobiling Hazards, 11/00, reaffirmed 5/04, 1/07, 6/10

Swimming Programs for Infants and Toddlers (joint with Committee on Sports Medicine and Fitness), 4/00, reaffirmed 5/04

The Teen Driver (joint with Committee on Adolescence), 12/06, reaffirmed 6/10

Transporting Children With Special Health Care Needs, 10/99, reaffirmed 1/03, 1/06, 3/13

COUNCIL ON SCHOOL HEALTH (FORMERLY COMMITTEE ON SCHOOL HEALTH AND SECTION ON SCHOOL HEALTH)

Active Healthy Living: Prevention of Childhood Obesity Through Increased Physical Activity (joint with Council on Sports Medicine and Fitness), 5/06, reaffirmed 5/09, 8/12

Climatic Heat Stress and Exercising Children and Adolescents (joint with Council on Sports Medicine and Fitness), 8/11

Corporal Punishment in Schools, 8/00, reaffirmed 6/03, 5/06, 2/12

Creating Healthy Camp Experiences, 3/11

The Crucial Role of Recess in School, 12/12

Disaster Planning for Schools, 10/08, reaffirmed 9/11

Guidance for the Administration of Medication in School, 9/09, reaffirmed 2/13

Head Lice (Clinical Report) (joint with Committee on Infectious Diseases), 7/10

Home, Hospital, and Other Non–School-based Instruction for Children and Adolescents Who Are Medically Unable to Attend School, 11/00, reaffirmed 6/03, 5/06

Honoring Do-Not-Attempt-Resuscitation Requests in Schools (joint with Committee on Bioethics), 4/10, reaffirmed 7/13

The Inappropriate Use of School "Readiness" Tests (joint with Committee on Early Childhood, Adoption, and Dependent Care), 3/95, reaffirmed 4/98, 1/04, 4/10

Medical Emergencies Occurring at School, 10/08, reaffirmed 9/11

Organized Sports for Children and Preadolescents (joint with Committee on Sports Medicine and Fitness), 6/01, reaffirmed 1/05, 6/11

Out-of-School Suspension and Expulsion, 2/13

Preventing and Treating Homesickness (Clinical Report), 1/07, reaffirmed 5/12

Returning to Learning Following a Concussion (Clinical Report) (joint with Council on Sports Medicine and Fitness), 10/13

Role of the School Nurse in Providing School Health Services, 5/08

Role of the School Physician, 12/12

The Role of Schools in Combating Illicit Substance Abuse (joint with Committee on Substance Abuse), 12/07

School-Based Health Centers and Pediatric Practice, 1/12

School Health Assessments, 4/00, reaffirmed 6/03, 5/06, 10/11

School Health Centers and Other Integrated School Health Services, 1/01

School Readiness (Technical Report) (joint with Committee on Early Childhood, Adoption, and Dependent Care), 4/08, reaffirmed 9/13

School Transportation Safety (joint with Committee on Injury, Violence, and Poison Prevention), 7/07, reaffirmed 10/11

School-Based Mental Health Services, 6/04, reaffirmed 5/09

Soft Drinks in Schools, 1/04, reaffirmed 1/09

Testing for Drugs of Abuse in Children and Adolescents: Addendum—Testing in Schools and at Home (joint with Committee on Substance Abuse), 3/07

COUNCIL ON SPORTS MEDICINE AND FITNESS (FORMERLY COMMITTEE ON SPORTS MEDICINE AND FITNESS AND SECTION ON SPORTS MEDICINE AND FITNESS)

Active Healthy Living: Prevention of Childhood Obesity Through Increased Physical Activity (joint with Council on School Health), 5/06, reaffirmed 5/09, 8/12

Athletic Participation by Children and Adolescents Who Have Systemic Hypertension, 5/10, reaffirmed 5/13

Baseball and Softball, 2/12

Boxing Participation by Children and Adolescents (joint with Canadian Paediatric Society), 8/11

Cheerleading Injuries: Epidemiology and Recommendations for Prevention, 10/12

Climatic Heat Stress and Exercising Children and Adolescents (joint with Council on School Health), 8/11

Human Immunodeficiency Virus and Other Blood-borne Viral Pathogens in the Athletic Setting, 12/99, reaffirmed 1/05, 1/09, 11/11

Injuries in Youth Soccer (Clinical Report), 1/10, reaffirmed 5/13

In-line Skating Injuries in Children and Adolescents (joint with Committee on Injury and Poison Prevention), 4/98, reaffirmed 1/02, 1/06, 1/09, 11/11

Intensive Training and Sports Specialization in Young Athletes, 7/00, reaffirmed 11/04, 1/06, 5/09

Knee Brace Use in the Young Athlete (Technical Report), 8/01, reaffirmed 1/07, 4/10, 5/13

Medical Concerns in the Female Athlete, 9/00, reaffirmed 5/05, 5/08

Medical Conditions Affecting Sports Participation (Clinical Report), 4/08, reaffirmed 5/11

Organized Sports for Children and Preadolescents (joint with Committee on School Health), 6/01, reaffirmed 1/05, 6/11

Overuse Injuries, Overtraining, and Burnout in Child and Adolescent Athletes (Clinical Report), 6/07, reaffirmed 3/11

Promotion of Healthy Weight-Control Practices in Young Athletes, 12/05

Protective Eyewear for Young Athletes (joint with American Academy of Ophthalmology), 3/04, reaffirmed 2/08, 6/11

Returning to Learning Following a Concussion (Clinical Report) (joint with Council on School Health), 10/13

Safety in Youth Ice Hockey: The Effects of Body Checking, 3/00, reaffirmed 1/06, 5/09

Sport-Related Concussion in Children and Adolescents (Clinical Report), 8/10

Sports Drinks and Energy Drinks for Children and Adolescents: Are They Appropriate? (Clinical Report) (joint with Committee on Nutrition), 5/11

Strength Training by Children and Adolescents, 4/08, reaffirmed 6/11

Swimming Programs for Infants and Toddlers (joint with Committee on Injury and Poison Prevention), 4/00, reaffirmed 5/04

Trampoline Safety in Childhood and Adolescence, 9/12

Use of Performance-Enhancing Substances, 4/05, reaffirmed 5/08

JOINT COMMITTEE ON INFANT HEARING

Supplement to the JCIH 2007 Position Statement: Principles and Guidelines for Early Intervention After Confirmation That a Child Is Deaf or Hard of Hearing, 3/13

Year 2007 Position Statement: Principles and Guidelines for Early Hearing Detection and Intervention Programs, 10/07

MEDICAL HOME INITIATIVES FOR CHILDREN WITH SPECIAL NEEDS PROJECT ADVISORY COMMITTEE

Identifying Infants and Young Children With Developmental Disorders in the Medical Home: An Algorithm for Developmental Surveillance and Screening (joint with Council on Children With Disabilities, Section on Developmental and Behavioral Pediatrics, and Bright Futures Steering Committee), 7/06, reaffirmed 12/09

The Medical Home, 7/02, reaffirmed 5/08

NEUROMOTOR SCREENING EXPERT PANEL

Motor Delays: Early Identification and Evaluation (Clinical Report), 5/13

NEWBORN SCREENING AUTHORING COMMITTEE

Newborn Screening Expands: Recommendations for Pediatricians and Medical Homes—Implications for the System (Clinical Report), 1/08

RETAIL-BASED CLINIC POLICY WORK GROUP

AAP Principles Concerning Retail-Based Clinics, 12/06, reaffirmed 1/11

SECTION ON ALLERGY AND IMMUNOLOGY

Allergy Testing in Childhood: Using Allergen-Specific IgE Tests (Clinical Report), 12/11

Effects of Early Nutritional Interventions on the Development of Atopic Disease in Infants and Children: The Role of Maternal Dietary Restriction, Breastfeeding, Timing of Introduction of Complementary Foods, and Hydrolyzed Formulas (Clinical Report) (joint with Committee on Nutrition), 1/08

Management of Food Allergy in the School Setting (Clinical Report), 11/10

Self-injectable Epinephrine for First-Aid Management of Anaphylaxis (Clinical Report), 3/07

SECTION ON ANESTHESIOLOGY AND PAIN MEDICINE

Premedication for Nonemergency Endotracheal Intubation in the Neonate (Clinical Report) (joint with Committee on Fetus and Newborn), 2/10, reaffirmed 8/13

Recognition and Management of Iatrogenically Induced Opioid Dependence and Withdrawal in Children (Clinical Report) (joint with Committee on Drugs), 12/13

Relief of Pain and Anxiety in Pediatric Patients in Emergency Medical Systems (Clinical Report) (joint with Committee on Pediatric Emergency Medicine), 10/12

SECTION ON BREASTFEEDING

Breastfeeding and the Use of Human Milk, 2/12

WIC Program, 11/01

SECTION ON CARDIOLOGY AND CARDIAC SURGERY

ACCF/AHA/AAP Recommendations for Training in Pediatric Cardiology (joint with American College of Cardiology Foundation and American Heart Association), 12/05, reaffirmed 1/09

Cardiovascular Health Supervision for Individuals Affected by Duchenne or Becker Muscular Dystrophy (Clinical Report), 12/05, reaffirmed 1/09

Cardiovascular Monitoring and Stimulant Drugs for Attention-Deficit/Hyperactivity Disorder (joint with Black Box Working Group), 8/08

Echocardiography in Infants and Children, 6/97, reaffirmed 3/03, 3/07

Endorsement of Health and Human Services Recommendation for Pulse Oximetry Screening for Critical Congenital Heart Disease, 12/11

Guidelines for Pediatric Cardiovascular Centers, 3/02, reaffirmed 10/07

Pediatric Sudden Cardiac Arrest, 3/12

Role of Pulse Oximetry in Examining Newborns for Congenital Heart Disease: A Scientific Statement from the AHA and AAP (joint with Committee on Fetus and Newborn and American Heart Association Congenital Heart Defects Committee of the Council on Cardiovascular Disease in the Young, Council on Cardiovascular Nursing, and Interdisciplinary Council on Quality of Care and Outcomes Research), 8/09

Ventricular Fibrillation and the Use of Automated External Defibrillators on Children (joint with Committee on Pediatric Emergency Medicine), 11/07, reaffirmed 6/11

SECTION ON CLINICAL PHARMACOLOGY AND THERAPEUTICS

Fever and Antipyretic Use in Children (Clinical Report) (joint with Committee on Drugs), 2/11

SECTION ON COMPLEMENTARY AND INTEGRATIVE MEDICINE (FORMERLY PROVISIONAL SECTION ON COMPLEMENTARY, HOLISTIC, AND INTEGRATIVE MEDICINE)

Sensory Integration Therapies for Children With Developmental and Behavioral Disorders (joint with Council on Children With Disabilities), 5/12

The Use of Complementary and Alternative Medicine in Pediatrics (Clinical Report) (joint with Task Force on Complementary and Alternative Medicine), 12/08, reaffirmed 10/12, 1/13

SECTION ON CRITICAL CARE

Admission and Discharge Guidelines for the Pediatric Patient Requiring Intermediate Care (Clinical Report) (joint with Committee on Hospital Care and Society of Critical Care Medicine), 5/04, reaffirmed 2/08, 1/13

Guidelines for the Determination of Brain Death in Infants and Children: An Update of the 1987 Task Force Recommendations (Clinical Report) (joint with Section on Neurology, Society of Critical Care Medicine, and Child Neurology Society), 8/11

Guidelines for Developing Admission and Discharge Policies for the Pediatric Intensive Care Unit (joint with Committee on Hospital Care and Society of Critical Care Medicine), 4/99, reaffirmed 5/05, 2/08, 1/13

Management of Pediatric Trauma (joint with Section on Orthopaedics, Committee on Pediatric Emergency Medicine, Section on Surgery, Section on Transport Medicine, and Pediatric Orthopaedic Society of North America), 4/08, reaffirmed 4/13

Pediatric Organ Donation and Transplantation (joint with Committee on Hospital Care and Section on Surgery), 3/10

SECTION ON DERMATOLOGY

Ultraviolet Radiation: A Hazard to Children and Adolescents (joint with Council on Environmental Health), 2/11

Ultraviolet Radiation: A Hazard to Children and Adolescents (Technical Report) (joint with Council on Environmental Health), 3/11

SECTION ON DEVELOPMENTAL AND BEHAVIORAL PEDIATRICS

Early Childhood Adversity, Toxic Stress, and the Role of the Pediatrician: Translating Developmental Science Into Lifelong Health (joint with Committee on Psychosocial Aspects of Child and Family Health and Committee on Early Childhood, Adoption, and Dependent Care), 12/11

Identifying Infants and Young Children With Developmental Disorders in the Medical Home: An Algorithm for Developmental Surveillance and Screening (joint with Council on Children With Disabilities, Bright Futures Steering Committee, and Medical Home Initiatives for Children With Special Needs Project Advisory Committee), 7/06, reaffirmed 12/09

The Lifelong Effects of Early Childhood Adversity and Toxic Stress (Technical Report) (joint with Committee on Psychosocial Aspects of Child and Family Health and Committee on Early Childhood, Adoption, and Dependent Care), 12/11

SECTION ON ENDOCRINOLOGY

Bone Densitometry in Children and Adolescents (Clinical Report), 12/10

Congenital Adrenal Hyperplasia (Technical Report) (joint with Committee on Genetics), 12/00, reaffirmed 10/04

Prevention and Treatment of Type 2 Diabetes Mellitus in Children, With Special Emphasis on American Indian and Alaska Native Children (Clinical Report) (joint with Committee on Native American Child Health), 10/03, reaffirmed 10/08

Screening for Retinopathy in the Pediatric Patient With Type 1 Diabetes Mellitus (Clinical Report) (joint with Section on Ophthalmology and American Association for Pediatric Ophthalmology and Strabismus), 7/05, reaffirmed 1/09

Update of Newborn Screening and Therapy for Congenital Hypothyroidism (Clinical Report) (joint with Committee on Genetics, American Thyroid Association, and Lawson Wilkins Pediatric Endocrine Society), 6/06, reaffirmed 12/11

SECTION ON GASTROENTEROLOGY, HEPATOLOGY, AND NUTRITION

Gastroesophageal Reflux: Management Guidance for the Pediatrician (Clinical Report), 4/13

Probiotics and Prebiotics in Pediatrics (Clinical Report) (joint with Committee on Nutrition), 11/10

SECTION ON HEMATOLOGY/ONCOLOGY

Evaluating for Suspected Child Abuse: Conditions That Predispose to Bleeding (Technical Report) (joint with Committee on Child Abuse and Neglect), 3/13

Evaluation for Bleeding Disorders in Suspected Child Abuse (Clinical Report) (joint with Committee on Child Abuse and Neglect), 3/13

Guidelines for Pediatric Cancer Centers, 6/04, reaffirmed 10/08

Health Supervision for Children With Sickle Cell Disease (joint with Committee on Genetics), 3/02, reaffirmed 1/06, 1/11

Long-term Follow-up Care for Pediatric Cancer Survivors (Clinical Report) (joint with Children's Oncology Group), 3/09, reaffirmed 4/13

Preservation of Fertility in Pediatric and Adolescent Patients With Cancer (Technical Report) (joint with Committee on Bioethics and Section on Surgery), 5/08, reaffirmed 2/12

SECTION ON HOME CARE

Financing of Pediatric Home Health Care (joint with Committee on Child Health Financing), 8/06

SECTION ON HOSPICE AND PALLIATIVE MEDICINE

Pediatric Palliative Care and Hospice Care Commitments, Guidelines, and Recommendations (joint with Committee on Hospital Care), 10/13

SECTION ON HOSPITAL MEDICINE

Guiding Principles for Pediatric Hospital Medicine Programs, 9/13

Medical Staff Appointment and Delineation of Pediatric Privileges in Hospitals (Clinical Report) (joint with Committee on Hospital Care), 3/12

Physicians' Roles in Coordinating Care of Hospitalized Children (Clinical Report) (joint with Committee on Hospital Care), 9/10

SECTION ON INTERNATIONAL CHILD HEALTH

Increasing Antiretroviral Drug Access for Children With HIV Infection (joint with Committee on Pediatric AIDS), 4/07, reaffirmed 4/10

SECTION ON MEDICAL STUDENTS, RESIDENTS, AND FELLOWSHIP TRAINEES

Parental Leave for Residents and Pediatric Training Programs (joint with Committee on Early Childhood), 1/13

SECTION ON NEUROLOGICAL SURGERY

Prevention and Management of Positional Skull Deformities in Infants (Clinical Report) (joint with Committee on Practice and Ambulatory Medicine), 11/11

SECTION ON NEUROLOGY

Guidelines for the Determination of Brain Death in Infants and Children: An Update of the 1987 Task Force Recommendations (Clinical Report) (joint with Section on Critical Care, Society of Critical Care Medicine, and Child Neurology Society), 8/11

SECTION ON OPHTHALMOLOGY

The Eye Examination in the Evaluation of Child Abuse (Clinical Report) (joint with Committee on Child Abuse and Neglect), 7/10

Eye Examination in Infants, Children, and Young Adults by Pediatricians (joint with Committee on Practice and Ambulatory Medicine, American Association of Certified Orthoptists, American Association for Pediatric Ophthalmology and Strabismus, and American Academy of Ophthalmology), 4/03, reaffirmed 5/07

Instrument-Based Pediatric Vision Screening Policy Statement (joint with Committee on Practice and Ambulatory Medicine, American Academy of Ophthalmology, American Association for Pediatric Ophthalmology and Strabismus, and American Association of Certified Orthoptists), 10/12

Learning Disabilities, Dyslexia, and Vision (joint with Council on Children With Disabilities, American Academy of Ophthalmology, American Association for Pediatric Ophthalmology and Strabismus, and American Association of Certified Orthoptists), 7/09

Learning Disabilities, Dyslexia, and Vision (Technical Report) (joint with Council on Children With Disabilities, American Academy of Ophthalmology, American Association for Pediatric Ophthalmology and Strabismus, and American Association of Certified Orthoptists), 3/11

Ophthalmologic Examinations in Children With Juvenile Rheumatoid Arthritis (Clinical Report) (joint with Section on Rheumatology), 5/06

Red Reflex Examination in Neonates, Infants, and Children (joint with American Association for Pediatric Ophthalmology and Strabismus, American Academy of Ophthalmology, and American Association of Certified Orthoptists), 12/08

Screening Examination of Premature Infants for Retinopathy of Prematurity (joint with American Academy of Ophthalmology, American Association for Pediatric Ophthalmology and Strabismus, and American Association of Certified Orthoptists), 12/12

Screening for Retinopathy in the Pediatric Patient With Type 1 Diabetes Mellitus (Clinical Report) (joint with Section on Endocrinology and American Association for Pediatric Ophthalmology and Strabismus), 7/05, reaffirmed 1/09

SECTION ON ORAL HEALTH (FORMERLY SECTION ON PEDIATRIC DENTISTRY AND SECTION ON PEDIATRIC DENTISTRY AND ORAL HEALTH)

Oral Health Care for Children With Developmental Disabilities (Clinical Report) (joint with Council on Children With Disabilities), 2/13

Oral Health Risk Assessment Timing and Establishment of the Dental Home, 5/03, reaffirmed 5/09

Preventive Oral Health Intervention for Pediatricians, 12/08

SECTION ON ORTHOPAEDICS

Management of Pediatric Trauma (joint with Committee on Pediatric Emergency Medicine, Section on Critical Care, Section on Surgery, Section on Transport Medicine, and Pediatric Orthopaedic Society of North America), 4/08, reaffirmed 4/13

SECTION ON OTOLARYNGOLOGY—HEAD & NECK SURGERY

Cochlear Implants in Children: Surgical Site Infections and Prevention and Treatment of Acute Otitis Media and Meningitis (joint with Committee on Infectious Diseases), 7/10

Follow-up Management of Children With Tympanostomy Tubes, 2/02

Hearing Assessment in Infants and Children: Recommendations Beyond Neonatal Screening (Clinical Report) (joint with Committee on Practice and Ambulatory Medicine), 9/09

SECTION ON RADIOLOGY

Diagnostic Imaging of Child Abuse, 4/09

Radiation Risk to Children From Computed Tomography (Clinical Report), 9/07

SECTION ON RHEUMATOLOGY

Ophthalmologic Examinations in Children With Juvenile Rheumatoid Arthritis (Clinical Report) (joint with Section on Ophthalmology), 5/06

SECTION ON SURGERY

Assessment and Management of Inguinal Hernia in Infants (Clinical Report) (joint with Committee on Fetus and Newborn), 9/12

Do-Not-Resuscitate Orders for Pediatric Patients Who Require Anesthesia and Surgery (Clinical Report) (joint with Section on Anesthesia and Pain Medicine and Committee on Bioethics), 12/04, reaffirmed 1/09, 10/12

Management of Pediatric Trauma (joint with Section on Orthopaedics, Committee on Pediatric Emergency Medicine, Section on Critical Care, Section on Transport Medicine, and Pediatric Orthopaedic Society of North America), 4/08, reaffirmed 4/13

Pediatric Organ Donation and Transplantation (joint with Committee on Hospital Care and Section on Critical Care), 3/10

Postdischarge Follow-up of Infants With Congenital Diaphragmatic Hernia (Clinical Report) (joint with Committee on Fetus and Newborn), 3/08, reaffirmed 5/11

Preservation of Fertility in Pediatric and Adolescent Patients With Cancer (Technical Report) (joint with Committee on Bioethics and Section on Hematology/Oncology), 5/08, reaffirmed 2/12

Prevention and Management of Pain in the Neonate: An Update (joint with Committee on Fetus and Newborn and Canadian Paediatric Society), 11/06, reaffirmed 5/10

SECTION ON TELEHEALTH CARE (FORMERLY SECTION ON TELEPHONE CARE)

Payment for Telephone Care (joint with Committee on Child Health Financing), 10/06

SECTION ON TRANSPORT MEDICINE

Management of Pediatric Trauma (joint with Section on Orthopaedics, Committee on Pediatric Emergency Medicine, Section on Critical Care, Section on Surgery, and Pediatric Orthopaedic Society of North America), 4/08, reaffirmed 4/13

SECTION ON UNIFORMED SERVICES

Health and Mental Health Needs of Children in US Military Families (Clinical Report) (join with Committee on Psychosocial Aspects of Child and Family Health), 5/13

STEERING COMMITTEE ON QUALITY IMPROVEMENT AND MANAGEMENT

ADHD: Clinical Practice Guideline for the Diagnosis, Evaluation, and Treatment of Attention-Deficit/ Hyperactivity Disorder in Children and Adolescents (Clinical Practice Guideline) (joint with Subcommittee on Attention-Deficit/Hyperactivity Disorder), 10/11

Classifying Recommendations for Clinical Practice Guidelines, 9/04

Developmental Dysplasia of the Hip Practice Guideline (Technical Report), 4/00

Diagnosis and Management of Acute Otitis Media (Clinical Practice Guideline) (joint with American Academy of Family Physicians), 5/04

Diagnosis and Management of Childhood Obstructive Sleep Apnea Syndrome (Clinical Practice Guideline) (joint with Subcommittee on Obstructive Sleep Apnea Syndrome), 8/12

Diagnosis and Management of Childhood Obstructive Sleep Apnea Syndrome (Technical Report) (joint with Subcommittee on Obstructive Sleep Apnea Syndrome), 8/12

Early Detection of Developmental Dysplasia of the Hip (Clinical Practice Guideline), 4/00

An Evidence-Based Review of Important Issues Concerning Neonatal Hyperbilirubinemia (Technical Report), 7/04

Febrile Seizures: Clinical Practice Guideline for the Long-term Management of the Child With Simple Febrile Seizures (Clinical Practice Guideline) (joint with Subcommittee on Febrile Seizures), 6/08

Management of Hyperbilirubinemia in the Newborn Infant 35 or More Weeks of Gestation (Clinical Practice Guideline), 7/04

Management of Sinusitis (Clinical Practice Guideline), 9/01

Otitis Media With Effusion (Clinical Practice Guideline), 5/04

Principles for the Development and Use of Quality Measures (joint with Committee on Practice and Ambulatory Medicine), 2/08

Principles of Pediatric Patient Safety: Reducing Harm Due to Medical Care (joint with Committee on Hospital Care), 5/11

Toward Transparent Clinical Policies, 3/08

Urinary Tract Infection: Clinical Practice Guideline for the Diagnosis and Management of the Initial UTI in Febrile Infants and Children 2 to 24 Months (Clinical Practice Guideline) (joint with Subcommittee on Urinary Tract Infection), 8/11

SUBCOMMITTEE ON ATTENTION-DEFICIT/ HYPERACTIVITY DISORDER

ADHD: Clinical Practice Guideline for the Diagnosis, Evaluation, and Treatment of Attention-Deficit/ Hyperactivity Disorder in Children and Adolescents (Clinical Practice Guideline) (joint with Steering Committee on Quality Improvement and Management), 10/11

SUBCOMMITTEE ON CHRONIC ABDOMINAL PAIN

Chronic Abdominal Pain in Children (Clinical Report) (joint with North American Society for Pediatric Gastroenterology, Hepatology, and Nutrition), 3/05

Chronic Abdominal Pain in Children (Technical Report) (joint with North American Society for Pediatric Gastroenterology, Hepatology, and Nutrition), 3/05

SUBCOMMITTEE ON DIAGNOSIS AND MANAGEMENT OF BRONCHIOLITIS

Diagnosis and Management of Bronchiolitis (Clinical Practice Guideline), 10/06

SUBCOMMITTEE ON FEBRILE SEIZURES

Febrile Seizures: Clinical Practice Guideline for the Long-term Management of the Child With Simple Febrile Seizures (Clinical Practice Guideline) (joint with Steering Committee on Quality Improvement and Management), 6/08

Febrile Seizures: Guideline for the Neurodiagnostic Evaluation of the Child With a Simple Febrile Seizure (Clinical Practice Guideline), 2/11

SUBCOMMITTEE ON OBSTRUCTIVE SLEEP APNEA SYNDROME

Diagnosis and Management of Childhood Obstructive Sleep Apnea Syndrome (Clinical Practice Guideline) (joint with Steering Committee on Quality Improvement and Management), 8/12

Diagnosis and Management of Childhood Obstructive Sleep Apnea Syndrome (Technical Report) (joint with Steering Committee on Quality Improvement and Management), 8/12

SUBCOMMITTEE ON URINARY TRACT INFECTION

Diagnosis and Management of an Initial UTI in Febrile Infants and Young Children (Technical Report), 8/11

Urinary Tract Infection: Clinical Practice Guideline for the Diagnosis and Management of the Initial UTI in Febrile Infants and Children 2 to 24 Months (Clinical Practice Guideline) (joint with Steering Committee on Quality Improvement and Management), 8/11

SURGICAL ADVISORY PANEL

Guidelines for Referral to Pediatric Surgical Specialists, 7/02, reaffirmed 1/07

TASK FORCE ON CIRCUMCISION

Circumcision Policy Statement, 8/12

Male Circumcision (Technical Report), 8/12

TASK FORCE ON COMPLEMENTARY AND ALTERNATIVE MEDICINE

The Use of Complementary and Alternative Medicine in Pediatrics (Clinical Report) (joint with Provisional Section on Complementary, Holistic, and Integrative Medicine), 12/08, reaffirmed 10/12, 1/13

TASK FORCE ON GRADUATE MEDICAL EDUCATION REFORM

Graduate Medical Education and Pediatric Workforce Issues and Principles, 6/94

TASK FORCE ON MENTAL HEALTH

The Future of Pediatrics: Mental Health Competencies for Pediatric Primary Care (joint with Committee on Psychosocial Aspects of Child and Family Health), 6/09, reaffirmed 8/13

TASK FORCE ON SUDDEN INFANT DEATH SYNDROME

The Changing Concept of Sudden Infant Death Syndrome: Diagnostic Coding Shifts, Controversies Regarding the Sleeping Environment, and New Variables to Consider in Reducing Risk, 11/05, reaffirmed 5/08

SIDS and Other Sleep-Related Infant Deaths: Expansion of Recommendations for a Safe Infant Sleeping Environment, 10/11

SIDS and Other Sleep-Related Infant Deaths: Expansion of Recommendations for a Safe Infant Sleeping Environment (Technical Report), 10/11

TASK FORCE ON TERRORISM

The Pediatrician and Disaster Preparedness (joint with Committee on Pediatric Emergency Medicine and Committee on Medical Liability), 2/06, reaffirmed 6/09, 9/13

Psychosocial Implications of Disaster or Terrorism on Children: A Guide for the Pediatrician (Clinical Report) (joint with Committee on Psychosocial Aspects of Child and Family Health), 9/05

WORK GROUP ON SEDATION

Guidelines for Monitoring and Management of Pediatric Patients During and After Sedation for Diagnostic and Therapeutic Procedures: An Update (Clinical Report) (joint with American Academy of Pediatric Dentistry), 12/06, reaffirmed 3/11

WORKING GROUP ON SLEEPINESS IN ADOLESCENTS/ YOUNG ADULTS

Excessive Sleepiness in Adolescents and Young Adults: Causes, Consequences, and Treatment Strategies (Technical Report) (joint with Committee on Adolescence), 6/05

JOINT STATEMENTS

Joint Statement of the American Academy of Pediatrics and the American Academy of Child and Adolescent Psychiatry

Psychological Maltreatment (Clinical Report), 7/12

Joint Statement of the American Academy of Pediatrics, the American Academy of Child and Adolescent Psychiatry, and the National Center for Child Traumatic Stress

Understanding the Behavioral and Emotional Consequences of Child Abuse (Clinical Report), 9/08

Joint Statement of the American Academy of Pediatrics and the American Academy of Family Physicians

Diagnosis and Management of Acute Otitis Media (Clinical Practice Guideline), 5/04

Joint Statement of the American Academy of Pediatrics, the American Academy of Family Physicians, and the American College of Physicians

Supporting the Health Care Transition From Adolescence to Adulthood in the Medical Home (Clinical Report), 7/11

Joint Statement of the American Academy of Pediatrics, the American Academy of Family Physicians, and the American College of Physicians-American Society of Internal Medicine

A Consensus Statement on Health Care Transitions for Young Adults With Special Health Care Needs, 12/02

Joint Statement of the American Academy of Pediatrics and the American Academy of Ophthalmology

Protective Eyewear for Young Athletes, 3/04, reaffirmed 2/08, 6/11

Joint Statement of the American Academy of Pediatrics, the American Academy of Ophthalmology, the American Association for Pediatric Ophthalmology and Strabismus, and the American Association of Certified Orthoptists

Instrument-Based Pediatric Vision Screening Policy Statement, 10/12

Screening Examination of Premature Infants for Retinopathy of Prematurity, 12/12

Joint Statement of the American Academy of Pediatrics and the American Academy of Pediatric Dentistry

Guidelines for Monitoring and Management of Pediatric Patients During and After Sedation for Diagnostic and Therapeutic Procedures: An Update (Clinical Report), 12/06, reaffirmed 3/11

Oral and Dental Aspects of Child Abuse and Neglect (Clinical Report), 12/05, reaffirmed 1/09

Joint Statement of the American Academy of Pediatrics, the American Association of Certified Orthoptists, the American Association for Pediatric Ophthalmology and Strabismus, and the American Academy of Ophthalmology

Eye Examination in Infants, Children, and Young Adults by Pediatricians, 4/03, reaffirmed 5/07

Learning Disabilities, Dyslexia, and Vision, 7/09

Learning Disabilities, Dyslexia, and Vision (Technical Report), 3/11

Joint Statement of the American Academy of Pediatrics, the Society of Critical Care Medicine, and the Child Neurology Society

Guidelines for the Determination of Brain Death in Infants and Children: An Update of the 1987 Task Force Recommendations (Clinical Report), 8/11

Joint Statement of the Federation of Pediatric Organizations

Pediatric Fellowship Training, 7/04

ENDORSED CLINICAL PRACTICE GUIDELINES AND POLICIES

(The AAP endorses and accepts as its policy the following clinical practice guidelines and policies that have been published by other organizations.)

Advisory Committee on Immunization Practices

General Recommendations on Immunization: Recommendations of the Advisory Committee on Immunization Practices (ACIP), 12/06

Advisory Committee on Immunization Practices and Centers for Disease Control and Prevention

A Comprehensive Immunization Strategy to Eliminate Transmission of Hepatitis B Virus Infection in the United States, 7/06

Ambulatory Pediatric Association

Report of the National Consensus Conference on Family Presence during Pediatric Cardiopulmonary Resuscitation and Procedures, 9/03

American Academy of Child and Adolescent Psychiatry and Child Welfare League of America

Foster Care Mental Health Values, 2002

Mental Health and Substance Use Screening and Assessment of Children in Foster Care, 2003

American Academy of Emergency Medicine, American Association of Critical Care Nurses, American College of Emergency Physicians, Association of periOperative Registered Nurses, Emergency Department Practice Management Association, Emergencies Nurses Association, and National Association of EMS Physicians

Consensus Statement: Definitions for Consistent Emergency Department Metrics (2/10)

American Academy of Family Physicians, American Academy of Orthopaedic Surgeons, American College of Sports Medicine, American Medical Society for Sports Medicine, American Orthopaedic Society for Sports Medicine, and American Osteopathic Academy of Sports Medicine

Selected Issues for the Adolescent Athlete and the Team Physician: A Consensus Statement, 11/08

American Academy of Neurology and Child Neurology Society

Evidence Report: Genetic and Metabolic Testing on Children With Global Developmental Delay, 9/11

Evidence-Based Guidelines Update: Medical Treatment of Infantile Spasms, 6/12

American College of Emergency Physicians

Clinical Policy: Evidence-Based Approach to Pharmacologic Agents Used in Pediatric Sedation and Analgesia in the Emergency Department (Clinical Practice Guideline), 10/04

American College of Obstetricians and Gynecologists

Timing of Umbilical Cord Clamping After Birth, 12/12

American College of Rheumatology

Guidelines for Referral of Children and Adolescents to Pediatric Rheumatologists, 6/02, reaffirmed 5/07

American Diabetes Association

Diabetes Care for Emerging Adults: Recommendations for Transition From Pediatric to Adult Diabetes Care Systems, 11/11

Safe at School Campaign Statement of Principles, endorsed 2/06

Type 2 Diabetes in Children and Adolescents, 3/00

American Heart Association

Cardiovascular Risk Reduction in High-Risk Pediatric Populations, 12/06

Diagnosis, Treatment, and Long-Term Management of Kawasaki Disease: A Statement for Health Professionals (Clinical Report), 12/04

Dietary Recommendations for Children and Adolescents: A Guide for Practitioners, 9/05

Genetic Basis for Congenital Heart Defects: Current Knowledge, 6/07

Importance and Implementation of Training in Cardiopulmonary Resuscitation and Automated External Defibrillation in Schools, 2/11

Long-term Cardiovascular Toxicity in Children, Adolescents, and Young Adults Who Receive Cancer Therapy: Pathophysiology, Course, Monitoring, Management, Prevention, and Research Directions: A Scientific Statement From the American Heart Association, 9/13

Neurodevelopmental Outcomes in Children With Congenital Heart Disease: Evaluation and Management: A Scientific Statement From the American Heart Association, 7/12

Noninherited Risk Factors and Congenital Cardiovascular Defects: Current Knowledge, 6/07

Prevention of Infective Endocarditis: Guidelines From the American Heart Association (Clinical Practice Guideline), 5/07

Prevention of Rheumatic Fever and Diagnosis and Treatment of Acute Streptococcal Pharyngitis, 2/09

Response to Cardiac Arrest and Selected Life-Threatening Medical Emergencies: The Medical Emergency Response Plan for Schools. A Statement for Healthcare Providers, Policymakers, School Administrators, and Community Leaders, 1/04

American Medical Association

Gifts to Physicians From Industry, 8/01

American Pediatric Surgical Association

Best Practice for Infant Surgery: A Position Statement From the American Pediatric Surgical Association, 9/08

American Society for Parenteral and Enteral Nutrition
Defining Pediatric Malnutrition: A Paradigm Shift Toward Etiology-Related Definitions, 3/13

American Thoracic Society and Centers for Disease Control and Prevention
(*The AAP endorses and accepts as its policy the sections of this statement as they relate to infants and children.*)
Targeted Tuberculin Testing and Treatment of Latent Tuberculosis Infection, 4/00

American Urological Association
Report on the Management of Primary Vesicoureteral Reflux in Children (Clinical Practice Guideline), 5/97

Canadian Paediatric Society
Skiing and Snowboarding Injury Prevention, 1/12

Centers for Disease Control and Prevention
Guidelines for Field Triage of Injured Patients, 1/12
Managing Acute Gastroenteritis Among Children: Oral Rehydration, Maintenance, and Nutritional Therapy (Clinical Practice Guideline), 11/03
Prevention and Control of Meningococcal Disease: Recommendations of the Advisory Committee on Immunization Practices (ACIP), 3/13
Prevention of Perinatal Group B Streptococcal Disease: Revised Guidelines from CDC, 2010 (Clinical Practice Guideline), 11/10
Recommendations for Using Fluoride to Prevent and Control Dental Caries in the United States (Clinical Practice Guideline), 8/01
Update on Japanese Encephalitis Vaccine for Children—United States, May 2011, 8/11

Centers for Disease Control and Prevention, Infectious Diseases Society of America, and American Society of Blood and Marrow Transplantation
Guidelines for Preventing Opportunistic Infections Among Hematopoietic Stem Cell Transplant Recipients (Clinical Practice Guideline), 10/00

Emergency Nurses Association
Weighing Pediatric Patients in Kilograms, 3/12

The Endocrine Society
Congenital Adrenal Hyperplasia Due to Steroid 21-hydroxylase Deficiency: An Endocrine Society Clinical Practice Guideline (Clinical Practice Guideline), 9/10

Family Violence Prevention Fund
Identifying and Responding to Domestic Violence: Consensus Recommendations for Child and Adolescent Health, 9/02

Guidelines for the Management of Adolescent Depression in Primary Care Steering Group
Guidelines for Adolescent Depression in Primary Care (GLAD-PC): I. Identification, Assessment, and Initial Management (Clinical Practice Guideline), 11/07
Guidelines for Adolescent Depression in Primary Care (GLAD-PC): II. Treatment and Ongoing Management (Clinical Practice Guideline), 11/07

Infectious Diseases Society of America
Clinical Practice Guidelines by the Infectious Diseases Society of America for the Treatment of Methicillin-Resistant *Staphylococcus aureus* Infections in Adults and Children (Clinical Practice Guideline), 2/11
Seasonal Influenza in Adults and Children—Diagnosis, Treatment, Chemoprophylaxis, and Institutional Outbreak Management: Clinical Practice Guidelines of the Infectious Diseases Society of America (Clinical Practice Guideline), 4/09

Institute of Medicine
Dietary Reference Intakes for Calcium and Vitamin D, 2011

International Consensus Conference on Intersex (Lawson Wilkins Pediatric Endocrine Society and the European Society for Paediatric Endocrinology)
Consensus Statement on Management of Intersex Disorders, 8/06

Joint Committee on Infant Hearing
Supplement to the JCIH 2007 Position Statement: Principles and Guidelines for Early Intervention After Confirmation That a Child Is Deaf or Hard of Hearing, 3/13

National Association of Neonatal Nurses
The Management of Hypotension in the Very-Low-Birth-Weight Infant: Guideline for Practice, 2011

National Association of School Nurses
Emergency Equipment and Supplies in the School Setting, 1/12

National Athletic Trainers' Association
Appropriate Medical Care for the Secondary School-Age Athlete Communication, 2004
Lightning Safety for Athletics and Recreation (Position Statement), 12/00

National Athletic Trainers' Association, National Interscholastic Athletic Administrators Association, College Athletic Trainers' Society, National Federation of State High School Associations, American College Health Association, American Orthopaedic Society for Sports Medicine, National Collegiate Athletic Association, American Medical Society for Sports Medicine, National Association of Collegiate Directors of Athletics, and National Association of Intercollegiate Athletics
Inter-Association Consensus Statement on Best Practices for Sports Medicine Management for Secondary Schools and Colleges, 7/13

National Diabetes Education Program
Helping the Student with Diabetes Succeed: A Guide for School Personnel, 6/03

National Heart, Lung and Blood Institute
Expert Panel on Integrated Guidelines for Cardiovascular Health and Risk Reduction in Children and Adolescents: Summary Report, 3/12

National Institute of Allergy and Infectious Diseases
Guidelines for the Diagnosis and Management of Food Allergy in the United States: Report of the NIAID-Sponsored Expert Panel (Clinical Practice Guideline), 12/10

National Institutes of Health, Centers for Disease Control and Prevention, HIV Medicine Association of Infectious Diseases Society of America, and Pediatric Infectious Diseases Society
Guidelines for the Prevention and Treatment of Opportunistic Infections in HIV-Exposed and HIV-Infected Children (Clinical Practice Guideline), 11/13

North American Society for Pediatric Gastroenterology, Hepatology, and Nutrition
Guideline for the Evaluation of Cholestatic Jaundice in Infants (Clinical Practice Guideline), 8/04

Guidelines for Evaluation and Treatment of Gastroesophageal Reflux in Infants and Children (Clinical Practice Guideline), 2001

Helicobacter pylori Infection in Children: Recommendations for Diagnosis and Treatment (Clinical Practice Guideline), 11/00

Pediatric Infectious Diseases Society and Infectious Diseases Society of America
The Management of Community-Acquired Pneumonia (CAP) in Infants and Children Older Than 3 Months of Age (Clinical Practice Guideline), 10/11

Pediatric Orthopaedic Society of North America/ American Academy of Orthopaedic Surgeons/ Scoliosis Research Society
Screening for Idiopathic Scoliosis in Adolescents, 1/08

Quality Standards Subcommittee of the American Academy of Neurology and Child Neurology Society
Diagnostic Assessment of the Child with Cerebral Palsy (Clinical Practice Guideline), 3/04

Diagnostic Assessment of the Child With Status Epilepticus (An Evidence-based Review) (Clinical Practice Guideline), 11/06

Neuroimaging of the Neonate (Clinical Practice Guideline), 6/02

Pharmacological Treatment of Migraine Headache in Children and Adolescents (Clinical Practice Guideline), 12/04

Screening and Diagnosis of Autism (Clinical Practice Guideline), 8/00

Treatment of the Child With a First Unprovoked Seizure (Clinical Practice Guideline), 1/03

Quality Standards Subcommittee of the American Academy of Neurology, Child Neurology Society, and American Epilepsy Society
Evaluating a First Nonfebrile Seizure in Children (Clinical Practice Guideline), 8/00

Renal Physicians Association
Shared Decision-Making in the Appropriate Initiation of and Withdrawal from Dialysis, 2nd Edition (Clinical Practice Guideline), 10/10

Society for Academic Emergency Medicine
Pediatric Care in the Emergency Department, 11/03

Society for Adolescent Medicine
Executing Juvenile Offenders: A Fundamental Failure of Society, 10/04

Expedited Partner Therapy for Adolescents Diagnosed With Chlamydia or Gonorrhea: A Position Paper of the Society for Adolescent Medicine, 9/09

Protecting Adolescents: Ensuring Access to Care and Reporting Sexual Activity and Abuse, 11/04

Society of Critical Care Medicine, Infectious Diseases Society of America, Society for Healthcare Epidemiology of America, Surgical Infection Society, American College of Chest Physicians, American Thoracic Society, American Society of Critical Care Anesthesiologists, Association for Professionals in Infection Control and Epidemiology, Infusion Nurses Society, Oncology Nursing Society, Society of Cardiovascular and Interventional Radiology, American Academy of Pediatrics, and Healthcare Infection Control Practices Advisory Committee of the Centers for Disease Control and Prevention
Guidelines for the Prevention of Intravascular Catheter-Related Infections (Clinical Practice Guideline), 2002

US Department of Health and Human Services
Guidelines for the Prevention and Treatment of Opportunistic Infections in HIV-Exposed and HIV-Infected Children (Clinical Practice Guideline), 11/13

Treating Tobacco Use and Dependence: 2008 Update (Clinical Practice Guideline), 5/08

World Health Organization
(The AAP endorses the recommendation pertaining to the use of thimerosal in vaccines.)

Meeting of the Strategic Advisory Group of Experts on Immunizations, April 2012–Conclusions and Recommendations, 5/12

AFFIRMATION OF VALUE CLINICAL PRACTICE GUIDELINES AND POLICIES
(These guidelines are not endorsed as policy of the American Academy of Pediatrics [AAP]. Documents that lack a clear description of the process for identifying, assessing, and incorporating research evidence are not eligible for AAP endorsement as practice guidelines. However, such documents may be of educational value to members of the AAP.)

American Society of Anesthesiologists
Practice Guidelines for the Perioperative Management of Patients with Obstructive Sleep Apnea (Clinical Practice Guideline), 5/06

National Environmental Education Foundation
Environmental Management of Pediatric Asthma: Guidelines for Health Care Providers (Clinical Practice Guideline), 8/05

National Hospice and Palliative Care Organization
Standards of Practice for Pediatric Palliative Care and Hospice (Clinical Practice Guideline), 2/09

Turner Syndrome Consensus Study Group
Care of Girls and Women With Turner Syndrome: A Guideline of the Turner Syndrome Study Group (Clinical Practice Guideline), 1/07

APPENDIX 2

PPI: AAP Partnership for Policy Implementation

· ·

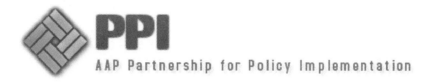

AAP Partnership for Policy Implementation

BACKGROUND

The American Academy of Pediatrics (AAP) develops policies that promote the attainment of optimal physical, mental, and social health and well-being for all infants, children, adolescents, and young adults. These documents are valued highly not only by clinicians who provide direct health care to children, but by members of other organizations that share similar goals, and also by parents, payers, and legislators. Unfortunately, AAP policy documents vary widely in terms of how they are written, and some find these documents difficult to implement. Pediatricians who have expertise in medical informatics found AAP policy documents particularly challenging when they tried to convert policy recommendations into items that could be easily programmed into an electronic system. In June 2005, with initial funding support from the federal Maternal and Child Health Bureau, the AAP launched the Partnership for Policy Implementation (PPI), a pilot program to create changes in the development of policy statements, clinical reports, technical reports, and clinical practice guidelines—specifically, how they are written. Unofficially, collaboration began that resulted in this project to demonstrate the feasibility of integrating health information technology (HIT) functionalities into AAP policy. The PPI is currently funded by the AAP Child Health Informatics Center (CHIC).

VISION

The vision of the PPI is for all AAP policy statements, clinical reports, technical reports, and clinical practice guidelines to have medically sound content, a transparent evidence base, and clearly stated, actionable recommendations that can be implemented in practice and incorporated into electronic systems to support the delivery of high-quality care for children and youth and their families.

MISSION

The mission of the PPI is to facilitate implementation of AAP recommendations at the point of care by ensuring that AAP documents are written in a practical, action-oriented fashion with unambiguous recommendations.

WHAT IS THE PPI?

It is a network of pediatric informaticians who work with AAP authors and guideline subcommittees throughout the writing process.

Contributions of the PPI to the AAP writing process include disambiguation and specification; development of clear definitions; clearly defined logic; implementation techniques; action-oriented recommendations, including clinical algorithms; transparency of evidence basis for recommendations; and health information technology (HIT) standard development.

WHAT HAS THE PPI ACCOMPLISHED?

Since its inception, over 20 statements have been published using the PPI process covering child health topics as diverse as identifying developmental disorders through surveillance and screening (*Pediatrics.* 2006;118:405–420); diagnosis and management of bronchiolitis (*Pediatrics.* 2006;118:1774–1793); prevention of influenza (*Pediatrics.* 2007;119:846–851 and subsequent annual updates); identification, evaluation, and management of autism (*Pediatrics.* 2007;120:1162–1182 and *Pediatrics.* 2007;120:1183–1215); recommendations for and implications of newborn screening (*Pediatrics.* 2008;121:192–217); hearing assessment (*Pediatrics.* 2009; 124:1252–1263); enhancing pediatric mental health care (*Pediatrics.* 2010;125:S109–S125); and the diagnosis and management of childhood obstructive sleep apnea syndrome (Pediatrics. 2012; 130: e714–e755).

One example of how a statement developed using the PPI process has gained broader acceptance is the influenza statement published in April 2007. The Centers for Disease Control and Prevention chose to adopt components of the PPI statement (specifically, the clinical algorithm) within its own statement on the same topic. In addition, the Childhood Influenza Immunization Coalition posted an interactive version of the influenza algorithm on its Web site (www.preventchildhoodinfluenza.org/resource/algorithm.swf).

WHAT IS THE PPI DOING NOW?

In addition to creating practical, action-oriented documents that pediatricians can use, the PPI is also working to make it easier for these documents to be incorporated into electronic systems. To date, the PPI has focused its involvement on the statement development process. The involvement of the PPI during the writing process helps to produce a clear, more concise document. As these standards of care become well documented, the PPI can begin to focus on building or mapping pediatric vocabulary; once solidified, this vocabulary can be built into electronic health record (EHR) systems. The standards of care can also be matched to the various logical and functional HIT standards that already exist today. Through this work, the PPI hopes to improve AAP policy documents by providing specific guidance to pediatricians at the point of care, to help ensure that EHRs are designed to assist pediatricians in providing optimal care for children.

For more information about the PPI, please visit the Web site (http://www2.aap.org/informatics/PPI.html) or contact Lisa Krams (lkrams@aap.org or 847/434-7663).

APPENDIX 3

American Academy of Pediatrics Acronyms

AMERICAN ACADEMY OF PEDIATRICS

Acronyms

AACAP	American Academy of Child and Adolescent Psychiatry
AAFP	American Academy of Family Physicians
AAMC	Association of American Medical Colleges
AAOS	American Academy of Orthopaedic Surgeons
AAP	American Academy of Pediatrics
AAPD	American Academy of Pediatric Dentistry
ABMS	American Board of Medical Specialties
ABP	American Board of Pediatrics
ACBOCCSA	Advisory Committee to the Board on Community, Chapter, and State Affairs
ACBOCSP	Advisory Committee to the Board on Community and Specialty Pediatrics
ACBOE	Advisory Committee to the Board on Education
ACBOF	Advisory Committee to the Board on Finance
ACBOFA	Advisory Committee to the Board on Federal Affairs
ACBOGCH	Advisory Committee to the Board on Global Child Health
ACBOIT	Advisory Committee to the Board on Information Technology
ACBOM	Advisory Committee to the Board on Membership
ACBOMP	Advisory Committee to the Board on Marketing and Publications
ACBOP	Advisory Committee to the Board on Practice
ACBOR	Advisory Committee to the Board on Research
ACBOSP	Advisory Committee to the Board on Strategic Planning
ACBOSPe	Advisory Committee to the Board on Specialty Pediatrics
ACCME	Accreditation Council for Continuing Medical Education
ACEP	American College of Emergency Physicians
ACGME	Accreditation Council for Graduate Medical Education
ACIP	Advisory Committee on Immunization Practices
ACMG	American College of Medical Genetics
ACO	Accountable Care Organization
ACOG	American Congress of Obstetricians and Gynecologists
ACOP	American College of Osteopathic Pediatricians
ACP	American College of Physicians
ADAMHA	Alcohol, Drug Abuse, and Mental Health Administration
AG-M	Action Group—Multidisciplinary (Section Forum)
AG-M1	Action Group—Medical 1 (Section Forum)
AG-M2	Action Group—Medical 2 (Section Forum)
AG-S	Action Group—Surgical (Section Forum)
AHA	American Heart Association
AHA	American Hospital Association
AHRQ	Agency for Healthcare Research and Quality
ALF	Annual Leadership Forum
AMA	American Medical Association
AMCHP	Association of Maternal and Child Health Programs
AMSA	American Medical Student Association
AMSPDC	Association of Medical School Pediatric Department Chairs
AMWA	American Medical Women's Association
APA	Academic Pediatric Association
APHA	American Public Health Association
APLS	Advanced Pediatric Life Support
APPD	Association of Pediatric Program Directors
APQ	Alliance for Pediatric Quality
APS/SPR	American Pediatric Society/Society for Pediatric Research
AQA	Ambulatory Care Quality Alliance
ASHG	American Society of Human Genetics
ASTM	American Society of Testing and Materials
BHP	Bureau of Health Professions
BIA	Bureau of Indian Affairs
BLAST	Babysitter Lessons and Safety Training
BOD	Board of Directors
BPC	Breastfeeding Promotion Consortium
CAG	Corporate Advisory Group
CAMLWG	Children, Adolescents, and Media Leadership Workgroup
CAP	College of American Pathologists
CAQI	Chapter Alliance for Quality Improvement
CATCH	Community Access to Child Health
CDC	Centers for Disease Control and Prevention
CESP	Confederation of European Specialty Pediatrics
CFMC	Chapter Forum Management Committee
CFT	Cross Functional Team
CHA	Children's Hospital Association
CHCA	Child Health Corporation of America

CMC	Council Management Committee	CPS	Canadian Paediatric Society
CME	Continuing Medical Education	CPTI	Community Pediatrics Training Initiative
CMS	Centers for Medicare & Medicaid Services	CQN	Chapter Quality Network
		CSHCN	Children With Special Health Care Needs
CMSS	Council of Medical Specialty Societies	DHHS	Department of Health and Human Services
CnF	Council Forum		
COA	Committee on Adolescence	DOD	Department of Defense
COB	Committee on Bioethics	DVC	District Vice Chairperson
COCAN	Committee on Child Abuse and Neglect	EBCDLW	Early Brain and Child Development Leadership Workgroup
COCHF	Committee on Child Health Financing		
COCIT	Council on Clinical Information Technology	EC	Executive Committee
		EMSC	Emergency Medical Services for Children
COCM	Council on Communications and Media	EPA	Environmental Protection Agency
COCME	Committee on Continuing Medical Education	eQIPP	Education in Quality Improvement for Pediatric Practice
COCN	Committee on Coding and Nomenclature	eTACC	Electronic Translation of Academy Clinical Content
COCP	Council on Community Pediatrics		
COCWD	Council on Children With Disabilities	FCF	Friends of Children Fund
COD	Committee on Drugs	FDA	Food and Drug Administration
CODe	Committee on Development	FOPE II	Future of Pediatric Education II Project
COEC	Council on Early Childhood	FOPO	Federation of Pediatric Organizations
COEH	Council on Environmental Health	FTC	Federal Trade Commission
CoF	Committee Forum	GME	Graduate Medical Education
COFCAKC	Council on Foster Care, Adoption, and Kinship Care	HAAC	Historical Archives Advisory Committee
		HBB	Helping Babies Breathe
COFGA	Committee on Federal Government Affairs	HCCA	Healthy Child Care America
		HEDIS	Health Plan Employer Data and Information Set
CoFMC	Committee Forum Management Committee		
		HHS	Health and Human Services
COFN	Committee on Fetus and Newborn	HIPAA	Health Insurance Portability and Accountability Act of 1996
COG	Committee on Genetics		
COGME	Council on Graduate Medical Education (DHHS/HRSA)	HMO	Health Maintenance Organization
		HQA	Hospital Quality Alliance
COHC	Committee on Hospital Care	HRSA	Health Resources and Services Administration
COID	Committee on Infectious Diseases		
COIVPP	Committee on Injury, Violence, and Poison Prevention	HTC	Helping the Children
		HTPCP	Healthy Tomorrows Partnership for Children Program
COM	Committee on Membership		
COMLRM	Committee on Medical Liability and Risk Management	IHS	Indian Health Service
		IMG	International Medical Graduate
COMSEP	Council on Medical Student Education in Pediatrics (AMSPDC)	IOM	Institute of Medicine
		IPA	International Pediatric Association
CON	Committee on Nutrition	IPC	International Pediatric Congress
CONACH	Committee on Native American Child Health	IRB	Institutional Review Board
		JCAHO	Joint Commission on Accreditation of Healthcare Organizations
COPA	Committee on Pediatric AIDS		
COPACFH	Committee on Psychosocial Aspects of Child and Family Health	LLLI	La Leche League International
		MCAN	Merck Childhood Asthma Network
COPAM	Committee on Practice and Ambulatory Medicine	MCH	Maternal and Child Health
		MCHB	Maternal and Child Health Bureau
COPE	Committee on Pediatric Education	MCN	Migrant Clinicians Network
COPEM	Committee on Pediatric Emergency Medicine	MHICSN-PAC	Medical Home Initiatives for Children With Special Needs Project Advisory Committee
COPR	Committee on Pediatric Research		
COPW	Committee on Pediatric Workforce		
COQIPS	Council on Quality Improvement and Patient Safety	MHLWG	Mental Health Leadership Work Group
		MRT	Media Resource Team
CORS	Committee on Residency Scholarships	NACH	National Association of Children's Hospitals
COSA	Committee on Substance Abuse		
COSGA	Committee on State Government Affairs	NACHC	National Association of Community Health Centers
COSH	Council on School Health		
COSMF	Council on Sports Medicine and Fitness		

NACHRI	National Association of Children's Hospitals and Related Institutions
NAEMSP	National Association of Emergency Medical Physicians
NAEPP	National Asthma Education and Prevention Program
NAPNAP	National Association of Pediatric Nurse Practitioners
NASPGHAN	North American Society for Pediatric Gastroenterology, Hepatology, and Nutrition
NAWD	National Association of WIC Directors
NBME	National Board of Medical Examiners
NCE	National Conference & Exhibition
NCEPG	National Conference & Exhibition Planning Group
NCQA	National Committee for Quality Assurance
NHLBI	National Heart, Lung, and Blood Institute
NHMA	National Hispanic Medical Association
NHTSA	National Highway Traffic Safety Administration
NIAAA	National Institute on Alcohol Abuse and Alcoholism
NICHD	National Institute of Child Health and Human Development
NICHQ	National Initiative for Children's Healthcare Quality
NIDA	National Institute on Drug Abuse
NIH	National Institutes of Health
NIMH	National Institute of Mental Health
NMA	National Medical Association
NMS	Neuromotor Screening Expert Panel
NNC	National Nominating Committee
NQF	National Quality Forum
NRHA	National Rural Health Association
NRMP	National Resident Matching Program
NRP	Neonatal Resuscitation Program
NSC	National Safety Council
NVAC	National Vaccine Advisory Committee
ODPHP	Office of Disease Prevention and Health Promotion
OED	Office of the Executive Director
OHISC	Oral Health Initiative Steering Committee
OLW	Obesity Leadership Workgroup
P4P	Pay for Performance
PAC	Project Advisory Committee
PAHO	Pan American Health Organization
PALS	Pediatric Advanced Life Support
PAS	Pediatric Academic Societies
PCO	*Pediatric Care Online*™
PCOC	Primary Care Organizations Consortium
PCPCC	Patient-Centered Primary Care Collaborative
PCPI	Physician Consortium on Performance Improvement
PEAC	Practice Expense Advisory Committee
PECOS	Pediatric Education in Community and Office Settings

PECS	Pediatric Education in Community Settings
PEPP	Pediatric Education for Prehospital Professionals
PIR	*Pediatrics in Review*
PLA	Pediatric Leadership Alliance
PMO	*Practice Management Online*
PPAAC	Private Payer Advocacy Advisory Committee (COCHF Subcommittee)
PPAC	Past President's Advisory Committee
PPAC	Practicing Physicians' Advisory Council
PPC-PCMH	Physician Practice Connections—Patient-Centered Medical Home (NCQA)
PPI	Partnership for Policy Implementation
PREP	Pediatric Review and Education Program
PROS	Pediatric Research in Office Settings
PSOLGBTHW	Provisional Section on Lesbian, Gay, Bisexual, and Transgender Health and Wellness
PSOTCo	Provisional Section on Tobacco Control
PUPVS	Project Universal Preschool Vision Screening
QA	Quality Assurance
QI	Quality Improvement
QuIIN	Quality Improvement Innovation Network
RBPE	Resource-Based Practice Expense
RBRVS	Resource-Based Relative Value Scale
RCE	Richmond Center of Excellence
RRC	Residency Review Committee (ACGME)
RUC	AMA/Specialty Society Relative Value Scale Update Committee
RVU	Relative Value Unit
SAM	Society for Adolescent Medicine
SAMHSA	Substance Abuse and Mental Health Services Administration
SCHIP	State Children's Health Insurance Program
SDBP	Society for Developmental and Behavioral Pediatrics
SF	Section Forum
SFMC	Section Forum Management Committee
SOA	Section on Anesthesiology and Pain Medicine
SOAC	Subcommittee on Access to Care
SOAH	Section on Adolescent Health
SOAI	Section on Allergy and Immunology
SOAPM	Section on Administration and Practice Management
SOATT	Section on Advances in Therapeutics and Technology
SOB	Section on Bioethics
SOBr	Section on Breastfeeding
SOCAN	Section on Child Abuse and Neglect
SOCC	Section on Critical Care
SOCCS	Section on Cardiology and Cardiac Surgery
SOCPT	Section on Clinical Pharmacology and Therapeutics
SOD	Section on Dermatology
SODBP	Section on Developmental and Behavioral Pediatrics

SOEM	Section on Emergency Medicine	SOPPSM	Section on Pediatric Pulmonology and Sleep Medicine
SOEn	Section on Endocrinology	SOPS	Section on Plastic Surgery
SOEp	Section on Epidemiology	SORa	Section on Radiology
SOGBD	Section on Genetics and Birth Defects	SORh	Section on Rheumatology
SOGHN	Section on Gastroenterology, Hepatology, and Nutrition	SOSM	Section on Senior Members
SOHC	Section on Home Care	SOSu	Section on Surgery
SOHM	Section on Hospital Medicine	SOTC	Section on Telehealth Care
SOHO	Section on Hematology/Oncology	SOTM	Section on Transport Medicine
SOHPM	Section on Hospice and Palliative Medicine	SOU	Section on Urology
SOICH	Section on International Child Health	SOUS	Section on Uniformed Services
SOID	Section on Infectious Diseases	SOYP	Section on Young Physicians
SOIM	Section on Integrative Medicine	SPR	Society for Pediatric Research
SOIMP	Section on Internal Medicine/Pediatrics	SPWG	Strategic Planning Work Group
SOMP	Section on Medicine-Pediatrics	TA	Technical Assistance
SOMSRFT	Section on Medical Students, Residents, and Fellowship Trainees	TA	Technology Assessment
SONp	Section on Nephrology	TFOA	Task Force on Access (also known as Task Force on Health Insurance Coverage and Access to Care)
SONS	Section on Neurological Surgery	TFOC	Task Force on Circumcision
SONu	Section on Neurology	TFOI	Task Force on Immunization
SOOb	Section on Obesity	TIPP	The Injury Prevention Program
SOOH	Section on Oral Health	TJC	The Joint Commission
SOOHNS	Section on Otolaryngology/Head & Neck Surgery	UNICEF	United Nations Children's Fund
SOOp	Section on Ophthalmology	UNOS	United Network for Organ Sharing
SOOPe	Section on Osteopathic Pediatricians	USDA	US Department of Agriculture
SOOr	Section on Orthopaedics	WHO	World Health Organization
SOPPe	Section on Perinatal Pediatrics	WIC	Special Supplemental Nutrition Program for Women, Infants, and Children

Subject Index

· · · · · · · · · · · · · · ·

C

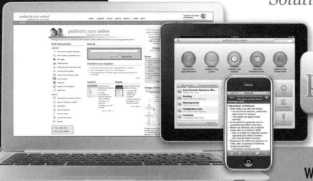
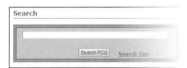